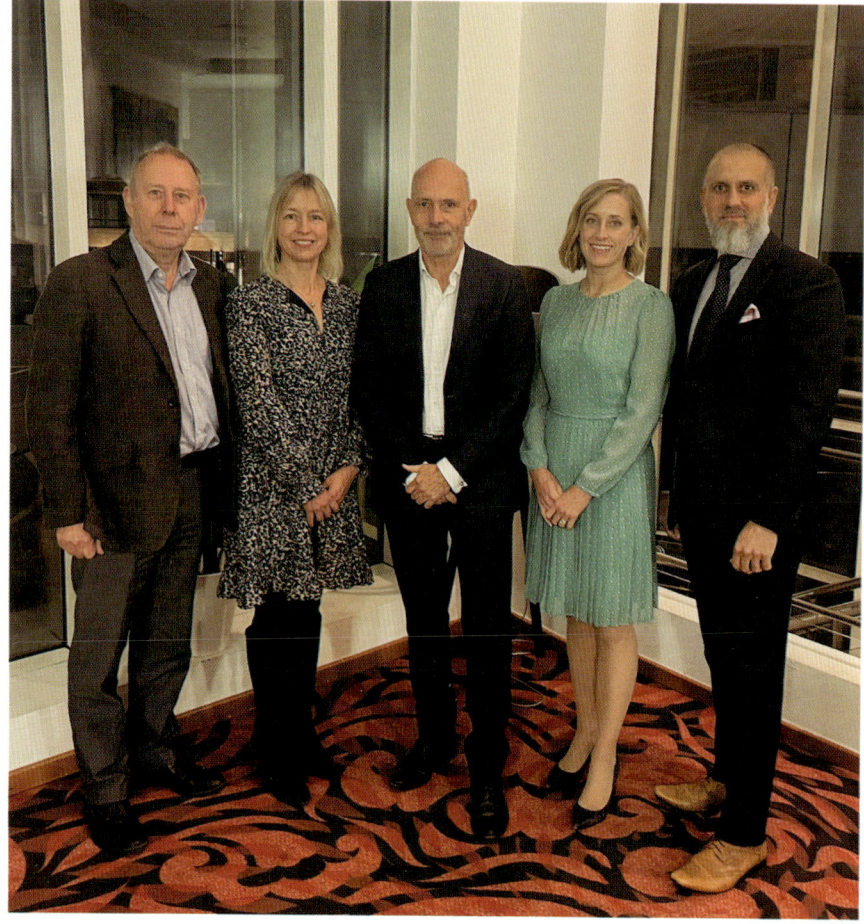

The Editors
From left to right: Jonathan Barker, Tanya Bleiker, Christopher Griffiths, Rosalind Simpson, Walayat Hussain

Rook's Textbook of Dermatology

TENTH EDITION

EDITED BY

Christopher Griffiths OBE, MD, FMedSci
Emeritus Professor of Dermatology
The University of Manchester
Manchester, UK

Adjunct Professor & Consultant Dermatologist
King's College London
London, UK

Jonathan Barker MD, FRCP
Professor of Medical Dermatology
St John's Institute of Dermatology
Faculty of Life Sciences and Medicine
King's College London
London, UK

Tanya Bleiker FRCP
Consultant Dermatologist
University Hospitals of Derby and Burton NHS Foundation Trust
Derby, UK

Walayat Hussain FRACP
Consultant Dermatological & Mohs Micrographic Surgeon
Dermatology Surgical & Laser Unit
Chapel Allerton Hospital
Leeds, UK

Rosalind Simpson MRCP, PhD
Associate Professor and Consultant Dermatologist
Centre of Evidence Based Dermatology
University of Nottingham
Nottingham, UK

IN FOUR VOLUMES

VOLUME 4

WILEY Blackwell

This edition first published 2024
© 2024 John Wiley & Sons Ltd

Edition History
John Wiley & Sons Ltd (9e, 2016); Blackwell Publishing, Ltd (1e, 1968, 2e, 1972, 3e, 1979, 4e, 1986, 5e, 1992, 6e, 1998, 7e, 2004, 8e, 2010)

All rights reserved. No part of this publication may be reproduced, stored in a retrieval system, or transmitted, in any form or by any means, electronic, mechanical, photocopying, recording or otherwise, except as permitted by law. Advice on how to obtain permission to reuse material from this title is available at http://www.wiley.com/go/permissions.

The right of Christopher E. M. Griffiths, Jonathan N. W. N. Barker, Tanya O. Bleiker, S. Walayat Hussain, Rosalind C. Simpson to be identified as the authors of the editorial material in this work has been asserted in accordance with law.

Registered Office(s)
John Wiley & Sons, Inc., 111 River Street, Hoboken, NJ 07030, USA
John Wiley & Sons Ltd, The Atrium, Southern Gate, Chichester, West Sussex, PO19 8SQ, UK

Editorial Office(s)
9600 Garsington Road, Oxford, OX4 2DQ, UK
The Atrium, Southern Gate, Chichester, West Sussex, PO19 8SQ, UK

For details of our global editorial offices, customer services, and more information about Wiley products visit us at www.wiley.com.

Wiley also publishes its books in a variety of electronic formats and by print-on-demand. Some content that appears in standard print versions of this book may not be available in other formats.

Limit of Liability/Disclaimer of Warranty
The contents of this work are intended to further general scientific research, understanding, and discussion only and are not intended and should not be relied upon as recommending or promoting scientific method, diagnosis, or treatment by physicians for any particular patient. In view of ongoing research, equipment modifications, changes in governmental regulations, and the constant flow of information relating to the use of medicines, equipment, and devices, the reader is urged to review and evaluate the information provided in the package insert or instructions for each medicine, equipment, or device for, among other things, any changes in the instructions or indication of usage and for added warnings and precautions. While the publisher and authors have used their best efforts in preparing this work, they make no representations or warranties with respect to the accuracy or completeness of the contents of this work and specifically disclaim all warranties, including without limitation any implied warranties of merchantability or fitness for a particular purpose. No warranty may be created or extended by sales representatives, written sales materials or promotional statements for this work. The fact that an organization, website, or product is referred to in this work as a citation and/or potential source of further information does not mean that the publisher and authors endorse the information or services the organization, website, or product may provide or recommendations it may make. This work is sold with the understanding that the publisher is not engaged in rendering professional services. The advice and strategies contained herein may not be suitable for your situation. You should consult with a specialist where appropriate. Further, readers should be aware that websites listed in this work may have changed or disappeared between when this work was written and when it is read. Neither the publisher nor authors shall be liable for any loss of profit or any other commercial damages, including but not limited to special, incidental, consequential, or other damages.

Library of Congress Cataloging-in-Publication Data has been applied for.

Set ISBN (4 Volumes): 9781119709213

Cover Design: Wiley
Cover Image: © khamkula/Adobe Stock

Set in 9.5/12pt, Palatino LT Std by Straive, Chennai, India

Printed in Great Britain by Bell & Bain Ltd, Glasgow

10 9 8 7 6 5 4 3 2 1

Contents

List of Associate Editors, x

List of Contributors, xi

Preface to the Tenth Edition, xxi

Preface to the First Edition, xxii

About the Companion Website, xxiii

VOLUME 1

Part 1 Foundations of Dermatology

1. History of Dermatology, 1.1
   Nick J. Levell

2. Structure and Function of the Skin, 2.1
   John A. McGrath and Jouni Uitto

3. Histopathology of the Skin: General Principles, 3.1
   Eduardo Calonje and John Mee

4. Diagnosis of Skin Disease, 4.1
   Ian H. Coulson, Emma C. Benton and Stephanie Ogden

5. Epidemiology of Skin Disease, 5.1
   Hywel C. Williams and Sinéad M. Langan

6. Health Economics and Skin Disease, 6.1
   Matthias Augustin

7. Global Health Dermatology, 7.1
   L. Claire Fuller

8. Genetics and the Skin, 8.1
   John A. McGrath

9. Inflammation, Immunology and Allergy, 9.1
   Muzlifah Haniffa

10. Photobiology, 10.1
    Antony R. Young

11. Cutaneous Response to Injury and Wound Healing, 11.1
    Edel A. O'Toole

12. Topical Drug Delivery, 12.1
    Richard H. Guy and Adrian F. Davis

13. Clinical Pharmacology, 13.1
    Richard T. Woolf and Catherine H. Smith

14. Adverse Immunological Reactions to Drugs, 14.1
    Michael R. Ardern-Jones

Part 2 Management

15. Psychological and Social Impact of Long-Term Conditions and Principles of Holistic Management, 15.1
    Sandy R. McBride and Alexandra Mizara

16. Principles of Measurement and Assessment in Dermatology, 16.1
    Andrew Y. Finlay and Faraz M. Ali

17. Principles of Evidence-based Dermatology, 17.1
    Michael Bigby and Hywel C. Williams

18. Principles of Topical Therapy, 18.1
    Deirdre A. Buckley

19. Principles of Systemic Therapy, 19.1
    Andrew E. Pink, Richard T. Woolf and Catherine H. Smith

20. Principles of Skin Surgery, 20.1
    S. Walayat Hussain, Christopher J. Miller and Timothy S. Wang

21. Principles of Phototherapy, 21.1
    Kevin McKenna and Sally Ibbotson

22. Principles of Photodynamic Therapy, 22.1
    Sally Ibbotson and Kevin McKenna

23. Principles of Cutaneous Laser Therapy, 23.1
    Vishal Madan and Jill S. Waibel

24. Principles of Radiotherapy, 24.1
    Charles G. Kelly, John Frew and Najibah Mahtab

Part 3 Infections and Infestations

25. Viral Infections, 25.1
    Catherine A. Harwood and Jane C. Sterling

26. Bacterial Infections, 26.1
    Catriona Wootton and Ivo Elliott

27 Mycobacterial Infections, 27.1
Stephen L. Walker and Richard O. Phillips

28 Leprosy, 28.1
Diana N. J. Lockwood and Stephen L. Walker

29 Syphilis and Congenital Syphilis, 29.1
George R. Kinghorn and Rasha Omer

30 Non-syphilitic Bacterial Sexually Transmitted Diseases, 30.1
George R. Kinghorn and Nadi K. Gupta

31 HIV and the Skin, 31.1
Christopher B. Bunker and Vincent Piguet

32 Fungal Infections, 32.1
Roderick J. Hay

33 Parasitic Diseases, 33.1
Austinn C. Miller, Alfredo Siller Jr. and Stephen K. Tyring

34 Arthropods, 34.1
Charlotte Bernigaud, Gentiane Monsel, Pascal Delaunay and Olivier Chosidow

Index

VOLUME 2

Part 4 Inflammatory Dermatoses

35 Psoriasis and Related Disorders, 35.1
Brian Kirby and A. David Burden

36 Pityriasis Rubra Pilaris, 36.1
Curdin Conrad

37 Lichen Planus and Lichenoid Disorders, 37.1
Felix Lauffer and Kilian Eyerich

38 Graft-versus-host Disease, 38.1
Tanya N. Basu

39 Eczematous Disorders, 39.1
Avad A. Mughal and John R. Ingram

40 Seborrhoeic Dermatitis, 40.1
Sarah Wakelin and Anastasia Therianou

41 Atopic Eczema, 41.1
Michael R. Ardern-Jones, Carsten Flohr and Nick J. Reynolds

42 Urticaria, 42.1
Clive E. H. Grattan and Alison V. Sears

43 Recurrent Angio-oedema without Weals, 43.1
Clive E. H. Grattan and Marcus Maurer

44 Urticarial Vasculitis, 44.1
Karoline Krause and Clive E. H. Grattan

45 Autoinflammatory Diseases Presenting in the Skin, 45.1
Dan Lipsker, Clive E. H. Grattan and Christopher R. Lovell

46 Mastocytosis, 46.1
Clive E. H. Grattan and Deepti H. Radia

47 Reactive Inflammatory Erythemas, 47.1
Ruth Murphy

48 Adamantiades–Behçet Disease, 48.1
Christos C. Zouboulis

49 Neutrophilic Dermatoses, 49.1
Philip J. Hampton and Stephanie Ball

50 Immunobullous Diseases, 50.1
Enno Schmidt and Richard Groves

51 Lupus Erythematosus and Antiphospholipid Syndrome, 51.1
Jan Dutz and Touraj Khosravi-Hafshejani

52 Dermatomyositis, 52.1
Patrick Gordon and Daniel Creamer

53 Undifferentiated and Mixed Connective Tissue Disease and Dermatological Manifestations of Rheumatoid Disease, 53.1
Philip M. Laws

54 Systemic Sclerosis, 54.1
Catherine H. Orteu and Christopher P. Denton

55 Morphoea and Allied Scarring and Sclerosing Inflammatory Dermatoses, 55.1
Catherine H. Orteu

Part 5 Metabolic and Nutritional Disorders Affecting the Skin

56 Cutaneous Amyloidoses, 56.1
Stephan Schreml

57 Cutaneous Mucinoses, 57.1
Franco Rongioletti

58 Cutaneous Porphyrias, 58.1
Robert P. E. Sarkany

59 Calcification of the Skin and Subcutaneous Tissue, 59.1
Johnny Bourke and Matthew Murphy

60 Xanthomas and Abnormalities of Lipid Metabolism and Storage, 60.1
Paul D. Flynn

61 Nutritional Disorders Affecting the Skin, 61.1
Albert C. Yan and Netravali Michelle Oboite

62 Skin Disorders in Diabetes Mellitus, 62.1
Johnny Bourke and Matthew Murphy

Part 6 Genetic Disorders Involving the Skin

63 Inherited Disorders of Cornification, 63.1
Vinzenz Oji, Kira Süßmuth, Dieter Metze, Angela Hernandez Martin and Heiko Traupe

64 Inherited Acantholytic Disorders, 64.1
Mozheh Zamiri

65 Ectodermal Dysplasias, 65.1
Peter Itin

66 Inherited Hair Disorders, 66.1
Eli Sprecher

67 Genetic Defects of Nails and Nail Growth, 67.1
Samantha Gordon and Amy S. Paller

68 Genetic Disorders of Pigmentation, 68.1
Fanny Morice-Picard and Alain Taïeb

69 Genetic Blistering Diseases, 69.1
John A. McGrath

70 Genetic Disorders of Collagen, Elastin and Dermal Matrix, 70.1
Nigel Burrows

71 Disorders Affecting Cutaneous Vasculature, 71.1
Anne Dompmartin, Nicole Revencu, Laurence M. Boon and Miikka Vikkula

72 Genetic Disorders of Adipose Tissue, 72.1
George W. M. Millington

73 Congenital Naevi and Selected Naevoid Conditions, 73.1
Veronica A. Kinsler and Neil J. Sebire

74 Chromosomal Disorders, 74.1
Neil Rajan, Alan D. Irvine and Jemima E. Mellerio

75 Poikiloderma Syndromes, 75.1
Alan D. Irvine and Jemima E. Mellerio

76 DNA Repair Disorders with Cutaneous Features, 76.1
Hiva Fassihi

77 Syndromes with Premature Ageing, 77.1
Alan D. Irvine and Jemima E. Mellerio

78 Inherited Skin Tumour Syndromes, 78.1
Neil Rajan, Jemima E. Mellerio and Alan D. Irvine

79 Inherited Metabolic Diseases, 79.1
Andrew A.M. Morris

80 Inherited Immunodeficiency, 80.1
Tim Niehues and Andrew R. Gennery

Part 7 Psychological, Sensory and Neurological Disorders and the Skin

81 Pruritus, Prurigo and Lichen Simplex, 81.1
Sonja Ständer and Gil Yosipovitch

82 Mucocutaneous Pain Syndromes, 82.1
Jon Goulding and Anthony Bewley

83 Neurological Conditions Affecting the Skin, 83.1
Andrew G. Affleck

84 Psychodermatology, 84.1
Anthony Bewley and Ruth E. Taylor

85 Acquired Disorders of Epidermal Keratinisation, 85.1
Matthew J. Scorer and Graham A. Johnston

Index

VOLUME 3

Part 8 Skin Disorders Associated with Specific Cutaneous Structures

86 Acquired Pigmentary Disorders, 86.1
Nanja van Geel and Reinhart Speeckaert

87 Acquired Disorders of Hair, 87.1
Matthew J. Harries, Susan Holmes, Amy McMichael and Andrew G. Messenger

88 Acne, 88.1
Alison M. Layton, Christos C. Zouboulis and Heather Whitehouse

89 Rosacea, 89.1
Esther J. van Zuuren, Jerry Tan, Mireille M. D. van der Linden and Martin Schaller

90 Hidradenitis Suppurativa, 90.1
John R. Ingram, Hessel H. van der Zee and Gregor B. E. Jemec

91 Acquired Non-infective Disorders of the Pilosebaceous Unit, 91.1
Kapil Bhargava, Evangelos Christou and Christos Tziotzios

92 Disorders of the Sweat Glands, 92.1
Ian H. Coulson and Niall J. E. Wilson

93 Acquired Disorders of the Nails and Nail Unit, 93.1
Marcel C. Pasch, Bertrand Richert and Matilde Iorizzo

94 Acquired Disorders of Dermal Connective Tissue, 94.1
Caoimhe M. R. Fahy and Christopher R. Lovell

95 Granulomatous Disorders of the Skin, 95.1
John W. Frew and Saleem M. Taibjee

96 Sarcoidosis, 96.1
Joaquim Marcoval and Juan Mañá

97 Panniculitis, 97.1
Luis Requena and Lorenzo Cerroni

98 Non-inflammatory Disorders of Subcutaneous Fat, 98.1
Grace L. Lee, Amit Garg and Amy Y.-Y. Chen

Part 9 Vascular Disorders Involving the Skin

99 Purpura, 99.1
Nick J. Levell

100 Cutaneous Vasculitis, 100.1
Nick J. Levell and Chetan Mukhtyar

101 Dermatoses Resulting from Disorders of the Veins and Arteries, 101.1
Portia C. Goldsmith and Christina George

102 Ulceration Resulting from Disorders of the Veins and Arteries, 102.1
Jürg Hafner and Eberhard Rabe

103 Disorders of the Lymphatic System, 103.1
Peter S. Mortimer and Kristiana Gordon

104 Flushing and Blushing, 104.1
Elizabeth Keeling and Síona Ní Raghallaigh

Part 10 Skin Disorders Associated with Specific Sites, Sex and Age

105 Dermatoses of the Scalp, 105.1
Paul Farrant, Megan Mowbray and Anita Takwale

106 Dermatoses of the External Ear, 106.1
Cameron Kennedy and Ashish Sharma

107 Dermatoses of the Eye, Eyelids and Eyebrows, 107.1
Valerie P. J. Saw and Stuart N. Cohen

108 Dermatoses of the Oral Cavity and Lips, 108.1
Barbara Carey and Jane Setterfield

109 Dermatoses of the Male Genitalia, 109.1
Christopher B. Bunker and Richard E. Watchorn

110 Dermatoses of the Female Genitalia, 110.1
Fiona Lewis

111 Dermatoses of Perineal and Perianal Skin, 111.1
Eleanor Mallon

112 Cutaneous Complications of Stomas and Fistulae, 112.1
Calum Lyon

113 Dermatoses of Pregnancy, 113.1
Amy Stanway

114 Dermatoses of the Neonate, 114.1
Timothy H. Clayton and Jennifer C. Harrison Sharif

115 Dermatoses of Infancy, 115.1
Lea Solman and Mary T. Glover

116 Haemangiomas and Other Non-malignant Tumours of Infancy, 116.1
Lea Solman and Mary T. Glover

Index

VOLUME 4

Part 11 Skin Disorders Caused by External Agents

117 Benign Cutaneous Adverse Reactions to Drugs, 117.1
Michael R. Ardern-Jones

118 Severe Cutaneous Adverse Reactions to Drugs, 118.1
Daniel Creamer, Sarah Walsh and Haur Yueh Lee

119 Cutaneous Side Effects of Chemotherapy and Radiotherapy, 119.1
Louise Fearfield and Charlotte Edwards

120 Dermatoses Induced by Illicit Drugs, 120.1
Anthony Bewley and Iyas Assalman

121 Dermatological Manifestations of Metal Poisoning, 121.1
Rabindranath Nambi

122 Mechanical Injury to the Skin, 122.1
Saqib J. Bashir and Ai-Lean Chew

123 Pressure Injury and Pressure Ulcers, 123.1
Emily Haesler and Jan Kottner

124 Cutaneous Reactions to Cold and Heat, 124.1
Saqib J. Bashir and Ai-Lean Chew

125 Burns and Heat Injury, 125.1
Marc G. Jeschke

126 Cutaneous Photosensitivity Diseases, 126.1
Sally Ibbotson

127 Allergic Contact Dermatitis, 127.1
David Orton and Natalie Stone

128 Irritant Contact Dermatitis, 128.1
Jonathan M. L. White

129 Occupational Dermatology, 129.1
Jonathan M. L. White

130 Stings and Bites, 130.1
Alfredo Siller Jr., Austinn C. Miller and Stephen K. Tyring

Part 12 Neoplastic, Proliferative and Infiltrative Disorders Affecting the Skin

131 Benign Melanocytic Proliferations and Melanocytic Naevi, 131.1
Irene Stefanaki, Dimitris Sgouros and Alexander Stratigos

132 Benign Keratinocytic Acanthomas and Proliferations, 132.1
Edward Seaton and Vishal Madan

133 Cutaneous Cysts, 133.1
Vishal Madan and Edward Seaton

134 Lymphocytic Infiltrates, 134.1
Fiona Child and Sean J. Whittaker

135 Cutaneous Histiocytoses, 135.1
Thai Hoa Tran, Elena Pope and Sheila Weitzman

136 Soft-tissue Tumours and Tumour-like Conditions, 136.1
Eduardo Calonje and Zlatko Marušić

137 Tumours of Skin Appendages, 137.1
Eduardo Calonje and Zlatko Marušić

138 Kaposi Sarcoma, 138.1
Kenneth Y. Tsai

139 Cutaneous Lymphomas, 139.1
Sean J. Whittaker

140 Basal Cell Carcinoma, 140.1
Carl Vinciullo and Vishal Madan

141 Squamous Cell Carcinoma and its Precursors, 141.1
Girish Gupta and Thomas Dirschka

142 Melanoma Clinicopathology, 142.1
Jean Jacques Grob and Caroline Gaudy-Marqueste

143 Melanoma Surgery, 143.1
Noah R. Smith, Kelly B. Cha, Timothy M. Johnson and Alison B. Durham

144 Systemic Treatment of Melanoma, 144.1
Reinhard Dummer and Simone M. Goldinger

145 Dermoscopy of Melanoma and Naevi, 145.1
Natalia Jaimes and Ashfaq A. Marghoob

146 Merkel Cell Carcinoma, 146.1
Jürgen C. Becker, Isaac Brownell and Thibault Kervarrec

147 Skin Cancer in the Immunocompromised Patient, 147.1
Catherine A. Harwood, Rubeta N. Matin and Charlotte M. Proby

Part 13 Systemic Disease and the Skin

148 Cutaneous Markers of Internal Malignancy, 148.1
Lennart Emtestam and Karin Sartorius

149 The Skin and Disorders of the Haematopoietic and Immune Systems, 149.1
Tanya N. Basu and Austin Kulasekararaj

150 The Skin and Endocrine Disorders, 150.1
Ralf Paus and Yuval Ramot

151 The Skin and Disorders of the Heart, 151.1
Sonja Molin and Thomas Ruzicka

152 The Skin and Disorders of the Respiratory System, 152.1
Sonja Molin and Thomas Ruzicka

153 The Skin and Disorders of the Digestive System, 153.1
Sonja Molin and Thomas Ruzicka

154 The Skin and Disorders of the Kidney and Urinary Tract, 154.1
Sonja Molin and Thomas Ruzicka

155 The Skin and Disorders of the Musculoskeletal System, 155.1
Christopher R. Lovell

Part 14 Aesthetic Dermatology

156 Skin Ageing, 156.1
Elisabeth A. Pedersen, Gary J. Fisher, John J. Voorhees and Dana L. Sachs

157 Cosmeceuticals, 157.1
Neera R. Nathan, Eubee Koo, Alexandra B. Kimball and Molly Wanner

158 Soft-Tissue Augmentation (Fillers), 158.1
Berthold Rzany

159 Aesthetic Uses of Botulinum Toxins, 159.1
Nicholas J. Lowe and Philippa L. Lowe

160 Chemical Peels, 160.1
Chee-Leok Goh and Joyce Teng Ee Lim

161 Lasers and Energy-based Devices, 161.1
Nazanin Saedi and Christopher B. Zachary

Index

PART 11
Skin Disorders Caused by External Agents

CHAPTER 117

Benign Cutaneous Adverse Reactions to Drugs

M. Ardern-Jones

Sir Henry Wellcome Laboratories, Clinical and Experimental Sciences, Faculty of Medicine, University of Southampton, Southampton General Hospital, Southampton, UK

Drug-induced exanthems, 117.1	Drug-induced urticaria, angioedema and anaphylaxis, 117.5	Lichen planus-like drug eruptions and drug-induced lupus erythematosus, 117.7
Drug-induced pruritus, 117.2		
Drug-induced eczema, 117.3		Key references, 117.9

Drug-induced exanthems

Definition and nomenclature
Exanthematic eruptions can be caused by a variety of drugs and resemble in appearance the classical rash of viral infection for which the paradigm is the morbilliform rash associated with measles. Typically, exanthematic drug reactions do not show systemic involvement, but a mild fever and eosinophilia, which would characterise a viral reaction, may be seen [1,2].

> **Synonyms and inclusions**
> - Morbilliform drug eruption
> - Maculopapular drug eruption is a term that is frequently used but many eruptions are often not papular

Introduction and general description
There is no consensus definition of an exanthem, but it is generally considered to represent an acutely spreading eruption, hence the derivation of the name from the Latin/Greek exanthem 'to burst forth' [3]. These types of eruptions are the most frequent of all cutaneous reactions to drugs and can occur after almost any drug at any time up to 3 (but usually 2) weeks after administration; they may be accompanied by fever, pruritus and eosinophilia. It is not possible to identify the offending drug by the nature of the eruption.

Epidemiology
Exanthematous reactions are the most frequent presentation of non-immediate (non-IgE) drug allergy. The epidemiology of such reactions is not well characterised, but a French study identified 3.6 cutaneous allergic reactions per 1000 hospitalised patients, of which 56% showed exanthematous reactions [4] and a later study showed similar results [5]. Approximately 5% of those with Epstein–Barr virus infection who are prescribed aminopenicillins will develop a drug-induced exanthem [6].

Pathophysiology
The mechanism of cutaneous inflammation is mediated by drug-specific T cells (Chapter 14).

Pathology
Histology is generally non-specific. However, some histological features are used to discriminate drug-induced exanthems from non-drug exanthems including apoptotic keratinocytes, eosinophils within the inflammatory infiltrate, papillary oedema, and vascular changes [7].

Clinical features
These eruptions are often pruritic and the clinical features are variable; the lesions may be scarlatiniform, rubelliform or morbilliform, or may consist of a profuse eruption of small papules showing no close resemblance to any infective exanthem (Figures 117.1 and 117.2). Less common are eruptions with large macules, polycyclic and gyrate redness, reticular eruptions and sheet-like redness. The distribution is also variable but is generally symmetrical. The trunk and extremities are usually involved, and not uncommonly intertriginous areas may be favoured, but the face may be spared. Palmar and plantar lesions may occur, and sometimes the eruption is generalised. Purpuric lesions, especially on the legs, and erosive stomatitis may develop. There may be relative sparing of pressure areas.

Differential diagnosis
Viral infection is the most important differential diagnosis. Classical viral exanthems such as measles and chickenpox are readily identifiable [8]. In a recent series of atypical exanthems, morphology and laboratory investigations led to an aetiological diagnosis in 77% of cases [9]. Drugs were responsible for 25% of the exanthems (more commonly in adults) of which antibiotics and non-steroidal anti-inflammatory drugs (NSAIDs) were most frequently implicated. It is useful, in differentiating exanthematic drug eruptions from viral exanthems, to remember that viral rashes may start on the face and acral sites with subsequent progression to involve the

Rook's Textbook of Dermatology, Tenth Edition. Edited by Christopher Griffiths, Jonathan Barker, Tanya Bleiker, Walayat Hussain and Rosalind Simpson.
© 2024 John Wiley & Sons Ltd. Published 2024 by John Wiley & Sons Ltd.

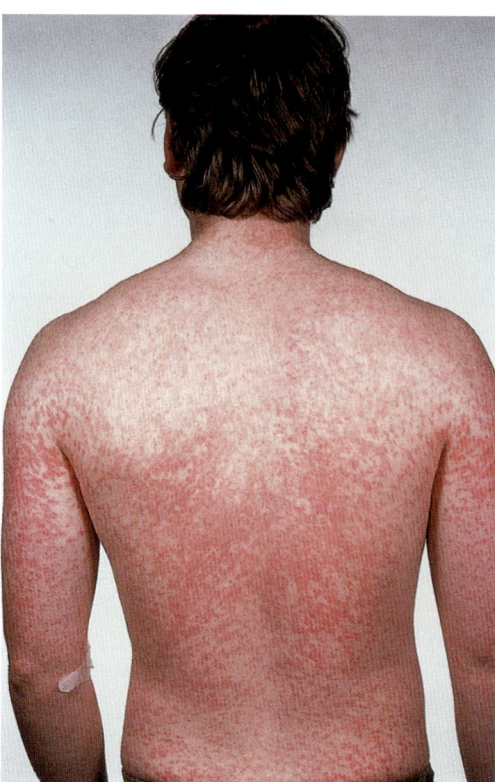

Figure 117.1 An exanthem caused by ampicillin.

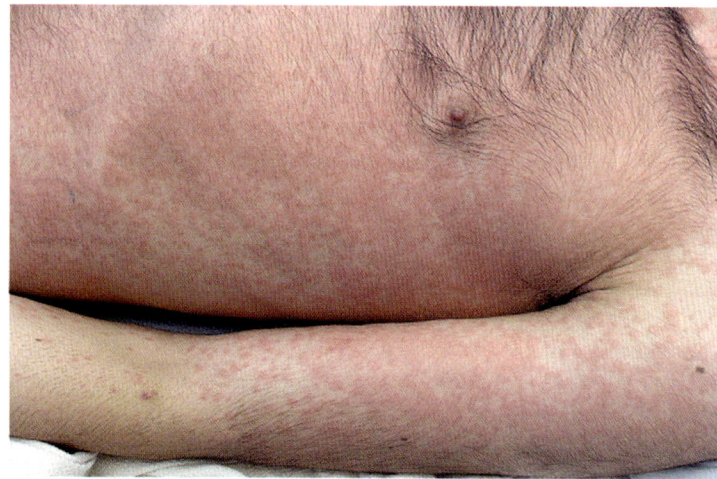

Figure 117.2 A drug-induced exanthem composed of macular and popular lesions, becoming confluent on the chest.

Table 117.1 Drugs causing exanthematic reactions.

Most common	Less common
Ampicillin and penicillin	Proton pump inhibitors
Carbamazepine	Cephalosporins
Sulphonamides	Thiazides
Phenytoin	Naproxen
Non-steroidal anti-inflammatory drugs	Isoniazid
Allopurinol	Phenothiazines
	Angiotensin-converting enzyme inhibitors

trunk, and are significantly more often accompanied by fever, sore throat, gastrointestinal symptoms, conjunctivitis, cough and insomnia [9]. Furthermore, enanthems (involving mucous membranes) were more commonly associated with an infectious aetiology. Pruritus was more commonly associated with drug causes in adults.

Drug reaction with eosinophilia and systemic symptoms (DRESS) is also important to exclude as the rash can be similar (Chapter 118). Stevens–Johnson syndrome or toxic epidermal necrolysis would not typically present in a similar manner. However, blisters, facial involvement, facial oedema, mucous membrane involvement and pyrexia should alert the clinician to the possibility of a severe cutaneous reaction [6].

Complications and co-morbidities

If the administration of the drug is continued, an exfoliative dermatitis may develop, although occasionally the eruption subsides despite continuation of the medication.

Disease course and prognosis

The illness follows a benign course and resolves without sequelae following cessation of the offending drug.

Investigations

Blood tests to exclude organ dysfunction and haematological abnormalities associated with DRESS are important. Viral serology/polymerase chain reaction may be useful to exclude viral infections. Skin histology is not routinely undertaken as it is not diagnostic of a drug cause, but may be useful to exclude other conditions where the clinical features are not characteristic.

Management

Cessation of the culprit drug is essential. On withdrawal of the drug, maculopapular drug eruptions usually fade with desquamation, sometimes with postinflammatory hyperpigmentation, and resolution is faster than for infectious exanthems.

Generally, symptomatic treatment only is required, and most cases benefit from emollients. Approximately 50% of exanthematous eruptions are pruritic and intermediate potency topical corticosteroids may be useful for these cases.

Morbilliform drug eruptions usually, but not always, recur on rechallenge. Commoner causes are listed in Table 117.1.

Drug-induced pruritus (Table 117.2)

Definition

Itch, which may be localised or generalised, caused by a drug.

Introduction and general description

Pruritus is generally a complication of systemic drugs, but is also associated with topical application, e.g. calcineurin inhibitors and beta-adrenergic blockers [10,11]. Drug-induced pruritus may be a primary neuronal/central nervous system interaction or through secondary mechanisms. Secondary pruritus includes direct skin effects such as hypersensitivity drug (allergy) rashes, xerosis and induction of inflammatory skin disease (such as lichen planus, psoriasis and eczema); alteration of biochemical profiles (e.g. renal or hepatic dysfunction); or other as yet unexplained mechanisms.

Table 117.2 Drugs causing pruritus.[a] Adapted from Reich et al. 2009 [22].

More frequent side effects	Less frequently reported
Opioids	Lapatinib
Statins	Quinolones
Paclitaxel	Metronidazole
Antimalarials	Cephalosporins
Granulocyte-macrophage colony-stimulating factor	Methyldopa
Interleukin-2	Tetracyclines
Matuzumab	Tiamphenicol
Angiotensin-converting enzyme inhibitors	Rifampin
Sulphonylurea derivates	Selective serotonin reuptake inhibitors
Non-steroidal anti-inflammatory drugs	Non-vitamin K oral anticoagulants

[a] Excludes those drugs in which the aetiology of pruritus is thought to be due to drug hypersensitivity or drug-induced cholestatic liver injury.

Epidemiology

Pruritus has been reported to arise in 13.3% of adverse reactions to prescribed drugs in general practice [12]. Opioid-induced pruritus is the most frequent and best recognised primary drug-induced pruritus and is reported to arise in 2–10% of patients treated with opiates [13].

Pathophysiology

The risk of drug-induced pruritus is increased with higher doses. Itching is usually first noted on the face, especially the perinasal area, but may become widespread. Opioids can induce mast cell degranulation and histamine release associated with an itchy urticarial rash. However, most opioid pruritus appears not to be histaminergic and likely involves binding of the drug to central μ-opioid pain receptors in the medullary dorsal horn [14], but serotonin and dopamine D_2 receptors, spinal inhibitory pathways and prostaglandins have also been implicated [15].

Chloroquine can cause mast cell-induced histamine pruritus. However, the precise cause of generalised pruritus seen in 60–70% of black African people treated with antimalarials is unclear and likely to be multifactorial, including μ-opioid receptor signalling as well as a genetic cause (it is less common in white people) [16,17]. Selective serotonin reuptake inhibitor (SSRI)-induced pruritus is also well recognised; these drugs can induce itching when injected into the skin [18]. Interestingly, SSRIs can also be used to treat psychogenic itching [19].

Hydroxyethyl starch (HES) is used for colloid fluid replacement in some settings and has been associated with chronic pruritus in approximately one-third of patients. HES-induced itch can arise even after small volumes, but the complication is more common with greater exposure. The symptoms typically arise after 1–6 weeks of HES infusion, which accounts for the relatively recent characterisation of this association in 1990 [20]. Furthermore, the itch can persist for 12–24 months [21] and is generally refractory to treatment [22].

Recently, the increased prescribing of non-warfarin oral anticoagulants has led to the recognition that these therapies may be common causes of drug-induced itch although the mechanism has not been elucidated [23].

Clinical features

Pruritus describes only the sensation of itch, which is purely subjective to the patient, and therefore there may be no skin changes evident. However, scratching may leave excoriations or purpura from recent-onset pruritus, or lichenification in more chronic cases.

Differential diagnosis

Pruritus is most commonly caused by dry skin and associated disorders such as eczema, so other conditions must be excluded (Chapter 81).

Disease course and prognosis

Although considered a mild adverse drug reaction, chronic pruritus can have a very significant negative effect on quality of life.

Investigations

Exclusion of other causes of itch is recommended (Chapter 81).

Management

Generally, cessation of the culprit drug brings rapid relief. However, as with HES, some drug-induced pruritus can be long-lived. Although antihistamine medications are frequently prescribed for drug-induced pruritus, they are rarely of benefit. Cooling emollients such as 0.5% menthol in aqueous cream may be of benefit.

In view of the direct involvement of opioid receptors in opiate-induced pruritus, the most effective means of treatment is reduction in dose or cessation of opiate treatment. Alternatively, introduction of naloxone, naltrexone (μ-receptor antagonists) or nalbuphine (partial κ-receptor agonist, μ-receptor antagonist) may be tried, but all of these approaches are likely to lead to loss of pain control. Other approaches including addition dopamine (D_2) receptor antagonists, serotonin (5-HT_3) receptor antagonists (ondansetron, dolasetron), antihistamines and preoperative gabapentin have been tried with varying success [22]. Interestingly, μ-receptor antagonists have also been utilised in other forms of pruritus especially where endogenous endorphins are thought to be pathogenic, such as in cholestatic pruritus, which has been proven in a double-blind randomised controlled clinical trial [24].

For more resistant cases of drug-induced pruritus, phototherapy and other therapeutic options may be of value (Chapter 81).

Drug-induced eczema

Definition and nomenclature

Allergic contact dermatitis is discussed in Chapter 127. This section concerns systemic allergic contact dermatitis (SACD) [25–27].

Synonyms and inclusions [28]
Systemic allergic contact dermatitis includes:
- Symmetrical drug-related intertriginous and flexural exanthema (SDRIFE)
- Baboon syndrome (BS)
- Allergic contact dermatitis syndrome
- Systemic nickel allergy syndrome

Table 117.3 Terms previously used for systemic allergic contact dermatitis and related conditions. Adapted from Pan et al. 2021 [**29**] and Hausermann et al. 2004 [30].

Internal-external contact type hypersensitivity (Ratner et al. 1974) [39]
Mercury exanthem (eczema rubrum) (Nakayama et al. 1983) [38]
Baboon syndrome – systemically induced allergic contact dermatitis (Andersen et al. 1984) [37]
Non-pigmenting fixed drug eruption (Shelley and Shelley 1987) [40]
Intertriginous drug eruption (Wolf et al. 1992) [41]
Drug-induced intertrigo (Wolf et al. 1993) [42]
Systemic contact dermatitis (Menne et al. 1994) [27]
Paraptic eczema (Happle 1994) [43]
Symmetric ptychotropic and non-pigmenting fixed drug eruption (Helmbold et al. 1998) [44]
Flexural (drug) eruption (Wakelin et al. 1999) [45]
Symmetrical drug-related intertriginous and flexural exanthema (SDRIFE) (Hausermann et al. 2004) [30]
Systemic allergic (contact) dermatitis (Thyssen and Maibach 2008) [46]

Introduction and general description

Systemic allergic contact dermatitis describes the elicitation of an eczematous reaction following topical sensitisation on subsequent systemic re-exposure to the same substance. Discussion of this condition in the literature is confused by the variety of names used to describe this problem (Table 117.3). A patient initially sensitised to a drug by way of allergic contact dermatitis may develop an eczematous reaction when the same, or a chemically related, substance is subsequently administered systemically. The eruption tends to be symmetrical, and may involve first, or most severely, the site(s) of the original dermatitis, before becoming generalised.

Epidemiology

Rare.

Pathophysiology

The eczematous response is mediated by drug-specific T-cell-induced inflammation in the skin. Recently, the possibility of sensitisation via other routes of exposure including implants and prostheses has been proposed [**29**] (Chapter 14).

Pathology

The histological features of drug-induced eczema (including BS and SDRIFE) are non-specific but show eczematous features including variable spongiosis and upper dermal infiltrates of mononuclear cells and including eosinophils. Apoptotic and necrotic changes in keratinocytes are reported in some cases but are uncommon [30].

Clinical features

Patients with a contact allergy to ethylenediamine may develop urticaria or systemic eczema following injection of aminophylline preparations containing ethylenediamine as a solubiliser for theophylline [31,32]. Patients with contact allergy to parabens may develop systemic eczema on medication with a drug containing parabens as a preservative [33]. Similarly, sensitised patients may develop eczema following oral ingestion of neomycin or hydroxyquinolines [34]. Diabetic patients sensitised by topical preparations containing *p*-amino compounds, such as *p*-phenylenediamine hair dyes, *para*-aminobenzoic acid (PABA) sunscreens and certain local anaesthetic agents (e.g. benzocaine), may develop a systemic contact dermatitis with the hypoglycaemic agents tolbutamide or chlorpropamide. Sulphonylureas may also induce eczematous eruptions in sulphanilamide-sensitive patients as a result of cross-reactivity. Phenothiazines can produce allergic contact dermatitis, photoallergic reactions and eczematous contact-type dermatitis, and may cross-react with certain antihistamines. Tetraethylthiuram disulphide (disulfiram, Antabuse) for the management of alcoholism can cause eczematous reactions in patients sensitised to thiurams via rubber gloves. Drugs given systemically have also been identified as causing eczematous drug reactions without prior contact sensitisation and approximately 50% of cases of SACD are due to penicillins or β-lactam antibiotics (Table 117.4). The term 'endogenic contact eczema' [35] refers to the occurrence of an eczematous contact drug reaction following primary sensitisation by oral therapy, as in the case of a patient with a drug-related exanthem who later develops localised dermatitis due to topical therapy. Such eczematous eruptions have been reported following therapy with penicillins, NSAIDs and others. Patients may have positive patch tests to the drug.

BS denotes a characteristic pattern of systemic allergic contact dermatitis [21,**22**,23] in which there is diffuse redness of the buttocks, upper inner thighs and axillae. There has been some debate regarding the exact pathomechanism of this pattern and although

Table 117.4 Systemic drugs associated with systemic allergic contact dermatitis[a]. Adapted from [46–52].

α-Blockers
8-Methoxypsoralen
5-Aminosalicylic acid
Aminophylline
Analgesics: non-steroidal anti-inflammatory drugs, opiates, paracetamol
Antibiotics: amoxicillin, ceftriaxone, chloramphenicol, clindamycin, erythromycin, fusidic acid, gentamicin, isoniazid, miconazole, neomycin, nystatin, quinolones, streptomycin, sulfamethoxazole-trimethoprim, terbinafine
Antihistamines: cetirizine, diphenhydramine, hydroxyzine
Antihypertensives: alprenolol, captopril, telmisartan-hydrochlorothiazide
Anti-inflammatories: acetyl salicylic acid, 5-aminosalicylic acid, corticosteroids, cyclo-oxygenase-2 inhibitors
Antivirals: acyclovir, valacyclovir
Biologic agents: cetuximab
Chemotherapy agents: 5-fluorouracil, mitomycin C
Clobazam
Clonidine
Doxepin
Ephedrine
Glyceryl trinitrate
Heparin
Hydroxycarbamide
Intravenous human immunoglobulins
Iodinated radio contrast media
Oestradiol
Phenobarbitol
Phenothiazines
Pseudoephedrine
Rivastigmine
Sulfonamides
Suxamethonium
Vitamin B6

[a] Including Baboon syndrome and SDRIFE.

initially reported as a systemic allergic contact dermatitis in which the rash evolves following systemic exposure to a known contact allergen, it has become clear that systemic drugs can also induce BS without prior skin sensitisation and without cross-reactivity to known contact allergens. Thus, the term SDRIFE was proposed to identify those cases of BS in whom exposure to a systemically administered drug induces BS [30]. Diagnostic criteria for SDRIFE stipulate a symmetrical, sharply demarcated redness of the buttocks/perineum and groin, with involvement of at least one other flexural site and absence of systemic symptoms and signs. SDRIFE is considered alongside other 'classical' systemic delayed-type T-cell-mediated drug hypersensitivity variants such as DRESS (Chapter 118).

BS/SDRIFE has been reported to be provoked by antibiotics (especially penicillins), nickel, heparin, mercury (including that found in a homeopathic medicine [36]), and more recently biologics (Table 117.4). Disulfiram therapy of a nickel-sensitive alcoholic patient may induce this syndrome, as the drug leads to an initial acute increase in blood nickel concentration [37]. Cases have been described from Japan under the name 'mercury exanthem' following inhalation of mercury vapour from crushed thermometers in patients with a history of mercury allergy [38].

Differential diagnosis
- Idiopathic eczematous reactions
- Allergic contact dermatitis
- Bacterial toxin reaction

Complications and co-morbidities
Following drug withdrawal, complications and co-morbidities are minimal.

Disease course and prognosis
On withdrawal of the offending drug, resolution of the clinical symptoms generally occurs in 1–3 weeks. Re-exposure at a later time would be expected to reproduce the same clinical picture.

Investigations
Patch tests are commonly positive and usually vesicular, although histology of the eruption itself may show leukocytoclastic vasculitis; oral challenge with the suspected antigen may be required to substantiate the diagnosis.

Management
The primary objective is cessation of the causative drug. Therapies utilised to treat eczematous dermatoses, such as topical corticosteroids, are usually effective. For severe reactions systemic treatment with prednisolone may be appropriate.

Drug-induced urticaria, angioedema and anaphylaxis

Definition and nomenclature
Urticaria and angioedema are physical signs that principally involve circumscribed skin oedema and redness and are described in detail in Chapter 42. Anaphylaxis is a constellation of clinical findings that describes respiratory and cardiovascular compromise (bronchoconstriction and hypotension) in a life-threatening manner and is described in Chapter 42. This chapter is concerned with drug-induced causes of these reaction patterns.

> **Synonyms and inclusions**
> - Pseudoallergy (non-immune mediated) describes a presentation which is clinically indistinguishable from true allergy (IgE mediated). Pseudoallergic urticaria, angioedema and anaphylaxis are commonly mediated by drugs as discussed here and these reactions are sometimes referred to as 'anaphylactoid'.

Introduction and general description
Drug-induced urticaria can be seen in isolation or in association with anaphylaxis and angioedema.

Epidemiology
Urticaria (Chapter 42) is the second most common type of adverse cutaneous drug eruption [53,54] (Figure 117.3). Drug-induced urticaria is seen in 0.16% of medical in-patients and accounts for 9% of chronic urticaria or angioedema seen in dermatology out-patient departments [53]. Urticaria develops in about 1% of patients receiving blood transfusions [55].

In children, food is the commonest cause of anaphylaxis, whereas in adults it is drugs. It has been estimated that 1 in 1500 of the population of England has experienced anaphylaxis at some point in their lives [56] and of the average 20 deaths recorded each year in the UK, at least half were due to drugs [57]. The incidence of anaphylaxis during general anaesthesia has been estimated to arise in 1:4000 to 1:25 000 cases [58].

Pathophysiology
The mechanisms underlying the localised superficial vasodilation, oedema and itch in urticaria are identical to that seen in the angioedema (deeper in skin) and anaphylaxis (systemic circulation). Classical reactions are mediated by the presence of drug-specific IgE. On exposure to the drug, cross-linking of IgE on the surface

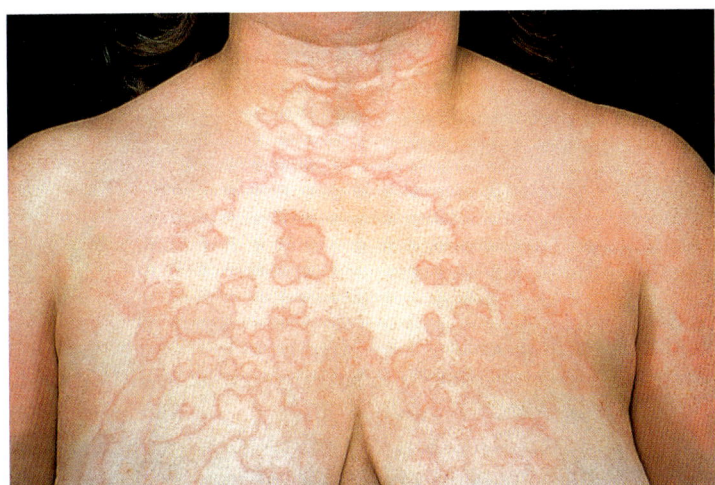

Figure 117.3 Urticaria induced by acetylsalicylic acid. Courtesy of St John's Institute of Dermatology, King's College London, UK.

of mast cells (and possibly basophils) is followed by inflammatory mediator release (including histamine), which induces vasodilatation, neuronal activation and smooth muscle contraction (Chapter 14).

Recent discovery of the Mas-related G protein–coupled receptor member X2 (MRGPRX2) [59] has helped explain pseudoallergic reactions. The MRGPRX2 receptor binds a variety of drugs and causes mast cell degranulation without involvement of adaptive immunity. Drugs which bind this receptor include morphine and contrast agents. NSAIDs are well-established inducers of pseudoallergic urticaria and angiodema, but as yet evidence does not support their interaction with MRGPRX2 [60].

Genetics
See Chapter 14.

Pathology
See Chapter 42.

Clinical features
Urticaria with or without angioedema and anaphylaxis typically arises within 24–36 h of drug ingestion on the first occasion. On rechallenge, lesions may develop within minutes. Angioedema, involving oedema of the deep dermis or subcutaneous and submucosal areas, usually arises with urticaria, but the combination is seen less frequently than urticaria alone.

Anaphylaxis and anaphylactoid reactions usually develop within minutes to hours (the vast majority within the first hour), are often severe and may be fatal [61]. In most cases, there are associated skin or mucosal changes.

There are different clinical features of anaphylaxis identified in different organs. In less severe cases, there may be premonitory dizziness or faintness, skin tingling and reddening of the bulbar conjunctiva, followed by urticaria, angioedema, bronchospasm, abdominal pain and vasomotor collapse. Intravenous administration is associated with more severe reactions and more rapid progression over minutes to cardiac arrest as compared with insect sting- and food-induced anaphylaxis which evolves more slowly [62]. Deaths are uncommon (<2%) and the major predisposing risk factor for poor outcome is coexistent severe asthma [63,64]. Anaphylaxis usually develops on second exposure to a drug as it is thought that prolonged treatments may induce tolerisation rather than allergy (in contrast to T-cell-mediated hypersensitivities) and are typically noted on the first dose of the second exposure.

Recent identification of anaphylaxis with the Covid-19 vaccine has highlighted the role of vaccines as unpredictable triggers in 2.5–11 per 10^6 doses. This may be as high as 2–8.5 times more frequent than that noted for routine vaccinations [65].

Differential diagnosis
Drug-induced urticaria needs to be distinguished from other causes of urticaria, especially infection. This distinction may require specialist testing. More than 90% of those investigated for penicillin allergy are subsequently found to be negative on testing. Drug allergy testing for local anaesthetics suggests that the frequency of allergy to these drugs is very rarely confirmed.

Drug-induced anaphylaxis needs to be distinguished from other causes of anaphylaxis (Chapter 42). Angiodema without urticaria induced by angiotensin-converting enzyme (ACE) inhibitors is not a true allergy and is usually mediated by ACE induced bradykinin accumulation. It arises in 0.1–0.7% of treated patients [66]. This may arise many months to years after commencing therapy. Other possibilities are not drug related and include hereditary angioedema, for which various screening tests are required [67].

Complications and co-morbidities
Anaphylaxis may result in death if untreated. With early intervention treatment outcomes are good. However, it is critical that causation is addressed and investigated as necessary to prevent accidental reoccurrence.

Disease course and prognosis
On withdrawal of the offending drug, clinical improvement arises within 24–48 h. It is important to recognise that after an initial improvement from anaphylaxis, late phase reactions may arise 5–6 h afterwards (Chapter 14).

Investigations
The investigation of immediate drug allergy reactions (characterised by urticaria, angioedema or anaphylaxis) is well established and various guidelines represent consensus approaches to the investigation of the culprit drug [68]. The general approach is based upon a careful documentation of the exposure history in the hours preceding the reaction to establish the most likely causative drugs. Careful record should be made of the timeline of clinical features, for example detailed examination of the anaesthetic chart for records of onset of hypotension in cases of perioperative anaphylaxis. Testing involves an escalation of exposures which is stopped if any positive result is identified, thereby minimising risk. In many circumstances it is more useful to prove a negative through testing than confirm a drug allergy through testing, so as to establish what is safe for the patient to take. The testing process involves plasma sampling for drug-specific IgE, skin prick testing, intradermal testing and challenge testing. Despite the availability of some antibiotic-specific IgE measurements (e.g. penicillin), it is to be emphasised that because the interpretation of the results requires detailed knowledge, such investigation is recommended to only be undertaken by those who have specialist experience in drug allergy investigation [69].

Aspirin and NSAIDS are the most frequently implicated drugs in allergic reactions and most frequently cause NSAID-induced urticaria [70] as well as exacerbating idiopathic urticaria [71] and physical urticarias. However, NSAID-induced urticaria is not thought to precipitate chronic urticaria [70]. Although cross-reactivity occurs throughout the NSAID class, selective COX-2 inhibitors are recommended in low-risk NSAID-sensitive patients where anti-inflammatory therapy is required [69]. In addition, an unsuspected agent, for example the yellow dye tartrazine, may really be responsible for an urticaria attributed to aspirin or another drug. The opiate analgesics are also a cause of urticaria by directly activating mast cells [72]. There have been numerous papers on the potential role of food and drug additives [73], including preservatives such as benzoic acid, butylated hydroxyanisole, butylated hydroxytoluene, sulphites and rarely aspartame, as well as tartrazine dyes, in the development of chronic urticaria. However, reports of the role of food additives in the pathogenesis of urticaria are conflicting [74,75]. Urticaria may follow alcohol consumption, but this is thought to be most commonly due to sulphite reactivity [76]. Other reports associate the reaction with intra-articular methylprednisolone [77] and even cetirizine and fexofenadine [78,79].

Other drugs, such as radiocontrast media, local anaesthetics and dextrans (in plasma expanders), may release mast cell mediators directly (see earlier). Cyclo-oxygenase inhibitors, such as aspirin and indomethacin, and ACE inhibitors, such as captopril and enalapril, may cause urticaria or angioedema by pharmacological mechanisms.

The most frequent drug causes are antibiotics (usually beta-lactams) and NSAIDs [58]. However, biologics are increasingly common culprits including anti-IgE therapy. Omalizumab causes anaphylaxis in approximately 0.09–0.2% of treated patients [58]. Infliximab is estimated to cause anaphylaxis or IgE-mediated reactions in 2–3% [80] and reaction to other tumour necrosis factor (TNF) antagonists is also recorded [81]. Anaphylaxis during general anaesthesia is also an important problem and can be difficult to investigate if intraoperative exposures are not well recorded. Furthermore, distinction between true immune-mediated and non-immune-mediated reactions can be challenging. Due to their similar formulation, increasing reports of anaphylaxis to excipients of injectable therapies are recognised. These are difficult to diagnose and usually come to light in individuals with reactions to multiple unrelated active medications, and therefore it is important to consider excipient allergy in multidrug-allergic individuals to avoid the possibility of a further reaction [82].

Common perioperative causes of anaphylaxis or anaphylactoid reactions include anaesthetic agents (especially thiopental), neuromuscular blocking agents (NMBA), analgesics (opioids are usually associated with non-IgE-mediated reactions), antibiotics, protamine and blood transfusions (mechanism unclear) [58]. The pholcodeine hypothesis suggests that NMBA cross-reactivity to pholcodeine, a common ingredient in cough medicines, has gained support from European countries that have banned its sale and noted subsequent decline in NMBA anaphylaxis, in contrast to countries where sale was permitted to continue [83]. Recently, anaphylaxis caused by drugs bioengineered onto medical equipment such as chlorhexidine-coated central venous catheters has been increasingly recognised [84]. The β-blockers enhance anaphylactic reactions caused by other allergens and may make resuscitation more difficult [62].

β-Lactam allergy reactions are due to IgE recognition of the drug bound to a carrier molecule (Chapter 14). Skin testing is undertaken with benzylpenicilloyl-polylysine 'major antigenic determinant' and 'minor determinants' (other penicillin antigens). Drug-specific IgE measured by ImmunoCAP™ (RAST) has a high specificity but low sensitivity and therefore should only be used by specialists with access to the full range of skin testing as well. Progression to intradermal testing and challenge if necessary is advocated by European and UK guidelines [68]. Multiple studies have shown the very low positive predictive value of labels of 'penicillin allergy' confirmed by negative testing including oral challenge. Although penicillin avoidance is not difficult for the majority of cases, adverse outcomes of mislabelling with penicillin allergy are increasingly recognised and confirmatory testing is recommended in specific groups [69]. Given the prevalence of mislabelling of penicillin allergy, false negatives and false positives, and cost of skin testing, some groups have promoted 'direct challenge' testing by non-allergists for both children [85] and adults [86]. This would require a validated questionnaire to de-risk the process and identify high-risk cases.

Patch testing is not useful in the investigation of anaphylaxis and caution should be employed when considering patch testing to allergens where the clinical reaction may have been IgE mediated. Anaphylaxis does occur after non-mucosal topical drug administration, especially to skin wounds or to skin with impaired barrier function [87].

Management
For evolving urticaria with or without angioedema or anaphylaxis, the key principal management step is to stop the offending drug and disease resolution occurs quickly. Oral/IV antihistamines, oral/IV corticosteroids and SC epinephrine/adrenaline may be required as per local guidelines [88].

Lichen planus-like drug eruptions and drug-induced lupus erythematosus

Definition
Lichen planus-like drug eruptions are clinically indistinguishable from normal lichen planus although they are more frequently severe and show similar lichenoid histology. Generally, this diagnosis is established by temporal association with drug exposure and disease resolution on drug withdrawal but distinction from idiopathic lichen planus can be challenging.

Drug-induced lupus shows the clinical and immunological features of idiopathic lupus erythematosus but is initiated by drug exposure and resolves on withdrawal of the offending drug.

Introduction and general description
Lichenoid skin eruptions are characterised by epidermal basal keratinocyte damage, with an associated dermal lymphoid infiltrate. Lichenoid drug eruptions may present as a variety of clinical patterns including fixed drug eruptions, lupus erythematosus (LE) and lichen planus (LP). It has been suggested that the different clinical patterns reflect lymphocyte 'cell rich' (e.g. LP) and 'cell poor' (e.g. LE) lichenoid patterns [89]. However, although it seems likely from the highly varied presenting features, there is no clear evidence that a different disease mechanism underlies the different conditions.

Epidemiology
Drug-induced LP reactions are less common than non-drug, and probably represent approximately 10% of cases. They are largely clinically indistinguishable from the non-drug reactions.

Table 117.5 Causes of drug-induced lupus erythematosus. Adapted from [103–105].

Important/widely used causes	Less widely used causes	Low-risk causes	Recent reports
ACE inhibitors (e.g. captopril)	Anti-thyroid drugs (e.g. propylthiouracil)	Anticonvulsants (e.g. carbamazepine)	Biologic anti-TNF monoclonal antibodies
β-Blockers (e.g. atenolol)[a]	Chlorpromazine	Ciprofloxacin	Cimetidine
Calcium channel blockers (e.g. diltiazem)[b]	Fluorouracil (systemic)[b]	D-penicillamine	Clobazam
Isoniazid	Hydralazine	Griseofulvin[b]	Clopidogrel
Statins[a]	Methyldopa	Hydroxycarbamide	Clozapine
Sulfasalazine	Procanamide	Lithium	Interferons
Terbinafine[b]	Quinidine	NSAIDs[b]	Interleukin-2
Thiazide diuretics	Minocycline	Penicillin	Ticlopidine
		Proton pump inhibitors (e.g. Omeprazole)[b]	Zafirlukast
		Rifampicin	

ACE, angiotensin-converting enzyme; NSAID, non-steroidal anti-inflammatory drug; SCLE, subacute cutaneous lupus erythematosus; SLE, systemic lupus erythematosus; TNF, tumour necrosis factor.
[a] More typically associated with SCLE-type reactions.
[b] May be associated with both SLE and SCLE-type reactions.

Pathophysiology

The mechanisms underlying lichenoid drug eruptions are essentially unknown, but they may develop as a result of autoreactive T cells directed against a drug–MHC antigen complex, such that keratinocytes and Langerhans cells are viewed by the immune system as 'non-self'. Genetic factors have been strongly linked with drug-induced lupus such as hydralazine (73% HLA-DR4) [90] and minocycline (HLA-DQB1) [91], which support the prevailing concept of a T-cell-mediated disease. Lage et al. showed a significant positive correlation between CD8 frequency and perforin expression in skin biopsies from drug-induced lichenoid eruptions versus classical LP, suggesting that cytotoxic CD8 T cells may be crucial for induction of keratinocyte apoptosis [92]. However, injection of autoreactive CD4 T cell clones has been shown to be sufficient to induce a lichenoid skin reaction in a murine model reaching maximal severity at day 5 [89]. The presence of epidermotropic T cells correlates with that of MHC class II (HLA-DR)-expressing keratinocytes and Langerhans cells in lichenoid eruptions [89]. The cross-reactive nature of herpes simplex virus (HSV)-specific T cells with drugs has recently been reported and the authors suggest that antiviral skin-resident CD8 memory T cells cross-reactive with drug antigens may represent an important disease mechanism in lichenoid drug eruptions [89].

Pathology

Lichenoid drug eruptions show typical histological evidence of lichenoid change including hyperkeratosis, hypergranulosis, 'saw tooth' acanthosis, and a band-like infiltrate in the superficial dermis. Although histological features such as a more pleomorphic and less dense infiltrate and the presence of focal parakeratosis, focal interruption of the granular layer and cytoid bodies in the cornified and granular layers have been reported to be suggestive of a drug cause [93], a recent study found that the only distinguishing characteristics were a statistically significantly higher frequency of necrotic keratinocytes (in clusters), and infiltrating plasma cells and eosinophils were associated with drug-induced LP [92]. Drug-induced LP may also show sparse eosinophils, often identified around blood vessels [94]. Later, there may be scarring, with destruction of the sweat glands.

Clinical features

The skin changes of LP-like drug eruptions may be non-specific or may resemble the classical small, shiny papules and plaques with Wickham striae as in idiopathic LP. Mucosal lichenoid reactions can similarly be caused by drugs. Oral LP is less frequently associated with drugs, and typically occurs on the buccal mucosa, tongue and gingivae (Chapter 37).

It is recognised that approximately 10% of LE cases are mediated by drugs, but the clinical pattern of drug-induced LE is more commonly like systemic LE than subacute LE [95].

Drug-induced LE is classically caused by drugs such as procainamide, methyldopa, quinidine and hydralazine (Table 117.5), but many of these are no longer widely used. Hyperpigmented lichenoid drug eruptions are more common in skin of colour and have been reported with a variety of medications including statins (Figure 117.4).

Photodistributed lichenoid lesions may occur with a number of drugs, including thiazide diuretics. More recent reports of biologics (especially anti-TNF-α inhibitors and immune checkpoint inhibitors) causing lichenoid eruptions suggest that this may become an increasing problem [96–98,**99**,100].

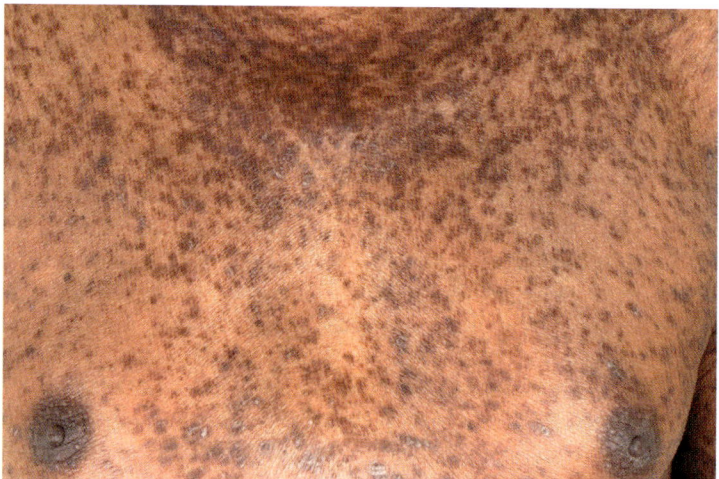

Figure 117.4 Pravastatin-induced lichenoid drug eruption with numerous hyperpigmented patches and plaques disseminated over the torso.

Table 117.6 Causes of drug-induced lichen planus. Adapted from [94,106,107].

Well-established causes	Less well-established causes
Antimalarials	Angiotensin-converting enzyme inhibitors
Gold	β-Blockers
Mercury amalgam	Lithium
Non-steroidal anti-inflammatory drugs	Methyldopa
Pencillamine	Quinidine
Anti-tumour necrosis factor drugs	Statins
Nivolumab; pembrolizumab	Sulfonylureas
Thiazide diuretics	Ethambutol

Differential diagnosis
- Idiopathic lichen planus
- Idiopathic lupus erythematosus

Complications and co-morbidities
If untreated these are the same as the idiopathic conditions (Chapters 37 and 51).

Disease course and prognosis
The diagnosis is proven by disease resolution on withdrawal of the offending drug.

Investigations
Skin histology is essential for the investigation of lichenoid drug eruptions (Chapter 37).

In drug-induced LE, immunological findings typically show positive antinuclear antigen and positive anti-Ro antibodies. Positive antihistone antibodies (90% ANA positive) are seen in 75% of patients [101].

Management
Diagnosis is confirmed by withdrawal of the offending drug and this is the essential step in management. Time to resolution will be modified by drug half-life and therefore biologics-induced lichenoid eruptions may resolve slowly. Therapy with topical corticosteroids, oral antihistamines, gabapentin and pregabalin have been used to modify the itch. Oral glucocorticoids may be required but should be employed cautiously because they may mask ongoing disease activity, should the diagnosis be incorrect. Only in rare circumstances would oral retinoids or methotrexate be considered if stopping the offending drug was not possible [102].

Common causes for drug-induced LE are represented in Table 117.5. Common causes for drug-induced LP are represented in Table 117.6.

Key references

The full list of references can be found in the online version at https://www.wiley.com/rooksdermatology10e

2 Peter JG, Lehloenya R, Dlamini S et al. Severe delayed cutaneous and systemic reactions to drugs: a global perspective on the science and art of current practice. *J Allergy Clin Immunol Pract* 2017;5:547–63.

3 Brockow K, Ardern-Jones MR, Mockenhaupt M et al. EAACI position paper on how to classify cutaneous manifestations of drug hypersensitivity. *Allergy* 2019;74:14–27.

22 Reich A, Stander S, Szepietowski JC. Drug-induced pruritus: a review. *Acta Derm Venereol* 2009;89:236–44.

29 Pan Z, Yang Y, Zhang L et al. Systemic contact dermatitis: the routes of allergen entry. *Clin Rev Allergy Immunol* 2021;61:339–50.

59 McNeil BD, Pundir P, Meeker S et al. Identification of a mast-cell-specific receptor crucial for pseudo-allergic drug reactions. *Nature* 2015;519(7542):237–41.

65 Sampath V, Rabinowitz G, Shah M et al. Vaccines and allergic reactions: the past, the current COVID-19 pandemic, and future perspectives. *Allergy* 2021; 76:1640–60.

69 Dworzynski K, Ardern-Jones M, Nasser S; Guideline Development Group Diagnosis and management of drug allergy in adults, children and young people: summary of NICE guidance. *BMJ* 2014;349:g4852.

99 Ellis SR, Vierra AT, Millsop JW, Lacouture ME, Kiuru M. Dermatologic toxicities to immune checkpoint inhibitor therapy: a review of histopathologic features. *J Am Acad Dermatol* 2020;83:1130–43.

104 Valeyrie-Allanore L, Sassolas B, Roujeau JC. Drug-induced skin, nail and hair disorders. *Drug Saf* 2007;30:1011–30.

CHAPTER 118

Severe Cutaneous Adverse Reactions to Drugs

Daniel Creamer[1], Sarah Walsh[1] and Haur Yueh Lee[2]

[1]Department of Dermatology, King's College Hospital, London, UK
[2]Department of Dermatology, Singapore General Hospital; DUKE-NUS Graduate Medical School, Singapore

Introduction, 118.1	Drug reaction with eosinophilia and systemic symptoms, 118.4	Stevens–Johnson syndrome/toxic epidermal necrolysis, 118.12
Acute generalised exanthematous pustulosis, 118.1		Key references, 118.22

Introduction

Phenotypic classification of the cutaneous adverse drug reactions can divide these disorders according to severity. Benign cutaneous adverse reactions (Chapter 117) tend not to have a systemic component whereas the severe cutaneous adverse reactions (SCARs) are characterised by significant systemic involvement causing considerable morbidity and a risk of mortality. The entities classified as SCARs are acute generalised exanthematous pustulosis (AGEP), drug reaction with eosinophilia and systemic symptoms (DRESS) and Stevens–Johnson syndrome/toxic epidermal necrolysis (SJS/TEN). The initial presentation of all of the SCAR disorders, however, may be similar to a drug-induced exanthem and therefore serial evaluation of the patient is necessary to monitor for progression or the emergence of a serious dermatosis. The clinician must be aware of the features ('red flags') that herald a more severe phenotype, therefore careful evaluation for a SCAR syndrome is essential in the assessment of any patient with a suspected drug-induced dermatosis.

Acute generalised exanthematous pustulosis

Definition and nomenclature

Acute generalised exanthematous pustulosis is one of the SCAR syndromes. It is characterised by the rapid appearance of sheets of non-follicular sterile pustules, usually localised to the major flexures, in response to a drug. It is a self-limiting phenomenon, which usually resolves without sequelae.

Synonyms and inclusions
- Exanthemic pustular psoriasis
- Toxic pustuloderma
- Pustular drug rash

These terms are now outmoded and in the interests of clarity, the term AGEP is preferred.

Introduction and general description

It is a drug-induced cutaneous reaction pattern first recognised in 1968 by Baker and Ryan who, in describing a series of patients with pustular psoriasis, identified a subgroup of five patients with a pustular eruption which was rapid in onset and in resolution, without a past history of psoriasis and in whom recurrence of the pustules was not seen [1]. There appeared to be a drug trigger in each of these cases, and the term exanthemic pustular psoriasis was coined. This term was later superseded by the terms toxic pustuloderma and pustular drug rash, which were variously used by authors to describe drug-related pustular eruptions which had a similar time course and characteristics; that is, short latency, rapid onset and resolution, and full recovery without recurrence [2,3]. In 1980, Beylot *et al.* suggested the term pustulose exanthemique aiguë généralisée (PEAG), and its English translation, AGEP, is now the accepted name for this phenomenon [4].

Epidemiology

The incidence of AGEP is estimated to be 1–5 per million per year [5].

Age

Acute generalised exanthematous pustulosis occurs more frequently in the adult population than in paediatric patients. A case–control study of 97 patients with a validated diagnosis of AGEP taken from the EuroSCAR registry demonstrated the mean age of onset to be 56 years [6].

Sex

The EuroSCAR registry study demonstrated a slight female preponderance, reporting a male to female incidence ratio of 0.8 [6].

Ethnicity

No ethnic variations have been described.

Rook's Textbook of Dermatology, Tenth Edition. Edited by Christopher Griffiths, Jonathan Barker, Tanya Bleiker, Walayat Hussain and Rosalind Simpson.
© 2024 John Wiley & Sons Ltd. Published 2024 by John Wiley & Sons Ltd.

Associated diseases

While 90% of cases of AGEP are thought to be drug related, there have been case reports associating the condition with a variety of underlying infections such as *Mycoplasma pneumoniae* [7], coxsackievirus [8], parvovirus B19 [9,10] and cytomegalovirus (CMV) [11]. Mercury exposure [12] and spider bites [13] have also been associated with AGEP in isolated case reports.

Pathophysiology

The pathophysiology of AGEP has not been fully elucidated, although some pathogenetic mechanisms have been proposed. Drug-specific CD4+ and CD8+ cells have been isolated from patch test sites and the peripheral blood of patients with AGEP [14,15]. These have demonstrated a high level of CXCL8 production. In addition, subtypes of T cells producing interleukin 8 (IL-8), a neutrophil-attracting chemokine, have also been identified in the peripheral blood of patients with AGEP [16,17]. These are proposed to be important in the pathogenesis of the sterile pustules seen in this disease process, by attracting neutrophils into the already oedematous skin and creating pustules. More recently, mutations in the *IL36RN* gene, which codes for the IL-36 receptor antagonist (IL-36Ra), have been identified in a subgroup of patients with AGEP [18]. Mutations in the *IL36RN* gene have been recognised to predispose to pustular psoriasis, particularly in patients who develop this condition without a preceding history of psoriasis vulgaris, as well as a number of other pustular phenotypes [19,20]. This indicates a possible mechanism of genetic predisposition to the development of AGEP.

Predisposing factors

Certain drugs are more closely associated with the development of AGEP (Box 118.1). In the largest study to date of this disease, the most commonly associated agents were pristinamycin, aminopenicillins, quinolones, chloroquine and hydroxychloroquine, sulphonamides, terbinafine and diltiazem [6]. Less commonly associated drugs were corticosteroids, other macrolide antibiotics, non-steroidal anti-inflammatory drugs of the oxicam class and antiepileptic medications (except valproate). Of note, this study also demonstrated that a number of commonly prescribed drugs which predispose to SJS/TEN do not appear to trigger AGEP. This included paracetamol, benzodiazepines, angiotensin-converting enzyme (ACE) inhibitors, β-blockers, aspirin, calcium-channel blockers, thiazide diuretics, angiotensin 2 receptor blockers ('-sartans'), allopurinol and cephalosporins [6].

Box 118.1 Commonest drugs causing acute generalised exanthematous pustulosis

- Aminopenicillins
- Chloroquine and hydroxychloroquine
- Diltiazem
- Pristinamycin
- Quinolones
- Sulphonamides
- Terbinafine

The EuroSCAR study examined other potential risk factors for AGEP and failed to find an association with infections, or past personal or family history of psoriasis [6].

Pathology

The histopathology of AGEP is characterised by marked spongiosis affecting the dermis and epidermis, accompanied by intraepidermal pustules and vesicles. A perivascular infiltrate occurs, which is usually neutrophilic. Occasional eosinophils may be seen but are not invariably present. There are infrequent necrotic keratinocytes (Figure 118.1). The classic histopathological features of psoriasis are absent, a fact which may be important in distinguishing the presentation of AGEP from its closest differential, pustular psoriasis.

A study of the histopathological features of 21 patients with AGEP demonstrated marked to moderate papillary dermal oedema and a mixed dermal inflammatory infiltrate in all biopsy samples [21]. Spongiform pustules were noted within the epidermis and occasional dyskeratotic cells with residual perivascular dermal oedema. Although no definitive vasculitis was seen, there was leukocytoclasis within the dermal infiltrate in the majority of biopsy specimens performed more than 48 h after the onset of the eruption.

Genetics

A genetic susceptibility common to AGEP and pustular psoriasis has been described in patients with mutations in the gene *IL36RN*, which codes for IL-36Ra, an anti-inflammatory cytokine. In a study examining a cohort of 96 patients with AGEP, one was found

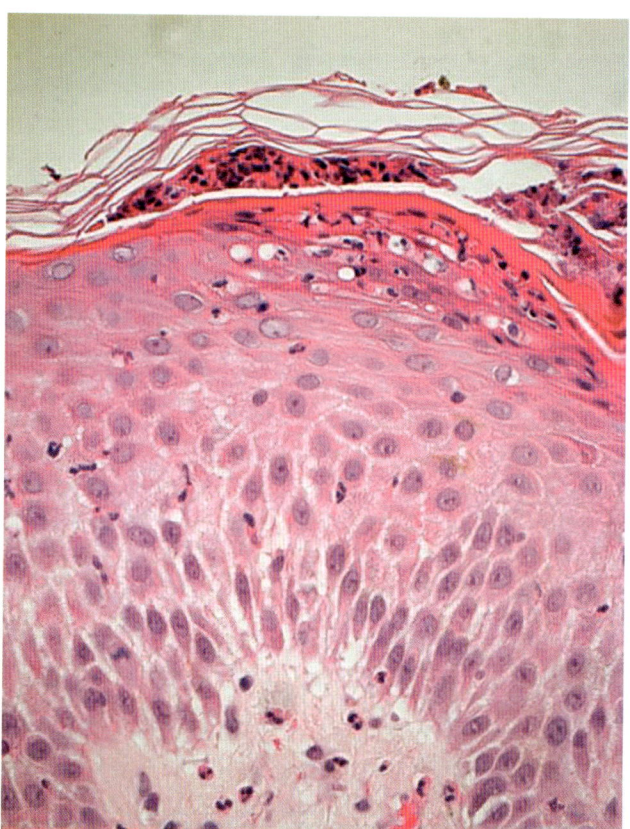

Figure 118.1 Histopathology of acute generalised exanthematous pustulosis.

to have a homozygous *IL36RN* mutation, and a further three to have heterozygous mutations in this gene [18]. It is proposed that *IL36RN* mutations may constitute a genetic predisposition to the development of a number of pustular phenotypes, including AGEP, and such mutations may be found in a subset of patients with this disease [22]. Similarly, the CARD14 mutation, associated with the pustular variant of psoriasis, has been detected in patients with AGEP, suggesting that this may represent a further common genetic susceptibility factor for pustular psoriasis and AGEP [23].

Clinical features
History
Exposure to the culprit drug typically occurs between 2 and 5 days prior to the onset of the eruption. This short latency is typical of AGEP. A prodrome of burning or itching in the skin may be described, and the patient may be asthenic. More than 90% of cases are caused by an identifiable drug, and therefore careful history taking should explore over-the-counter preparations which may have been ingested, as well as prescribed drugs.

Presentation
Sheets of hundreds of sterile, non-follicular pustules are seen arising most commonly in the major flexures such as the neck, axillae and inframammary and inguinal folds (Figures 118.2 and 118.3). However, non-flexural sites may be involved. The pustules typically arise on a background of oedema and reddening. Less commonly described clinical features include atypical targets, purpura, blisters and vesicles. Mucous membrane involvement is rare, and if present,

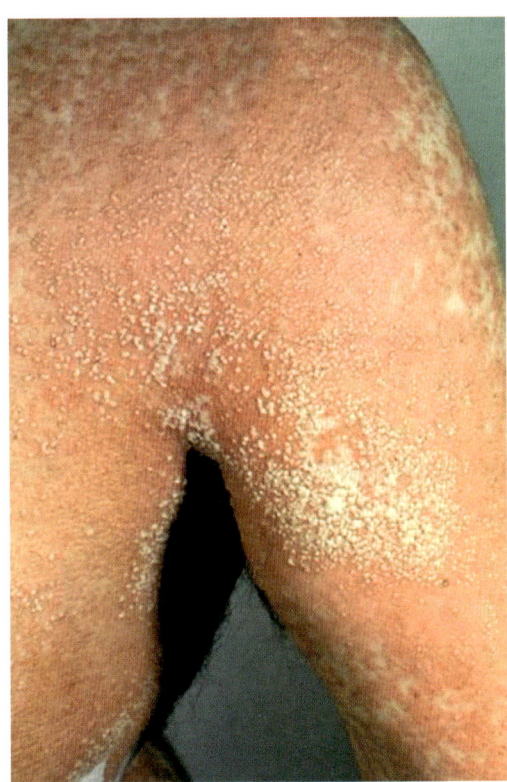

Figure 118.2 Acute generalised exanthematous pustulosis (AGEP): sheets of sterile, non-follicular pustules on the arm of a patient who developed AGEP 3 days after a dose of amoxicillin.

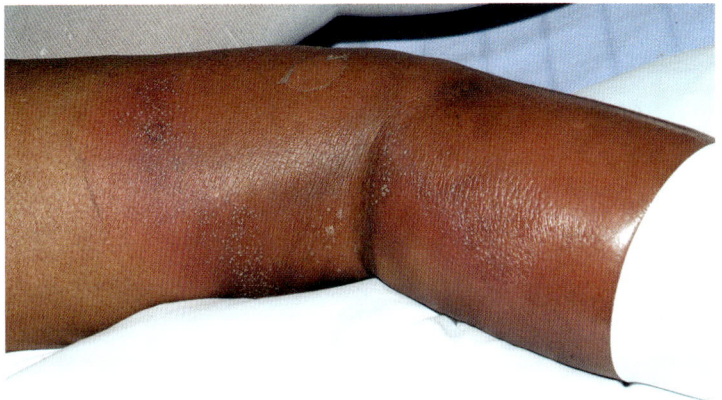

Figure 118.3 Acute generalised exanthematous pustulosis: similar appearance of pustules at the knee flexure.

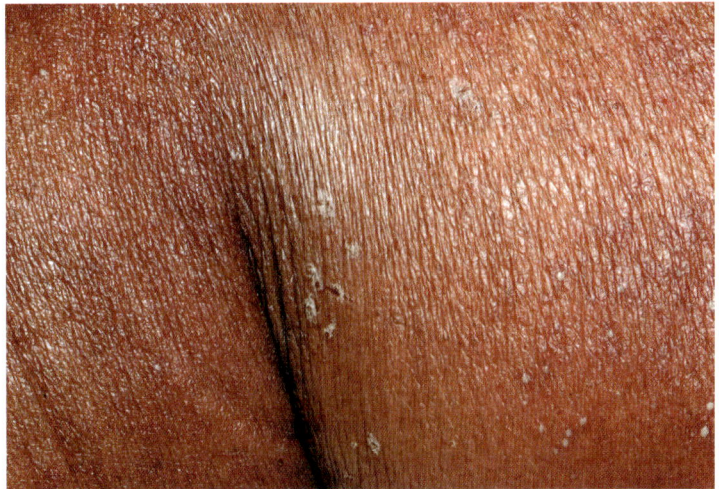

Figure 118.4 Acute generalised exanthematous pustulosis. The eruption typically resolves with postpustular desquamation.

is mild and generally limited to one site, usually the mouth. The Nikolsky sign has been described but arises in the minority of patients.

Systemically, the patient may be febrile. A leukocytosis, typically a neutrophilia, may be present. Eosinophils are less commonly elevated. A study of 58 patients with AGEP has suggested that involvement of internal organs may be present in up to 18% of patients with AGEP, including hepatic, renal and pulmonary dysfunction [24]. Agranulocytosis has also been described in a few cases, suggesting that bone marrow may be affected. Systemic involvement of this kind appears to be self-limiting and resolves spontaneously.

The disease resolves rapidly, within days, leaving postpustular desquamation (Figure 118.4).

A set of diagnostic criteria was proposed by Roujeau *et al*. in 1991 [25] as follows:
1 Appearance of hundreds of sterile, non-follicular pustules at flexural sites.
2 Histopathological changes of spongiosis and epidermal pustule formation.
3 Fever >38°C.

Table 118.1 Features that distinguish acute generalised exanthematous pustulosis (AGEP) from psoriasis.

	AGEP	Psoriasis
History of psoriasis	Possible	Common
Distribution pattern	Predominance in the folds	More generalised
Duration of pustules	Shorter	Longer
Duration of fever	Shorter	Longer
History of drug reaction	Usual	Uncommon
Recent drug administration	Very frequent	Less frequent
Arthritis	Rare	c.30%
Histology	Spongiform subcorneal and/or intraepidermal pustules, oedema of papillary dermis, vasculitis, exocytosis of eosinophils, single-cell necrosis of keratinocytes	Subcorneal and/or intraepidermal pustules, papillomatosis, acanthosis

4 Blood neutrophil count $>7 \times 10^9$/L.
5 Acute evolution.

This was then refined by Sidoroff *et al.* in 2001, as a series of criteria both to assist in the diagnosis of AGEP, as well as its distinction from pustular psoriasis (Table 118.1) [5].

Clinical variants
A localised form of AGEP, called acute localised exanthematous pustulosis (ALEP), is recognised and is characterised by pustules confined to a single body area, most commonly the neck. A similar clinical course of short latency, rapid recovery and lack of recurrence is seen. Since the first case was published in 2005 [26], nine further cases of ALEP have been reported [27–33].

Differential diagnosis
Pustular psoriasis (the Von Zumbusch variant) is the major differential of AGEP, and some difficulty may be encountered in distinguishing the two entities. A relevant drug history, the lack of a personal or family history of psoriasis and the absence of other stigmata of psoriasis on clinical examination may be helpful in directing the clinician to the diagnosis of AGEP rather than psoriasis (Table 118.1) [5].

Subcorneal pustular dermatosis (Sneddon–Wilkinson disease) may be distinguished by its less acute course, and the presence of flaccid pustules which demonstrate a hypopyon.

AGEP must also be distinguished from DRESS, as the latter disorder may feature pustules; however pustules will generally be less numerous in DRESS than in AGEP [34]. The former diagnosis will also invariably have systemic involvement of an internal organ, while this is less common in AGEP.

Candida infection can present with pustules in flexural sites, but can be distinguished by clinical context and the detection of yeast on microbiological samples.

Classification of severity
While classed as one of the SCAR syndromes, AGEP is generally rapid in both onset and resolution. While the patient may feel unwell during the acute episode, particularly in cases where systemic involvement is pronounced, supportive care is generally limited to topical therapy. Intensive care or organ support is not required.

Complications and co-morbidities
The patient must avoid the culprit drug and related compounds following the episode. No other sequelae are described.

Disease course and prognosis
The prognosis in AGEP is excellent and full recovery is to be expected.

Investigations
In most cases, a careful drug history is adequate to elucidate the culprit drug, which must be excluded as a matter of priority in the care of these patients. A skin biopsy should be taken early in the disease presentation as it will assist in the distinction from pustular psoriasis. Baseline haematological investigations, looking for neutrophilia and eosinophilia, should be undertaken. Biochemical investigations should be performed to rule out renal and liver dysfunction, as well as hypocalcaemia. Measurement of acute phase reactants such as C-reactive protein (CRP) may help to distinguish infection from the systemic involvement in AGEP. A septic screen may be instituted if suspicion of infection is high.

Management
Management of AGEP generally involves corticosteroid therapy, the route of administration being determined by the severity of the presentation. In cases where the patient appears systemically well, with limited areas of involvement, potent topical corticosteroid may suffice. In cases of more extensive involvement, or where systemic features such as fever, haemodynamic compromise or systemic upset are seen, oral corticosteroids may be required. Intravenous administration is not usually necessary. Emollient therapy should be prescribed, and continued throughout the phase of postpustular desquamation, until full skin integrity is restored.

In cases where systemic involvement such as renal impairment or liver function disturbance is noted, appropriate supportive care such as intravenous fluids and careful haemodynamic monitoring should be employed. If the patient is febrile, care should be taken to exclude an infective source, and if suspicion of this remains, then empirical antibiotic therapy should be considered.

Drug reaction with eosinophilia and systemic symptoms

Definition
Drug reaction with eosinophilia and systemic symptoms is one of the SCAR syndromes, characterised by cutaneous features, namely a rash, and systemic upset incorporating haematological and solid-organ disturbances [1].

Introduction and general description

There has been a proliferation of terms used to describe the entity discussed here as DRESS. This perhaps reflects the difficulties that have been encountered in defining the disorder. The first descriptions of the disease date from the 1940s, following the introduction of the first anticonvulsant drugs, hydantoin and its derivatives. Early in the use of these agents, reports emerged of a cutaneous adverse reaction pattern associated with lymphadenopathy, fever and systemic upset. The dermatopathological features of skin biopsies taken from these patients resembled cutaneous lymphoma, and the term drug-induced pseudolymphoma was coined [2]. The introduction of newer anticonvulsants such as carbamazepine led to a broadening of the definition and the suggestion of the term 'anticonvulsant hypersensitivity syndrome' [3]. When it was noted that a similar constellation of symptoms could be seen following exposure to other medicines such as allopurinol and antibiotics, the more generic term drug-induced hypersensitivity syndrome (DIHS) was introduced, and is preferred by some authors currently [4]. A further attempt to name the disease was made by Sontheimer in 1998, with drug-induced delayed multiorgan hypersensitivity syndrome (DIDMOHS), but this has not gained popular approval [5].

The acronym DRESS was proposed by Bocquet *et al.* in 1996, and is preferred by this author in that it has a mnemonic purpose, describing the component parts of the syndrome [6].

It is an idiosyncratic multisystem drug hypersensitivity disorder characterised by cutaneous features, namely a rash, which may be of variable morphology, and systemic involvement. The latter includes haematological disturbance, with eosinophilia being the most consistent finding. Leukocytosis, lymphopenia, lymphocytosis, thrombocytosis and thrombocytopenia are also described. Atypical lymphocytes are a common finding on blood film in DRESS patients, the presence of which is used as a component of the diagnostic criteria. Lymphadenopathy is found in more than 75% of patients, with involvement of two nodal basins required to meet diagnostic criteria.

Systemic disease typically comprises solid organs, most commonly the liver, although renal, lung, intestinal, myocardial, pericardial, splenic, pancreatic, thyroid and central nervous system involvement have also been described. The disease is usually accompanied by a fever.

Management in the acute phase is centred on the identification and withdrawal of the culprit drug; corticosteroid therapy, administered by topical, oral or intravenous routes, is guided by the severity of the disease. In most patients, the disease is of less than 4 weeks' duration, with few or no sequelae. However, it is recognised that a minority of patients enter a chronic phase of disease characterised by persistence either of the cutaneous features or of the systemic involvement.

Epidemiology
Incidence and prevalence
The incidence of DRESS was estimated to be 1 in 1000 to 1 in 10 000 in one study examining the risk of the disease in a population taking anticonvulsants [7].

Age
The largest study of validated cases to date demonstrated a mean age of onset of 48 years [7].

Sex
A slight female preponderance has been found, with a male to female ratio of 0.8 [7].

Ethnicity
No clear ethnic predisposition has been demonstrated, although certain human leukocyte antigen (HLA) types may confer added risk when particular medicines are administered. Many of these observations are ethno-specific (see Genetics section).

Associated diseases
While no specific disease entity has been associated with susceptibility to DRESS, the notoriety of certain drug classes such as anticonvulsants, antibiotics and allopurinol leads to an overrepresentation of cases in the neurology, neurosurgical and rheumatological settings, as well as acute hospital admissions of patients with fever. Patients with human immunodeficiency virus (HIV) infection may also be at higher risk of developing DRESS, in part no doubt due to the high notoriety of the drugs used to treat this disease.

Pathophysiology
A number of pathogenetic models have been proposed to explain the multisystem nature of DRESS; however, none is fully accepted. The two main theories are that of a drug-specific T-cell reaction, and that of viral reactivation [8,9]. In reality, it is likely that there are a number of mechanisms at play, acting synergistically to produce the clinical phenotype.

The drug-specific T-cell theory is based on the principle that a given drug may elicit a T-cell reaction specific to that medication. There are a number of proposed mechanisms for this, chief among which are the haptenisation theory, and secondly the p-i concept. Haptenisation describes the process whereby a small immunologically neutral molecule is rendered antigenic when bound to a protein. In order for this binding process to occur, the drug must first undergo enzymatic degradation. It is thought that one possible locus of susceptibility to DRESS might be polymorphisms in the genes that encode these enzymes; nevertheless, thus far no such variation has been discovered [10,11].

However, it has also been noted that drugs may stimulate production of T-cell receptors without undergoing haptenisation. A drug molecule may bind directly to the major histocompatibility complex (MHC) via a protein bound to the MHC, or may insert itself into the MHC groove. In each of these scenarios, the part of the antigen-presenting cell (APC) presented to the T-cell receptor has been reconfigured, thus provoking a T-cell response. If the drug-modified structure is subsequently recognised by a T cell in the context of co-stimulation, then a cascade effect of the T-cell response occurs. This putative mechanism by which T-cell responses are elicited by drugs bound to MHC molecules has been termed the p-i concept – 'pharmacological interaction of drugs with the immune receptor' [12].

Herpesvirus reactivation has been reproducibly demonstrated to occur in DRESS [13,14,**15**]. The implicated viruses have included human herpesvirus 6 (HHV-6), CMV, Epstein–Barr virus (EBV) and HHV-7 [8,16]. Virus reactivation appears to occur in a sequential fashion, with HHV-6 and EBV being detected earlier in the course of the disease, followed by HHV-7 and CMV [14]. It has been postulated that a drug-induced immunosuppressed state, characterised by hypogammaglobulinaemia, facilitates the initial reactivation of latent herpesvirus [17]. The sequential nature of viral reactivation suggests a correlation with the clinical phases of DRESS. Rash and fever are often the first presenting features, followed by lymphadenopathy and internal organ dysfunction. Some authors have hypothesised that it is the fluctuation of viral loads that gives rise to these 'waves' of disease in DRESS [18]. It has also been asserted that the persistence of viral reactivation explains the so-called chronic phase of DRESS experienced by some patients [18,19,20].

The detection of anti-HHV-6 immunoglobulin G (IgG) and HHV-6 viral DNA in blood and lesional skin of patients with DRESS led to the hypothesis that this agent was pivotal in disease pathogenesis [21]. However, it has proved difficult to consolidate this hypothesised relationship between the phenomenon of virus reactivation and the pathogenesis of the disease. Some authors believe that the virus is directly responsible for the disease manifestations of rash, fever and haematological and solid organ dysfunction, while others suggest that the virus reactivation is a bystander phenomenon, similar to that seen in graft-versus-host disease [14]. It seems likely that there is a complex interplay between the virus, the host immune response to the virus and a drug-specific immune response, which produces the clinical picture [15].

Predisposing factors
As mentioned, the high notoriety of certain drugs in the causation of DRESS has led to an overrepresentation of patients with coexisting neurological or rheumatological disease, as well as in patients with HIV infection. Certain genetic polymorphisms may also predispose DRESS to certain drug agents.

Pathology
The histopathological features of DRESS vary widely, but common features seen include spongiosis, a superficial perivascular lymphocytic infiltrate and an eosinophilic infiltrate in the dermis [21,22]. A lichenoid infiltrate may be seen (Figure 118.5). In some cases, basal cell vacuolar change with the presence of necrotic keratinocytes has been noted, with changes resembling erythema multiforme (EM) (Figure 118.6) [23]. Walsh *et al.* found a correlation between the presence of EM-like changes histopathologically and more severe liver dysfunction, and suggested that such features may be predictive of a higher mortality [24].

Genetics
The paradigm for genetic susceptibility to severe drug reactions was the observation in 2002 of an association between severe drug hypersensitivity to abacavir, and the expression of HLA-B*5701 in white HIV-positive patients [25]. Subsequently, susceptibility to reactions to carbamazepine has been noted in association with HLA-B*1502, a haplotype commonly expressed in South-East Asian populations [26–32]. Susceptibility to carbamazepine reactions in white and Chinese populations appears to be linked to expression of HLA-B*3101 [33,34]. This association has also been demonstrated in Japanese

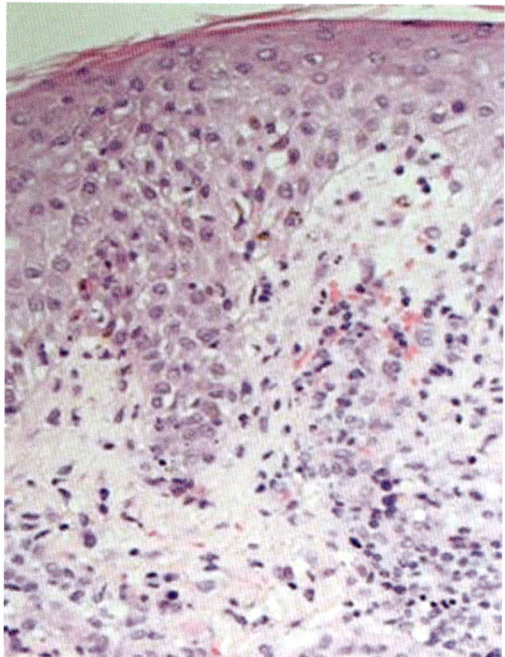

Figure 118.5 Drug reaction with eosinophilia and systemic symptoms (DRESS). Histopathology in a case of DRESS: spongiosis is seen in the epidermis, with a superficial perivascular lymphocytic infiltrate in the upper dermis, with some eosinophils.

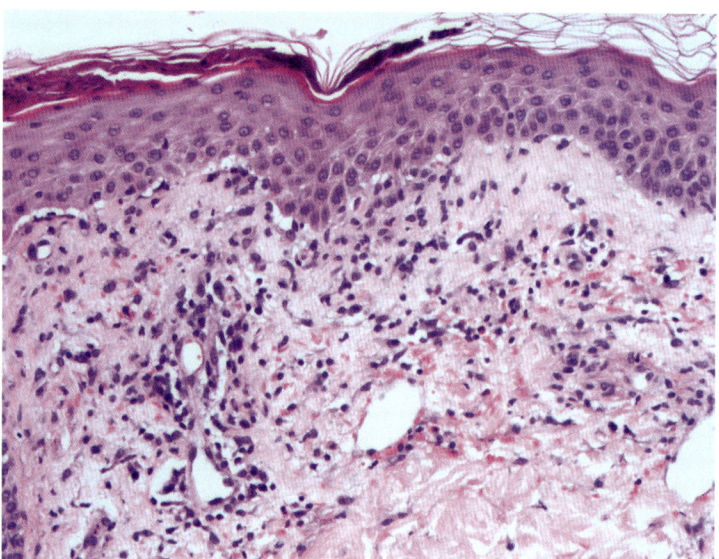

Figure 118.6 Drug reaction with eosinophilia and systemic symptoms (DRESS). Histopathology in a case of DRESS: this skin biopsy demonstrates features reminiscent of erythema multiforme, with basal cell vacuolation, and several necrotic keratinocytes. Courtesy of Dr Marianna Philippidou.

populations [35–37]. Pharmacogenetic investigations focusing on allopurinol hypersensitivity have demonstrated a susceptibility to reactions in Han Chinese [38,39] and Portuguese [40] populations expressing HLA-B*5801. More generically, HLA-DR3 and HLA-DQ2 have been linked to DRESS secondary to carbamazepine [41,42]. DRESS in response to vancomycin has been associated with HLA-A*32:01 [43].

Other authors have found an association between cytokine gene polymorphisms and heightened susceptibility to DRESS [44]. Allelic variants associated with low IL-10 production, as well as polymorphisms and differing haplotypes in IL-1 gene clusters, have been more frequently seen in patients with DRESS [44]. Putative mechanisms for this include a greater susceptibility to virus reactivation and a reduced drug tolerance [45].

Clinical features
History
The patient may present with a variety of non-specific symptoms in the early phase of the disease. The prolonged latency of DRESS following drug exposure adds to diagnostic difficulty for the non-specialist, and thus it is unsurprising that the constellation of presenting features may be misattributed to infection on initial presentation. Patients typically describe a prodromal phase characterised by asthenia, malaise and fatigue. They may have a fever. The appearance of a rash, accompanied by facial swelling, is usually the first clinical feature to emerge, and may provoke the patient to seek medical attention. The drug history should be elicited carefully in such patients, as a considerable period of time, between 2 and 6 weeks, may have elapsed between ingestion of the culprit drug and the onset of symptoms. The patient may not attach importance to a drug which they deem to have been taken too long ago to be relevant, and thus this aspect of the history must be explored thoroughly. Latencies towards the shorter end of this spectrum (less than 2 weeks) have been described with antibiotics and iodinated contrast media; more prolonged latencies have been described with anticonvulsants, allopurinol and sulfasalazine [46]. It is helpful to construct a timeline of drug ingestion as it relates to the onset of symptoms in order to demonstrate causality [6]. Some of the medicines with high notoriety for causing DRESS are displayed in Box 118.2.

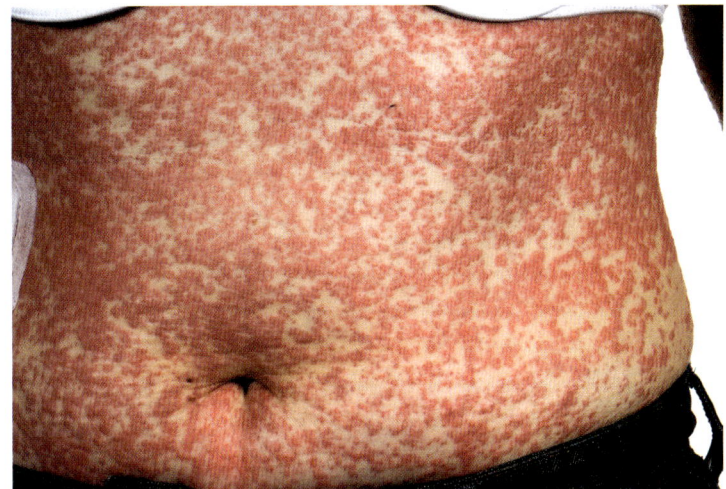

Figure 118.7 Drug reaction with eosinophilia and systemic symptoms (DRESS). The most common clinical phenotype is widespread papules and plaques accompanied by cutaneous oedema, seen here in a patient who developed DRESS to phenytoin.

> **Box 118.2 Commonest drugs causing drug reaction with eosinophilia and systemic symptoms (DRESS)**
> - Allopurinol
> - Antibiotics – vancomycin, amoxicillin, minocycline, piperacillin-tazobactam
> - Antiepileptics – carbamazepine, phenytoin, lamotrigine
> - Furosemide
> - Ibuprofen
> - Omeprazole
> - Sulpha drugs – sulphasalazine, dapsone, sulphadiazine

There is also value in exploring the family history for drug reactions of a similar nature. Familial cases of DRESS in reaction to carbamazepine, linked to HLA-A3101, have been described [47].

Presentation
By definition, DRESS is characterised by a rash suspected to be drug induced, accompanied by a fever, lymphadenopathy and systemic upset, the latter referring to derangement of the function of at least one organ system, and haematological abnormalities [6,48–50].

A clinical classification system for the cutaneous findings in DRESS has been proposed [24]. The most common variant appears to be the urticated papular exanthem. This consists of widespread

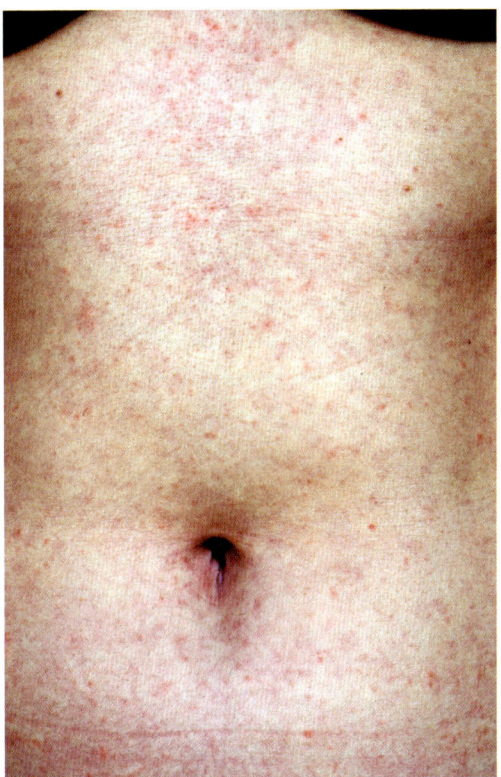

Figure 118.8 Drug reaction with eosinophilia and systemic symptoms (DRESS). A morbilliform eruption may occur.

papules and plaques, often accompanied by cutaneous oedema (Figure 118.7). A morbilliform eruption has been noted in a smaller proportion of patients, consisting of a pinkish macular rash resembling measles (Figure 118.8). In black skin, the eruption is red or reddish brown. Erythroderma may occasionally be the presenting cutaneous feature, characterised by a widespread exfoliative dermatitis (Figure 118.9). A number of patients with DRESS may present with EM-like features in the skin, developing dusky or purpuric atypical targets, not necessarily confined to acral sites

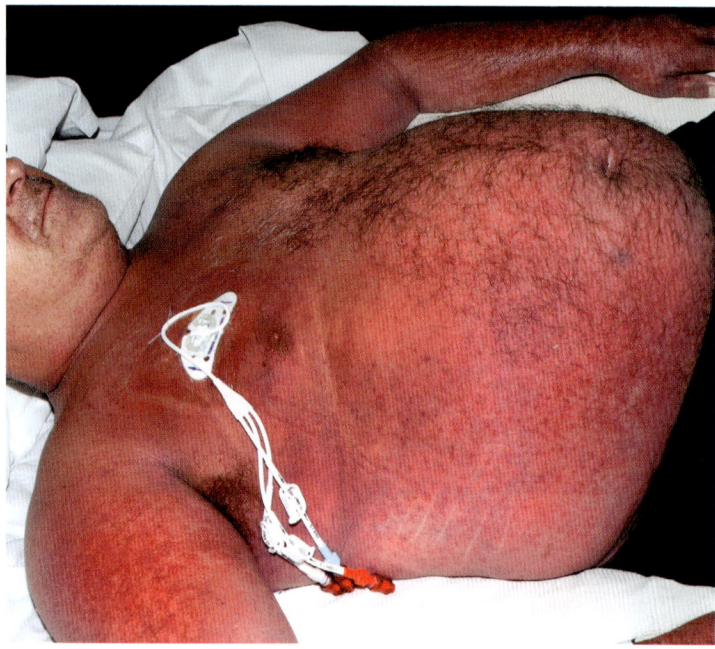

Figure 118.9 Drug reaction with eosinophilia and systemic symptoms (DRESS). A widespread exfoliative dermatitis seen in a patient with DRESS following allopurinol given as prophylaxis against tumour lysis syndrome.

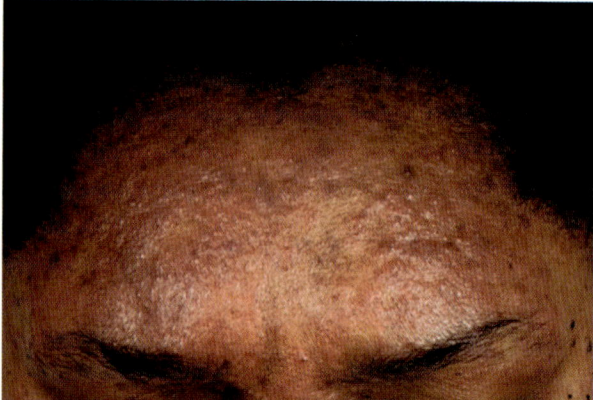

Figure 118.11 Drug reaction with eosinophilia and systemic symptoms (DRESS). Facial oedema is an important sign in patients with DRESS.

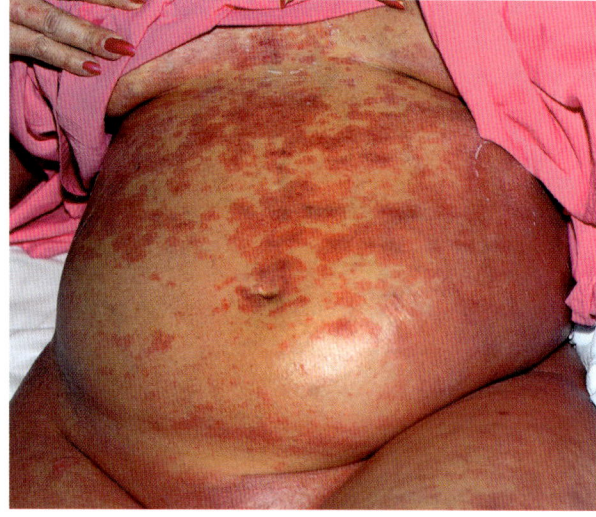

Figure 118.10 Drug reaction with eosinophilia and systemic symptoms (DRESS). The erythema multiforme-like phenotype in DRESS is often accompanied by more severe liver dysfunction; this patient went on to develop acute liver failure necessitating a liver transplant.

(Figure 118.10). The EM-like presentation may be associated with a more severe systemic phenotype [24].

An important clinical finding in the majority of patients with DRESS is head and neck oedema (Figure 118.11). This is often most noticeable when looking at the ears. It is worthwhile in cases where the clinician is unsure as to the presence of oedema to ask the patient themselves or a relative if they find the face is swollen compared with normal appearance. The face may be uniformly swollen, or have a more leonine appearance [1].

Other accessory cutaneous features have been noted in DRESS. Although frank mucous membrane involvement is a rarity (and indeed its presence should call the diagnosis of DRESS into question), cheilitis is a common finding. Pustules may be seen but are more sparse than the sheets of pustules seen in AGEP [7].

Clinical examination reveals lymphadenopathy in at least two sites in the majority of patients. One set of clinical criteria require the nodes to be at least 2 cm in diameter to be considered clinically significant [49].

Regarding haematological abnormalities, the most common seen is that of eosinophilia, with both modest and marked elevations noted by authors. The eosinophil level may fluctuate over the initial phase of disease progression, but in general settles in tandem with overall clinical improvement. Pancytopenia is seen in some cases, and is a negative predictive factor in terms of outcome [51]. IL-5 levels, which stimulate eosinophil release, have been noted to be elevated in DRESS [52,53]. It is also postulated that the protein content of the eosinophil granules may have a pathogenetic role in the visceral involvement in DRESS, being toxic to many tissues, including the liver [53]. A pronounced lymphocytosis may be seen, with levels rising to $>20 \times 10^9$ leukocytes/L. It is imperative in all cases for a blood film to be examined for the presence of atypical lymphocytes, which are frequently present in DRESS. Leukopenia, lymphopenia (possibly virally induced) and thrombocytopenia have been noted [18,51].

The liver is the most common viscera to be involved, with both hepatocellular and obstructive patterns of hepatitis reported. Between 70% and 95% of cases of DRESS demonstrate liver abnormalities [7,20,54]. Although any drug has the potential to cause liver dysfunction in the context of DRESS, phenytoin, minocycline and dapsone have been described as having a particular propensity to provoke this component of the disease complex. Severity of involvement varies widely, from mild and transient hepatitis, with alanine aminotransferase levels <250 iU/L, to fulminant hepatic failure requiring liver transplantation. Early identification of patients at highest risk has proved difficult, but there are indications that certain clinical markers (such as the presence of atypical targets and purpura at presentation) [24] and specific high-notoriety drugs (such as minocycline) [55] may confer a higher risk of more severe hepatic involvement. Liver dysfunction is the primary cause of mortality from DRESS [7].

Renal involvement in DRESS is well described, with up to 10% of patients manifesting this in the course of their illness [26,28,29]. Again, certain drugs are postulated to confer a higher risk of kidney injury, notably allopurinol. Any underlying renal dysfunction may be exacerbated by the syndrome, and prerenal causes of kidney impairment such as dehydration from fever in the prodromal phase may contribute. While structural abnormalities of the kidneys are not usually encountered on ultrasound, the patient may have haematuria, proteinuria and the presence of urinary eosinophils. Histologically, interstitial nephritis is seen. Severe renal impairment analogous to the fulminant liver failure described earlier is exceptionally rare, although dysfunction sufficient to require dialysis in the acute phase of illness has been described [56–58].

Cardiac involvement, both pericarditis and myocarditis, is reported in DRESS [59–61]. These are rare manifestations, but, where present, may have serious consequences. Cardiac complications are suggested by the presence of chest pain and dyspnoea. Examination may reveal tachycardia, hypotension and signs of a pericardial and/or pleural effusion. An electrocardiogram (ECG) may demonstrate T-wave abnormalities or other arrhythmias. Echocardiograms may demonstrate a pericardial effusion or reduced ejection fraction. Cardiac enzymes such as creatine kinase MB fraction and troponin I may be elevated. The majority of patients will demonstrate resolution of both pericarditis and myocarditis with standard therapy [59]. However, a clinical variant of myocarditis known as acute necrotising eosinophilic myocarditis (ANEM) has been described in the context of DRESS. This is a severe form of myocarditis which carries a high mortality (>50%). Diagnosis is suggested by more pronounced findings on echocardiogram, such as extreme impairment of ejection fraction and major systolic dysfunction [62].

Pulmonary involvement in DRESS is less fully described in the literature, but clinical symptoms of cough and dyspnoea should prompt examination and investigation of the respiratory system, looking for pleural effusion, pleuritis or acute interstitial pneumonitis [63]. Lung function tests may reveal a reduced diffusion gradient [20,54].

Central nervous system involvement in DRESS is again a more poorly elucidated aspect of the syndrome [64]. Rather subjective symptoms such as headache are described and are postulated to indicate inflammation of the meninges. There are isolated descriptions of more objective phenomena such as seizures and cranial nerve palsies, but these are in the authors' experience exceptional [20]. Objective assessments of neurological involvement in DRESS have been attempted; magnetic resonance imaging (MRI) of the brain of a patient with DRESS and symptoms of limbic encephalitis revealed symmetrical enhancement of the amygdala, cingulate gyrus and temporal lobes, with HHV-6 demonstrated by polymerase chain reaction (PCR) on the patient's cerebrospinal fluid (CSF) [65]. A presentation of inappropriate secretion of antidiuretic hormone in a patient with limbic encephalitis in the context of DRESS has also been described [66].

The incidence of gastrointestinal involvement in DRESS is unknown, but probably underreported. Endoscopic evaluation of this aspect of disease is sparse, but the symptom of diarrhoea, which may be bloody, is the most common presenting feature [54]. Authors who have examined this entity have described an ulcerative colitis with or without eosinophilic infiltrate on endoscopic biopsy [30,67–71]. Upper gastrointestinal tract involvement has also been described, with eosinophilic oesophagitis [68] and dysphagia [72,73].

Involvement of the endocrine system is more usual in the latter phase of DRESS than the acute phase, with the thyroid gland being most frequently involved. Both hyper- and hypothyroidism are recognised in the convalescent phase, both of which may have a chronic course, and therefore regular monitoring of thyroid function for a year after the acute event is advocated [74]. In a study of 27 patients with DRESS presenting to a tertiary referral centre for severe drug reactions over a 5-year period, five patients developed thyroid dysfunction, namely sick euthyroid syndrome, isolated increased free T4, low thyrotropin and thyroiditis [63].

Where pancreatitis has manifested as part of the DRESS constellation, pancreatic insufficiency may supervene, presenting as type 1 diabetes [75–77]. Type 1 diabetes occurring following DRESS does not appear to be accompanied by islet cell antibodies. However, the most common cause of diabetes in the context of DRESS is that arising secondary to corticosteroid therapy administered for the disease.

Other autoimmune phenomena such as alopecia areata, alopecia universalis [78] and systemic lupus erythematosus (SLE) have also been described in the aftermath of DRESS [18,79,80].

Clinical variants

The spectrum of disease in DRESS is broad. Diagnostic criteria have been proposed by a number of authors [49,50]; the preferred criteria of the authors are those proposed by the RegiSCAR group (Table 118.2) [49]. The onset of the components of disease may have a sequential nature and thus patients who do not initially reach the diagnostic criteria on admission may evolve such that they subsequently fulfil these requirements. There is a further cohort of patients who do not appear to ever reach the full diagnostic criteria

Table 118.2 RegiSCAR drug reaction with eosinophilia and systemic symptoms (DRESS) scoring system (abbreviated version).

Clinical feature	Score
Extent of rash >50% body surface area	1 point
Rash suggestive of DRESS	1 point
Systemic involvement: lymphadenopathy[a], eosinophilia[b], atypical lymphocytosis[b], organ involvement[c]	Maximum 6 points
Relevant negative serological tests[d]	1 point

<2 points: no case; 2–3 points: possible case; 4–5 points: probable case; >5 points: definite case.
[a] ≥2 sites, ≥1 cm. A maximum of 1 point gained from lymphadenopathy.
[b] Eosinophilia: 10–19% of total white cell count = 1 point; ≥20% = 2 points (if total leukocytes <4 × 10^9/L, an eosinophil count of 0.7–1.5 × 10^9/L will gain 1 point, an eosinophil count ≥1.5 × 10^9/L will score 2 points). Atypical lymphocytosis will gain 1 point.
[c] Liver: transaminases >2 × upper limit of normal (ULN) on two successive dates or bilirubin × 2 ULN on two successive days or aspartate aminotransferase, γ-glutamyltransferase and alkaline phosphatase >2 × ULN on one occasion. Renal: creatinine 1.5 × patient's baseline. Cardiac: echocardiographic evidence of pericarditis. Maximum of 2 points gained from internal organ involvement.
[d] ≥3 of the following performed and negative: hepatitis A, B and C; Mycoplasma/chlamydia; antinuclear antibody; blood culture (performed ≤3 days after hospitalisation). A maximum of 1 point is gained for relevant negative serological tests.

and yet clearly manifest a syndrome that is more complex than a simple drug exanthem. The term 'mini-DRESS' has been used to describe this phenomenon.

The concept of overlap syndromes within the sphere of DRESS has gained credence in recent years, with certain presentations acknowledged to have features of one of the other SCAR diagnoses such as AGEP or SJS/TEN. A study examining overlap cases recorded to a SCAR disease registry found this to be a rare entity, with only three cases (two SJS/TEN–DRESS and one AGEP–DRESS) out of 216 examined (2.1%) confirmed as being true overlap syndromes (i.e. simultaneously meeting the criteria for two diagnoses). However, a larger number of cases (45, 21%) were found to have one predominant SCAR diagnosis, and even more cases were found to have features of one or more of the other SCAR syndromes. While true overlap syndromes are rare, it would seem that features of other SCAR diagnoses may be seen more frequently in DRESS [81].

Differential diagnosis

Drug reaction with eosinophilia and systemic symptoms is most commonly mistaken for sepsis/infection, caused by virus or bacteria, and care must be taken to exclude this as a cause of the patient's symptoms. That infection may supervene during the course of a hospital admission for DRESS should also be remembered [82].

The other SCAR syndromes should be considered in the differential diagnosis of DRESS [83]. Certain clinical features are common to different SCAR syndromes, such as pustules, which when present should provoke consideration of AGEP as a differential diagnosis. However, the pustules in AGEP tend to be predominantly flexural, whereas in DRESS they are unlikely to be localised to these sites. Epidermal loss, purpura and target lesions of the skin may be present in DRESS, all of which may occur in EM, SJS or TEN. One of the most helpful features in distinguishing DRESS from the other SCAR syndromes is latency of onset of the eruption; this is classically shorter in AGEP (<5 days) and SJS/TEN (7–10 days) than in DRESS, where the latency may be 2–6 weeks after drug ingestion. As outlined earlier, overlap syndromes do exist and thus two diagnoses may not be mutually exclusive [81].

Where exfoliative erythroderma is the presenting cutaneous feature of DRESS, this may mimic the presentation of an acute severe eczema or psoriasis, or a cutaneous lymphoma. Where purpura and targets are present, the differential diagnosis of a systemic vasculitis should be considered. Angioimmunoblastic lymphoma is a rare differential of DRESS and may mimic its presentation [6,83,84].

Classification of severity

Prognostication has been attempted by several researchers in the domains of morphological features, drug characteristics and laboratory results. A prognostic scoring system, analogous to SCORTEN in SJS/TEN, has been described [85]. Application of the scoring system to a cohort of patients with a diagnosis of DRESS suggests that older age, longer exposure to the culprit drug, extent of rash involvement, duration of fever and appetite loss are predictive of a poorer outcome. Allopurinol as the culprit drug was also associated with a negative impact on prognosis. Laboratory markers form part of the score, with elevations of creatinine, liver enzymes and C-reactive protein all conferring a negative prognosis

Table 118.3 Scoring system for drug reaction with eosinophilia and systemic symptoms (DRESS).

Parameter[a]	Grade/extent	Score
Age (years)	≤40/41 to 74/≥75	−1/0/1
Duration of drug exposure after onset (days)	0–6/≥7	0/1
Allopurinol exposure	Yes	1
Pulsed prednisolone[b]	Yes	2
Skin involvement:		
Erythema %BSA	<70/≥70/erythroderma	0/1/2
Erosion %BSA	<10/10 to 29/≥30	0/1/3
Fever ≥38.5°C (days)	0–1/2 to 6/≤7	0/1/2
Appetite loss (≤70% regular intake) (days)	0–4/≥5	0/1
Creatinine (mg/dL)	<1.0/1.0 to 2.0/≥2.1 or dialysis	0/1/3
Alanine aminotransferase (iU/L)	<400/400 to 1000/>1000	0/1/2
CRP (mg/dL)	≤2/<2 to <10/≥10 to <15/≥15	−1/0/1/2

Reproduced from Mizukawa et al. 2019 [85].
<1 point: mild DRESS (may be managed with topical therapy only); 1–3 points: moderate DRESS (systemic corticosteroids indicated (≤50 mg/day)); ≥4 points: severe DRESS (systemic corticosteroids indicated (≥50 mg/day)).
[a] Each variable parameter was determined at early (days 0–3 after the initial presentation) and later times (2–4 weeks after the initial presentation), and on an as-needed basis.
[b] Intravenous methylprednisone use 500 mg/day for 3 days.
BSA, body surface area; CRP, C-reactive protein.

(Table 118.3). The score calculated early in the course of disease may be used to guide treatment choices.

Walsh et al. classified the eruption seen in DRESS morphologically into four categories: urticated papular exanthem, morbilliform erythema, exfoliative erythroderma and an EM-like reaction. The EM-like group demonstrated more pronounced liver dysfunction, and there was an overrepresentation of mortality in this group [24].

Some observers have associated cases of DRESS where allopurinol and minocycline were causative with increased severity of disease [51,55]. There is conflicting evidence as to whether or not higher viral titres are associated with a more severe course of disease [11,19]. A number of haematological markers such as eosinophilia, pancytopenia and thrombocytopenia have been proposed to be poor prognostic indicators. A further study linked lymphocytosis, eosinophilia, elevated ferritin and elevated creatinine with greater disease duration and higher mortality rates [5].

Putative biomarkers for DRESS have been described. Serum thymus and activation-related chemokine (TARC) levels have been proposed as markers of disease severity, but none has consistently and reproducibly shown an association [45,86,87]. High mobility group box 1 (HMGB1) has been demonstrated to be preferentially elevated in DRESS, and has been proposed as a marker of disease severity [10]. Polymorphisms in the genes coding for IL-1 and IL-10 have also been demonstrated as a predisposing factor in DRESS [44]. More recently, interferon-γ-induced protein 10 (IP10) levels have been demonstrated to be elevated in patients with DRESS who exhibited HHV6 reactivation; higher IP10 levels were associated with a higher probability of the development of long-term sequelae [88].

Complications and co-morbidities

The most severe and life-threatening complication of DRESS is fulminant liver failure, necessitating transplant or leading to death. Mortality has been estimated at 5–10%, with hepatic failure being the predominant cause of death. A delayed-onset interstitial nephritis is described [31] following cases of DRESS where kidney involvement has been prominent, and, analogous to this, a persistent interstitial pneumonitis is also described where pulmonary involvement has been present. Thyroid dysfunction may supervene in the convalescent phase of DRESS. Myocarditis, with associated cardiac insufficiency, has also been described.

Autoimmune phenomena may arise following DRESS, including lupus erythematosus and, as described earlier, autoimmune thyroid disease. One author has described the detection of autoantibodies in the convalescent phase in 44% of a series of 34 patients with DRESS syndrome. The autoantibodies detected were antinuclear antibody (ANA), antithyroglobulin antibody (ATGA) and antithyroperoxidase antibody (ATPOA). The authors demonstrated a preponderance of autoantibody positivity in the non-corticosteroid-treated group as compared with the group who received corticosteroid, suggesting a possible protective role for this treatment [20].

The development of fulminant type 1 diabetes has been described as a sequela in 27 cases of DRESS; blood glucose should be monitored actively in the acute and convalescent phases [89].

A small number of patients may experience a protracted course of cutaneous involvement, characterised by a chronic exfoliative dermatitis.

Disease course and prognosis

The majority of patients with DRESS will recover fully following withdrawal of the culprit drug and management of the acute episode as described. A number of organ-specific chronic sequelae may arise following involvement of these organs in the acute phase. In addition, a number of autoimmune phenomena such as alopecia areata and autoimmune thyroid disease are described.

Investigations

Investigations suggested in the acute phase are listed in Table 118.4. In both the acute and convalescent phases of illness, lymphocyte transformation tests and cytokine release assays have been used to assign culpability to triggering medications, but with variable degrees of sensitivity and specificity [90–92].

Management

The most important initial task once the diagnosis of DRESS is established is to identify and exclude the culprit medication. In some cases where polypharmacy has been in place this may not be straightforward, but all efforts must be made to ascribe causality to a likely culprit based on latency and notoriety data. A review of the patient's regular medication should be performed in order to exclude all unnecessary drugs. In all cases, supportive care should be prioritised, placing the patient in a clinical area equipped to provide an intensity of clinical care and monitoring appropriate to the severity of disease. This may involve intravenous fluids, thermoregulation, catheterisation to facilitate fluid balance management and supplemental oxygen. Extracorporeal membrane oxygenation (ECMO) has been used in cases of cardiac insufficiency secondary to myocarditis in DRESS [61]. Careful surveillance for coexisting infection, either in an organ or arising in the skin, should be undertaken. However, in the absence of indicators of infection, no empirical antibiotic therapy should be given. Skin-directed therapy should be prescribed by a physician with expertise in the management of DRESS, including topical emollient and, if appropriate, topical corticosteroid therapy.

Advice regarding the management of organ-specific involvement should be sought from appropriate specialties such as hepatology, cardiology, renal medicine and respiratory medicine.

The mainstay of active treatment is corticosteroid therapy, administered topically, orally or intravenously. In refractory cases, or where the disease enters a chronic phase, recourse to a steroid-sparing agent such as ciclosporin may be required. Although no definitive evidence is available, the active treatments outlined reflect recent literature based on case series and case reports.

First line

In cases of limited severity with minimal cutaneous involvement, or where administration of corticosteroid by other routes is

Table 118.4 Suggested investigations in drug reaction with eosinophilia and systemic symptoms (DRESS). Those in italics do not form part of the standard assessment of a patient with DRESS, but may be ordered when clinically indicated.

Body system	Investigation
Haematological	Full blood count to include white cell differential
Hepatic	Liver function tests
	Lactate dehydrogenase (LDH)
	Ferritin
	Coagulation screen (prothrombin time/international normalised ratio)
	Hepatitis B, C
	Epstein–Barr virus, cytomegalovirus, human herpesvirus 6 (HHV-6), HHV-7 titres
Cardiac	Electrocardiogram
	Echocardiogram
	Cardiac enzymes (creatine kinase, troponin)
Pulmonary	Chest X-ray
	Pulmonary function tests
Autoimmune	Antinuclear antibody
	Extractable nuclear antigens
	Complement
	Antineutrophil cytoplasmic antibody
Renal	Urea and creatinine
	Calcium
	Urinalysis
	Renal ultrasound
Neurological	Microscopy, culture and sensitivity of cerebrospinal fluid
	Computed tomography/magnetic resonance imaging of head
	Electroencephalogram
Endocrine	Thyroid-stimulating hormone
	T3/T4
	Blood glucose
Infection	Blood cultures
	Mycoplasma serology
	Polymerase chain reaction for herpes simplex virus
Gastrointestinal	Amylase
	Lipase
	Triglycerides
	Colonoscopy

contraindicated, the application of highly potent topical steroids may suffice as treatment. However, the majority of patients will require systemic corticosteroid therapy via either the oral route or the intravenous route, as guided by clinical state. An oral prednisolone dose of 1 mg/kg/day is recommended as initial treatment, with a tapering-off period varying from 1 to 3 months [21]. Where intravenous therapy is required, or where institution of oral therapy has failed to produce a satisfactory clinical improvement, methylprednisolone is indicated [15]. One study using 1 g/day methylprednisolone for 3 days demonstrated safety and improved clinical outcome with this dose [93].

Second line
Cases of DRESS refractory to steroid treatment may require alternative agents. Ciclosporin has been used in this capacity, and is useful in patients where a protracted course of illness (e.g. with persistent liver dysfunction or a chronic exfoliative dermatitis) supervenes [58]. The use of intravenous immunoglobulin (IVIg) as second line therapy has been described [94–99]. The rationale for IVIg is based on early observations that a fall in endogenous immunoglobulins is seen in DRESS, and this has a permissive effect on virus reactivation [17,100,101]. However, severe adverse reactions have been observed when the drug has been used in the setting of DRESS, and outcomes reported in the literature are conflicting [97,98].

Third line
The literature contains a number of case reports of other treatments used in refractory cases of DRESS. Plasmapharesis has been used [102,103], as has ECMO [61]. Alternative immunosuppressants such as cyclophosphamide [104] may be used for their steroid-sparing effect. Rituximab has been reported to have benefit in this setting [103]. Valganciclovir has been used, in theory to combat the virus reactivation described in this syndrome [105]. In cases of severe liver involvement, N-acetylcysteine has been used as an adjunct to other treatments [105].

Stevens–Johnson syndrome/toxic epidermal necrolysis

Definition and nomenclature
Stevens–Johnson syndrome (SJS) and toxic epidermal necrolysis (TEN) are severe mucocutaneous reactions, usually to drugs, characterised by blistering and epithelial sloughing. The two terms describe phenotypes within a severity spectrum, in which SJS is the less extensive form and TEN is the more extensive. Both names are used to describe the syndrome, thus SJS/TEN.

Synonyms and inclusions
- Lyell syndrome

Introduction and general description
Stevens and Johnson first reported their eponymous syndrome in 1922 by describing two boys, aged 7 and 8 years, who presented with a widespread eruption, fever, erosive stomatitis and severe ocular inflammation [1]. The original report suggested that the cutaneous lesions were indicative of EM, and as a consequence SJS was considered for many years to be a severe form of EM. In 1956, Lyell published a report of six patients presenting with a dermatosis characterised by extensive epidermal loss, similar to scalding, and associated with marked systemic upset [2]. Lyell coined the term toxic epidermal necrolysis to describe the new syndrome. Over time, it was recognised that severe forms of SJS could lead to extensive epidermolysis, and so in 1993 a group of clinician-experts suggested that SJS should be removed from the EM spectrum and added to TEN, therefore propounding a new spectrum of severe drug-induced dermatoses, SJS/TEN [3].

SJS/TEN presents as an acute eruption characterised by epidermal loss and multisite mucositis, accompanied by systemic disturbance. Although rare, SJS/TEN is a devastating disease; in severe cases, the acute phase is accompanied by a variety of systemic complications and may proceed to multiorgan failure. As well as it carrying an appreciable mortality during the acute illness, survivors often develop significant long-term sequelae [4].

Epidemiology
Incidence and prevalence
The incidence of SJS/TEN is approximately one to two cases per million per year [5,6].

Age
It occurs in all age groups including infants and children. There is an increased incidence in the elderly.

Sex
There is an increased incidence in women, the female to male ratio being 2 : 1 [4].

Ethnicity
It occurs in all ethnic groups.

Associated diseases
There is an increased risk of SJS/TEN in HIV-infected individuals [7]. There is a suggested association with SLE, however an extensive form of acute bullous lupus erythematosus can mimic TEN [8].

Pathophysiology
It is primarily a drug-induced phenomenon, with a culprit drug being demonstrated in approximately 85% of cases [9]. The disease is characterised by widespread epithelial keratinocyte necrosis of both the skin and mucous membranes, a process initiated by drug-induced cytotoxic T lymphocytes (CTLs) [10]. MHC class I-restricted drug presentation leads to clonal expansion of CD8+ CTLs [10] which infiltrate the skin, while soluble factors induce keratinocyte apoptosis [11]. Pro-apoptotic molecules, including tumour necrosis factor α (TNF-α), interferon γ and inducible nitric oxide synthase, may link drug-induced immune responses to keratinocyte damage [12]. Soluble Fas ligand, perforin and granzyme have all been implicated in triggering keratinocyte death [13,14], however current evidence favours granulysin as the key mediator

of apoptosis in SJS/TEN [15]. A study by Chung *et al.* demonstrated the presence of high concentrations of secretory 15 kDa granulysin in TEN blister fluid, while the injection of 15 kDa granulysin into mouse skin induced changes mimicking the clinical features of SJS/TEN [15]. A study by Saito *et al.* has indicated that keratinocyte necrosis (necroptosis) in SJS/TEN may be mediated by annexin A1 acting through the formyl peptide receptor 1 [16]. Overexpression of receptor-interacting protein kinase 3 (RIP kinase3) in lesional skin suggests that additional pathways of cytotoxicity and necroptosis regulation may be involved in SJS/TEN keratinocyte apoptosis [17].

Notoriety of specific drugs in causing SJS/TEN can be determined from population pharmacovigilance data and is useful in identifying a likely culprit [18]. Two multinational case–control studies have evaluated drug causation risk: the first, conducted from 1989 to 1995, included 372 cases and 1720 controls [19]; the second, carried out between 1997 and 2001, consisted of 379 cases and 1505 controls [18]. From these studies, a list of drugs has been identified which are strongly associated with the induction of SJS/TEN and are responsible for one-half of all cases (Box 118.3).

> **Box 118.3 Commonest drugs causing Stevens–Johnson syndrome/toxic epidermal necrolysis (SJS/TEN)**
>
> - Allopurinol
> - Carbamazepine
> - Lamotrigine
> - Nevirapine
> - Oxicam non-steroidal anti-inflammatory drugs
> - Phenobarbital
> - Phenytoin
> - Sulfamethoxazole and other sulfa antibiotics
> - Sulfasalazine

Histopathology

There is variable epidermal damage ranging from individual cell apoptosis to confluent epidermal necrosis [20]. Keratinocyte necrosis is also seen in mucosal biopsies. Epidermal changes are associated with basal cell vacuolar degeneration and subepidermal vesicle or bulla formation (Figure 118.12). Adnexal structures such as sweat ducts and hair follicles are occasionally involved. Within the dermis, there is usually only a mild perivascular infiltrate of lymphocytes and histiocytes. Dermal eosinophils occur in the minority of cases and, if present, tend to be few in number [20].

Causative organisms

In at least 15% of SJS/TEN cases a culprit drug is not identified. In SJS, some cases, especially in children, appear to be triggered by infections, most notably by *Mycoplasma pneumoniae* [21].

Genetics

Research in Taiwan has investigated SJS/TEN susceptibility in the Han Chinese people, who possess a high degree of genetic homogeneity. Investigations have demonstrated a strong genetic predisposition to the development of carbamazepine-induced SJS/TEN in individuals bearing HLA-B*1502 [22] and an association of HLA-B*5801 with allopurinol-induced SJS/TEN [23].

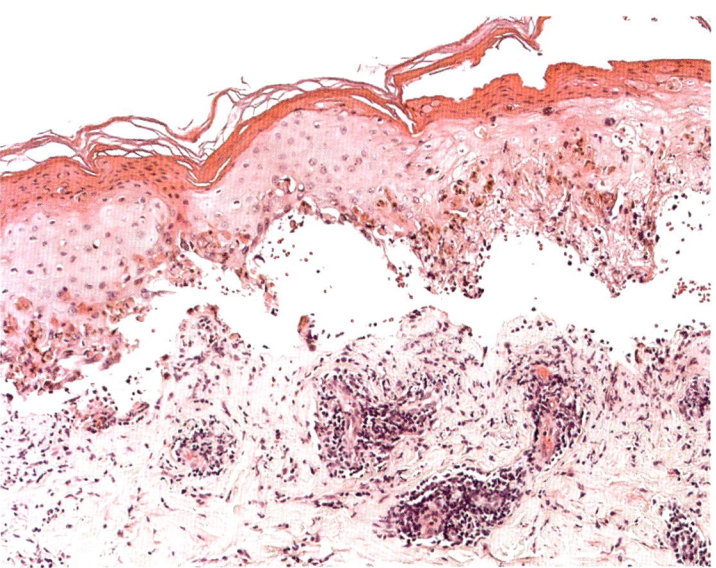

Figure 118.12 Stevens–Johnson syndrome/toxic epidermal necrolysis (SJS/TEN). Histopathology. There is parakeratosis overlying the epidermis which has separated from the papillary dermis. On the left, there are multiple Civatte bodies affecting the full thickness of the epidermis in a 'gunshot' distribution; on the right, there is full-thickness epidermal necrosis. Within the dermis, there is a superficial, predominantly lymphocytic perivascular infiltrate, vascular telangiectasiae and red cell extravasation. Courtesy of Dr Marianna Philippidou.

The same susceptibility to carbamazepine has been demonstrated with HLA-B*1502 in other Asian countries including Thailand and Malaysia [24]. The presence of this genetic association in any given ethnic population depends on the allele frequency within that population. These studies indicate that MHC-restricted presentation of the drug is central to the pathogenesis of SJS/TEN. Genetic markers have the potential to be used as pharmacogenetic tests to identify individuals at risk of SJS/TEN [25].

Clinical features

History

A latent period occurs between initiation of the culprit drug and onset of SJS/TEN. This latency is typically 7–10 days, but ranges from 5 to 28 days. A history of malaise, fever and upper respiratory tract symptoms often precedes the onset of the dermatosis by a few days (the prodrome). The rash of SJS/TEN commonly develops on the face and chest initially and disseminates widely over the ensuing days. Pruritus and cutaneous pain accompany the skin signs. Involvement of mucosal sites may occur before, after or simultaneously with the dermatosis. SJS/TEN involvement of the respiratory tract presents with cough, chest pain, dyspnoea or haemoptysis. Involvement of the bowel is characterised by diarrhoea.

Presentation

The patient with SJS/TEN is unwell with malaise, fever and, usually, prostration. The earliest skin lesions are atypical targets or purpuric macules which occur on the face, upper torso and proximal limbs (Figures 118.13 and 118.14). Subsequently, lesions spread to involve the rest of the trunk and limbs; involvement of the palms and soles with target lesions (usually atypical) is often prominent (Figure 118.15). Dusky redness of periungual skin is commonly seen. Lesions increase in size and number over 5–7 days, tending

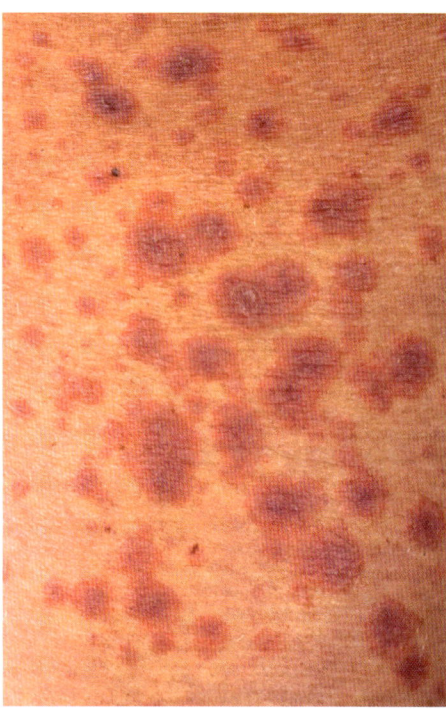

Figure 118.13 Stevens–Johnson syndrome/toxic epidermal necrolysis (SJS/TEN). Atypical targets. There are multiple discrete red macules – each has a darker centre and a slightly paler outer ring.

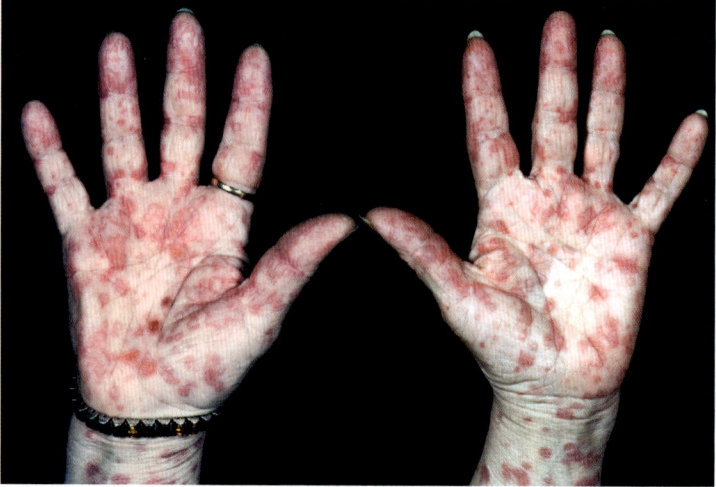

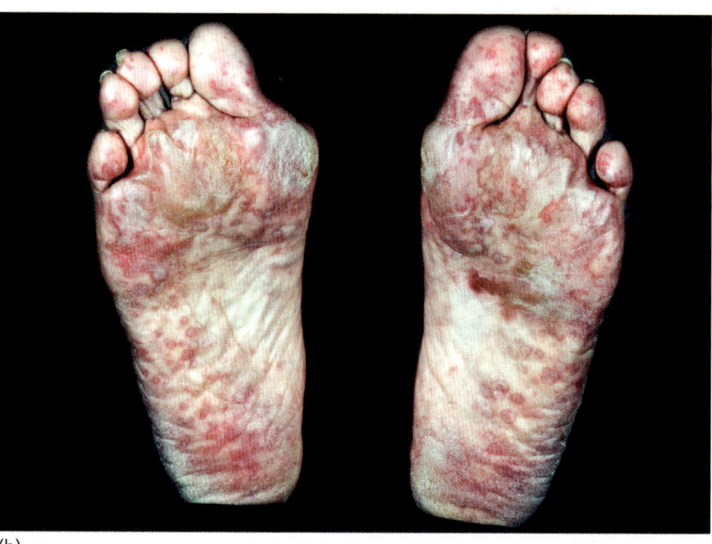

Figure 118.15 Stevens–Johnson syndrome/toxic epidermal necrolysis (SJS/TEN). Palmoplantar involvement. Multiple circular lesions are present on (a) the palms and (b) the soles. Blistering is occurring at both sites, but prominently on the feet.

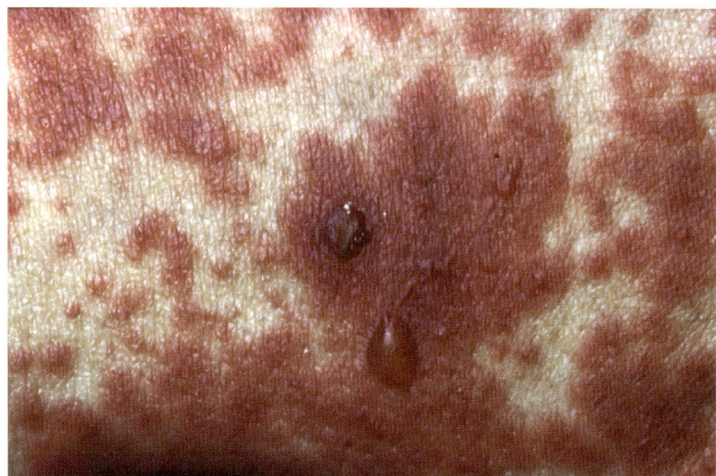

Figure 118.14 Stevens–Johnson syndrome/toxic epidermal necrolysis (SJS/TEN). Purpuric macules. The dusky, purpuric lesions on this patient's skin are coalescing and blistering.

to coalesce. Vesicles or fluid-filled blisters develop within lesional skin (Figure 118.16). Large areas of confluent redness may develop, either *de novo* or from confluence of discrete lesions (Figure 118.17). Detachable epidermis (as opposed to detached epidermis) is demonstrated by a positive Nikolsky sign, in which gentle lateral pressure causes lesional epidermis to slide over the dermis. Although not specific for SJS/TEN (it is also positive in pemphigus), the Nikolsky sign is a helpful clinical indicator of epidermal necrolysis. Shearing forces applied to the skin (typically from careless patient handling) will cause fragile lesional epidermis to peel back leaving areas of exposed dermis (Figure 118.18). The combination of necrolytic blistering and shearing-induced epidermal detachment will produce areas of denuded dermis which readily bleed and can become secondarily infected (Figure 118.19) [26].

Acute inflammation of the mucosal surfaces of the eye and eyelids is painful and causes visual impairment (Figure 118.20). The ocular signs are varied and include chemosis, conjunctivitis, pseudomembrane formation and corneal and conjunctival epithelial defects [27]. Compared with SJS, patients with TEN have more frequent but not more severe acute ocular involvement [27].

Oral involvement in SJS/TEN is usual and characterised by painful mucosal redness with subsequent blistering and ulceration. Similar changes to the vermillion of the lips progress to the retention of adherent haemorrhagic crusts (Figure 118.21). The tongue and palate are frequently affected. In severe cases, mucosal involvement may extend to the oropharynx, larynx, respiratory tract and oesophagus. Drinking and eating are usually compromised by oral involvement in acute SJS/TEN.

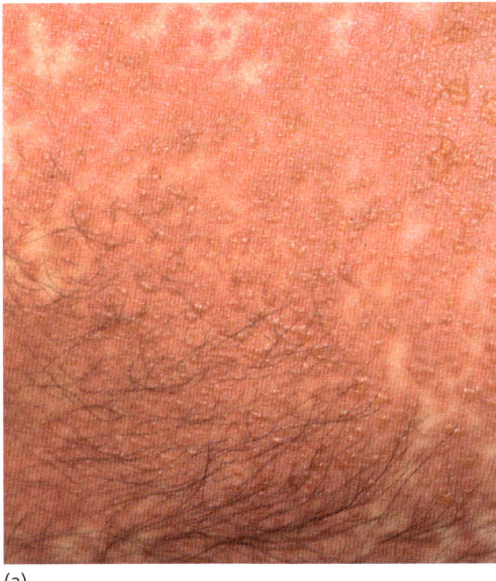

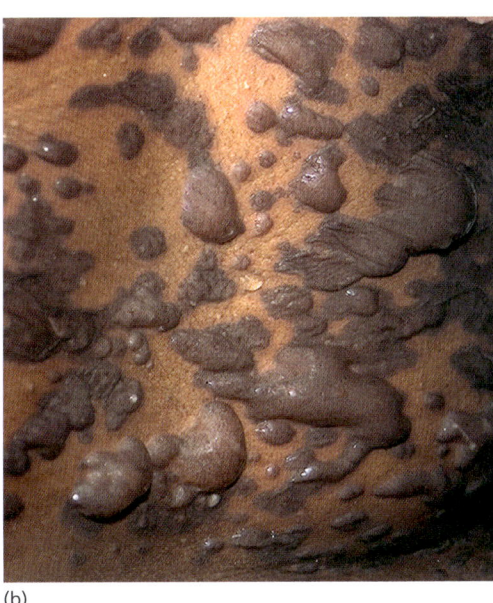

Figure 118.16 Stevens–Johnson syndrome/toxic epidermal necrolysis (SJS/TEN). Blistering. Lesional skin in SJS/TEN typically blisters forming both vesicles (a) and large flaccid bullae (b).

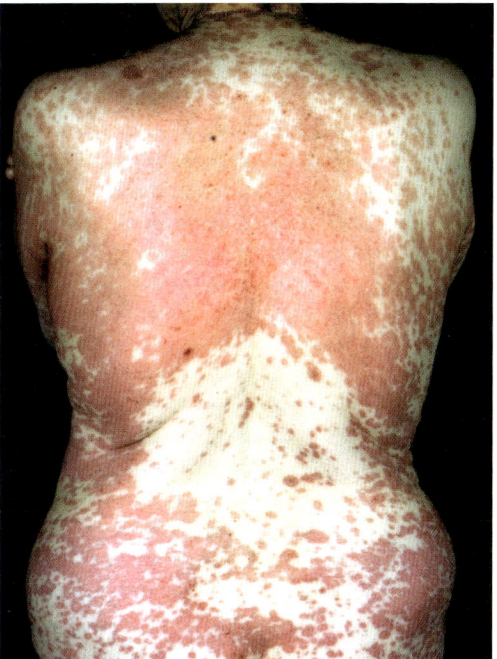

Figure 118.17 Stevens–Johnson syndrome/toxic epidermal necrolysis (SJS/TEN). Individual lesions may coalesce to form large areas of redness, as seen on this patient's back. In this case, blistering/epidermal detachment was negligible.

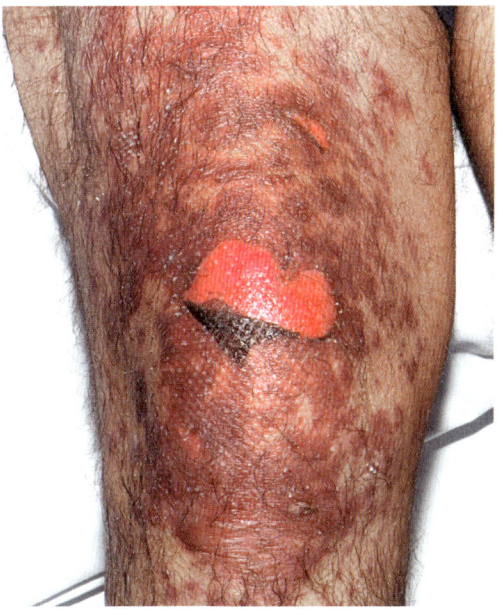

Figure 118.18 Stevens–Johnson syndrome/toxic epidermal necrolysis (SJS/TEN). Detached epidermis. In SJS/TEN, lesional necrolytic epidermis readily peels back to reveal the dermis.

Involvement of the uro-genital tract in SJS/TEN is characterised by mucosal redness, blistering and erosions (Figure 118.22). During the acute phase, uro-genital pain is prominent and urinary dysfunction (dysuria or retention) is common.

One-quarter of SJS/TEN patients develop pulmonary manifestations early in the disease characterised by dyspnoea, increased respiratory rate and bronchial hypersecretion [28]. Fibreoptic bronchoscopy reveals bronchial epithelial detachment and loss in the proximal airways [29].

Clinical variants

At the less severe end of the spectrum, differentiation of SJS from erythema multiforme major (EMM) is difficult. In both EMM and SJS there is mucous membrane involvement and cutaneous blistering with epidermal detachment of less than 10% body surface area (BSA). However, in EMM the lesions consist of typical targets or raised atypical targets, predominantly localised on the limbs and extremities; in SJS, the lesions are atypical targets with predilection for the torso. Distinguishing EMM from SJS/TEN has causality implications: EMM is mostly related to herpes simplex virus reactivation and rarely to drugs; SJS/TEN is usually triggered by a drug, rarely by an infection. *Mycoplasma*-induced SJS is reported,

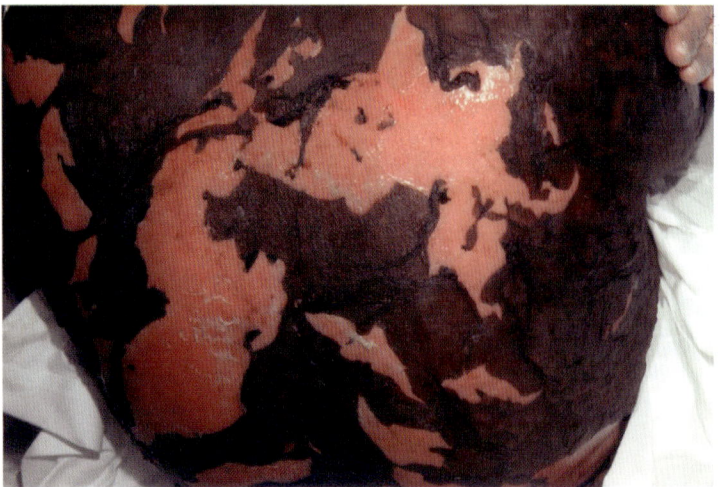

Figure 118.19 Stevens–Johnson syndrome/toxic epidermal necrolysis (SJS/TEN). Denuded skin. Extensive epidermal loss in TEN produces large areas of exposed dermis.

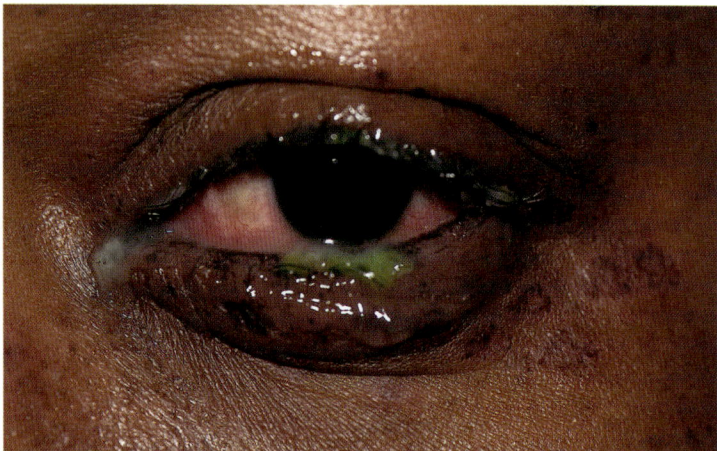

(a)

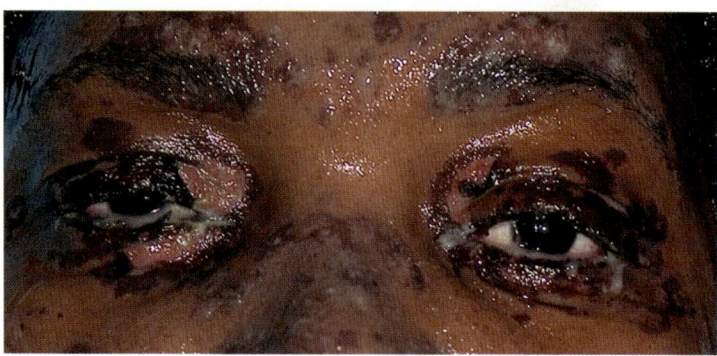

(b)

Figure 118.20 Stevens–Johnson syndrome/toxic epidermal necrolysis (SJS/TEN). Ocular involvement. (a) There is eyelid oedema, conjunctivitis and keratitis: the green material is exudate stained by fluorescein dye used for ophthalmic examination. (b) The same patient 5 days later: there is eyelid epidermal loss and a purulent ocular discharge.

and in some cases (mostly children) may be characterised by a predominance of mucous membrane involvement with little or no cutaneous lesions. This clinically atypical form of SJS has been termed *Mycoplasma pneumoniae*-associated mucositis (MPAM) [30].

Differential diagnosis

A number of disorders can present with blistering of the skin and mucosal erosions or a mucositis (Box 118.4).

> **Box 118.4 Differential diagnosis of Stevens–Johnson syndrome/toxic epidermal necrolysis (SJS/TEN)**
>
> - Erythema multiforme major
> - Pemphigus vulgaris
> - Mucous membrane pemphigoid
> - Bullous pemphigoid
> - Paraneoplastic pemphigus
> - Bullous lupus erythematosus
> - Linear IgA bullous dermatosis
> - Generalised bullous fixed drug eruption
> - Acute bullous acute graft-versus-host disease
> - Staphylococcal scalded skin syndrome
> - Acute generalised exanthematous pustulosis

Classification of severity

In a study from Bastuji-Garin *et al.*, a group of expert physicians reviewed the clinical photographs of more than 200 patients and categorised the cases according to type of cutaneous lesion and extent of maximal epidermal detachment [3]. From this study the following disease classification is used in clinical practice:
- SJS: epidermal detachment less than 10% BSA, plus widespread purpuric macules or flat atypical targets.
- Overlap SJS–TEN: detachment of 10–30% BSA, plus widespread purpuric macules or flat atypical targets.
- TEN with spots: detachment greater than 30% BSA, plus widespread purpuric macules or flat atypical targets.

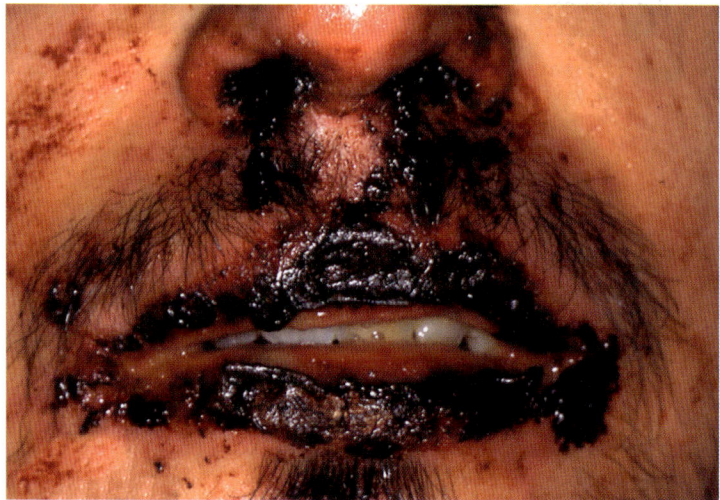

Figure 118.21 Stevens–Johnson syndrome/toxic epidermal necrolysis (SJS/TEN). Lip involvement. Severe cheilitis has produced thick haemorrhagic crusts. This SJS/TEN patient had a coagulopathy which resulted in bleeding from the involved mucosae of the mouth and nose.

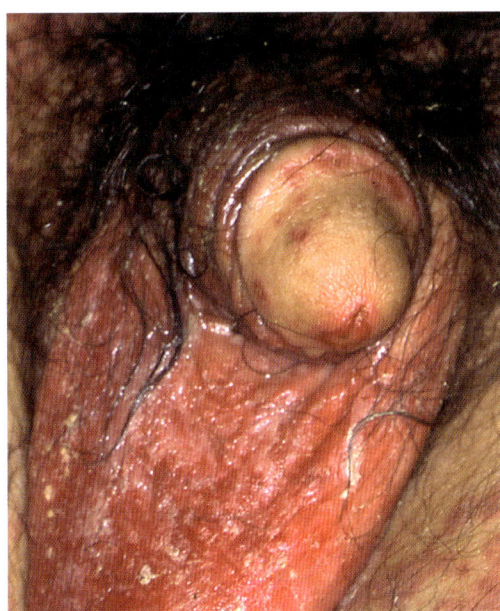

Figure 118.22 Stevens–Johnson syndrome/toxic epidermal necrolysis (SJS/TEN). Genital involvement. There is confluent redness of the scrotum and discrete lesions on the glans penis. Redness at the meatus indicates that urethral involvement is likely.

- TEN without spots: detachment greater than 30% BSA, with loss of large epidermal sheets without purpuric macules or target lesions.

A system has been devised by Power *et al.* to grade the severity of acute ocular SJS/TEN according to degree and extent of involvement [31].

Complications and co-morbidities

Acute. Extensive epidermal detachment in SJS/TEN is complicated by deranged thermoregulatory control leading to hypothermia. Skin failure also results in considerable transcutaneous fluid losses, compounded by decreased oral fluid intake due to disease involvement of the mouth. Epidermal detachment of 50% BSA will lead to a water loss of 2–3 L/day from exudation and evaporation. Fluid depletion can cause end-organ hypoperfusion leading to acute kidney injury. Haematological complications accompanying the acute phase of SJS/TEN are common, most notably anaemia and leukopenia. Abnormal liver function is typical during the early stage of the disease, but rarely leads to hepatic failure. Hypoalbuminaemia usually occurs in TEN. Hyperglycaemia may develop as a stress response in acute SJS/TEN. Extensive epidermal detachment is accompanied by a greatly increased metabolic demand [32].

Epithelial necrolysis may occur in the bronchi during the acute phase of SJS/TEN resulting in bronchial erosions and airway obstruction by sloughed epithelium. This occurs in up to 25% of patients and causes dyspnoea, haemoptysis, increased bronchial secretion and hypoxaemia [33]. Colonic involvement in SJS/TEN can occur, but is a rare complication [34].

The commonest life-threatening complication of acute SJS/TEN is septicaemia. The denuded dermis in SJS/TEN acts as a substrate for microbial colonisation, initially by *Staphylococcus aureus* and later by Gram-negative rods from the digestive flora, especially *Pseudomonas aeruginosa*. Systemic sepsis can quickly follow skin infection and lead to multiorgan failure [4].

Long-term. Survivors from an acute episode of SJS/TEN may develop delayed sequelae which are associated with significant morbidity and reduced quality of life. The most common sequelae involve the skin and mucous membranes; the most disabling complications are ocular. In the skin, postinflammatory dyspigmentation persists in darker skinned patients from months to years following resolution of the acute dermatosis [35]. Re-epithelialisation usually occurs without scarring but cicatricial healing may develop in areas that were infected during the acute phase, at sites of unrelieved pressure injury and in circumstances where skin grafts were used [36]. Eruptive melanocytic naevi occur occasionally in the recovery phase, more commonly in children and young adults [37]. Shedding of nails (onychomadesis) may occur a few weeks after the acute episode due to nail matrix arrest; occasionally, there is subsequent permanent anonychia [38]. Involvement of the scalp in acute SJS/TEN is extremely unusual, however telogen effluvium occurs in about 20% of patients in the post-acute phase [38]. Other skin complications include pruritus, abnormal photosensitivity, abnormal sweating and heterotopic ossification [38].

Long-term ocular sequelae are the most disabling complications of SJS/TEN. In a study of 49 patients with acute ocular involvement, 31 went on to develop chronic eye disease; the severity of the acute ocular involvement was found to be the only significant risk factor for late eye complications [39]. Chronic eye complications include corneal and conjunctival ulceration and scarring, dry eye, distichiasis, entropion, trichiasis and ocular surface failure [40]. Corneal erosions and ulcers are perpetuated by the loss of limbal corneal stem cells, as well as destruction of the conjunctival goblet cells, which impairs the tear film [40]. In the conjunctiva, scarring of the fornix obstructs the ductal openings of lacrimal glands thus aggravating ocular dryness. Bulbar and forniceal cicatricial changes lead to symblepharon or ankyloblepharon formation with limitation of ocular mobility and interference of the tear meniscus. Scarring of the eyelid margin leads to ectropion, entropion and misdirected eyelashes. Patients with chronic eye involvement require lifelong management for dryness, conjunctival inflammation and ocular discomfort; many suffer permanent visual impairment or blindness.

A range of long-term oral complications may occur resulting in functional impairments. Oral mucosal scarring can cause gingival synechiae resulting in food trapping and limitation of oral mobility [41]. A Sjögren-like syndrome has been reported (ANA/Ro/La-negative) and is believed to occur in up to 40% of survivors [42].

The most important late complication of pulmonary involvement is bronchiolitis obliterans, in which airway epithelial injury is followed by regeneration and scarring [43]. It leads to severe airway obstruction and progressive dyspnoea. Most cases present 3–4 months after the acute episode and are associated with a poor prognosis [43].

Long-term complications in the gastrointestinal tract are rare but oesophageal stricture is reported [44]. Intestinal ulceration may occur in acute SJS/TEN and usually heals along with skin re-epithelialisation, however in some patients small intestinal ulcers can be persistent causing diarrhoea and malabsorption. Vanishing bile duct syndrome, characterised by cholestasis and histological loss of interlobular bile ducts, has been reported [45].

Chronic uro-genital lesions in SJS/TEN are mostly adhesions: vaginal and introital adhesions may be associated with dyspareunia and, in one report, haematocolpos [46]. Other gynaecological complications include vaginal adenosis, which is the replacement of non-cornified vaginal epithelium with metaplastic epithelium of endocervical differentiation [47].

Although little is written on the subject, it appears that many survivors of SJS/TEN suffer psychological sequelae, including post-traumatic stress disorder [48]. In a qualitative study, it was found that many patients, following an episode of acute SJS/TEN, were fearful of taking medications [48].

Disease course and prognosis

During the acute phase of SJS/TEN the extent of skin involvement increases over the first 5–10 days. With appropriate supportive therapy, and intensive skin/mucous membrane-directed treatment, re-epithelialisation should start once the disease stops extending. Epithelialisation of involved mucous membranes tends to take longer than healing of lesional skin. Delayed healing will occur in the presence of skin sepsis, systemic complications or if the triggering agent (culprit drug) has not been removed. Uncomplicated re-epithelialisation will take 3–4 weeks to heal eroded areas fully.

The overall SJS/TEN mortality is about 22%; in SJS less than 10% of patients die from the acute illness, while in TEN the mortality is approximately 30% [49]. The cause of death in SJS/TEN is usually septicaemia-induced multiorgan failure. In 2000, Bastuji-Garin *et al.* published a validated prognostic scoring system for SJS/TEN, called SCORTEN (SCORe of Toxic Epidermal Necrolysis), which uses seven clinical parameters to predict probability of hospital mortality (Box 118.5) [50]. In SCORTEN, one point is attributed to each of the parameters, with increasing scores predicting higher mortality rates (Table 118.5). SCORTEN should be calculated on admission and again within the first 5 days of hospitalisation. Retrospective analysis of several SJS/TEN case series has confirmed SCORTEN's ability to predict mortality accurately [51,52]. Survivors of the acute illness often develop significant long-term sequelae.

Table 118.5 SCORTEN (SCORe of Toxic Epidermal Necrolysis) predicted mortality

Number of parameters	Predicted mortality (%)
0	1.2
1	3.9
2	3.9
3	32.4
4	62.2
5	85.0
6	95.1
7	98.5

Box 118.6 Blood tests needed at presentation in Stevens–Johnson syndrome/toxic epidermal necrolysis (SJS/TEN)

- Full blood count
- Urea and electrolytes
- Amylase
- Bicarbonate
- Glucose
- Liver function tests
- Erythrocyte sedimentation rate
- C-reactive protein
- Coagulation studies
- *Mycoplasma* serology
- Antinuclear antibody and extractable nuclear antigen
- Complement
- Indirect immunofluorescence

Box 118.5 The seven parameters used to calculate SCORTEN (SCORe of Toxic Epidermal Necrolysis)

- Age greater than 40 years
- Presence of malignancy
- Heart rate >120 beats/min
- Epidermal detachment >10% of body surface area at admission
- Serum urea >10 mmol/L
- Serum glucose >14 mmol/L
- Bicarbonate level <20 mmol/L

Investigations

If SJS/TEN is suspected clinically, a set of investigations is needed to (i) substantiate the diagnosis; (ii) exclude other blistering dermatoses; and (iii) identify any systemic complications. Important blood tests are listed in Box 118.6. A biopsy must be taken from lesional skin, just adjacent to a blister, for routine histopathology. A second biopsy taken from periblister lesional skin should be sent unfixed for direct immunofluorescence to exclude an immunobullous disorder.

At presentation, swabs should be taken from lesional skin and sent for bacteriology. A chest X-ray is mandatory. Clinical photographs of the skin should be taken to show the type of lesion and extent of involvement. The extent of redness and the extent of epidermal detachment should be recorded separately on a body map; for each parameter the percentage of BSA involved should be estimated.

Management

Evaluation of both cutaneous and systemic disease components of SJS/TEN should be undertaken immediately the diagnosis is suspected. It is also imperative to identify the culprit drug as soon as possible, and to discontinue it. The fundamental elements of patient management in SJS/TEN are meticulous care of lesional skin and mucous membranes, coupled with intensive supportive care for the systemic complications of acute skin failure. The patient must be managed in an appropriate care setting, usually an intensive care unit (ICU) or burns unit, by a team of clinicians experienced in treating SJS/TEN.

Currently, the efficacy of active pharmacological therapy in SJS/TEN is not clear; unambiguous data from therapeutic trials are lacking. Similarly, the role of surgical debridement of lesional epidermis in SJS/TEN has been challenged [4].

Culprit drug

As soon as a diagnosis of SJS/TEN has been made, discontinuation of the culprit drug is an essential and immediate intervention; this manoeuvre decreases the risk of death [53]. The patient's other regular medicines must be continued. In order to identify the culprit, the date of onset of the adverse reaction must be noted and a record made of all medicines taken by the patient over the previous 2 months. For each drug, delineate a timeline indicating the date of drug commencement in relation to the onset of SJS/TEN. A latent period between the drug initiation and onset of SJS/TEN always occurs; a latency of 7–10 days is typical, but this period can range from 5 to 28 days.

Identification of the causative agent may be straightforward in cases where a single drug is implicated, but difficulties are posed by the patient who has been exposed to multiple drugs. Although any medicine can, theoretically, cause SJS/TEN, certain drugs have a greater probability to trigger the reaction. A list of drugs has been identified that are strongly associated with the induction of SJS/TEN, and are responsible for one-half of all cases (see Box 118.3). Paracetamol, aspirin, ibuprofen and corticosteroid have an unclear association, but may be confounders used to treat prodromal symptoms of SJS/TEN. An algorithm, termed ALDEN (ALgorithm of Drug causality in Epidermal Necrolysis), has been developed to help define drug causality in SJS/TEN [9]. ALDEN is generally used as a tool for the retrospective assessment of drug causality, and not for use in the acute phase of illness.

No test currently available, either *in vitro* or *in vivo*, is able to rule out, categorically, a potential culprit drug so that the patient can undergo risk-free drug rechallenge. However, several testing methods are used and can be helpful in strengthening the clinical assessment. Patch testing is safe but has a low sensitivity in SJS/TEN. *In vitro* tests, such as lymphocyte-transformation test (LTT) or enzyme-linked immunospot assay (ELISPOT), offer the potential for a clinically useful biological assay in drug hypersensitivity.

Following a diagnosis of SJS/TEN the patient must carry a Medic Alert card, or wear a Medic Alert bracelet or amulet, which states the culprit drug.

Care environment and care provision

Patients with large areas of epidermal loss (greater than 10% of BSA) should be admitted to an ICU for critical care management and specialist nursing. Since the cutaneous defect in SJS/TEN is analogous to a large superficial burn, many patients are transferred to a burns unit that can deliver both intensive supportive management as well as skin-directed therapy. Rapid admission to a specialist unit improves survival, while a delay in transfer is accompanied by increased mortality [54,55].

A number of specialist services are needed to manage SJS/TEN cases effectively. A multidisciplinary team (MDT), coordinated by a specialist in acute skin failure (dermatologist or burns surgeon), should be convened to manage the patient. As well as dermatology and wound care expertise, the SJS/TEN MDT must include clinicians from intensive care, ophthalmology and skin care nursing. Additional clinical input is often required from thoracic medicine, gastroenterology, gynaecology, urology, oral medicine, microbiology, dietetics, physiotherapy and pharmacy. Within an ICU or burns care unit the patient must be barrier nursed in a side room on a pressure-relieving mattress with the ambient temperature raised to 25–28°C.

Skin handling, topical therapy and dressings

In SJS/TEN, necrolytic epidermis readily detaches from the underlying dermis and therefore careful handling of the skin is essential. Day-to-day bedside care should be delivered by specialist nurses familiar with skin fragility disorders [56]. Shearing forces applied to the skin are a particular problem; extreme care is required when handling and moving an SJS/TEN patient. Other sources of skin trauma to be avoided include the use of sphygmomanometer cuffs, adhesive ECG leads, adhesive dressings and identification wrist tags.

Despite careful nursing, lesional epidermis (referred to as 'detachable epidermis') in SJS/TEN often peels away, especially at pressure areas, to leave zones of denuded dermis. In the conservative approach, detached epidermis can be left *in situ* to act as a biological dressing for the underlying dermis. In cases where bullae are prominent, blisters can be decompressed by fluid aspiration and the blister roof retained to cover the underlying dermis. In the interventional approach, favoured by many burns surgeons, necrotic or infected epidermis which has fully detached is removed using a variety of surgical techniques. At present there are no comparative studies of conservative versus interventional regimens to support the universal adoption of one approach over the other.

The intact skin should be cleansed each day by gentle irrigation with warmed sterile water or sprayed with a weak solution of chlorhexidine (1/5000). If mobility permits, the patient may be bathed in a weak solution of chlorhexidine (1/5000). The whole skin, including denuded areas, should be treated with frequent applications of a greasy emollient, such as 50% white soft paraffin with 50% liquid paraffin (50/50 WSP/LP). Aerosolised formulations of 50/50 WSP/LP can be used to minimise shearing forces associated with the manual application of topical agents. A topical antibiotic ointment should be used only on sloughy or crusted areas, or at sites of proven bacterial infection.

The use of dressings on denuded areas in SJS/TEN will reduce fluid and protein loss, limit microbial colonisation, help pain control and accelerate re-epithelialisation. Silicone dressings are recommended for areas of exposed dermis, while an absorbent non-adherent dressing should be applied as a secondary layer to collect exudate and protect lesional skin. Smear the surface of dressings with 50/50 WSP/LP prior to contact with the patient.

In the surgical approach, favoured by burns specialists, biological dressings or skin grafts are applied to denuded areas under a general anaesthetic.

Local therapy for eyes, mouth and uro-genital tract

Eyes. The eyes should be examined by an ophthalmologist as a part of the initial assessment and daily thereafter during the acute phase. An ocular lubricant must be applied 2-hourly. Ocular hygiene, to remove inflammatory debris and break down conjunctival adhesions, must be carried out each day. A broad spectrum topical antibiotic should be used in the presence of corneal fluorescein staining or frank ulceration. The use of topical corticosteroid drops, supervised by an ophthalmologist, may reduce ocular surface damage in the acute phase of SJS/TEN. For patients in whom there is extensive loss of ocular surface epithelia, which is unresponsive to conservative measures, then amniotic membrane transplantation (AMT) can be considered [57,58]. The proposed benefits of AMT in the acute phase include reduced inflammation, enhanced re-epithelialisation and reduction of scarring and symblepharon formation [59,60].

Mouth. Regular examination of the mouth must be undertaken. WSP ointment should be applied frequently to the lips; protect ulcerated intraoral surfaces with a mucoprotectant mouthwash. Clean the mouth daily with warm saline mouthwashes or an oral sponge. Use an anti-inflammatory oral rinse containing benzydamine hydrochloride every 3 h, and an antiseptic mouthwash (e.g. chlorhexidine digluconate) twice per day. In the absence of secondary infection, consider using a topical corticosteroid four times per day (e.g. Betnesol mouthwash 0.5 mg in 10 mL of water as a 3 min rinse-and-spit preparation).

Uro-genital tract. Examine the uro-genital tract regularly throughout the acute illness. Use WSP ointment as an emollient frequently. Use silicone sheet dressings to eroded areas in the vulva and vagina. Consider applying a topical corticosteroid cream with additional antimicrobial activity to the involved but non-eroded surfaces. Catheterising all patients will prevent urethral strictures.

Fluid replacement and nutrition

Extensive epidermal detachment will result in large insensible transcutaneous fluid losses, compounded by decreased oral intake due to disease involvement of the mouth. During the acute illness, replace fluids intravenously, using a crystalloid fluid at 2 mL/kg body weight/% of BSA epidermal detachment, or alternatively use urine output to guide fluid replacement [61]. Establish peripheral venous access by inserting a cannula through non-lesional skin. Overaggressive fluid resuscitation may be associated with pulmonary, cutaneous and intestinal oedema.

In SJS/TEN cases with significant areas of skin involvement, a nutritional regimen must be initiated early to support metabolic disturbances, minimise protein losses and promote healing. Enteral nutrition is preferable to parenteral nutrition since this feeding route will reduce peptic ulceration and limit translocation of gut bacteria. Since buccal mucositis in SJS/TEN often precludes normal oral intake, naso-gastric feeding with a silicone tube should be instituted when necessary. During the early, catabolic phase of SJS/TEN 20–25 kcal/kg/day should be delivered, while requirements in the recovery, anabolic phase increase to 25–30 kcal/kg/day [62].

Respiratory support

Disease involvement of the bronchial epithelium can cause occlusion of airways and hypoxia. In this situation, bronchoscopic removal of necrotic debris is helpful [28]. Nonetheless approximately 25% of SJS/TEN patients require intubation and mechanical ventilation, an intervention which is associated with a worse outcome [29]. Sedation and ventilation are also indicated when cutaneous pain limits effective patient handling.

Analgesia

Stevens–Johnson syndrome/toxic epidermal necrolysis is characterised by cutaneous pain which is most severe at sites of epidermal detachment. Patients should receive adequate background simple analgesia to ensure comfort at rest, with the addition of opiates, as required, delivered either by patient-controlled analgesia (PCA) or infusion. Involvement of the skin of the hands may limit the ability of the patient to operate a PCA device. If the patient is in severe pain, then an opiate-based analgesia regimen using morphine delivered by an appropriate route should be considered. Additional analgesia is often needed to address increased pain associated with patient handling, repositioning, dressing changes and physiotherapy: a bolus of 0.1 mg/kg of morphine may be given intravenously 10–20 min before commencement of the procedure. Bolus ketamine analgosedation (0.5 mg/kg) may be useful for procedural analgesia. Adjuvants, including γ-aminobutyric acid (GABA) analogues, may have an opiate-sparing role. Topical anaesthesia of mucous membranes may facilitate placement of naso-gastric tubes and urinary catheters.

Additional supportive medication

Patients with SJS/TEN are subject to stress-related gastric or duodenal ulceration and, if immobile, are at risk of venous thromboembolism. Gastric protection with a proton pump inhibitor is recommended if the patient is not absorbing food. Prophylactic anticoagulation with low-molecular-weight heparin is necessary, unless contraindicated.

Anaemia and leukopenia are common complications of the acute phase of SJS/TEN. Neutropenia will increase the risk of sepsis and therefore the administration of recombinant human granulocyte colony-stimulating factor (G-CSF) has been used to resist infectious complications [63]. It has been suggested that G-CSF in SJS/TEN may also be immunomodulatory and enhance re-epithelialisation [63].

Monitoring for infection

Cutaneous infection, which is a common complication of SJS/TEN, will impair re-epithelialisation and may lead to systemic sepsis. Swabs for bacterial and *Candida* culture should be taken from multiple sites, particularly sloughy or crusted areas, throughout the acute phase of SJS/TEN. Prophylactic systemic antimicrobial therapy may increase skin colonisation, particularly with *Candida albicans*, therefore antibiotics should only be given if there are clinical signs of infection. The SJS/TEN disease process may be accompanied by a fever which complicates detection of secondary sepsis. Patients should be monitored carefully for other signs of systemic infection such as confusion, hypotension, reduced urine output and reduced oxygen saturation [64]. The detection of sepsis may also be indicated by a rise in CRP, elevated procalcitonin, a neutrophilia and an increase in skin pain. A monoculture of organisms from swabs taken at various sites indicates that one strain of bacteria has become predominant and increases the likelihood of invasive infection [64].

In a small proportion of cases, SJS/TEN is triggered by *Mycoplasma pneumoniae* infection. Typically the patient is a child, there is no culprit drug and the disorder is marked by high fever and cough at the outset. If *Mycoplasma* infection is considered, treat with a macrolide antibiotic while awaiting results from naso-pharyngeal PCR and serology.

Active therapy

Only one randomised controlled trial of an active treatment has been conducted in TEN: the anti-TNF agent thalidomide was compared with placebo. However, the study was discontinued prematurely because of an excess of deaths in the thalidomide treatment group [65]. A number of other immunomodulating drugs have been studied in SJS/TEN patients, most notably IVIg, systemic corticosteroid and ciclosporin [66]. Unfortunately, the nature of SJS/TEN is such that published studies have been sullied by ascertainment bias, low numbers of patients, variations in the timing and nature of intervention, diversity of case mix and setting and differences in supportive care. Trials have, thus far, failed to identify a therapy with unambiguous benefit. There is insufficient evidence, at the time of writing, to support unequivocally the use of any particular systemic intervention in SJS/TEN.

Intravenous immunoglobulin. Evidence for possible efficacy of IVIg in SJS/TEN came from a study indicating a role for Fas-Fas ligand (Fas-FasL) interaction in TEN keratinocyte apoptosis [13]. This study, from Viard et al., demonstrated that high concentrations of normal immunoglobulin inhibited Fas-FasL interaction and apoptosis through anti-Fas activity. The authors then reported an uncontrolled prospective open trial of 10 patients with TEN treated with IVIg, none of whom died [13]. Since this report in 1998, a number of studies of IVIg treatment in SJS/TEN have been published, with results that vary from benefit to harm [67,68–79]. In a systematic review and meta-analysis, published in 2012, a pooled estimate of mortality risk was determined, comparing IVIg and supportive care in patients with TEN [80]. The pooled odds ratio (OR) for mortality comparing IVIg and supportive care was 1.00 (95% confidence interval (CI) 0.58–1.75, $P = 0.99$) [80]. Paediatric patients treated with IVIg had significantly lower mortality than adults (0% versus 21.6%, respectively; $P = 0.001$). Adults treated with high-dose IVIg exhibited significantly lower mortality than those treated with low-dose IVIg (18.9% versus 50%, respectively; $P = 0.022$). However, multivariate logistic regression model adjustment indicated that IVIg dose does not correlate with mortality (high-dose versus low-dose: OR 0.494, 95%CI 0.106–2.300, $P = 0.369$) [80]. Two further studies (published after the meta-analysis) comprising a total of 87 SJS/TEN patients demonstrated no improved survival in subjects receiving IVIg [79,81].

Corticosteroids. Corticosteroids have been used in the management of SJS/TEN for many years. It has been suggested that high-dose systemic corticosteroid administered early in the disease may 'switch off' the inflammatory process [82]. However, it is also recognised that systemic corticosteroids used indiscriminately may increase the risk of sepsis and impair re-epithelialisation. The majority of studies of systemic corticosteroid treatment in SJS/TEN indicate benefit, however all are case series, none is a randomised controlled trial and most are retrospective [67,68,82,83]. Retrospective analysis of a large number of SJS/TEN patients in France and Germany (the EuroSCAR study) indicated a lower mortality in German patients (but not French patients) treated with corticosteroids compared with controls receiving supportive care alone [67]. Two studies have investigated the effects of pulsed intravenous high-dose corticosteroids [82,84]. In the study by Kardaun et al., 12 patients received 100 mg or 1.5 mg/kg of IV dexamethasone for 3 days and were reported to have a decreased mortality compared with the death rate predicted by SCORTEN [83]. Hirahara et al. presented a series of eight SJS/TEN patients who received 1000 mg of IV methylprednisolone on 3 consecutive days, followed by either a tapering course of oral prednisolone, or a further 2 days of half-dose IV methylprednisolone [81]. No patients died despite a SCORTEN-predicted mortality of 1.6 [81].

Ciclosporin. Inhibition of lymphocyte function should interfere with a key element in SJS/TEN pathogenesis; thus, ciclosporin is a drug with theoretical efficacy in SJS/TEN. Four cohort studies demonstrated that ciclosporin treatment in SJS/TEN may improve outcomes [85–88]. A study by Valeyrie-Allanore et al. from the dermatology ITU in Créteil, Paris, demonstrated that in 29 SJS/TEN patients given ciclosporin (3 mg/kg/day for 10 days, and then tapered) there were no deaths, despite a SCORTEN predicted mortality in this group of 2.75 [86]. Singh et al. reported 11 SJS/TEN patients treated with ciclosporin (3 mg/kg/day for 7 days, and then tapered) and compared their outcomes with six historical controls treated with systemic corticosteroids [87]. In the ciclosporin group there was a significantly enhanced speed of epithelialisation, a reduced length of hospital stay and a benefit in SCORTEN-predicted mortality [87]. A similar positive outcome was demonstrated by Kirchhof et al. in a group of ciclosporin-treated patients compared with a group treated with IVIg [88]. However, in a larger, single-centre, retrospective study of 174 patients the reduction of mortality and improvement in healing time with ciclosporin were not confirmed [89].

Other treatments used in the management of SJS/TEN. Other therapies have been tried in SJS/TEN, but studies contain small numbers of patients and are, generally, uncontrolled. Plasmapheresis has been used in SJS/TEN and reports suggest that it may provide a rapid benefit [90,91]. There is also interest in the therapeutic role of TNF-α inhibitors in SJS/TEN. Paradisi et al. reported an uncontrolled series of 10 SJS/TEN patients treated with a single 50 mg subcutaneous dose of etanercept. None of the patients died, despite a SCORTEN-predicted mortality rate of approximately 50% [92]. An uncontrolled, prospective study compared etanercept with corticosteroids in 96 patients (60% of the study population had SJS) and reported a quicker healing time with etanercept but a similar mortality rate in the two groups [93].

Treatment ladder for Stevens–Johnson syndrome/toxic epidermal necrolysis

First line
- Withdraw culprit drug
- If epidermal loss is >10% body surface area transfer to a specialist unit (intensive care unit or burns unit)
- Institute supportive care package, with particular attention to:
  - Heated environment
  - Fluid replacement

- Nutritional regimen
- Analgesia
- Preventing/treating infection
- Specialist skin care nursing is essential for delivery of topical therapy/dressings

Second line

In the early stages of the acute phase consider using:
- Intravenous immunoglobulin (0.5–1 g/kg daily for 3–4 consecutive days), *or*
- Systemic corticosteroid (e.g. prednisolone 0.5–1 mg/kg daily for 10 days, and tapered; or IV methylprednisolone 500 mg on 3 consecutive days), *or*
- Ciclosporin (3 or 4 mg/kg/day in divided doses for 10 days, and tapered)

Resources

Further information

SJS Awareness UK: www.sjsawareness.org.uk (last accessed June 2023).

Key references

The full list of references can be found in the online version at https://www.wiley.com/rooksdermatology10e

Acute generalised exanthematous pustulosis

5 Sidoroff A, Halevy S, Bavinck JN, Vaillant L, Roujeau JC. Acute generalized exanthematous pustulosis (AGEP) – a clinical reaction pattern. *J Cutan Pathol* 2001;28:113–19.
6 Sidoroff A, Dunant A, Viboud C et al. Risk factors for acute generalized exanthematous pustulosis (AGEP) – results of a multinational case–control study (EuroSCAR). *Br J Dermatol* 2007;157:989–96.
15 Britschgi M, Steiner UC, Schmid S et al. T-cell involvement in drug-induced acute generalized exanthematous pustulosis. *J Clin Invest* 2001;107:1433–41.
18 Navarini AA, Valeyrie-Allanore L, Setta-Kaffetzi N et al. Rare variations in IL36RN in severe adverse drug reactions manifesting as acute generalized exanthematous pustulosis. *J Invest Dermatol* 2013;133:1904–7.
24 Hotz C, Valeyrie-Allanore L, Haddad C et al. Systemic involvement of acute generalized exanthematous pustulosis: a retrospective study on 58 patients. *Br J Dermatol* 2013;169:1223–32.
25 Roujeau JC, Bioulac-Sage P, Bourseau C et al. Acute generalized exanthematous pustulosis. Analysis of 63 cases. *Arch Dermatol* 1991;127:1333–8.

Drug reaction with eosinophilia and systemic symptoms

1 Walsh SA, Creamer D. Drug reaction with eosinophilia and systemic symptoms (DRESS): a clinical update and review of current thinking. *Clin Exp Dermatol* 2011;36:6–11.
6 Bocquet H, Bagot M, Roujeau JC. Drug-induced pseudolymphoma and drug hypersensitivity syndrome (drug rash with eosinophilia and systemic symptoms: DRESS). *Semin Cutan Med Surg* 1996;15:250–7.
7 Kardaun SH, Sekula P, Valeyrie-Allanore L et al. Drug reaction with eosinophilia and systemic symptoms (DRESS): an original multisystem adverse drug reaction. Results from the prospective RegiSCAR study. *Br J Dermatol* 2013;169:1071–80.
15 Shiohara T, Inaoka M, Kano Y. Drug-induced hypersensitivity syndrome (DIHS): a reaction induced by a complex interplay among herpesviruses and antiviral and antidrug immune responses. *Allergol Int* 2006;55:1–8.
18 Chen Y-C, Chang C-Y, Cho Y-T, Chiu H-C, Chu C-Y. Long-term sequelae of drug reaction with eosinophilia and systemic symptoms: a retrospective cohort study from Taiwan. *J Am Acad Dermatol* 2013;68:459–65.
20 Ushigome Y, Kano Y, Ishida T, Hirahara K, Shiohara T. Short- and long-term outcomes of 34 patients with drug-induced hypersensitivity syndrome in a single institution. *J Am Acad Dermatol* 2013;68:721–8.
21 Chiou CC, Yang LC, Hung SI et al. Clinicopathological features and prognosis of drug rash with eosinophilia and systemic symptoms: a study of 30 cases in Taiwan. *J Eur Acad Dermatol Venereol* 2008;22:1044–9.
24 Walsh S, Diaz-Cano S, Higgins E et al. Drug reaction with eosinophilia and systemic symptoms: is cutaneous phenotype a prognostic marker for outcome? A review of clinicopathological features of 27 cases. *Br J Dermatol* 2013;168:391–401.
51 Chen Y-C, Chiu H-C, Chu C-Y. Drug reaction with eosinophilia and systemic symptoms: a retrospective study of 60 cases. *Arch Dermatol* 2010;146:1373–9.
81 Bouvresse S, Valeyrie-Allanore L, Ortonne N et al. Toxic epidermal necrolysis, DRESS, AGEP: do overlap cases exist? *Orphanet J Rare Dis* 2012;7:72.

Stevens–Johnson syndrome/toxic epidermal necrolysis

3 Bastuji-Garin S, Rzany B, Stern RS et al. Clinical classification of cases of toxic epidermal necrolysis, Stevens–Johnson syndrome, and erythema multiforme. *Arch Dermatol* 1993;129:92–6.
5 Roujeau JC, Guillaume JC, Fabre JP et al. Toxic epidermal necrolysis (Lyell syndrome). Incidence and drug etiology in France, 1981–1985. *Arch Dermatol* 1990;126:37–42.
6 Rzany B, Mockenhaupt M, Baur S et al. Epidemiology of erythema exsudativum multiforme majus, Stevens–Johnson syndrome, and toxic epidermal necrolysis in Germany (1990–1992): structure and results of a population-based registry. *J Clin Epidemiol* 1996;49:769–73.
10 Roujeau JC. Immune mechanisms in drug allergy. *Allergol Int* 2006;55:27–33.
11 Schwartz RA, McDonagh PH, Lee BW. Toxic epidermal necrolysis. Part I. *J Am Acad Dermatol* 2013;69:173.e1–13.
12 Viard-Leveugle I, Gaide O, Jankovic D et al. TNF-alpha and IFN-gamma are potential inducers of Fas-mediated keratinocyte apoptosis through activation of inducible nitric oxide synthase in toxic epidermal necrolysis. *J Invest Dermatol* 2013;133:489–98.
13 Viard I, Wehrli P, Bullani R et al. Inhibition of toxic epidermal necrolysis by blockade of CD95 with human intravenous immunoglobulin. *Science* 1998;282:490–3.
15 Chung WH, Hung SI, Yang JY et al. Granulysin is a key mediator for disseminated keratinocyte death in Stevens–Johnson syndrome and toxic epidermal necrolysis. *Nat Med* 2008;14:1343–50.
17 Kim SK, Kim W-J, Yoon J-H et al. Upregulated RIP3 expression potentiates MLKL phosphorylation-mediated programmed necrosis in toxic epidermal necrolysis. *J Invest Dermatol* 2015;13:2021–30.
18 Mockenhaupt M, Viboud C, Dunant A et al. Stevens–Johnson syndrome and toxic epidermal necrolysis: assessment of medication risks with emphasis on recently marketed drugs. The EuroSCAR-study. *J Invest Dermatol* 2008;128:35–44.
19 Roujeau JC, Kelly JP, Naldi L et al. Medication use and the risk of Stevens–Johnson syndrome or toxic epidermal necrolysis. *N Engl J Med* 1995;333:1600–7.
22 Chung WH, Hung SI, Hong HS et al. Medical genetics: a marker for Stevens–Johnson syndrome. *Nature* 2004;428:486.
26 Revuz J, Penso D, Roujeau JC et al. Toxic epidermal necrolysis. Clinical findings and prognosis factors in 87 patients. *Arch Dermatol* 1987;123:1160–5.
27 Gueudry J, Roujeau JC, Binaghi M et al. Risk factors for the development of ocular complications of Stevens–Johnson syndrome and toxic epidermal necrolysis. *Arch Dermatol* 2009;145:157–62.
50 Bastuji-Garin S, Fouchard N, Bertocchi M et al. SCORTEN: a severity-of-illness score for toxic epidermal necrolysis. *J Invest Dermatol* 2000;115:149–53.
67 Schneck J, Fagot JP, Sekula P et al. Effects of treatments on the mortality of Stevens–Johnson syndrome and toxic epidermal necrolysis: a retrospective study on patients included in the prospective EuroSCAR Study. *J Am Acad Dermatol* 2008;58:33–40.
80 Huang YC, Li YC, Chen TJ. The efficacy of intravenous immunoglobulin for the treatment of toxic epidermal necrolysis: a systematic review and meta-analysis. *Br J Dermatol* 2012;167:424–32.
89 Poizeau F, Gaudin O, Le Cleach L et al. Ciclosporin for epidermal necrolysis: absence of beneficial effect in a retrospective cohort of 174 patients – exposed/unexposed and propensity-score matched analyses. *J Invest Dermatol* 2018;138:1293–300.
93 Wang C-W, Yang L-Y, Chen C-B et al. Randomized, controlled trial of TNF-α antagonist in CTL-mediated severe cutaneous adverse reactions. *J Clin Invest* 2018;128:985–96.

CHAPTER 119

Cutaneous Side Effects of Chemotherapy and Radiotherapy

Louise Fearfield and Charlotte Edwards
Chelsea & Westminster, London, UK

Toxic erythema of chemotherapy, 119.1	Chemotherapy-induced hypertrichosis, 119.6	Photosensitivity, 119.10
Papulopustular eruptions, 119.3	Chemotherapy-induced nail changes, 119.6	Recall reaction dermatitis, 119.12
Chemotherapy mucositis, 119.5	Dyspigmentation, 119.9	Radiotherapy-associated skin side effects, 119.13
Chemotherapy-induced hair changes, 119.5	Chemotherapy-induced hyperpigmentation, 119.9	Other skin side effects of radiotherapy, 119.14
Chemotherapy-induced alopecia, 119.5	Chemotherapy-induced hypopigmentation, 119.10	Key references, 119.15

Toxic erythema of chemotherapy

Definition and nomenclature
Toxic erythema of chemotherapy is the term used to describe a variety of overlapping cutaneous reactions to chemotherapy agents.

> **Synonyms and inclusions**
> - Palmoplantar erythrodysaesthesia
> - Intertriginous eruption associated with chemotherapy
> - Neutrophilic eccrine hidradenitis

Introduction and general description
Although several distinct dermatoses are described it has been suggested that the term 'toxic erythema of chemotherapy' (TEC) should be used to encompass the spectrum of eruptions triggered by anticancer drugs [1]. TEC includes entities such as palmoplantar erythrodysaesthesia, intertriginous eruption associated with chemotherapy and neutrophilic eccrine hidradenitis [1]. The drugs that are most commonly associated with the induction of TEC are listed in Box 119.1.

> **Box 119.1 Cancer chemotherapy agents associated with toxic erythema of chemotherapy**
> - Cytarabine
> - Clofarabine
> - Anthracyclines (e.g. doxorubicin)
> - Carboplatin
> - Cyclophosphamide
> - 5-Fluorouracil
> - Capecitabine
> - Taxanes (e.g. docetaxel)
> - Methotrexate

It is important for clinicians to recognise that TEC is a non-allergic reaction. An understanding of this concept avoids erroneously labelling patients as having a drug allergy.

Epidemiology
Incidence and prevalence
There are no reliable data for the incidence or prevalence of TEC in patients exposed to chemotherapy.

Age and sex
Toxic erythema of chemotherapy affects both sexes equally, and all ages.

Pathophysiology
It has been proposed that TEC is caused by direct toxicity of a chemotherapeutic agent after it is excreted through the straight portion of the eccrine duct, the acrosyringium and the epidermis [1]. The high density of eccrine glands in the palms and soles may explain, in part, the predilection of TEC to these sites. Other factors, including temperature gradient, friction, trauma and vascularity, may play a role in the distribution of skin signs in TEC [1,2]. TEC reactions are dose dependent.

Pathology
The histopathology of TEC will depend on the timing of the skin biopsy. Early histological features (within the first 24 h of the eruption) include hyperplastic eccrine ducts with mitotic figures and multiple necrotic duct cells without associated keratinisation. Late histological features (within 72–96 h of the eruption) include syringosquamous metaplasia, in which there is non-inflammatory metaplastic transformation of the eccrine cuboidal epithelium into two or more layers of squamous cells with intraductal keratinisation [3–5].

Rook's Textbook of Dermatology, Tenth Edition. Edited by Christopher Griffiths, Jonathan Barker, Tanya Bleiker, Walayat Hussain and Rosalind Simpson.
© 2024 John Wiley & Sons Ltd. Published 2024 by John Wiley & Sons Ltd.

Clinical features

TEC usually presents between 2 days to 3 weeks after the administration of chemotherapeutic agents with pain, pruritus, paraesthesia and tenderness over the hands and feet and/or intertriginous areas [1,2]. Patients present with red patches or oedematous plaques, typically distributed on the acral skin and at the major flexures (axillae, groins and inframammary folds). Less often it can involve the elbows, knees and ears. In some areas the redness may become dusky or contain petechiae. Occasionally, lesional skin in TEC may blister.

A delayed onset of TEC, up to 2–10 months after the onset of treatment, can be seen in patients receiving continuous, low-dose intravenous infusions of chemotherapy [1,2].

Clinical variants

Prior to the adoption of the umbrella term of TEC, several distinct entities were described and appear in the dermatological literature.

Palmoplantar erythrodysaesthesia. This describes a reaction of acral reddening, which starts 24 h to 3 weeks after the initiation of chemotherapy. Patients initially complain of a tingling or burning sensation that precedes the eruption. When the skin signs appear, there is well-demarcated palmoplantar reddening with oedema. Lesional skin can become bullous and may erode (Figure 119.1). The reaction generally resolves 1–2 weeks after stopping chemotherapy treatment [6,7]. Doxorubicin, cytarabine, docetaxel, fluorouracil and capecitabine are the most commonly implicated agents. The combination of a taxane (especially docetaxel) with capecitabine is associated with an increased incidence of palmoplantar erythrodysaesthesia. Dose reduction of the culprit agent(s) usually ameliorates the symptoms.

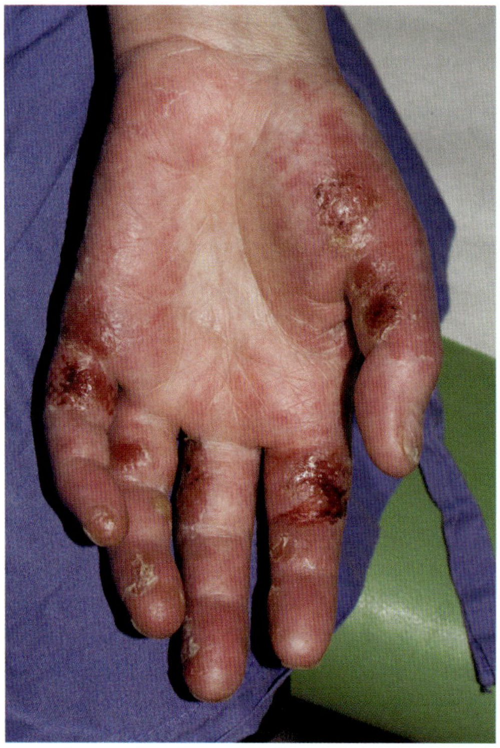

Intertriginous eruption associated with chemotherapy. This eruption appears between 1 and 25 days following the onset of the chemotherapy cycle. It is characterised by dusky red papules coalescing into patches and plaques. The redness of lesional skin may become dusky. The eruption predominates in the major flexures, especially in the axillary and inguinal folds and antecubital fossae. It can also be seen in areas of occlusion. Histologically there is eccrine squamous syringometaplasia. The eruption resolves spontaneously with postinflammatory pigmentation and desquamation [8,9].

Neutrophilic eccrine hidradenitis. This is characterised by red papules, nodules or plaques that typically involve the extremities, trunk, face and palms. It usually appears between 2 days and 3 weeks following the start of chemotherapy and may be preceded by a fever. Patients are often neutropenic at the time skin signs appear. Pustules, purpura and urticarial lesions have also been described [10,11]. Neutrophilic eccrine hidradenitis is caused by a variety of chemotherapeutic agents, particularly cytarabine, and usually resolves spontaneously within 4 weeks of discontinuing the culprit drug. Histologically there is usually a dense neutrophilic inflammation around the eccrine glands, and secretory coils with associated necrosis of the eccrine coils and glands in the deeper reticular dermis or subcutaneous fat. If patients are neutropenic then lower numbers of neutrophils will be seen.

Differential diagnosis

Main differentials include drug hypersensitivity reaction or graft-versus-host disease. Intertriginous eruption associated with chemotherapy can be mistaken for an infective intertrigo or symmetrical drug-related intertriginous and flexural exanthem (Chapter 116). Neutrophilic eccrine hidradenitis can be mistaken for erysipelas.

Disease course and prognosis

TEC can recur if the patient is rechallenged to the same dose of the chemotherapeutic agent, or there may be a more intense skin reaction with higher doses of the same agent. Recurrence can be reduced by dose reduction and a lengthening of the interval between cycles of chemotherapy.

TEC usually resolves spontaneously with desquamation without any specific treatment.

Investigations

A skin biopsy can be helpful in cases of diagnostic difficulty.

Management

There is no standardised treatment regimen for TEC. The treatment is symptomatic as the reaction usually spontaneously resolves with intense desquamation [1]. Discontinuing treatment is needed if the skin reaction is severe.

Figure 119.1 Severe palmoplantar erythrodysaesthesia secondary to docetaxol treatment demonstrating reddening, desquamation and erosions.

Papulopustular eruptions

Definition and nomenclature
Papulopustular eruptions are drug-induced acneform dermatoses that resemble acne vulgaris in lesion morphology and distribution, but generally lack a comedonal component.

Synonyms and inclusions
- Acneform eruption

Introduction and general description
Papulopustular eruptions are a side effect of many of the targeted agents now used in cancer therapy, especially epidermal growth factor receptor (EGFR) and mitogen-activated protein kinase (MEK) inhibitors. The drugs that are most commonly associated with the induction of papulopustular eruptions are listed in Box 119.2.

Epidemiology
Incidence and prevalence
Papulopustular eruption of any toxicity grade can occur in up to 90% of patients receiving an EGFR inhibitor and up to 10% for grade 3. Third generation EGFR-TKI inhibitors (osimertinib) have been reported to have significantly less skin side effects; 58% compared with 78% of standard EGFR inhibitors (gefitinib or erlotinib) [1].

Age and sex
Patients of any age may be affected. With erlotinib there is an increased risk of developing a severe papulopustular eruption in patients aged over 70 years; with cetuximb there is an increased risk of developing severe papulopustular eruption in male patients aged under 70 years.

Box 119.2 Commonest drug triggers for papulopustular eruptions

EGFR-targeting monoclonal antibodies
- Cetuximab (for treating colo-rectal, head and neck cancers)
- Panitumumab (for treating colo-rectal cancer)
- Necitumumab (for treating lung cancer)

EGFR-tyrosine kinase inhibitors
- Erlotinib (for treating lung and pancreatic cancer)
- Gefitinib (for treating lung cancer)
- Lapatinib (for treating breast cancer)
- Osimertinib (for treating lung cancer)
- Dacomitinib (for treating lung cancer)

Mitogen-activated protein kinase inhibitors
- Trametinib (for treating *BRAF* mutated melanoma)
- Selumetinib (for treating lung cancer)

EGFR, epidermal growth factor receptor.

Pathophysiology
The pathophysiology of EGFR and MEK inhibitor induced rash remains poorly understood. It has been proposed that inhibition of signal transduction pathways play a role in papulopustular development as EGFR is expressed in undifferentiated, proliferating keratinocytes in the basal epidermis and hair root sheath [2]. EGFR inhibitors interfere with EGFR-mediated signalling, causing growth arrest and premature differentiation of keratinocytes. The subsequent release of inflammatory cell chemoattractants recruits leukocytes and induces a folliculocentric inflammatory response [3]. Also, reduced inhibition of *Staphylococcus aureus* colony formation by the supernatant produced by EGFR inhibitor keratinocytes has been implicated in the increased risk of secondary infections found in a third of patients on EGFR and MEK inhibitors [4].

Pathology
The histopathology of EGFR inhibitor-induced papulopustular eruption demonstrates a superficial neutrophilic suppurative folliculitis with ectatic follicular infundibula and rupture of the epithelial lining [5].

Clinical features
The papulopustular eruption typically occurs within the first 2 weeks of treatment. Prior to the appearance of the dermatosis, patients may complain of a burning pain and pruritus. Lesions occur in a seborrhoeic distribution on the scalp, face, chest and back; other sites which may be involved include the extremities, abdomen and buttocks.

The eruption consists of sterile follicular pustules and papules, without comedones (Figure 119.2). The evolution of the eruption passes through four phases: (i) sensory disturbance with redness and oedema on the face and upper trunk; (ii) papulopustular lesions; (iii) crusting lesions; and (iv) persistent xerosis, redness and telangiectasis [6].

Patients with fair skin (skin phototype I/II) are at particular risk of EGFR inhibitor-induced papulopustular eruption.

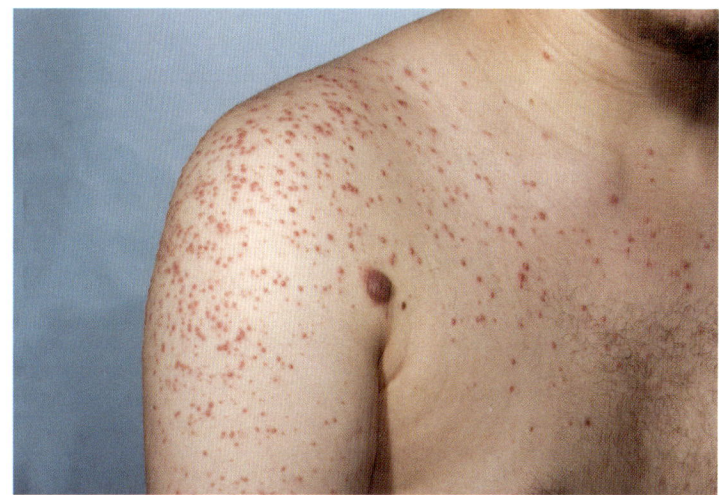

Figure 119.2 Papulopustular eruption, secondary to an epidermal growth factor receptor inhibitor, involving the trunk.

Differential diagnosis

Differential diagnoses include drug-induced acne, *Malassezia* folliculitis, *Staphylococcus* folliculitis, eosinophilic folliculitis and tinea barbae.

Classification of severity

The National Cancer Institute Common Terminology Criteria for Adverse Events (CTCAE) has published a widely used severity grading scale for papulopustular eruptions (Table 119.1). The Multinational Association of Supportive Care in Cancer (MASCC) Skin Toxicity Study Group has created a grading scale specific to EGFR inhibitor-induced dermatological toxicities (Table 119.2) [7].

Table 119.1 The National Cancer Institute Common Terminology Criteria for Adverse Events (CTCAE) severity grading scale for papulopustular eruptions.

Grade	Adverse event
Grade 1	Papules and/or pustules covering <10% BSA, which may or may not be associated with symptoms of pruritus or tenderness
Grade 2	Papules and/or pustules covering 10–30% BSA, which may or may not be associated with symptoms of pruritus or tenderness; associated with psychosocial impact; limiting instrumental ADL; papules and/or pustules covering >30% BSA with or without mild symptoms
Grade 3	Papules and/or pustules covering >30% BSA with moderate or severe symptoms; limiting self-care ADL; associated with local superinfection with oral antibiotics indicated
Grade 4	Life-threatening consequences; papules and/or pustules covering any % BSA, which may or may not be associated with symptoms of pruritus or tenderness and are associated with extensive superinfection with IV antibiotics indicated
Grade 5	Death

Definition: a disorder characterised by an eruption of papules and pustules, typically appearing in face, scalp, upper chest and back. ADL, assisted daily living; BSA, body surface area.
From National Cancer Institute, Cancer Therapy Evaluation Program. CTCAE v5, Nov 2017. https://ctep.cancer.gov/protocoldevelopment/electronic_applications/docs/CTCAE_v5_Quick_Reference_5x7.pdf (last accessed February 2023).

Table 119.2 The Multinational Association of Supportive Care in Cancer (MASCC) Skin Toxicity Study Group severity grading scale for papulopustular eruptions due to epidermal growth factor receptor inhibitors.

Grade	Adverse event
Grade 1A	Number of papules or pustules <5 *Or* one area of erythema or oedema <1 cm in size
Grade 1B	Number of papule or pustules <5 *Or* one area of erythema or oedema <1 cm in size *and* pain or pruritus
Grade 2A	Number of papules or pustules 6–20 *Or* 2–5 areas of erythema or oedema <1 cm in size
Grade 2B	Number of papules or pustules 6–20 *Or* 2–5 areas of erythema or oedema <1 cm in size *and* pain, pruritus or effect on emotions or functioning
Grade 3A	Number of papules or pustules >20 *Or* >5 areas of erythema or oedema <1 cm in size
Grade 3B	Number of papules or pustules >20 *Or* >5 areas of erythema or oedema <1 cm in size *and* pain, pruritus, or effect on emotions or functioning

Adapted from [7].

Table 119.3 The Multinational Association of Supportive Care in Cancer (MASCC) Skin Toxicity Study: papulopustular rash recommendations.

Preventative management
Topical	Hydrocortisone 1% cream, with moisturiser and sunscreen twice daily
Systemic	Minocycline 100 mg daily/doxycycline 100 mg BD

Treatment
Topical	Fluocinomide 0.05% cream BD/alclometasone 0.05% cream/clindamycin 1%
Systemic	Doxycycline 100 mg BD/minocycline 100 mg daily. Low-dose isotretinoin 20–30 mg daily

Adapted from [8].

Disease course and prognosis

The severity of the skin eruption can vary, with clinically more severe reactions seen with the monoclonal antibodies compared with the EGFR and EGFR-TK inhibitors [8]. An EGFR inhibitor-related papulopustular eruption may wax or wane and typically resolves without scarring within 2 months of therapy discontinuation provided there was no superadded skin infection [6]. Postinflammatory hyperpigmentation can be prominent.

There is growing evidence to suggest that the presence and severity of the skin eruption may correlate with improved tumour response to the targeted agent. An early phase II study of erlotinib used in 57 patients with advanced non-small cell lung cancer (stage IIIB or IV) demonstrated that median survival improved with the severity of the papulopustular eruption: grade 0 rash, 1.5 months median survival; grade 1 rash, 8.5 months median survival; and grade 2–3 rash, 19.6 months median survival [7,9]. Several other retrospective analyses of phase II and III studies on EGFR inhibitors in other tumour types including colo-rectal, ovarian cancer and pancreatic cancer have confirmed this correlation [9,10]. The skin eruption is the best surrogate marker for clinical response to EGFR inhibitors.

Investigations

Skin biopsy can be useful in demonstrating the histopathology but is not mandatory. Skin swabs should be taken to exclude an infective folliculitis and/or superadded infections.

Management

Prior to the initiation of an EGFR inhibitor, the potential dermatological side effects should be discussed with the patient. Avoidance of excessive sun exposure while on the treatment is advised since UV radiation can trigger an eruption. A high protection factor topical sunscreen should be applied to uncovered skin 1–2 h prior to sun exposure and reapplied every 2 h.

Prophylactic skin treatments started 24 h prior to initiating the EGFR inhibitor (including moisturiser, sunscreen, hydrocortisone 1% and oral doxycycline 100 mg BD) are beneficial in reducing the incidence of grade 2 reactions by 50% at 6 weeks (Table 119.3) [8,11]. A randomised, double-blind, controlled trial of prophylactic oral minocycline 100 mg reduced the number of papulopustular lesions during the first 8 weeks on cetuximab therapy [12]. Effective prophylaxis with topical dapsone gel has also been reported [13].

Active measures to treat EGFR inhibitor-induced skin reactions include the use of potent topical steroids and tetracycline antibiotics (Table 119.3). Topical EGF creams have recently been reported to be effective [14].

Low-dose isotretinoin (20–30 mg/day) is recommended for the management of severe EGFR inhibitor-induced eruptions that fail to respond to standard therapy [15].

Resources

Further information

National Cancer Institute, Cancer Therapy Evuaulation Program. Common Terminology Criteria for Adverse Events (CTCAE) v5, Nov 2017. https://ctep.cancer.gov/protocoldevelopment/electronic_applications/docs/CTCAE_v5_Quick_Reference_5x7.htm (last accessed February 2023).

Chemotherapy mucositis

See Chapter 108.

Chemotherapy-induced hair changes

Chemotherapy-induced alopecia

Definition
This is a loss of scalp and body hair caused by the cytostatic effect of chemotherapy on hair follicles.

Introduction and general description
Chemotherapy-induced alopecia (CIA) is a common and distressing manifestation that is seen with most chemotherapeutic agents. The hair is an innocent bystander since chemotherapy drugs target dividing cells and in so doing interrupt the cell division of the hair matrix cells. Up to 90% of scalp hair is in the anagen, proliferative phase at any given time and therefore the pattern of alopecia is known as anagen effluvium. The degree of alopecia is, however, dependent on the specific chemotherapeutic drug, the dose regimen, the duration of treatment and the route of administration [1]. Combination therapy consisting of two or more agents usually produces a greater incidence of more severe CIA compared with single-agent therapy [2]. The drugs that are most commonly associated with CIA are listed in Box 119.3.

Epidemiology
Incidence and prevalence
The overall incidence of CIA is estimated to be 65% [2]. The frequency of CIA differs for the four major drug classes: >80% for antimicrotubule agents; 60–100% for topoisomerase inhibitors; >60% for alkylators; and 10–50% for antimetabolites.

Age and sex
CIA affects all ages and both sexes equally.

Pathophysiology
Cytostatic drugs act preferentially on follicles in the proliferative, anagen phase of the hair cycle. This results in anagen effluvium with the shedding of fully pigmented hair shafts. However, telogen effluvium also occurs as a response to chemotherapy and contributes to hair loss in these patients.

> **Box 119.3 Cancer chemotherapy agents associated with alopecia**
>
> - Antimicrotubule agents (e.g. paclitaxel, docetaxel)
> - Topoisomerase inhibitors (e.g. etoposide, doxorubicin)
> - Alkylators (e.g. cyclophosphamide, ifosfamide)
> - Antimetabolites (e.g. 5-fluorouracil)

Much of our understanding of the pathogenesis of CIA is derived from human and C57BL/6 mouse model studies of cyclophosphamide-induced alopecia. These studies showed that hair follicular damage is dose dependent, and is accompanied by dystrophic anagen and catagen response pathways [3].

Pathology
Histopathological features include the disruption of melanin accumulation, an irregular banding pattern of the hair shaft, an irregular follicular diameter, widened hair canal and distortion of the hair follicle. Permanent alopecia is characterised by an increased vellus to terminal hair ratio, an increased ratio of telogen to anagen follicles and the appearance of basaloid epithelium without scarring or inflammation [3].

Clinical features
CIA usually presents suddenly within days to weeks of initiating therapy. The hair is usually lost first over the vertex and the sides of the head above the ears. By 2–3 months a more established, diffuse or patchy pattern of alopecia is seen, which continues throughout the treatment.

Differential diagnosis
The speed of onset of hair loss discriminates CIA from telogen effluvium.

Disease course and prognosis
On discontinuing therapy, the alopecia is usually reversible and spontaneously recovers within 1–3 months and is fully recovered by 6 months [1]. Mild to moderate hair follicle damage initiates the dystrophic anagen pathway, whereas the dystrophic catagen pathway is triggered with severe hair follicle damage. These pathways determine the clinical appearance and the subsequent speed and quality of hair regrowth. Dystrophic anagen hairs recover more slowly, are of poor hair shaft quality and have pigmentary defects. In comparison, dystrophic catagen pathway is associated with the fastest and most complete recovery of damaged hair follicles.

Sometimes after chemotherapy the hair may grow back with a different texture, colour and thickness. A rare adverse effect of permanent CIA can occur with incomplete and absent hair regrowth at 6 months post therapy. It is most commonly seen with bulsulphan, cyclophosphamide and taxane therapy.

Investigations
None are needed.

Management
The management of CIA consists of careful explanation, psychological support and providing access to wigs.

Scalp cooling methods are the most widely used preventative measure for CIA. Data suggests a relative risk reduction of between one-third and two-thirds depending on chemotherapy regimen [4–6]. A cooling agent (air or liquid) applied to the scalp via a cooling cap is thought to reduce the cytotoxic effect of the drug by causing local vasoconstriction, thus slowing cellular uptake of the drug and limiting toxicity.

Currently there is no pharmacological treatment for CIA. Scalp compression alone and topical minoxidil 2% lotion have not been shown to be helpful as prophylaxis in preventing CIA; it has, however, been shown to be a safe accelerator of hair regrowth after CIA [2].

Chemotherapy-induced hypertrichosis

Definition
This is excessive growth of scalp and body hair caused by chemotherapeutic agents.

Introduction and general description
Hypertrichosis as a side effect of cancer treatment is encountered most frequently with the EGFR inhibitors but also reported in newer pan-FGFR inhibitors [1–3]. These drugs are associated with a number of hair changes at different body sites including: (i) facial hypertrichosis; (ii) slow-growing, brittle, curly hair; and (iii) increased thickness, length and curvature of eyebrow hair and eyelashes (trichomegaly) [4]. The EGFR inhibitors can also cause diffuse non-scarring alopecia over the scalp and body. The multitargeted receptor TK inhibitors, including sunitinib and dasatinib, may cause reversible hair depigmentation. The drugs that are most associated with chemotherapy-induced hypertrichosis are listed in Box 119.4.

Pathophysiology
Epidermal growth factor receptor is physiologically expressed in the outer root sheath of the hair follicle. EGFR functions as a biological on–off switch guarding the entry and exit from the anagen growth phase.

Clinical features
Patients notice a change in the texture, length and thickness of the hair in various body sites. Hair changes tend to occur from 2 to 6 months after initiation of EGFR inhibitor therapy [3,5]. Trichiasis is a complication of trichomegaly; eyelash hairs grow towards the eye, inducing corneal abrasions and posing a risk for conjunctivitis [6].

Differential diagnosis
The differential diagnosis includes paraneoplastic hypertrichosis.

Disease course and prognosis
The hair changes are usually reversible and disappear within a month of stopping treatment.

There are rarely any significant long-term problems arising from chemotherapy-induced hypertrichosis.

> **Box 119.4 Cancer chemotherapy agents associated with hypertrichosis**
>
> - Interferon α
> - Cetuximab
> - Erlotinib
> - Gefitinib

Investigations
No investigations are needed.

Management
Stop the culprit chemotherapeutic agent. Facial hirsutism with EGFR inhibitors can be treated with temporary or permanent hair removal methods, including topical eflornithine or laser hair removal.

Chemotherapy-induced nail changes

Definition
These are any nail changes caused by chemotherapeutic drugs.

Introduction and general description
Nail abnormalities are a common side effect of systemic chemotherapy and can cause significant morbidity especially when long-term maintenance treatment is required, as with the EGFR inhibitors. The clinical presentation of drug-induced nail changes depends on the duration and severity of the toxic damage, as well as on the nail constituent involved. The drugs most implicated in causing chemotherapy-induced nail changes, and their effects, are listed in Table 119.4. Newer agents such as the selective pan-FGFR (fibroblast growth factor receptor) 1–4 tyrosine kinase inhibitors have recently been associated with severe nail toxicity.

Epidemiology
Incidence and prevalence
A meta-analysis of published nail changes associated with EGFR inhibitors revealed an overall incidence of all-grade nail toxicity to be 17.2% and high-grade nail toxicity to be 1.4% [1]. The published incidence of taxane-induced nail toxicity ranged from 0% to 44% [2]. Peri-ungual toxicity has been observed in 5–46% of patients on anticancer mTOR inhibitors (everolimus, temsirolimus) [3].

A single centre study, at the Gustave Roussy (Paris, France), demonstrated that 235 (39%) of 607 patients who were referred to the dermatology unit for any chemotherapy-associated cutaneous toxicities presented with nail changes [4].

Age and sex
Chemotherapy-induced nail changes can affect all ages and both sexes equally.

Table 119.4 Effects of cancer chemotherapy agents associated with nail changes [5–8].

Drug	Nail changes
Docetaxol, paclitaxel	Onycholysis, Beau lines, pigmentation, onychomadesis, subungual haemorrhage
Sorafenib, sunitinib	Subungual haemorrhage
Trametinib	Onycholysis, paronychia
Cetuximab, pamitumumab	Onycholysis, paronychia
Bleomycin	Onycholysis, dystrophy
Cyclophosphamide	Beau lines, onycholysis
Dactinomycin	Beau lines
Daunorubicin	Transverse leuconychia (Mees lines)
Doxorubicin	Onycholyis, Beau lines
Fluorouracil	Onycholysis, dystrophy, onychomadesis
Gefitinib	Paronychia
Hydroxyurea	Onycholysis, dystrophy
Lapatinib	Paronychia
Melphalan	Transverse leuconychia (Mees lines)
Methotrexate	Paronychia, onycholysis

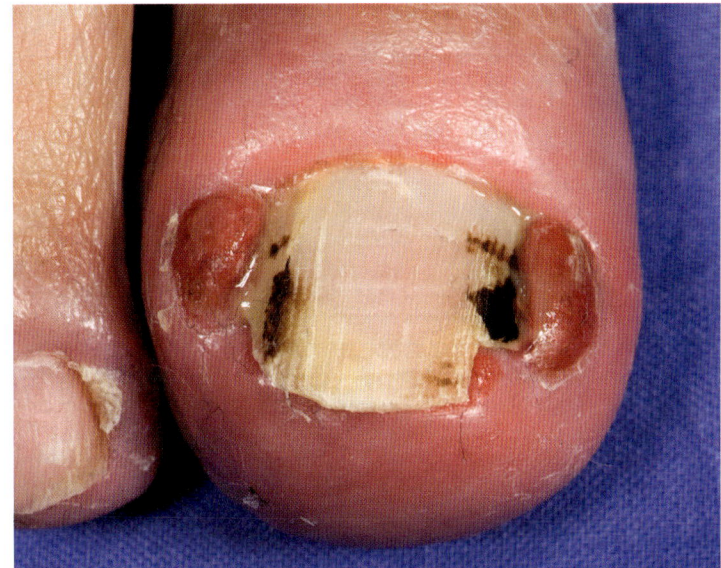

Figure 119.3 Grade 3 reaction with periungual pyogenic granulomas secondary to erlotinib.

Pathophysiology

Nail changes occur in the majority of cases because of direct toxicity to the nail plate. The nail matrix epithelium, which is formed from proliferating cells that differentiate and keratinise, is highly susceptible to damage from cytotoxic agents that cause defective nail plate production. The most typical changes are Beau lines and onychomadesis (reflecting arrest in epithelial proliferation) or leukonychia (indicating abnormal keratinisation). Toxicity to the matrix epithelium can also result in melanocyte activation with nail plate pigmentation and melanonychia.

The nail bed epithelium is very thin and is mainly responsible for the adhesion of the nail plate to the underlying structures. Onycholysis can result from toxic damage to this epithelium, which causes nail plate detachment.

Drugs that interfere with the integrity of the proximal nail fold may cause exposure of the nail matrix, leading to disordered nail growth.

Pathology

Nail biopsies are rarely performed to assess chemotherapy-induced nail changes.

Clinical features

The nail changes that occur as a side effect of chemotherapeutic agents include dystrophy, onycholysis, onychomadesis, Beau lines, transverse leuconychia (Mees lines), melanonychia, subungual erythema, subungual haemorrhage and paronychia.

Cytotoxic chemotherapy-induced nail changes tend to occur mostly in the nail plate or matrix, with nail plate colour abnormalities (chromonychia), transverse grooves on the nail plate (Beau lines) and decreased linear nail growth as the most common associated changes. MEK, EGFR and mTOR inhibitors treated patients can also develop mild to moderate changes of the nail bed and matrix characterised by mild onycholysis, brittle nails and a slower nail growth rate usually after 1–2 months of treatment. However, EGFR and MEK inhibitors may also cause damage to nail folds, with paronychia and periungual pyogenic granuloma. The risk is independent of the EGFR inhibitor being used [1]. Patients complain of nail plate and nail fold tenderness and pain, which may be associated with bleeding, crusting and discharge. The nails can be slow growing and brittle; the surrounding skin tends to be dry and fissured. EGFR inhibitor-related paronychia is often suppurative and painful; it usually affects the thumbs and great toes. When severe, periungual pyogenic granulomas can develop with friable granulation tissue involving the lateral nail folds (Figure 119.3). Subsequent onycholysis and onychodystrophy may develop. Similar changes are also seen in patients receiving MEK inhibitors.

Lichenoid nail changes can also be observed in patients on checkpoint inhibitors characterised by nail plate thinning, which may then become grooved and ridged. The nail may eventually darken, thicken or lift off the nail bed (onycholysis).

Differential diagnosis

The differential diagnosis includes psoriasis, tinea infection, trauma and vasculitis. When nail pigmentation is involved, the differential diagnosis includes idiopathic melanonychia, melanocytic naevus and melanoma.

Classification of severity

Changes in the nail apparatus induced by anticancer therapies are classified using the CTCAE v5.0 and include paronychia, nail loss, nail ridging, nail discoloration and nail infection. However, this does not capture all the nail changes observed with anticancer therapies and the significant effects that such symptoms can have on a patient's quality of life. Table 119.5 shows the grading scale of the adverse effects to the nail plate and nail folds caused by EGFR inhibitors (can be extended to include MEK and mTOR inhibitors) developed by the MASCC group [9].

Furthermore, according to CTCAE v5.0 paronychia is classified under the infectious group of toxicities as 'a disorder characterised by an infectious process involving the soft tissues around the nail', whereas it is in fact inflammatory, although secondary infection

Table 119.5 The Multinational Association of Supportive Care in Cancer (MASCC) Skin Toxicity Study Group grading scale for nail changes due to epidermal growth factor receptor inhibitors [9].

Grade	Adverse event nail plate changes	Nail fold changes	Digit tip
Grade 1	Onycholysis or ridging without pain	Disruption or absence of cuticle Or erythema	Xerosis and/or erythema without pain
Grade 2	Onycholysis with mild/moderate pain; any nail plate lesion interfering with instrumental ADL	Erythematous/tender/painful nail fold changes Or pyogenic granuloma Or crusted lesion or any fold lesion interfering with instrumental ADL	Xerosis and/or erythema with mild/moderate pain or stinging Or fingertip fissures or any digit tip lesion interfering with instrumental ADL
Grade 3	Nail plate changes interfering with self-care ADL	Periungual abscess or fold changes interfering with self-care ADL	Digit tip lesions interfering with self-care ADL

ADL, activities of daily living.

often occurs. Pyogenic granuloma is also not mentioned in this grading.

Disease course and prognosis

The nail changes secondary to EGFR and MEK inhibitors are usually evident by 1–2 months and can persist for several months even after stopping the EGFR inhibitor treatment. Xerosis and fissures are evident within 30–60 days of EGFR inhibitor therapy. Beau lines can occur after each cycle of chemotherapy and resolve once the chemotherapy has stopped. Dyspigmentation of nails may persist once treatment has stopped.

Most nail changes reverse after the causative chemotherapeutic agent is stopped. However, full resolution generally takes many months and rarely does not resolve.

Investigations

Skin swabs should be taken to exclude secondary infection of EGFR, MEK or mTOR inhibitor paronychia [10]. Clippings of dystrophic nails must be sent to mycology to exclude a tinea infection.

Management

Most nail changes caused by chemotherapeutic agents can be managed conservatively. Preventative measures should include advice on avoidance of any damaging or irritating regimen including drying nails carefully after wet work, avoiding excessive immersion in water, smoothing nail edges with a file, regular use of emollients and in some cases application of nail lacquers is sometimes advised to restrict water evaporation from the nail plate. Recommendations for managing EGFR inhibitor-related paronychia are summarised in Table 119.6 [11].

Drug withdrawal is not recommended as it would take several months for the nail changes to improve, given the relatively long half-life of EGFR inhibitors and the slow growth of nails. Preventative measures to reduce periungual trauma include wearing comfortable shoes and avoiding aggressive nail manicuring. Measures to reduce superinfection include the use of topical antimicrobial washes, topical steroids and oral tetracyclines for least 4–6 weeks. Brittle nails can be treated with biotin. Excessive granulation tissue can be removed by cautery or topical silver nitrate. Recent

Table 119.6 The Multinational Association of Supportive Care in Cancer (MASCC) skin toxicity study: paronychia recommendations [11].

	Recommend	Not recommended	Level of evidence	Recommendation grades	Comments
Preventive					
Topical	Diluted bleach soaks Avoid irritants		II[a]	A	Recommend final concentration of approximately 0.005% (approximately 1/4–1/8 cup of 6% bleach for 3–5 gal water)
Treatment					
Topical	Corticosteroids Calcineurin inhibitors	Antifungals Antibiotics	II[a]	A	Recommend usage of ultrapotent topical steroids as first-line therapy given cost and availability of these agents
Systemic	Tetracyclines	Empiric antibiotics—employed without culturing lesional skin	IV[b]/II[a]	D/A	
	Antimicrobials: reserved for culture proven infection	Antifungals			
Systemic	Biotin for brittle nails		III[a]	B	
Other	Silver nitrate chemical cauterization weekly Electrodesiccation Nail avulsion		IV[a]	D	Reserved for pyogenic granulomata; consensus of experts

[a] Non-EGFRI noncancer treatment study
[b] EGFRI study

studies have demonstrated that topical timolol (beta blocker) can be helpful to treat periungual pyogenic granulomas [12].

Dyspigmentation

Skin, mucosa and nail pigmentary changes are well recognised as side effects of anticancer medication [1]. Both hyperpigmentation and hypopigmentation have been described.

Chemotherapy-induced hyperpigmentation

Definition and nomenclature
This is an increase in skin pigmentation caused by cancer chemotherapy [2].

> **Synonyms and inclusions**
> - Hypermelanosis
> - Postinflammatory hyperpigmentation
> - Flagellate dermatosis

Introduction and general description
The anticancer drugs that are most commonly associated with the induction of hyperpigmentation are listed in Table 119.7.

Epidemiology
Incidence and prevalence
Flagellate hyperpigmentation in patients treated with bleomycin has a reported incidence of between 8% and 22% [3].

Age and sex
There is no specific association with either age or sex.

Pathophysiology
Postulated mechanisms of drug-induced hyperpigmentation include: (i) a direct pigmentary effect of the deposited drug in the skin; (ii) a direct toxic effect on epidermal melanocytes stimulating increased melanin production; (iii) the suppression of adrenal function leading to increased adrenocorticotrophic hormone and melanocyte-stimulating hormone causing hyperpigmentation; and (iv) a depletion of tyrosinase inhibitors resulting in increased pigmentation.

Bleomycin-induced flagellate hyperpigmentation appears to be induced by minor trauma to the skin causing increased blood flow and local accumulation of the drug. Tissues contain a cysteine proteinase capable of inactivating bleomycin; however, reduced concentration of this enzyme in the skin may lead to a local adverse effect causing hyperpigmentation [5].

Pathology
The histopathological changes of flagellate pigmentation include hyperkeratosis of the basal layer, focal parakeratosis and spongiosis within the epidermis. There is a characteristic increase in melanin pigmentation in the basal epidermal layer. Dermal oedema and perivascular lymphocytes can also sometimes be seen.

Clinical features
Hyperpigmentation can occur locally at the site of infusion or diffusely [1]. Flagellate hyperpigmentation of bleomycin is characterised by multiple, macular, linear streaks, which are initially red and subsequently become pigmented (Figure 119.4). The stripes often form a criss-cross pattern, giving the appearance of a scourging or whipping. Fluorouracil, vinorelbine and daunorubicin can cause pigmentation which, although not flagellate in nature, can follow the distribution of the veins and is termed serpentine supravenous hyperpigmentation. Chemotherapy-induced hyperpigmentation is more typically patchy and widespread. The nails, mucous membranes and teeth have all been reported sites of discoloration.

Table 119.7 Cancer chemotherapy agents associated with hyperpigmentation [1,4].

Drug	Type of hyperpigmentation	Incidence
Bleomycin	Flagellate, nails	Frequent
Busulfan	Generalised, mucous membrane	Frequent
Capecitabine	Generalised, nails	Occasional
Carmustine	Localised to injection site	Occasional
Cyclophosphamide	Generalised	Occasional
Daunorubicin	Generalised, nails	Occasional
Doxorubicin	Generalised, nails, mucous membrane	Frequent
Epirubicin	Nails	Frequent
5-Fluorouracil	Generalised, nails, mucous membrane	Frequent
Hydroxyurea	Generalised	Occasional
Ifosfamide	Localised to injection site	Occasional
Methotrexate	Generalised, nails	Occasional
Vinorelbine	Generalised, nails, mucous membrane	Occasional

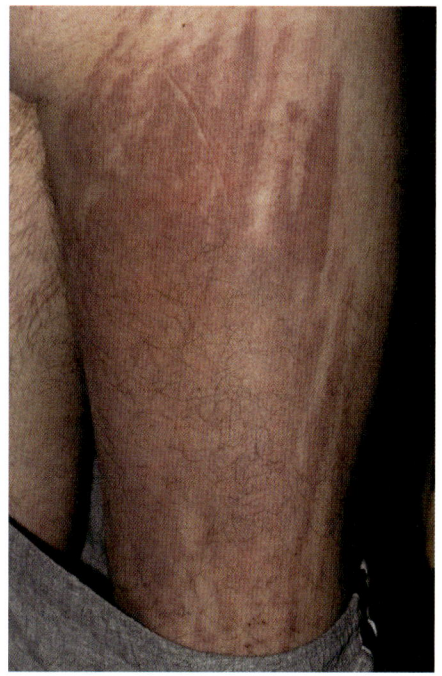

Figure 119.4 Flagellate hyperpigmented dermatitis on a patient's leg induced by bleomycin.

Differential diagnosis
The differential diagnosis includes postinflammatory hyperpigmentation, haemochromatosis, Addison disease (adrenocorticoid insufficiency) and hypermelanosis in patients with metastatic melanoma.

Disease course and prognosis
Hyperpigmentation can progress further if the patient continues on the chemotherapeutic agent or may remain limited to the initial site of involvement.

Some hyperpigmentation may be irreversible, but most often it resolves after discontinuation of the culprit chemotherapeutic agent.

Investigations
Generally, the diagnosis can be made after taking a good clinical history, identifying the likely culprit drug and examining the patient. A skin biopsy can be taken if the diagnosis is in doubt.

Management
There is no specific treatment for chemotherapy-induced hyperpigmentation. When the chemotherapy drug is stopped, the pigmentation can be expected to slowly disappear. Patients should be counselled about the risk of developing pigment changes when starting any of the chemotherapeutic agents listed in Table 119.7.

Chemotherapy-induced hypopigmentation

Definition and nomenclature
This is a decrease in skin pigmentation (partial or complete) caused by cancer chemotherapy.

> **Synonyms and inclusions**
> - Post-inflammatory hypopigmentation
> - Hypomelanosis

Introduction and general description
A variety of chemotherapeutic medications have been demonstrated to cause pigment loss or vitiligo. The anticancer drugs that are most associated with the induction of hypopigmentation are listed in Box 119.5. Checkpoint inhibitor associated vitiligo or vitiligo-like depigmentation is the newest addition to this list and occurs in 8% on anti-PD1 therapy and 5% on anti-CTLA-4 therapy and has been observed to be a good prognostic feature [4].

Pathophysiology
In most cases of chemotherapy-induced hypopigmentation the pathogenesis is unknown. Several hypotheses have been proposed to explain the pathogenesis, including genetic factors, neurological factors, toxic metabolites and lack of melanocyte growth factors. In tyrosine kinase inhibitors the proto-oncogene c-Kit mutations, along with blockade of the stem cell factor ligand and inhibition of the c-Kit signal transduction pathway of melanocytes, have been postulated in the pathogenesis of drug-induced hypopigmentation [6].

Pathology
Histopathological examination of skin affected by drug-induced hypopigmentation has shown the absence of melanin using the Fontana–Masson stain and the absence of melanocytes using S-100 and melan A stains [7].

Clinical features
Chemotherapy-induced hypopigmentation results from the destruction of melanocytes and clinically manifests as partial and/or total loss of skin pigment. Hypomelanotic and amelanotic macules develop symmetrically in a similar manner to idiopathic vitiligo. Affected areas often include distal digits and peri-orificial sites.

Differential diagnosis
This includes idiopathic vitiligo and post-inflammatory hypopigmentation.

Disease course and prognosis
The onset of chemotherapy-induced hypopigmentation has been found to occur as early as a couple of days to as long as 6 months after the associated medication has been started. In most patients the chemotherapy is continued despite the progression of hypopigmentation. Hypopigmentation may persist after discontinuation of the associated drug.

Investigations
Wood's light examination can be helpful to distinguish between the diagnosis of chemotherapy-induced hypopigmentation and post-inflammatory hypopigmentation. A skin biopsy may also be performed if the diagnosis cannot be made clinically.

Management
Patients should be advised to wear sunblock.

> **Box 119.5 Cancer chemotherapy agents associated with hypopigmentation** [8,9]
> - Doxorubicin
> - Imatinib
> - Dasatinib
> - Gefitinib
> - Vemurafenib
> - Imiquimod
> - Interferon α
> - Interferon β
> - Interleukin 2
> - Interleukin 4
> - Mitoxantrone
> - Survivin inhibitor
> - Checkpoint inhibitors – anti-PD1 (anti-Programmed Cell Death) and anti-CTLA-4 (anti-cytotoxic T lymphocyte associated protein 4)

Photosensitivity

Definition
This is abnormal photosensitivity induced by a chemotherapy agent.

Introduction and general description
Photosensitive drug eruptions occur after exposure to a drug or its metabolite and then to either ultraviolet light (UVA, UVB) and/or visible light [1,2]. Chemotherapy associated with photosensitivity reactions can be divided into phototoxic, photoallergic and UV recall reactions. A phototoxic reaction is the most common reaction pattern with chemotherapeutic agents; it is non-immunologically mediated and is characterised by an exaggerated sun burn reaction [3]. Drug-induced phototoxicity requires three essential steps: (i) the drug or metabolites must reach the viable cells in the skin; (ii) light of an appropriate wavelength must penetrate the skin; and (iii) a photon of light must be absorbed by photosensitising chemicals [4]. Photoallergic reactions occur in a minority of individuals and require immune sensitisation. UV recall reaction is a rare, unique phenomenon that can occur with certain chemotherapeutic agents. The chemotherapeutic agents most commonly associated with abnormal photosensitivity are listed in Box 119.6.

Pathophysiology
Chemotherapy-associated photosensitivity can involve the absorption of radiation (UVA, UVB and visible light) by a photosensitising drug or drug metabolite within the skin to cause a phototoxic or photoallergic reaction [1]. Phototoxic reactions are a dose-dependent phenomenon involving both the drug and amount of light exposure. Ultimately the reaction is due to the damaging effects of photoactivated chemicals on cell membranes and DNA. Photoallergic reactions are cell-mediated responses whereby UV radiation converts the drug into an immunologically active compound (a photo-antigen) which subsequently induces a T-cell-mediated inflammatory skin response.

Pathology
The histology of a phototoxic reaction reveals spongiosis and necrotic keratinocytes associated with dermal oedema and a mononuclear cell infiltrate. The histology of a photoallergic reaction is similar to allergic contact dermatitis with spongiosis and an intense lymphocytic perivascular infiltrate in the dermis [9].

Clinical features
A phototoxic reaction is characterised by redness, which can be categorised according to its onset as immediate, delayed (12–24 h) or late-onset redness (24–120 h), the latter often referred to as 'exaggerated sunburn'. Reactions usually occur in light-exposed sites over the face, neck, anterior 'V' of the chest and forearms. It can present with painful, well-demarcated redness and oedema progressing to blistering and desquamation. The reaction resolves with hyperpigmentation over several months. Photo-onycholysis is a form of phototoxicity that involves the distal one-third of the nail and can be associated with tenderness. It is seen with mercaptopurine therapy [5].

Photoallergic reactions can present with an eczematous reaction over sun-exposed sites which spread beyond the exposed irradiated areas. It has been described with flutamide and tegafur [5]. They do not occur until 24–72 hours after exposure and as it is a cell-mediated type IV hypersensitivity reaction it can only occur in previously sensitised patients.

Differential diagnosis
The differential diagnosis includes other photosensitivity diseases, such as chronic actinic dermatitis.

Box 119.6 Cancer chemotherapy agents associated with photosensitivity [5–7,8]

Type of drug			
Alkylating	Hydroxyurea	Dacarbazine	Chlorambucil
	Procarbazine		
Antimetabolite	Methotrexate	Pentostatin	Thioguanine
	Mercaptopurine	Tegafur/uracil	Tegafur/gimeracil/oteracil
	Capecitabine	Tegafur	Fluorouracil
Antimicrotubule	Vinblastine	Docetaxel	Paclitaxel
Anthracycline	Epirubicin		
Small molecule inhibitors	Vemurafenib	Cobimetinib	Regorafenib
	Vandetanib	Crizotinib	Erlotinib
	Dabrafenib	Dasatinib	Imatinib
	Gefitinib	Canartinib	Alectinib
	Lapatinib	Trametinib	
Topoisomerase inhibitor	Irinotecan		
Monoclonal antibodies	Nivolumab	Cetuximab	Trastuzumab
	Eculizumab	Panitumumab	Mogamulizumab
		Ipilumumab	Pembrolizumab
Others	Flutamide	Bicalutamide	Rucaparib
	Midostaurin	Mitomycin	Anagrelide
	PEG interferon	Interferon alpha	Mercatopurine

Disease course and prognosis
Phototoxic reactions usually subside within a week, whereas photoallergic reactions may last up to 3 weeks.

Chemotherapy-induced photosensitivity usually resolves over weeks; however, the subsequent hyperpigmentation may last several months.

Investigations
Laboratory investigations are usually not necessary. Suspected phototoxic and photoallergic drug reactions can be investigated with phototesting, photopatch testing or re-challenge testing to determine the wavebands involved, the degree of photosensitivity and the reaction to the suspected drug [1,2].

Management
The treatment of chemotherapy-induced photosensitivity is symptomatic. Discontinuing the culprit chemotherapeutic agent may be necessary if the skin reaction is severe. Alternatively, dose reduction can sometimes be helpful. The use of topical steroids, broad spectrum sunscreens and UV light-protective clothing is recommended [4,9].

Recall reaction dermatitis

Definition
Recall reaction dermatitis is a rare phenomenon characterised by a drug-induced inflammatory eruption confined to an area of skin that has previously been irradiated.

Introduction and general description
Recall reaction dermatitis represents the 'recalling' of an effect similar in appearance to that of an acute radiation reaction in a previously irradiated field. The recall is initiated by a culprit medication given days to years after exposure to ionising radiation. Anticancer agents, in particular cytotoxics, are the most common causes of radiation recall, but other drugs have been implicated including antibiotics and simvastatin [1,2,3]. It can also develop, albeit infrequently, in areas of skin that have been previously sunburnt. Rarely, radiation recall phenomena have been described in different internal organs with concomitant radiation recall dermatitis affecting the skin as the presenting symptom [4]. The most common drugs that can cause recall reactions are listed in Box 119.7.

Epidemiology
Incidence and prevalence
Few systematic reports have examined the incidence of radiation recall. However, radiation recall was reported in 8.8% of patients receiving a range of chemotherapeutic agents after completion of radiotherapy in an observational study of 91 patients undergoing palliative treatment for metastatic disease [7].

Age and sex
There is no specific association with either sex or age.

Box 119.7 Cancer chemotherapy agents associated with recall reactions [5,6]

- Gemcitabine
- Methotrexate
- Docetaxel
- Paclitaxel
- Hydroxyurea
- Etoposide
- Doxorubicin
- Capecitabine
- Tamoxifen
- Vemurafenib

Pathophysiology
The mechanism of recall reactions is unknown. Various hypotheses have been proposed including the notion that radiotherapy-induced mutations in skin yield cells that are vulnerable to cytotoxic therapies [1,2,3]. Others propose that local vascular permeability or proliferative change induced by the radiotherapy may affect the subsequent pharmacokinetics of certain drugs. Camidge and Price have also proposed that cutaneous radiation recall reactions are caused by idiosyncratic drug hypersensitivity reactions which are analogous to a fixed drug eruption [3]. It has been suggested that this mechanism could be mediated by continued low-level secretion of the inflammation-mediating cytokines induced by radiation. The presence of a precipitating chemotherapy agent may then up-regulate these cytokines, resulting in a radiation recall reaction.

There is no relationship between the occurrence of radiation recall and the applied radiation dose. Therapeutic schedules well below 20 Gy can elicit radiation recall [3].

Pathology
Specimens from eight patients with radiation recall dermatitis showed ballooning degeneration of epidermal keratinocytes with a mixed inflammatory infiltrate [8]. Others have reported a histological picture mimicking the pattern of a graft-versus-host reaction of the skin or cutaneous drug allergies [9].

Clinical features
One of the important features of cutaneous radiation recall is that the reaction affects skin that was previously quiescent and apparently normal (Figure 119.5). The area affected clearly corresponds to an area previously irradiated, although may occasionally spread or become generalised. Clinically the reaction can range from a red maculopapular eruption through to vesicle formation, desquamation and rarely severe skin necrosis. Patients who experience radiation recall reactions may or may not have experienced acute radiation reactions.

The interval between radiotherapy and recall reaction after drug administration should be more than 7 days. Most recall reactions occur when radiotherapy and chemotherapy are separated by fewer than 2 months [10]; the median interval is 40 days [3]. However, there are several reports of radiation recall occurring many years after completion of radiation treatment. Skin reactions appear to be more severe when the period between the radiation and exposure to the recall-triggering drug is shorter.

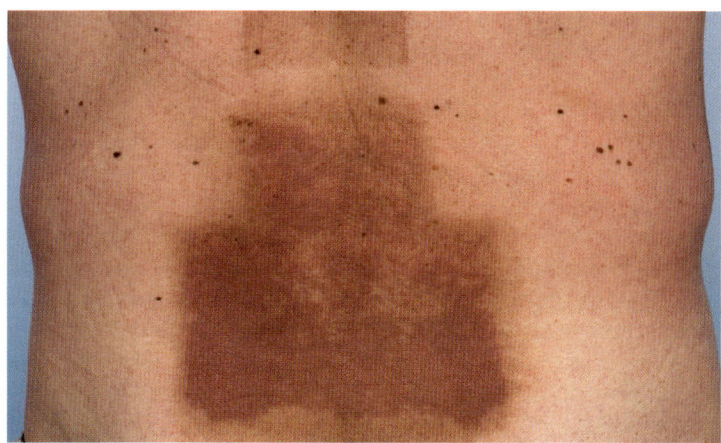

Figure 119.5 Radiation recall reaction secondary to vemurafenib confined to the previously irradiated site.

The skin reaction develops within minutes to days of taking the drug. The time to develop the reaction may be slightly longer for oral than intravenously administered drugs, reflecting differences in bioavailability. Recall usually occurs on first exposure to a particular recall-triggering drug.

Differential diagnosis
Acute or chronic radiodermatitis should be considered within the differential diagnosis. Contact dermatitis and photosensitivity reactions may also cause a similar reaction.

Disease course and prognosis
Skin reactions usually settle within a few days of stopping the triggering drug. Re-challenge does not always result in the recurrence of the skin reaction.

Investigations
A careful history is needed to establish the link between the drug and the radiation recall phenomenon. A skin biopsy may be helpful.

Management
Severe reactions should be treated with systemic or topical steroids, non-steroidal anti-inflammatory agents and antihistamines [2]. Treatment should also involve minimising exposure to the sun. Once the reaction has occurred it is advisable to discontinue the triggering drug.

Uneventful rechallenge may be achievable with prophylactic oral corticosteroids or dose reduction of the culprit chemotherapeutic agent.

Radiotherapy-associated skin side effects

Definition and nomenclature
Radiotherapy consists of using high energy ionising radiation, usually X-rays and similar rays such as electrons, to target and kill cancer cells in the area treated. There are two ways of giving radiotherapy – either external beam radiotherapy or internal radiotherapy. Radiotherapy is associated with a number of skin side effects.

Synonyms and inclusions
- Radiation dermatitis

Introduction and general description
Skin side effects from radiation therapy are common and can be divided into those occurring early (days to weeks) during the treatment and those occurring late (months to years). Most reactions are due to radiation-induced dermatitis. Radiation dermatitis is a side effect of external beam ionising radiation. It can rarely result from exposure to radiation during interventional procedures such as coronary angiography, embolisation procedures and indwelling catheter placements [1]. Cutaneous side effects are the main dose-dependent effects of ionising radiation. They result from direct damage to the irradiated tissue and have known threshold doses. Specifically, the threshold doses for the development of redness, permanent epilation, moist desquamation and necrosis are 3–10, 7–10, 12–25 and 25 Gy, respectively [2].

Epidemiology
Incidence and prevalence
The development of radiation dermatitis is common. For example, during the course of breast cancer radiotherapy the vast majority of patients (74–100%) will experience radiation dermatitis [3]. Radiation dermatitis has also been reported to occur in the majority of patients undergoing radiotherapy for loco-regionally advanced head and neck cancer [4]. In most patients, the radiation dermatitis is mild to moderate (grades 1 and 2), but 20–25% of patients experience severe reactions (grade 3 and 4) [5].

Certain risk factors have been found to be associated with a higher rate of development of radiation dermatitis including obesity, poor nutrition, existing skin disease and prolonged or multiple procedures requiring radiation exposure. Also, underlying concomitant diseases and syndromes increase the risk of radiation dermatitis including porphyria, connective tissue disease, ataxia telangiectasia, HIV and diabetes.

Pathophysiology
Irradiation of the skin leads to a complex pattern of direct tissue injury and inflammatory cell recruitment, involving damage to epidermal basal cells, endothelial cells and vascular components and a reduction in Langerhans cells [6]. Radiation-induced keratinocyte damage induces DNA injury repair via activation of the p53 pathway and a simultaneous release of inflammatory cytokines as a consequence of the generation of free radicals. The main cytokines involved in this reaction are tumour necrosis factor α, interleukins 1 and 6 and transforming growth factor β [7].

Significant infiltration of the epidermis with neutrophils and associated apoptosis is seen in severe radiation dermatitis. Recovery of the epidermis is limited by the nature of the treatment, which is repeated, usually daily, thereby leading to further cumulative damage. Chronic radiation-induced changes in the skin are characterised by the disappearance of follicular structures, an increase in dermal collagen and damage to elastic fibres.

Clinical features

Radiation dermatitis generally manifests within a few days to weeks after the start of radiotherapy. It is confined to areas of skin that have been irradiated, and the skin changes are usually sharply demarcated. Its onset varies depending on the radiation dose intensity and the normal tissue sensitivity of individuals. As the cumulative dose of radiation increases, the transient redness occurring during the first weeks of radiotherapy may evolve into more persistent redness to dry or even moist desquamation, which reflects the damage to the basal cell layer and the sweat and sebaceous glands.

Radiation dermatitis can be classified as acute or chronic.

Acute radiation dermatitis. Acute radiation dermatitis occurs within 90 days of exposure to radiation. The initial symptoms are usually redness of the skin, which can be associated with oedema. Further progression to desquamation and in severe cases skin necrosis and ulceration can also occur. Mucositis can develop if mucosal surfaces are included within the treatment zone.

Chronic radiation dermatitis. The onset of chronic radiation dermatitis may occur from 15 days to 10 years or more after the beginning of radiation therapy. It is an extension of the acute process and involves further inflammatory changes in the skin. Changes result from an increase in collagen and damage to elastic fibres with the loss of follicular structures (alopecia), appearance of telangiectasia and in some cases pigmentation. The skin often appears hypopigmented and atrophic.

Differential diagnosis

A Koebnerisation phenomenon may occur in sites of radiation, and therefore a differential diagnosis of psoriasis should be considered. If recurrent tense bullae develop then bullous pemphigoid should be excluded and a biopsy taken. Radiation recall may also occur confined to the radiotherapy site, but this will be triggered by concomitant use of a chemotherapeutic agent not with radiotherapy alone. Infection and contact dermatitis should also be considered.

Classification of severity

Table 119.8 gives the criteria for grades 1 to 5 of the CTCAE definition of radiation dermatitis.

Investigations

Careful history taking and timing of the eruption should in most cases be enough to make a clinical diagnosis. Where there is doubt as to the diagnosis a skin biopsy can be taken. A skin swab may be helpful if infection is thought a possibility.

Management

There is currently no evidence that prophylactic treatments, beyond keeping the irradiated area clean and dry, are effective in reducing the incidence or severity of radiation dermatitis. However, emollients and soap substitutes are generally instituted early on during treatment [8]. Patients being irradiated should be advised to avoid sun exposure, cover up and using broad spectrum sun protection. Grade 1 reactions require no specific treatment although the use of a regular, unperfumed, emollient therapy with careful drying of the area after washing with a soap substitute can be helpful for symptomatic relief.

In grades 2 and 3 radiation dermatitis, as with grade 1, the irradiated area should be cleaned and dried, even when ulcerated. A number of topical applications can be used including antiseptic-based creams (e.g. silver sulfadiazine), hydrophilic dressings and moderate or strong topical steroids. These topical agents are generally applied in the evening after cleaning the area first.

If infection is suspected a swab should be taken and, depending on the severity, either topical or systemic antibiotics given. Severe desquamation is associated, in a number of cases, with a risk of septicaemia. Grades 2 and 3 radiation dermatitis are best managed by an integrated team comprising the radiation oncologist, medical oncologist (where appropriate), nurse and dermatologist, as required. Skin reactions should be assessed at least once a week. Grade 4 radiation dermatitis is relatively rare, generally occurring in <5% of patients receiving radiotherapy for squamous cell carcinoma of the head and neck [4]. This stage of radiation dermatitis requires specialised wound care and should be treated on a case-by-case basis.

Other skin side effects of radiotherapy

Chronic ulcers may develop after many years as a result of necrosis in areas previously treated with radiotherapy (Figure 119.6). Often these need to be biopsied to exclude a second malignancy. Both basal cell and squamous cell carcinomas have been reported to occur in previous radiotherapy sites.

Radiation-induced cutaneous vascular neoplasms occur infrequently and comprise benign, so-called atypical vascular lesions and angiosarcomas, the latter being high-grade malignant tumours [9]. Both arise most frequently within previously irradiated skin in cancer patients with breast-conserving treatment. Whether an atypical vascular lesion is a precursor of angiosarcoma is much debated and unresolved to date.

Post-irradiation morphoea is a potential complication after radiotherapy, particularly radiotherapy for breast cancer [10,11]. It can

Table 119.8 Common Terminology Criteria for Adverse Events (CTCAE): definition of the five grades of radiation dermatitis. Version 5. Published 2017.

Grade 1	2	3	4	5
Faint erythema or dry desquamation	Moderate to brisk erythema; patchy, moist desquamation, mostly confined to skin folds and creases; moderate oedema	Moist desquamation in sites other than skin folds and creases; bleeding induced by minor trauma or abrasion	Skin necrosis or ulceration of full thickness of dermis; spontaneous bleeding from involved site; skin graft indicated.	Death

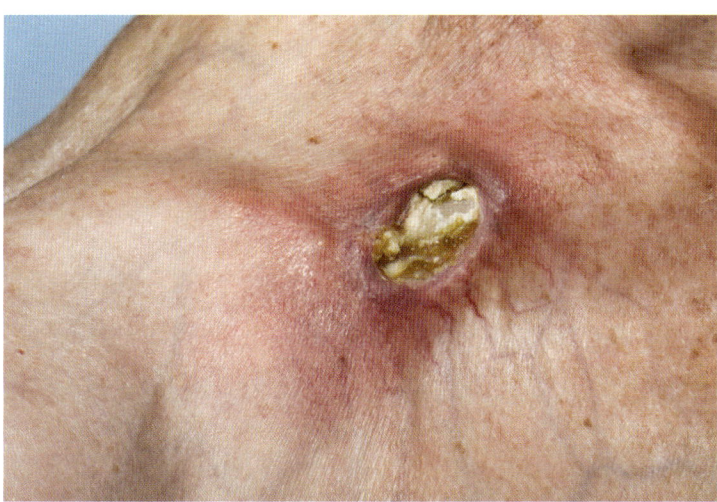

Figure 119.6 Radionecrosis causing ulceration over the clavicle occurring 20 years after radiotherapy treatment.

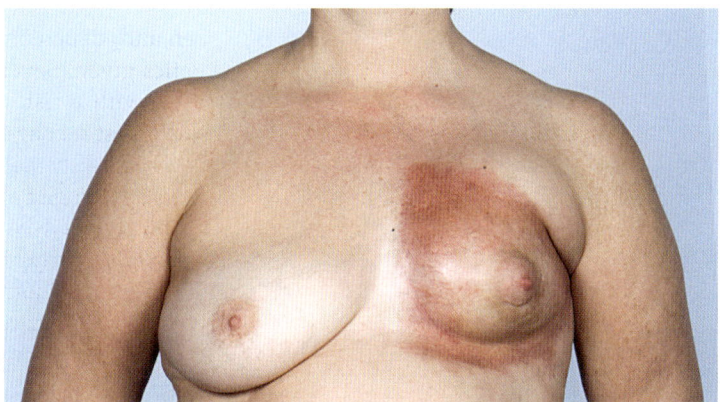

Figure 119.7 Morphoea affecting the left breast confined to the radiotherapy zone for breast cancer treatment.

occur months to years after treatment, and is associated with considerable morbidity and pain as well as being cosmetically disfiguring (Figure 119.7). Treatment is very difficult, with poor results reported from all modalities tried including topical and systemic steroids and phototherapy. Sclerosing post-irradiation panniculitis is a rare condition presenting as subcutaneous nodules in previous irradiated sites.

Erythema nodosum has also been reported to occur as a result of radiotherapy treatment [12].

Vitiligo and depigmentation have been reported in association with radiotherapy [13–15]. It can occur in patients with or without a previous history of vitiligo. The suggested mechanism for the hypopigmentation is radiation-induced apoptosis of susceptible melanocytes. In patients with previous vitiligo, the risks and benefits of radiation therapy should be carefully weighed in order to prevent undesired cosmetic results, particularly if an alternative therapy is available. Repigmentation rarely occurs.

Key references

The full list of references can be found in the online version at https://www.wiley.com/rooksdermatology10e

Toxic erythema of chemotherapy
1 Bolognia JL, Cooper DL, Glusac EJ. Toxic erythema of chemotherapy: a useful clinical term. *J Am Acad Dermatol* 2008;59:524–9.

Papulopustular eruptions
7 Lacouture ME, Maitland ML, Segaert S et al. A proposed EGFR inhibitor dermatologic adverse event-specific grading scale from the MASCC Skin Toxicity Study Group. *Support Care Cancer* 2010;18:509–22.
8 Lacouture ME, Anadkat MJ, Bensadoun RJ et al. Clinical practice guidelines for the prevention and treatment of EGFR inhibitor-associated dermatologic toxicities. *Support Care Cancer* 2011;19:1079–95.

Chemotherapy-induced hair changes
Chemotherapy-induced alopecia
1 Chon SY, Champion RW, Geddes ER, Rashid RM. Chemotherapy-induced alopecia. *J Am Acad Dermatol* 2012;67:e37–47.

Chemotherapy-induced hypertrichosis
6 Choi JN. Chemotherapy induced iatrogenic injury of skin: new drugs and new concepts. *Clin Dermatol* 2011;29:587–601.

Chemotherapy-induced nail changes
4 Robert C, Sibaud V, Mateus C et al. Nail toxicities induced by systemic anticancer treatments *Lancet Oncol* 2015;16:e181–9.

Dyspigmentation
1 Alley E, Green R, Schuchter L. Cutaneous toxicities of cancer therapy. *Curr Opin Oncol* 2002;14:212–16.

Photosensitivity
8 Hofman GA, Weber B. Drug-induced photosensitivity: culprit drugs, potential mechanisms and clinical consequences. *J Dtsch Dermatol Ges* 2021;19:19–29.

Recall reaction dermatitis
3 Camidge R, Price A. Characterizing the phenomenon of radiation recall dermatitis. *Radiother Oncol* 2001;59:237–45.

Radiotherapy-associated skin side effects
6 Hymes SR, Strom EA, Fife C. Radiation dermatitis: clinical presentation, pathophysiology, and treatment 2006. *J Am Acad Dermatol* 2006;54:28–46.

CHAPTER 120

Dermatoses Induced by Illicit Drugs

Anthony Bewley[1] *and Iyas Assalman*[2]

[1] Department of Dermatology, Barts Health NHS Trust, London; Queen Mary College of Medicine, University London, London, UK
[2] East London NHS Foundation Trust, London, UK

Introduction, 120.1	Cannabis, 120.4	Dermatoses caused by intravenous and subcutaneous drug administration, 120.6
Recreational drug usage and dermatology, 120.2	Inhalants, 120.4	Scarring, ulceration, popping and necrosis, 120.6
Alcohol use in dermatology patients, 120.3	Ecstasy, 120.4	Skin and soft-tissue infections, 120.7
Recreational and pharmaceutical drug interactions, 120.3	Methamphetamine, 120.4	Management of skin diseases associated with recreational drug use, 120.8
Legal aspects of drug use, 120.3	Cocaine, 120.5	
Drug-induced dermatoses, 120.4	Heroin, 120.5	Key references, 120.9

Introduction

The use of psychoactive drugs or narcotic drugs and psychotropic substances without medical supervision is associated with significant health risks. For this reason, international treaties regulate the production, sale, distribution and use of many of these substances with the aim of preventing negative effects that could significantly undermine health and security. Traditionally, psychoactive drugs were mainly plant-derived substances, such as cocaine, heroin and cannabis. However, in recent decades, new psychoactive substances synthetised in illicit laboratories have become more widely available and are consumed in every region [1].

Far from being an exceptional and 'deviant' behaviour, the use of illicit drugs is relatively common and is found among all sections of society. The misuse of drugs is often thought of as mainly a problem among adolescents and young adults but it also occurs among children and older adults, although patterns of use tend to differ in different age groups.

The terms used to describe recreational drug use are often vague and poorly defined, and this is especially true of the terms 'misuse' and 'abuse' which have no precise medical or scientific meaning. Drug-taking behaviours may occur as experimental use, occasional and recreational use, or as regular and dependent use of drugs. Drug taking may be conceptualised in terms of three dimensions. These are: (i) consumption behaviours (e.g. frequency of use, dose levels, route of administration); (ii) substance-related problems (intoxication, accidents and injury, overdose, infections); and (iii) severity of dependence (withdrawal symptoms, impaired behavioural control). These three dimensions can be regarded as being conceptually distinct and separate. In reality, of course, they may be related (sometimes closely) in a number of ways. Drug dependence (addiction) differs fundamentally from the mere use of drugs: it is manifested, psychologically and behaviourally, in feelings of compulsion to use drugs and difficulty in resisting those urges, and these changes are underpinned by neurophysiological changes in the brain.

Many forms of drug use, but especially drug dependence, can cause a wide range of serious health and social problems, and the use of medical health services among persons with substance use disorders is far higher than for the general population. All doctors can expect to see substantial numbers of patients who use illegal drugs, although this will often not be made explicit at the time of seeking treatment. In a UK study of treatment outcomes for individuals receiving treatment for drug addiction, about half of them were found to have attended an accident and emergency department in the 2 years prior to starting addiction treatment, and a quarter had at least one admission to a hospital for a medical problem; more than-two thirds had also visited a general practitioner [2]. Physicians should bear in mind that drug users' concerns about problems with their physical health are often an important motivating factor that may lead them to seek substance use treatment. Drug deaths in the UK in 2021 were the highest on record (over 4800), 6.2% higher than the rate in 2020. Heroin and morphine are the most commonly mentioned drugs, alongside an 8% increase in deaths involving cocaine or crack cocaine [3].

The United Nations Office on Drugs and Crime (UNODC) *World Drug Report 2019* estimates that around 271 million people, or 5.5% of people aged 15–64 years worldwide, used an illicit drug at least once in 2017. Some 35 million of the people who used drugs (0.7% of the adult population) have drug use disorders [4]. The overall prevalence of drug use reported in the UK has remained relatively stable throughout the last decade. Approximately 1 in 11 adults aged 16–59 years (9.2%: approximately 3 million adults) and approximately 1 in 5 adults aged 16–24 years

---

Rook's Textbook of Dermatology, Tenth Edition. Edited by Christopher Griffiths, Jonathan Barker, Tanya Bleiker, Walayat Hussain and Rosalind Simpson.
© 2024 John Wiley & Sons Ltd. Published 2024 by John Wiley & Sons Ltd.

(18.6%: approximately 1.1 million adults) reported drug use in the year ending June 2022; there was no change compared with the year ending March 2020 [5]. The most commonly used drugs have not changed over time. Cannabis is the most prevalent, followed by powder cocaine, ecstasy/N-methyl-3,4-methylenedioxymethamphetamine (MDMA), ketamine and amphetamine. Synthetic cannabinoid receptor agonists, such as Spice, are widely used in prisons; they were detected in more random drug tests than cannabis in England and Wales in 2018–19. In Scotland, buprenorphine was the most commonly detected drug in addiction prevalence tests carried out in prisons in 2018–19 [6].

In the UK, taking the health and criminal justice costs together (alongside associated costs to families and society), the total cost of the illicit drugs trade is now estimated to be over £19 billion a year, which is more than double the estimated value of the illicit drugs market itself [7]. An estimate in the USA suggested that in 2007 recreational drug use cost the US economy more than $193 billion [4]. Health costs include the treatment of a wide range of medical problems as well as the treatment of psychiatric and addiction problems. Medical care costs associated with heroin addiction and its associated medical complications account for a large proportion of the treatment costs. Other costs are incurred by social services, and for policing, interdiction and processing offenders within the criminal justice system.

For the dermatologist, skin eruptions induced by recreational drugs may be encountered in a variety of clinical settings. Dermatoses in this group of patients may range from pharmacological side effects of the drug to cutaneous complications of drug administration (Table 120.1) [8].

Some 'recreational' drugs may be used for iatrogenic purposes (e.g. opiates or even substances such as ketamine) by health care professionals (HCPs) such as anaesthetists working in pain clinics. This may be relevant to the clinical picture.

There is a growing body of (albeit of variable quality) research indicating that some recreational drugs may be *beneficial* in the management of some inflammatory dermatoses such as psoriasis. Patients may access these (especially 'medicinal' cannaboids) from partly or totally unregulated sources.

Recreational drug usage and dermatology

Recreational drug usage in dermatology is common and is more usual in specific scenarios. It is likely that recreational drug usage will increase over the next decades and so dermatologists will need to be familiar with the use of recreational drugs, the dermatological implications of their use and how to detect when they are being used. It is clear also that patients who use (abuse) recreational substances will not always admit that they have a recreational drug habit (for a variety of reasons). Therefore, having a lower threshold of suspicion about the use of recreational drugs may be relevant to dermatologists. Dermatologists may need to consider asking for consent to test patients for their use even when a patient denies their usage [1].

Psychodermatology
In the Chapter 84 on psychodermatology it is clear that there are several psychodermatological conditions which are very much

Table 120.1 Recreational drugs with potential dermatological and non-dermatological complications.

Substance	Dermatology-specific complications	Non-dermatology-specific complications
Cannabis	Arteritis Delusional infestation Pruritus Dysaesthesia Vasculitis Cutaneous necrosis Contact dermatitis	Neglect Interaction with medicines Psychosis Affective disorders
Cocaine	Acneform facial rash (no comedones) Delusional infestation Pruritus Dysaesthesia Vasculitis Cutaneous necrosis IV drug use dermatological syndromes	Neglect Interaction with medicines Psychosis Affective disorders
Amphetamines	Oral disease (dry mouth, caries, ulceration) Delusional infestation Dysaesthesia Pruritus Vasculitis Cutaneous necrosis Tactile hallucinations	Neglect Interaction with medicines Psychosis Affective disorders
Ecstasy/MDMA	Acneform facial rash (no comedones) Delusional infestation Pruritus	Neglect Interaction with medicines Psychosis Affective disorders
Opiates	Delusional infestation Dysaesthesia Pruritus Cutaneous necrosis Pemphigus vegetans Fixed drug eruptions Toxic epidermal necrolysis Necrolytic migratory erythema Phlebitis (from IV use) Limb ischaemia Cutaneous embolic disease IV drug use dermatological syndromes Tactile hallucinations	Neglect Interaction with medicines Psychosis Affective disorders
Inhalants	Irritant dermatitis	Neglect Interaction with medicines Psychosis Affective disorders

MDMA, N-methyl-3,4-methylenedioxymethamphetamine.

associated with the use of recreational drugs, in particular delusional infestation. Patients with a recreational drug habit may not admit to it.

ChemSex
There is an increasing trend of ChemSex, especially in the men who have sex with men (MSM) community. ChemSex is a term that is used when people are having sex that involves using one or more of three specific drugs ('chems') in any combination. People take part in ChemSex for a number of different reasons: some find it increases

sexual stimulation, for other people it can reduce their inhibitions. ChemSex can take place in groups, and it can often last for days or over a weekend. Drugs commonly used in ChemSex include cocaine, mephedrone and γ-hydroxybutyric acid (GHB). Asking about ChemSex practice may be relevant for conditions described in this chapter and Chapter 84 and for the chapters related to genital dermatoses and infections.

Sexually transmitted diseases

Gamma-hydroxybuyrate is one of the newer recreational drugs which may be used in ChemSex meetings (often in MSM). This is a difficult drug as the therapeutic window is narrow, so overdose (with a risk of coma and death) is relatively common. There is an increased risk of sexually transmitted diseases (Chapters 29–31) in MSM and other individuals who use GHB (and other drugs), and there is an increased risk of anal intraepithelial neoplasia in human immunodeficiency virus (HIV) infected MSM who use GHB [2].

Psoriasis

It has been known for some time that patients with psoriasis are more likely to abuse alcohol and to smoke than patients who do not have psoriasis. Recent research has shown that patients with psoriasis may abuse other substances in addition to alcohol and tobacco when compared with patients who do not have psoriasis (Chapter 35). It is expedient, then, for clinicians who work with patients living with psoriasis to ask about recreational drug use as well as alcohol and tobacco usage.

Testing for recreational drug use

It is becoming increasingly important, for the reasons discussed, for health care professionals working in dermatology to ask patients routinely about recreational drug use. Even then patients may not own up to taking recreational drugs, and so dermatology HCPs may need to ask for a recreational drug screen. This involves:

1 Consent. Verbal consent to test for recreational drugs is necessary. HCPs should record in the patient notes that they have asked the patient's permission to check for recreational drugs via a urine/blood/hair sample.
2 Urine screens for recreational drugs can be performed with a screening strip or with a sample formally sent to the biochemistry laboratory.
3 Other tests for recreational drugs (usually used in specific circumstances such as in child or vulnerable adult protection issues) may include blood samples and hair/nail samples (these samples may indicate past recreational drug use).

Alcohol use in dermatology patients

See Chapter 84 on psychodermatology.

Recreational and pharmaceutical drug interactions

There is a paucity of evidence regarding the metabolism and pharmacokinetic interactions with illicit substances, and further research is needed. Despite the absence of comprehensive data on the subject, the available information indicates that the use of illicit substances may have a significant impact on medications used to treat co-morbid conditions. Alternatively, those medications may affect the kinetics of recreationally used substances. For example, marijuana may have serious interactions with drugs including warfarin (increased international normalised ratio and risk of bleeding), clobazam (increased risk of benzodiazepine toxicity), central nervous system depressants and sympathomimetics (additive effects) and theophylline, clozapine and olanzapine (reduced efficacy). Patients should be advised about possible increased cannabinoid effects with concomitant CYP3A4 and -2C9 inhibitors [1,2]. There is also an interaction between cocaine and β-blockers by direct and indirect action, particularly at postsynaptic levels on dopamine and norepinephrine reuptake, sympathetic activation and increase of heart rate, blood pressure and cardiovascular toxicity. Cocaine also induces an increase in serotonin synaptic activity leading to the development of a serotoninergic syndrome when used with drugs that affect the serotonin pathway [3].

Legal aspects of drug use

The laws controlling drug use are complicated but there are three main statutes regulating the availability of drugs in the UK: the Misuse of Drugs Act (1971), the Medicines Act (1968) and the Psychoactive Substances Act (2016) [1].

Misuse of Drugs Act 1971

This act is intended to prevent the non-medical use of certain drugs. For this reason it controls not just medicinal drugs (which will also be in the Medicines Act) but also drugs with no current medical use. Drugs subject to this act are known as 'controlled' drugs. The law defines a series of offences including: unlawful supply, intent to supply, import or export and unlawful production. The main difference from the Medicines Act is that the Misuse of Drugs Act also prohibits unlawful possession.

The Misuse of Drugs Act (MDA) divides drugs into three classes as follows:

1 *Class A*. These include: cocaine and crack, ecstasy (added in the January 2021 sentencing guidelines), heroin, lysergic acid diethylamide (LSD), methadone, methamphetamine (crystal meth) and fresh and prepared magic mushrooms.
2 *Class B*. These include amphetamine (not methamphetamine), barbiturates, codeine, ketamine, synthetic cannabinoids such as Spice and cannabis (medicinal cannabis is now legal in the UK and can be prescribed by specialist doctors, since 1 November 2018), γ-butyrolactone (GBL) and GHB (available since April 2021) and synthetic cannabinoid receptor agonists (SCRAs) (added in the January 2021 sentencing guidelines). All cathinone derivatives, including mephedrone, methylone, methedrone and methylenedioxypyrovalerone (MDPV) were brought under control as class B substances in 2010.
3 *Class C*. These include anabolic steroids, minor tranquillisers or benzodiazepines, khat and benzylpiperazine (BZP).

Class A drugs are treated by the law as the most dangerous.

Psychoactive Substances Act 2016
The Psychoactive Substances Act received Royal Assent on 28 January 2016. The act applies across the UK and came into force on 26 May 2016. The act excludes legitimate substances, such as food, alcohol, tobacco, nicotine, caffeine and medical products, from the scope of the offence, as well as controlled drugs, which continue to be regulated by the Misuse of Drugs Act 1971. Exemptions include health care activities and approved scientific research on the basis that persons engaged in such activities have a legitimate need to use psychoactive substances in their work.

Medicines Act 1968
This law governs the manufacture and supply of medicine. It divides medical drugs into three categories: prescription-only medicines, pharmacy medicines and general sales list medicines.

Drug-induced dermatoses

Cannabis
Cannabis is the most widely used of the recreational drugs, and a conservative estimate suggests that about 78 million Europeans (about 20% of all 15–64-year-olds) have used cannabis on at least one occasion, and an estimated 22.5 million have used it in the previous year [1].

Cannabis, or marijuana, is prepared from the plant *Cannabis sativa* and can be eaten, drunk or, as is most common in Europe and America, smoked. Pharmacologically, cannabis is a complex substance; the main active components are the cannabinoids, tetrahydrocannabinol being the most psychoactive constituent. The subjective effects of cannabis include a sense of relaxation, coupled to a heightened sensory awareness.

The short-term side effects of cannabis include a reddening of the eyes, dry mouth and a slight rise in blood pressure. If a large dose is taken then the user may develop intense anxiety, which can be misinterpreted as an acute psychiatric illness.

Cannabis-induced dermatoses
Chronic cannabis use can cause cannabis arteritis, a subtype of thromboangiitis obliterans, which may lead to peripheral necrosis, most often of the lower limbs [2] (Chapter 101). It is thought to be caused by the vasoconstrictive effects of Δ-9-tetrahydrocannabinol and other unidentified contaminants. Cannabis arteritis presents with Raynaud phenomenon and, if neglected, digital necrosis. Duplex ultrasound can differentiate between cannabis arteritis and atherosclerosis [2]. Revascularisation and reperfusion of an affected extremity should occur with discontinuation of cannabis along with antiplatelet and vasodilator therapies. Other cannabis-induced dermatoses include delusional infestation, pruritus, dysaesthesia, vasculitis and cutaneous necrosis.

Contact and irritant dermatitis has also been reported from topical use (e.g. for treatment of inflammatory dermatoses) and handling of cannabis. The use of over-the-counter and Internet-acquired cannabinoid oils is likely to increase both for non-dermatological reasons (e.g. psychiatric disease) and for skin disease (e.g. psoriasis) [3].

Short term and longer term use of cannabis is also a potent cause of both anxiety and/or depression and other affective disease, and is one of the commoner causes of secondary delusional infestation [4].

Inhalants
The misuse of volatile substances (sometimes, though inaccurately, referred to as 'glue sniffing') may involve the inhalation of aerosols, glues, lighter fuel, thinners and other solvents, and is primarily a problem found among children and young adolescents. Reliable prevalence estimates are difficult to obtain. However, it is thought that between 3.5% and 10% of adolescents may have at least experimented with volatile substances [5]. Solvent fumes are normally inhaled through the nose ('sniffing') or via a plastic bag held tightly around the mouth ('bagging') or with a solvent-soaked rag placed in the mouth ('huffing'). Aerosolised cleaning products for electronic equipment can be inhaled by placing the canister nozzle straw into a nostril ('dusting').

Inhalant-induced dermatoses
A characteristic perioral or perinasal papular eruption with pustules, known as 'glue sniffer's rash', is caused by a non-specific contact reaction and may be encountered in chronic users of inhalants [6]. The abuse of aerosolised cleaning fluid has been associated with cutaneous and mucosal blistering, and also with angioedema [7]. Chemical burns around the nose and mouth caused by solvent irritancy have been also reported [8].

Ecstasy
Ecstasy is the name given to MDMA, a drug which is taken orally. It is mainly used as a 'dance drug' and has widespread usage in the 'dance', 'rave' and 'techno' scenes. Ecstasy has unique psychoactive properties, producing a controllable emotional state of relaxation and happiness. Doses are generally in the range of 75–150 mg, the effects starting within 30 min of taking the drug by mouth. The peak effects tend to occur during the next hour, and then diminish over the following 2 h.

Among the more common side effects of ecstasy are tension in the jaw and grinding of the teeth (bruxism). Anxiety, palpitations and an increase in blood pressure may also occur. Acute hepatotoxicity is recognised, while the exertion that follows fast dancing may compound the pharmacological effects of ecstasy resulting in collapse, convulsions and acute kidney injury [9]. Hyperthermia is another potentially life-threatening side effect that may be mediated by increased dopamine release acting on D1 receptors [10].

Ecstasy-induced dermatoses
'Ecstasy pimples' describe a facial dermatosis occurring in individuals shortly after the consumption of ecstasy [11]. The dermatosis consists of inflammatory papules and pustules, but no comedones, similar to perioral dermatitis.

Methamphetamine
Crystal methamphetamine (meth) is made by the reduction of ephedrine or pseudoephedrine through a toxic and flammable process, often in mobile 'meth labs', using batteries and fertilisers. It can be injected, smoked or snorted. Methamphetamine induces euphoria and gives the user a feeling of increased energy; the 'high' lasts for up to 10 h.

Cocaine

Cocaine is extracted from the *Erythroxylum coca* plant in the form of a paste. It is then purified into a water-soluble powder that can be inhaled, ingested orally or mixed with water and injected. It can only be smoked as 'crack cocaine', a free base, hard, brittle substance produced after neutralisation with sodium bicarbonate or ammonia mixed with water. Cocaine is a sympathomimetic that causes euphoria within minutes or seconds if smoked.

Inhalation of cocaine results in nasal inflammation, while the local vasoconstrictor effect may lead to mucosal necrosis. Cocaine-induced midline destructive lesions are exacerbated by microtraumas to the nasal mucosa complicated by *Staphylococcus aureus* infections [17]. The continuous consumption of high doses of cocaine is associated primarily with psychological side effects: the user may experience feelings of persecution or, in extreme cases, develop a toxic psychosis [18].

Cocaine-induced dermatoses

Formication may occur with cocaine usage and, as in other similar situations, may result in skin picking [19]. A few case reports have identified long-term cocaine abusers who have developed pyoderma gangrenosum (PG). In one report, PG occurred on the legs in conjunction with cavitating chest lesions; investigations revealed a positive level of perinuclear antineutrophil cytoplasmic antibodies (ANCA), indicating a Wegener granulomatosis-like syndrome [20]. In this patient, episodes of PG were associated with periods of cocaine use, while remission from PG coincided with cocaine abstinence.

Since 2010 there have been case reports of cocaine users developing cutaneous vasculitis [21] (Chapter 100). The causative substance is an adulterant, levamisole, used as a cocaine-bulking agent. Levamisole-induced vasculitis presents with purpuric retiform lesions, typically on the ears, cheeks, nose and extremities (Figure 120.2). Lesional skin may become confluent to produce large areas of cutaneous necrosis or haemorrhagic bullae [22]. Histologically, lesions demonstrate a leukocytoclastic vasculitis and/or thrombotic vasculopathy involving small or medium-sized vessels [23]. Many patients are found to have a positive ANCA, as well as other autoantibodies [24].

Heroin

Heroin (chemical name, diacetylmorphine) is synthesised from morphine, which is a naturally occurring substance extracted from the seed pod of the Asian opium poppy plant. The most common forms of heroin are a white powder or a black sticky substance (called 'black tar'). The heroin base (common in Europe) must be mixed with an acid such as lemon juice to dissolve it in water; the hydrochloride salt (common in the USA) only requires water to be dissolved. Heroin is usually injected but can be smoked or snorted. Intravenous injection of heroin induces an instantaneous sensation of ecstasy (the 'rush') followed by a period of detached and dreamy relaxation (the 'high').

'Krokodil' is the jargon term for an opiate drug being used increasingly in eastern Europe and elsewhere. It is manufactured by boiling codeine tablets with a number of other substances to yield a suspension containing desomorphine [25]. Krokodil has a swift onset and short half-life.

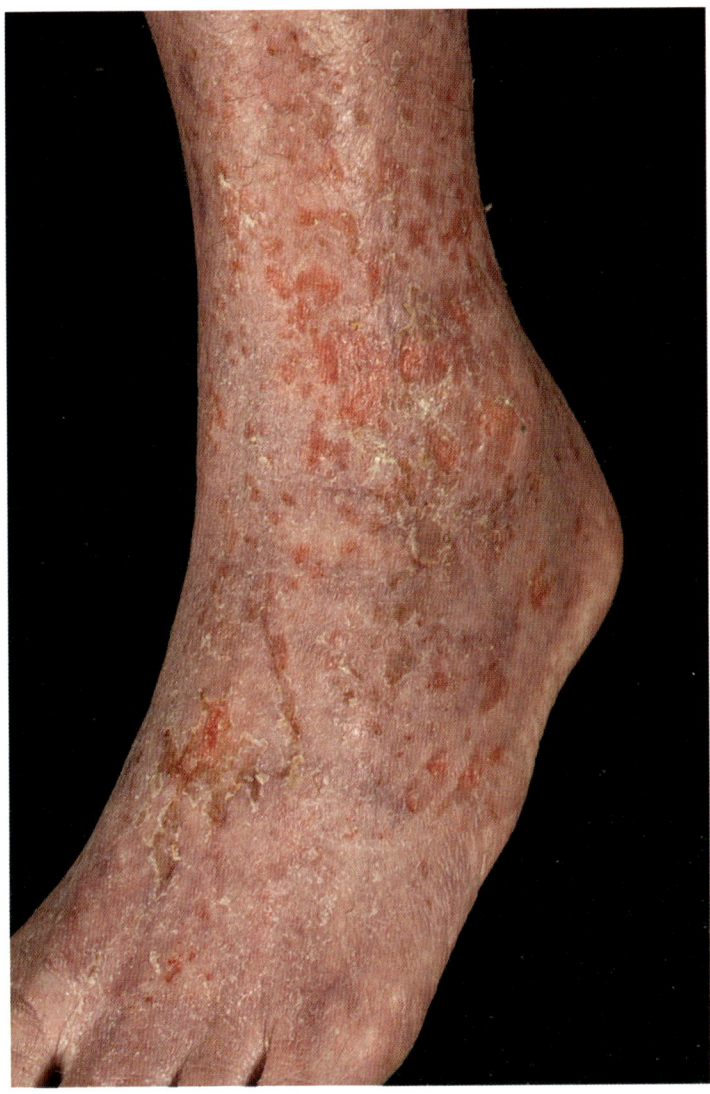

Figure 120.1 A patient with intractable itch and excoriations from using amphetamines.

The side effects of crystal meth are predominantly psychological or psychiatric. Anxiety and irrational fear is a short-term problem. Prolonged, heavy use of meth may be accompanied by persecutory symptoms resembling those of paranoid schizophrenia [12].

Recreational amphetamine use also commonly causes tactile hallucinations and delusional infestation [13]. Patients may seem agitated, and unable to concentrate or focus on the consultation.

Methamphetamine-induced dermatoses

The commoner cutaneous side effects of crystal meth abuse are xerosis and pruritus (Figure 120.1). Pruritus and formication ('meth mites') are well recognised and can lead to skin picking, especially on the face [14]. A florid form of tooth decay, 'meth mouth', is also well recognised and characterised by severe caries, excessive tooth wear and gum disease [15]. It is caused by poor oral hygiene, bruxism, xerostomia and, perhaps, a reduction in saliva pH. Resorption of gingival bone from tooth decay and gum disease contributes to a loss of volume of the lower face, which exaggerates the premature ageing characteristic of crystal meth abuse [16].

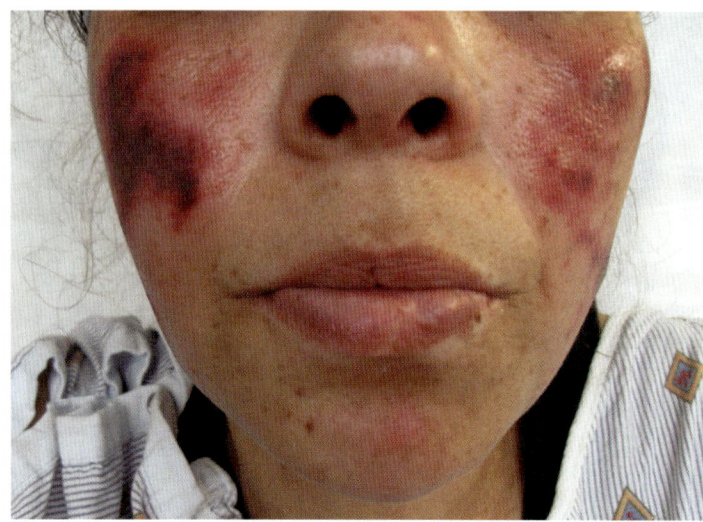

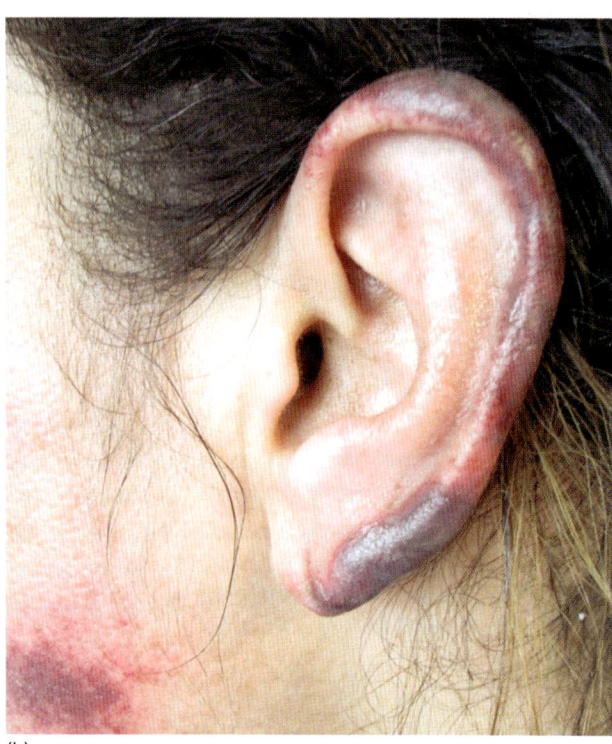

Figure 120.2 (a) Characteristic retiform purpuric lesions on both cheeks in levamisole-associated vasculitis. (b) Involvement of the helices and pinna is typical in patients with levamisole-associated vasculitis. Reproduced from Massera *et al.* 2012 [28] with permission of BMJ Publishing Group Ltd.

vegetans, fixed drug eruptions, toxic epidermal necrolysis and necrolytic migratory erythema (not associated with glucagonoma) have all been described with long-term heroin consumption [27]. Krokodil contains numerous toxic contaminants that cause damage to the blood vessels and soft tissues. Thrombophlebitis, abscesses and skin and soft-tissue necrosis are all common with krokodil and produce widespread cicatricial and scaly skin changes reminiscent of crocodile skin, hence the name.

Dermatoses caused by intravenous and subcutaneous drug administration

Scarring, ulceration, popping and necrosis

The skin is the tissue most prominently affected by injecting drug use [1]. The commonest cutaneous stigma of drug use is a line of

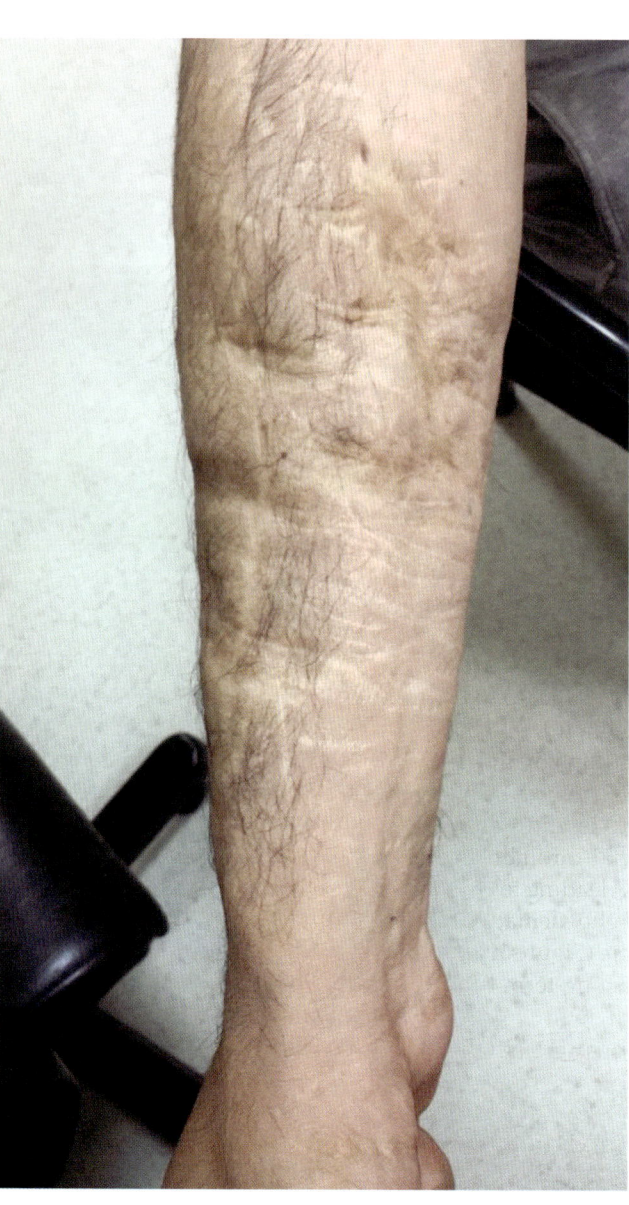

Figure 120.3 Scarring, subcutaneous atrophy and fibrosis as a consequence of skin popping with recreational drugs when venous access is difficult. Courtesy of Professor Ilknur Altunay, Istanbul.

The major side effects of heroin use relate to the dangers of drug injection, most notably the risk of infection with HIV and hepatitis viruses. However, the drug itself is recognised to impair sexual drive and to cause impotence.

Heroin-induced dermatoses

Itching at the site of the injection, the central face and genital skin is common with heroin use. However, in a blinded cross-over study, itch and urticaria were more severe in 39 injecting drug users when given morphine compared with heroin [26]. Pemphigus

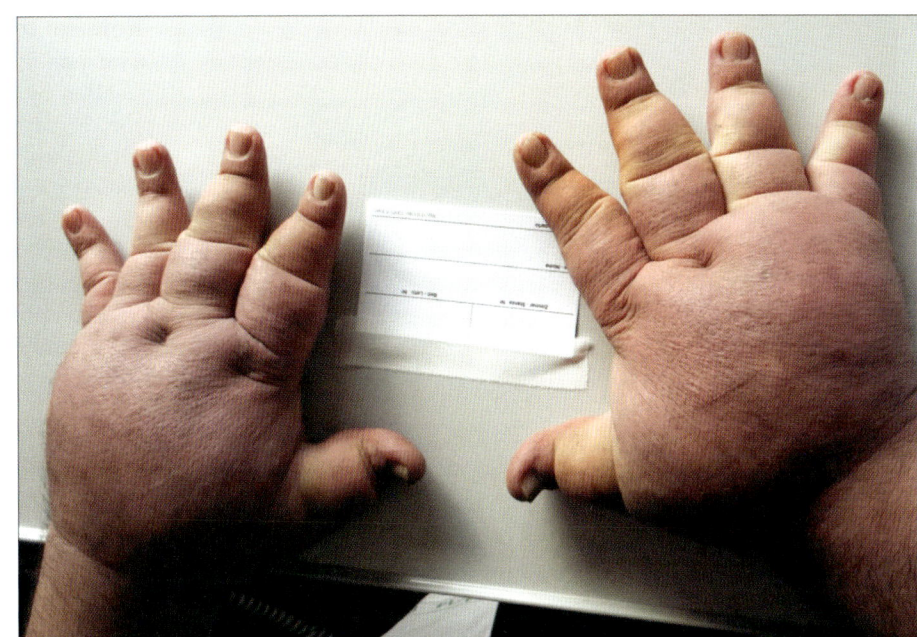

Figure 120.4 Puffy hand syndrome caused by injection of sublingual buprenorphine to the wrists. Oedema of the hands is seen extending to the forearm bilaterally, characterised by loss of visibility of the tendons and veins, small scars and symmetrical cyanosis of the dorsum of both hands with no cyanosis of the fingers. Reproduced from Vivaldelli et al. 2017 [21] with permission of Elsevier.

puncture scars distributed over a vein, or parallel to it. The typical progression of venous access sites used over time starts with the antecubital fossae followed by the upper arms and then the hands. As accessible veins become sclerosed, the drug user will utilise veins in the neck, feet, legs, groins, digits and even the penis [2]. Postinflammatory hyperpigmentation occurs at sites of injections; more specifically 'soot tattooing' may occur from flamed needles [3]. When all the veins have been destroyed, users may inject subcutaneously or intramuscularly, known as 'skin popping' (Figure 120.3), which results in circular, pale, atrophic (or hypertrophic) scars measuring 1–2 cm in diameter, or to large areas of thickened woody skin (sclerodema-like changes) [4]. Necrotising ulcers may also develop as a consequence of skin popping, and are caused by infection or the irritant properties of the drug or adulterant. Injection of the analgesic drug pentazocine may cause ulceration, panniculitis, sclerosis and hyperpigmentation [5]. Large areas of cutaneous fibrosis interspersed with ulceration can complicate methadone injection [6].

Injection by the intra-arterial route may occur once venous access is no longer obtainable and is accompanied by postinjection pain, cyanosis and oedema [7]. Cutaneous necrosis may be caused by arterial thrombosis or by particulate material within the injected drug, leading to embolic infarction. Irreversible, non-pitting oedema (lymphoedema) of the dorsum of the hands, the puffy hand syndrome (Figure 120.4), is caused by damage to cutaneous lymphatics from long-term IV drug use [8].

Skin and soft-tissue infections

Cutaneous infections are a common complication of IV drug abuse. A retrospective study in a London teaching hospital over a 5-year period identified a cohort of 124 injecting drug users requiring 191 admissions. Skin and soft-tissue infections were the commonest reason for admission (58%) [9]. Abscesses, cellulitis and necrotising lesions occur frequently [10]. One study of IV drug users found that 11% of subjects reported having at least one abscess in the past 6 months [11], and a fivefold higher risk associated with 'skin popping' in comparison with IV injection [12]. Most bacterial infections are caused by the subject's own skin flora, with *Staphylococcus aureus* and *Streptococcus* species being the most common pathogens [13]. A number of factors contribute to skin infection, including contamination of drugs, non-sterile equipment, lack of aseptic technique, HIV positivity, intradermal injection and 'booting', which is the jargon term for repeatedly flushing and pulling back during injection [14]. Injecting 'speedballs' (a mixture of cocaine and heroin) is a recognised risk factor for skin abscesses; it has been suggested that the vasoconstrictive effect of cocaine may enhance the risk of skin sepsis [15]. Other bacterial pathogens isolated in skin infections include Gram-negative and anaerobic organisms, which may originate from the mouth since drug addicts are known to use saliva as a skin cleanser and as a drug diluent.

Over the past 20 years cases of wound botulism have been reported occurring among injecting drug users in the USA and Europe [16]. Injection sites become infected with the anaerobic, spore-forming bacterium *Clostridium botulinum*, which releases a neurotoxin causing cranial nerve palsies and descending flaccid paralysis (botulism). In many of these cases *C. botulinum* has been isolated from the drugs used, particularly black-tar heroin. Many of the patients had injected the drug subcutaneously, suggesting the role of skin popping. There has also been a cluster of tetanus cases in the UK among drug users, suggesting contamination of drugs with *Clostridium tetani* [17]. Necrotising fasciitis due to clostridial infection is also seen. In a US study of necrotising fasciitis in injection drug users, all 32 patients were injecting black-tar heroin; it was caused by clostridial infections in 24 of the cases, eight of which were *C. sordelli* [18]. Skin infections caused by other virulent organisms have been reported, including *Candida* [19] and Panton–Valentine leucocidin-elaborating *S. aureus* [20]. Finally, deep tissue fungal infections are more common in intravenous drug use and skin popping patients, especially where there is immunocompromise from HIV and neglect.

Referral to drug and alcohol services

The management of recreational drug use can start with psychoeducation by dermatology health care professionals as the treatment for recreational drug use is mainly psychological. However, it is vital to utilise the psychiatric liaison services available locally when facing a complex or what is considered to be a high-risk presentation. Dermatology health care professionals can ask the primary care services to initiate a referral to the local drug and alcohol services. However, having a positive therapeutic relationship with patients plays a significant role in signposting to the right services. Information about the local services is readily available in the UK through the NHS website or by visiting the FRANK website to find local drug treatment services. There are charities and private drug treatment options which can be accessed by visiting the Adfam website to see a list of useful organisations. Patients can approach their local drug and alcohol services without the need of referral. There are different tiers of therapeutic interventions, starting from giving information and psychoeducation to in-patient specialist rehabilitation treatment. It is the responsibility of the specialist services to decide the intervention level a patient requires. In the USA, information about the drug and alcohol services are available from the Substance Abuse and Mental Health Services Administration (SAMHSA), which is the agency within the US Department of Health and Human Services that leads public health efforts to advance the behavioural health of the nation.

Management of the skin

Management of the skin may include:
- Stop and/or manage the recreational drug use.
- Consider investigating for blood-borne diseases (e.g. HIV, hepatitis).
- Consider a multidisciplinary approach (usually via drug and alcohol rehabilitation services).

Specific treatments are given in Table 120.2.

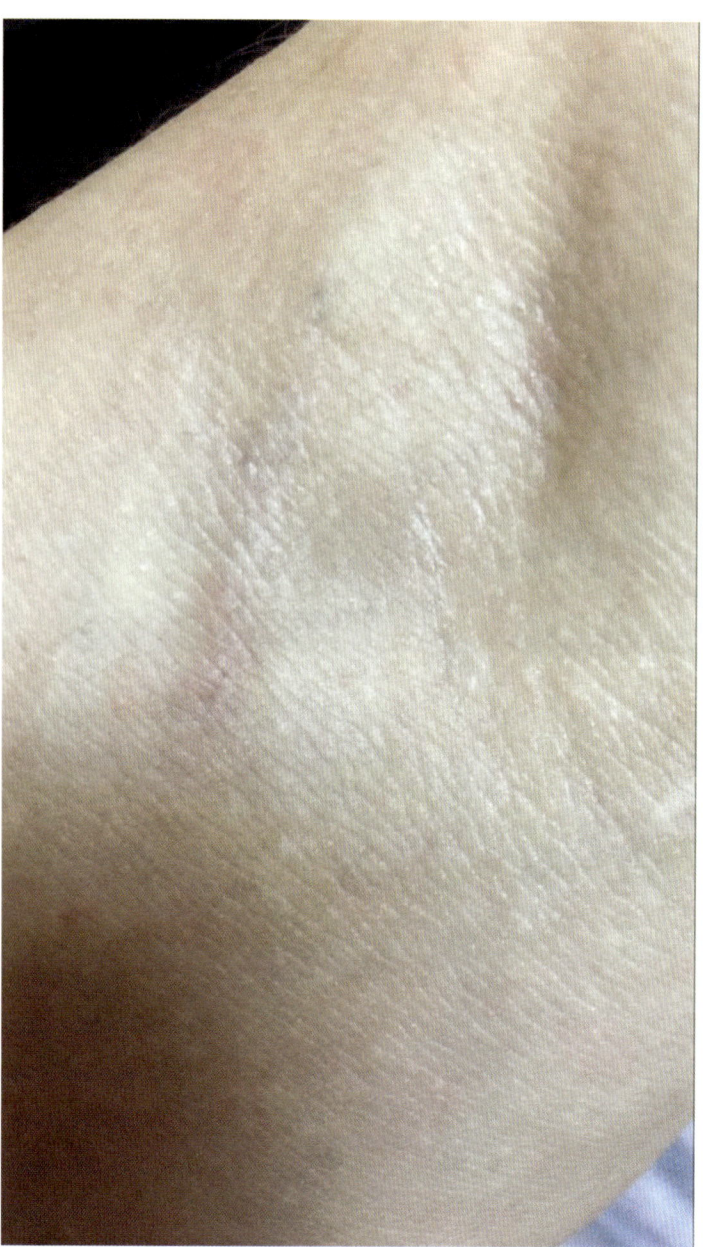

Figure 120.5 Track marks in the antecubital fossa from intravenous drug use. Courtesy of Professor Ilknur Altunay, Istanbul.

Management of skin diseases associated with recreational drug use

Managing the *patient* who uses recreational substances and who has skin disease is similar to managing patients with any psychodermatological disease. It is important to manage the skin disease while managing the recreational drug habit as well.

Assessment and management of psychosocial co-morbidities

Assessment and management of anxiety and/or depression, or other psychosocial co-morbidities including recreational drug use can be and should be initiated by dermatology health care professionals if they are the primary source of contact with the patient (Chapter 84). Signposting to psychological and/or psychiatric services can also be initiated by dermatology staff.

Table 120.2 Management of the skin following recreational drug use.

Skin manifestation	Management
Track marks (Figure 120.5)	Rotate injections sites Clean needles Consider topical steroid/antibiotic combination
Skin infections	As above Consider systemic antibiotics according to microbiology advice
Skin popping	As above Suggest patients stop 'popping' Antibiotics Systemic steroids Lasers
Necrosis	As above Systemic steroids Immunosuppresants Surgery See Chapter 102
Vasculitis	As above Systemic steroids Immunosuppresants Surgery See Chapter 100

Resources

Further information

Substance Abuse and Mental Health Services Administration: www.samhsa.gov/about-us.

Patient resources

Adfam: https://adfam.org.uk/.
FRANK: https://www.talktofrank.com/.
NHS website, getting help for drug addition: https://www.nhs.uk/live-well/healthy-body/drug-addiction-getting-help/.
(All last accessed June 2023.)

Key references

The full list of references can be found in the online version at https://www.wiley.com/rooksdermatology10e

Introduction

2 Gossop M, Marsden J, Stewart D et al. Substance use, health and social problems of service users at 54 drug treatment agencies: intake data from the National Treatment Outcome Research Study. Br J Psych 1998;173:146–71.

8 Hennings C, Miller J. Illicit drugs: what dermatologists need to know. J Am Acad Dermatol 2013;69:135–42.

Drug-induced dermatoses

16 Liu SW, Lien MH, Fenske NA. The effects of alcohol and drug abuse on the skin. Clin Dermatol 2010;28:391–9.
19 Brewer JD, Meves A, Bostwich JM, Pittelkow MR. Cocaine abuse: dermatologic manifestations and therapeutic approaches. J Am Acad Dermatol 2008;59:483–7.
21 Strazzula L, Brown KK, Brieva JC et al. Levamisole toxicity mimicking autoimmune disease. J Am Acad Dermatol 2013;69:954–9.
25 Gahr M, Freudenmann RW, Hiemke C et al. Desomorphine goes 'crocodile'. J Addict Dis 2012;31:407–12.

Dermatoses caused by intravenous and subcutaneous drug administration

1 Del Giudice P. Cutaneous complications of intravenous drug abuse. Br J Dermatol 2004;150:1–10.
9 Marks M, Pollock S, Morris-Jones S et al. Needles and the damage done: reasons for admission and financial costs associated with injecting drug use in a Central London teaching hospital. J Infect 2013:66:95–102.
13 Gordon RJ, Lowy FD. Bacterial infections in drug users. New Engl J Med 2005;353:1945–54.
16 Yuan J, Inami G, Mohle-Boetani J, Vagia DJ. Recurrent wound botulism among injection users in California. Clin Infect Dis 2011;52:862–6.

CHAPTER 121

Dermatological Manifestations of Metal Poisoning

Rabindranath Nambi

University Hospitals of Derby and Burton NHS Foundation Trust, Derby, UK

Introduction, 121.1	Reactions to lead, 121.4	Reactions to thallium, 121.8
Reactions to antimony, 121.1	Reactions to mercury, 121.5	Reactions to other metals, 121.9
Reactions to arsenic, 121.2	Reactions to selenium, 121.6	
Reactions to gold, 121.3	Reactions to silver, 121.7	Key references, 121.9

Introduction

An excessive exposure to any metal can result in cutaneous and systemic toxicity. Cutaneous manifestations of metal poisoning vary from acute skin problems to longstanding, chronic dermatoses, and occur with or without signs of internal involvement. Contact with metal compounds may be from environmental sources, through contaminated air, water or soil (and thus food), or can be encountered in an occupational setting. Iatrogenic sources, usually from an alternative form of medicine, need to be considered in certain situations: natural health food supplements may contain metals and trace elements in toxic doses [1,2]. A patient can also present with the signs of metal toxicity occurring as a consequence of deliberate poisoning. The exponential rise of internet shopping allows easy access to markets in countries where manufacturing practices are less stringently regulated. Cosmetic products, such as eyebrow pencils, containing excessive lead (kohl) have been obtained via the internet, their use resulting in lead poisoning. Complementary medicines are also frequently affected: one study demonstrated that 20% of 231 complementary medicines purchased over the internet contained higher than permitted levels of mercury, arsenic and lead. The percentage did not vary between products manufactured in the USA and those produced in developing countries [3].

Measurement of abnormal levels of metals in the body is an integral assessment in situations where toxicity is being considered. The main routes of metal elimination are the urinary and biliary system, but skin and its appendages also play a role. The natural presence of various metals in the skin means that quantification for toxicity purposes is meaningless unless compared with control levels.

The easy accessibility of hair has encouraged its use as a tissue for assaying the presence of metals: palladium, arsenic, cadmium and mercury are metals for which normal and toxic values can be assessed in hair [4]. Nails can also be used to measure metal content. The usual growth pattern of a nail allows a 3-month time-frame for analysis following exposure to the culprit substance. Toenails are preferred since levels of external contamination are low: lead, chromium and manganese levels measured in this fashion provide a reasonable record of exposure.

Reactions to antimony

Antimony (Sb)
- Atomic number: 51
- Atomic weight: 125.75 Da
- Normal concentrations: serum = 3 µg/L

Synonyms and inclusions
- Antimony poisoning

Introduction and general description

Antimony is a semimetallic chemical which, along with arsenic, once enjoyed a reputation of being a universal panacea for multiple diseases.

Antimony is a metalloid existing as a lustrous silver-white, brittle, hard metal which is easily converted into antimony oxide or antimony trioxide. The origin of its name suggesting 'anti-monos' ('enmity to solitude' or 'not alone') is due to the fact that antimony is usually found with other metals.

The usage of antimony as a therapeutic agent dates to around the third to fourth millennium BC and closely parallels arsenic with similar broad historical indications. Antimony has been used to treat syphilis, whooping cough, leprosy, epilepsy and pneumonia. Antimony is still used in the treatment of leishmaniasis and schistosomiasis [1].

Antimony exposure is a hazard in the enamel and ceramic industries. Smelting workers may also be occupationally exposed. Inadvertent toxicity via medical usage may occur in areas where leishmaniasis and schistosomiasis remain endemic.

Rook's Textbook of Dermatology, Tenth Edition. Edited by Christopher Griffiths, Jonathan Barker, Tanya Bleiker, Walayat Hussain and Rosalind Simpson.
© 2024 John Wiley & Sons Ltd. Published 2024 by John Wiley & Sons Ltd.

Pathophysiology
Antimony, like lead, has an affinity for sulfhydryl groups and phosphates, and thus interferes with multiple metabolic functions [2].

Pathology
No specific features on pathology are attributable to antimony.

Clinical features
Acute exposure results in a pustular rash with crusting resembling varicella. In some patients there may be vesicles along the lips, gingivitis, stomatitis, conjunctivitis and keratitis. Perforation of the nasal septum may occur; nodules can develop in the flexures.

Chronic antimony exposure can result in a flexural eczematous rash with sparing of the face, hands and feet [3]. 'Antimony spots' are due to airborne contamination with antimony resulting in a pustular eruption on the trunk and limbs. These are seen close to sweat and sebaceous glands, and resemble miliaria rubra. A cooler environment results in the rash clearing up within 2 weeks [4]. Recently, antimony trioxide has been reported to cause contact eczema among enamellers and decorators in the ceramic industry [5].

Investigations
A 24-hour urinary antimony concentration can be used to assess toxicity, with normal levels ranging from 0.5 to 6.2 μg/L.

Management
Treatment of skin involvement is symptomatic, with supportive care as the mainstay of antimony poisoning. Chelation experience has been limited in view of the rarity of case reports. Dimercaprol (British anti-lewisite or BAL) may help patients with acute severe antimony toxicity [6].

Reactions to arsenic

Arsenic (As)
- Atomic number: 33
- Atomic weight: 74.92 Da
- Normal concentrations: whole blood <5 μg/L (<0.067 μmol/L), urine <50 μmol/g (<13.3 μmol/g creatinine)

Synonyms and inclusions
- Arsenical poisoning

Introduction and general description
Arsenic or arsenic trioxide is a metalloid with the trivalent and pentavalent forms being the most prevalent.

Human arsenic exposure may occur from various sources. The commonest routes are from medicines (including traditional remedies), the workplace (occupational) or environmental sources [1]. Typically, people are exposed to the inorganic form, pentavalent arsenic, through soil and water. The safe level of arsenic in drinking water, recommended by the World Health Organization (WHO), is a maximum concentration of around 10 ppb. Arsenic is used in fertilisers and can be found in fish and algae. It is used in the semi-conductor industry. Arsenic can be found in the minerals arsenopyrite, loellingite and arsenic trioxide. Exposure to arsenic is a worldwide problem as it is ubiquitously present in small amounts in drinking water. Hydroarsenicism (contamination of water with arsenic) has been reported in many countries. In Bangladesh alone it has been estimated that 40 million people are at risk [2]. Chile, Taiwan, Brazil, India, Mexico and Argentina have also reported cases of hydroarsenicism [1].

Arsenic is a favoured poison since it is virtually tasteless and lacks a specific odour.

Pathophysiology
The toxicity of arsenic occurs through the inhibition of adenosine triphosphate (ATP) synthesis with an effect on oxidative phosphorylation. Arsenite has an affinity with thiol groups in molecules such as keratin. As a result of this affinity, the metabolites have a predilection for the skin, hair and nails. There is also a direct effect on DNA damage with p53 mutations being reported [3]. Methylation in the liver is a major route of metabolism for arsenic and pre-existing liver disease consequently results in increased toxicity. The presence of inflamed skin can cause increased absorption when arsenic is topically applied to the skin. The comparison of subjects who develop cutaneous malignancies versus normal controls has led to suggestions that increased absorption and retention of arsenic occurs in individuals predisposed to arsenic toxicity [4]. A genome-wide association study has identified a gene, *AS3MT*, which codes for the enzyme arsenite methyltransferase, at the chromosome 10q24.32 region. Mutations in this gene impact on metabolism efficiency and subsequent toxicity risk [5].

Pathology
The diffuse pigmentation seen in arsenic toxicity is due to increased melanin production with no increase in melanocytes. The pre-cancers and malignancies due to arsenic show no special features.

Clinical features
Acute toxicity features include alopecia, oral herpetiform ulcers and diaphoresis (diffuse sweating state). Acute arsenical dermatitis is a pruritic, red, papular eruption that can blister and may lead to erythroderma [6]. Acute contact dermatitis due to arsenic as an occupational contact allergen has been reported [7]. Mee's lines are transverse white bands on the nails (transverse striate leukonychia) that occur in arsenic poisoning. Mee's lines also occur in thallium poisoning (Figure 121.1) [8]. Toxic epidermal necrolysis has been reported after 3 weeks of usage with a topical herbal cream containing high levels of arsenic [9].

Features of chronic arsenic poisoning include arsenical keratoses on the palms and soles, which usually occur after approximately 2 years and are premalignant in nature (Figures 121.2 and 121.3). Peripheral neuropathy can be prominent in chronic arsenicism. Intraepidermal carcinomas, basal cell carcinomas (BCC) and squamous cell carcinomas (SCC) have all been reported. Latency periods of between 1 and 40 years have been reported for the development of SCC [10,11].

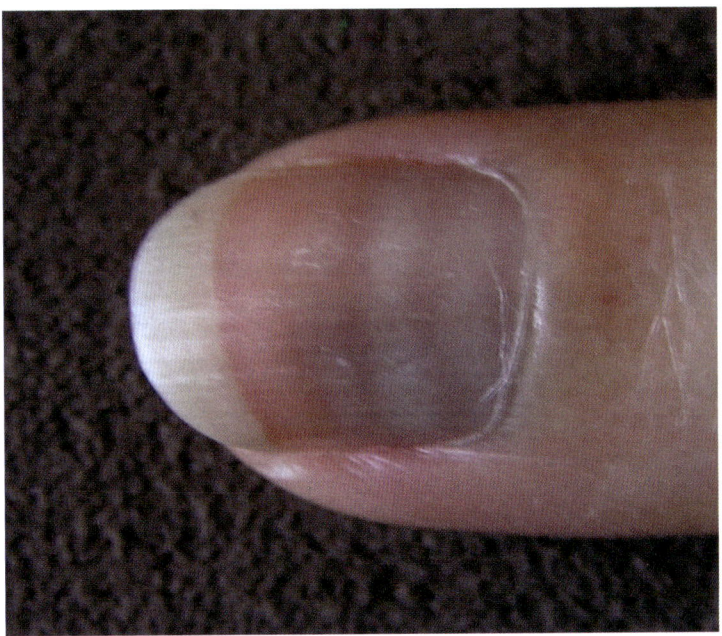

Figure 121.1 Mees lines caused by chemotherapy. Source: Yannick Trottier/Wikimedia Commons/CC BY-SA 3.0.

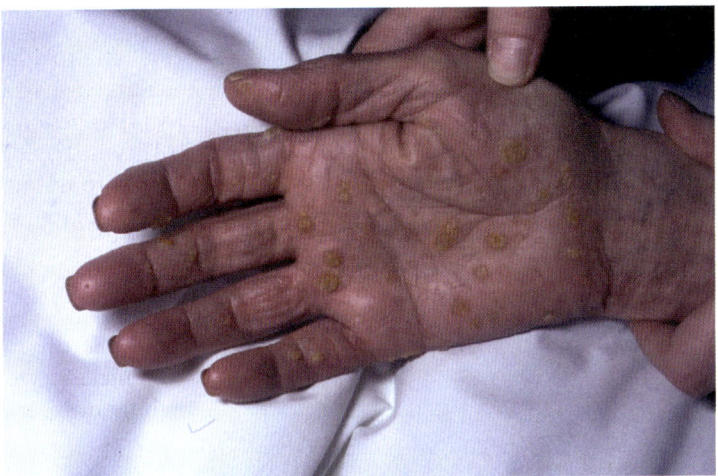

Figure 121.2 Multiple discrete punctate keratoses on the palm due to chronic arsenic exposure. Courtesy Dr S. Evans.

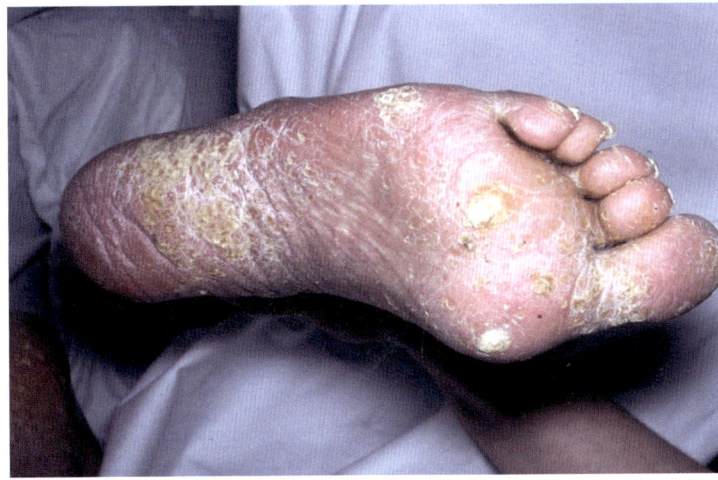

Figure 121.3 Diffuse scaling and keratoses on the sole in chronic arsenicism. Courtesy Dr S. Evans.

Diffuse pigmentation with macular areas of depigmentation within the hyperpigmented skin may result from long-term arsenic exposure. There may be flexural predominance [12]. This pigmentary anomaly has been described as 'rain drops on a dusty road'. Both alopecia and a palmoplantar vesicular dermatitis have been reported as manifestations of arsenic toxicity.

Blackfoot disease describes the presence of gangrenous feet secondary to chronic arsenic toxicity. In the past this was more prevalent in southwest Taiwan [13].

Patients with chronic arsenicism features should be screened for liver, lung and bladder malignancies [14–16].

Investigations
To assess the presence of excess arsenic, a spot urine test or a 24-hour urine test for arsenic is available. The 24-hour urine test is more reliable and is considered positive if arsenic levels exceed 50 µg/L, 100 µg/g creatinine or 100 µg of total arsenic [1].

Management
Acute arsenic toxicity is treated with BAL 5 mg/kg with a maximum of 300 mg intramuscularly along with 2,3 dimercaptopropane sulphonic acid (DMPS) intravenously followed by long-term monotherapy with oral DMPS [17,18].

Nicotinamide has been shown to play a role in repair of arsenic and ultraviolet radiation induced DNA damage and its use may be considered in cases of chronic arsenicism [19].

In a phase 3 randomised controlled ONTRAC study performed in Australia, high-risk individuals – defined by patients with two or more non-melanoma skin cancers (NMSC) in the last 5 years – were given nicotinamide 500 mg BD for 1 year. Overall, a 23% reduction in NMSC was noted, with a specific reduction of 30% in SCC and a 20% reduction in BCC at 1 year [20].

Reactions to gold

Gold (Au)
- Atomic number: 79
- Atomic weight: 196.96 Da
- Normal concentrations: whole blood = 0.055 ng/mL

Synonyms and inclusions
- Gold poisoning
- Chrysiasis

Introduction and general description
Elemental gold is inert; however, mono- and trivalent forms combine with electron donors. These ions bind strongly with sulfhydryl groups [1].

Gold is an inert substance present throughout the world and exposure is predominantly through the mining industry and as a therapeutic agent. Introduction of gold into the skin can also occur from tattoos, piercings, dental restorations and prolonged wearing of gold jewellery [2]. Gold has been used to treat rheumatoid arthritis, pemphigus and psoriatic arthritis. As an isotope ^{198}Au has been used to treat cancers. Edible gold leaf is used in liqueurs and as a flavourless wrap in expensive foods [3].

Pathophysiology
A wide variety of immune reactions to gold are recognised; most typical is a type 4 cell-mediated hypersensitivity, resulting in a lichenoid eruption. Type 1 (immediate) and type 3 (immune complex) reactions also occur.

Gold, after being engulfed by macrophages, is stored in lysosomes (aureosomes). It inhibits lysosomal enzyme activity, histamine release from mast cells, phagocytosis and the inflammatory effects of prostaglandins [4]. Gold also reduces the production of proinflammatory cytokines including tumour necrosis factor α (TNF-α), interleukin-1 (IL-1) and IL-6 [4]. There has been an association between human leukocyte antigen (HLA) types and cutaneous gold reactions, particularly with HLA-DRW3, HLA-DR5, HLA-B7, HLA-B8 and HLA-B27 [5–8]. A study has shown that gold dermatitis in patients with rheumatoid arthritis is associated with both HLA-B35 and disease duration [9]. Antibodies to the Ro 52-kDa antigen are associated with skin eruptions in rheumatoid arthritis patients treated with gold [10].

Pathology
The histology of a gold-induced eczematous and lichenoid eruption is characterised by a sparse dermal perivascular infiltrate, predominantly of CD4$^+$ HLA-DR-positive helper T lymphocytes, an increase in the number of dermal Langerhans cells and epidermal macrophage-like cells, and Langerhans cell apposition to mononuclear cells [11]. Metallic gold particles can be demonstrated in dermal macrophages and around blood vessels [12].

Clinical features
The use of gold in rheumatoid arthritis is associated with a 23–30% incidence of reactions [3,13,14]; most of these are minor, but about 15% may be severe or even fatal [15]. Rashes and mouth ulcers are common [2,3,16–21], representing about 50% of all complications with parenteral gold and 35% of those with oral gold. Localised or generalised pruritus is an important warning sign of potential toxicity. Gold reactions may simulate exanthematic eruptions [22], erythema annulare centrifugum [23], seborrhoeic dermatitis or lichen planus [24,25]. A mixture of these patterns, sometimes with discoid eczematoid lesions, is characteristic. Lichen planus is often of the hypertrophic variety especially on the scalp, and severe and irreversible alopecia may follow [26]. There may be striking and persistent postinflammatory hyperpigmentation. Permanent nail dystrophy has followed onycholysis [27]. Yellow nails have been described [28].

In one study, eczematous or lichenoid rashes persisted for up to 11 months after cessation of therapy [21]. A patient with a lichenoid and seborrhoeic dermatitis-like rash on gold sodium thiomalate therapy had a positive intradermal test to gold thiomalate; patch tests were positive to thiomalate (the thiol carrier of gold thiomalate) but negative to gold itself [29]. Interestingly, the same patient subsequently developed a seborrhoeic dermatitis-like eruption, but not a lichenoid eruption, while on auranofin. This time, patch tests were positive to both auranofin and gold.

A previous contact dermatitis from gold jewellery may be reactivated [30]. Other reactions documented include erythema nodosum [31], severe hypersensitivity reactions [32], vasculitis [33], polyarteritis, a systemic lupus erythematosus-like syndrome, generalised exfoliative dermatitis and toxic epidermal necrolysis. Psoriasis was reported to be exacerbated in a patient with arthritis treated with gold [34]. Prolonged administration of gold may cause a distinct grey, blue or purple pigmentation of exposed skin (chrysiasis), which is a dose-dependent reaction that occurs above a threshold of 20 mg/kg; gold granules are seen within dermal endothelial cells and macrophages [35–39]. Even in the absence of pigmentation, gold can be detected histochemically in the skin up to 20 years after therapy. Localised argyria with chrysiasis has been caused by acupuncture needles [40]. An unusual late cutaneous reaction involved the appearance of widespread keloid-like angiofibromatoid lesions [41]. Oral lesions due to gold include red eroded areas and lichenoid reactions. Stomatitis may be seen as a result of gold reactions [42]. The gold cyanidation process used in the gold industry causes irritant reactions on the skin with discoloration of fingernails [43].

A benign vasodilatory 'nitritoid' reaction, consisting of flushing, light-headedness and transient hypotension, may occur immediately after the first injection of gold [2,44]. It occurs in roughly 5% of patients taking gold sodium thiomalate. Non-vasomotor effects including arthralgia, myalgia and constitutional symptoms within the first 24 h are recognised. Mucous membrane symptoms include loss of taste, metallic taste, stomatitis, glossitis and diarrhoea. Punctate stomatitis may occur with or without skin lesions. Gold is also deposited in the cornea and may cause keratitis with ulceration.

Eosinophilia is common, and serum IgE may be raised [45]. Other immunological reactions are rare, although pulmonary fibrosis is recorded [46]. Blood dyscrasias, especially thrombocytopenic purpura, and occasionally fatal neutropenia or aplastic anaemia, occur in a small proportion of cases and usually present within the first 6 months of therapy. Jaundice occurs in about 3% of cases and may result from idiosyncratic intrahepatic cholestasis [47]. Proteinuria and renal damage are well recognised.

Management
Generally, there are no effective treatments for chrysiasis – localised or generalised. Recently, a case of localised chrysiasis was successfully treated with a long-pulsed ruby laser [48].

Dimercaprol has been used with varied success. Acetyl cysteine and granulocyte colony-stimulating factor have been used mainly to reduce the haemopoietic side effects [3].

Reactions to lead

Lead (Pb)
- Atomic number: 82
- Atomic weight: 207.0 Da
- Normal concentrations: whole blood <10 μg/dL (<0.48 μmol/L)

Synonyms and inclusions
- Plumbism
- Colica pictorum
- Devon colic
- Painter's colic
- Saturnism

Introduction and general description

Lead is a silvery grey metal with trivalent and pentavalent forms.

Lead poisoning represents an important health issue, both as an environmental and occupational hazard. Exposure to lead in the environment can be from dust or from contaminated soil and water. In the past, lead used in paints was a cause of poisoning, particularly in children licking painted toys. In 2007 millions of toys produced in China were withdrawn due to their high lead content. Imported diaper powder has been linked with lead poisoning in an infant [1]. 'Kajal', an eye cosmetic, has repeatedly been reported to be contaminated with lead in multiple countries [2]. Lead in engine fuel was another important source. However, leaded fuel has now been withdrawn from most countries. Occupations with high risk of exposure include automobile mechanics, ceramic workers, lead smelters, those working in storage battery manufacturers, painters and construction workers [3].

Pathophysiology

Lead competes with calcium, thus affecting various metabolic pathways. Even though lead forms complexes with several elements, the most important toxicological combination is with the sulfhydryl group [4]. A direct carcinogenic effect on cells has also been postulated [5]. Three genetic polymorphisms have been reported to influence the toxicokinetics of lead in humans: a gene coding for δ-aminolaevulinic acid dehydratase, the vitamin D receptor gene and the HFE protein gene [6].

Pathology

There are no histological features unique to lead-induced dermatoses.

Clinical features

Chronic lead poisoning results in a typical, waxy 'lead hue' with pallor on the skin. Kohl pencils sold in the Middle East and Asian countries, used as eyeliners, have been shown to have high lead content. These may result in periocular pigmentation [7]. An eczematous eruption on the left chest has been reported as being due to lead pencils [8]. Greenish discoloration of the skin, due to embedded lead fragments in the skin, from bullets used in the Second World War, has been described in one patient [9].

Burton's lead line is a bluish line on the gingival margin, seen in lead poisoning, and is due to the deposition of lead sulphite resulting from a reaction between sulphur from the oral flora and lead [10].

Oral erosions on the lips mimicking paraneoplastic pemphigus has been reported in a 61-year-old patient working in a tin foil factory [11].

Exposure to lead has effects on multiple organs including peripheral neuropathy, problems with learning and memory function, erythrocyte fragility, Fanconi-like syndrome, plumbism gout (saturnine gout), increased blood urate concentrations and urate crystals in the joints, hypertension, altered cardiac electrophysiology, infertility, hypothyroidism, hypopituitarism, lead lines in the bones, impaired bone growth, shortened stature and gastrointestinal toxicity resulting in lead colic and lead-induced constipation.

Investigations

To determine lead toxicity, whole blood lead levels can be performed. Radiographical studies may also show lead lines in the bones.

Management

Three chelation agents – dimercaprol, ethylenediaminetetra-acetic acid (EDTA) and succimer – have been used for lead toxicity.

Reactions to mercury

Mercury (Hg)
- Atomic number: 80
- Atomic weight: 200.59 Da
- Normal concentrations whole blood <10 µg/L (<50 µmol/L), urine <20 µg/L (<100 µmol/L)

Synonyms and inclusions
- Hydrargyria
- Mercurialism

Introduction and general description

Mercury is a trace metal that occurs in the elemental form or in organic and inorganic compounds. It is the only metal that exists as a liquid at room temperature. Restrictions on its usage have been imposed due to concerns about toxicity. Three main forms exist: metallic mercury found in thermometers and paints; inorganic salts of mercury found in laxatives, pesticides and antiseptics; and organic mercurials used as commercial fungicides.

The three forms of mercury – elemental, organic and inorganic – have varied toxic effects on the gastrointestinal, renal and central nervous system. Effects on the skin are primarily due to inorganic mercury salts. Mercury is widely used in alternative medicines. Multiple episodes of accidental mercury exposure have been reported. In the 18th century, 'hatter's shakes' were described among the hat industry workers in Danbury, USA, who used mercury in the production of felt, and led to the origin of the phrase 'mad as a hatter' [1,2]. Later on, in the 19th century, acrodynia, or pink disease, was reported in children who were given calomel (mercurous chloride) as a universal panacea [3]. The most recent mass episode of mercury poisoning was in Iraq in 1971 when seeds earmarked for cultivation were mistakenly used in making bread. These seeds had been treated with methyl mercury as a fungicidal agent. This calamity was thought to have caused at least 400 deaths [4]. Replacement of old mercury thermometers with digital thermometers has resulted in decreased exposure. Fluorescent lamps, dental amalgams, barometers, old paints and seeds treated with the now banned mercurous chloride are significant exposure risks. Incorrect disposal of paints, batteries, lights and coal power plants pollutants may result in water contamination with mercury [5].

Pathophysiology

Mercury binds predominantly with sulfhydryl groups but also retains an affinity to phosphoryl, carboxyl and amide groups, resulting in the disruption of multiple cellular mechanisms and resultant widespread organ toxicity.

Pathology

The histology of mercury skin deposition shows brown-black granules within macrophages and in the dermis. In most situations, the granules are around the superficial blood vessels and are also distributed along the connective tissue fibres [6]. Mercury granulomas have been described as spherical, opaque globules of varying sizes with a zone of necrosis around them. Granulomatous inflammation with a mixed infiltrate along with epidermal or dermal necrosis may also be seen [7]. Subcorneal pustules with dermal oedema are a feature of generalised mercury-induced exanthematous eruption. A few patients may also show leukocytoclastic vasculitis [8]. Cutaneous hyperpigmentation due to mercury results partly from increased melanin production in the epidermis and partly from the presence of multiple mercury granules in the papillary dermis [9]. Eccrine hyperplasia with a non-specific infiltrate is seen in cases of acrodynia [10].

Clinical features

Acute mercury exposure results in a symptom complex that may include gingivostomatitis, hypersalivation (ptyalism) and erethism. Erethism consists of facial blushing and tremors. Individuals have a specific emotional state including shyness, anxiety, emotional lability and delirium.

A fatal episode of mercury toxicity in an adult female patient has been described after usage of a topical herbal cream containing high levels of mercuric bromide for eczema of the chest [11].

Mercury exanthem has been reported due to exposure to mercury or its metabolic compound. Fifteen patients have been described with a typical inverted triangular or V-shaped redness involving both inner thighs. Other major flexures were also affected with purpura and pustules on a red background. Previous sensitisation with mercurochrome during its use as a topical disinfectant and subsequent exposure to mercury either due to the use of a thermometer or with dental treatment resulted in the onset of the exanthematous rash [12].

Repeated exposures may result in acrodynia, which was first described in 1903 by Selter, who termed this trophodermatoneurose or vegetative neurose [13–15]. It was first described in children with significant redness, scaling and induration of the extremities, and hyperkeratosis on the palms, soles and face. There may be ulceration of the extremities. Acrodynia can feature an exanthematous rash that may have urticarial, vesicular and haemorrhagic components. Other features include hyperhidrosis, irritability, photophobia, alopecia, loss of nails and scarlet cheeks, ears and nose. Eleven patients have been described with a distinct, mildly pruritic eruption, predominantly on palms and forearms. These patients had high blood levels of mercury, ingested via a diet high in seafood. All patients responded to either restrictions in diet or chelation therapy [5].

The chronic application of mercury-containing creams used as skin bleachers can paradoxically result in an accumulation of mercury compound in the skin resulting in a slate grey hyperpigmentation. Face and flexures are common sites to be affected. Histology in these situations shows multiple mercury granules deposited in the upper dermis [16]. Baboon syndrome has been reported as a result of mercury toxicity [17]. Membranous fat necrosis has been described in a 21-year-old after subcutaneous and intramuscular injections of mercury [18]. Mercury has also been reported as a contact allergen due to its incorporation into dental mercury fillings. Oral lichenoid lesions have been reported with dental amalgams. In the original study by Laine *et al.* involving 118 patients with oral lichenoid plaques, 68% had positive patch tests to related metal compounds. Replacement of the fillings caused complete healing in 45% of patients [19]. Since then, other studies have shown patch testing to be of limited value [20,21]. A more pragmatic approach to correlate the site of oral lichenoid reactions with the dental restoration materials has been recommended [19]. Mercuric sulphide in tattoos causes a distinctive red colour in the case of lichenoid or granulomatous reactions (Chapter 122).

Investigations

In acute poisoning, increased levels of mercury can be demonstrated in whole blood and in urine samples. Hair can be assessed in suspected cases of chronic mercury toxicity [22]. Skin biopsies may be useful in identifying mercury granules.

Management

The treatment of rashes caused by mercury is mainly symptomatic and dependent on presentation, and the extent of mercury toxicity documented by investigations. In acute mercury toxicity, chelation is appropriate, and may be combined with plasma exchange or dialysis (peritoneal or haemodialysis). The two main chelation agents are dimercaptosuccinic acid (DMSA) and dimercaptopropane sulfonate (DMPS).

Reactions to selenium

Selenium (Se)
- Atomic number: 34
- Atomic weight: 78.96 Da
- Normal concentrations:
  whole blood = 0.1–0.34 mg/L (<1.27–4.32 μmol/L)
  serum = 0.040.06 mg/L (0.51–7.6 μmol/L)
  urine (24 h) <0.03 mg/L (<0.38 μmol/L)

Synonyms and inclusions
- Selenium poisoning
- Selenosis

Introduction and general description

Selenium is an essential trace element with a recommended daily intake of 55 μg. Discovered by Jons Berzilius in 1817, as a contaminant in sulphuric acid wax, its chemical activity closely resembles that of sulphur and tellurium [1].

Named after the moon Selene, selenium is unusual in that it has good photovoltaic and photoconductive properties. This has resulted in wide usage in electronics and in the glass industry. Sodium selenite is also found in animal feeds and food supplements. Toxicity is usually due to industrial exposure, inadvertent high-dose selenium supplement ingestion or excessive intake of paradise nuts (*Lecythis ollaria*). Selenium occurs naturally in the environment and is present in grains, cereals and meat. Exposure to excessive selenium can also occur via water. Chronic selenium toxicity has been described in China and Venezuela in seleniferous areas, resulting in eczematous and bullous skin changes, alopecia, onychodystrophy and nail changes [2].

Pathophysiology

In selenium deficiency, glutathione peroxidase levels are lowered. This interferes with the detoxification of reactive oxygen species. In selenium toxicity, it has been proposed that oxidative stress causes tissue damage and is due to excessive levels of pro-oxidant selenite and ions. Molecular mimicry between selenium and sulphur in cellular enzyme cycles could cause disruption of mitochondrial functions. Selenium also interferes with the disulphide bridges in structural proteins, such as keratin, causing tissue damage [3].

Pathology

Histological findings are non-specific and relate to the lesion being biopsied.

Clinical features

Acute exposure on the skin to selenious acid or selenium dioxide causes considerable tissue necrosis resulting in a chemical burn [4]. Inorganic selenium ingestion results in toxic effects in the gastrointestinal tract and cardiovascular system and can cause fulminant damage resulting in death from circulatory collapse, in some cases within an hour. In these patients, a typical garlicky odour has been reported [5,6].

Excessive ingestion of certain nutritional supplements can cause chronic selenosis or selenium toxicity [7]. In a study of 201 patients who ingested a supplement with 200 times the stated selenium dose, multiple skin problems were noted [8]. Alopecia was common (70%), as was greyish nail discoloration and brittleness (61%); 26% of patients also reported a non-specific cutaneous eruption, with 37% reporting garlicky breath. Intentional fatal overdose with selenium has been reported, with death occurring within a few hours. A striking orange-brown staining of skin and viscera was noted at autopsy [9].

Selenosis has also been reported after excessive ingestion of paradise nuts [10]. In this report a 55-year-old woman presented with headaches, dizziness, nausea and abdominal pain for 5 days. There was quite significant hair loss and a trichogram showed anagen hairs with dystrophic follicles with progression to complete alopecia on day 2. Generalised greyish discoloration of the skin was noted. Red eczematous plaques on the limbs, which can blister and ulcerate, may also be a feature in some cases [2]. Dental caries have been reported [11].

Nail changes in chronic selenosis include leukonychia (which can be transverse or longitudinal) associated with paronychia. Leukonychia has been described in a patient with Crohn disease induced by selenium deficiency [12]. In this report a 30-year-old patient presented with leukonychia affecting the proximal half of the nails on the fingers and toes. After 14 weeks of selenium substitution the nails returned to normal. Haemorrhagic onychomadesis has been reported in eight adults and two children due to consumption of wheat contaminated by selenium. In these cases, initial splinter haemorrhages were noted, which then progressed to subungual and in late stages led to haemorrhagic onychomadesis [13].

Investigations

Increased selenium levels can be demonstrated by serum concentrations greater than 2 mg/L. Hair levels have been extensively studied. However, in patients who use selenium sulphide as a shampoo, this may be misleading.

Management

Acute selenium exposure to skin and nail beds may cause pain and may be treated with 10% sodium thiosulphate solution, which converts selenium dioxide to elemental selenium [1]. Decontamination is essential in acute exposure. In some patients, haemodialysis has been tried. Dimercaprol and EDTA have been used unsuccessfully and may, paradoxically, worsen the toxic effects of selenium.

Reactions to silver

Silver (Ag)
- Atomic number: 47
- Atomic weight: 107.9 Da
- Normal concentrations: serum <1 μg/L (<9 μmol/L), urine (24 h) <2 μg/L (<18.0 μmol/L)

Synonyms and inclusions
- Silver poisoning
- Argyria
- Argyrosis

Introduction and general description

Silver is a rare but naturally occurring precious metal. The antibacterial properties of silver have been exploited in medicine and as a water purifier.

Silver is a commonly used brilliant white, highly ductile and malleable metal. It has been shown to have excellent electrical and thermal conductivity with little contact resistance. It is used as a bactericidal agent and has been incorporated into metal containers for transporting water as well as into surgical appliances. Silver has also been used as a medicament to treat various illnesses and still enjoys a reputation as an alternative to antibiotics. Silver plays a large role in various industries including health, engineering and science. The use of silver as a photographic reagent has reduced due to the ascendancy of digital photography. Silver iodide crystals are used to make rain by 'cloud melting' exercises in drought-hit areas. The crystals induce freezing in clouds and allow the water held in them to fall as rain [1].

Silver exposure is predominantly occupational in the photographic, medical and pharmaceutical industries. Cutaneous exposure also occurs in mining and manufacturing industries. Colloidal silver proteins are widely available as a 'natural health antibiotic supplement'.

Pathophysiology

Activated silver causes electron displacement in bacterial membranes and has an affinity to sulfhydryl, carboxyl and phosphate groups, resulting in significant protein denaturation and precipitation [2]. This activity accounts for silver's bacteriocidal action. Large doses of silver can block Na^+-K^+-ATPase activity with severe effects on the heart, liver and bone marrow. A single dose of 50 mg of silver is fatal in humans [1,3].

The photoreduction of silver nanoparticles to elemental silver and stimulation of melanin production by photoactivated silver is thought to be the basis for the increased pigmentation seen in argyria [4,5,6,7]. Ingested silver is transformed by stomach acid into an activated nano silver form and transported to the skin. Here it is converted to elemental silver by a process akin to a photochemical process used in old black and white photographs. The scientific basis has been described elaborately by Liu *et al.*, while Shelley *et al.* have eloquently and concisely described it as an *intradermal photograph* [5,7].

Pathology

Silver granules in the dermis can be seen close to the vasculature and in the basement membranes in close approximation to dermal elastic fibres [8]. The colour has been described as brown-black.

Silver particles may also be found lying free within the cytoplasm of the epithelial cells, in the secretory segment of eccrine sweat glands and in mast cells.

Silver granules are readily visible with dark-field illumination. Electron microscope and X-ray dispersive microanalysis studies have also been used to visualise the silver granules [9].

Clinical features

Argyria is the main manifestation of cutaneous silver toxicity. Argyria is divided into localised argyria and generalised argyria.

Localised argyria, due to repeated direct exogenous contact with silver particles, results in the silver particles being embedded into the skin. This appears as bluish grey discoloration due to silver elements in the dermis. Localised argyria can also be present in the mucous membranes and cornea [10,11]. Corneal argyrosis is due to the use of silver eye drops. The incidence has now reduced because silver-containing eye drops have largely been discontinued. Unilateral conjunctival and corneal argyrosis mimicking melanoma has been reported in a photographer who repeatedly used the same cloth contaminated with a photographic fixing agent to wipe his tears [12]. The commonly used silver sulfadiazine agent can produce localised argyria around wounds. In one study, after 4 weeks of using silver-containing dressings for leg ulcers, levels of silver in the blood increased in 50% of patients. This indicates a high propensity for absorption in granulating wounds. Therefore, silver dressings should only be used for short periods and for small ulcers [13]. Blue argyria macules have been noted to appear at the sites of acupuncture needles [14]. Silver earrings may also cause localised argyria. Localised argyria may be mistaken for a blue naevus if sufficiently small [15].

The use of silver dental amalgams can result in argyria being present in the tongue and gingiva [16]. Argyria may be present in the gingiva as a bluish line due to the presence of metallic silver and silver sulphide.

Generalised argyria is due to systemic absorption of silver. The dermatosis usually occurs in a photosensitive distribution affecting the face, neck, back and dorsal aspect of the hands [4]. The 'Blue Man' presented at the Barnum and Bailey circus in New York was a case of generalised argyria. Generalised argyria may be due to cutaneous absorption over a large area of skin or mucous membranes, or from ingestion of silver as a health supplement. This results in a generalised pigmentation appearing as a bluish grey tint on the skin. The sclera, mucous membranes and nails may become hyperpigmented. Permanent bluish discoloration of the lunula of the nails (azure lunulae) has been reported with argyria [17]. Nasal sprays containing silver have been reported to cause argyria, which is more marked on exposed areas [18,19].

Four cases of argyria have been reported after chewing betel nut covered with silver. It has been proposed that as exposure to silver in the diet is common in Asian countries, argyria is underdiagnosed as a cause of photosensitive pigmentation in this population [20].

Investigations

Skin biopsies with electron microscopic and X-ray diffraction studies may be useful in unusual cases to identify silver granules. Urine and serum concentration of silver may aid in the diagnosis of silver toxicity.

Management

Treatment with depigmenting preparations may be tried but they are not usually effective. Sunscreens should be advised for all patients with generalised argyria. The Q-switched 1064 nm Nd:YAG laser has been used successfully in the treatment of argyria in patients with a history of colloidal silver protein ingestion [21,22].

Reactions to thallium

Thallium (Tl)
- Atomic number: 81
- Atomic weight: 204.37 Da
- Normal concentrations: whole blood <2 µg/L (<978.9 µmol/L), urine (24 h) <2 thin>µg/L (<24.5 thin>µmol/L)

Synonyms and inclusions
- Thallium poisoning
- Thallotoxicosis

Introduction and general description

Thallium is a soft metal that is generally non-toxic; however, conversion to monovalent thallous and trivalent thallic salts results in a highly toxic version.

Thallium has a long history of being used to treat various disorders including syphilis, tuberculosis and tinea capitis. A case study of thallium usage in tinea capitis listed 46 deaths in 700 cases [1]. Thallium is an efficient rodenticide. As a result of its odourless and tasteless nature, human accidental and intentional poisonings were common until 1972, when commercial use was banned in most countries. Contamination of homeopathic medications and substance abuse products with thallium has also been reported with resultant toxicity [2,3]. Homicidal use is well recognised.

Pathophysiology

Thallium competes with potassium for its metabolism and has a tendency to be substituted as a physiological mimicker. This is predominantly in the central and peripheral nervous systems, liver and striated muscle [4]. As a substitute for potassium, thallium stimulates potassium-dependent enzymes in low doses, but is inhibitory in high doses. Along with other heavy metals, thallium has a high affinity to sulfhydryl groups, resulting in altered enzyme function and denaturation of proteins. In hair, thallium interferes with the keratin bonds resulting in alopecia, with a similar mechanism in nails leading to defective nail growth and the appearance of Mees lines [5,6].

Clinical features

Alopecia and peripheral neuropathy are striking features of thallium poisoning. Alopecia is considered to be highly typical of thallium toxicity and usually occurs around 10 days after exposure to thallium. The delay of alopecia onset can cause misdiagnosis in its early stages. Careful examination of the hair reveals hyperpigmentation of the hair roots [7–10]. Multiple alternating bands on the hair shaft may also be present. 'Bayonet hairs' with tapering points may be seen in thallium intoxication. Alopecia may be irreversible after considerable thallium toxicity. Acne, xerosis and redness of the palms have also been reported [10]. Red scaly patches on the face that later became acneform have been described [11]. Mees lines are homogenous, white, horizontal bands traversing the entire nail plate. Multiple nails may be affected, a feature also seen in arsenic poisoning.

Cardiovascular effects include tachycardia and hypertension. Peripheral neuropathy is usually painful, progressive and associated with paraesthesia. Other features include nephrotoxicity and optic neuritis.

Investigations

Elevated thallium concentrations may be found in the hair, nails, saliva, blood and urine. Hair analysis should be performed 7–10 days following exposure, to eliminate false negative results, which may occur if analysis is undertaken before this interval.

Management

Decontamination after immediate exposure has been recommended. Activated charcoal has also been used in acute thallium poisoning. Prussian blue is widely used in thallium poisoning, and is administered three or four times a day, with a total dose of 250 mg/kg/day, orally through a nasogastric tube [12]. Recently, Prussian blue, along with haemodialysis, has been recommended in severe thallium poisoning [13].

Reactions to other metals

Beryllium

Beryllium is a light, alkaline, rare metal that was used until 1950 in multiple industries including the manufacture of fluorescent lamps. The usage of beryllium has now been reduced, resulting in fewer cases of beryllium toxicity. Beryllium exposure to intact skin does not cause any significant toxicity, although soluble beryllium salts readily penetrate inflamed and damaged skin causing hypersensitivity reactions and allergic contact dermatitis [1].

Beryllium hypersensitivity is permanent and significant re-exposure can cause recurrence of beryllium dermatitis [2,3]. The Koebner phenomenon has been reported in beryllium dermatitis [4]. Beryllium is also added to copper and exposure to this alloy can result in beryllium dermatitis. Beryllium usage in dental material has resulted in beryllium stomatitis and hypersensitivity reactions [5].

Beryllium nodules are non-tender and persistent; excision has been recommended [6–9].

Molybdenum

Molybdenum toxicity is primarily from high exposure in foundry industries and molybdenum mines. Molybdenum sensitivity can result in an eczematous response as well as urticarial responses [1]. Generalised urticaria has been reported due to dental implants [2]. Molybdenum has been implicated in orthopaedic implants, resulting in systemic sensitisation. Newer alloys have now been employed reducing the usage of molybdenum [3].

Platinum

Platinum is an inert material; however, platinum salts can be absorbed in tetra- and hexachloro-palatinate forms. This results in platinum salt sensitivity known as platinosis.

The main features are contact urticaria, asthma, cyanosis, rhinoconjunctivitis and in severe cases anaphylaxis [1,2]. A case of occupational argyrosis and platinosis has been reported [3].

Key references

The full list of references can be found in the online version at https://www.wiley.com/rooksdermatology10e

Introduction

2 MacFarquhar JK, Broussard DL, Melstrom P *et al*. Acute selenium toxicity associated with a dietary supplement. *Arch Intern Med* 2010;3:256–61.

Reactions to antimony

1 Tarabar AF. Antimony. In: Nelson LS, Lewin NA, Howland MA *et al.*, eds. *Goldfrank's Toxicologic Emergencies*, 9th edn. New York: McGraw-Hill, 2011:1207–11.

Reactions to arsenic

10 Wong SS, Tan KC, Goh Cl. Cutaneous manifestations of chronic arsenicism: review of seventeen cases. *J Am Acad Dermatol* 1998;139:1092–6.
20 Chen AC, Martin AJ, Choy B *et al*. A phase 3 randomized trial of nicotinamide for skin-cancer chemoprevention. *N Engl J Med* 2015;373:1618–26.

Reactions to gold

1 Guy RH, Hostýnek JJ, Hinz RS, Lorence CR. Gold. In: *Metals and the Skin: Topical Effects and Systemic Absorption*. New York: Marcel Dekker, 1999:75–87.
3 Schonwald S. Gold. In: Dart RC, Caravati EM, Mcguigan MA *et al.*, eds. *Medical Toxicology*, 3rd edn. Philadelphia: Lippincott Williams and Wilkins, 2004:1048–50.

Reactions to mercury

9 Granstein RD, Sober AJ. Drug- and heavy metal-induced hyperpigmentation. *J Am Acad Dermatol* 1981;5:1–18.

Reactions to silver

5 Liu J, Wang Z, Liu FD *et al*. Chemical transformations of nanosilver in biological environments. *ACS Nano* 2012;6:9887–99.
7 Shelley WB, Shelley ED, Burmeister V. Argyria: the intradermal 'photograph,' a manifestation of passive photosensitivity. *J Am Acad Dermatol* 1987;16:211–17.
13 Brouillard C, Bursztejn AC, Latarche C *et al*. Silver absorption and toxicity evaluation of silver wound dressings in 40 patients with chronic wounds. *J Eur Acad Dermatol Venereol* 2018;32:2295–9.

Reactions to thallium

7 Moore D, House I, Dixon A. Thallium poisoning: diagnosis may be elusive but alopecia is the clue. *BMJ* 1993;306:1527–9.

CHAPTER 122

Mechanical Injury to the Skin

Saqib J. Bashir[1] and Ai-Lean Chew[2]

[1] King's College Hospital, King's College Hospital NHS Foundation Trust, London, UK
[2] Beckenham Beacon Hospital, King's College Hospital NHS Foundation Trust, London, UK

Overview of skin injury, 122.1
Determinants of the response to injury, 122.1
Isomorphic (Koebner) response, 122.2
Nikolsky sign, 122.2
Utilisation of mechanical stimuli, 122.3
Biomechanical considerations, 122.3
Mechanical properties of the skin, 122.4
Determinants of mechanical properties of the skin, 122.4
Physiological variation, 122.5
Pathological variation, 122.5
Modifying biomechanical properties of the skin, 122.5
Effects of friction, 122.6
REACTIONS TO MECHANICAL INJURY, 122.7

Callosities, corns and calluses, 122.7
Friction blisters, 122.9
Black heel and palm, 122.10
Skin reactions to musical instruments, 122.11
Hypothenar hammer syndrome, 122.13
Achenbach syndrome, 122.13
Spectacle-frame acanthoma, 122.14
Semicircular lipoatrophy, 122.15
Acne mechanica, 122.15
Dermatoses due to traumatic effects of sports, 122.16
REACTIONS TO FOREIGN MATERIALS, 122.17
Foreign-body reactions, 122.17
Paraffinoma, 122.19

Sclerodermiform reaction to vitamin K and vitamin B_{12} injections, 122.19
Pentazocine ulcers, 122.19
Reactions to intralesional corticosteroids, 122.19
Reactions to silicone, 122.21
Fibreglass dermatitis, 122.21
Complications of tattoos, 122.21
Hair as a foreign body, 122.22
OTHER SKIN INJURIES, 122.24
Hand–arm vibration syndrome, 122.24
Piezogenic pedal papules, 122.26

Key references, 122.27

Overview of skin injury

The skin is constantly subjected to both internal and external mechanical forces, so that for experimental purposes it may be impossible to determine what constitutes the normal resting state. These forces are likely to be as important in the maintenance of the structural integrity of the connective tissues of the dermis [1,2,3] and the keratin intermediate filament network of the epidermis [4] as they are with bone, which becomes demineralised during the protracted absence of normal gravitational force during space travel [5]. Mechanical stretching of keratinocytes induces a hyperproliferative response via the activation of extracellular signal-related kinase [6]. In contrast to events in the whole organism, isolated human dermal fibroblasts in culture make more collagen when subjected to reduced gravity [7]. Many normal biochemical functions of the skin are dependent on appropriate mechanical forces, and when these become excessive, as in lymphoedema, protease inhibitors are released with many deleterious consequences [8].

Healthy skin is well adapted to resist the adverse effects of a wide range of mechanical injuries [9]. These include friction, pressure, contusion, laceration, suction and vibration. The clinical consequence of injury will depend on characteristics of the noxious stimulus, such as its intensity and duration. Factors related to the skin also influence the response; thus, the same degree of friction may produce a blister in one person but no visible change in another. Time is required for adaptive responses, such as callus formation and lichenification, to occur.

When skin is subjected to mechanical stress its properties may be altered, and these changes may make disease more likely. For example, stretched skin can have a higher transepidermal water loss [10].

Determinants of the response to injury

It is likely that racial and genetic factors have a major role in determining the responses to mechanical forces. At extremes of age, the skin has a reduced ability to withstand shear and other forces. Body site can determine how the skin responds, for example friction blisters do not occur on loose skin. The presence and degree of subcutaneous fat will influence the effect of pressure on the skin.

The physiological status of the skin that is being subjected to injury can have a major effect. For example, a moderate degree of sweating hydrates the stratum corneum and increases the coefficient of friction, whereas higher levels of sweating sufficient to produce free fluid on the surface markedly reduce the coefficient of friction. Environmental temperature is also important, as is humidity, the stratum corneum becoming brittle and inelastic when humidity is reduced. The withdrawal response to noxious stimuli is impaired by neurological disorders, such as syringomyelia, and as a result burns and other injuries are common in patients with neurological deficits. Some systemic diseases can result in a qualitatively different response to injury, for example the dermopathy of diabetes, and debilitating disease will increase susceptibility to pressure. The defective organisation of the dermal–epidermal junction or of the superficial dermis seen in the mechanobullous disorders predisposes to blister formation with trivial trauma, and individuals with disorders of the connective tissue, such as Ehlers–Danlos syndrome and Marfan syndrome, show abnormal fragility to mechanical injury. Some drugs, notably corticosteroids, can modify the structural integrity of the skin. Occasionally, structural changes in the skin protect patients from mechanical injury. In amyotrophic lateral sclerosis, pressure ulcers occur less than in comparably bedridden patients, probably because of more dense packing of collagen fibrils [1]. Finally, there seem to be reproducible differences in response between individuals that are poorly understood.

The discussion of mechanical injury to the skin in this chapter is limited to those effects that may concern the dermatologist.

Isomorphic (Koebner) response
Introduction and general description
Koebner originally described the localisation of psoriasis to skin injured by a wide range of stimuli [1] but the term has been used for a similar phenomenon in other diseases [2].

The isomorphic response is the development of lesions in previously normal skin that has been subjected to trauma [1,2]. The response should be reproducible and not limited to one type of trauma. The term Koebner response is best not used when a dermatosis results from the spread of an infective agent (e.g. molluscum contagiosum or warts); for this phenomenon, the term 'pseudo-Koebner' could be used. In the 'reverse' Koebner response, trauma to a lesion results in it resolving. It differs from the isotopic response [3,4], in which a dermatosis occurs at the site of a previous healed and unrelated dermatosis.

Pathophysiology
Many forms of physical trauma, including friction, pressure, incision and laceration, skin grafting, bites, vaccination skin tests, burns, freezing and ultraviolet (UV) and ionising radiation, have been implicated. In addition, many infections of the skin and dermatoses have been associated with the Koebner response.

Pathogenesis
The underlying mechanisms have been most intensively studied in psoriasis (Figure 122.1) [5], in which it seems that the epidermis and dermis both contribute [6] but that epidermal damage is probably a critical event [7]. There is an increased influx of CD4 lymphocytes [8], and the local production of cytokines and adhesion molecules are likely to be important. Little is known about the pathogenesis in other conditions in which the Koebner phenomenon occurs.

Clinical features
A dermatosis develops at a site of trauma. In psoriasis, the Koebner response occurs in about 20% of patients but reported series vary widely [5]. The latency is about 10–14 days, and a Koebner response is more likely to occur when the disease is active. As well as in psoriasis [9], the Koebner response is often seen in lichen planus [2] and vitiligo (Figure 122.2) [10,11–13]. It has been well recorded in many other diseases, some of which are shown in Table 122.1 [14–29].

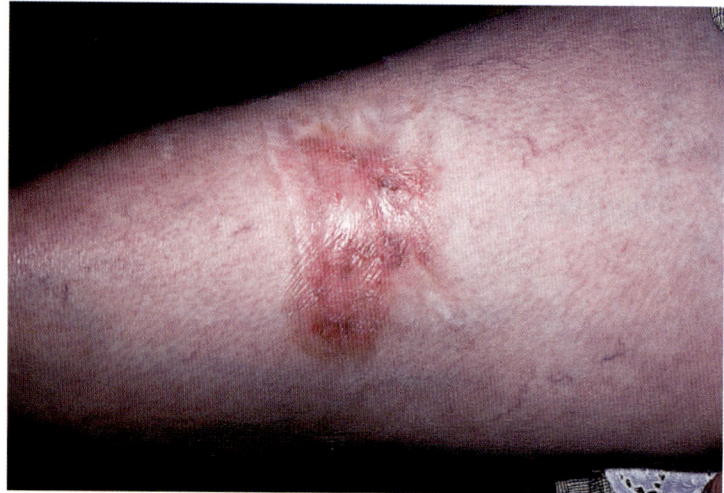

Figure 122.1 Histologically proven psoriasis appearing in a split-skin donor site. Courtesy of Southmead Hospital, Bristol, UK.

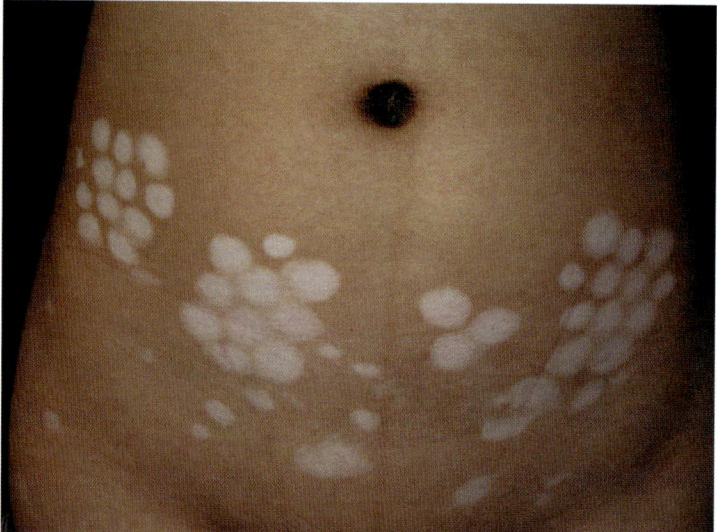

Figure 122.2 Multiple nummular depigmented macules in the donor areas of the abdomen of a 14-year-old girl with vitiligo. Reproduced from Liu and Ma 2019 [30].

It is controversial whether it is appropriate to use the term Koebner phenomenon for the pustular response to injury in Behçet disease and pyoderma gangrenosum; this is usually termed pathergy (Chapter 48). Sacroidosis is known to appear in scars and in some tattoos, however it is not clear that this is a true Koebner response as there may be a long delay of years between the tattoo and the development of the sarcoidosis, or the sarcoidal granulomas may only appear in one colour of the tattoo and spare the remaining tattoo area.

Nikolsky sign
This well-known effect of shearing trauma was originally described as evoking lesions of pemphigus foliaceus (Chapter 50) but may be positive in other bullous diseases such as Stevens–Johnson syndrome and toxic epidermal necrolysis (Chapter 118).

Table 122.1 Diseases showing the Koebner response.

Disease	Reference
Carcinomas	Fisher et al. 1967 [14]
Darier disease	Penrod et al. 1960 [15]
Erythema multiforme	Huff and Weston 1983 [16]
Granuloma annulare	Borgia et al. 2004 [17]
Hailey–Hailey disease	Morales et al. 1966 [18]
Leukaemia	Koizumi et al. 1991 [19]
Lichen planus	See Chapter 37
Lichen sclerosus	Todd et al. 1994 [20]
Lupus erythematosus	Ueki 2005 [21]
Scleromyxoedema	Durani et al. 2001 [22]
Multicentric reticulohistiocytosis	Aldridge et al. 1984 [23]
Necrobiosis lipoidica	Gebauer and Armstrong 1993 [24]
Pemphigus foliaceus	Rotunda et al. 2005 [25]
Perforating collagenosis and folliculitis	Jelinek 1986 [26]
Psoriasis	Farber et al. 1965 [9]
Myxoedema, pretibial	Missner et al. 1998 [27]
Vasculitis	Green and Narajan 1986 [28]
Vitiligo	Sweet 1978 [**10**]
Xanthoma	Miwa and Kanzaki 1992 [29]

Utilisation of mechanical stimuli

Selective use may be made of mechanical stimuli to confirm the diagnosis or to allow for the biopsy of early lesions in conditions in which dynamic changes and secondary effects occur rapidly [1]. Simple frictional trauma, such as that caused by twisting a rubber-tipped pencil on the skin, can be used to facilitate accurate diagnosis of mechanobullous diseases.

The Nikolsky and Koebner phenomena may be used to study the early changes in diseases in which they are characteristic and can be of value in the diagnosis of pemphigus when patients are already on treatment and immunofluorescent techniques are not available [2]. The pustular reaction to skin puncture (including venesection) is evidence of an active stage of Behçet disease. Suction [3,4] evokes bullous diseases and may produce petechiae in scurvy, etc. It has also been used to study vasculitis [5,6].

Firm stroking of the skin may elicit purpura in amyloidosis, is routinely used to diagnose dermographism, and has also been used to study the early lesions of vasculitis [7] and to confirm a diagnosis of delayed pressure urticaria [8].

Biomechanical considerations

Resistance to various mechanical stimuli, both external and arising within the body, is a fundamental property of the skin [**1**,2,3,**4**]. External forces include friction, stretching, compression, vibration and penetration. The major mechanical properties of skin are stiffness (resistance to change of shape), elasticity (ability to recover the initial shape after deformation) and viscoelasticity. Quantification of the behaviour of skin subjected to mechanical forces is complicated by many factors. The skin is composed of not one but multiple and interrelated functional components, and its behaviour is subject to the confounding effects of physiological phenomena, such as the previous experience of the tissue, nutritional status, sweating and sebum excretion. Other variables of practical relevance [5] are related to body site, age, sex and disease – not only cutaneous disease but also systemic (e.g. diabetes). In addition, the mechanical properties of the skin may be profoundly influenced by environmental factors such as UV and heat radiation.

The generation of mechanical forces within the skin and subcutis has long been of interest to surgeons, with early contributions by Langer on the oval shapes produced when round punctures are made in the skin, and the recognition of relaxed skin tension lines [6]. The mechanical qualities of skin, especially creep, are critical to understanding the expansion techniques used in dermatological surgery [7]. The effects of mechanical forces have also been studied extensively in relation to wound healing and the consequences of excess fluid in tissues [8].

In vitro studies have shown that the application of mechanical stress results in increased DNA synthesis [9], the production of collagen and proteoglycans [10] and non-collagenous proteins [11] and cytoskeleton formation. The application of mechanical force intermittently results in more cellular activity than a constant force [12]. Wounds that heal under some stress have greater strength than those where there is no stress [13].

The importance of weight bearing on bones for their normal structural integrity was recognised long ago, and the stress imposed by gravitational forces is also important for the maintenance of dermal constituents [14].

A quantitative analysis of the mechanical properties of skin and subjacent tissues must begin from engineering principles [**1**,15]. Most studies involve the measurement over time of deformation produced by a given constant force. The force is standardised as force per unit area or 'stress'. Stresses perpendicular to the surface are termed normal, whereas those in other directions are termed shearing stresses. The change in dimensions may be expressed as 'strain' and is the ratio between the deformation and the original length. Many elastic materials show a linear relationship between stress and strain, for example:

Stress = Young modulus × strain

Similarly, linear viscous liquids obey the Newton law in which stress is directly proportional to the rate of strain but independent of the strain itself. Many biological materials combine the characteristics of elastic solids and viscous liquids and are termed viscoelastic. Skin, in common with other viscoelastic materials, has non-linear stress–strain properties and has time-dependent behaviour even with low loads [16]. The best known of these are the properties of hysteresis (in which the stress–strain relationships are different between loading and unloading), stress relaxation (the stress resulting from a constant strain decreases with time) and 'creep' (increasing strain or length of the material when a constant stress is maintained). These time-dependent properties are thought in part to be a function of the ground substance. Furthermore, skin shows anisotropic properties; there is a systematic and regular directional variation in its mechanical and viscoelastic properties. The elastic component is broadly analogous to a linear spring and the viscous component to a dashpot shock absorber.

Much of the earlier work on the mechanical properties of the skin was carried out on tissues or their components (collagen, elastin, etc.) *in vitro* [**1**,17]. Strength-related values such as breaking strain, time-dependent creep and non-time-dependent parameters, such as elasticity and viscosity, have been measured, but these studies can be unhelpful in predicting the behaviour of whole skin *in vivo*.

The principal source of mechanical strength in the skin and subcutis is the reticular dermis. The papillary and periadnexal dermis (often known as the adventitial dermis) and the connective tissue running between fat lobules to deeper structures have a somewhat similar although lesser capacity to resist deformation [18], and it is likely that the epidermal components are only relevant in resisting relatively minor forces [2]. At a molecular level, it is the properties of collagen, usually of types I and III, and its relationship with elastic fibres and ground substance that determine the mechanical responses of skin.

Mechanical properties of the skin
Methods of evaluation
Many methods have been used to derive information about the mechanical properties of the skin [1,2,**3**,**4**]. Some have included subcutaneous tissue [5,6]. Most methods measure properties of the dermis, although some give information predominantly about the stratum corneum [7,8], and all have limitations. The following are the main test methods.

1. Tensile tests, in which the skin is extended by applying a force parallel to the surface [9–17].
2. Torsional tests, in which force is used to rotate a disc glued to the skin [**3**,18–20].
3. Vertical traction [7,21–23].
4. Indentation [8,24–26] and nano-indentation [27].
5. Suction within a cup pressed on the skin [28–34].
6. Vibration, for example using the hammer of a ballistometer [35–38].
7. Elastic wave propagation [39].
8. Hardness, using a durometer [40,41].

Because of problems with the standardisation of methods, results are not usually comparable between investigators. Details of methodology, such as the area of skin subjected to suction, are of great importance in understanding which zone of the skin is being evaluated. Results should always be standardised for skin thickness [42,43]. One of the few studies that directly compared different methods concluded that the suction cup device mainly measures elasticity, whereas the ballistometer predominantly measures stiffness [44].

Some of the measurements that can be derived from *in vivo* methods such as torsion [42] and suction [43] can be expressed as ratios, obviating the dependence on skin thickness, and give useful information about the elastic and viscoelastic properties of the skin (Figure 122.3). Despite their shortcomings, the various methods used have led to a general understanding of the mechanical properties of the skin, and quantification of some of these properties has proved useful in the recognition of pathological changes in connective tissues before they have become clinically apparent.

Determinants of mechanical properties of the skin
Stratum corneum
The main function of the stratum corneum is to provide a limited barrier across which exchanges occur with the environment. It consists of dead corneocytes embedded in an extracellular lipid matrix. *In vivo* it is criss-crossed by a series of depressions outlining

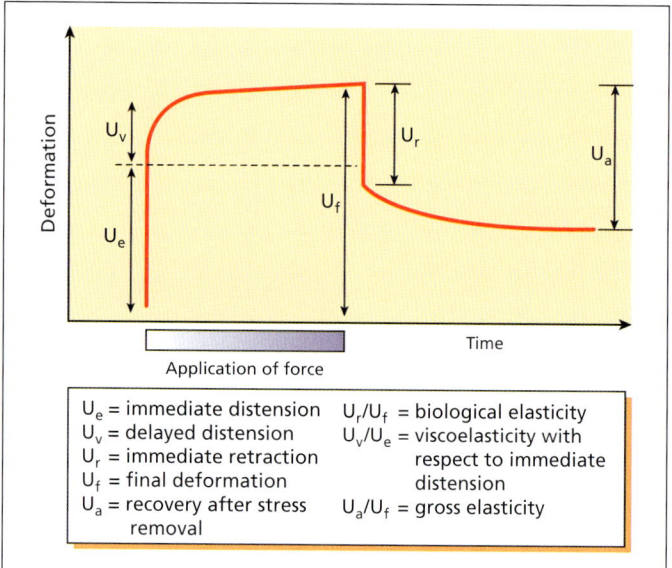

Figure 122.3 Deformation of skin by an applied force showing how elastic and viscoelastic properties can be deduced from ratios of measurements.

polygonal zones. This pattern is anisotropic and related to the anisotropy of the underlying dermis. When subjected to stretch it is only slightly extensible [1], deformation occurring by flattening out or redistribution of these depressions [2]. These changes cause secondary alterations in the shape of the cells in the Malpighian layer and the underlying papillary dermis [2]. The elastic modulus of the individual corneocyte is far higher than of the complete stratum corneum, suggesting that the biomechanical properties of the latter are largely a function of the substances binding the cells to each other [3,4]. Direct measurements of the biomechanical properties of the stratum corneum using nanotechnology methods have recently been published [5].

The extensibility of the stratum corneum is greatly influenced by the relative humidity and its state of hydration [4,6,7–9].

Frictional contact with the stratum corneum is an essential prerequisite for tactile sensation and many physical activities. It is also a cause of a variety of acute and chronic injuries to the skin. The stratum corneum behaves as a viscoelastic membrane when subjected to frictional force. The major component producing friction is a tendency to adhesion at the surface. In general, frictional resistance increases with the state of hydration, although free water or sebum on the surface reduces resistance. The contribution of the stratum corneum towards skin biomechanics can be seen in studies evaluating the effect of moisturisers and emollients. Extensibility and creep were both rapidly increased when water and paraffin oil were applied, and more slowly with glycerine; water only had a very short-term effect [10]. Chemical modification of stratum corneum proteins (e.g. by glutaraldehyde) can also reduce frictional resistance [11].

The important property of the stratum corneum to resist forces that would tend to separate its layers, as occurs with Sellotape stripping, has been studied in various ways [12].

Basement-membrane region
This has been evaluated mainly by suction devices, which can split the skin in this region. It is likely that the basement-membrane

region has a relatively minor role in the overall mechanical integrity of the skin [13], although abnormalities of structural components such as laminin 5 in the lamina lucida cause marked weakening of the skin in some types of junctional epidermolysis bullosa.

Dermis
The dermal collagen bundles are an intermeshing network of undulating fibres (Chapter 3). Although electron microscopic studies show the bundles running in all directions, in the reticular dermis the predominant direction is parallel with the skin surface, and in the adventitial dermis and subcutis the alignment is perpendicular to the surface. The initial response to deformation is a straightening of the collagen bundles and realignment of the straightened fibres in the direction of the applied force. Beyond this, extension may occur through slip between fibrils, a process opposed by the closely associated glycosaminoglycans (Chapter 3). Elastic fibres are responsible for returning the collagen to its predeformation state, particularly with low levels of load [14]. Elastin is the only mammalian protein with truly elastic properties. The interdependence of elastic tissue and collagen has been demonstrated in experiments using selective removal [15]. In addition to collagen, elastin and glycosaminoglycans, α and β integrins are essential for mechanical integrity, and contribute to fibroblast homeostasis [16].

Physiological variation
Age
From about the age of 35 years in women and 45 years in men, the thickness of skin decreases with ageing on light-protected sites and the dermal–epidermal junction becomes flatter [1,2,**3**,**4**]. Many studies, using a variety of techniques, have evaluated the skin at different ages (reviewed in [5]). Although there are some conflicting results, overall there is agreement that there is a decrease in elastic properties with age. It seems likely that there is increasing resistance by the dermis to traction parallel to the skin surface, at least until the age of 60 years, but vertical resistances at the dermal–epidermal junction and within the dermis and subcutis progressively fall. Using a device for the propagation of low-amplitude shear disturbances it has been shown that there is a progressive increase in viscosity of the skin with age [6].

Sex
Again, no clear answer emerges as to whether there is a difference between sexes, except for a decrease in skin thickness and elasticity after menopause. Some methods have shown that female skin is more extensible [7,8,**9**], although others have failed to confirm this [1,10,11]. The increase in extensibility from hydration of the stratum corneum may be greater in women than men [**12**]. Hormone replacement therapy appears to alleviate the loss of elasticity associated with the menopause [13,14].

Body site
There are great differences between body sites, mainly because of differences in skin thickness [**3**,15]. When this is corrected for, skin distensibility and elasticity are lower in the acral areas than centrally, and are subject to diurnal variation, with elasticity increasing in the evening [16]. Elasticity is greater across the epidermal ridges of the fingerpads, a feature that may contribute to their specialised sensory function [17]. These properties contribute resistance to gravitational oedema formation, and are diminished in the elderly.

Using a small suction device, the ratio between viscous deformation and elastic deformation and the biological elasticity (i.e. the ratio between immediate recovery and total deformation) was lower in vulval than in forearm skin [18].

Light exposure
Chronic sun exposure produces a decrease in extensibility, elastic recovery and elastic modulus. The higher the melanin content, the lower the differences between sun-exposed compared with sun-protected sites [**19**]. Sun-exposed facial dermis has both increased thickness and decreased parameters of elasticity [20].

Pathological variation
Various *in vivo* techniques have been used to measure the mechanical properties of the skin in disease states over a period of time. In some situations, the abnormalities predate the clinical changes (as in Raynaud phenomenon when preceding scleroderma [1]). Such measurements clearly have application for monitoring therapy [2]. Examples include scleroderma [3–7] and its treatment [8,9]; the decreased distensibility but unaltered elasticity of scleroderma of Buschke [10,11]; the consequences of corticosteroid atrophy [12,13]; the waxy skin of diabetics [14]; the increased elasticity in acromegaly, broadly related to insulin-like growth factor 1 (IGF-1) levels [15]; the reduced extensibility (photosclerosis) resulting from psoralen and UVA (PUVA) therapy [**16**,17,18]; and an acute increase in elasticity during radiotherapy [19] and in the gravitational syndrome [20]. In neurofibromatosis the skin is hyperextensible, even clinically normal skin to some extent [21]. In lymphoedema there is reduced viscoelasticity [22]. Chronic haemodialysis produces some impairment of the viscous properties of the skin similar to those of ageing [23]. Useful correlations have emerged between biomechanical and genetic differences in diseases of connective tissue such as pseudoxanthoma elasticum [24] and Ehlers–Danlos syndrome [25–27]. Smoking can cause facial wrinkling [28] but the biomechanical correlates have not been defined.

Piérard *et al.* [**16**] have studied the ability of skin to be elongated (skin extensibility) and its capacity to regain the initial position after deformation (biological elasticity) in a number of disease states. Their findings are used in Figure 122.4 to illustrate the principles outlined in this section.

Modifying biomechanical properties of the skin
Understanding these mechanical properties can lead to strategies of modifying them for the treatment of disease or ageing (Chapter 156). This may be possible through dietary manipulation through nutrients or through external treatments such as injectables and laser (Chapters 158 and 161).

One promising method to improve the biomechanical properties of the skin could be the injection of small amounts of hyaluronic acid. Several studies have shown that serial injections of small molecules of hyaluronic acid can increase the elasticity of the skin. This can be seen with both cross-linked and non-cross-linked hyaluronic acid. The injections are typically given in monthly intervals for 3 months, with some of the benefits lasting 4 months or more, but declining with time [1].

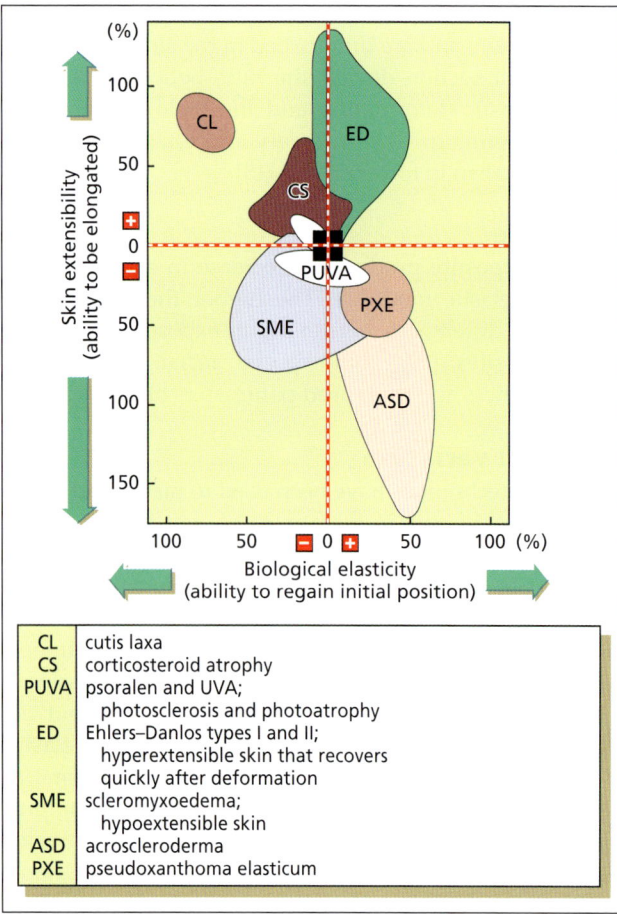

Figure 122.4 Rheological properties of some conditions affecting the dermis. Each area represents data from several patients. From Piérard et al. [16]. Reproduced with permission of MTP Press.

Another emerging method is the ingestion of collagen peptide supplements. These treatments are based on the premise that a large proportion of the skin (and other connective tissues) is composed of collagen. Collagen, while the most abundant molecule, is closely associated with other key skin components, such as hyaluronic acid, elastin, reticulin and cellular components such as immune cells, keratinocytes and melanocytes. Animal- and marine-based collagens, sometimes on their own or supplemented with other vitamins or nutrients, have been shown to bring about measurable changes in the skin's properties. The properties most consistently improved are skin hydration, elasticity, skin density and a reduction in wrinkles. This can be seen with collagen supplementation alone, or combined with a variety of vitamins and nutritional supplements. For example, hydrolysed collagen can combine with coenzyme Q10, which in itself can lead to a reduction in skin wrinkles and increased smoothening. The effect of the collagen supplements may be through increased collagen synthesis by dermal fibroblasts, but may also be due to an increase in hydration as there is also an increased production of hyaluronic acid. These benefits last while the supplements are being taken, up to 90 days in studies, but may decrease 30 days after disontinuation. More studies are required to clarify if there are long-term increases in collagen deposition [2]. It is also possible that the improvements seen are because the collagen peptides have an affect on regulatory T lymphocytes and M2 macrophages, which may suppress an immune response to endogenous collagen [3].

Lasers, both non-ablative and ablative, can increase the amount of collagen and elastin in the dermis, with sustained benefits measured at 12 months. These benefits can be seen as increased elasticity and not just increased extracellular matrix components [4]. As with hyaluronic acid injections and oral collagen supplements, more data are needed about the long-term benefits and in which patient groups these supplements are best targeted.

Effects of friction

Friction is defined as the resistance that any body meets in moving over another. Humans cannot function without friction between themselves and the environment, although even mild degrees of friction can cause distress, as in the unpleasant sensation that wool can induce for an atopic subject. Excessive frictional forces will cause injury, which may be acute, occurring in seconds or minutes, or chronic, as a result of repeated, lesser degrees of friction. The response of the skin will depend on the magnitude and duration of the frictional force applied and properties of the skin itself. Abrasions and friction blisters are examples of acute frictional trauma, but blisters can only form if the stratum corneum is tough and thick enough to form a blister roof. Friction blisters are therefore difficult to produce except on the palms and soles [1]. The chronic effects of friction are dependent on adaptive responses, in particular a steady rate of increase in epidermal turnover, and perhaps the laying down of thickened, vertically orientated collagen bundles in the papillary dermis, as seen in lichenification. The best-defined clinical consequences of chronic frictional injury are calluses and corns, but various forms of dermatitis are perpetuated and perhaps initiated by friction.

The scientific study of friction-induced injury has largely been directed towards understanding friction blister formation. The laws of static friction state that frictional resistance is (i) directly proportional to load; and (ii) independent of the area of contact between the surfaces [2]. The ratio between the force necessary to move one surface over the other and the load between the two surfaces is thus a constant, called the coefficient of friction. The static coefficient of friction is the force required to start one object in motion past another, and the dynamic coefficient is the force required to sustain the motion of one object past another. Because of its viscoelastic properties, skin deviates from the Amonton laws. Several different techniques have been used to measure friction [1,2,3–9,10,11,12,13]. Coefficients of static and dynamic friction have been determined for a number of materials in contact with human skin, with and without lubricants, but there is great individual variation [1,2,14,15]. Of the various anatomical sites measured, the palm of the hand has the highest coefficient of friction [16]. A number of machines to simulate repetitive rubbing have been devised, but there is no entirely satisfactory model for chronic frictional injury [6].

Physiological changes, such as the degree of hydration, have a large effect – very dry or wet skin having a much lower frictional resistance than moderately hydrated skin [17] for most sites but not for the dorsal forearm or lower back [18]. Skin surface lipids have relatively little effect [19]. Petrolatum initially decreases the coefficient of friction because of its lubricating property but then increases it because of its occluding effect on the skin, causing increased hydration [15]. Age and sex have no significant effect on the frictional properties of the skin, but body site is important: the forehead and behind the ear have the highest dynamic coefficient of friction, and the abdomen the lowest [18]. The rough skin in atopics has a lower coefficient of friction than normal [10].

REACTIONS TO MECHANICAL INJURY

Callosities, corns and calluses

Definition and nomenclature
A callosity is a plaque of hyperkeratosis caused by repeated friction and/or pressure. A corn is a sharply demarcated callosity occurring over a bony prominence, usually on the hand or foot, and is painful. A soft corn occurs between the toes. Podiatrists often refer to a corn as a heloma (Greek *helus*, a stone wedge). A callus is a broad-based diffuse area of hyperkeratosis of *relatively* even thickness, usually under the metatarsal heads (Figure 122.5) [1].

Introduction and general description
Calluses and corns on the feet are usually the result of deformity, sometimes associated with dynamic changes in the function of the foot. They are more common in the elderly, in particular in those with high pressures exerted on the plantar skin [2]. They are often made worse or even caused by unsuitable footwear.

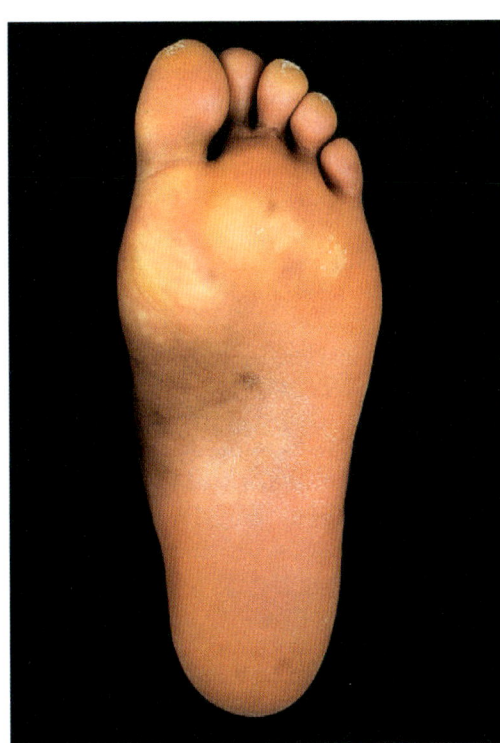

Figure 122.5 Calluses of the forefoot.

Perhaps the most extreme example of footwear causing gross abnormalities is the Chinese foot-binding syndrome, although some western shoe fashions, such as 'winkle-pickers' and high-heeled shoes, can be similarly damaging albeit on a lesser scale [3]. Various intrinsic abnormalities of the foot predispose to callosities. These include bony prominences such as occur with hallux valgus, a prominent condylar projection or malunion of a fracture.

Epidemiology
Age
Calluses may form in all age groups, depending on the predisposing factors to which the patient is exposed.

Sex
Both sexes are prone to callus formation, although the distribution and presentation may vary with social factors such as occupation and hobbies.

Pathophysiology
Predisposing factors
In some rheumatic diseases (e.g. rheumatoid arthritis) there are distinctive patterns of callosity formation which can be predicted from the joints involved [4]. Diabetic subjects, especially those with neuropathy, are prone to callus formation, and high mechanical pressure is strongly associated with ulceration [5]. Faulty foot mechanics can occur when there is a toe deformity (e.g. claw, hammer or mallet toe), a short first metatarsal or hallux rigidus. The dermatologist should be aware of the effects of deformity throughout the foot. In the hindfoot, a varus or valgus position of the heel as an anatomical abnormality will lead to a failure of the foot to absorb loads applied to it during the stance phase of gait. The net result is that excessive loads are applied to the plantar skin, leading to callosities. The pattern of these changes can be very distinctive. With the hindfoot anomaly, there is often an associated forefoot deformity with excessive pronation or supination of the metatarsals, hallux valgus and fixed deformities of the lesser toes. Calluses on the edges of the weight-bearing area of the sole are often caused by shoes that are too loose.

The biomechanics of the foot that lead to callosities have been investigated in detail [6–8]. A variety of measuring devices are available to document the abnormal forces and assist in the design of appropriate orthoses [9].

On the dorsum of the foot, factors provoking callosities include footwear and a habit of sitting with the foot tucked under the body [10,11], with or without a prominent underlying talus. A soft corn usually occurs when tight shoes press the condyle of a metatarsal or phalanx against the base of a phalanx on the adjacent toe.

On the hands and at other sites, callosities generally reflect repeated frictional injury which will be apparent from the history.

Pathology
In a callus, there is epidermal hyperplasia. The stratum corneum is thickened and compact, sometimes with parakeratosis over the dermal papillae, and there may be expansion of the granular layer. The underlying dermis may show an increase in dermal collagen and fibrosis around neurovascular bundles. An increased expression

of adhesion molecules such as corneodesmosin, desmoglein 1 and desmoglein 3, and an increase in the number of proliferating stratum basale cells, are suggested mechanisms for callus formation [12].

A corn differs in that there is a thick parakeratotic plug set in a cup-shaped depression of the epidermis, usually with loss of the granular cell layer.

Genetics

An inherited disposition to callosities has been described, with an autosomal dominant inheritance [13,14].

Clinical features

History

Patients present with thickened areas of skin, gradually progressing over time, which are usually very well localised to the affected area. In some cases, the areas may be tender on direct pressure.

Presentation

Feet [1,5,10,11,13]. On the plantar surface, the most common site for corns and callosities is over the metatarsal heads (Figure 122.5), although the sides of the arches and heel can be involved. A callus is an ill-defined area of waxy, often yellowish, thickening over which the dermatoglyphic markings may become indistinct. A corn is smaller, usually very painful, and may have a glassy centre. Corns can occur within an area of callus. On the dorsum of the foot, corns and calluses are particularly found over the interphalangeal joints and tips of the toes. A distinctive variety of callus occurs over the talus, anteromedial to the lateral malleolus [13]. Calluses and corns can be painful, interfere with mobility and can damage deeper tissues, even causing ulceration.

In the autosomal dominant 'hereditary callosities', blisters occur at the periphery of hyperkeratotic skin [13]. This is distinct from epidermolysis bullosa, epidermolytic hyperkeratosis and blistering sometimes associated with palmoplantar keratodermas.

Soft corns are usually between the fourth and fifth toes, are typically very painful and exhibit hyperkeratosis that becomes white from maceration. A small sinus may be present, and secondary bacterial infection can then present as cellulitis.

Hands. Callosities on the hands most commonly occur as distinctive occupational stigmata in many trades and professions [15,16]. Areas of thickening most commonly occur on the palmar surface and over the metacarpo-phalangeal joints. The site of the callosity may be highly specific [17]. They are rarely complained of, as was shown in a survey of solid-waste handlers in whom there was a 75% prevalence of palmar calluses [18]. Unless they become fissured or infected, they should be considered as an adaptation rather than a disability.

The habit of biting or chewing the side or knuckle of the finger is not uncommon in children ('gnaw warts'). Larger callosities are sometimes seen in those with intellectual disability.

Callosities on the hands caused by frictional injury against the teeth have been described in patients with bulimia nervosa as a result of repeated manual stimulation of the gag reflex [19,20]. A distinctive hyperkeratosis on the side of the thumb can occur with use of a cigarette lighter [21].

Callosities from clothing and appliances. Trusses, especially if ill fitting, may cause circumscribed patches of hyperkeratosis and pigmentation. Pressure from calipers or reinforced shoes may cause calluses in those wearing them.

Clinical variants

Prayer nodules are seen on the forehead of Muslims from repeatedly touching the forehead on a prayer stone [22–24,**25**]. They may also occur on the knees, ankles and dorsa of feet from the squatting position adopted by worshippers. A similar pattern has been described on the ankles from sitting cross-legged [10].

Differential diagnosis

The differential diagnosis includes viral warts, keratoderma, granuloma annulare and knuckle pads.

Investigations

Skin biopsy is rarely indicated.

Management

The major difficulties with diagnosis lie with foot callosities. The patient's footwear and any orthoses, the gait and the alignment of the feet should all be examined. Palpation may reveal abnormal bony prominences. There may be a past history of surgery. Radiography can be helpful. Pressure studies (pedobarographs) can be helpful in evaluating foot biomechanics (reviewed in [**9**,26]).

The aims of treatment are to:
1 Provide symptomatic relief.
2 Determine the source of the abnormal mechanical stress.
3 Relieve the cause by conservative means.
4 Consider surgery if these fail.

Relief of symptoms caused by corns and calluses can usually be achieved by careful and regular paring. Regular paring reduces the pressure induced by corns [27]. The initial procedure is often best done with a scalpel and subsequent treatment with an abrasive device. For soft corns, the use of a toe separator (felt, foam or silicone) can provide rapid relief. Salicylic acid (10–20%) keratolytic preparations can be of some help, but care is needed to avoid irritancy.

The role of the patient's shoes in producing callosities should be carefully assessed, and appropriate corrective steps taken. Extra width may be needed, especially with the toebox. A softer upper may be needed. With marginal calluses, the shoe is likely to be too loose. The shoe may need to be adapted to receive an orthosis – a cushioning device designed to redistribute the mechanical forces causing the callosity. Examples are the metatarsal pad for localised plantar callus, and a medial wedge for the cavovarus foot. Customised shoe inlays can be moved from shoe to shoe. Another useful orthosis is the silicone sleeve that can be used on deformed toes that have corns on them.

Sometimes, conservative measures are insufficient or fail. The surgical correction of toe deformities and resection of prominent condyles causing soft corns can be rewarding. Surgery for other bony causes should only be undertaken after careful study of radiographs and pedobarographs by an orthopaedic surgeon with expertise in the field [28,29]; results can be encouraging [30,**31**], but can also be disappointing [32]. When there is loss of subcutaneous fat, silicone injections are sometimes used [33].

The principles outlined here can be applied to symptomatic callosities elsewhere, for example at sites of abnormal pressure from a limb prosthesis. Occasionally, excision is justified on cosmetic grounds, for example for athlete's nodules [34]. However, surgical debridement of painful calluses in a randomised, blinded study showed no significant improvement in pain scores compared with a sham intervention in elderly patients [35]. Similarly, no improvement was found in rheumatoid arthritis patients undergoing debridement of plantar callosities [36]. In this study, pain scores did not improve compared with sham treatment and localised pressure or gait function was not significantly improved. A multicentre randomised controlled trial of rheumatoid arthritis patients compared standard foot care comprising education, bespoke orthoses and/or provision of footwear with standard care plus scalpel debridement. There was no additional benefit seen in the scalpel debridement group [37].

Nevertheless, simple debridement in combination with a topical application of 1% cantharidin, 30% salicylic acid and 5% podophyllin has been shown to treat calluses effectively, with a 1.4% recurrence rate. This treatment, applied under occlusion, leads to blister formation in about 2 days, with the callus peeling off at day 5. Seventy-nine per cent (57/72) of patients were treated in one session, with the remainder responding to multiple sessions [38].

Friction blisters

Definition
These are blisters that form in response to frictional force applied across the skin surface.

Introduction and general description
In order for friction blisters to occur, the stratum corneum must be strong enough not to be rubbed away. Usually, friction blisters do not form on lax or thin skin but are common on the palm (Figure 122.6), sole, heel or dorsum of the fingers. Frictional force and the number of times an object moves across the skin determine the likelihood of blister development; the greater the force, the fewer the number of cycles of movement needed.

Epidemiology
Incidence and prevalence
The incidence may increase in populations where there is increased mechanical trauma particularly on acral skin. For example, athletes such as long-distance runners or skaters may experience horizontal shearing forces that may split the stratum granulosum [1].

In a study of 872 military personnel serving in Iraq, with a 97% response rate, blister prevalence was self-reported at 33% of which 11% sought medical treatment [2]. The US military study found a 1.55 female : male prevalence ratio, which may be related to wearing boots that were not sufficiently broken in. Other factors identified were age 26–34 years, a past history of blisters and greater than 6 months on active service.

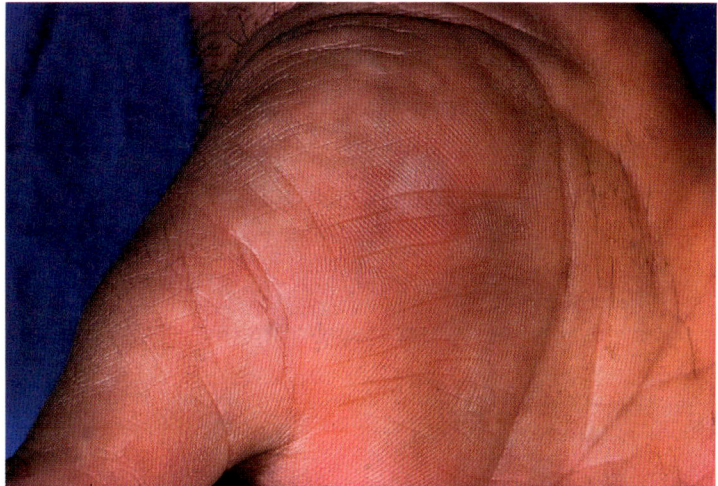

Figure 122.6 Friction blister on the palm mimicking a target lesion of erythema multiforme. This patient had generalised pruritus caused by biliary cirrhosis, and he repeatedly rubbed his thenar eminence on his skin to relieve the itch.

Pathophysiology
Any form of friction applied to the skin with sufficient intensity may cause a blister to form. In the feet, friction between socks and the skin can lead to blistering. This may be exacerbated by increased skin moisture.

Pathology
The blister usually forms in the spinous layer, just beneath the stratum granulosum. The keratinocytes in the base of the blister show variable oedema and perhaps degenerative changes. Mitotic activity commences in the base within 30 h [3,4].

Genetics
Patients with epidermolysis bullosa have a genetic susceptibility to friction-induced blisters (Chapter 69).

Environmental factors
Skin hydration and increased skin temperature may increase the risk of blistering.

Clinical features
History
A careful history of appropriate frictional trauma will usually enable the diagnosis to be made. There are often specific aspects to the circumstances in which blisters occur that are relevant to occupational causes [5]. Other situations, such as sporting activities, may also be relevant.

Presentation
These are usually self-evident and seldom present diagnostic problems when the cause is known. However, a patient may seek advice when a bulla appears unexpectedly or under inappropriate circumstances. It then becomes important for the dermatologist to consider whether the trauma was merely a localising factor in a hitherto undiagnosed congenital or acquired disease (Figure 122.6). As well as blister formation, there may be other consequences of the inciting trauma such as callus formation, petechiae, etc.

Trauma may induce lesions in both acquired and hereditary epidermolysis bullosa. Skin fragility can occasionally be a presenting feature of systemic amyloidosis. The blisters seen in patients comatose from neurological lesions or drug overdose can clinically resemble those caused by friction; however, they differ histologically. Occasionally, bullous insect-bite reactions and other bullous diseases can be confused with friction blisters.

Differential diagnosis
The differential diagnosis includes epidermolysis bullosa, epidermolysis bullosa acquisita and bullous diseases.

Disease course and prognosis
Uncomplicated blisters heal rapidly.

Investigations
These are not usually required.

Management
Preventative measures include the use of antiperspirants [6]; some case studies have shown that these may reduce blistering in epidermolysis bullosa simplex (Weber–Cockayne disease) [7] and in pachyonychia congenita [8]. Although most controlled trials have not shown convincing evidence of benefit [9,10], 20% aluminium chloride hexahydrate in anhydrous ethyl alcohol used for 3 days before hiking can reduce blistering [11], but such preparations may cause irritant dermatitis. Foot powders with the aim of absorbing moisture are another traditional approach [12], but again controlled trials show lack of efficacy [13–15].

By contrast, certain types of synthetic insole can absorb frictional force and reduce blistering, for example Spenco, a closed-cell neoprene material [16,17], and the polyurethane product Poron® [18]. Acrylic socks [19] and the use of a thin polyester sock under a thick, dense, outer sock [20] can reduce blistering. It is likely that subthreshold exposure of the feet to friction reduces the likelihood of blistering [21].

When blistering has occurred, drainage so as to allow the roof to adhere to the base provides relief of symptoms and optimises healing [22]. If the blister has burst and the roof has torn away, the wound should be treated with a non-adherent dressing and protective padding. Hydrocolloid dressings have been used with success [23,24]. There is no evidence to support the use of cyanoacrylate glue in the management of friction blisters [25].

Black heel and palm

Definition and nomenclature
This is pigmentation of the heel or palm secondary to extravasation of red blood cells.

Synonyms and inclusions
- Talon noir
- Calcaneal petechiae

Introduction and general description
The condition results from shear–stress rupture of the papillary capillaries, for example during violent sport, particularly where repeated jumping and sudden stopping or twisting of the heel occur. Similar circumstances explain the occurrence on the palm.

Epidemiology
Age
Young adolescents may be more prone, in addition to athletes and sportspersons.

Sex
Either sex may be affected.

Pathophysiology
Black heel occurs when the repeated shearing force of the epidermis sliding over the dermal papillae results in damage to the papillary dermal capillaries, resulting in intraepidermal haemorrhage.

Pathology
Extravasated erythrocytes may be found in the dermal papillae [1], but often the histological changes are limited to the stratum corneum, where amorphous yellow-brown material may be found in rounded collections having undergone transepidermal elimination. This material is often negative with Perls stain (which stains haemosiderin) but gives a positive benzidine reaction, showing that it is derived from haemoglobin [2,3].

Clinical features
History
The patient may not recall the precise onset, and may therefore not relate the blue-black pigmentation to their own activities. However, a history of participation in sports or other traumatic exposures to the heel will often be elicited.

Presentation
Closely aggregated groups of bluish black specks occur suddenly at the back or side of the heel (Figure 122.7), just above the hyperkeratotic edge of the foot. The metatarsal area has, rarely, been involved. The lesion may resemble a tattoo [4] or even a melanoma [2,5]. Either sex may be affected [2], but the condition is virtually confined to athletic adolescents [6]. Football, basketball, lacrosse and, less often, tennis and squash players are mainly affected. The condition can occur on the hands of weightlifters [7]. Dermoscopy may help visualise subcorneal haemorrhage, revealing a red-black homogeneous pattern or red-black globules at the periphery of the lesion. In cases where a black pigment is seen from haemorrhage, this can be removed by scratching the stratum corneum (Figure 122.8) [8].

When there is a history of a sudden appearance of the pigmented lesions at a typical site, diagnosis is rarely in doubt. Occasionally, melanoma or atypical melanocytic hyperplasia [9] will need to be excluded.

Differential diagnosis
This includes malignant melanoma (acral type) and viral warts which can be haemorrhagic.

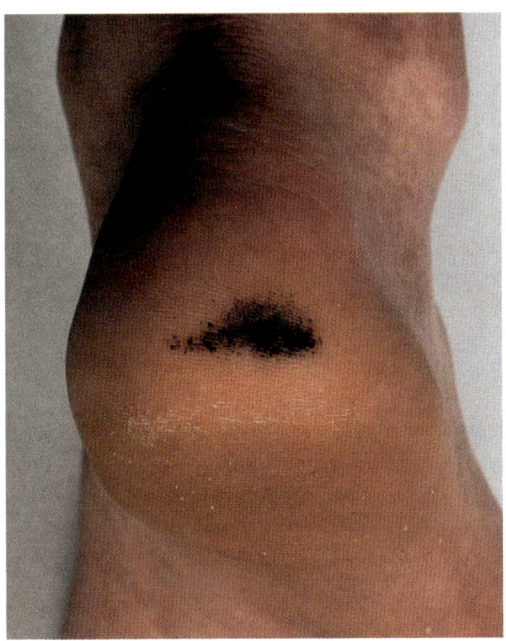

Figure 122.7 Black heel showing stippled pigmentation within the stratum corneum.

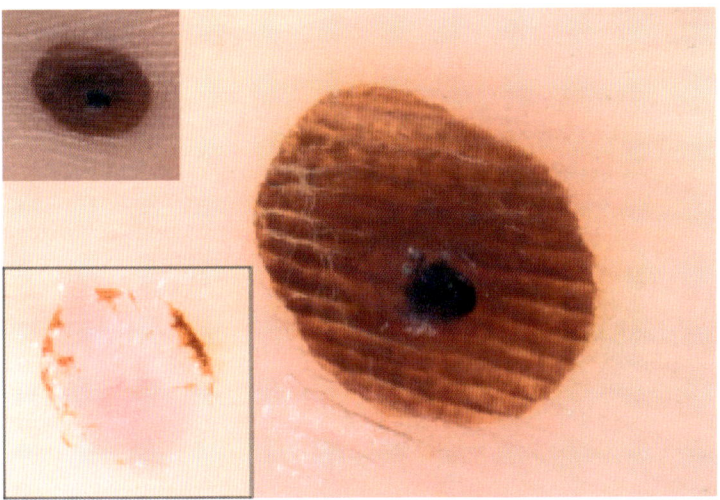

Figure 122.8 Dermoscopy of a subcorneal haematoma showing a parallel-ridge pattern. This is typified by a brownish pigmentation aligned along the ridges of the skin markings that are thicker than the non-pigmented furrows. A blotch of black homogeneous pigmentation is also seen in the centre. Scratching of the stratum corneum, performed using a scalpel, allowed an almost complete removal of the pigmentation (bottom inset). The clinical appearance of the lesion is shown in the upper inset (original magnification 10×). Reproduced from Zalaudek et al. 2004 [8] with permission of John Wiley & Sons.

Investigations

By epiluminescence microscopy, black heel has highly specific features [10]. Sharply demarcated reddish brown or reddish black pigmentation may be seen. This can appear as pebble-like droplets, in the ridges of the skin, with no pigment network.

A skin biopsy may be required to rule out melanoma, depending on the clinical history and appearance.

Management

The condition is asymptomatic, and its importance lies in its resemblance to malignant melanoma. When in doubt as to the diagnosis, carefully paring away the stratum corneum is generally sufficient to remove the pigment.

Skin reactions to musical instruments

Definition and nomenclature

These are skin surface changes that may occur following the repetitive movements made by musicians.

Synonyms and inclusions
- Clarinettist's cheilitis
- Fiddler's neck

Introduction and general description

The prolonged hours of practice required of musicians, whether professional or amateur, predispose them to a variety of medical complaints, such as musculoskeletal overuse injuries. Dermatologically, the repetitive movements required in instrument practice may result in skin changes caused by or exacerbated by repetitive friction or pressure, although contact allergy should not be overlooked. Differences in presentation depend on the instrument and the body site involved.

Epidemiology

Incidence and prevalence

In a self-reported questionnaire study of German university-level music students, 22% (89/412) of respondents reported skin changes related to their instrument [1]. Callosities were seen in 58%, contact dermatitis in 19% and skin reactions of the neck in 19%. In this group, 26% of respondents reported that this slightly or moderately altered their music making, with only 2% reporting severe disease.

Sex

In the German university study, the greatest difference between the sexes was noted in the string/plucking instrument group, where the female : male ratio was 42 : 19, but this may simply represent the demographic of the responders (115 female to 66 male) [1].

Pathophysiology

The pathophysiology of most skin reactions to musical instruments is callosities, lichen simplex chronicus-type reaction or irritant contact dermatitis with repeated friction or pressure at the site of contact as an exacerbating factor. Allergic contact dermatitis is an important differential diagnosis.

Predisposing factors

The predisposition depends on the instrument being played and individual susceptibility. Faulty technique, sweating or excessive hours of playing are aggravating factors.

Clinical features

History
Patients present with lichenificaton, hyperpigmentation, redness, swelling, papules, pustules and, occasionally, cysts, depending on the instrument and the body site.

Presentation
These have been reviewed by type of instrument [2,3,4] and by type of causative injury [5,6]. One study was prospective [7]. Mechanical injuries can be acute (e.g. redness, blisters and erosions) but are more commonly chronic, resulting from repetitive friction and/or pressure between the musician and the instrument. In some situations, cutaneous reactions to musical instruments can be aggravated by sweating, faulty technique or excessive hours of playing. Not only the skin but also bony and soft tissues can be affected, and in younger wind instrument players there can be permanent distortion of dentition and palatal morphology. Trauma to the fingers can also damage nails and associated tissues.

Contact allergies in musicians are usually to rosin (string instruments), exotic woods (string instruments, woodwind instruments, chin rests), nickel (flute, brass instruments), cane reeds (saxophones, clarinets) or to propolis (violin varnish) [4,8].

Violin and viola players may develop 'fiddler's neck' [9], characterised by localised plaques of lichenification, often with hyperpigmentation, redness, inflammatory papules, pustules and sometimes cysts. Marked oedema may be associated in some cases [10]. The condition occurs at the site where the chin rest of the instrument presses against the skin over the angle of the jaw (Figure 122.9). The mode of grip on the instrument and the fitting of the chin rest are likely causative factors and a soft cloth may ameliorate a poor fit in the short term [11]. Violinists are also subject to developing thickened pads over the interphalangeal joints (Garrod pads or 'fiddler's fingers'). These are areas of thickening over the dorsal aspect of the left second and third proximal interphalangeal joints. They may result from the intermittent relaxation and contraction of the extensor tendon over an interphalangeal joint that is held in extreme flexion [12]. Thrombosis of the axillary and subclavian veins has occurred from pressure from a viola [13]. Pizzicato paronychia is another hazard for string players.

Finger callosities occur on the pulps of the fingers of many musical instrument players. A typical example is 'harpist's fingers', which usually show paronychia and calluses on the sides and tips of the fingers, often together with onycholysis and subungual haemorrhage [14].

Piano paronychia is associated with long hours of piano playing, and nails can be loosened by repetitive glissando (gliding of fingers over the keys).

'Guitar nipple' is usually found in young girls and presents as an inflamed cystic swelling at the base of the nipple [15]. Deep-vein thrombosis has been described in guitarists as a result of a combination of flexion of the left leg with pressure from the belly of the guitar on the medial aspect of the thigh [16]. Acro-osteolysis has been described in the digits of the left hand, the only symptom being tenderness in relation to pressure on the nails [17].

Cellists can develop a condition known as 'cellist's chest' [18] from pressure, producing redness, oedema and pigmentation over the sternal area. There may be changes similar to those found on violinists' necks. 'Cellist's knee' and even 'cello scrotum' have been described, although the validity of the latter has been questioned [19]. In fact, Baroness Murphy and her husband confessed that this was a hoax, publishing a retraction in 2008 [20] and themselves casting doubt on the aforementioned 'guitarist's nipple'.

'Clarinettist's cheilitis' [21,22] is a localised eczematous condition of the middle portion of the lower lip, under the reed of the clarinet. Patch testing is usually negative, ruling out an allergy, and is thought to be secondary to friction, pressure, shearing forces and occlusion.

'Flautist's chin' [23] is probably similar to 'fiddler's neck'.

Wind instrument players can develop permanent laxity of the cheeks, and forceful blowing of the trumpet can rupture the orbicularis oris (Satchmo syndrome) [24].

'Drummer's digit' is an erosion or blister on the left ring finger [25].

Black dermographism of the lip has been described in a flute player using a lotion containing zinc oxide, titanium dioxide, iron oxides and talc [26].

Differential diagnosis
This includes allergic contact dermatitis and localised skin infection.

Management
A period of refraining from playing is recommended if possible. Patch testing may be required to identify potential allergens. In many cases, modification of technique may be all that is required to resolve skin reactions in musicians. For more recalcitrant cases, particularly in irritant or allergic contact dermatitis, topical corticosteroids or topical calcineurin inhibitors may be used. In cases of allergic contact dermatitis, substitution of the allergenic component of the instrument may be possible. Callosities may be reduced by emollients, keratolytics and gentle abrasion with a pumice stone.

Resources

Gambichler T, Boms S, Freitag M. Contact dermatitis and other skin conditions in musicians. *BMC Dermatol* 2004;4:3.

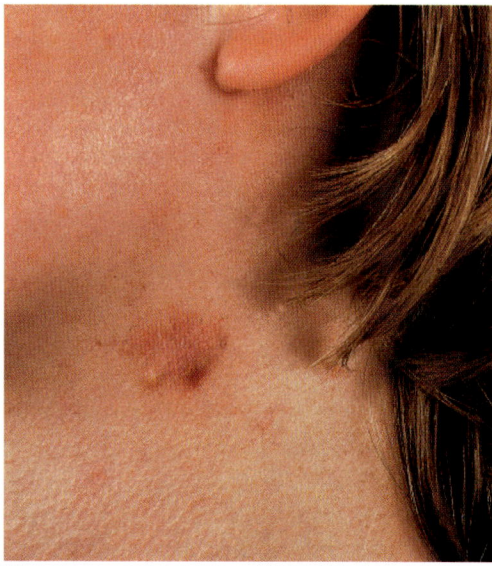

Figure 122.9 'Fiddler's neck'. Lichenification and cysts on the neck of a violinist. Courtesy of Dr R. D. G. Peachey, Bristol Royal Infirmary, Bristol, UK.

Hypothenar hammer syndrome

Definition
Hypothenar hammer syndrome is ischaemic and neurological changes in the digits in the distribution of the ulnar artery, following repetitive trauma.

Introduction and general description
This condition is brought about by the effects on the ulnar artery and associated soft tissues of repetitive trauma to the hypothenar eminence [1]. It is typically associated with actions that use the hand to hammer, push or squeeze.

Epidemiology
This syndrome is mainly found among individuals in certain craft occupations, such as mechanics and carpenters, but can also occur as a sporting injury (e.g. in golf and badminton) [2] and may present in those using a vibrating tool [3].

Age
The condition tends to present in the mid-forties [4].

Sex
Among manual workers, most patients are male.

Associated diseases
Surprisingly, common risk factors for peripheral vascular disease, such as hypertension, diabetes and hyperlipidaemia, are not over-represented in affected cohorts.

Pathophysiology
The proposed pathogenesis is that the superficial palmar branch of the ulnar artery is compressed against the hook of the hamate and this can lead to stenosis, occlusion or aneurysm, with thrombosis or emboli ensuing. Although the condition typically presents unilaterally, the presence of bilateral abnormalities when patients are investigated suggests that there is an underlying predisposition [5].

Clinical features
Presentation
Patients present with pain or paraesthesia and variable degrees of ischaemic change, including blackened eschar formation on the ends of the second, third, fourth or fifth digits of the dominant hand. There may be surrounding hyperkeratotic changes [6]. Fingers affected by the underlying vascular pathology are cooler, and may show other signs of chronic ischaemia.

Differential diagnosis
The condition is often misdiagnosed as hand–arm vibration syndrome [7] (see section later in this chapter), a connective tissue disease or some other vaso-occlusive disorder.

Complications and co-morbidities
Some patients have co-morbidity factors such as smoking and cold exposure.

Investigations
Investigations should include arteriography, which can demonstrate stenosis, occlusion, aneurysm, etc. and provide essential information for vascular surgical repair. Magnetic resonance angiography is proving to be a highly informative and minimally invasive method of evaluation [8].

The Allen test may be used to demonstrate signs of chronic ishaemia: the ulnar and radial artery are both compressed, while the fist is repeatedly clenched and relaxed to drain blood from the hand. One of the ateries is released and the rate of reperfusion of the hand can be observed. This is repeated so both the ulnar and radial arteries are tested. A 'negative' test indicates poor perfusion from that vessel. This serves as a quick clinical assessment but can be enhanced with the addition of pulse oximetry to look for loss of the waveform, or more advanced tests such as Doppler ultrasound, computed tomography or magnetic resonance angiography.

Management
First line
Management includes counselling to avoid repetitive trauma, to minimise exposure to the cold and to stop smoking.

Second line
Aspirin and calcium-channel blockers may be helpful.

Third line
Vascular surgical expertise will generally be required for thrombolytic measures or resection of the abnormal vasculature and appropriate reconstruction.

Achenbach syndrome

Definition and nomenclature
This is a sudden, painful, bluish discoloration and swelling of a finger or fingers (or sometimes the palm of the hand), often after a physical effort of gripping or twisting [1].

> **Synonyms and inclusions**
> - Paroxysmal finger haematoma
> - Finger apoplexia

Epidemiology
Sex
A female preponderance has been reported [2], with some reports of familial links spanning two generations [3].

Associated diseases
Raynaud phenomenon may be associated.

Pathophysiology
It is probably caused by the rupture of a small vein.

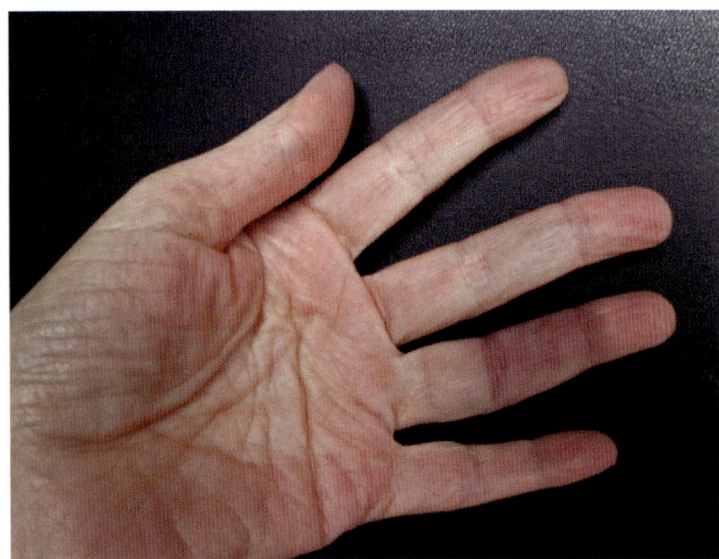

Figure 122.10 Typical appearance of Achenbach syndrome with blue discoloration and swelling localised to a single finger. Reproduced from Moss and Cohen 2022 [5].

Clinical features
History
Patients may present with a sharp pain in the hand, particularly the volar aspect of the finger, accompanied by a rapid bluish discoloration of the affected digit (Figure 122.10). This may occur after minor trauma or light manual work, but may be recurrent and force the patient to withdraw from work involving manual tasks.

Prominent phlebectasia may be seen on the volar aspects of the fingers, over the interphalangeal joints.

Differential diagnosis
Its importance is that it may be confused with the Raynaud phenomenon.

Disease course and prognosis
The condition is self-limiting and resolves within a few days.

Investigations
There may be angiographic abnormalities in some patients [4] but generally invasive investigations are not warranted in uncomplicated self-limiting cases.

Management
Rest the affected limb and cool the area to reduce the swelling. Avoid trigger activities.

Spectacle-frame acanthoma

Definition and nomenclature
This condition is a skin change at the site of contact with the spectacle frame, often with a lesion that mimics basal cell carcinoma.

Synonyms and inclusions
- Granuloma fissuratum of the ear
- Acanthoma fissuratum

Introduction and general description
Spectacle-frame acanthoma is characterised by localised skin thickening in response to low-grade, chronic pressure from spectacle frames [1]. It is often unilateral and occurs in the postauricular groove, or on the bridge of the nose, and is commonly mistaken for a basal cell carcinoma.

Epidemiology
Sex
In a review of 27 published cases, males predominated [2].

Pathophysiology
Friction between the skin and spectacles frame at the postauricular fold, or the lateral nose, can lead to localised epidermal hyperplasia.

Predisposing factors
Factors that contribute to the pathogenesis include the weight of the spectacles, minor derangement in local anatomy and maceration.

Pathology
Histology shows acanthosis and hyperkeratosis of the epidermis, with a central depression and occasionally ulceration. In the dermis, there is often hyalinisation of the collagen and a mild, mixed inflammatory infiltrate [2]. Granulomatous change is not usually present.

Clinical features
Presentation
The typical lesion occurs behind the ear or on the side of the nose [3–5] as a soft, flesh-coloured papule, nodule or plaque, often with a groove at the site where there is contact with the spectacle frame (Figure 122.11). Cases with bilateral involvement are uncommon [6].

Differential diagnosis
Basal cell carcinoma should be considered as a differential diagnosis.

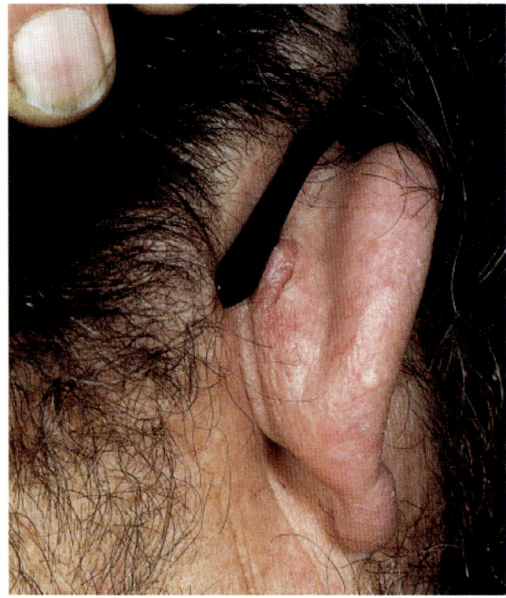

Figure 122.11 Spectacle-frame acanthoma showing a soft plaque, which may mimic basal cell carcinoma, caused by pressure and friction from the spectacle frame.

Investigations
A biopsy to exclude basal or squamous cell carcinoma should be undertaken if there is clinical suspicion.

Management
First line
Spectacle-frame acanthoma usually resolves after a few weeks or months if the patient discontinues wearing spectacles or changes are made to obviate the mechanical trauma. For example, a thin hydrocolloid or silicone dressing may be applied to the overlying skin as a cushion.

Second line
Corticosteroids may be injected intralesionally.

Third line
If necessary, the condition can be treated by surgical excision, electrosurgery and curettage.

Semicircular lipoatrophy

Definition and nomenclature
Semicircular lipoatrophy is caused by mechanical injury to the subcutaneous fat inducing band-like depressions in the skin.

Synonyms and inclusions
- Lipoatrophia semicircularis

Introduction and general description
It should be noted that mechanical injury to the subcutaneous fat, especially on the lower legs, can be a primary cause of fat injury [1,2]. It is often followed by atrophic changes. Since the initial report [3], relatively few cases of semicircular lipoatrophy have been reported, but it is asymptomatic so may be underreported; several authors have commented that it may well not be rare [4].

Epidemiology
Age and sex
It mainly occurs in women, aged between 20 and 40 years.

Clinical features
History
Repetitive mild trauma has been suggested as causative in most cases. In one series, seven women of different heights and body mass index working in the same office all developed the condition at the same vertical distance from the floor, corresponding to the height of the edge of their desks; pressure against this edge was postulated to have caused the semicircular lipoatrophy [5]. Pressure from folds in trousers has also been implicated [6]. Leaning on the edge of a table/desk while working/passing files to colleagues seems to be a common theme in many of the reported cases. Semicircular lipoatrophy on the thighs can also occur following therapeutic injections [7].

Presentation
Semicircular lipoatrophy is characterised by one or more partial, horizontal, band-like depressions, usually on the anterolateral thigh or thighs.

Management
When a cause is identified and remedial action taken, spontaneous resolution generally occurs [5], in most cases after 9 months to 4 years.

Acne mechanica

Definition and nomenclature
Acne mechanica is a localised acneform eruption induced by occlusion or friction [1].

Synonyms and inclusions
- Stump acne

Introduction and general description
Most cases of acne mechanica in the literature refer to patients who are using a medical device such as a prosthetic stump or crutches, or to athletes who are experiencing friction from the use of equipment and protective clothing.

Pathophysiology
Friction with heat, increased humidity and maceration may cause an acneform folliculitis in susceptible individuals. The effect of occlusion has been proposed to lead to the rupture of microcomedones that are not ordinarily clinically visible [1].

Clinical features
Presentation
Right-handed students may have predominantly left-handed facial acne from pressure of the left hand. High-necked jerseys, shoulder pads, seat backs in trucks or even adhesive plasters may produce the required mechanical stress. Some athletes are prone to this condition [2]. Acne mechanica has also been described in other circumstances, for example on the backs of young patients lying in hospital beds for several weeks, and on the face following jaw splinting [3] and with the use of orthopaedic crutches [4]. The resultant acne can be severe (e.g. acne conglobata occurred on the buttocks in a trans-Atlantic rower) [5].

Management
Devices in contact with the skin should be removed as soon as they are not in use. For example, sports equipment should be removed immediately after the activity is over. Benzoyl peroxide, applied for 5 min, can be used to clean the skin prior to being rinsed off [2]. Topical retinoids may be applied at night [6]. Other keratolytics may be useful, such as 3% salicylate and 8% resorcinol in 70% ethanol [2].

Dermatoses due to traumatic effects of sports

Definition
Skin conditions related to sport include mechanical injuries and other direct consequences of the sporting activity.

Introduction and general description
The traumatic dermatoses induced by sports have been usefully reviewed in terms of disease processes [1] and the causative sports [2,3]. While the professional sportsperson and trainer may be well aware of these skin conditions, the amateur may not recognise any connection and even the dermatologist may at times be puzzled. Some of the clinical entities are highly characteristic. The skin adapts to training, developing a higher degree of 'elastic efficiency', but this requires time and continuity in the chosen sport. Many traumatic effects occur in the 'weekend jogger' or the summer holiday activist. The wheelchair athlete is particularly prone to blisters and pressure injury [4,5].

Some of the dermatoses affecting those engaged in sports are an indirect consequence of trauma. These include infections commonly transmitted by contact [6,7], such as herpes simplex [8], molluscum contagiosum [9] and tinea corporis [10,11]. Other infections that appear to be more common include viral warts [12], impetigo and furunculosis [13]. The sport of mud-wrestling has been associated with Gram-negative folliculitis [14]. Tinea pedis, often in a mixed infection with Gram-negative bacteria, is a common problem particularly in those using swimming pools. Otitis externa is also an important problem for the swimmer (Chapter 106). Trauma together with heat and moisture are likely contributory factors to contact dermatitis acquired during various sporting activities [15,16].

The sports enthusiast is often at significant risk from sunburn and skin cancer or cold injury. In hot conditions, miliaria and hyperhidrosis can be problems. There are many circumstances in which contact dermatitis can occur – from sports equipment, environmental allergens, etc. [3,16,17]. Sporting activities can exacerbate pre-existing skin disease, such as atopic dermatitis, psoriasis, acne and other skin diseases. The spectrum of sports-related skin disorders also includes the consequences of anabolic steroid misuse, physical urticarias, exercise-induced anaphylaxis [18] and leukocytoclastic vasculitis [19].

Clinical features

Blisters. These usually result from violent or unaccustomed localised friction, and are most common on weight-bearing surfaces; in the wheelchair athlete, this includes the back [5]. Heat and humidity favour the development of blisters. Preventative measures and the management of friction blisters are discussed earlier in this chapter.

Haemorrhagic effects. Black heel (calcaneal petechiae) [20] is described earlier in this chapter. It is particularly common after sports where there are sudden stops, such as basketball. A similar condition, 'black palm', can occur in weightlifters [21] and is occasionally seen in golf and tennis players. Petechiae around the ankle in a long-distance runner have been described [22]. Annular purpura can occur when the skin is struck by a table tennis ball ('ping-pong patch') [23]. Annular purpura of a different type has been described in association with step aerobics, where annular purpuric lesions developed on the legs [24]. Subungual haematoma, sometimes preceded by redness, oedema and a throbbing pain, is common among racket-sport enthusiasts ('tennis toe') [25] and runners ('jogger's toe') [26]. Splinter haemorrhages have been seen in golfers [27]. Tennis toe most often affects the first or second toe, whichever is the longer, and the symptoms and signs may mimic a fracture. Jogger's toe tends to involve the third, fourth or fifth toe. Hyperpigmentation resulting from small ecchymoses of the skin on either side of the upper portion of the gluteal cleft is a distinctive finding in long-distance runners, and has been called 'runner's rump'. It is caused by contact between the buttocks while running [28]. Auricular haematoma may affect athletes in close contact, for example in wrestling, boxing and judo. This is caused by shearing forces separating the perichondrium and cartilage leading to the accumulation of blood and serum.

Abrasions. These are common in many sports but are particularly associated with contact with wrestling mats [29,30] and artificial turf, which can also produce 'turf toe'. Abrasions from the use of skateboards are also common [31].

Acute inflammation. 'Turf toe', a painful condition in which there is oedema and redness over the dorsal aspect of the great toe with acute tendonitis of the flexor and extensor tendons, frequently occurs in athletes playing on artificial turf [32,33]. 'Jogger's nipples' occurs in women who run without brassieres [34], but also in men who wear shirts consisting of coarse fibres. It may be more prevalent when ambient conditions are cool, making the nipples erect, and when the skin is moist from sweating, increasing frictional resistance. A similar condition can be seen in competitive cyclists, but it has been suggested that the injury is thermal rather than the result of friction [35].

Corns and calluses. Many sporting activities result in calluses and corns. Some special examples include 'pulling boat hands' [36] in which there is an additional effect of cold injury, and 'rower's rump' [37]. When calluses or corns are a problem on the feet in runners, it is important to consider basic biomechanical principles of the foot, which may require specialist orthopaedic intervention.

Athlete's nodules. An entity sometimes known as 'surfer's nodules' or 'athlete's nodules' can present on the anterior tibial prominence [38], dorsa of the feet or knuckles [39]. These asymptomatic nodules show dermal fibrosis as well as epidermal hyperplasia. Knuckle pads can occur at this site but these fail to resolve when the athletic activity is discontinued [40]. A similar ovoid, largely dermal nodule occurring in the sacro-coccygeal area of Japanese students has been attributed to pressure from the bicycle saddle over a distinctive abnormally posteriorly projecting sacrum [41,42].

Other frictional effects. Acne mechanica is common in many participants in sports [43] and may precede acne keloidalis nuchae in football players [44]. This may be caused by protective clothing such as helmets, masks and pads and lead to a localised acneform eruption caused by a combination of pressure, friction, occlusion and heat [45].

'Swimmer's shoulder' is a transient red plaque caused by friction from an unshaven face during freestyle swimming [46].

Intertrigo of the groins is a frequent problem in the heavily muscled athlete. 'Judo jogger's itch' [47] occurred while jogging following vigorous judo, but may be a manifestation of a dry skin subjected to abnormal physical and climatic trauma. A distinctive eruption of symmetrical, red, linear plaques on the palms has been described in children, resulting from grabbing the floor and walls of the pool while swimming underwater [48].

'Mogul skier's palm' consists of hypothenar ecchymoses from repetitive planting of ski poles [49]. 'Hooking thumb' is unique to competitive weightlifters and consists of abrasions, haematomas and calluses on the distal third of the thumb [50].

Miscellaneous. Striae distensae have been associated with weightlifting [51,52]. The areas of skin most frequently involved are the anterior shoulders, lower back and thighs. Painful piezogenic pedal papules and muscle herniation have been ascribed to sporting activities [53,54]. 'Bicyclist's vulva' is a unilateral lymphoedema resulting from repeated chafing and folliculitis; investigations showed previously unrecognised abdomino-pelvic lymphatic abnormalities [1].

REACTIONS TO FOREIGN MATERIALS

Foreign-body reactions

Definition
This is a host immune response, typically granulomatous, to exogenous material within the skin.

Introduction and general description
The term foreign-body reaction is used for this tissue response but may also be used for other patterns of pathological response to extraneous materials that become deposited in the skin or deeper tissues. This is usually as a result of direct penetration of the skin by the material itself, during surgery or by injection. Epidermis, hair and nail can induce a 'foreign-body' response if implanted in or beneath the dermis.

Some extraneous materials (e.g. silica, zirconium) incite a characteristic pattern of granulomatous reaction in which a distinctive type of multinucleate giant cell, the foreign-body giant cell, is prominent.

Pathophysiology
The biological response to a foreign body will depend on its composition, how it enters the body, the body site, the quantity of material and its physical form. In some instances (e.g. mercury and some animal and vegetable matter), a toxic or allergic reaction can occur as well as a later foreign-body reaction. Some reactions are complicated by infection, especially traumatic inoculation of wooden splinters and vegetation spines, which can introduce sporotrichosis and deep mycotic organisms as well as more common pyogenic infections. Infection may also localise to sites of inert foreign bodies during bacteraemia [1]. When material has penetrated the skin there is usually a phase of acute inflammation in response to the injury. This may be necrotising if there is significant trauma, toxin release or bacterial infection. Persistence of foreign material results in the accumulation of monocytes, the evolution of these into tissue macrophages, epithelioid histiocytes and giant cells (Langhans and foreign-body type) and a fibroblastic reaction with laying down of new connective tissue around the area of foreign-body deposition.

Penetration injury can also result in implantation cysts mixed with granulomatous response.

Polarisable foreign bodies can be seen in biopsies of otherwise typical sarcoidosis, and if adequate criteria are met for a diagnosis of sarcoidosis, such foreign-body material does not alter the diagnosis [2].

Pathology
The classic histopathology of a foreign-body reaction consists of foreign-body granulomas, containing multinucleate giant cells, with haphazardly arranged nuclei, interspersed with neutrophils and necrotic debris (Figure 122.12). The granulomas may contain foreign bodies such as suture material, talc, tattoo pigment, hair, etc. Polarised light microscopy and special stains should be considered when a foreign-body reaction is suspected.

Clinical features
Presentation
The clinical presentation will depend on the mode of entry and nature of the foreign body, the tissue response to it and whether there is associated infection. In some instances, there may be characteristic toxic effects (e.g. absorption of mercury from a broken thermometer) [3], pharmacological effects (e.g. resulting from alkaloids in blackthorn) [4] or allergic responses (e.g. to oils and resins in some woods).

Retained foreign bodies are commonly associated with bacterial infection, which tends to be resistant to antibiotic therapy. Vegetative foreign bodies may be associated with fungal infection. Soft-tissue infections may manifest as cellulitis, an abscess or a draining sinus. A wound that fails to heal or continues to cause pain with movement may suggest the presence of a foreign body, as can the persistence of a purulent discharge.

Many types of foreign body elicit a granulomatous response, seen clinically as reddish brown or purple papules, nodules or plaques. The lesions often become harder over time because of fibrosis. Some materials result in discharge even when there is no infection (e.g. paraffins and other oils).

The implanted material may produce pigmentary change (e.g. carbon and metals result in a tattoo-like, black or bluish black colour). A metallic foreign body rich in iron can present as a black skin lesion and be mistaken for a melanoma [5].

Clinical presentation can be modified by epidermal cyst formation, resulting from pieces of epidermis being carried in by a penetrating foreign body. It is important to recognise that even small external signs of entry of a foreign body can denote significant damage to deeper structures, such as tendons, joints and bones. This

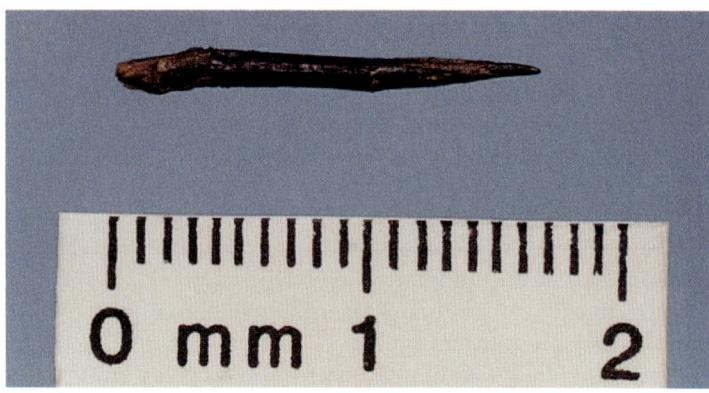

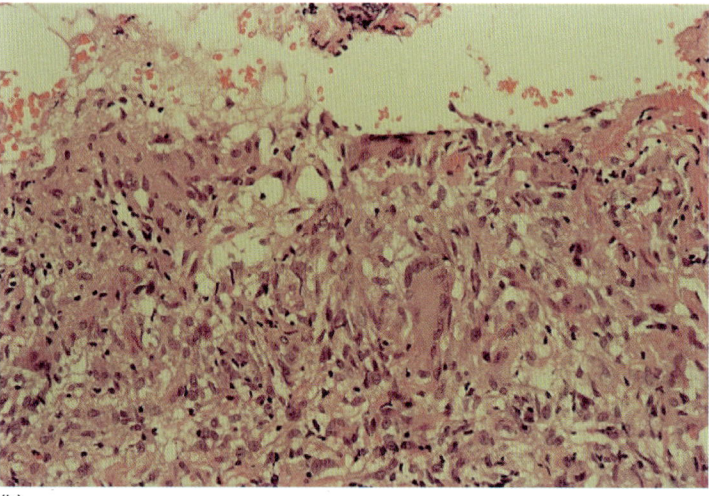

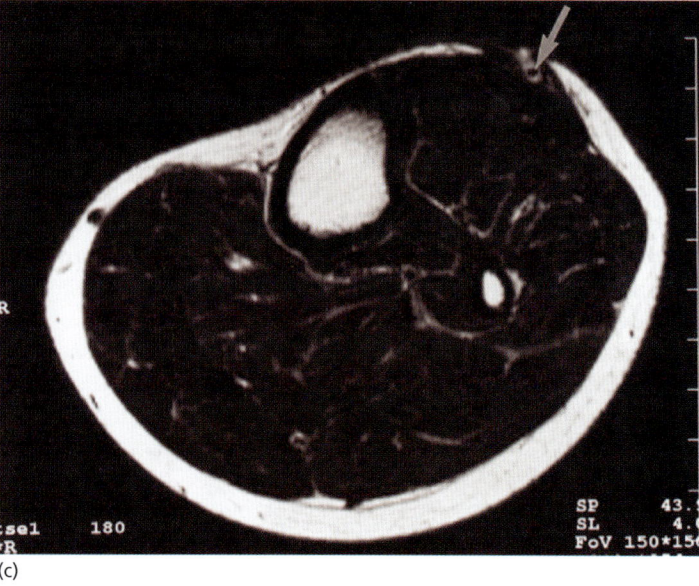

Figure 122.12 Foreign-body reaction caused by a deeply embedded thorn. The patient presented with a chronic leg ulcer. (a) Thorn that eventually emerged spontaneously. (b) Mixed inflammatory and granulomatous reaction from the ulcer bed. (c) Magnetic resonance imaging scan showing the sinus tract containing the thorn (in cross-section, at tip of arrow).

is especially true of high-pressure injection (grease, paint, water and some firearm injuries).

A careful history surrounding any suspected penetrating injury is essential, taking into account the timing and the type of material involved. Patients with a foreign body implanted into the skin may have discomfort at the wound site. Lacerations should be carefully examined for foreign bodies, using instruments rather than the gloved finger if there might be a sharp object in the wound. Palpation of a mass may justify extending the wound so as to explore it adequately.

When there is strong suspicion that all or part of a foreign body is in or beneath the skin, imaging techniques should be considered.

Investigations
Plain radiography
A plain X-ray will often detect a foreign body, but visualisation depends on the object's density, configuration, size and orientation. Metal, bone, teeth, pencil graphite, some plastics, glass and gravel are radio-opaque but may not be visible if located over a radiologically dense background such as bone. Some materials that are less dense than tissue can be seen as filling defects (e.g. white pine) [6], but very often organic foreign bodies are not visible on plain radiographs, especially 48 h or more after entry [7]. Plain films, using multiple projections, can enhance localisation.

Ultrasonography
Ultrasound imaging is often helpful for vegetative foreign bodies that are not visible on plain X-ray. However, there are a number of pitfalls in interpretation, especially in the hand where tendons produce their own echogenic images [8,9]. Wooden splinters can be obscured by surrounding granulomatous tissue [10], and old scar tissue, small bones, fresh bleeding and sutures can produce false positive echo patterns [11].

Computed tomography
Computed tomography (CT) scanning, which can visualise wooden material, has the advantage of producing images in multiple planes, which can aid localisation and can relate a foreign body accurately to nearby structures. However, there is a greater radiation dose than plain radiography, so CT is best avoided as a screening procedure.

Magnetic resonance imaging
Magnetic resonance imaging (MRI) is comparable to CT for materials of similar density to soft tissue (Figure 122.12c) and may be superior for the detection of plastics [12], but must not be used for metal fragments. Gravel produces a severe artefact.

Histopathological techniques
For foreign bodies below the limits of detectability by imaging techniques, it may be possible to make a diagnosis on material taken at biopsy by microscopic or ultrastructural techniques [13]. Some foreign materials have a distinctive microscopic structure, for example the regular arrays of plant cells in some vegetative material, such as wooden splinters and thorns. The presence of particulate material in phagocytic cells can often be seen on routine haematoxylin and eosin (H&E) stained sections. The periodic acid–Schiff (PAS) stain often shows up splinters, talc, starch and

fungi. Dark-field illumination can help visualise some metallic materials. Polarisation microscopy can demonstrate silica, talc, suture material, wood and plant matter [14].

In suitably processed material the elements present can be ascertained by electron-dispersive X-ray analysis (EDXA) and for lower-molecular-weight substances electron energy loss spectroscopy (EELS) may be appropriate [15]. The application of different methods is indicated in Table 122.2.

Management
First line
It can be difficult to judge whether or not to remove a foreign body [16]. Some indications for the removal of a foreign body are shown in Box 122.1. Reactive material, especially if organic in nature (e.g. thorns, spines), should be removed so as to prevent infection and inflammation. Non-reactivity, small size and inaccessibility may weigh in favour of leaving a foreign body. All wounds should be clean and tetanus immunisation provided if necessary.

> **Box 122.1 Indications for the removal of a foreign body**
>
> - Reactivity of the material (e.g. thorns, spines, clothing)
> - Heavy bacterial contamination (e.g. teeth, soil)
> - Toxicity (e.g. spines with venom, heavy metals)
> - Proximity to tendons, vessels, nerves or fractured bone
> - Impairment of mechanical function (e.g. abnormal gait from foreign body in foot)
> - Intra-articular location
> - Potential for migration towards an important anatomical structure
> - Intravascular location
> - Persistent pain
> - Established infection or inflammation
> - Allergic reaction
> - Cosmetic or psychological considerations
>
> Adapted from Lammers and Magill 1992 [16].

The best approach to removing a foreign body will depend on the size, location and nature of the material, and length of time it has been there. A simple method for locating a radio-opaque foreign body is to insert two or three needles of different sizes angled at 90° to each other. Using radiographs in multiple projections, ultrasound or CT, the needle closest to the foreign body is identified, and tissue dissected along its path [17]. It may be possible to pull out the foreign body intact, or slide out a long pointed object along the axis it entered. Material likely to be dealt with by the dermatologist may often be excised as a block of tissue.

After removal, the wound should be irrigated and debrided if necessary. If the foreign body was radio-opaque, and there is any doubt about completeness of removal, a postoperative film can be carried out.

Paraffinoma
Some vegetable oils containing triglyceride can be digested by lipases, but others, and mineral oils, greases and wax, cannot be broken down, and elicit a foreign-body reaction. Most instances of paraffinoma nowadays are caused by misguided attempts at tissue augmentation, often self-administered. The penis is the most common site [1]; other sites include the male breast [2], gluteal regions and extremities. Paraffin gauze that was used to pack the nasal passages and sinuses has caused chronic inflammatory paraffinoma of the periorbital tissues [3,4]. A study of 11 patients with periocular deposition of petrolatum-based material demonstrated a range of iatrogenic causes, including ointment being applied to the eyelid skin, to the canaliculi and to the ethmoid cavities following surgery [5].

The pathology of paraffinoma shows rounded, clear spaces of varying sizes surrounded by fibrous tissue and a mixed inflammatory reaction, including foamy macrophages and multinucleated giant cells – the 'Swiss cheese' appearance. A study of paraffinomas of the female breast reported MRI appearances that can reliably distinguish a mass caused by paraffin injection from a breast cancer [6].

Treatment is by excision and may require a local or distant flap reconstruction.

Sclerodermiform reaction to vitamin K and vitamin B_{12} injections

The intramuscular injection of preparations of vitamin K has been followed by a red plaque in the lumbo-sacral area, which takes on a dusky colour and becomes infiltrated and itchy after 10–15 days. After some months, it resembles a patch of scleroderma, ivory white in colour with a surrounding lilac ring. Confluence of plaques in the trochanteric and lumbo-sacral area produces the so-called 'cowboy's belt' appearance, complete with holsters. The distribution of these changes reflects the sites of vitamin K injections. A case has been reported of similar changes occurring on the upper arms, where intramuscular injections of vitamin K had been administered [1]. Histopathology demonstrated dermal and pannicular sclerosis [1]. A case resembling eosinophilic fasciitis has also been described [2]. All the nine cases studied by Texier [3] had received other vitamins, liver extract or iron injections and no case resulted from vitamin K alone, but this ingredient was a common factor. There is a tendency for sclerotic reactions to resolve slowly following withdrawal of vitamin K injections [1,4]. Intradermal testing with vitamin K produced redness and induration at 2 days in one reported case [4].

Localised sclerodermoid skin reactions have also been reported occurring at the site of intramuscular injections of vitamin B_{12} [5,6].

Pentazocine ulcers

A distinctive woody induration with overlying ulceration is characteristic of repeated intramuscular or subcutaneous use of the analgesic pentazocine (Figure 122.13) [1]. Such reactions are usually found in narcotic abusers. Longstanding changes occurring around major joints can lead to myofibrosis with contractures [2].

Reactions to intralesional corticosteroids

Occasionally, deposits of injected insoluble corticosteroids have been associated with a granulomatous response [1,2] and in one instance a reaction resembling rheumatoid nodule was

Table 122.2 Foreign bodies: their sources and investigation techniques.

Source	Material	Pathological features	Reference
Traumatic	Metals	H, EDXA as appropriate (e.g. mercury)	
	Glass	P, EDXA (silicone)	
	Graphite, e.g. carbon fibre	P, characteristic heat resistance up to 600°C	Young et al. 1995 [18]
	Thorns, wood splinters		Mehregan and Faghri 1974 [19]
	Other vegetation	P, H&E; rectangular cell walls	Hirsh and Johnson 1984 [20]
	Cactus spines	PAS; may be concurrent bacterial and/or fungal infection	Winer and Zeilenga 1955 [21]
			Snyder and Schwartz 1983 [22]
			Lindsey and Lindsey 1988 [23]
			Iwatsu and Miyaji 1984 [24]
			Connor and Gibson 1985 [25]
	Sea-urchin spines		Kinmont 1965 [26]
	Arthropod mouth parts		Allen 1948 [27]
	Grease gun injury	H&E; extensive necrosis and thrombosis	Schon et al. 1980 [28]
	Blast injury	EDXA (silicone)	Mesquita-Guimaraes et al. 1987 [29]
			Hanke et al. 1987 [30]
	Amalgam tattoo	EDXA (usually mercury, aluminium, tin)	Hatch et al. 1984 [31]
			Hartman et al. 1986 [32]
	Synthetics:		
	Plastics		Cortez Pimentel 1977 [33]
	Fibres	P, H, FTIRM	Centeno et al. 1992 [34]
	Epidermis		Stein 1985 [35]
	Hair	P, H&E appearance	Hogan 1988 [36]
	Nail		Brown et al. 1993 [37]
Occupational	Beryllium	EELS	Jones Williams 1988 [38]
	Silica	P, EDXA (silicone)	Mowry et al. 1991 [39]
	Hair	P, H&E appearance	Hogan 1988 [36]
	Fibreglass	P	See Fibreglass dermatitis in this chapter
Cosmetic	Tattoos	H&E appearance, EDXA (appropriate elements)	See Complications of tattoos in this chapter
	Silicone		Travis et al. 1985 [40]
	Collagen	IRS or EDXA (silicone), H&E; vacuoles	Swanson et al. 1983 [41]
		Immunoperoxidase using antibovine type I collagen antibody	Kligman 1988 [42]
			Morgan 1995 [43]
	Paraffins		Oertel and Johnson 1977 [44]
	Vegetable oils	H&E; 'Swiss cheese' cavities	Alagaratnam and Ong 1983 [45]
		FDMS	Nakamura et al. 1985 [46]
	Zirconium	EDXA (zirconium)	Hirsh and Johnson 1984 [47]
Surgically implanted	Suture materials	P, H&E	Postlethwaite et al. 1975 [48]
	Talc	P, EDXA	Terzakis et al. 1978 [49]
	Starch	?P, PAS crystals with Maltese cross appearance on polaroscopy	Leonard 1973 [50]
	Absorbable gelatine		Jaworsky 1991 [51]
Injected drugs	Insulin	H&E appearance of acellular sponge material	Jordaan and Sandler 1989 [52]
	Vaccines		Slater et al. 1982 [53]
		EDXA (zinc)	Garcia-Patos et al. 1995 [54]
		EDXA (aluminium)	Morgan 1995 [55]
	Calcium salts	H, EDXA (calcium)	
	Intralesional corticosteroid		Goldman 1962 [56]
		H&E; granular, amorphous, acellular material	Weedon et al. 1982 [57]
			Bhawan 1983 [58]
			Morgan 1995 [55]
	Polyvinylpyrrolidone		Kossard et al. 1980 [59]
			Morgan et al. 1989 [60]
	Vitamin K		Texier 1975 [61]
Self-inflicted	Narcotic and analgesic abuse, e.g. pentazocine (Figure 122.12), meperidine	H&E (P if talc from tablets is used); thrombosis and fibrosis	Padilla et al. 1979 [62]
			Posner and Guill 1985 [63]
	Talc in fillers used by intravenous drug abusers	EDXA	Hirsch 1972 [64]
	Dermatitis artefacta using injections of faeces, milk, etc.	H&E; necrosis, abscesses	Sullivan 1949 [65]

EDXA, electron-dispersive X-ray analysis; EELS, electron energy loss spectroscopy; FDMS, field desorption mass spectroscopy; FTIRM, Fourier transform infrared microscopy; H, histochemical reaction available; H&E, haematoxylin and eosin; IRS, infrared spectrophotometry; P, birefringence by polarisation microscopy; PAS, periodic acid–Schiff stain.

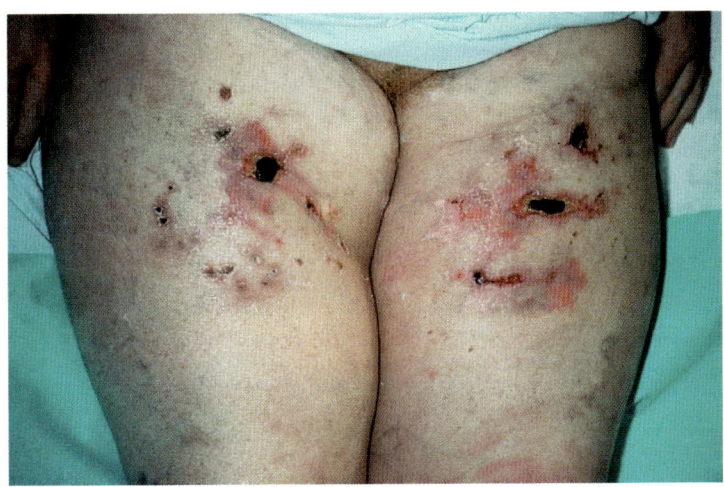

Figure 122.13 Pentazocine ulcers.

described [2]. Another case of a bodybuilder using anabolic steroids has been described, with granulomatous inflammation and ossification [3].

Reactions to silicone

Silicone (polydimethyl siloxane) is used medically in three forms: liquid for soft-tissue augmentation, bag-gel implants for augmentation mammoplasty and as a solid elastomer in joint prostheses. In tissues, it has a tendency to migrate both locally and via the lymphatics. Many of the reported adverse effects are likely to have been a result of adulterants, although even medical-grade silicone can produce a granulomatous reaction [1,2].

When silicone bag-gel material ruptures, it can migrate along fascial planes and gravitate into the skin, producing indurated inflammatory subcutaneous masses [3].

Following liquid or gel silicone injections, the histological appearance is of varying sized vacuoles similar to paraffinoma, but with less fibrosis and usually an absence of granulomatous response if medical-grade silicone is used [4]. Sometimes, however, granulomatous reactions do occur [5], including cases of multiple silicone-containing granulomas at the site of entry of acupuncture needles coated in silicone oil [6,7]. A case has been reported of widespread granulomatous papules developing many years after liquid silicone injection into the face [8]. In the facial lesions, silicone was demonstrated by EDXA, while extrafacial lesions did not contain foreign material but were histologically consistent with sarcoidosis [8]. It was suggested that the granulomatous response to silicone in this case occurred as a manifestation of sarcoidosis [9].

If adulterants are present, a more inflammatory reaction is described. Particles of rubbery silicone elastomer can elicit a vigorous foreign-body granulomatous response.

The Si–C chemical bond, characteristic of silicone and not found in nature, can be detected by infrared spectroscopy, and silicone can be demonstrated by EDXA.

Silicone reactions can be treated by surgery, where amenable. Amelioration of the inflammatory response by treatment with minocycline has been reported [10]; however, a variety of topical and system agents have been thought to be useful in case reports [11].

Fibreglass dermatitis

Reactions to glass fibre are usually caused by physical injury, although allergic contact dermatitis resulting from residual epoxy resin on the fibres has been described [1]. The fibres that cause reactions are generally greater than 4 µm in diameter [2]. Pruritus is very common and may occur with or without skin lesions, which, if present, usually consist of transient red papules that are often follicular. The forearms, hands, face, neck and flexural folds are common sites. Covered sites can be affected because the fibres can penetrate clothing. Fair-skinned, blue-eyed individuals seem to be more susceptible [3]. The fibres only penetrate the more superficial epidermis, yet the histopathological changes include subcorneal pustules, spongiosis and a mixed upper dermal infiltrate [4]. The mechanisms underlying these changes remain speculative. Glass fibres are often difficult to see in biopsy specimens but can be recovered by Scotch tape stripping and this may be of use in diagnosis [5].

With prolonged exposure, a form of hardening can occur, with the pruritus but not the visible signs of dermatitis reducing in intensity [3].

Complications of tattoos

The term tattoo, derived from the Tahitian *tatau* [1], is used for both the deliberate introduction of permanent colours into the skin through punctures, and for accidental entry of pigmented material [2]. The latter is common after abrasion injuries, for instance in cyclists and coal miners. Cases have been described of tattooing from close exposure to black gunpowder, as used in replica firearms [3]. Accidental tattooing from Monsel solution or ferric chloride [4,5] provides rare iatrogenic causes. Tattooing can occur from contact with jewellery (e.g. earrings) [6]. The placement of tattoos for cosmetic reasons has increased in recent years; a US survey from 2004 showed that 24% of adults aged 18–50 years had at least one tattoo [7].

For body art, the most common method of tattooing uses an electric tattoo machine, in which a group of oscillating needles injects ink into the skin 80–150 times a second. Since tattoo instruments come in contact with blood, infectious diseases may be transmitted if appropriate precautions are ignored. A properly equipped tattoo studio will have a sharps container for used needles, biohazard containers and an autoclave for sterilising equipment. In certain states in the USA, tattoo artists are required to pass a test of health and safety understanding to gain a licence. The potential infection risk has led to the prohibition of blood donation for 12 months after receiving a tattoo in the USA (unless the procedure was done in a state-regulated and licensed studio) and for 6 months in the UK.

Modern tattooing inks are carbon-based pigments and have uses outside tattoo applications. Many of the brighter tattoo pigments available are derived from the plastic acrylonitrile butadiene styrene (ABS). ABS is ground down to particles less than 1 µm in diameter and these are introduced into tattoo inks to produce vivid colours that are less likely to fade. The traditional pigments are carmine, indigo, vermilion, India ink, chrome green, cobalt blue, cinnabar (red) and cadmium sulphide (yellow). Ferrous oxide is used to pigment the eyebrow area [8]. A study using energy-dispersive spectrometry analysed the constituents of 30 tattoo inks and found that the most commonly identified elements were aluminium, oxygen, titanium and carbon [9]. Histologically, tattoo pigments are refractile and found in macrophages and fibroblasts clustered around vessels in the upper and mid dermis [10]. Deposits of pigment can also be visualised between collagen bundles [10].

Immediately after tattooing there is a local traumatic response with the formation of a scab. Although pyogenic infection as a postprocedure complication is generally uncommon, one US study identified unlicensed tattooists as the source of six unlinked clusters of community-acquired meticillin-resistant *Staphylococcus aureus* (MRSA) skin infection [11]. The tattooists were found to be using non-sterile equipment and poor infection control procedures [11]. Hepatitis infection has also been attributed to tattooing [12], however a US study was unable to identify an increased risk for hepatitis B or C virus infection in low-risk adults who had received a tattoo [13]. In a study of 345 Brazilian subjects, a positive association between tattooing and hepatitis C infection was demonstrated but no relationship with respect to hepatitis B, human immunodeficiency virus (HIV) or syphilis [14]. Transmission of molluscum contagiosum [15] and of viral warts [16] by tattoos has been reported.

Aside from infectious complications, other adverse effects of tattoos include the induction of skin diseases via the Koebner phenomenon, such as lichen planus, psoriasis, Darier disease and discoid lupus erythematosus. Sarcoidal granulomatous inflammation can also develop in tattoos (Figure 122.14) and may occur in conjunction with systemic sarcoidosis [17,**18**,19,20]. Hypersensitivity reactions to the tattoo inks are most commonly seen with the red pigment cinnabar (mercuric sulphide) [21,**22**], but also with inks containing cobalt, chrome, manganese [23] and aluminium (purple) [24]. Histologically, there is a diffuse lymphohistiocytic infiltrate in the dermis with an admixture of plasma cells and eosinophils [9]. Other histological patterns reported include lichenoid reactions [25,26] and a pseudolymphomatous infiltrate [27,28]. B-cell lymphoma has been recorded as evolving from a tattoo-induced pseudolymphoma [29]. Abnormal photosensitivity in tattoos has been observed and is considered to be triggered by photoreaction to pigments containing cadmium yellow [30,31]. Perforating granuloma annulare can also complicate tattooing [32].

Traumatic tattooing (e.g. from an explosion) is amenable to laser treatment (e.g. with erbium:yttrium-aluminium-garnet (Er:YAG) laser) [33]. The treatment of decorative tattoos is discussed in Chapter 161.

Hair as a foreign body

Fragments of hair may penetrate the skin and cause a variety of reactions, according to the site and depth of penetration, ranging from slight redness to the formation of abscesses and sinuses. Chronic reactions take the form of foreign-body granulomas, which may present as subcutaneous nodules or with hypertrophy of the overlying epidermis. The clinical syndromes encountered are very diverse and their cause is often unsuspected.

Barbers' hair sinus. Interdigital sinuses are common in men's barbers, presumably because of the short, sharp hair fragments generated from cutting men's hair [**1**,2]. They also occur in female hairdressers [3] and those who cut animal hair [**1**]. The sinuses usually affect the first or third left or second right finger web. The lesions are tender nodules within the affected finger web containing a central sinus that may intermittently discharge. Barbers' hair sinuses are relatively inconspicuous and may be disregarded by the patient. Hair can also cause inflammation when implanted into the finger pulp [4] and beneath the fingernails [5], probably when there is an abnormality of the nail or a pre-existing dermatosis [6].

Hair sinuses of the feet. Hair fragments may penetrate the skin of the feet. Long, curved hairs embedded in the toes or ankles have been recorded in ladies' hairdressers [**7**]. Deeper penetration may provoke tender nodules or abscesses. A distinctive syndrome, seldom recognised, may follow the penetration by a hair of the toe cleft skin, usually the fourth. The patient complains of pain and tenderness, which is usually attributed to other causes. There is oedema of the dorsum of the foot above the involved cleft. A pinhole sinus is found beneath the accumulated interdigital debris. Surgical excision may be necessary. The hair-thread tourniquet syndrome may also involve the feet.

Creeping hair. Loose, individual hairs can penetrate the skin and migrate superficially, producing a wave-like linear redness with the hair at the leading end. This eruption has been called 'creeping hair' and clinically resembles cutaneous larva migrans. Two reported cases have involved pubic hairs penetrating the lower abdominal or pubic skin and migrating along the Langer lines to the iliac region [**8**,9]. The hair can be easily removed by extracting it through a shallow incision.

Milkers' sinuses. Milkers' sinuses are now uncommon but are more disabling. Fragments of cow hair may penetrate deeply,

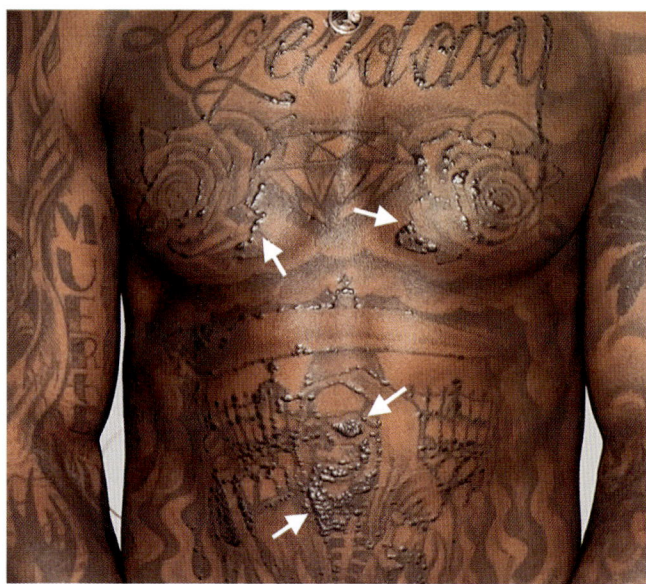

Figure 122.14 Cutaneous sarcoid-like reactions secondary to tattoo ink. Examination shows linear raised papules confined to the tattoo ink on the patient's torso (arrows). Reproduced from Mathis and Johnson 2023 [34].

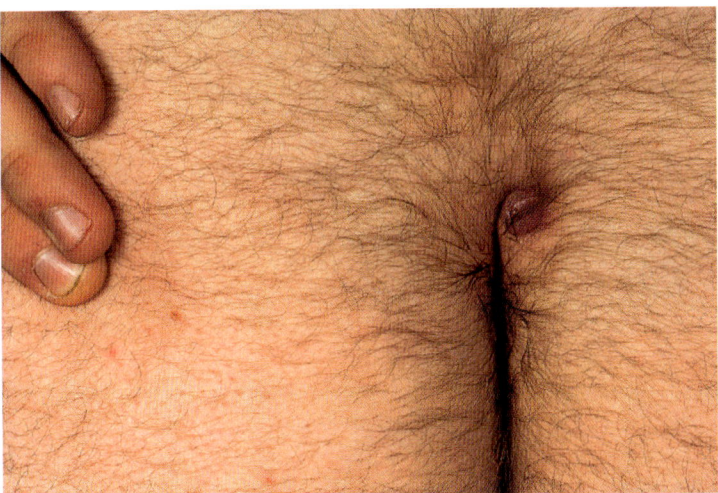

Figure 122.15 Pilonidal sinus.

involving even the tendon sheaths. Secondary infection often follows, sometimes by dermatophytes [10]. Most lesions involve the second or third web of the right hand, forming tender nodules and discharging sinuses [11]. Recurrent episodes of cellulitis follow. Spontaneous cure may eventually take place, but may be so long delayed that surgical intervention is advisable.

Ano-genital pilonidal sinus. Ano-genital pilonidal sinus is discussed more fully in Chapter 111. Some cases are of developmental origin but many follow the penetration of the skin by hair(s) by the root end, through the action of the cuticular cells. The sinus itself does not have hair follicles. The penetrating hair(s) may cause a foreign-body giant cell reaction, sometimes with secondary bacterial infection, which can cause a sudden onset of pilonidal abscess. In addition to the primary track resulting from the initiating hair(s), there may be secondary tracks opening from the cavity. Presentation is usually as a midline opening or series of openings in the natal cleft about 5 cm from the anus. Pilonidal disease usually starts at the onset of puberty. Males are affected much more commonly than females. The peak age of onset is 15–24 years and it is rare over the age of 45 [12]. It occurs more commonly in individuals with stiff dark or auburn hair.

Half of affected patients present as emergencies with an acute pilonidal abscess; the remainder have chronic, fluctuating discomfort associated with a foul-smelling discharge from one or more sinus openings [12]. Examination reveals the characteristic opening in the natal cleft (Figure 122.15) through which a tuft of hair is often seen emerging.

There is no uniform approach to management. A small sinus can sometimes be treated by removal of the hairs and regular shaving of the surrounding skin. A phenol injection technique has been used, either alone, with curettage or combined with excision [12]. Most patients are treated either by excision and primary closure [13], or by laying open and healing by secondary intention or repair with skin flaps [14]. Primary closure or flap repair produces more rapid healing and shorter time off work [14,15]; wound breakdown after suturing may be lessened by prophylactic use of clindamycin [16]. Modifications of direct closure can be used to flatten the natal cleft and thereby reduce the risk of recurrence [17], but there may be greater morbidity if such techniques fail [12].

A pilonidal abscess is probably best treated by incision, drainage, curettage of the hair and granulation tissue, and leaving open for secondary intention healing.

Squamous cell carcinoma has been described as a rare complication of pilonidal sinus [18,19]. The high rate of metastasis and mortality in reported cases indicates that pilonidal sinus-related squamous cell carcinoma tends to be aggressive [20,21].

Miscellaneous hair-filled sinuses. The penis can occasionally be the site for a pilonidal sinus-like lesion [22]. Pain, tenderness and discharge in the umbilicus have been associated with the presence of hair, perhaps in association with a hirsute abdomen and poor umbilical hygiene [23]. A hair sinus originating on the chin has resulted in the loss of a tooth resulting from penetration of the sinus through into the incisor tooth socket [24]. Trauma was reported to account for a hair sinus over the mandible [25].

Hair-thread tourniquet syndrome. A foreign-body reaction to hair and hair-like fibres has been described following the encirclement of the fingers, toes and penis, usually as an accidental event [26] but also as an instance of child abuse. The affected area presents as a dusky swelling, sometimes with focal discharge, and the hair may be completely buried and only evident after surgery [27]. Removal of the constricting fibre is usually sufficient to solve the problem [26,28].

Pseudofolliculitis barbae. This foreign-body reaction to the ingrowth of obliquely cut, often tightly curled hair causes an eruption of red papules in the beard area [29,30]. It is especially common in dark-skinned people. Stretching of the skin and shaving against the 'lie' of the hair increase the tendency. The pubic hair has also been involved. A similar condition has been described in Iraqi women who pluck the hairs of their legs, leaving some broken stumps that curl back into the follicle [31]. Pseudofolliculitis vibrissae [32] represents a variant caused by the close cutting of nasal hairs that may be confused with perforating folliculitis of the nose.

Preventative measures include discontinuing shaving and the use of a clipper to maintain a beard hair length of 1 mm.

Treatment is generally unsatisfactory; reported symptomatic remedies include topical retinoids, α-hydroxyacids and antibiotics. Depilation techniques modify the physical trigger in pseudofolliculitis barbae, and laser hair removal may offer the best approach thus far [33,34]. A variety of lasers and light devices are suitable: alexandrite and Nd:YAG lasers, in addition to intense pulsed light.

Complications of artificial hair implantation. Although the use of synthetic fibres implanted in the scalp has been known for many years to produce severe foreign-body reactions [35–37], baldness sufferers continue to undergo implantation procedures with synthetic materials. Although some fibres, such as polyester, have been promoted as less liable to produce reactions [38], chronic purulent foreign-body reactions remain a typical consequence [39,40].

OTHER SKIN INJURIES

Hand–arm vibration syndrome

Definition and nomenclature
Vibration is defined as a repetitive movement about a point of equilibrium. Transmission of vibration energy to the skin has been associated with a number of chronic biological consequences, the best defined of which is the hand–arm vibration syndrome.

> **Synonyms and inclusions**
> - Vibration white finger
> - Vibration syndrome

Introduction and general description
The term 'vibration white finger' has long been used for Raynaud phenomenon resulting from the use of hand-held vibratory tools. Recognition that there are also neurological and musculoskeletal consequences of vibration exposure in the affected limb has led to the now preferred term hand–arm vibration syndrome (HAVS) [1,2–4]. Vibration-related changes can also occur in the feet [5].

The most common tools causing HAVS are percussive metal-working machines, such as riveting and fettling tools, drills, impact wrenches, jack hammers, road-breaking tools and chainsaws. In many other occupations there is some risk, albeit less well studied [6]. The condition has even been described in a teenager making prolonged use of a hand-held vibrating computer game [7].

It is also recognised that vibration can induce localised hyperhidrosis, callus formation, vibratory angioedema and a condition characterised by pain, swelling and erythrocyanosis [8]. Vibration may be a contributory factor to the hypothenar hammer syndrome. Potentially beneficial effects have been ascribed to short-term exposure to vibration, such as the elevation of skin temperature and increased lymphatic clearance [9]. The monographs by Griffin [10] and Pelmear et al. [11] deal comprehensively with the study of vibration and its medical consequences.

Epidemiology
Incidence and prevalence
In the UK approximately 500 000 workers are exposed to vibration and of these about 20 000 suffer moderate to severe HAVS [3]. In high-risk occupations, the incidence and prevalence can be 90% or more [12,13].

The time of exposure to vibrations may be as little as 1 month to more than 30 years, but increased exposure is associated with an increased risk. A longitudinal study of Swedish car mechanics showed a prevalence of HAVS rising from 15% to 25% after 20 years' exposure [12].

Pathophysiology
Predisposing factors
There are numerous variables that determine whether or not the condition occurs [14]. Some relate to the equipment, some to the environment and others to the individual [15]. Thus, low ambient temperature, firm gripping of the equipment and smoking are risk factors [16,17].

Pathology
Almost any vibratory source within the range 4000–5000 Hz can produce HAVS if sufficiently intense. Under experimental conditions a vibration frequency of 125 Hz has been shown to induce greater changes in finger circulation than lower or higher frequencies [18]. A study of vibration transmission at various frequencies has shown that, at low frequencies (<25 Hz), energy absorption into the palms is greater than into the fingers, but is similar at higher frequencies (>100 Hz) [19]. The same study demonstrated that vibration energy absorption by fingers is independent of the type of hand–handle coupling [19]. There is some evidence to suggest that exposure to intermittent vibration has a less severe effect than continuous vibration [20]. Existing vascular disease and vasoconstrictive medications may be risk factors in some cases [21]. HAVS was thought not to occur in hot climates; a study of quarry workers in Vietnam found no evidence of vibration white finger among rock drill operators [22]. However, it is recognised that there are differences in presentation in tropical climates, with white finger being less of a feature compared with neurological changes [23].

The initial events are not well understood [24]. The following documented changes are likely to be important: (i) damage to mechanoreceptor nerve endings and non-medullated fibres [25]; (ii) a more generalised loss of neuronal activity than occurs in primary Raynaud phenomenon [26]; and (iii) selective damage to α_1-adrenergic receptors in vessels causing an excessive vasoconstrictor response from the predominant α_2-receptors [16,27,28]. There is also a reduction of cutaneous nerve fibres that express calcitonin gene-related peptide, a powerful vasodilator [29]. An ultrastructural study of forearm skin biopsies demonstrated a significant reduction in epidermal nerve density in workers exposed to hand-transmitted vibration compared with controls [30]. Nerve conduction velocity along the distal part of the radial nerve is reduced in patients with HAVS when compared with normal controls, again identifying a putative neurogenic pathophysiology [31]. Other structural neural changes noted include loss of myelin, increased numbers of Schwann cells and fibrosis [32].

Vascular lumina are reduced, probably by both internal thickening and smooth muscle hypertrophy [25,33,34,35]. There is an increase in fibrous tissue within and around blood vessels [36] and arterial thrombosis can occur [37]. Laser Doppler flowmetry studies demonstrated a longer time to maximal reactive hyperaemia after a standard provocation in HAVS compared with primary Raynaud phenomenon. This finding suggests the involvement of arterial occlusive disease in addition to microcirculatory vasospasm [38]. An in vivo study demonstrated a decreased vasodilator response in the finger skin of patients with HAVS when challenged with histamine and endothelin 1 [39]. These findings are in contrast to asymptomatic vibration-exposed workers who showed normal responses to both mediators, while patients with primary Raynaud disease had a normal histamine-induced flare, but a reduced vasodilatation with endothelin 1 [39]. Soluble intercellular adhesion molecule 1 (ICAM-1) levels are increased, as in scleroderma, suggesting that neutrophils may adhere and contribute to the microvascular damage [40]. Whole blood viscosity may be elevated [41], although the importance of this is uncertain.

A generalised abnormality in the autonomic nervous system [42] may cause orthostatic hypotension [43] and vasoconstriction of limbs not directly exposed to vibration [44]. There is an association with hearing loss in HAVS that is not explained purely by occupational exposure to noise [45]. Auditory impairment may be caused by ischaemia in the inner ear [46], via damage to the central nervous system [47], and exacerbated by the effects of vibration on the autonomic nervous system [48,49].

As well as damage to nerves, there is evidence of damage to muscles, especially the intrinsic muscles of the hand [50]. Bone cysts have been described in HAVS but may be a coincidental finding and not purely a result of vibration injury [51].

Clinical features
Presentation
There are three possible major components to HAVS: circulatory, neural and musculoskeletal [52].

After a highly variable latent period, the initial symptom is usually tingling and/or numbness in one finger. This often occurs directly after using the vibrating tool and also at night. This sensory change is followed by episodes of blanching, initially of the tip of the finger most exposed to the vibration source, with progression towards the base, and then increasing numbers of digits are affected. The thumb below the tip is usually spared. The pattern of digits affected reflects the subject's grip on the tool, and extent of involvement increases with cumulative vibration exposure. Attacks are usually precipitated by cold and sometimes damp conditions, most common early in the morning and during rest periods rather than during work. However, many patients experience attacks that are unprovoked and unpredictable. The attacks may last 15–120 min followed by painful reactive hyperaemia. With progression of the disease there is reduction in touch sensation, and difficulty doing fine manual work. Muscle fatigue and weakness are common, probably because of incomplete muscle contraction.

Late in the disease, attacks of pallor wane but there is persistent dusky cyanosis, swelling and stiffness of the digits and focal areas of necrosis of the fingertips. When the latent period is short, the symptoms and signs of HAVS tend to be more severe and more rapidly progressive.

The toes can be affected, either directly (e.g. from exposure to a vibrating platform) or by reflex sympathetic spasm.

Other changes attributed to vibration injury include carpal tunnel syndrome [53,54], although this may be more a result of mechanical and ischaemic factors [55].

Differential diagnosis
This includes primary Raynaud disease, thoracic outlet syndrome, syringomyelia, spinal cord compression, connective tissue disease, peripheral vascular disease and vasoconstrictive drugs [2,57,58].

Classification of severity
Patients with HAVS should be staged as part of the assessment of their disability, for each hand separately. The Stockholm Workshop Scales [1,56] are most widely used (Table 122.3).

Table 122.3 The Stockholm Workshop Scales for assessing vibration injury.

	Stage	Grade	Description
Vascular component	0V		No attacks
	1V	Mild	Occasional attacks affecting only the tips of one or more fingers
	2V	Moderate	Occasional attacks affecting the distal or middle (rarely also proximal) phalanges of one or more fingers
	3V	Severe	Frequent attacks affecting all the phalanges of most fingers
	4V	Very severe	As in stage 3, with trophic changes in the fingertips
Sensorineural	0SN		Vibration exposed but no symptoms
	1SN		Intermittent numbness with or without tingling
	2SN		Intermittent or persistent numbness, reduced sensory perception
	3SN		Intermittent or persistent numbness, reduced tactile descrimination and/or manipulative dexterity

Clinical variants
Other vasomotor symptoms. This is a condition in which pain, swelling and erythrocyanosis is induced by high-speed electrical tools (frequency 166–833 Hz) and was described many years ago [8]. This syndrome is not provoked by exposure to cold.

Vibratory angioedema. Unlike the other dermatological phenomena induced by vibration, vibratory angioedema tends to occur at low frequencies (approximately 10 Hz) [59], such as are produced by handling a power lawnmower or by rubbing or towelling the skin. The condition may be quite common among mountain bikers [60].

Disease course and prognosis
The early stages of HAVS are reversible, but advanced stages in patients aged over 45 years are irreversible and may progress despite withdrawal from vibration [9,61]. One observational study demonstrated that 43% of patients with stage 2 HAVS at first examination and 70% of patients with stage 3 still suffered from finger blanching attacks 15 years after presentation [62]. However, if measures are taken early in the course of disease, improvement is possible [63].

Investigations
The diagnosis of HAVS is based on a history of vibration exposure before the onset of symptoms. A variety of tests have been used in the diagnosis and assessment of vascular, neurological and musculoskeletal abnormalities [58,64]. For the purposes of assessing a claim for industrial injury compensation, certain tests may be regarded as the most reliable [65]. Thus, in the UK, the following are recommended: (i) finger systolic blood pressure following cooling to assess vascular abnormalities; (ii) either vibrometry or aesthesiometry for neurological dysfunction; and (iii) grip strength [66,67]. These tests are likely to be available only in centres specialising in the evaluation of HAVS. In general, a reduced finger systolic blood pressure following cooling is indicative of HAVS, whereas zero finger systolic blood pressure suggests Raynaud phenomenon [68].

Laser Doppler flowmetry can be used to assess skin blood flow after cold provocation and can discriminate between patients with HAVS who demonstrate significantly lower perfusion compared with controls [69].

Even with a battery of tests it may be difficult to determine which patients will benefit from carpal tunnel release [70].

Management
Because the more advanced stages of HAVS are irreversible, preventative measures and surveillance of at-risk workers are widely regarded as essential. Various steps can be taken to reduce exposure, for example automation [71], shorter shifts, antivibration gloves and pads on the tools. Much effort has been made to redesign equipment so as to reduce vibration [72,73] and the need for excessive grip strength. In a large Finnish study of forestry workers, HAVS decreased from 13% to 4% over a 19-year period during which time antivibration chainsaws were introduced [74]. Workers should be informed of the hazards of their occupation, and should wear warm antivibratory gloves, avoid smoking and undergo regular medical surveillance. It is best for those at risk to avoid medications that can cause vasoconstriction (e.g. β-blockers).

Current industry standards in the USA and Europe are reviewed in [75].

First line
It is important to maintain central body temperature and to avoid allowing the hands to become cold. Mittens are preferable to gloves. Smoking should be strongly discouraged. If possible, further vibration exposure should be avoided; if this is not feasible, frequent work breaks should be allowed.

Second line
Calcium-channel antagonists such as nifedipine can help the vascular symptoms. Other drugs that may be useful include α-adrenoreceptor antagonists such as thymoxamine and some prostanoids. A case report has indicated a positive response to iloprost infusions in a patient with severe HAVS [76]. Other remedies used in the Raynaud syndrome are given in Chapter 123. Sympathectomy is not generally effective.

Resources
UK Health and Safety Executive, hand–arm vibration at work: http://www.hse.gov.uk/vibration/HAV/ (last accessed September 2023).

Piezogenic pedal papules

Definition
These are soft, skin-coloured papules and nodules that appear on the side of the heel, usually the medial aspect, when the subject is standing, and disappear when weight is taken off the foot (derived from 'piesis' meaning pressure) [1].

Introduction and general description
Observation of healthy subjects has shown that such papules are common, although painless and indeed often unnoticed [2,3,4,5,6].

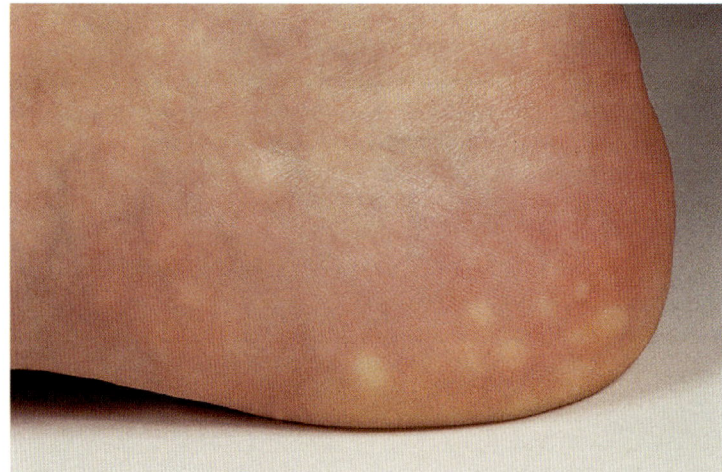

Figure 122.16 Piezogenic pedal papules.

The frequency of the condition makes it difficult to assess the assertion that piezogenic pedal papules can be familial [7] and also that there is an increased frequency in some diseases such as Ehlers–Danlos syndrome [8]. In a population study, there was no association with hypermobile joints [5]. It has also been described in several patients with Prader–Willi syndrome [9].

Pathophysiology
Painless papules consist of normal fat tissue [3], but when pain occurs it has been attributed to herniation of the fat into the dermis with a resultant reduction in dermal thickness [10,13]. Postulated reasons for this pain include a defect in septation of the adipose tissue [13] and ischaemia resulting from the extrusion of fat within its vascular supply and associated nerves [14].

Clinical features
Presentation
Piezogenic pedal papules are transient, soft, skin-coloured papules or nodules that appear on standing and disappear on lying. They most typically occur on the medial side of the heel (Figure 122.16). Pain on standing is the usual reason for presentation, although some patients do express curiosity about the papules even when they are symptomless.

Similar papules have also been noticed on the lateral edge of the hand [10] and wrist [11], and piezogenic palmar papules have recently been described as a physical sign of suprafascial palmar lipoma [12].

Investigations
Clinical assessment is usually sufficient. Ultrasound can demonstrate fat globules protruding into the dermis.

Management
First line
When piezogenic pedal papules of the feet are painful, improvement of the symptoms can sometimes be achieved by avoidance of prolonged standing and, when relevant, loss of weight.

Second line

Compression hosiery [15], electroacupuncture [16] and injections of equal parts of betamethasone with bupivacaine [17] have been reported to relieve symptoms. Supportive rubber footpads and heel cups can also be helpful.

Third line

If conservative measures fail, small excisions of the papules can be curative [18].

Key references

The full list of references can be found in the online version at https://www.wiley.com/rooksdermatology10e

Overview of skin injury

1 Smith DW. Mechanical factors in the normal and abnormal development of the skin and its derivatives. *Birth Defects* 1981;17:61–6.
8 Ryan TJ. Biochemical consequences of mechanical forces generated by distension and distortion. *J Am Acad Dermatol* 1989;21:116–30.
9 Suskind RR. Environment and the skin. *Med Clin North Am* 1990;74:307–24.
10 Pedersen L, Jemec GB. Mechanical properties and barrier function of healthy human skin. *Acta Derm Venereol* 2006;86:308–11.

Isomorphic (Koebner) response

1 Köbner H. Zur aetiologie der psoriasis. *Vierteljahresschr Dermatol Syph* 1876;3:559–61.
2 Boyd AS, Neldner KH. The isomorphic response of Köbner. *Int J Dermatol* 1990;29:401–10.
5 Mohla G, Brodell RT. The Köbner phenomenon in psoriasis: a common response to skin trauma. *Postgrad Med* 1999;106:39–40.
6 Miller RAW. The Köbner phenomenon. *Int J Dermatol* 1982;21:192–7.
10 Sweet RD. Vitiligo as a Köbner phenomenon. *Br J Dermatol* 1978;99:223–4.

Utilisation of mechanical stimuli

1 Shelley WB. Experimental disease in the skin of man. *Acta Derm Venereol Suppl (Stockh)* 1983;108:5–32.
2 Hameed A, Khan AA. Microscopic Nikolsky's sign. *Clin Exp Dermatol* 1999;24:312–14.

Biomechanical considerations

1 Tregear RT. *The Physical Functions of Skin*. New York: Academic Press, 1966.
4 Serup J, Jemec GBE, Grove GL, eds. *Handbook of Non-invasive Methods and the Skin*, 2nd edn. Boca Raton, FL: CRC Press, 2006.
5 Kligman AM. The chronic effects of repeated mechanical trauma to the skin. *Am J Ind Med* 1985;8:257–64.

Mechanical properties of the skin

3 Elsner P, Berardesca E, Wilhelm K-P, Maibach HI, eds. *Bioengineering of the Skin: Skin Biomechanics*. Boca Raton, FL: CRC Press, 2001.
4 Serup J, Jemec GBE, Grove GL, eds. *Handbook of Non-invasive Methods and the Skin*, 2nd edn. Boca Raton, FL: CRC Press, 2006.

Determinants of mechanical properties of the skin

1 Park AC, Baddiel CB. Rheology of stratum corneum: a molecular interpretation of the stress–strain curve. *J Soc Cosmet Chem* 1972;23:3–12.
2 Schellander FA, Headington JT. The stratum corneum: some structural and functional correlates. *Br J Dermatol* 1974;91:507–15.
5 Yuan Y, Verma R. Measuring microelastic properties of stratum corneum. *Colloids Surf B Biointerfaces* 2006;48:6–12.
6 Blank IM. Factors which influence the water content of the stratum corneum. *J Invest Dermatol* 1952;18:433–40.
12 Marks R, Nicholls S, Fitzgeorge D. Measurement of intracorneal cohesion in man using in vivo techniques. *J Invest Dermatol* 1977;69:299–302.

Physiological variation

3 Cua AB, Wilhelm KP, Maibach HI. Elastic properties of human skin: relation to age, sex and anatomical region. *Arch Dermatol Res* 1990;282:283–8.
4 Lévêque JL, Agache PG. *Ageing Skin: Properties and Functional Changes*. New York: Marcel Dekker, 1993.
9 Piérard G, Lapière CM. Physiopathological variations in the mechanical properties of skin. *Arch Dermatol Res* 1977;260:231–9.
12 Auriol F, Vaulant L, Machet L *et al*. Effects of short-term hydration on skin extensibility. *Acta Derm Venereol (Stockh)* 1993;73:344–7.
19 Berardesca E. Racial differences in skin function. *Acta Derm Venereol Suppl (Stockh)* 1994;185:44–6.

Pathological variation

16 Piérard GE, de la Brassine M, Lapière CM. Effects of long term photochemotherapy on the dermis. *J Invest Dermatol* 1977;68:249–50.

Effects of friction

1 Sulzberger MB, Cortese TA, Fishman L *et al*. Studies on blisters produced by friction. I. Results of linear rubbing and twisting techniques. *J Invest Dermatol* 1966;47:456–65.
2 Comaish S, Bottoms E. Skin and friction: deviations from Amonton's laws, and the effects of hydration and lubrication. *Br J Dermatol* 1971;84:37–43.
10 Loden M, Olsson H, Axell T, Linde YW. Friction, capacitance and transepidermal water loss (TEWL) in dry atopic and normal skin. *Br J Dermatol* 1992;126:137–41.
12 Elsnau WH. Skin friction measurement. In: Berardesca E, Elsner P, Wilhelm K-P, Maibach HI, eds. *Bioengineering of the Skin: Methods and Instrumentation*. Boca Raton, FL: CRC Press, 1995:120–3.
18 Cua AB, Wilhelm K-P, Maibach HI. Frictional properties of human skin: relation to age, sex and anatomical region, stratum corneum hydration and transepidermal water loss. *Br J Dermatol* 1990;123:473–9.

Reactions to mechanical injury

Callosities, corns and calluses

1 Singh D, Bentley G, Trevino SG. Callosities, corns and calluses. *BMJ* 1996;312:1403–6.
2 Menz HB, Zammit GV, Munteanu SE. Plantar pressures are higher under callused regions of the foot in older people. *Clin Exp Dermatol* 2007;32:375–80.
9 Orlin MN, McPoil TG. Plantar pressure assessment. *Phys Ther* 2000;80:399–409.
12 Kim SH, Kim S, Choi HI *et al*. Callus formation is associated with hyperproliferation and incomplete differentiation of keratinocytes, and increased expression of adhesion molecules. *Br J Dermatol* 2010;163:495–501.
13 Baden HP, Bronstein BR, Rand RE. Hereditary callosities with blisters. *J Am Acad Dermatol* 1984;11:409–15.
25 Abanmi AA, Al Zouman AY, Al Hussaini H, Al-Asmari A. Prayer marks. *Int J Dermatol* 2002;41:411–14.
27 Pitei DL, Foster A, Edmonds M. The effect of regular callus removal on foot pressures. *J Foot Ankle Surg* 1999;38:251–5.
31 Okuda R, Kinoshita M, Morikawa J *et al*. Surgical treatment for hallux valgus with painful plantar callosities. *Foot Ankle Int* 2001;22:203–8.
38 Akdemir O, Bilkay U, Tiftikcioglu YO *et al*. New alternative in treatment of callus. *J Dermatol* 2011;38:146–50.

Friction blisters

1 Tlougan BE, Mancini AJ, Mandell JA *et al*. Skin conditions in figure skaters, ice-hockey players and speed skaters: part I – mechanical dermatoses. *Sports Med* 2011;41:709–19.
3 Brehmer-Andersson E, Goransson K. Friction blisters as a manifestation of pathomimia. *Acta Derm Venereol (Stockh)* 1975;55:65–71.
5 Pigatto PD, Legori A, Bigardi AS. Occupational dermatitis from physical causes. *Clin Dermatol* 1992;10:231–43.
6 Darrigrand A, Reynolds K, Jackson R *et al*. Efficacy of antiperspirants on feet. *Mil Med* 1992;157:256–9.

Black heel and palm
1 Crissey JT, Peachey JC. Calcaneal petechiae. *Arch Dermatol* 1961;83:501.
2 Kirton V, Wheatley-Price M. Black heel. *Trans St John's Hosp Derm Soc Lond* 1965;51:80–4.
10 Saida T, Oguchi S, Ishihara Y. In vivo observations of magnified features of pigmented lesions on volar skin using video microscope. *Arch Dermatol* 1995;131:248–304.

Skin reactions to musical instruments
1 Gamblicher T, Uzun A, Boms S *et al*. Skin conditions in instrumental musicians: a self-reported survey. *Contact Dermatitis* 2008;58:217–22.
2 Rimmer S, Spielvogel RL. Dermatologic problems of musicians. *J Am Acad Dermatol* 1990;22:657–63.
4 Gambichler T, Boms S, Freitag M. Contact dermatitis and other skin conditions in instrumental musicians. *BMC Dermatol* 2004;4:3.

Hypothenar hammer syndrome
1 Conn J, Bergan JJ, Bell JL. Hypothenar hammer syndrome: post-traumatic digital ischaemia. *Surgery* 1970;68:1122–8.

Achenbach syndrome
2 Thies K, Beschorner U, Noory E *et al*. Achenbach's syndrome revisited. *Vasa* 2012;41:366–70.

Spectacle-frame acanthoma
2 Benedetto AV, Bergfeld WF. Acanthoma fissuratum: histopathology and review of the literature. *Cutis* 1979;24:225–9.

Semicircular lipoatrophy
4 Nagore E, Sanchez-Motilla JM, Rodriguez-Serna M *et al*. Lipoatrophia semicircularis: a traumatic panniculitis – report of cases and review of literature. *J Am Acad Dermatol* 1998;39:879–81.

Acne mechanica
1 Mills DH, Kligman AM. Acne mechanica. *Arch Dermatol* 1975;111:481–3.

Dermatoses due to traumatic effects of sports
1 Adams BB. Dermatologic disorders of the athlete. *Sports Med* 2002;32:309–21.
2 Metelitsa A, Barankin B, Lin AN. Diagnosis of sports-related dermatoses. *Int J Dermatol* 2004;43:113–19.
3 Mailler-Savage EA, Adams BB. Skin manifestations of running. *J Am Acad Dermatol* 2006;55:290–301.
6 Beck CK. Infectious diseases in sports. *Med Sci Sports Exerc* 2000;32:431–8.
16 Kockentiet B, Adams BB. Contact dermatitis in athletes. *J Am Acad Dermatol* 2007;56:1048–55.
20 Wilkinson DS. Black heel: a minor hazard of sport. *Cutis* 1977;20:393–6.
26 Sher RK. Jogger's toe. *Int J Dermatol* 1978;17:719–20.
28 Basler RSW. Skin injuries in sports medicine. *J Am Acad Dermatol* 1989;21:1257–62.
30 Birrer RB, Halbrook SP. Martial arts injuries: the results of a 5 year national survey. *Am J Sports Med* 1988;16:408–10.
32 Clanton TO, Ford JJ. Turf toe injury. *Clin Sports Med* 1994;13:731–41.
43 Basler RSW. Acne mechanica in athletes. *Cutis* 1992;50:125–8.

Reactions to foreign materials
Foreign-body reactions
13 Jaworsky C. Analysis of cutaneous foreign bodies. *Clin Dermatol* 1991;9:157–78.
14 Bloom W, Fawcett DW. *A Textbook of Histology*, 10th edn. Philadelphia: Saunders, 1975:21–30.

Paraffinoma
1 Claudy A, Garcier F, Schmitt D. Sclerosing lipogranuloma of the male genitalia: ultrastructural study. *Br J Dermatol* 1981;105:451–6.
3 Feldman R, Harms M, Chavaz P *et al*. Orbital and palpebral paraffinoma. *J Am Acad Dermatol* 1992;26:833–5.

Sclerodermiform reaction to vitamin K and vitamin B_{12} injections
1 Alonso-Llamazares J, Ahmed I. Vitamin K-induced localised scleroderma (morphea) with linear deposition of IgA in the basement membrane zone. *J Am Acad Dermatol* 1998;38:322–4.
6 Ho J, Rothchild YH, Sengelmann R. Vitamin B12-associated localized scleroderma and its treatment. *Dermatol Surg* 2004;30:1252–5.

Pentazocine ulcers
1 Prasad HRY, Khaitan BK, Ramam M *et al*. Diagnostic clinical features of pentazocine-induced ulcers. *Int J Dermatol* 2005;44:910–15.

Reactions to intralesional corticosteroids
1 Goldman L. Reactions following intralesional and sublesional injections of corticosteroids. *JAMA* 1962;182:613–16.

Reactions to silicone
1 Ellenbogen R, Ellenbogen R, Rubin L. Injectable fluid silicone therapy: human morbidity and mortality. *JAMA* 1975;234:308–9.
4 Selmanovitz VJ, Orentreich N. Medical-grade fluid silicone: a monographic review. *J Dermatol Surg Oncol* 1977;3:597–611.
10 Senet P, Bachelez H, Ollivaud L *et al*. Minocycline for the treatment of cutaneous silicone granulomas. *Br J Dermatol* 1999;140:985–7.

Fibreglass dermatitis
3 Bjornberg A. Fiberglass dermatitis. *Am J Ind Med* 1985;8:395–400.

Complications of tattoos
7 Laumann AE, Derick AJ. Tattoos and body piercings in the United States: a national data set. *J Am Acad Dermatol* 2006;55:413–21.
10 Goldstein AP. Histologic reactions in tattoos. *J Dermatol Surg Oncol* 1979;5:896–900.
12 Limentani AE, Elliott LM, Noah ND *et al*. An outbreak of hepatitis B from tattooing. *Lancet* 1979;ii:86–8.
18 Sowden JM, Cartwright PH, Smith AG *et al*. Sarcoidosis presenting with a granulomatous reaction confined to red tattoos. *Clin Exp Dermatol* 1992;17:446–8.
22 Mortimer NJ, Chave TA, Johnson GA. Red tattoo reactions. *Clin Exp Dermatol* 2003;28:508–10.

Hair as a foreign body
1 Price SM, Popkin GL. Barbers' interdigital hair sinus. *Arch Dermatol* 1976;112:523–4.
7 Schroder CM, Merk HF, Frank J. Barber's hair sinus in a female hairdresser: uncommon manifestion of an occupational dermatosis. *J Eur Acad Dermatol Venereol* 2006;20:209–11.
8 Sakai R, Higashi K, Ohta M *et al*. Creeping hair: an isolated hair burrowing in the uppermost dermis resembling larva migrans. *Dermatology* 2006;213:242–4.
12 Jones D. Pilonidal sinus. *BMJ* 1992;305:409–12.
21 Matsushita S, Ohtake N, Mochitomi Y *et al*. A case of squamous cell carcinoma arising in a pilonidal sinus. *J Dermatol* 2002;29:757–8.
30 Perry PK, Cook-Bolden FE, Rahman Z *et al*. Defining pseudofolliculitis barbae in 2001: a review of the literature and current trends. *Am Acad Dermatol* 2002;46:113–19.
40 Kelly RI, Marsden RA. Complications of artificial hair implantation. *J R Soc Med* 1994;87:291–2.

Other skin injuries
Hand–arm vibration syndrome
1 Gemne G, Pyykkö I, Taylor W *et al*. The Stockholm Workshop Scale for the classification of cold-induced Raynaud's phenomenon in the hand–arm vibration syndrome (revision of the Taylor–Pelmear Scale). *Scand J Work Environ Health* 1987;13:275–8.
6 Palmer KT, Griffin MJ, Syddall H *et al*. Risk of hand–arm vibration syndrome according to occupation and sources of exposure to hand-transmitted vibration: a national survey. *Am J Ind Med* 2001;39:389–96.
11 Pelmear PL, Taylor W, Waiserman DE. *Hand–Arm Vibration: A Comprehensive Guide for Occupational Health Professionals*. New York: Van Nostrand Reinhold, 1992.

23 Su AT, Darus A, Bulgiba A *et al*. The clinical features of hand-arm vibration syndrome in a warm environment – a review of the literature. *J Occup Health* 2012;54:349–60.

25 Takeuchi T, Imanishi H. Histopathologic observations in finger biopsy from 30 patients with Raynaud's phenomenon of occupational origin. *J Kumamoto Med Soc* 1984;58:56–70.

28 Ekenvall L, Lindblad LE, Norbeck O *et al*. Alpha-adrenoreceptors and cold-induced vasoconstriction in human finger skin. *Am J Physiol* 1988;255:1000–3.

31 Hirata M, Sakakibara H, Abe M. Reduced sensory nerve conduction velocity of the distal part of the radial nerve among patients with vibration syndrome. *Electromyogr Clin Neurophysiol* 2002;42:113–18.

34 Takeuchi T, Futatsuka M, Imanishi H *et al*. Pathological changes observed in the finger biopsy of patients with vibration induced white finger. *Scand J Work Environ Health* 1986;12:280–3.

37 Noel B. Pathophysiology and classification of the vibration white finger. *Int Arch Occup Environ Health* 2000;73:150–5.

52 Pelmear PL, Taylor W. Hand–arm vibration syndrome. *J Fam Prac* 1994;33:180–5.

65 Bilgi C, Pelmear PL. Hand–arm vibration (HAVS): a guide to medical impairment assessment. *J Occup Med* 1993;35:936–42.

75 Pelmear PL, Leong D. Review of occupational standards and guidelines for hand–arm (segmental) vibration syndrome (HAVS). *Appl Occup Environ Hyg* 2000;15:291–302.

Piezogenic pedal papules

1 Cohen HJ, Gibbs RC, Minkin W *et al*. Painful piezogenic pedal papules. *Arch Dermatol* 1970;101:112–13.

3 Schlappner OLA, Wood MG, Gerstein W *et al*. Painful and non-painful piezogenic pedal papules. *Arch Dermatol* 1972;106:729–33.

5 Van Straaten EA, van Langen IM, Oorthuys JWE *et al*. Piezogenic papules of the feet in healthy children and their possible relation with connective tissue disorders. *Pediatr Dermatol* 1991;8:277–9.

15 Boni R, Dummer R. Compression therapy in painful piezogenic pedal papules. *Arch Dermatol* 1996;132:127–8.

16 Woodrow SL, Brereton-Smith G, Handfield-Jones S. Painful piezogenic pedal papules: response to local electro-acupuncture. *Br J Dermatol* 1997;136:628–30.

17 Doukas DJ, Holmes J, Leonard JA. A nonsurgical approach to painful piezogenic pedal papules. *Cutis* 2004;73:339–40, 346.

18 Ronnen M, Suster S, Huszar M *et al*. Solitary painful piezogenic pedal papule in a patient with rheumatoid arthritis. *Int J Dermatol* 1987;6:240–1.

CHAPTER 123

Pressure Injury and Pressure Ulcers

Emily Haesler[1,2] *and Jan Kottner*[3,4]

[1] Curtin Health Innovation Research Institute, Curtin University, Perth, Western Australia, Australia
[2] Australian Centre for Evidence Based Aged Care, School of Nursing, La Trobe University, Melbourne, Victoria, Australia
[3] Charité-Universitätsmedizin Berlin, Institute of Clinical Nursing Science, Berlin, Germany
[4] Ghent University, Faculty of Medicine and Health Sciences, Ghent, Belgium

Definition and nomenclature, 123.1	Predisposing factors, 123.3	Risk assessment, 123.6
Introduction and general description, 123.1	Clinical features, 123.4	Prevention of pressure ulcers, 123.6
Epidemiology, 123.1	Classification, 123.4	Treatment of pressure ulcers, 123.9
Pathophysiology, 123.2	Management, 123.6	Key references, 123.12

Definition and nomenclature

A pressure ulcer may be defined as localised damage to the skin and/or underlying tissue as a result of pressure or pressure in combination with shear. Pressure injuries/ulcers usually occur over a bony prominence but may also be related to a medical device or other object [1]. A pressure ulcer can involve damage to the epidermis, dermis and subcutaneous tissues, including fat, muscle and tendon.

> **Synonyms and inclusions**
> - Pressure ulcer (UK/English-speaking community Europe)
> - Pressure injury (US/Canada/Australia/Asia)

Previous terms that are still used include 'decubitus ulcers' and 'bed sores' (both terms that refer to lying in bed, which is just one potential mechanism for tissue damage) and 'ischaemic ulcers' (a term which implies an overly limited aetiological pathway) [1,2]. In the latest *ICD-11* the term 'pressure ulceration' is used [3].

Introduction and general description

Pressure ulcers present a significant health concern for patients, their families and health care systems. They are associated with increased morbidity and mortality [4], pain and discomfort. There is also a negative impact on quality of life, including increased anxiety and depression [5,6], and decreased autonomy [6] and social function [7]. Economic evaluations show high financial costs associated with increased hospitalisation and care cost [8,9], approaching $11.6 billion annually in the USA [9] and up to 4% of NHS budget in the UK [10].

Pressure ulcers occur most often in individuals with multiple risk factors, including age over 65 years, spinal cord injuries, other mobility-related deficits (e.g. fractured hip and extended surgical procedure), chronic neurological conditions, diabetes mellitus, and requiring critical or trauma care [1].

Pressure ulcers primarily occur on bony prominences. Based on data from almost 80 European clinical studies, pressure ulcers are shown to occur most often at the sacrum and heels (Figure 123.1) [11].

As pressure ulcers are largely preventable, identifying patients who exhibit risk factors and developing a prevention plan that addresses these risks are essential [12]. Strategies including an appropriate support surface, a skin care regimen and regular repositioning of the patient are key preventative measures [1] alongside regular skin assessment to ensure early identification of localised skin and/or tissue damage.

Once a pressure ulcer is suspected, differential diagnosis followed by an assessment of the extent of skin and/or tissue damage using a pressure ulcer classification system should be undertaken, followed by appropriate management by a multidisciplinary team.

Epidemiology

Estimates of prevalence and incidence of pressure ulcers vary widely depending on the clinical setting, population and methodology used to measure and report pressure ulcer proportion and rates. While prevalence provides an overview of the burden of pressure ulcers, incidence rates provide an indication of new events over time. So called facility-acquired pressure ulcers are also reported, indicating pressure ulcerations that occur during an individual's facility stay [1]. Table 123.1 provides estimates of pressure ulcer prevalence and incidence in a range of populations, based on pooled meta-analysis when available.

Rook's Textbook of Dermatology, Tenth Edition. Edited by Christopher Griffiths, Jonathan Barker, Tanya Bleiker, Walayat Hussain and Rosalind Simpson.
© 2024 John Wiley & Sons Ltd. Published 2024 by John Wiley & Sons Ltd.

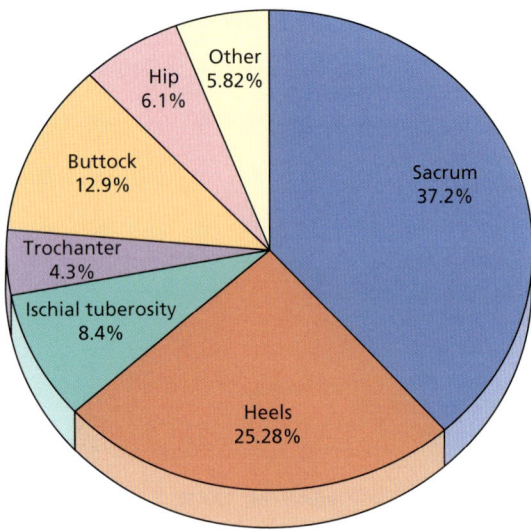

Figure 123.1 Indicative pressure ulcer prevalence by anatomical site.

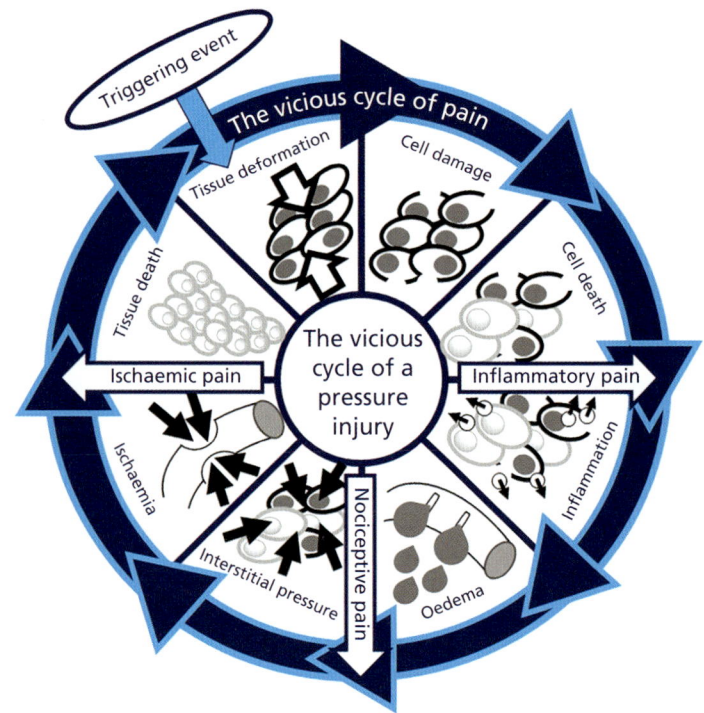

Figure 123.2 Cycle of cell damage and pain experience in pressure ulcer development. Developed by Gefen and Soppi (2020) [37], reproduced with permission from Cambridge Media.

Additionally, many pressure ulcers are associated with medical devices (e.g. monitors, leads, tubes, splints and braces, catheters, etc.), particularly in populations with more vulnerable skin such as neonates and children. In intensive care units (ICUs) where medical device use is almost ubiquitous, estimates of the prevalence of medical device-related pressure injuries is estimated at 6.46% (95% confidence interval [CI] 1.97–13.11%), while the incidence of medical device-related pressure injuries in ICU is estimated at 3.85% (95%CI 0–16.71%) [28].

Pathophysiology

Pressure ulcers occur due to prolonged exposure to mechanical load increasing internal stresses and strains exceeding the resistance of the skin and/or underlying soft tissues, such as subcutaneous fat and muscle tissues [29]. Damage is more likely to occur when the patient's damage threshold is reduced due to morphological properties of the tissue or bone anatomy, mechanical properties of the skin and tissue and/or their circulatory supply, and other unknown highly individual intrinsic susceptibility to mechanical loading [30–32].

Mechanical load refers to forces that are applied to the skin and soft tissues due to contact between the skin and a supporting surface (for example, a bed or chair). These forces are pressure, friction and shear. They may occur either as an external load or as a force transferred through bony structures and the soft tissue to the supporting surface (i.e. bodyweight). External loads can occur as forces that are either perpendicular (normal force) or parallel to the skin surface (shear force); in real-world clinical situations both normal and shear forces always occur together [33]. Mechanical loads are usually highest near to bony prominences or other stiff internal anatomical structures (e.g. tendon or joint capsules), where pressure ulceration is most likely to start.

Prolonged deformation of skin and underlying soft tissues leads to a number of pathophysiological processes (represented in Figure 123.2). Very high strains (e.g. when lying on a hard spine board) may lead to *direct tissue deformation damage* in very short periods of time (e.g. minutes) [29,33,34]. The mechanical deformation may directly cause cell membrane failure and/or the disruption of the cytoskeleton [34].

Irrespective of the primary triggering event, the initial cell damage and necrotic area cause local inflammation, oedema and further changes in the mechanical properties of the affected soft tissues, leading to a possible damage cycle [33,35]. Depending on the duration and degree of strain, blood and lymph vessels may also be occluded, limiting perfusion (*ischaemia*). This causes metabolic changes, including accumulation of waste products and acidosis in the affected tissues. If this ischaemic process continues for several hours, cell damage and local necrosis may occur [29]. Unloading of the compressed tissue helps to restore perfusion (reactive hyperaemia); however, unloading may also result in increased inflammatory responses known as *reperfusion injury* [29,33,36].

Because mechanical loads are highest near bony prominences and muscle tissue is most susceptible to ischaemic and direct deformation damage, initial necrotic regions usually occur near bony prominences under intact skin [30,38,39]. If the initial necrotic area is small, there is complete perfusion, no other mechanical deformation occurs and there is sufficient healing capacity [35,40], this injury can resolve quickly, sometimes unnoticed by clinicians [41]. However, if the necrotic region exceeds an absorbable size, perfusion is reduced and/or other direct or indirect risk factors apply, deep pressure ulcers may develop. This is referred to as the 'bottom-up' or 'inside-out' pathway of pressure ulceration [41] and may take up to two weeks from initial damage to fully visualise the extent of the pressure ulcer [42–44]. Even if only superficial clinical signs are visible (ie. a Category I or II pressure ulcer as

Table 123.1 Prevalence and incidence by population and clinical setting.

Population and setting		Prevalence	Incidence/facility-acquired
Adult care	By setting		
	Acute care	12.8% (95%CI[a] 11.8–13.9%) [13]	8.4% (95%CI 7.6–9.3%) [13]
	Intensive care	10.0–25.9% [14]	16.9–23.8% [14]
	Aged care	3.4–32.4% [15]	1.9% [16] to 59% [17]
	Palliative care	12.4% (range 9.9–54.7%) [18]	11.3% (range 0–37.5%) [18]
	Mixed settings	10.8% (SD[b] 7%, range 4.6–27.2%) [11]	—
Paediatric care	By age		
	Neonates	27.0% (95%CI 22.1–33.1%) [19]	9.8% (95%CI 2.9–19.8%) [19]
	<1 year old	19.2% (95%CI 9.4–31.3%) [19]	11.3% (95%CI 4.4–20.7%) [19]
	1–18 years old	12.3% (95%CI 2.3–27.9%) [19]	—
	By setting		
	Primary health care	1.75% [20]	0.57% [21] to 21.4% [22]
	General acute care	1.8–4.0% [22]	0.25% [23] to 27% [24]
	Critical care	32.8% [22]	0.29% [25] to 27.7% [26]
	Rehabilitation	4.40% [27]	0.86% [27]
	Mixed settings	2.25% [27]	1.41% [27]

[a] 95%CI = 95% confidence interval.
[b] SD = standard deviation.

Table 123.2 Pressure ulcer risk factors: mechanisms and level of associated risk [1,46].

Risk factors	Risk factor mechanism[a]	Risk[b]
Activity and mobility limitations		
General activity and mobility limitation	MBC	High
Time spent immobilised before surgery	MBC	Moderate
Duration of surgery	MBC	Moderate
Skin status		
Having a Category/Stage I pressure ulcer	ST	High[c]
Having pressure ulcer of any category/stage	ST	Weak[d]
Skin maturity in neonates and children	ST	Moderate
Perfusion, circulation and oxygenation factors		
Diabetes mellitus	ST	Moderate
Perfusion and circulation deficits	ST	Moderate
Oxygenation deficits	ST	Weak
Impaired nutrition	ST	Moderate
Moist skin	MBC; ST	Weak
Increased body temperature	ST	Weak
Older age	MBC; ST	Weak
Sensory perception limitations	MBC	Weak
Blood markers	ST	Weak
General and mental health status	MBC; ST	Weak

[a] MBC, mechanical boundary conditions; ST, individual's susceptibility and tolerance.
[b] Likelihood that risk factor presence will increase pressure ulcer risk based on systematic review of prognostic studies.
[c] Risk of developing a more serious pressure ulcer.
[d] Risk of developing another pressure ulcer.

described in Table 123.3), deeper soft tissues are also likely to be affected [45].

Predisposing factors

Risk for pressure ulcers is influenced by a range of factors that affect either the level of damage associated with exposure to mechanical load, or the individual's susceptibility and ability to tolerate that load (Figure 123.3) [46].

Risk factors (Table 123.2) that influence the type, magnitude and duration of the mechanical load contribute to increased internal strain and stress that could lead to a pressure ulcer. This is more likely to occur in the presence of risk factors that influence the susceptibility and tolerance of the patient to tissue loading [1,46]. The factors in Table 123.2 often occur in combination leading to more complex pathophysiological processes that increase pressure ulcer risk.

Mechanical boundary-related risk factors. Reduced mobility and/or activity are necessary conditions for pressure ulcers [1]. When a person moves around regularly, they probably will not develop a pressure ulcer (unless associated with medical devices). Reduced mobility influences the mechanical boundary conditions by increasing exposure to friction and shear and increasing the duration of exposure to mechanical load [1,46]. Patients who are bed- or chairbound are at specific risk [47,48]; other examples include critically unwell, neurological impairment, or undergoing anaesthesia.

Moisture, temperature, humidity and airflow at the skin/surface interface are referred to as the *microclimate* [49]. Changes in these conditions, particularly increased hydration of the stratum corneum, affect mechanical boundary conditions by influencing the frictional properties of skin, the magnitudes of frictional forces and the level of frictional sliding movement and shear force between the skin and surface. Additionally, skin structural changes associated with hydration can influence its protective ability and therefore the patient's tolerance and susceptibility to forces. Numerous conditions increase skin hydration and are therefore considered risk factors, including incontinence and increased perspiration [1].

Sensory deficits, common sequelae of neurological impairment, reduce the patient's ability to detect pain and discomfort from pressure, reducing the natural response to reposition and thereby increasing duration of exposure to the mechanical load [50].

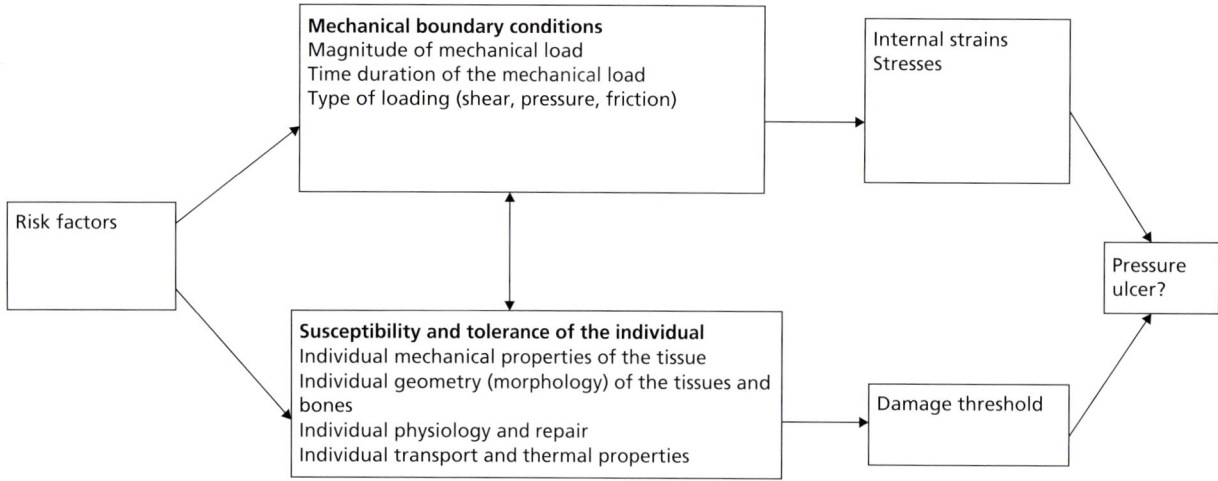

Figure 123.3 Factors influencing risk of developing a pressure ulcer/injury [46]. Reproduced from [46] with permission from John Wiley & Sons.

Susceptibility and tolerance-related risk factors. Logistic models indicate that a previous pressure ulcer is indicative of increased risk of future ulceration or scar tissue breakdown [51]. Patients with an existing pressure ulcer have a high propensity to developing a deeper or a new pressure ulcer [1,46]. Other cutaneous changes including xerosis may also increase pressure ulcer risk. In neonates, skin immaturity is considered as an additional risk [52]. More recently, skin pain at pressure points has been identified as a potential risk factor [53].

Perfusion, circulation and oxygenation factors are indicators of cardiovascular supply to the skin. Diabetes mellitus is a surrogate indicator of underlying cardiovascular dysfunction and can also contribute to neurological and sensory impairment [1]. Deficits in perfusion, circulation and oxygenation are identified and measured via numerous indicators including smoking status, pulse pressure, blood pressure, ankle-brachial pulse index, oedema and diagnosed vascular or respiratory disease [1,46,54]. For patients receiving critical care, use of both vasopressors and mechanical ventilation are additional risks [55].

Impaired nutritional status, measured as food intake, diagnosis of malnutrition, anthropometric measurements or score on a nutrition assessment tool, is associated with a moderate increase in pressure ulcer risk [1,46,56]. Other factors commonly recognised to increase risk include age, general health and mental status and impaired laboratory blood tests (e.g. lymphopenia, albumin levels and inflammatory markers) [57], which are de facto measures of disease and inflammation [1].

Clinical features

Following a baseline risk assessment, regular assessment of the skin is required to identify early signs of a pressure ulcer. Changes to the characteristics and appearance of skin and underlying tissues can provide an early indicator of pressure damage [58]. Pay particular attention to skin folds, skin over bony prominences, skin around and under medical devices and, in children, the occiput [1].

Differential diagnosis from other types of skin ulcer or skin conditions (particularly so-called moisture-associated skin damage [59]) is required.

Redness is the most significant indicator of pressure damage; it is important to differentiate persistent, non-blanchable redness (an indicator of pressure damage) from blanchable redness. Non-blanchable redness persists with the application of pressure and suggests structural damage to the capillary bed/microcirculation, and is an indication of a Category 1 pressure ulcer [60]. Blanchable redness goes white under light pressure and may be either a normal hyperaemic response or an inflammatory response without damage to the microcirculation. When evaluating darker skin tones, redness may be more subtle and it is important to assess for tissue oedema, cooler skin temperature and areas of discoloration in relation to surrounding skin [1,61,62].

Skin temperature may be assessed using either the hand, a thermographic imaging device or an infrared thermometer [1,63]. Tissue oedema can be assessed by palpation, paying attention to changes in consistency, or using instrumental devices (e.g. instruments *measuring the water content of soft tissues based on the electrical capacitance*) [1,64]. Poorer prognosis of a pressure injury, and detection of deep tissue injury, is associated with cooler areas of skin [61] and increase in tissue oedema [62].

Classification

To document, interpret and compare morbidity and mortality data [2] and, to a lesser extent, to assist in selecting treatment options, pressure ulcers are classified according to the type and extent of skin and tissue involvement that can be visually observed (and felt/palpated). Different classification systems have evolved as the conceptualisation of pressure damage has changed over time.

Two of the most commonly used pressure ulcer classification systems are the National Pressure Injury Advisory Panel/European Pressure Ulcer Advisory Panel (NPIAP/EPUAP) International Classification System (2009, 2014, 2019) [1,65,66] and the World Health Organization International Statistical Classification of Diseases and Related Health Problems, edition 11 (WHO ICD-11) (2018) [3] (Table 123.3).

Table 123.3 Two commonly used pressure ulcer classification systems. With permission from National Pressure Injury Advisory Panel, © 2020.

NPIAP/EPUAP International PU Classification (2009, 2014, 2019) [1,65,66]	WHO ICD-11 (2018) [3]	Graphic	Indicative photograph
Category/Stage I pressure ulcer: non-blanchable erythema Intact skin with non-blanchable redness of a localised area usually over a bony prominence. Darkly pigmented skin may not have visible blanching; its colour may differ from the surrounding area. The area may be painful, firm, soft, warmer or cooler as compared with adjacent tissue. Category/Stage I may be difficult to detect in individuals with dark skin tones. May indicate 'at risk' individuals (a heralding sign of risk).	**EH90.0 Pressure ulceration grade 1** Pressure ulceration grade I is a precursor to skin ulceration. The skin remains intact but there is non-blanchable redness of a localised area, usually over a bony prominence. The area may be painful, firm, soft, warmer or cooler as compared with adjacent tissue. It can be difficult to detect in individuals with dark skin but affected areas may differ in colour from the surrounding skin. The presence of pressure ulceration grade 1 may indicate persons at risk of progressing to frank ulceration.	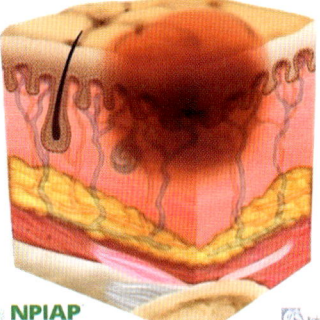	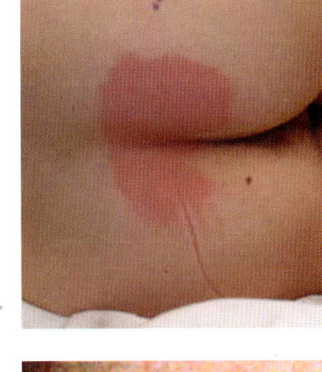
Category/Stage II pressure ulcer: partial-thickness skin loss Partial-thickness loss of dermis presenting as a shallow open ulcer with a red/pink wound bed, without slough. May also present as an intact or open/ruptured serum-filled blister. Presents as a shiny or dry shallow ulcer without slough or bruising.* This category/stage should not be used to describe skin tears, tape burns, perineal dermatitis, maceration or excoriation. *Bruising indicates suspected deep tissue injury.	**EH90.1 Pressure ulceration grade 2** Pressure injury with partial-thickness loss of dermis. It presents as a shallow open ulcer with a red or pink wound bed without slough or as a serum-filled or serosanguinous blister which may rupture. This category should not be used to describe skin tears, tape burns, incontinence associated dermatitis, maceration or excoriation.	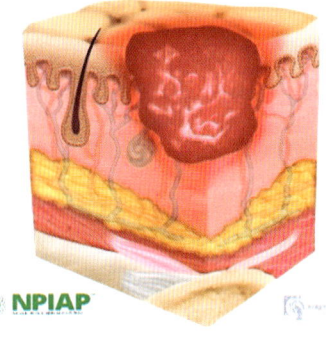	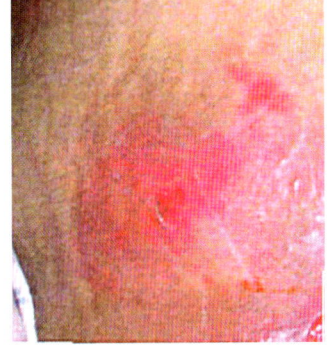
Category/Stage III pressure ulcer: full-thickness skin loss Full-thickness tissue loss. Subcutaneous fat may be visible, but bone, tendon or muscle is not exposed. Slough may be present but does not obscure the depth of tissue loss. May include undermining and tunnelling. The depth of a Category/Stage III pressure ulcer varies by anatomical location. The bridge of the nose, ear, occiput and malleolus do not have subcutaneous tissue and Category/Stage III ulcers can be shallow. In contrast, areas of significant adiposity can develop extremely deep Category/Stage III pressure ulcers. Bone/tendon is not visible or directly palpable.	**EH90.2 Pressure ulceration grade 3** Pressure ulcer with full-thickness skin loss. Subcutaneous fat may be visible but bone, tendon or muscle is not exposed. Slough may be present but does not obscure the depth of tissue loss. There may be undermining and tunnelling into adjacent structures. The depth varies by anatomical location: grade 3 pressure ulcers can be shallow in areas with little or no subcutaneous fat (e.g. bridge of the nose, ear, occiput and malleolus). In contrast, grade 3 pressure ulcers can be extremely deep in areas of significant adiposity.	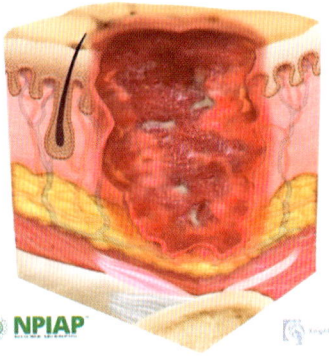	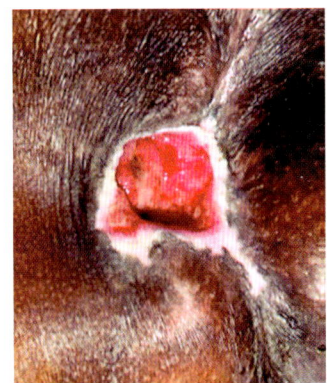
Category/Stage IV pressure ulcer: full-thickness tissue loss Full-thickness tissue loss with exposed bone, tendon or muscle. Slough or eschar may be present on some parts of the wound bed. Often include undermining and tunneling. The depth of a Category/Stage IV pressure ulcer varies by anatomical location. The bridge of the nose, ear, occiput and malleolus do not have subcutaneous tissue and these ulcers can be shallow. Category/Stage IV ulcers can extend into muscle and/or supporting structures (e.g. fascia, tendon or joint capsule) making osteomyelitis possible. Exposed bone/tendon is visible or directly palpable.	**EH90.3 Pressure ulceration grade 4** Pressure ulcer with visible or directly palpable muscle, tendon or bone as a result of full-thickness loss of skin and subcutaneous tissue. Slough or eschar may be present. The depth varies by anatomical location: grade IV pressure ulcers can be shallow in areas with little or no subcutaneous fat (e.g. bridge of the nose, ear, occiput and malleolus) but are typically deep and often undermine or tunnel into adjacent structures.	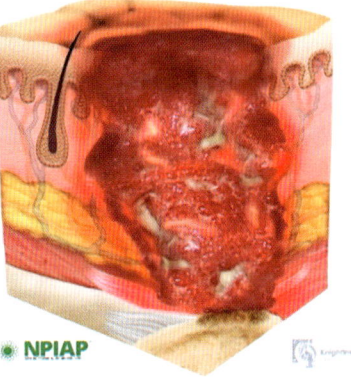	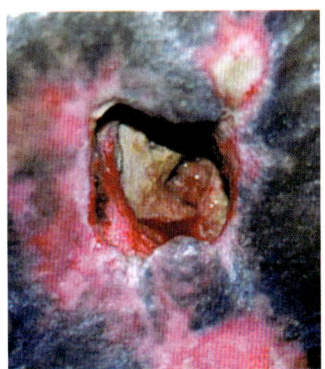

(continued overleaf)

Table 123.3 (continued)

NPIAP/EPUAP International PU Classification (2009, 2014, 2019) [1,65,66]	WHO ICD-11 (2018) [3]	Graphic	Indicative photograph
Unstageable: depth unknown Full-thickness tissue loss in which the base of the ulcer is covered by slough (yellow, tan, grey, green or brown) and/or eschar (tan, brown or black) in the wound bed. Until enough slough and/or eschar is removed to expose the base of the wound, the true depth, and therefore category/stage, cannot be determined. Stable (dry, adherent, intact without redness or fluctuance) eschar on the heels serves as 'the body's natural (biological) cover' and should not be removed.	**EH90.5 Pressure ulceration, ungradable** Pressure ulcer with full-thickness skin loss in which actual depth of the ulcer is completely obscured by slough (yellow, tan, grey, green or brown) and/or eschar (tan, brown or black) in the wound bed. Until enough slough and/or eschar are removed to expose the base of the wound, it is not possible to determine whether the ulcer is grade 3 or grade 4.	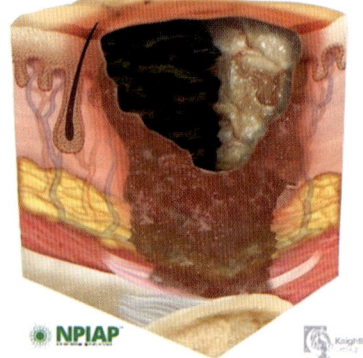	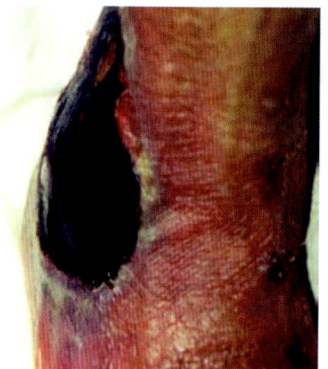
Suspected deep tissue injury (SDTI): depth unknown Purple or maroon localised area of discoloured intact skin or blood-filled blister due to damage of underlying soft tissue from pressure and/or shear. The area may be preceded by tissue that is painful, firm, mushy, boggy, warmer or cooler as compared with adjacent tissue. Deep tissue injury may be difficult to detect in individuals with dark skin tones. Evolution may include a thin blister over a dark wound bed. The wound may further evolve and become covered by thin eschar. Evolution may be rapid exposing additional layers of tissue even with optimal treatment.	**EH90.6 Suspected deep pressure-induced tissue damage, depth unknown** An area of soft tissue damage due to pressure or shear which is anticipated to evolve into a deep pressure ulcer but has not yet done so. The affected skin is typically discoloured purple or maroon and may display haemorrhagic blistering. It may be painful and oedematous. It can be either warmer or cooler than adjacent tissue. Evolution into a deep ulcer may be rapid even with optimal treatment.	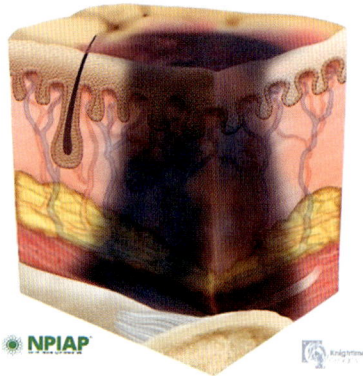	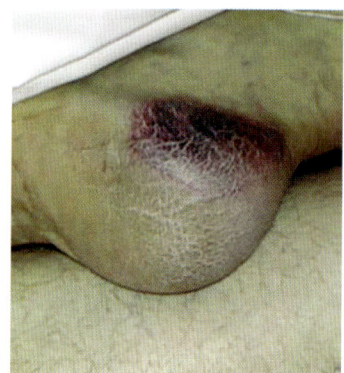

Other classification systems [67] are used in some geographic regions or clinical settings.

Management

Risk assessment

Every patient should be rapidly screened for pressure ulcer risk on admission using clinical knowledge of the risk factors, noting that impairment to mobility/activity or skin integrity are strong predictors of a high risk [1,68,69]. A more comprehensive risk assessment should follow, using a structured approach based on clinical judgement [69,70], which could be facilitated using a risk assessment tool [71] (Table 123.4). Assessment tools offer a structured approach to risk assessment, but are neither comprehensive, nor do they replace clinical judgement [70,71]; using them alone does not reduce the risk of a pressure ulcer [1,71]. In addition to questionable clinical relevance, the measurement properties depend on cut-off scores and are highly dependent on the setting and unlikely to improve clinical decision making.

Once assessed the health care professional should develop an individualised plan to mitigate and minimise risks specific to the patient [1].

Prevention of pressure ulcers

Figure 123.4 provides an overview algorithm for prevention and treatment of pressure ulcers.

Repositioning. Repositioning is one of the most important preventative interventions because it reduces the duration once anatomical location is exposed to mechanical load. This is particularly important for people who are unable to reposition themselves, and/or who are unable to detect or respond to stimulus that indicates exposure to pressure (e.g. pain) [73]. Repositioning should be done in such a way and using appropriate manual handling equipment to avoid exposure to unintentional friction and shear from dragging [1]. Assess the patient after repositioning to ensure that medical devices are correctly positioned, no items are inadvertently left under the patient and pressure points are fully offloaded [1]. More recently, real-time continuous bedside pressure mapping has become available in some regions and this may be used to evaluate pressure redistribution on the support surface [1].

Frequency of repositioning should be individualised [1] and based on level of activity/mobility [74], response of the skin and tissue [53,75] to the time spent in one position, general condition, sleep requirements [76], comfort and pain [53]. Using repositioning reminder systems (e.g. wearable sensors, musical

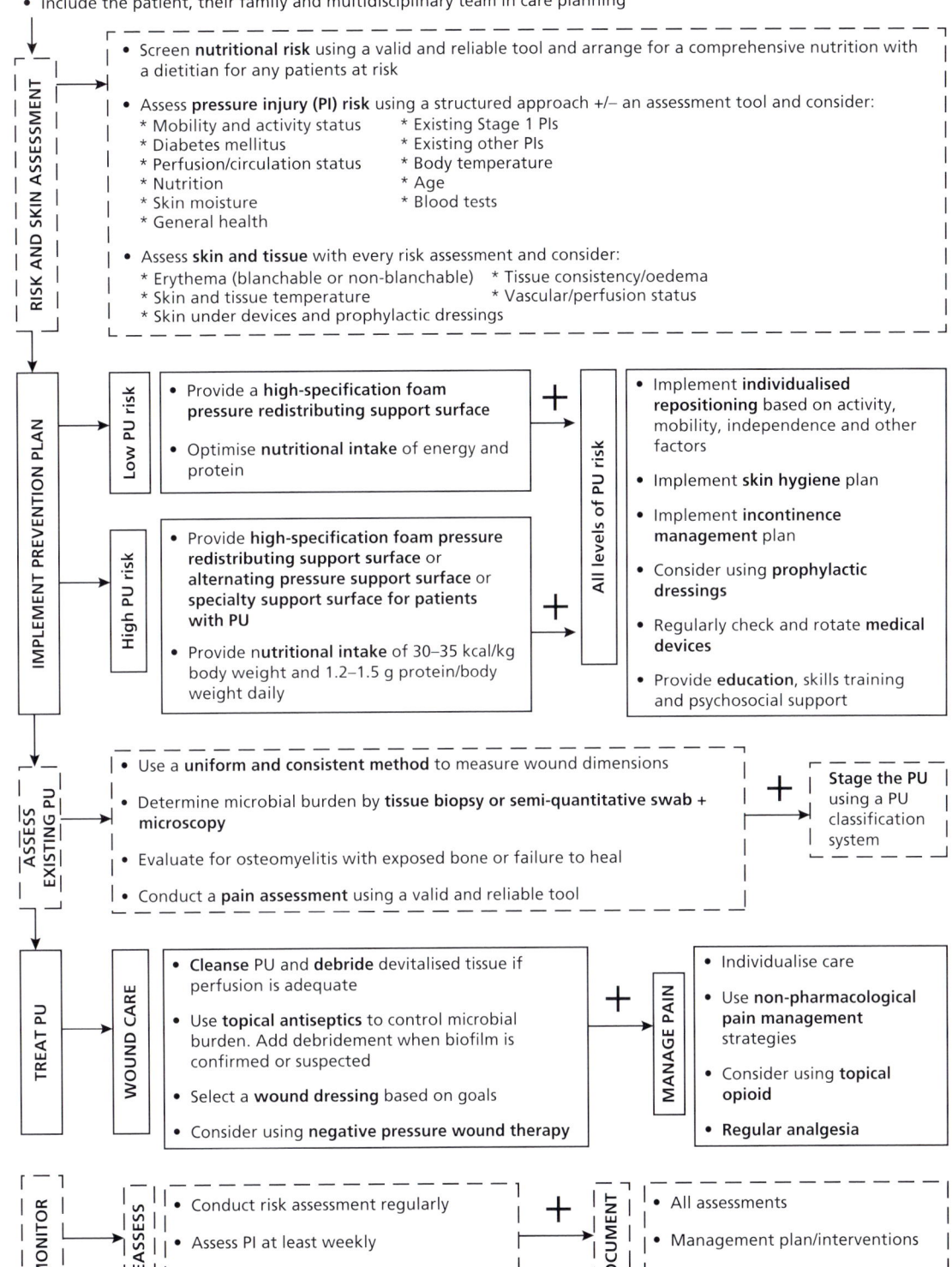

Figure 123.4 Algorithm for assessment, prevention and treatment of pressure ulcers. Adapted from [72].

Table 123.4 Characteristics of pressure ulcer risk assessment tools, adapted with permission from EPUAP/NPIAP/PPPIA International Pressure Ulcer/Injury Guideline (2019) [1].

Risk tool	Risk factors on tool		Sensitivity median (range)	Specificity median (range)
Braden Scale (all adults)	Mobility Activity Friction-shear	Nutrition Moisture Sensory perception	0.74 (0.33–1.0)	0.68 (0.34–0.86)
Norton Scale (all adults)	Mobility Activity Food intake Fluid intake	Incontinence Physical condition Mental condition	0.75 (0–0.89)	0.68 (0.59–0.95)
Waterlow Scale (all adults)	Mobility Skin type Special risk Appetite Build (weight for height)	Continence Gender/age Neurological deficit Major surgery/trauma Medications	0.88–1.00	0.13–0.29
Cubbin-Jackson Scale (critically ill adults)	Mobility General skin condition Hygiene Oxygen requirements Respiration Haemodynamics	Weight/tissue viability Nutrition Incontinence Mental condition Past medical condition	0.72	0.68
SCIPUS (adults with spinal cord injury)	Mobility Level of activity Complete SCI Autonomic dysreflexia/severe spasticity Blood glucose levels Tobacco use Cardiac disease	Urine incontinence or moistness Age Albumin Haematocrit Respiratory disease Renal disease Cognitive function	0.85	0.38
Braden Q (children)	Mobility Activity Friction-shear	Tissue perfusion oxygenation Sensory perception	0.86 (0.76–0.96)	0.59 (0.55–0.63)

chimes or visual cues) has been shown to increase adherence of both patients and health professionals to repositioning regimens [77,78].

The way in which the patient is repositioned is as important as repositioning frequency. Avoid positioning the patient on areas of existing non-blanchable erythema [1]. Use support pillows to promote offloading and ergonomic positioning, paying particular attention to the heels. Heel lifts or heel supports that provide support along the full length of the calf, avoiding pressure on the Achilles tendon, are recommended [1,79]. When positioned in supine, maintain the bed as flat as possible to reduce shear and friction [80]. In lateral position, a 30-degree tilt reduces pressure on the trochanter more effectively than a 90-degree tilt [81]. Prone position should be minimised unless the patient's clinical condition requires. Use facial pillows and prophylactic dressings to reduce pressure ulcer risk when using this vulnerable position [1,82]. For patients sitting out of bed, reduce time spent seated upright and reduce the mechanical load on the sacrum by using reclined seating with the legs supported, and tilt-in-space options when available [83,84]. This prevents the person from sliding forward, causing friction and shear [1].

Support surfaces. A support surface is a specialised device designed to redistribute pressure through the management of the mechanical load (Table 123.5). A pressure redistributing support surface distributes the forces applied to the body across a larger surface area, which reduces the mechanical load sustained to pressure susceptible anatomical locations. Redistribution of pressure occurs through immersion and/or envelopment of the patient in the support surface [1]. In most advanced countries, the standard foam mattress that is supplied in a health care setting has technical characteristics that are classified as high specification. However, some facilities still provide mattresses that do not adequately redistribute pressure.

Strong evidence shows that using a foam mattress with high-specification pressure redistributing characteristics is more effective in preventing a pressure ulcer than a standard foam mattress [88]. Individual patient needs and preferences may require consideration of other support surfaces. Reactive air support surfaces are comparable to high-specification foam mattresses [1,89]; less evidence is available on effectiveness of other constant lower-pressure surfaces. Contemporary alternating air pressure mattresses and low air loss beds are considered specialty support surfaces because they have more technical features that optimise the microclimate, which is a priority for some patients. Alternating pressure air mattresses are more effective than a standard foam mattress but have also been shown to be less comfortable [87], as have low

Table 123.5 Types of support surfaces, their characteristics and clinical use.

Type of surface	Characteristics	Clinical use
Reactive support surfaces High-specification single-layer foam mattress/cushion/overlay	Constant lower pressure Immerses and/or envelops the body Made from high-resilience foam and with a density >35 kg/m^3 [1] Sufficient thickness to prevent bottoming out [1]	Select for patients at risk of pressure ulcers who can independently reposition [1]
Static air mattress/cushion/overlay without alternating air features	Constant lower pressure Immerses and/or envelops the body Requires regular inspection to ensure it is functional May require power and regular maintenance If powered, may be noisy and generate heat and motion	An option for patients at risk of pressure ulcers who can independently reposition [1] Consider other options if noise, heat or motion is disruptive [1]
Water, gel or bead surfaces Medical grade sheepskin (Australian Standard AS4480.1)	Constant lower pressure Immerses and/or envelops the body Can become overly warm Requires specialty laundering [85]	An option for patients at risk of pressure ulcers who can independently reposition [1,85] Consider other options for people with incontinence or heavy wound exudate [1]
Air fluidised beds	High immersion and envelopment High moisture vapour transmission rate, which can increase humidity between the surface and the skin [1] Reduces patient mobility	An option for patients with pressure ulcers [1]
Active support surfaces Low air loss surfaces (may be combined with an active or reactive surface)	Ambient air is circulated below the mattress to control temperature and moisture, maintaining a constant microclimate Noisy and generates heat and motion May be uncomfortable [1,86]	An option for patients with or at risk of pressure ulcers regardless of whether they can independently reposition [1] An option for people with obesity who require superior control of the microclimate [1] Consider other options if noise, heat or motion is disruptive [1]
Alternating pressure air mattress or overlay or cushion	Periodic redistribution of pressure across surface of the body as different mattress cells inflate and deflate Control of microclimate achieved by the changing cell contact with the body continually replacing air at the skin surface Noisy and generates heat and motion Can be difficult to get in/out of bed Less comfortable than a standard hospital mattress [87]	

air loss beds [1,86]. Regardless of the support surface chosen, the patient still requires regular repositioning [1].

Nutrition. The patient requires macro- and micronutrients for maintenance and repair of the skin and tissues. Inadequate nutritional intake and undernutrition are associated with the development, severity and duration of pressure ulcers [90]. All patients should be screened using a population-specific nutrition screening tool, and those identified as having a nutrition risk should be referred to a dietitian for a comprehensive nutritional assessment [1,91–93].

Skin protection and hygiene. Maintaining skin integrity and the barrier function is important. Increased skin hydration, as well as the mechanical damage of the stratum corneum and underlying skin layers, increases the risk of pressure ulcers [1]. Ensure that excess moisture on the skin surface is reduced through regular hygiene, use of high-absorbency incontinence products [94] and application of skin protection products. Minimise exposure to irritants (including faeces and urine) and promote the skin's integrity through use of mild soaps or cleansers [95], and avoid friction from excessive rubbing [96].

Prophylactic soft silicone multilayered foam dressings are used to protect individuals with higher pressure ulcer risk. A prophylactic dressing should be initiated early in the care pathway and used at anatomical sites most vulnerable for the specific patient (e.g. heels or sacrum) [1,97]. Prophylactic dressings made of multiple layers reduce the interface pressure, friction and shear between and within the skin and the support surface [98,99]. It is important to assess the skin underneath the dressing regularly [1]; prophylactic dressings are transparent and/or designed to be easily lifted for skin inspection [97,100,101].

Treatment of pressure ulcers

Continue and escalate preventative strategies. Review and reinforce preventative measures discussed earlier.

The nutrition management plan should ensure intake meets general energy, protein and micronutrient requirements, plus additional requirements associated with wound healing [102]. For adults

Table 123.6 Aspects of wound care and associated local wound care strategies.

Aspect of wound care	Goals of wound care	Clinical strategies to achieve goals
Tissue management	Removing devitalised or necrotic tissue	Wound assessment Cleansing Debridement
Inflammation and infection	Control of inflammation Treatment of microbial burden Treatment of biofilm	Wound assessment Control of inflammation Topical antimicrobial treatment Debridement
Moisture balance	Promoting moist wound healing	Wound assessment Wound dressings Debridement
Epithelial edges	Reducing the wound size	Wound monitoring Control of inflammation Topical antimicrobial treatment Debridement Wound dressings Negative pressure wound therapy
Repair and regeneration	Stimulating wound healing process	Advanced stimulating therapies Surgical repair Negative pressure wound therapy Electrical stimulation
Social and patient factors	Addressing individual contexts that influence healing	Psychosocial assessment Education Psychosocial support

with a pressure ulcer who are at risk of being or are malnourished, general recommendations are for an intake of 30–35 kcal/kg of body weight/day and 1.25–1.5 g protein/kg of body weight/day [1]. Supplementation, usually with high-calorie, high-protein oral nutritional supplements containing arginine, zinc and antioxidants, may be required for adults who are unable to meet these needs through dietary intake [103]. For neonates and children with pressure ulcers, nutritional requirements should be individualised and monitored by a paediatric dietitian [1,104,105].

Repositioning and the support surface require re-evaluation. Patients should not be repositioned on an existing pressure ulcer, unless unavoidable [1]. Frequency of repositioning and feasibility of positions should be reviewed. For individuals with ischial pressure ulcers, optimal healing will occur by avoiding seated positions. The benefits of complete pressure avoidance should be weighed against the risks associated with prolonged bed rest [106].

The patient should be supplied with a pressure redistributing support surface. If available and tolerated, a specialty support surface (with additional technology such as alternating pressure, air fluidised or loss air loss features) could be considered [1,107].

Pain management. Pain includes nociceptive pain (e.g. gnawing, aching and/or throbbing) and neuropathic pain (e.g. burning and/or stinging) [37]. Pain assessment tools should be used to develop an individualised pain management plan.

Local wound care. Six major aspects of wound care are involved in managing hard-to-heal, chronic wounds such as pressure ulcers [108]. These concepts are outlined in Table 123.6.

Wound cleansing and debridement. Cleanse the wound and peri-wound surface to remove exudate, debris and fibrinous material; for most pressure ulcers cleansing with potable water is acceptable unless local wound care guidelines require a sterile fluid [1,109]. If infection is suspected or confirmed cleanse with a topical antiseptic solution [1,109].

Non-viable tissues (dead cells and debris) along with slough (fibrin, cells and proteinaceous material) can form on the surface of wounds, promoting inflammation and the growth of microorganisms, and affecting the moisture balance. This leads to slower or delayed healing of the pressure ulcer [1,109]. Debridement, the removal from the wound bed of non-viable tissue, should be undertaken (excepting stable, dry eschar present on ischaemic limbs and heels that should be left undisturbed) [1,109,110]. Different methods are summarised in Table 123.7.

Wound infection. Due to the ischaemic processes that may be involved in their development, pressure ulcers are highly susceptible to infection that can delay healing. Moreover, biofilms, which are synergistic collections of microorganisms of varying species and strains that have mechanisms to increase their virulence when developing in a microbial community, are commonly present in chronic wounds [110,111]. Wound infection is recognised as occurring on a continuum in which more severe signs and symptoms

Table 123.7 Debridement techniques [1,109].

Debridement technique	Description and characteristics
Surgical sharp	Removes non-viable tissue rapidly Removes biofilm Stimulates healing Can be painful Causes bleeding
Mechanical	Physical methods to remove non-viable tissue including brushes, ultrasound therapies and wet-to-dry gauze Can be painful Non-selective, may damage healthy tissue
Autolytic	Utilises endogenous enzyme to break down non-viable tissue Takes more time Painless
Enzymatic	Application of enzyme treatment to break down non-viable tissue Examples include papain/urea, fibrinolysin/DNAase, streptokinase/streptodornase combination and subtilisin
Biological	Laval (sterilised fly maggots) destroy non-viable tissue Highly selective Not painful

become apparent as the microbial burden increases in quantity or virulence, overwhelming the host response [110,112].

Local wound infection may present as covert signs and symptoms. This includes hypergranulation, friable granulation, delayed wound healing or large areas of wound breakdown, pocketing and epithelial bridging. As infection develops, overt signs of infection including increased redness, local warmth, swelling, purulent discharge, pain and wound odour become apparent [110,112]. Without adequate management, infection can spread to other local structures or systemically [110]. Because pressure ulcers frequently occur over bone and joint structures, osteomyelitis is a risk [1].

Definitive diagnosis of wound infection is made based on tissue biopsy or semi-quantitative swab technique using the Levine technique and microscopy. High-resolution microscopy is required to identify biofilm [110,111]. Plain film X-rays, nuclear bone scan and magnetic resonance imaging are appropriate for confirming osteomyelitis [1,113,114].

Topical antiseptics used at tissue-appropriate strengths prevent and treat wound infection. If possible, antiseptic choice should be based on sensitivity and culture results, and the chosen antiseptic should be used for 2 weeks before evaluating its effect (unless deterioration is evident earlier) [1,110]. Topical antiseptics should be used in combination with regular debridement to address biofilm [1,110,115].

Wound dressings. Contemporary wound dressings are designed to protect the wound and surrounding skin and to optimise wound bed moisture, with some including an antimicrobial component to treat infection. Advanced wound dressings are universally effective in achieving these goals [1,109]. Selection should be based on the diameter/shape/depth of the wound, moisture balance requirements, condition of the wound bed and peri-skin, presence of microbials, pain, resources and the patient's preferences [1,109]. A summary of wound dressings available in most advanced health care systems is provided in Table 123.8.

Surgery. Surgical management may be an option. The two most common reconstructive procedures are the musculocutaneous and the fasciocutaneous flap that provide vascularised tissue for closure of deep pressure ulcers [116,117]. Rates of complete healing following surgery are generally high [118]; however, recurrence is a significant concern, particularly in patients who have a high pressure ulcer risk (e.g. people with spinal cord injury). This risk should be discussed with surgery candidates, together with the strict

Table 123.8 Wound dressing selection [1,109].

Dressing type	Uses in pressure ulcers	Cautions
Basic wound dressings		
Transparent film	Secondary dressing Autolytic debridement when enzymatic options unavailable	Cannot contain heavy exudate Avoid skin trauma on removal
Moist gauze	Used when advanced wound dressings are unavailable Soaked in saline or topical antiseptic Packing deeper cavities and sinuses	Monitor moisture to prevent drying of the wound bed or skin maceration
Advanced wound dressings		
Foams (including hydropolymers)	Stage 2 pressure injuries with moderate to heavy exudate Secondary dressing	
Hydrogels	Uninfected Stage 2 pressure ulcer Uninfected Stage 3 or 4 pressure ulcer with minimal exudate Autolytic debridement	Protect peri-skin to prevent maceration
Hydrocolloids	Uninfected Stage 2 pressure ulcer Locations where wound dressing is unlikely to roll	Avoid skin trauma from removal Protect peri-skin to prevent maceration
Polymeric membrane	Moderate to heavy exudate Reduce inflammation and oedema	
Calcium alginates	Stage 3 or 4 pressure ulcer with moderate to heavy exudate	Avoid use in narrow sinuses Irrigate to facilitate removal
Antimicrobial dressings		
Iodine (povidone or cadexomer) impregnated	Infected pressure ulcers Suspected biofilm	Avoid use for people with iodine sensitivity
Honey impregnated	Infected pressure ulcers Suspected biofilm Low or moderate exudate	Avoid products that are not gamma irradiated
Silver	Infected pressure ulcers Suspected biofilm	Change regularly in presence of heavy exudate

postoperative repositioning, rehabilitation and skin assessment requirements. Appropriate candidate selection [117], adequate preoperative education and high motivation to adhere to management are associated with superior long-term outcomes [1,116].

Key references

The full list of references can be found in the online version at https://www.wiley.com/rooksdermatology10e

1 European Pressure Ulcer Advisory Panel, National Pressure Injury Advisory Panel, Pan Pacific Pressure Injury Alliance. *Prevention and Treatment of Pressure Ulcers/Injuries: Clinical Practice Guideline*. Haesler E, ed. EPUAP/NPIAP/PPPIA, 2019.
2 Kottner J, Cuddigan J, Carville K *et al*. Pressure ulcer/injury classification today: an international perspective. *J Tissue Viability* 2020;29:197–203.
12 Kottner J, Hahnel E, Lichterfeld-Kottner A, Blume-Peytavi U, Büscher A. Measuring the quality of pressure ulcer prevention: a systematic mapping review of quality indicators. *Int Wound J* 2018;15:218–24.
33 Gefen A, Brienza D, Cuddigan J, Haesler E, Kottner J. Our contemporary understanding of the aetiology of pressure ulcers/pressure injuries. *Int Wound J* 2022;19:692–704.
46 Coleman S, Nixon J, Keen J *et al*. A new pressure ulcer conceptual framework. *J Adv Nurs* 2014;70:2222–34.
49 Kottner J, Black J, Call E, Gefen A, Santamaria N. Microclimate: a critical review in the context of pressure ulcer prevention. *Clin Biomech* 2018;59:62–70.
71 Moore ZEH, Patton D. Risk assessment tools for the prevention of pressure ulcers. *Cochrane Database Syst Rev* 2019;Issue 1: CD006471.
87 Shi C, Dumville JC, Cullum N. Support surfaces for pressure ulcer prevention: a network meta-analysis. *Plos One* 2018;13:e0192707.
109 Wounds Australia. *Standards for Wound Prevention and Management*. Osborne Park, WA: Cambridge Media, 2016.
110 International Wound Infection Institute (IWII). *Wound Infection in Clinical Practice*. Wounds International, 2022. https://woundinfection-institute.com (last accessed February 2023).

CHAPTER 124

Cutaneous Reactions to Cold and Heat

Saqib J. Bashir[1] and Ai-Lean Chew[2]

[1] King's College Hospital, King's College Hospital NHS Foundation Trust, London, UK
[2] Beckenham Beacon Hospital, King's College Hospital NHS Foundation Trust, London, UK

Introduction, 124.1	Acrocyanosis, 124.6	Experimental effects, 124.14
Physiological reactions to cold, 124.1	Erythrocyanosis, 124.7	DISEASES CAUSED BY HEAT AND INFRARED RADIATION, 124.14
DISEASES CAUSED OR AGGRAVATED BY COLD, 124.1	Livedo reticularis, 124.8	
	Raynaud phenomenon, 124.10	Erythema ab igne, 124.14
Frostbite, 124.2	Cryoglobulinaemia, 124.13	Key references, 124.16
Trench foot, 124.4	Cold agglutinins, 124.13	
Perniosis, 124.5	Physiological reactions to heat and infrared radiation, 124.14	

Introduction

Human exposure to cold and warm environments has occurred throughout millennia. Human skin responds physiologically to environmental temperature; however, pathological responses may occur to extremes of temperature in those who have an underlying predisposition. This chapter details the pathophysiological responses to cold and heat, the resultant disease processes and the treatment plans used to manage patients injured by cold or heat.

Physiological reactions to cold

The maintenance of a steady core body temperature is achieved by various thermoregulatory mechanisms, not least of which is control of the skin's blood flow. Exposure to cold causes constriction of the arterioles and veins by a direct mechanism mediated in part by endothelial synthesis of the vasoconstrictor peptide endothelin-1 [1]. A reflex increase in sympathetic tone is triggered by cold receptors in the skin and, if the blood temperature falls, by the hypothalamic heat-regulating centre. Heat conservation is further enhanced by a counter-current exchange system between the arteries and veins in the limbs. Cold-induced vasoconstriction causes shunting of blood to the deep venous system which allows heat to be transferred from the arteries to veins. Consequently, arterial blood passing into the limbs is cooler, venous blood returning to the body is warmer and less heat is lost to the outside environment.

Persistent exposure of fingers to cold leads to the 'hunting reaction' of Lewis in which there are repeated cycles of vasodilatation following periods of vasoconstriction [2]. Cold-induced vasoconstriction is a heat-preserving, protective mechanism but prolonged vasospasm may jeopardise the vitality of the skin. Therefore, a transient vasodilatory response, mediated by the opening of arteriovenous anastamoses, protects against skin necrosis. With continued cold exposure, there is a phasic increase and decrease in blood flow through the cutaneous microvasculature. However, when core temperature is under threat the hunting reaction stops and vasoconstriction persists [2].

Cold-induced vasoconstriction causes a rise in intracapillary pressure and increased filtration of fluid into the interstitium, resulting in haemoconcentration and a reduction in plasma volume. Other physiological effects of cold include increased blood viscosity, slowing of the dissociation of oxyhaemoglobin to haemoglobin, diminished conduction velocity in cutaneous nerves and changes in platelet adhesiveness [3].

DISEASES CAUSED OR AGGRAVATED BY COLD

The ambient temperature and duration of exposure will determine the type and degree of injury sustained by all people when exposed to severe cold. However, there is a variable endogenous susceptibility to cold; certain individuals suffer cold-related disorders on exposure to modest degrees of cold that would be tolerated without ill effect by other normal individuals. Hence, cold-induced diseases can be divided into two groups: (i) diseases of cold exposure; and (ii) diseases of abnormal susceptibility to cold (Box 124.1).

Rook's Textbook of Dermatology, Tenth Edition. Edited by Christopher Griffiths, Jonathan Barker, Tanya Bleiker, Walayat Hussain and Rosalind Simpson.
© 2024 John Wiley & Sons Ltd. Published 2024 by John Wiley & Sons Ltd.

> **Box 124.1 Diseases caused by or aggravated by cold**
>
> **Diseases of cold exposure**
> - Frostbite
> - Trench foot
>
> **Diseases of abnormal susceptibility to cold**
> - Raynaud phenomenon (Chapter 54)
> - Livedo reticularis (Chapters 99 and 100)
> - Cryoglobulinaemia (Chapters 99 and 100)
> - Cold agglutinins
> - Cold haemolysis
> - Cold urticaria (Chapter 42)
> - Perniosis
> - Acrocyanosis
> - Erythrocyanosis
> - Cold erythema
> - Cold panniculitis (Chapter 97)
> - Neonatal cold injury (Chapter 114)

Frostbite

Definition and nomenclature

Frostbite is the term used to describe tissue damage caused by freezing. Skin and subcutaneous tissues are at risk of frostbite when exposed to cold air, liquids or metals.

> **Synonyms and inclusions**
> - Frostnip – this is a milder form of cutaneous cold damage than frostbite and is characterised by reversible redness of the skin

Introduction and general description

Frostbite, and its precursor, frostnip, can lead to varying degrees of tissue damage, ranging from redness to necrosis of soft tissue, muscle and bone. Most cases of frostbite are seen in winter sports enthusiasts and climbers who have been stranded in exposed sites in cold weather. Frostbite also occurs in soldiers, homeless people and those who work outdoors in cold climates.

Pathophysiology

Predisposing factors

The risk of frostbite increases with alcohol use and smoking [1].

Pathology

Freeze-induced damage results largely from the formation of ice in both the intracellular and extracellular compartments [2]. Fast freezing tends to produce intracellular ice, while slow freezing causes the formation of extracellular ice. Ice crystals not only injure cellular architecture but also disturb the flux of electrolytes and water across cell membranes [3]. The degree of cryodamage is also influenced by the rate of thawing. Slow rewarming causes the formation of larger, more destructive ice crystals and the development of greater osmotic stresses. As well as the direct effects on cells, tissue damage in frostbite is compounded by cold-induced vascular and haematological responses. Reflex vasoconstriction in the extremities results in decreased capillary perfusion, which is aggravated by cold-induced hyperviscosity and a tendency to thrombus formation [4].

Clinical features

Presentation

The parts of the body that can be least protected from cold are affected – the toes, feet, fingers, ears, nose and cheeks. Frostnip involves the skin only and is characterised by painful red patches, which normalise with rewarming. In superficial frostbite there is involvement of the skin and subcutis with redness accompanied initially by pain and then a sense of warmth. The affected skin becomes waxy and white. The injury in deep frostbite extends to the subcutaneous tissues and may involve the nerves, major vessels, muscle and bone, resulting in joint immobility and paralysis [5]. The cold exposure is fairly evident at presentation, but the degree of damage may take many weeks to become apparent (Figure 124.1).

Classification of severity

A method of classifying frostbite severity has been proposed. In first-degree frostbite there is partial skin freezing, with redness, oedema and hyperaemia, but no blisters or necrosis. Desquamation develops 5–10 days later, leading to complete recovery. Second-degree frostbite is a full-thickness skin freeze, with reddening, substantial oedema, vesiculation, blistering and a black eschar, requiring soft-tissue amputation only. Third-degree frostbite requires bone amputation. Fourth-degree frostbite necessitates major amputation and is complicated by systemic effects [6].

Complications and co-morbidities

The extent and severity of tissue damage become apparent on rewarming. Redness and mild pain lasting for a few hours occur following mild frostbite. Blistering, full-thickness skin necrosis and gangrene can be seen in severe cases [7]. Damage to nerves and blood vessels can lead to paraesthesiae, abnormal sensitivity to cold and hyperhidrosis, which may last for months to years [7].

Prognosis

The prognosis of frostbite injury only becomes apparent over a period of weeks, as the demarcation between viable and non-viable tissue becomes evident.

Investigations

Technetium-99 bone scintigraphy may be helpful in evaluating outcome in frostbite injury and indicating the level of amputation needed in severe cases (Figure 124.2) [8]. Magnetic resonance angiography may also be beneficial, with the ability to visualise directly any vascular occlusion and simultaneously image the surrounding soft tissues (Figure 124.3).

Bone scintigraphy can be performed early at day 2–4 with a comparison study at day 7–10 after exposure. This imaging method can be performed in three phases which allow evaluation of the vasculature, soft tissues and bone uptake of technetium. Technetium binds to viable hydroxyapatite in bone, with a reported 99% specificity and 96% sensitivity for ischaemic bone [9]. These studies can allow for early debridement of non-viable areas.

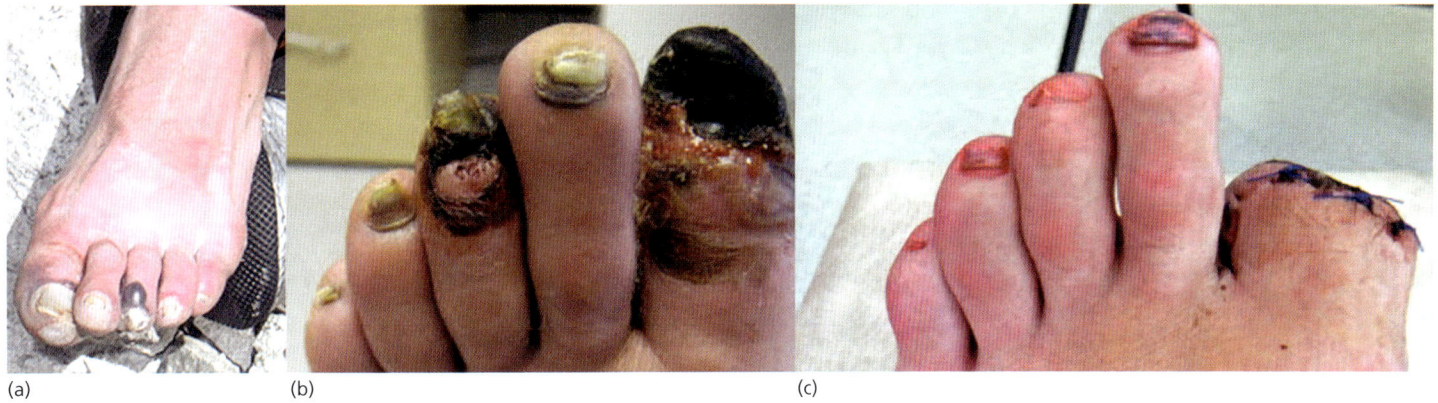

Figure 124.1 Typical frostbite affecting the hallux and third left toes showing the initial injury at (a) presentation at base camp on Everest, (b) at 6 weeks and (c) at 10 weeks. Reproduced from Hallam et al. 2010 [15] with permission of BMJ Publishing Group.

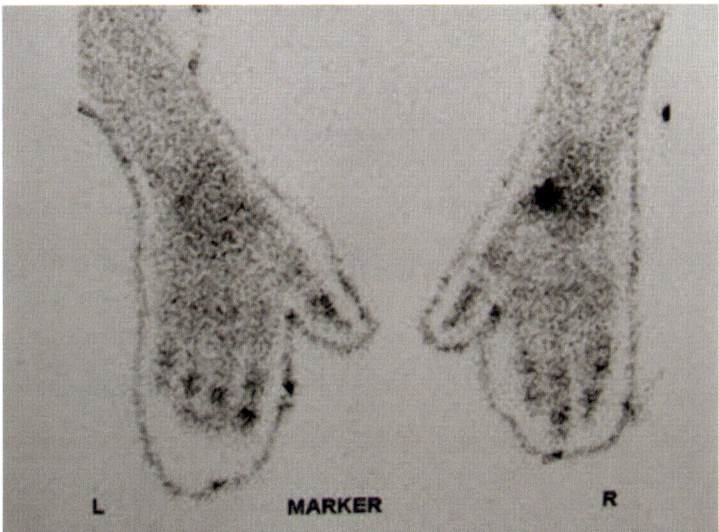

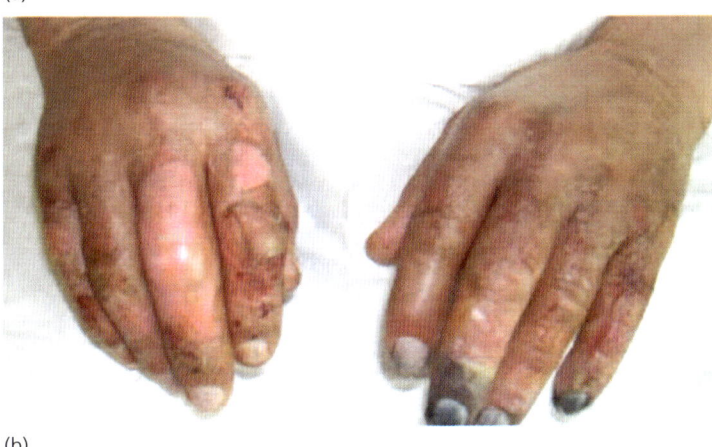

Figure 124.2 (a) Technetium-99 scans of the hands of a patient with frostbite (b). Reproduced from Hallam et al. 2010 [15] with permission of BMJ Publishing Group.

Management

First line

It is important that immediate warming techniques are instituted. Debridement surgery should be delayed until the full extent of the recovery/persisting damage is clear.

Rapid rewarming by immersion in water at 37–39°C is recommended. Use a thermometer to measure water temperature, or a caregiver's hand, to ensure that an additional thermal burn injury is not imparted. As the water will cool rapidly, it will need to be topped up to maintain the temperature, and circulated around the limb. Rapid rewarming has been shown to be more effective than slow rewarming and the tissue can be considered completely rewarmed when it takes on a red/purple appearance and is soft and pliable to the touch. Further additional rewarming does not add additional benefit. The area should be air dried or patted dry to avoid shearing forces damaging tissue [10]. Other authors have advocated a higher-temperature rewarming for at least 30 min at 40–41°C until tissues are soft and pliable, with continuing twice daily warming.

Non-steroidal anti-inflammatory drugs (NSAIDs) such as ibuprofen have been recommended although the evidence for their use is weak. The Wilderness Medicine Society recommends their use at 12 mg/kg body weight twice daily in order to reduce levels of prostaglandins and thromboxanes that may contribute to vasoconstriction, ischaemia and tissue damage [10]. Also, NSAIDs may help alleviate the pain of rewarming. Topical aloe vera gel has been suggested on the basis that it may also reduce inflammatory prostaglandins; however there is a lack of strong clinical evidence or animal studies to confirm efficacy. It is recommended that non-haemorrhagic blisters should be aspirated as the blister fluid may also contain prostaglandins and thromboxanes. The blister roof should be kept intact and not debrided.

Second line

In the hospital setting, other pharmacological interventions can be beneficial. A retrospective study has indicated a reduction in the need for digital amputation if intra-arterial infusion of tissue plasminogen activator (tPA) is given within 48 h of the injury [11]. In this study, the incidence of amputation reduced from 41% (untreated) to 10% in those treated within 24 h of injury. Vasodilator drugs may also improve outcome [12] – in addition to vasodilatation, they may also inhibit microvascular occlusion and platelet aggregation. In a study of aspirin with buflomedil versus aspirin plus iloprost, or aspirin plus iloprost and tPA, no amputations were seen in the iloprost group (0/16) versus 3/16 patients when combined with tPA or 9/15 patients treated with buflomedil. The authors recommend aspirin with iloprost for third-degree

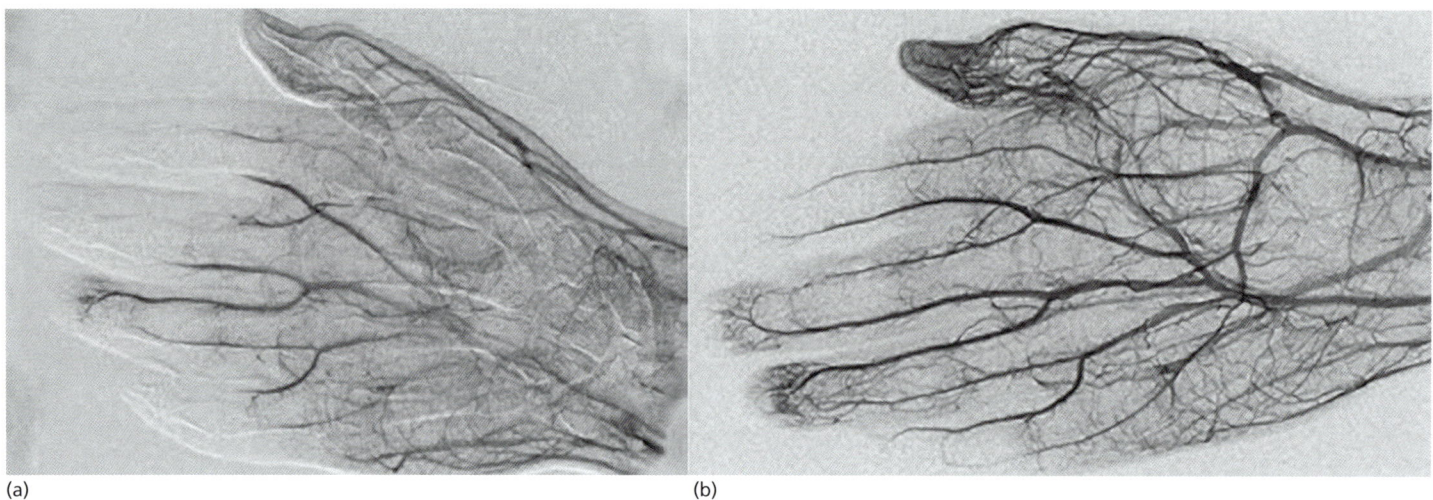

Figure 124.3 Digital subtraction angiography showing thrombotic occlusion of the terminal digits in a major frostbite injury of the hand (a) and reperfusion after urgent thrombolysis (b). Reproduced from Hallam *et al.* 2010 [15] with permission of BMJ Publishing Group.

frostbite, with consideration of tPA on a case-by-case basis for fourth-degree frostbite [13]. Following tPA, patients are treated with low-moelcular-weight heparin for a week and then aspirin 325 mg daily for 1–3 months [14].

Third line
Surgical removal of gangrenous tissue should be delayed until there is a distinct demarcation between viable and non-viable tissue, a process that usually takes several weeks.

Trench foot

Definition and nomenclature
Trench foot describes a combination of stasis, non-freezing cold injury and wet conditions leading to numbness and skin changes on the distal legs and feet.

Synonyms and inclusions
- Immersion foot

Introduction and general description
Trench foot and immersion foot are regarded as similar processes. Trench foot was a common problem suffered by soldiers in the early years of trench warfare in the First World War [1] but is now mostly encountered among the homeless population [2]. A similar entity, tropical immersion foot, is a warm water immersion injury and is less severe.

Pathophysiology
Predisposing factors
Smoking and peripheral vascular disease probably contribute to the severity of the tissue damage, with variation in vasoconstriction and vasodilatation leading to local tissue damage.

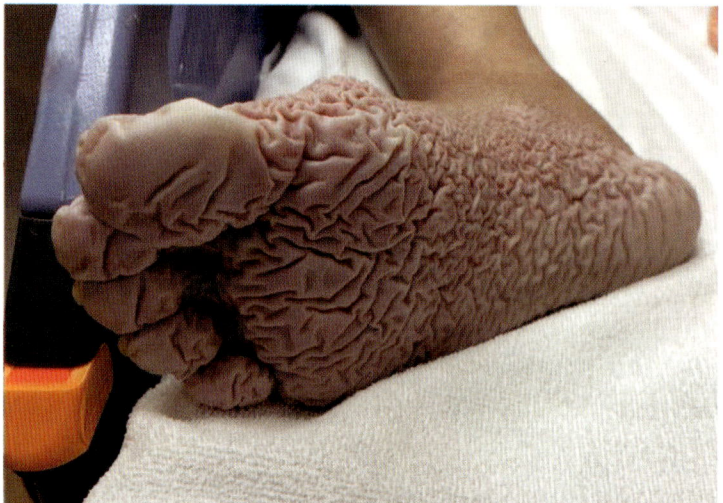

Figure 124.4 A 91-year-old patient who had been trapped in the bath for 4 days. The foot is grey, with maceration and wrinkling of the skin. Reproduced from Matsuura and Nakazawa 2019 [4] with permission of Oxford University Press.

Pathology
The pathological changes are those of dependent oedema and lymphovenous stasis. Perivascular inflammation occurs and in severe cases arterial occlusion and ischaemic necrosis. There is damage to both myelinated and unmyelinated nerve fibres [3].

Clinical features
Affected individuals develop numbness of the feet and distal legs accompanied by skin changes caused by non-freezing cold injury. This is compounded by wet conditions and aggravated by leg dependency, immobility and constrictive footwear.

Affected legs and feet are cold and anaesthetic (Figure 124.4). There is redness, oedema, tenderness and, in severe cases, areas of superficial gangrene. On rewarming there is worsening oedema, hyperaemia and painful paraesthesiae.

Differential diagnosis
Other causes of limb ulceration should be considered, such as diabetes mellitus, arterial and venous insufficiency, autoimmune disease, inflammatory disease such as pyoderma gangrenosum and infections.

Prognosis
Initially the ability to sweat is lost but with time there is hyperhidrosis, cold sensitivity and vasomotor instability. Changes may persist for months or years.

Investigations
The investigations required depend on the clinical presentation. Usually there is a clear history of cold water immersions and no specific investigations are required.

Management
The best approach is prevention, but once the condition has occurred bed rest, elevation and analgesics are helpful. Conservative excision of necrotic tissue may be necessary and antibiotics should be given if there is evidence of infection.

Perniosis

Definition and nomenclature
Perniosis describes localised inflammatory lesions on the acral skin, which occur as an abnormal reaction to cold in susceptible individuals [1].

Synonyms and inclusions
- Chilblains

Introduction and general description
Perniosis lesions are cold induced and affect areas of the skin vulnerable to cold exposure, such as the digits, nose and ears.

Epidemiology
Age and sex
Presentation is typically in the late thirties, with a large female preponderance (79%) [2].

Associated diseases
Aetiological factors include poor nutrition, anorexia nervosa and systemic diseases, most typically lupus erythematosus (LE) and haematological malignancy [3–5]. The Covid-19 pandemic (SARS-CoV-2 viral infection) saw an increases in cases but the relationship to viral infection remains controversial (Chapter 25).

Pathophysiology
Pathology
In perniosis there is a persistent, cold-induced vasoconstriction of the deep cutaneous arterioles with concomitant dilatation of the smaller, superficial vessels. This is in contrast with normal subjects, in whom cold exposure induces cutaneous vasoconstriction succeeded by vasodilatation, a homeostatic mechanism necessary for the maintenance of reperfusion. Investigation of the cutaneous nerves in patients with perniosis demonstrated no quantitative or qualitative difference in immunoreactivity for substance P, neuropeptide Y, calcitonin gene-related peptide or vasoactive intestinal peptide compared with controls [6]. However, in the affected skin of patients with acral perniosis, who also had a past history of very low body weight, immunohistochemistry revealed a great increase in nerve bundles in the papillary dermis, some with an abnormal morphology [6]. This indicates that in uncomplicated perniosis the neuronal supply to the microvasculature is normal and suggests that the pathology involves the microvessels themselves.

Although there may be a temporal relationship between Covid-19 infection and the clinical appearance of chilblains, or 'Covid toes', the evidence for a causal relationship remains weak. Despite immunohistochemistry suggesting SARS-CoV-2 spike protein stains positive in the lesion in some studies, authors report inconsistencies in immunostaining, with positive stains seen in control samples from normal skin and negative stains in affected skin. Also, many of the patients with the clinical presentation of 'Covid toes' were negative on both serology or reverse transcription polymerase chain reaction (RT-PCR) for present or past infection with the virus. There may be a relationship with levels of interferon type I, but this is also inconclusive [7,8]. Another postulated mechanism is the sedentary lifestyle imposed by the Covid-19 lockdowns, which may also be related to the acrocyanosis seen in this condition.

Histopathology
The histopathology of perniosis usually demonstrates dermal oedema with superficial and deep dermal inflammation [9]. The mononuclear cell infiltration, mostly T cells, is primarily perivascular but also occurs in a perieccrine distribution [10]. Epidermal changes in chilblains consist mainly of necrotic keratinocytes and spongiosis. Perniosis occurring on the lateral thigh is characterised by an intense mononuclear cell infiltrate extending throughout the dermis and into the subcutaneous fat, with 'fluffy oedema' of the blood vessel walls [9]. In these cases of deep perniosis, dermal oedema is not a prominent feature. Inflammation occurring in the deeper dermis and subcutis may be explained by the combined effects of external cooling together with insulation from internal warming [9].

Genetics
There may be a genetic influence in perniosis since several generations within a family can be affected [1].

Environmental factors
Perniosis occurs in susceptible individuals during the autumn or winter in a climate that is both cold and damp.

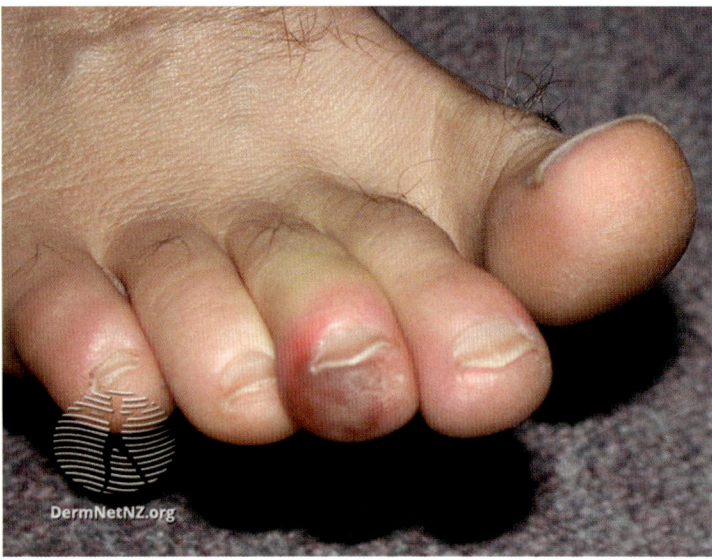

Figure 124.5 Perniosis over the distal right middle toe. Reproduced from DermNet New Zealand Trust/https://dermnetnz.org/assets/Uploads/reactions/pernio1__WatermarkedWyJXYXRlcm1hcmtlZCJd.jpg (last accessed August 2023).

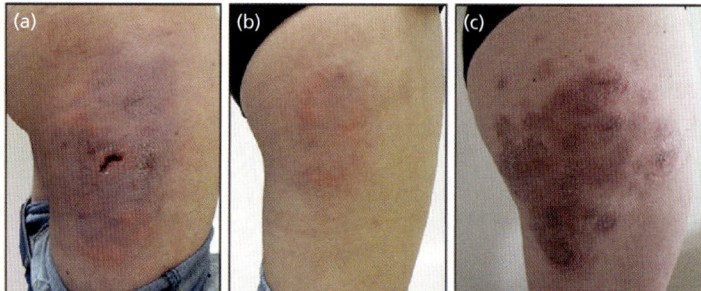

Figure 124.6 (a–c) Red and violaceous plaques of the upper thigh in horse riders. From Karkouche et al. 2017 [18] with permission of John Wiley & Sons.

Clinical features
Presentation
The lesions are red-purple and usually macular, papular or nodular (Figure 124.5). Plaque-like perniosis also occurs, as do lesions with an annular morphology. Perniosis develops symmetrically on the acral skin, in particular the fingers and toes, but other body extremities may also be involved including the heels, lower legs, nose and ears. Pruritus and burning pain are common, although some lesions may be asymptomatic. In severe cases blistering and ulceration may occur. Each lesion tends to undergo spontaneous resolution after 2–3 weeks; however, in some patients perniosis persists throughout the winter and occasionally continues to develop in the summer.

Chilblain LE (also known as Hutchinson lupus) is a form of cutaneous LE that presents in a similar way to idiopathic perniosis. Erythrocyanotic papules, located on the fingers and toes, develop in cold weather and tend to persist, in some cases becoming ulcerated [11]. Chilblain LE may be accompanied by discoid LE or other forms of cutaneous LE. Up to 20% of patients with chilblain LE develop systemic LE [12] (Chapter 51).

Perniosis may also complicate haematological malignancy, typically myelodysplastic syndrome and chronic myelomonocytic leukaemia (Chapter 149). Cyanotic swelling of acral digital skin, particularly the toes, has been reported in these patients [13]. The onset of perniosis may coincide with a blast crisis, which can be demonstrated on skin biopsy by the presence of large, atypical mononuclear cells in the perivascular infiltrate [14].

Clinical variants
There are various less common variants. In papular perniosis, crops of small lesions develop on the sides of the fingers often on a background of acrocyanosis [15]. Perniosis occurring on the outer thighs has been reported in women who are horse-riding enthusiasts ('equestrian panniculitis') (Figure 124.6) [11]. Clinically, these lesions are composed of clustered papules or plaques, which may ulcerate. Tight-fitting trousers, such as riding breeches, have been implicated aetiologically [11]. In chronic perniosis, especially in the presence of arterial disease or prolonged cold exposure, irreversible changes of fibrosis, lymphoedema and hyperkeratosis may occur, altering the physical signs.

Differential diagnosis
This includes granuloma annulare, peripheral vascular insufficiency and vasculitis.

Prognosis
The prognosis depends on the underlying cause. Most patients will experience good disease control when steps are taken to prevent cold exposure.

Investigations
Investigations should be guided by the clinical presentation of the patient but may include a full blood count and/or blood film, protein electrophoresis, an autoimmune screen, cryoglobulins and cold agglutinins. Investigations were positive in 11/20 tested patients from a Mayo Clinic series [2].

Management
Warm clothing and central heating generally prevent perniosis. Susceptible individuals must avoid cold, damp conditions and should not smoke. A double-blind, placebo-controlled study demonstrated the efficacy of nifedipine in clearing existing lesions and preventing the development of new ones [16]. A study has demonstrated the successful treatment of chilblain LE with mycophenolate mofetil [17].

Acrocyanosis

Definition
Acrocyanosis is a persistent cyanotic or erythrocyanotic mottled discoloration of the hands and, less commonly, feet and face.

Introduction and general description
Acrocyanosis may be idiopathic or secondary to a number of systemic disorders, including an underlying malignancy (Box 124.2) [1]. Sometimes there is a family history, indicating a genetic basis. Rarely, it is drug induced.

Box 124.2 Aetiology of acrocyanosis

Idiopathic

Secondary
- Autoimmune:
  - Connective tissue disorders
  - Primary and secondary antiphospholipid antibody syndrome
- Neoplastic:
  - Benign and malignant paraproteinaemias
  - Paraneoplastic syndrome
- Cold agglutinin disease
- Cryoglobulinaemia
- Eating disorders:
  - Anorexia nervosa
  - Bulimia nervosa
- Orthostatic disorders:
  - Chronic orthostatic intolerance
  - Postural orthostatic tachycardia syndrome of adolescents
  - Adolescent chronic fatigue syndrome
- Neurological disorders:
  - Brachial plexus neuropathy
- Chronic arsenic poisoning
- Drugs:
  - Butyl nitrate
  - Interferon α (2a)
- Metabolic diseases:
  - Fucidosis
  - Ethylmalonic encephalopathy
- Psychiatric:
  - Intellectual disability
  - Schizophrenia
- Essential thrombocythaemia

remits. Acrocyanosis must be distinguished from the Raynaud phenomenon, which occurs episodically with triphasic colour changes and often involves just a few digits. Arterial and venous occlusion must be excluded. In cases of acrocyanosis developing for the first time in adult life a secondary cause should be sought (Box 124.2).

Differential diagnosis
This includes Raynaud phenomenon, arterial occlusion and venous occlusion.

Prognosis
The prognosis varies with the underlying disorder. Primary acrocyanosis in young adults may disappear spontaneously by middle age.

Investigations
Capilleroscopy has been used to demonstrate dilated and congested capillary loops at the base of the fingernail. However, the usefulness of this technique in distinguishing primary acrocyanosis from connective tissue disease has yet to be firmly established. Duplex vascular ultrasound can be used to exclude intravascular thrombosis.

Management
There is no effective medical treatment for acrocyanosis. Vasodilator therapies, such as the calcium-channel antagonists, do not appear to be beneficial. Drug-induced acrocyanosis will be improved by cessation of the culprit drug. Treatment of an underlying systemic disorder may improve the appearance in secondary acrocyanosis.

Epidemiology
Age and sex
Presentation is typically in adolescence, with a reported female preponderance [2].

Pathophysiology
There is vasospasm of peripheral arterioles, aggravated by cold, and dilatation of the subpapillary venous plexus [3]. The condition is most probably a primary vascular defect since studies have not demonstrated a deficit of neuronal supply to the cutaneous vessels [4]. Decreased acral blood flow may be further compromised by plasma hyperviscosity. In ethylmalonic encephalopathy – a rare metabolic disorder with neuromotor delay, hyperlactic acidaemia and orthostatic acrocyanosis – a mutation has been demonstrated in *ETHE1*, a gene encoding a mitochondrial matrix protein [5].

Clinical features
Presentation
Idiopathic acrocyanosis usually starts in adolescence and persists into adult life. The changes may be transient after cold exposure but usually persist during the winter and even throughout the summer months. Clinically there is a painless mottled duskiness of both hands in the presence of normal peripheral pulses. Similar changes may be seen on the feet and face. Trophic changes, such as ulceration, are absent. In some individuals acrocyanosis spontaneously

Erythrocyanosis

Definition
Erythrocyanosis is a persistent, dusky redness of the skin occurring at sites with a thick layer of underlying subcutaneous fat, such as the thighs and lower legs. Erythrocyanosis is seen less commonly on the buttocks and arms.

Introduction and general description
Erythrocyanosis is a condition that predominantly affects the lower legs, distinguishing it from acrocyanosis, which affects peripheral areas such as digits and appendages [1].

Epidemiology
Age and sex
Erythrocyanosis occurs most commonly in adolescent girls and middle-aged women.

Pathophysiology
It has been hypothesised that the subcutaneous fat in these sites acts to insulate the superficial vessels from the warmth of the underlying blood supply, thus rendering them susceptible to cold exposure. It is exacerbated by cold and therefore usually more prominent during the winter.

Clinical features
Presentation
Erythrocyanosis is seen on the lower legs of adolescent girls, the thighs and buttocks of overweight boys and the thighs and lower legs of middle-aged women. Very occasionally it can occur on the forearms of infants. It is characterised by dusky discoloration of the skin and may be accompanied by keratosis pilaris, angiokeratomas and telangiectases. The area is cold to touch. Nodular perniotic lesions occurring after cold exposure may complicate erythrocyanosis. Oedema and fibrosis may be seen as chronic manifestations of erythrocyanosis.

Differential diagnosis
While the diagnosis is often clinically apparent, other vascular disorders and livedo reticularis may be considered in the differential.

Prognosis
The disorder may persist indefinitely but spontaneous improvement can occur in adolescent patients.

Investigations
None is required.

Management
Warm clothing, exercise, weight reduction and elastic support hosiery may be helpful. Vasodilators, such as calcium-channel antagonists, are of limited value.

Livedo reticularis

Definition and nomenclature
Livedo reticularis is a mottled, cyanotic discoloration of the skin, which has a characteristic network pattern. It is accentuated by cold.

Synonyms and inclusions
- Livedo racemosa
- Livedo annularis

Introduction and general description
Livedo reticularis is a lace-like pattern on the surface of the skin created by low blood flow within anastomoic areas of the skin.

Pathophysiology
Pathology
The blood supply of the skin is arranged in cones, the bases of which measure 1–4 cm in diameter and lie on the skin's surface [1]. Each cone is supplied by an arteriole, which passes through the dermis perpendicular to the surface. When blood flow through the feeding arterioles is diminished, deoxygenated blood at the anastamotic junctions produces a cyanotic network pattern on the skin which is livedo reticularis (Figure 124.7). Livedo reticularis may be physiological, idiopathic or secondary to intravascular obstruction or vessel wall disease (Box 124.3).

Box 124.3 Classification of livedo reticularis

Physiological livedo reticularis
- Cutis marmorata

Idiopathic or primary livedo reticularis
- Congenital:
  - Cutis marmorata telangiectatica congenita
- Acquired idiopathic:
  - Uncomplicated
  - With winter ulceration
  - With summer ulceration
  - With systemic vascular involvement

Secondary livedo reticularis
- Intravascular obstruction:
  - Stasis:
    - paralysis
    - cardiac failure
    - amantadine therapy
  - Occlusive disease:
    - emboli [8,9]
    - oxalosis (primary hyperoxaluria) [10,11]
    - compressed air
    - bismuth, pentazocine, non-steroidal anti-inflammatory drugs, minocycline [12]
  - Thrombocythaemia [13,14]
  - Cryoglobulins
  - Cold agglutinins
- Vessel wall disease:
  - Arteriosclerosis
  - Arteritis:
    - polyarteritis nodosa
    - systemic lupus erythematosus
    - antiphospholipid syndrome
    - rheumatoid arthritis
    - dermatomyositis
    - lymphoma
    - pancreatitis
  - Infections:
    - tuberculosis
    - syphilis
    - hepatitis C
    - brucellosis
    - *Coxiella burnetii*
  - Metabolic disease:
    - hyperparathyroidism and hypercalcaemia [15]
    - calciphylaxis [16]

There is hyperkeratosis, red blood cell aggregates and vessel wall thickening in the deep dermis. If the livedo reticularis is caused by vasculitis, there will be vascular inflammation and arterial obliteration in the deep dermis and the subcutaneous tissue. There is no difference in the histological features between the blanched and red areas [2].

Clinical features
Presentation
Livedo reticularis most commonly occurs on the legs but the arms and trunk may also be affected. Cold usually exacerbates the

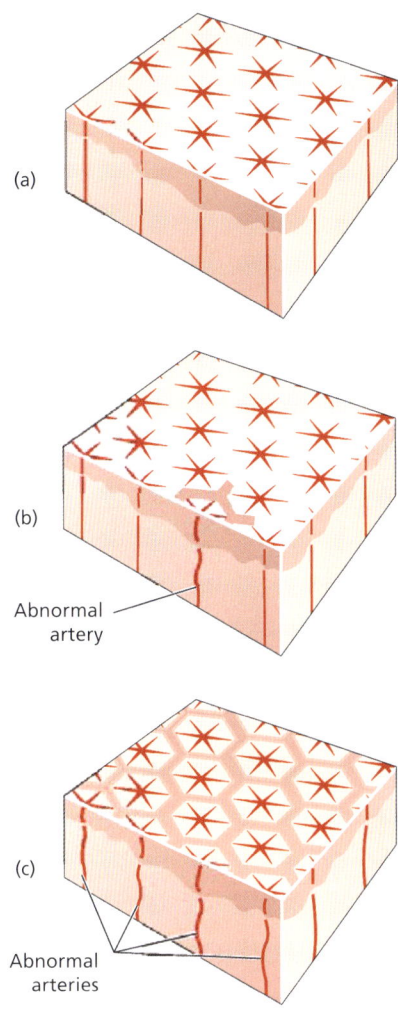

Figure 124.7 (a) Normal vasculature. (b) Livedo racemosa due to patchy arterial pathology. (c) Livedo reticularis due to diffuse arterial pathology.

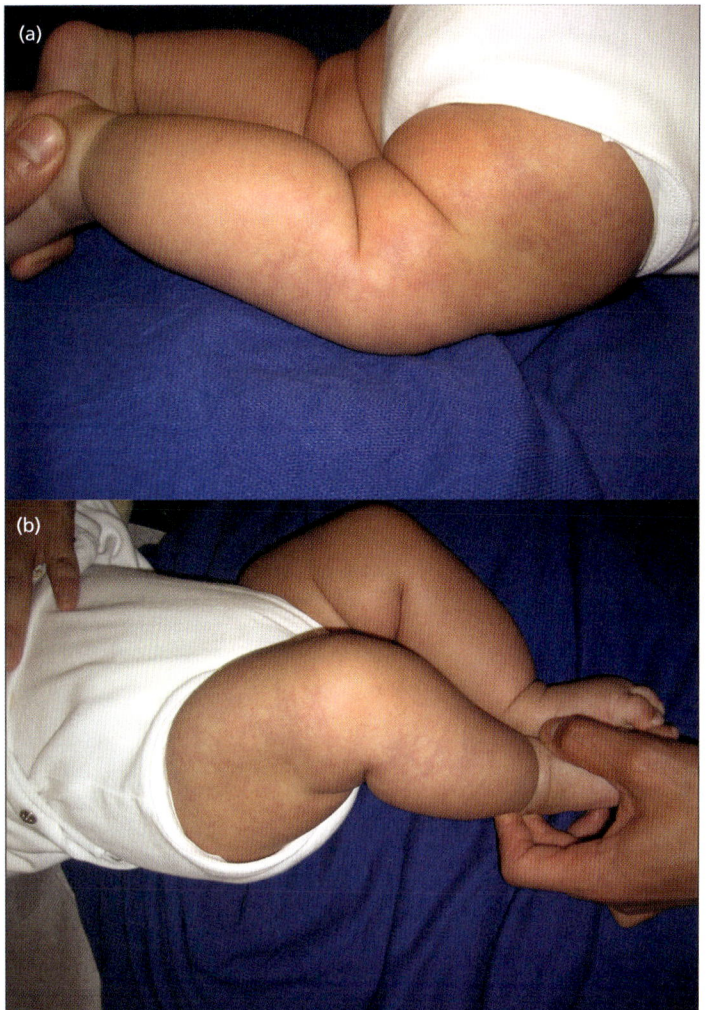

Figure 124.8 (a,b) A reticular red patch and subtle cutaneous atrophy over the right thigh extending to the midsection of the shin, consistent with cutis marmorata telangiectatica congenita, in a 3-month-old girl. Reproduced from Levy and Lam 2011 [17] with permission of CMA Impact Inc.

cyanotic discoloration, while leg elevation tends to decrease the intensity of the colour changes. Diffuse arterial disease or hyperviscosity problems give rise to diffuse livedo reticularis; limited arterial disease leads to patchy mottling. In many cases livedo reticularis forms a complete network, in other cases there is a branching configuration known as livedo racemosa. Ulceration of the dark areas occurs rarely but, if present, suggests significant large-vessel vasculitis or intraluminal thrombosis. The appearance of livedo reticularis is initially reversible if the underlying cause is treated, but with chronic problems permanent telangiectases develop.

Clinical variants

Physiological livedo reticularis. Also known as cutis marmorata, this is a transient cyanotic mottling of the skin that occurs as a physiological response to cold exposure and disappears with warming. It is usually encountered in healthy infants and resolves during the first year of life. Involvement of the trunk as well as the limbs is common. Physiological livedo reticularis rarely occurs in adults, but in this situation is often associated with a disorder that causes stasis within blood vessels, for example paralysis.

Congenital livedo reticularis. Also known as cutis marmorata telangiectatica congenita, this is a rare developmental defect, present at birth, characterised by a red-purple vascular network [3–5]. Lesions are usually asymmetrical, typically on a limb (Figure 124.8), less often involving the torso or head. The reticulated area is persistent and enhanced by cold, crying and exercise. Skin atrophy may accompany the livedo. Usually congenital livedo reticularis occurs in isolation but it may be associated with a variety of other congenital abnormalities. In most cases the condition gradually resolves, with most improvement occurring during the first 2 years of life.

Acquired idiopathic livedo reticularis. This occurs predominantly in young adult and middle-aged women. Mild degrees are harmless, while more severe cases are associated with ulceration, usually in the winter. The mottling is at first transient and occurs on exposure to cold (Figure 124.9). Permanent livedo may develop with time. Tingling and numbness of the skin, and sometimes oedema, may be present. The diagnosis is clinical and can only be made once other

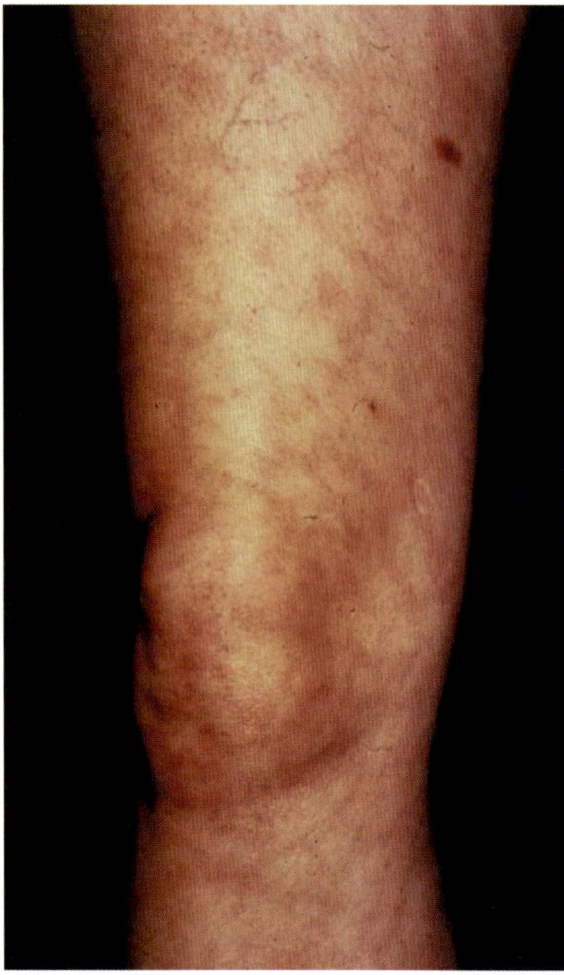

Figure 124.9 Livedo reticularis. Macular, reticulate, violaceous discoloration of the thigh. Reproduced from Gibbs et al. 2005 [18] with permission from Elsevier.

disorders have been ruled out, including erythema ab igne, capillary naevi and angioma serpiginosum and causes of secondary livedo reticularis. Livedo reticularis occurs in 20–25% of migraine sufferers and in this subset stroke is more frequent, raising the possibility that livedo reticularis can be used as a clinical marker to identify those migraine sufferers with an increased risk of stroke [6].

Livedoid vasculopathy. This may be a distinct entity, presenting with broken livedo, forming incomplete circles in the livedo racemosa pattern (Figure 124.10). Histologically, a true vasculitis is not seen, although there may be mild leukocytoclasis and hyalinisation of the vessels. The predominant feature is that of vascular occlusion by intraluminal thrombi in the upper and mid dermis. Therefore, besides the primary (idiopathic) form, many cases can be considered secondary to underlying diseases that promote vascular occlusion [7].

Differential diagnosis
This includes erythema ab igne, capillary naevi and angioma serpiginosum.

Prognosis
Prognosis is related to the underlying cause, if one is present.

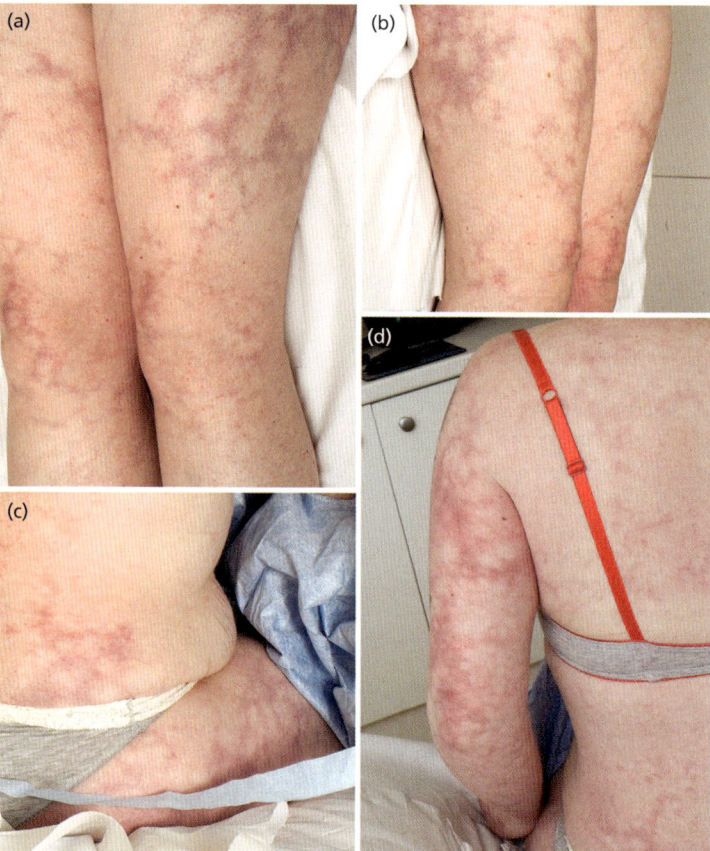

Figure 124.10 (a–d) Clinical photographs demonstrating widespread livedo racemosa with persistant, violaceous, mottled discoloration of the skin. Reproduced from Timoney et al. 2019 [19] with permission of BMJ Publishing Group.

Investigations
Laboratory studies should be directed by the underlying medical presentation. Typical investigations would include a thrombophilia screen, autoimmune screen, full blood count, metabolic panel and serum protein electrophoresis. Further investigations such as ultrasound and echocardiography may be required to look for sources of emboli.

Skin biopsies should be performed from both the central blanched areas and the purplish livedo areas to increase the diagnostic yield as changes may be present in either or both areas.

Management
The management is directed to the underlying condition, if one is identified.

Raynaud phenomenon

Definition
Raynaud phenomenon is defined as episodic digital ischaemia occurring in response to cold or emotional stimuli.

Introduction and general description
Raynaud phenomenon is characterised by sequential colour changes: white (pallor), blue (cyanosis) and red (rubor). Pallor

is essential for the diagnosis. However, in severe recalcitrant Raynaud phenomenon, particularly in association with a connective tissue disease, attacks of long duration may occur in which the initial pallor is short-lived and succeeded by prolonged cyanosis. Primary Raynaud phenomenon (also called Raynaud disease) is idiopathic and occurs as an isolated innocuous disorder (Box 124.4). Secondary Raynaud phenomenon occurs in association with underlying diseases, or is caused by physical factors or drugs (Box 124.5).

> **Box 124.4 Criteria for the diagnosis of primary Raynaud phenomenon**
>
> - Intermittent attacks of discoloration of the extremities
> - No evidence of organic peripheral arterial occlusion
> - Symmetrical or bilateral distribution
> - Exclusion of any disease, occupation, trauma or drug ingestion that could give rise to vasospastic abnormalities
> - Absence of immunological abnormalities
> - Commoner in female sex, age under 25 years
> - History of cold intolerance since childhood
> - Normal nail fold capillaries

The sequential colour changes were first described by Maurice Raynaud in 1862 [1]. In 1901, Jonathan Hutchinson reported that there were several causes for the phenomenon [2] and, subsequently, Allen and Brown established clinical criteria to distinguish innocent primary Raynaud phenomenon from secondary Raynaud phenomenon [3]. The advent of immunological tests for the connective tissue diseases has helped refine the diagnosis of primary Raynaud phenomenon (Box 124.4).

Epidemiology
Incidence and prevalence
Studies of prevalence of the Raynaud phenomenon have been hampered by differences in diagnostic criteria and survey technique. Population-based surveys have reported a prevalence of between 6% and 20% in women, and between 3% and 12.5% in men [4]. There is some evidence for an increased prevalence of Raynaud phenomenon in family members of affected individuals, suggesting a genetic susceptibility [5]. A genome linkage study of affected individuals within a family indicated five candidate regions with possible linkage, of which three were potential candidate genes: the beta subunit of the muscle acetylcholine receptor and the serotonin 1B and 1E receptors [6].

Age
The age of onset is usually under 40 years, but it may occur over this age.

Sex
Primary Raynaud phenomenon is commoner in women, in the proportion of at least 5 : 1 [7].

Pathophysiology
The pathogenesis of Raynaud phenomenon is centred on a functional unit composed of vascular endothelium, smooth muscle cells and nerve endings. This integrated neurovascular system responds to a range of soluble mediators and physical stimuli, which determine the balance between vasoconstriction and vasodilatation. In primary Raynaud phenomenon the vascular changes are considered to be functional. In contrast, in secondary Raynaud

> **Box 124.5 Aetiology of Raynaud phenomenon**
>
> **Primary Raynaud phenomenon (Raynaud disease)**
>
> **Secondary Raynaud phenomenon**
> - Trauma or vibration:
>   - Reflex sympathetic dystrophy
>   - Vibration exposure
>   - Arteriovenous fistula
>   - Hypothenar hammer syndrome (ulnar artery thrombosis)
>   - Intra-arterial drug administration
> - Connective tissue disease and vasculitis:
>   - Systemic sclerosis
>   - Systemic lupus erythematosus
>   - Rheumatoid arthritis
>   - Sjögren syndrome
>   - Mixed connective tissue disease
>   - Dermatomyositis
>   - Temporal arteritis
>   - Hepatitis B antigen vasculitis
> - Obstructive arterial disease:
>   - Atherosclerosis
>   - Thromboangiitis obliterans (Buerger disease)
>   - Hypothenar hammer syndrome (ulnar artery thrombosis)
> - Neurological disease:
>   - Thoracic outlet syndrome (cervical rib)
>   - Carpal tunnel syndrome
>   - Hypothenar hammer syndrome
>   - Reflex sympathetic dystrophy
> - Haematological disease:
>   - Cryoglobulinaemia
>   - Cold agglutinins
>   - Paroxysmal haemoglobinuria
>   - Waldenström macroglobulinaemia
> - Drugs and toxins:
>   - Ergot
>   - β-Blockers
>   - Methysergide
>   - Bleomycin
>   - Amphetamines
>   - Imipramine
>   - Bromocriptine
>   - Clonidine
>   - Ciclosporin
>   - Oral contraceptives
>   - Vinyl chloride
>   - Nitroglycerin withdrawal
>   - Heavy metals
> - Miscellaneous:
>   - Paraneoplastic syndrome
>   - Chronic renal failure
>   - Primary pulmonary hypertension
>   - Hypothyroidism
>   - Anorexia nervosa

phenomenon there are structural vascular changes, most clearly delineated in patients with systemic sclerosis. Severe intimal hyperplasia consisting of collagen deposits is often associated with intravascular thrombi, which can completely occlude the lumen [8]. In systemic sclerosis there is also distorted nail fold capillary architecture with dilated loops and areas of vessel drop-out.

Aberrant expression of endogenous vasodilatory substances (nitric oxide, prostacyclin, prostaglandin and leukotrienes) and vasoconstrictors (endothelin, angiotensin II and thromboxane A2) has been implicated in the pathogenesis of the Raynaud phenomenon [9]. A disturbance in vascular homeostasis may lead to uncontrolled vasoconstriction and studies have demonstrated downregulation of nitric oxide and upregulation of endothelin-1 in Raynaud phenomenon patients [10,11]. Investigation into the innervation pathways of vascular smooth muscle have highlighted a prominent role for α_{2c}-adrenoreceptors in cold-induced vasoconstriction [12]. Studies of Raynaud phenomenon patients have demonstrated that, compared with normal controls, the increased contractile response to cold and α_2-adrenergic agonists is associated with increased activity of protein tyrosine kinase and tyrosine phosphorylation in vascular smooth muscle [13].

Clinical features
Presentation
The Raynaud phenomenon affects the hands and, less often, the feet; changes elsewhere are exceptional, although the tongue can be involved [14].

A typical attack consists of sudden pallor of one or more digits, followed after a few minutes by cyanosis or sometimes by redness. In primary Raynaud phenomenon the condition is usually symmetrical and involves several digits. In secondary Raynaud phenomenon only one or a few digits are affected and asymmetry is not unusual. Attacks are usually precipitated by cold, either local or of the whole body, or by psychological stimuli. Episodes may occur infrequently or many times each day. Severe cases, which are usually of the secondary type, may be complicated by telangiectases of the nail fold, thinning and ridging of the nail and atrophy or sclerosis of the fingers (sclerodactyly). Skin necrosis is extremely rare in primary Raynaud phenomenon but not uncommon in secondary Raynaud phenomenon and may result in destruction of the digits.

The disease tends to run a variable course. In primary Raynaud phenomenon the outcome is good in 80% of cases, but some disability occurs in 20%. In secondary Raynaud phenomenon the prognosis is that of the underlying disease.

Differential diagnosis
This includes acrocyanosis, hand–arm vibration syndrome, heavy metal intoxication, ergot intoxication, thoracic outlet syndrome and cervical rib, and Buerger disease and other arterial diseases.

Prognosis
Prognosis varies with the underlying disease, if one is present.

Investigations
Investigations are directed towards detecting an underlying cause for the Raynaud phenomenon. A variety of vascular imaging studies have been employed but are not specifically useful in clinical diagnosis.

Management
Conservative management includes taking measures to keep the hands and feet warm and reducing cold exposure and also emotional stress. Hand and feet warmers may be useful. With drug treatment, the clinician must balance the beneficial effects versus drug-related adverse effects [15].

First line
Calcium-channel antagonists can be useful in decreasing the frequency, duration and severity of attacks. A meta-analysis of 18 randomised, placebo-controlled, double-blinded trials assessed the efficacy of calcium-channel blockers against placebo in patients with primary Raynaud phenomenon and found a decrease in attacks and reduction in symptom severity [16]. Recommended doses of nifedipine range from 30 to 180 mg daily and for amlodipine between 5 and 20 mg daily. Slow-release or long-acting preparations are recommended to improve compliance and reduce side effects; nonetheless discontinuation occurs in approximately 15% of subjects because of headaches and leg oedema [17].

Second line
In a double-blind, placebo-controlled study of 16 patients with secondary Raynaud phenomenon, sildenafil 50 mg twice daily demonstrated significant improvement in mean attack rates and duration [18]. Sildenafil is a phosphodiesterase inhibitor and acts by increasing the vasodilatory effect of both nitric oxide and prostacyclin. A variety of newer phosphodiesterase inhibitors are being investigated that may increase perfusion but with variable efficacy on duration and severity of attacks.

Third line
Intravenous infusion of vasodilatory prostaglandins can reverse ischaemic complications in Raynaud phenomenon. Iloprost, a prostacyclin analogue, is commonly administered to patients with severe digital ulceration. In a randomised, placebo-controlled, double-blind study of 131 patients with systemic sclerosis, the mean weekly number of Raynaud phenomenon attacks significantly decreased on iloprost compared with placebo [19]. Repeated treatment with iloprost over 1 year was found to be more effective than nifedipine in reducing the severity score of Raynaud phenomenon in patients with systemic sclerosis [20].

A study of bosentan, an endothelin receptor antagonist, demonstrated a marked reduction in new digital ulcers in systemic sclerosis patients but did not decrease the frequency or severity of Raynaud attacks [21]. A randomised controlled trial demonstrated that the angiotensin II receptor antagonist losartan significantly reduced the frequency and severity of vasoconstrictive episodes in patients with primary Raynaud phenomenon and in Raynaud phenomenon secondary to systemic sclerosis [22].

Topical glyceryl trinitrate, a nitric oxide donor, significantly reduced the number and severity of Raynaud attacks in individuals with primary Raynaud phenomenon and secondary Raynaud phenomenon compared with placebo [23]. Glyceryl trinitrate 2% was associated with headaches whereas glyceryl trinitrate 1% reduced the incidence of side effects but maintained a similar improvement in Raynaud phenomenon symptoms [23]. A systematic review of typical nitrate use suggests that improvements are seen in both primary and secondary Raynaud phenomena, with the response being greater in secondary cases [24]. Botulinum toxin A, injected into the hand, can also cause vasodilatation; its role in the treatment of Raynaud phenomenon has yet to be established [25]. Several studies have shown decreased pain, decreased ulceration and improvement in Raynaud symptoms with either botulinum toxin A or botulinum toxin B. The dose range used in studies is variable, but can be as low as 10 units of botulinum toxin A [26,27].

Cryoglobulinaemia

Definition
Cryoglobulinaemia refers to the presence of immunoglobulin complexes that precipitate *in vitro* when cooled below body temperature [1].

Introduction and general description
Cutaneous features in cryoglobulinaemia occur as a consequence of intravascular precipitation of cryoglobulins in the small vessels of the skin or as an immune complex disease (Chapters 99 and 100). In the demonstration of cryoglobulins, venous blood is drawn into a warm syringe and allowed to clot at 37°C. The serum (or plasma if cryofibrinogen is suspected) is cooled to 4–5°C and any precipitate noted. This should redissolve on warming. The amounts of cryoglobulin reported to cause symptoms are very variable: less than 25 mg/dL may rarely be associated with symptoms, however much higher levels may be symptomless. Levels as high as 80 g/L have been recorded.

Epidemiology
Incidence and prevalence
There are few epidemiological data on the prevalence of cryoglobulinaemia. However, a population study of a small town in Italy, Origgio, demonstrated a prevalence of mixed cryoglobulinaemia affecting 8.5/10 000 in the general population, or 26/10 000 in those aged over 50 years. In this study, the main underlying association was hepatitis C [2].

Age
The mean age of onset of symptoms in mixed cryoglobulinaemia is reported as being 53 years, with a mean age at diagnosis of 56 years [3].

Pathophysiology
Type I cryoglobulins are single monoclonal immunoglobulins usually associated with haematological disorders, such as multiple myeloma, macroglobulinaemia and lymphoma. These precipitate in blood vessels, leading to ischaemia from vascular occlusion.

Type II mixed cryoglobulins are composed of a monoclonal component (usually immunoglobulin M κ (IgM-κ)) with rheumatoid factor activity against polyclonal IgG. In type III mixed cryoglobulins, all the components are polyclonal [3]. Mixed cryoglobulinaemia is most commonly associated with hepatitis C virus (HCV) infection and is mainly of type III [4]. Other infections are also implicated in mixed cryoglobulinaemia, including hepatitis B and human immunodeficiency virus (HIV), and cases are also seen in conjunction with autoimmune diseases such as Sjögren syndrome, systemic LE and rheumatoid arthritis [5]. Mixed cryoglobulinaemia causes a systemic vasculitis with multiorgan involvement, mainly of the skin, joints, kidneys and peripheral nerves.

Clinical features
The most usual skin manifestation is purpura on the lower legs, which may develop after cooling of the extremities. In cryoglobulinaemia of all types, other skin signs are livedo reticularis, Raynaud phenomenon, atypical ulceration of the legs, digital skin necrosis and cold urticaria [6].

Differential diagnosis
Other causes of vascular occlusion such as hypercoagulable states, embolic disease and vasculitides need to be included in the differential diagnosis.

Investigations
Investigations include a skin biopsy to look for vascular occlusion or vasculitis, immunoglobulin titres and plasma protein electrophoresis, and hepatitis B and C serology. Serology for autoimmune disease should also be performed.

If cryoglobulinaemic vasculitis is suspected clinically, investigations should demonstrate circulating cryoglobulins, high rheumatoid factor titre and low C4 levels.

Histology may show a leukocytoclastic vasculitis of the small blood vessels on a skin biopsy. Histopathology of cryoglobulinaemia without vasculitis will reveal homogeneous eosinophilic material within the vascular lumina of dermal vessels, which corresponds to cryoglobulin deposits.

Management
Treatment of mixed cryoglobulinaemia is aimed at reducing immune complex activity by immunosuppression (with prednisolone and cyclophosphamide) and plasmapheresis. In the presence of HCV infection, therapy should also be directed at viral eradication with pegylated interferon and ribavirin. Recently, reports have demonstrated benefit from the use of rituximab, a chimeric monoclonal anti-CD20 antibody, that exerts a selective B-cell control [7]. Similarly, for hepatitis B virus infection, a step-wise approach with antiviral therapy (oral nucleot(s)ide analogues, B-cell depletion (rituximab), steroids, plasmapharesis and non-steroidal drugs has been proposed [8].

Cold agglutinins

Cold agglutinin disease is a disorder of autoimmune haemolysis in which cold-sensitive immunoglobulins react against erythrocyte surface antigens. In primary cold agglutinin disease, a bone marrow monoclonal CD20+ κ+ B-lymphocyte population is often demonstrated, while lymphoplasmacytic lymphoma may underlie the production of cold agglutinins in other patients [1]. Cases may also be secondary to a variety of diseases, notably *Mycoplasma* and

Epstein–Barr virus infections. Cutaneous features occur mainly on acral sites and include Raynaud phenomenon, acrocyanosis and skin necrosis.

Fatigue is one of the dominant symptoms of cold agglutinin disease, affecting about 90% of patients. This can vary with time but has a marked impact on physical, emotional and financial well-being [2].

Non-pharmacological treatments involve avoiding or mitigating against cold exposures. This may include wearing gloves for example when accessing fridges or freezers, making sure patients have a warm environment on hospital wards and warming intravenous infusions. The results of therapy with corticosteroids, alkylating agents and interferon α have been poor. However, studies of the chimeric anti-CD20 antibody rituximab have produced good response rates [3]. This may be further enhanced when combined with fludarabine or bendamustine [4].

Physiological reactions to heat and infrared radiation

The physical and biochemical effects of infrared (IR) radiation, comprising approximately 40% of solar irradiation, have been relatively neglected [1], but are the subject of a comprehensive review [2].

IR is the segment of the electromagnetic spectrum that extends between red visible light and microwaves and radiowaves. The wavelengths range from 0.75 μm (750 nm) to 100 μm. As with ultraviolet (UV) radiation, there is an arbitrary subdivision into near IR (0.75–3 μm), middle IR (3–30 μm) and far IR (30–100 μm). Energy is inversely proportional to wavelength, therefore most biological effects are seen at shorter wavelengths. IR causes molecular vibration, the most obvious effect of which is to raise temperature. Radiation from 0.75 to 0.8 μm can cause photochemical reactions. Some wavelengths of IR are strongly absorbed by water – both in the atmosphere and in the hydrated stratum corneum. Transmitted IR can penetrate up to 30 mm [3].

The major sources of IR radiation are the sun and IR lamps, but in clinical practice various forms of radiant heater in the home and workplace, hot water bottles, heating pads, etc. are important. Most experimental work into the effects of IR radiation on the skin has used sources that emit UV and/or visible radiation as well, and the data are conflicting.

Experimental effects
Acute effects
Infrared radiation alone produces redness, which disappears by 6 h [4]. Histological studies have shown vasodilatation and mast cell degranulation [5]. The mediators have been studied in suction blisters and are essentially similar to those found in UVB-induced skin changes: free arachidonic acid, prostaglandins PGD_2, PGE_2, PGF_2 and 6 oxo-$PGF_{1\alpha}$. The free arachidonic acid level is still high after 72 h [6]. Epidermal proliferation is reduced by IR and does not become normal until after 7 days [7].

Prior heating with IR radiation reduces the phototoxic response to methoxypsoralen and UVA [8]. The interaction between UV and IR radiation has been evaluated but with conflicting results [8–10] and further studies are needed.

Chronic effects
In a mouse model, over a 45-week period, the histological effects of radiation were studied, using a visible plus IR source, either alone, in combination with UVA and UVB, or with UV followed by IR [11]. There was deposition of fibres with the staining properties of elastin in animals receiving only visible plus IR radiation, and an augmentation of the elastosis was attributable to UV radiation. As with clinical solar elastosis, there was also an increase in ground substance.

Carcinogenesis
Infrared radiation can coagulate protein and nucleic acid and is synergistic with UV radiation in denaturing DNA. The production of UVB-induced cyclobutane dimers is temperature dependent [12], therefore this tumour-initiating event is likely to be augmented by IR radiation. DNA repair after UV- and X-ray-induced damage is slower at 41–43°C than at 37°C, as occurs with heating resulting from IR [13]. It has been shown that mice heated to 35–38°C had a shorter latent period for UVR-induced tumours than controls [14,15]. Heat, wind and humidity have been shown to enhance UV carcinogenesis [16].

DISEASES CAUSED BY HEAT AND INFRARED RADIATION

Erythema ab igne

Definition
This is a characteristic reticular telangiectatic and pigmented dermatosis, resulting from repeated or prolonged exposure to IR radiation, insufficient to produce a burn.

Introduction and general description
The condition, once common in the UK, has become rare since the introduction of central heating, although it is still sometimes seen in rural areas among elderly people who stand or sit closely over fires (Granny's tartan), or who are habituated to the use of hot water bottles. It may be a valuable sign of hypothyroidism. A resurgence of the condition in the USA affects not only the elderly but also impecunious students [1], because of the high cost of central heating.

Sources other than domestic heating may be responsible for erythema ab igne at other body sites. Examples include the repeated application of hot water bottles or heated pads for chronic backache, recliner chairs with built-in heaters [2] and even bathing in hot water [3]. Among occupations, foundry workers and bakers and the various tasks that involve carrying heated coals are sometimes relevant. Car heaters may also be a cause [4]. Erythema ab igne has been found on the thighs of laptop computer users [5–8]. It has been reported as a useful marker of chronic pancreatitis because local heat relieves the abdominal pain [9] but also occurs when heat is applied for other real and imagined pains [10], including cancer [11]. In mentally disturbed patients with thermophilia, bizarre areas of erythema ab igne are sometimes encountered.

Epidemiology
Sex
Erythema ab igne most commonly affects the legs of women.

Pathophysiology
Pathology
In the early stages, epidermal atrophy, dermal pigmentation and vasodilatation are evident. Basophilic degeneration of the connective tissue, focal hyperkeratosis and epithelial cellular atypia occur later, closely resembling the changes induced by actinic damage [12]. Electron microscopy shows similar changes in the elastic fibres as found in chronic sun exposure [13]. There can be loss of type IV collagen from the basement membrane zone [14]. Keratoses and eventually squamous cell carcinomas may form [15–17].

Clinical features
In most cases, a heat source explaining the dermatosis is readily identified in the clinical history, although some patients may deny heat exposure. Any surface of the body is susceptible [18] and the condition can occur at all ages including in children [19]. Following a single exposure to IR radiation of a subthreshold intensity, a mild and transient reticular redness occurs. Further or repeated exposure causes a more marked redness with noticeable hyperpigmentation (Figure 124.11) and, sometimes, superficial epidermal atrophy. Subepidermal blistering [20] can occur in the affected skin (Figure 124.12). The cumulative effects of the small and repeated thermal exposures often clear during the summer months but involution gradually becomes less complete. The changes caused by repeated and prolonged exposure to IR radiation eventually resemble those of poikiloderma, with reticulate telangiectasia, atrophy, melanosis and diffuse hyperkeratosis.

The distribution of the dermatosis depends not only on the direction of the incident radiation, but also on the contour of the skin and the interposition of clothing. When erythema ab igne results from sitting in front of the fire, people may sit sideways, causing the outer aspect of one leg and the inner aspect of the other to be particularly affected. Others habitually sit directly in front, and a strictly symmetrical eruption is seen. In severely affected individuals the reticular pattern is lost, a wide area of skin becoming pigmented and atrophic, with only the periphery showing the characteristic pattern.

An unusual variant has been described in elderly immobile females with lymphoedema in which there are reticulate ridges of tissue that can be compressed [21].

Rarely, lichen planus, psoriasis or chilblain lupus may appear as a Koebner phenomenon in the affected area.

While often the heat source is a heater or warming pad, increasing reports of laptop computer-related erythema ab igne are appearing in the literature. A cluster of paediatric erythema ab igne cases has even been reported in children being home schooled in the Covid-19 lockdown, while sitting next to a space heater [22].

Heat-associated carcinomas
Squamous carcinomas of the skin occurring in areas of heat damage have been known from ancient times; they have often been regarded as exotic curios and their significance overlooked [23].

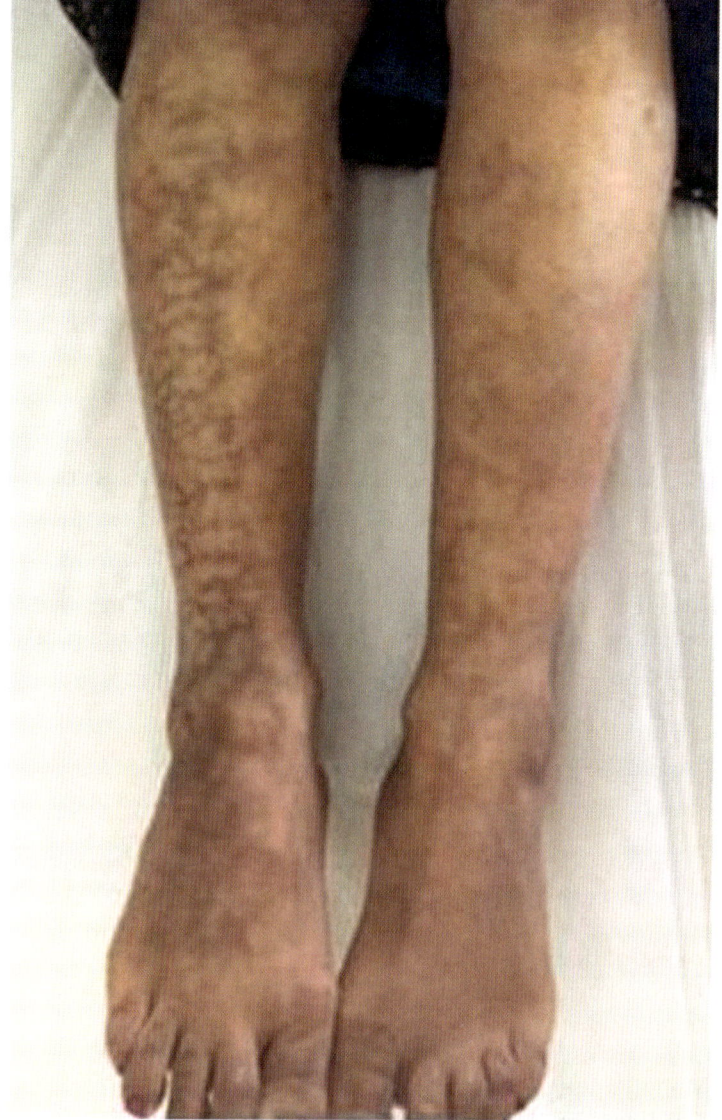

Figure 124.11 Reticular hyperpigmentation on the anterior aspect of both legs. Reproduced from Ozturk and An 2020 [34] with permission from John Wiley & Sons.

They include the Kang cancer of northern China [24] and Japan [25] from sleeping on beds of hot bricks, the Kangri cancer of Kashmir [26,27] from wearing pots of hot coals and the Kairo cancer of Japan caused by carrying metallic benzene-burning flasks – all devices used to counteract the cold. 'Turf' cancer of the legs of rural Irish women has been associated with standing for long periods of time over peat fires [28]. Simultaneous occurrence of Merkel cell carcinoma with squamous carcinoma has been recorded [29,30]. Basal cell carcinomas and actinic keratoses have been reported at a site on the cheeks of those wearing rimless glasses, where the temperature is higher than the surrounding skin because of focusing of the sun's rays [31,32].

Differential diagnosis
Although diagnosis is usually straightforward, there may be confusion with livedo reticularis, in which changes are strictly symmetrical and telangiectatic rather than pigmented.

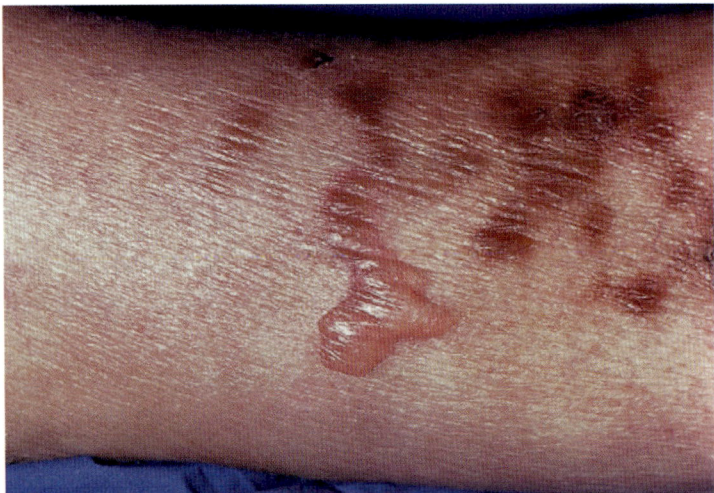

Figure 124.12 Erythema ab igne with subepidermal bulla formation.

Complications and co-morbidities

There may be associated hypothyroidism, explaining the need for warmth in some cases. When heat is being used to control pain, for example on the abdomen, the relevant underlying causes of pain should be investigated.

Prognosis

Milder cases of erythema ab igne will settle spontaneously. However, in more severe cases the pigmentation and atrophy may persist. The increased risk of skin cancer means that long-term monitoring either by the patient or a physician may be required.

Investigations

Thyroid function tests and ultrasound of the abdomen can be used if appropriate.

Management

Removing the heat source from the skin and investigating for underlying causes of pain, where appropriate, are the mainstay of management. Hypothyroidism should be excluded. In elderly women living alone, erythema ab igne may be a sign of hypothermia. The help of ancillary social services may be needed. Advice should be given on clothing and efforts made to improve the microvascular circulation. 5-Fluorouracil cream has been used to eliminate the dyskeratotic keratinocytes [33].

Key references

The full list of references can be found in the online version at https://www.wiley.com/rooksdermatology10e

Diseases caused or aggravated by cold
Frostbite
1 Golant A, Nord RM, Paksima N, Posner MA. Cold exposure injuries to the extremities. *J Am Acad Orthop Surg* 2008;16:704–15.

10 McIntosh SE, Freer L, Grissom CK *et al*. Wilderness Medical Society clinical practice guidelines for the prevention and treatment of frostbite: 2019 update. *Wilderness Environ Med* 2019;30:S19–32.
13 Cauchy E, Cheguillaume B, Chetaille E. A controlled trial of a prostacyclin and rt-PA in the treatment of severe frostbite. *N Engl J Med* 2011;364:189–90.
14 Zaramo TZ, Green JK, Janis JE. Practical review of the current management of frostbite injuries. *Plast Reconstr Surg Glob Open* 2022;10:e4618.

Trench foot
3 Irwin MS, Sanders R, Green CJ, Terenghi G. Neuropathy in non-freezing cold injury (trench foot). *J Roy Soc Med* 1997;90:433–8.

Perniosis
2 Cappel JA, Wetter DA. Clinical characteristics, etiologic associations, laboratory findings, treatment, and proposal of diagnostic criteria of pernio (chilblains) in a series of 104 patients at Mayo Clinic, 2000 to 2011. *Mayo Clin Proc* 2014;89:207–15.

Acrocyanosis
4 Goldsmith PC, Leslie TA, Polak JM, Dowd PM. Acrocyanosis and perniosis: an investigation of cutaneous neural and endothelial peptides in digital skin. *Skin Pharmacol* 1994;7:563–73.

Livedo reticularis
2 In SI, Han JH, Kang HY, Lee ES, Kim YC. The histopathological characteristics of livedo reticularis. *J Cutan Pathol* 2009;36:1275–8.

Raynaud phenomenon
15 Boin F, Wigley FM. Understanding, assessing and treating Raynaud's phenomenon. *Curr Opin Rheum* 2005;17:752–60.
18 Fries R, Shariat K, von Wilmowsky H, Bohm M. Sildenafil in the treatment of Raynaud's phenomenon resistant to vasodilatory therapy. *Circulation* 2005;112:2980–5.
25 Jenkins SN, Neyman KM, Veledar E, Chen SC. A pilot study evaluating the efficacy of botulinum toxin A in the treatment of Raynaud's phenomenon. *J Am Acad Dermatol* 2013;69:834–5.

Cryoglobulinaemia
2 Monti G, Francesco S, Laura C *et al*. Prevalence of mixed cryoglobulinaemia syndrome and circulating cryoglobulins in a population-based survey: the Origgio study. *Autoimmun Rev* 2014;13:609–14.

Cold agglutinins
1 Berentsen S, Beiske K, Tjonnfjord GE. Primary chronic cold agglutinin disease: an update on pathogenesis, clinical features and therapy. *Haematology* 2007;12:361–70.

Physiological reactions to heat and infrared radiation
1 Kligman LH, Kligman AM. Reflections on heat. *Br J Dermatol* 1984;110:369–79.
11 Kligman LH. Intensification of ultraviolet induced dermal damage by infrared radiation. *Arch Dermatol Res* 1982;272:229–38.

Diseases caused by heat and infrared radiation
Erythema ab igne
1 Kligman LH, Kligman AM. Reflections on heat. *Br J Dermatol* 1984;110:369–79.

CHAPTER 125

Burns and Heat Injury

Marc G. Jeschke

Hamilton Health Sciences, Hamilton; McMaster University, Hamilton; Department of Surgery, Division of General Surgery, Plastic Surgery, Department of Immunology, University of Toronto, Toronto, Ontario, Canada

Introduction, 125.1	Evaluation of burn depth, 125.6	**Hypermetabolism, 125.11**
Initial assessment, pre-hospital care and emergency treatment, 125.1	Choice of topical dressings, 125.10	Treatment of the hypermetabolic response, 125.13
	Escharotomy, 125.10	Nutrition, 125.13
Burn shock and resuscitation, 125.3	Operative management, 125.10	Other non-pharmacological strategies, 125.14
Inhalation injury, 125.5	**Infection control, 125.10**	Pharmacological modalities, 125.14
Background, 125.5	Clinical management of burn wound infection, 125.10	**Summary and conclusions, 125.15**
Diagnosis, 125.5	Central line-associated infections, 125.11	**Acknowledgement, 125.15**
Treatment, 125.6	Ventilator-associated pneumonia, 125.11	
Evaluation and early management of the burn wound, 125.6	Sepsis, 125.11	**Key references, 125.15**

Introduction

There is no greater trauma than major burn injury, which can be classified according to different burn causes and depths. Over half a million burn injuries occur in the USA yearly [1]. These injuries are typically not severe, but 40 000–50 000 burn patients require admission and treatment at a burn centre or burn hospital. The debilitating effects of burns have led to the dedication of considerable amounts of resources, which have greatly improved outcomes [2,3,4]. Improved outcomes can be attributable to specialised burn centres, advances in resuscitation, protocolised and specialised critical care, better coverage of wounds, improved treatment of infections and inhalation injury, and enhanced management of the burn-induced hypermetabolic response [4,5]. Another major advance is the recent initiative by burn care providers to hold consensus conferences and implement specific definitions of disease processes in severely burned patients, allowing for the conduct of appropriate multicentre trials [6] and comparative studies. All these changes have significantly improved post-burn morbidity and mortality. Indeed, in a recent study in *The Lancet*, it was shown that the burn size associated with an enhanced risk of mortality in a specialised centre increased from 40% total body surface area (TBSA) burned to over 60% TBSA in children [5], while it increased from 20% TBSA to 30–40% TBSA in adults [7].

Despite advances in burn care, severe burns still inflict damage on almost every organ in the body resulting in profound debilitating complications or even death [2,3,4,5,7,8]. Of all burn cases, nearly 4000 people die of complications related to thermal injury [2,9,10]. Burn deaths generally occur either immediately after the injury or weeks later as a result of infection/sepsis, multisystem organ failure or hypermetabolic catabolic responses [5,11]. Over the last decade, the cause of death has changed profoundly [11]. The major cause of death in severely burned patients admitted to a burn centre used to be due to anoxic brain injury, followed by sepsis and multiple organ failure. Now, the major cause of death in burned patients is sepsis followed by multiple organ failure and anoxic brain injury [11]. This shift in the cause of death requires the development of novel paradigms and treatment approaches to improve post-burn morbidity and mortality further. The quality of the complex care that burn patients receive is directly related to patient outcome and survival. Key aspects of care are as follows:

- *Initial care at the scene, pre-hospital care and the early hospital phase:* adequate and timely response, evaluation of the burns, resuscitation and admission to a burn centre; escharotomies/fasciotomies, resuscitation and treatment of inhalation injury.
- *Later hospital phase:* wound care including burn surgeries, infection control, maintaining organ function and attenuation of hypermetabolism.
- *Long-term phase:* persistent hypermetabolism, reconstruction and rehabilitation.

Four aspects appear to be central for survival and are interrelated: burn shock and resuscitation, inhalation injury, wound closure and burn hypermetabolism. Therefore, in this chapter, standards of care and novel treatment avenues in these areas will be discussed.

Initial assessment, pre-hospital care and emergency treatment

The initial assessment and management of a burn patient begin with pre-hospital care. There is a great need for efficient and accurate

---

Rook's Textbook of Dermatology, Tenth Edition. Edited by Christopher Griffiths, Jonathan Barker, Tanya Bleiker, Walayat Hussain and Rosalind Simpson.
© 2024 John Wiley & Sons Ltd. Published 2024 by John Wiley & Sons Ltd.

Guidelines for Burn Patient Referral

(Advice on Transfer and Consultation)

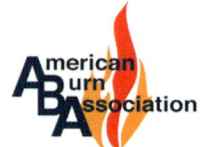

- These guidelines are designed to be used to aid in clinical decision making. If you have sustained a burn injury, please seek medical advice from a medical professional.
- Local and regional infrastructure, resources, and relationships may determine the necessity and timeliness of burn center referral.
- These guidelines are not meant to be definitive care recommendations. They may facilitate building the proper referral network within the local healthcare community.

	Immediate Consultation with Consideration for Transfer	Consultation Recommendation
Thermal Burns	• Full thickness burns • Partial thickness ≥10% TBSA* • Any deep partial or full thickness burns involving the face, hands, genitalia, feet, perineum, or over any joints • Patients with burns and other comorbidities • Patients with concomitant traumatic injuries • Poorly controlled pain	• Partial thickness burns <10% TBSA* • All potentially deep burns of any size
Inhalation Injury	• All patients with suspected inhalation injury	• Patients with signs of potential inhalation such as facial flash burns, singed facial hairs, or smoke exposure
Pediatrics (≤14 years, or <30 kg)	• All pediatric burns may benefit from burn center referral due to pain, dressing change needs, rehabilitation, patient/caregiver needs, or non-accidental trauma	
Chemical Injuries	• All chemical injuries	
Electrical Injuries	• All high voltage (≥1,000V) electrical injuries • Lightning injury	• Low voltage (<1,000V) electrical injuries should receive consultation and consideration for follow-up in a burn center to screen for delayed symptom onset and vision problems

Burn Severity Determination

SUPERFICIAL
- Dry, red, easily blanching, sometimes painful
- Example: Sunburn
- NOT counted in calculations of total burn surface area (TBSA)

SUPERFICIAL PARTIAL THICKNESS
- Moist, red, blanching, blisters, very painful
- Counted in calculations of total burn surface area (TBSA)

DEEP PARTIAL THICKNESS
- Drier, more pale, less blanching, less pain
- Counted in calculations of total burn surface area (TBSA)

FULL THICKNESS
- Dry, leathery texture, variable color (white, brown, black), loss of pin prick sensation
- Counted in calculations of total burn surface area (TBSA)

Percentage Total Body Surface Area (TBSA)

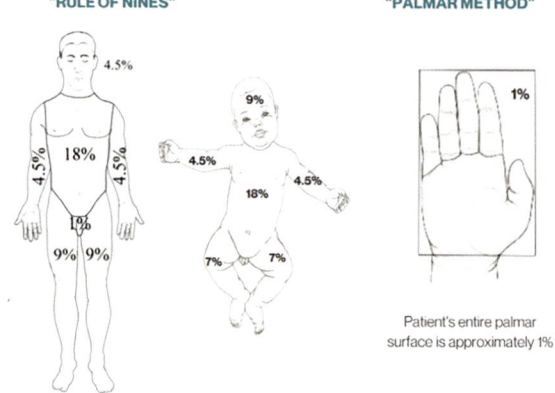

For more information visit **ameriburn.org/burnreferral**

Figure 125.1 ABA guidelines for burn patient referral. Reproduced with permission of the American Burn Association.

assessment, transportation and emergency care for these patients in order to improve their overall outcome. Once the initial evaluation has been completed, transportation to the appropriate care facility is of utmost importance. It is imperative that the patient is transported to a facility with the capacity to provide care for the thermally injured patient; however, at times, patients need to be transported to the nearest care facility for stabilisation (i.e. airway control, establishment of intravenous access, etc.).

Once in the emergency room, the assessment as with any trauma patient is composed of primary and secondary surveys (Box 125.1). As part of the primary survey, the establishment of a secure airway is paramount. An expert in airway management should accomplish this as these patients can rapidly deteriorate from airway oedema. Once this initial assessment is complete, the clinical status of the patient will be determined by the American Burn Association (ABA) criteria for burn unit referral (Figure 125.1).

Table 125.1 Typical clinical appearances of burn depths (see also Figure 125.3).

First-degree burns	Involve only the epidermis and never blister Appear as a 'sun burn' Are not included in the % total body surface area calculation
Second-degree burns (dermal burns)	Superficial: pink, homogeneous, normal capillary refill, painful, moist, intact hair follicles Deep: mottled or white, delayed or absent capillary refill, dry, decreased sensation or insensate, non-intact hair follicles
Third-degree burns	Dry, white or charred, leathery, insensate

Burn shock and resuscitation

Once the patient is assessed and evaluated at a burn centre, the management of a burn patient starts. A central aspect of this phase is determining if the patient's injury is 'survivable' or futile. Futility in adults or elderly burn patients is usually determined by the sum of age (years) plus burn size (%) plus presence or absence of inhalation injury (±14) being greater or equal to 140–150 [12]. In paediatric patients, the philosophy of many paediatric burn centres is that there is no futility in children except in very rare instances, for example a 100% TBSA full-thickness burn. Once the decision to treat is made, the initial management and therapeutic goal is preservation of limbs and prevention of organ failure, which begins with well-established recognition of injury severity, first care protocols and surgical interventions [2,4].

Resuscitation formula

A central aspect of the clinical response is adequate resuscitation [13–16]. Many formulae have been studied, with all having the same goal: maintenance of organ perfusion during burn shock with restoration of intravascular volume. The most commonly used formulae are the Parkland formula [14] and modified Parkland formulae:

Parkland

$$4\,\text{mL} \times \%\text{TBSA} \times \text{weight (kg)} = 24\,\text{h fluid requirement, with half given over the first 8 h and the remainder over the following 16 h}$$

Modified Parkland

$$2\,\text{mL} \times \%\text{TBSA} \times \text{weight (kg)} = 24\,\text{h fluid requirement, with half given over the first 8 h and the remainder over the following 16 h}$$

Recent analyses indicate that the modified formula is superior to the traditional 4 cc and the recent ABLS ABA recommendation uses the modified 2 cc/kg.

However, recent evidence suggests that the Parkland formula may not be as accurate as previously thought in providing estimates of fluid requirements in patients with large/deeper burns, inhalation injury, delays in resuscitation, obesity, alcohol or drug use, and electrical injury, resulting in inadequate/inappropriate resuscitation [13,17–19]. The catastrophic events associated with underresuscitation include multiple organ failure and death. Over-resuscitation induces 'fluid creep' with its inherent complications such as pulmonary oedema, pleural effusions, pericardial effusions,

---

Box 125.1 Initial assessment of a burned patient

Primary survey
- Airway
  - Endotracheal tube placed orally
  - Always be prepared for possible surgical airway
- Breathing
  - Ensure proper placement of endotracheal tube by auscultation/X-ray
  - Bronchoscopic assessment for inhalation injury
- Circulation
  - Establish adequate intravenous access (large-bore intravenous placed peripherally in non-burned tissue if possible, central access would be required but can wait)
  - Begin resuscitation based on the Parkland formula

Secondary survey
- Complete head to toe assessment of patient
- Obtain information about the patient's past medical history, medications, allergies, tetanus status
- Determine the circumstances/mechanism of injury
  - Entrapment in closed space
  - Loss of consciousness
  - Time since injury
  - Flame, scald, grease, chemical, electrical
- Examination should include a thorough neurological assessment
- All extremities should be examined to determine possible neurovascular compromise (i.e. possible compartment syndrome) and need for escharotomies
- Burn size and depth should be determined at the end of the survey

---

In determining the % TBSA burn, the 'rule of 9s' can be used; however, it is not as accurate as the Lund and Browder chart (Figure 125.2) which further subdivides the body for a more accurate calculation. First-degree burns are not included. Assessment of burn depth can be difficult even for experts in the field. There are some basic principles, which can help in evaluating the burn depth (Table 125.1 and Figure 125.3). Always be aware that burns are dynamic and burn depth can progress or convert to being deeper. Therefore, reassessment is important in establishing burn depth.

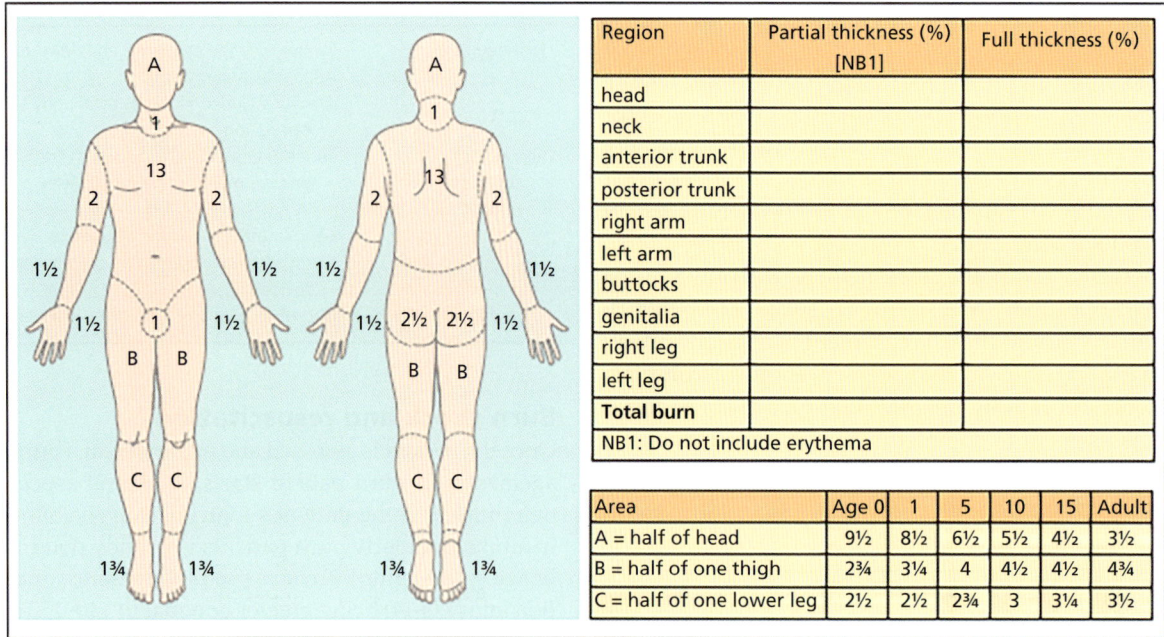

Figure 125.2 Lund and Browder chart to calculate body surface area burned.

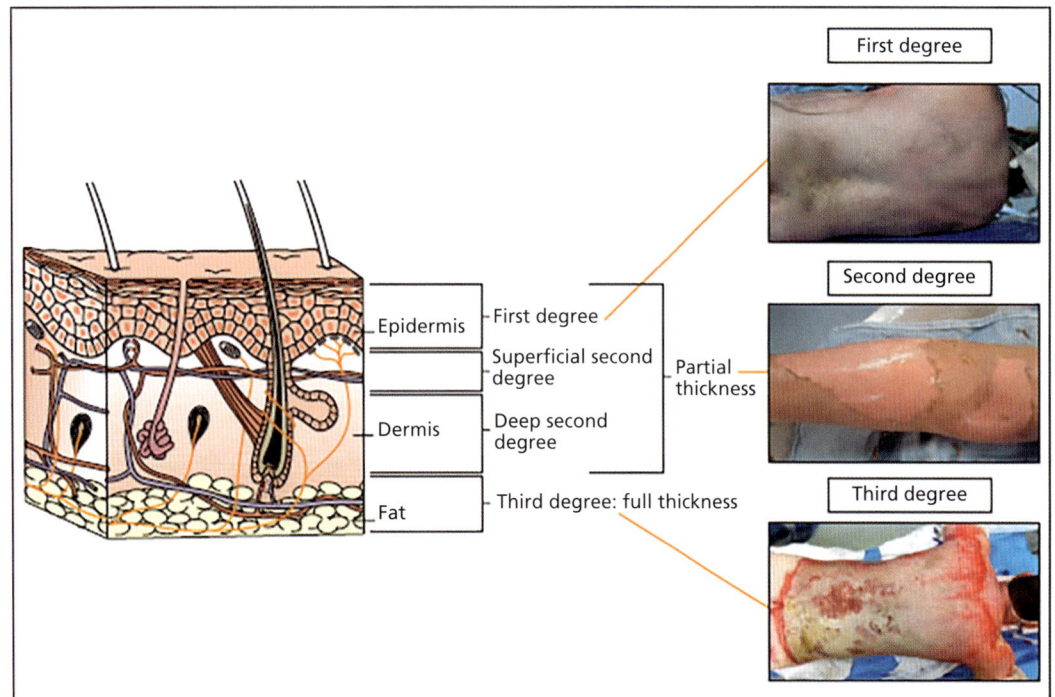

Figure 125.3 First-, second- and third-degree burn levels in the skin.

abdominal compartment syndrome, extremity compartment syndrome and conversion of burns to deeper wounds [6]. In addition, providing greater fluid than required in burn patients significantly increases the risk of developing acute respiratory distress syndrome, pneumonia, bloodstream infections, multiple organ failure and death [20].

Resuscitation goal

One of the greatest challenges in resuscitation is monitoring whether it is adequate and effective. The traditional end points of urine output (0.5–1 cL/kg body weight/h), mean arterial pressure (>60–65 mmHg), normal base excess and lactate levels are not always accurate and can be misleading [14,17,18,20]. However, there are currently no better physiological markers that enable adequate resuscitation, and therefore these parameters remain the 'gold standard'. New attempts to improve and individualise resuscitation include use of thermal dilution catheters (e.g. PiCCO®) [15,21] and computer-assisted closed loop resuscitation [22,23]. These technologies hold promise but have not been fully established in the clinic.

Type of resuscitation fluid

Current literature is related not only to the amount of fluid used in resuscitation but also the type of fluid. Crystalloids have been compared with colloids or other means of resuscitation (e.g. hypertonic saline). To date, no large prospective randomised trial has been conducted to determine whether crystalloids are superior to colloids. However, the majority of specialist burn surgeons use crystalloids (e.g. Ringer lactate) and add colloids (e.g. albumin) as a rescue modality [14,24]. Fresh frozen plasma is being used in trauma patients but is not currently used in burn patients, and its use should be limited to experimental clinical trials. Hypertonic saline showed some promise in small studies of burn patients [25], but failed to improve outcome in patients with traumatic brain injury [26]. Recently two resuscitation adjuncts gained interest in the burn community. First, the use of high doses of vitamin C and second, the addition of antioxidants and trace elements. Vitamin C has been discussed over the last decade and is controversial. Recent evidence in critically ill patients led a large group of collaborators to launch the VICToRY (Vitamin C in Thermal injuRY) trial, a feasibility and pilot study led by Dr Daren Heyland (personal communication) [27].

This will hopefully give burn care providers an answer as to whether vitamin C is beneficial or not during acute resuscitation. The addition of antioxidants and trace elements is another aspect that may improve outcomes of burn patients. A recent study by Rehou *et al.* [28] indicated that antioxidants and trace elements dampen the inflammatory response in burn patients. While the aforementioned study was not sufficiently powered to detect differences in clinical outcomes, it is believed that this modality can be of further benefit in decreasing inflammation and hypermetabolism after burn. In general, resuscitation has profoundly evolved over the last two decades and will continue to do so, because it plays a central role in initial post-burn survival.

Inhalation injury

Background

A total of 20–30% of all major burns are associated with a concomitant inhalation injury, with a mortality of 25–50% when patients required ventilatory support for more than 1 week post-injury [2,4,29]. A significant portion of fire-related deaths result not from burn injury but from inhalation of the toxic products of combustion [17,29–31]. Many of these compounds may act together and can increase mortality. This is especially true of carbon monoxide (CO) and hydrogen cyanide where a synergism has been found to increase tissue hypoxia and acidosis, and may also decrease cerebral oxygen consumption and metabolism. Cyanide (CN) toxicity associated with inhalation injury remains a diagnostic dilemma because markers for CN toxicity (i.e. elevated blood lactate, elevated base deficit or metabolic acidosis) can also represent underresuscitation, associated trauma, CO poisoning or hypoxia. Regardless, aggressive resuscitation and administration of 100% oxygen remains a mainstay of treatment. Controversy continues as to the need for specific antidotes in CN poisoning [32]. The use of hydroxycobalamine (a standard of pre-hospital care in some European centres) has not been as widely accepted in North America. There is minimal evidence for the role of CN antidotes in smoke inhalation injury. Therefore, aggressive supportive therapy aimed at permitting hepatic clearance of CN without specific antidotes should be the first line of treatment. Other possible contributing toxic substances are hydrogen chloride (produced by polyvinyl chloride degradation), nitrogen oxide or aldehydes, which can result in pulmonary oedema, chemical pneumonitis or respiratory irritability. Direct thermal damage to the lung is seldom seen except as a result of high-pressure steam, which has 4000 times the heat-carrying capacity of dry air. Laryngeal reflexes and the efficiency of heat dissipation in the upper airway prevent heat damage to the lung parenchyma.

The clinical course of patients with inhalation injury is divided into three stages:
- First stage: acute pulmonary insufficiency. Patients with severe lung injuries show acute pulmonary insufficiency from 0 to 36 h after injury with asphyxia, CO poisoning, bronchospasm, upper airway obstruction and parenchymal damage.
- Second stage: pulmonary oedema. This stage occurs in 5–30% of patients, usually from 6 to 72 h post-burn, and is associated with a high mortality rate.
- Third stage: bronchopneumonia appears in 15–60% of these patients and has a reported mortality of 50–86%. Bronchopneumonia occurs typically 3–10 days after burn injury and is often associated with the expectoration of large mucous casts formed in the tracheobronchial tree. Those pneumonias appearing in the first few days are usually due to penicillin-resistant *Staphylococcus* species, whereas after 3–4 days the changing flora of the burn wound is reflected in the appearance in the lung of Gram-negative species, especially *Pseudomonas* species.

Diagnosis

Early detection of bronchopulmonary injury is critical in improving survival after a suspected inhalation injury. Clinical signs include the following [17,29]:
- History of exposure to smoke in a closed space (patients who are stuporous or unconscious).
- Physical findings of facial burns/singed nasal vibrissae/bronchorrhoea/sooty sputum/auscultatory findings (wheezing or rales).
- Laboratory findings: hypoxaemia and/or elevated levels of CO.
- Chest X-ray (insensitive method because admission studies are very seldom abnormal and may remain normal as long as 7 days post-burn).
- Bronchoscopy should be the standard diagnostic method on every burn patient. Inhalation injury can be graded using the scale of Endorf and Gamelli [31] as follows:
  - *No inhalation injury (grade 0)*: absence of carbonaceous deposits, erythema, oedema, bronchorrhoea or obstruction.
  - *Mild injury or (grade I)*: minor or patchy areas of erythema, carbonaceous deposits in proximal or distal bronchi (any or combination).
  - *Moderate injury (grade II)*: moderate degree of erythema, carbonaceous deposits, bronchorrhoea with or without compromise of the bronchi (any or combination).

- *Severe injury (grade III)*: severe inflammation with friability, copious carbonaceous deposits, bronchorrhoea, bronchial obstruction (any or combination).
- *Massive injury (grade IV)*: evidence of mucosal sloughing, necrosis, endoluminal obliteration (any or combination).
- To define parenchymal injury, the most specific method is ^{133}Xe lung scanning, which involves intravenous injection of radioactive xenon gas followed by serial chest scintiphotograms. This technique identifies areas of air trapping from small airway partial or total obstruction by demonstrating areas of decreased alveolar gas washout.
- Additionally, pulmonary function test can be performed and could show an increased resistance and decreased flow in those with abnormal ^{133}Xe scans.

Treatment

The treatment of inhalation injury should start immediately, with the administration of 100% oxygen via face mask or nasal cannula. This helps reverse the effects of CO poisoning and aids in its clearance, as 100% oxygen lowers its half-life time from 250 to fewer than 50 min. Maintenance of the airway is critical. If early evidence of upper airway oedema is present, early intubation is required because the upper airway oedema normally increases over 8–12 h. Prophylactic intubation without good indication, however, should not be performed.

Several clinical studies have shown that pulmonary oedema could not be prevented by fluid restriction. Indeed, fluid resuscitation appropriate for the patient's other needs results in a decrease in lung water, has no adverse effect on pulmonary histology and improves survival. Although overhydration could increase pulmonary oedema, inadequate hydration increases the severity of pulmonary injury by sequestration of polymorphonuclear cells and leads to increased mortality.

Prophylactic antibiotics for inhalation injury are not indicated, but clearly are indicated for documented lung infections. Empirical choices for the treatment of pneumonias prior to culture results should include coverage of meticillin-resistant *Staphylococcus aureus* in the first few days post-burn (these develop within the first week after burn) and of Gram-negative organisms (especially *Pseudomonas* or *Klebsiella*) which mostly occur after 1 week post-burn. Systemic antibiotic regimes are based on serially monitored sputum cultures, bronchial washings or transtracheal aspirates.

Pharmacological management

- Bronchodilators: every 2 h.
- Nebulised heparin: 5000–10 000 units with 3 mL normal saline 4 hourly which alternates with:
  - Nebulised acetylcysteine: 20%, 3 mL 4 hourly.
- Hypertonic saline: to induce effective coughing.
- Racemic epinephrine: to reduce mucosal oedema.

The theoretical benefits of corticosteroid therapy include a reduction in mucosal oedema, reduced bronchospasm and the maintenance of surfactant function. However, in several animal and clinical studies, mortality increased with the administration of corticosteroids and bronchopneumonia showed a more extensive abscess formation. Thus the use of corticosteroids is contraindicated.

Evaluation and early management of the burn wound

Evaluation of burn depth

Closure of the burn wounds determines the length of hospital stay, risk of infection and ultimately survival, while failure to get the wounds closed is equivalent to death. Treatment strategies for superficial wounds must be differentiated from treatment plans for deeper wounds. The most significant factor improving patient outcome has been the implementation of early excision and grafting of burn wounds, which was first described by Janzekovic and colleagues in the 1970s [33]. Subsequent studies clearly demonstrated that if the source of stress and inflammation is removed early, survival is significantly improved [34–36]. The challenge that came along with this approach was how to best cover the excised burn wounds. Currently, the gold standard is to cover these wounds with autografts, either in combination with allograft, when the autograft is meshed widely (1:3, 1:4 or larger), or just autografting as a sheet, or when meshed 1:1.5 or 1:2. There are several new strategies on the horizon that may change the surgical care for burn patients.

First-degree burns are of minimal concern. They only involve the epidermis with erythema and no blisters and do not require medical attention.

Second-degree burns (dermal burns) and beyond are those that will require medical attention. Dermal burns are divided into superficial and deep. Their clinical characteristics are summarised in Table 125.1 (and see Figure 125.3). The depth of the burn determines not only the requirement for admission but also the management – operative versus conservative. The ideal treatment for all burns which will not heal between 14 and 21 days is operative excision and skin grafting. All others can be treated conservatively. The conservative management of burns includes appropriate wound care and therapy aimed at maintaining range of motion and overall function.

Partial-thickness burns

Partial-thickness burns can be categorised as superficial or deep burns. Superficial wounds usually heal in between 7 and 14 days. Conversely, complete re-epithelialisation of deep dermal burns can take up to 4–6 weeks, with scarring often resulting from the loss of dermis. A large variety of topical creams and agents are available for treatment, and many are silver-based for anti-infective effects (summarised in Table 125.2). Recent studies support the use of synthetic and biosynthetic membranes (e.g. Biobrane® and Suprathel® [37]). These membranes decrease the number of dressing changes and the amount of pain medication associated with these dressing changes. Several studies have been conducted on Biobrane, which was established in 1982, and they have shown that this membrane is efficacious for superficial burns [38–40]. Suprathel is a synthetic copolymer containing >70% lactic acid. Prospective randomised clinical studies of partial-thickness burns and split-thickness donor sites have shown that Suprathel is associated with less pain than other commercially available membranes, though wound healing times and long-term scar qualities are comparable between this synthetic membrane and other membranes [37].

Another approach to burn wound coverage is the use of biological membranes. Human amniotic membrane has a long history of

Table 125.2 Topical therapy for treatment of cutaneous burns.

Antimicrobials	Agent	Description
Solutions	Mafenide acetate	Available as 11% water-soluble cream or 5% solution for deep dermal and full-thickness burns
		Painful application and when used over large areas may cause severe systemic metabolic acidosis
		Broad antibacterial spectrum (poor against *Staphylococcus aureus*). Good eschar penetration. Useful on full-thickness infected or unexcised burns
		Good eschar penetration. Useful on full-thickness infected or unexcised burns. Topically applied cream to ears and nose
	Chlorhexidine	Concentrations vary from 0.02% to 4%. Can be found in alcoholic or aqueous solution
		High concentrations are not proven to be more effective than lower concentrations. Toxicity is dose dependent
		Broad spectrum against Gram-positive and Gram-negative organisms, facultative anaerobes, aerobes and yeast
		Indicated for superficial burns. May produce skin hypersensitivity
	Povidone	Available commercially as solutions, creams and impregnated dressings
		Used for disinfection of inanimate objects and intact skin, and as an antimicrobial agent for all types of wounds
		Spectrum against Gram-positive and Gram-negative organisms, fungi and protozoa
		Toxic to fibroblasts, reduces cell proliferation. Contraindicated in extensive lesions or a known allergy to iodine. Use cautiously on pregnant women, children, diabetics and patients with known thyroid disorders, compromised renal function or receiving lithium therapy
	Acetic acid	Antiseptic, topical agent often used in a diluted form as an adjunct in the setting of *Pseudomonas aeruginosa*
		Effective against Gram-negative bacteria including *Pseudomonas aeruginosa*
		High concentrations inhibit epithelialisation, polymorphonuclears and fibroblasts
		Superficial burns have been described when not used properly
	Sodium hypochloride	Topical antiseptic used to irrigate, cleanse or as a component in wet-to-dry dressings to treat or prevent skin and soft tissue infections. Concentration varies: full strength at 0.5%, half strength at 0.25% and quarter strength at 0.125%.
		Broad-spectrum antimicrobial activity includes MRSA, Vancomycin-resistant *Enterococcus* (VRE) and other antibiotic-resistant bacteria
		Loses its antiseptic properties rapidly after application. Gauze sponges soaked with the antiseptic applied once a day are recommended
		May produce redness, swelling, skin irritation and impaired wound healing with higher concentrations
Silver-containing dressings	Aquacel® Ag	Methylcellulose dressing with ionic silver for superficial dermal burns
		Can be left intact until wound fully healed
		Wound base needs to be clean for dressing adherence
	Silver sulfadiazine	1% cream for deep dermal and full-thickness burns
		Has broad spectrum of activity
		Intermediate eschar penetration
		Has broad spectrum of activity, but minimal activity against *Staphylococcus* species
		Excellent eschar penetration
	Acticoat®	Sheet of thin, flexible rayon/polyester bonded with silver crystal embedded polyethylene mesh
		Can be left on the wound for 3–7 days
		Has broad spectrum of activity
	Silver nitrate	Available as 0.5% solution, applied through a soaked gauze dressing
		Broad antimicrobial spectrum, stains black, makes a flaky crust on unburned skin and has no eschar penetration
		Also used for cauterisation of wounds and removal of granulation tissue
		Over larger areas produces hyponatremia and hypochloremia
	UrgoTul™	Non-adherent petrolatum and hydrocolloid impregnated dressing
		Treatment of partial-thickness burns
		No adherence to the wound, expect pain-free and non-traumatic removal
	Mepilex® Ag	Silicone contact layer and silver-impregnated foam
		Broad-spectrum antimicrobial activity
		Designed to absorb exudate and maintain a moist wound environment. Protects surrounding skin
		Atraumatic removal and minimal pain at dressing change
Ointments	Bacitracin/polymyxin B	Ointment for superficial burns
	Mupirocin	2% ointment for superficial burns
		Activity against MRSA
	Neomycin	Use limited to small burn areas as spray or ophthalmic ointment. Frequently mixed with bacitracin and polymyxin to reduce absorption
		Caution in patients with impaired renal function. It may cause nephrotoxicity and neurotoxicity

(continued overleaf)

Table 125.2 (continued)

Antimicrobials	Agent	Description
Other		
	Biobrane®	Artificial skin substitute bilayer – silicone film with a nylon fabric outer layer and a tri-filament thread with collagen-bound inner layer
		For treatment of superficial dermal burns can be left intact until wound fully healed
		Reduces pain and evaporative losses
	Bismuth-containing petrolatum gauze	Preferred dressing for skin graft donor sites and for covering fresh skin grafts. May use on small superficial partial-thickness burns. Antimicrobial properties
		Applied as a single layer over the burn and then covered with a bulky dressing. Will separate from the wound when it has re-epithelialised. Useful in children
	Medihoney®	Consists of *Leptospermum* honey
		Exerts antimicrobial activity due to a low pH, high osmolarity, presence of phytochemicals, hydrogen peroxide and blocking cell adhesion
		Anti-inflammatory properties, reduces malodour, debrides slough and keeps moisture
	Enzymatic debridement	Collagenase derives from a strain of *Clostridium histolyticum*. Papain derives from papaya and bromelain derives from pineapple
		Effectiveness is questionable. High cost. Relatively slow acting
		Good option in patients who require debridement but are not surgical candidates

MRSA, meticillin-resistant *Staphylococcus aureus*.

use as a wound dressing. However, amnion can be used only as a temporary wound covering, not as a skin transplant. Over the last two decades, an increasing amount of data has accumulated with regard to the use of amnion in burn wound coverage. Some of the benefits of amnion are that it is thin, pliable, adhesive but not prone to sticking and is easily removed. In a recent prospective study of paediatric burns by Branski *et al.* [41], amnion exhibited outstanding wound healing properties and produced excellent long-term cosmetic results. Because amnion is complicated to harvest, process and store, various companies who recognise the potential of amnion have now added it to their repertoire. The most fascinating aspect of amniotic membrane is that it contains stem cells, which can be applied in various ways to create new treatment approaches. These approaches await further evaluation in prospective clinical trials.

Bioengineered approaches have also been tested for use in partial-thickness burns. Examples include keratinocyte-fibrin sealant sprays, fibrin sealant-containing growth factors and cell suspensions. An autologous cell suspension known as ReCell® has gained recent interest. This spray contains autologous keratinocytes, melanocytes, fibroblasts and Langerhans cells that are harvested from a split-thickness biopsy. Small clinical studies indicate that ReCell improves time of wound healing and quality of wound healing. These results led to a prospective randomised multicentre trial comparing ReCell to autologous skin grafting [42,43].

Full-thickness burns

Full-thickness burns will not heal and are treated by excision and coverage with autograft. If autografting is not possible due to a large burn size, allograft or other dermal/epidermal substitutions are required. The scientific and commercial community agrees that harvesting autograft is the gold standard, though this is an ancient approach. Hence, several new approaches have surfaced over the last two decades.

The oldest and best studied dermal substitute is Integra® which was developed by a team led by surgeon John Burke from the Massachusetts General Hospital and by scientist Ioannis V. Yannas from the Massachusetts Institute of Technology [44,45]. Integra is composed of bovine collagen and glucosaminoglycans which allow fibrovascular ingrowth. Various clinical trials have demonstrated that Integra is an effective tool for burn surgeons and results in excellent cosmetic and functional outcomes [46,47]. Another dermal analogue available for the treatment of full-thickness burns is Alloderm®. Alloderm consists of cadaveric dermis devoid of cells and epithelial elements. Its use is very similar to that of other dermal analogues, and it has shown favourable results [48].

After the potential of dermal substitutes became understood, a trend emerged to produce epithelial skin substitutes with or without a dermis. Cultured epithelial autografts (CEA) became a surgical option in the management of patients with massive injuries involving more than 90% TBSA burned. CEAs are created *in vitro* from autologous keratinocytes and, as the name indicates, consist of a pure layer of keratinocytes. The promise of this technique has not been fully realised because of costs and the low quality of the neo-skin [49]; however, it is currently considered a rescue modality for massive burns. A possible improvement over CEA is ReCell. ReCell is sprayed onto the wound, which is usually grafted with widely meshed autograft, and this spray contains an epidermal cell mix that may be superior to CEA. Positive findings from small animal studies and clinical trials need to be confirmed in larger randomised trials [42,43]. A very promising bioengineered approach is the combination of autologous keratinocytes and Integra, known as cultured skin substitute (CSS). Boyce *et al.* first described this method in the 1990s [50–53]. The healing and take were very good, but CSS had several negative features: it had no or spotty pigmentation, it took a long time to produce and was highly expensive. Since then, the group has added melanocytes, shortened the time of production and, with novel manipulation, introduced hair follicle and sweat glands [54,55]. The addition of skin appendages may make this a highly promising tool for the future care of burn patients. Studies are also investigating the possibility of using porcine dermis as a dermal substitute. Porcine dermal matrices are very similar to human dermal matrices. Although they have the disadvantages of xenografts, they represent the first choice among non-human-derived natural biological dermal substitutes and many researchers consider them to be the best substitute for acellular human dermal matrices in the future [56,57]. Currently, there are three acellular porcine dermal matrices on the market: Permacol®, Strattice™ and Xenoderm®, and their efficacy needs to be proven in clinical trials.

Stem cells represent a new hope in the management of burns. These cells play an important role in wound healing, both locally and systemically, and several of the mechanisms underlying their actions in wound healing have been described. In humans, stem cells can be found in adipose tissue, bone marrow, umbilical blood and the blastocystic mass of embryos [58,59]. Stem cells have a multitude of promising features. Given their clonicity and pluripotency, they can be used to regenerate dermis and expedite re-epithelialisation. Another important characteristic of stem cells is their lack of immunogenicity, which would allow them to be transplanted with relative ease [60,61]. Stem cells present in the bone marrow migrate to tissues affected by injury and aid in the healing and regeneration process [59]. Embryonic human stem cells can be differentiated into keratinocytes *in vitro* and stratified into an epithelium that resembles human epidermis [62]. This graft can then be applied to open wounds on burn patients as a temporary skin substitute while autograft or other permanent coverage means become available.

Table 125.3 gives a more conclusive listing of all available skin substitutes for significant burn wounds [7].

Table 125.3 Skin substitutes for full-thickness burns.

Name (manufacturer)	Composition	Advantages	Disadvantages
Epicel® (Genzyme Tissue Repair Corp, Cambridge, MA, USA)	CEA from human keratinocytes embedded in fibrin mesh	Autologous coverage of epidermis	High cost; limited reliability; fragile; increased susceptibility to infections; complex postoperative care; tendency for blistering; poor healing
ReCell® (Avita Medical, Woburn, MA, USA)	Autologous skin suspension produced using minimal donor skin and applied as a cell spray	Induces acceleration re-epithelialisation and wound healing; for wide meshes, most likely to improve appearance of scar	High cost; no dermal substitute; limited to more superficial burns
Myskin® (Regenerys, Cambridge, UK)	Suspended CEA delivered as a spray	Promotes re-epithelialisation	No RCT data
SkinGun™ (RenovaCare, Inc., New York, USA)	Epidermal cells and stem cells	Expansion ratio of skin donor site to treatment surface area of ≈1 : 20	No RCT data
KeraHeal™ (MCTT, Seoul, Korea)	Suspension formed of cultured epithelial cells plus fibrin glue	Facilitates epithelial cell attachment	No RCT data
OASIS® Wound Matrix (Healthpoint Ltd, Fort Worth, TX, USA)	Derived from the submucosal layers of the porcine intestine; contains glycosaminoglycans and growth factors	Dermal element to improve scar appearance	Porcine composition; high cost
MatriDerm® (Skin and Health Care AG, Billerbeck, Germany)	Made of type I collagen fibre coated with 3% α-elastin hydrosylate matrix	Can be used as single-stage procedure with split-thickness skin grafts; very good outcomes in initial clinical trials	Possible increased susceptibility to infections
Biodegradable Temporizing Matrix, BTM (PolyNovo, Melbourne, Australia)	Biodegradable polyurethane foam plus a temporary non-biodegradable polyurethane seal; fully synthetic	Low cost; improves appearance; good results in initial clinical trials	No RCT data
MatriStem™ (Acell, Inc., Columbia, MD, USA)	Composed of extracellular matrix derived from porcine urothelium	Provides barrier protection	No RCT data
Integra® (LifeSciences, Plainsboro, NJ, USA)	Bovine collagen matrix with a silicone layer	Most-studied dermal replacement matrix; improves scarring and skin appearance; used in acute and reconstructive surgery; efficacy shown in RCT	High cost; possible increased susceptibility to infections
AlloDerm™ (Allergan, Coolock, Dublin, Ireland)	Human cadaveric acellular matrix	Improved scarring	High cost
Suprathel® (PolyMedics Innovations GmbH, Denkendorf, Germany)	Synthetic copolymer >70% DL-lactide polymerised with ε-caprolactone and methylenecarbonate	Promising results in initial clinical studies	No RCT data
NovaDerma (Regenicis, New York, USA)	Autologous fibroblasts and keratinocytes embedded with collagen and glycosaminoglycan substrates	Autologous epidermal and dermal skin substitute	No RCT data; limited information
Self-Assembled Skin Substitute (SASS) (Loex, Quebec, Canada)	Reconstruction of a fully autologous bilayered skin substitute	No exogenous scaffold or biomaterial needed; good scar development; autologous	Requires a 31-day production period; very high cost; limited clinical data
Epifix® (MiMedx Group, Marietta, GA, USA)	Composed of dehydrated amniotic and chorionic membrane containing collagen, connective tissue, cytokines and growth factors	Improves wound healing and regeneration	Not a skin substitute *per se*; no RCT data
Cultured Skin Substitute (Cincinnati, OH, USA)	Autologous keratinocytes and fibroblasts from patient biopsy, combined into a bilayer with bovine collagen matrix	Good scarring; epithelial and dermal elements	High cost; long production time; does not include melanocytes

RCT, randomised clinical trial.

Choice of topical dressings

There are various topical agents that are available for the management of burns. Typically, the topical management of deep burns requires an antimicrobial agent to minimise bacterial colonisation and hence infection. For superficial burns, the goal of the topical agent is to reduce environmental factors causing pain and provide the appropriate environment for wound healing. Table 125.2 summarises some of the agents available for the topical treatment of burns; the choice of agent is dependent on their availability and the comfort and knowledge of the caregivers. The choice of burn dressing needs to take into account the following factors:

- The need to eliminate the environmental factors causing pain.
- Acting as a barrier to environmental flora.
- Reducing evaporative losses.
- Absorbing and containing drainage.
- Providing splinting to maintain position and function.

Escharotomy

In the evaluation of wounds, consideration also needs to be given to the possible need for escharotomy. All deep circumferential burns to the extremity have the potential to cause neurovascular compromise and therefore benefit from escharotomy. The typical clinical signs of impaired perfusion in the burned extremity/hand include cool temperature, decreased or absent capillary refill, tense compartments with the hand held in the claw position and, as a late sign, absence of pulses. On occasion, non-circumferential deep burns or circumferential partial-thickness burns might require a prophylactic escharotomy as the patient might require large resuscitation volumes due to overall injury or the inability to perform serial reassessments. Escharotomies of the extremities are performed along the medial and lateral lines, with the extremity held in the anatomical position. For the hand, the escharotomy is performed along the 2nd and 4th metacarpals and for the fingers care is taken to prevent any neurovascular damage; therefore, escharotomies are typically not performed along the ulnar aspect of the thumb or the radial aspect of the index finger.

Operative management

Once the thermally injured patient has been admitted, resuscitated, all wounds assessed and managed appropriately with escharotomy and dressing, the surgeon needs to determine the most efficient course of action in regard to excision of burn and coverage. This needs to be undertaken as soon as the patient is resuscitated, usually within 24–48 h post-injury.

Infection control

Infections remain one of the leading causes of death in burn patients [11]. This is not only the result of loss of the environmental barrier function, but also due to a combination of immunosuppression, inflammation, hypermetabolism and catabolism, all of which contribute to the immune dysfunction of burn patients [2,3]. To improve the morbidity and mortality of burn patients, early diagnosis and treatment are of paramount importance. The pathophysiological progression of burn wound infection runs the spectrum from bacterial wound colonisation to infection to invasive wound infection [63]. The characteristics of each are as follows:

- *Bacterial colonisation:*
  - Bacterial levels of $<10^5$.
  - Does not necessarily prevent wound healing.
- *Bacterial infection:*
  - Bacterial levels $>10^5$.
  - Can result in impaired wound healing and graft failure.
  - Can lead to systemic infection.
- *Invasive wound infection:*
  - Clinically, can have separation of the eschar from the wound bed.
  - Appearance of focal dark brown, black or violaceous discoloration of the wound.
  - Presence of pyocyanin (green pigment) in subcutaneous fat.
  - Erythema, oedema, pain and warmth of the surrounding skin.
  - Associated with signs of systemic infection/sepsis and positive blood cultures.

Not every burn centre uses this differentiation. Some centres believe in qualitative measurements and do not quantitate. In general, the organisms causing burn wound infection/invasion have a chronological appearance with initial Gram-positive organisms, while Gram-negative organisms become predominant 5–7 days post-burn injury. Yeast and fungal colonisation/infection follow, and finally multiresistant organisms appear typically as a result of broad-spectrum antibiotics or inadequate burn excision or patient response to therapy. Recently, burn care providers have had to face not only common pathogens (Table 125.4) but also very uncommon and multidrug-resistant organisms [63].

Clinical management of burn wound infection

Early excision and wound coverage not only remove the inflammatory source but are also the best method of minimising burn wound infection. Any delay in the surgical treatment of burn wounds leads to increased bacterial loads, and any wound with bacterial counts exceeding 10^5 organisms per gram of tissue can develop burn wound sepsis. Beside the burn wound excision, the treatment of burn wound infections involves both local and systemic therapy [2,4,63].

Table 125.4 Common pathogens of burn wound infection.

Organism	Common species
Gram-positive bacteria	*Staphylococcus* and *Streptococcus* spp.
Gram-negative bacteria	*Pseudomonas aeruginosa, Acinetobacter baumannii, Escherichia coli, Klebsiella pneumoniae, Enterobacter cloacae*
Yeast	*Candida* spp.
Fungi	*Aspergillus, Penicillium, Rhizopus, Mucor, Rhizomucor, Fusarium* and *Curvularia* – have greater invasive potential
Virus	*Herpes simplex* virus, cytomegalovirus
Multiresistant bacteria	MRSA, VRE, MDR pseudomonal and *Acinetobacter* spp.

MDR, multidrug-resistant; MRSA, meticillin-resistant *Staphylococcus aureus*; VRE, vancomycin-resistant enterococci.

Table 125.5 Extract of topical agents and the antimicrobial activity.

Agent	Affective against
Silver sulfadiazine	Gram-positives, Gram-negatives, yeast
Mafenide acetate (5%)	Gram-positives, Gram-negatives
Silver nitrate (0.5%)	Gram-positives, Gram-negatives, yeast, fungi
Acetic acid (0.5%, 2%)	Gram-positives, Gram-negatives, *Pseudomonas* at higher concentration
Dakin solution (0.25% or 0.5% sodium hypochlorite)	Gram-positives, Gram-negatives, yeast, fungi
Acticoat®	Gram-positives, Gram-negatives, yeast, fungi, MRSA, VRE

MRSA, meticillin-resistant *Staphylococcus aureus*; VRE, vancomycin-resistant enterococci.

Local/topical
- Early excision of burn wound.
- Aggressive excision of necrotic/infected tissue.
- Bacterial or fungal invasion of viable tissue needs to be treated as a 'cancerous' process and excised from healthy non-infected tissue.
- Topical agents and their antimicrobial targets are shown in Table 125.5; their goal is to minimise bacterial colonisation. The use of any particular topical agent should be based on the suspected organism in the wound but is at times guided by the availability of the agent on the hospital formulary. These are not a substitute for aggressive surgical management of wound infections.

Systemic
- Use of antibiotics and antifungals should be reserved for patients demonstrating systemic signs of severe infection or sepsis, or are profoundly immunosuppressed. Prophylactic administration of antibiotics is controversial; although the use of systemic prophylaxis can reduce rates of surgical wound infection, it can also increase bacterial antimicrobial resistance.
- The choice of antimicrobials needs to be based on each institution's antibiogram and needs to be tailored specifically to the organism.
- Yeast species (e.g. *Candida*) are typically sensitive to fluconazole, while fungal infections would most likely require treatment with amphotericin or caspofungin.
- Viral infections, often herpes simplex virus, cytomegalovirus or HIV, should be treated with aciclovir.

Burn wound infection occurs in 30–40% of all burn patients and represents a common complication. The usual organisms remain *Staphylococcus* and *Pseudomonas*; however, more 'exotic bacteria' and dangerous multidrug-resistant strains are becoming prevalent. The key to improved outcomes of burn wound infection and sepsis is prevention, but if prevention fails early recognition and treatment are paramount.

Central line-associated infections
Central catheters inserted into veins and arteries are common practice in the management of the burn patient and are necessary but are associated with an increased risk of infection and thrombosis. Infection rates have been reported from 1.5% to 20%. Recently, the introduction of central line insertion bundles by the Centers for Disease Control and Prevention (CDC) has significantly reduced these infection rates. The full description of these bundles is available via the CDC. The diagnosis of catheter-related infection (CRI) is based on clinical and microbiological criteria. Following the diagnosis of CRI, prompt treatment is essential as delay in catheter removal or in the start of appropriate antimicrobial therapy can result in increased morbidity and mortality. Currently, there is no clear evidence that routine exchange of lines decreases the rate of catheter-related bloodstream infections (CRBSI); however, all catheters need to be removed once a CRBSI is diagnosed or once they are no longer needed. As already indicated, the CDC also provides guidelines for central line care and replacement.

Ventilator-associated pneumonia
Ventilator-associated pneumonia (VAP), as defined by the CDC, is an infection that occurs in a mechanically ventilated patient with an endotracheal or tracheostomy tube (by definition >48 h after hospital admission). The diagnosis of VAP in burn patients can be challenging, as the symptoms such as fever, leukocytosis, tachycardia and tachypnoea are typically present due to the inflammatory response. The organisms also have a temporal pattern: community-acquired organisms (*Streptococcus pneumoniae* and *Haemophilus influenzae*) are dominant in the early phase of VAP and Gram-negative and multiresistant organisms (i.e. meticillin-resistant *Staphylococcus aureus* (MRSA)) are the common pathogens in late-stage VAP. Regardless of the organisms, early antimicrobial treatment guided towards the likely organism based on the onset of VAP (early versus late) is beneficial in the overall outcome for patients. Broad spectrum antimicrobials would need to be de-escalated as culture and sensitivities become available.

Sepsis
The incidence of burn sepsis has been described at a rate between 8% and 40% with a mortality of 28–65%. Burn care providers recognise the presence of sepsis, but the definition of burn sepsis has been challenging. The ABA criteria for the definition of burn sepsis have been described by an ABA expert panel [6]. However, Mann-Salinas *et al.* have challenged the predictive ability of ABA criteria, demonstrating that their multivariable model (heart rate >130, mean arterial pressure < 60 mmHg, base deficit ≤6 mmol/L, temperature <36°C, use of vasoactive medications and glucose >150 mg/dL) is capable of outperforming the ABA model [64]. Recently, Yan *et al.* [65] compared the ABA definition, Man-Salinas definition and Sepsis-3 definition in terms of sensitivity and specificity. The authors showed that sepsis-3 is the best performing definition even for burn patients and suggested that sepsis-3 should be used. There are new initiatives, however, to adjust and edit the ABA sepsis definition to improve its sensitivity and specificity. As much as the diagnosis of burn sepsis is difficult, the treatment of burn sepsis is very straightforward. Burn sepsis treatment follows the guidelines as recommended by the Surviving Sepsis Campaign committee [66].

Hypermetabolism

A key cause of poor outcomes after burn injury is the hypermetabolic response, which is associated with severe alterations in glucose, lipid and amino acid metabolism [3,7,67,68]. Hypermetabolism leads to vast catabolism that is associated with protein breakdown in muscle and specific organs, leading to multiple organ dysfunction. Therefore, hypermetabolism, organ function and, consequently, survival are likely closely linked with one another. The burn-induced hypermetabolic response is profound, extremely complex and most likely induced by stress and inflammation [3,7,67,68]. The reason for this response is not entirely clear, but persistent elevations in catecholamines, glucocorticoids, glucagon and dopamine secretion are thought to participate in activating cascades that trigger the hypermetabolic response and subsequent catabolism [69,70–76]. In addition, coagulation and complement cascades as well as cytokines, endotoxin, neutrophil-adherence complexes, reactive oxygen species and nitric oxide may modulate the hypermetabolic response [77]. After activation, the pathways upstream of the hypermetabolic response seem to contribute to prolonging hypermetabolism with changes in glucose, lipid and amino acid metabolism [7,67].

Burn-induced changes in metabolism occur in two separate phases [78] (Figure 125.4). The 'ebb phase' usually occurs within 48 h of burn [78,79] and is associated with a reduction in cardiac output, oxygen consumption and metabolism. It is also associated with

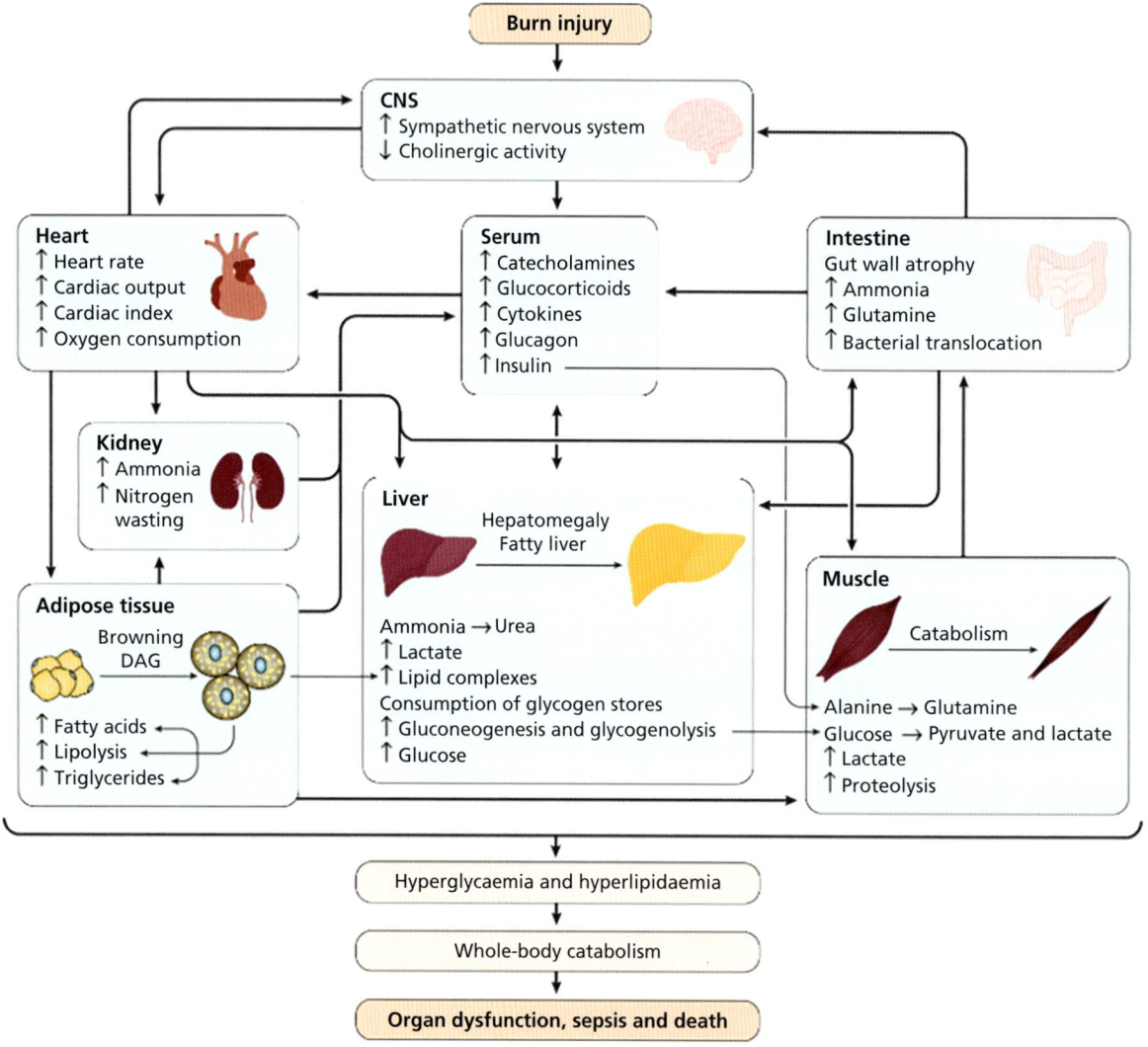

Figure 125.4 Hypermetabolic state in burn injury. Severe burn injury induces a unique and remarkably complex response that involves the release of stress hormones and pro-inflammatory mediators. The immediate response leads to a hypometabolic response that lasts for ≈72–96 hours (ebb phase), but then rapidly turns into the flow phase that can persist for years after the initial injury. Stress mediators, such as catecholamines, glucocorticoids and cytokines, are released into the system and cause a plethora of systemic responses. The heart goes into a hyperdynamic overdrive, increasing circulation and blow flow to increase oxygen and nutrient delivery. However, increased stress signalling causes changes in organ function and metabolic demand. Protein is degraded to deliver energy for hepatic function, and the gut develops mucosal atrophy to absorb more nutrients but also enables bacterial translocation. The kidneys are hyperperfused but oxygen delivery is decreased, leading to acute kidney injury and stress signals from the kidney. The interplay between these organs accumulates, leading to conversion to this metabolic and inflammatory overdrive subsequently causing white adipose tissue change to brown adipose tissue. Brown adipose tissue releases energy and induces substantial lipolysis and with the accompanying appearance of lipotoxic intermediates, such as triglycerides, free fatty acids and diacylglycerols (DAG), all of which are transferred to the liver. The liver is unable to metabolise all of the accumulating substances and develops hepatomegaly. In turn, hyperlipidaemia and hyperglycaemia with insulin resistance are present, which worsen the hypermetabolic and inflammatory state. If hypermetabolism cannot be diminished or decreased this response leads to holistic catabolism and, subsequently, to multiple organ failure and death. CNS, central nervous system. Reproduced from Jeschke et al. [7] with permission from Springer Nature.

diminished glucose tolerance and a hyperglycaemic state. After the ebb phase, the metabolic rate slowly increases within the first 5 days after injury to a plateau or 'flow' phase. This phase is associated with hypermetabolism and hyperdynamic circulation. The flow phase is also associated with insulin resistance (IR) [80,81], as seen by a twofold increase in insulin release in response to glucose load [82,83] and elevated blood glucose levels. In addition, lipolysis is tremendously increased, leading to elevated levels of free fatty acids and triglycerides. These metabolic changes have previously been thought to resolve shortly after wound closure is complete. However, burn-induced hypermetabolism appears to last a much longer time, as seen by a 3-year elevation in energy requirements, catecholamines, urine cortisol and serum cytokines, and impairment in glucose metabolism and insulin sensitivity [7,67,84]. These results underscore the importance of long-term follow-up and treatment of the seriously burned. The hypermetabolic response involves a vast number of pathways; however, two in particular appear to most profoundly affect post-burn outcomes: (i) glucose metabolism with IR and hyperglycaemia [85–87,**88**] and (ii) lipid metabolism with increased lipolysis [**89**,90–92].

Treatment of the hypermetabolic response

Various studies suggest that hypermetabolism is a major contributor to poor outcome post-burn and that treatment or alleviation of the hypermetabolic response is beneficial for patient outcomes. Treatment options include pharmacological and non-pharmacological strategies (Figure 125.5).

Nutrition

The primary goal of nutritional support is to provide an adequate energy supply and the nutrients necessary to maintain organ function and survival. Early adequate enteral nutrition alleviates catabolism and improves outcomes [93]; however, overfeeding in the form of excess calories and/or protein is associated with hyperglycaemia, carbon dioxide retention, fatty infiltration of organs and azotaemia [94]. Therefore, nutrition is an essential component of alleviating hypermetabolism, but too much feeding is detrimental. Consequently, calculating caloric requirements as accurately as possible is imperative. Currently, resting energy requirements of burned patients are commonly estimated using equations that incorporate body mass, age and sex. Although these equations are based on patient-specific factors, caloric requirements still may be significantly overestimated, increasing the risk of overfeeding [95,96]. The adapted Toronto equation seems to be the best formula for calculating resting energy expenditure, as the calculated results very closely match the measured values [97]. In general, adequate nutrition is an essential component of burn care and should be initiated within 12 h after injury [98].

No ideal nutrition or gold standard for burn patients exists. Many experts recommend using high-glucose, high-protein/amino acid and low-fat nutrition with some unsaturated fatty acids [4]. Carbohydrates and amino acids should serve as the chief energy source, sparing protein from oxidation for energy and allowing it to be effectively used by the skin and organs. Supplementation of single amino acids, especially alanine and glutamine, is controversial. After burn injury, glutamine is quickly depleted from serum and muscle [99,100]. However, this depletion mainly occurs intracellularly; effective delivery of glutamine to the cells is very difficult. Small studies in burn patients indicate that glutamine supplementation decreases the incidence of infection, length of stay and mortality [90,100]. Therefore, glutamine supplementation may be beneficial. A multicentre trial (REducing Deaths due to OXidative Stress (REDOXS)) is addressing this question, and the results are expected over the next 4–5 years. The literature on alanine is even sparser, and there are no data related to whether alanine should be administered. Finally, dietary components that have

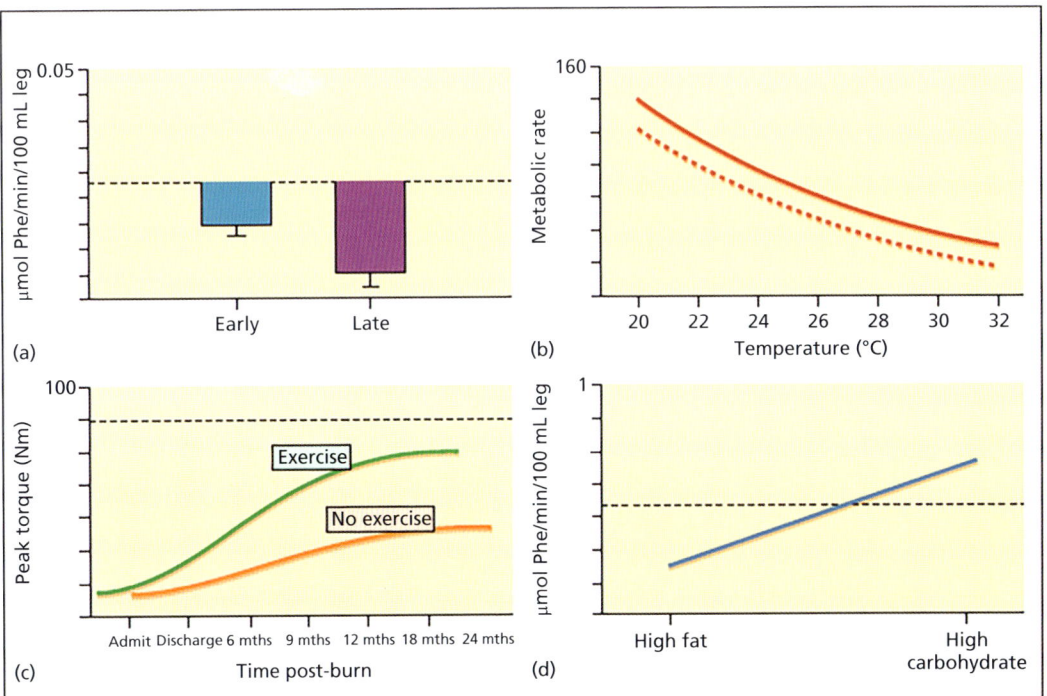

Figure 125.5 Early excision and grafting (a), high ambient temperatures (b), exercise (c) and diet (d) can all alleviate the hypermetabolic response improving post-burn outcomes. LBM, lean body mass; Phe, phenylalanine. Reproduced from Williams FN, Jeschke MG, Chinkes DL, Suman OE, Branski LK, Herndon DN. Modulation of the hypermetabolic response to trauma: temperature, nutrition and drugs. *J Am Coll Surg* 2009 Apr;208(4):489–502; reproduced with permission from *JACS* and Elsevier.

gained more recent attention are vitamins, micronutrients and trace elements [101]. Plasma levels of vitamins and trace elements are significantly depressed for prolonged periods after the acute burn injury due to increased urinary excretion and significant cutaneous losses. Replacement of these micronutrients reduces morbidity in severely burned patients [102–108]. Therefore, a complete daily multivitamin/mineral supplement should be given.

Other non-pharmacological strategies

Of the advances in burn care occurring over the past few decades, early wound excision and closure has been the greatest. It has considerably reduced basal energy expenditure, mortality and costs [3,34–36,109]. Excising burn wounds early and covering the excised areas with temporary cover materials or autologous skin is imperative. This will diminish burn-induced inflammatory and stress responses, in turn decreasing hypermetabolism.

The hypermetabolic response is thought to occur, at least in part, to compensate for dissipation of heat resulting from water loss. Accordingly, the skin and core body temperatures are elevated by 2°C. It is not often realised that increasing ambient room temperature is a simple approach to counteracting this response to burn injury [110]. In fact, a change in temperature from 25°C to 33°C has been shown to reduce resting energy expenditure in seriously burned patients [3].

Providing burn patients with physical therapy is a crucial yet easy intervention that can ameliorate metabolic disruptions and prevent contractures of the burn wound. Progressive resistance exercises have been shown to promote muscle protein synthesis, increase body mass, strengthen muscles and build endurance [95,111]. Resistance exercises are safe for burned children who do not have exercise-related hyperpyrexia [95,111].

Pharmacological modalities

Beside non-pharmacological interventions various pharmacological agents have been used in an attempt to reduce the hypermetabolic response and improve outcomes in burn patients.

Recombinant human growth hormone

Acute administration of recombinant human growth hormone (rhGH) (0.1–0.2 mg/kg/day IM) has been shown to have a host of beneficial effects. It increases donor site healing and quality of wound healing [112], diminishes stress responses and inflammation [113,114], elevates levels of insulin-like growth factor 1 (IGF-1) [115], decreases basal energy expenditure and cardiac output [116] and augments muscle protein and preserves muscle growth [117,118]. Nonetheless, a large multicentre trial showed that morbidity and mortality were higher in critically ill patients taking high doses of rhGH (0.10 ± 0.02 mg/kg) than in patients receiving placebo [119]. Growth hormone treatment has also been linked to hyperglycaemia and IR [120,121]. Despite these findings, rhGH was not found to affect survival in paediatric patients with severe burns when given for a brief or prolonged time [72,122].

Insulin-like growth factor

Given that IGF-1 is an effector of growth factor, it is not surprising that administering IGF-1/binding protein-3 (BP-3) complex (i.e. equimolar amount of recombinant human IGF-1 and IGFBP-3) ameliorates protein metabolism in burned children and adults with fewer episodes of hypoglycaemia than rhGH [123]. IGF-1/BP-3 reduces muscle protein breakdown, ameliorates gut mucosal integrity, improves immune function, attenuates the acute-phase response, elevates constitutive proteins in the serum and decreases inflammatory responses [123–126]. However, unpublished data have revealed that IGF-1/BP-3 increases neuropathies in severely burned patients and it is, therefore, on hold for clinical use. Various studies by other investigators indicate that, when used by itself, IGF-1 alone is ineffective in non-burned critically ill patients.

Oxandrolone

Oxandrolone is structurally similar to testosterone but, for the most part, lacks the virilising effects of this hormone. This anabolic agent has been shown to stimulate muscle protein synthesis [127], reduce weight loss and promote wound healing [128]. Oxandrolone (10 mg, twice daily) has also been shown to decrease hospital stay, morbidity and mortality [49]. When given at a dose of 0.1 mg/kg (BD), oxandrolone decreases hospitalisation, preserves lean body mass, improves body composition and enhances protein synthesis in the liver [129]. The effects of oxandrolone are comparable among patients of all ages [130,131]. Finally, long-term treatment with oxandrolone decreases hypermetabolism and promotes weight gain, with lean body mass and bone mineral content increasing from 6 to 12 months post-burn [132,133]. A recent long-term study in severely burned children found significant benefit for long-term oxandrolone administration over 5 years [134].

Propranolol

Of the anticatabolic therapies for burns, the β-adrenergic blocker, propranolol, is perhaps the most effective [135]. When administered acutely, propranolol exerts anti-inflammatory and antistress effects [136]. In burn patients, propranolol counters loss of skeletal muscle, augments lean body mass [137,**138**] and decreases IR [139]. Long-term propranolol treatment significantly reduces predicted heart rate and resting energy expenditure, decreases accumulation of central mass and central fat, prevents bone loss and improves lean body mass accretion [**140**]. Very few adverse effects were noted with the dose of propranolol used [**140**].

Insulin

Burn patients with stress-induced hyperglycaemia have a greater incidence of bacteraemia/fungaemia, poorer wound healing, more pronounced protein catabolism and lower likelihood of survival than burn patients with adequate glucose control [85,86]. Normalisation of blood glucose levels with insulin is an effective therapy for stress-induced diabetes and coincident IR and hyperglycaemia. Insulin administration also promotes muscle protein production, helps prevent decreases in lean body mass, blocks the acute phase response and speeds wound healing [73,141–147]. In a recent study, patients receiving insulin exhibited better wound healing and organ function than controls [**88**]. These results are in agreement with two other cohort studies demonstrating that insulin administration is beneficial to burn patients [87,148]. The ideal glucose concentration to be targeted in severely burned children is 130 mg/dL, as this concentration falls below 150–160 mg/dL while avoiding detrimental hypoglycaemia [149]. Care must be taken to avoid hypoglycaemia at any cost. In a large paediatric burn population, patients who suffered more than one episode of hypoglycaemia (blood glucose <60 mg/dL) had an almost 5–10-fold greater incidence of morbidity and mortality [150]. Together, the above data show that hyperglycaemia associated with IR is a clinically significant problem in burn patients and that insulin administration improves morbidity and mortality.

Other options

Ongoing trials are investigating other agents for treating post-burn hyperglycaemia. These include glucagon-like peptide-1 (GLP-1), agonists of peroxisome proliferator-activated receptor (PPAR-γ) (e.g. pioglitazone and thioglitazones), and combinations of diabetic medications. In diabetic patients, the PPAR-γ agonist fenofibrate reduces IR. This finding has been confirmed by a blinded placebo-controlled trial, which also showed that fenofibrate increases mitochondrial glucose oxidation, ultimately reducing blood glucose concentrations [151]. Fenofibrate has also been shown to promote insulin receptor signalling, as seen by its ability to stimulate tyrosine phosphorylation of the insulin receptor and its downstream effector, insulin receptor substrate-1, following hyperinsulinaemic–euglycaemic clamp [151]. GLP-1 has been shown to reduce glucose levels in severely burned individuals; however, GLP-1 may not be sufficient to decrease glucose by itself and insulin needs to be given as an adjunct therapy. The biguanide metformin (Glucophage®) suppresses gluconeogenesis and increases peripheral insulin sensitivity, making it a candidate for the treatment of hyperglycaemia associated with severe burns [152,153]. To date, no large randomised controlled trials have been conducted in burn patients; however, two small studies have shown that metformin decreases glucose production, speeds glucose removal and improves muscle protein synthesis/net muscle protein balance [152,154]. Although metformin has clear advantages, it and other biguanides often produce lactic acidosis [155]. Metformin is an interesting agent that may or may not have a place in the treatment of post-burn metabolism.

Summary and conclusions

Burn injury triggers pronounced metabolic changes accompanied by prolonged impairments in glucose metabolism, both of which lead to detrimental outcomes. Progress in diminishing the hypermetabolic response has led to a clinically significant improvement in patient outcomes; however, developing strategies to counteract long-lasting hypermetabolism and associated hyperglycaemia still remain a challenge. Prompt wound excision and closure remains the most important development in burn care over the last 20 years, with this advance considerably reducing basal energy expenditure and increasing survival. Currently, the β-adrenergic blocker propranolol appears to be the most effective pharmacotherapy for countering catabolism in burn patients. Other drugs available for easing burn-induced hypermetabolism include growth hormone, oxandrolone and IGF. Intensive insulin management aimed at maintaining glucose at <130 mg/dL has also lessened morbidity and increased survival in the critically ill, though hypoglycaemia associated with this approach has prompted the search for better substitutes such as metformin and PPAR-γ agonists. Additional studies are needed to identify ideal glucose ranges and determine if the abovementioned agents are safe for the critically ill.

Acknowledgement

This chapter was supported by National Institutes of Health R01-GM087285, the CFI Leader's Opportunity Fund (project no. 25407), CIHR grant no. 123336.

Key references

The full list of references can be found in the online version at https://www.wiley.com/rooksdermatology10e

4 Jeschke MG, Kamolz L, Sjoeberg F, Wolf SE. *Handbook of Burns*, Vol. 1. Vienna, New York: Springer, 2012.
5 Kraft R, Herndon DN, Al-Mousawi AM, Williams FN, Finnerty CC, Jeschke MG. Burn size and survival probability in paediatric patients in modern burn care: a prospective observational cohort study. *Lancet* 2012;379(9820):1013–21.
6 Greenhalgh DG, Saffle JR, Holmes JH *et al.* American Burn Association consensus conference to define sepsis and infection in burns. *J Burn Care Res* 2007;28:776–90.
7 Jeschke MG, van Baar ME, Choudhry MA, Chung KK, Gibran NS, Logsetty S. Burn injury. *Nat Rev Dis Primers* 2020;6:11.
8 Jeschke MG, Chinkes DL, Finnerty CC *et al.* Pathophysiologic response to severe burn injury. *Ann Surg* 2008;248:387–401.
66 Dellinger RP, Levy MM, Rhodes A *et al.* Surviving Sepsis Campaign: international guidelines for management of severe sepsis and septic shock: 2012. *Crit Care Med* 2013;41:580–637.
67 Jeschke MG, Gauglitz GG, Kulp GA *et al.* Long-term persistence of the pathophysiologic response to severe burn injury. *PLOS One* 2011;6:e21245.
69 Hart DW, Wolf SE, Chinkes DL *et al.* Determinants of skeletal muscle catabolism after severe burn. *Ann Surg* 2000;232:455–65.
88 Jeschke MG, Kulp GA, Kraft R *et al.* Intensive insulin therapy in severely burned pediatric patients: a prospective randomized trial. *Am J Respir Crit Care Med* 2010;182:351–9.
89 Barrow RE, Wolfe RR, Dasu MR, Barrow LN, Herndon DN. The use of beta-adrenergic blockade in preventing trauma-induced hepatomegaly. *Ann Surg* 2006;243:115–20.
138 Herndon DN, Hart DW, Wolf SE, Chinkes DL, Wolfe RR. Reversal of catabolism by beta-blockade after severe burns. *N Engl J Med* 2001;345:1223–9.
140 Herndon DN, Rodriguez NA, Diaz EC *et al.* Long-term propranolol use in severely burned pediatric patients: a randomized controlled study. *Ann Surg* 2012;256:402–11.

CHAPTER 126
Cutaneous Photosensitivity Diseases

Sally Ibbotson

Photobiology Unit, Dermatology Department, Ninewells Hospital and Medical School, University of Dundee, Dundee, UK

Introduction, 126.1

IDIOPATHIC (IMMUNOLOGICAL) PHOTODERMATOSES, 126.2
Polymorphic light eruption, 126.2
Juvenile springtime eruption, 126.8
Actinic prurigo, 126.10
Chronic actinic dermatitis, 126.13
Solar urticaria, 126.21
Hydroa vacciniforme, 126.24

DRUG- AND CHEMICAL-INDUCED PHOTOSENSITIVITY, 126.27
Exogenous drug- and chemical-induced photosensitivity, 126.27

PHOTOAGGRAVATED DERMATOSES, 126.32

CLINICAL ASSESSMENT AND MANAGEMENT OF A PATIENT WITH SUSPECTED PHOTOSENSITIVITY, 126.32

History, 126.32
Examination, 126.34
Differential diagnosis, 126.34
Investigation, 126.34
Management, 126.36

Key references, 126.37

Introduction

Cutaneous erythema (skin reddening) develops as a normal response following exposure to ultraviolet radiation (UVR) and this is termed photosensitivity (Figure 126.1). Abnormal photosensitivity occurs when an individual's cutaneous responses to sunlight (UVR and/or visible radiation) fall outside the ranges for healthy subjects. This includes the development of skin reddening at lower doses than those required in the normal population. Abnormal photosensitivity also encompasses cutaneous reactions to sunlight of abnormal morphology, that is, a rash developing during or following sun exposure.

The photosensitivity diseases can be broadly categorised as shown in Box 126.1. The idiopathic (immunological) photodermatoses are the commonest due to the high prevalence of polymorphic light eruption (PLE) [1,2]. The genophotodermatoses are rare (Chapters 75 and 76). Drug and chemical photosensitivity may be due to excess endogenous photoactive chemicals, as in the porphyrias, or photosensitisation by exogenous drugs or chemicals. Photoaggravated diseases are relatively common and are often hard to distinguish from the specific photodermatoses on clinical grounds, emphasising the importance of phototesting.

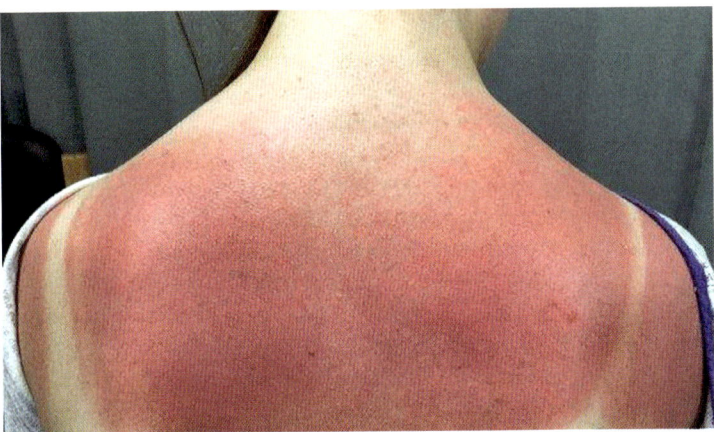

Figure 126.1 Skin reddening (erythema) following acute UV radiation (intense natural sunlight) exposure ('sunburn').

Box 126.1 The cutaneous photosensitivity diseases

- Idiopathic (immunological):
  - Polymorphic light eruption (PLE)
  - Juvenile spring eruption (JSE)
  - Actinic prurigo (AP)
  - Chronic actinic dermatitis (CAD)
  - Solar urticaria (SU)
  - Hydroa vacciniforme (HV)
- Genophotodermatoses (Chapter 76)
- Metabolic (Chapter 61)
- Drug- or chemical-induced photosensitivity:
  - Endogenous – porphyrias (Chapter 58)
  - Exogenous – systemic or topical drug/chemical photosensitivity
- Photoaggravated skin diseases

Rook's Textbook of Dermatology, Tenth Edition. Edited by Christopher Griffiths, Jonathan Barker, Tanya Bleiker, Walayat Hussain and Rosalind Simpson.
© 2024 John Wiley & Sons Ltd. Published 2024 by John Wiley & Sons Ltd.

IDIOPATHIC (IMMUNOLOGICAL) PHOTODERMATOSES

Polymorphic light eruption

Definition and nomenclature
PLE is a recurrent, delayed-onset, abnormal reaction to sunlight (or artificial UVR source) that resolves without scarring. There are several morphological variants [3–8], hence the term 'polymorphic'.

Synonyms and inclusions
- Polymorphous light eruption (PMLE)
- Juvenile springtime eruption: arguably a variant of PLE [9]
- Spring and summer eruption of the elbows: probably a variant of PLE [10]
- Benign summer light eruption: probably a variant of PLE [11–13]
- Taiwanese solar dermatitis: probably a variant of PLE [14]

Introduction and general description
PLE is common and can vary widely in severity and can markedly affect quality of life [15–17,**18**,19–21], and so should not be disregarded. The diagnosis is usually straightforward and based on history. Investigations to exclude alternative or concomitant diagnoses are not usually required [22,23]. Management involves photoprotection and advice on natural hardening, and prophylactic topical or systemic corticosteroid therapy, sometimes also with prophylactic phototherapy. Uncommonly, other immunosuppressive therapy is necessary.

Historically, actinic prurigo was sometimes considered within PLE but is now recognised as a distinct entity [24,25].

Epidemiology
Incidence and prevalence
In many parts of the world PLE is the commonest cause of photosensitivity. Studies have shown high point prevalence (10–20%) in selected northern European and North American populations [2,26–28]. The frequency in a population survey of photodermatoses in China produced lower prevalence figures, although it was still the most common photodermatosis diagnosed [29]. Although it may occur more frequently in places further from the equator, PLE has been reported in many countries, including those near the equator.

Age
It usually starts before 30 years of age, although onset was later in 25% of 545 patients investigated in Dundee [**30**].

Sex
PLE is much commoner in females [31,32].

Ethnicity
PLE is most frequently reported in Northern Europe and North America but has also been described among African, African American [7,33,34,**35**], Chinese and Indian [36] populations in addition to those of western European background.

Associated diseases
Associations with PLE have been described but are probably mainly coincidental. Positive reported associations include the following:
- *Lupus erythematosus (LE: systemic, subacute cutaneous and discoid)*. A questionnaire survey of LE patients in Sweden and Finland found that 49% of respondents might have PLE as well as LE [37]. Another questionnaire survey appeared to corroborate these findings [38]. However, prospective follow-up of 94 PLE patients did not detect an increased risk of developing LE [39]. If PLE patients are at increased risk of developing LE, the risk is small.
- *Actinic prurigo (AP)*. PLE may be more common in AP patients; 35% of AP patients also reported PLE symptoms [40].
- *Photosensitive psoriasis*. There is no evidence that PLE and psoriasis occur together more than would be expected due to chance. However, PLE is the most frequent trigger for photosensitive psoriasis [41].

In one report, the coexistence of hepatitis C and PLE was observed [42], with an apparent beneficial effect of interferon α2a (IFN-α2a) (for hepatitis C) on PLE. However, another case report described an eruption occurring on covered injection sites of IFN-α2a that shared histological features with PLE and developed simultaneously with classic photo-exposed site PLE [43]. Other probably coincidental associations have been reported between PLE and solar urticaria [22,44–47] and, in a separate case, with aquagenic urticaria [48]. Other coexistent conditions have been reported because of unusual localisation of PLE on sites of vitiligo [49] and naevoid telangiectasia [50]. The coexistence of common variable hypogammaglobulinaemia was noted because of an improvement in PLE when the patient was treated with intravenous immunoglobulins [51]. The coexistence of PLE and autoimmune thyroid disease has also been observed, although as both conditions are common a genuine association has not been confirmed [52,53].

Pathophysiology
PLE is believed to be a delayed-type hypersensitivity response to a UV-induced allergen (photoallergen). This is supported by (i) the nature of the lymphocytic infiltrate, which comprises mainly T-helper cells early on but is predominantly T-suppressor cells at 72 h [54], and (ii) the pattern of adhesion molecule expression, which also resembles that of contact dermatitis [55,56].

It is not known what causes PLE, although increasing evidence suggests a multifactorial pathogenesis [16]. It may be an autoimmune disorder, with an abnormal delayed hypersensitivity to an undetermined endogenous molecule. Impaired apoptotic cell clearance may facilitate photo-induced autoantigen development and with impaired UV-induced immunosuppression then enabling the manifestation of PLE lesions [16,57]. Pro-inflammatory cytokines from the interleukin (IL)-1 family (particularly IL-36 α and γ) and IL-31, altered regulatory T cells and dermal dendritic cells, differential antimicrobial peptide expression and IL-15 expression, have also been implicated in the pathogenesis of PLE [58–64], although the pathways and processes involved need further clarification [16,65].

The relative intensity of wavelengths at different latitudes may play a part in determining whether PLE occurs or not, but it is not certain that relatively greater exposure to longer wavelengths at higher latitudes is important in the initiation of the disorder, or whether this just unmasks it. Some investigators have an impression that it begins after particularly intense UVR exposure, such as experienced during sunbathing or sunbed use. Perhaps such exposure leads to autosensitisation [66].

There is evidence that in people with PLE there is less UVR suppression of the induction phase of delayed hypersensitivity responses than in those without PLE [67,68]. This may be the factor predisposing some people to the presumed autosensitisation of PLE as proposed above [16]. This would fit with the fact that people with PLE appear less prone to skin cancer than would be expected due to sunlight avoidance alone [69]; perhaps those who show easier induction of skin antigen recognition after UVR exposure are better immunologically protected against skin cancer but more prone to PLE.

Predisposing factors
The occurrence of PLE is more frequent at higher latitudes. Although not confirmed, there is an impression that previous greater sunlight exposure followed by more intermittent, less intense exposure might predispose to PLE development.

Pathology
In most cases there is a superficial and deep, predominantly perivascular, dermal inflammatory cell infiltrate (Figure 126.2). The cells of this infiltrate are mainly T lymphocytes [70–72], usually CD4+ in early lesions and CD8+ later [54]. Upper dermal oedema is common [73]. It has been suggested that an absence of dermal deposits of acid mucopolysaccharides may help distinguish it from LE [74], but in practice this may not be useful. Some basal liquefaction is not uncommon but is not as marked as in LE. Spongiosis may be found, especially in papulovesicular PLE [75]. Direct immunofluorescence is negative in PLE.

Causative organisms
The previous suggestion that PLE might be triggered by *Chlamydia* has not been substantiated [76].

Genetics
Many patients diagnosed with PLE have close relatives with a similar problem. Percentages with a positive family history have ranged from 12% to 46% [28,77,78]. We would expect at least 10–20% (the same as the general population prevalence) of relatives to have PLE. However, 15% of monozygotic twin pairs compared with 5% of dizygotic twin pairs had PLE [77], helping to confirm an inherited component to the predisposition to PLE [79]. Genetic modelling of abnormal photosensitivity suggestive of PLE, in families of patients with PLE or AP, further confirmed a significant inherited component to the disorder [78].

Environmental factors
UVR and occasionally visible light [80] exposure are important in the manifestation of PLE. There is one report suggesting that in China, PLE occurs more commonly at higher altitudes [29]; however, this study may have included cases of AP, a photodermatosis that is considered to have an altitude association [29]. The contraceptive pill, once considered as possibly relevant [81,82], is not implicated [83,84]. One study indicated that disease may be less severe post menopause, although any causal association has not been proven and this may reflect the natural history of the condition, with an overall tendency to diminish in severity over time [85].

Clinical features
History
The trigger time for PLE induction can be from as little as 10 min of exposure through to several hours of sunlight (or occasionally other UVR source) exposure. Typically, there is then a delay until an intensely itchy photo-exposed site eruption develops. Some, particularly those who only have a significant problem during sunny holidays, describe a 'priming phenomenon' – the need for 2 or 3 days of initial exposure before PLE occurs. The delay after exposure until onset is usually 6 or more hours. Often, the symptoms or rash are not noted until the evening or night after midday sunlight exposure, or not until the following day. However, there is an early-onset PLE variant, with onset as soon as 30 min after first exposure, which may cause diagnostic confusion with solar urticaria.

With subsequent sunlight avoidance, the eruption usually resolves within a few days to 2 weeks of onset. Occasionally, patients describe a longer duration. Reasons for this include (i) unclear history causing confusion between postinflammatory changes and the original rash; (ii) true persistence due to inadequate avoidance measures; and (iii) secondary 'eczematisation', particularly in atopic patients, although the possibility of contact and photocontact reactions to sunscreens should be considered. An unexplained, unusually prolonged rash raises suspicion of LE or AP.

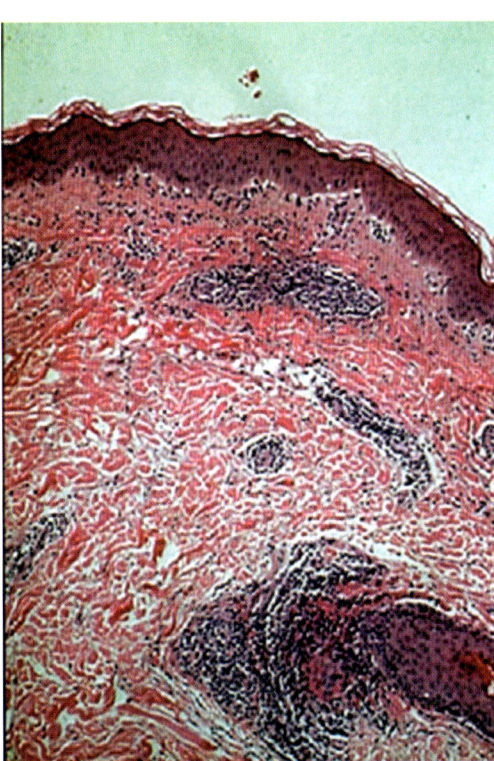

Figure 126.2 Histopathology of polymorphic light eruption showing a superficial and deep, predominantly perivascular, lymphohistiocytic, dermal inflammatory infiltrate.

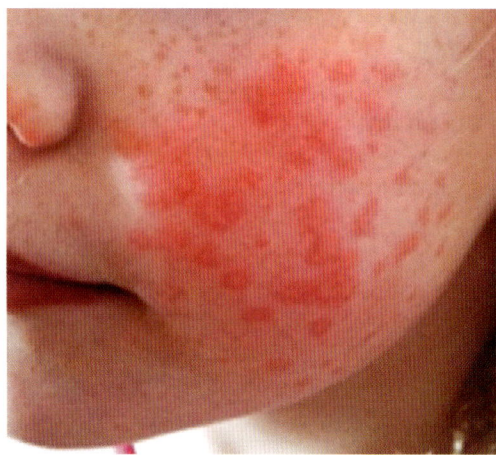

Figure 126.3 Papulovesicular polymorphic light eruption in a child; facial involvement is seen more commonly in children.

Presentation

Affected sites. PLE typically affects only sunlight-exposed sites. The occasional exceptions to this can usually be explained by UV transmission through clothing. Sparing of the face (in 28% of 549 patients in one series) [30] and of the dorsal hands is quite common, and presumably due to tolerance induced by repeated perennial UVR exposure. This is akin to the 'hardening' phenomenon, characterised both by the decline of PLE susceptibility after repeated sunlight exposure, and by the tendency of PLE to be less troublesome towards the end of summer. Facial involvement is more commonly seen in children with PLE (Figure 126.3). Localised forms, such as PLE described at sites of a brachial neuropathy, have also been reported [86]. PLE is generally non-scarring unless secondary excoriation is prominent.

Exposure source. This is usually sunlight, whether direct or transmitted through window-glass or thin clothing. Sunbed irradiation can also be responsible and has been reported as the only trigger in a patient who developed PLE just on a site exposed to pressure while irradiated [87]. If questioned directly about sunbed use (this information is often not volunteered), many patients will describe sunbed-induced episodes. Many use sunbed exposure in the hope this will have a prophylactic effect, and descriptions of this causing the 'worst ever' PLE are frequent. Arc welding and photocopying equipment are occupational irradiation sources that have been reported to provoke PLE [88–90].

Clinical variants

One recent series found the mixed papulovesicular type to be most frequent (Figure 126.4a), closely followed by plaque (Figure 126.4b) and papular/micropapular morphologies (Figure 126.4c); vesiculobullous and erythema multiforme-like variants were uncommon (Figure 126.4d) [35,91]. An insect bite-like PLE variant (strophula), a form without a rash ('sine eruptione' with a typical time course but no visible eruption) and purpuric/haemorrhagic subtypes are rarely reported (Figure 126.4e, f) [3–6,92,93]. It has been suggested that some of these morphological variants, such as papulovesicular [94] or purpuric [92,93] PLE, should be regarded as distinct entities [95]. However, currently, as we do not know if the different subtypes have differing aetiologies, and as the treatment approach is the same it may be best to continue to regard them as variants of one condition. PLE is often said to be monomorphic within individuals – it looks similar each time it occurs. However, some individuals have different morphologies on different sites, for example oedematous plaques on the face and a papulovesicular eruption on the forearms [30]. Severe photosensitivity as part of the clinical features of the PLE spectrum (Polymorphic Light Eruption with Severe Abnormal Phototesting Sensitivity, PLESAPS) is also recognised and these patients may be referred for photodiagnostic investigations as it is important to exclude chronic actinic dermatitis (CAD) [96]. However, the characteristics and time course of the photosensitive eruption and response to UVB desensitisation phototherapy in PLESAPS are more typical of PLE than of CAD.

Differential diagnosis

It is usually straightforward to diagnose PLE. If the suspected PLE starts almost immediately after sunlight exposure, then solar urticaria (idiopathic or secondary to drugs, lupus or porphyria) should be considered in the differential. Cutaneous LE should be excluded if lesions last for more than 3 weeks. Jessner lymphocytic infiltrate may also be a differential but the distinction is usually clear. AP can be distinguished by its typical early age of onset and involvement of the dorsal nose and, frequently, lips and conjunctivae. Occasionally, CAD needs to be considered, such as in the situation of a patient with pre-existing atopic eczema in whom the main differential is between PLE-triggered photoaggravated eczema and CAD.

Classification of severity

The effect on an individual's quality of life is the key issue and will vary according to whether it only occurs occasionally on holidays, or is recurrent throughout the spring and summer months or, uncommonly, may occur on sunny winter days. Various PLE severity scores have been developed for use in clinical trials.

Complications and co-morbidities

Sunscreen allergy and photoallergy can complicate PLE [97–99]. Patients can be reassured that they are not at increased risk of developing skin cancers; in fact, they have a lower skin cancer risk than people without PLE, even when the confounding factor of increased sun avoidance is accounted for [69].

Disease course and prognosis

Follow-up of 94 Finnish patients (by questionnaire, supplemented by repeat clinical assessments of a subgroup) up to a mean of 32 years after onset found 24% to have experienced resolution of PLE, and 51% to have milder disease [39]. A more recent registry study also indicated that PLE usually follows a long-term course, but that symptoms usually improve over time [100]. One report suggested that those with negative provocation tests would be more likely to enter remission than those with positive provocation tests [101]. In view of the differences in provocation test procedures between centres, and the variation in patients referred to different

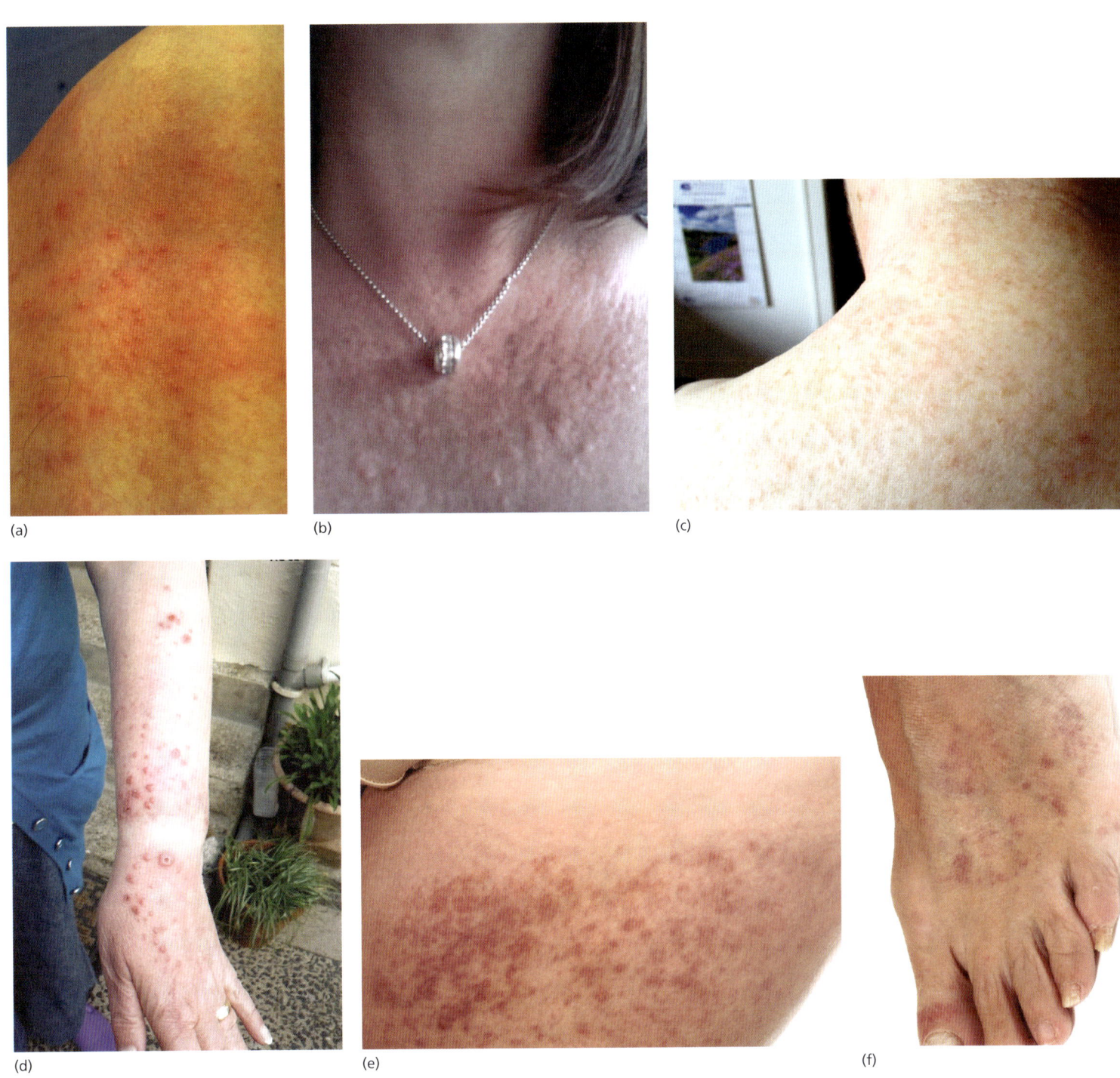

Figure 126.4 Polymorphic light eruption (PLE) subtypes. (a) Mixed papulovesicular PLE in an adult with vesicles predominating. (b) Plaque PLE showing variably sized red papules, which have merged to form plaques (patient's own photograph). (c) Micropapular/papular PLE. (d) Erythema multiforme-like PLE; note sparing under the watch strap. (e, f) Purpuric/haemorrhagic PLE of the anterior thigh, showing sparing at bikini line, and dorsum of the foot; note sparing under the sandal straps.

photodiagnostic units, it will be interesting to see if this finding is replicated. If so, provocation testing might provide valuable prognostic information for newly diagnosed patients. In Dundee, Scotland, a substantial proportion of those with PLE severe enough to require repeated yearly prophylactic phototherapy, after several years, experienced resolution, or marked improvement, so that they could stop attending for treatment [102]. It is not known whether this is spontaneous resolution or a result of repeated treatment courses.

Investigations

Monochromator phototesting. The majority of people with PLE do not need phototesting. Those that do are generally patients with more severe disease or atypical features, thus raising diagnostic doubt and the need for referral to a photodiagnostic centre [1,103]. Most patients have normal minimal erythema doses (MEDs) [30], but moderately reduced thresholds occur to UVA and/or UVB in about one-third of patients tested. In an uncommon subset of patients with PLE, there can be severe abnormal photosensitivity

(PLESAPs) on monochromator phototesting and in these cases it is important to distinguish from CAD [96].

Provocation testing. PLE can occasionally be provoked by irradiating very small areas of skin with a monochromator, or when determining the MED before UVB phototherapy or the minimal phototoxic dose (MPD) before psoralen and UVA (PUVA) treatment. In this setting, a papular response is noted at the threshold erythema dose (and sometimes at a lower dose). However, to provoke it in most patients, larger areas – ranging from a 4–6 cm diameter square field [91] to the whole body [13] – must be irradiated.

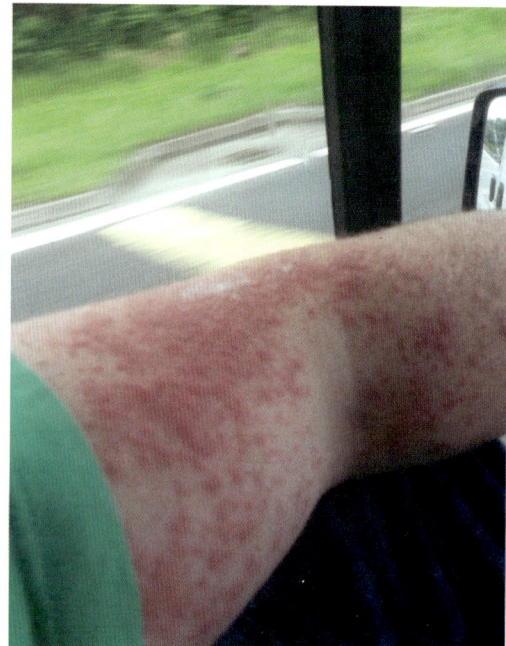

Figure 126.6 Polymorphic light eruption provoked on the extensor forearm by window glass-transmitted light (patient's own photograph).

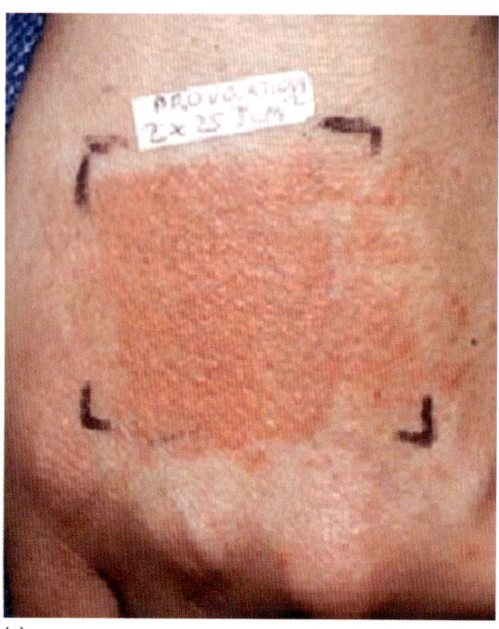

(a)

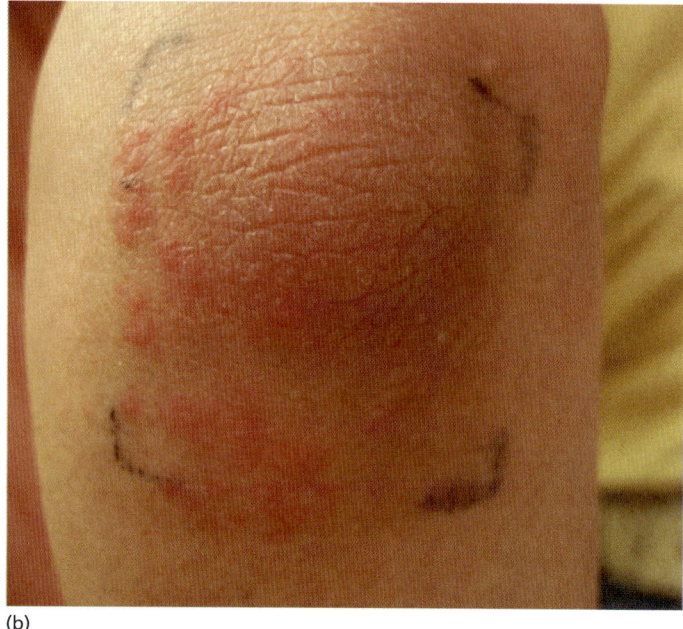

(b)

Figure 126.5 Artificially provoked polymorphic light eruption (PLE). (a) Back of the hand after iterative UVA photoprovocation (2 × 25 J/cm^2). (b) Erythema multiforme-like PLE provoked on the elbow.

Often, iterative testing with repeated daily exposures is required (Figure 126.5) [31,104,105]. Up to four successive daily doses were needed to reach a 90% positive provocation test in one series of PLE patients [106]. High UVA doses, close to the erythema threshold, may be necessary [107–109]. The choice of irradiation site is another factor to be considered: most centres use sites on the arms or legs where the eruption occurs naturally (Figure 126.6) [110]. However, it is possible that testing on sites not usually exposed, and thus not usually affected, may be more useful in providing prognostic information [101], although perhaps less helpful in making the initial diagnosis. In most series UVA has induced PLE (Figure 126.7a) in more patients than UVB, but there is no doubt from localised provocation testing [111], and experience in whole-body UVB treatment, that UVB can also reproduce PLE in many patients (Figure 126.7b) [102,112].

Photopatch testing. This may reveal relevant coexistent contact or photocontact allergy to sunscreen agents [97–99].

Autoantibody screen. Autoantibody screens (antinuclear antibody (ANA), anti-Ro and anti-La) should always be done if phototherapy or PUVA is considered, or if there are atypical features raising suspicion of LE. Unfortunately, ANA screening is not very specific, although reasonably sensitive: in other words, a negative ANA is reassuring, but if positive at a low titre (as it often is in PLE patients) it may be hard to interpret [113]. In general, it is acceptable to disregard a low-titre ANA if unaccompanied by positive anti-Ro or anti-La antibodies and without clinical pointers towards LE (e.g. unusually persistent skin lesions or systemic symptoms). High ANA titres, unless explained, for example by Sjögren syndrome, should usually mean avoidance of phototherapy unless UVA1 treatment, which can also be used in LE, is available [114,115].

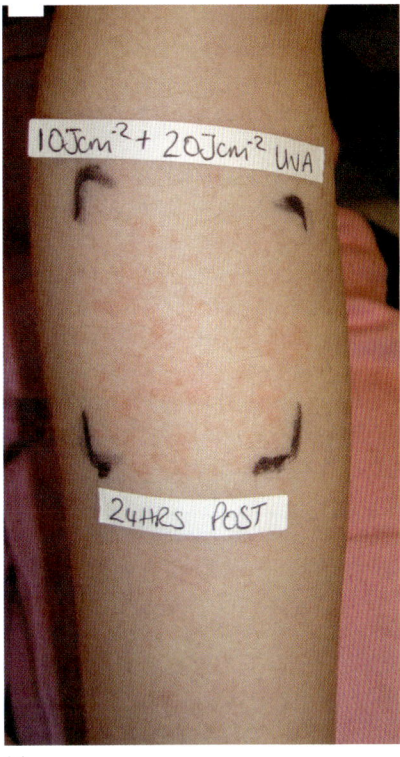 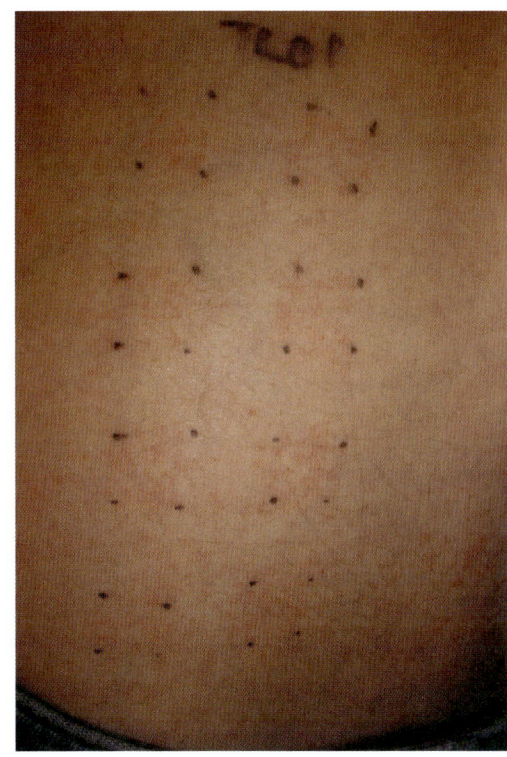

Figure 126.7 Artificially provoked papular polymorphic light eruption. (a) On the extensor forearm (two UVA exposures: 10 and 20 J/cm²). (b) At narrow-band UVB (TL-01) MED test sites.

Porphyrin screen. Occasionally porphyria cutanea tarda (PCT) will be considered in the differential diagnosis for a patient with vesiculobullous PLE, or erythropoietic protoporphyria (EPP) in a patient with early-onset PLE. Plasma spectrofluorimetry screening is quick to perform, so is worth requesting even if the index of suspicion is low.

HLA class II typing. This may be useful if AP is suspected. Based on the determination of likelihood ratios for the presence of AP versus PLE with positive and negative tests we can say, in a UK population (based on summated London and Dundee data) [40,116], that the absence of HLA-DR4 helps to rule out AP (and supports a diagnosis of PLE) whereas the presence of the subtype HLA-DRB1*0407 helps to confirm a diagnosis of AP (rather than PLE).

Histopathology of a skin biopsy. This is usually unnecessary but can help in atypical cases.

Management

Once the diagnosis of PLE has been made and discussed with the patient, management depends on disease severity, the patient's wishes and other factors that influence risk–benefit considerations. In those patients who are only affected a few times each year, such as on holidays, photoprotection – sometimes supplemented by infrequent prophylactic topical or systemic corticosteroid use – usually suffices. Patients may sometimes be able to induce natural 'hardening' or tolerance by repeated low levels of natural sunlight exposure. For those more severely affected, who are repeatedly affected throughout at least the spring and summer months, one of the second line phototherapy approaches is indicated [**102**,103–111,**112**]. For those who remain severely affected despite prophylactic phototherapy/photochemotherapy, systemic immunosuppression is occasionally appropriate.

First line

Sun avoidance and protective measures are sufficient for most mild/moderately affected people. Many who are affected sufficiently severely enough to be referred to a dermatologist require other treatment as well, but sunlight avoidance remains important for all patients. Avoidance of unnecessary environmental exposure, such as intense exposure on holidays in sunny climates, is recommended. However, total avoidance is to be avoided as low-level sub-triggering levels of exposure can help to induce a degree of natural hardening. For some severely affected individuals, advice on the use of UV-absorbing window film on car and house windows is appropriate [117]. Patients should avoid middle of the day sun (11 a.m. to 3 p.m.) and wear appropriate clothing (tightly woven fabrics). Broad-spectrum high SPF sunscreens [118–122] should be used and applied correctly (thickly, evenly and frequently) [123]. Advice should be provided regarding dietary vitamin D intake and supplementation because despite sun avoidance measures, knowledge and awareness of the risks of vitamin D deficiency are often lacking and highlighting this through patient education is important [**124**].

Second line

Prophylactic phototherapy/photochemotherapy is the main second line therapy used. There is randomised, double-blind, controlled trial evidence that narrow-band (TL-01) UVB is as effective as PUVA [**112**], although PUVA is more effective than broad-band UVB [125]. UVA1 therapy can also be used [126], although this phototherapy has also been reported as triggering unusually prolonged

PLE [127]. UVA 'rush hardening' may also be beneficial in some cases [128], although it is a time-intensive regimen for patients and phototherapy services and is not generally required.

Courses given in the spring serve to 'harden' the skin (by tanning and epidermal thickening and/or effects on immune responses) and are beneficial in most patients. No treatment is sufficient to allow unlimited exposure. Nevertheless, it is prudent to limit prophylactic treatment as far as possible, and it is certainly worth considering a trial without 'desensitisation' for those patients who have previously responded [102].

How treatment is given is important. Factors to consider in optimising it include time of year of administration (too early in the year may lead to loss of effect before it can be topped up by natural UVR exposure), whether to treat the whole body or normally exposed sites only, how to deal with PLE provoked during therapy, how many exposures are given, and what advice is given following the course [102,129,130]. A typical regimen would be narrowband UVB three times per week for 5 weeks in springtime [102,129], although the optimal methodology has not been rigorously investigated. In one retrospective study in 15 patients with severe PLE, 88% experienced sustained benefit from desensitisation using narrowband UVB twice a week for a month, so shorter courses may also be effective [131]. PLE is provoked during desensitisation phototherapy in the majority of patients, whereas it will only be provoked in the minority of patients receiving phototherapy for other indications, such as psoriasis [132]. However, use of lower dose increments and topical corticosteroids after each treatment usually enables patients to complete a phototherapy course [102,129].

Prednisolone tablets taken at the first onset of PLE in a population only affected by holiday-type exposure slightly, but significantly, shortened the duration of the eruption [133]. Although not fully supported by published studies, the use of a potent to very potent topical corticosteroid applied daily from the day before to the third day of a holiday can also be helpful for prevention of PLE on holiday [134].

Experimental second line systemic therapies
- β-Carotene has proved disappointing. A randomised crossover trial found 15% of patients to have an 'excellent' response (no skin symptoms despite extensive sun exposure), whereas none had an 'excellent' response during their years when they received placebo capsules [135]. Lesser degrees of improvement were similar regardless of therapy. So, possibly β-carotene has a small effect. However, despite attempts at blinding, as β-carotene changes skin colour this would have been challenging, potentially influencing the reliability of interpretation of these studies. Another controlled study suggested a small beneficial effect [136] but attempts at replication with a larger β-carotene dose failed.
- Controlled trials using antimalarial drugs showed only minimal, if any, benefit [135,137–139].
- A preliminary study using omega-3 polyunsaturated fatty acids from fish oil showed a statistically significant effect [140]. However, it is not known whether reduced PLE provocation experimentally will translate into a clinically useful therapeutic approach.
- Encouraging early studies of *Escherichia coli* filtrate [141–143] and of nicotinamide have not been replicated [142,144] and are not used in clinical practice.
- An extract of the tropical fern *Polypodium leucotomos*, which has antioxidant and anti-inflammatory effects, may, according to uncontrolled studies, be of value [145–147].
- A randomised controlled study suggested that prophylactic application of a vitamin D analogue can have a beneficial effect [148].

Third line
Long-term immunosuppressive drugs, such as azathioprine [149] and ciclosporin [150], have been used for refractory cases.

Juvenile springtime eruption

Definition and nomenclature
This is typically a recurrent blistering eruption affecting the upper pinnae of boys and young men occurring with intense sunlight exposure during spring [1].

> **Synonyms and inclusions**
> - Benign springtime eruption
> - 'Lambing ears'
> - Dermatitis vernalis aurium
> - Spring perniosis

Introduction and general description
This is a characteristic condition which is far more common than is typically recognised. It is usually a nuisance rather than a severe problem and the relationship between this condition and sunlight exposure is normally clear-cut. These factors mean that medical advice is often not sought.

Epidemiology
Juvenile springtime eruption (JSE) appears common, at least among boys and young men exposed to intense sunlight [2–5]. It was found in 12% of a group of school-age New Zealand boys examined in springtime [6]. It has been reported among school children, farmers during the lambing season in spring [7] and military personnel [5,8,9].

Sex
Although it has been reported in females it is typically a condition of males. This may be due to differences in hairstyles between males and females meaning that the upper pinnae of boys and men are more often exposed to intense sunlight.

Ethnicity
It has mainly been reported among those of European ancestry.

Associated diseases
It can occur concomitant with PLE and some categorise it as a variant of PLE.

Pathophysiology
The pathophysiology of the condition is not well defined but considered to be similar to that of PLE.

Predisposing factors
It is more common in males with short hair and prominent ears.

Pathology
A dermal, perivascular, mononuclear cell infiltration is seen on biopsies taken from recent-onset lesions. Later, epidermal ulceration and acanthosis are found.

Causative organisms
It has been reported in outbreaks, such as among military conscripts. However, shared hairstyles and sunlight exposure probably explain these outbreaks rather than there being an infectious aetiology. An association with Parvo-B19 was reported in one case [10]. However, these observations have not been replicated and a causative organism has not been identified.

Genetics
No strong genetic component has been identified.

Environmental factors
JSE eruption seems more common in countries with typically separate seasons rather than similar weather year-round.

Clinical features
History
The typical history is of blisters, sometimes coalescing, but usually unilocular on the upper pinnae, often occurring after a few days of sunlight exposure (Figure 126.8). Pruritus and papules are usually also present.

Presentation
Blisters and papules appear on the upper pinnae.

Differential diagnosis
This may be a variant of PLE. Erythema multiforme [11] can appear similar as, rarely, can erythropoietic protoporphyria, hydroa vacciniforme and bullous LE.

Classification of severity
There is no standard severity scoring scheme. Measures of disease-related quality of life, including the DLQI (dermatology life quality index), have been used.

Complications and co-morbidities
None has been described.

Disease course and prognosis
No good-quality follow-up studies have been reported but JSE, while sometimes recurring over a few years, does appear to spontaneously resolve.

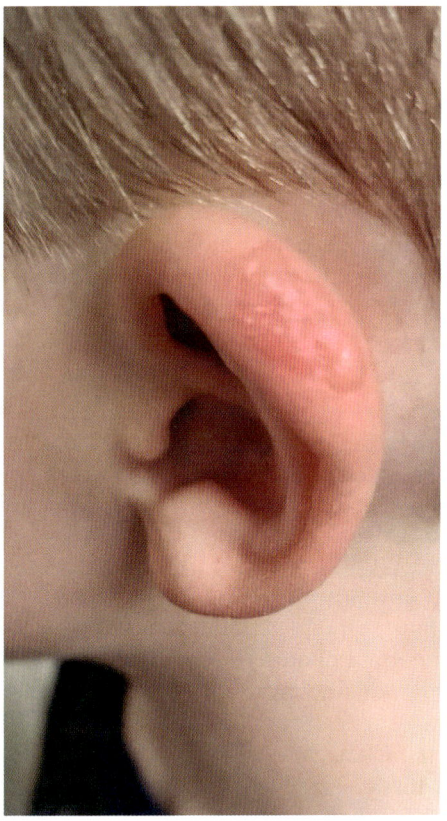

Figure 126.8 Juvenile spring eruption: sunlight-induced blisters on the prominent pinna of a young male.

Investigations
Diagnosis is based on history and examination findings. Rarely, in atypical presentations, the exclusion of other diagnoses such as porphyria or lupus is required. Phototesting is not usually undertaken but, if it is, monochromator responses are typically normal, and iterative UVA provocation testing may be positive [8].

Management
Advice on its benign nature and expected spontaneous resolution can be given. Where possible, depending on occupational requirements, advice to grow hair long enough to cover upper pinnae is usually all that is required.

Treatment ladder

First line
- Sunlight avoidance – best by hair cover

Second line
- Topical broad-spectrum sunscreen
- Desensitisation may be achieved naturally by repeated low-level, less intense sunlight exposure

Third line
- Rarely, prophylactic (desensitisation) phototherapy, usually with narrow-band UVB as administered for PLE, may be appropriate

Actinic prurigo

Definition and nomenclature
Actinic prurigo (AP) is a distinct photodermatosis, diagnosed on the basis of characteristic clinical features including perennial (although typically worse in summer) itchy papules and vesicles during acute flares, persistent eroded nodules and/or dermatitic patches (sometimes affecting covered sites), scarring, dorsal nose involvement and, frequently, cheilitis and conjunctivitis [1,2].

> **Synonyms and inclusions**
> - Hereditary polymorphous light eruption of American Indians
> - Hutchinson's summer prurigo
> - Photodermatitis in North American Indians
> - Hydroa aestivale (this term has also included other photodermatoses)

Introduction and general description
AP is rare in Europe but is common among some populations in the Americas. Abnormal photosensitivity (UVA, UVB) is often severe, but generally gradually improves, especially when (as is usual, at least in Native American and European cases) it presents before the age of 10 years. Classic AP is clinically distinct but there is some overlap in features with severe PLE. In general, it can be managed similarly to PLE. When severe, an additional treatment that may be required is thalidomide.

Epidemiology
Incidence and prevalence
AP ranges in prevalence from about 3 per 100 000 population in Scotland [3] to around 10% of the population among some isolated susceptible populations. AP probably occurs in most parts of the world [3–5,**6**,**7**,8–14].

Age
Most commonly AP starts in childhood.

Sex
AP is commoner in females.

Ethnicity
It is more common among those of Native American ancestry than in other populations [7,8,15,16].

Associated diseases
AP can, like the other photodermatoses, be complicated by sunscreen allergy.

Pathophysiology
UVR exposure is important in AP and the action spectrum for abnormal photosensitivity is usually in the UVB and UVA wavelengths (rarely UVA only). There is a possibility that AP and PLE share pathomechanisms, with some considering AP essentially as a persistent form of PLE in those who are genetically susceptible. The underlying mechanism is considered to be immunological: a delayed hypersensitivity reaction; although as with PLE the chromophore(s) and/or photo-induced antigen(s) are unknown. A lack of Langerhans cell migration after UV irradiation in patients with AP who have abnormal phototesting supports the hypothesis of aberrant UV-induced immunosuppression in AP [15].

Pathology
A dermal, perivascular, mononuclear cell infiltration is seen on biopsies taken from recent-onset lesions. Later, epidermal ulceration, acanthosis and fibrosis occur. Histopathology of cheilitis is said to be characteristic [17], with a follicular pattern of cheilitis predominating [18], although changes elsewhere are not specific to AP.

Genetics
There is strong evidence of a genetic component with inheritance occurring within families. The majority of AP patients have the HLA-DR4 tissue type, which is common in most populations; more than two-thirds of AP patients express the DRB1*0407 subtype, which is usually rare [**6**,19,20,**21**,**22**,23–27]. Other allele associations have been reported, such as an association with HLA DRB1*03:01 in Singaporean Chinese AP patients [4].

Environmental factors
AP is more frequent in populations living at high altitude although there are exceptions such as the high prevalence among Chimila Native American people living near sea level in Columbia [20].

Clinical features
History
AP may begin at any age but most commonly starts in childhood, although late-onset variants have been reported, particularly in Asia [5]. Patients with AP typically present with symptoms in the first decade, have chronic and perennial disease and most affected people are aware of distinct flares related to UVR exposure, usually from sunlight. These features are common to all ethnicities and geographical locations [**6**,**7**,28]. It is commonly very itchy, with early pink papules or small nodules and plaques, and sometimes vesicles, which usually become rapidly excoriated, crusted and scabbed (Figure 126.9), not infrequently with associated 'eczematisation' and subsequent scarring. Ocular symptoms and soreness and inflammation of the lips are also common.

Presentation
The face (including dorsal nose) (Figure 126.10) and distal limbs are most affected, with lesser involvement of more frequently covered sites. The buttocks may be affected in severe cases. There may be hypo- or hyperpigmented resolving lesions and scars (Figure 126.11). There may also be cheilitis and conjunctivitis (Figure 126.10) – these features are considered more common in Native American populations with AP than among those of western European and Asian ancestry [**6**,**7**]. These features are more frequent, and often more severe, in those of indigenous American background.

Clinical variants
Some have considered the Native American form of AP to be distinct from AP in other populations. It is true that the frequency,

Idiopathic (immunological) photodermatoses

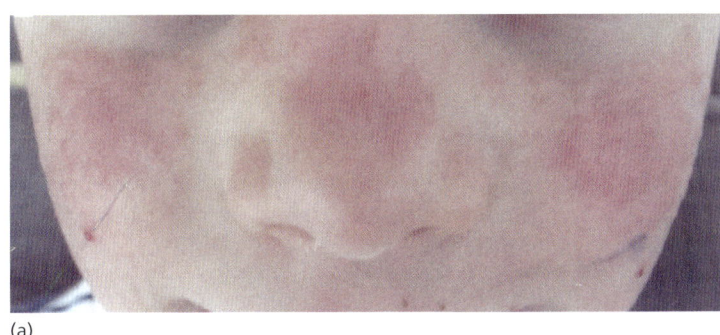
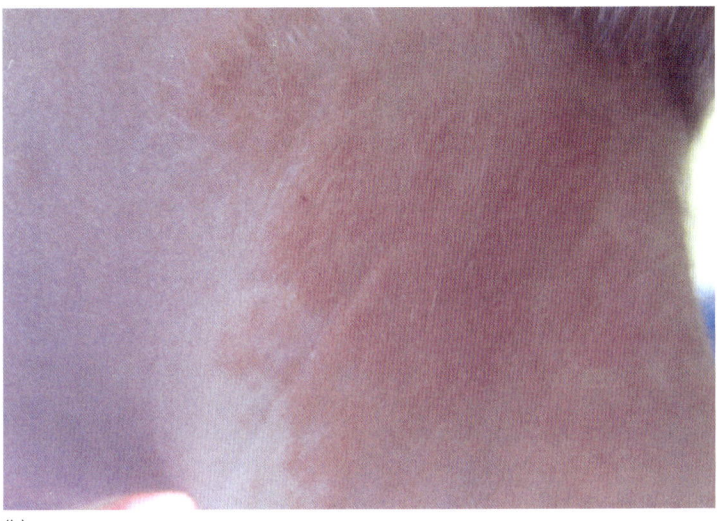
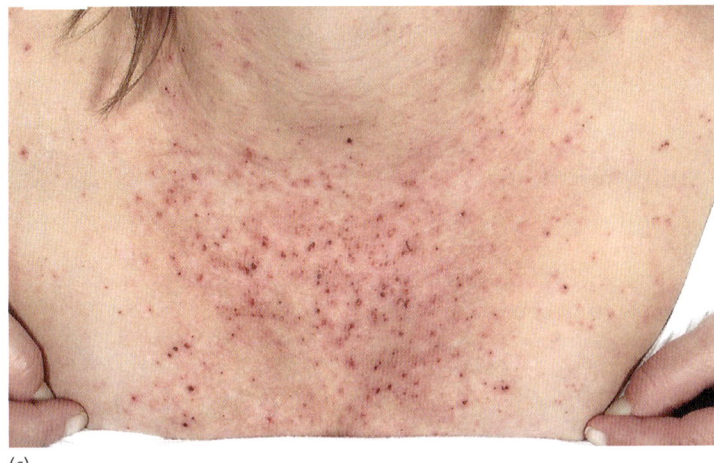

Figure 126.9 Papules and plaques on photo-exposed sites during an acute flare of actinic prurigo (AP). (a) On the cheeks and nose; note distal nose involvement. (b) On the mastoid area of the neck. (a and b are patient's own photographs.) (c) Excoriated papules on a photo-exposed part of the chest in AP.

and probably the severity, of cheilitis and conjunctivitis is greater in Native American populations.

Differential diagnosis

Severe PLE, especially in a patient who also has atopic eczema, can appear similar. Widespread, florid, insect bite reactions may have similar features to early AP. Photoaggravated atopic eczema, nodular prurigo and hydroa vacciniforme should also be considered.

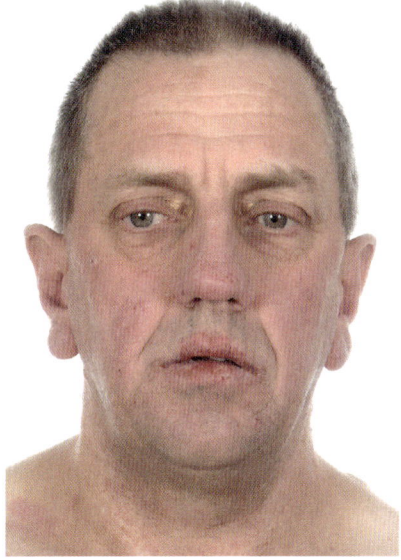
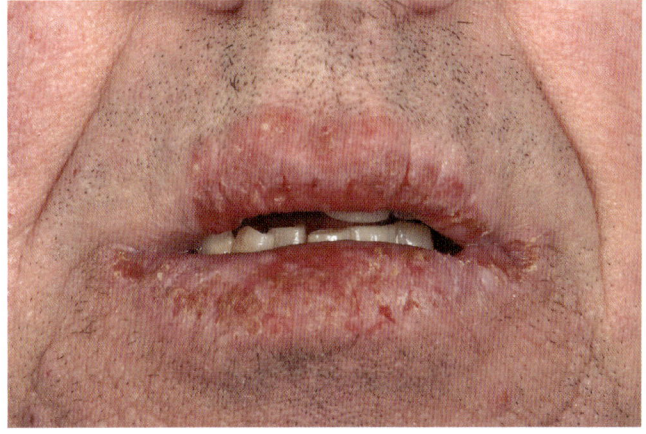
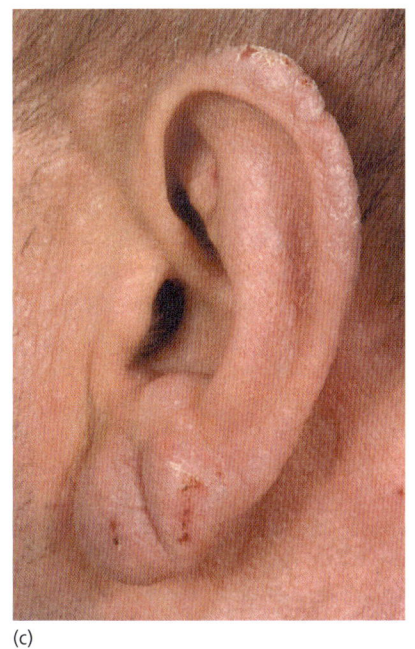

Figure 126.10 Persistent actinic prurigo in an adult. (a) Note inflammation of the lower eyelids, distal nose involvement and cheilitis (with coincidental xanthelasma). (b) Close-up of the cheilitis. (c) Close-up of the photo-exposed sites of the ear.

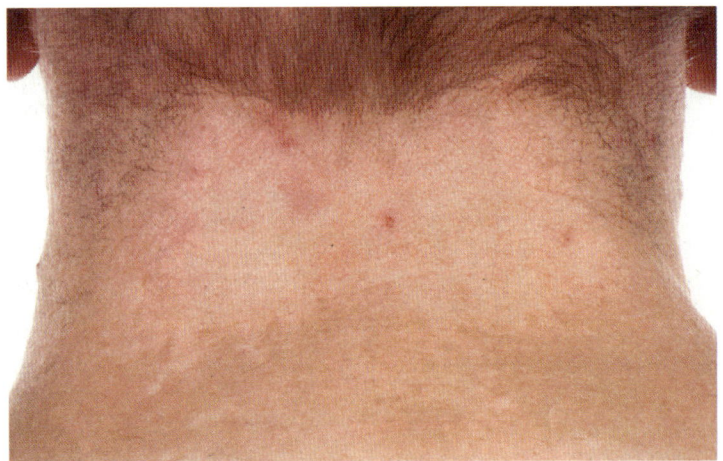

Figure 126.11 Scarring and hypopigmentation on the chronically photo-exposed site of the back of the neck in actinic prurigo.

Classification of severity
There is no standard severity scoring scheme. Measures of disease-related quality of life, including the DLQI, have been used [29].

Complications and co-morbidities
Secondary infection with staphylococci and sometimes streptococci can occur. Scarring may also occur with chronic disease.

Disease course and prognosis
While AP typically spontaneously improves and may resolve by teenage years or early adulthood, the precise proportion among whom this occurs is unknown. Persistence of disease into adult life can also occur and it is advisable to be cautious about prognosis in the early stages of the disease course.

Investigations
Diagnosis is based largely on history, particularly age of onset and distribution, with a history of dorsal nose involvement often being a helpful clue to the diagnosis. This is supported by examination findings. Monochromator phototesting is important, showing severe abnormal photosensitivity in most cases, sometimes as marked as that typically found in CAD, and with far more prominent abnormal sensitivity than in most patients with PLE (Figure 126.12a). Iterative UVA provocation testing can usually provoke an abnormal papular response (Figure 126.12b). Abnormal photosensitivity may also be evident on narrowband UVB MED testing and on exposure to compact fluorescent lamps (Figure 126.12c, d). HLA typing is not a diagnostic test for AP but can be helpful in cases of doubt. The absence of HLA-DR4 makes AP unlikely whereas the presence of the DRB1*0407 subtype (rare in most populations) is supportive of an AP diagnosis [25]. To help exclude other diseases, which occasionally mimic AP, antinuclear and extractable nuclear antibodies and porphyria biochemical screening are usually indicated. Lesional histopathology can also be helpful [17]. Photoaggravated atopic eczema and nodular prurigo may be distinguished on clinical grounds and insect bites by their shorter time course and asymmetry; phototesting would be normal in these conditions.

The diagnosis of AP may be uncertain early on and may require follow-up of disease evolution.

Management
Once the diagnosis is established, initial treatment consists of advice on sunlight avoidance measures (behavioural, clothing, hats, sunscreen, window film) and the use of potent or very potent topical corticosteroids. The UV-absorbing properties of window film may be reduced due to photodegradation and may, depending upon the construction of the window film, need replacing every 5 years or so [30]. If this approach alone is insufficient, the addition of springtime narrow-band UVB or PUVA therapy may be required; usually only photo-exposed sites need to be treated. Application of a potent topical steroid to the treated areas immediately after each exposure reduces the risk of disease flares. Vitamin D supplements are commonly required.

In Scotland, systemic treatment is uncommonly needed. Systemic treatment is more often necessary where the availability of phototherapy is limited and in countries with more intense year-round sunlight exposure. Antimalarials and β-carotene are sometimes tried but are of uncertain value. Thalidomide may be more useful, but its use is restricted by teratogenicity and the risk of irreversible peripheral neuropathy. However, low-dose thalidomide may be more safely used in children with AP than for example in adults with lupus and thus may occasionally be required in severe disease, with appropriate monitoring [31,32]. Pentoxifylline has anti-tumour necrosis factor α (anti-TNF-α) effects and may be worth considering before thalidomide because of its more attractive safety profile. Efficacy of ciclosporin or dupilumab has also been reported in single case reports of children with AP [32,33,**34**].

> **Treatment ladder**
>
> **First line**
> - Sunlight avoidance: environmental, behavioural, clothing, sunscreen, window film [35]
> - Potent/very potent topical corticosteroids [2,36]
> - Narrow-band (TL-01) UVB phototherapy [37]
>
> **Second line**
> - Psoralen–UVA photochemotherapy [38]
> - Thalidomide in those who are not of child-bearing potential [2,**31**,32,39–47]
>
> **Third line**
> - β-carotene [48]
> - Pentoxifylline [49]
> - Tetracycline and vitamin E [50]
> - Oral corticosteroids
> - Azathioprine [51]
> - Chloroquine [**52**]
> - Topical ciclosporin [53,54]
> - Oral ciclosporin [33]
> - Dupilumab [**34**]

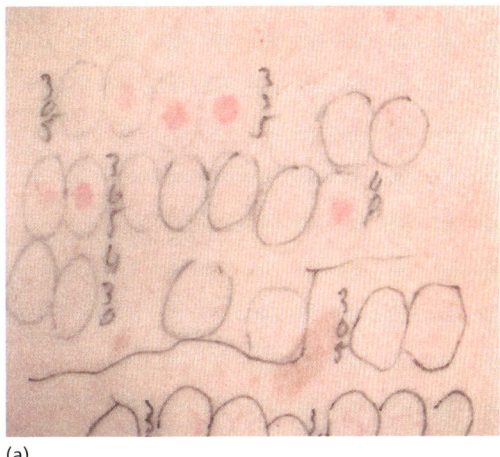
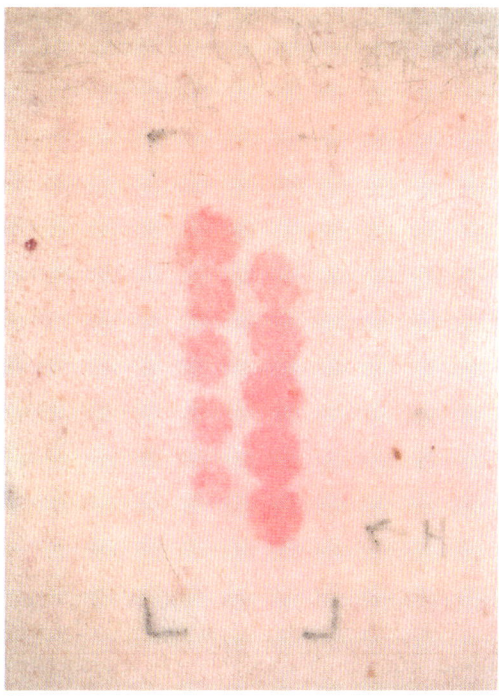
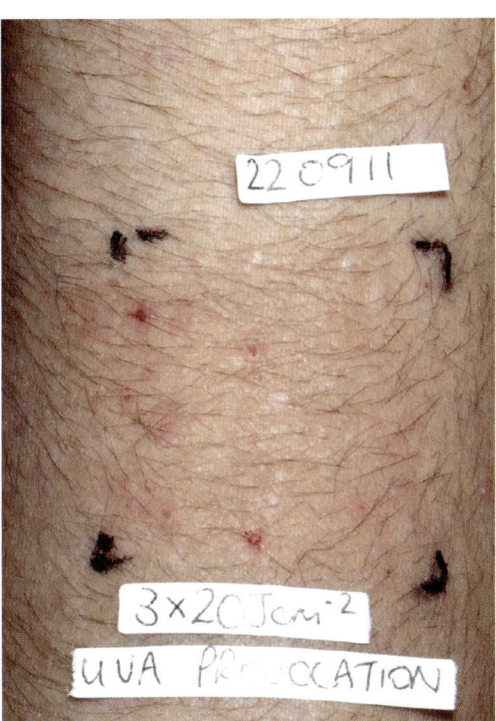
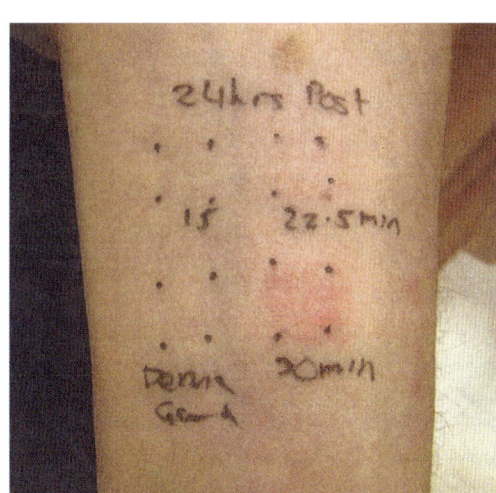

Figure 126.12 Abnormal phototesting in actinic prurigo (AP). (a) Monochromator phototesting showing broad-band UVB and UVA photosensitivity. (b) A positive UVA photoprovocation site on the forearm in AP. (c) Abnormal UVB photosensitivity confirmed by erythema at all narrow-band UVB (TL-01) MED test sites. (d) Abnormal erythema at sites exposed to a compact fluorescent lamp. Note that the site irradiated through Dermagard film (which blocks all UV transmission) is negative.

Chronic actinic dermatitis

Definition and nomenclature
CAD is a chronic dermatitis mainly affecting photo-exposed sites, in association with abnormal photosensitivity. The clinical picture and phototesting abnormalities of dermatitis morphology are required for the diagnosis.

Synonyms and inclusions
- Actinic reticuloid
- Photosensitive eczema
- Photosensitivity dermatitis/actinic reticuloid
- Persistent light reaction

Introduction and general description
CAD is a persistent or recurring dermatitis predominantly affecting photo-exposed sites, in association with objective evidence of photosensitivity. The photosensitivity is usually to broad-band, predominantly UVB, wavelengths [1,2]. The term CAD [3,4] encompasses four previously reported diagnoses: (i) actinic reticuloid, which described the pseudolymphomatous infiltrative changes seen in patients with broad-band photosensitivity [5]; (ii) photosensitive eczema, which described patients with a photo-exposed site dermatitis [6] and UVB photosensitivity; (iii) photosensitivity dermatitis/actinic reticuloid, which was the term applied to patients with features of both photo-exposed-site dermatitis and actinic reticuloid in association with broad-band photosensitivity [7]; and (iv) persistent light reactors, who were patients with photocontact allergy and positive photopatch tests, usually to halogenated

salicylanilides or musk ambrette, who developed persistent photosensitivity without ongoing exposure to photoallergen [4,8–10]. The consensus view was that these four conditions were all part of the same disease, CAD, supporting the heterogeneous nature of the condition between and within patients [3,4].

Epidemiology
Incidence and prevalence
CAD occurs worldwide, although it is commoner in temperate climates [2,3,7,11–14,15]. Generally, in photodiagnostic units CAD is the second most commonly diagnosed idiopathic (immunological) photodermatosis, after PLE, accounting for 7–17% of patients investigated [13,16–21]. In Tayside, Scotland, CAD occurred in 1 in 2000 of those aged ≥75 years [22]. The estimated overall prevalence is 1–5 per 10 000.

Age
It typically occurs in elderly males [2,3,7,22,23], although onset in younger life and females is observed [15,24–27], usually in association with atopic eczema. Three separate studies in New York/Japan, Melbourne and Dundee showed a mean age at diagnosis of 60–62.7 years [12,13,28].

Sex
Male to female ratios of 2.6–7.1 : 1 are reported [12,13,28], although in CAD arising in those of higher skin phototypes, a female to male ratio of 2 : 1 is reported [15].

Ethnicity
The condition can occur in patients of any skin phototype and in CAD presenting at a younger age, higher skin phototypes are over-represented [7,11–14,15,20,24–27,29].

Associated diseases
CAD is associated with contact and/or photocontact allergy in most patients [30]. It is uncommon to develop CAD in the absence of a pre-existing dermatitis [7]. There may also be a lengthy prodrome of dermatitis before photosensitivity develops. Indeed, in one study of 34 patients with CAD, 23% had a prior history of persistent dermatitis for more than 20 years [7]. The occurrence of CAD in young patients with atopic eczema is increasingly recognised, particularly in patients with skin phototypes IV–VI [15,24–27]. An association with HIV is reported [12,31,32,33–35]. The concurrence of CAD and solar urticaria was seen in three patients, and although this may be coincidental it seems unlikely given the rarity of the two diagnoses [36].

Pathophysiology
The pathophysiological mechanisms underlying CAD are not fully understood, although the condition is considered to have an immunological basis. This is supported by associations with contact/photocontact allergy, atopic eczema, response to immunosuppressive drugs and HIV. A role for photoactive drugs has been considered but not substantiated [3,4,8,9,37,38]. The existence of a prolonged prodrome, such as atopic or allergic eczema, before the development of photosensitivity suggests a requirement for persistent T-cell activation to trigger photosensitivity, although this does not explain its occurrence in some patients in whom it arises *de novo*. Light exposure alone appears to suffice as a trigger, without an identifiable photoallergen/allergen(s). The most plausible hypothesis is of a delayed cell-mediated hypersensitivity reaction to unknown endogenous photo-induced antigen(s), similar to the mechanisms in allergic contact dermatitis [39–44].

There is a paucity of recent studies but early investigations of induced lesional skin demonstrated a predominance of CD8 cytotoxic suppressor T cells, similar to that seen in established allergic contact dermatitis, although in the early stages CD4 helper T cells are increased [40,41,43–46]. Further support for a delayed cell-mediated hypersensitivity mechanism was provided by mediator studies. Upregulation of adhesion molecules (E-selectin, VCAM1, ICAM1) and IL-1, -6 and -8 occurs in both CAD and allergic contact dermatitis [43].

Knowledge of the nature of the antigen/photoantigen(s) is lacking, although photochemical modification of an endogenous protein rendering it antigenic seems plausible [4]. Studies *in vitro* showed that the photoallergen tetrachlorosalicylanilide was able to photo-oxidise histidine and modify the carrier protein albumin, rendering this weakly antigenic [47]. As contact/photocontact allergy is not a prerequisite in CAD, the relevance of these findings *in vivo* remains unclear. Other theories of retained photoallergen [48], altered kynurenic acid metabolism [49] and abnormal handling of oxidative stress [50–54] have not been substantiated, and the role of cutaneous Langerhans cells is not defined [40]. A report of photoreactivity of lactones to thymidine is of interest as it may go some way to explaining the evolution of contact allergy and photosensitivity, but it does not explain CAD arising in the absence of lactone allergy and this requires further study [55]. Antibody-mediated immunity appears normal. While serum total IgE levels can be raised in some cases, this is not a prerequisite and therefore its place in the pathophysiology of CAD is unclear [56,57].

Predisposing factors
Dermatitis of various types is a predisposing factor.

Pathology
The histology of CAD is not specific. Epidermal spongiosis, acanthosis and an upper dermal perivascular lymphohistiocytic infiltrate occur acutely (Figure 126.13a). Epidermal hyperplasia, a deep, dermal, inflammatory infiltrate and increased numbers of perivascular histiocytes and granulomatous changes occur chronically [58]. Mast cells may be observed in early lesions, and eosinophils, plasma cells, atypical large, hyperchromatic, convoluted nuclei and mitoses may be evident, and Langerhans cells can be increased [59]. In the chronic phase, lichenification and pseudolymphomatous (actinic reticuloid) changes can emerge, with epidermotrophism and atypical lymphocytes (Figure 126.13b), which may be difficult to distinguish from mycosis fungoides [5,7]. Atypical circulating cells can occur but distinction from Sézary syndrome can usually be made by immunophenotyping [60–63] and T-cell-receptor rearrangement studies. There are occasional reports of lymphoma occurring in patients with CAD but in a longer-term follow-up study no increased risk of lymphoreticular or other malignancy was

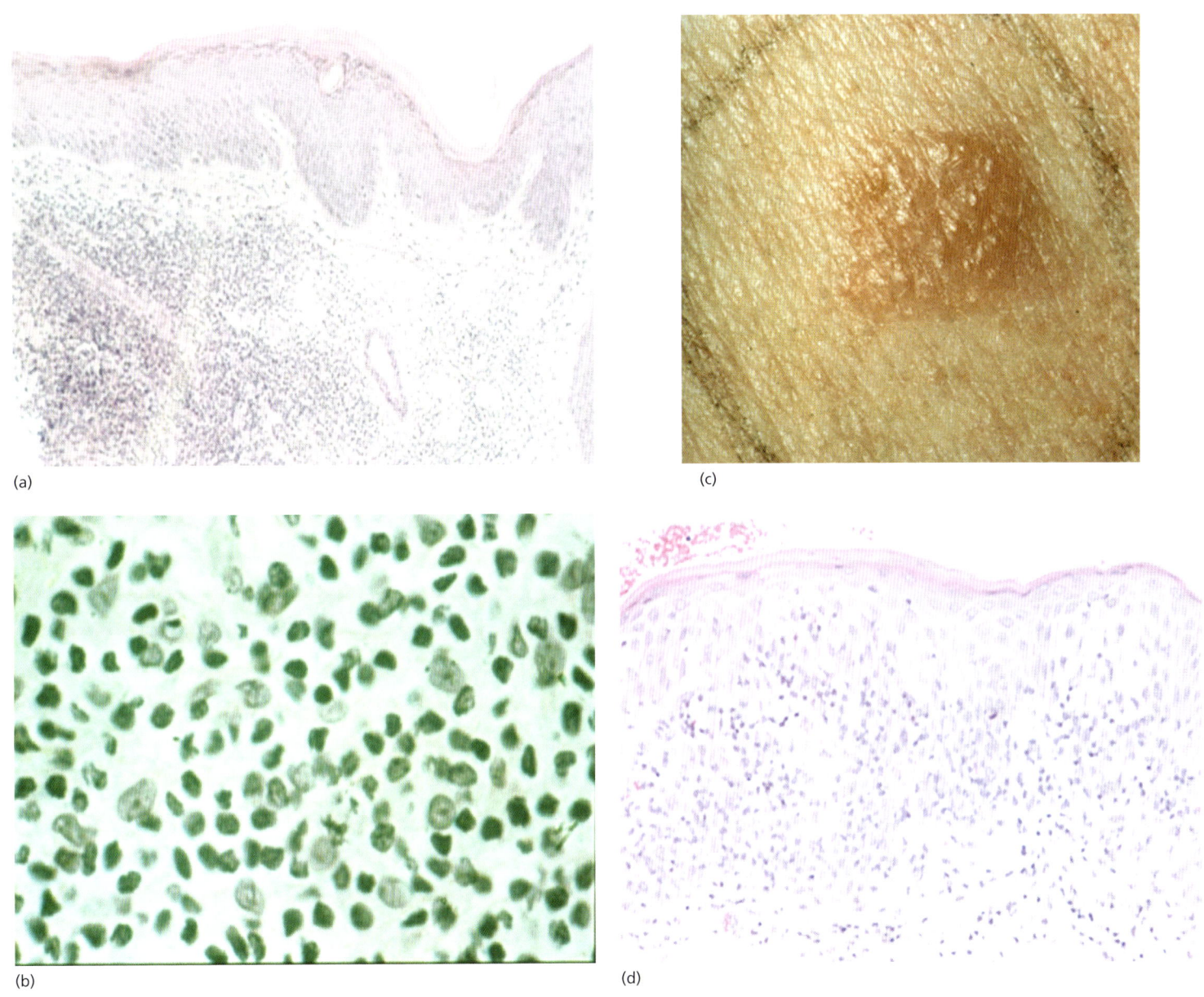

Figure 126.13 Histopathology of chronic actinic dermatitis. (a) Epidermal spongiosis, acanthosis and an upper dermal lymphohistiocytic inflammatory infiltrate (seen in the acute phase). (b) Atypical lymphocytes can be seen chronically with a pseudo-lymphomatous picture. (c, d) An acute spongiotic dermatitis will be seen if an eczematous abnormal phototest site is biopsied.

seen [64,65,66]. If an abnormal eczematous phototest site is biopsied then an acute spongiotic dermatitis will be seen (Figure 126.13c, d).

Genetics
CAD is a sporadic disease and no genetic factors have been identified to date [67]. Differential gene expression in CAD patients compared with controls has been observed, with emphasis on genes involved in inflammation and immunity. However, the clinical relevance of these findings is unclear at present although future work may help identify therapeutic targets [68].

Environmental factors
CAD is more common in patients with multiple contact allergies [7,30]. A recent association between increased incidence of CAD in Korea with climate change, indicated by increased sun exposure hours and air humidity, requires further study [69].

Clinical features
History
The classic features are of a pruritic, recurrent or persistent dermatitis predominantly affecting photo-exposed sites, which is worse in summer (Figure 126.14). Some patients are not aware of the association with sunlight exposure [1,7]. This may be because there is pre-existing dermatitis, for example a patient with atopic eczema who develops a change in pattern of involvement, with the head and neck affected, or a change in season, being worse in summer. It may also occur if there are perennial symptoms because of broad-band photosensitivity, and covered site involvement.

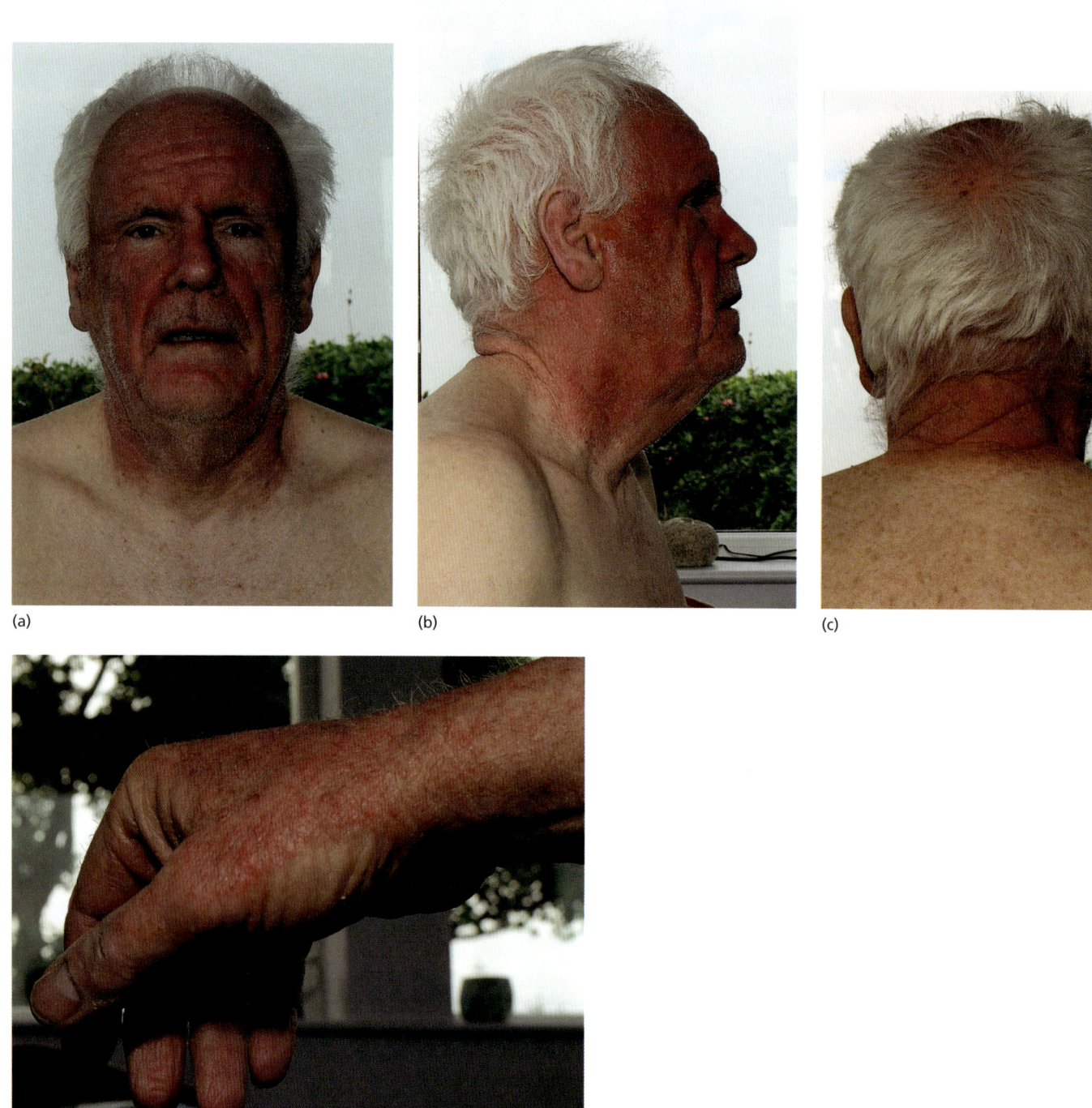

Figure 126.14 Chronic actinic dermatitis presenting with a photo-exposed-site dermatitis. (a, b) Note the prominent head and neck involvement and sharp cut-off at the collar line. There was sparing of the upper eyelids, and under the eyes and in the shaded areas under the lower lip and chin. (c) Involvement of the back of the neck with a cut-off at the collar line. Also note involvement of the bald scalp. (d) Note the prominent involvement of the thenar eminence and extensor surfaces of the hand and the sharp cut-off at photoprotected sites.

Only 21% of patients will have no preceding history of dermatitis. Most patients have a history of atopic, contact allergic, seborrhoeic or endogenous hand eczema, often over many years, and it may be difficult to pinpoint from the history when photosensitivity began [7].

Presentation

Presentation can be diverse, and features may also vary within the same patient. For example, with persistent, uninterrupted inflammation, pseudo-lymphomatous areas [5,7] can develop; these may be the only sites of activity seen in winter, whereas in summer a more

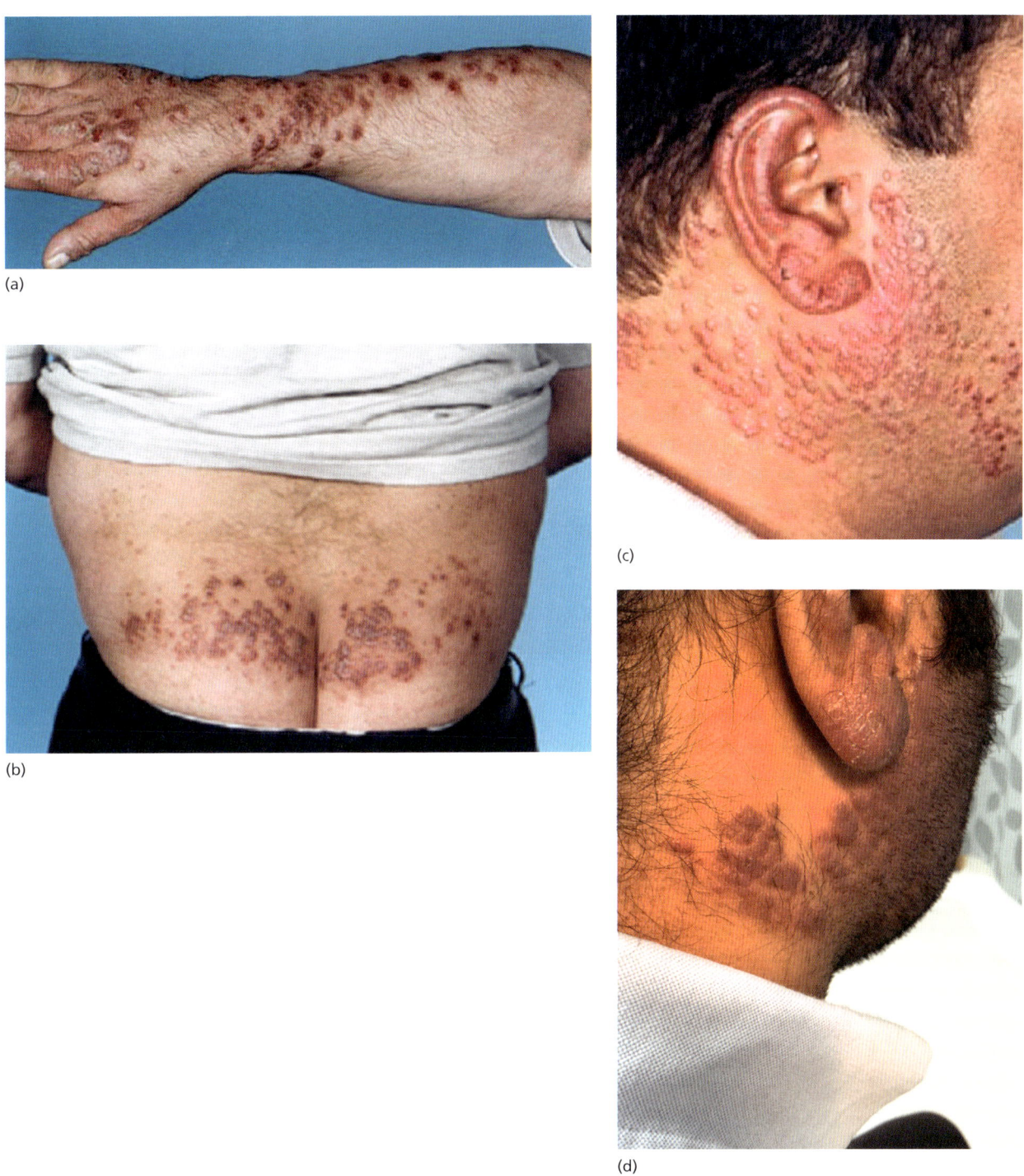

Figure 126.15 In patients of higher skin phototypes (IV–VI) with chronic actinic dermatitis, a nodular prurigo-like morphology may be apparent. (a) Prominent involvement of photo-exposed sites of the extensor forearm. (b) This patient worked as a builder and similar involvement was seen at photo-exposed sites on the lower back between the shirt and trousers. (c) Note the involvement of photo-exposed sites of the ears and side of neck. (d) The relative sparing behind the ear (Wilkinson's triangle should be examined by pulling the ear forward) is clearly seen in this patient of skin phototype V with CAD.

extensive photo-exposed-site dermatitis can occur (Figure 126.14). Acutely, there may be redness, exudation and vesicular dermatitis on photo-exposed sites; chronicity lichenification, pseudo-lymphomatous infiltrative plaques, alopecia, ectropion and hyper-/hypopigmentation (which can appear vitiliginous [70]) can occur. In patients of higher skin phototype (IV–VI) there can be a nodular prurigo-like morphology (Figure 126.15) and lichenoid and pigmentary changes [71]. Examination may show prominent involvement of photo-exposed sites of the head, neck and limbs. The removal of clothes, hats, watches and spectacles is important as a lack of involvement and sharp cut-off at sites of protection may be seen. In one study of 34 patients, 44%

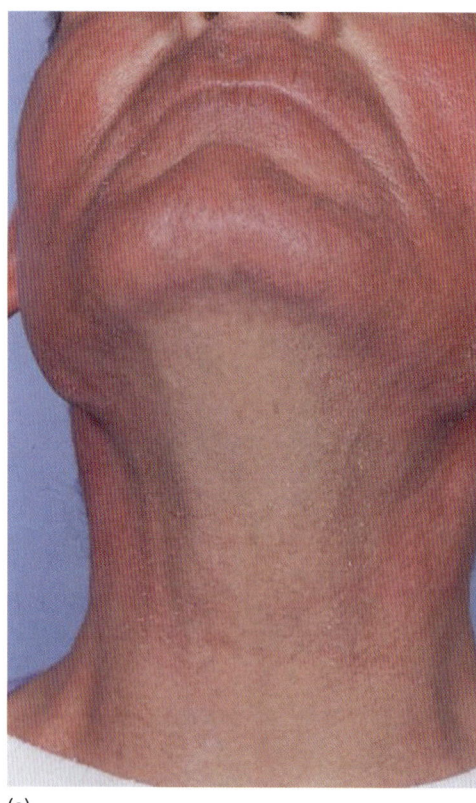
(a)

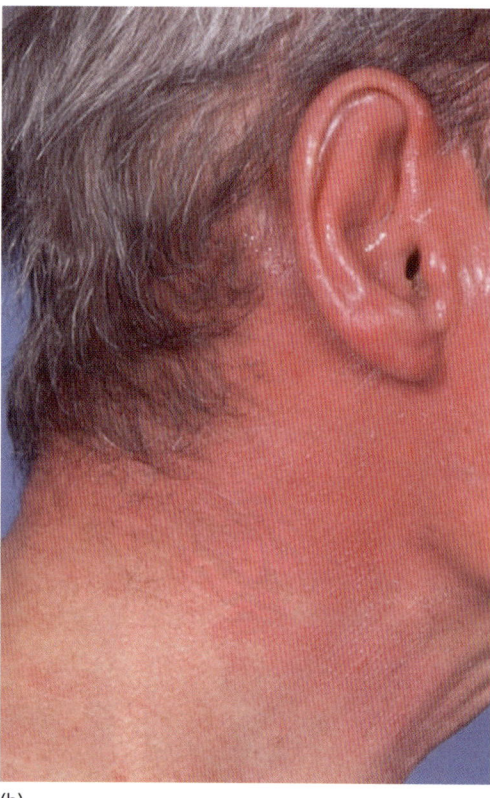
(b)

Figure 126.16 This patient presented with unexplained erythroderma. Slight sparing is seen (a) under the chin and (b) at the collar line and within the scalp. Chronic actinic dermatitis was confirmed by phototesting once the patient had received intensive in-patient treatment of the erythroderma.

presented with covered site involvement and 15% with erythroderma (Figure 126.16) [7]. Patients may also have concurrent palmar and/or plantar dermatitis.

Clinical variants

The morphology of presentation may vary from a typical photosensitive presentation to a more contact allergic dermatitis picture. Pseudo-lymphomatous (actinic reticuloid) [5,7] and nodular prurigo-like changes may occur. CAD can present as an unexplained erythroderma [7].

Classification of severity

There is no specific objective measure of CAD severity and impact, although the DLQI is a useful tool [15,72]. The wavelength dependence and degree of photosensitivity on monochromator phototesting and presence of multiple allergens provide some information on disease severity and prognosis [28]. One study of 51 patients with CAD showed an association between total IgE level and chemokine CCR4 expression and disease severity. An association between total IgE, eosinophil count and a shift to Th2 immunity was also shown in another study of 72 patients with CAD, although as serum IgE is not raised in all cases, the clinical significance of these findings needs further investigation [56,57].

Differential diagnosis

Airborne contact dermatitis typically involves the upper eyelids and under the nose and chin, while the back of the neck is spared. Photoaggravated atopic or seborrhoeic eczema may be impossible to distinguish from CAD on clinical grounds (Figure 126.17).

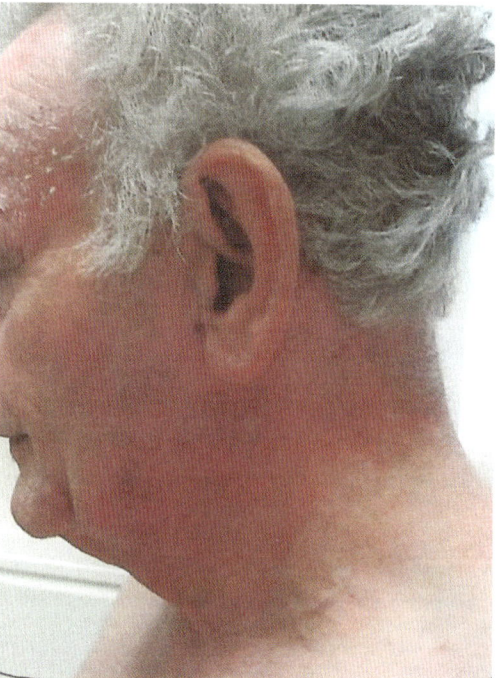

Figure 126.17 This patient presented with a photo-exposed site dermatitis but phototesting was normal and this was photoaggravated seborrhoeic dermatitis (patient's own photograph).

Likewise, drug-induced photosensitivity and cutaneous T-cell lymphoma, the latter especially if there is erythroderma, must be considered [73]. A case of CAD presenting as cutis verticis gyrata has also been documented [74].

Complications and co-morbidities

Most patients have pre-existing or concurrent eczema: endogenous, atopic, seborrhoeic or contact allergic. Sunscreen allergy/photoallergy may occur.

Disease course and prognosis

Once patients receive the diagnosis there is generally symptomatic improvement due to light and allergen avoidance. One retrospective study in Scotland showed that by 5-year follow-up, abnormal photosensitivity had resolved in one in ten patients, rising to one in five at 10 years, and one in two by 15 years [28]. If UVB photosensitivity is severe at diagnosis and there are two or more separate contact allergens there is a poorer prognosis for resolution of photosensitivity [28]. Contact allergies usually, but not always [75], persist [28,76] and it is unclear whether the prognosis is different for patients presenting at a young age [77]. In the absence of erythroderma, life expectancy is normal and there is no evidence of increased risk of lymphoreticular or other malignancies [66,78].

Investigations
Phototesting

Monochromator phototesting to UV and visible wavelengths across the solar spectrum is the investigation of choice (Figure 126.18a) [1,2,22,79–81]. Abnormal erythemal responses (assessed by MED at each waveband tested) will be most apparent 24 h after phototesting and will become dermatitic (Figure 126.18b). Most patients with CAD will have predominant UVB sensitivity, although many will also have UVA and visible wavelengths involved (100% UVB, 88% UVA, 59% at 400 nm, 26% at 500 nm) [7]. Isolated UVA sensitivity has been reported in CAD [13,14] but is rare and, if seen, drug photosensitivity should be suspected [82,83–85]. The action spectrum for the induction of abnormal dermatitis responses in CAD is similar to that of normal erythemal 'sunburn' responses but reactions occur at much lower doses [86].

Monochromator phototesting can only be undertaken if there is sufficient clear skin on the back. If there is limited clear back skin, phototesting using a solar simulator may be undertaken as an initial screen [87]. Provocation testing with broad-band UV sources provides less information on the wavelength dependency of photosensitivity than monochromator phototesting [88]. CAD may also be unexpectedly picked up by MED testing prior to phototherapy [89–91], for example in a patient with suspected photoaggravated atopic eczema (Figure 126.18c). If the MED is abnormally low then CAD should be suspected and monochromator phototesting should be performed (Figure 126.18d). This highlights the importance of routine MED or small area phototesting prior to phototherapy as a safety measure [92].

If a patient has used potent topical corticosteroids on the back in the week prior to phototesting, this may suppress the responses [93] and should be avoided. Likewise, although one study showed no suppression of erythemal responses to monochromator phototesting in healthy volunteers taking 30 mg per day prednisolone [94], a dose as low as 10 mg per day may suppress abnormal phototesting responses in CAD so this should be taken into account [95]. The effect of other systemic immunosuppressants on abnormal phototesting in CAD is not known.

Patch and photopatch testing

Patch testing is an essential investigation in a patient with suspected CAD, and photopatch testing can be helpful when practicable to perform [15,56]. Of 86 patients with CAD, positive patch and/or photopatch tests were seen in 74% and to a diverse range of common allergens (Figure 126.19) [30]. Young patients with CAD also commonly have positive patch tests [15,24–27]. Allergens, often multiple, include fragrances, rubber additives, nickel, colophony, medicaments and sunscreens [30,96]. Plant contact allergy in CAD is also very common, notably to Asteracea (Compositae), lichens and oleoresins [30,97–99]. In one study 36% of patients with CAD had a positive patch test to sesquiterpene lactone [30]. However, this screen can miss significant plant allergy, for example to daisy, dandelion and thistle, which if tested may be positive in up to 23% of CAD patients [100,101]. In addition to Asteraceae being contact allergens, they are also phototoxic, although not photoallergic, so they do not need to be included in photopatch test series [102,103].

Patients with CAD regularly use sunscreens so it is unsurprising that allergic and photoallergic reactions to sunscreens occur [15,56,104,105]. The UV-absorbing sunscreen chemicals such as the benzophenones, dibenzoylmethanes and octycrylene are the most likely culprits but this allergen profile changes with time and exposure patterns [106]. The investigation of choice is photopatch testing [107–111], although this can be difficult or impossible to undertake and interpret in patients with significant photosensitivity, and the relevance of positive results may be unclear. In four separate studies of patients with CAD, positive reactions occurred in 12–33% so photopatch testing should always be considered if there is unexplained deterioration of the condition [12,15,30,104]. There may be a prodrome of contact/photocontact allergy, which lasts for years before photosensitivity develops [112].

In photoaggravated atopic or seborrhoeic eczema, phototesting will be normal (Figure 126.17). In airborne contact allergy or in photocontact allergy, phototesting is normal but patch and/or photopatch testing are positive. In drug-induced photosensitivity there will usually be predominant UVA sensitivity in a patient taking a photoactive drug and the morphology of the eruption is usually not eczematous. In erythrodermic CAD, Sezary syndrome/T-cell lymphoma needs to be excluded and phototesting in the latter, if feasible, is usually normal. Occasionally, a few atypical circulating cells can occur in erythrodermic CAD. If in doubt, T-cell receptor gene rearrangement studies can be undertaken to confirm the polyclonal nature of CAD. Although cutaneous lupus and porphyrias generally do not present confusion clinically with CAD, these should be excluded.

Management

Establishing the diagnosis, excluding drug photosensitivity and defining the action spectrum for abnormal photosensitivity are all paramount [1,2,113]. The impact on day-to-day life must be considered [15,71,114,115]. If a patient is taking a photoactive drug such as thiazide or quinine this should be stopped, if feasible, and phototesting should be repeated 3–6 months later [83–85]. Management involves the prevention of flares and the suppression of active disease [1,2,12]. Careful avoidance of UVR, and when necessary visible light, by photoprotection using behavioural modification, hats,

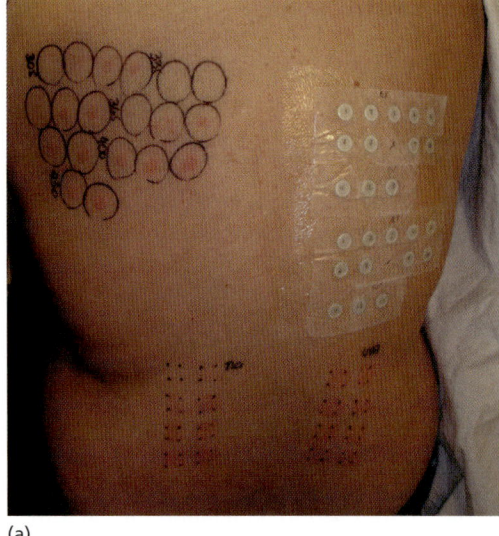
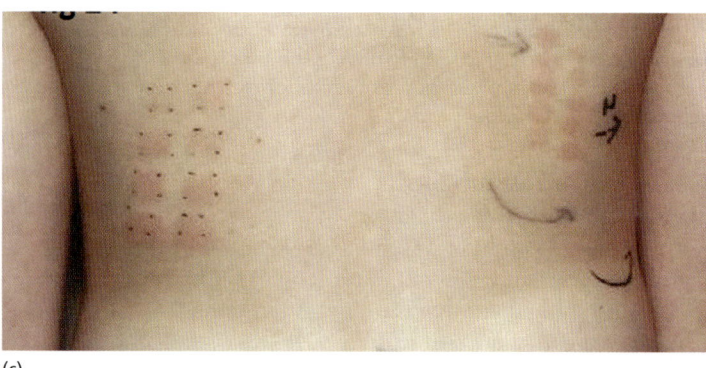
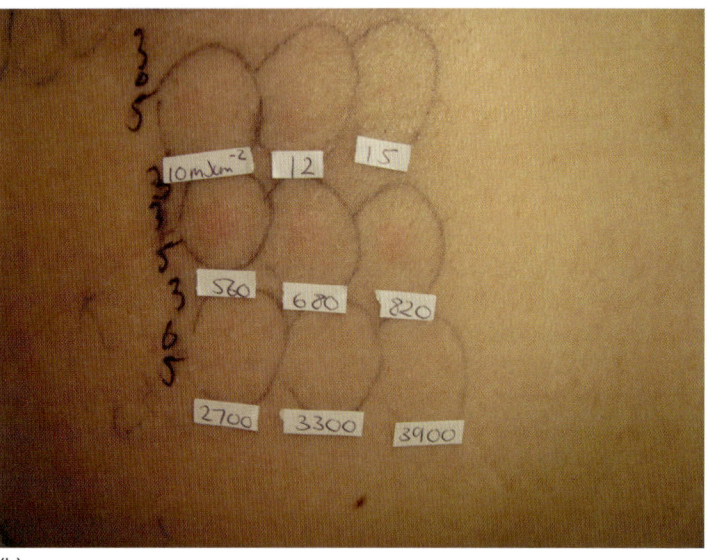
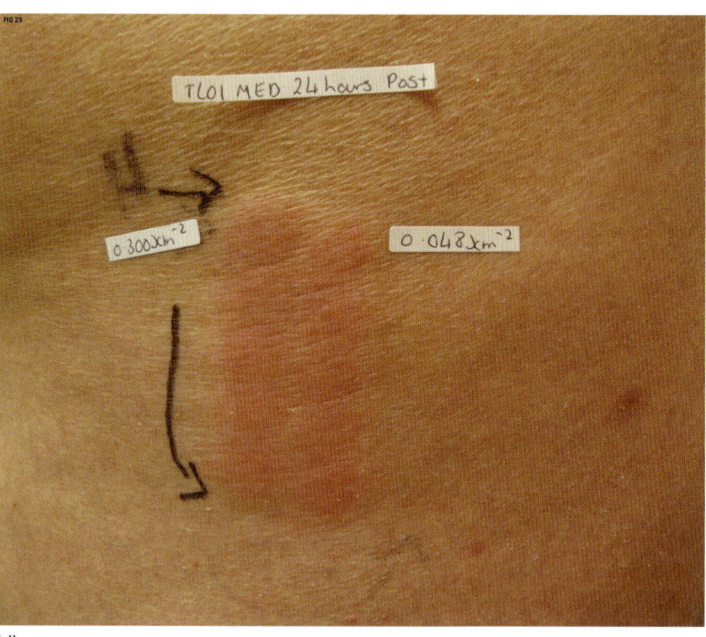

Figure 126.18 Abnormal monochromator phototesting in chronic actinic dermatitis (CAD) showing broad-band UVB, UVA and visible light photosensitivity. (a) This patient with CAD also had abnormally low narrow-band UVB (TL-01) (left side of back) and broad-band UVA (right side of back) MEDs. The patient was also being photopatch tested as part of the investigation, although irradiation and interpretation of photopatch tests are difficult in the presence of severe photosensitivity. (b) Close-up showing the abnormal eczematous morphology at the phototest sites in CAD. (c) CAD in a child with atopic eczema. Abnormal photosensitivity was picked up on MED testing prior to phototherapy for a presumed diagnosis of photoaggravated atopic eczema. Abnormal erythema at narrow-band UVB MED (right of back) and broad-band UVA MED (left of back, as part of photopatch testing) test sites. Phototesting can be undertaken in a child if they are able to sit still and have sufficient back space. (d) This patient was referred for a narrow-band UVB MED prior to phototherapy and abnormal erythema was seen at all test sites. The patient was subsequently diagnosed with CAD after monochromator phototesting confirmed broad-band photosensitivity. MED testing prior to phototherapy is important as a safety measure to detect unsuspected photosensitivity.

clothing [116–118], education and high-factor, broad-spectrum, non-fragranced, low-allergenic sunscreens are fundamentally important [119]. For patients who are abnormally sensitive to visible light, the addition of a large-particle, pigmentary-grade, reflectant sunscreen (e.g. Dundee cream, Tayside Pharmaceuticals) to the broad-spectrum product can provide additional protection [120]. For patients who are UVA sensitive, UV-absorbing window film can be helpful. Watching television [121], using computers and artificial lighting exposure are not a problem for most patients, although the introduction of compact fluorescent lamps, which emit more UV, can pose a risk for severely photosensitive patients, including those with CAD [121–123], and the risk of sources of artificial light exposure should be considered, particularly for those with visible light photosensitivity [124,125]. Allergens and photoallergens must be identified and avoided indefinitely. Patients should also be aware of the need to optimise dietary vitamin D intake and if necessary to take supplements [126,127]. Repeat phototesting at intervals, and if indicated patch/photopatch testing, should be considered in order to ascertain if there are changes in photosensitivity and to identify new allergens/photoallergens.

First line

The treatment of established disease involves the use of very potent/potent topical corticosteroids [1,**2**,12].

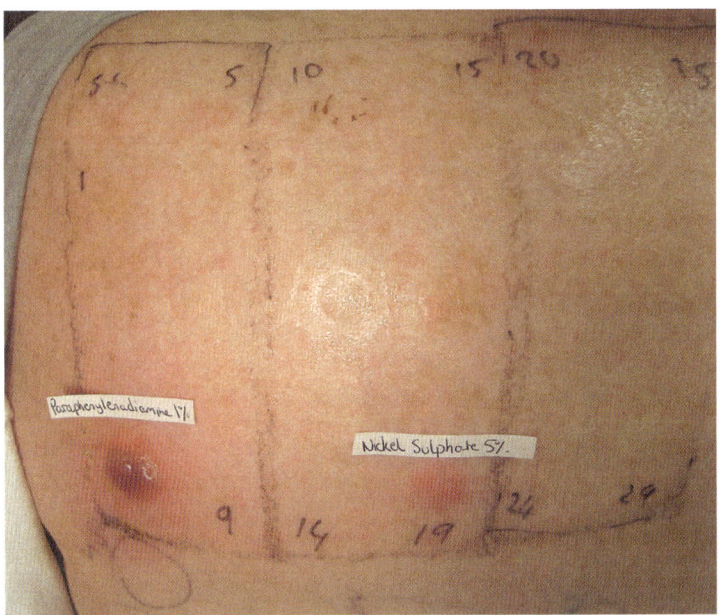

Figure 126.19 Strong positive patch tests in a patient with chronic actinic dermatitis. Patch testing is an essential investigation to undertake in this patient group.

Second line
In some cases, in-patient nursing behind visible- and UV-absorbing window film may be required if feasible [128,129]. Topical tacrolimus or pimecrolimus can be effective [130–135]. If topical measures are inadequate, systemic glucocorticoids may be used in acute flares. PUVA may also be effective if tolerated and systemic glucocorticoid may be required to prevent flares during treatment [**136**,137,140]. UVB phototherapy may be effective [41,138] but is often not feasible because of the degree of UVB photosensitivity, although it may be possible in patients with CAD who are of higher skin phototype [141]. UVA rush hardening may also be considered [142]. Phototherapy or PUVA often requires systemic glucocorticoid cover in the early stages to prevent disease flares [143].

Third line
A randomised placebo-controlled trial showed clinical benefit (not assessed by phototesting) with azathioprine 150 mg/day, which can be used as a steroid-sparing agent, following thiopurine methyltransferase (TPMT) measurement pre-treatment [**144**,145–148]. Hydroxychloroquine [12,145], ciclosporin [12,149–153], mycophenolate mofetil [154,155], hydroxyurea [156], etretinate [12], danazol [157], thioguanine [158], topical nitrogen mustard [159], thalidomide [160,161], infliximab [162], apremilast [163], INF-α [164,165] and colostrum-macrophage-activating factor [166] have been reported to be effective but only in case reports or small case series. The avoidance of combined photo(chemo)therapy and systemic immunosuppressants, particularly ciclosporin, is advised due to photocarcinogenic risk [150,151,167]. Emerging data relating to dupilumab use in CAD indicate that some patients may show a good or partial clinical response, although improvement in photosensitivity of CAD may be less marked, but can be significant, so this drug should be kept in mind for some patients with CAD and concomitant atopic dermatitis [168–173]. Jak inhibitors, such as tofacitinib, may also be therapeutic options but need further evaluation [174,175].

Solar urticaria

Definition and nomenclature
Solar urticaria (SU) can be primary (idiopathic) or secondary to drugs, chemicals, porphyria or lupus. Idiopathic SU is an immunological photodermatosis based on a type 1 immediate hypersensitivity reaction [1] to poorly defined photo-induced antigen(s). It is characterised by the immediate development of urticaria following exposure to UVA, visible and less commonly UVB radiation [2].

> **Synonyms and inclusions**
> - Solar angio-oedema

Introduction and general description
SU is an uncommon immunological photodermatosis, which is usually idiopathic and characterised by urticaria occurring on exposed sites within minutes of exposure to UVR and/or visible light, with resolution occurring within an hour or so [3,4–14,**15**].

Epidemiology
Incidence and prevalence
Idiopathic SU is uncommon, representing 2.2–17.8% of diagnoses made at tertiary photodiagnostic centres, with the lower figures being seen in centres where patients are of higher skin phototype (IV–VI), indicating that this condition may be more commonly diagnosed in lighter-skinned populations [8,9,16–19]. However, there are reports of SU worldwide [20–25,**26**,27]. One study in Scotland estimated the prevalence to be 3.1 per 100 000 of the population [**3**]. Estimated overall prevalence is 1–5 per 10 000. While it has been suggested that there is a trend to increasing prevalence, this is not substantiated [21,28].

Age
SU can occur at any age, with a peak incidence between the third and fifth decades [3,13,20–23,25–27,29–31]. In one case series, five paediatric cases were reported, with onset ranging from 1 month to 2 years of age [24] and disease characteristics and treatment responses were similar to those reported for adults with SU.

Sex
It is more common in females [3,6,13,20–23,**26**].

Ethnicity
It can occur in all ethnic groups, although one study in the USA indicated a difference in relative frequency with racial group, being higher in white people than in black people [**15**,16,20–25,**26**,27].

Associated diseases
SU may coexist with other types of urticaria [32–35] and with other photodermatoses, notably PLE [**15**,36–38], CAD [39] or AP [40]. There does not seem to be an increased prevalence of atopy.

Pathophysiology
Idiopathic SU may, in some cases, be an allergic type 1 hypersensitivity response, mediated at least in part by histamine and

other agents [1,41–45]. The proposed pathway is likely that of photochemical alteration of an endogenous chromophore by UVR and/or visible light, resulting in antigen. This is then recognised by specific IgE on mast cells, with subsequent mast cell degranulation, histamine and other mediator release causing increased vascular permeability and dermal oedema. In secondary SU, the drug or porphyrin presumably acts as the chromophore. Some patients have a detectable circulating factor 'photoallergen'; early studies demonstrated passive transfer of this circulating factor to normal individuals (not done in practice for ethical reasons). The factor behaves like a globulin, with molecular weight 25–1000 kDa. Provocation wavelengths vary between and within patients, indicating that a range of photoallergens activated by UVR and visible light may be implicated. The mechanisms of photoaugmentary and photoinhibitory wavelengths are poorly understood [46,47,48], although recent investigations of augmentation spectra indicate the induction of an urticaria-forming factor, with potential for provocation of severe SU or anaphylaxis in these cases [15,48,49]. Infrared radiation may also exacerbate SU responses [50]. Heterogeneous therapeutic responses between and within patients indicate that several pathways may be involved.

Histamine is implicated since antihistamines are at least partially effective in most cases. However, other mediators in SU are likely to be involved; possible candidates include leukotrienes, platelet-activating factor, substance P, serotonin and acetylcholine. The role of non-histamine mediators is not fully defined. The mechanism of effect for the induction of tolerance using wavelengths that the patient can tolerate, such as narrow-band UVB, is unclear but probably involves immunomodulation (as when using phototherapy for other chronic urticarias), immunosuppression, stratum corneum thickening and pigmentation.

Pathology
Within minutes of irradiation, a cutaneous perivascular infiltrate of neutrophils, eosinophils and mast cells occurs [51]. This is followed by swelling of the endothelial cells of dermal vessels and dermal oedema. Occasionally vasculitic features may be seen. The histology of SU is not significantly different from that of other causes of urticaria and biopsy is only undertaken if there is diagnostic doubt.

Genetics
SU is sporadic and genetic factors have not been identified. However, molecular genetic analysis is planned [25].

Clinical features
History
Onset is typically sudden and clearly recalled. Most (63%) have perennial symptoms due to UVA/visible light photosensitivity. Itch, burning sensation, redness and weals typically occur within seconds to minutes of exposure (Figure 126.20). In the minority, pruritic skin reddening alone may occur (urticarial weals may be elicited on phototesting) [52,53]. Any photo-exposed site can be affected and in most patients (76%) lightly clothed sites can also be involved since loose-weave fabric will not protect against UVA and visible light transmission. Sparing under layered clothes, watches and footwear may occur. Most patients (83%) will also

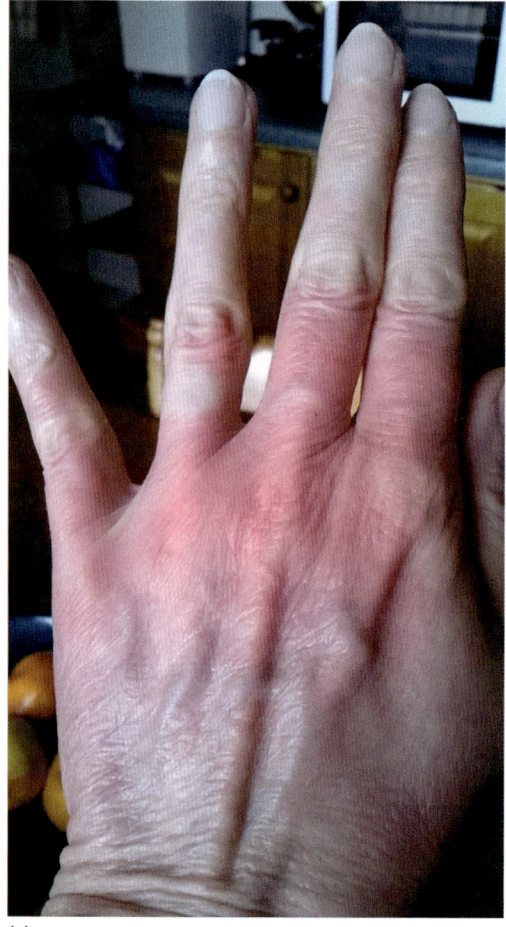
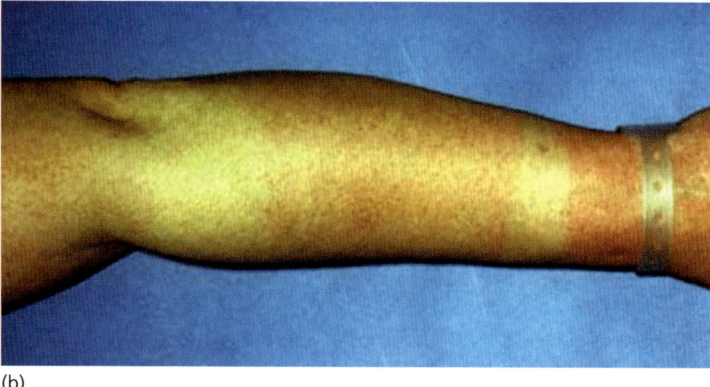

Figure 126.20 Solar urticaria. (a) Acute erythema on the back of the hand after 2 min of wintertime daylight exposure. Note sparing of the distal phalanges and under the wedding ring. (b) Solar urticaria occurring within a few minutes of sunlight exposure. Note sparing under the watch strap and sleeve on the upper forearm.

be troubled with SU triggered by UVA and visible light transmitted through window glass. Hardening is not typically reported in SU, although some patients do have lesser involvement of the face and back of hands. Additionally, there may be a refractory period when, after an acute episode, affected skin may be more resistant to further involvement for a few hours. In most patients, urticarial lesions resolve within 2 h, although a degree of abnormal erythema at exposed sites may persist for 24 h. Triggering of SU

Idiopathic (immunological) photodermatoses

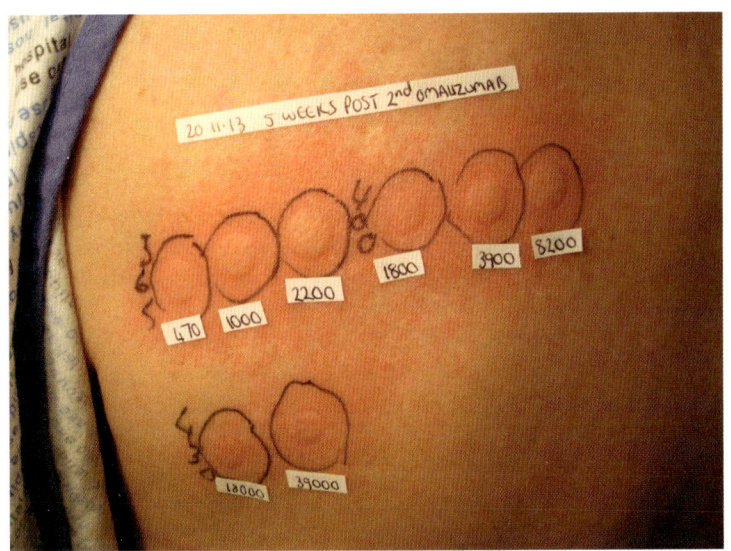

Figure 126.21 Abnormal immediate photosensitivity to UVA (365 nm) and visible (400 and 430 nm) wavelengths in a patient with treatment-resistant solar urticaria. Note the erythema, oedema, weal and flare, which developed within 5 min of phototesting.

by sunbed exposure can occur and if patients have large areas exposed, systemic symptoms of malaise, headache, photophobia, wheeze, nausea, dizziness and rarely hypotension and anaphylaxis may occur [20,**48**,49]. Exacerbation by internal lighting, particularly the low-energy compact fluorescent sources [54–57], and rarely by infrared radiation [58] may occur.

Presentation
If assessed during an acute episode, skin reddening and urticaria will be evident on photo-exposed or lightly clothed sites (Figure 126.21). There may be no abnormal signs if the patient is not seen acutely.

Clinical variants
There are infrequent reports of delayed-onset [59,60] and more persistent SU [61]. In these cases, phototesting is essential to distinguish SU from early-onset PLE. Changes of leucocytoclastic vasculitis can occasionally be seen [62]. There are also reports of SU occurring only at fixed reproducible sites or sites of bruising, although these are rare [60,63–66]. Systemic symptoms and rarely anaphylaxis may occur [67]. Solar angio-oedema has been reported and appears to be a variant of SU [68,**69**,70,71].

Differential diagnosis
The exclusion of secondary causes is essential as SU can occur secondary to drugs such as tetracyclines [72], fluoroquinolones, chlorpromazine [73,74], some non-steroidal anti-inflammatory drugs (NSAIDs) (notably benoxaprofen [75,76], which is no longer available), repirinast [77], topical tar, pitch [78], atorvastatin [79] and some sunscreens, such as the benzophenones [80]. An association with progesterone has been reported in a single case report [81] but not substantiated further. Porphyria (both erythropoietic protoporphyria [31,82,83] and PCT [82,84], particularly if there is photosensitivity at 430–460 nm) and lupus must be excluded. Other causes of urticaria should be considered, in particular heat-induced urticaria.

Classification of severity
There is no formal classification of severity. The impact on quality of life should be assessed by DLQI.

Complications and co-morbidities
Anxiety and depression can occur in SU [26]. Patients may also have other urticarias, particularly physical [34]. SU has been reported with concomitant PLE [36–38], CAD [39] and AP [40]. An association with Churg–Strauss syndrome was reported in one case and given the rarity of both diseases this may be significant [85]. Contact/photocontact sunscreen allergy may occur [26].

Disease course and prognosis
Idiopathic SU is a chronic disease in the majority. One report indicated that the chance of disease resolution was 58% by 5 years after onset [13], but a second report in 87 patients in whom 60 were followed up indicated resolution of only 12% by 5 years and 36% by 15 years [3]. In one large review of 224 patients in Spain, those with only visible or natural light sensitivity were more likely to have complete resolution on follow-up [21].

Investigations
Secondary causes of SU are uncommon but must be considered. A detailed drug history is important and porphyria and lupus must be considered [31,82–84]. Monochromator phototesting is the investigation of choice; skin reddening, oedema, weal and flare will occur within minutes at phototest sites (Figure 126.21) and will resolve over an hour or so, often with associated delayed abnormal skin reddening at 24 h [14]. The immediate minimal urticarial dose (MUD) and the MED at 24 h should be ascertained at each waveband. Most patients have a fairly broad action spectrum for abnormal immediate photosensitivity, with the longer UVA and shorter visible wavelengths being most commonly involved [2,**3**,5,13,20–23,**26**,27,38,86]. If SU is strongly suspected but not detected on monochromator phototesting, phototesting with broader spectrum sources, such as the solar simulator or even natural sunlight, may be advised as, rarely, SU is only provoked by an interaction of wavelengths [26]. Augmentation and inhibition spectra are reported, and these may be useful regarding management and awareness of risk of severe SU or anaphylaxis [46,47,**48**,49,87–89]. Detailed knowledge of the wavelength dependency of photosensitivity is critical for patient management and monitoring of responses. The action spectrum may change within patients over time, reinforcing the need for follow-up phototesting [90,91]. If the condition is severe and unresponsive to treatment, intradermal testing with irradiated autologous serum and/or plasma may help indicate whether there might be a beneficial response to plasmapheresis but is only positive in the minority [3].

Management
Anxiety and depression are common in SU as impact on quality of life is considerable and psychological support may be needed [26,92,93]. Photoprotection alone is usually inadequate, unless the symptoms are mild, but is nevertheless important [3,27]. Behavioural sun avoidance and the use of layered, tightly woven, dark clothing and broad-brimmed hats are advised. Window film may be useful at home, work or on car windows. Photoprotective

window film blocks UVA transmission but as many patients are also sensitive to visible light [54–57], it may not suffice. Attention to dietary vitamin D intake and, if necessary, supplementation is important. The majority of patients gain some benefit from broad spectrum, high protection factor sunscreens, although the addition of reflectant sunscreens such as Dundee cream (Tayside Pharmaceuticals), which offer protection in the shorter parts of the visible spectrum, may be helpful [3,94].

First line
One-third of patients respond completely, and one-third partially, to non-sedating H_1 antihistamines, with the remainder having no response [10,21,95–100]. Antihistamines are most effective at reducing or abolishing weal and flare, although not immediate or delayed skin reddening [97,101]. Antihistamines may need to be used at higher dose and in combination and there may be a synergistic benefit with sunscreens [20,94,102–104]. The addition of an H_2 antagonist and/or a leukotriene receptor antagonist may provide additional benefit [102,104]. There is variation between patients in responses to the different antihistamines and often several must be tried and at higher doses than those required to block histamine alone, in order to find an effective regimen.

Second line
Doxepin [43], ketotifen, chromoglycate and montelukast may have some beneficial effects in individual patients although, due to the rarity of the condition, these agents have not been thoroughly evaluated [102]. Dihydroxyacetone 'sunless tan' products have been explored but are of limited use [105].

It may be possible to undertake desensitisation using natural or artificial light and this will be determined by the wavelength dependency and severity of photosensitivity [88,106,107]. It may also be feasible for a patient to induce natural tolerance by graded exposure to daylight, although many patients are too sensitive to be able to manage this approach. Phototherapy, if it can be tolerated, can be beneficial [108,109,**110**,111–114]. As most patients have maximal sensitivity in the UVA1 and visible spectrum, narrow-band UVB responses are often normal and this can be successfully used [**110**,111,112,115–118]. However, a baseline MED prior to phototherapy should be performed as 24h MED may be reduced [119]. Effective desensitisation with narrow-band UVB, UVA and PUVA is reported, although benefit may be short-lived and home desensitisation may be considered [109,**110**,111,120–124]. UVA rush hardening, using frequent sub-urticaria-triggering broad-band UVA exposures, usually several times per day, either prior to the introduction of PUVA or alone, may also be beneficial [23,67,121,125–128] and rarely cautious UVA1 hardening may be successful [23,129]. Phototesting to determine the SU action spectrum, and the immediate MUD and delayed MED (or MPD for PUVA) prior to desensitisation, is essential. Treatment should be combined with antihistamines throughout the course and would usually be administered to photo-exposed sites only. Following a course of desensitisation, some natural daylight exposure is required to prolong tolerance.

Third line
Other approaches may be required for severe recalcitrant disease, although there is no good evidence base to support these therapies, most having been used in single cases or small case series. Ciclosporin, systemic glucocorticoids and other immunosuppressants may be considered [130,131]. β-Carotene [132] and hydroxychloroquine are unlikely to be effective. Intravenous immunoglobulins may be effective in some patients and ineffective in others [133–139]. For severely affected patients, particularly if the intradermal test is positive, plasmapheresis may be beneficial, although even in responders sustained remission cannot be guaranteed and this procedure is only undertaken in specialist centres and is not without risks [140–146]. Increasingly, experience with efficacy of the anti-IgE monoclonal antibody omalizumab has been reported in SU, with evidence of clinical and phototesting improvement or resolution and long-term efficacy feasible, although there are also reports of lack of effect [33,147–152,**153**,154,155,**156**,157,158,**159**,160–166]. Response may be immediate and life-changing, although in some cases higher doses and prolonged treatment may be needed. Oral polypodium leukotomos and α-melanocyte stimulating hormone (α-MSH) analogues have been used experimentally in small numbers but require further study [167–171]. Thus, it does seem that the disease is heterogeneous and that one treatment approach does not suit all.

Hydroa vacciniforme

Definition and nomenclature
Hydroa vacciniforme (HV) is a rare acquired photodermatosis, which usually occurs in children and has a characteristic clinical presentation of photo-exposed site vesicles, crusts and varioliform scars.

Synonyms and inclusions
- Hydroa aestivale

Introduction and general description
HV was described by Bazin in 1862 [1]. This condition usually presents in the first decade of life and is typified by the development of vesicles, crusting (which is often haemorrhagic) and subsequently varioliform scars on photo-exposed sites.

Epidemiology
Incidence and prevalence
HV is rare. One review of 17 Scottish patients with HV estimated the prevalence to be at least 0.34 cases per 100 000 population [2], although our impression is that this may be reducing over the years. Estimated overall prevalence is 1–9 per 1 000 000.

Age
It typically occurs in children, with a bimodal age distribution with onset either between 1 and 7 years or 12 and 16 years, with a mean age of onset of 7.9 years (range 1–16 years) reported in one study ($n = 17$) [2]. There are exceptional cases presenting in infancy [3] or of later onset [4] and persisting in the elderly [5–7,**8**].

Sex
Initial reports suggested that HV was commoner in females, although a more recent review indicated that both sexes were equally affected. However, the disease may present earlier (mean age 6.7 years) and be of shorter duration in females compared with males (mean age 8.7 years) [2,3].

Ethnicity
HV can occur in all ethnic groups.

Pathophysiology
The aetiology of HV is unknown. UVA wavelengths are implicated in the provocation of lesions which are induced either by spring and summer sunlight or by artificial UV. The chromophore(s) have yet to be defined. A role for Epstein–Barr virus (EBV) infection has been proposed as latent virus was found in the dermal inflammatory infiltrate of patients with HV in South-East Asia. However, this may be an HV-like clinical presentation of EBV [6,9–19]. An HV-like presentation has also been reported in an aggressive form of T-cell lymphoma in children, which may be EBV driven, although the clinical presentation is usually distinct from that of classical HV [18–27]. However, there have been increasing reports clarifying the role of chronic EBV in patients with HV-like T-/NK-cell lymphoproliferative disorder (HVLPD), particularly in Latin America and Asia [28,**29**,30,**31**,32–37]. HVLPD is extremely rare in Europe and America and in one study of 16 patients with HVLPD reported over an 11-year period, those who presented at an older age, were non-white and had markedly elevated EBV DNA levels were more likely to develop systemic disease and have a poorer prognosis [38]. An association with HLA-DR4 tissue typing has also been suggested for familial cases, although not confirmed due to the rarity of such presentations [2]. Earlier reports of impaired DNA repair *in vitro* [39] and of the implication of pyridoxine photoproducts [40,41] in the production of tissue damage have not been confirmed.

Pathology
A biopsy of a lesion at a positive UVA provocation site may show non-specific histology acutely, with reticulate keratinocyte degeneration, spongiosis and a perivascular inflammatory cell infiltrate, consisting of lymphocytes, histiocytes and neutrophils. However, lesional histology a few days later is usually diagnostic with ulceration, epidermal necrosis, papillary oedema, upper dermal necrosis and subsequent scarring (Figure 126.22). Direct immunofluorescence is typically negative [3,**42**].

Causative organisms
A possible role of EBV in classical HV is not fully defined.

Genetics
The condition is usually sporadic, although familial cases are reported, including in identical twins [43,44].

Clinical features
History
Patients typically present with seasonal symptoms in spring/summer. Following 15 min to a few hours of direct or window

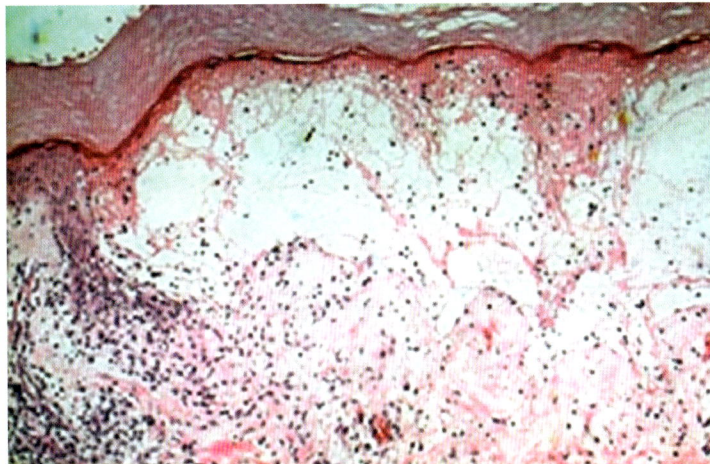

Figure 126.22 Histopathology of hydroa vacciniforme showing epidermal necrosis, dermal oedema and a lymphohistiocytic inflammatory infiltrate.

glass-transmitted light, intensely pruritic crops of papules and vesicles, often arising on a background of skin reddening and oedema, occur on exposed sites within 12–24 h. A burning sensation and pain may occur. Vesicle fluid often becomes haemorrhagic. There may be systemic malaise and fever during acute episodes.

Presentation
The commonest sites affected are the cheeks, nose, ears and back of hands (Figure 126.23a, b). As the vesicles resolve, haemorrhagic crusting develops and as this detaches, varioliform scarring remains and can be severe (Figure 126.23c) [45]. Subungual haemorrhage can occur [46]. There may rarely be cartilage destruction, for example of the ears [47] or nose, or contractures of the digits. The eyes can also be affected, with photophobia, conjunctivitis, keratitis, anterior uveitis [48], corneal clouding and neovascularisation, scarring and visual impairment [49,**50**,51–53]. Oral mucosal involvement is rare but can occur [11,54].

Differential diagnosis
It is important to exclude bullous LE [55], EPP [55] and Hartnup disease [56]. It is also important to consider and rule out HVLPD, particularly in non-white patients and if there are other features of systemic disease and/or ocular or oral involvement [19,38,57–60]. AP may also be in the differential.

Classification of severity
There is no specific classification of severity. The DLQI may be helpful [**61**].

Complications and co-morbidities
There may be significant scarring [45], ocular complications [48,49,**50**,51–53] and, rarely, cartilage destruction [47].

Disease course and prognosis
In classical HV, the condition usually improves and resolves in later teenage years, with a mean disease duration of 9 years [2].

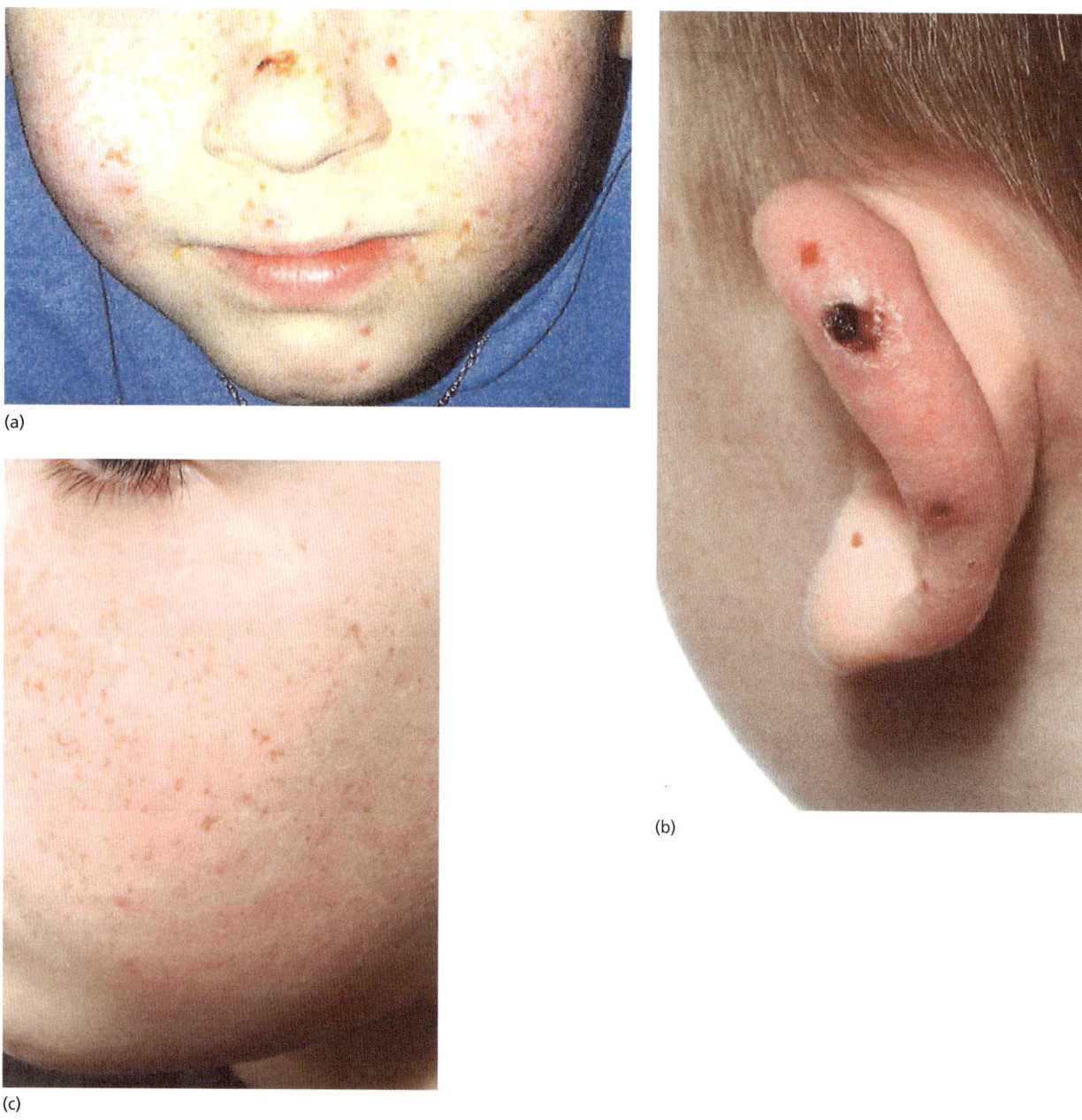

Figure 126.23 Hydroa vacciniforme. (a) Papules, vesiculation and haemorrhagic crusting on the cheeks (patient's own photograph). (b) Papules on the ears. (c) Subtle but definite vacciniforme scarring on the cheek at sites of previous inflammatory lesions.

However, persistence of disease into middle age may also occur [5,6,8].

Investigations

Full blood count, ANAs, extractable nuclear antigens and porphyrin biochemistry should be undertaken. EBV DNA levels should be measured as markedly elevated levels may be associated with the possibility of progression to HVLPD, particularly in non-white patients and atypical disease. Urinary amino acids may also be requested. These investigations are normal in classical HV [2,3]. Monochromator phototesting may be normal or more typically shows predominantly UVA sensitivity (Figure 126.24a) [2,3,62].

Repeated artificial UVA provocation will usually induce lesions (Figure 126.24b), typically papules, vesicles and sometimes purpura [8], which are indistinguishable from those provoked by natural sunlight [55,62]. Negative photoprovocation with artificial sources has been suggested to be a good prognostic factor [63].

Management

Photoprotection by behavioural modification, use of clothing, hats, sunglasses, UV-absorbing window film and a broad spectrum high SPF sunscreen is important. Dietary vitamin D intake should be optimised and, if necessary, supplements considered. Psychological support may be required [61].

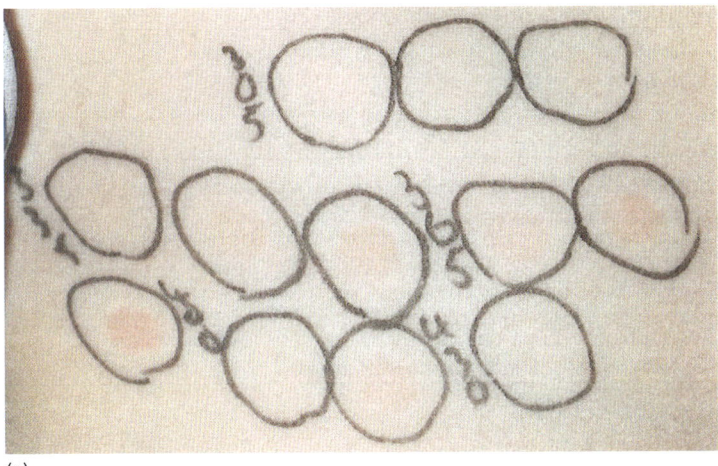

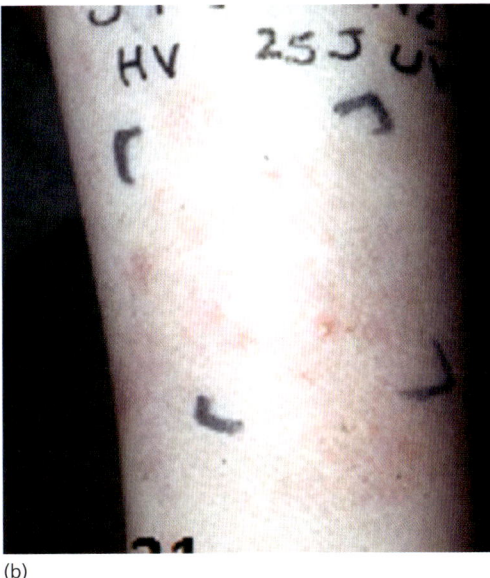

Figure 126.24 (a) Monochromator phototesting showing abnormal UVA photosensitivity. (b) Positive UVA photoprovocation in hydroa vacciniforme.

First line
Photoprotection and topical corticosteroid use in active disease are indicated.

Second line
Springtime desensitisation with narrow-band UVB phototherapy can be successful, with 60% of patients finding this beneficial in one study [64]. PUVA is used less often as most patients are typically children [3,55].

Third line
Given the rarity of HV, the evidence base for therapeutic options is limited to case reports and case series. Oral glucocorticoids, β-carotene [2,3,52,55], azathioprine [7], ciclosporin [7] and antimalarials [3] have been tried, although their benefits are unproven. Dietary fish oil may be helpful but is generally poorly tolerated [65–67]. Thalidomide appears to be ineffective [3]. The role of drugs with systemic toxicity must be weighed up against their use in a disease, which although associated with significant morbidity, usually resolves with time.

DRUG- AND CHEMICAL-INDUCED PHOTOSENSITIVITY

Exogenous drug- and chemical-induced photosensitivity

Definition and nomenclature
These are abnormal cutaneous reactions to UVR and visible radiation induced by photosensitising drugs and chemicals. They are subdivided according to whether the drug/chemical is administered systemically or topically [1–7,**8**,9–11,**12**,13].

> **Synonyms and inclusions**
> - Phototoxicity
> - Exaggerated sunburn
> - Photoallergy
> - Pseudoporphyria
> - Skin fragility
> - Photo-induced telangiectasia
> - Topical photocontact allergy
> - Drug-induced lupus

Introduction and general description
Drug- and chemical-induced photosensitivity may have diverse presentations, although phototoxicity ('exaggerated sunburn') is most common [1–7,**8**,9–11,**12**,13,14]. It is important *not* to miss this diagnosis as it is reversible if drug exposure is stopped.

Epidemiology
Incidence and prevalence
Drug phototoxicity can theoretically occur in anyone and on first exposure, although idiosyncratic and probably genetic factors exist, which means that not all those exposed to photoactive drugs become photosensitive. Systemic drug-induced photosensitivity may account for 2–15% of cases diagnosed in tertiary photodiagnostic units [**8**,13,14,**15**,16–21]. In one questionnaire-based study of patients with cystic fibrosis who had received ciprofloxacin, 48.4% reported increased sun sensitivity compared with approximately 2.4% of the control population [22]. Topical drug- and chemical-induced photosensitivity is more likely to occur in regular sunscreen users or those who use topical NSAIDs [23–31,**32**,33–36]. The latter are most commonly used in continental Europe, particularly France, Portugal and Spain.

Age
Older patients, whose polypharmacy often includes photoactive drugs, are thus more at risk for developing drug-induced photosensitivity.

Sex
Sex does not appear to be a determinant of susceptibility.

Ethnicity
Patients of all ethnicities and skin phototypes may be affected [16–21,23].

Pathophysiology
There are several mechanisms of drug- and chemical-induced photosensitivity and most require oxygen, resulting in toxic photosensitiser and substrate species [2,6,8,11,37]. Most systemic drug photosensitivity is phototoxic, that is non-immunological. The clinical manifestations of such drug photosensitivity will depend on the subcellular localisation of the drug and photoactive metabolites and may be diverse. Drugs/chemicals applied topically may also cause phototoxicity. A wide variety of drugs and chemicals, both systemically and topically administered, may cause photosensitivity [7,8,9–11,12,13,14,15,38–40]. Box 126.2 details the most common culprits in the UK and elsewhere in Europe. The classical phototoxic drugs (thiazides, NSAIDs, quinine) remain the most common culprits, but many diverse drugs have been reported in association with photosensitivity and vigilance must also be kept with respect to more recently introduced drug culprits [7,8,9–11,12,13,14,15,38–40].

Other less common mechanisms include pseudoporphyria, drug-induced lupus, lichenoid reactions, erythema multiforme, pellagra and photoallergy (Box 126.3 and Table 126.1) [7,8,11,37]. Awareness of the potential of photoactive drugs to induce photosensitivity via multiple mechanisms is also important. For example, both thiazides and proton pump inhibitors may cause photosensitivity via either phototoxic or drug-induced lupus routes. Photoallergy is uncommon and poorly defined with systemic drugs and most frequently seen with topical sunscreens, NSAIDs and, less commonly now, certain fragrances [23–31,32,33–36]. Sunscreens are the commonest topical photoallergens [31,32,33,34,36]. Topical phototoxicity can occur to dyestuffs and psoralen-containing plants (phytophotodermatitis) [30,41,42]. Knowledge of drug-induced photosensitivity is derived from anecdotal reports, postmarketing surveillance and, more recently, controlled trials required by regulatory authorities [2,38,43,44,45,46,47].

Pathology
The commonest histological picture is of a phototoxic reaction, with epidermal necrosis, apoptotic keratinocytes and mild inflammation [48]. Lesional histology may show interface lupus-like or lichenoid changes, erythema multiforme or may be indistinguishable from PCT in some of the less frequent clinical presentations. Spongiotic dermatitis can occur but is not typical except in photoallergy, which is usually due to topical agents.

Genetics
There are likely to be genetic factors that predispose individuals to drug photosensitisation to specific agents but these are not defined [8,11,49].

Clinical features
History
The symptoms of drug phototoxicity are usually an immediate burning sensation on sun-exposed sites, often with skin reddening and sometimes urticaria. There is commonly also a delayed skin reddening and sometimes blistering. Depending on the drug this may follow the same time course as sunburn, peaking at 24 h, although psoralens produce delayed skin reddening peaking between 72 and 120 h after exposure.

Box 126.2 Selective list of exogenous photosensitisers

Systemic
- Diuretics: thiazides, furosemide, nalidixic acid
- Antibiotics: fluoroquinolones, tetracyclines[a], sulphonamides
- Non-steroidal anti-inflammatory drugs[b]
- Quinine
- Hydroxychloroquine [52]
- Antipsychotics: phenothiazines (chlorpromazine[b])
- Cardiology: amiodarone, calcium antagonists, ACE inhibitors, statins
- Hypoglycaemics: sulphonylureas
- Retinoids
- Psoralens[b]
- Antifungals: voriconazole, itraconazole, ketoconazole [53,54,55–59]
- Pirfenidone [8,60–71]
- Proton pump inhibitors [15,72]
- Antihepatitis C drugs [73,74]
- Leflunomide [75]
- Venlafaxine
- Escitalopram
- Celecoxib
- Exogenous porphyrins for photodynamic therapy [76,77]
- Azathioprine
- Fibrates [78]
- Pyridoxine B6
- Targeted anticancer drugs: vemurafenib, dabrafenib, encorafenib, nivolumab, vandetanib, imatinib [15,79,80,81,82,83–85]
- Biologics: anti-TNF, denosumab [15]

Topical
- Psoralens (phototoxic)
- Polycyclic aromatic hydrocarbons (phototoxic)
- Dyes (phototoxic)
- Phenothiazines (chlorproethazine) (phototoxic and photoallergic)
- Halogenated salicylanilides (mainly photoallergic)
- Fragrances (phototoxic and photoallergic)
- Sunscreens (phototoxic and photoallergic)
- Non-steroidal anti-inflammatory drugs (phototoxic and photoallergic)

[a] Doxycycline and demeclocycline are phototoxic and minocycline may cause drug-induced LE.
[b] Can also cause photosensitivity via topical application.
ACE, angiotensin-converting enzyme.

Box 126.3 Mechanisms of photosensitivity

- Phototoxicity
- Pseudoporphyria
- Photoallergy
- Lichenoid
- Lupus
- Pellagra

Table 126.1 Patterns of presentation of drug- and chemical-induced photosensitivity and examples of culprit drugs.

Pattern of presentation	Examples
Immediate burning, prickling and subsequent pigmentation	Amiodarone, chlorpromazine, Photofrin, Foscan, topical tars, pitches
Exaggerated sunburn	Thiazides, fluoroquinolones, quinine, tetracyclines, amiodarone, chlorpromazine
Delayed skin reddening and pigmentation	Psoralens
Pseudoporphyria	Non-steroidal anti-inflammatory drugs (particularly naproxen, diclofenac and piroxicam), frusemide, nalidixic acid, tetracyclines, fluoroquinolones, retinoids
Photo-exposed site telangiectasia	Calcium antagonists
Lupus	Chapter 117
Lichenoid	Chapter 117

Although it is more common for photosensitivity to develop if a drug is new or the dose increased, it can also occur after a prolonged period of being on the drug. This is particularly true for the calcium antagonists, where photo-exposed-site telangiectasia may only develop after several months to years of drug ingestion [50]. Other drugs have also been associated with photo-distributed telangiectasia, so a thorough drug history is essential [51]. Detailed history taking is essential, including probing about non-prescribed drugs and supplements.

Presentation

The patterns of presentation of drug- and chemical-induced photosensitivity are listed in Table 126.1. Reddening, blistering, oedema and even urticaria may be seen on photo-exposed sites in an acute episode of drug phototoxicity (Figure 126.25). Uncommonly, photo-distributed purpura can be seen, as reported with levofloxacin photosensitivity [86]. Occasionally there may be extension of the eruption and erythroderma can follow. A lichenoid dermatitis may occur, for example with thiazides or NSAIDs [87,88]. Pseudoporphyria typically presents with photo-exposed-site fragility, blistering, milia and scarring and can be indistinguishable from PCT or variegate porphyria, although porphyrins are normal and it is thought to occur due to chronic drug-induced phototoxic damage at the dermal–epidermal junction [83,89–92]. NSAIDs are common culprits for pseudoporphyria [91]. Drug-induced lupus is uncommon but can occur, for example with thiazides [93] and other drugs, including proton pump inhibitors [72,94]. Pellagra is rare but can be triggered by isoniazid, phenytoin and other drugs. Drug-induced photo-distributed telangiectasia and angiomas have been reported with calcium antagonists and venlafaxine [50,51,95]. Photo-onycholysis has been reported in association with the use of some photosensitising drugs, such as doxycycline and psoralens [96–100].

Topical drug- and chemical-induced photosensitisation can be caused by a diverse range of topical drugs and chemicals, notably tars, pitches [101,102], plants, dyes [103], NSAIDs, fragrances, halogenated salicylanilides [104,105], phenothiazines [35,106] and sunscreen chemicals [30,31,**32**,33,34,36]. In particular, skin contact with the psoralen-containing sap of the Umbelliferae and Rutaceae plant families and/or citrus fruits and subsequent UVA exposure from sunlight will result in a phototoxic reaction, with linear and angular skin reddening becoming apparent 48–72 h later at the sites of plant, fruit, sap or juice contact, with blistering and subsequent pigmentation (phytophotodermatitis) (Figure 126.26). This should be recognised clinically as it may be confused with non-accidental injury [8,41,42,107–114]. This may follow a specific clinical pattern, such as strimmer's dermatitis or Berloque dermatitis, depending on the type of exposure. Organic sunscreen chemicals, fragrances and NSAIDs can be both phototoxic and photoallergic. With the latter, prior sensitisation is required, so the clinical presentation will not be on first exposure, and while occurring predominantly on the sites exposed to the drug/chemical and light, may extend beyond these sites and become more of a generalised dermatitis, particularly with continuing exposure to the drug/chemical and light.

Although there are reports of 'persistent light reaction' occurring following oral or topical drug/chemical photosensitivity, most of these cases would fall within the spectrum of CAD and there is no convincing evidence to support the case of long-term continued

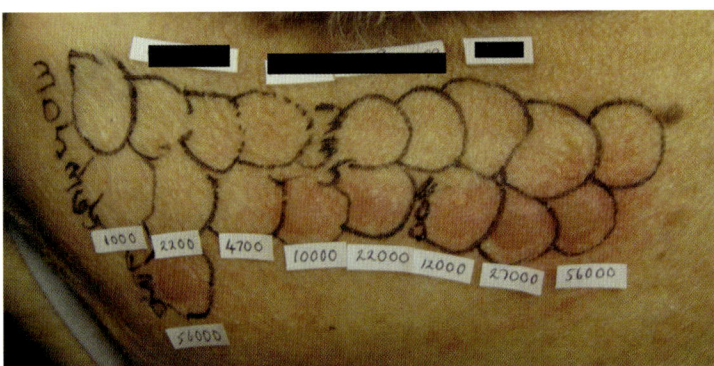

Figure 126.25 Phototoxicity to demeclocycline. There is predominant UVA and visible light photosensitivity. Acute erythema, oedema and urticaria were seen at the test sites within 15 min of phototesting and abnormal delayed erythema was still present at 24 h.

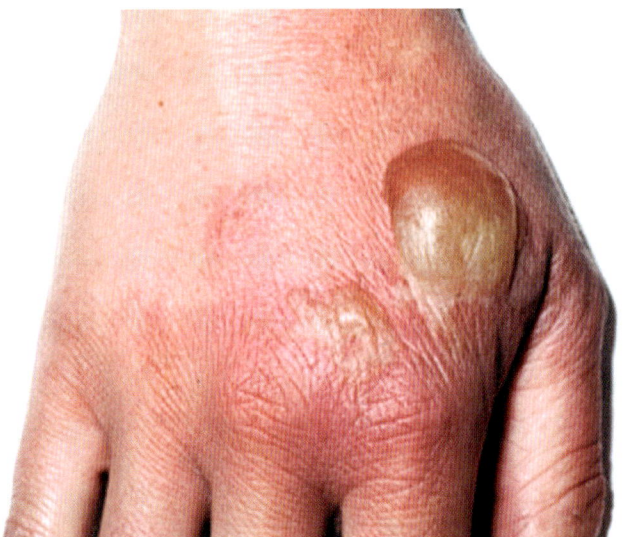

Figure 126.26 Phytophotodermatitis. Erythema and blistering are seen on sites immersed in psoralen-rich lime marinade during barbeque preparations and subsequently exposed to sunlight. Erythema and blistering will usually be maximal 72–96 h after exposure.

photosensitivity following cessation of a drug photosensitiser [104,105,115,116]. Prolonged pigmentation can occur after systemic or topical drug- and chemical-induced phototoxicity. For example, linear streaks of hyperpigmentation often persist for months after an episode of phytophotodermatitis. Reticulate hyperpigmentation has been reported with photosensitivity due to the calcium antagonist diltiazem [117]. Leucomelanoderma may occur as a consequence of drug phototoxicity, particularly with thiazides or quinine, although it is also reported with other phototoxic drugs, such as pirfenidone, and these pigmentary changes appear to be due to dysfunction of melanocytes [63,118]. Chlorpromazine and amiodarone photosensitivity is often complicated by prolonged pigmentation (Figure 126.27) [119,120], and an acneiform eruption on photo-exposed sites can occur with amiodarone.

Clinical variants
See Box 126.3 and Table 126.1.

Differential diagnosis
Depending on the clinical presentation, this may include CAD, PCT, variegate porphyria, LE and idiopathic SU, and cutaneous T-cell lymphoma if there is erythroderma.

Classification of severity
There is no formal classification.

Complications and co-morbidities
The role of drug- and chemical-induced photosensitisation in photocarcinogenesis is unclear, although there is recent evidence to support possible associations between photosensitising drug use and risk of squamous cell carcinoma (SCC), basal cell carcinoma (BCC) and melanoma [8,121–134,**135**]. Undoubtedly psoralens are photomutagenic and with repeated PUVA exposures skin cancer risk is increased [136]. A role for other photoactive drugs in photocarcinogenesis is unclear [**137**], although abnormal lentigines and increased skin cancers, both SCC and melanoma, have been observed in patients taking the photoactive drug voriconazole (Figure 126.28) [53,**54**,55] and skin tumours are induced in mice exposed to fluoroquinolones and light. Azathioprine can cause UVA photosensitivity and is photomutagenic [138]. Interestingly, photosensitivity has been reported in patients receiving BRAF inhibitors for melanoma [139] and these patients are also at markedly increased risk of developing SCC [140]. Potential acute or chronic ocular damage should also be considered as most drug photosensitivity involves UVA/visible light wavelengths. Furthermore, photodegradation of the drug may potentially also reduce drug efficacy [141]. It is important to establish whether patients are taking photoactive drugs prior to and during a course of UV phototherapy as some drugs may increase the risk of skin reddening episodes during the treatment course [8,142–144].

Disease course and prognosis
The time course for the resolution of photosensitivity off the drug will depend on its bioavailability and the half-life of any photoactive metabolites. Psoralen photosensitivity undergoes strong saturable first-pass metabolism but will clear within a few hours [2,145,146],

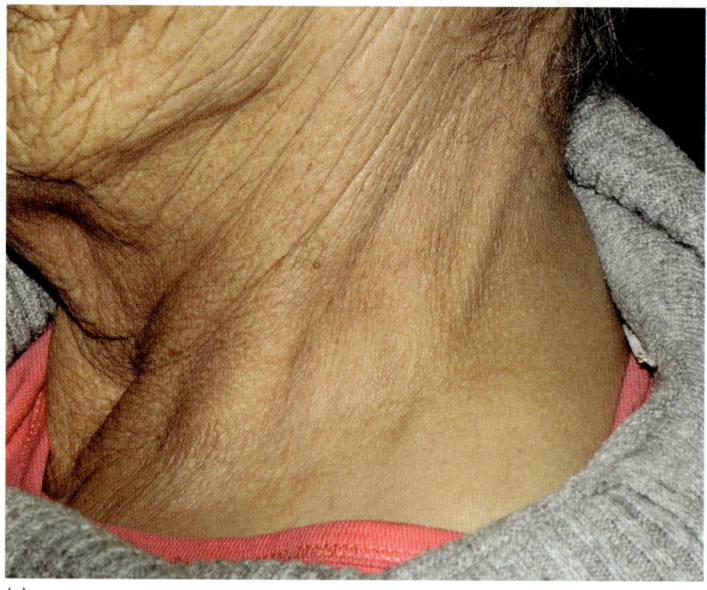
(a)

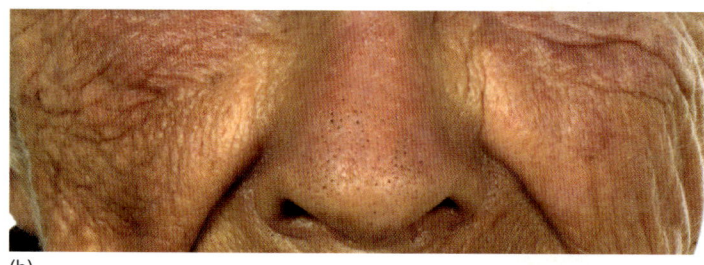
(b)

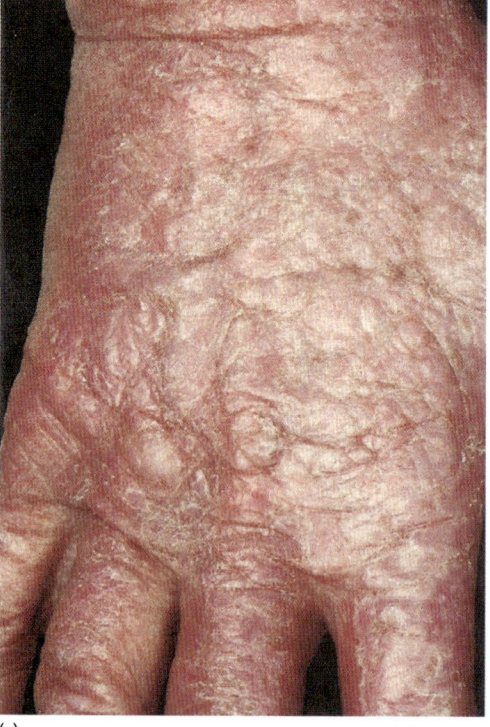
(c)

Figure 126.27 Chlorpromazine phototoxicity. (a) Characteristic brown-grey pigmentation associated with chronic photosensitivity secondary to chlorpromazine. (b) Violaceous erythema on photo-exposed sites of the face. (c) Brawny erythema and oedema on photo-exposed sites of the back of the hands.

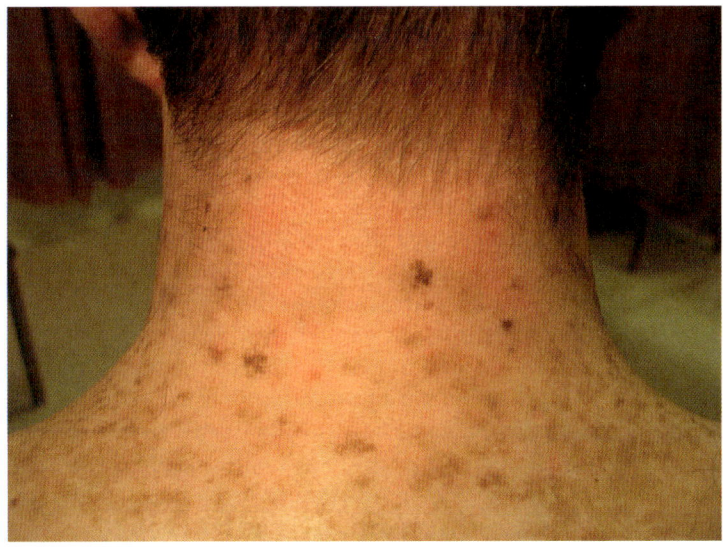

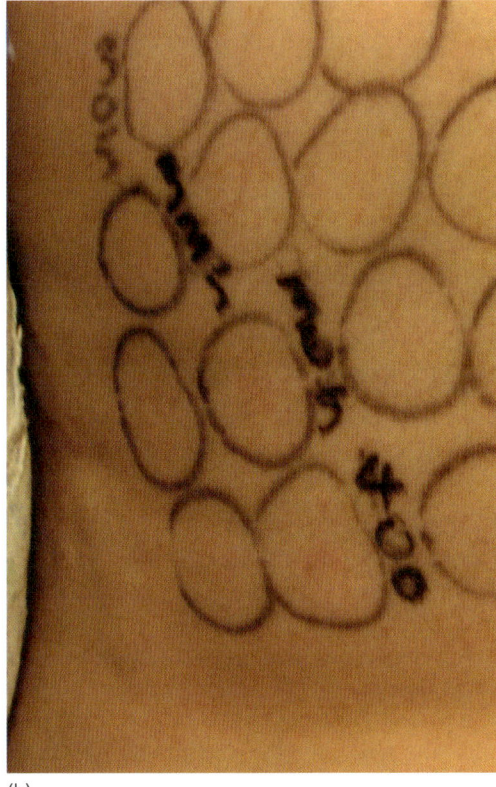

Figure 126.28 Voriconazole photosensitivity. (a) Abnormal stellate lentigines developed on photo-exposed sites in this patient who had been taking voriconazole for several months. Note also the erythema on the back of the neck. (b) Abnormal UVA photosensitivity on monochromator phototesting.

the drug [2,119,149,150]). Hydroxychloroquine photosensitivity may also be of long duration after drug cessation [52]. Skin fragility may persist for many months and pigmentation and telangiectasia can remain for longer [50].

Investigations

Monochromator phototesting should be undertaken while on the drug and repeated after a period off the drug, the interval depending on the kinetics of the drug and its metabolites. Most photoactive drugs have maximal absorption in the UVA waveband and therefore photosensitivity is usually either restricted to UVA wavelengths or disproportionately involves the UVA region [7,8,151]. Some drugs, such as quinine and thiazides, have an extension of their action spectrum into the UVB region [1,88,93,150,152] and others, such as the fluoroquinolones and systemic porphyrin drugs used in PDT, cause visible light photosensitivity. Indeed, some drugs, notably NSAIDs, phenothiazines and calcium antagonists, may lower the narrow-band UVB MED in patients referred for phototherapy. Screening for porphyria and lupus should always be undertaken. Histology may be informative [48]. Photopatch testing is the investigation of choice for suspected topical photocontact allergy (Figure 126.29) [25–31,32,33–36] but is not reliable for investigating systemic drug photosensitivity. *In vitro*, *ex vivo* and controlled healthy volunteer drug phototoxicity studies are increasingly important and requested by regulatory authorities such as the US Food and Drug Administration and the European Union [2,8,43,45,46,47,153].

Management

Recognition of the diagnosis and cessation of the suspected drug/chemical is essential. Vigilance about considering possible new culprits is important [154]. The distinction between drug photosensitivity and CAD may be a challenge, although disproportionate UVA sensitivity favours a drug cause and disproportionate UVB sensitivity favours CAD. If in doubt, a suspected drug should be stopped and phototesting repeated at an interval off the drug [151]. For most drugs, non-phototoxic alternatives exist. However,

and fluoroquinolones [5,45,147,148] and chlorpromazine [2] within 48 h. Other drugs may take much longer, for example thiazide photosensitivity may last 3–6 months [6], systemic porphyrins used for photodynamic therapy (PDT) can still be detected at 3 months [76] (although clinical photosensitivity may resolve within a few weeks [77], quinine photosensitivity may last for several months and amiodarone effects may last for a year or more after stopping

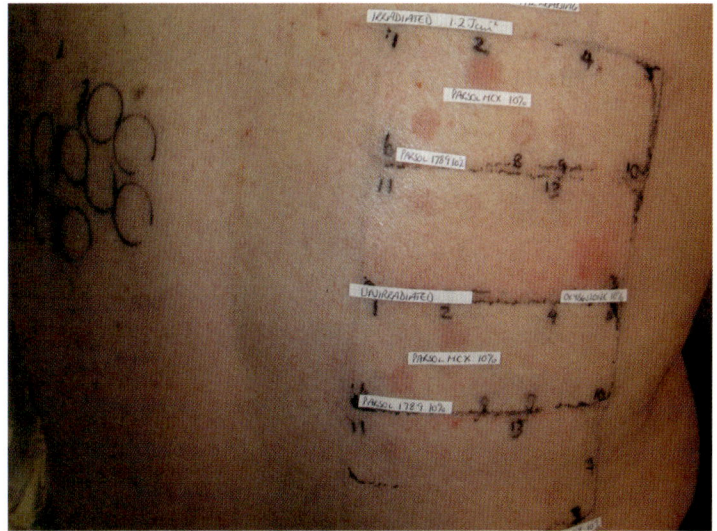

Figure 126.29 Positive photopatch testing to sunscreen chemicals.

if a drug cannot be stopped, dosage reduction may be beneficial [155,156]. Photoprotection including broad spectrum and reflectant sunscreens is important until photosensitivity has resolved [157].

First line
Stop the drug, improve photoprotection and initiate symptomatic treatment with emollients and topical corticosteroids.

Second line
If a drug, such as amiodarone [158], cannot be stopped, the induction of tolerance using narrow-band UVB or PUVA may be helpful [**159**].

PHOTOAGGRAVATED DERMATOSES

Synonyms and inclusions
- Light-exacerbated, photo-exacerbated dermatoses

A range of skin diseases can be aggravated or exacerbated by natural or artificial UV or visible radiation, although they also occur in the absence of sun exposure (Box 126.4) [1,2–4]. Photoaggravated skin diseases are relatively common and may represent almost a third of patients diagnosed at tertiary photodiagnostic units [5–8]. These conditions are heterogeneous and generally only a proportion of patients experience photoaggravation and they may or may not be aware of the triggering role of sunlight. For example, psoriasis and eczema generally improve with sun exposure, but in a minority (approximately 10% or fewer) [**9**] there is worsening of the dermatosis with sun exposure (Figure 126.30a, b) [10]. This may manifest as a disease flare at photo-exposed sites initially, followed by the spread of cutaneous inflammation to covered skin. This may be attributed to the heat of the sunlight or, as is often the case for psoriasis and eczema, a flare of the disease at sites where PLE (or other photosensitivity diseases) has been induced [11,12]. Some photoaggravated conditions that are generally phototherapy responsive, including psoriasis and eczema, may be successfully treated by cautious use of UVB phototherapy or PUVA. This should usually be avoided in other photoaggravated conditions such as bullous pemphigoid, dermatomyositis or cutaneous lupus (Figure 126.30c).

Box 126.4 Photoaggravated skin diseases

- Psoriasis [13–15,**16**,17,18]
- Eczema – atopic [**9**,10,**19**], seborrhoeic [20], allergic contact [21–24,**25**,**26**], pompholyx [27,28]
- Acne vulgaris [29]
- Actinic folliculitis [30–32]
- Rosacea and facial telangiectasia [33]
- Herpes simplex and other viral exanthems [34,35]
- Erythema multiforme [36–38]
- Lupus erythematosus (LE) [**39**,40–42]
- Jessner lymphocytic infiltrate/LE tumidus [**1**,43]
- Lymphocytoma cutis [**1**]
- Lichen planus [44–48,**49**]
- Bullous pemphigoid [50–52]
- Pemphigus and Hailey-Hailey disease [53]
- Linear IgA disease [**1**]
- Dermatitis herpetiformis [**1**]
- Dermatomyositis [54,55]
- Darier and transient acantholyic dermatosis [56–58]
- Disseminated superficial actinic porokeratosis [59–62]
- Pellagra [63]
- Mycosis fungoides [64,65]
- Melasma [66–68]
- Vitiligo [69]
- Pityriasis rubra pilaris [**70**,71]
- Reticular erythematous mucinosis [72]
- Urticaria [**1**]
- Actinic granuloma [73]
- Keratosis pilaris [**1**]
- Sweet syndrome [74–76]

Photoprotection and treatment of the underlying disorder are the mainstay approaches to management of these conditions.

CLINICAL ASSESSMENT AND MANAGEMENT OF A PATIENT WITH SUSPECTED PHOTOSENSITIVITY

History

Detailed history taking is essential. For many patients the relationship with sunlight is clear-cut, particularly if only affected in spring/summer and on sun-exposed sites, such as in PLE. However, in patients with perennial photosensitivity, or in those with covered site involvement or in erythroderma, there may be no awareness of the role of light.

Important information includes age at disease onset and duration, sex, presence of atopy, occupation and hobbies, family history and drug/chemical (systemic and topical) exposure. Some conditions are most likely to present in childhood, such as xeroderma pigmentosum (XP), EPP, AP and HV, whereas CAD is more likely in older males, although it may occur at a young age with coexistent atopic eczema. A positive family history is likely in XP and EPP. Details of the exposure required to trigger the eruption are informative. Is it perennial or seasonal? What are the type and duration of exposure (i.e. direct sunlight, window glass-transmitted light, artificial internal lighting, sunbed exposure or a combination)? A triggering of the rash by window glass-transmitted light indicates a role for UVA and/or visible light and is seen in several of the photodermatoses, particularly drug photosensitivity, PLE and solar urticaria, but is not usual in XP or indeed as a normal sunburn response. The duration of time from the triggering exposure to occurrence of the eruption (the latent period) is also helpful. The time course of the eruption – when it peaks and how long it takes to resolve – is important. For example, in typical PLE, a few hours of exposure may be required to trigger a rash later that day, peaking the next day and resolving within 2–3 days. In contrast, in SU, typically a few minutes of exposure will trigger immediate urticaria on exposed sites that will resolve within an hour or two. It is also important to determine whether there is hardening – the rash being less likely to

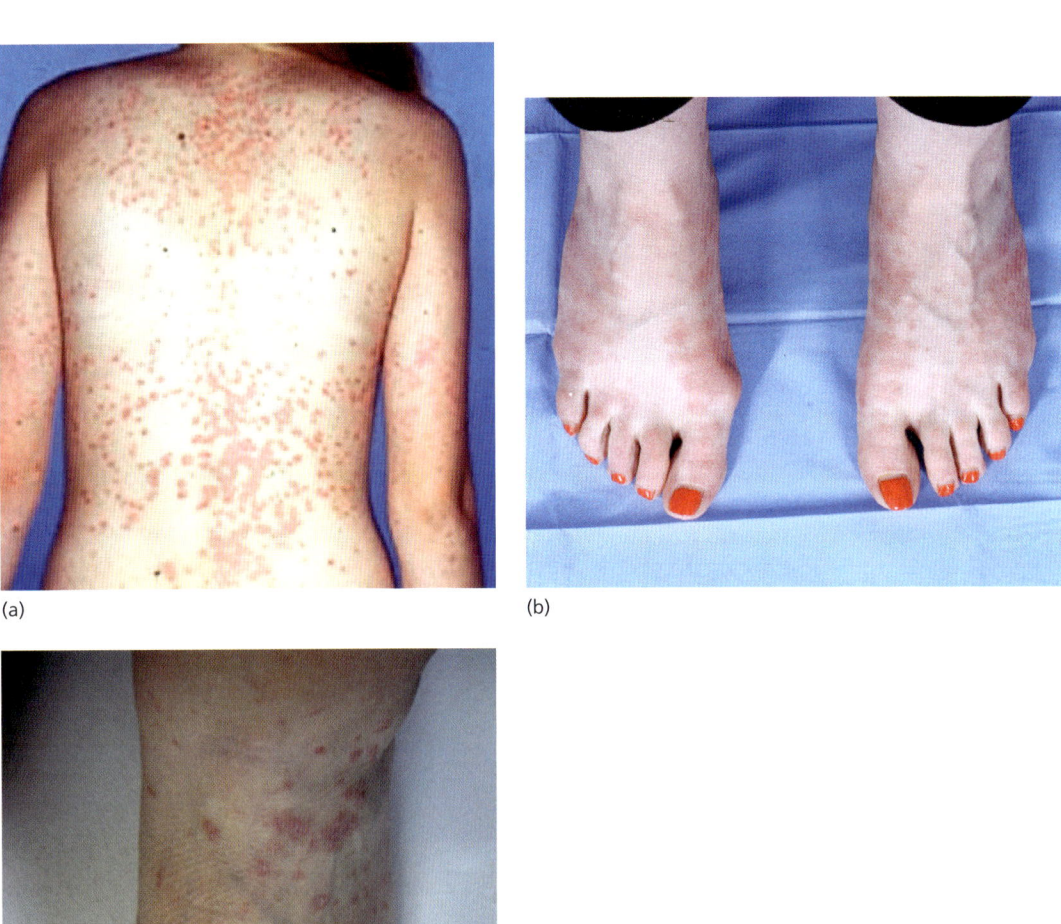

Figure 126.30 (a) Photoaggravated guttate psoriasis. Note the sparing at photoprotected sites under the crop top. (b) This patient had atopic eczema and systemic lupus erythematosus, with predominant involvement on photo-exposed sites of feet and sparing under footwear. (c) Note the predominantly photo-exposed sites of involvement in this patient with cutaneous lupus. Sparing under the sandals was evident.

occur on habitually exposed sites of the face and back of hands or less easy to provoke in later summer – as is often seen in PLE.

Symptoms are important. Pruritus occurs in many photodermatoses, such as PLE or CAD. Pain or burning on sun exposure should raise the possibility of EPP or drug photosensitivity. The distribution of the eruption is important: does it only occur on photo-exposed sites or are covered sites also involved, as is common in AP and CAD? Can it occur through clothing, as in SU? It is critical to establish from the history the morphology of the rash as patients may have no physical signs if they present in wintertime. For example, a papulovesicular rash is characteristic of PLE, whereas urticated weals are the hallmark of SU. Haemorrhagic vesicles and crusts are seen in HV. Scarring occurs in HV, AP and EPP. Exaggerated 'sunburn' skin reddening may occur in drug photosensitivity and in XP, with a delayed peak at 2–3 days or later. However, it is also important to be aware that increased 'sunburning' susceptibility does not always occur in XP and these patients may present earlier with skin cancers. It is also important to elicit whether there are systemic features, which may be relevant diagnostically, for example in SLE, HV or SU. The possibility of concomitant contact/photocontact allergy, which may modify the clinical presentation, should be considered by enquiring about a possible history of adverse effects to sunscreens, although patients may not necessarily be aware of this.

Examination

Prominent photo-exposed sites to examine are the bald scalp, forehead, malar surfaces, nose, chin, rims of ears, mastoid and sternomastoid sites, and anterior, sides and back of neck (Figures 126.9, 126.14, 126.15 and 126.23), which are commonly affected. Sparing may occur in shadows cast by sideburns, spectacles, hairline, deep skin creases on the forehead, under the nose, chin (Figure 126.16a) and lower lip, behind the ears (Wilkinson triangle) (Figure 126.15c, d) and on the upper eyelids. The dorsa of hands, especially the thenar (Figures 126.4d, 126.14d, 126.20a, 126.26 and 126.27c), and feet (Figures 126.4f, 126.30b and 126.30c) and the extensor surfaces of the limbs may also be involved (Figures 126.4d, 126.6, 126.15a and 126.20b). In these locations, there may be sparing of the web spaces and distal phalanges of the fingers and under watch straps (Figure 126.4d and 126.20b), rings (Figure 126.20a) and footwear (Figures 126.4f and 126.30b, c). If covered sites are affected this is usually to a lesser extent. The distribution and nature of the eruption are important – for example, is it papulovesicular (Figures 126.3, 126.4 and 126.8) as in PLE or JSE; eczematous as in CAD (Figure 126.13c, 126.14 and 126.15); is there fragility as in PCT or pseudoporphyria; are there associated features, such as cheilitis (Figure 126.10b) and conjunctivitis in AP (Figure 126.10a)? Even if the patient does not have active disease at the time of examination it is important to look for scarring, such as in HV (Figure 126.23c), EPP, PCT or AP; other relevant signs include lentigines and/or hypopigmented macules in the earlier stages of XP, with premalignant dysplastic changes and skin cancer as the disease progresses, and pigmentation in drug photosensitivity (Figures 126.27 and 126.28). It is also important to be aware that skin reddening may be less obvious in patients with skin phototypes IV–VI and that in patients with skin phototype V and VI, a dermatitis may more commonly present with a papular, lichenoid or nodular prurigo-type morphology than would otherwise be the case in patients of lower skin phototypes.

Differential diagnosis

Based on the clinical assessment through history and examination it should be possible to have a good idea of diagnosis, or at least a narrow differential diagnosis. However, it is usually not possible to have absolute confidence in the diagnosis on clinical grounds and patients with suspected photosensitivity should be referred for further investigation.

Investigation

Investigation is usually undertaken at specialist photodiagnostic centres because quality control of the optical equipment used for phototesting, with calibrated metering and spectroradiometry, is essential [1,2,3,4,5,6–8]. The investigations undertaken will be tailored to the patient's presentation and suspected diagnosis.

Narrow-waveband phototesting. The mainstay investigation is narrow-waveband testing, typically monochromator phototesting, which employs a filtered high-pressure xenon arc lamp to deliver relatively monochromatic UV and visible light across the solar spectrum, at very precise dose ranges, to skin on the back (Figure 126.31a) [1,2,3,4]. Phototesting is usually feasible in children as well if there is sufficient space on the back and they can sit still for the necessary time (Figure 126.31b); even babies can undergo limited testing (Figure 126.31c). Immediate and delayed erythemal responses are assessed based on the MEDs at each waveband and are compared with normal population data. MEDs below the normal range indicate abnormal photosensitivity. It is thus important that the normal range data used are those relevant to the skin phototype distribution of the local population [9,10–12]. It is also important to be aware that skin reddening induced on phototesting may be less obvious in patients of skin phototypes IV–VI and that good lighting and the angle of the lighting are critical. Furthermore, palpation of phototest sites is essential as just palpable subtle oedema without obvious reddening may be the only indicator of abnormal responses on phototesting in patients of higher skin phototypes. Phototesting enables a diagnosis of abnormal photosensitivity to be made and provides information on wavelength dependency and degree of photosensitivity. In general, the 24 h MEDs are the main assessment point, but for SU the immediate MUDs would be defined. The morphology of phototesting responses is important, for example in CAD these become eczematous. Thus, the diagnosis can be confirmed.

Phototesting is also an important investigation to be used at follow-up to assess a patient's response to treatment or to ascertain whether the condition has improved spontaneously [13,14].

Iterative provocation testing. Larger area iterative provocation testing, using a broad-band source (often UVA), at a site where rash is provoked with natural sunlight exposure, may induce the dermatosis and can be particularly useful in PLE and AP (Figure 126.32) [15]. Phototesting with a solar simulator may also have a role, particularly if there is limited back space due to disease activity [16]. However, the emission of this source is such that induced skin reddening is mainly due to UVB and it is therefore a cruder screen for photosensitivity, providing less detailed information on which wavelengths are involved. It is important that the emission characteristics of any light source used are well characterised as, for example, the presence of infrared radiation may influence the ease of photodermatosis provocation [17].

Other phototesting methods. If phototherapy is to be considered, it is always recommended that the MED (or MPD for PUVA) for a light source (e.g. narrow-band UVB) is determined to exclude abnormal photosensitivity (Figure 126.33). It has recently been identified that compact fluorescent lamps, which have replaced tungsten filament sources for internal lighting, emit more UV and pose a risk for severely light-sensitive patients (Figure 126.34) [18–21]. Phototesting can be undertaken with these sources to define risk for an individual patient, although it is not used routinely.

Photopatch and patch testing. If a patient has a photo-exposed site eczematous eruption and/or is also suspected to have contact allergic dermatitis, then patch and photopatch testing should additionally be undertaken. Thus, patch testing is an essential investigation for a patient with CAD. Photopatch testing is undertaken

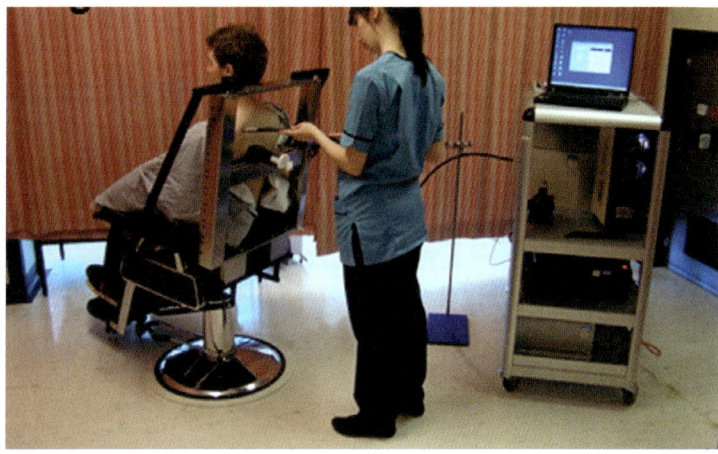

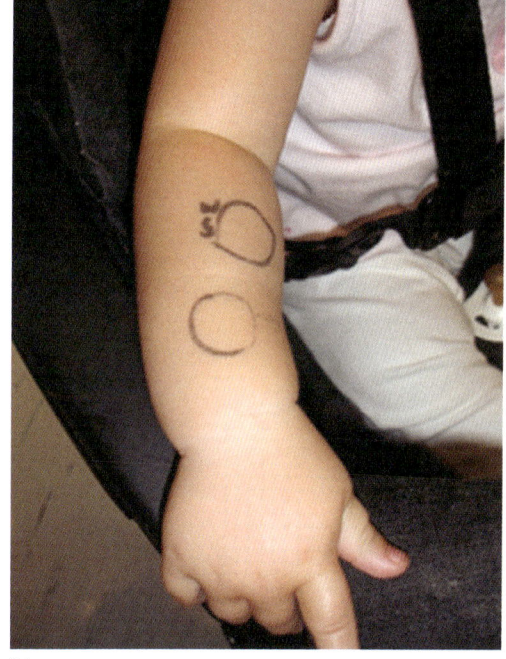

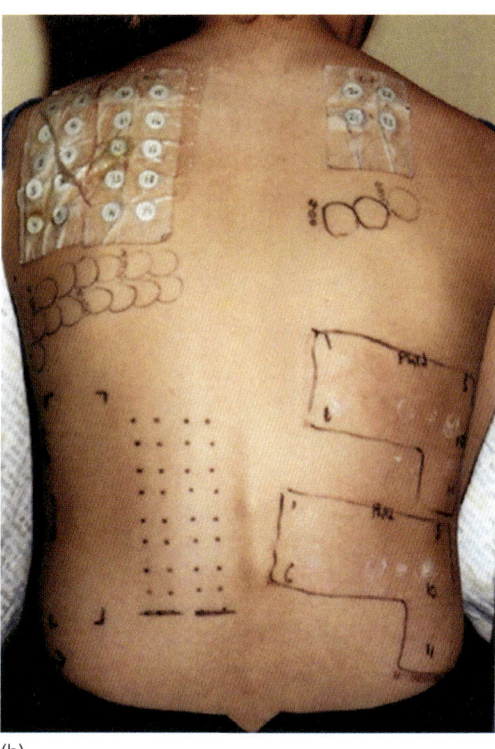

Figure 126.31 (a) Monochromator phototesting using a fibreoptic light guide. (b, c) Phototesting and other photo-investigations should be possible in most children. The amount of testing that is feasible will be influenced by how long they can sit still or sleep for and the size of the child's back.

using standardised European methodology to investigate suspected photocontact allergy (Figure 126.30) [22–25,26,27], which may mimic or complicate other photodermatoses [28]. The commonest photoallergens are sunscreen chemicals and to a lesser extent topical NSAIDs and occasionally topical phenothiazines. Further confirmation of this through reports from Europe, North and South America, New Zealand and Thailand indicates that these remain the most prevalent photoallergens, although this requires regular review [29–35]. Photopatch testing should be considered based on clinical presentation and in photosensitive patients, such as those with CAD, who are regular sunscreen users and who develop unexplained deterioration in their condition. In photopatch testing a duplicate series of photoallergens is applied; one set is irradiated 24–48 h later with a suberythemal UVA dose, the readings being undertaken 48 h after irradiation. The value of additional delayed readings at 96 h has not been fully investigated, but may be relevant for some photoallergens [34,35]. This ensures that photocontact allergy, as opposed to contact allergy, is not missed, as some sunscreen chemicals are only allergenic when irradiated. In practice this investigation may be difficult to perform and interpret if the patient is severely photosensitive, but it should be undertaken if possible.

Other investigations. These will be determined by the individual patient's presentation. The exclusion of lupus is important in a patient with suspected photosensitivity, and serology for antinuclear factor and extractable nuclear antigens (anti-SSA (Ro) and anti-SSB (La)) should be determined. When indicated, porphyria

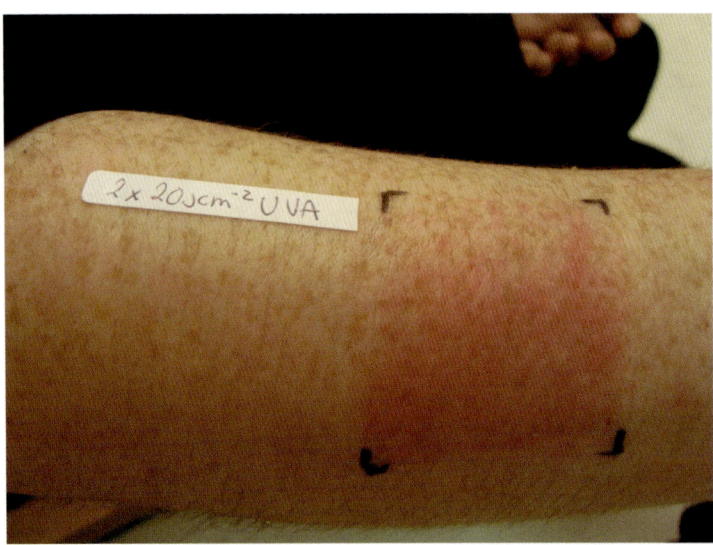

Figure 126.32 Iterative photoprovocation, usually using a broad-band UVA source, can be particularly useful in confirming a diagnosis of polymorphic light eruption, as shown here.

should be excluded, and if there is a low index of clinical suspicion spectrofluorimetry of plasma will usually suffice, with a more detailed quantitative analysis of blood (plasma and red cells), urine and faeces when indicated. If AP is suspected, HLA typing should be requested. The histology of an existing or provoked rash may be informative, for example in HV, but is rarely diagnostic. If a genophotodermatosis is suspected, the necessary skin and blood samples should be taken for DNA repair activity and genetic studies (Chapter 76). Rare disorders with metabolic, biochemical or nutritional abnormalities may also occasionally need to be ruled out, such as with amino acidurias, Smith–Lemli Opitz syndrome or pellagra. For patients who are strictly photoprotecting due to photosensitivity, vitamin D levels should be measured and replacement advised for those who are deficient (≤ 25 nmol/L).

The ability to undertake deep phenotyping through photodiagnostic investigations guided by the clinical presentation is invaluable in characterising the photodermatoses and has facilitated the identification of new diagnostic entities, such as actinic folliculitis, PLESAPS and broadspectrum abnormal localised photosensitivity syndrome (BALPS) [36,**37**,38].

Management

Photoprotection. The management of a patient with photosensitivity rests on establishing the correct diagnosis and having knowledge of the action spectrum for abnormal photosensitivity. General approaches to photoprotection apply, with emphasis on behavioural modification, seeking out the shade and avoiding direct sun exposure between 11 a.m. and 3 p.m. Patients should be advised that relative exposure can be increased due to reflection from sand, water, snow and lightly coloured pavements and that significant UVR exposure can still occur on cloudy days. Covering up with tightly woven, dark and, if necessary, layered clothing and wearing hats with wide brims is beneficial. Regular and liberal use of broad spectrum high-factor sunscreens applied every 2–3 h

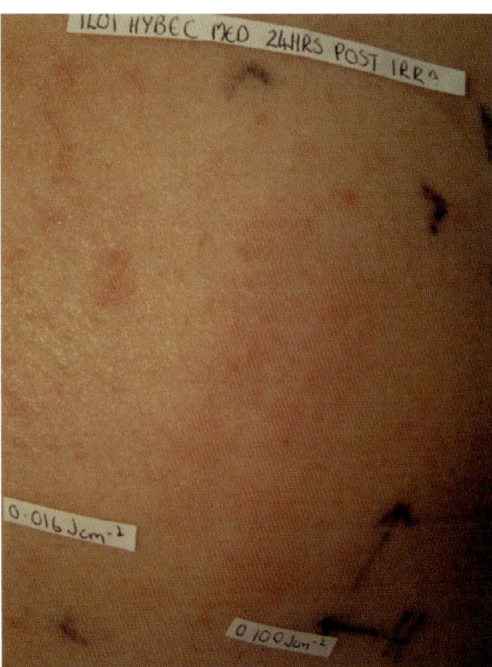

(a)

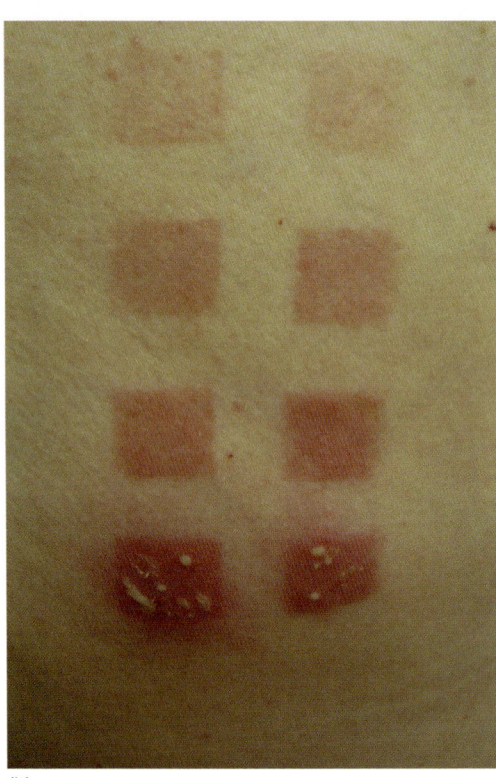

(b)

Figure 126.33 Abnormal erythemal responses on (a) narrow-band UVB (TL-01) MED and (b) psoralen–UVA (PUVA) MPD testing.

is advised. In practice, sunscreens offer 25–33% of the protection stated against normal sunburn, thus an SPF30 will in reality offer SPF10 and patients must be aware of the limitations of sunscreens [39–43]. In particular, advice on sunscreens should be tailored to the nature of the abnormal photosensitivity. For example, if a patient has visible light sensitivity, such as in SU, CAD or a cutaneous

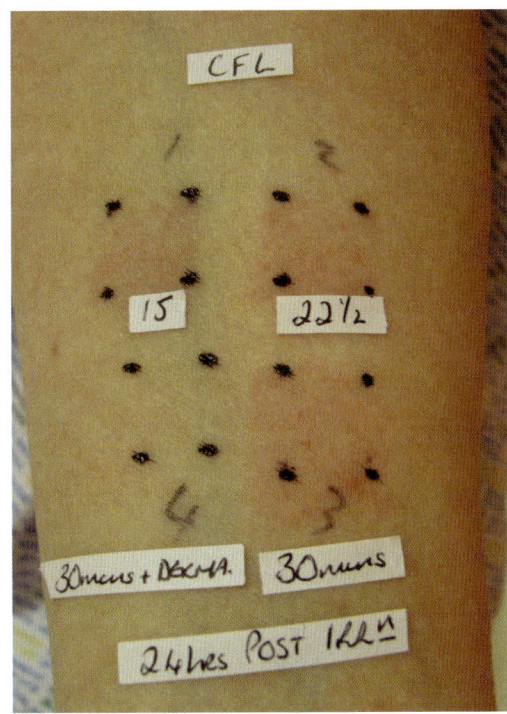

Figure 126.34 Abnormal erythemal responses on phototesting to compact fluorescent lamps. Note the negative response at the site irradiated through window film (Dermagard), which blocks all UV transmission. This patient had chronic actinic dermatitis.

porphyria, the additional use of a reflectant sunscreen (such as Dundee cream, Tayside Pharmaceuticals) that offers additional visible light protection is recommended [44]. For patients with UVA sensitivity, UV-blocking window film that absorbs UVR can be applied to car windows and at home or work [45]. This can lose some of its protection after 5 years due to photodegradation, so may need replacement [46].

Natural hardening. Complete sun avoidance is generally not advisable, other than in XP, as this can have a major adverse impact on health and well-being. In some of the photodermatoses, particularly PLE, threshold photosensitivity can be improved through natural hardening (tolerance), achieved by regular sub-triggering low-level sun exposure.

Vitamin D. Advice should be provided with respect to optimising vitamin D dietary intake and supplements where necessary.

Quality of life. The major adverse impact of photosensitivity on quality of life, particularly when chronic and severe, should not be underestimated and psychological support may be required [47,48]. Recognition and management of anxiety and depression are essential [49,**50**,51].

Overall approach. In general management is subdivided into prevention and treatment, with prevention being the main goal. Active disease should be treated in the conventional way, often using topical glucocorticoids, for example for PLE or CAD suppression.

Light-based therapies. Photo(chemo)therapy may be used in an attempt to induce tolerance, when this is not possible to achieve through natural exposure, and is most commonly used for the idiopathic (immunological) photodermatoses, such as PLE, although it can also be used in other disorders. Knowledge of the characteristics of the abnormal photosensitivity is essential in selecting the most appropriate desensitisation regimen. Systemic therapies, often with immunosuppressants or immunomodulatory agents, may be required in severe disease [52].

Specific therapeutic measures. These are disease-specific and discussed in the relevant sections of this chapter.

Key references

The full list of references can be found in the online version at https://www.wiley.com/rooksdermatology10e

Introduction, Idiopathic (immunological) photodermatoses and polymorphic light eruption

2 Rhodes LE, Bock M, Janssens AS et al. Polymorphic light eruption occurs in 18% of Europeans and does not show higher prevalence with increasing latitude: multicenter survey of 6,895 individuals residing from the Mediterranean to Scandinavia. *J Invest Dermatol* 2010;130:626–8.

18 Richards HL, Ling TC, Evangelou G, Brooke RCC, Fortune DG, Rhodes LE. Evidence of high levels of anxiety and depression in polymorphic light eruption and their association with clinical and demographic variables. *Br J Dermatol* 2008;159:439–44.

30 Frain-Bell W. The idiopathic photodermatoses. In: Frain-Bell W, ed. *Cutaneous Photobiology*. Oxford: Oxford University Press, 1986:24–59.

35 Wadhwani AR, Sharma VK, Ramam M, Khaitan BK. A clinical study of the spectrum of photodermatoses in dark-skinned populations. *Clin Exp Dermatol* 2013;38:823–9.

69 Lembo S, Fallon J, O'Kelly P, Murphy GM. Polymorphic light eruption and skin cancer prevalence: is one protective against the other? *Br J Dermatol* 2008;159:1342–7.

91 Mastalier U, Kerl H, Wolf P. Clinical, laboratory, phototest and phototherapy findings in polymorphic light eruptions: a retrospective study of 133 patients. *Eur J Dermatol* 1998;8:554–9.

102 Man I, Dawe RS, Ferguson J. Artificial hardening for polymorphic light eruption: practical points from ten years' experience. *Photodermatol Photoimmunol Photomed* 1999;15:96–9.

112 Bilsland D, George SA, Gibbs NK, Aitchison T, Johnson BE, Ferguson J. A comparison of narrow-band phototherapy (TL-01) and photochemotherapy (PUVA) in the management of polymorphic light eruption. *Br J Dermatol* 1993;129:708–12.

124 Orekoya O, Rhodes LE, Osman JE, Webb AR, Farrar MD. A qualitative study of knowledge, behaviour and attitudes regarding vitamin D acquisition among patients with photosensitivity disorders. *Photodermatol Photoimmunol Photomed* 2020;36:378–83.

132 Gruber-Wackernagel A, Hofer A, Legat F, Wolf P. Frequency of occurrence of polymorphic light eruption in patients treated with photohardening and patients treated with phototherapy for other diseases. *Photodermatol Photoimmunol Photomed* 2019;35:100–5.

Juvenile springtime eruption

1 Lava SA, Simonetti GD, Ragazzi M, Guarino Gubler S, Bianchetti MG. Juvenile spring eruption: an outbreak report and systematic review of the literature. *Br J Dermatol* 2013;168:1066–72.

2 Anderson D, Wallace HJ, Howes EI. Juvenile spring eruption. *Lancet* 1954;266(6815):755–6.

3 Berthjones J, Norris PG, Grahambrown RAC, Burns DA. Juvenile spring eruption of the ears. *Clin Exp Dermatol* 1989;14:462–3.

4 Requena L, Alegre V, Hasson A. Spring eruption of the ears. *Int J Dermatol* 1990;29:284–6.

5 Kılıç Sayar, S. Juvenile spring eruption among soldiers: a report of a large outbreak. *Australas J Dermatol* 2021;62:e265–6.
6 Tan E, Eberhart-Phillips J, Sharples K. Juvenile spring eruption: a prevalence study. *N Z Med J* 1996;109(1027):293–5.
7 Heathcote K, Theaker JM, Gibbins N, Healy E, Heathcote GB, Friedmann PS. 'Lambing ears': a blistering disorder affecting farmers at lambing time. *Br J Dermatol* 2008;158:134–7.
8 Stratigos AJ, Antoniou C, Papadakis P et al. Juvenile spring eruption: clinicopathologic features and phototesting results in 4 cases. *J Am Acad Dermatol* 2004;50(Suppl.):S57–60.
10 Kreuter A, Koushk Jalali B, Tigges C, Silling S, Lehmann P, Wieland U. Juvenile spring eruption associated with parvovirus B19 infection. *JAMA Dermatol* 2018;154:1356–7.
11 Pérez-Carmona L, Vaño-Galvan S, Carrillo-Gijón R, Jaén-Olasolo P. Photosensitive erythema multiforme presenting as juvenile spring eruption. *Photodermatol Photoimmunol Photomed* 2010;26:53–4.

Actinic prurigo
1 Addo HA, Frain-Bell W. Actinic prurigo – a specific photodermatosis? *Photodermatol* 1984;1:119–28.
6 Macfarlane L, Hawkey S, Naasan H, Ibbotson S. Characteristics of actinic prurigo in Scotland: 24 cases seen between 2001 and 2015. *Br J Dermatol* 2016;174:1411–14.
7 Pardo-Zamudio AC, Valbuena MC, Jiménez-Torres HD, Colmenares-Mejía CC. Actinic prurigo in a dermatological reference center in Colombia: 108 cases. *Biomedica* 2020;40:487–97.
21 Sheridan DP, Lane PR, Irvine J, Martel MJ, Hogan DJ. HLA typing in actinic prurigo. *J Am Acad Dermatol* 1990;22:1019–23.
22 Duran MM, Bernal J. HLA typing in actinic prurigo. *J Am Acad Dermatol* 1992;26:658.
31 Palmieri T, Arujuna N, Sarkany R, Fassihi H. Efficacy and tolerance profile of thalidomide in photodermatoses: a retrospective analysis of 20 patients with actinic prurigo and lupus erythematosus. *Br J Dermatol* 2019;181(S1):98.
34 Eickstaedt JB, Starke S, Krakora D, Hinshaw M, Arkin LM. Clearance of pediatric actinic prurigo with dupilumab. *Pediatr Dermatol* 2020;37:1176–8.
37 Collins P, Ferguson J. Narrow-band UVB (TL-01) phototherapy – an effective preventative treatment for the photodermatoses. *Br J Dermatol* 1995;132:956–63.
38 Farr PM, Diffey BL. Treatment of actinic prurigo with PUVA: mechanism of action. *Br J Dermatol* 1989;120:411–18.
52 Crouch R, Foley P, Baker C. Actinic prurigo: a retrospective analysis of 21 cases referred to an Australian photobiology clinic. *Australas J Dermatol* 2002;45:128–32.

Chronic actinic dermatitis
2 Ibbotson S, Dawe RS. Chronic actinic dermatitis. In: Lebwohl MG, Heymann WR, Coulson I, Murrell D, eds. *Treatment of Skin Disease*, 6th edn. Philadelphia: Elsevier, 2021:154–7.
4 Norris PG, Hawk JLM. Chronic actinic dermatitis – a unifying concept. *Arch Dermatol* 1990;126:376–8.
7 Frain-Bell W, Lakshmipathi T, Rogers J, Willock J. The syndrome of chronic photosensitivity dermatitis and actinic reticuloid. *Br J Dermatol* 1974;91:617–34.
15 Tan K, Haylett AK, Ling TC, Rhodes LE. Comparison of demographic and photobiological features of chronic actinic dermatitis in patients with lighter vs darker skin types. *JAMA Dermatol* 2017;153:427–35.
28 Dawe RS, Crombie IK, Ferguson J. The natural history of chronic actinic dermatitis. *Arch Dermatol* 2000;136:1215–20.
30 Menage H, Ross JS, Norris PG, Hawk JL, White IR. Contact and photocontact sensitization in chronic actinic dermatitis: sesquiterpene lactone mix is an important allergen. *Br J Dermatol* 1995;132:543–7.
32 Pappert A, Grossman M, DeLeo V. Photosensitivity as the presenting illness in 4 patients with human immunodeficiency viral infection. *Arch Dermatol* 1994;130:618–23.
66 Bilsland D, Crombie IK, Ferguson J. The photosensitivity dermatitis and actinic reticuloid syndrome – no association with lymphoreticular malignancy. *Br J Dermatol* 1994;131:209–14.
72 Rizwan M, Reddick CL, Bundy C, Unsworth R, Richards HL, Rhodes LE. Photodermatoses: environmentally induced conditions with high psychological impact. *Photochem Photobiol Sci* 2013;12:182–9.
82 O'Reilly FM, McKenna D, Murphy GM. Is monochromatic irradiation testing useful in the differentiation of drug-induced photosensitivity from chronic actinic dermatitis? *Clin Exp Dermatol* 1999;24:118–21.
136 Chee SN, Novakovic L, Fassihi H, Garibaldinos T, Sarkany R. Chronic actinic dermatitis: successful treatment with psoralen-ultraviolet A photochemotherapy. *Br J Dermatol* 2018;178:e189–90.
144 Murphy GM, Maurice PDL, Norris PG, Morris RW, Hawk JLM. Azathioprine treatment in chronic actinic dermatitis – a double-blind controlled trial with monitoring of exposure to ultraviolet-radiation. *Br J Dermatol* 1989;121:639–46.

Solar urticaria
3 Beattie PE, Dawe RS, Ibbotson SH, Ferguson J. Characteristics and prognosis of idiopathic solar urticaria – a cohort of 87 cases. *Arch Dermatol* 2003;139:1149–54.
15 Uetsu N, Miyauchi-Hashimoto H, Okamoto H, Horio T. The clinical and photobiological characteristics of solar urticaria in 40 patients. *Br J Dermatol* 2000;142:32–8.
26 Haylett AK, Koumaki D, Rhodes LE. Solar urticaria in 145 patients: assessment of action spectra and impact on quality of life in adults and children. *Photodermatol Photoimmunol Photomed* 2018;34:262–8.
48 Uetsu N, Nomura Y, Matsuyama Y, Okamoto H. Characteristics and clinical significance of augmentation spectra in solar urticaria. *J Dermatol* 2020;47:369–77.
50 de Galvez MV, Aguilera J, Sanchez-Roldan C, Herrera-Ceballos E. Infrared radiation increases skin damage induced by other wavelengths in solar urticaria. *Photodermatol Photoimmunol Photomed* 2016;32:284–90.
69 Calzavara-Pinton P, Sala R, Venturini M et al. Local angioedema following sun exposures: a report of five cases. *Int Arch Allergy Immunol* 2010;153:315–20.
93 Rizwan M, Reddick CL, Bundy C, Unsworth R, Richards HL, Rhodes LE. Photodermatoses: environmentally induced conditions with high psychological impact. *Photochem Photobiol Sci* 2013;12:182–9.
110 Calzavara-Pinton P, Zane C, Rossi M, Sala R, Venturini M. Narrowband ultraviolet B phototherapy is a suitable treatment option for solar urticaria. *J Am Acad Dermatol* 2012;67:e5–9.
153 Morgado-Carrasco D, Giácaman-Von der Weth M, Fustá-Novell X, Podlipnik S, Pérez-Ferriols A, Aguilera P. Clinical response and long-term follow-up of 20 patients with refractory solar urticaria under treatment with omalizumab. *J Am Acad Dermatol* 2023;88(5):1110–11.
156 Snast I, Kremer N, Lapidoth M et al. Omalizumab for the treatment of solar urticaria: case series and systematic review of the literature. *J Allergy Clin Immunol Pract* 2018;6:1198–204.
159 Griffin LL, Haylett AK, Rhodes LE. Evaluating patient responses to omalizumab in solar urticaria. *Photodermatol Photoimmunol Photomed* 2019;35:57–65.

Hydroa vacciniforme
2 Gupta G, Man I, Kemmett D. Hydroa vacciniforme: a clinical and follow-up study of 17 cases. *J Am Acad Dermatol* 2000;42:208–13.
3 Sonnex TS, Hawk JLM. Hydroa vacciniforme: a review of ten cases. *Br J Dermatol* 1988;118:101–8.
8 Livideanu CB, Lamant L, Calonje E et al. Purpuric lesions induced by UVA1 spectrum (340–400 nm) phototesting in an adult with persistent and severe hydroa vacciniforme. *Photodermatol Photoimmunol Photomed* 2010;26:104–6.
29 Chen C-C, Chang K-C, Medeiros LJ, Lee JY-Y. Hydroa vacciniforme and hydroa vacciniforme-like lymphoproliferative disorder: a spectrum of disease phenotypes associated with ultraviolet irradiation and chronic Epstein–Barr virus infection. *Int J Mol Sci* 2020;21:9314.
31 Liu Y, Ma C, Wang G, Wang L. Hydroa vacciniforme-like lymphoproliferative disorder: clinicopathologic study of 41 cases. *J Am Acad Dermatol* 2019;81:534–40.
42 Eramo LR, Garden JM, Esterly NB. Hydroa vacciniforme: diagnosis by repetitive ultraviolet-a phototesting. *Arch Dermatol* 1986;122:1310–13.
50 Zeng R, Du L, Wang D. Ocular involvement preceded the onset of cutaneous lesions in hydroa vacciniforme-like lymphoproliferative disorder: a case report. *Ocul Immunol Inflamm* 2022;30:320–3.
61 Huggins RH, Leithauser LA, Eide MJ, Hexsel CL, Jacobsen G, Lim HW. Quality of life assessment and disease experience of patient members of a web-based hydroa vacciniforme support group. *Photodermatol Photoimmunol Photomed* 2010;25:209–15.
64 Collins P, Ferguson J. Narrow-band UVB (TL-01) phototherapy – an effective preventative treatment for the photodermatoses. *Br J Dermatol* 1995;132:956–63.

Drug- and chemical-induced photosensitivity
Exogenous drug- and chemical-induced photosensitivity
8 Ibbotson S. Drug and chemical induced photosensitivity from a clinical perspective. *Photochem Photobiol Sci* 2018;17:1885–903.

12 Kim WB, Shelley AJ, Novice K, Joo J, Lim HW, Glassman SJ. Drug-induced phototoxicity: a systematic review. *J Am Acad Dermatol* 2018;79:1069–75.

15 Alrashidi A, Rhodes LE, Sharif JCH, Kreeshan FC, Farrar MD, Ahad T. Systemic drug photosensitivity – culprits, impact and investigation in 122 patients. *Photodermatol Photoimmunol Photomed* 2020;36:441–51.

22 Tolland JP, Murphy BP, Boyle J, Hall V, McKenna KE, Elborn JS. Ciprofloxacin-induced phototoxicity in an adult cystic fibrosis population. *Photodermatol Photoimmunol Photomed* 2012;28:258–60.

32 Kerr AC, Ferguson J, Haylett AK et al. A European multicentre Photopatch Test Study (EMCPPTS). *Br J Dermatol* 2012;166:1002–9.

45 Dawe RS, Ibbotson SH, Sanderson JB, Thomson EM, Ferguson J. A randomized controlled trial (volunteer study) of sitafloxacin, enoxacin, levofloxacin and sparfloxacin phototoxicity. *Br J Dermatol* 2003;149:1232–41.

54 Haylett AK, Felton S, Denning DW, Rhodes LE. Voriconazole-induced photosensitivity: photobiological assessment of a case series of 12 patients. *Br J Dermatol* 2013;168:179–85.

80 Ciccolini KT, Kim J, Chaudhari SP et al. Incidence and risk of developing photosensitivity with targeted anticancer therapies. *J Am Acad Dermatol* 2019;81:1009–11.

82 Lembo S, Raimondo A, Conti V, Venturini M. Photosensitivity and cancer immune-targeted therapies. *Photodermatol Photoimmunol Photomed* 2020;36:172–8.

135 Adalsteinsson JA, Muzumdar S, Waldman R et al. Association between hydrochlorothiazide and the risk of in situ and invasive squamous cell skin carcinoma and basal cell carcinoma: a population-based case-control study. *J Am Acad Dermatol* 2021;84:669–75.

137 O'Gorman SM, Murphy GM. Photosensitizing medications and photocarcinogenesis. *Photodermatol Photoimmunol Photomed* 2014;30:8–14.

151 O'Reilly FM, McKenna D, Murphy GM. Is monochromatic irradiation testing useful in the differentiation of drug-induced photosensitivity from chronic actinic dermatitis? *Clin Exp Dermatol* 1999;24:118–21.

159 Collins P, Ferguson J. Narrow-band UVB (TL-01) phototherapy – an effective preventative treatment for the photodermatoses. *Br J Dermatol* 1995;132:956–63.

Photoaggravated dermatoses

1 Dawe R. Photoaggravated dermatoses. In: Ferguson J, Dover J, eds. *Photodermatology*. London: Manson Publishing, 2006:57–65.

9 ten Berge O, van Weelden H, Bruijnzeel-Koomen CAFM, de Bruin-Weller MS, Sigurdsson V. Throwing a light on photosensitivity in atopic dermatitis: a retrospective study. *Am J Clin Dermatol* 2009;10:119–23.

16 Rutter KJ, Watson REB, Cotterell LF, Brenn T, Griffiths CEM, Rhodes LE. Severely photosensitive psoriasis: a phenotypically defined patient subset. *J Invest Dermatol* 2009;129:2861–7.

19 Ellenbogen E, Wesselmann U, Hofmann SC, Lehmann P. Photosensitive atopic dermatitis – a neglected subset: clinical, laboratory, histological and photobiological workup. *J Eur Acad Dermatol Venereol* 2016;30:270–5.

25 Trokoudes D, Banerjee P, Fityan A et al. Photoaggravated contact dermatitis caused by methylisothiazolinone. *Contact Derm* 2017;76:303–4.

26 Adler BL, Houle MC, Pratt M. Photoaggravated contact dermatitis to methylisothiazolinone and associated photosensitivity: a case series. *Dermatitis* 2022;33:e60–3.

39 Foering K, Chang AY, Piette EW, Cucchiara A, Okawa J, Werth VP. Characterization of clinical photosensitivity in cutaneous lupus erythematosus. *J Am Acad Dermatol* 2013;69:205–13.

49 Wadhwani AR, Sharma VK, Ramam M, Khaitan BK. A clinical study of the spectrum of photodermatoses in dark-skinned populations. *Clin Exp Dermatol* 2013;38:823–9.

70 Evangelou G, Murdoch SR, Palamaras I, Rhodes LE. Photoaggravated pityriasis rubra pilaris. *Photodermatol Photoimmunol Photomed* 2005;21:272–4.

Clinical assessment and management of a patient with suspected photosensitivity

2 Naasan H, Dawe RS, Moseley H, Ibbotson SH. A review of photodiagnostic investigations over 26 years: experience of the National Scottish Photobiology Service (1989–2015). *J R Coll Physicians Edinb* 2017;47:345–50.

4 MacKenzie LA, Frain-Bell W. The construction and development of a grating monochromator and its application to the study of the reaction of the skin to light. *Br J Dermatol* 1973;89:251–64.

5 O'Reilly FM, McKenna D, Murphy GM. Is monochromatic irradiation testing useful in the differentiation of drug-induced photosensitivity from chronic actinic dermatitis? *Clin Exp Dermatol* 1999;24:118–21.

9 Welti M, Ramelyte E, Dummer R, Imhof L. Evaluation of the minimal erythema dose for UVB and UVA in context of skin phototype and nature of photodermatosis. *Photodermatol Photoimmunol Photomed* 2020;36:200–7.

17 de Gálvez MV, Aguilera J, Sánchez-Roldán C, Herrera-Acosta E, Herrera-Ceballos E. Water-filtered infrared radiation decreases the generation of photodermatoses dependent on ultraviolet and visible radiation. *Photochem Photobiol* 2019;95:874–8.

26 Kerr AC, Ferguson J, Haylett AK et al. A European Multicentre Photopatch Test Study (EMCPPTS). *Br J Dermatol* 2012;166:1002–9.

37 Butt S, Khalid A, Alani A et al. Broadspectrum abnormal localised photosensitivity syndrome. *J Am Acad Dermatol* 2021;85:1298–300.

44 Petersen B, Thieden E, Philipsen PA, Heydenreich J, Young AR, Wulf HC. A sun holiday is a sunburn holiday. *Photodermatol Photoimmunol Photomed* 2013;29:221–4.

50 Rizwan M, Reddick CL, Bundy C, Unsworth R, Richards HL, Rhodes LE. Photodermatoses: environmentally induced conditions with high psychological impact. *Photochem Photobiol Sci* 2013;12:182–9.

CHAPTER 127

Allergic Contact Dermatitis

David Orton[1] and Natalie Stone[2]

[1] OneWelbeck Skin Health and Allergy, London, UK
[2] Aneurin Bevan University Health Board, Newport, Wales, UK

Introduction, 127.1
Allergic contact dermatitis, 127.2
Specific allergens, 127.36
Metals, 127.36
Fragrances, balsams, flavouring agents and spices, 127.41
Applied medicaments, 127.45
Cosmetics, 127.47

Antimicrobial agents and preservatives, 127.49
Vehicles and other cosmetic excipients, 127.58
p-Phenylenediamine and related dyes, 127.60
Methacrylate nail systems, 127.61
Ultraviolet filters, 127.62
Rubber, 127.62
Clothing, 127.65

Shoes, 127.67
Resins and plastics, 127.68
Plants, 127.71
Woods, colophony, turpentine and propolis, 127.74
Photoallergic contact dermatitis, 127.78
Allergic contact urticaria, 127.82
Key references, 127.86

Introduction

Contact dermatitis is a subspecialty of dermatology dealing with environmental and occupational dermatoses, including both irritant and allergic types.

The term 'allergie' was first coined by the scientist von Pirquet in 1906 [1,2]. The word was derived from the Greek *allos* and *ergon*, meaning other or different work [3]. However, idiosyncratic reactions to various substances had been recognised since the 17th century [2]. In 1829, Dakin observed the selectivity of *Rhus* dermatitis [4] and Fuchs suggested that 'dermatitis venenata' was an expression of constitutional idiosyncrasy in 1840 [5]. The word 'idiosyncrasy' was again applied by Neisser in his descriptions of iodoform dermatitis in 1884 [6].

Allergic sensitisation of the skin was first proved experimentally by Bloch and Steiner-Woerlich using *Primula* extract on human skin [7]. Thereafter, research on the pathogenesis of allergic dermatitis has largely involved animal experiments using guinea pigs. Landsteiner and Jacobs [8] performed a basic experiment that showed that a simple chemical capable of causing contact dermatitis must be combined with proteins in order to sensitise. Up to 1940 it was not known whether sensitisation depended on a factor localised in the skin, but in 1942 Landsteiner and Chase [9] succeeded in transmitting sensitivity from one guinea pig to another by the use of a mainly mononuclear peritoneal exudate from sensitised guinea pigs. In the same year, Haxthausen's transplantation experiments [10] finally proved that allergy was due to a factor supplied to the skin from within.

Patch testing is the tool for diagnosing allergic dermatitis and Josef Jadassohn is generally accepted as the founder of this technique in 1895, while working at Breslau University, publication taking place the following year [11]. Nevertheless, anecdotal observations of a similar nature had been made prior to this, usually by applying the suspected causative agent to intact skin [12]. By 1847 Stadeler had developed a rudimentary patch test using blotting paper to reproduce lesions provoked by *Anacardium occidentale* [13].

Bruno Bloch was a dermatological pioneer who was able to expand and enhance Jadassohn's technique while working in Basel in 1911, when he produced a grading system for patch test reactions [14]. He then moved to Zurich where he introduced the concept of a standard series of allergens [15]. He furthermore conceived important ideas about both cross-sensitisation and systemic allergic contact dermatitis [1]. Marion Sulzberger had been an assistant to both Bloch and Jadassohn before returning to New York where he introduced the patch test technique and was a strong advocate and promoter of its use in the USA. Another former assistant of Bloch's, Paul Bonnevie, Professor of Occupational Medicine in Copenhagen, expanded the standard series to what could be considered the prototype of our present-day series.

By the early 1960s, Scandinavian dermatologists were developing a standardised protocol for patch testing and their group was expanded to involve, initially, other European members before it finally evolved into the International Contact Dermatitis Research Group (ICDRG) [1]. The group disseminated an informal newsletter among interested parties for 8 years which culminated in the first 2-day international symposium on contact dermatitis held in Copenhagen in 1974. The group was also pivotal in the foundation of the specialist journal, *Contact Dermatitis*, first published in 1975 with Dr Charles Calnan as Editor.

The European Environmental and Contact Dermatitis Research Group (EECDRG) was founded in 1984, having its first meeting in the UK 1 year later, during 1985. Its initial goals were the

---

Rook's Textbook of Dermatology, Tenth Edition. Edited by Christopher Griffiths, Jonathan Barker, Tanya Bleiker, Walayat Hussain and Rosalind Simpson.
© 2024 John Wiley & Sons Ltd. Published 2024 by John Wiley & Sons Ltd.

formation of the European Society of Contact Dermatitis, conducting joint studies to help validate the allergens in various patch test series, the publication of a new textbook in the field of contact dermatitis and writing review articles for *Contact Dermatitis*.

Further national and international research groups have proliferated during the last 30 years – a fitting recognition of the significance of the findings and research of these pioneers [16].

Allergic contact dermatitis

Definition and nomenclature

Allergic contact dermatitis is an eczematous reaction that occurs as an immunological response following exposure to a substance to which the immune system has previously been sensitised.

Synonyms and inclusions
- Contact allergy
- Allergic contact eczema

Introduction and general description

Contact allergy is caused by skin contact with low-molecular-weight haptens and may evolve into allergic contact dermatitis if exposure exceeds the individual threshold.

The diagnosis of allergic contact dermatitis can only be confirmed by patch testing and should always be used to exclude contact allergy as a complicating factor in stubborn cases of eczematous diseases, as well as cases where allergic contact dermatitis is suspected from the pattern or distribution of the eczema. During the last few decades much effort has been put into the standardisation of allergens, vehicles, concentrations, tapes and the scoring of test reactions. Despite this, both the investigator's knowledge and experience are crucial factors in providing accurate information to patients.

Constant surveillance allows for trends to be determined and for epidemics to be recognised, which in turn have shaped the response of regulatory authorities. Examples of this include the epidemics of biocide contact dermatitis caused by methyl dibromoglutaronitrile and methylisothiazolinone resulting in the withdrawal and partial withdrawal, respectively, of such chemicals from cosmetics.

Allergens exist in the home environment and the occupational setting. Prevention strategies include primary, secondary and tertiary prevention. In primary prevention the focus is on minimising the risk of inducing sensitisation in workers and consumers. Secondary and tertiary prevention aims at reducing the risk of elicitation and morbidity among those with dermatitis. In the workplace, primary prevention includes pre-employment screening, minimising contact between allergens and the skin, and education to employees in at-risk occupations. These strategies have all been reported as effective.

The quantitative risk assessment (QRA) procedure currently developed by the cosmetic industry for fragrances as a means of evaluating the risk of skin sensitization before market entry (primary prevention) has a major flaw as it is not able to predict the elicitation risk of chemicals. Hence the 'acceptable exposure level' does not protect those already sensitised. About a third of all allergies against cosmetic products are caused by fragrances.

In recent years Europe has successfully implemented a whole set of regulations aimed at reducing the exposure of the workforce and consumers to contact allergens. Examples are the 'Nickel directive' [1] and the 'Chromium directive', [2] and more recently the 2015 European Union (EU) 'Leather regulation' limiting chromium VI (CrVI) exposure from leather articles placed on EU markets. The directive on detergents requires the listing of preservatives and certain fragrances if their content in detergents and similar household products exceeds 100 ppm [3]. Detergents are thus treated as rinse-off cosmetics. Furthermore, details of the product formulation have to be released when necessary, to allow investigation of adverse reactions. Following implementation of the 'Nickel directive', nickel allergy rates among young patients showed a substantial decline in several countries including Germany [4], Sweden [5] and Denmark [6]. In Denmark, the frequency of nickel allergies dropped from 26.9% before the EU directive to 12.4% thereafter [6].

Allergic contact dermatitis to CrVI was recognised as a significant problem in the occupational setting, for example affecting an estimated 17% of cement workers during the construction of the Channel Tunnel connecting Europe with the UK [7]. In 2005, the EU therefore regulated the content of CrVI in cement and sensitisation to chromate in construction workers has since declined [8,9]. However, this regulation does not include leather products such as shoes, where an increasing incidence has been recognised [10].

Product labelling may be one method of handling allergic contact dermatitis but as significant numbers of the sensitised population are unlikely to be diagnosed, and those who are diagnosed may find it difficult to read the labelling and identify the allergens to which they are allergic, this way of preventing allergic contact dermatitis may not be efficient.

It is not the remit of this chapter to detail past *in vivo* systems used to identify potential allergens or to discuss *in vitro* tests being developed to replace them. However, all these systems require validation, not only against other methods but also against human observational data from clinical epidemiological surveillance systems. Such validation is the gold standard for any predictive safety assessment.

In this context, clinical data and the epicutaneous patch test, as described by Jadassohn over 100 years ago [11], remain invaluable, as they continue to highlight substances and problems missed by other approaches.

Epidemiology [1]
Incidence and prevalence

Methodologies. Epidemiological studies may be undertaken on the general population or on selected groups, for example those referred for patch testing or those with a specific occupation. Follow-up studies select individuals on the basis of the presence or absence of a defined risk factor such as 'wet work'. The relative risk of developing hand dermatitis can then be calculated as the ratio of those developing dermatitis in the exposed population compared with the unexposed population. The attributable risk is the difference in incidence rates between the two populations. Case–control studies select individuals based on the presence or absence of a particular disease. By comparing the frequency of exposure to a factor such as 'wet work' in the two populations, an odds ratio can be calculated that expresses the relative contribution of the exposure to the development of the disease. In such studies the choice of controls is critical if the results are not to be biased. In cross-sectional studies, all individuals are studied irrespective of exposure or disease status (in contrast with the above).

Data collection. The method of data collection in studies on the general population, which need to be large to gain useful information and are challenging to perform, can significantly influence the results. For reasons of expediency, questionnaires have been used, but when performed alone will underestimate those suffering from dermatitis because accuracy of recall fades with time. The validity of the results also depends on the extent to which those who respond to the questionnaire differ from those who do not. As a rough guide, studies in which the response rate is below 70% may be unrepresentative.

Population assessments concerning individuals attending a general practitioner or referred to a dermatologist may be unreliable, particularly in the UK where prompt access to a dermatologist is limited. In a UK survey, only 21% of individuals with skin disease thought to justify medical care had seen their general practitioner about the condition in the previous 6 months [2]. In another large-scale study of a Swedish population of over 107 000, only 50% of the patients with dermatitis had seen a doctor within the previous year [3].

The reporting of contact dermatitis also varies according to the method of collection and the type of person collecting the data. Results from the UK EPIDERM occupational dermatoses surveillance study show how reports of occupational dermatoses differ according to whether the returns are made by dermatologists or by occupational health physicians (Table 127.1) [4]. The differences probably reflect the different types of occupational population accessed by the two groups. Occupational physicians will relate to large industries and collective working groups, whereas dermatologists will mainly receive individual referrals, accounting for the comparatively high representation of, for example, hairdressers, florists and beauticians seen by them.

Case definition. Studies of the epidemiology of dermatitis may be further confounded by the fact that it is commonly multifactorial in origin. It is therefore difficult to analyse the relative prevalence of irritant versus allergic contact dermatitis because the two commonly coexist, and constitutional eczema may also be involved. Ideally, all those studied should be examined and patch tested, but this is not always a practical proposition when large numbers of an unselected group are being assessed.

Standardisation. Apparent differences in overall sensitisation frequencies may be due to differences in population structure, especially in relation to age and sex. This can be compensated for, either by using standardised populations or by reporting results within specified age bands, and by reporting results for each sex separately. However, in a particular clinic the incidence of allergic contact dermatitis is reflected not only by the sex and age of the patients but also by the industrial development in the area and the degree of interest dermatologists take in the various facets of contact dermatitis (e.g. occupational dermatitis, medicament allergy, leg ulcers). Furthermore, local prescribing habits can influence patch test results. It has been suggested that all comparative patch test data should include an analysis of patient details – the MOAHLFA index (where M is the percentage of males tested, O is percentage occupational, A is percentage of atopics, H is percentage with hand eczema, L is percentage with leg ulcers or stasis eczema, F is percentage with facial eczema and A those aged over 40 years) [5]. The percentage of atopics is important, particularly in relation to irritant contact dermatitis. Certain body sites, especially the lower legs in those with stasis eczema or leg ulcers and the ears, eyelids and perineum, have a particularly high level of allergic contact dermatitis from medicaments; and facial eczema from higher levels of cosmetic allergens. Inclusion of a significant number of any such cases in a patch test series will affect the overall sensitivity rates for various allergens. Guidelines for the presentation of contact allergy data have been produced [6].

General population studies. Contact dermatitis is common, accounting for 4–7% of all dermatological consultations [1]. Skin disease, chiefly dermatitis, accounts for almost half of all reported cases of occupational disease. Thyssen *et al.* have reviewed 36 previous studies of hand eczema prevalence in the general population from around the world. They estimated hand eczema to have a point prevalence of 4%, 1-year prevalence of 10% and lifetime prevalence of 15% in the general population. Atopic dermatitis was the single most strongly associated risk factor, followed by female sex, contact allergy and wet work [7].

A recent cross-sectional study analysed data from the general adult population in five different European countries ($n = 12\,377$); 27% were reported to have at least one positive patch test reaction to an allergen on the European baseline, suggesting a diagnosis of contact allergy in one-quarter of the European general population. As with other studies, prevalence was higher in women and nickel the most common allergen. Reactions to thiomersal were, however, included in this study. This is a controversial allergen, causing frequent positive patch test reactions often of no clinical relevance. This may have falsely elevated the contact allergy prevalence figure [8].

A systematic review and meta-analysis has been performed looking at a total of 28 consecutive studies assessing the prevalence of

Table 127.1 Occupational skin disease: estimated rate per 100 000 workers as reported by dermatologists and occupational doctors to EPIDERM (Occupational Dermatoses Surveillance Scheme, University of Manchester).

Reporting group	Rate per 100 000
Dermatologists	
Hairdressers and barbers	116.3
Printers	85.8
Beauticians	76.8
Other chemical operatives	69.1
Window dressers, floral arrangers	68.1
Occupational physicians	
Other chemical operatives	183.8
Glass product and ceramic makers	101.2
Vehicle and metal assemblers	94.8
Engineering labourers	82.4
Machine tool operatives	67.9

contact allergy in the general population over a 10-year period. The studies all looked at unselected individuals, presented absolute percentages of contact allergy, tested with a wide range of haptens, and excluded reactions to thiomersal. Combined, the 28 studies included 20 107 patch-tested individuals. The results gave a pooled allergic contact dermatitis general population prevalence of 20.1%. There was a lower prevalence of 16.5% reported in children and adolescents. In keeping with other studies, contact dermatitis prevalence was significantly higher in women (27.9%) than in men (13.2%). The most common contact allergens in the general population were also in keeping with previous studies, with nickel (11.4%) being the most common, followed by fragrance mix 1 (3.5%), cobalt (2.7%), *Myroxylon pereirae* (1.8%), chromium (1.8%), *p*-phenylenediamine (PPD) (1.5%), methylchloroisothiazolinone/methylisothiazolinone (1.5%) and colophonium (1.3%) [9].

Selected population studies. Most epidemiological studies are based on patients already attending dermatology clinics, or involve either specific occupations or other population groups. The selective nature of patients patch tested in dermatology clinics for the investigation of contact allergy is not necessarily representative of the general population. Nevertheless, the findings may reflect the relative frequency of the causes of allergic contact dermatitis in that population. Patch testing can be used to generate information for individuals, groups of patients and allergens, as well as to assess risk factors in particular subgroups of the population.

Occupational studies. The incidence of occupational dermatitis in most western European countries is in the range of 0.5–1.9 cases per 1000 workers per year; skin diseases account for 13–34% of all occupational diseases and contact dermatitis constitutes 90–95% of this [1]. Risk reflects both constitutional susceptibility (atopy) and exposure. Skin disease is a significant occupational problem, accounting for 5.73 claims per 100 000 workers, with 47% having job tenure of less than 1 year [2710]. The average disability time in this US study was 23.9 days at a cost of $3552 [11]. Twenty-two per cent of occupational skin disease may be attributable to atopy [12].

Occupational disease surveillance and compensation registries identify occupations at high risk of dermatitis (Table 127.1). Most are unable to distinguish between irritant and allergic dermatitis. Some countries have mandatory reporting. In the UK, EPIDERM is a scheme accepting reports made on a voluntary basis from dermatologists and occupational physicians [4]. In a study covering the years 1993–99, 52% of dermatitis cases reported by dermatologists and 30% of those reported by occupational physicians had allergic contact dermatitis as the primary cause or as a contributory factor [20]. The higher rate reported by dermatologists might be a reflection of their more frequent use of patch testing. The most common allergens were rubber chemicals, nickel and epoxy resins. The numbers and proportion of cases of contact dermatitis within occupations remained fairly constant over the 6-year reporting period, although nursing personnel showed an increase, perhaps as a result of increased exposure to agents required to reduce infectious disease transmission. In a recent study of 5265 cases reported to the Finnish register of occupational disease, 42% had irritant contact dermatitis, 35% allergic contact dermatitis, 11% contact urticarial and 9% skin infections (mainly scabies). The total incidence rate of occupational skin disease was 18.8 cases/100 000 person-years [11].

The Covid-19 pandemic has led to a significant surge in occupational dermatoses among health care workers. The first report from Wuhan, China, where Covid-19 is thought to have originated, suggested an enormous 97% of all frontline health care workers to have self-reported skin problems linked with occupational infection control measures [13]. A recent UK-based multicentre audit reported 315 health care workers with occupational dermatoses during the Covid-19 pandemic. The most common diagnosis was irritant contact dermatitis (59%) on a background of atopic eczema present in 40%. This was most commonly seen in nurses and health care assistants requiring frequent hand washing and use of personal protective equipment (PPE). Facial acne/rosacea associated with wearing of masks affected 16%, and 3% reported facial pressure injury due to use of tight-fitting masks, often worn for prolonged periods of time [14]. The Covid-19 pandemic caused an unprecedented, urgent, increased demand for all types of PPE, including gloves, masks and surgical gowns. It is therefore not surprising that, in addition to significant irritant contact dermatitis, the pandemic has also been associated with cases of occupational allergic contact dermatitis. These reports include allergy to isocyanates within the polyurethane sponge strip inside a mask, thiuram in the elastic mask ear straps, formaldehyde within mask materials and aluminium in the mask nose clip [15–18].

Social, cultural and environmental factors

The percentage of patients with positive reactions to many standard test substances remains largely constant [1], and although some allergens such as colophony, thiuram mix and nickel in women have become less common, this has been balanced by an increase in other sensitisers such as *Myroxylon pereirae* and PPD. The prevalence of allergy to specific allergens in patch-tested patients is discussed later in the chapter. It should be noted that the presence of sensitisation does not imply the presence of dermatitis. In addition, variations in the reading or interpretation of patch test results can affect the perceived prevalence of allergic contact dermatitis.

In general, the most common allergens are similar from one country to another, although there are differences in rank order. Some environmental allergens are widely dispersed and the level of sensitivity remains fairly constant, but cosmetics and fragrance materials are becoming increasingly important sources of sensitivity. Medicament allergens, such as benzocaine, neomycin and lanolin, have traditionally been common in all countries. Benzocaine within medicaments is, however, being substituted for lidocaine or cinchocaine in some countries which may lead to differences in allergy rates [2]. There may be differences in prescribing habits even within the same country, which can be reflected by the pattern of medicament sensitisation. For example, corticosteroid allergy has been shown to have a very different profile in Oxford compared with Manchester, UK, by virtue of differences in prescribing habits leading to a greater usage of non-fluorinated corticosteroids in the latter catchment [3].

Young females tend to have more cosmetic and occupational sensitivities. In older people, many sensitivities will be of past relevance only, and there tends to be a higher prevalence of medicament sensitivity. Nickel allergy is more common in women and, unless allowance is made for this, false occupational associations may be inferred. Allergens can come and go [4], with the prevalence of sensitivity to an individual substance depending on many variables, including the selection of individuals tested, exposure levels, fashion, environment, introduction of new materials and loss of others, maximum permitted concentrations and usage.

The incidence and prevalence of allergic reactions will parallel the extent of environmental exposure, and occasionally this may lead to localised 'epidemics' of sensitivity to a particular allergen. Cosmetic and preservative exposure varies from country to country and from region to region, according to the degree of usage. This principle may extend to other allergenic sources, so there is a rationale for each centre and country developing its own epidemiological base.

Patterns also change with fashion, as shown by the virtual disappearance of suspender dermatitis from nickel, which was replaced by an increase in dermatitis from earrings, watches and jeans studs. With the introduction of controls on nickel release from jewellery, the association of ear piercing with nickel allergy was then lost [5]. More recent sources of nickel include mobile phones, lap-top computers and vaping pens [6–8]. Differences in environmental exposures influence the nature of sensitisers; for instance *Toxicodendron* species dermatitis is extremely common in the USA but virtually absent in Europe, whereas *Primula* dermatitis was well recognised in the UK. The introduction of primin-free *Primula* species then led to a decline in primin allergy such that primin has now been removed from the British baseline series. Preservatives show the classic 'Dillarstone effect' with increasing allergy levels with the introduction of new sensitisers such as methylisothiazolinone, with a subsequent decrease on their withdrawal [9,10].

Technological advances have led to new and more widespread exposures to allergens, such as epoxy and acrylic resins in the occupational setting [11], although the potential for contact allergy may be reduced by improved PPE, better containment of sensitising chemicals and allergen substitution. Similarly, in the domestic environment, acrylates are an increasingly common cause of allergy through the popular use of acrylic nail polish. In contrast, phosphorus sesquisulphide is an historic domestic allergen as 'strike anywhere' matches are no longer available.

Cultural factors are important, and not always fully appreciated as a predisposing cause for contact allergy, particularly the use of sensitising traditional herbal medicines and balms to treat skin disorders in the Middle and Far East [12,13]. Furthermore, ingested herbal folk remedies containing *Toxicodendron* have caused outbreaks of systemic allergic contact dermatitis in Korea [14].

Hair dyes are used more commonly by men in the Middle East and the Indian subcontinent, including use on the beard [15]. Indian women may become sensitised to dyes and adhesives used in kumkum and bindis applied to the forehead [16]. Afro-Caribbean hair can require specific hair products for maintenance. The allergen content of products marketed for different hair types have been compared and significant differences found [17].

Age

The process of ageing alters T-cell immunity. The number of patch test positive reactions increases with age [1], likely due to the accumulation of exposure and sensitivities over a lifetime. However, there is a significant age-related decline in the ability to mount a significant immune response to viral infections and vaccinations, termed 'immunosenescence' [2].

Young adults are more likely to have occupation- or cosmetic-related allergies, whereas elderly people are more liable to medicament [3] and 'historic' sensitivities. Children seem to be sensitised as easily as adults, with poison ivy (*Toxicodendron* spp.) dermatitis being very common in American children [4]. Reported lower contact allergy rates in children may be due to the simpler environment of childhood, having less time to develop sensitivities and a reluctance to patch test children. Susceptibility to sensitisation with dinitrochlorobenzene (DNCB) declines after the age of 70 years but is otherwise constant, and sensitivities may fade with time [5].

Lynch *et al*. evaluated the age dependency of positive patch test reactions to allergens in the baseline series in 45 110 patients over a 30-year period. They interestingly suggested three different patterns of allergy trend with age for different allergens. Nickel and cobalt showed a peak incidence in the early twenties and then a subsequent decline, fragrance mix 1 and PPD showed a peak in the late fifties and a third group, including thiuram and fragrance mix 2, showed a progressive increase over time [6]. It is recognised that different haptens are likely to sensitise by different immune pathways [7]. The three age-related allergy patterns could possibly be explained by differences in immunsenescence of different immune pathways.

Contact dermatitis in children seems to be increasing, either because a child's environment is now more complex or dermatologists increasingly patch test younger children. Paediatric patch test series results have been summarised by Goossens and Morren [8]. The increased prevalence of sensitivity in children has been associated with increased exposure to nickel-containing objects and an earlier age of ear piercing [9]. The most common allergens are nickel (especially in girls), fragrance, thimerosal, medicaments, rubber chemicals, chromate and resins in footwear [10]. As previously mentioned, relevance of the high number of reactions to thimerosal remains obscure, but has been blamed on vaccines and inoculations [11]. Nickel allergy rates have, however, fallen significantly particularly in younger patients since the introduction of the European 'Nickel directive' [12]. The use of PPD-contaminated henna tattoos on children has resulted in increasing numbers of cases of contact allergy from this source [13].

Small children pose practical problems with patch testing. There is a limited area to which a series of patch tests can be applied and they may become restless once the tests are applied, creating problems with adhesion. It is advised that more than one session of patch tests should be undertaken if necessary and a stronger adhesive used to keep the patches in place [14]. The use of lower concentrations for certain allergens has been suggested, but most published reports have advocated no change. Removal of the patches can cause significant discomfort for younger children. Medical adhesive remover products can help to minimise traction forces.

Attempts have been made to identify clinical patterns to indicate which children should be patch tested, but recent studies suggest that, like adults, any child with persistent eczema should be considered for patch testing [15,16]. Although an abbreviated standard series based on previous published results has been suggested for children [17], many centres perform a full adult standard series, plus relevant extra tests whenever possible.

Sex

Women have stronger cell-mediated immune responses than men [1,2] and yet, at least experimentally, women do not appear to be more susceptible to sensitisation [3]. However, sensitisation is accomplished more easily with some allergens, for example lanolin, fragrance and PPD, perhaps as a result of prior 'conditioning' exposure and subclinical sensitisation [4]. In one study, women were found to have greater reactivity to DNCB than men [5] whereas, in another, men were more susceptible than women [6]. The reason for the female preponderance in clinical patch test studies is mainly explained by exposure [1] – for instance the large number of metal-sensitive women may largely be the result of ear piercing [7] and the greater exposure to fragrances, cosmetics and hair dyes. Multiple allergies are found most frequently in elderly women [8]. It is of interest that nickel sensitivity seems to be less common in men even if they wear earrings [9].

Hormones have some effect on contact dermatitis [10]. In one study the response to DNCB was enhanced in women taking an oral contraceptive [11]. Pregnancy and the use of progestogens may, unpredictably, either improve or aggravate contact dermatitis [12,13]. Contact dermatitis may flare premenstrually and cutaneous reactivity to patch testing may vary according to the stage of the menstrual cycle [14], with patch tests to nickel being less intense during the ovulatory than the progestogenic phase [15]. Premenstrual exacerbation of nickel allergy has been described [16].

Ethnicity

Racial differences appear to exist, judging from experimental sensitisation to poison ivy and DNCB, with Afro-Caribbean skin generally less easily sensitised than white skin [1]. This may, however, be complicated as redness may be subtle and overlooked in more pigmented skin. Differences in the prevalence of sensitisation to individual allergens among racial groups is generally felt to be a reflection of exposure rather than predisposition [2,3].

Associated diseases

Patients with acute or debilitating diseases, such as cancer, Hodgkin disease or mycosis fungoides, have impaired capacity for contact sensitisation [1–3]. This may also apply to patients who for other reasons have impaired T-lymphocyte function.

Impact of drugs on patch test reactions

Drug influences on skin test reactivity have been reviewed by Schopf [1]. Antihistamines and sodium cromoglicate (disodium cromoglycate) appear to have little effect, whereas both prednisolone (dose >15 mg/day) [2] and potent topical steroids [3] suppress allergic patch test reactions. Similarly, other immunomodulators such as ciclosporin and azathioprine may reduce the intensity of allergic contact reactions [4]. Therapeutic ultraviolet B (UVB) or psoralen and UVA (PUVA) therapy may also temporarily reduce contact allergic reactions [5,6]. Dupilumab acts as a specific Th2 cell-specific immunosuppressive agent and does not seem to have significant dampening effects on patch test reactions [7].

Pathophysiology

The immune mechanisms of allergic contact dermatitis remain only partially understood. It clearly involves a complex interplay between dendritic cells, keratinocytes, activating T cells and suppressing regulatory T cells. The original pathways for allergic contact dermatitis were suggested from mouse models involving potent skin sensitisers, such as DNCB, which are not of clinical relevance. Other studies focused on nickel allergy and presumed a single common pathway for all allergens. It is increasingly recognised that the pathophysiology of allergic contact dermatitis is much more complex than previously presumed, with different allergens able to trigger different inflammatory pathways [1]. Regulatory T cells are recognised to have a fundamental role [2] and the innate immune system to have a wider influence in both sensitisation and elicitation phases [3].

Sensitisation and elicitation

The immunology of skin disease is discussed in detail in Chapter 9. There are two main processes involved in allergic contact dermatitis: (i) sensitisation (induction or afferent limb of sensitivity); and (ii) elicitation (or efferent limb) of contact dermatitis. Four different types of delayed-type hypersensitivity reactions to exogenous chemicals, of which allergic contact dermatitis is one form, have been proposed [1]:

1 Th1-mediated, with the release of interferon γ (IFN-γ) and tumour necrosis factor α (TNF-α), and the activation of monocytes and macrophages in allergic contact dermatitis, bullous exanthema and the tuberculin skin test.
2 Th2-mediated, with the release of interleukin 5 (IL-5), IL-4, IL-13 and eotaxin, resulting in eosinophilic inflammation seen in maculopapular and bullous exanthema.
3 Mediated by cytotoxic CD4+ and CD8+ T cells, with the release of perforin, granzyme and Fas ligand, resulting in allergic contact dermatitis and maculopapular, pustular and bullous exanthema.
4 Release of CXCL-8 and granulocyte–macrophage colony-stimulating factor (GM-CSF) by T cells, resulting in the recruitment of neutrophils in pustular exanthema.

Sensitisation. The induction of sensitivity is the primary event, which has to take place before the clinical expression of dermatitis can occur. The main events are described here.

1 *Penetration of the sensitiser through the stratum corneum*. Broadly speaking, chemicals that result in sensitisation are either metal ions or low-molecular-weight chemicals that are able to penetrate the stratum corneum. A cut-off size for a sensitising chemical of <500 Da had previously been presumed but larger chemicals of up to 2000 Da molecular weight are now recognised to have sensitising potential [2]. Sensitising chemicals have also been thought to be required to be hydrophilic in order to cross the skin barrier, but this has also now been refuted [3]. Molecules may be modified by chemical or physical factors prior to penetrating the skin to become more allergenic (pre-haptens). Chemicals may enter the epidermis through three routes, either between the epidermal cells through the intercellular matrix, transcellularly through the epidermal cell cytoplasm or via structures such as hair follicles or sweat glands. Factors that disrupt the skin barrier tend to enhance the risk of sensitisation.
2 *Binding of allergen to skin components*. Having passed through the skin barrier allergens covalently bind with endogenous proteins (haptenisation). Some molecules are altered by biotic or enzymatic activity after passing through the skin barrier to become

more allergenic (pro-haptens). The hapten–protein complexes are able to be recognised by the immune system and bind with major histocompatibility complex (MHC) class II molecules on the surface of dermal dendritic cells or Langerhans cells [4]. The metal ions nickel, palladium and cobalt are able to directly ligate and trigger Toll-like receptor 4 (TLR-4) on the surface of dermal dendritic cells. The direct stimulation of this strong danger signal to dermal dendritic cells is likely to be an important factor in explaining why nickel is our most common allergen [5]. In contrast, non-metal sensitisers are thought to trigger the release of reactive oxygen species (ROS) in the skin, leading to the degradation of hyaluronic acid into pro-inflammatory fragments, which act as damage-associated molecular patterns (DAMPs), that indirectly trigger TLRs 2 and 4 [6]. Direct or indirect stimulation of TLRs leads to pro-inflammatory cytokine release.

3 *Pro-inflammatory cytokine milieu*. In response to antigens entering the epidermis, keratinocytes release 'stress' cytokines, IL-1β, TNF-α, IL-8 and GM-CSF, which activate antigen-presenting cells (APCs). 'Danger signals' from pro-inflammatory cytokines are essential for the full activation of immature dendritic cells and the triggering of an adaptive immune response. Cytokines additionally activate mast cells and neutrophils, resulting in upregulation of endothelial adhesion molecules and downregulation of epidermal adhesion factors, such as E-cadherin, allowing the migration of APCs to the regional lymph nodes [7]. In the absence of inflammation, tolerance is likely to occur.

4 *Antigen-presenting cell migration to regional lymph nodes*. Sensitisation is possible only if the connection to the regional lymph nodes is intact [8]. The APCs travel via the afferent lymphatics to the paracortical areas of the regional lymph nodes, where they become apposed to naïve T lymphocytes. The binding is assisted not only by physical factors – the ruffled membrane and dendritic nature of the Langerhans cells and the intricate structure of the paracortical areas – but also by specialist cellular adhesion molecules (CAMs). These CAMs act at different loci to encourage binding. For example, leukocyte functional antigen 1 (LFA-1) on CD4 helper cells interacts with intercellular adhesion molecule 1 (ICAM-1) on Langerhans cells, and CD2 on T cells binds to LFA-3 in plasma membranes on most nucleated cells. With recognition of the antigen, many mediators or cytokines are released by this apposition, most importantly IL-1 by APCs and IL-2 by T lymphocytes.

5 *Proliferation of sensitised T lymphocytes*. The cytokines cause blast formation in the lymph nodes and proliferation of antigen-specific cytotoxic CD8+ (Tc1), CD4+ (Th1) and Th17 lymphocytes [9,10]. The type of T-cell response generated is now thought to be dependent on the specific allergen involved. Nickel generates the traditional Th1 and Th17 response. Fragrance is thought to generate a skew towards a Th2 and Th22 response, with a smaller Th1 signal [**11**]. There is a simultaneous generation of antigen-specific skin resident memory T cells and lymph node central memory T cells which are important for later elicitation reactions.

6 *Dissemination of activated T cells*. The T cells disseminate via the efferent lymphatics throughout the body and interact with Langerhans cells and residual antigen in the skin. Contact hypersensitivity is mediated through a subset of T cells that express cutaneous lymphocyte-associated antigen (CLA). Localisation to areas of inflammation occurs via the production of the chemokine CCL27 by basal keratinocytes, which binds to dermal glycoprotein. CLA-positive lymphocytes also express CCR10, the receptor for CCL27 [12]. The cytotoxic T cells induce keratinocyte death through the release of Fas ligand and perforin-mediated pathways [13].

7 *Downregulation of the inflammatory response*. To avoid tissue damage several regulatory mechanisms are triggered after allergen exposure to limit the inflammatory response. This role is mainly played by regulatory T cells (Tregs), which are stimulated by IL-10 from Langerhans cells [14]. B cells additionally secrete IL-10 [15].

Elicitation. On first exposure to a strong sensitiser such as DNCB, most subjects develop a local reaction after 5–25 days. During this period, sensitisation has been accomplished, and the residues of the allergen in the skin react with the newly formed, sensitised T lymphocytes. Such a response has been termed a 'late' reaction. There is evidence to suggest that allergen-specific T lymphocytes persist at the site of original contact for some months following an initial sensitisation exposure, and this may explain the 're-test' or 'flare-up' reactions that are sometimes observed during patch testing, following re-exposure at a distant site [16].

If a sensitised person is re-exposed to a specific allergen in sufficient concentration, the clinical reaction subsequently develops much more quickly, usually within 24–48 h. However, depending on the degree of sensitivity, penetration and other factors, this may vary from a few hours to many days. Antigen may be presented not only by antigen-presenting Langerhans cells but also by IL-1-secreting keratinocytes that acquire Ia/HLA-DR status, augmenting the cascade of cytokine, immune cell and inflammatory response. This cascade is autoregulating, and although the mechanism of this is not well understood it probably involves CD4+ T cells.

A delayed reaction time describes a delayed elicitation response following antigenic challenge in persons who are already sensitised. There has been confusion over the use of this term, as it has been used not only to describe reactions that have taken more than the usual 4 days to develop, but also acute primary sensitisation reactions which, in normal clinical practice, often present as more sudden and florid reactions around 21 days after challenge. A delayed reaction time is found with low degrees of sensitivity (when there are very few memory T cells), following exposures to small amounts of allergen (when it takes longer to augment the T-cell response) and in situations of delayed penetration of allergens (e.g. neomycin in petrolatum).

Predisposing factors

Pre-existing or concomitant constitutional and/or irritant contact dermatitis damages the skin, affecting its barrier function and producing increased opportunities for allergen absorption and secondary sensitisation. It is known that hand eczema predisposes to nickel sensitivity and vice versa [1], and that the prevalence of chromate, cobalt and balsam sensitivity is increased in men with hand eczema [2]. The longer the duration of the eczema, the greater is the chance of sensitisation. Occlusion greatly promotes percutaneous absorption and probably contributes to the high incidence of medicament dermatitis in stasis eczema, otitis externa and perianal dermatitis, and is also a factor in dermatitis from shoes and rubber gloves.

As sensitivity is more easily acquired if an allergen is applied to damaged skin, concomitant irritant contact dermatitis will promote sensitisation and lower the threshold for the elicitation of an allergic contact dermatitis in those exposed to associated allergens [3]. In experimental sensitisation, skin damage may be produced by a previous application of sodium lauryl sulphate. The enhanced risk of sensitisation may be due to: (i) increased absorption of the allergen as a result of skin barrier disruption; (ii) priming of the immunological response with prior recruitment of immunocompetent cells, cytokines, etc.; or (iii) accumulation of mononuclear cells. Furthermore, by adapting the Matzinger 'danger model' concept for sensitisation [4], it has been suggested that contact allergy can *only* develop in the presence of cytokine release from non-immune skin cells (principally keratinocytes) provoked by a coexisting irritant (often the same as the allergen) or trauma [5,6]. If there is no concomitant irritancy, then tolerance rather than allergy is likely to follow.

In guinea pigs, sensitisation is facilitated by acanthosis induced by detergents or paraffins, even in the absence of dermatitis [7]. Although the mechanism for this promotion of sensitisation by acanthosis is unknown, it may be relevant to burns and other types of skin damage known to increase the chance of sensitisation [8].

Once allergy is established, it seems reasonable to suppose that an allergen may be able to reactivate or maintain dermatitis at a low concentration. However, even when such exposure seems to have ceased, hand eczema that started as a contact dermatitis may continue as an apparently 'constitutional' postinsult form of dermatitis [9].

Chemical factors. Skin cells, especially their nucleic acids and proteins, are composed of molecules that contain nucleophilic atoms that are negatively charged and electron rich. Most allergens (haptens) are 'simple' chemicals of low molecular weight (less than 500–1000 Da) that contain electrophilic atoms [10,11] that are positively charged and electron deficient. Interaction between these two types of atoms leads to strong covalent bonding to form a hapten–protein complex or 'complete antigen'. Metal and metal salts can bond to electron-rich atoms (ligands) by taking some of the electrons and forming coordinate bonds. Haptens can be grouped according to their chemical reactivity in relation to putative carrier proteins or according to functional groups (Table 127.2).

Thus, the potential of a low-molecular-weight compound to become a hapten is determined by its chemical reactivity towards skin proteins. Some compounds react directly (e.g. nickel), while others require activation, either metabolically inside the skin or externally. The latter are classified either as pro- or pre-haptens, depending on the mode of activation. Non-sensitising compounds that require metabolic activation are pro-haptens, while pre-haptens are compounds with no or low sensitising potential that are activated externally.

Pro-haptens are metabolically activated in the skin and thus activation could vary depending on the individuals' enzymatic expression patterns. Well-known examples of pro-haptens are cinnamyl alcohol (3-phenyl-2-propen-1-ol) and urushiols.

Table 127.2 Classification of haptens based on functional grouping.

Hapten group	Example
1 Acids	Maleic acid
2 Aldehydes	Formaldehyde
3 Amines	Ethylenediamine, p-phenylenediamine
4 Diazo compounds	Bismark brown, Congo red
5 Esters	Benzocaine
6 Ethers	Benzyl ether
7 Epoxides	Epoxy resin
8 Halogenated compounds	Dinitrochlorobenzene, picryl chloride
9 Quinones	Primin, hydroquinone
10 Metals	Ni^{2+}, Co^{2+}, Cr^{3+}, Hg^{2+}, etc.
11 Unsaturated compounds	Δ^3-carene (turpentine)

Examples of pre-haptens are the common fragrance terpenes, the diterpenes in colophony and ethoxylated surfactans. Patch tests revealed some of these substances to be potent skin sensitisers following their activation by auto-oxidation. Auto-oxidation of limonene (from citrus) and linalool (from lavender), two frequently used fragrances, results in the formation of the corresponding hydroperoxides. Multicentre studies imply that oxidised limonene and oxidised linalool are among the most common causes for allergic contact dermatitis, while the compounds themselves rarely cause sensitisation [12].

Cutaneous enzymatic transformation of a chemical into many different metabolites, depending on the pathway taken, makes determination of the allergenicity of the original chemical more difficult. It also explains the difficulty in deciding if multiple sensitivities are cross-reactions or concomitant sensitisation.

Enzymatic systems may also play a preventative role, as with glutathione in some drug-induced reactions [13].

Assessment of sensitisation potential. The sensitisation potential is the relative capacity of a given agent to induce sensitisation in a group of humans or animals [14]. Both in guinea pigs and humans, an estimate of the sensitising index requires patch test exposures modified to increase the sensitising impact. Such predictive patch tests are used to compare the sensitising properties of new products or chemicals with those of known substances. Many test procedures have been developed over the last 40 years to evaluate the sensitising properties of new chemicals. Kligman and Basketter [15] have critically evaluated the various methods of predictive testing. Most previous methods could not reveal even potent sensitisers. Kligman and Epstein have described a 'maximisation test', based on the application of a high concentration of the chemical to be studied on a skin area previously irritated by sodium lauryl sulphate [14]. This method was later modified by Marzulli and Maibach, who used repeated patch tests with high concentrations of the allergen to be studied. Jordan and King have have shown that some substances giving negative reactions in maximisation tests in males sometimes sensitise females. This may reflect previous subliminal exposure to substances such as the ingredients of cosmetics.

Ethical considerations may prevent experimental sensitisation in humans. The guinea pig maximisation test described by Magnusson and Kligman gives results that compare favourably with predictive patch tests in humans. To enhance sensitisation, the guinea pig maximisation test employs a combination of patch testing and intradermal injection of allergen in a simple solution of Freund adjuvant. Other tests, such as the Buehler test and the open epicutaneous test, use the epicutaneous route only, whereas the Draize test and Freund complete adjuvant test use a purely intradermal method of sensitisation. There is, however, no absolute conformity in the sensitising potential of a substance in the mouse, guinea pig or human.

The 6th Amendment of the EC Cosmetic Directive, which came into effect in January 1997, is committed to banning all animal testing. The local lymph node assay is a mouse model that has gained regulatory approval. A logarithmic scale is used to classify the potential of chemicals to induce sensitisation, from strong to non-sensitising, depending on the dose needed to induce lymphocyte proliferation [16]. The mouse ear swelling test [17] avoids postmortem examination of tested animals.

The theoretical allergenicity [11,18] of a compound may be studied by reference to databases of cases of reported sensitivity and the results of previously performed guinea pig maximisation tests. By comparing the structure of known allergens and reactive groups with that of any new compound, an expert system can be developed to predict a compound's likely sensitisation potential. Molecular modelling using structure–activity relationships has been used with the sesquiterpene lactones and primin and a relative alkylation index for sultones to test such a model.

Reconstituted 3D human epidermis models, which are very similar to human skin with respect to histology and metabolic activity, are now commercially available. This has enabled further research into the reactivity of cutaneous allergens in an ethical manner [19].

Sensitisation risk. The risk of sensitisation depends not only on the sensitisation potential of the substance applied, but prior to stimulating the immune system a chemical must penetrate the epidermis. Subsequently, the log dose applied per unit area, where the area of application is greater than 1 cm^2, appears to be the most important determinant of the risk of sensitisation, with the reactivity showing a sigmoid dose–response curve [20]. In practice, the conditions of exposure are also important: the duration of exposure (rinse-off or leave-on product), if the exposure is repeated [21] and the condition of the skin (the presence of pre-existing dermatitis predisposing to the presence of accessory signals in the sensitisation process).

There are also individual factors; studies in individuals already sensitised indicate that those with more contact allergies have a greater susceptibility to sensitisation by other allergens compared with those who do not demonstrate any pre-existing contact allergy. With high concentrations of a strong allergen such as DNCB, individual susceptibility is of little importance; nearly everyone is capable of being sensitised.

In personal care products the concentration of any allergen is adjusted so that the risk of inducing sensitisation is small, although there may still be sufficient to induce dermatitis in an individual already sensitised. An approach to sensitisation risk assessment for such products has been described [22]. This involves an assessment of both exposure (including knowledge of skin absorption) and sensitisation potential, based on literature review and known structure–activity relationships. If *in vivo* testing is needed, various animal tests or human repeat-insult patch tests would then be performed. Legislative measures have been introduced in an attempt to reduce the prevalence of contact dermatitis [23].

Development of dermatitis. Some persons sensitive to a substance may tolerate normal contact with it, and are said to have a latent sensitivity. There is no immunological difference between latent and expressed sensitivity. Whether sensitivity is manifest or latent is determined partly by the threshold of sensitivity, which is the lowest concentration of allergen giving a positive patch test response. The dose at induction determines, in part, the strength of response at challenge – higher induction doses resulting in greater reactions at challenge [20]. Persons who are clinically sensitive to poison ivy invariably have a positive reaction to 1 : 10 000 pentadecylcatechol (PDC), but many who react only to 1 : 100 PDC are clinically immune. Patch test sensitivity and clinical sensitivity are not necessarily proportional. The threshold determined by patch tests depends on a number of technical factors, such as the base used and the region where the tests are applied. It also varies from time to time in the same person. The threshold may fall after repeated contact with an allergen, and positive test reactions in latent allergy may reveal candidates for future allergic contact dermatitis.

Patch testing with a new substance may reveal that some people are already sensitive to it, either from contact with related substances or from exposure to the compound in other forms. Negative reactions in 200 people do not exclude the possible occurrence of sensitivity in 1 of 38 consumers (99.5% level). This frequency would immediately preclude any practical use of the substance. It has been calculated that negative patch tests in 5300 subjects indicate that sensitivity would be liable to occur in less than one of 1000 consumers.

Immunological tolerance. Recent studies have highlighted that allergic contact dermatitis has been associated with defective Tregs and indeed it has become clear that Tregs influence sensitisation as well as elicitation. Originally, Tregs were defined as CD4+ CD25+ T cells and were mainly associated with self-tolerance. We now know that this definition comprises a heterogeneous cell population that includes natural and inducible Tregs. The skin contains predominantly inducible Tregs, which can be triggered by Langerhans cells as well as dermal dendritic cells. However, the precise phenotypes of Tregs involved in allergic contact dermatitis are still not known. Finally, Tregs are involved in the control and eventual termination of the inflammatory response [2].

The sensitisation reaction induces effector T cells and suppressor T cells, the latter curtailing the immune response so that the epidermal reaction regresses and does not continue indefinitely [24]. Theoretically, therefore, preferential stimulation of suppressor cells could lead to antigen unresponsiveness. This can be achieved by administering the allergen (in previously unsensitised individuals) by non-cutaneous routes, such as intravenously, orally or peritoneally [25], thereby bypassing epidermal Langerhans cells. This tolerance is also achieved by applying the allergen to skin with no Langerhans cells, for example mouse tails, or skin in which the Langerhans cells have been inhibited by UV radiation or depleted by glucocorticoids. Suppressor T cells, or their precursors, are sensitive to cytostatic drugs, so that the administration of cyclophosphamide can reverse a tolerant state.

Pathology

Biopsies are of limited help in contact dermatitis. Most types of eczema show identical pathological changes, and allergic and primary irritant contact dermatitis cannot be distinguished with certainty. The only sure way to distinguish irritant from allergic contact dermatitis is by study of the very early events of the inflammatory process, because the remainder of the inflammatory cascade is similar in the two processes [1].

Causative organisms

Fauna are not a major cause of contact allergy, although European fishermen are liable to contact dermatitis of exposed skin during the summer when handling nets containing marine organisms known as bryozoans. The disorder is known as 'Dogger Bank itch' in the UK [1]. The allergen has been identified as the (2-hydroxyethyl) dimethylsulphoxonium ion [2].

Genetics

Allergic contact dermatitis, like so many conditions, is likely to be caused by a complex interplay between environmental and genetic factors. Genetic influence has long been suspected, with family studies suggesting first degree relatives of sensitised patients to have increased risk [1]. Twin study results have, however, been conflicting [2,3]. Several immunogenetic markers associating nickel allergy with major histocompatibility loci have been suggested [4,5]. Genetic influence is, however, suggested to be 'overruled' if potent allergens or siginificant allergen exposure occurs [1].

Genetic polymorphisms may influence antigen uptake through the skin barrier, the antigen-specific response by immune cells and metabolism of antigens by cutaneous enzymes [1]. The following proteins display genetic polymorphisms that have been linked with a possible role in contact allergy:

- Filaggrin is epidermal protein, important for cutaneous structure and barrier function. Loss-of-function filaggrin mutations are associated with dry skin, reduced skin barrier function and increased risk of atopic dermatitis. The possible role of filaggrin mutations in contact allergy is, however, debated with conflicting results from different studies [6,7]. There does seem to be a link with polysensitised individuals [8].
- N-acetyltransferases (NATs) are enzymes that catalyse acetylation of PPD, among other chemicals, within the epidermis. Studies found a relationship between genetic polymorphisms for these phase II enzymes and risk for contact dermatitis. Different studies have again yielded contrary results, linking rapid acetylating NATs to both higher and lower susceptibility for PPD sensitisation [9,10].
- Glutathione-S-transferases (GSTs) are a large family of phase II enzymes that have a role in toxification and detoxification of chemicals. GST polymorphisms have been investigated with respect to mercury and chromate allergy [11]. Low GST activity appears generally associated with increased ROS damage [12].
- Angiotensin-converting enzyme (ACE) is a well-recognised enzyme responsible for catalysing the conversion of angiotensin I to angiotensin II. Animal models suggest a role for ACE in modulating Langerhans cell and T-lymphocyte functions and degradation of bradykinin and substance P produced by the allergic inflammatory response [13]. ACE polymorphisms have been linked with allergy risk.
- Tumour necrosis factor is a pro-inflammatory cytokine recognised to play an important role in both the sensitisation and elicitation phases of allergic contact dermatitis, particularly involved in promoting Langerhans cell migration to draining lymph nodes. The TNF-α-308 polymorphism is linked with polysensitised subjects, suggesting an influence on susceptibility to contact allergy [14].
- Interleukin-16 polymorphisms have also been suggested as a link with polysensitised individuals [15,16].

The relationship of atopy, particularly atopic eczema, to predispose to allergic contact dermatitis has prompted much debate. Patients with severe atopic eczema are shown to have a diminished capacity for DNCB sensitisation [17]. Clinical studies are conflicting, some showing an increase in the prevalence of contact allergy, especially to medicaments [18], others the same [19] and others a decrease [20,21]. In a study of 101 sets of twins, no correlation was found between positive patch tests and atopy and the prevalence of allergic contact dermatitis in atopics was found to be similar to that in patients suffering from discoid or seborrhoeic eczema. An increased level of nickel sensitisation noted in one study [22] contrasts with another where there was no increase [23].

These studies are, however, complicated by the relative irritant nature of many allergens, particularly nickel, cobalt and chromate in atopic skin, which may lead to overinterpretation of patch test positive results in atopic cohorts. The term 'atopy' is also used in some studies to mean a history of atopic dermatitis, or simply 'eczema in childhood', or may include atopic asthma and hayfever.

A recent large, single-centre study looked at 46 250 patients patch tested over 30 years' duration. It found statistically significant differences for nine allergens between the atopic and non-atopic groups. Nickel, cobalt and primin allergy were less common in the atopic group (with nickel being highly significant; $P < 0.0001$) but sesquiterpene lactone mix, fragrance mix 1, tixocortol pivalate, neomycin, imidazolidinyl urea and lanolin allergy were more common in atopic individuals [24].

There are many reasons why atopic dermatitis should predispose to development of allergic contact dermatitis:
- Skin barrier function is reduced.
- Increased exposure to topical medicaments.
- Increased tendency to irritant dermatitis and therefore DAMPs [25].
- Increased tendency to cutaneous infection and therefore pathogen-associated molecular patterns (PAMPs) [26].
- The Th2 immune response may reduce filaggrin levels.

Atopic individuals, however, downregulate Th1 lymphocytes, which may play a significant role in protecting patients with atopic dermatitis from developing allergic contact dermatitis [27,28]. Different allergens have been recognised to now trigger allergy through different pathways [29]. At present no certain conclusion can be made about the relative risk of contact sensitisation in atopic patients. The answer is likely to be that atopic eczema may increase the risk of developing allergic contact dermatitis to some allergens (such as the moderately sensitising non-metal allergens present within medicaments and personal care products) but may reduce the risk for other allergens such as nickel which particularly stimulate via a Th1 skewed pathway.

Environmental factors

By definition, the environment will influence exposure to potential allergens, which in turn will affect liability to contact allergy. For the individual, certain immediate environments, including those encountered in the home, at work and during spare-time activities, are particularly relevant. However, more general influences are important, including climatic, geographic, ecological, socio-economic and cultural factors. Some of these may also affect the individual's response to allergen exposure. Climate, geography and ecology are often interrelated.

Climate. Climate, by virtue of varying UV exposure, heat and relative humidity, may play a part in liability to contact allergy. UVB exposure has been shown to diminish the skin's immune response to contact allergens [1,2]. UVA exposure, however, does not appear to have the same effect, and there is evidence that the reduction in immune responsiveness is transient, perhaps due to an adaptive mechanism [2]. UVB exposure from the sun may therefore temporarily reduce contact allergic reactions, although there is conflicting evidence about the effect of sunshine on patch test reactions [3,4]. Conversely, chapping of the skin during winter predisposes to irritant contact dermatitis and also increases the incidence of false positive patch test reactions to substances such as formaldehyde [4] and propylene glycol [5]. Occlusion and increased sweating may increase allergy from shoes and clothing. Exposure to UV-absorbing chemical filters increases where there is a higher exposure to sunshine, with a consequent increase in contact and photocontact allergy from this source during the summer months, when photoallergy from other causes would also be anticipated to be more of a problem.

Flora and fauna. Plant dermatitis commonly shows a distinct seasonal pattern, the allergenicity of some plants such as *Primula obconica* varying considerably with light and season [6]. Many allergenic plants, especially those belonging to the Compositae (Asteraceae) family, are destroyed by cold and frosty weather but return during the warmer spring and summer months. Global warming is also felt to be an issue, with evidence that *Toxicodendron* species may become more abundant and allergenic as a result [7]. Distribution of allergenic plant material will be facilitated by dry and windy climates. Similarly, geographic location is a very important influence. Exposure to *Toxicodendron* species is mainly confined to North America. Compositae allergy is seen in many parts of the world but the plants responsible vary: in the USA ragweed is the main cause, in Europe it is chrysanthemums and garden weeds, in India the weed *Parthenium*, and in Australia a number of wild Compositae found in the 'bush'. Occupational contact allergy from plants is often seasonal, for instance in lichen pickers [8] and from plant and vegetable cultivation [9,10].

Clinical features
History

Contact dermatitis can mimic or be associated with any type of eczematous eruption. The diagnosis is based on a careful history combined with a sound knowledge of common allergens and irritants in a patient's environment. A comprehensive history is essential to identify contact with allergens, and some knowledge of chemistry and industrial processes is of value. Sensitisation and subsequent contact dermatitis can result from a single exposure [1], although usually several or many exposures are necessary before sensitisation and dermatitis occur.

Primary site. This must be ascertained by questioning the patient carefully. By definition, contact dermatitis must begin in sites where contact has taken place with the responsible agent(s), and the sites of origin are an important clue to the cause. Patients are frequently assessed at a stage when there has been worsening and secondary spread of the dermatitis, obscuring the original pattern.

Duration and behaviour. Once the date of onset and the primary site(s) have been identified, it is necessary to establish the subsequent behaviour of the dermatitis. In particular, did the rash spread and if so where? Has the problem been persistent or intermittent? Repeated sudden exacerbations may point to an allergic contact dermatitis. Are there any obvious exacerbating factors? In contrast, irritant contact dermatitis does not tend to spread.

Improvement of dermatitis during weekends or holidays may indicate an occupational origin. Relapse at weekends may favour a hobby or non-occupational allergen. However, this history could prove to be misleading if there are multiple sources of exposure. Seasonal variation (worsening when light intensity is greatest) may suggest a plant allergen, perhaps with photoaggravation, or photoallergy. Plant dermatitis may recur in atypical patterns. Dermatitis around a wound, especially leg ulcers, suggests sensitisation to medicaments (Figure 127.1) and exacerbations and recurrences induced by particular medicaments or cosmetics suggest contact

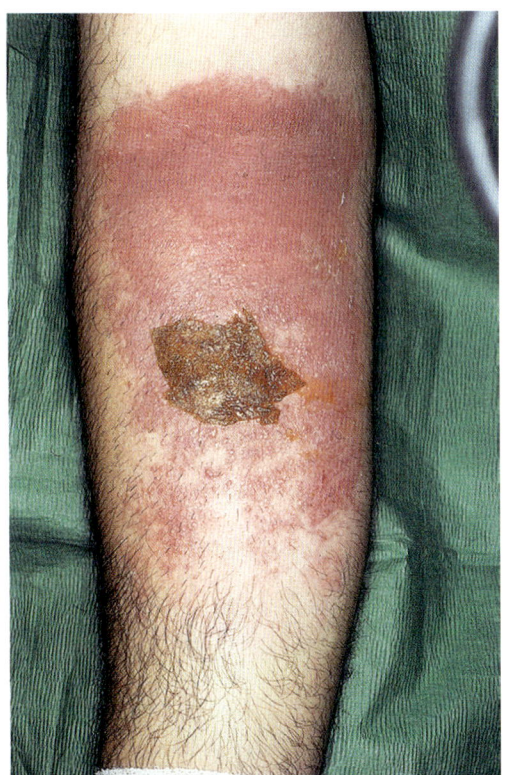

Figure 127.1 Medicament contact dermatitis. Courtesy of Dr J. D. Wilkinson.

allergy from these sources. Dermatitis occurring during or following a holiday should include an assessment whether different personal care products might have been used including the use of sunscreens.

Previous history. A history of previous dermatitis may provide a clue to the origin of a relapse. For example, earring dermatitis may precede nickel dermatitis of the hands by several years. Previous dermatitis, especially if localised to the lower legs, may have been caused or complicated by the repeated use of medicaments containing sensitisers. It may be useful to ask specifically about skin reactions to costume jewellery, perfume and adhesive plasters.

A history of infantile or childhood flexural eczema, asthma or seasonal allergic rhinoconjunctivitis may point to an atopic diathesis. Atopic eczema also predisposes to irritant contact dermatitis of the hands, and in such cases constitutional factors may be a major, but not necessarily the sole, cause.

Sources of allergy. A search for possible sources of allergic contact dermatitis should include a review of all the patient's activities, but initially should concentrate on: (i) occupation, present and past; (ii) hobbies; (iii) use of cosmetics including nail cosmetics, clothing and personal objects; (iv) home environment (including cooking, gardening and painting and decorating); and (v) current and previous topically applied medicaments both prescribed and over-the-counter. Most patients believe that newly encountered items are the cause of dermatitis, whereas in fact those that have been in use for a long time are commonly responsible.

Occupation. A precise history backed up by a thorough knowledge of the materials handled at work, the machinery operated and the PPE in use will all be necessary when occupational dermatitis is suspected (Figure 127.2). However, no dermatologist can rely entirely on their knowledge of industrial processes, and a factory visit may be required to become familiar with the process described, especially if it is new. Material safety data sheets must be examined as these may give the chemical names of materials used, as well as an indication of their irritancy or allergenicity. A telephone number or email address may be given for further enquiries, if required. The presence of other similar cases will alert one to an increased probability of occupational dermatitis.

Problems associated with housework should not be overlooked. The amount of housework performed and methods employed are extremely variable. The number and age of children and availability of labour-saving devices should also be determined. Few people volunteer information about domestic work outside their own home, and all must be directly questioned about this. Patients who are unemployed or students may, in fact, be engaged in casual work, and even employed persons should be asked about second jobs.

Hobbies. Common sensitisers, recognised as occupational allergens, are introduced into most homes for do-it-yourself work. Adhesives and paint are handled by many householders. Another important source of hobby dermatitis is gardening. Other pursuits, such as sports and cookery should also be considered.

Personal objects and medicines. Such items include those worn or applied to the skin such as cosmetics, toiletries, fragrances, medicaments, textiles, footwear, protective clothing and gloves, jewellery, spectacles, hearing aids and medical appliances. Adverse reactions to cosmetics, toiletries and topical medicaments are among the commonest reasons for hospital referral with suspected allergic contact dermatitis. The number of products used may be large, and some may be used only intermittently. Often, only prescribed therapies are declared, and repeated specific enquiry must be made about over-the-counter preparations, including cosmetics used as moisturisers, herbal treatments and borrowed medicaments. Often patients will not mention 'hypoallergenic' products in the mistaken belief that they could not be responsible. Applied cosmetics may be removed from the skin by employing creams, lotions or wipes, the use of which may easily be overlooked. Patients should be specifically asked about the use of nail varnish, methacrylate nails and hair dyes. Skin cleansing and hair products that are 'rinse off' as opposed to 'leave on' may also be responsible. Many patients have a poor recollection of products used, and most forget some items. They should be invited to bring all their topically applied items when they attend for patch testing and these can be specifically tested if indicated, and examined for ingredient listings when appropriate.

Presentation

Eczematous responses (dermatitis). The severity of the dermatitis is determined by the intensity of exposure and the level of sensitivity. The clinical picture is also to some extent dependent upon the site of dermatitis and on the causative agent. The distribution of the dermatitis may suggest a cause, for example that due to nickel or textiles.

The primary signs in acute contact dermatitis are redness, swelling, papules and papulovesicles, which reflect the sequence of inflammatory changes in the dermis and the intracellular and intercellular oedema in the epidermis. In more acute and severe cases this may progress to disruption of the intercellular bridges and the development of larger vesicles or blisters; if they burst, a weeping dermatitis results. The dominant symptom is itching.

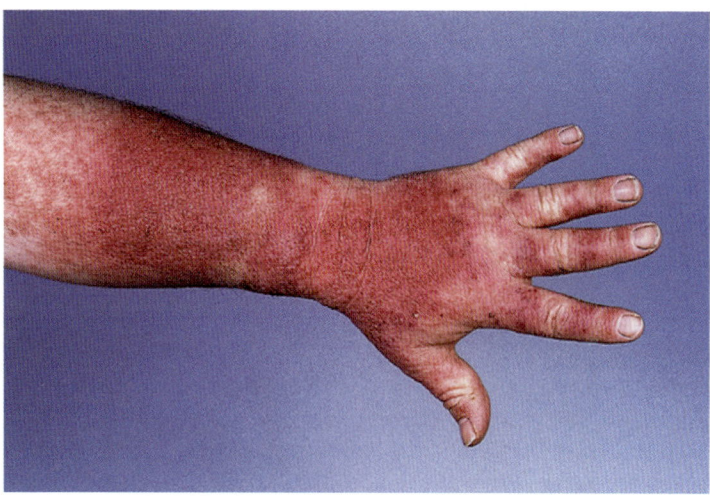

Figure 127.2 Acute allergic contact dermatitis in a patient allergic to acrylates used in the printing industry. Courtesy of Dr J. D. Wilkinson.

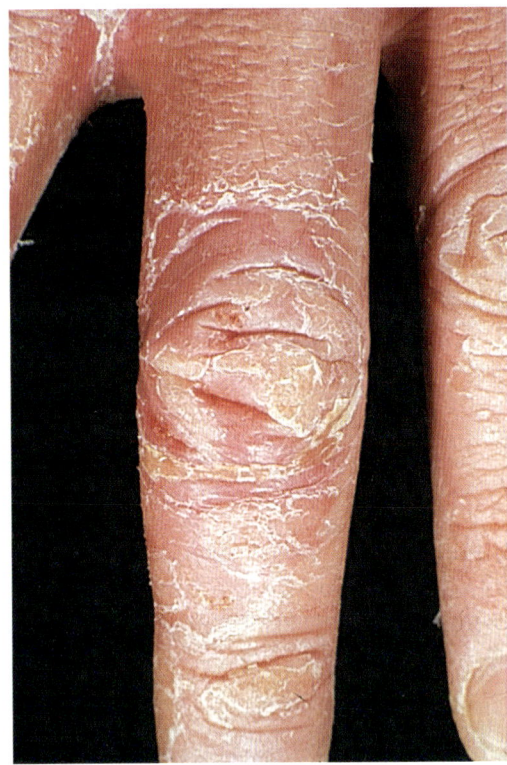

Figure 127.3 Dry, scaling, thickened skin with fissuring due to chronic contact dermatitis.

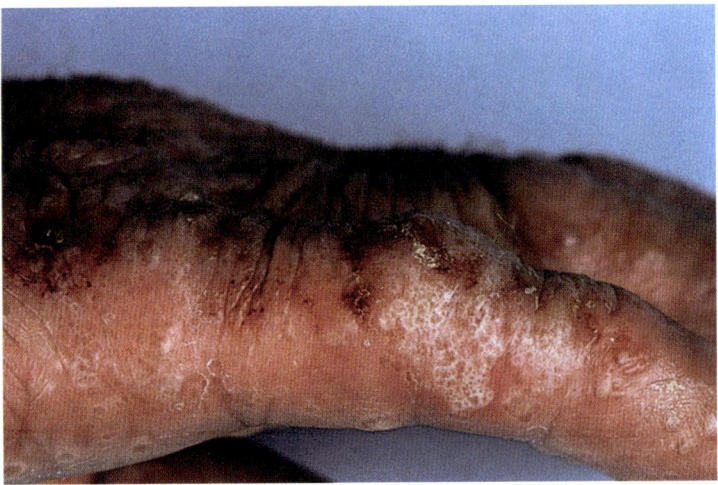

Figure 127.4 Acute vesicular eczema in a patient allergic to 1,2-benzisothiazolin-3-one mimicking constitutional pompholyx. Courtesy of Dr J. D. Wilkinson.

If contact dermatitis persists, it may be due to continued or repeated exposure to the allergen or to secondary irritants or allergens. The skin becomes dry, scaly and thicker as a result of acanthosis, hyperkeratosis, oedema and cellular infiltration in the dermis. Lichenification and fissuring may develop later (Figure 127.3). These clinical features of chronic allergic contact dermatitis cannot always be distinguished from constitutional (Figure 127.4) or irritant contact dermatitis, and the aetiology may often be mixed.

The distribution of the dermatitis is of diagnostic importance but its morphology is usually of no help in identifying the cause.

There may be some exceptions, for example exceptionally strong allergens may provoke a bullous eruption even after brief contact and dermatitis from plant leaves may provoke a linear pattern of dermatitis.

Primary patterns. Anatomical patterns of dermatitis often suggest a specific cause, but in other cases the pattern merely indicates a range of possible allergens, such as in shoe dermatitis. Sometimes, the dermatitis is sharply limited to the usual site of contact, but because the area of contact with most objects varies, the distribution may be more erratic. Some allergens may be spread locally by the fingers or be carried to distant body regions. Even when there is no eruption on the hands, allergens on the fingertips may cause dermatitis elsewhere, for example the genital area, eyes, or face and neck.

Once the primary site has been established, questioning should focus on those allergens that are particularly frequent causes of dermatitis in that region.

Hands and arms. Hand dermatitis is usually multifactorial. About two-thirds of all cases of contact dermatitis involve the hands, which are the most important site for both irritant and allergic contact dermatitis [1,2]. No pattern of hand eczema is characteristic of a particular aetiology, and it is important to emphasise that allergic contact dermatitis may mimic constitutional patterns. The Danish Contact Dermatitis Group has proposed a classification of hand eczema and identified that allergic contact dermatitis is more common in vesicular-type dermatitis [3]. 'Homemaker's dermatitis' and most occupational dermatitis remain confined to the hands. Although the majority of cases are primarily irritant in nature, the yield of relevant positive patch test reactions is high [1]. Allergens may be traced by relating the shape and site of the eczematous patches to the items handled. Rubber gloves may induce a clear pattern of dermatitis over the sites where they are worn, particularly involving the dorsa of the hands with a sharp line of demarcation at the wrists.

Vesicular palmar contact dermatitis may mimic constitutional eczema and may result not only from contact with, but also from ingestion of, an allergen to which the person is already sensitised.

Streaky dermatitis on the fingers, dorsa of the hands and forearms is typically caused by plants (Figure 127.5), and may be allergic (e.g. *Primula obconica* and poison ivy), irritant (e.g. *Dieffenbachia* and spurge) or phototoxic (e.g. giant hogweed and rue).

Dermatitis of the hands in those involved with agriculture, animals and food preparation may be associated with immediate-type hypersensitivity to animal and plant proteins [4,5]. Allergic contact dermatitis of the fingertips is seen with plant allergens such as tulipalins in horticulturists and florists ('tulip fingers') [6]. Garlic allergy in chefs typically affects the non-dominant thumb and fore and middle fingers (Figure 127.6) [7].

Methacrylate allergic contact dermatitis from sculptured and UV-cured nails and UV-cured nail polish commonly affects the nail unit, and is often accompanied by facial and eyelid involvement (Figure 127.7). Onychodystrophy, paronychia and onycholysis may also accompany eczematous reactions of the nail unit.

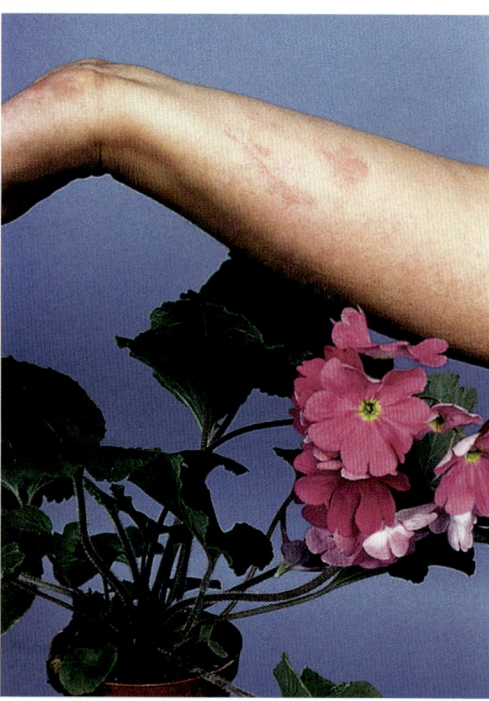

Figure 127.5 Characteristic 'streaky' contact dermatitis on the wrists in a patient allergic to *Primula obconica*. Courtesy of Dr J. D. Wilkinson.

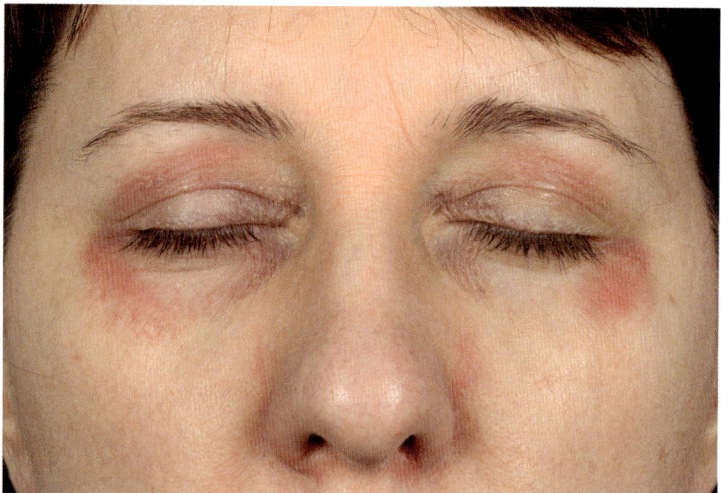

Figure 127.7 Periocular allergic contact dermatitis from nail methacrylate chemicals. Courtesy of Dr N. Stone.

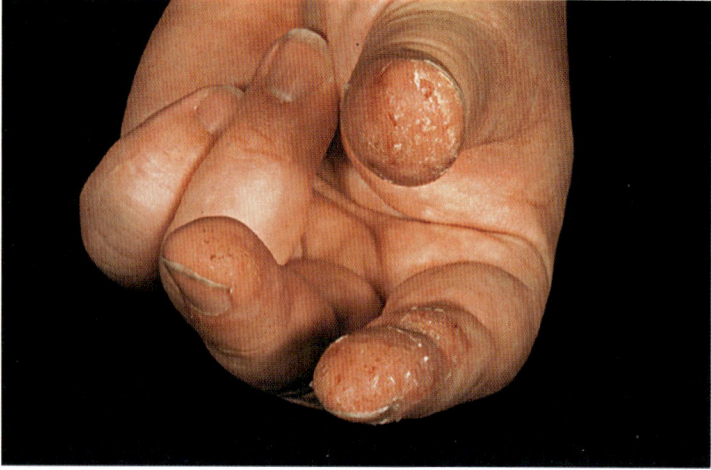

Figure 127.6 Fingertip pattern of allergic contact dermatitis from garlic affecting the non-dominant thumb, forefinger and middle fingers.

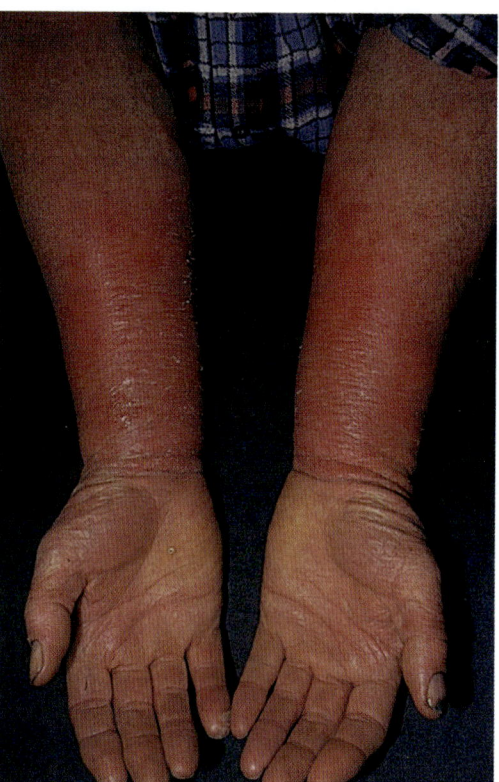

Figure 127.8 Contact allergy to epoxy resin and hardener affecting unprotected forearms.

The arms are affected by the same allergens as the hands, but usually later on in the process. If the hands have been protected by gloves at work, the forearms may be the major sites of occupational dermatitis (Figure 127.8). Allergy to nickel, chromate and *p*-tert-butylphenol (PTBP) formaldehyde resin may develop at the wrists from sensitivity to the metal, leather and glue, respectively, in watchstraps containing these allergens. Dust (exotic woods, cement), nickel and textiles produce dermatitis in the elbow flexures, which must be distinguished from atopic eczema.

Head and neck. Allergic contact dermatitis of the head and neck can occur from multiple exposure routes including direct application, airborne exposure, hand to face and neck, by proxy and by systemic and mucosal exposure.

Face. Dermatitis of the face may occur alone or in association with eczema elsewhere. Facial allergic contact dermatitis from fragrances, hair dyes, preservatives and other constituents of skincare products and cosmetics, including nail varnish, is common.

Dermatitis due to a cosmetic may start with dryness, tightness and itching. Most consumers change to another brand at this stage and are never assessed by a dermatologist. They are referred only

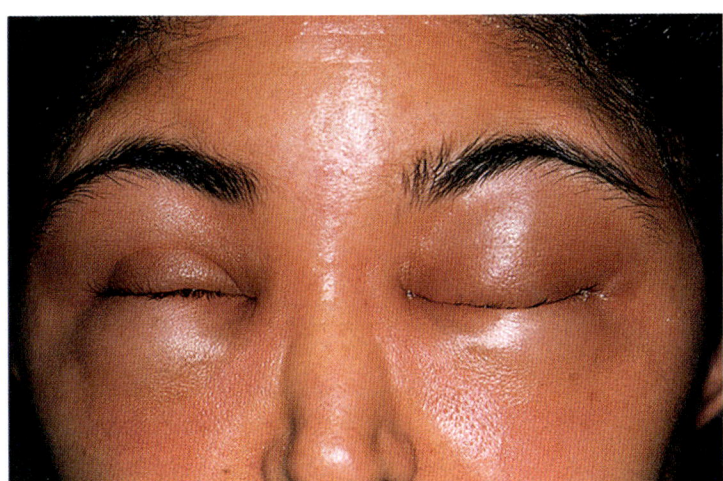

Figure 127.9 Contact dermatitis presenting as acute oedema, as seen in patients sensitive to *Primula* and *p*-phenylenediamine-type hair dyes and in those with volatile patterns of contact dermatitis. Courtesy of Dr J. D. Wilkinson.

if symptoms persist or are severe. Some allergens, for example hair dyes, may provoke acute oedema (Figure 127.9) and intense pruritus – but not eczema – followed by desquamation. Nail varnish allergy often affects the face in well-localised patches, and may be associated with eyelid dermatitis and more extensive involvement of the neck, chest and even further afield [8]. It is important to note that these nail varnish allergens may also be present in other nail cosmetics such as nail strengtheners and hardeners. The clinical presentation can suggest artefact because the affected sites are so well demarcated [9]. A similar distribution may be seen from allergy to acrylic-based artificial nails and rubber sponge applicators [10]. The forehead is affected by allergy to anything applied to the hair and also to chromate or clothing dyes in leather hatbands. Spectacle frames containing nickel or plastics may cause dermatitis on areas of contact with the cheeks, nose, eyelids and ears.

The patterns of dermatitis caused by airborne or volatile allergens [11] and photosensitisers can often be distinguished by involvement of the eyelids in the former, and by triangles of relatively spared skin below the chin and behind and below the ear lobes in the latter.

Facial allergic contact dermatitis must be distinguished from cosmetic intolerance, irritant contact dermatitis and constitutional eczemas, but it is sometimes multifactorial.

Eyelids. Allergens affecting the face may initially produce eyelid dermatitis [12,13] as the skin of the eyelids is thin, sensitive and may be contaminated by the fingers (e.g. nail varnish [8]), airborne droplets (e.g. fragrance sprays) or volatile substances (e.g. epoxy resin). Eye creams, eye shadows, mascara and eye make-up removers may be responsible, often for irritant dermatitis, but patch testing may reveal relevant allergens.

Cyanoacrylate-induced dermatitis from the use of false eyelash glue or PPD contact allergy from the use of eyebrow or eyelash tints have been reported as responsible for severe oedematous allergic reactions [14,15].

Dermatitis can also be caused by medicaments for ocular disorders. Sensitisers in eye drops and ointments include neomycin, framycetin, gentamicin, tobramycin, chloramphenicol, fucidin, sulphonamides, local anaesthetics, antihistamines, β-blockers, anticholinergics and sympathomimetics. Eye drops and contact lens solutions often contain preservatives (e.g. benzalkonium chloride, ethylenediamine tetracetate (EDTA), mercurials), which may also sensitise.

Lips or perioral area. Sensitivity may occur from lipsticks and salves, nickel, medicaments, flavourings, garlic [16], shellac [17] and cosmetic excipients. Lipstick dermatitis may be limited to the vermilion border, which appears dry, scaling or cracked; but the perioral area may also be affected. Eosin was a common sensitiser in lipsticks before 1960 [18] but since its allergenicity was found to be due to impurities there have been no further reports of adverse effects, and lipstick dermatitis is less common.

Allergy to toothpaste is a recognised cause of cheilitis and perioral eczema. Flavours (fragrances) are the usual cause, such as cinnamic aldehyde [19], spearmint oil, peppermint oil, anethole and *l*-carvone [20]. Colophonium and derivatives may be found in chewing gum but rarely cause allergic contact cheilitis [21]. Allergy to other food additives such as sodium metabisulphite, preservatives, colours and antioxidants may have a potential to cause cheilitis. In Europe, their presence can be determined by identifying the relevant E number on the ingredient label of the foodstuff packaging. Lip cosmetics with sun protection factor (SPF) may also contain sunscreen agents and even photoallergic contact cheilitis has been described [22]. Other important allergens to consider in patch testing cheilitis patients are the antioxidant gallates used in lip cosmetics and propolis [23,24].

Allergic reactions to dentures and fillings are considered in the section on mucous membranes later in this chapter. Angular cheilitis is usually due to badly fitting dentures, but cheilitis may exceptionally be caused by sensitisers habitually carried to the mouth, such as nail varnish or nickel-plated objects (e.g. keys, pins, musical instruments) [25].

Allergy to PPD contained in dyes for moustaches have also been reported as causing lip and perioral dermatitis.

Ears. External otitis has a complex aetiology (Chapter 106) and usually runs a chronic relapsing course. Neurodermatitis (lichen simplex chronicus) is also common, and may be superimposed on seborrhoeic eczema. Secondary medicament contact dermatitis, which is often unsuspected, is particularly common in the ear [26]. Dermatitis can also be both caused and maintained by habitual scratching with hairpins (nickel) or fingertips (nail varnish).

Although dermatitis from hearing aids occurs it is often a non-specific consequence of occlusion [27]. Hearing aids may contain acrylates and plasticising and stabilising chemicals. Headsets may contain urea and phenol-formaldehyde resins, or rubber in earphones.

Spectacle-frame dermatitis may be of irritant origin, especially behind and over the ears. Metals, particularly nickel and palladium, may cause allergy, and some frames responsible for dermatitis have been wrongly described as being nickel-free or made of titanium [28,29]. Plastic components, including epoxy resins, acrylates, plasticisers, UV inhibitors and dyes, have also been identified as the cause of the dermatitis. Earplugs for noise protection may contain antiseptics, dyes, rubber and plastic chemicals and finishes including formaldehyde resins.

Earrings and clips commonly cause dermatitis on the ear lobes as a result of the presence of nickel or, less commonly, gold. Piercing of the ear lobe may be the sensitising event in nickel dermatitis, leading to a chronic contact dermatitis. Granulomatous contact allergy to nickel, palladium and gold has been seen after ear piercing [30].

Scalp. The scalp tends to be relatively spared from involvement of allergic contact dermatitis. Dermatitis caused by fragrances, preservatives and amphoteric detergents in hair cosmetics is usually limited to the ears, neck and face, but may be preceded by persistent itching of the scalp. Permanent hair dye allergens, PPD and related oxidative dye chemicals still remain an important source of dermatitis. Correctly used, permanent hair dyes are applied to the hair and not the scalp, followed by oxidation and rinsing. Bleaches contain ammonium persulphate, which can cause peculiar urticarial eruptions as well as contact dermatitis. Glyceryl monothioglycolate, used for acid or cold perms, is a significant sensitiser in hairdressers but only occasionally causes problems in their clients. Hair-styling products such as mousses, gels, waxes and holding sprays often contain fragrances and preservatives that may be allergenic, but they also contain conditioning quaternary ammonium compounds, which are often irritant. Medicated shampoos may contain tar extracts, zinc pyrithione or other agents, and many shampoos contain formaldehyde, formaldehyde releasers or isothiazolinones added as preservatives. Some sources of cocamidopropylbetaine, found in many shampoos, may contain the sensitising impurity dimethylaminopropylamine. All these materials may potentially sensitise, although allergic subjects may tolerate them because of the short duration of contact, provided the hair is thoroughly rinsed after washing. Topical minoxidil lotion, prescribed to promote hair growth, will sensitise occasionally [31]. A European hair cosmetic series has been suggested [32].

Neck. Nickel in the clasps of necklaces or zip fasteners can produce a small area of dermatitis on the nape of the neck. Nail varnish (Figure 127.10) or nail methacrylates from fingertips may be the cause of a patchy and asymmmetrical allergic dermatitis, as can direct contact from fragrance allergens in perfumes. Hair dye allergens can elicit reactions in this region from certain hairstyles. Textiles (finishes in collars, dyes) and necklaces (nickel, exotic wood) may cause a collar-like dermatitis, or eruptions on the sides of the neck. Dermatitis from airborne allergens and photosensitisers is sharply limited by the collar to the 'V' of the neck if blouses or open-necked shirts are worn.

Axillae. Many cases of dermatitis are due to irritation from sweating, occlusion and the use of antiperspirants, which often contain aluminium salts to block the sweat glands. Allergic sensitivity may occur to fragrances used to mask odour, and to antiseptics intended to reduce the bacterial flora. The dermatitis produced by textiles tends to be periaxillary.

Trunk. The distribution of a clothing dermatitis may provide a clue to the responsible garment. In both sexes, nickel buttons and zip fasteners cause dermatitis localised to where they are worn, but a more widespread secondary spread rash may often occur. This is now less

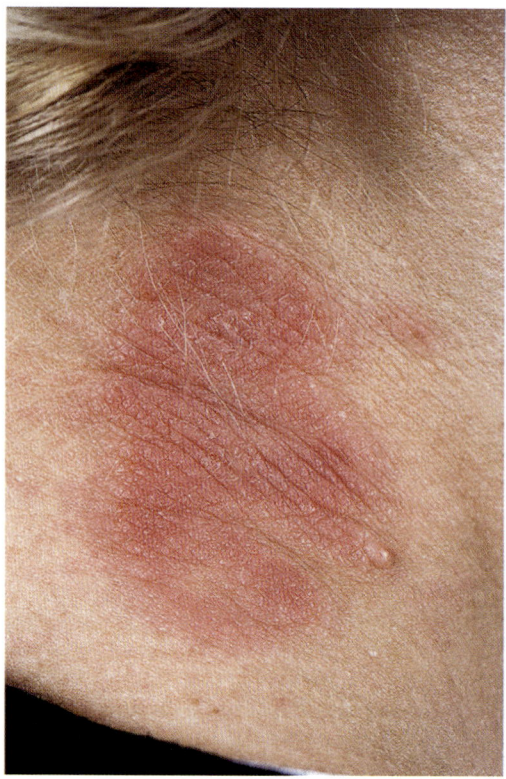

Figure 127.10 A patch of lichen simplex-like eczema on the nape of the neck associated with allergy to tosylamide formaldehyde resin (nail varnish). Courtesy of Dr J. D. Wilkinson.

often seen in Europe due to the 'Nickel directive'. Chromate, cobalt and octylisothiazolinone sensitivity from leather [33], and rubber allergy from elastic, may present as truncal eczema. Dermatitis from dresses, blouses and sweaters predominantly affects the neck and folds of the axilla, and spare areas of skin covered by underwear. The allergens are usually textile dyes or finishes.

Outdoor workers sensitised to Compositae (Asteraceae) plants may have a diffuse dermatitis or dermatitis of an airborne pattern, which affects all the exposed areas, including the trunk if they remove their clothing to work.

Detergents and fabric conditioners are commonly blamed for truncal skin eruptions but objective confirmation is usually lacking [34]. Diffuse papular eczema may be a feature of medicament sensitivity with secondary spread.

Ano-genital. The ano-genital region is a common site for medicament sensitisation. There is often experimentation with a wide range of prescribed and over-the-counter medicaments for pruritus, skin eruptions and haemorrhoids, and many of these contain sensitisers, most commonly fragrance, local anaesthetics and balsam of Peru (*Myroxylon pereirae*). Other sensitisers prescribed by the medical profession include neomycin, hydroxyquinolines, corticosteroids and topical antifungals. Some moist toilet tissues and wipes used to contain high levels of preservatives, which were associated with an increased prevalence of contact allergy (e.g. methylisothazolinone) [35]. Ectopic contact dermatitis from nail varnish may also affect this site [36].

The ingestion of contact allergens may cause pruritus ani, particularly if they are excreted unchanged. Spices and medicaments may occasionally be suspected.

Many studies in women have not distinguished an ano-genital pattern from dermatitis confined to the perianal or vulval area, but allergic contact dermatitis confined to the vulva appears to be less common [37]. Medicaments used for vaginitis rarely provoke allergic reactions on the mucosa but sometimes produce a rash on the adjacent skin, and may cause connubial dermatitis in sexual partners. Medicament allergy has frequently been associated with vulval dermatitis [38,39].

In a relatively recent study, 9% of patients suffering from lesions in the (peri)anal/genital area had positive patch test results to topical drug preparations and/or their ingredients, sometimes in association with cosmetics for intimate hygiene. The most frequent sensitising active principles were local anaesthetics and corticosteroids, while wool alcohols and to a minor extent benzoic acid were the most frequent culprits among the vehicle components and preservative agents, respectively [40]. Perfumes or antiseptics in soaps, sprays or sanitary pads are rare causes of genital dermatitis, although feminine hygiene sprays may cause both irritant and allergic reactions. Vulvodynia does not appear to be frequently associated with contact allergy [41]. Rubber accelerators in condoms can be a cause of genital eczema or pruritus vulvae. Delayed hypersensitivity to semen has also been reported [42]. Genital dermatitis from the transfer of material carried on the hands may occur in carpenters and cabinet makers and those who work with resins.

Thighs. Textile-related dermatitis may start at the edge of underwear, and is usually more pronounced in the popliteal spaces or gluteal folds. Finishes in the material of the pockets or objects kept in the pockets (e.g. nickel coins/keys) may provoke a patch of dermatitis on the underlying skin (Figure 127.11). Allergens may penetrate work clothes and should always be considered in relevant occupational cases.

Lower legs. The lower leg is particularly prone to contact allergy. Allergic contact dermatitis from medicaments and dressings predominate, especially in those with varicose eczema and ulcers. The common medicament allergens are topical antibiotics and components of creams and paste bandages, such as lanolin, cetostearyl alcohol and preservatives [43]. Allergy seems to occur readily to materials that are rarely problematic in other sites (e.g. parabens). Rubber allergy may be associated with compression bandaging and elastic hosiery. Allergy to colophony and derivatives may occur from dressing adhesives.

Rubber boots provoke dermatitis either at their upper edge or on the calf in areas of greatest friction.

Feet. Dermatitis may result from shoe materials including leather, rubber, glues and nickel, topical medicaments, antiseptics and antiperspirants.

Generalised. Generalised erythroderma may be the result of a chronic contact dermatitis maintained by continued exposure to a wide range of allergens, including components of topical medicaments. Patch testing is not possible until the skin has cleared.

Exposed sites. Contact dermatitis from dust, sprays, pollens or volatile chemicals is typically confined to the exposed surfaces of the hands, arms, face and neck. The first attack often originates from direct handling of an allergen, but recurrences may be seen despite avoidance of direct contact. There is great diversity in the nature of airborne reactions, which may be irritant, allergic, phototoxic, photoallergic or contact urticarial. Some agents may cause more than one type of reaction.

Lists of airborne allergens have been published and updated. Presently, most of the airborne allergens (and irritants) identified occur in occupational settings. Drugs and preservatives have recently become more important causes of airborne dermatitis [1].

Historically, plants, natural resins and woods were among the commoner causes of this distribution of contact allergy. In the USA, the oleoresins of ragweed commonly cause allergic contact dermatitis. A similar pattern in the UK during the summer months is caused by other Compositae (Asteraceae) weeds which, when they occur in other parts of the world, also produce an 'airborne' pattern of dermatitis. In India and Pakistan, *Parthenium* has been associated with widespread epidemics of severe dermatitis and even deaths [2]. Dermatitis from wood dust is common in carpenters and cabinet makers. It normally starts on the eyelids or the lower half of the face, and is often preceded by a period of itching. Swelling and redness spread to the neck, hands and forearms. By the time the patient attends for treatment, a diffuse dermatitis may have developed, distinctly limited at the margins of the sleeves and collar. Due to the accumulation of dust and sweat, the elbow flexures and the skin under a tight collar are often lichenified. Cabinet makers frequently develop a genital dermatitis from the accumulation of sawdust on the clothes during sawing and planing, and by hand contact. Swelling and redness of the eyelids may be the only signs of recurrence. Exotic woods are more likely to sensitise than fir or spruce, although the latter may cause dermatitis in patients sensitive to colophony and turpentine. Dermatitis in woodworkers may additionally be caused by liverworts and lichens on the bark of trees. Colophony can also result in an exposure pattern of dermatitis

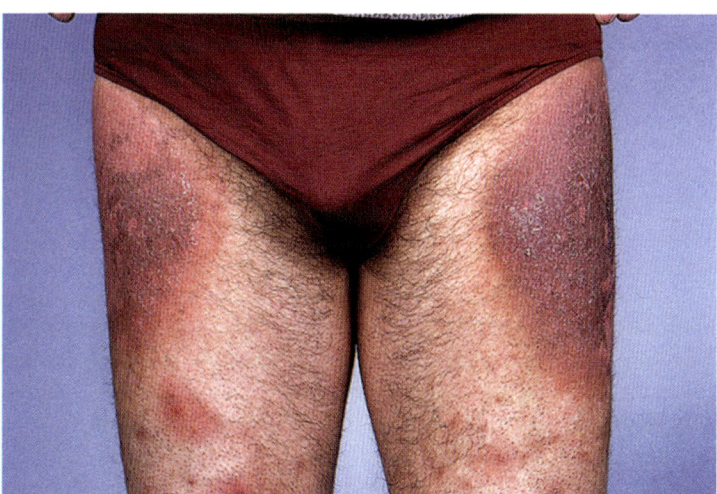

Figure 127.11 Allergic contact dermatitis due to items kept in trouser pockets. Courtesy of Dr J. D. Wilkinson.

from its presence in solder fluxes, paper dust, polish and linoleum flooring [3,4]. Resin systems, particularly epoxy resins, including the more volatile amine hardeners, may induce an airborne pattern of allergy, especially in the occupational setting. Other causes of this pattern include perfumes, metals, many industrial and pharmaceutical chemicals, pesticides, fungicides and animal feed additives [1]. Equivalent patterns of airborne dermatitis may be seen with type I allergens, such as house-dust mite antigens in atopics [5]. Photocontact allergy causes a similar distribution and is discussed in a separate section later in this chapter.

Mucous membranes. The application of DNCB to the oral mucosa may, in some cases, induce a low degree of contact sensitivity, but more often an immunological tolerance to later sensitisation [1]. Similarly, prior exposure to nickel and chromate in orthodontic appliances seems to reduce the risk of later sensitisation [2,3].

Contact inflammation of the mucous membranes is uncommon, and is often secondary to skin sensitisation with the same substances. Reactions may be allergic or irritant in nature. Both immune and non-immune immediate-type contact urticarial reactions can also occur.

The skin and mucous membranes differ in both anatomy and environment. In the mouth, except on the gums and hard palate, there is no horny layer with a barrier function and storage capacity. There is no lipid secretion, but instead a continuous flow of saliva, which washes away foreign substances. The penetration of water-soluble substances is rapid. It is not known whether these differences are relevant to the paucity of allergic contact reactions in mucous membranes. The oral mucosa of sensitised animals has been shown to have an identical cellular phenotype and cytokine expression as the skin when challenged by an allergen [4].

Allergic reactions in the mouth show redness and swelling, but vesicles are rarely seen, except on the vermilion border. Intraoral blistering has been seen from cinnamon allergy [5]. The symptoms are soreness and burning, and itching is uncommon. Eczematous reactions of the adjacent skin may occur, and these may be the only signs of an allergic contact dermatitis.

The burning mouth syndrome is an entity in which psychological factors may be important. Sometimes, allergens such as metals, rubber, food additives and flavourings have been identified and the symptoms relieved by contact avoidance [6], but return from investigations is often disappointing [7].

Oro-facial granulomatosis has been associated with contact allergy to food additives and some individuals suffering from this may obtain a favourable response, often only partial, to dietary elimination of the identified allergens – usually cinnamates and benzoates [8] (Chapter 108).

Dentures are frequently incriminated as the cause of oral symptoms and lesions. Allergic reactions to denture materials have been found in some cases [9] due to traces of residual acrylic monomer following the wearing of new dental appliances or following their repair with cold-curing resins. Most cases are the result of irritation from ill-fitting dentures. Candidal infection may also play a role [10], and is often present in angular cheilitis. Acrylate allergy is rarely seen after dental restorative work [11], but may be seen secondary to primary sensitisation from their use in artificial nails.

Mercury from amalgam fillings may cause local mucosal [12] or lichenoid [13,14] reactions; perioral dermatitis after dental filling may also occur, as may generalised skin eruptions [15]. Contact reactions to other metals have also been reported, especially gold used in dental restorative materials and nickel and palladium in orthodontic appliances [16,17]. Gingivitis is reported from eugenol in dental cement [18]. Toothpaste flavours can cause stomatitis, glossitis, gingivitis, cheilitis and perioral eczema [19].

The nasal mucosa may react to medications containing antibacterial agents and antihistamines. Corticosteroid allergy from nasal sprays has been reported, with one case of associated perforation of the nasal septum [20]. In the conjunctivae, various drugs are reported to have elicited allergic contact reactions, for example β-blocking compounds for the treatment of glaucoma, antibiotics and preservatives in both topical drugs and contact lens solutions [21].

Genital mucous membranes may be affected by allergens, particularly medicaments, causing dermatitis on the surrounding skin [22].

There remains debate as to whether materials sensitise via the mucosal route or whether there is only elicitation in those already sensitised and the induction of tolerance in those who have not already been sensitised [3,4].

Specific allergens

For information on specific allergens in ACD, see the separate section later in this chapter.

Clinical variants

Systemically reactivated contact dermatitis [1]. Systemically reactivated allergic contact dermatitis, where ingestion or other systemic exposure to a contact allergen takes place in an already sensitised person, may result in a number of different patterns of skin eruption. The threshold of reaction varies in each individual case and depends on the dose given and the level of sensitivity. Reactions may occur not only after systemic exposure to the primary allergen but also to closely related allergens.

The most frequent types of reaction are focal flares of previous patch tests and sites of previous dermatitis, sometimes with additional urticarial features. In severe cases vasculitis [2], erythema multiforme [3] and systemic upset may occur. Involvement of the eyelids, body folds and buttocks induced by oral challenge with nickel in allergic subjects led to this reaction being labelled the 'baboon syndrome' [4]. This is often also the pattern seen in patients with a mercury exanthem [5] and is now referred to as SDRIFE (systemic drug-related intertriginous and flexural exanthema). In some patients following widespread reactions, and in others following attempts at 'desensitisation', the level of patch test reactivity appears to be reduced [6].

Probably all contact allergens can cause systemic reactions provided the patient has a sufficient degree of pre-existing sensitivity and the dose administered is sufficiently large. The causes are many and include medicaments that may have been given not only by mouth but also parenterally, rectally, intravesically or as an inhalant. Dietary causes include metals, plants and spices.

Systemic contact dermatitis from medicaments [7] has decreased as a result of reduced use of topical sensitisers such as the antibiotics streptomycin, sulphonamides and penicillin, and topical antihistamines such as promethazine. Nevertheless, exposure to other topical and systemic medicament sensitisers continues to give problems. Standard allergens responsible for these reactions include neomycin, quinolines, local anaesthetics, ethylenediamine and corticosteroids. In subjects with contact allergy to ethylenediamine, parenteral and oral administration of aminophylline (which contains ethylenediamine) has resulted in widespread eczematous eruptions. Ethylenediamine is structurally related to some antihistamines (e.g. hydroxyzine, cetirizine, levocetirizine) and may therefore also trigger a systemic flare [8]. A positive patch test to tixocortol pivalate is an indication of hydrocortisone allergy, and the systemic administration of hydrocortisone has induced the recurrence and extension of dermatitis [9]. Furthermore, the administration of parenteral adrenocorticotrophic hormone, thereby raising endogenous hydrocortisone, has resulted in flares in hydrocortisone-allergic individuals. Other systemic steroids have also induced systemic contact dermatitis. Inhalation of budesonide has been associated with reactivation of positive patch tests, and continued exposure to budesonide from this source may therefore maintain dermatitis in sensitised subjects [10].

The persistence of dermatitis, especially vesicular hand eczema in metal-allergic subjects, has been blamed on dietary intake, particularly of nickel. Traces of metal dissolved by cooking acid or salty food in stainless steel may be of consequence in the persistence of dermatitis due to metals, such as chromium, nickel and cobalt [11]. In one study, the dietary restriction of nickel helped about one-quarter of selected nickel-sensitive patients with resistant dermatitis. However, the role of ingested or dietary nickel in hand dermatitis remains controversial, especially as a percentage of patch test-negative patients also appear to have flares of vesicular hand eczema following oral metal challenge, and the challenge dosage has been artificially high. A recent meta-analysis suggests that 1% of nickel-allergic subjects will develop systemic allergic contact dermatitis from normal daily exposure to nickel in drinking water and the diet.

Balsam of Peru, garlic, certain ingested food colours, preservatives and antioxidants have also been reported as causing flares of vesicular hand eczema [12–14].

Members of the Compositae family of plants can cause allergic contact dermatitis and systemic contact dermatitis in this group of patients is easily overlooked [15]. Sesquiterpene lactones are found in food and herbal remedies containing laurel, chamomile and goldenrod. Paulsen has thoroughly reviewed the literature on systemic contact dermatitis from sesquiterpene lactones in plants [16].

Cutaneous reactions to implanted metals. Orthopaedic metallic prosthetic implants [17] are made from a variety of metals, often alloys and especially stainless steel. Stainless steel – as given by ISO 5832-1 – consists mostly of iron and approximately 18% chromium (Cr), 15% nickel (Ni), and 3% molybdenum (Mo). However, nickel release from stainless steels, apart from those containing sulphur, is very low [18]. Titanium-based implants may either be used as (99%) pure titanium according to ISO 5832-2 or as alloy consisting of approximately 87% titanium (Ti) and 6% aluminium (Al) with further 4% vanadium (Va) or 7% niobium (Nb). In arthroplasty, CoCrMo-based alloy is predominantly used and has over 60% Co as the main constituent. Vitallium, a cast cobalt/chromium alloy, and titanium may also be used for implants.

Orthopaedic implants may be static (e.g. plate and screws) or dynamic (e.g. artificial hips). There are two potential concerns in relation to metal allergy and these implants: namely allergic skin disorders and loosening. There is little doubt that static implants can be associated with localised eczema over the site of implantation and more extensive skin eruptions in sensitised subjects, sometimes only resolving after removal [19]. The delay between the insertion of the prosthesis and the onset of dermatitis may be days or years. Similar eruptions were reported in the early days of hip replacements when metal heads articulated with metal cups. This problem seemed to have largely disappeared following the introduction of plastic joint surfaces, and prospective studies of hip joint replacements in known metal-allergic subjects are reassuring.

There is evidence of increased metal sensitisation associated with the loosening and failure of joints, particularly when these joints involve metal–metal contact. It is suggested that the increased allergy is caused by, rather than being responsible for, the loosening. Furthermore patch testing, although valuable in cutaneous contact allergy, cannot prove a causal relationship between implant failure and a dermal reaction.

In recent years there has been a return to metal-on-metal hip prostheses because it is felt that they produce less wear debris. Consequently, the issue of metal allergy in relation to these procedures has re-emerged [19,20]. As allergy is common in the general population, prospective controlled studies will be required to assess whether there is a genuine risk of dermatitis and loosening as a result. It is suggested by some authors that patch testing is undertaken preoperatively where requested to guide the choice of a suitable prosthesis. Postoperatively, where a problem has occurred, removal of an implant in a sensitised patient results in a resolution of symptoms in the majority [20]. A late reading at day 6 or 7 is strongly recommended since the yield of positive test reactions is increased.

Titanium allergy is virtually unknown, and thus titanium is an alternative for patients with extreme sensitivity to other metals. The patient should be told that the metal is not thought to be as long lasting as stainless steel.

Reactions have also been reported to sternotomy wires, shrapnel, mitral valve prostheses, dental prostheses and fillings, pacemakers, atrial septal occluders, infusion and acupuncture needles and implanted gynaecological devices [21]. While the release of metal ions from stents has been shown, the clinical relevance in restenosis of the coronary artery after stenting has yet to be definitively proven [22]. However, there is evidence of an increased rate of restenosis and allergy to gold after the stenting procedure when using gold-plated stents [23].

A diagnostic algorithm for use where a reaction to a metal implant is suspected has been proposed [24].

Non-eczematous responses.
Erythema multiforme-like reactions. The characteristic presentation is that of a spreading eruption from the primary site, which may also involve distant sites. The rash has features of erythema multiforme, in that single lesions appear target-like, but the distribution is not necessarily acral as in classic erythema multiforme nor is the

histology characteristic. There is sometimes a vasculitic purpuric element to the rash and, although the mechanism is unknown, it appears to represent an immune complex (type III) reaction as well as a delayed hypersensitivity (type IV) reaction. Many of these patients will give a very strong patch test response to the causative allergen, often accompanied by a flare of their dermatosis.

It is often precipitated by strong allergens, such as quinones in exotic woods [1], and *Primula*. Contact with other plant materials may cause this reaction, including poison ivy (*Toxicodendron* spp.), Compositae (Asteraceae) and tea tree oil. The ingestion of herbal remedies containing *Toxicodendron* and sesquiterpene lactones by sensitised persons has also induced erythema multiforme-like eruptions.

Topical medicaments, especially antimicrobials, corticosteroids and anti-inflammatories, have all caused erythema multiforme-like eruptions. A nitroglycerin patch has also induced erythema multiforme at the applied site, with a secondary spread eruption. Medicaments applied to mucosal surfaces may sensitise and may also be absorbed, causing systemic erythema multiforme-like reactions, for example sulphonamide in vaginal creams and ocular preparations.

PPDs in hair dye and temporary tattoos, rubber chemicals and clothing dyes are also recognised causes of this reaction pattern.

Erythema annulare centrifugum of the trunk has been linked to contact allergy to nickel and cobalt in clothing hooks and studs.

Purpuric reactions. Originally described in association with khaki uniforms, although the precise cause was not established, pigmented purpuric reactions are uncommon and have mostly been described recently from textile azo dyes [2] and textile resins. The presence of the rubber chemical IPPD in footwear, diving suits, bandages and bras is also reported as a cause of allergic contact purpura [3]. Purpuric reactions have been described with allergy to diphenylthiourea in heat retainers, PPD in black hats and as a secondary spread eruption from balsam of Peru.

Lichen planus and lichenoid reactions. These were historically described following contact with colour developers used in the photographic industry [4]; the developers are PPD derivatives. PPD-induced allergic lichenoid contact reactions from hair dye have been reported from India [5]. *Primula obconica* allergy has also produced a lichen planus-like eruption of the hands [6].

Lichen planus-like reactions of the buccal mucosa may represent allergy to metals [7], other materials used in dental treatments, cinnamal and spearmint. Some patients have had improvement in their lichen planus following the removal of some or all of their fillings [8]. Oral lichen planus is more apparent where there is evidence of corrosion and the aetiology of lichenoid lesions is likely to be multifactorial. The histology may show features compatible with lichen planus or a non-specific, chronic, superficial perivascular dermatitis.

Lichenoid reactions to tattoo pigments are discussed in the section on granulomatous reactions.

Lymphomatoid eruptions. Occasionally, contact dermatitis presents with cutaneous lymphoma-like plaques and histopathology suggestive of cutaneous T-cell lymphoma. These plaques have been seen at the site of ear piercing in those sensitised to gold. The reaction tends to persist for months, even when contact with metallic gold is avoided. The patch test reaction to gold sodium thiosulphate in these patients is papular and very strongly positive. The histology of both the papular eruption and the patch test reaction shows a dense T-cell infiltrate. Other reported causes include nickel, dental amalgam, medicament components, PPD, MCI/MI, parabens, isopropyl-diphenylenediamine and PTBPFR. A review of the literature has been published [9].

Pigmented dermatitis. Contact dermatitis may induce postinflammatory hyperpigmentation, and distinctive patterns of pigmented dermatitis without a lichenoid appearance or histopathology are recognised. These patterns are much more commonly seen in the Far East [10] but have been seen in Europe. The hyperpigmentation occurred mainly on covered areas, with or without dermatitis, and was traced to an optical whitener in washing powder, Tinopal CH 3566. Another outbreak was described in textile workers and traced to contact with naphthol AS, an azo dye coupling agent. Cases also occurred on covered sites from garments in Japan, and this led to a systematic search for other causes of textile dermatitis. Chemicals implicated included the fungicide Biochek 60, an impurity of colour index blue CI Blue 19, and textile finishes.

Pigmented cosmetic dermatitis is seen mainly in Asian women [11]. Slight dermatitis may precede or coexist with the hyperpigmentation, which occurs mainly on the cheeks. The allergens associated with this have been found to be fragrances and pigments, especially D and C Red 31 (from an impurity) and Yellow 11 in cosmetics and soaps. Pigmented cheilitis has occurred from allergy to ricinoleic acid in castor oil used in lipsticks [12]. Components of kumkum, applied as a cosmetic to the forehead, commonly cause a pigmented dermatitis [13].

Oral ingestion of flavourings allied to the fragrances, such as cinnamon, may cause not only a focal flare but also diffuse hyperpigmentation on the body [10].

Environmental agents, possibly pesticides and fungicides, have sometimes been thought to be a factor. In one study, most pigmented dermatitis cases were found to have positive patch tests to chlorothalonil used as a fungicide in banana plantations. It is used in other parts of the world as a preservative for wood and paint [14].

Depigmentation. Irritant and allergic contact dermatitis can induce hypopigmentation as a postinflammatory effect or by koebnerisation of vitiligo. This must be distinguished from the direct melanocytotoxic effect of certain quinones and substituted phenols, which most commonly present as an occupational vitiligo. This effect occurs independently of their sensitising potential.

A number of cases of persistent leukoderma following allergic contact dermatitis have been reported. In some it has been difficult to be certain whether the cause was postinflammatory or melanocytotoxic. In particular, it is reported from hair dyes and is commonly seen from temporary tattoos; persistence of hypopigmentation for longer than 2 years has been seen [15].

Epoxy resin components, methacrylates, perfumes, *Alstroemeria* and chloroxylenol are also reported as causes. *Primula* allergy has resulted in the extension of pre-existing vitiligo to sites affected by

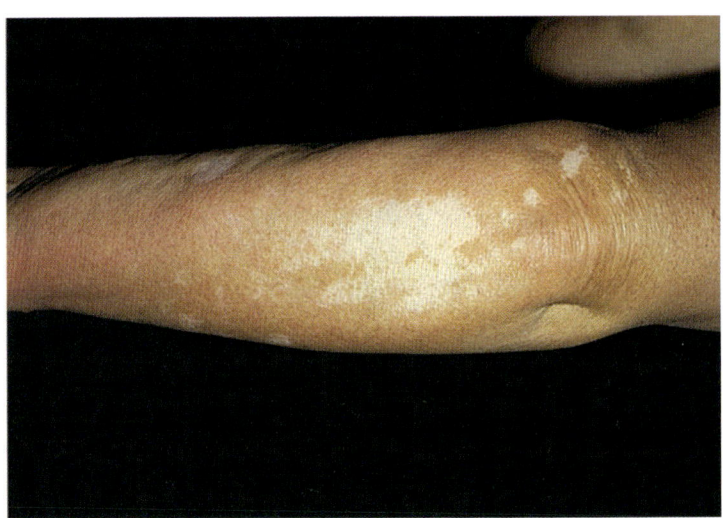

Figure 127.12 Koebnerisation of vitiligo as a result of previous *Primula obconica* allergy.

the dermatitis (Figure 127.12). The allergic reaction to primin was followed by vitiligo at the positive patch test sites [16].

Granulomatous reactions. Some topically applied metal salts produce non-allergic granulomatous skin reactions, for example zirconium in deodorants. Granulomas occurring at the site of previous immunisation with aluminium-adsorbed vaccines, or following the use of parenteral hyposensitisation preparations, are often due to aluminium allergy [17]. Patch tests are positive either to aluminium chloride 2% aqueous or an empty Finn chamber. Granulomatous reactions have also been found in association with allergy to gold and palladium in earrings [18].

Pigments in tattoos may cause allergic granulomatous and lichenoid reactions. Historically, metal salts have been identified as culprits: mercury (red colour), chromium (green colour), cobalt (blue colour) and cadmium (yellow colour). However, in our experience most reactions are in the red areas, and patch testing with mercurials is negative, suggesting another cause. Unfortunately, tattooists are extremely secretive about the nature of the pigments they use but an analysis has been undertaken of a series of pigments obtained from 20 tattoo parlours [19]. This has shown that a wide range of metallic salts, pigments and dyes may be used, and a suitable patch test series for tattoo reactions has been suggested as a result of this investigation.

Oro-facial granulomatosis has been associated with allergy to gold crowns and mercury fillings [20]. In one study 22% of patients with this condition had allergy to one or more food additives on patch testing, and most of these improved with an elimination diet. The authors concluded that the cause of the disorder was multifactorial and that patch testing had been helpful for a subgroup of those affected [21].

Onycholysis. Onycholysis may be the only presenting feature in contact dermatitis to hairdressing chemicals. It can occur as an isolated finding in nail varnish allergy. More commonly, it is found in subjects sensitised to multifunctional acrylates in anaerobic sealants and methacrylate nail cosmetics when there may be concomitant dystrophy and persistent paraesthesiae.

Systemic non-eczematous reactions. Extensive allergic contact dermatitis is not uncommonly associated with systemic upset from the metabolic effects of the disorder itself and secondary infection, particularly in those who are erythrodermic. Sultones occurring as impurities in lauryl ethyl sulphate have in the past caused several outbreaks of contact dermatitis characterised by intense oedema accompanied by general malaise [22].

Differential diagnosis

It should always be remembered that allergic contact dermatitis can mimic or complicate other types of eczema and other dermatoses. Sensitisation to topical applications may be a complication of almost any dermatosis that leads to specialist referral. The diagnostic problem differs according to the site of the dermatitis. Patch testing will often be required before confirming the cause in its entirety.

Head. Allergic and photoallergic conditions of the face must be distinguished from a number of disorders. Atopic eczema may be confined to the face, especially around the eyes and particularly the medial aspects. A previous or family history of infantile or childhood flexural eczema, asthma, allergic conjunctivitis, hay fever or immediate skin reactivity to animals and certain foods may point to the patient's atopic status. Associated flexural eczema, ichthyosis or xeroderma may be features. Multiple positive specific IgE tests or prick tests to common environmental allergens are used by some to confirm an atopic diathesis.

Seborrhoeic eczema, which commonly starts around the alae nasi, is usually accompanied by dandruff or seborrhoeic eczema in the scalp and eyebrows and by blepharitis. Involvement of the presternal region, the external auditory meati and the retro-auricular areas is common. Older patients frequently develop a flexural pattern of seborrhoeic eczema. Allergic contact dermatitis may imitate seborrhoeic eczema [1].

Psoriasis is normally easy to distinguish as there is evidence elsewhere on the body, although psoriasis in and around the ears and scalp margins may mimic a dry, scaly contact dermatitis.

Photosensitivity, including reactions to ingested drugs, cannot always be distinguished from photoallergic contact dermatitis, and may also simulate contact dermatitis from airborne sensitisers. Lupus erythematosus may be confused both clinically and histologically with contact allergy [2]. Dermatomyositis may initially appear identical to allergic contact dermatitis. The purple-mauve hue of the eyelids is a major clue, and the hands, fingers and nail folds must be carefully examined. The characteristic associated muscle pains and weakness may not always be present.

Angioedema, especially of the eyelids, is notoriously difficult to differentiate from contact allergy. The swelling would be expected to resolve within 24–48 h. Patch tests are helpful in reaching a conclusion.

Cellulitis and erysipelas may be difficult to distinguish from an acute allergic contact dermatitis, but the former are usually accompanied by pyrexia and systemic symptoms.

Herpes simplex may be simulated by *Primula obconica* dermatitis affecting the face and elsewhere. Haemorrhage into the blisters seems to be more common with the latter.

Basal cell carcinoma has been simulated by nickel allergy from spectacle frames [3].

Hands and arms. Allergic and irritant contact dermatitis and constitutional eczema of the hands may only be distinguishable by a careful history and patch testing. They commonly coexist. Superimposed irritant contact dermatitis from home and work exposures is common.

Indicators of atopic eczema are discussed elsewhere in the chapter. The eczema may be confined to the hands, especially in later life. A nummular pattern of eczema is commonly constitutional but may be a feature of irritant and allergic contact dermatitis, particularly from chromate exposure.

Recurrent vesicular eczema of the palms may indicate constitutional pompholyx, although contact allergy can produce an identical appearance. Some contact allergies, for example from IPPD and BIT, seem to induce a palmar pattern of dermatitis preferentially. *Primula* allergy often induces a haemorrhagic vesicular dermatitis of the palmar surfaces and fingertips. The relationship of pompholyx to the ingestion of contact allergens, especially nickel, by sensitised subjects is controversial [4]. There is evidence that oral intake of balsams and garlic can induce palmar vesicular eczema in patch test-positive subjects [5,6]. Tinea pedis can induce palmar pompholyx as an id eruption. Papules and vesicles on the hands and fingers are a feature of scabies, and this disorder must always be excluded by a careful history and examination for diagnostic burrows. The condition is normally associated with a more generalised pruritus and rash.

Psoriasis of the palms and hyperkeratotic eczema are often confused. Differentiation is sometimes somewhat arbitrary. Often, hyperkeratotic plaques are localised at points of contact, for example with tools, but not all frictional hyperkeratosis is necessarily an expression of psoriasis. The possibility of psoriasis koebnerising into areas of contact dermatitis should not be forgotten [7].

Tinea manuum is classically unilateral or asymmetrical. An inflammatory edge may be seen extending on to the dorsum of the hand. Nail dystrophy may be an association. Scaling palms should be scraped for mycology. These appearances may be complicated by a vesicular id eruption.

Lichen planus confined to the palms can be difficult to distinguish from a palmar dermatitis, but usually there are more typical changes elsewhere on the skin or in the mouth.

Porphyria cutanea tarda may simulate a bullous contact dermatitis such as plant dermatitis. The formation of bullae after minor trauma and the presence of white atrophic scars and milia suggest the diagnosis, which can be confirmed by porphyrin assays.

Flexures and ano-genital region. Seborrhoeic eczema and psoriasis may preferentially involve the flexures and be difficult to distinguish from allergic contact dermatitis, but there is often evidence of these conditions elsewhere. Tinea is usually asymmetrical or unilateral and has an inflammatory edge. Scrapings for mycology should be taken from inflammatory flexural rashes. The typical coral-pink fluorescence under Wood light will help to distinguish erythrasma from other flexural rashes.

Legs and feet. Persistent varicose eczema is an indication for patch testing as it is often complicated by sensitivity to topical medicaments and dressings, including rubber in support bandages and stockings. Vesicular and vesiculobullous areas may occur in tinea pedis, and mycological specimens should be taken if this is suspected. In common with the hands, scabies affecting the feet may induce a papulovesicular eruption and must be considered in the differential diagnosis.

Trunk. Papular drug eruptions or scabies may sometimes be difficult to distinguish from nickel or textile dermatitis. Dermatomyositis and mycosis fungoides sometimes show eczematous features.

Exposed sites. Photosensitive dermatoses and phototoxic drug eruptions must be distinguished from contact allergy to volatile and airborne materials. Although not always reliable, sparing in certain sites – behind the ears and under the chin – might indicate a photosensitive eruption. Nevertheless, some patients will require thorough investigation with phototesting, patch and photopatch testing before a diagnosis can be made.

Generalised. Erythroderma is rarely primarily due to contact allergy, and other causes such as drug eruptions, constitutional eczema and psoriasis should be considered; the possibility of secondary contact allergy from topical medicaments must not be forgotten. Skin biopsy may be helpful in these cases. Scabies can easily be overlooked as a cause of a widespread pruritic rash, especially as skin lesions may look classically eczematous. Careful examination of the hands, feet and genitals for diagnostic lesions is required.

Complications and co-morbidities

Complications of allergic contact dermatitis include those of eczema in general. Contact dermatitis may start at one site, but commonly other sites are subsequently involved, and sometimes several regions simultaneously. By the time the patient has been sensitised, many body regions may have been in contact with the allergen, some indirectly by contamination from the fingertips. Heavily contaminated areas, or those that were exposed last, tend to be the ones to react first, other sites flaring later. This has been shown experimentally with poison ivy, and is an obvious clinical feature in *Primula obconica* dermatitis. Regions close to the primary site of allergic contact dermatitis are easily contaminated by the allergen.

Such a simple explanation cannot account for the frequent spread of dermatitis from the feet to the hands and *vice versa*. This occurs primarily in constitutional eczema but may occur in contact dermatitis. Sometimes, a common allergen is found that could explain occurrence at both sites, yet often it is a pattern of secondary spread. No precise explanation exists. Because of the similarity to Darier trichophytids and eczematids, dissemination to distant regions has been termed an 'id-like' spread. Local aggravation may precede secondary spread by several days.

The pattern of spread is largely determined by the primary site. Dermatitis of the hands commonly spreads to the arms and face; dermatitis of the feet tends to spread to the legs and hands. Many patients with stasis dermatitis have secondary eruptions by the time they are seen by a dermatologist, and are referred because of the alarming dissemination. This may be due to an 'id' reaction or secondary contact dermatitis. Dissemination from leg eczema commonly involves the arms and shoulders in a patchy fashion before becoming generalised, often beginning with pruritus and sometimes progressing to generalised erythroderma. On the face, diffuse redness and oedema are common. Eyelid dermatitis or a diffuse dry dermatitis of seborrhoeic type may be seen.

Severe nickel allergy may induce extensive patchy eczema, which is slow to respond to treatment. This will not settle unless strict nickel avoidance measures are undertaken.

Contact allergy to components of topical treatments presents special difficulties. The allergen may be an active ingredient or an excipient. If the dermatitis spreads further in spite of treatment, it may wrongly be assumed to be an endogenous process. In contact dermatitis caused by topical steroid preparations, the action of the steroid may partially suppress the local reaction. The sensitivity becomes clinically manifest only as 'failure to heal' of the original eczema or with the development of a secondary eruption.

Constant alertness is therefore a prerequisite for the diagnosis of allergic contact dermatitis in which dissemination is a dominant feature. Patch tests should be delayed until the acute eruption has settled.

Disease course and prognosis

The prognosis of allergic contact dermatitis depends on its cause and the feasibility of avoiding repeated or continued exposure to the causative allergen. Associated irritant dermatitis and constitutional factors are also important. Some studies suggest that the age of onset is not important prognostically for occupational dermatitis but others suggest a poorer outlook in older age [1,2]. In the USA, patients with allergic contact dermatitis were found to tend to have a poorer quality of life if they were non-white, younger or industrial workers but sex was not important [3]. In Sweden, skin atopy was the factor that carried the worst outlook, followed by contact allergy, especially to nickel, and female sex [2].

The prognosis is generally relatively poor for those allergic to nickel [4] and chromate [5] probably as a result of their ubiquity in the environment, even though most chromate studies have involved those with occupational dermatitis, which is a selective group. It has been suggested that dietary nickel [6] and chromate [7] exposure might be responsible for the chronicity, but this is disputed [8].

There is a better outlook for those allergic to materials that are easy to identify and avoid, and often the dermatitis will resolve within a few weeks if conscientious avoidance measures are taken. This was exemplified by a European joint study where the sources of contact with allergens could be traced in only 35% of those who reacted to colophony, but in 85% of those sensitive to tetramethylthiuram disulphide. The reason for the limited success with colophony was probably lack of knowledge of the sources of this sensitiser. However, in a small Australian study, workers with epoxy resin allergy had a worse outlook than might be expected in spite of avoidance [9]. Greater age, associated atopy and longer duration and severity of dermatitis at diagnosis correlated with poorer prognosis in this survey. It is clear from a number of other studies that poor compliance and understanding results in a higher rate of ongoing exposure to the causative allergen, and is associated with a worse prognosis [10–12].

As the skin integrity is compromised there are enhanced opportunities for new sensitivities to medicaments or other substances to develop during the course of dermatitis. During a long course of relapsing dermatitis, sensitivity to various allergens may accumulate, and this increases the risk of recurrence or persistence [13].

Contact dermatitis of the hands is often of mixed origin, with alternating or simultaneous exposure to allergens and irritants. In one study of the prevalence of dermatitis of the hands, half the patients had suffered from their dermatitis for more than 5 years. Follow up after 6–22 months revealed one-quarter had healed completely, half had improved and one-quarter were unchanged or worse. There was no difference in prognosis between irritant and allergic dermatitis. A change of occupation does not necessarily alter the prognosis of occupational hand dermatitis, particularly if the change is inappropriate [14]. The concept of persistent postoccupational dermatitis despite avoidance of the original cause(s) is now well established, and may occur following both irritant and allergic contact dermatitis [15].

Once acquired, contact sensitivity tends to persist [16]. The degree of sensitivity may decline unless boosted by repeated exposure, but with a high initial level of sensitivity it often remains demonstrable even several years later [17]. Sensitivity to ubiquitous allergens, such as nickel and chromate, and to strong allergens, such as primin and PPD, is reported to persist, whereas sensitivity to other weaker and avoidable allergens may disappear. Patterns of cross-sensitisation tend to persist.

Relapse or chronicity is due not only to unavoidable or unrecognised re-exposure to allergens and irritants but also to other contributory mechanisms.

1 The barrier function of the skin is impaired for months after an attack of dermatitis. Recovery is prevented by exposure to allergens or irritants in concentrations that might well be tolerated by normal skin.
2 Inappropriate treatment, including the overzealous use of cleansers and antiseptics, and the use of sensitising popular or herbal remedies may also prolong the course of dermatitis.
3 The ingestion of allergens.
4 Secondary infection, especially with dermatitis of the hands. Microbial allergy may also be a factor in some eczemas.
5 Contact sensitivity has been thought in some cases to involve sensitisation to the protein moiety ('protigen') of the hapten–protein conjugate. On this assumption, autosensitisation might account for chronicity [18].
6 Stress is common in chronic dermatitis and may be both a consequence of, and a trigger for, eczema.
7 Constitutional factors predispose to chronicity.
8 There appears to be an 'inherent tendency' in almost any eczema to become continuous and chronic, but the factors causing this are unknown.

Investigations: patch tests
Background

The diagnosis of allergic contact dermatitis is made by patch testing. The techniques have evolved into a standardised methodology worldwide, although there are some variations, particularly with regard to reading times and test units [1]. Patch testing relies on the observation that primed antigen-specific T lymphocytes will be present throughout the body, and hence allergen in the patch test can be applied to normal skin, usually on the upper back where the tests are least likely to be disturbed. Other sites may be considered when this is not practicable, for example when there is pre-existing inflammation or other skin changes are on the back.

The test relies on the allergen being absorbed in sufficient quantity to induce a reproducible inflammation of the skin at the site of application in sensitised subjects. A positive reaction to a correctly prepared and applied patch test confirms the person has an allergic contact sensitivity, although this does not necessarily mean that the substance is the cause of the presenting clinical dermatitis and its relevance should always be carefully considered.

Indications

It is well established that aimed patch testing with a few suspected allergens is suboptimal. The reason is that even experienced dermatologists are poor predictors of the outcome of patch tests; they are more likely to be correct for common allergens such as nickel (50–80%) and less likely for less common allergens (<10%) [2].

An audit of patch testing has suggested that the investigation is underused, and consequently important opportunities to improve or resolve potentially disabling and wrongly classified eczema/dermatitis are lost [3]. The audit concluded that facilities should be available to patch test at least 142 per 100 000 population annually. The indications for patch testing are listed in Box 127.1. Dermatology-specific quality of life has been shown to improve significantly more in those patients who are patch tested because of more accurate diagnosis and earlier intervention [4,5,6]. Furthermore, the investigation has been shown to be cost-effective and to reduce the cost of therapy in patients with severe allergic contact dermatitis [4,7].

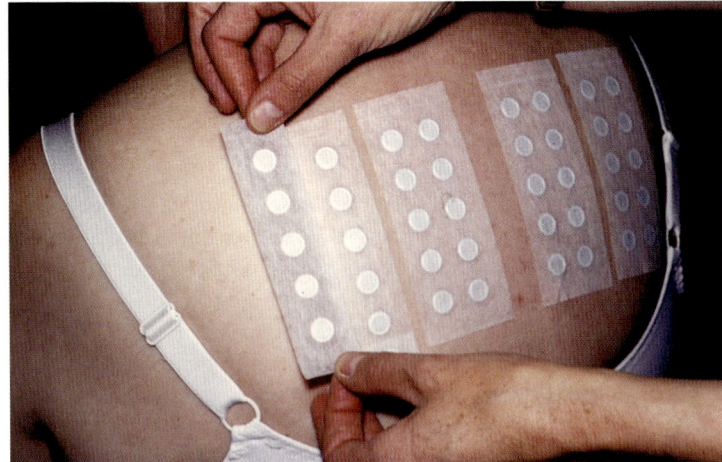

Figure 127.13 Finn patch test chambers being applied to back.

> **Box 127.1 Indications for patch testing**
>
> - Eczematous disorders where contact allergy is suspected or is to be excluded (including occupational)
> - Eczematous disorders failing to respond to treatment as expected (including occupational, stasis, atopic, seborrhoeic and discoid)
> - Chronic hand and foot eczema
> - Persistent or intermittent eczema of the face, eyelids, ears and perineum
> - Certain drug eruptions
> - Mucous membrane reactions (conjunctivitis, stomatitis or vulvitis)
> - Implants
> - Also includes other morphological presentations that may represesent a contact allergic reaction, e.g. erythema multiforme like, lymphomatoid or granulomatous presentations

Methods

Updated guidelines have been prepared by the European Society of Contact Dermatitis [1]. The basis of this *in vivo* test aims to reproduce the elicitation phase of the reaction to a contact allergen. The amount of test allergen is defined by its concentration in the vehicle and the amount applied. By testing the same allergens in parallel, the technique has been confirmed to be generally reproducible [8,9].

Chambers or discs are used to ensure occluded contact with the skin (Figure 127.13). The fixing tape should be non-occlusive, non-allergenic and non-irritant. If the adhesive tapes peel off, the test should be repeated. Ideally, patch testing should not be carried out in patients with active eczema because it may reduce the threshold of activity and cause non-specific reactions, although in practice this is usually not possible. The procedure ideally should be delayed until the test site has been clear of eczema for at least a fortnight. Patch testing should be delayed for 4 weeks following sunbathing, and the patches should not be exposed to the sun or other sources of UV light. This information should be given to the patients before they book their appointments. Corticosteroids and other immunosuppressive drugs should be stopped (if this is feasible) before patch testing as they may reduce or extinguish positive patch tests in sensitised subjects. Nevertheless, this is unlikely at doses below 15 mg prednisolone daily [10], and we have identified relevant positive patch tests in patients who could only be investigated while they were taking other immunomodulators.

Some prefer not to patch test pregnant patients in case an adverse event is blamed on the test, although we are unaware of any proven problem. Young children, even infants, can be patch tested when indicated, but the number of allergens tested may have to be reduced because of lack of space [11].

Test materials. Commercially prepared test allergens are obtainable from the following manufacturers or from their local distributors: SmartPractice (https://www.smartpractice.com last accessed July 2023), which markets allergEAZE® allergens, and Chemotechnique Diagnostics (https://www.chemotechnique.se/patch-testing//; last accessed July 2023). The materials should be of pharmaceutical quality and in some countries they may be registered as drugs.

The commonest system used to apply allergens is the Finn chamber (Epitest Ltd, Tuusula, Finland) on Scanpor tape (Norgesplaster, Vennesia, Norway). These are also available from local distributors. The chambers are supplied in strips of five or 10 (two rows of five), and consist of small, occlusive aluminium discs. They are mounted on non-occlusive tape with an acrylic-based adhesive backing that has been chosen for its hypoallergenicity. Other systems consist of square plastic chambers (Van der Bend chambers), and systems continue to be developed (e.g. IQ Ultra™) to improve adhesion and comfort and also to impart water resistance to enable brief showering during the tests.

There is also a prepackaged, ready to use patch test system, the T.R.U.E. test®, based on a dispersion of allergen in a hydrophilic polymer. This is currently available as a series of 35 allergens and a negative control. This system has been tested in parallel with the established Finn chamber system and there was close correlation of results [12]. It is a consistent, convenient, portable method for those wishing to test only a few allergens, but supplementary tests are necessary to achieve a comprehensive range of investigations [13]. It has been estimated that by using preprepared tests alone between 60% and 70% of relevant allergic reactions may be missed.

Patch test vehicles. Few substances can be applied to the skin as they are. In order to avoid an irritant effect, they must be mixed or dissolved in a vehicle to achieve a suitable test concentration. The test substance should, if possible, be soluble in the vehicle. If a dispersion of allergen in petrolatum is used, contact with the skin depends on the size of the particles and on their solubility or dispersion in petrolatum. Uniform dispersion and particle size are important. Many substances can also be dissolved in water, alcohol, acetone, methylethylketone or olive oil, as appropriate. Irritant solvents must not be employed. False positive or false negative reactions may occur when inappropriate vehicles are used. Petrolatum is generally more reliable, and has the added advantage of being occlusive, which helps to prevent oxidation and prolongs shelf-life. Allergic reactions to petrolatum itself are very rare [14].

Patch test concentrations. The choice of a suitable concentration is of fundamental importance. Excessive concentrations result in false positive reactions because of their irritant effect, and may even sensitise patients; insufficient concentrations produce false negative results. The concentration of allergen routinely employed for patch tests may, under some conditions and in some individuals, give rise to false negative or false positive reactions. The choice of concentration is thus a compromise, but most have been chosen by long experience with commonly used allergens. The concentrations used for patch testing are usually much higher than those encountered during the development of dermatitis. To demonstrate the existence of nickel dermatitis produced by the minute amounts dissolved from nickel-plated objects, a 5% concentration of nickel sulphate in petrolatum is necessary. Neomycin should be tested at 20% despite only being at 0.5% concentration in many topical medicaments.

Lists of suitable concentrations and vehicles are provided in the text by De Groot (see 'Resources' later in this chapter). Metal salts in particular are tested at the margins of irritancy and may give false positive, irritant patch test reactions, especially in atopic individuals. Weak reactions may not be allergic. In important cases of doubt the patient can be retested later with serial dilutions. Other standard allergens such as fragrance mix, parabens mix and wool alcohols may also be marginally irritant. On rare occasions, active sensitisation may still occur even at the concentrations recommended. Irritant reactions are rarer with other substances used in the baseline series. They are potentially much more common with materials brought to the clinic for testing. Many industrial or domestic chemicals, if undiluted, will give irritant false positive reactions which may be severe. No chemical or substance should be applied to the skin until full details of its composition and potential irritancy or toxicity are known.

If substances from work or other materials are brought, a number of factors should be considered before they are used for patch testing. Is it appropriate to test with the material? Some materials are strong irritants and not allergens (e.g. strong acids and alkalis), and others may be contaminated or of uncertain or mixed composition (e.g. dust or grime from a working environment). The product may be intrinsically dangerous (e.g. explosive or produces toxic fumes) and requires special handling. Some patients bring foods in the mistaken belief that the test will diagnose ingested food allergy.

The precise nature of the material should be ascertained by questioning the patient and examining the product label. In the UK, employers are required by law to have material safety data sheets for all materials handled at work. These provide key information and a contact point with the manufacturing company. They must be scrutinised carefully, particularly with regard to irritancy, allergenicity, stability and solubility of the product and its components. Named chemical substances may be recognised as irritants or allergens and their concentrations documented. Substances can be checked for pH and neutralised if necessary [15]. It should be remembered that a data sheet is only as good as the individual writing it and may not be comprehensive or completely accurate. Consequently a degree of scepticism is helpful in their interpretation.

An initial patch test concentration can often be selected either by reference to standard texts or by contacting the manufacturer for details of toxicological testing data. A range of differing test concentrations is advised where there is no literature on the material. It is advisable to start low (0.01% or less) and increase the concentration gradually if there is doubt about the optimum level for testing. It may be advisable to perform open tests before proceeding to closed patch tests because the effect of irritants is enhanced by occlusion. Materials intended to be left on the skin, such as medicaments and cosmetics, can be tested 'as is', rinse-off products at 5%, and soaps, shampoos and detergents at 1% or less. However, the dermatologist administering a patch test will need to refer to standard references for guidance on dilutions and vehicles when testing finished products or specific chemicals.

If a positive reaction to an unknown substance occurs, it should not be immediately accepted as allergic. Volunteers, who are not suffering from dermatitis related to the same agent, should be tested at the same concentration and using the same methods. If any reaction occurs among up to 50 controls, the substance should be regarded as a primary irritant at that concentration, and subsequent tests should be performed with decreasing concentrations.

Patch test dose. If petrolatum is used as the vehicle and disposable syringes are the containers, a length of 5 mm of test substance in a vehicle will suffice. For an 8 mm Finn chamber, 20 mg of allergen as a petrolatum dispersion has been shown to be the optimum dose [16]. If the vehicle is a fluid, a digital pipette should be used to deliver 15 µL to a filter paper in the 8 mm Finn chamber. These figures have been calculated to be 25 mg and 20 µL resepctively for an IQ Ultra chamber. Dropper bottles supplied by the allergen manufacturers tend to overfill the chambers. A surplus should be avoided, as it may contaminate neighbouring test sites. With the T.R.U.E. test, the patches are preprepared. The risk of patch test sensitisation increases with the concentration and amount of test substance applied.

Storage of allergens. Shelf-life is prolonged if test substances not in daily use are stored in the dark in a refrigerator at 4°C. Many substances are unstable if exposed to light. Commercially available allergens are labelled with an expiry date which should

Table 127.3 Reactivity of various test sites.

Test site	Irritant (%)	Allergic (%)
	Type of reaction	
Upper back	100	100
Lower back	50	95
Upper arm	52	72
Forearm	38	74
Thigh	36	50

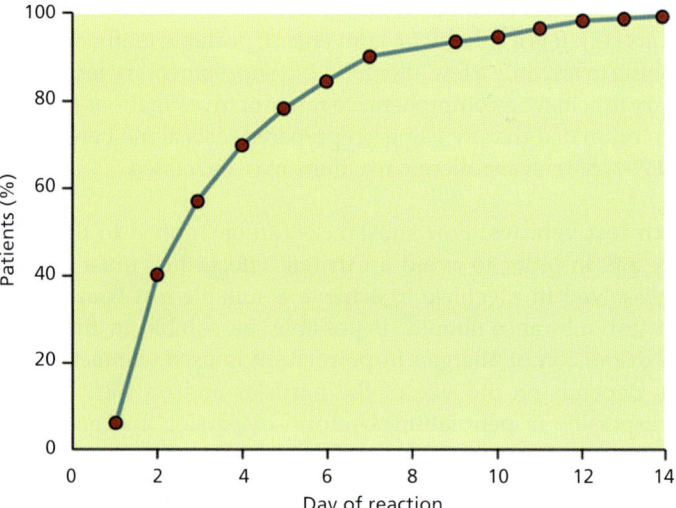

Figure 127.14 Patch tests with neomycin 20% in petrolatum: positive reaction times after application.

be continually reviewed. With potentially volatile allergens, the allergen may be lost over time even when refrigerated so substances should be regularly replaced. For some materials such as isocyanates, freezing is essential to prevent the loss of allergen [17]. Homogeneity of patch test allergens may be lost, especially in hot climates, if they are not refrigerated.

Many centres preprepare their allergens prior to application. However, care must be taken, particularly with volatile allergens such as fragrances and isocyanates, where it has been shown that following application, even with refrigeration, the allergen is rapidly lost from the test chamber [18]. It is preferable to prepare test allergens on the day, and apply immediately to avoid consequent false negative reactions.

Test site. For practical reasons the upper back is preferably used (Figure 127.13). Both allergic and irritant reactions are most easily provoked on the upper back (Table 127.3) [19]. Reactions on the lateral aspect of the upper arm are stronger than on the medial aspect. Sites other than the back and lateral aspect of the upper arm are generally less suitable as test areas, although it is considered reasonable to use the thighs when absolutely required.

Marking. Test sites must be marked with indelible ink or stratum corneum stains. Marking materials can be obtained from allergen suppliers. It is necessary to repeat marking before removal of the patches because their positions cannot be distinguished once the pressure effects have subsided. The patient should be instructed not to bathe or shower for the duration of the tests, and to avoid exercise or other activity likely to dislodge the patches.

Occlusion time

Few formal studies on the relationship of exposure time, dose and elicitation have been undertaken. Work with PPD and isoeugenol has shown that elicitation is dependent not only on exposure time but also on concentration and number of applications of the allergen [20,21].

Well-established allergens, however, are conventionally tested in such concentrations that a 48 h exposure under an occlusive patch will generally allow penetration of an amount sufficient to provoke a reaction. With low sensitivity, low concentration of allergen or poor absorption of a particular agent, there may be a long period of latency.

Reading times

Immediately after removal of the patch tests, there may be redness from the stripping action of the tape, especially in dermographic subjects, and this must be allowed to settle. Furthermore, some reactions may take up to 1 h to develop once the pressure of the strips has been released, and the infiltration allowed to swell the dermis.

A typical regimen is a 48 h application time, with readings taken 1 h after removal and again 48 h later (that is, day 2 and day 4), with preferably the same observer performing each reading. Others have suggested that a second reading on day 5 is better. A single day 2 reading is not advised as it may lead to the labelling of some marginal irritants as allergens, and positive reactions to more poorly absorbed allergens may be missed. Variations to this schedule are made for expediency, to fit in with clinic times, and for the convenience of patients travelling long distances. If only one patch test reading is possible, a day 4 reading has been recommended [22] although, according to some authors, a single day 4 reading is also associated with the risk of missing some significant positive reactions. A third reading on day 5, 6 or 7 seems to identify a small proportion of additional relevant positive allergies where sensitivity is weak or partially 'forgotten', or where there is poor absorption of the allergen [23]. Neomycin, some metals and corticosteroids are particularly liable to give late reactions (Figure 127.14).

Therefore, in preference at least two readings of reactions are required ideally performed on day 2, 3 or 4 and around day 7.

Morphology and interpretation

It is important that patch test readings are scored according to the reactions seen and not according to the interpretation placed on the reaction by the reader. As the strength of a reaction is not always reproducible, an overdetailed quantification should be avoided. The scoring system devised by the ICDRG in 1970 is shown in Table 127.4 [24]. There are drawbacks to the ICDRG system in that it confuses morphology with interpretation. The ideal system is to record what is seen on days 2 and 4 and then to decide if this represents an allergic or irritant response. This is done by assessing the morphology and skin type, combined with knowledge and experience of the substance and the patient's history. Patch test results should be recorded

Table 127.4 Recording of patch test reactions according to the International Contact Dermatitis Research Group scoring system.

Score	Description
–	Negative
?+	Doubtful reaction; faint erythema only
+	Weak positive reaction; palpable erythema, infiltration, possibly papules
++	Strong positive reaction; erythema, infiltration, papules, vesicles
+++	Extreme positive reaction; intense erythema and infiltration and coalescing vesicles
IR	Irritant reaction of different types
NT	Not tested

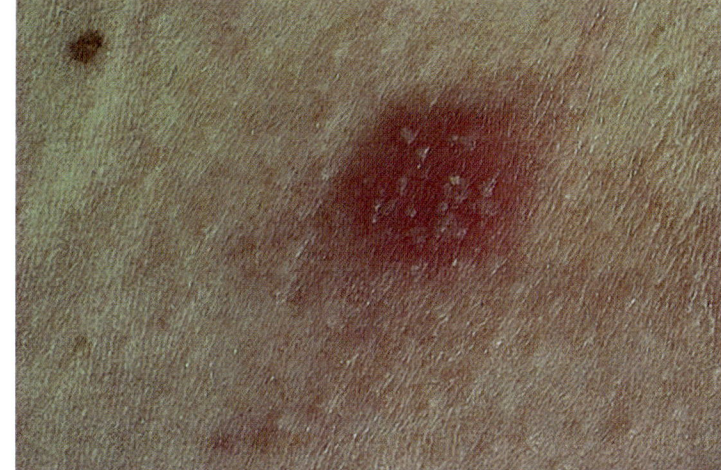

Figure 127.16 Pustular patch test reactions to metals are common in patients with atopy and are often irritant in type.

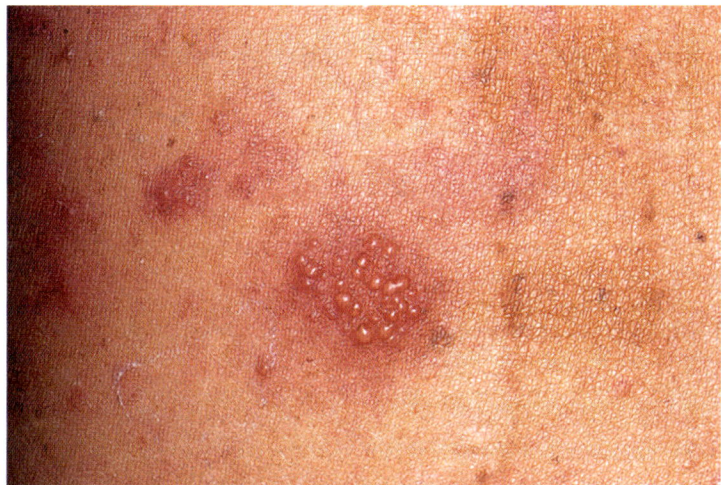

Figure 127.15 A positive allergic (++) patch test response in a patient sensitive to neomycin. Courtesy of Dr J. D. Wilkinson.

objectively, and the interpretation of the results should be recorded separately. In this way raw data remain available for re-examination.

Once they have developed, positive allergic reactions often persist for several days. The strength of the reaction depends on barrier function, the presence or absence of sweating, atmospheric humidity, test material, technique and the reactivity of the individual.

Strong reactions of an allergic nature are erythematous and infiltrated, commonly with minute papules or vesicles (Figure 127.15), which in severe reactions coalesce into bullae. The infiltration causes a thickening in the dermis that is palpable and can be distinguished from surface changes in the epidermis. The reaction may extend beyond the margins of the patch, and there is often some itching. Nevertheless, sometimes true allergic reactions can be weaker than this, making interpretation more difficult.

Morphologically positive patch test reactions (+, ++ or +++) at day 3 or later are usually assessed as allergic.

In most instances there is little difficulty for the experienced clinician in identifying true positive allergic patch test reactions. Nevertheless, there are occasions when distinguishing an allergic from a false positive non-allergic irritant reaction can be difficult, or even impossible. There may be clues: no infiltration, lack of itching, deep redness or a brown hue, and sharp delineation corresponding to the margins of the patch test all point to an irritant reaction. Some irritants provoke a 'soap effect', with a well-localised, glistening, finely wrinkled surface. Patch tests with nickel may cause pustular reactions that are often false positive (Figure 127.16), although some progress to more typical allergic reactions. Cobalt also produces a distinctive false positive purpuric reaction that may result from poor dispersion of the allergen in the petrolatum base. In our experience these tend to occur much more in atopic individuals and need to be distinguished from allergic follicular reactions consisting of papules without pustules or purpura.

False positive irritant reactions are liable to induce stronger reactions at day 2 than at day 4, the so-called crescendo–decrescendo effect. However, this is not always the case and the reverse can happen in our experience. Difficulties in evaluation are particularly common with substances brought in by the patient for testing. It may be necessary to apply several concentrations at the first visit; controls should be performed with any substances giving positive reactions.

There is no substitute for a thorough knowledge and experience of the allergens used for patch testing. Even some standard allergens may be liable to induce weak false positive reactions (e.g. metal salts, fragrance mix, parabens mix, wool alcohols, carba mix). Repeat patch testing, especially with a breakdown of the mixes or testing with dilutions, may be helpful.

Interobserver variability has been observed, especially differentiating between doubtful and irritant reactions and doubtful and weak positive reactions. Continued reading training has been advised [25].

Relevance of patch tests

Once a decision has been reached that a patient has an allergic positive patch test, it is then important to establish relevance by systematically re-examining the patient's history, distribution of the rash and materials with which there has been contact including reviewing ingredient labelling. In many cases relevance can be clearly established and avoidance advice given. In some instances, the relevance may be in the past and may no longer apply. In other cases the relevance may be uncertain or impossible to ascertain. If a material 'cross-reacts' with a diagnosed allergen, previous exposure and sensitisation to this cross-reacting material is not necessary.

Patients will need to be advised on the potential sources of all their allergies for future reference, and if their problem is ongoing, it may be necessary to reassess their exposures. A person may react to a patch test but still tolerate contact with the allergen. However, confusion can occur if they are given extensive avoidance advice for materials of no relevance to their dermatitis, and therefore advice should be targeted.

Non-invasive measurement techniques

There are several non-invasive techniques that can be used to quantify and delineate patch test reactions, including measurements of changes in the skin surface, epidermal hydration and water barrier function and parameters of inflammation. At present, these are more useful to the investigator than to the clinician. They include transepidermal water loss, skin reflectance, laser Doppler flowmetry, thermography and high-frequency ultrasound. Attempts have been made to use some of these techniques to differentiate irritant from allergic patch test reactions but they have not superseded the combination of human brain, eye and hand in the assessments of patch tests.

Sources of error

False positive reactions (Box 127.2). Irritant reactions occur if a chemical is tested at excessive concentration. Incorrectly interpreted false positive reactions may lead to the wrong conclusions about the cause of dermatitis, and this may result in inappropriate career or medicolegal advice. Recent or active dermatitis in the test area lowers the threshold for irritant reactions, as does dermatitis in other areas; non-specific reactions can also occur. Secondary non-specific reactions close to genuine positive ones have been termed 'angry back' or the 'excited skin syndrome' [26], and this may be an important cause of false positive patch test reactions. The phenomenon has been extensively investigated by Bruynzeel [27].

> **Box 127.2 Causes of false positive reactions**
>
> - Excessive concentration
> - Impure substance (contaminants)
> - Irritant vehicle
> - Excess allergen applied
> - Uneven dispersion
> - Current or recent dermatitis at patch test site
> - Current dermatitis at distant sites
> - Pressure effect of hard materials
> - Adhesive tape reactions
> - 'Angry back' reaction causing intensification of weak irritants
> - Artefacts

If there is any doubt, the patch tests should be repeated some weeks later, preferably with individual agents and at various dilutions, as false positive irritant reactions tend to stop abruptly below a certain concentration whereas allergic responses tend to persist, albeit proportionally weaker, at lower concentrations. Testing the same substance on a panel of controls, using the ROAT on the elbow flexure or usage tests, may help to differentiate allergic from irritant responses. Controls should be tested at the lowest concentration of a positive test to avoid interpreting a false positive irritant reaction as allergic.

False negative reactions (Box 127.3). Sometimes a patch test fails to provoke a positive reaction in a person who is sensitive to the substance tested. The dermatitis therefore persists because of continued exposure to the allergen. The most common cause of false negative reactions is insufficient penetration through the skin. A low degree of sensitivity or poor penetration sometimes results in a long period of latency before a positive reaction develops, so that up to 7.5% of allergic positive patch tests do not become apparent until after 4 days and may go unnoticed unless read 7–14 days after application. This particularly applies to neomycin and corticosteroids.

> **Box 127.3 Causes of false negative reactions**
>
> - Insufficient concentration
> - Insufficient amount applied
> - Poor adhesion of patches
> - Patches applied at wrong site
> - Inappropriate vehicle
> - Readings performed too early
> - Substance degraded
> - Pretreatment of patch test site with topical corticosteroids
> - UV irradiation of patch test site
> - Systemic treatment with immunosuppressants

The apparent discrepancy between the concentration of allergen needed to elicit clinical dermatitis and the occasional failure of a patch test to elicit a reaction can be explained by many factors. A single exposure on normal skin is probably not representative of the accumulation of the allergen during repeated exposure conditions and chronic usage on already primed skin.

False negative reactions are common when testing with textiles, cosmetics, medicaments, leather and rubber, as some ingredients are present in very low concentrations. False negative reactions also occur when allergens are present in irritant products. Because of irritancy, a product may have to be diluted to such an extent before it can be safely tested that the allergen is present in insufficient concentration to elicit a response. Such products include cutting oils and washing materials. Sensitivity to finished products and topically applied preparations is best confirmed and revealed by testing with the individual components.

An allergy may be missed on patch testing if the test material has been wrongly diluted in a material in which it is immiscible or insoluble. Furthermore, an incorrect diluent may change the allergen into another substance altogether. Partition coefficients are also important, because oil/water solubility may be a significant factor in skin penetration and allergenic potential.

Local treatment with topical corticosteroids, and systemic treatment with immunosuppressants including ciclosporin, azathioprine, methotrexate and corticosteroids such as prednisolone (at a dose above 15–20 mg/day), may diminish or abolish reactions [28], as does preceding sunbathing [29]. Negative reactions, despite clinical sensitivity, also occur in photocontact dermatitis if appropriate allergens are not photopatch tested.

In practice, it may be difficult or impossible for patients to stop their immunosuppressants and under such circumstances patch testing should be undertaken but the clinician should be aware of the possibility of a false negative investigation. However, there is no doubt that positive reactions occur even under these circumstances.

Compound allergy. Compound allergy occurs when a positive allergic patch test reaction is seen to a finished product but tests with the ingredients are negative [30]. Hence, the product and the constituents should be patch tested when allergy is suspected.

New compounds may be formed within a product, and their presence can be confirmed by the finding of incongruous peaks on spectrometry. This was elegantly demonstrated in Hirudoid cream, where a new allergen was formed as a reaction product of two preservatives in the medicament [31]. The additive effect of multiple weak sensitisers [32], or the additive effect of weak allergens and irritants, should be considered [33].

There are several possible alternative explanations. The reaction to the finished product may be irritant. A product's irritancy is not merely the sum of the irritancy of the ingredients, but an expression of the hydrophilic–hydrophobic balance of its ingredients. This can change with varying manufacturing techniques, for example changing the temperature or manipulating the proportion of one of the ingredients. A constituent allergen may be an undeclared ingredient or there may be batch/source differences between the original compound and the subsequently provided components. The allergen may be in the container, for example a rubber stopper, and not in the product. The allergen may not have been tested in the correct vehicle or at the correct concentration, and testing it in its own base may reveal the allergy.

Quenching. Theoretically, just as there may be potentiation of allergic and irritant responses, so a combination of chemicals may lead to a quenching effect. This phenomenon has been investigated mostly in fragrance material aldehydes. It might be explained by the combined compounds changing available bonding sites for class II molecules or forming a compound that does not follow the same detoxification pathway. However, some authors have been unable to demonstrate any physicochemical interaction, and its existence has been questioned [34].

Other observed quenching effects may be due to one of the compounds having anti-inflammatory properties [35], such as triclosan having a 'quenching' effect on nickel allergic contact dermatitis.

Other factors. The interpretation of patch test reactions can be affected by the presence or absence of impurities or degradation products, hidden additives, batch differences and the fact that some chemicals may undergo reactive metabolic changes in the skin. Natural products vary according to source, season and method of extraction. Storage or 'ageing' of a product may also affect its allergenicity and irritancy; limonene and linalool must be tested as hydroperoxides and only elicit allergic reactions in this state. Patients should therefore always be tested with their own product. Season may also influence patch test results, but whether this is due to UV radiation suppression of test reactions in the summer or an enhancement of irritant-type reactions in the winter remains uncertain [36].

Errors may occur in the registration of the relative sites of the tests. It is therefore advisable to repeat the test if in doubt.

Selection of test substances

The decision about what to test is dependent on a sound knowledge of the common sensitisers, in conjunction with a thorough history of exposure. Fortunately, a high proportion of cases of contact dermatitis are caused by sensitivity to a small number of contactants, although there are potentially thousands of these. In relatively few cases of contact dermatitis are the clinical appearances and history so typical that an allergen can be incriminated readily.

It is therefore essential to test with a baseline series of common contact allergens. Many investigation clinics have extra allergens and some of these may be grouped into additional special test series or 'batteries' (e.g. for certain occupations or affected sites). Furthermore, it may be necessary to test with materials encountered in a patient's working and domestic environments, and with any medicaments and cosmetics applied to affected areas.

Baseline series

The principle of screening all patients with a series of allergens commonly encountered in their environment is now well established. Aimed patch testing is ill advised. The decision as to what should be in the standard series has now generally devolved from the ICDRG to other national and international groups. At the time of writing the recommended European baseline series contains 30 allergens, the BSCA baseline series has 50 allergens and the North American baseline series includes 50 allergens (Table 127.5). As some allergens disappear from a given environment and others attain significance, it is important that a baseline series evolves and necessarily there will be national variation. An allergen is generally suggested for inclusion in the baseline series when routine (consecutive) patch testing of patients with suspected contact dermatitis results in a proportion of contact allergy to the substance exceeding 0.5–1.0% or when this allergen is ubiquitous and/or clinically highly relevant or if without it a significant number of unsuspected allergic reactions would be missed [37].

In the past, several common sources of contact dermatitis were overlooked until they were included in a baseline series. Nowadays, fragrance materials are familiar contact allergens but were virtually unknown 40 years ago [38]. Conversely, others (e.g. wood tars, turpentine) were removed from the baseline series some years ago. In the UK the addition of 2-hydroxyethyl methacrylate shadows the increased use of artificial nails [39]. At one time, the European standard series identified 75–80% of all allergies diagnosed in one multicentre study [40].

In some studies as many as half of the relevant positive reactions were unexpected. Obviously, if patch testing is carried out for very wide indications, the percentage of negative reactions will increase, but at the same time unexpected positive reactions will correct misdiagnoses of constitutional or irritant dermatitis.

The selection of substances for a baseline patch test series must be based on local experience, but several substances are universally recognised allergens. Unless a permanent record is kept, a number of substances will continue to be included despite a low yield of positive reactions. The results of testing to a standard series of allergens vary from one part of a country to another and the European

Table 127.5 Comparative lists of allergens in European and British standard series.

Allergen	European	BSCA	North American	Vehicle
Potassium dichromate	0.5%	0.5%	0.25%	pet.
Neomycin sulphate	20.0%	20.0%	20.0%	pet.
Thiuram mix	1.0%	1.0%	1.0%	pet.
p-Phenylenediamine	1.0%	1.0%	1.0%	pet.
Cobalt chloride	1.0%	1.0%	1.0%	pet.
Caine mix III	Not present	10.0%	Not present	pet.
Benzocaine	5.0%	Not present	Not present	pet.
Formaldehyde	2.0%	2.0%	2.0%	aq.
Colophony	20.0%	20.0%	20.0%	pet.
Clioquinol or quinoline mix (BSCA)	5.0%	6.0%	Not present	pet.
Myroxylon pereirae (balsam of Peru)	25.0%	25.0%	25.0%	pet.
N-isopropyl-N-phenyl-4-phenylenediamine	0.1%	0.1%	Not present	pet.
Lanolin alcohol	30.0%	30.0%	Not present	pet.
Mercapto mix	2.0%	2.0%	Not present	pet.
Epoxy resin, bisphenol A	1.0%	1.0%	1.0%	pet.
Parabens mix	16.0%	16.0%	12.0%	pet.
4-Tert-butylphenol formaldehyde resin	1.0%	1.0%	1.0%	pet.
Fragrance mix I	8.0%	8.0%	8.0%	pet.
Quaternium 15 (Dowicil 200)	1.0%	1.0%	2.0%	pet.
Nickel (II) sulphate hexahydrate	5.0%	5.0%	2.5%	pet.
Cl+Me-isothiazolinone	0.02%	0.02%	0.02%	aq.
2-Mercaptobenzothiazole	2.0%	2.0%	Not present	pet.
Amerchol L101	Not present	50.0%	50.0%	pet.
Sesquiterpene lactone mix	0.1%	0.1%	0.1%	pet.
p-Chloro-m-cresol	Not present	1.0%	Not present	pet.
2-Bromo-2-nitropropane-1,3-diol	Not present	0.5%	0.5%	pet.
Cetearyl alcohol	Not present	20.0%	Not present	pet.
Sodium fusidate	Not present	2.0%	Not present	pet.
Tixocortol-21-pivalate	0.1%	1.0%	0.1%	pet.
Budesonide	0.01%	0.1%	0.1%	pet.
Imidazolidinyl urea (Germal115)	Not present	2.0%	2.0%	pet.
Diazolidinyl urea (Germal 11)	Not present	2.0%	1.0%	pet.
Methyldibromo glutaronitrile	0.5%	0.3%	0.5%	pet.
Tree moss absolute	Not present	1.0%	Not present	pet.
4-Chloro-3,5-xylenol (PCMX)	Not present	0.50%	Not present	pet.
Carba mix	Not present	3.0%	3.0%	pet.
Disperse blue mix 106/124	Not present	1.0%	1.0%	pet.
Fragrance mix II	14.0%	14.0%	14.0%	pet.
Hydroxyisohexyl-3-cyclohexenecarboxaldehyde	5.0%	5.0%	Not present	pet.
Compositae mix	Not present	2.5%	5.0%	pet.
Methylisothiazolinone	0.2%	0.2%	0.2%	aq.
Sodium metabisulphite	Not present	1.0%	Not present	pet.
Hydroperoxides of linalool	Not present	0.5%	Not present	pet.
Hydroperoxides of linalool	Not present	1.0%	1.0%	pet.
Hydroperoxides of limonene	Not present	0.2%	Not present	pet.
Hydroperoxides of limonene	Not present	0.3%	0.3%	pet.
2- Hydroxyethyl methacrylate	Not present	2.0%	2.0%	pet.
Benzisothiasolinone	Not present	0.1%	Not present	pet.
Octylisothiazolinone	Not present	0.1%	Not present	pet.
Decyl glucoside	Not present	5.0%	5.0%	pet.
Lauryl polyglucose	Not present	3.0%	Not present	pet.
2-Methoxy-6-n-pentyl-4-benzoquinone	0.01%	Not present	Not present	pet.
Textile dye mix	6.6%	Not present	6.6%	pet.
Cinnamal	Not present	Not present	1.0%	pet.
Ethylenediamine dihydrochloride	Not present	Not present	1.0%	pet.
Ylang ylang oil	Not present	Not present	2.0%	pet.
1,3-Diphenylguanidine	Not present	Not present	1.0%	pet.
DMDM hydantoin	Not present	Not present	1.0%	pet.
Bacitracin	Not present	Not present	20.0%	pet.
Mixed dialkyl thiourea	Not present	Not present	1.0%	pet.
Glutaral	Not present	Not present	0.5%	pet.
Propylene glycol	Not present	Not present	30.0%	aq.
Propolis	Not present	Not present	10.0%	pet.
Iodopropynyl butylcarbamate	Not present	Not present	0.2%	pet.
Ethyl acrylate	Not present	Not present	0.1%	pet.
Toluenesulfonamide formaldehyde resin	Not present	Not present	10.0%	pet.
Methyl methacrylate	Not present	Not present	2.0%	pet.
Oleamidopropyl dimethylamine	Not present	Not present	0.1%	aq.
Cocamidopropyl betaine	Not present	Not present	1.0%	aq.

aq., aqueous; BSCA, British Society of Cutaneous Allergy; DMDM, 1,3-dimethylol-5,5-dimethylhydantoin; pet., petroleum.

Standard Series continues to be monitored in multinational studies [41,42].

Additional series

There are many situations in which additional series of allergens are useful, for example in the investigation of dermatitis occurring in certain sites liable to medicament allergy (eyes, ears, perineum and venous ulcers/eczema) or cosmetics or sensitisation from components of shoes or clothing. Some occupational groups, for example hairdressers, florists, dentists and metal machinists, are exposed at work to a variety of potential allergens not found in the standard series. Others may handle a specific group of allergenic chemicals, for example epoxy or acrylic resins. The main patch test allergen producers now market additional series, although these may have to be further adapted to local habits or occupational exposures. Allergens provided by commercial allergen manufacturers tend to be of pharmaceutical grade and may be negative when the actual sensitiser is an impurity in a commercial-grade product. These series should also be subjected to regular scrutiny and review [43].

Other materials

Commercially produced patch test allergens, either singly or in small numbers, may be applied where relevant. Patients may bring a wide variety of materials from their own home or work for testing and, as mentioned previously, these must be thoroughly assessed and diluted appropriately before being tested. In those units with access to thin-layer chromatography there is the opportunity to patch test with extracted components of textiles, plastics, plants and other materials [44].

Concentrations and vehicles for patch testing

Recommended patch test concentrations and vehicles for many different materials, including specific chemicals, chemical groups and substances and finished products, have been collated in a number of standard contact dermatitis references given in the resources list at the end of this section. Most (but not necessarily all) of these lists are reliable, in that the stated concentrations do not usually give an irritant effect. Before patch testing with any unfamiliar material, the appropriate vehicle and concentration should be sought from one or more of these databases.

Complications of patch and photopatch tests

Generally, the risks of patch testing when it is performed correctly are minimal, but there are a number of potential complications (Box 127.4).

> ### Box 127.4 Potential complications of patch testing
>
> - Pruritus
> - Folliculitis
> - Leakage of materials on to clothing, especially dyes
> - Localised flare of dermatitis and other skin disorders
> - Flare of dermatitis at previous contact sites
> - Generalised flare of dermatitis
> - Irritant reactions from patients' own inappropriately diluted products
> - Active sensitisation
> - Pigmentation or depigmentation
> - Persisting reaction
> - Scarring
> - Anaphylaxis (very rare)

Positive reactions may spread locally and cause a flare of contact dermatitis at the original site or more generally. The long strips of adhesive semiocclusive tape, which preclude bathing for several days, may lead to eczema, itching or folliculitis, especially with high temperatures and humidity. In warm weather there may be leakage of the test materials on to clothing, and patients should be advised to wear old clothing during the test. Irritants at excessive concentrations may induce caustic burns and scarring, and even a strong allergic reaction that could cause a scar on extremely rare occasions. Secondary infection of a positive reaction is virtually never a problem.

Short-term postinflammatory hypopigmentation does occur occasionally following positive patch tests, but more permanent hypopigmentation may develop, including koebnerisation of vitiligo (Figure 127.17). Postinflammatory hyperpigmentation may also develop, although this is usually temporary. Phototoxic substances may cause pigmentation if exposed to UV light from photopatch tests or natural sunlight.

Significant epidermal detachment has been seen in patients with blistering disorders including pemphigus foliaceus and Hailey–Hailey disease after removal of the patch test units [45,46].

Short-lived, non-immunological, urticarial reactions are common, particularly from cinnamates and sorbic acid. More importantly, anaphylactic reactions are a potential risk when patch testing with some materials, especially natural rubber latex [47] and penicillin. A history of immediate hypersensitivity to rubber should be sought before patch testing with latex.

Rarely, persistence of patch test reactions may continue for several weeks unless treated. This has been especially noted with gold sodium thiosulphate [48].

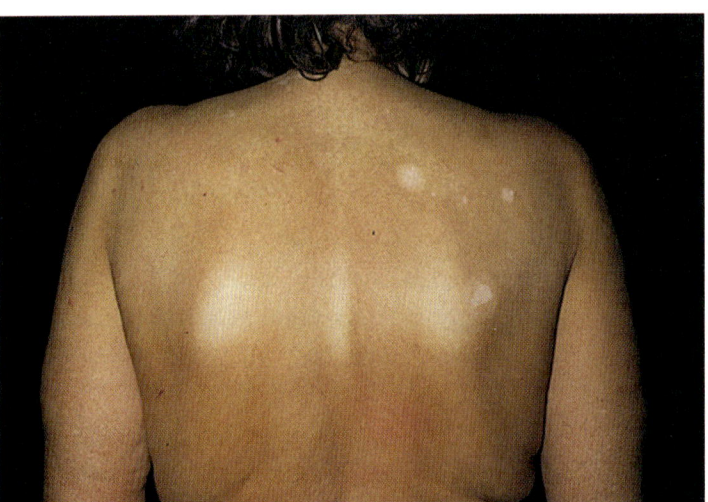

Figure 127.17 Persistent hypopigmentation after patch tests.

Active sensitisation

Patch testing involves a small risk of sensitisation (active sensitisation). A reaction appearing 7 or more days after the application may indicate either delayed expression of a pre-existing sensitivity or active sensitisation. However, some late reactions, occurring up to 14 days after the application of patch tests, are weak sensitivities from poorly penetrating allergens. Active sensitisation usually presents as a strong positive patch test occurring generally beyond 2 weeks. Few clinics observe their patients long enough to note such reactions, but patients report them. The true incidence of sensitisation is therefore difficult to establish because even re-examination of a random sample of the patients tested cannot differentiate between those sensitised by patch testing and those whose pre-existing subliminal sensitivity has been boosted by further exposure from patch testing. Active sensitisation from most routinely tested substances is very uncommon, and occurs more frequently when new substances are being investigated to ascertain the correct patch test concentration. To confirm the diagnosis of active sensitisation, repeat patch testing can be performed whereby a positive reaction within the 'usual' latency period (one to a few days) supports the diagnosis.

Multiple patch test reactions

The finding of multiple positive patch tests is common, and it is important to consider the reasons for this so that the correct advice can be given to the patient. The main explanations are:
1 Non-specific hyperreactivity.
2 Multiple primary hypersensitivities.
3 Cross-reactions (true and false).

Non-specific hyperreactivity. Ideally, patch tests should be applied at a concentration that always identifies the allergen and never induces false positive reactions. Unfortunately, some allergens have to be applied at a concentration that is marginally irritant in some subjects in order that allergic positive reactions are not missed. The threshold at which a false positive irritant reaction develops differs from individual to individual and may even be variable in the same subject. During active dermatitis, uninvolved skin, even at distant body sites, exhibits increased susceptibility to irritant reactions. This 'status eczematicus' may lead to false positive patch test results. It has become an established tenet that 'eczema creates eczema', and that a strongly positive patch test reaction may induce other non-specific false positive patch test reactions [49]. Such reactions occur more readily with marginally irritant chemicals. When this affects adjacent patch test sites it is often referred to as 'spillover', 'excited skin' or 'angry back'. Rietschel [50] has proposed that 'stochastic resonance' may be involved. This suggests that there is signal amplification of immune-mediated events by neurological influences. The incidence has been variously assessed as between 8.6% and 63.5% [51]. In view of these findings, it has been proposed that repeat patch tests should be undertaken in all individuals with three or more strong positive allergic reactions, with exclusion of the strongest reactants. However, some studies have not found evidence to support a concept of non-specific hypersensitivity [52].

The occurrence of weak false positive patch test reactions can be reduced by delaying patch testing until all active eczema has settled. As skin hyperirritability may persist for some weeks or months, even when the dermatitis has resolved, this is often impractical.

Multiple primary hypersensitivities. Multiple primary specific (or concomitant) sensitivities to substances that are unrelated chemically are frequent among patients with contact dermatitis. Among 5000 Scandinavian patients, they occurred in 20% of all persons tested. The reason why some patients develop multiple sensitivities and others do not is not clear. Patients with a long history of dermatitis are those most likely to accumulate several primary sensitivities, because of the opportunities to encounter new allergens under conditions favourable for sensitisation. Patients with leg ulcers are especially prone to developing multiple allergies, as are patients with chronic actinic dermatitis. One sensitivity may predispose to the acquisition of another, and there may be a genetic or constitutional predisposition to acquire sensitivities [53].

Sensitisation is facilitated if an allergen is applied on injured (e.g. eczematous) skin [54], particularly if it is occluded, and such local factors may be sufficient to explain the frequency of sensitivity to topical medicaments and simultaneous sensitivity to several constituents. In dermatitis from applied medicaments, concomitant sensitivity to both an antibiotic and an unrelated component of the vehicle is quite common. Similarly, in rubber dermatitis, sensitivity to unrelated vulcanising agents is not unusual.

In dermatitis of the feet, concomitant sensitivity to chromate, rubber and dyes in shoes or stockings presents a particularly difficult clinical problem; one allergen may be primarily responsible but others are important in maintaining the eczematous state. The inflammatory response to allergens has been shown to be additive [55], as has the response to an allergen and an irritant [56].

Cross-reactions. Cross-sensitisation is defined as the phenomenon where sensitisation engendered by one compound, the primary allergen, extends to one or more other compounds, the secondary allergens, as a result of structural similarity [57]. The proposal is that the primary and secondary allergens are so closely related that sensitised T cells are unable to distinguish between them and therefore react as if the compounds were identical. Aromatic compounds with a 'para' group, for example PPD, benzocaine, procaine, sulphonamides, mesalazine, diaminodiphenylmethane and PABA UV filters, may all cross-sensitise. Aminoglycosides may do the same to a varying degree. Other examples include chlorocresol and chloroxylenol, as well as corticosteroids of a similar structure.

Contaminants may cause 'false' cross-sensitivity as one substance may contain traces of another. In studies of cross-sensitivity, absolutely pure test substances must be used. Few investigations in the past have fulfilled these requirements, and most should be repeated using modern methods of separation.

In simultaneous sensitivity to natural products such as perfumes, balsams and wood tars, it is impossible to decide whether reactions to several of the substances may be due to related or identical chemicals. Cinnamic aldehydes, for example, may occur in them all. The same applies to plants such as Compositae (Asteraceae), *Frullania* and *Toxicodendron* species.

Investigations: other tests

Occlusive patch testing has stood the test of time. Although it is an artificial procedure, it has not been superseded. Nevertheless, alternatives continue to be sought and some of these may be useful adjunctive investigations.

Open tests

Patch testing is usually performed with the test site occluded in order to increase percutaneous absorption. This is an artificial procedure, and clinical exposure might be more closely simulated by simple application of the sensitiser to uninvolved skin. However, few allergens provoke dermatitis with a single exposure on normal skin.

The technique involves dripping the product 'as is' or dissolved in water or organic solvent onto a 1 cm diameter area of skin and then allowing it to dry. The volar aspect of the forearm is commonly used. There is no occlusion [1]. The time for reading and the characteristics of the reaction are the same as for closed patch testing. The reaction can be followed from the start and may develop sooner than with a closed patch test reaction. It is often weaker and a positive reaction, especially in the initial phase, may consist of isolated papules only.

One situation where open testing has been widely used and advocated is prior to dyeing hair. Application of the dye to the retroauricular area and examination of the site 2 days later was shown to be an accurate method of detecting sensitised subjects [2]. However, hairdressers and individual users tend to do this only once and not each time the hair is tinted, and often they mistakenly undertake a 30 min reading. They may therefore miss the allergy if it develops subsequently.

With irritants, the reactions are also usually fewer and weaker in open than in closed patch testing because of reduced absorption. Open tests are therefore sometimes used as a preliminary screening procedure with less well-known substances to reduce the risk of severe reactions. They can give some confidence that one can proceed with occlusive patch testing. However, experience with open tests is limited and the risk of sensitisation cannot always be estimated.

Semi-open tests

These have been suggested as useful for testing patient-supplied products with suspected irritant properties such as shampoos, detergents, paints and some cosmetics. A small volume of the product (15 µL) is applied with a cotton swab to a 1 cm diameter area of skin and allowed to dry completely. It should then be covered with permeable tape. Readings are performed in the same way as for occlusive patch tests.

Usage tests

In cases of doubt, when either a closed patch test or open test is negative yet the history suggests a contact dermatitis, the patient can be asked to use the preparation again. This is especially helpful with cosmetic and clothing dermatitis. Because it reproduces all the other factors associated with the original dermatitis, for example sweating, friction and application of allergen on damaged or presensitised skin, it is sometimes positive when conventional patch tests fail to reveal sensitivity. However, it is not always possible to differentiate between an allergic and a non-specific or irritant response. With cosmetic preparations or medicaments, a repeat 'dab' test may be performed on previously affected skin.

Repeat open application tests

These are standardised exposure tests mimicking a use situation and they aim to elicit allergic contact dermatitis at the test site although reactions often start with follicular papules. In the ROAT, substances are applied twice daily for up to 2 weeks (sometimes extended up to 4 weeks in cases where suspicion is high) or until an eczematous reaction develops [3]. The most appropriate site is the upper arm or flexor surface of the forearm near the antecubital fossa, as patients can perform the test and observe any developing reaction. They should be told to discontinue the application if eczema occurs. An area of at least 5 cm^2 should be employed. The test may be used to determine the relevance of doubtful positive patch test reactions to preparations in which the putative allergen is present in a low concentration, although false negative results may occur. It may also establish the clinical relevance of such products and confirm the source of the allergy. A scale for recording ROAT reactions has been proposed and advocated [4].

Extracts and chromatograms

Ultrasonic bath extracts can be used as an alternative to testing with solid materials. Here, small samples of material are placed in water or organic solvent (ethanol, acetone or ether) and extracted in an ultrasonic device and then filtered. In addition, patch testing with thin-layer chromatograms can be particularly useful for testing textiles, plastics, foods, plants and drugs [5].

In vitro tests

The principle of diagnosing contact allergy by *in vitro* testing is attractive although the use of peripheral blood as a routine investigation for contact dermatitis may not be viable, not only from the budgetary point of view but also for logistical and practical reasons. Nevertheless, attempts continue to be made to achieve this, albeit with single or small numbers of allergens. A number of different techniques including migration inhibition tests and lymphocyte transformation tests have been tried [6,7].

As yet, none of these tests is a substitute for the *in vivo* system of the patch test. However, they may be helpful in elucidation of the immune cascade as they are based on measurements of products from T-cell activation. They may also have a role in looking at cross-sensitivity patterns.

Spot tests

Three spot tests are of particular practical value in the patch test clinic as the materials are easy to handle and store.

Dimethylglyoxime test for nickel [8]. A commercial 'one step' solution is now available for using directly on test surfaces. One study showed a sensitivity of the test at 0.5 µg/cm^2/week of about 60% and a specificity of about 98%, showing that the test works well for screening purposes, but in some cases there is a risk of false negative values [9]. A pink coloration on the cotton bud denotes the presence of nickel (Figure 127.18). It is a very useful test, and patients can be given kits to test items in the home and at work.

Cobalt spot test. For the detection of cobalt ions, a spot test may be prepared using the reagent disodium-1-nitroso-2-naphthol-3,6-disulphonate (nitroso-R salt). This is also commercially available. The release of cobalt may be detected by rubbing a cotton-tipped applicator against the test material (e.g. metal, pigments or leather)

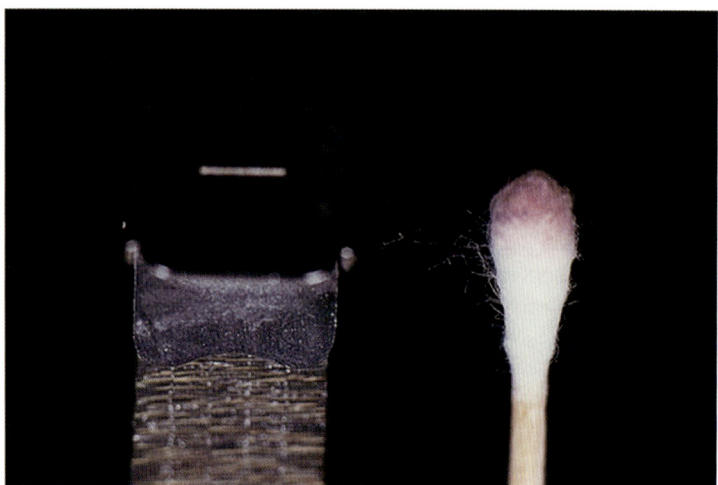

Figure 127.18 Dimethylglyoxime test: a pink colour is detected when metals release a significant amount of nickel. Courtesy of Dr J. D. Wilkinson.

and upon the release of cobalt ions, the yellow test solution turns orange-red. A detection limit of about 1.5 ppm has been found for the test [10].

Acetylacetone method for formaldehyde [11]. The reagent is prepared by dissolving 15 g of ammonium acetate, 0.2 mL of acetylacetone and 0.3 mL of glacial acetic acid in 100 mL of distilled water. It can then be stored in a refrigerator. A sample (1 mL or 1 mg) of the product to be tested is put in a disposable glass test tube and 2.5 mL of the reagent is added. The mixture is shaken and stoppered and then placed in a water bath at 60°C for 10 min. A yellow colour is produced in the presence of formaldehyde, due to the formation of 3,5-diacetyl-1,4-dihydrolutidine. The alternative chromotropic acid method is less specific.

Management
General principles of management

Avoidance advice. A diagnosis of allergic contact dermatitis is reached on the basis of a detailed history and examination followed by patch tests, with an assessment of the relevance of any positive reactions. Once a diagnosis has been made, possible sources of exposure to the causative allergen(s) should be identified and avoidance advice given. In some instances, particularly in work-related problems, appropriate protective clothing or changes in handling technique may be advised. Materials used for protection, especially gloves, should not allow penetration of the allergen responsible for the dermatitis.

The first principle of management is to give advice on avoidance tailored to an individual. Examples of specific avoidance measures include plastic instead of rubber gloves, cosmetics and medicaments free of an identified allergen, and clothing free of nickel-containing studs, zips, etc. More general written information on the allergen sources may be helpful, but may also be confusing if information is not relevant to that person.

The ESCD, the BSCA and the American Contact Dermatitis Society as well as the manufacturers of patch test allergens all provide patient information leaflet resources. There is some evidence that written information is superior to verbal information alone [1].

Ideally, the result of this advice will be a resolution of the dermatitis, but this does not always occur, and other factors such as the possible contribution of irritant or constitutional factors should be considered and discussed with the patient. The possibility of non-compliance with avoidance advice should also be considered. Factors affecting compliance include the social and educational status of the individual and lack of resources [2]. This is also complicated by the fact that there are variable rules on labelling. European cosmetics must include full ingredient labelling (excluding partial labelling of fragrance substances). The nomenclature used in Europe for such purposes is the INCI, yet labelling on European medicinal products use the international non-proprietary name (INN). Therefore, in cases of allergic contact dermatitis it may be important to provide both the INCI and INN names for the same chemical to patients (e.g. parabens and hydroxybenzoates, respectively). Both the INCI and INN names are complex.

Patients should be made aware that ingredient labelling can be misleading and not reveal all potential sensitisers in a product [3]. It may also include unhelpful 'marketing' terms like 'hypoallergenic', 'organic' and 'dermatologically tested'.

Reassessment and reinforcement of avoidance measures is often required, in order that patients are fully aware of what action they should take.

In some patients continued exposure is unavoidable but can be reduced to a sufficient degree to keep the dermatitis at an acceptable level. It is advisable to stress that allergy does not disappear when the dermatitis clears but that the risk of relapse after further contact with the allergen persists throughout life.

To aid patients identify personal care products free from allergens to which they are sensitised, various databases have been developed in the USA and Europe. These are costly and resource intensive to run and may not always keep pace with product reformulations and batch numbers.

To underscore the challenge of educating patients about contact allergy, one UK study showed that, among 135 patch-tested patients, about 25% could not even recall having received any information about their test results 2–3 months later [4]. A US survey, including 757 patch-tested patients identified that only 50% of patients with positive patch test reactions to one or two allergens remembered their allergies [5]. There was a tendency for there to be better recall of allergens among those aged >50 years of age and among women. If feasible it might be useful to repeat information at a new appointment, for example some months later.

Active treatment. The mainstay of treatment of allergic contact dermatitis is avoidance of the causative factor(s), although topical corticosteroids will be required in most instances to control the disorder. Potent steroids are typically used on the hands [6]. The general principles of treatment are the same as for other forms of eczema. In particular, the regular and liberal use of hydrating emollients and soap substitutes is recommended. Fissures of the fingers, palms and soles can be covered with hypoallergenic tape.

Recalcitrant, disabling cases may require consideration of systemic therapy such as alitretinoin, azathioprine and ciclosporin. Phototherapy, both PUVA and UVB, is helpful in some subjects, including Compositae-allergic individuals with photosensitivity [7].

The use of barrier creams as preventatives in already sensitised persons is generally unsatisfactory. Other barrier creams containing active agents (e.g. chelating agents) against specific allergens may have future potential [8,9]. In one study clioquinol was the most effective agent at preventing nickel dermatitis [10]. It has also been shown that pretreatment of the skin with the antioxidant ascorbic acid reduces the elicitation reaction to a PPD-containing hair dye in sensitised subjects [11].

It has been reported that certain patterns, especially vesicular palmar eczema, have benefited from dietary avoidance or reduction in the intake of allergen, most notably nickel and balsams, in sensitised subjects [12,13]. The effects of a low-nickel diet have been disappointing in our experience; nevertheless, there are strong advocates of these measures. Dietary chelation of nickel has also been attempted [14] but is not widely used in practice because of side effects.

Dietary manoeuvres have been reported to be helpful for cheilitis and oral symptoms, particularly in those with positive patch tests to balsam of Peru, cinnamates, eugenol, colophony, flavours and antioxidants [15]. Diets for other food-related preservative allergens have been developed [16]. However, the relationship between 'burning mouth' and contact allergy is questionable [17].

Hyposensitisation [18]. Many attempts have been made to down-regulate the immune response to allergens in an already sensitised individual. This has proved difficult to realise in practice. The degree of hyposensitisation achieved by oral doses of allergens is limited and transient, for example DNCB and chromate in guinea pigs and poison ivy in humans. Although it has been attempted for *Toxicodendron* spp. allergy [19], oral hyposensitisation is not routinely recommended. Some success has nevertheless been claimed in India for hyposensitisation against *Parthenium hysterophorus* [20].

Prevention

Many statutory bodies have a role in the prevention of contact dermatitis, including medical personnel, legislative bodies, governments, industry, the media, consumer bodies and patient support groups. Principles of prevention can be related to two categories, individual and collective, and further divided into primary, secondary and tertiary [21]. Primary prevention focuses on the induction of contact sensitisation and control of exposure. Secondary prevention relates to elicitation, and tertiary to measures for established and continuing dermatitis. Some of the more important elements of prevention are discussed here.

Allergen containment and replacement [22]. Potent allergens encountered in industry can be kept in closed systems, thereby avoiding the potential for direct skin contact. In other instances, products can be kept in special containers that allow a no-touch technique when using the contents. Replacement and elimination of potential allergenic hazards can be helpful in both the domestic and working environments, for example by using perfume-free cosmetics and medicaments, and non-latex gloves.

European legal and other regulatory measures [23]. Regulatory measures can influence the incidence of dermatitis [24]. They may be legally or voluntarily enforced. The EU has passed a number of directives relating to contact dermatitis, particularly in relation to nickel, chromate and cosmetics – the impact of which can be seen in the earlier relevant sections.

The EU Regulation 1223/2009 on cosmetic products [25] lists materials as allowed, not allowed and restricted in European cosmetics and details the requirements for labelling. Enforced ingredient labelling on the packaging of cosmetics, which is also a requirement in the USA, has been a major factor in enabling the avoidance of cosmetic allergens by sensitised consumers. Since 2005, in the EU, labelling of certain fragrance substances (26 in all), at levels of >10 ppm for leave-on products and >100 ppm for wash-off products, has also been required.

REACH (Registration, Evaluation, Authorisation and Restriction of Chemicals) Regulation (EC) No. 1907/2006 [26] is a regulation of the EU adopted to improve the protection of human health and the environment from the risks that can be posed by chemicals. In principle, REACH applies to all chemical substances, not only those used in industrial processes by certain occupational groups but also in products for consumer use (e.g. in cleaning products, paints, clothes, furniture, electrical equipment and jewellery). The CLP Classification, Labelling and Packaging) Regulation (EC) No. 1272/2008 aligns the EU system of classification, labelling and packaging of chemical substances and mixtures to the Globally Harmonised System (GHS). In practice, the burden of responsibility for the completion of REACH and CLP assessments of chemicals and any subsequent risk assessment has, deliberately, been placed on industry. Test methods for the identification and classification of skin sensitisers (H317, formerly R43 'may cause sensitisation by skin contact') are set out within the legislation, but it also encourages a wide range of other evidence to be taken into account including chemical structure and human evidence [27].

Corporate responsibility. Although legal measures can influence the incidence of dermatitis, few have been introduced. In many instances governments will not intervene with legislation, relying instead on self-regulation, and this includes the cosmetic and pharmaceutical industries. The withdrawal of musk ambrette is an example of cosmetic industry self-regulation. Manufacturers of all goods should ensure that their products are safe to use, including the performance of pre- and postmarketing risk assessments. A risk assessment programme involves hazard identification, dose–response assessment, exposure assessment and risk characterisation, including any potential for allergenicity [28,29]. A product must be clearly labelled to ensure that it is handled safely.

Dermatologists and consumers have a pivotal role in alerting authorities to the emergence of both new and existing allergens within communities. National groups, surveillance systems, particularly of occupational dermatitis, or more comprehensive data networks such as the ESSCA, can feed back their findings to responsible agencies who can then respond to any concerns [30]. Rapid computerised analysis of epidemiological information, with feedback to interested parties, can provide early warning of new allergens and sources of work-related dermatoses, as it did with the MI epidemic.

Work. The preventative aspects of occupational contact dermatitis are discussed in detail in Chapter 129.

Domestic. The availability of modern domestic equipment should significantly reduce skin contact with irritants and potential sensitisers in the home; however, homemakers are still one of the greatest 'at-risk' groups as far as the development of hand dermatitis is concerned. Cotton-lined gloves should be worn when the hands are in contact with irritants, including food, cleaning agents and polishes. Plastic gloves are less allergenic than rubber but are less pliable and malleable.

Education. Education of the community and workforces through the media, courses, lectures and wall charts in public places and at work will help to promote awareness of the problem of contact dermatitis. Skin protection courses and education have been shown to reduce occupational dermatitis [31]. Patient support groups have played an increasing role in education of the general public as well as those suffering from dermatitis.

Resources

Further information

De Groot AC. *Patch Testing*, 4th edn. Wapserveen: Acdegroot Publishing, 2018.
Johansen JD, Frosch PJ, Lepoittevin J-P, eds. *Contact Dermatitis*, 6th edn. Berlin: Springer, 2020.
Johansen JD, Thyssen J, Lepoittevin JP. *Quick Guide to Contact Dermatitis*. Berlin: Springer, 2016.
Lovell CR. *Plants and the Skin*. Oxford: Blackwell Science, 1993.
Rietschel RL, Fowler JF. *Fisher's Contact Dermatitis*, 6th edn. Hamilton: BC Decker, 2008.
Rustemeyer T, Elsner P, John SM, Maibach HI, eds. *Kanerva's Occupational Dermatology*, 2nd edn. Berlin: Springer, 2012.

Patient resources

American Contact Dermatitis Society, patient information leaflets: https://www.contactderm.org/.
British Society of Cutaneous Allergy, patient information leaflets: https://cutaneousallergy.org/.
DermNetz, NZ, contact urticaria: http://dermnetnz.org/reactions/contact-urticaria.html.
European Society of Contact Dermatitis, patient information leaflets: https://escd.org/. (All last accessed July 2023.)

Specific allergens

Metals

Nickel [1–3]

Chemistry. In common with cobalt, but unlike chromium, the metal itself sensitises and is, in practice, the most frequent source of sensitisation [2]. Most salts, for example nickel chloride ($NiCl_2$) and nickel sulphate ($NiSO_4$), are readily soluble in water and sweat and have strong sensitising properties. Some oxides (e.g. Ni_2O_3) and the hydroxide ($Ni(OH)_2$) can elicit contact dermatitis, but heated NiO does not.

Incidence and prevalence. Nickel is the commonest contact allergen in most industrialised countries worldwide. In Europe, the prevalence of nickel allergy has declined in some countries following implementation of the EU 'Nickel directive' [4,5]. The prevalences are approximately 8–19% in adults [6] and 8–10% in children and adolescents in the general population [7–9] with a strong predominance in women as compared with men (4–10 times) and in girls as compared with boys. The prevalence of nickel sensitivity in patch test clinics lies between 15% and 30%, and is influenced by the relative number of females tested [10]. The prevalence may be higher in some occupational groups, for example hairdressers, in whom studies have shown that 27–38% are nickel allergic [11,12].

The European 'Nickel directive' primarily based on a Danish regulation was introduced in 1994 and came into full force in 2001 and was revised in 2005 (Table 127.6).

Occurrence. Nickel is primarily used in stainless steel and other alloys; it is also used in its pure form in plating and in a large variety of products, owing to its high ductility, resistance to oxidation and corrosion, high melting point, ferromagnetism and low cost. The most important factor for the induction and elicitation of cutaneous nickel allergy is the amount of nickel per unit area present in the epidermis over time ($\mu g/cm^2$ over time) [13]. Exposure to free nickel ions may occur following skin contact with various metallic items, corroded by human sweat [14]. High rates of corrosion have been documented from nickel-plated items, nickel-iron, coins and several other alloys [15]. Chromium-plated metal is often first nickel-plated, and after long use the nickel may reach the surface, for example on water taps. Stainless steels contain nickel but most are incapable of releasing sufficient quantities to elicit allergic contact dermatitis. Quantitative studies indicate that repeated exposure to occluded metal items releasing nickel at a rate greater than 0.5 $\mu g/cm^2$/week involves a significant risk of nickel sensitisation [16], but thereafter very small amounts of nickel are sufficient to elicit dermatitis in sensitised persons. Jewellery and metal clothes fasteners/components are the usual sources of nickel in prolonged contact with the skin. Transient but potentially frequent and repeated exposure may occur from handling coins, keys, scissors, knitting needles, thimbles and other metallic tools and utensils. Platers and some metal machinists are necessarily at risk of occupational nickel allergy. Other sources include pigments in glass, pottery and enamel, electrocautery plates [17], mobile phones [18], laptop computers [19], electronic cigarettes [20], bindi [21], intravenous cannulae [2], tattoo pigment [23] and orthodontic appliances [24]. Nickel has also been identified in some eye cosmetics [25,26] but the importance of this exposure is less well studied. The safe limit in pigmented make-up products such as eye shadow and mascara has been estimated to be <5 ppm, although discrepant results exist regarding the clinical implications of such exposure [27–29].

Systemic nickel exposure is possible from inhalation, oral ingestion, transcutaneous absorption or exposure from metallic implants (e.g. joint replcements or dental braces).

Elicitation of allergic nickel dermatitis has been described, including vesicular hand eczema, flexural eczema, flare-up reactions at earlier sites of contact dermatitis and the 'baboon syndrome' [30,31]. Certain foods and plants contain much higher concentrations than others, as can particular sources of domestic water [32], and nickel may also be a contaminant in fertilisers [33] and fungicides. Stainless steel saucepans release negligible nickel, but cooking acid fruit in them, particularly when they are new, has the potential to contribute to dietary intake [34].

Table 127.6 European Union 'Nickel directive' (summary).

Part	Nickel may not be used	CEN standard for control of limit
1	*To September 2005*: In post assemblies used during epithelisation, unless they are homogeneous, and the concentration of nickel is less than 0.05%	EN 1810 (nickel content by atomic absorption spectrometry)
1 rev.	*From September 2005*: In all post assemblies which are inserted into pierced ears and other pierced parts (not only during epithelisation), unless the nickel release is less than 0.2 µg/cm²/week	EN 1811 (nickel release in artificial sweat)
2	In products intended to come into direct and prolonged contact with the skin, such as earrings, necklaces, wristwatch cases, watch straps, buttons, tighteners, zips and mobile phones, if the nickel release is greater than 0.5 µg/cm²/week	EN 1811 (nickel release in artificial sweat) CR 12471 (screening test by dimethylglyoxime)
3	In coated products such as those in part 2, unless coating is sufficient to ensure that the nickel release will not exceed 0.5 µg/cm²/week after 2 years of normal use	EN 12472 (wear and corrosion test)

From Thyssen *et al.* 2021 [1].

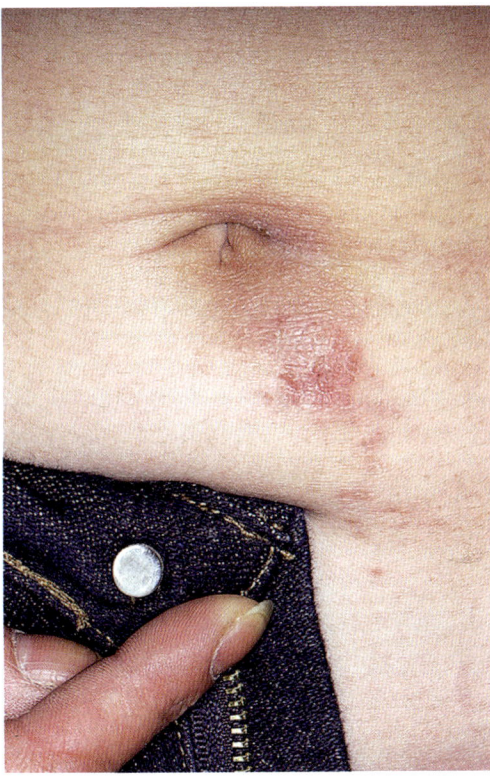

Figure 127.19 Allergic contact dermatitis to nickel in metal studs on jeans. Courtesy of Dr J. D. Wilkinson.

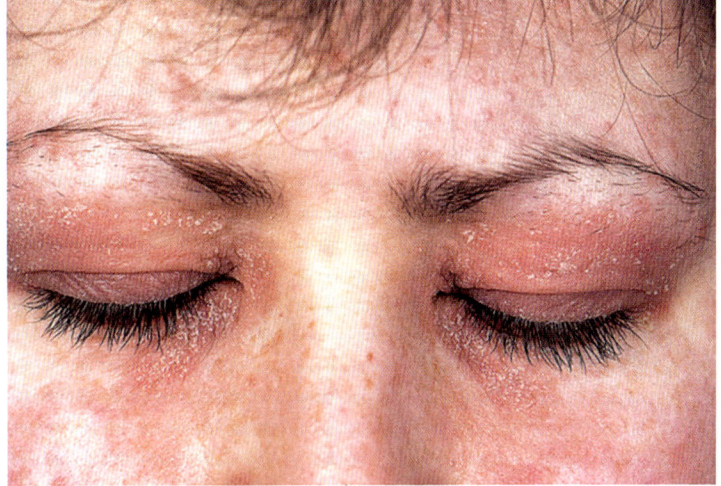

Figure 127.20 Secondary eyelid dermatitis in a patient sensitive to nickel. Courtesy of Dr J. D. Wilkinson.

Systemic exposure from implanted metals is considered in the section 'Cutaneous reactions to implanted metals' later in this chapter.

Clinical features. Classic nickel allergy is identified by patches of dermatitis at sites of contact with metal objects, most commonly the ears from earrings, the wrists from watches and bracelets, the neck from necklaces and their clasps, the central abdomen from belt buckles, studs and zips in trousers (Figure 127.19) and the dorsa of the feet from shoe buckles. Lesions on the upper cheeks and sides of the nose and face may relate to metal-framed spectacles, and on the eyelids to eyelash curlers.

The eruption may be papular, nummular, diffuse or consist only of excoriated papules on almost normal-looking skin. Some patients have a spread of dermatitis to distant regions. These secondary eruptions used to be a characteristic feature of nickel dermatitis [35], but now seem to be less common. The secondary rash normally starts shortly after, or at the same time as, the primary eruption. It affects the neck, face (especially the eyelids; Figure 127.20), the elbow flexures and the flexor surfaces of the arms; the ano-genital area may also be affected, and the rash may be generalised. Flexural lesions may resemble textile dermatitis or atopic eczema.

The relationship between hand eczema and nickel sensitivity remains complex [36]. However, well-controlled statistical studies support a connection between hand eczema and nickel allergy [37–40], and nickel-sensitive women do appear to have a predilection for hand eczema [41]. Nickel allergy in childhood did not seem to predispose to hand dermatitis later in life in one study. However, hand eczema is often multifactorial, and is particularly common in women who have a heavy burden of housework or who are employed in occupations that expose the skin regularly to trauma or 'wet work'. There may be a vesicular palmar (dyshidrotic) pattern, but other distributions occur without being diagnostic. Wet work, atopy and nickel sensitivity are associated with an increased risk of hand dermatitis [42], although atopy is probably the most important factor.

Sometimes, nickel allergy is purely occupational in origin, and in more than half of these cases it starts on the hands. It is normally associated with the metal and nickel-plating industries, although considerable skin deposition of nickel has also been found on the hands following repeated contact with items such as tools, keys and coins at work [43]. Spread occurs to the elbow flexures, eyelids and face in the same manner as described earlier.

A recurrent vesicular palmar (dyshidrotic) pattern of eczema has been related to dietary intake of nickel. Ingestion of nickel sulphate caused a flare of vesicular hand eczema in 9 of 12 patients studied by Christensen and Möller [44]. The significance of this has been disputed, as similar results have been demonstrated in non-sensitised patients and the challenge dose was artificially high [45–47]. There is a clear tendency toward a dose–response relationship, with few persons reacting at a dose below 0.5 mg elemental nickel, and the majority reacting at 5.6 mg [48]. Experimental provocation doses have traditionally been higher than the daily nickel intake in food, which ranges between 100 and 300 µg/day. Under normal circumstances, a number of factors can interfere with the amount of nickel absorbed; including alcohol intake, atopy drugs and the composition of food. A further meta-analysis of 17 relevant studies has concluded that 1% of those exposed to a normal dietary nickel intake will develop systemic contact dermatitis [49].

Avoidance. Most people think of their environment in terms of objects rather than materials, and it is important to realise that they find it difficult to identify nickel unless the possible causes of contact are specifically listed. Many dermatologists provide all nickel-sensitive patients with a list of possible contact items. A dimethylglyoxime test kit (see 'Spot tests' later in this chapter) may also be of use in identifying nickel-containing objects among a patient's personal items at work or in the home [50].

Nickel cannot be entirely avoided in daily life, but the elimination of nickel from clothing and the avoidance of nickel-containing jewellery may be sufficient to clear dermatitis. In our experience, initial compliance with avoidance advice is poor, particularly with clothing, and repeated explanations may be necessary. Waterproof tape and metal lacquer can be used to cover nickel-plated objects that cannot be replaced, although nickel can leach out if the contact site is sweaty and prone to friction. Contact may be difficult to avoid in certain occupations. Protection with rubber gloves may be insufficient as nickel solutions may penetrate them [51]. Heavy-duty vinyl gloves have been suggested as an alternative.

Prognosis. The prognosis of dermatitis due to nickel in jewellery and clothing is excellent if further use of nickel-plated objects is avoided. Once the hands are involved, the eczema may remain chronic, persistent or intermittent. Ingestion of nickel remains a possible cause of chronicity.

Specific therapies. Barrier creams and cleansers containing chelating agents may have potential benefit, and a number have shown promise under experimental conditions [52–54]. Clioquinol is known to chelate nickel [55], and a topical clioquinol–steroid combination can be considered as a treatment.

Dietary reduction of nickel intake is recommended, by some, for those nickel-allergic subjects with recurrent palmar vesicular eczema. Knowledge of the nickel content of foods is imprecise, and the prescription of a low-nickel diet [56] is often not practical. Nevertheless, there are strong advocates for this approach and a trial of dietary reduction may be worthwhile, although this is frequently disappointing in our experience.

Treatment with tetraethylthiuram disulphide (disulfiram; Antabuse), which chelates nickel, has been reported as helpful [57] but has a significant number of potential adverse effects [58].

Patch tests. Nickel sulphate 5% in petrolatum is used for patch tests. False negative reactions are common with 2.5% nickel in petrolatum or 2% aqueous nickel [59]. False negative reactions may also occur with 5% nickel sulphate in petrolatum because nickel ions penetrate the skin slowly [60]. Testing with nickel sulphate may produce irritant false positive reactions with a deep redness and pustulation, especially in atopics. Some follicular reactions are irritant, but those with raised papules are often truly allergic in our experience.

Cobalt [1]

Chemistry. Cobalt metal and its oxides (e.g. Co_2O_3 and CoO) and salts (e.g. $CoCl_2$ and $CoSO_4$) are sensitisers. Also, heated CoO elicits positive patch test reactions (unlike NiO).

Prevalence. It is estimated that 1–3% of adults, and probably a larger proportion of younger females in the general population, are allergic to cobalt [2]. Studies suggest that 5–8% of patch-tested dermatitis patients in Europe and North America have contact allergy to cobalt with a higher proportion in females [3,4].

Occurrence. Metallic cobalt is present in 'hard metal' used for metal cutting and drilling. The salts are seldom used for plating, unlike nickel salts. It is also used in the production of jewellery, superalloys, rechargeable batteries and magnets. Cobalt blue is widely used in paints and for ceramics and glassware. It is almost always present as a contaminant in nickel [5]. Cobalt oxides, present in trace amounts in cement, are sensitisers; however, isolated cobalt allergy from cement is much rarer than chromate allergy. Cobalt exposure is therefore traditionally described as occurring in hard metal, glass and pottery workers. It is also used in a wide range of metallic and non-metallic products and materials to which consumers are exposed such as dental alloys, electronic devices, jewellery, magnetic materials, orthopaedic implants, pigments in cosmetics and leather, putty, siccatives in paints and tools. Leather is an emerging source of sensitisation [6,7] where the cobalt is used as a mordant to bind dyes onto leather. The proportion of leather goods that contain (and possibly release) cobalt is unclear but may reach 15–20% [8].

Clinical features. As cobalt is an invariable contaminant of nickel, the clinical features of cobalt allergy can be identical to those of nickel allergy. Cobalt sensitivity might explain why some women with dermatitis typical of that provoked by nickel have a negative patch test reaction to the latter. Furthermore, its presence in cement may induce a clinical pattern identical to allergy from chromate in this source. Isolated cobalt allergy is seen in hard-metal workers and in the pottery and glass industries, when it is usually associated with hand dermatitis. Stomatitis has been reported from dentures. Allergic granulomatous reactions to tattoo pigment are recognised, but are rare in our experience. Animal feed may induce contact allergy [9], and photocontact dermatitis has been reported from this source, as well as from cement [10]. Vitamin B_{12} is a cobalt-containing compound and cheilitis has been reported from oral vitamin B_{12} ingestion, and dermatitis from its parenteral use [11]. An oral lichenoid eruption due to a chrome/cobalt prosthesis has been reported [12]. It can sometimes be difficult to identify the source of allergy when there is an isolated positive cobalt patch test.

The relationship of cobalt allergy to metal implants is discussed in 'Cutaneous reactions to implanted metals' later in this chapter.

Avoidance. This will depend on identifying a relevant cause and eliminating contact. In those with a nickel-allergic pattern, the advice is the same as for nickel-allergic subjects. Reduction of the dietary intake of cobalt (monitoring plasma vitamin B_{12} if prolonged) may possibly benefit some cobalt-sensitive patients [13]. A cobalt spot test has also been developed and is now commercially available [14,15].

Prognosis. Concomitant cobalt and chromate sensitivity is associated with more troublesome dermatitis than that which occurs with chromate allergy alone. Possibly the same applies to a combined nickel and cobalt sensitivity because of the increased number of contact sources, which may cause recurrence of the dermatitis.

Patch tests. Cobalt chloride 1% in petrolatum is reliable for testing. False positive, irritant, purpuric reactions are common, especially in atopics.

Chromium [1,2]

Chemistry. Chromium has several different valencies (oxidation states). The two most common stable states are its trivalent form (Cr(III)) and its hexavalent (Cr(VI)) form. Chromium contact allergy is first and foremost associated with exposure to Cr(VI) in the form of chromate ions (CrO_4^{2-}) in alkali solutions, and/or dichromate ions ($Cr_2O_7^{2-}$) in acid solutions.

The question whether there is one or more chromium haptens is not firmly resolved. Cr(III) is considered to be the actual hapten at the cellular level [3]. Cr(VI) is a more potent skin sensitiser than Cr(III) as it can pass more easily through the skin barrier due to its water solubility [4,5]. It is thought that it is reduced enzymatically to Cr(III), which combines with protein to act as the hapten [3]. It is known that both Cr(III) and Cr(VI) can elicit allergic contact dermatitis in previously sensitised individuals [6]. However, the concentration of Cr(III) required to elicit a reaction is estimated to be 6–2000 times higher than that of Cr(VI) [6].

Incidence and prevalence. In Europe, chromate was for many years a frequent cause of occupational allergic contact dermatitis and chronic incapacity from cement exposure.

Patch test data for several European countries show that contact allergy to chromium has decreased to 3–4%, particularly among male dermatitis patients [7,8]. Although the overall prevalence of chromium allergy in dermatitis patients has been decreasing in Europe over the past decades, several reports demonstrate that chromium allergy remains significant. The current overall prevalence of contact allergy to chromium in the European general population is under 1% [9].

Historically, allergic chromium dermatitis mainly affected the hands of male construction workers because of cement exposure, resulting in a high degree of occupational disability [10]. However, prompted by a highly effective regulatory intervention in 2005 by the EU, the addition of ferrous sulphate to cement became compulsory to reduce the amount of water-soluble hexavalent chromium to no more than 2 ppm [11]. In countries where cement is not manufactured in this way, this trend may not be observed.

While there has also been a decrease in chromate allergy in parts of Europe attributed to the replacement of Cr(VI) in bleaches and detergents [12], this may be partially offset by an increased rate of allergic contact dermatitis caused by chromate from leather products [13]. Since 2015 the EU has restricted Cr(VI) in leather articles coming into contact with the skin above 3 ppm (via Annex XVII of the REACH regulation (EU) No. 301/2014). However, test protocols in current use do not take into account important storage conditions (temperature and relative humidity) which have been shown to be crucial for the level of Cr(VI) release. Equally, no restriction of Cr(III) in leather has been formally discussed and the release of Cr(III) from leather may also significantly higher (>10-fold) than that of Cr(VI) [14].

Occurrence. The main source of hexavalent chromium was cement [15]. Other important sources are antirust paints (lead chromate and zinc chromate) [16], including dust liberated by drilling, cutting or sandpapering of painted metals which may cause contact dermatitis on the hands, arms and face. Further rarer sources are plating salts, metal alloys, lithography/offset printing materials, anticorrosive oil, cutting oils, cooling water [17], foundry sand, polysulphide sealants [18], wood preservatives, wood ashes, wood pulp [19], mordant in wool dyeing, stains in glass, glazing enamels [20], catgut, violin strings [21], coating on zinc-galvanised iron sheets [22], textiles [23], glass polishing [24], soaps and detergents [25] and dental prostheses [26]. Chromate sensitivity in some European women was found to be related to chromate in household bleach [27], which was subsequently removed. An emerging important source of sensitisation is from leather. During the leather tanning procedure Cr(III) is used to give the leather properties such as smoothness/softness, flexibility and water resistance. In contact with air, Cr(III) in some leathers can be oxidised to Cr(VI), so skin exposure to Cr(VI) is possible even if it is not used during tanning [28,29]. Chemical analyses of leather articles have shown that the concentrations of Cr(VI) have often been above known elicitation thresholds. Also, a recent use test study showed that Cr(III), the dominating form of chromium released from new leather articles, can elicit allergic reactions in chromium-allergic individuals for leather articles that are used for a prolonged period [30].

Clinical features. Acute weeping dermatitis is unusual in patients allergic to chromate in cement; more commonly there is a dry insidious eruption, which tends to fissure, particularly on the hands. Secondary lichenification is often a feature. There is frequently a concomitant irritant element, because cement is alkaline, hygroscopic and abrasive. Primary irritant dermatitis, discoid eczema and atopic dermatitis may be mimicked, and a palmar distribution may be difficult to distinguish from chronic tinea manuum. Widespread eruptions may occur from cement dust, with flexural accentuation and involvement of the ankles and dorsa of the feet. Palmar vesicular eruptions have been blamed on traces of chromate in the diet [31]. Contact with leather footwear, gloves, belts and other clothing, or even handbags, purses and leather steering wheels, may produce dermatitis in those areas in contact with the material. Exposure to leather furniture has induced eczematous flares on the back, calves, arms and feet in sensitised subjects [32]. An oral lichenoid eruption to a chrome/cobalt prosthesis has been reported [33].

Avoidance. Avoidance of contact with sources of chromate, including leather footwear and gloves, will be necessary, although those cement workers with hardening may be able to stay at their work, remembering that there is a poor prognosis. In patients sensitised to chromium from leather footwear it is possible to source 'vegetarian shoes' and replace leather inners with cork insoles; it is also usually necessary to replace contaminated hosiery. Primary prevention strategies including the addition of ferrous sulphate to cement has already significantly reduced chromium sensitisation by cement. It is not known whether reduction of the dietary intake of chromate might benefit chromate-sensitive patients [34].

Prognosis. Historically, occupationally cement-induced chromate sensitivity persisted [35], and the prognosis of occupational dermatitis was poor as a result of its chronicity and the associated social and financial handicap [36]. Few of those affected gave up their work despite the long-term nature of the condition [37]. Changing work to avoid contact with cement did not seem to improve the prognosis [38]. Many chromate-sensitised cement workers develop hardening and are able to continue at work, albeit with ongoing but manageable dermatitis. Insufficient knowledge of the occurrence of chromate in the environment may account for the poor prognosis.

Patch tests. Sensitivity is demonstrated by a closed patch test with potassium dichromate 0.5% in petrolatum. At this concentration, weak irritant reactions are quite common, especially in atopics, but lower concentrations will miss relevant positives. Nevertheless, in the USA, a concentration of 0.25% is recommended because of the potential for false positive results. A compromise (0.375%) has been suggested although there may still be a risk of false positive and false negative reactions [39]. Dilutions can be tested to assist in distinguishing allergic from irritant reactions.

Palladium [1]

Chemistry. Palladium is a relatively inexpensive metal of the platinum group of elements.

Prevalence. Of patients undergoing routine patch testing to palladium chloride, 3–8% were shown to be allergic [2]. The sensitisation rate is reported to be increasing [3]. Nearly always there is concomitant sensitivity to nickel, and guinea pig and clinical studies have suggested this may be a true cross-reaction [4,5]. There are, however, mixed views as to whether this association is concomitant sensitivity, cross-reactivity or contamination of palladium chloride by nickel sulphate [6–8]. Of nickel-sensitive individuals, 30–40% are also patch test positive to palladium chloride [9].

Occurrence. Palladium is increasingly used in dental alloys, prostheses and industry [3]. It can be used as a whitener in white gold. Occupationally, its main uses are in electrical components and as a catalyst.

Clinical features. The clinical relevance of a positive palladium chloride patch test reaction is questionable in many instances, and may just be a reflection of nickel allergy. Stomatitis and lichen planus have nevertheless been related to palladium in dental materials [10–12]. The removal of prostheses or dental alloys containing palladium may need to be considered in these instances. A granulomatous reaction after ear piercing has also been seen with palladium allergy [13].

Patch tests. Palladium chloride is normally tested at 1% in petrolatum.

Gold [1]

Chemistry. Metallic gold is soft, malleable and ductile. It is stable and resistant to corrosion. Its strength is increased when alloyed with other metals. Gold salts, such as gold trichloride and potassium dicyanoaurate, are recognised as sensitising as well as irritant.

Occurrence. Metallic gold is mainly encountered in jewellery, stents and dental materials. Gold salts are used in the plating, electronics, photographic, glass and porcelain industries [1].

Prevalence. Metallic gold has, until fairly recently, been regarded as safe and very unlikely to sensitise. However, when gold sodium thiosulphate was added to the standard patch test series, positive reactions were obtained in 8.6% of a series of Swedish patients [2], and subsequent surveys of various selected subgroups recorded a frequency of positive reactions ranging from 1% to 23% [1]. There is a female predominance, and where relevance has been found it has usually been in the context of jewellery or gold dental work [3]. However, the allergic mechanisms behind the positive patch tests, and their relevance, have been questioned [3–5]. There is a relationship between the amount of dental gold and frequency of allergy [6]. There is also evidence of an increased rate of allergy to gold after the use of gold-plated cardiac stents [7] (see 'Cutaneous reactions to implanted metals' later in this chapter).

Clinical features. In our experience a relevance for a gold sodium thiosulphate positive patch test is found infrequently, and generally these patients can wear gold jewellery and have gold dental fillings without problems [2,3]. Nevertheless, analysis of the involved anatomical sites has been undertaken by others who have found that involvement of fingers, ear lobes and eyes by dermatitis predominates [3]. A seborrhoeic eczema pattern has been described [8], as have persistent papules and nodules on the ear lobes, with lymphomatoid or granulomatous histology [9,10]. Reported oral manifestations of allergy have included redness, burning mouth, erosions, ulceration, oro-facial granulomatosis and lichen planus-like lesions [11–14].

Sodium aurothiomalate injections for rheumatoid arthritis have induced systemic contact dermatitis and 'fever' in those previously sensitised to gold [15].

Acral dermatitis has been described from allergy to gold salts in the gilding industry [16]. A statistically significant association was also found between contact allergy to stent material and restenosis of the coronary arteries [17]. The risk for restenosis was three-fold increased when the patient was gold allergic and stented with a gold-plated stent.

Patch tests. Many gold salts have been used for patch testing, but most centres now use gold sodium thiosulphate 0.5% in petrolatum. Late reactions are common and an additional 7-day or even 2- or 3-week reading has been advised [18]. The appearance of a positive patch test may be 'dermal', with redness and oedema but no vesiculation, and persistent patch test reactions are well recognised. The controversy over the debatable relevance has led many to advise against routine standard series screening for gold allergy [5].

Mercury [1]
Chemistry. The metal and its inorganic salts, for example corrosive sublimate ($HgCl_2$), calomel ($HgCl$), fulminate ($Hg(CNO)_2$) and ammoniated mercury ($HgCl \cdot 2NH_4Cl$), as well as organic compounds (e.g. mercurochrome, thimerosal and phenylmercuric salts), may all sensitise.

Occurrence. The metal is used in instruments and dental amalgam (alloy of silver or copper and mercury) for filling teeth. Mercury and inorganic mercurials were more historically used in disinfectants, fungicides, herbicides, insecticides, detonators, emulsion paints and jewellery, as well as in the production of caustic soda and chlorine. Red mercuric sulphide (cinnabar, HgS) is used in red tattoos and in artists' paints.

Organic mercurials may be found in topical and parenteral medicaments.

Clinical features. Contact dermatitis is only rarely seen on the skin from mercury and inorganic mercurials in the UK but amalgam fillings in patients already sensitised to mercury have caused local mucosal reactions and stomatitis, which settled when they were removed [2]. Hypertrophic amalgam dermatitis simulating carcinoma of the tongue has been described in one patient [3]. Perioral dermatitis after dental filling may also occur [2].

There are many reports of oral lichen planus in association with amalgam fillings [4,5] but the relationship is not consistent [6,7]. Patch tests to mercury are frequently positive when lichen planus is adjacent to amalgam fillings, but less so when there is not a close anatomical relationship [5]. The disorder is more apparent when there is corrosion [8]. In many sensitised subjects the condition will improve or settle when the amalgam is removed [5,9]. The causes of lichen planus are nevertheless likely to be multifactorial [5].

The relationship between oral inflammation, burning mouth syndrome and mercury allergy is contentious [6,10,11], but some individuals with mercury allergy have responded to amalgam removal. Oro-facial granulomatosis has also been seen in association with mercury allergy and has resolved after removal of amalgam fillings [6,12].

Generalised exanthems and erythema multiforme have been reported from mercury exposure, including inhalation, dental fillings, following the breakage of thermometers in the mouth and also the use of an antiparasitic powder for the treatment of crab lice [13,14]. Recalcitrant eczemas in mercury-sensitised individuals are recorded as clearing after the removal of mercury amalgam fillings [15], although in most cases systemic reactions from amalgam seem to develop a few hours after insertion or removal and settle after 10–14 days [16]. In our view, malaise and general ill health are not related to allergy to mercury in amalgams.

Red mercuric sulphide (cinnabar) in a tattoo may induce granulomatous reactions in allergic subjects [17]. We have seen several granulomatous and lichenoid reactions confined to the red parts of tattoos but none of our patients has been allergic to mercurials.

Patch tests. Mercury is normally tested at 0.5% in petrolatum, mercurochrome 2% in petrolatum or aqueous, mercuric chloride 0.1% in petrolatum and ammoniated mercury 2% in petrolatum (pet.). However, mercury compounds can be irritant, and aqueous solutions of mercury salts may react with aluminium in Finn chambers to cause false positive reactions [2]. Patch testing with both mercury and ammoniated mercury is suggested if allergy is suspected [2]. Patch testing to amalgam is also possible and is available commercially at 5% pet.

Aluminium
Occurrence and clinical features. Aluminium is widely used but contact allergy is very rare. Most reported cases are from aluminium-adsorbed vaccines and parenteral solutions used for hyposensitisation, with granulomatous reactions at the injection site [1–3]. It is found in antiperspirants, and axillary dermatitis (usually irritant) may occur. Allergy in a child with chronic otitis externa treated with aluminium acetate ear drops has been seen [4].

Patch tests. As Finn chambers are aluminium, a positive patch test, often annular in configuration, may develop under every single test site in sensitised persons. Patch testing is best undertaken with plastic chambers if this diagnosis is suspected. Pure aluminium metal or salts, for example aluminium acetate 10% aqueous or aluminium chloride 2% aqueous, can be used for testing.

Other metals
Copper is a ubiquitous metal found especially in coinage, jewellery, pipes, electrical equipment and wiring. Its salts are used in insecticides, fungicides, wood preservatives, food processing, fertilisers and fur dyes. Contact allergy is very rare [1]. Dermatitis has been reported from copper intrauterine contraceptive devices and proven by patch testing and resolution of the dermatitis after removal [2,3].

Other metals used in dentistry may have the potential to cause contact allergy, including platinum, rhodium, indium and iridium [4–6].

Fragrances, balsams, flavouring agents and spices
Perfumes are blends of fragrance chemicals producing an odour intended to be aesthetically pleasant or to mask other less pleasant odours. The components are either of natural origin or produced synthetically. Natural sources include extracts from plants, trees, lichens and animals (e.g. musk, civet) [1,2]. Commercially available perfumes are mixtures of essential oils from these sources and

synthetic compounds, with usually at least 10, and up to several hundred, ingredients [3]. The scent or 'note' is determined by the mixture of volatile substances. 'Fixatives' are added to delay evaporation, influencing the quality and persistence of the perfume. Common 'fixatives' are balsams, benzyl benzoate, benzyl salicylate and synthetic musks.

Tree balsams contain many different fragrance and flavouring components. Balsam of Peru is one such material that has been studied in depth [4]. It comes from the tree *Myroxylon pereirae* that grows in Central America (not Peru!). The balsam was given its name because it was packed in, and shipped from, Peru to Europe [5]. It was widely used earlier this century for treating scabies and wounds [4]. As a natural substance its composition is complex but contains benzyl benzoate, benzyl cinnamate, cinnamic acid alcohol and aldehyde, benzoic acid, vanillin, farnesol and nerolidol [6]. It may cross-sensitise with resorcinol monobenzoate used in cellulose ester plastics [7]. Other related balsams include balsam of Tolu, balsam of spruce, gum benzoin and storax.

Flavours may similarly be of natural or synthetic origin. Examples of natural flavours include citrus fruit peel, peppermint oil, spearmint and vanilla. Natural spices include nutmeg, mustard, cinnamon, cloves and oil of juniper. In the modern food industry a large number of synthetic flavouring agents are used. As with perfumes, flavours may be complicated mixtures.

A European Scientific Committee on Consumer Safety (SCCS) review of fragrances in 2011 (SCCS/1459/11) listed 82 substances that can be classified as established fragrance contact allergens. Of these, 54 are single chemicals and 28 are natural extracts, which in turn include all those that are required to be listed on consumer products. In the past fragranced products have been simply labelled as containing 'parfum' or 'fragrance'. Since 2005 it has been mandatory in the EU for 26 well-established fragrance allergens to be individually named on the ingredients label if present at >10 ppm in leave-on products or >100 ppm in rinse-off products. This has been a significant step forward in the evaluation and surveillance of fragrance allergy and is of great benefit to individuals living with fragrance allergy.

Prevalence. In general, as measured by the frequency of allergic reactions in routinely patch-tested patients, fragrances are the second most common allergen (after nickel). Fragrance allergy affects in the region of 1.9% of the general adult European population [8]. In dermatitis patients, reported fragrance allergy rates vary between 5.7% and 17.4%, with roughly 10% being average for European patch test clinics. The prevalence of perfume allergy seems to be increasing [1,9], although this may be skewed by the increased numbers of fragrance chemicals now routinely tested [10]. Several studies suggest a preponderance of females affected, likely linked with increased exposure to leave-on fragranced products in women [8–12]. There are also links with self-reported 'sensitive skin' and increasing prevalence with age [9,12]. Occupational fragrance allergy is a significant problem, particularly for beauticians, hairdressers and allied professions [13].

The pattern of fragrance allergy continues to change. In one UK centre, although the level of allergy to the test allergen Fragrance mix I (FMI) remained stable, a significant reduction of cinnamic aldehyde and cinnamic alcohol allergy occurred within components of the mix, mirroring decreasing commercial use of these chemicals in cosmetics [11]. In 2004, the SCCS recommended the future ban of the highly sensitising fragrance chemicals chloroatranol and atranol from consumer products. Chloroatranol and atranol are the most sensitising components in extracts of oak moss (*Evernia prunastri*) and tree moss (*E. furfuracea*). Additionally, in 2011, the synthetic fragrance hydroisohexyl-3-cyclohexenecarboxaldehyde (HICC or Lyral®), was recommended for removal. These changes have been enforced by EU law from August 2021. There is evidence that the industry reduced the use of these chemicals prior to this date reflected in decreasing allergy rates to these individual fragrances [14,15].

Occurrence. Fragrances are ubiquitous. Perfumes, cosmetics, moisturisers, deodorants, aftershaves, soaps, bath additives, aromatherapy oils and toilet tissues and wipes are all typical sources. Medicaments, work creams and occupational cleansers often contain perfume. In the domestic environment cleansers, fabric conditioners, candles, pot pourri, air fresheners and polishes may all be scented. At work some materials (e.g. coolant oils) may contain a masking perfume [16]. Limonene is used in industrial and histology solvents and degreasing agents. D-limonene and other terpenes have been shown to act as allergens when they become oxidised and may therefore only be allergenic with prolonged exposure to air [17]. Auto-oxidation of terpenes is likely to make a significant contribution to the allergenicity of perfumes [18].

Flavours and spices are found in foods, beverages, lipsalves and dental products, including toothpastes, which will often use the term 'aroma' to denote their presence.

Clinical features. The analysis of common patterns of perfume dermatitis has shown a tendency to involve the hands, face and neck in women (Figure 127.21); the hands, face and lower legs in men; and the axillae in both sexes [19]. A streaky pattern may be observed. There is evidence that allergy to more than one perfume component may result in a synergistic effect [1].

Connubial (consort) allergy is well recognised [20], and allergy to lavender applied to a pillow has been described (Figure 127.22)

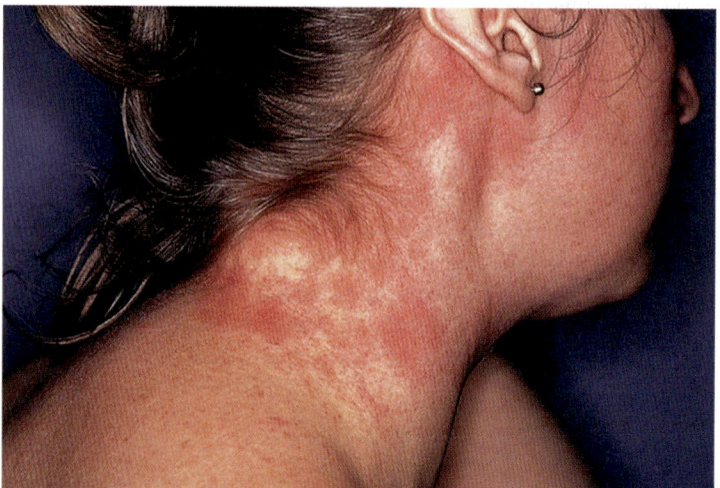

Figure 127.21 An urticated contact dermatitis in a patient allergic to fragrance. Courtesy of Dr J. D. Wilkinson.

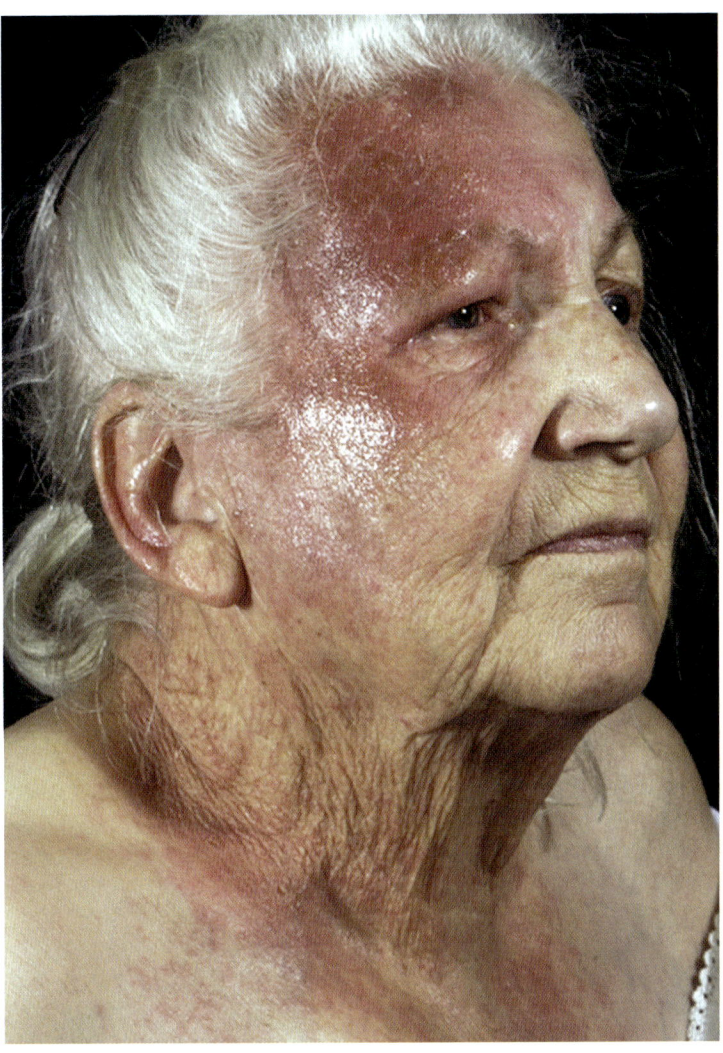

Figure 127.22 Allergic contact dermatitis from lavender essential oil on pillow. Courtesy of Dr N. Stone.

[21]. Many affected subjects suspect their allergy, but a substantial number do not. Furthermore, those who are aware of their allergy may continue to suffer dermatitis by failing to take appropriate avoidance measures, for example by unwittingly applying perfumed medicaments and cosmetics to their skin. Aromatherapists and their clients are liable to sensitisation in sites where there is contact with essential oils [22,23].

D-limonene in its oxidised state may cause allergic occupational hand dermatitis [17], which can also develop in bakers and chefs as a result of contact with sensitising flavouring agents [24]. Peeling of citrus fruit in the domestic environment may also induce allergic hand dermatitis.

Cheilitis may be a reflection of allergy to flavouring agents in toothpastes [25,26], lipsalves [27] and food and drink [28]. Gingivitis has occurred from allergy to eugenol in dental cement [29] and cinnamon has induced oral blisters, erosions and lichen planus [30,31].

Balsam of Peru is still used as a medicament, particularly in haemorrhoid preparations, and allergy is therefore relevant to perianal problems. Sensitising balsams are used in medicaments and balms for wounds, sprains and joint pains, particularly in the Far East [32]. Tincture of benzoin is used in a similar way, and may also be used under orthopaedic plaster casts [33]. Vesicular hand dermatitis has been related to dietary intake of flavours related to balsam of Peru [34].

Musk ambrette is a synthetic perfume component responsible for photoallergy, and although its use has been discontinued in the western world it may still be present in perfumed materials from other parts of the world.

Fragrance-allergic subjects appear to be at an increased risk of more frequent and more severe eye and respiratory symptoms than would be expected by chance [35].

Avoidance. Perfumes are marketed as concentrated liquids and in more diluted forms such as eau de toilette, or as sprays, and all should be avoided. The application of perfume to clothing may still cause problems in allergic subjects, who often believe they will only react if perfume is applied directly to the skin. Occasionally, affected subjects are able to use a specific perfume without any problem. Other perfumed skin products to be avoided include deodorants, aftershaves, talcum powders, soaps and bath additives.

In addition to the 26 named fragrance chemicals, the presence of perfume in a cosmetic or wet wipe within the EU is denoted by the International Nomenclature of Cosmetic Ingredients (INCI) term 'parfum', and the presence of balsam of Peru by the INCI term '*Myroxylon pereirae*'. Patients should be warned that some cosmetics' labels may suggest they are fragrance-free, yet the products are found to contain perfume when the full ingredient label is studied, reinforcing the need to avoid unlabelled products. Some plant extracts may potentially be a hidden source of fragrance in cosmetics as the INCI nomenclature may use the plant's Linnaean name rather than the word parfum. Some extracts, however, may only contain traces of fragrance chemicals. Within some personal care products the term 'fragrance' may also be replaced by the word 'aroma'. Patients need to be made aware that the ever-increasingly popular range of products containing 'botanicals' can also act as a source of fragrance chemical exposure and would be best avoided.

Surprisingly, some prescribable moisturisers, emollients, bath additives and corticosteroids, as well as over-the-counter medicaments, contain perfume. Menthol, lavender oil and peppermint oil are the top allergens in patients reacting to a medicated cream [36]. Fragrance-allergic patients with ongoing problems should also be counselled carefully about avoidance of these sources in medicaments.

In the domestic situation, perfume-containing sprays such as air fresheners, insect repellents and hairsprays should be avoided, as should skin contact with perfumed household cleansing products and polishes. Unperfumed soaps or soap substitutes are required for washing the skin. The levels of perfume residues from washing powders and fabric conditioners for clothes are probably too low to cause clinical problems [37], but in those with a clothing pattern of eczema, extra rinsing and avoidance of fabric conditioners can be considered. Peeling citrus fruit with the bare hands should be avoided by those with hand eczema and an allergy to balsam of Peru.

Furthermore, if a fragrance material has a second function in a formulation, such as a preservative (benzyl alcohol) or emollient (methyl benzoate), it can still be included in 'fragrance-free' products by unscrupulous manufacturers. Therefore, a review of the patient's own personal care products may be very useful.

In the occupational environment many cleansers, conditioning creams and barrier creams are perfumed, and similar avoidance measures are needed. Some work materials, including cutting oils and paints, may contain masking perfume and enquiries may be necessary to establish their components.

Dietary measures may be helpful not only for oral and perioral allergy from flavours but have been suggested for those with vesicular palmar eczema associated with balsam of Peru allergy. However, the response can be disappointing [38,39].

Patch tests. Patch testing for fragrance allergy is complex. The chemicals themselves are volatile and petrolatum preparations may not be stable over time. Patch test chambers should be freshly prepared and used quickly, with allergens stored in a fridge with caps tightly applied [40]. Many fragrance chemicals, including the fragrance mixes, are irritant such that care must be taken in patch test readings. Most importantly, the complexity of commercially produced perfumes are such that there is not a perfect screening patch test for all perfume allergy. Fragrance allergy patch testing recommendations have changed significantly over time and are being continually updated.

Before 1977, the main recommended marker for perfume allergy was balsam of Peru, which is still part of the standard series. It is tested at 25% in petrolatum, but was thought to identify only 50% of perfume-allergic subjects [41]. Screening for perfume allergy was significantly advanced by the development of the first fragrance mix of eight common fragrance sensitisers (Table 127.7) [42,43]. FMI contains an emulsifier, sorbitan sesquioleate at 5%, which is reported to have improved the bioavailability of the fragrance chemicals [44]. Sorbitan sesquioleate is an allergen in its own right and is also the emulsifier in the commercial preparations of *Myroxylon pereirae* resin and 2-hydroxyethyl methacrylate. Adding sorbisan sesquioleate to the baseline series has therefore been suggested to reduce the risk of misinterpretation of patch test reactions to these three allergens [45].

The next fragrance chemical introduced for routine testing was HICC (Lyral). It was noted as a common perfume sensitiser that would be missed if reliance was placed on FMI and balsam of Peru testing alone [46]. This and five other fragrances (citral, farnesol, coumarin, citronellal and α-hexyl-cinnamaldehyde) were combined

Table 127.7 Ingredients of Fragrance mix I.[a]

Substance	Concentration (%)[b]
Cinnamaldehyde	1
Cinnamyl alcohol	1
Eugenol	1
Amyl cinnamaldehyde	1
Hydroxycitronnellol	1
Geraniol	1
Isoeugenol	1
Oak moss absolute (*Evernia prunastri*)	1

[a] Fragrance mix allergens contain sorbitan sesquioleate (5% in petrolatum) as an emulsifier.
[b] All ingredients are diluted in petrolatum.

Table 127.8 Ingredients of Fragrance mix II.

Substance	Concentration (%)[a]
Alpha-hexyl cinnamaldehyde	5
Citral	1
Citronellal	0.5
Farnesol	2.5
Coumarin	2.5
Hydroxy-methylpentyl-cyclohexene carboxyaldehyde (Lyral)	2.5

[a] All ingredients are diluted in petrolatum.

to make a further mix for patch testing known as Fragrance mix II (FMII) (Table 127.8). Since 2008 the European Society of Contact Dermatitis (ESCD) has recommended using FMII in the baseline series and for Lyral to also be tested as a separate allergen at 5% pet. Allergy rates to Lyral were however declining prior to its ban from European consumer products from August 2021. It has now been suggested for possible removal as a single allergen from the baseline series [15].

Both FMI and FMII may give false positive irritant reactions, which testing the ingredients separately may help to avoid. However, when individual materials are mixed they may combine in such a way as to produce a compound allergy, or other synergistic effects inducing a true allergic reaction, despite the components themselves being negative. The reverse situation (quenching) – that is the mix is negative and one or more of the components positive – has also been reported, but questioned [47]. Nevertheless, it is worthwhile testing with the breakdown allergens in addition to the fragrance mixes when perfume allergy is suspected. It should be noted that the individual allergens from FMI are tested at 1% (as opposed to higher concentrations for FMII allergens with the exception of citral). It has recently been suggested that the FMI individual allergen concentrations should be increased to minimise false negative reactions [48].

The oxidised terpenes, hydroperoxides of limonene (HO-limonene) and linalool (HO-linalool), have now emerged as leading causes of fragrance allergy and can be tested for using commercially available allergens. Linalool is found in more than 200 natural oils including lavender, ylang ylang, bergamot, jasmine and geranium oils. Studies show that it might also be present in 90–95% of prestige perfumes. Limonene is found in many oils including rosemary, eucalyptus, lavender, lemongrass and peppermint [49]. High rates of positive reactions to both HO-limonene and HO-linalool in dermatitis patients are reported (9.4% and 11.7%, respectively, in one study), with the majority being of clinical relevance [50]. Both limonene and linalool are pre-haptens, requiring preoxidation to become allergenic. In 2017 HO-limonene 0.3% and HO-linalool 1.0% were recommended for addition to the British baseline series [10]. Patch test readings from these allergens are, however, notoriously difficult to interpret due to their irritancy, such that many centres also test with HO-limonene 0.1% and HO-linalool 0.5% to allow for more accurate reading. Limonene and linalool are currently the most commonly used fragrance chemicals in personal care and household cleaning products in the UK [14]. HO-limonene and HO-linalool were added to the European baseline series as single allergens in 2018.

Evernia furfuracea (tree moss) is the latest individual fragrance chemical to be suggested for inclusion in the standard series [51]. A recent cross-sectional study of 6004 patients patch tested with FMI and FMII as well as all of the 26 EU-labelled fragrance allergens, revealed allergy to one or more fragrance chemicals in 15.7%. 'Non-fragrance-mix' chemicals were the most common sensitisers. Individual fragrance chemicals with the highest sensitisation rates were HO-linalool (3.9%), *E. furfuracea* (3%), HO-limonene (2.5%) and HICC (2.1%). Tree moss is a lichen that grows on the bark of conifers, in particular pine and cedar trees. Tree moss and the similar lichen, oak moss, have been used by the fragrance industry for many years and share chemicals which are degraded to the potent allergens atranol and chloroatranol. Positive patch test reactions to tree moss and oak moss therefore often coincide. Tree moss allergy also often coincides with colophonium allergy, thought to be related to their common pine tree origin, with resin acids of colophony occurring in tree debris and migrating into the tree lichen. A recent study of 632 patients tested with tree moss 1% showed a positive result in 3.5%, with eight patients showing no other fragrance reactions and 75% having a relevant associated reaction to colophony. Colophony-allergic patients should be alerted to the possible need to also avoid products containing tree moss as a precaution [52].

Following on from the recognition that HO-limonene and HO-linalool are significant causes of relevant fragrance allergy, recent reports have suggested that hyperoxides of both citronellol and geraniol may also be significantly more allergenic [53,54]. Further studies will be required to investigate whether the oxidised versions of these fragrances should also be routinely tested. There are suggestions that all 26 EU-labelled fragrance allergens should be tested on a more regular basis due to the high frequency and relevancy of fragrance allergy [55]. This would obviously increase patch test numbers significantly, but may be important for targeted patients.

The pattern of fragrance allergy will continue to change over time with industry developments, changing fashion trends and new regulatory interventions. Investigation of fragrance allergy has similarly adapted to these changes and will continue to progress.

Applied medicaments [1,2]

Prevalence and incidence. Of all allergic contact dermatitis cases, about 15% are caused, or complicated, by sensitivity to medicaments, although this may be higher in susceptible patient populations [2]. The literature on contact dermatitis abounds with reports of reactions to medicaments, and it is not possible to review all of these. It is doubtful whether the incidence has changed significantly, although the incidence of sensitivity to a particular allergen varies from country to country and from decade to decade, according to both local prescribing habits and the number of patients who are at high risk, for example with leg ulcers and stasis eczema, included in any series. Contact allergy to medicaments is also more common in an elderly population, particularly to fragrance, lanolin, local anaesthetics, neomycin and corticosteroids [3]. Cases will be missed unless patch tests are routinely performed and if locally used medicaments are not included in a medicament series. Owing to the increased use of antiseptic hand washes both in the occupational setting and home setting, testing for sensitisation to benzalkonium chloride and chlorhexidine should also be considered. Meaningful sensitisation indices for the various medicaments can be calculated only if the prevalence of sensitivity is correlated with the usage.

Antibiotics (neomycin and aminoglycosides, bacitracin, polymyxin B, fusidic acid) and antiseptics (chlorhexidine, povidone-iodine, quaternary ammonium compounds) are among the main culprits, followed by local anaesthetics (dibucaine, amethocaine, lidocaine, benzocaine), corticosteroids (budesonide) and non-steroidal anti-inflammatory drugs (NSAIDs) (ketoprofen, etofenamate, piroxicam, diclofenac, benzydamine), but many other drugs can induce contact reactions. Contact photosensitivity occurs mostly with promethazine and NSAIDs, like ketoprofen, in this case with cross-reactivity to benzophenones, octocrylene and oral fenofibrate [4].

Most cases represent iatrogenic contact dermatitis, but connubial and occupational cases in, for example, health personnel, workers from the pharmaceutical industry or veterinarians are also reported.

Clinical features. Certain sites appear to be prone to the development of allergic contact dermatitis from medicaments. This is probably the result of frequent medicament usage at these sites, occlusive skin conditions such as the flexures and pre-existing skin damage. Sensitisation to medicaments is particularly common in patients with leg ulcers or eczema of the lower legs (Figure 127.23), and is found in about half of those with chronic stasis eczema. Even weak allergens appear to sensitise if used on the lower leg. In one French prospective multicentre study 59.6% of patients with chronic leg ulcers had at least one positive patch test reaction to a 'modern dressing' [5].

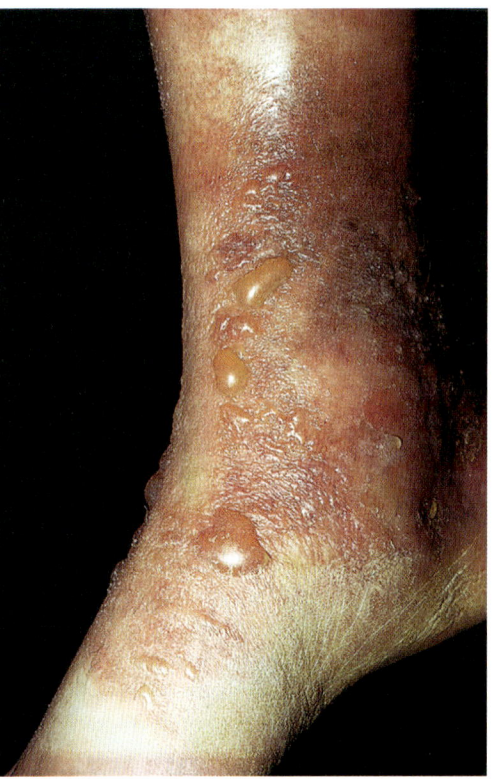

Figure 127.23 Medicament allergic contact dermatitis superimposed on stasis eczema. Topical antibiotics/antibacterials, preservatives, lanolin and other constituents of the medicament base are often to blame. Courtesy of Dr J. D. Wilkinson.

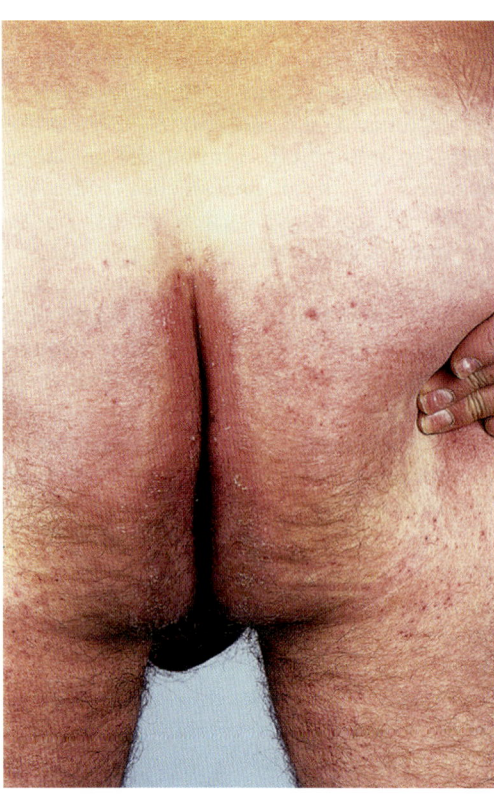

Figure 127.24 Pruritus ani is often complicated by secondary contact dermatitis to local anaesthetics or other medicaments. Courtesy of Dr J. D. Wilkinson.

Contact dermatitis is also common in patients with chronic perianal inflammatory disorders (Figure 127.24), pressure sores, chronic otitis externa [6,7] and in those who frequently use ocular medicaments [8].

Mucosal exposure (e.g. to chlorhexidine) may promote the development of immediate-type skin reactions, which can be severe and life-threatening.

However, dermatitis from applied medicaments can develop anywhere. Sometimes, the sensitivity is obvious but often it is occult and easily overlooked, and it will then only be detected by patch testing. In burns, the damaged skin may be incapable of reacting, and dermatitis may only be apparent at the periphery of the burn site.

Sensitivity to a topically applied medicament may result in several types of reaction.

1 Local aggravation, with increased itching and redness.
2 Spread to other regions, in most cases preceded by local aggravation. This is especially common in patients with stasis eczema or leg ulcers.
3 A local reaction may not develop, and dissemination may be the only sign of sensitivity. This typically occurs with creams and ointments containing a potent steroid capable of suppressing the reaction locally, but not in other regions.
4 Sensitisation can also manifest merely as failure to respond to treatment. The original condition may worsen or fail to improve, without there being any acute flares or spread to arouse suspicion. This is seen mainly when there is a low degree of sensitivity and low concentration of allergens, typically with parabens and lanolin, or where the contact allergen is a corticosteroid.
5 Persistent generalised erythroderma is a rare manifestation of allergic contact sensitisation to medicaments.
6 Contact urticarial, phototoxic and photoallergic reactions have also been reported.

Systemic reactions. Patients sensitised by the topical use of a drug may develop systemic reactions if that drug, or one that is closely related, is then given systemically. Systemic contact dermatitis usually presents with dermatitis or redness of the buttocks and flexural involvement elsewhere. It is also called symmetrical drug-related intertriginous and flexural exanthema (SDRIFE) or the 'baboon syndrome' [9]. Widespread dermatitis or generalised exfoliative dermatitis has been reported following challenge with a systemic drug to which the patient already has contact allergy.

Other patients may develop a systemic reaction after topical application of a medicament. Anaphylactic reactions have been reported, for example following the topical use of bacitracin, cephalosporins, rifamycin and chlorhexidine. Erythema multiforme-like reactions to topical medicaments have also been reported. Some patients have positive patch test reactions to a topically applied drug, having previously been sensitised by its systemic use.

Patients who have been sensitised by the topical use of promethazine hydrochloride may develop serious photosensitivity if the drug is given systemically. Care must always be taken in prescribing an antihistamine systemically if the patient is known to have been exposed to the same or a chemically similar drug topically.

Avoidance and prognosis. Sensitisation from a single constituent may lead to recurrent dermatitis due to its inclusion in several proprietary formulations. In only a few countries are the contents of a proprietary medicament stated on the package or listed on the data sheet and, even then, the information is often insufficient, constituents sometimes being given as trade names or only 'active' ingredients listed. In order to reduce the risk of relapse, the ingredients of all topical medicaments should be established. Ideally, all topical medicaments, whether prescribed or purchased without a prescription, would display full ingredient labelling.

It is also necessary to consider cross-sensitivity to other, untested medicaments. This has received particular study in relation to contact sensitivity to the aminoglycoside group of antibiotics. A similar situation may develop in patients sensitive to the 'para' group of chemicals, with cross-sensitisation between local anaesthetics, dyes, sulphonamides, UV filters, etc.

Patch tests. Patients with suspected contact dermatitis should be tested with all their medicaments. The information obtained in the history may be incomplete so commonly used medicaments should also be routinely tested. It is often helpful to have a vehicle and medicament series or several 'site' series with the ingredients of the most commonly used topical preparations in that geographic location. Testing to the medicament ('as is') may miss allergens because they may be present in insufficient concentration. Where there is a high index of suspicion, the individual components should be obtained and appropriately diluted for patch testing.

It is important not to forget self-prescription of over-the-counter preparations. Popular habits of self-treatment vary from country to country and region to region. Knowledge of these habits is obtained by experience, but local pharmacists can often supply information. Certain remedies may be popular in one country but almost unknown in another. 'Natural' or herbal treatments are increasing in popularity. Some of these are irritant, and others, such as Chinese herbal remedies [10] and tea tree oil [11], contain allergens.

Medicament allergens included in the EECDRG recommended European standard series include the following:

- *Neomycin 20% in petrolatum.* Neomycin has two active components, neomycin B and neomycin C, which are stereoisomers. It cross-reacts with other aminoglycoside antibiotics. The pattern of cross-sensitivity has been studied in guinea pigs. Clinically, neomycin is known to cross-react frequently with kanamycin and framycetin (Soframycin®), which would be anticipated with the latter as it consists almost entirely (99%) of neomycin B. Cross-sensitivity also occurs to a varying degree with gentamicin and tobramycin. Neomycin classically produces late reactions (beyond 96 h readings).
- *Clioquinol 3% in petrolatum.* In areas where there is high use of chlorquinaldol, the retention of the quinoline mix may be of value due to the lack of cross-reactions between it and clioquinol.
- *Benzocaine 5% in petrolatum.* Experience suggests that, in the UK at least, the replacement of benzocaine with a mixture containing cinchocaine (dibucaine) 2.5% and amethocaine (tetracaine) 2.5% will double the yield of allergic-positive reactions. Local anaesthetics are either of the ester or amide type, and cross-reactions can occur within groups. Although cinchocaine is an aminoalkylamide and lidocaine (lignocaine) is an aminoacylamide, most individuals do not cross-react. Ideally, any reaction to the mix should be followed up by testing to the constituents and to lidocaine. Not all reactions to local anaesthetics are detected by the mix and patch tests should always be dictated by the particular exposure of the patient.
- *Corticosteroids* (tixocortol pivalate 1.0% in petrolatum and budesonide 0.1% in petrolatum in the British baseline series) [12,13]. When testing with corticosteroids it is not unusual to see reflex vasodilatation following the steroid-induced vasoconstriction and this should not be interpreted as a positive reaction. Conversely, an annular response is frequently allergic, as a result of central suppression of the reaction by the corticosteroid.

A reaction to tixocortol pivalate almost invariably means that the patient is allergic to hydrocortisone. The British Society of Cutaneous Allergy (BSCA) recommends that tixocortol pivalate is tested at 1.0% [13]. In the UK, a reaction to budesonide almost certainly represents a cross-reaction to another corticosteroid, most likely an 'ester' such as hydrocortisone 17-butyrate or an 'acetonide' such as triamcinolone acetonide. A reaction to either of these steroids in the standard series should prompt further testing to an extended steroid series, as 50% of tixocortol pivalate-positive and 90% of budesonide-positive individuals react to other corticosteroids. According to the literature, the prevalence of allergic reactions to corticosteroids is extremely variable, with a range between 0.2% and 5%, with 85% of these patients having multiple steroid allergies [14]. Our experience suggests that although intradermal testing may have a role, testing other corticosteroids at 1% in ethanol is more sensitive although these test preparations are not available commercially at present.

Together with knowledge of cross-reaction patterns [15], this helps in deciding what topical steroid to use as an alternative. Empirically, fluocinolone acetonide (Synalar®) preparations react least frequently, and are available in a range of potencies. In view of the potential cross-reactivity between these two markers of corticosteroid allergy and prednisolone and its derivatives, it seems prudent to advise the use of either betamethasone or dexamethasone if a systemic steroid is needed, in order to reduce the risk of inducing a generalised dermatitis.

Although steroids are also applied topically to mucosal surfaces in the treatment of respiratory diseases, reports of contact allergy are rare. Indeed, individuals challenged with inhaled steroid to which they are sensitised, typically develop a cutaneous but not a respiratory response. In contrast, there are reports of both immediate and delayed-type allergic reactions following various other systemic routes of administration.

Cosmetics [1,2]

Cosmetics have been defined as any preparation applied to the skin, mouth, hair or nails for the purpose of cleansing, enhancing appearance, giving a pleasant smell or providing protection [1]. There is consequently a considerable range of products that can be included within this definition, for example perfumes, deodorants, aftershaves, hairsprays, lipsticks, nail varnishes and (meth)acrylate-based nails, moisturisers, cleansers and wipes, mascara, eye shadow, make up, make-up removers, sunscreens, hair colours and styling agents, depilatories, soaps, shampoos, shower gels, bath oils and toothpastes.

Good manufacturers aim to eliminate known sensitisers and irritants. However, because all cosmetics and toiletries have to be protected against bacteriological contamination and decomposition, and as most consumers require their cosmetics to have a pleasing smell, there are potentially sensitising preservatives and fragrances in most cosmetic products. The substitution of one allergen by an alternative component may lead to the introduction of perhaps an even more sensitising substance [3]. When entirely new products or ingredients are used on a large number of consumers, unexpected allergic or irritant reactions may occur, and it may be some time before the cause is identified.

The range of cosmetic allergens is considerable. The more frequently detected allergens are discussed in the specific sections relating to fragrances, preservatives, vehicles and excipients, PPD and related dyes and UV filters.

(Meth)acrylate-related contact allergy in gel nails, acrylic nails and gel-polish products have been on the rise across Europe in the past decade, mirroring their use among consumers [4].

There is an increasing vogue for including natural plant-based ingredients in cosmetics, for example tea tree oil (*Melaleuca alternifolia*), and these may be potentially allergenic [5–7].

Hairdressers (and their clients) are exposed to a wide range of allergens in dyes, bleaches (ammonium persulphate), permanent wave solutions (thioglycolates), shampoos and hairsprays, etc. [8,9]. Depilatory waxes may contain colophony derivatives, which can induce allergic dermatitis [10].

Labelling of cosmetic ingredients has been required for over 35 years in the USA, but only since 1997 in Europe. The nomenclature used within the EU is the INCI, which is based on the US Cosmetic, Toiletry and Fragrance Association nomenclature [1].

Incidence and prevalence. Contact dermatitis to ingredients of cosmetics and toiletries is common in patients attending patch test clinics; approximately 10% of patients investigated for contact dermatitis in a multicentre European study were allergic to cosmetic products [11]. The exact incidence and prevalence of sensitivity in the population is difficult to establish. In a UK study of 1022 persons, 8.3% had experienced some sort of adverse reaction to a cosmetic or toiletry in the preceding year; most reactions were irritant rather than allergic in nature [12]. In one American survey comprising 30 000 consumers, 700 reactions had occurred during 1 year [13]. Some reactions are transient, such as stinging and smarting, and contact urticarial. Most people simply change brand and do not report adverse reactions to the manufacturer. It is nevertheless estimated that 1–3% of the population is allergic to a cosmetic or cosmetic ingredient [14], with a female predominance.

Studies have shown that there is significant variation in practice in screening with allergens for cosmetic allergy across Europe [15], which has also led to an attempt to develop a European cosmetic screening series [**16**].

Cosmetic ingredients can be classified into several categories: fragrances, preservatives (including antimicrobials and antioxidants), UV light absorbers, excipients (vehicles), emollients, surfactants (including detergents and emulsifiers), hair styling products and dyes and nail products.

The most common cosmetic allergens are fragrances and preservatives. Also of importance are PPD, UV filters and (meth)acrylates, but there are potentially many others [**16**].

Clinical features [1]. Cosmetic allergy is unsuspected in about half of those in whom it is subsequently diagnosed [17]. Apart from hair dye allergy, acute weeping and oedematous reactions are unusual. More commonly, there are red scaly patches or a more diffuse redness. Differentiation from atopic and seborrhoeic eczema and lupus erythematosus may be difficult, especially on the face.

Sites of involvement are varied, and depend on the type of product containing the allergen(s) and where it has been applied. Patterns of perfume allergy are described in the section on fragrances, and hair dye allergy in the section on PPD and related dyes. The eyelids, face and neck (Figure 127.25) are sites commonly involved in cosmetic allergy, but hand involvement and more widespread dermatitis are seen. It is not always appreciated how often cosmetics, particularly moisturisers, are applied not only to dry skin but also to pre-existing eczemas, including constitutional forms. Flares may wrongly be blamed on the underlying disorder, and cosmetic allergy may go undetected unless

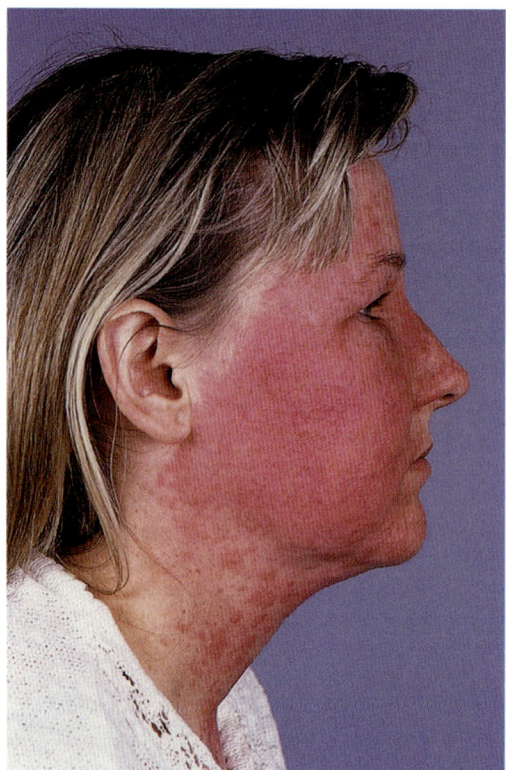

Figure 127.25 Facial allergic contact dermatitis, often due to fragrance, preservatives or other ingredients of cosmetics. Courtesy of Dr J. D. Wilkinson.

appropriate patch testing is undertaken. In general, leave-on products are more likely to sensitise than wash-off cosmetics, although dermatitis may be maintained from the latter source in allergic subjects [1].

Cheilitis is seen from lipstick, lipsalve and toothpaste allergy. Hair cosmetic allergy may cause a scalp margin pattern as well as periorbital swelling. A similar distribution is seen in hairdressers' clients allergic to permanent wave chemicals (usually glyceryl monothioglycolate) but perms are currently not fashionable so this is now rarer.

Nail varnish allergy is often ectopic, with patches and streaks on the face, neck (see Figure 127.10) and behind the ears, and episodic periorbital swelling. The allergen is usually tosylamide formaldehyde resin, but phthalic anhydride/trimellitic anhydride/glycols copolymer and adipic acid/neopentyl glycol/trimellitic anhydride copolymer are increasingly being reported as nail cosmetic allergens [18]. Nail (meth)acrylate chemicals may also cause dystrophy and paronychia [19]. A similar, potentially widespread, ectopic pattern of contact allergy may occur from (meth)acrylates in nail cosmetics. Passive transfer of allergy from cosmetics used by partners (connubial or consort allergy) and relatives [20–22] should not be forgotten.

Occupational allergic hand dermatitis associated with hairdressing materials is described elsewhere.

Avoidance. Full ingredient labelling of cosmetics in Europe has made a major contribution to avoidance measures. It is important to give the patient the INCI name of the material to which they are allergic as this is the nomenclature used on cosmetic ingredient labels. There is still potential for confusion, particularly with plants which, when used in cosmetics, are identified by their Latin name in the Linnaean system. Some plant extracts may potentially contain or cross-react with fragrances, and it may be difficult for the patient and the dermatologist to be absolutely sure if a product containing natural plant extracts is safe for fragrance-allergic subjects. Unlabelled products should not be used. The reader is referred to the sections on individual cosmetic allergens for more details.

A complete list of INCI names for substances can be obtained from https://ec.europa.eu/growth/sectors/cosmetics/cosing_en (last accessed July 2023).

Patch tests. The ESCD baseline series contains a number of cosmetic allergens, including FMI and FMII, balsam of Peru (*Myroxylon pereirae*), HICC (Lyral), parabens mix, lanolin, quaternium-15, methylchloroisothiazolinone-methylisothiazolinone (MCI/MI), MI, formaldehyde, PPD, propolis and colophonium (colophony). The BSCA include additional cosmetic chemicals in their recommended baseline series: Amerchol L101, 2-bromo-2-nitropropane-1,3-diol, imidazolidinyl urea, diazolidinyl urea, HO-limonene, HO-linalool, *Evernia furfuracea*, hydroxyethyl (meth)acrylate, decyl glucoside and lauryl glucoside (https://cutaneousallergy.org/; last accessed July 2023).

However, a wider screen of allergens is advised when investigating cosmetic allergy, in particular nail cosmetic allergens (tosylamide formaldehyde resin, the newer anhydride copolymers and nail (meth)acrylates). Patch testing with a series of UV filters may also be advised. In addition, the main allergen suppliers have a range of other potential allergens, including more preservatives, antioxidants, surfactants, emulsifiers and other cosmetic excipients [16].

It is also important to consider patch testing with the cosmetics used by the patient. As a general rule, leave-on products and perfumes can be tested 'as is' but, because of irritancy, soaps and shampoos should be diluted to 1% aqueous. There is still a risk of false positive reactions and also, because of the dilution, false negatives. Mascara and nail varnish are often irritant, and should be applied to a chamber and the solvents left to evaporate before applying them as a patch test.

Allergy cannot be totally ruled out unless all the ingredients of all cosmetics have been tested individually at appropriate concentration and in a suitable vehicle. In practice, however, most cosmetics are initially tested 'as is', but false negative reactions and marginal irritant reactions are common. Ideally, each component of a suspect cosmetic should be tested individually and where there is a high index of suspicion the individual components should be obtained from the manufacturer if they are willing to provide them. Ideally, the raw material should be the same as that used in the suspect product, because batch differences, source and purity may all be important. Sometimes the allergy is to the substance itself, and sometimes to an impurity. The concentration necessary to test an individual substance is often greater than its concentration in the product. Manufacturers' patch test kits, which may contain ingredients at the concentration in which they are present in the product, are likely to be misleading and should not be used.

Testing with hair dyes is discussed in the section on PPD and related dyes.

Other tests. If cosmetic allergy is still suspected despite negative patch test reactions to a cosmetic containing sunscreen chemicals, then the possibility of photoallergy should also be considered and, if clinically indicated, photopatch tests should be undertaken [23].

ROATs may also be useful to try and identify the offending cosmetic, although these will not necessarily differentiate between irritant and allergic reactions. Finally, after discussion with the patient, a usage test can be considered, with reintroduction of the suspected products, one at a time, and using each for up to 3 days.

Antimicrobial agents and preservatives

One of the greatest challenges facing cosmetic industry formulators at present is the choice of preservative(s) to use in their products. The palette of available chemicals is rapidly diminishing following regulatory control, mainly for reasons other than contact allergy issues, although there have been some recent examples such as with methyldibromoglutaronitrile (MDBGN) and methylisothiazolinone. Therefore, on the basis of possible regulatory-led withdrawal of commoner preservatives in Europe it will be important to monitor the use of the less commonly used ones.

Formaldehyde [1]

Chemistry. Formaldehyde (HCHO) is a gas, and formalin is a solution of the gas in water (about 38%). Methylol groups can be combined with other compounds to form formaldehyde releasers, which are widely used as preservatives. Formaldehyde may combine with other chemicals to produce resins, which may sensitise (see the section on resins and plastics later in this chapter).

Prevalence. The introduction of textile finishing resins low in formaldehyde and the replacement of formaldehyde with formaldehyde releasers in cosmetics have greatly contributed to a decline in sensitisation. Nevertheless in individuals routinely patch tested for the investigation of contact dermatitis, the frequency of allergic-positive reactions to formaldehyde is near 5% in North America, and in Europe near 1% [2,3].

Occurrence. In the USA, exposure to free formaldehyde still often occurs from cosmetics, whereas in Europe sensitisation to free formaldehyde is believed to occur mainly from occupational exposure (e.g. laboratory technicians, haemodialysis nurses, embalmers, housekeepers, hairdressers, beauticians, machinists, metal workers). Free formaldehyde is still present in up to 0.1% of cosmetic products in the USA, whereas in Europe its use is low (or even forbidden such as in Sweden), although notably nail hardeners may still contain up to a 5% concentration [1]. Nevertheless, formaldehyde in cosmetics, 'as is' or hidden as an impurity or derived from formaldehyde releasers, still causes allergic contact dermatitis.

Box 127.5 gives an idea of the wide variety of potential sources of formaldehyde.

Box 127.5 Formaldehyde sources
- Antiperspirants
- Colouring agents
- Cosmetic preservatives
- Cotton clothing (wash and wear, crease resistant)
- Disinfectants and deodorisers
- Dry-cleaning materials
- Embalming fluids and tissue fixative
- Fertilisers
- Fibreboard/chipboard
- Fumigators
- Glues
- Hardeners
- Household cleaning products
- Hyperhidrosis treatment
- Industrial biocides
- Insecticide (flypapers)
- Metal-working fluids
- Orthopaedic casts
- Paints/lacquers
- Photographic plates and solutions
- Plywood
- Polishes
- Preservatives
- Printing chemicals
- Rayons
- Renal dialysis
- Reusable gloves
- Shampoos and soaps
- Smoke from tobacco, coal and wood
- Tanning agents for leather
- Wart treatment
- Water-resistant papers and tissues

It can often be difficult to find relevance for a positive patch test, but more commonly identified causes are cosmetic ingredients and less commonly now clothing resins. In this regard, some authors have advised the use of ROATs as well as formaldehyde detection by the chromotropic acid method [4] to be applied to products used by the patient, although this is not always feasible in clinical practice.

Shampoos may contain formaldehyde, although this is more likely to be of relevance in the context of hairdressers' hand dermatitis than in relation to transient use on the hair. Some textile resins will release formaldehyde, and free formaldehyde may be found in treated cotton clothing and rayons. Paints/lacquers, printing inks and cleaning products, filling agents and glues were the most frequently registered products containing formaldehyde marketed in Denmark [5]. Formaldehyde is used for the preservation of anatomical and pathological specimens, and those working with such specimens, for example histopathologists and embalmers, are at risk of allergy from free formaldehyde. It is used medically in renal dialysis and may be found in orthopaedic casts.

In cosmetics and industry (e.g. cutting oils), formaldehyde has largely been replaced by formaldehyde-releasing preservatives

Table 127.9 Formaldehyde-releasing preservatives in cosmetics and medicaments.

Substance	Patch test concentration
Quaternium-15	1% in petrolatum
Imidazolidinyl urea	2% in petrolatum (or 2% aqueous)
Diazolidinyl urea	2% in petrolatum (or 2% aqueous)
2-Bromo-2-nitropropane-1,3-diol	0.25% in petrolatum (or 0.5% in petrolatum)
DMDM hydantoin	2% aqueous

DMDM, 1,3-dimethylol-5,5-dimethylhydantoin.

which exert the same broad spectrum activity against bacteria, notably Gram-negative bacteria such as *Pseudomonas aeruginosa*, yeasts and fungi (Table 127.9).

Many of these releasers not only sensitise simultaneously with, but also independently of, formaldehyde [6–9].

Clinical features. The presenting dermatitis will depend on the source of contact, for instance a clothing pattern, a cosmetic pattern or involvement of the hands in occupational dermatitis. Formaldehyde allergy is often only diagnosed retrospectively by finding a positive patch test and relating this to the distribution of the problem by identifying formaldehyde or formaldehyde-releasing chemicals that come into contact with the affected site.

Avoidance. Avoidance may be difficult, bearing in mind the wide exposure possibilities, but it is important to recognise that avoidance steps are only required if the individual has skin problems that are relevant to the exposure. If cosmetics, medicaments and moisturisers come into contact with the affected sites their ingredient labels should be carefully assessed in order that those containing not only formaldehyde but also the formaldehyde-releasing preservatives listed in Table 127.9 are avoided. It may also be necessary to contact manufacturers or check the material safety data sheet to establish the presence of formaldehyde in their products, particularly cutting oils. The difficulties faced by patients in identifying formaldehyde in products is highlighted by the fact that in one study of sensitised persons with persistent dermatitis, all were still using at least one product containing formaldehyde. Only by detailed enquiries and access to product databases could the presence of formaldehyde be demonstrated [10].

Undeclared free formaldehyde in cosmetics continues to pose a particular problem for example the addition of formaldehyde to detergents at source by suppliers, which are then used in formulations and since no further formaldehyde may be added to the product its presence goes unlabelled.

Formaldehyde release from other chemicals in the formulation, such as emulsifiers and surfactants, as well as from materials used in packaging (melamine or carbamide-formaldehyde resins) has also been described [11].

A number of tests can be used to detect the presence of formaldehyde. The chromotropic acid test may give false positive reactions, and the alternative acetylacetone method may be more sensitive and specific (see 'Spot tests' earlier in this chapter).

Prognosis. In a follow-up study of 57 patients with formaldehyde dermatitis, 29 (51%) still had frequent or persistent dermatitis several years later. Formaldehyde was identified in cosmetics, toiletries, household cleaners and other materials still being used by 38 of these patients. The authors concluded that patients who paid attention to their allergy had statistically significantly fewer eruptions than those who did not [12].

Patch tests. Patch testing is recommended with formaldehyde 2% aqueous [13]. It is generally recommended as a baseline test allergen.

Formaldehyde-releasing preservatives/biocides [1]

The five most relevant formaldehyde releasers (in declining order of their potential to release formaldehyde) are: quaternium-15, diazolidinyl urea, dimethylol dimethyl (DMDM) hydantoin, imidazolidinyl urea and 2-bromo-2-nitropropane-1,3-diol (bronopol) [2]. As patients may become sensitised to formaldehyde releasers themselves, without necessarily being sensitised to formaldehyde, their addition to the European baseline series has been proposed [3]. In a recent study, the high percentage of isolated reactions to formaldehyde releasers showed that co-reactivity to formaldehyde 2% aqueous is virtually non-existent for 2-bromo-2-nitropropane-1,3-diol (BNPD) whereas a weak concordance for quaternium-15 was detected. The results suggested that patch testing with formaldehyde 2% aqueous was an inadequate screen to identify independent contact sensitisation to formaldehyde releasers [4]. A study looking at the 10-year trends in contact allergy to formaldehyde releasers in Denmark showed that contact allergies to formaldehyde and formaldehyde releasers overall continue to remain frequent [5].

Quaternium-15

Quaternium-15 is also known as Dowicil 75, 100 or 200, chlorallyl methenamine chloride, N-(3-chlorallyl)-hexaminium chloride and 1-(3-chlorallyl)-3,5,7-triaza-1-azoniondamantane. It is water soluble, odourless and colourless. Its broad antimicrobial activity is independent of the pH of the product.

Prevalence. Quaternium-15 can sensitise either independently or via formaldehyde release, or both. The prevalence of positive patch tests in those attending for routine testing in pan-European studies is just below 1% [6] although much higher levels are observed in North America [7].

Occurrence. Quaternium-15 was infrequently used in European cosmetics (<0.5%), in contrast to the USA where it was still included in up to 1.5% of leave-on formulations. It may also be found in (topical) pharmaceuticals, household detergents, cleansers and laundry soaps, paints, adhesives, glues and a variety of industrial products, such as metal working fluids, paper board, polyurethane resins and paper (e.g. for the packaging of food), textiles and gloves [8]. In 2019, European legislation came into force that banned the use of formaldehyde and quaternium-15 in cosmetics. All finished products that release formaldehyde listed in Annex V of the EU cosmetic regulation must be labelled with the warning 'contains formaldehyde' if the concentration of formaldehyde in the finished product exceeds 0.05%.

Clinical features. These are discussed in the sections on allergy to cosmetics and medicaments.

Avoidance. The INCI name is quaternium-15. Only ingredient-labelled products should be used, and any product shown to contain it should be avoided. Knowledge of its synonyms is helpful, particularly as non-cosmetic products, including medicaments, may not adhere to INCI terminology.

Patch tests. For quaternium-15, 1% in petrolatum is the generally recommended concentration and vehicle. It is recommended as a standard test allergen in Europe and North America.

Diazolidinyl urea

Diazolidinyl urea is also known as Germall II. It is a broad spectrum biocide, soluble in water and effective at various pH levels.

Prevalence. Studies in the UK on routinely patch-tested individuals showed that 0.7% of 3062 patients were patch test positive [9], similar to the finding of 0.79% in a multicentre Spanish study [10], whereas in North America 3.1% were positive [11].

Occurrence. Diazolidinyl urea has been used since 1982, predominantly in cosmetics. It is found in up to 8% of cosmetics, both in Europe and in the USA, in concentrations varying between 0.1% and 0.5%. It can also be present in detergents, topical pharmaceuticals (e.g. corticosteroid creams) and to a lesser extent in occupational products [1].

Clinical features. These are discussed in the section on allergy to cosmetics earlier in this chapter.

Avoidance. The INCI name is diazolidinyl urea. Only ingredient-labelled cosmetics and creams should be used, and any product shown to contain it should be avoided. ROATs confirm that formaldehyde-allergic subjects should also avoid creams preserved with diazolidinyl urea [11].

Patch tests. Patch testing at 1% and 2% aqueous has been advised [12], but it is generally supplied at 2% in petrolatum, which we have found satisfactory. Although not a frequent sensitiser in the UK, the BSCA has recommended its inclusion in the baseline series [13].

Imidazolidinyl urea

Imidazolidinyl urea is also known as Germall 115. It has broad spectrum antimicrobial activity and is colourless, water soluble and not pH dependent. It acts synergistically with other preservatives and will kill *Pseudomonas aeruginosa*. It releases only small amounts of formaldehyde, and may therefore possibly be less of a problem than other formaldehyde releasers for formaldehyde-sensitive subjects [14].

Prevalence. It is not a common allergen in most pan-European studies, with positive reactions occuring in 0.5% of routinely patch-tested persons [6].

Occurrence. Imidazolidinyl urea is commonly used in cosmetics, shampoos and hand creams, including barrier and other work creams.

Clinical features. These are discussed in the section on allergy to cosmetics.

Avoidance. Imidazolidinyl urea is the INCI name. Only ingredient-labelled cosmetics should be used, and any product shown to contain it should be avoided. In UK medicaments its presence may be denoted by the word 'imidurea'.

Patch tests. Although patch testing with 2% aqueous has been advised [15], 2% in petrolatum is generally used. Its inclusion in the baseline series is recommended by the BSCA in the UK [13].

2-Bromo-2-nitropropane-1,3-diol

2-Bromo-2-nitropropane-1,3-diol is also known as bronopol and BNPD. It has broad spectrum antimicrobial activity and is particularly effective against *Pseudomonas aeruginosa*. It is soluble in water, alcohols, glycols and, to a lesser degree, oils. Its (often formaldehyde-independent) sensitising properties, as well as concerns related to the formation of nitrosamine carcinogens, make it a less attractive preservative for continued use.

Prevalence. The reported prevalence of positive reactions to BNPD in routinely patch-tested individuals in North America in 2001–02 was 3.3% [7]. In the UK, 0.8% of individuals were positive in a 1986 study [16] and in a pan-European study just under 1% [6].

Occurrence. BNPD can be found in a wide range of cosmetics, moisturisers, shampoos, medicaments and hand creams. It may also be found in a number of chemical products, especially paints, lacquers and cleaning agents [17].

Clinical features. These are discussed in the section on allergy to cosmetics. In the occupational setting the usual site of involvement is the hands.

Avoidance. The INCI name is 2-bromo-2-nitropropane-1,3-diol. The simpler name of bronopol may be used in other products. Only ingredient-labelled cosmetics should be used, and any product shown to contain it should be avoided.

Patch tests. The two recommended concentrations are 0.5% and 0.25% in petrolatum; 0.5% may occasionally give false positive reactions. It is recommended by the BSCA for inclusion in the baseline series at 0.5% (pet.) [13].

Dimethylol dimethyl hydantoin

Dimethylol dimethyl hydantoin is also known as Glydant® and is a colourless liquid that contains 0.5–2% free formaldehyde and over 17% combined formaldehyde.

Prevalence. In pan-European studies <0.5% of patients routinely patch tested to DMDM hydantoin showed allergic reactions and the the North American Contact Dermatitis Group (NACDG) reported 2.8% positivity [7]. Testing with formaldehyde has demonstrated poor concomitant sensitivity [4].

Occurrence. DMDM hydantoin can be found in cosmetics, topical pharmaceuticals, glues and adhesives, paints and a wide range of industrial products such as herbicides, cutting oils, papers and inks.

Clinical features. These are discussed in the section on allergy to cosmetics.

Avoidance. DMDM hydantoin is the INCI name, and it can be identified in a product provided this is fully labelled with ingredients. There is evidence from ROATs that formaldehyde-allergic patients should avoid products containing DMDM hydantoin [18].

Patch tests. Patch tests have been undertaken at 1–3% aqueous and 1% in petrolatum. We have found 2% aqueous satisfactory.

Other biocides

The above formaldehyde releasers are encountered particularly in cosmetics, including shampoos and other hair care products. A much broader series of formaldehyde releasers is to be found in materials such as industrial and household cleaning agents, colouring agents, paints and lacquers, polishes and especially metalworking fluids [19–21]. A number of formaldehyde-releasing biocides in these fluids will sensitise, and a special series of allergens should be used for testing in those exposed, as well as the material itself [22].

Formaldehyde-releasing preservatives. cross-reactivity and concomitant reactions: advice for patients

Although studies reveal that patch test reactions to formaldehyde releasers show poor co-reactivity to formaldehyde 2% aqueous in many instances [4], the question as to whether patients sensitised to formaldehyde may tolerate products preserved with formaldehyde releasers is difficult to resolve.

It is generally accepted that if sensitisation to formaldehyde occurs, both formaldehyde and strong releasers – such as quaternium-15, diazolidinyl urea and DMDM hydantoin – should be avoided. In selected cases, the use of products containing BNPD (and to a lesser extent imidazolidinyl urea), due to a low effective formaldehyde content, might still be tolerated, especially on healthy skin. Nevertheless, as a precaution, avoidance of all formaldehyde releasers is usually advised.

If a patient is sensitised to only one releaser, especially when it concerns a weak releaser, such as BNPD or imidazolidinyl urea, and not to formaldehyde, then contact allergy was most likely induced by the releaser itself and not related to formaldehyde. Consequently, only this particular releaser should then be avoided. However, if a patient is sensitised to two or more releasers, it is likely that the most common sensitiser is formaldehyde, and therefore formaldehyde and all releasers would be better avoided.

Other cosmetic preservatives

Non-formaldehyde-releasing preservatives are also an important cause of contact allergy from cosmetics. These include parabens, MI, MCI/MI, MDBGN, phenoxyethanol, iodopropynyl butylcarbamate and sodium metabisulphite among others. The parabens paradox illustrates that they rarely cause contact allergy from cosmetic usage (see the section on parabens later in this chapter). Similarly, due to legislative changes, MDBGN use in cosmetics has been reduced and even banned within the EU.

Isothiazolinones [1]

Isothiazolinone preservative systems have effective broad spectrum activity against both bacteria and fungi. They have therefore been widely used for more than 30 years in water-based products such as household detergents, paints, glues and industrial biocides, and also in cosmetics. Other unusual sources of cosmetic, non-cosmetic and occupational exposures to isothiazolinone derivatives have been published including textiles, leather, plastics (spectacle frames), medical devices (ultrasound gel, wound dressings, vacuum-assisted closure sponges), pet cosmetics and homemade slime [2].

A number of different formulations have been shown to be sensitising to the skin.
1. Mixture of 5-chloro-2-methyl-4-isothiazolin-3-one and 2-methyl-4-isothiazolin-3-one in a 3 : 1 ratio by weight. The INCI name is methylchloroisothiazolinone and methylisothiazolinone (MCI/MI). This mixture has various other names, including Kathon CG, Kathon WT, Euxyl K 100 and Acticide.
2. Methylisothiazolinone by itself was also introduced as a cosmetic preservative in 2005 but its use in Europe has now been substantially restricted due to an epidemic of contact allergy.
3. 1,2-Benzisothiazolin-3-one (BIT). This is used under the commercial name Proxel in a range of biocides.
4. 2-n-Octyl-4-isothiazolin-3-one (OIT). This is also known as Kathon 893, Kathon LP and Skane M-8.

Although there is a structural similarity between the different derivatives, particularly the isothiazolinone ring common to all of them, and potential cross-reactivity has been suggested, this does not appear to be the case. No immunological cross-reaction is to be expected between chlorinated and non-chlorinated derivatives. Most observations rely on case reports, small case series or retrospective, observational studies, often using different (sometimes low) patch test concentrations.

Approximately 40% of Belgian patients with a positive patch test to OIT, for whom no relevant OIT-containing allergen source could be found, were shown to be primarily sensitised to cosmetics containing MI, suggesting the possibility of, at least partial, cross-reactivity between both molecules [3]. Alternatively, BIT reactions most often occur independently of other isothiazolinones, probably as a result of independent sensitisation [4]. In line with animal data, most epidemiological studies show that the majority of patients sensitised to MI will also show a patch test reaction to MCI/MI, suggesting cross-reactivity.

Methylchloroisothiazolinone and methylisothiazolinone [1].

Prevalence. Since it was first marketed in 1980, there have been many reports of MCI/MI allergy, particularly from Europe, with a prevalence of positive reactions as high as 8.3% in routinely tested patients in the first few years after its introduction [5]. This level had stabilised in Europe to around 2.5% until recently [6].

Levels below 15 ppm are considered unlikely to induce sensitisation [7], and in those already sensitised this concentration has been shown to be insufficient to elicit a dermatitis in many instances. Due to the high rates of allergy to MI seen across Europe, over the last decade the rates of cutaneous allergy to the mix of MCI/MI are similarly increased [8].

Occurrence. MCI/MI is used in cosmetics, mainly in rinse-off products, including liquid soaps and cleansers, shower gels, bubble baths and shampoos. Nevertheless, leave-on cosmetics may also contain it. However, this biocide can be found in other situations, most notably soluble cutting oils, paints, wallpaper pastes, glues, spin finishes, military fuel, household cleansers, printing inks and fountain solution, latex emulsions, water cooling systems and as a slimicide in paper mills.

Clinical features. These are discussed in the section on allergy to cosmetics. Shampoos do not usually cause problems from washing hair, but allergy may be associated with hairdressers' hand dermatitis. A positive patch test to MCI/MI associated with perianal dermatitis suggests the possibility of moist toilet paper or wipes as a cause [9]. This source of MCI/MI can also provoke allergic dermatitis of the hands and elsewhere [10]. Hands are the usual sites for occupational allergic dermatitis, although spread to other parts of the body, including an airborne exposure pattern, may occur [11]. A chemical burn from a spillage of concentrated MCI/MI on to any part of the skin may be followed by a secondary delayed dermatitis from active sensitisation [12,13].

Patch tests. The recommended patch test concentration and vehicle is now 200 ppm in water as there is evidence that this may identify sensitised subjects missed by the 100 ppm patch test [14,15]. MCI/MI is generally recommended as a baseline allergen.

Methylisothiazolinone. The sensitising properties of MCI/MI were attributed to MCI, whereas MI was considered a weak sensitiser, unable to sensitise individuals in concentrations below 1000 ppm [16,17]. After 2000, MI was introduced in industrial products (paints, glues, lacquers, varnishes, cooling fluids) due to its weaker biocide effects – at higher concentrations.

Prevalence. The first case report of occupational allergic contact dermatitis to MI appeared in 2004 [14] and in 2005 MI was allowed to be used independently of MCI as a cosmetic preservative in Europe, at a maximum permitted level of 100 ppm (Cosmetic Directive 2005/42/EC). This initial permitted usage level in cosmetics is what was ultimately responsible for the epidemic of sensitisation that was to follow. Several cases of occupational allergic contact dermatitis to MI were then observed from paints, followed in 2010 by the first case reports following cosmetic exposure [15]. Further case reports then emerged due to its presence in wet wipes, hair cosmetics, facial cosmetics, deodorants and sunscreens. These showed a wide range of presentations according to the causative products including ano-genital eczema, facial eczema and hand eczema. Furthermore, cases of airborne exposure to MI causing severe airborne and generalised dermatitis from recently painted walls and even from toilet cleaners were described.

In the UK, France, Denmark, Portugal, Germany and Spain there were steeply rising rates of allergy to MI recorded [19,20,**21**] with an exponential increase in prevalence among 14 UK patch test centres from 1.7% to 11.1% [22]. The relevant exposures identified in the patients were predominantly from cosmetic exposure. Studies showed that facial involvement, female sex and age >40 years were particularly associated with MI allergy [23]. Photoallergic contact dermatitis to MI and/or photoexacerbation of allergic contact dermatitis to MI is the subject of current debate [24]. Both the increase in the number of European cosmetics containing MI and a shift toward using it more in leave-on products were also considered important factors behind this epidemic. Since its removal from leave-on cosmetic products in the EU as of February 2017 and limitation to 15 ppm in rinse-off products, a decline has been noted although it still remains an important allergen [25,26]. Indeed, paints and detergents may still contain high concentrations of MI, and thus remain a problematic source of this allergen. In patients sensitised from cosmetic usage, the median duration necessary to enable entering a freshly painted room without recurrence of dermatitis was 5.5 weeks [27].

Patch tests. The recommended patch test concentration and vehicle is now 2000 ppm in water in the European baseline series [28].

European legislation on MCI/MI and MI. In the EU, MCI/MI and MI are no longer allowed in leave-on cosmetics and are limited to a maximum of 15 ppm (0.0015%) in rinse-off products, whereas OIT and BIT continue to be banned from use in any cosmetic product. In the USA, the use of MCI/MI in cosmetic leave-on products up to a usage level of 7.5 ppm is somewhat unusual when compared with most other parts of the world. However, the continued use of MI in leave-on cosmetic products up to a usage level of 100 ppm in the USA is presently in keeping with legislation in both Canada and Japan.

However, even in Europe, isothiazolinone usage in non-cosmetic products such as medical devices, detergents, textiles/leather, chemical (industrial) products (e.g. paints and glues) is still largely unregulated, and much higher usage concentrations can be found.

For chemical (industrial) products, MI, as with MCI/MI, has been recognised as a skin sensitiser 1A, H317, meaning that products containing ≥15 ppm should carry a warning concerning the risk of sensitisation, either on the product or in the safety data sheets.

1,2-Benzisothiazolin-3-one.
Occurrence. Sensitisation normally occurs from manufacturing or handling the raw material, for example paint manufacture, water treatment or in the laboratory. Painters and decorators may be exposed to BIT not only from paints but also wallpaper pastes. Allergy has been reported in the pottery industry from its presence in mould-release agents. Other potential sources include soluble cutting oils, laundry detergents and fabric softeners, varnishes, dyes, printing materials, water softener and air-freshener manufacture. Allergy to polyvinyl chloride gloves has been traced to BIT used in their manufacture [29].

Clinical features. Classically, with hand dermatitis, a low-grade palmar psoriasiform or pompholyx pattern occurs (see Figure 127.5). In more severe cases an exposed-site pattern develops [30]. Sensitised workers involved in manufacture may complain of a burning sensation of the eyes and face within the factory environment without there being observable dermatitis.

Patch tests. A number of patch test concentrations in petrolatum have been suggested, varying from 0.05% to 1%. False positive reactions have been reported with 0.1% in petrolatum [31]; as our experience is that false positive reactions occur above 500 ppm or 0.05% in petrolatum, we advocate the use of this concentration.

2-n-Octyl-4-isothiazolin-3-one.
Occurrence. OIT may occur in leather, textiles, soluble cutting oils, paints and polishes, adhesives, floor cleaning agents, wood preservatives and plastic manufacture.

Clinical features. Reports of contact allergy tend to be sporadic and anecdotal, and these include hand dermatitis associated with its presence in paints [32]. Contact allergy to leather in footwear and from a leather sofa have been reported [33–35].

Patch tests. OIT is usually patch tested at 0.1% in petrolatum.

Newer isothiazolinone preservatives. Industry has started using newer isothiazolinone derivatives including dichloro-octylisothiazolinone (DCOIT, CAS 64359-81-5), butyl-benzisothiazolinone (BBIT, CAS no. 4299 07 4), and methyl-benzisothiazolinone (MBIT, CAS 2527-66-4). DCOIT is used as a biocide in paints, construction products, silicone materials, plastics and wood processing. It has been reported as a cause of occupational dermatitis and also a cause of consumer dermatitis after wearing black trousers [36]. A case of occupational dermatitis caused by BBIT-containing cooling fluid and has also been published [37].

Parabens (hydroxybenzoates) [1]
Parabens are esters of *p*-hydroxybenzoic acid. The four main esters used are methyl-, ethyl-, propyl- and butyl-paraben (hydroxybenzoate). They may have a synergistic effect when used in combination and are often combined with other preservatives to broaden antimicrobial cover. They are more active against Gram-positive than Gram-negative bacteria (including poor activity against *Pseudomonas*). They are also active against moulds and yeasts. They are stable, colourless, odourless and poorly soluble in water [1].

Prevalence. There is a relatively low prevalence of positive reactions in routinely patch-tested patients, and rates between 0.5% and 1.7% are typical [2–4].

Occurrence. Parabens are very widely used preservatives in topical and parenteral medicaments, paste bandages, ultrasound gels, condoms and foods. In many respects for formulators of cosmetics products they are the 'preferred' preservatives. However, due to the so-called 'paraben phobia' concerning endocrine disruption [5], they have largely been replaced in positively marketed 'paraben-free' cosmetics. Nevertheless they continue to be used (often at higher concentrations) in topical medicaments where they are termed hydroxybenzoates.

Clinical features. The striking feature of allergy to parabens is its relative infrequency compared with the degree of usage and exposure in the general population. Relevant allergies are mainly from sensitisation to medicaments (including paste bandages) used on compromised skin such as venous ulcers and eczema, but contact allergy may be superimposed on other inflammatory dermatoses, particularly on high-risk sites such as the ano-genital region. Relevant problems from parabens in cosmetics are rare [1]. Interestingly, many individuals allergic to parabens in medicaments can use cosmetics containing them on normal skin without any problem, the so-called 'paraben paradox' [6]. However, there are exceptions, and sometimes cosmetics containing parabens have to be abandoned [7]. Flares from parabens in food and medicaments [8] have been reported in sensitised subjects, but a low-paraben diet did not help two patients whose eczema flared with oral challenge [9].

Avoidance. The INCI name for this group of preservatives ends in '-paraben' according to the ester used. In individuals in whom cosmetic allergy may be relevant, the full ingredient label must be examined in order that they may be avoided. Terminology for medicaments may be different, and the name may end in '-hydroxybenzoate'. Cross-reactivity between different parabens is often observed and it is advisable to avoid all parabens even if only one or two are positive in breakdown testing.

Patch tests. Parabens are normally tested as a mix of the four esters, each at 3% in petrolatum. The mix is marginally irritant, and testing with each ester individually will help to confirm whether the patch test reaction is truly allergic. Often more than one ester will react, which may be a marker of both concomitant sensitisation and cross-sensitisation. Parabens mix 12% in petrolatum is generally advised for the baseline series.

Methyldibromoglutaronitrile [1]

Methyldibromoglutaronitrile, also known as dibromocyanobutane, is to be found in the preservative system Euxyl K400 (also called Tektamer 38), which is a mix of MDBGN and phenoxyethanol in a ratio of 1 : 4. Euxyl K400 is a broad spectrum preservative with activity against fungi and bacteria. MDBGN is nearly always the allergen when sensitisation to Euxyl K400 occurs.

Prevalence. Until the European ban, increasing rates of sensitisation were reported throughout Europe and the USA. Of particular significance was the finding of a multicentre European study monitoring rates of preservative allergy, where the frequency of MDBGN allergy between 1991 and 2000 rose from 0.7% to 3.5%, whereas the level of all other cosmetic preservative allergies had remained stable [2]. In consequence, EU countries have banned the use of this preservative, initially in leave-on cosmetics (2003) and later in rinse-off cosmetics (2008). Since then, European sensitisation rates have fallen [3]. Rates reported by the NACDG have varied from 2.7% to 7.6% according to the test concentration used [4].

Occurrence. MDBGN was historically widely used in cosmetics, sunscreens, shampoos, liquid soaps and barrier and moisturising creams used at work. The EU ban has reduced these exposures very significantly and nowadays positive patch tests in EU consumers might represent historical sensitisation. However, positive patch tests are still observed and suggest that other non-regulated sources of exposure remain important (e.g. metalworking fluids, glues, adhesives, detergents, medical devices (ultrasound gels) and cosmetics bought outside the EU) [5].

Clinical features. These are discussed in the section on allergy to cosmetics. However, hand dermatitis is a frequent finding as a result of exposure to hand creams and liquid soaps [6]. Irritant hand dermatitis may be suspected prior to patch testing but the demonstration of allergy and withdrawal of the incriminated products often resolves the dermatitis [7,8].

Avoidance. Methyldibromoglutaronitrile is the INCI name that should be sought on the full ingredient label. In some instances its presence may be identified by its synonym 1,2-dibromo-2,4-dicyanobutane or Euxyl K400 (Tektamer 38). Many producers of work cleansers and creams now give a full ingredient list on the health and safety data sheet. Skin products whose ingredients are not known should not be used. Other potentially allergenic sources may require specific enquiry as to the nature of the biocide/preservative used.

Patch tests. There has been much discussion about the optimal patch test concentration. We prefer to test MDBGN at 0.3% in petrolatum, although this has been found by ourselves to be marginally irritant. Others have advised 0.2% as the optimum concentration [9], and 0.1% has been used, but may give false negative reactions [10]. Conversely, positive ROAT findings and some relevant allergies have only been confirmed by testing with 0.5% or 1% concentrations [11]. At present it is still recommended for the BSCA baseline series at a concentration of 0.3% [12] but is included at 0.5% in the European baseline series.

Chloroxylenol [1]

Chloroxylenol (parachlorometaxylenol, PCMX) is a halogenated aromatic compound used not only as a preservative but also as an active disinfectant. It is water and oil soluble, and active against Gram-positive and Gram-negative bacteria.

Prevalence. Generally, reports of chloroxylenol allergy have been sporadic, with few large-scale studies. In one UK study 1.8% of 951 routinely tested persons were patch test positive, with a high level of current or previous relevance [1]. A more recent British study yielded a lower prevalence rate of 0.4% [2]. Reports from the USA document seven patients sensitised by medicated Vaseline® or electrocardiogram paste and two with allergy to soap and hand cream [3,4].

Occurrence. Chloroxylenol is a potential allergen for the UK as it is found in Dettol®, a widely used household disinfectant. Chloroxylenol may also be found in a number of over-the-counter pharmaceutical preparations for cuts, grazes and infections [1]. Other sources include foot and talcum powders, soaps and cleansers, work creams, coolant oils, electrocardiograph pastes and, rarely, cosmetics. Further studies are required in the UK to check its current status with regard to usage and sensitisation rates.

Clinical features. In many cases there is a localised skin eruption at the site where a product containing chloroxylenol has been applied,

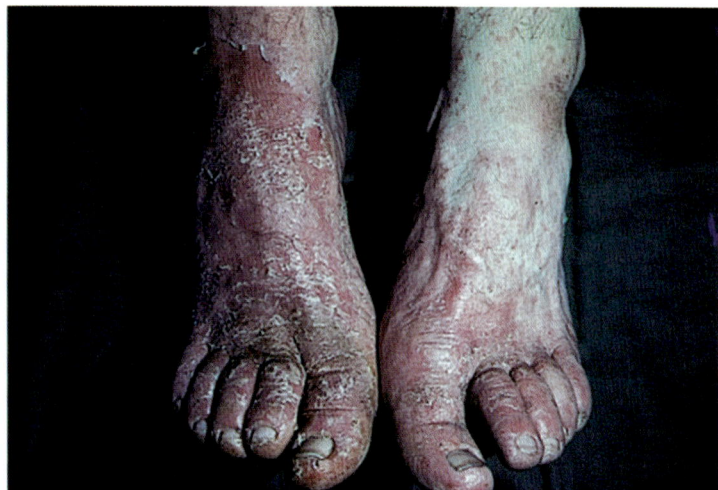

Figure 127.26 Allergy to chloroxylenol from washing with Dettol. Courtesy of Geoffrey Auckland Collection.

or allergy may present as an unexpected exacerbation of pre-existing dermatitis.

Hand dermatitis is a potential problem for cleaners coming in contact with disinfectants when their hands are unprotected. Allergy to chloroxylenol in other work materials (e.g. coolant oils) may give a similar distribution of rash. More widespread eruptions may be associated with its use for washing and bathing (Figure 127.26), and also when applied to clothing. Recently, widespread hypopigmentation following contact allergy to chloroxylenol added to bath water has been reported [5]. Often, the source is only identified retrospectively after finding a positive patch test.

Avoidance. Chloroxylenol is the INCI name. Cosmetics and work creams that contain it can usually be identified from the full ingredient label or data sheet. Labels on medicated foot powders and talcs generally acknowledge it as an ingredient, but specific enquiries may be necessary to establish its presence in some topical medicaments and disinfectants.

Patch tests. Chloroxylenol is generally patch tested at 1% in petrolatum. It may cross-sensitise with chlorocresol [6]. It has been recommended as a baseline allergen for the UK [2].

Chlorocresol

Chlorocresol (parachlorometacresol, PCMC) is identical with chloroxylenol, except for the absence of a methyl group on the benzene ring. It is active against Gram-positive and Gram-negative bacteria, and is water and oil soluble.

Prevalence. Chlorocresol is a rare allergen. A multicentre UK survey of routinely patch-tested patients confirmed a low rate of 0.6% [1].

Occurrence. The major source is corticosteroid creams. We have only seen it as a sensitiser from topical medicaments, although it may be used in hand cleaners, metalworking fluids, glues and occasionally cosmetics.

Clinical features. These are discussed in the section on medicament allergy. Erythroderma has occurred in a diabetic patient known to be allergic to chlorocresol when given insulin preserved with *m*-cresol, and this improved on changing to a parabens-preserved insulin [2].

Avoidance. It is helpful to give a sensitised patient a list of corticosteroid creams that indicates their constituents and which are free from chlorocresol. Moisturisers should not be used unless they are fully ingredient labelled or known to be free from this preservative. The INCI name is chlorocresol.

Patch tests. The recommended test concentration and vehicle is 1% chlorocresol in petrolatum. Although contact allergy is rare, its use in many popular corticosteroid creams available in the UK has prompted the BSCA to recommend its inclusion in the baseline series [3]. Cross-sensitivity with chloroxylenol is well recognised [4].

Sodium metabisulphite and related sulphites [1]

Sodium sulphite, sodium bisulphite and sodium metabisulphite (SMS) are widely used preservatives and antioxidants in foods, cosmetics and pharmaceuticals.

Prevalence. Although many studies of consecutively patch-tested patients show high rates of sensitisation to SMS exceeding a 1% level [2], concerns have been raised that some of these might be irritant, false positive reactions. This, coupled with difficulty determining relevance, has meant that it has only recently been included on the European baseline series (2019) and the BSCA baseline series [3]. Nevertheless there has been an argument that with careful evaluation, relevance rates might actually be much higher [2,4]

Occurrence. Sulphites are widely used in foods (E220–E224, E226–228, E150b,d), cosmetics (hand cleansers, bleaching agents, hair dyes, sunscreens, self-tanning lotions, antiageing products) and pharmaceuticals (topical steroids, antibacterials, injectable anaesthetics).

Clinical features. Features of sulphite allergy comprise a range of different symptoms following ingestion or inhalation, including immediate reactions,(such as flushing, urticaria, asthma, rhinoconjunctivitis and anaphylactoid reactions/anaphylaxis) and allergic contact dermatitis following skin contact. Besides hand and facial dermatitis, vulval and ano-genital dermatitis (from antifungal medicaments) have been highlighted by some authors [4].

Avoidance. The INCI name for SMS is sodium metabisulphite, and due to cross-reactivity sodium sulphite should also be avoided although patch testing to the specific sulphite derivative used may exceptionally still be necessary.

Patch tests. SMS is recommended to be tested at 1% (pet.) and is considered as a good screening agent for sulphite sensitisation.

Ethylhexylglycerin [1]

Ethylhexylglycerin, also known as octoxyglycerin or 3-(2-ethylhexyloxy)propane-1,2-diol, is a pale to colourless liquid. It is used for its surfactant, skin conditioning, emollient and antimicrobial properties in a wide variety of cosmetics (although according to EU regulations it is classified as having skin conditioning and deodorant properties only).

Occurrence. It may be used in many cosmetics including eye shadows, mascaras, lip gloss, cleansers and make-up removers, shampoos, shower gels, intimate hygiene products and 'antiageing' creams. It may particularly be found in products marketed as 'preservative free' or in products for 'sensitive' skin.

Prevalence. Several cases reports of allergic contact dermatitis have been reported from Europe [2] and North America [3] where it has been included in a core allergen series [4].

Clinical features. These are discussed in the section on allergy to cosmetics.

Avoidance. The INCI name is ethylhexylglycerin.

Patch tests. Patch testing at 5% (pet.) is recommended.

Iodopropynyl butylcarbamate [1]

Iodopropynyl butylcarbamate (IPBC) is a preservative with a wide spectrum of fungicide and bactericide properties,

Occurrence. IPBC was originally used as a paint and wood preservative, but is now found in a variety of other industrial products (building materials, metalworking fluids and cooling tower water), but also in both leave-on and rinse-off cosmetics, including alcohol hand rubs for hospital use.

Prevalence. There seems to be some disparity in rates of sensitisation in North America versus Europe, with sensitisation rates up to 4.2% in 2011–12 versus 1.2% in 2009–12 [2], respectively. This may partially be explained by different patch test concentrations and stricter regulations in the use of IPBC in cosmetics within Europe. Nevertheless an increasing trend in Europe has been observed mainly due to its use in cosmetics.

Clinical features. These are discussed in the section on allergy to cosmetics. Several case reports of allergic contact dermatitis from this preservative have been published, from moisturisers, wet wipes, treated wood and airborne exposure to paints.

Avoidance. The INCI name is iodopropynyl butylcarbamate.

Patch tests. The recommended test concentration of IPBC in Europe is 0.2% (pet.).

Benzalkonium chloride [1]

Benzalkonium chloride (BAC) or *N*-alkyl-*N*-benzyl-*N*,*N*-dimethylammonium chloride is the most frequently used quaternary ammonium compound.

Occurrence. It is used as a disinfectant and as a preservative in (mainly) rinse-off cosmetics (e.g. hand soaps, shampoos and conditioners, antiseptic bath oils, toothpastes, mouth washes), leave-on products (e.g. deodorants, moisturisers, body lotions), pharmaceuticals (e.g. mainly ophthalmic solutions, but also nasal sprays, throat lozenges, asthma nebulisers, antifungal treatments, spermicides, wound antiseptics, impregnated bandages, plaster of Paris, first-aid products) and cleaning agents (e.g. detergents, surface cleaning wipes, cleaning solutions for endoscopes and surgical instruments) [2].

Prevalence. Some studies have shown high rates of sensitisation of up to 10% of the study population [3], but caution must be exercised with interpretation as it is a recognised irritant at patch test concentration.

Clinical features. These are discussed in the section on allergy to cosmetics. However, manifestations of BAC-related contact allergy include eyelid dermatitis (typically related to the use of BAC in eye medicaments), cheilitis and stomatitis and hand dermatitis, also from occupational exposure (e.g. hand soaps, wipes) [3]. A few cases of flexural and ano-genital irritant and/or contact allergic dermatitis have been reported in the UK, related to the use of a highly concentrated (6%) BAC-containing antiseptic bath oil [4]. Specific occupations at risk relate to the use of products containing BAC as a disinfectant (i.e. at higher use concentrations) and comprise, among others, health care workers such as nurses and dental assistants [2].

Avoidance. The INCI name is benzalkonium chloride.

Patch tests. BAC is usually patch tested at 0.1% aqueous.

Chlorhexidine [1]

Chlorhexidine (CH) is a biguanide and well-known disinfectant for the skin and mucous membranes. It is effective against bacteria, yeasts and some viruses and is available in three different salts: digluconate, diacetate and dihydrochloride. Although chlorhexidine digluconate is probably most frequently used, all three salts have been approved for use in cosmetic and pharmaceutical products.

Occurrence. CH is most commonly found in products used perioperatively and prior to procedures, but it is also used in hair care products (shampoos, conditioners, hair dyes, treatments and styling products) and also face washes, toners, moisturisers, make-up removers and wet wipes [2]. Also, mouth washes, dental gels, eye drops and contact lens solutions may contain it.

Prevalence. In a Danish study, 1.0% of all patients patch tested between 2003 and 2013 had a positive reaction to CH, predominantly involving patients with leg ulcers and medicament allergy [3], which is supportive of other studies [4].

Clinical features. A range of reactions may be seen from (mild) irritant contact dermatitis to life-threatening anaphylaxis (seen intraoperatively), with allergic contact dermatitis in some cases preceding the latter [3,4]. It may also cause allergy among health care workers through occupational exposure. In adults with atopic dermatitis, the use of CH-based treatments may result in secondary contact allergy, complicating their eczema. Contact lens solutions containing CH have been reported to cause conjunctivitis in CH-sensitised patients; moreover, CH-containing mouth washes can trigger contact stomatitis. It has been recommended that, once delayed hypersensitivity to CH has been established, it is necessary to also test for immediate-type hypersensitivity [3].

Avoidance. The INCI name is chlorhexidine.

Patch tests. The optimal patch test concentration for CH salts remains unknown. Both chlorhexidine digluconate/diacetate are available commercially at 0.5% aqueous. Some patients have shown a positive test result to one salt and a negative test result to another salt, so it has been advised, in cases of suspected contact allergy, to test with appropriate salts. In suspected cases of allergic contact dermatitis it is preferable to test with both [3].

Other preservatives/biocides [1]

Many other antimicrobial agents have been used as preservatives and biocides, and have been reported to sensitise. These include sorbic acid (SA), triclosan (Irgasan DP300) benzyl alcohol, chlorphenesin and EDTA. SA and potassium sorbate (PS) have broad antimicrobial properties and can be used on their own, or in combination with other preservatives. They are used in rinse-off and leave-on cosmetics (including wet wipes and specifically baby products) and pharmaceutical products (including compounded ointments and creams and bandages). They are considered only weak and rare sensitisers. Interestingly, both can cause concentration-dependent, transient, non-specific redness and frank (non-immunological) contact urticaria (especially observed in consumers with concurrent rosacea).

Triclosan (2,4,4′-trichloro-2′-hydroxydiphenyl ether; Irgasan DP300) has broad spectrum antimicrobial properties against bacteria, particularly Gram-positive bacteria, yeasts and dermatophytes. It is used in cosmetics (e.g. shampoos, cleansers, hand soaps, deodorants, toothpastes, mouth washes), topical pharmaceuticals, household detergents, sportswear, textiles (e.g. compression stockings), bedding and toys. It is a weak sensitiser.

Benzyl alcohol (BA) is a preservative, solvent, antipruritic and viscosity-decreasing agent. It is used in cosmetics (including fragrances, sunscreens, hair care products including dyes), pharmaceuticals (notably corticosteroid preparations, but also antibacterial, antimycotic preparations and injectable medications), medical devices (e.g. hearing aids), household detergents and chemical (industrial) products (e.g. hardeners, paints, lacquers, photographic developers, binders). BA is a component (1–2%) of balsam of Peru (*Myroxylon pereira*) and is present in essential oils such as hyacinth, jasmine and ylang-ylang oils. Since it displays fragrance properties it also belongs to the EU list of 26 fragrances that need to be labelled within cosmetics. It may be a 'covert' fragrance chemical, even present in 'fragrance-free' formulations. Despite its widespread use, it is a weak and rare sensitiser. BA may also, similar to sorbic acid, produce non-immunological contact urticaria and true type I hypersensitivity.

Vehicles and other cosmetic excipients
Lanolin [1]

Lanolin is a natural product obtained from sheep fleece. It is a complex and variable mixture of sterols, fatty alcohols, fatty acids and their esters. Wool wax alcohols are obtained by hydrolysis of the oily wax fraction of the fleece. Although they are not all known, it is thought the allergens are in this fraction [2].

Attempts to reduce allergenicity include modification by acetylation, hydrogenation, ethylenation, transesterification and removal of the allergenic fractions by a purification process [1]. Allergenicity has been shown virtually to disappear by removing detergent residues and reducing the level of alcohols to below 3% (w/w) [3].

Prevalence. The prevalence of lanolin allergy in the general population is thought to be low [4]. The belief that lanolin is a frequent sensitiser has been questioned by Kligman [**5**], and there are grounds for this since experimental sensitisation of animals and humans has not been achieved [6]. The annual proportion of positive patch test reactions to lanolin has varied, for instance in North America the prevalence of patch test reactivity to lanolin alcohol 30% pet. significantly decreased from 3.7% in 1994–96 to 1.8% in 2005–06 [7]. The overall prevalence of contact allergy to lanolin alcohols in a large study from a centre in the UK was 1.7%, and appeared to be constant during 1982–96 [8]. Notably, the prevalence of positive reactions to lanolin increased from 1.05% (when only lanolin alcohols 30% pet. was tested) to 6.29% (when multiple lanolin derivatives were tested), emphasising the putative benefit of comprehensive testing [9]. This shows the difficulties in detecting lanolin contact allergy with only one marker in the baseline series. Several studies have shown the benefit of including Amerchol L101 (a commercial product obtained from hydrolysis of wool fat, containing 10% wool wax alcohols in mineral oil) in detecting lanolin contact allergy [9–11]. Caution needs to be taken with interpreting reactions to Amerchol l101 as it is a recognised irritant. Nevertheless, there is good evidence of a high prevalence of allergy to lanolin in medicaments applied to varicose eczema [12,13]. However, usage on normal skin rarely seems to be associated with significant problems [**14**].

Occurrence. Lanolin is most commonly encountered in medicaments, emollients, bath additives and cosmetics. Other sources include polishes, waxes, inks, adhesive tapes and bandages, anti-corrosive coatings, sealants and cutting oil emulsions.

Clinical features. These are discussed in the sections on allergy to cosmetics and medicaments.

Avoidance. Lanolin alcohols is the INCI name for lanolin, and its presence in cosmetics can be established by examining the full ingredient label. However, prescribed and over-the-counter medicaments are not always fully ingredient labelled in the UK. This also applies to other potential domestic and work exposures such as polishes, waxes, coatings and oils.

Patch tests. Standard testing with wool alcohols 30% (pet.) is advised, and the BSCA has added Amerchol L 101 50% (pet.) to its baseline series.

Cetearyl alcohol

Cetearyl alcohol has emulsifying and stabilising properties, and is also known as cetylstearyl alcohol and Lanette O. It is essentially a mixture of two long-chained stereoisomers, cetyl and stearyl alcohol. These alcohols are components of lanolin.

Prevalence. Reports of allergy are often anecdotal, although there is evidence of it being a significant allergen complicating varicose eczema and ulcers, with up to 16% positive reactions in patients with these conditions attending for patch testing [1]. In the UK, a level of 0.8% was seen in routinely patch-tested patients [2].

Occurrence. Cetearyl alcohol is widely used in steroid creams, emollients and cosmetics. Sometimes only one of the stereoisomers is used. It is a component of emulsifying wax and therefore found in emulsifying ointment and aqueous cream BP.

Clinical features. These are discussed in the sections on allergy to cosmetics and medicaments.

Avoidance. Cetearyl alcohol is the INCI name, but cosmetics labelled as containing cetyl or stearyl alcohol should also be avoided. Avoidance of medicaments, including emollients, is more difficult as they are not always fully ingredient labelled. Even when they are, they may not follow the rules for cosmetics. Emulsifying wax is an ingredient that may be listed without it being clear that the preparation contains cetearyl alcohol. The designations cetylstearyl alcohol or Lanette O may be used instead of the INCI name.

Patch tests. Although it is an uncommon allergen, its ubiquitous presence in dermatological therapies means that identification of allergy is important. The BSCA has therefore recommended its inclusion in the standard series for the UK [3]. Patients suffering from varicose eczema should always be patch tested with it. It is normally tested at 20% in petrolatum.

Other excipients

There is potential for virtually any vehicular component of a cosmetic or medicament to cause sensitisation. If allergy is suspected, it may be necessary to widen the range of allergens tested. Examples include antioxidants (e.g. butylated hydroxyanisole, butylated hydroxytoluene, *t*-butylhydroquinone, gallates), surfactants (e.g. cocamidopropyl betaine, which may cause hand dermatitis in hairdressers from shampoos, cocamide diethanolamide, alkyl glucosides) and humectants (e.g. propylene glycol).

Antioxidants prevent the deterioration of unsaturated fatty acids in cosmetics and are occasionally a cause of cosmetic allergy. They include butylated hydroxyanisole (BHA) and butylated hydroxytoluene (BHT) and *t*-butylhydroquinone (TBHQ). TBHQ and BHA are used in cosmetic products, particularly in lipsticks and hair dyes, where they have been reported to cause contact allergy.

The gallates (dodecyl, octyl, propyl) are antioxidant chemicals commonly used as preservatives in food products and cosmetics. These may be found in antibiotic creams, lipsticks, moisturises, topical steroids and eye cosmetics. In a recent systematic review of gallate-positive patch tests, the most commonly reported allergen was propyl gallate present in both foods and personal care products – especially lipsticks [1].

Tocopherol (vitamin E) and its ester (tocopherol acetate) have been described as rare allergens but are increasingly being used in anti-ageing products. It has been suggested to include them in a supplementary European cosmetic series for further investigation and clarification of their importance [2].

Surfactants lower the surface tension between two liquids or between a liquid and a solid. They can act as detergents, wetting agents, emulsifiers, foaming agents and dispersants. Examples include cocamidopropyl betaine (the actual allergen is likely to be an impurity including dimethylaminopropylamine) and most cases of allergy are related to shampoos. Prevalence rates of sensitisation to cocamidopropyl betaine range from 3.7% to 5%. Cocamide diethanolamide is a non-ionic surfactant frequently used in industrial, household and cosmetic products for its foam-producing and foam-stabilising properties. Contact allergy has been reported quite rarely in the past, but recently several cases have been published, raising the question of an increase in the frequency of allergic dermatitis caused by this substance [3].

The alkyl glucosides constitute a family of mild, non-ionic surfactants synthesised through the condensation of glucose with long-chain fatty alcohols and are completely biodegradable. Alkyl glucosides have gained favour in recent years because of their eco-friendly properties and they are used for their cleansing, foaming and emulsifying properties. Since the 1990s they have been used in both rinse-off products, (e.g. shower gels, shampoos, soaps, cleansers, hair dyes) and leave-on cosmetics (e.g. sunscreens, fragrances, tanning products, emollients, deodorants). They can also be found in certain baby products such as wipes and cleansers. Although alkyl glucosides are considered to have lower irritancy and allergenicity, a recent study concluded that the prevalence of alkyl glucoside-induced allergic contact dermatitis is relatively high, and there are frequent concomitant reactions between different alkyl glucosides necessitating its inclusion in a patch test cosmetic series [4].

Humectants include propylene glycol. This is an odourless, viscous liquid, readily miscible with water, and essential oils. It is a widely used vehicle for topical therapeutics and cosmetics. Allergic contact reactions are uncommon. However, a recent European study suggests that it should be included in a cosmetic series at 20% aqueous [2].

This list is by no means exhaustive. Many excipient allergens are available from the main allergen suppliers, suitably prepared for patch testing, but others may need to be sought from the material's manufacturer and diluted appropriately for patch testing.

Miscellaneous cosmetic allergens

Propolis (or bee glue) is a natural substance extracted from the buds of poplar or other trees, including evergreens. Its composition varies, depending on the geographic location and variety of trees. It is frequently found in in lip balms and lipsticks. It is an important allergen to include in patients presenting with cheilitis. A global increase in allergic contact dermatitis from propolis has been reported since 2002 [1,2].

Dexpanthenol (INCI name panthenol) is the alcohol analogue of pantothenic acid. It is widely used in the pharmaceutical and cosmetic industries for its moisturising and soothing properties. Although allergic contact dermatitis caused by dexpanthenol is considered to be rare, it may be frequently overlooked; one study found a relatively high frequency in relevant cases [3].

p-Phenylenediamine and related dyes [1,2]

p-Phenylenediamine and toluene-2,5-diamine (PTD) are aniline derivatives, whose main use is for dyeing hair. These chemicals are colourless until oxidised by hydrogen peroxide in the presence of ammonia, and polymerised by a coupler, often in the presence of other intermediates, to produce a variety of shades of colour that stay fast within the hair shaft [1]. Once oxidised and polymerised, PPD is no longer allergenic [3]. Semipermanent hair dyeing may be undertaken with related dyes, for example *o*-nitro-*p*-phenylenediamine (ONPPD).

There is structural similarity to some azo dyes (e.g. *p*-aminoazobenzene). Many disperse dyes used to dye synthetic clothing and fibres are azo dyes and these are discussed in the section on clothing.

Prevalence. The use of hair colours has increased greatly in recent years. Large population-based studies suggest over 50% of the European population have used hair dyes in the past (78% female and 20% male), and 6% actively avoid contact with hair dye due to previous skin reactions. A random sample of 2739 subjects from the general population of five European countries patch tested to PPD showed a positive result in 0.8% [4]. There is clear evidence of increasing frequency of allergy in the UK. PPD allergy in referred dermatitis patients in one clinic almost doubled to 7.1% over a 6-year period [5]. Of those patch tested in the early 2000s in North America, 4.8% were allergic to PPD [6]. Similarly, 4.8% have been shown to be allergic to PPD in Germany and Austria, where there was considerable geographic variation in frequency (2.8–7.1%) [7]. In a large Belgian study of over 5000 routinely tested patients, 7.2% were allergic to PPD, 1.6% were allergic to PTD and 1.8% were allergic to ONPPD [8]. The median prevalence of PPD allergy among dermatitis patients is reported to be 4.3% in Asia, 4% in Europe and 6.2% in North America. Relevant positive PPD reactions are most often associated with hair dye exposure, although some positive reactions may be the result of cross-sensitisation [9,10]. Black henna tattoo exposure is also an important risk factor [4]. PPD is the second most common allergen of relevance for hairdressers in Europe [11].

Occurrence. PPD and PTD are found in permanent hair dyes, and ONPPD in semipermanent hair dyes whose colour will persist for 5–10 washes. In the EU, PPD is allowed in hair dyes up to a maximum concentration of 6% free base [12]. PPD has also been used to dye fur. PPD may be mixed with henna and used on the skin as a temporary tattoo (black henna tattoo). The concentration of PPD within temporary tattoos may vary greatly with some containing concentrations >10% [13]. The use of these has become very popular among children, adolescents and young adults in Europe, usually being applied in holiday resorts. A proportion of these patients will become actively sensitised to PPD through the application of the tattoo and characteristically will develop severe allergic reactions to hair dyes containing PPD or related chemicals [14].

Allergy to PPD has also been reported from a violin chin-rest and cello bowstring stain [15,16]. PPD derivatives are used as rubber antioxidants, particularly in heavy duty black rubber.

Azo dyes are mainly encountered as disperse dyes for synthetic clothing. Allergy to azo dyes in maggots used for fishing bait has been reported [17].

Clinical features. PPD and related hair dye allergy can result in extremely severe skin reactions. The scalp is often relatively spared, but severe oedema and weeping of the scalp margin, ears and eyes, with more extensive secondary spread eruptions, may be seen. However, there can be lower grade reactions, usually around the scalp margin. The patient does not always recognise the relationship of the skin eruption to dyeing the hair. Allergic contact dermatitis from hair, including connubial allergy from a partner's dyed hair, has been described. This is probably the result of the presence of unoxidised residue when there is poor dyeing technique, which is more likely with self-application of the dye [18,19].

Although banned in the EU, permanent hair dye products are readily available for use on eyelashes and eyebrows. Severe reactions including blindness have been reported [20].

The possibility of contact allergy from the use of permanent hair dyes on the beard should not be overlooked [21]. Lichen planus-like presentations of hair dye allergy have been reported from the Indian subcontinent [22]. An overrepresentation of PPD allergy has been identified in African Americans [23]. Lymphomatoid eruptions are also described [24].

Hairdressers can become sensitised by the dyeing process, resulting in hand dermatitis. A pre-existing irritant hand dermatitis may predispose to this. Styling of dyed hair should theoretically not present a problem in view of the reported non-allergenicity of the oxidised dye.

As previously stated, allergy to PPD within black henna tattoos has been reported frequently in recent years [14]. Reactions at the site of application of temporary tattoos may be delayed for about 2 weeks while sensitisation takes place, but the subsequent reaction can be severe and persistent. Erythema multiforme-like and lichenoid eruptions are described, and both postinflammatory hypopigmentation and hyperpigmentation can be a feature [25–27]. If affected individuals dye their hair at a later date there may be a major recrudescence of allergic contact dermatitis [28]. Subsequent clothing dye allergy is also possible [29].

Immediate-type hypersensitivity presenting as an urticarial reaction to PPD is also recognised [30], and contact anaphylaxis and anaphylactoid reactions are described [31,32].

Clinical presentation of clothing dye allergy is described in the section on clothing.

Avoidance. Permanent hair dyes should be clearly marked 'contains phenylenediamines'. Industry currently recommends that consumers perform a 'self test' of hair dye or its constituents to a small area of skin on the arm or behind the ear prior to use of the dye. This is suggested to be an accurate method of identifying sensitised individuals [33], however significant concerns have been raised about this advice. Instructions provided by manufacturers on how to test vary significantly and the application of a potent sensitiser such as PPD directly onto the skin, on a repeated basis, brings a siginificant risk of active sensitisation [34].

Once PPD allergy is diagnosed, the hair should not be permanently dyed. Semipermanent dyes might be tolerated, but approximately 25% of PPD-allergic subjects are likely to have problems due to cross-sensitivity [1]. Other alternatives include pure henna and colour rinses with temporary (non-PPD related) dyes.

A new 'less sensitising' variant of PPD has been developed and marketed (2-methoxymethyl-*p*-phenylenediamine (ME-PPD)). Cross-reactivity with PPD, however, does occur with 48% of PPD-sensitised subjects reacting to an open test with a 2% ME-PPD-containing hair dye [35]. At present ME-PPD is therefore aimed to simply reduce the number of consumers who might become sensitised. Further novel alternative hair dye chemicals are in development [36]. Disperse azo clothing dye avoidance is discussed in the section on clothing.

Cross-sensitivity. Molecules with a similar structure may cross-sensitise with PPD, for example benzocaine, procaine, sulphonamides, mesalazine, diaminodiphenylmethane, *para*-aminobenzoic acid (PABA), UV filters and certain azo dyes. PPD allergic patients should be counselled about this possibility.

Patch tests. PPD is tested as PPD base 1% in petrolatum as part of the standard series. A significant drop in the frequency of positive allergic reactions was noted when the test allergen preparation was temporarily switched to PPD dihydrochloride with many relevant positive cases missed [37]. PPD base is again the preferred baseline test allergen.

Concern has arisen over the risk of active sensitisation from routine patch testing with PPD [38,39]. Most data on this issue have been reassuring [40,41]. PPD 1% is regarded as an important standard allergen as it is highly relevant and allergy is not always suspected from the history [42]. Testing PPD with concentrations of less than 1% carries a significant risk of false negative results [43].

In some individuals, close examination of the patch test site is required, as a positive reaction may be obscured by the black colour left by the patch test. Fierce '+++' reactions to PPD are seen on occasions. In those with a recent and severe presumed hair dye allergic dermatitis, and particularly those with a temporary tattoo reaction, some centres undertake an initial PPD test concentration of 0.5% in petrolatum; a more conservative step-wise increase starting at 0.01%, increasing to 0.1% before progressing to 1% has also been advocated [44]. Other strategies include shorter contact times by applying the 1% PPD patch in an accessible site, for the patient to remove early if symptoms occur. Related hair dye chemicals are also usually tested at 1% in petrolatum. Where permanent hair dye allergy is suspected it is important to test also with PTD, as many dyes contain this and not PPD. It has been shown that about 9% of PTD-allergic subjects are patch test negative to PPD [45].

Azo dyes will normally be incorporated into a larger series of allergens for the investigation of textile dermatitis (see the section on clothing). They are also tested at 1% in petrolatum.

Methacrylate nail systems

At present, three main systems are in use.
1 Acrylic nails, consisting of a powder polymer and a liquid monomer that polymerise in the presence of catalyst molecules.
2 Gel nails consisting of acrylic materials requiring UV light to polymerise them.

Both acrylic and gel nails are designed to rebuild a damaged nail or to be sculpted into a nail extension past the edge of the natural nail. They are usually applied on a mould, which is removed at the end of the procedure, or on a plastic tip glued onto the nail plate with a cyanoacrylate-based glue. Moulds and tips are clipped and filed into shape before application of the acrylic material.
3 Gel polish directly applied with a brush to the consumer's nail plate or as a finish on top of acrylic or gel nails, like a traditional nail lacquer, but more durable. At least three layers are usually applied. The first and final layers (base coat and top coat, respectively) are transparent, whereas the intermediate layers contain the pigments responsible for the final colour. All layers contain methacrylates and, after application of each layer, exposure to a UV or an LED source is required for polymerisation.

A trained beautician is able to apply a long-lasting nail polish in 15–30 min. On the other hand, it takes a trained professional 1–2 h to apply acrylic or gel nail manicures, which is why consumers have to pay more. For these reasons, the application of gel polish has become more widespread. This coupled with the fact that the products can also be purchased directly by consumers for non-professional use are likely to be contributory reasons behind the increased prevalence of methacrylate allergy [1].

Prevalence. Within the last decade, nail aesthetics has become the main occupation in which workers suffer from acrylate allergy [2–4] but now allergic contact dermatitis caused by nail acrylates are also frequently affecting consumers [5–7] at near epidemic proportions.

Clinical features. The methacrylates do not polymerise completely after mixing, with or without UV light. Typically, the allergy results in nail dystrophy and hand (fingertip) dermatitis (Figure 127.27), although it can present with ectopic site involvement, such as the face. Development of allergy to methacrylates may have other adverse health consequences for the consumer such as a reaction to uncured monomers in dental composite fillings [4] although some authors dispute this liklihood if direct mucosal contact is avoided [8]. Later in life, the use of acrylate-containing bone cement for hip prostheses has been associated with loosening and failure of the implant [9]. Acrylates may also cause allergy in the context of medical dressings and adhesives [10].

Patch tests. In light of the increasing number of cases seen in the UK, the BSCA has adopted testing 2-hydroxyethyl methacrylate 2% (pet.) in their baseline series [11]. Previous studies have aimed to establish a screening patch test series that would allow the identification of the majority of cases of ACD caused by methacrylates [12–16]. One is now also available commercially.

Management. For consumers who become sensitised to nail methacrylate chemicals, it is essential to avoid all the nail systems outlined here. Preformed plastic nails glued with cyanoacrylates should be safe due to the lack of cross-reactivity as well as the use of non-methacrylate-based varnishes. They should also be advised about the possibility of problems following other health

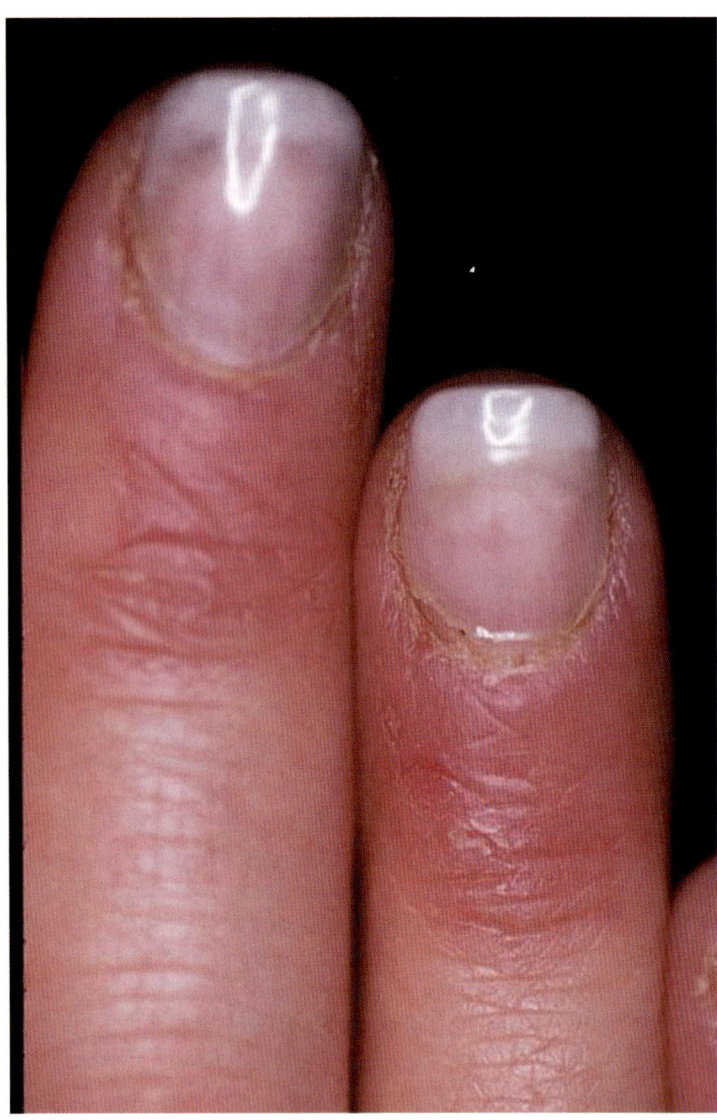

Figure 127.27 Periungual allergic contact dermatitis from nail methacrylates. Courtesy of Dr D. Orton.

care exposures such as dental restorative materials, bone cement and wound dressings.

For nail technicians, the primary prevention strategies to reduce risks include education and safer working 'no touch' practice, and the use of appropriate protective gloves (4H or nitrile) and frequent changes of these gloves [4].

Ultraviolet filters

Epidemiology. UV filters work by absorbing light chemically or by acting as a physical block. The latter agents are usually based on titanium or zinc oxide, which are not sensitisers. However, some chemical UV filters may be contact allergens, photocontact allergens or both. The pattern of usage of UV filters varies, and prevalence figures will reflect this. Current data are provided in the section on photoallergic contact dermatitis.

Some of the classic chemicals (PABA and its derivatives, salicylates, camphor derivatives, phenylbenzimidazole sulphonic acid, cinnamates, dibenzoylmethanes, benzophenones, octocrylene) have been partially replaced by more photo-stable filters with wider protection, namely terephthalylidene dicamphor sulphonic acid (Mexoryl SX), drometrizole trisiloxane (Mexoryl XL), methylene-bis-benzotriazolyl tetramethylbutylphenol or bisoctrizole (Tinosorb M), bis-ethylhexyloxyphenol methoxyphenyl triazine or bemotrizinol (Tinosorb S), disodium phenyl dibenzimidazole tetrasulphonate (Neo Heliopan EP), diethylamino hydroxybenzoyl hexyl benzoate (Uvinul A Plus), ethylhexyl triazone or octyl triazone, diethylhexyl butamido triazone or iscotrizinol (Uvasorb HEB) and polysilicone-15 (Parsol SLX) [1]. A European photopatch test baseline series has been suggested [1].

Clinical features. Allergy and photoallergy from UV filters may coexist or occur separately. Clinical features are discussed under photoallergic contact dermatitis and in the cosmetics section. It is important to appreciate that other photodermatoses can be complicated by photoallergy to UV filters being used in treatment, and this may easily go unrecognised. The possibility of allergy and photoallergy to UV filters must be considered before individuals are diagnosed as having an idiopathic photodermatosis such as polymorphic light eruption.

Investigations. These chemicals are not confined to sunscreens. They may be added to cosmetics in small quantities to prevent photodegradation and as an 'antiageing' agent [2]. UV light absorbers may also be added to plastics. Allergy from this source is unusual but has been reported, most notably from 2-(2-hydroxy-5-methylphenyl)-benzotriazole (Tinuvin P) [3,4]. UV filters are generally tested at 10% in petrolatum, although 5% has also been advocated. Sunscreens and cosmetics containing UV filters should also be patch tested, and if necessary photopatch tested at the same time. The photopatch testing investigation is described elsewhere in this chapter.

Management. Once allergy or photoallergy has been demonstrated, patients should be apprised of the need to avoid sunscreens and cosmetics containing the allergen, which will be identified by its INCI name. They should only use fully ingredient-labelled cosmetics. In addition, a list of synonyms should be given to the patients as they may encounter sunscreens labelled differently in other countries.

Rubber [1]

Rubber products, comprising natural rubber latex or synthetic elastomers such as nitrile and neoprene, are widely used in everyday and working life. Rubber additives, either as remnants from the production process (such as accelerators) or those deliberately added to enhance the product characteristics (such as antioxidants), constitute an important group of contact allergens. The most frequent rubber exposures leading to sensitisation to rubber components are from protective gloves often used in an occupational context. A list of potential sensitisers in rubber is shown in Box 127.6. It is important to note that type I mediated allergy to latex proteins (requiring diagnosis with skin prick tests or specific immunoglobulin E (IgE) measurements) and type IV mediated allergy to rubber chemicals can coexist and may need evaluating together.

Box 127.6 Common sensitisers in rubber[a]

Mercapto mix
- Mercaptobenzothiazole (MBT)
- Cyclohexylbenzothiazyl sulphenamide (CBS)
- Dibenzothiazyl disulphide (MBTS)
- Morpholinylmercaptobenzothiazole
  Patch test concentration: 0.5% each = total 2% in petrolatum

Thiuram mix
- Tetramethylthiuram disulphide (TMTD)
- Tetramethylthiuram monosulphide (TMTM)
- Tetraethylthiuram disulphide (TETD)
- Dipentamethylenethiuram disulphide (PTD)
  Patch test concentration: 0.25% each = total 1% in petrolatum

Black rubber mix
- Phenylcyclohexyl-p-phenylenediamine (CPPD)
- Phenylisopropyl-p-phenylenediamine (IPPD) (identical to isopropylaminodiphenylamine)
- Diphenyl-p-phenylenediamine (DPPD)
  Patch test concentration: 0.25% of CPPD and DPPD, 0.1% of IPPD = total 0.6% in petrolatum

Carba mix
- 1,3-Diphenylguanidine (DPG)
- Bis-(diethyldithiocarbamato) zinc (ZDC)
- Bis-(dibutyldithiocarbamato) zinc (ZBC)
  Patch test concentration: 1% each = total 3% in petrolatum

[a] The mixtures mentioned are commercially available.

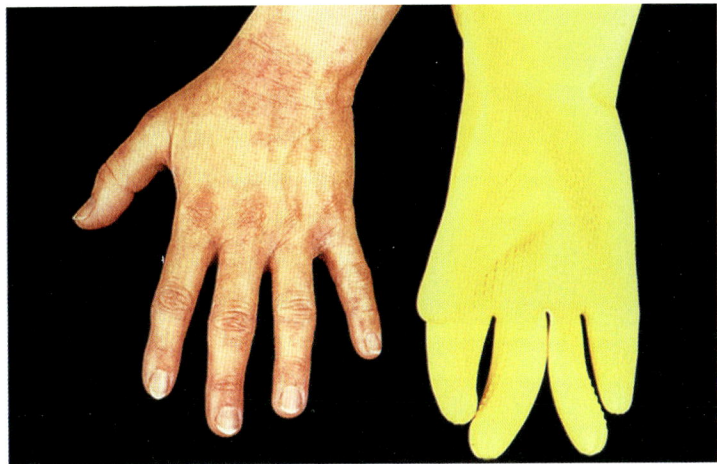

Figure 127.28 Contact dermatitis from rubber gloves. Courtesy of Dr J. D. Wilkinson.

Prevalence. At present, four of 30 allergens recommended in the European baseline series are rubber additives, namely thiuram mix 1% (pet.), 2-mercaptobenzothiazole (MBT) 2% (pet.), mercapto mix (with four constituents, including MBT) 2% (pet.) and N-isopropyl-N-phenyl-p-phenylenediamine (IPPD) 0.1% (pet.).

In comparison to the findings from the European Surveillance System on Contact Allergies (ESSCA) survey in 2007–08, recent multinational surveys from 12 European countries showed a certain decline of contact allergy to thiuram mix (with an overall prevalence of 1.87% (ESSCA 2013–14) versus 2.03% (ESSCA 2009–12), whereas the prevalence of allergy to carba mix was significantly increased (2.29% (ESSCA 2009–12) versus 2.68% (ESSCA 2013–14)) [2,3]. This might reflect that thiuram usage in manufactured gloves has largely been replaced by dithiocarbamates [4]. Positive patch test reactions to thiurams are frequently combined with positive patch test reactions to dithiocarbamates since they constitute a redox pair. However, positive patch test reactions to thiurams have been found to be more common than positive reactions to dithiocarbamates [5,6]. Thiurams are considered to be better markers for sensitisation to the dithiocarbamate/thiuram redox pair than the dithiocarbamates.

The prevalence of positive reactions to carba mix is steadily increasing with some experts calling for its inclusion in the European baseline series [7]. 1,3-Diphenylguanidine (DPG) is now more frequently used in rubber glove production, and there are increasing numbers of cases of true allergic sensitisation [3,8,9], although it is a recognised irritant at its present patch test concentration.

For assessing benzothiazole contact allergy, the mercapto mix is tested along with MBT. Their use in glove production has increased during the last decades but MBT remains the most widely used accelerator for industrial rubber [10]. Sensitisation rates have been recorded at 0.6% for MBT and 0.7% for mercapto mix in a recent European study [3]. The frequency of sensitisation to mercapto mix have been found to be most common in patients with allergic contact dermatitis of the feet [11] and MBT is found to be a frequent sensitiser in patients with shoe dermatitis [3].

Thioureas are used in the production of synthetic rubbers, particularly neoprene products and foam rubbers. The most frequent source of relevant positive patch test reactions have been reported to be shoes and medical devices and the prevalence of sensitisation even with aimed testing is usually <1% [3]. The most important antidegradant sensitisers are phenylenediamine derivatives: N-isopropyl-N'-phenyl-4-phenylenediamine (IPPD), N-phenyl-N'-cyclohexl-4-phenylenediamine (CPPD), N,N'-diphenyl-4-phenylenediamine (DPPD) and N-(1-3 dimethylbutyl)-N'-phenyl-4-phenylenediamine (DMPPD). They are found in industrial rubber and 'black' rubber materials. IPPD is included in the baseline series with a European sensitisation prevalence at 0.6% [12].

Clinical features. Rubber sensitivity may be the primary cause of a dermatitis or it may become superimposed on an existing dermatitis, as sometimes occurs following the use of protective rubber gloves (Figure 127.28). It is not always obvious, and many cases will be missed if patients are not routinely patch tested with a series of the more common rubber chemicals. A positive patch test reaction to a rubber chemical is usually relevant.

Dermatitis from rubber gloves [13] may be diffuse, but is more often localised to the dorsa of the hands, especially over the knuckles and the wrist, where a sharp proximal margin is often evident. The use of alcoholic disinfectant prior to polyisoprene glove donning increases the amount of DPG recovered from the hands.

Shoe dermatitis occurs in both adults and children, and in the latter group needs to be differentiated from juvenile plantar dermatosis [14]. Rubber chemicals may occur in almost any part of the shoe, and a rubber adhesive is commonly used to glue parts together. The dermatitis may occur on the dorsum of the foot, soles or toes, usually with sparing of the web spaces and instep.

Antioxidants related to PPD are used in car tyres and wear-resistant rubber products. IPPD allergy is strikingly more often

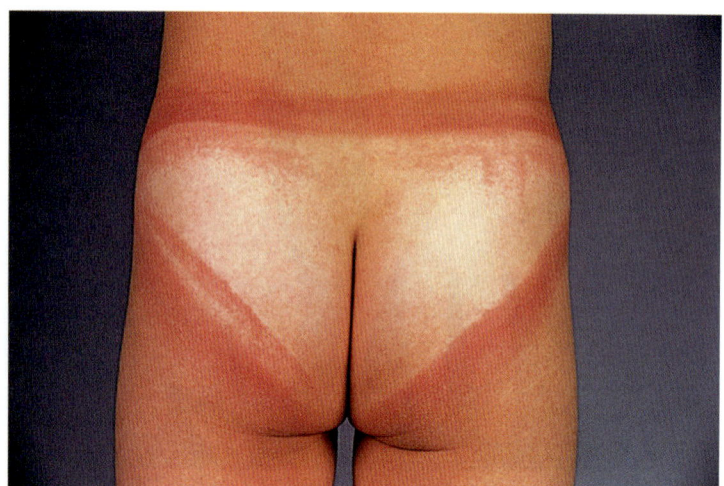

Figure 127.29 Allergic contact dermatitis to elastic in clothing. Courtesy of Dr J. D. Wilkinson.

found in patients with allergic contact dermatitis of the head and upper extremities (arm and hand) than in those with dermatitis of the trunk and lower extremities [11]. Although sometimes causing allergic contact dermatitis on the feet because of its presence in heavy boots, not all cases have an occupational origin. Black rubber flexes or cables, hoses, grips and even scuba masks or squash balls may be responsible. The ensuing dermatitis may sometimes be purpuric, and an erythema multiforme-like presentation has also been reported.

In some cases, the site of dermatitis may provide a clue as, for instance, when the dermatitis is due to a rubber finger-stall used when counting money or rubber bands under a wristwatch. Rubber dermatitis may also occur at the site of contact with rubber in clothing (Figure 127.29) or dressings, between the thighs or on the abdomen from hot water bottles and on the knees from kneeling mats. Genital dermatitis or pruritus vulvae may occur following the use of condoms and diaphragms, and may also result from rubber catheters, when the dermatitis also spreads down the thighs. An apparent worsening of venous eczema may be related to allergy to rubber in elastic bandaging, and such patients are prone to develop a secondary generalised eczema. A generalised dermatitis may occur after sleeping on a rubber mattress or using rubber pillows, or the dermatitis may be predominantly on the side on which the patient sleeps.

Investigations. Contact allergy to rubber is assessed by using the thiuram mix 1% (pet.), MBT 2% (pet.), mercapto mix (with four constituents, including MBT) 2% (pet.) and IPPD 0.1% (pet.). The thiurams included in the thiuram mix comprise tetramethylthiuram monosulphide (TMTM), tetramethylthiuram disulphide (TMTD), tetraethylthiuram disulphide (TETD) and dipentamethylenethiuram disulphide (PDT). Approximately 20% of thiuram-sensitised patients are missed by the mix. Therefore, it is advisable to patch test not only with the thiuram mix included in the baseline series but also with the rubber series in cases of suspected rubber (glove) allergy [5].

Dithiocarbamates include zinc diethyldithiocarbamate (ZDEC) and zinc dibutyldithiocarbamate (ZDBC). Both are tested alongside DPG as part of the carba mix in some centres. Almost all patients with a contact allergy against dithiocarbamates are also allergic against thiurams; vice versa, however, this ratio was only one-fifth [15]. DPG is not a carbamate, despite its inclusion in the carba mix; this is a source of potential confusion. To avoid this it may be preferable to patch test carba mix together with its three ingredients. Changing patterns of allergy to rubber chemicals in Europe has led to calls to add carba mix to the European baseline series. It is presently part of the BSCA baseline series.

For assessing benzothiazole contact allergy, the mercapto mix at 2% pet. (comprising MBT, N-cyclohexyl-2-benzothiazyl sulphenamide (CBS), dibenzothiazyl disulphide (MBTS) and morpholinyl mercaptobenzothiazole (MOR) is used along with MBT at 2% pet., tested separately. Since a high rate of false negative results was repeatedly demonstrated when testing with the mix or MBT alone [15–17] patch testing should be done in parallel with mercapto mix as well as with MBT. As a rule, if positive test reactions are found to a mix, subsequent patch testing of its components is recommended to clarify the relevant contact allergen to advise the patient accordingly.

In cases of suspected rubber allergy, additional rubber allergens should be tested. In particular, neoprene items such as gloves, shoes and wet suits frequently contain thioureas (Figure 127.30). These include dibutyl thiourea (DBTU), diethyl thiourea (DETU), diphenyl thiourea (DPTU) and ethylene thiourea (ETU). The mix of two thiourea chemicals (DETU and DBTU), also referred to as mixed dialkyl thioureas (MDTU), tested 1% in petrolatum, will detect 75% of relevant thiourea reactions [4,18]. Black rubber mix is no longer included in the European standard series, having been replaced by IPPD. Testing with IPPD alone will potentially miss 10% of individuals allergic to this group of antioxidants.

A 'European rubber series' including supplementary allergens has been proposed especially for cases of suspected occupational rubber contact allergy, particularly aimed to detect antioxidant allergens [19].

It is also often very useful to test directly to a patient's own rubber items such as their gloves (moistened with 96% ethanol for best results). By patch testing a patient's own materials novel rubber compounds with allergenic potency may be identified, for example dimethylthiocarbamylbenzothiazole sulphide (DMTBS) was recently found in canvas shoes [20].

Management. Sensitivity to a certain rubber chemical does not necessarily indicate any specific source, although sensitivity to carbamates and thiurams suggests rubber gloves, mercapto compounds suggests shoes, and the PPD group is mainly associated with black rubber products such as tyres. Although it may be impossible to avoid contact with rubber entirely, many patients remain clear of dermatitis, and others may only have intermittent symptoms if they take simple precautions to avoid contact. In many cases, hand eczema improves or clears if patients can be persuaded to change from rubber gloves to cotton-lined vinyl gloves. 'Accelerator-free' medical grade gloves are produced with varying production techniques, and are also becoming more widely available [21].

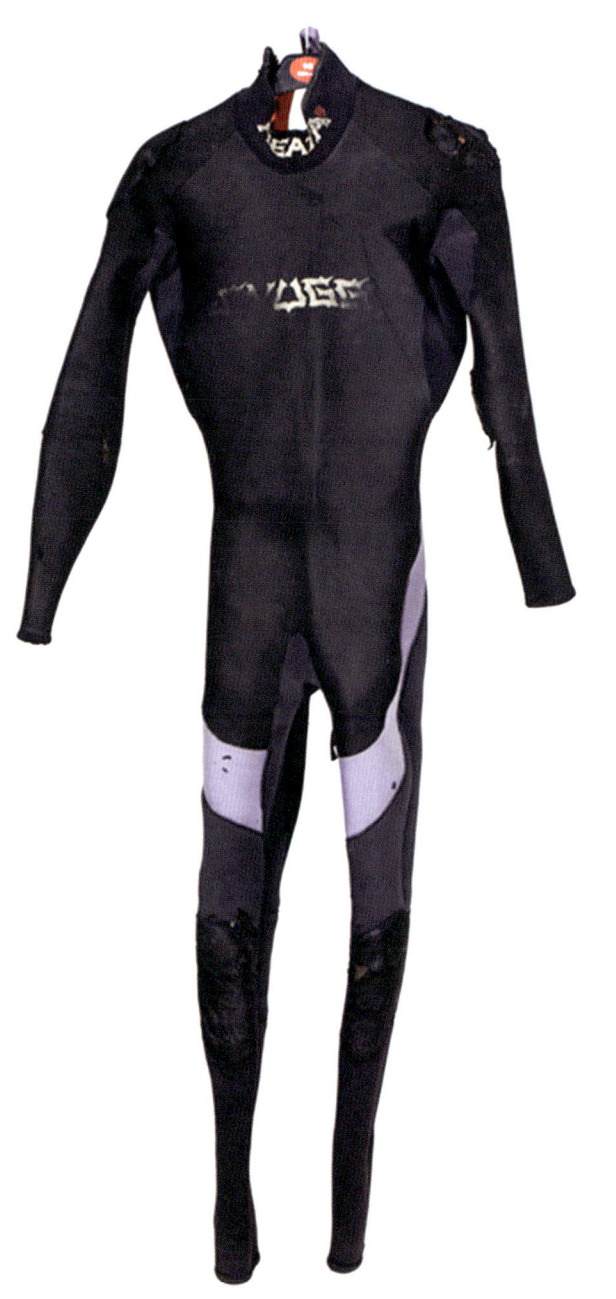
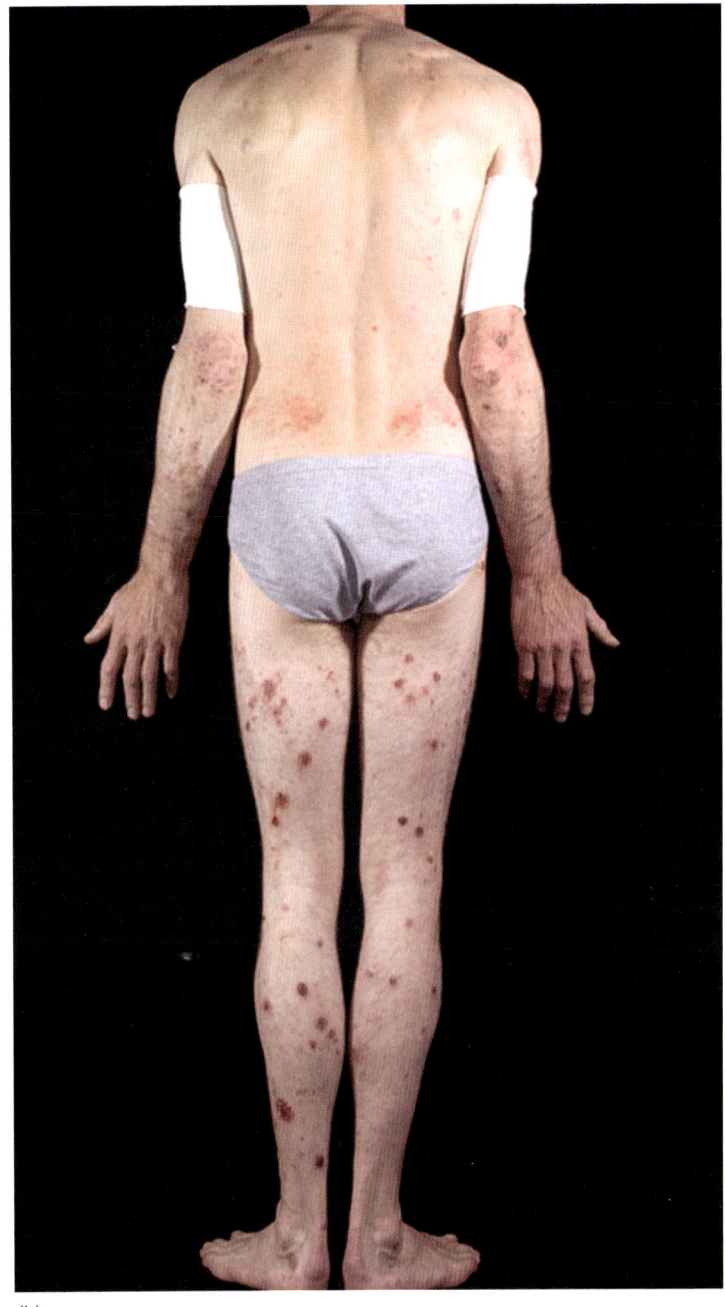

Figure 127.30 (a, b) Allergic contact dermatitis from thioureas in a wet suit. Courtesy of Dr N. Stone.

Clothing [1]

Epidemiology. Textile fibres may be natural, for example cotton, wool, silk, linen and rubber, or they may be synthetic, for example cellulose derivatives (rayon), polyamides such as nylon, polyesters, acrylics and elastomers. Apart from rubber, they rarely sensitise in their own right.

More common allergens in clothing include textile dyes, nickel, chromate (in leather and as a dyeing mordant), rubber, glues, biocides (triclosan, zinc pyrithione, MCI/MI, dimethyl fumarate, silver particles) and, in the past, formaldehyde and resins.

The main dye allergens belong to disperse dyes which are used for colouring synthetic textile fibres. They are principally anthroquinone and azo dyes. Disperse dyes may contain more than one fraction, as well as impurities, all of which can sensitise [2]. A mixture of several different dyes may be responsible for the final colour. Fibre-reactive dyes are covalently bound to the fibre and unlikely to cause problems from clothing, but may sensitise those handling the dye powder [3]. However, if the clothing is not adequately rinsed during the production process, reactive dye residue in new unwashed garments may then cause allergic dermatitis [4]. Clothing dermatitis has also been reported from acid, basic, direct, vat and solvent dyes, as well as coupling agents.

It is generally considered that formaldehyde, urea-formaldehyde resin and melamine-formaldehyde resin contact allergy may be of

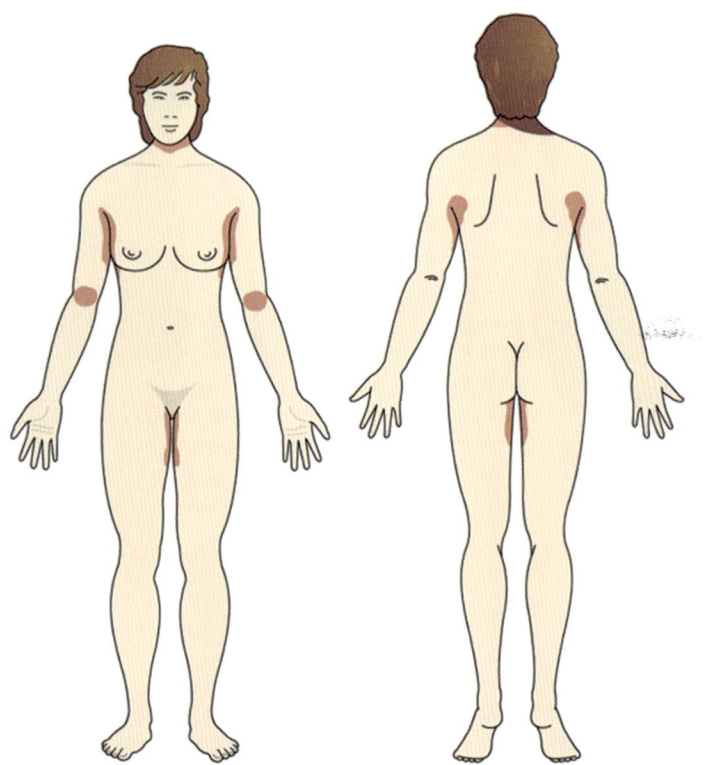

Figure 127.31 Pattern of textile dermatitis.

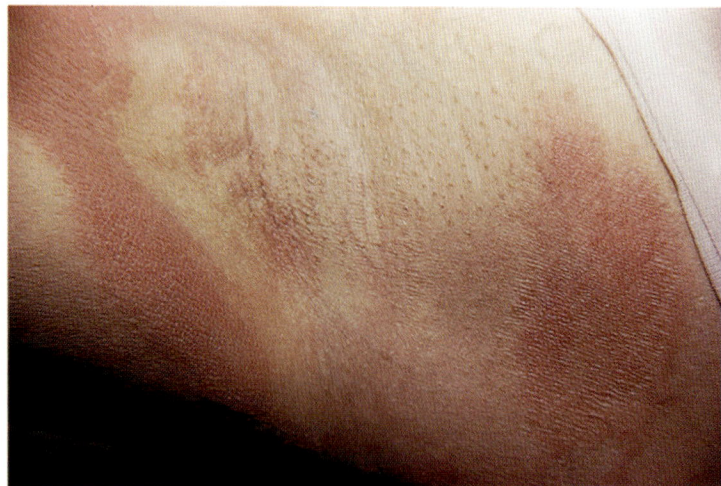

Figure 127.32 Axillary dermatitis (sparing the axillary vault). The characteristic pattern of eczema seen in patients allergic to textile dyes and finishes. Courtesy of Dr J. D. Wilkinson.

more historical importance [5] apart from a few isolated case reports in disposable surgical and military uniforms [6]. This might be due to the regulations and the use of newer finishes. These new resins may be less sensitising [7]. The prevalence of textile dermatitis is unknown. Only contact allergy to textile dyes (mainly disperse azo) has been evaluated in epidemiological studies. In a study based on routine patch tests, mainly from Europe, frequencies of sensitisation to textile dyes ranged from 0% to 5.8% [8].

Clinical features. The distribution of contact dermatitis in areas of sweating and friction is the same for dyes and finishes (Figure 127.31). The eruption typically starts in the axillae, sparing the hairy part of the vault (Figure 127.32), and forms a crescentic patch on the anterior chest wall sharply limited by the underwear. The anterior and posterior folds are also affected. Long sleeves cause eruptions in the elbow flexures, and collars provoke a rash around the neck. Later in the course of the disease, the chest and upper back may be involved. The dermatitis is often sheeted, and the inner posterior thighs, popliteal fossae and lower leg may be involved when trousers or tights are the responsible garments. Nevertheless, a high index of suspicion is required as the clinical presentation might not always indicate the cause [9]. In a majority of cases, textile contact dermatitis presents as typical pruritic eczematous dermatitis. However, approximately 20% of cases can present as atypical dermatitis (lichenoid, purpuric, dyshydrosiform, psoriasis-like, seborrhoeic, nummular, erythema multiforme-like, pustular) [10]. Up to 5% of textile dermatitis cases have an appearance of folliculitis, contact urticaria, excoriations due to itching or eczematid-like purpura.

Hand dermatitis may be a feature of textile allergy from occupational exposure [11].

Investigations. A PPD-positive patch test may alert one to clothing dye allergy, but it is an inadequate screen. Formaldehyde is a standard-series allergen but not sufficient to detect contact allergy to formaldehyde-based resins, if these are still suspected. Therefore, these should be additionally tested in appropriate circumstances. Textile dyes are commercially available as test allergens, although their purity is questioned.

As various azo dyes and PPD are structurally similar there is a risk of multiple strong positive reactions in allergic patients screened for clothing dye allergy. Patients investigated with a series of textile azo dyes should be warned of this risk [12].

In 2015 a textile dye mix was recommended for inclusion in the European baseline series [13]. The composition of the 6.6% wt/wt pet. mix is as follows: D Blue 35, D Yellow 3, D Orange 1, D Orange 3, D Red 1 and D Red 17, all at 1.0% wt/wt, and D Blue 106 and D Blue 124, both at 0.3% wt/wt. Patch testing with the suspected clothing can be undertaken, although there is a high risk of obtaining a false negative reaction. Soaking 1 cm^2 of the fabric in water for 10 min before testing might increase the return, and extraction techniques have also been suggested [14] as well as testing with thin layer chromatograms [15]. For most patch test centres further chemical investigation of textiles that are patch test positive is not possible. However, such testing can prove clinical relevance, and new emerging allergens may be detected.

Management. Patients sensitive to formaldehyde or one of the formaldehyde resins should be advised to avoid treated fabrics, for example drip-dry, crease-resistant or durable-press cotton, cotton mix and rayon clothes.

Disperse dyes are used to colour artificial fibres such as polyester, acetate, acrylic and nylon. Both azo and anthraquinone dyes may cause dermatitis from modern artificial fibres, and non-disperse azo dyes from natural fibres. Reactive dyes will combine with protein and cellulose in natural fibres and polyamides. A precise knowledge of the dye responsible for an individual's allergy is not helpful as cross-sensitivity is common and the finished colour is commonly a mix of several dyes. Strongly coloured synthetic clothing should be avoided, but lightly coloured garments may sometimes be tolerated. Pure natural fibres, such as cotton, wool, linen and silk of any colour, can generally be worn.

Shoes

Epidemiology. Chromium salts and cobalt, but also preservative agents in leather, colophonium and *para*-tert-butylphenol-formaldehyde resin (PTBPFR) in glues and rubber chemicals (mercaptobenzothiazole and derivatives, and to a lesser extent thiurams), as well as dyes, such as PPD and related compounds, are the most important causes of shoe dermatitis. However, other allergens may also be involved, for example shoe contaminants from topical pharmaceutical or other products contacted. The prevalence of shoe allergy has ranged between 3% and 11% in patients referred for routine patch testing. The highest frequencies of dermatitis have been reported from hot climates, which will promote sweating and leaching out of allergenic shoe chemicals [1].

Clinical features. Allergic contact dermatitis due to footwear should always be considered in the differential diagnosis in cases of persistent foot dermatitis. Sweating causes allergens in shoes to leach out and migrate, and as a result of this, the pattern of dermatitis is often not distinctive. It may be patchy or superimposed on a pre-existing constitutional eczema. Nevertheless, in many instances the distribution will reflect whether the sensitiser is present in the upper or sole of the shoe [1]. Dermatitis from the upper commonly starts over the dorsal surface of the big toes and spreads to the dorsa of the feet and the other toes. The interdigital spaces are normally spared. The heels may be involved, but less frequently than the toes. On the heels, patches of dermatitis may correspond to the heel cap, and on the dorsum of the foot they may correspond to the tongue of the shoe. Adhesives and rubber components may cause localised areas of dermatitis limited to the toe cap [2]. Nickel allergy from shoe buckles and eyelets may cause a localised dermatitis on the adjacent skin. Rubber chemical allergy has an increased tendency to affect the soles. Involvement of the sole usually affects only the weight-bearing areas – the instep is frequently spared. In sports shoes, the sole is usually moulded to fit into the instep and the dermatitis may affect the whole sole [3]. Sometimes, only the forefoot is involved (Figure 127.33), and in children the condition must be differentiated from juvenile plantar dermatosis by patch testing.

Surprisingly, not all cases are bilateral [4], but the great majority are. Patients with shoe dermatitis often have evidence of dermatitis elsewhere, especially on the hands.

Boots produce a pattern similar to shoe dermatitis, sometimes with an additional eruption on the calves.

Allergy to socks and stockings, agents such as perfumed sprays, talcs and antifungal powders used in shoes, and medicaments applied to the skin may simulate footwear dermatitis [5]. Shoe fabrics may become reservoirs for materials applied to the skin of the feet and act as a source for continued exposure even though the items are no longer being actively applied.

Investigations. Many of the commoner shoe allergens are found in the standard series, including dichromate, cobalt, certain rubber accelerators and antioxidants, PTBPFR, colophony and nickel. In

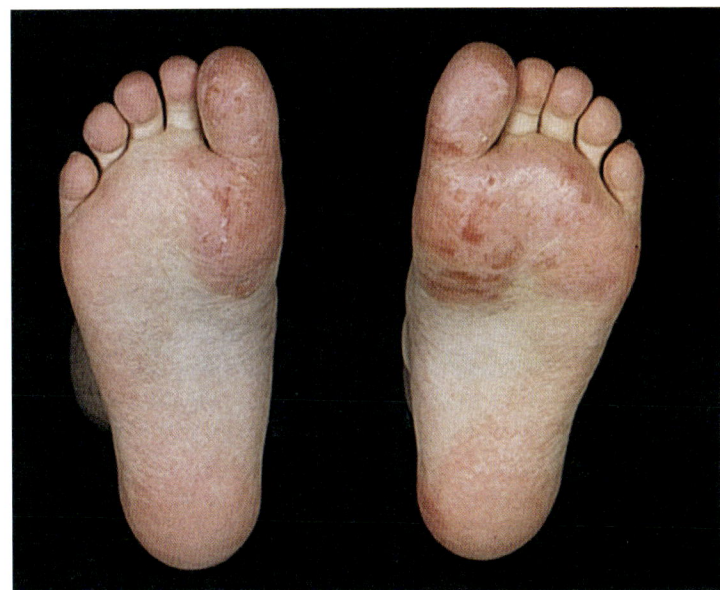

Figure 127.33 Forefoot dermatitis from shoe allergy.

addition, a special shoe series should be used, and commercial allergen suppliers have such a series of allergens. Non-standard allergens of emerging importance include biocides such as OIT [6], dimethylfumarate [7], dodecylmercaptan [8] and acetophenone azine [9].

Some allergies have only been identified by testing with pieces of the shoe itself. Ideally, pieces for patch testing should be taken from the parts of the shoe in contact with the dermatitic area. They should be thin and 1 cm^2 or larger. Some have suggested testing the pieces under a special large Finn chamber, whereas others recommend occlusive tape. Further suggestions have been to soak the pieces in water for 15 min before they are applied, and to leave the test pieces in place for 4–5 days [10]. False positive reactions may be seen from pressure, particularly around the edge, and false negative reactions are common. Patch testing with ultrasonic bath extracts (or extracts after soaking for 24 h) of shoe pieces might be the best method to identify contact allergy, which would otherwise go unrecognised.

Management. A typical shoe will be formed from an upper, a sole, an insole and heel and toe counters to stiffen the shoe and give it shape. Adhesives may be required throughout the shoe.

Uppers tend to be made of leather, rubber or synthetic material. Leather is tanned, usually with chromate, but other tanning agents, including vegetable tans, colophony, formaldehyde and glutaraldehyde, may be used. Formaldehyde is associated with the tanning of white or water-resistant leather and is tightly bound, making sensitisation less likely. After tanning, the leather may be oiled, dyed and finished. Biocides such as OIT may be added to the oils and finishes. Uppers may be made from, or be lined with, dyed fabric. Polyurethane, rubber and neoprene foams are used in the uppers, particularly of sports footwear. Neoprene is a synthetic rubber to which phenolic resins, most notably PTBPFR, thioureas, carbamates and other accelerators and additives, may be added.

Shoe soles are made from similar materials and more solid forms of rubber. Insoles can also be made of a similar range of materials. Fibreboard used for insoles is a composite of fibres, usually paper but occasionally wood or leather in a glue matrix, which may contain biocides. Insoles may also contain allergenic deodorisers, including formaldehyde and fragrances.

Counters may be made from many different potentially allergenic materials, including natural rubber, formaldehyde resins, biocides and pine oil.

The main adhesives are hot melt, urethane, neoprene and natural rubber. Hot melt adhesives do not tend to cause allergy but the others may, particularly rubber accelerators and PTBPFR. Additives include isocyanates, epoxy resins and biocides. Tackifiers may contain formaldehyde resins and colophony.

Individuals who are allergic to leather tanning agents and additives can be advised to wear synthetic fabric or rubber footwear. Some specialised outlets sell 'vegetarian' shoes that should not be leather.

However, with other allergens avoidance is often difficult. Manufacturers and distributors will not generally guarantee their shoes are free of rubber chemicals and PTBPFR in adhesives, and may know even less about other sensitisers. Patients allergic to rubber, PTBPFR and colophony should consider all-leather stitched footwear with no insoles, or injection-moulded plastic shoes, moccasins or wooden shoes. Certain manufacturers will produce bespoke shoes free of the allergen(s) but these are expensive. Sometimes, orthotists advising hospital orthopaedic departments are helpful in making special shoes.

Those allergic to dyes will need to avoid dyed fabric and nylon-lined footwear, as well as coloured nylon socks and stockings. Old socks may act as a reservoir of allergen and should be discarded with the incriminated shoes, medicaments, etc.

Hyperhidrosis is common in shoe dermatitis, and the dermatitis may be helped by treatment with iontophoresis, or by other means, and by wearing cotton socks to absorb the sweat.

Follow-up (average 3 years) of 48 patients after they had employed a number of strategies to avoid contact with the allergens responsible for their dermatitis revealed that 87.5% were clear or significantly better, 10% the same and only one person was worse [10].

Resins and plastics

Plastics comprise synthetic polymers that are produced from raw materials through polymerization. The two main types of plastics are thermoplastics and thermosets. Most plastic-related contact allergens are reactive raw materials for thermoset plastics, for example, acrylic, epoxy, phenolic, and urethane plastics and occur in the occupational setting (e.g. construction including painting, tiling and floor laying and the manufacturing sector including vehicles, aircraft, electronics and paints). Many products are bicomponent comprising a resin part and a hardener that are mixed to start polymerization. Thermoplastics seldom cause skin problems other than irritation, because they are usually handled as large polymers. Additives are used in the manufacture of all types of plastic to modify their properties, and they can also cause contact allergy.

Epoxy resins

Epidemiology. Approximately 75% of the epoxy resins currently used worldwide are derived from diglycidyl ether of bisphenol A (DGEBA) [1] although contact allergies to other epoxy resins, hardeners and modifiers, such as reactive diluents, also occur. Epoxy resin of the bisphenol A type is a standard allergen. However, figures for the prevalence of allergy in patch-tested patients will reflect the degree of occupational interest of the clinic, and also the local industry. Series of relatively unselected patch-tested patients have reported rates of 0.4–3% positive reactions, with a male preponderance. However, higher rates are recorded for occupational referrals. Annually, approximately 1% of exposed workers are believed to develop an epoxy resin allergy [2].

Allergy to other components of epoxy systems is commonly concomitant with resin sensitisation but may also occur by itself [3,4]. Detailed analysis of 182 cases in Finland showed that 80% were allergic to DGEBA epoxy resins, 23% to polyamine hardeners, 16% to reactive diluents and 9% to non-DGEBA epoxy resins.

A high incidence of allergy among exposed individuals has been reported in factory outbreaks, for example 56% in an aircraft construction factory, 45% in marble workers, 27% in ski factory workers and 21% in paint factory workers [5–7]. The epoxy resins are among the most sensitising substances that have been introduced to industrial work in recent years. Coatings, including paints and varnishes, account for roughly 45% of all epoxy resin use. They are widely used in the construction industry, in cement to make it waterproof and in floorings, grouts and filling materials, including those for marble and window frames. They are commonly used as binders and coatings for fibreglass and carbon fibre, for example in car body repairs, wind turbine rotor blades and aircraft construction. In the electronics industry they are used for insulation and in printed-circuit boards. They are efficient glues for metals, rubber, polyester resins and ceramics. Cardiac pacemakers and hypodermic needles may contain them. Dental personnel and their patients sensitised by epoxy acrylates in filling materials often also react to epoxy resin. In the laboratory they have been found as sensitisers in microscopy immersion oil.

High-molecular-weight resins, which may contain residual low-molecular-weight resin, are used for coating metal or wood. Occasionally, uncured epoxy resins are used as stabilisers and plasticisers in, for example, polyvinyl chloride plastic and spectacle frames. Thus, contact dermatitis may be elicited in consumers as well as occupationally and has also been reported from 'hobby' materials [8].

Diglycidyl ether of bisphenol F (DGEBF novolac) resins are also quite commonly used in epoxy products; these have lower viscosity and better chemical resistance than DGEBA. Non-DGEBA epoxy resins have found increasing use in electron microscopy, electronics and carbon and glass fibre composite materials, especially in the aerospace construction industry. Cycloaliphatic epoxy resin in hydraulic fluid and neat metalworking oil has also sensitised.

Clinical features. Dermatitis is predominantly occupational. It usually affects the hands and arms (see Figure 127.8), and often the face and eyelids from airborne contact. Facial and periorbital involvement may be indicators of associated or isolated allergy to the more volatile epoxy diluents and hardeners [9]. Partially cured epoxy resin dusts from sanding and drilling may induce dermatitis with a similar distribution.

Severe oedematous and weeping eruptions are not uncommon, and widespread generalised eruptions can develop if exposure continues. Erythema multiforme-like reactions have been described [10].

Localised dermatitis can sometimes be attributed to traces of free epoxy monomer found in a wide range of products, such as twist-off caps, coated door knobs, tool handles, microscopy immersion oil, stoma bags, clothing labels, portable infusion pumps, spectacle frames, plastic tubing in medical devices and gloves. A flare-up of hand eczema has been reported from an implanted epoxy resin-containing needle [11]. Other body sites, especially the genitals, may be affected following hand contact. Gingivitis and stomatitis may result from the use of epoxy acrylates in dental materials [12].

Contact allergy to epoxy components may rarely cause vitiligo [13].

Investigations. Epoxy resin of the bisphenol A type is included in the standard series at 1% in petrolatum; other components of epoxy resin systems are not. Extra patch test reagents, which incorporate the commoner amine hardeners and reactive diluents, are available from the commercial allergen suppliers, although these are not all inclusive. Allergy to non-DGEBA epoxy resins and other components may still be missed unless the worker's own materials are tested.

Epoxy resins may be reacted with other resins, for example acrylates and formaldehyde resins, to produce new resins that may have an allergic profile different from their parent resins [14].

Higher-molecular-weight resins may contain small amounts of the oligomers or monomer but rarely sufficient for the induction of sensitivity. However, they can elicit clinical and patch test reactions in those already sensitised.

Sometimes, 'reactive diluents' in the resins used to reduce viscosity are responsible for their sensitising capacity. These diluents are usually glycidyl ethers or, occasionally, glycidyl esters, and are thought to be present in over 50% of epoxy resin products. Bisphenol A and epichlorhydrin themselves are seldom responsible for allergy from epoxy resin.

The commonest sensitisers among the hardeners are amines, for example the aliphatic amines ethylenediamine, diethylenetetramine, triethylenetetramine, dipropylenetriamine and dimethylaminopropylamine. Triethylenetetramine is a particularly strong sensitiser [15]. There are also sensitising cycloaliphatic amines (e.g. isophoronediamine) and aromatic amines, such as *m*-xylenediamine, diaminodiphenylmethane (methylene dianiline) and 2,4,6-*tris*-(dimethylaminomethyl) phenol.

Hardeners of the polyaminoamide type are much less likely to sensitise, and so are anhydrides (e.g. phthalic anhydride). They are used for thermal hardening.

A rough guide to patch test concentrations (all in petrolatum) is 0.5% for non-DGEBA epoxy resins, 0.25% for reactive diluents and 1% for most polyamine hardeners, but a literature search should also be undertaken, and lower concentrations considered initially if in doubt.

Additives include colours, fillers, UV light absorbers, flame retardants and plasticisers.

Management. Redeployment away from contact with epoxy resin is usually required for occupational dermatitis but even so the prognosis is not always favourable [16]. The use of epoxy (usually two-part) adhesives and fillers in domestic and spare-time activities (e.g. car body repairs) should be avoided. The identification of epoxy chemicals in suspect materials by chromatography techniques may be helpful in confirming a suspected source of epoxy resin [17].

The prevention of epoxy dermatitis is important, and includes education, instructions and warning notices for the workforce, stressing the need for 'good housekeeping'. High-molecular-weight epoxy resins and diluents are less sensitising and, where possible and appropriate, are to be preferred. Aliphatic and aromatic amines may be replaced by polyaminoamides or amine epoxy adducts. If feasible, automation or a 'two in one' mixing package is advised or, if not, mixing should be done in disposable containers. Protective impermeable, preferably disposable, clothing and gloves should be worn. Epoxy resin will nevertheless penetrate plastic and rubber gloves [18]. Heavy-duty vinyl gloves or multilayered gloves of folio type (4H-Glove; Safety 4, Denmark) provide the best protection [19].

Acrylate resins [1]

Epidemiology. Acrylates are esters of acrylic acid, and methacrylates are esters of methacrylic acid. They are the main monomers in acrylic resin systems. However, acrylic resins also include esters of cyanoacrylic acid (cyanoacrylates), acrylamides and acrylonitrile. Acrylic resins can be combined with other types of resins such as epoxies, polyurethanes, polyesters and polyethers. The term 'acrylate' is often used for all acrylic compounds including of cyanoacrylic and methacrylic acid. Many acrylic resin systems are cured by radiation (e.g. UV light), especially many dermatologically important products. Polymerisation of acrylic resins can also be initiated by heat, peroxides or *N,N*-dimethyl-*p*-toluidine and inhibited by stabilisers such as the monomethyl ether of hydroquinone or hydroquinone itself. These additives only occasionally cause contact allergy. Acrylate allergy is not routinely sought, and levels of allergy used to reflect the referral pattern to a particular clinic – in particular with relevance to occupational dermatitis (e.g. dental personnel, beauticians, printers). However, this has all changed as detailed in the methacrylate nails section.

Clinical features. It is the uncured acrylic monomers that cause sensitisation. Cured products are usually safe even for strongly sensitised patients. The commonest sites of occupational allergy are the fingertips and hands (see Figure 127.2), but the face, arms and eyelids may also be involved. Manicurists may develop hand dermatitis, and sometimes a more extensive exposure pattern dermatitis from dust generated by nail filing. Associated rhinitis has concomitantly been reported [2], and acrylates may also induce occupational asthma. Workers with fingertip dermatitis should always be asked about contact with screwlocks and glues, as this is a typical distribution of allergic dermatitis from this source. A similar distribution may be seen in dentists and dental technicians. Localised dermatitis is seen from limb prostheses, the use of diathermy plates during surgery and incontinence pads. There may also be secondary spread of the eruption.

Dermatitis from artificial nails may be associated with painful onycholysis, nail dystrophy, periungual dermatitis, paraesthesiae and an ectopic dermatitis of the face, neck and elsewhere. Paraesthesiae can persist for some months after patients stop wearing the nails [3].

Stomatitis has been blamed on incompletely cured acrylate in newly made or repaired dentures, and gingivo-stomatitis from acrylates in a temporary crown. Oral problems may arise in those previously sensitised to acrylic nails [4].

Investigations. Methyl acrylate is mainly used for acrylic fibres, ethyl acrylate for paint polymers and textiles and butyl acrylate and 2-ethylhexyl acrylate for paint polymers and adhesives. Methyl methacrylate (MMA) is probably the most used acrylic monomer. Poly-MMA is transparent glass-like material (Perspex) that is used, for example, in automotive lamps, signs and displays. MMA is also used for dental prostheses, bone cement and two-component floor coatings with epoxy hardeners. 2-Hydroxyethylmethacrylate (2-HEMA) is an important small monofunctional methacrylate. It is used in most UV-cured dental restorative materials together with ethyleneglycol dimethacrylate, a bifunctional methacrylate, and bisphenol A-glycidyl methacrylate (bis-GMA), an epoxy methacrylate. 2-HEMA is also used as a primer in UV-cured structure nails (gel nails) and gel nail polishes. 2-hydroxypropylmethacrylate has a chemical structure closely similar to 2-HEMA, and it is often present in anaerobic sealants. Hydroxyethyl acrylate and 2-hydroxypropyl acrylate are particularly used as cross-linking agents, for example in heat-cured paints and adhesives. Isobornyl acrylate occurs in many industrially used acrylic glues and in adhesives of medical devices such as insulin pump infusion sets and glucose sensors [5]. Cyanoacrylates are utilised as instant adhesives. Various 2-cyanoacrylates (e.g. 2-ethyl cyanoacrylate, octyl cyanoacrylate) are available for a wide field of applications. They are used in the electrical and electronics industries, as well as in many areas of mechanical engineering such as automobile, ship and aircraft construction. In addition, 2-cyanoacrylates are used in medicine to close wounds and glue artificial nails [6] and eye lash extensions. Cyanoacrylate-based adhesives are also used in some medical devices such as glucose sensors. Epoxy acrylates are formed when epoxy resins are reacted with acrylic acid or methacrylic acid. These composite resins are extensively used in dentistry, for example bis-GMA (also named epoxy dimethacrylate), 2,2-bis(4-(methacryl-oxyethoxy)phenyl) propane (bis-EMA) and 2,2-bis(4-(methacryloxy)phenyl) propane (bis-MA).

Allergen suppliers produce three methacrylate series aimed at the main sources of exposure: adhesives, nails and printing. In general, methacrylated monomers are tested at 2% in petrolatum and acrylated monomers at 0.1% in petrolatum. The lower 0.1% concentrations have reduced the incidence of the previously noted problem of active sensitisation [6]. Multiple positives may be seen if the full series is tested as a consequence of complex cross-reaction patterns. As a result of retrospective analyses shorter screening series have been suggested [7].

Cyanoacrylates are tested at 10% in petrolatum.

Sometimes, additives such as dimethyl-*p*-toluidine, benzoyl peroxide, hydroquinone, *p*-methoxyphenol, pyrogallol, resorcinol or pentaerythritol tetrakis 3-mercaptopropionate may elicit contact dermatitis.

Management. Once identified, avoidance should be possible by removal of the cause, redeployment, adequate protection or altered work practice. Acrylates penetrate latex and vinyl gloves [8]. The 4H multilayer glove (Safety 4, Denmark) [9] is the best protection, but may be impractical for some activities. Double gloving, polyethylene gloves and nitrile gloves are possible, but potentially less effective alternatives.

Education, instructions on handling, printed warning notices and 'good housekeeping' are important preventative measures.

Formaldehyde resins

Epidemiology. Phenol formaldehyde resins are polymers that are manufactured from various phenols and formaldehyde. The most widely used resins are based on phenol or PTBPFR. Apart from allergy associated with adhesives used in shoes and other leather products and nail varnish, formaldehyde resin allergy is uncommon. Many cases of phenol formaldehyde resin (PFR) allergy are sporadic. It is not a common occupational sensitiser although laminate manufacturers in Sweden were found to have a high frequency of allergy [1]. In a recent review, 17 cases of PFR allergy were seen in one clinic over a 15-year period. More common occupational associations were friction material (e.g. brake linings) production, work with fibreglass and contact with foundry sand [2]. The prevalence of contact allergy to PTBPFR in patch-tested patients seems to be decreasing: the prevalence in 2013–14 had halved compared with 2004 in a study of the ESSCA [3]. The literature includes consumer contact allergy to PTBPFR in a lower limb prosthesis [4], a neoprene orthopaedic knee brace [5] and athletic tapes [6]. In many instances it is difficult to find relevance for a positive patch test.

Clinical features. Dermatitis from formaldehyde resins in clothing, shoes and nail varnish is discussed in the relevant sections. In most other cases of PTBPFR allergy, dermatitis is localised under leather watchstraps and limb prostheses, although the hands may be affected by contact with glues in the working and domestic environments.

Investigations. PTBPFR patch testing is discussed in the section on shoes, amine formaldehyde resin in the section on clothing and tosylamide formaldehyde resin in the section on cosmetics. PFRs are variable in composition and allergenicity [7].

'Phenoplastics' are condensation products of formaldehyde and phenolic compounds, for example phenol, cresol, *p*-tertiary-butylphenol and resorcinol. There are two main types of PFR: resol (phenol reacted with excess formaldehyde in alkaline conditions) and novolac (formaldehyde reacted with excess phenol in acid conditions). The two types of PFR do not necessarily cross-sensitise and neither of them seems to cross-sensitise to any significant degree with PTBPFR.

A resol resin based on phenol and formaldehyde (PFR2) that is commercially available (1% pet.) is a good marker of contact allergy to various phenol formaldehyde resins.

However, testing with the patient's own resin at 1% and 5% in petrolatum, followed by testing controls if positive, is probably the most reliable method.

Management. Once identified, avoidance should be possible by removal of the cause, redeployment, adequate protection or altered work practice.

PFRs have electrical resistance and binding properties, resulting in their widespread use in electrical appliances, glues, laminated floorboards, plywood, fibreglass (including insulation), brake linings, clutch facings, grinding wheels, foundry sand moulds, abrasive cloths and papers, plastic moulds, telephones and steering wheels. Finished plastics are often brown or black and of the Bakelite type.

PTBPFR is used as an adhesive and is found in sealants and neoprene glues. Contact may occur directly following its use as a glue, particularly in shoemakers and cobblers. Other sources include furniture and upholstery glue and marking pen ink.

Amino formaldehyde resins occur in textiles, plywood and waterproof paper. They are also used for finishing parquet floors, gluing wood and in orthopaedic casts. Tosylamide formaldehyde resin was extensively used in nail varnish. Formaldehyde, which is continuously liberated from formaldehyde resins in floors and walls, may elicit contact dermatitis in very sensitive people.

Other plastics

Other plastics are rarely the cause of allergic contact dermatitis outside industry. Other resin systems, most notably unsaturated polyesters and their hardeners, and isocyanates in polyurethanes (PUs) may sensitise. Allergic contact dermatitis from isocyanate-based products occurs in work places where isocyanates or PU resins are manufactured and processed. Risk occupations include spray painting, floor coating, laboratory work, manufacture of PU paints and other PU products, motor vehicles and electronics as well as construction work.

Co-polymers are emerging as sensitisers in cosmetics, sunscreens and nail varnish [1]. Additives in cellulose acetate spectacle frames have caused dermatitis. The literature contains many case reports of allergens traced to specific products, for example spectacle frames [2], hearing aids, ballpoint pens and other plastic items. Other plastic additives such as plasticisers, antioxidants, UV light absorbers, initiators, cross-linking agents, flame retardants and pigments may sometimes sensitise during the manufacturing process or during use.

Plants [1–3]

Epidemiology. Plant life is exceedingly diverse, with much geographic and seasonal variation. Consequently, the range of reported allergens is huge, with considerable differences worldwide in incidence and prevalence of allergy. Here we concentrate only on those plant families frequently associated with contact allergy. Accurate statistics for the prevalence and incidence of plant allergy as a whole are not available but it has been estimated that 5–10% of all cases of contact allergy seen in European dermatology clinics are caused by plants or their products. These parameters vary from country to country and depend on the local flora and the population's way of life. Occupational dermatitis to plants is common in gardeners, horticulturists, florists, farmers, cooks, foresters, undertakers and people involved in food processing [4].

Approximately 50–60% of North Americans are sensitive to poison ivy and other members of the Anacardiaceae family. The main allergens found in the oleoresin (or urushiol) are derivatives of catechol, particularly pentadecylcatechols, phenol, resorcinol and salicylic acid. Cross-reactions occur with cashew nut oil, which may be used industrially in resins, mucilages, printers' inks and electrical insulation. Haitian voodoo dolls and swizzle sticks made from cashew nut shells have also sensitised. Further cross-sensitivity is found with mangoes, gingko tree fruit, indelible laundry marking ink from the marking nut tree in India, furniture lacquer from the Japanese lacquer tree, *Lithraea* trees in South America and trees of the *Grevillea* genus found in Australia. Although poison ivy is not a native European plant it has been reported to have been brought back from North America and planted. Isolated cases of contact sensitisation have been seen from this source. Localised outbreaks of dermatitis from contact with the Japanese lacquer tree have occurred in the UK.

English ivy (*Hedera helix*) is not related to poison ivy but is becoming increasingly recognised as a common and likely underdiagnosed cause of plant allergy [5]. The causative allergen in *H. helix* is thought to be falcarinol which unfortunately is not currently available as a commercial patch test allergen.

In Europe the Compositae (Asteraceae) family of plants is the most common cause of phytoallergic contact dermatitis. Compositae are one of the largest flowering plant families in the world, with over 25 000 species described, of which over 200 are reported to cause allergy. The family includes decorative plants (e.g. chrysanthemums, dahlias, sunflowers), weeds (e.g. ragweed, dandelion, tansy, marsh elder, feverfew, chamomile, yarrow, arnica, *Parthenium*) and foods (e.g. lettuce, endive, artichoke). Herbal teas, medicines and cosmetics commonly contain Compositae plants or extracts. The allergenic chemicals are sesquiterpene lactones (STLs), which are low molecular weight, highly reactive and chemically based on a common alpha-methylene-gamma-butyrolactone ring. STLs are also present in other plant families including Frullania (liver worts), Lauraceae and Magnoliaceae.

Garlic allergy is particularly frequent in Spain, with a prevalence of 2% in patch test clinics, mainly associated with domestic food preparation [6]. Other countries where garlic is used frequently in cooking might have a similar prevalence. In the UK, curry chefs are an at-risk group.

Tea tree oil (*Melaleuca alternifolia*) is being increasingly used in cosmetics and medicaments and has caused allergic reactions in adults and children [7,8].

Primin, found in *Primula obconica*, was in the past a significant cause of plant allergic contact dermatitis and was tested in the baseline series. The development of allergen-free *Primula* species has led to a significant fall in frequency of reactions such that it is now simply tested as part of a specialist plant series [9].

Clinical features. Anacardiaceae: *Toxicodendron* spp. dermatitis occurs after contact with the sap of the plant. Classically the rash is streaky, with redness, papules and vesiculobullous lesions on exposed sites. The hardened sap may leave a black spot on the skin in the areas of dermatitis and this may be helpful diagnostically [10]. Distant spread is common, particularly facial and genital involvement from contaminated hands. More profound erythema multiforme-like, exanthematous and urticarial eruptions, and even renal damage, may occur from systemic absorption. Stomatitis and proctitis have occurred after chewing the leaves, and with hyposensitisation. Contamination of clothing, animals, garden tools, firewood, fishing rods and golf clubs may also act as sources of contact. Phytophotodermatitis (Chapter 126) and allergy to *Primula* and other plants has to be considered in the differential diagnosis. Plants from this family have caused more contact allergy than all other plants combined. Much of this sensitisation relates to poison ivy, sumac and oak, which are species of *Toxicodendron* found extensively in North America. The plants are generally found outdoors and are recognised by their three-leafed configuration. Their diverse morphology and various habitats have been described by Guin *et al.* [11].

Compositae (Asteraceae): a recent Danish review of patients monosensitised to Compositae reported the majority to present with hand dermatitis, classically in a vesicular, volar pattern. It was noted that localised dermatitis may progress, with continued allergen exposure, to a classic airborne or generalised Compositae dermatitis pattern [12]. Eight patterns of dermatitis are described, which are generally worse during the summer months in temperate climates [13].

1 *Pseudophotodermatitis*. Exposed sites are involved, including both eyelids, and photoprotected areas under the chin and behind the ears. In hot regions, during summer months, dry dead plant material contributes to the airborne pattern of dermatitis. In the USA, many Compositae weeds, including ragweed (*Ambrosia* spp.), induce this pattern of dermatitis, almost exclusively in males. A similar pattern is seen in Europe from Compositae flowers and weeds, in India from *Parthenium hysterophorus* and in Australia, where it is known as bush dermatitis. Chronic cases may produce a marked thickening of the facial skin – a leonine facies. Photosensitivity quite commonly coexists with Compositae allergy (Figure 127.34). In one UK study, 22% of the Compositae-allergic patients were also photosensitive. True photoallergy to Compositae is, however, generally not a feature.

2 *Atopic eczema-like*. Compositae allergy may mimic late-onset atopic eczema, with a flexural accentuation of involvement, which may include the groins and genital area.

3 *Erythrodermatous exfoliative*. This pattern is classically seen from the weed *P. hysterophorus*, which was transported to India from the USA in contaminated seed wheat. Unfortunately, the weed has spread over much of the subcontinent, including urban areas. It has become markedly allergenic in these environmental conditions, which also enhance the spread of dry plant dust and pollen. Severe incapacity and even fatalities have resulted from *Parthenium* dermatitis.

4 *Hand eczema*. This pattern is seen particularly in gardeners after contact with weeds. A palmar distribution often predominates. Dermatitis of the hands is also associated with handling lettuce.

5 *Localised dermatitis*. Dermatitis may be confined to one or more localised areas, although this pattern is unusual in our experience. Facial dermatitis has occurred from steaming chamomile tea, and hand and arm dermatitis from herbal compresses.

6 *Oral*. Oral swelling and soreness after eating lettuce has been reported in sensitised persons [14].

7 *Erythema multiforme*. This has been reported when it recurred after patch testing [15].

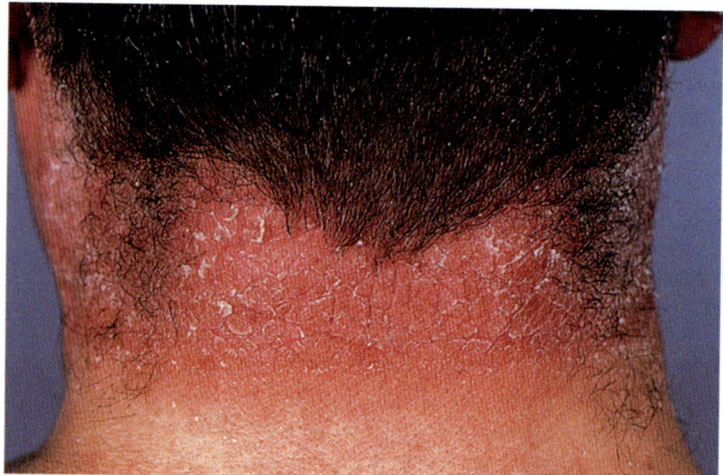

Figure 127.34 Photosensitive eczema in a patient also allergic to Compositae (sesquiterpene lactones). A similar pattern may be seen in woodcutters sensitive to lichens, and in others with photosensitive eczema, including photocontact allergy. Courtesy of Dr J. D. Wilkinson.

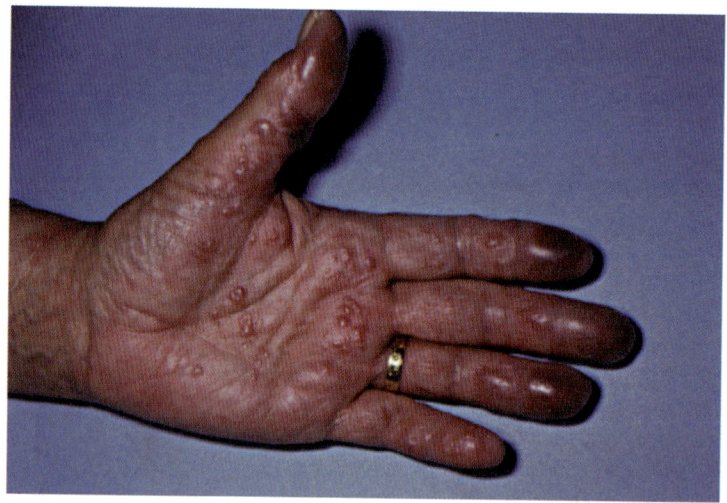

Figure 127.35 Haemorrhagic blisters on the palm from *Primula* allergy.

8 *Systemic*. Oral swelling, perianal pruritus and dermatitis of the trunk and arms have been reported after a sensitised subject drank chamomile tea [16]. A recent experiment giving chamomile tea to known STL-positive patients however failed to demonstrate induction of systemic allergic dermatitis [17].

Primulaceae: the classic appearance of *Primula* allergy is linear papulovesicles, oedema and blisters, which may be haemorrhagic, on the palms, dorsa of the hands and forearms (Figures 127.35). Transfer of the allergen via the fingers to the face, or more widely, is common. In some patients palpebral oedema is the presenting feature, but half of cases have other patterns, and the diagnosis is easily missed unless the possibility of *Primula* dermatitis is kept in mind. Misdiagnoses include constitutional pompholyx, urticaria or recurrent angioedema and disseminated herpes simplex. Erythema multiforme, a lichen planus-like eruption and toxic erythema as a result of *Primula* allergy can also cause diagnostic difficulty. *Primula obconica* is the most important allergenic plant, although other *Primula* species may also cause allergic contact dermatitis [18]. *P. obconica* is a decorative indoor plant. Contact occurs particularly when dead leaves and plant heads are removed manually. Primin levels are at their highest between April and August. Primin-free strains have now been developed [19] and allergy rates have dropped significantly [9].

Alstroemeriaceae and Liliaceae: dermatitis from tulip bulbs may cause a painful, dry, fissured and hyperkeratotic allergic dermatitis, at first underneath the free margins of the nails and then on the fingertips. Tulips are members of the Liliaceae family, and dermatitis is a particular risk for bulb collectors, sorters and packers, as well as florists. A similar pattern of dermatitis is seen in florists sensitised to *Alstroemeria*, and this may be followed by depigmentation. *Alstroemeria* (Peruvian lily) is a highly decorative plant commonly displayed as a spray with other flowers. The damaged plant's sap is allergenic to florists when the stems are wired and leaves stripped, in preparation for making the spray [20].

Alliaceae: garlic and onion are both members of this family and may sensitise, but do not seem commonly to cross-sensitise mutually. Classically there is fingertip involvement in those allergic to garlic (see Figure 127.6) and onion. This may preferentially affect the non-dominant hand, as this is the one that holds the vegetable while it is being cut with an implement held by the dominant hand. Cheilitis and photoallergic contact dermatitis have also been reported [21]. Systemic contact allergy, including pompholyx, caused by ingestion of garlic has been described [22].

Lichens and liverworts: a pattern similar to pseudophotodermatitis from Compositae has been seen in woodcutters' dermatitis caused by sensitivity to lichens and liverworts. Erythroderma may ensue in severe cases. Even walking through a forest may cause an exposed-site pattern of dermatitis in sensitised individuals [23]. Lichens consist of a fungus and an alga. They are found on trees, rocks, roofs and walls. Forestry workers, gardeners, lichen pickers and woodcutters are particularly liable to come in contact with them. Liverworts (Frullania) are small red-brown plants often growing with lichens and mosses.

Hedera helix (common ivy): *H. helix* allergy classically causes a vesiculobullous streaky eruption on exposed areas of skin, typically the hands and forearms. Dramatic facial swelling and progression to widespread dermatitis can occur. The blisters have led to misdiagnosis as disseminated herpes simplex infection. Associated allergy to carrot, parsley and celery, which also contain the allergen falcarinol, is reported. *H. helix* is also a recognised cause of contact urticaria [24].

Investigations. Specific allergen mixes have been developed to investigate Compositae allergy. Sesquiterpene lactone mix (SLM) contains alantolactone 0.033%, dehydrocostus lactone 0.033% and costunolide 0.033% emulsified with sorbitan sesquioleate. SLM is reported to detect only between 35% and 65% of Compositae sensitised patients [25]. Dandelion allergy may be missed by the SLM patch test [26]. An alternative 'Compositae mix' was developed consisting of a combination of arnica, yarrow, tansy, German chamomile and feverfew extracts with a higher detection rate than SLM. The initial Compositae mix I at 6% was, however, thought to yield false positive reactions and to cause active sensitisation [27]. Compositae mix II, containing extracts of Roman chamomile, German chamomile, yarrow, tansy, arnica and parthenolide, was then developed at 5% and a screening version at 2.5% [28]. Additional individual testing with parthenolide 0.1% is thought to increase pick-up rates by 10%. Individual extracts are suggested for testing if Compositae allergy is suspected. SLM and Compositae mix II 2.5% are both part of the current British baseline series.

Diallyl disulphide, the main allergen in garlic, is tested at 1% in petrolatum, and α-methylene-γ-butyrolactone (tulipalin A), the allergen in tulips and *Alstroemeria*, is tested at 0.01% in petrolatum.

Oak moss (*Evernia prunastri*) and other tree mosses are perfume ingredients derived from lichens. Chloroatranol and atranol are the main allergens [29]. They are common components of perfumed materials. Other allergenic components include atranornin, usnic acid and evernic acid. Lichen acid mix consists of atranornin, usnic acid and evernic acid, each at 0.1% in petrolatum. The allergens in liverworts are sesquiterpene lactones, explaining their cross reactivity with Compositae.

Oxidised tea tree oil is available at 5% but recent work suggests that 10% may be the concentration of choice [8]. Tea tree has been added to the updated recommended British facial/cosmetic allergen series [30].

Primin is the major allergen in *Primula obconica*. It is a quinone found in the tiny breakable hairs on the leaves, stem and flowers of the plant; however, it may occasionally fail to detect *Primula* allergy [31] as another potential allergen is miconidin [32]. The allergen in other *Primula* species is more likely to be miconidin. Allergy to *P. auicular* and *P. dendiculata* may need to be tested using a leaf. The diminishing number of cases of allergy has led to primin being removed from the standard series.

Where commercial preparations are not available, fresh plant extracts, preferably of known concentration, can be used for patch testing. Dipping the plant in diethyl ether for 60–90 s, evaporating to dryness and resuspending in petrolatum (1–10%) is a suggested method, although there are many alternative approaches [33]. Patch testing with fresh plant materials carries a risk of false positive irritant reactions and active sensitisation. Multiple tests with plants and plant allergens could lead to the development of an 'angry back' and subsequent false positive reactions to other allergens. Ideally, before patch testing with a plant, it should be identified. If it is a known irritant then testing may not be advisable. A textbook on plant dermatitis is a useful reference source. Several parts of one plant may contain the same allergen, in which case 1 cm^2 of leaf bruised gently with an orange stick may be sufficient for patch testing. Sometimes, however, the allergen is concentrated in one organ of the plant (e.g. orange peel, cinnamon bark) or the concentration of the allergen may vary from one part to another. When testing with unknown plants, several parts should be tested. Half of the material should be kept in a refrigerator for later botanical identification. Any plant that has given positive allergic reactions should be properly identified by its Linnaean name. In order to prevent registration of irritant tests, control testing with plants and their extracts is important.

Management. Patients who know of their sensitivity may manage to avoid further contact if taught to recognise the plants to which they are allergic. This is fairly straightforward for *Primula obconica*, *Alstroemeria*, tulips, Alliaceae, lichens and liverworts. In North America the recognition of *Toxicodendron* spp. is particularly important. Although the classic three-lobed leaves are a helpful feature, clusters of five or more leaves can occur. As there is considerable regional variability in the morphology of these species, it is preferable that sensitised persons become familiar with the appearance of *Toxicodendron* spp. in their own region. *Toxicodendron* oleoresin may remain under the fingernails and on the clothes, resulting in continuing problems. Detergents, soap and water will inactivate the residual unreacted allergen. After exposure, thorough washing of the hands, fingers and the rest of the body should be carried out as soon as possible, ideally within 10 min. Clothes should be changed. Contaminated tools and clothing, including shoes, should be washed in detergent. Specific creams, containing quaternium-18 bentonite and other barriers, have been developed and these may help prophylactically to a varying but incomplete extent [34,35]. Heavy-duty vinyl gloves afford better protection than rubber gloves.

Patients should be made aware that tulipalin A, in tulips and alstroemeria, penetrates vinyl gloves. Nitrile gloves are more satisfactory for handling bulbs and the plants [36]. Diallyl disulphide in garlic penetrates most glove materials [37].

Seasonal Compositae exposure may be difficult to avoid. Severe Compositae allergy may necessitate changing occupation (e.g. florists, gardeners) or avoiding pastimes such as flower arranging and gardening. It may be necessary to avoid handling lettuce, chicory, artichokes and endives in food preparation. Compositae-allergic patients should also be reminded to avoid personal care products with added plant extracts and to think of unusual sources such as handling plants to feed pets such as rabbits and guinea pigs. Those with associated photosensitivity may have significant problems over the summer months requiring a high-protection broad spectrum sunscreen. Where contact with *Toxicodendron* spp. and certain Compositae such as ragweed is unavoidable (e.g. outdoor workers), hyposensitisation has been attempted, with limited success. There is a risk of unpleasant side effects, including extensive skin eruptions and perianal dermatitis [38]. This treatment does not have the approval of the Food and Drug Administration in the USA.

Those sensitised to lichens may also be allergic to certain perfumes, particularly those containing oak moss (*Evernia prunastri*) or tree moss (*E. furfuracea*). Perfume avoidance advice may also have to be followed.

Woods, colophony, turpentine and propolis [1,2,3]

Epidemiology. The incidence and prevalence of wood allergy is unknown, but it is most commonly reported as an occupational allergen, for example in woodworkers, carpenters and wooden floor layers. Occupational allergic contact dermatitis is more frequently associated with hardwoods, especially among cabinet makers, carpenters and instrument makers. Some tropical hardwoods are especially allergenic. In many instances the precise allergens are not known, but some have been identified. Chemically, these include quinones (including dalbergiones and lapachol), phenols, terpenes, stilbenes and anthothecol. Softwoods, apart from pines and other conifers, are not commonly associated with contact allergy.

Colophony (syn. colophonium or rosin) is a resin derived from softwood coniferous trees. It is a common contact allergen with a prevalence of 2–6% in patch-tested populations. Colophony has significant industrial applications in the manufacture of paper, inks and adhesives, as well as ubiquitous domestic uses in cosmetics, sticky tapes, dressings, polish and tall oil soap. It is both an important occupational and non-occupational allergen [4]. Turpentine is a natural oil derived from spruce and pine trees, often used as a solvent. Its use in industry has now mainly been replaced by petroleum-based white spirit and allergy prevalence rates have dropped significantly. Propolis (bee glue) is a natural substance produced by honeybees, derived from resinous plant materials, in particular poplar trees. It was traditionally an occupational allergen of beekeepers but now is a common domestic allergen as is added to many 'natural' and 'herbal' cosmetics, lozenges, creams and pharmaceutical products. The reported frequency of propolis allergy in patch-tested patients has varied significantly between centres from 1.2% to 6.6% [5].

Clinical features. Most cases of wood allergy present in the occupational setting and are related to contact with airborne sawdust [6]. The pattern of dermatitis therefore affects exposed sites, with the scalp of bald men being typically involved. Differentiation from a photosensitive eczema may be difficult, but light-protected sites (e.g. under the chin, behind the ears) are more likely to be equally affected in wood dermatitis. However, sawdust can gain access inside clothing to produce dermatitis predominating in the flexures. Genital involvement is a particular feature, in part from transfer of allergens during urination. Severe erythema multiforme-like eruptions have been described, particularly caused by *Machaerium scleroxylon* allergy [7]. Localised dermatitis may occur under contact with exotic hardwoods, for example from a violin chin-rest or wooden adornments and utensils [8]. A classic linear dermatitis on the dorsal, upper thigh or circular buttock distribution has been noted due to the repopularisation of wooden toilet seats (Figure 127.36) [9].

Colophony allergy may present in many ways because it is ubiquitous. Over 300 potential allergenic colophony sources have been identified. An exposed-site pattern may be seen after machining pine and cutting down branches when gardening. Sensitivity to

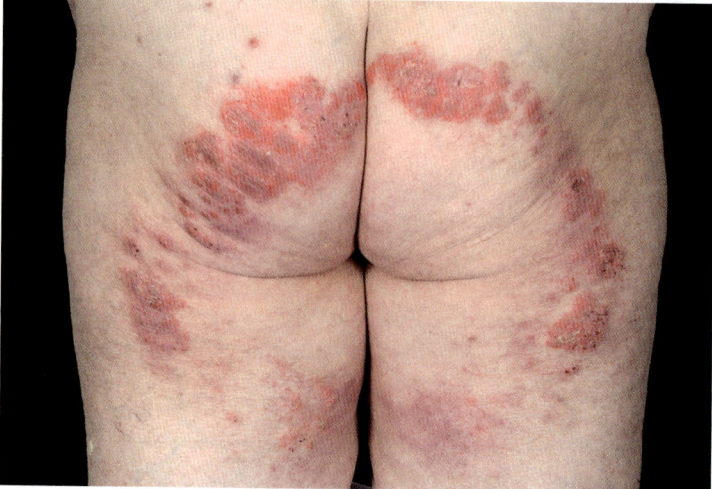

Figure 127.36 Allergic contact dermatitis from a hardwood toilet seat. Courtesy of Dr N. Stone.

Cupressocyparis leylandii trees have been associated with concomitant colophony allergy. Allergy to colophony in solder fumes can give a similar exposed-site distribution, or dermatitis may be confined to the face. Other sources for an exposed-site pattern have included linoleum flooring, paper dust and floor polish [10].

Localised facial and eye dermatitis can develop from contact with colophony-containing cosmetics, particularly mascara [11]. Reactions to sticky tapes and plasters, and colophony-containing medicaments, are often confined to the site of application, but secondary spread may be a feature from allergy to both colophony and colophony derivatives (e.g. ester gum resin) used as adhesives for lower leg dressings. This may be confused with varicose eczema and secondary medicament sensitisation [12]. Adhesive plasters are sometimes used to cover painful fissures on the hands and feet. These may have been caused by a pre-existing eczema or psoriasis, which may consequently be perpetuated or exacerbated by colophony allergy. Adhesive depilatory strips may contain colophony or derivatives and cause localised dermatitis [13], as may topical colophony-containing medicaments, including wart treatments or sanitary pads.

Colophony may induce hand dermatitis due to contact with a diverse range of colophony-containing materials such as glues, polishes, paper, rosin, antislip powders, topical medicaments, waxes and tall oils in metal-machining coolants. Perioral dermatitis and cheilitis have been related to colophony in chewing gum. Dental materials, including floss, fluoride varnish, dressings and impression materials, may contain colophony, but rarely sensitise in the mouth. A case of widespread dermatitis has been recorded after dental treatment in an allergic individual. Colophony can also be present in adhesives in footwear. It has also been incorporated, in a modified form, in footwear in an impregnated cloth.

Propolis-sensitised beekeepers may develop problems on the face and around the eyes. Allergy to propolis in cosmetics and medicaments is manifest at their sites of application. Ingestion of propolis has been reported to cause stomatitis due to propolis candy, cheilitis from propolis chewing gum and also fixed drug eruption [14,15]. An erythema multiforme-pattern of propolis delayed allergy is also reported [16].

Investigations. Woods are normally of two types, hard and soft. The same woods may have many different names, and sometimes an incorrect name is mistakenly or deliberately applied. The situation is complicated further by the occasional introduction of 'rogue' timbers into batches of hardwoods. The most common allergenic woods are listed in Table 127.10.

Patch testing with freshly made, uncontaminated sawdust 10% in petrolatum is recommended but may carry the risk of false positive and false negative patch tests, and active sensitisation. Apparent allergic-positive reactions should only be confirmed after testing on controls. It is advisable to ask the patient to bring a piece of unmachined wood at the same time as the sawdust. If a positive allergic reaction develops, the piece can be sent to a wood anatomist who may be able to correctly identify the wood. If the allergen for that wood is known, it is sometimes possible to patch test with it at the appropriate concentration, however most wood allergens are not commercially available.

Pine trees are the source of two significant allergenic materials, colophony and turpentine. Turpentine is the balsam from species of *Pinus*. Oil of turpentine is the volatile oil distilled from this balsam. Swedish and Finnish turpentine is made in the processing of paper pulp from wood. Venice turpentine is the balsam from larch trees. Colophony is the non-volatile part of the balsam and is known as gum rosin.

Colophony is also extracted as a distillate from pine tree stumps, when it is known as wood rosin, and as a by-product of pulping pine wood, known as tall oil rosin. As a natural product the specific chemical composition varies according to geographic source, production method and storage conditions. It is composed of approximately 90% resin acids and 10% neutral substances. Auto-oxidation products of abietic and dehydroabietic acids, including peroxides, hydroperoxides, epoxides and ketones, have all been proposed as allergens. The most potent allergen has been shown to be 15-hydroperoxyabietic acid. Colophony may also be modified, altering its allergenicity with the development of new allergens [17,18]. Maleopimaric acid and glyceryl monoabietate have been identified as allergens in modified colophony rosins.

Colophony is a standard allergen tested at 20% in petrolatum. A mixture of Chinese and Portuguese gum rosin is presently used in the commercial patch test allergen. The allergen profile may, of course, differ according to the specific source of the colophony; particularly if it has been modified, and consequently false negative reactions can occur. Where modified colophony allergy is suspected a wider series of patch tests should be considered, for example additionally testing ester gum resin, Granuflex®, as well as the suspected product [19].

The major sensitiser in turpentine is the hydroperoxide of Δ3-carene, which is also an auto-oxidation product. Swedish and Finnish turpentine contains more of this substance than, for example, French and American turpentine. Turpentine oil is tested at 10% in petrolatum. Oxidised limonene (D or L) and pinene (α or β) can also sensitise [20]. The term 'mineral turpentine' is used for the non-sensitising, but irritant, white spirit that is a petroleum product. Turpentine was in the past a standard patch test allergen, but allergy rates have fallen, mainly due to its replacement by industry with the petroleum product white spirit.

Propolis is patch tested at 10% in petrolatum. It may also be found contaminating beeswax [21]. The allergens include caffeates and benzyl isoferulate [22].

Lichens, liverworts and sensitising plants may cause allergic sensitisation by virtue of their coexistence with trees. Additives to wood such as varnishes, dyes, glues or preservatives may also sensitise at work.

Management. A demonstration of allergy to a wood should be followed by anatomical confirmation of its botanical name and, ideally, by testing with the known allergen(s) for that wood. Subsequent avoidance of the wood and related timbers may be necessary.

Table 127.10 Principal timbers causing dermatitis.[a]

Botanical name	Common name[b]	Origin	Uses
Apocynaceae			
Dyera costulata	Jelutong	South-East Asia	Model making
			Woodwork teaching
Boraginaceae			
Cordia gerascanthus R. Br.	Canalete	Venezuela	Furniture
			Interior construction
			Joinery
Cordia goeldiana Huber	Freijo	Brazil	Boat building
	Frei jorge		Furniture
			Interior construction
			Joinery
Cordia millenii Baker	Cordia	West Africa	Furniture
			Interior construction
			Joinery
Cordia platythyrsa Baker	Cordia	West Africa	Furniture
			Interior construction
			Joinery
Cupressaceae			
Calocedrus decurrens (Torrey) Florin	Incense cedar	USA	Fence posts
			Furniture
			Interior construction
			Pencils
Cupressocyparis leylandii	Leyland cypress	Temperate	Garden shrub
			Hedges
Thuja plicata Donn ex D. Don	Western red cedar Arbor vitae	USA	Boat building
			Construction
Ebenaceae			
Diospyros celebica Bakh.	Macassar	Indonesia	Cabinet and inlay work
			Musical instruments
			Rulers
Diospyros crassifolia Hiern	African ebony	Africa	Cabinet and inlay work
			Musical instruments
Diospyros ebenum Koenig	Ceylon ebony	Sri Lanka, India, Indonesia	Cabinet and inlay work
	East Indian ebony		Musical instruments
Diospyros melanoxylon Roxb.	Coromandel	Sri Lanka, India, Indonesia	Cabinet and inlay work
			Musical instruments
Leguminosae			
Caesalpiniaceae			
Distemonanthus benthamianus Baillon	Ayan	West Africa	Coffins
	Movingui		Floors
	Nigerian satinwood		Furniture
			Window frames
Mimosaceae			
Acacia melanoxylon R. Br.	Australian blackwood	Western Australia	Boat building
			Construction
			Furniture
			Musical instruments
Papilionaceae			
Bowdichia nitida Spruce ex Benth.	Sucupira	Brazil	Construction
			Floors
			Furniture
Brya ebenus	Cocus	West Indies	Handles
	Jamaica ebony		Musical instruments
			Plates
Dalbergia iatifolia Roxb.	East Indian rosewood	India, Indonesia	Furniture
	Bombay blackwood Sissoo		Handles
			Musical instruments
			Veneers
			Wooden jewellery
Dalbergia melanoxylon Guillemin & Perrottet	African blackwood	Africa	Handles
	Grenadil		Musical instruments

(continued)

Table 127.10 (continued)

Botanical name	Common name[b]	Origin	Uses
Dalbergia nigra All.	Brazilian rosewood Rio-Palisander Grenadilla Jacaranda	Brazil	Furniture Handles Musical instruments Veneers Wooden jewellery
Dalbergia retusa Hemsley	Cocobolo	Central America	Handles Scientific instruments Wooden jewellery
Machaerium scleroxylon Tul.	Pao ferro Santos palisander Caviuna vermelha	Brazil	Furniture Handles Veneers
Pterocarpus soyauxii Taub.	Red African padauk	West Africa	Furniture Handles Musical Instruments Veneers
Malvaceae (L.) Sol.			
Thespesia populnea (L.) Sol.	Milowood	USA	Bracelets Carved utensils Furniture
Meliaceae			
Khaya anthotheca C. DC	African mahogany Krala	West Africa	Furniture
Khaya grandiflora DC	Big leaf mahogany	West Africa	Furniture
Khaya ivorensis A. Chev.	Khaya mahogany	West Africa	Furniture
Khaya senegalensis (Desr.) A. Juss.	Dry zone mahogany	West Africa	Furniture
Moraceae			
Chlorophora excelsa Benth. & Hook.	Iroko Kambala African teak	West Africa	Construction Laboratory benches Shipbuilding
Pinaceae			
Picea spp.	Spruce Fir	Northern temperate areas	Construction Furniture General
Pinus spp.	Pine	Northern temperate areas	Construction Furniture General
Proteaceae			
Grevillea robusta Cunn. ex R. Br.	Australian silky oak	Australia (planted elsewhere)	Floors Furniture Plywood Telegraph poles
Sterculiaceae			
Mansonia altissima A. Chev.	Mansonia African black walnut Bété	West Africa	Furniture Walnut substitute
Verbenaceae			
Tectona grandis L.	Teak	India, South-East Asia	Construction Floors Furniture Shipbuilding

Adapted from Hausen 1981 [1].
[a] Lichens on the wood may also sensitise.
[b] There is no accepted international nomenclature.

Detection of the origin of colophony allergy requires careful appraisal of potential sources. The most common sources of colophony and its modifications are identified in Box 127.7. The use of traditional sticking plasters should be replaced by 'hypoallergenic' tapes. Insulating tapes may also contain colophony, as may certain adhesive leg ulcer dressings. Contact with pine and other coniferous trees, and probably *Cupressocyparis leylandii*, should be avoided. In those with extreme sensitivity, felling and removing the offending trees may be necessary. Occupationally, it may be possible to change the allergenic product to an alternative.

Box 127.7 Sources of colophony

- Adhesive dressings
- Adhesive plasters and tapes
- Balms and salves
- Chewing gum
- Clear and brown soaps
- Cosmetics (eye shadow, mascara)
- Dental dressings
- Depilatory strips
- Flypaper
- Glues, adhesives and sealants
- Herbal medicaments
- Insulating and jointing tapes
- Linoleum
- Metalworking fluids (tall oils)
- Ostomy appliances
- Paper
- Pine trees and wood
- Printing inks
- Rosin (grip/antislip materials)
- Shoe adhesives and counters
- Shoe and floor polishes
- Solder flux
- Spruce trees and wood
- Varnishes and coatings
- Wart treatments
- Wood wool

Colophony and derivatives can be identified in fully ingredient-labelled cosmetics. The INCI term colophonium is used. Derivatives that may be used in cosmetics include abietic acid, hydroabietic acid and hydroabietyl alcohol. Transparent colophony-containing soap should be avoided for washing. Wart paints incorporating collodion should also be avoided, along with colophony-containing topical medicaments and balms. Colophony allergy from paper has been implicated in hand dermatitis, and the use of cotton gloves is suggested if this is a possibility [23]. However, the list of potential exposures is so extensive that it will often be a case of establishing whether any of the sources identified in Box 127.7 are relevant and tailoring avoidance advice accordingly.

Turpentine substitutes are now readily available for sensitised subjects. Turpentine is present in balsams and sawdust from pine and spruce. It was used as an industrial solvent but has now largely been replaced by petroleum derivatives and D-limonene. It is still used by artists and in ceramic decoration. In certain producing countries such as Spain and Portugal, turpentine is still more widely used than elsewhere, and it remains a common allergen there. In the USA it is still commonly used as a paint remover.

Propolis is encountered not only by beekeepers but also in both systemic and topically applied agents used in 'natural' products from health food stores and mainstream cosmetic outlets. Solid propolis can be chewed. Propolis may also contaminate beeswax (cera alba) and is used in cosmetic and pharmaceutical products, as well as a food additive (E901), coating for sweets, in candles and as a varnish [24]. Beeswax may be allergenic in its own right [25]. Propolis-sensitive patients should ideally avoid both propolis and beeswax as a precaution.

Photoallergic contact dermatitis

Definition and nomenclature

Photoallergic contact dermatitis (PACD) is a classic type IV cell-mediated hypersensitivity reaction of the skin in response to a hapten in a person who has been previously been sensitised to the same chemical or one that cross-reacts with it. The hapten is produced following UV exposure, resulting in a photoactivated chemical or a photoproduct.

Synonyms and inclusions
- Photoallergy
- Photoallergic contact eczema

Introduction and general description

Photocontact dermatitis can be divided into photoallergic and phototoxic (irritant) dermatitis. In both cases exposure to the causative chemical and light energy are required to cause the reaction. In line with allergic and irritant contact dermatitis, PACD is much less common than phototoxic (irritant) dermatitis. PACD is a delayed type IV hypersensitivity reaction requiring prior exposure to the photoallergen for sensitisation. Many chemicals can cause both PACD as well as phototoxic reactions. Clinically distinguishing between the two can be difficult but clues from the history and examination are described. PACD requires photopatch testing for diagnosis.

Photoallergens are most commonly chemicals that absorb UV light, such as sunscreen chemicals and topical NSAIDs. Both topically applied and systemic drugs can produce photoallergic reactions. Systemic reactions are reviewed elsewhere, with this section focusing on photoallergic reactions from topical agents.

Historically the first significant recognised problems from photoallergy were related to the use of chlorinated salicylanilides in germicidal soaps in the early 1960s, with many thousands of individuals affected. Regulatory elimination of these photoallergens resulted in the disappearance of the allergy, but some affected individuals developed long-term photosensitivity known as 'persistent light reactors' [1]. By the mid-1980s the most important photoallergen was the fragrance musk ambrette. It was used in men's aftershave lotions and colognes and caused a characteristic patchy pattern of facial photosensitive dermatitis. Use of musk ambrette is now prohibited [2]. Since the 1990s and 2000s sunscreen chemicals and topical NSAIDs are now the current leading causes of PACD.

Epidemiology

Incidence and prevalence

The incidence of PACD is not known but it is thought to be uncommon. It is estimated to affect between 2% and 10% of patients referred with exposed-site dermatitis [3]. The 2012 European Multicentre Photopatch Test Study (EMCPPTS) expanded the number of screened photoallergens and reported PACD reactions in 200 (19.4%) of the 1031 patients tested [4]. A follow-on, single centre, retrospective study from Spain reported PACD reactions in 27% of patients tested with the European recommended photoallergen series [5]. Photopatch testing is not as readily available as standard patch testing and it therefore may be that PACD is a relatively underdiagnosed condition.

Age
There is no particular age group associated with PACD but it is noted to be occurring in increasingly younger patients. This is thought to be due to the rising use of sunscreens in children to reduce sun-induced skin damage [6]. Contact allergy to octocrylene has been particularly associated with paediatric sunscreens.

Ethnicity
Sunscreen use is greater in individuals with Fitzpatrick type I and II skin, making sunscreen PACD more common in lighter skinned ethnic groups.

Associated diseases
Patients with photosensitive disorders require the long-term, regular use of sunscreen are therefore considered to be at increased risk of developing PACD. Investigation with photopatch testing is important in this patient group. The EMCPPTS suggested that, in particular, patients with chronic actinic dermatitis were at increased risk of concomitant PACD to sunscreen chemicals [4].

Pathophysiology
The basic mechanisms of photosensitisation have been reviewed by Thune [7]. The initial phase of all photoreactions is dependent upon absorption of photons by light-sensitive chemicals. Following absorption, a higher state of energy (excited state) is induced in the molecule (photoactivation). Some of the energy may be released as fluorescence – that is emission of radiation at a longer wavelength. Alternatively, there may be phosphorescence, heat or other energy transfer to another molecule, or photochemical alteration of the molecule [8].

Photoactivation is a physical phenomenon and may occur *in vitro*. When it occurs *in vivo* the activation may have a phototoxic (non-immunological) or photoallergic (immunological) action. The photoactivated molecules may be transformed into new substances capable of acting as irritants or haptens. Photoallergic reactions are based on immunological mechanisms, and can be provoked by UV radiation only in a small number of individuals who have been sensitised by previous exposure to the photosensitiser. The reaction to a photoallergen is based on the same immunological mechanism as contact allergic reactions. In guinea pigs the sensitivity can be transferred with mononuclear cells [9]. The action spectrum for photoallergy is generally in the UVA range but some elicit reactions in both the UVA and UVB range, as is the case with diphenhydramine hydrochloride and NSAIDs [10].

Newly formed haptens may, by virtue of the excited state and free radical formation, be able to combine chemically with other substances, for example proteins, to produce a complete antigen. The photoallergen tribromosalicylanilide has been shown to change into dibromosalicylanilide and monobromosalicylanilide [11], and with sulphonamides it has been suggested that an oxidation product is formed [12]. Some photosensitisers may, in the presence of UV radiation, produce only short-lived reactive molecules [13]. The duration of the response to light irradiation after stopping the application of a known photoallergen is variable and depends on the photoallergen.

In sunscreens, for example, it is probably less than 4–6 days [14]. However, NSAIDs such as ketoprofen may cause subjects to react to sunlight up to several weeks after stopping its local application. This is most probably due to retention of the molecule in the epidermis [15].

Several photoallergic substances simultaneously produce phototoxic reactions when applied in high concentrations and with a sufficient amount and type of radiation. Thus, in an individual case, the two reactions may be clinically indistinguishable.

Pathology
The histological changes are identical to those of other forms of contact dermatitis.

Environmental factors
Photoallergic contact dermatitis will only occur in the event of exposure to potential photoallergens in the environment. In the present era, UV-absorbing chemical filters and topical NSAIDs are the main substances causing clinical photoallergic problems. In the EMCPPTS of 1031 'exposed site dermatitis' patients, PACD was most commonly caused by the topical NSAIDs ketoprofen (128 subjects) and etofenomate (59 subjects). Octocrylene, benzophenone-3 and butylmethoxydibenzoylmethane were the most common organic sunscreen chemicals to cause PACD [4]. The newer organic sunscreen chemicals, with larger molecular weights, showed very few reactions. This was suggested to perhaps be due to their reduced ability to penetrate the stratum corneum.

UV filters are encountered in the environment not only in sun protection products but also in personal care products such as face creams, shampoos and hairsprays. Their presence in cosmetics may be aimed to prolong shelf-life and/or to support 'antiageing' claims for the product. Shampoos and conditioners marketed as 'colour protect' often contain benzophenones, designed to reduce photodegradation of the consumer's dyed hair. Sunscreen chemicals have also been found added to miscellaneous rubber and plastic items. PACD to benzophenone-10 within plastic swimming goggles and in three cases to benzophenones within plastic wrist bands have recently been reported [16,17]. Of note the three cases of wrist band PACD all occurred in teenagers who had previously been sensitised to a topical ketoprofen-impregnated tape. Ketoprofen is the most frequently reported topical NSAID cause of PACD. Ketoprofen may cross-sensitise with the UV filter benzophenone-3 and octocrylene (Figure 127.37) [18]. Connubial cases of ketoprofen allergy have been reported [19].

Other groups of topical photocontact allergens have been identified with varying degrees of confirmatory evidence, and are summarised below:

- Fragrance chemicals: musk ambrette and 6-methyl coumarin, although now prohibited in Europe and the USA, caused significant problems in the 1980s. These products have now virtually disappeared. Lavender PACD is also reported [20].
- Halogenated salicylanilides: tribromosalicylanilide and tetrachlorosalicylanilide, used as antibacterials in soaps and detergents, caused many outbreaks of photosensitive eczema in the 1960s [1]. Fentichlor (bis(2-hydroxy-5-chlorphenyl)sulphide and bromosalicylchloranilide) is used as a topical antifungal agent

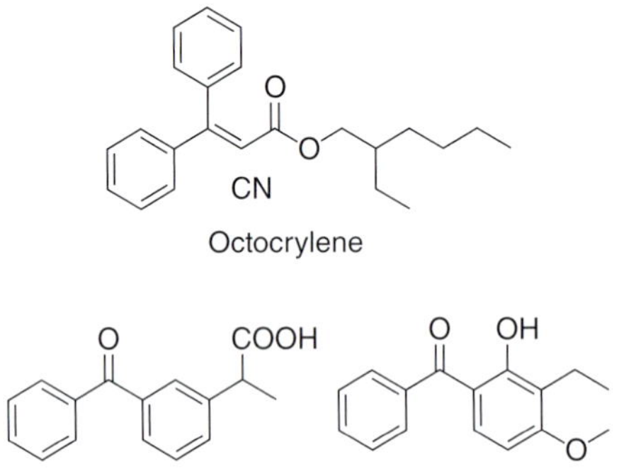

Figure 127.37 Structures of cross-reacting photoallergens. Adapted from Karlsson et al. 2011 [18].

in Australia and is used domestically in Sweden. It is a known photosensitiser.
- Phenothiazines: tranquillisers causing occupational dermatitis in hospital personnel, topical antihistamines and insecticides. Examples include topical promethazine, oral promazine and oral chlorpromazine [21].
- Sulphonamides: used for topical treatment.
- Bithionol and hexachlorophene: used in toilet soaps, shampoos and deodorants.
- N-butyl-4-chlorosalicylamide: for example the antifungal Jadit.
- Quinines: hair tonic, quinidine, quindoxin and olaquindox used in animal feeds [22]. Olaquindox is structurally similar to chlorpromazine. Quinidine has recently been reported to cause hand eczema in a carer who prepared the drug for administration [23].

Clinical features
History
Photoallergic contact dermatitis reactions require prior exposure for sensitisation to develop and usually occur 24–72 h after exposure to the combination of photoallergen and UV light. Typically, only small quantities of the photoallergen are required to provoke a reaction. The reaction typically starts on a sun-exposed site but can then spread to covered areas of skin. This is in contrast to photo-irritant reactions which can occur on first exposure, develop more quickly (<24 h) and usually remain limited to the exact area of exposure without spread to covered sites.

Presentation
Photoallergic reactions can initially urticate and resemble sunburn, but usually show the same spectrum of features as seen with allergic contact dermatitis. The dermatitis appears first localised to exposed areas of the skin, usually with well-demarcated margins where the skin is covered by clothing, for example at the collar and 'V' of the neck, below the end of sleeves on the backs of the hands and on the ankles below the trouser legs. Sites which are naturally shaded such as the folds of the neck, nasolabial/submental areas and the retroauricular skin (Wilkinson triangle) are usually spared. Gradual spread to covered sites often occurs. Asymmetry may result from increased UV exposure to one side of the body, for example those who drive with the vehicle windows open. The photoallergen may be transferred from one body site to another, for example to the contralateral areas, or may be due to a cross-leg effect or transfer by the hands.

Connubial contact can cause unusual patterns such as a reported eczematous 'hand print' from use of a ketoprofen containing gel by a dance partner [19].

Photoallergy to UV filters in cosmetics may be clinically identical to that seen from conventional allergy to cosmetics. It may be widespread when related to liberal use of sunscreen agents. Furthermore, it may simulate sunburn and other causes of photosensitivity.

The intensity of the response to photoallergens depends upon a number of factors:
- The nature and concentration of the substance applied.
- The duration of exposure to the substance.
- Percutaneous absorption.
- The intensity and wavelength of the radiation.
- The duration of radiation exposure.
- Radiation absorption in the skin, depending on the thickness of the stratum corneum as well as the amount and distribution of melanin.
- Extraneous matter and secretions on the skin.

Chelitis is reported as a potential presentation on PACD to toothpaste and mouthwash photoallergens [24], as well as to sunscreen chemicals added to lipsticks and lipsalves. Photopatch testing is recommended for this patient group.

Differential diagnosis
Photoallergy may simulate other photosensitive dermatoses and airborne contact allergy, and vice versa. Furthermore, a combination of these disorders may affect the same individual. It is important to recognise that photoallergy may sometimes fail to follow the typical pattern of sparing of light-protected sites and airborne contact allergy may paradoxically induce the classic photosensitivity distribution. Combined airborne and photoaggravated contact allergy is seen particularly with Compositae (Asteraceae) (see Figure 127.34) [25] and lichens [26]. A similar pattern of dermatitis may also be seen in patients sensitive to colophonium, pine and spruce. It is therefore important to identify every potential component of these clinical presentations by screening for contact allergy using patch tests (especially to plants), for photoallergy with photopatch tests and also for photosensitivity using phototesting.

Complications and co-morbidities
In some individuals, photoallergic reactions may progress to produce a light sensitivity that can persist a long time after the elimination of the sensitiser. This is known as a persistent light reaction [27]. The phenomenon has been reported with many different substances, including chlorpromazine [28], halogenated salicylanilides, musk ambrette, promethazine hydrochloride, ketoprofen [29], quindoxin [30] and olaquindox. This chronic photosensitive dermatitis presents as chronic eczematous changes on light-exposed areas with or without spread elsewhere. On monochromator testing, patients have abnormal responses to UV radiation with a shift to UVB sensitivity [31].

Patients with established photosensitivity who have a flare of their dermatitis may have reacted to an increase in light levels or re-exposure to their primary allergen or a cross-reacting allergen by airborne contact. Alternatively, they may have developed a secondary allergic or photoallergic contact sensitivity to their sunscreen or to one of their other medicaments.

Table 127.11 Photopatch test protocols.

Protocol	Day				
	0	1	2	3	4
Protocol 1	Phototest Apply allergens	Read phototest results Remove patches and irradiate allergens		Read results	
Protocol 2	Apply allergens		Remove patches, read results and irradiate allergens		Read results
Protocol 3	Apply allergens	Phototest	Read phototest results Remove patches, read results and irradiate allergens		Read results

From British Photodermatology Group 1997 [32].

The disorder of chronic actinic dermatitis (Chapter 126) may be associated with contact allergy, particularly to Compositae. Often, there are multiple contact allergies. Phototesting reveals abnormal results but photopatch tests to Compositae and other allergens are generally normal. Nevertheless, persistent light reactivity following photoallergy may progress to chronic actinic dermatitis.

Disease course and prognosis
Typically, with avoidance of the cause, the dermatitis will resolve.

Investigations
Photopatch testing
Indications. The main clinical indications for photopatch tests include the investigation of patients with eczematous rashes predominantly affecting light-exposed sites and a history of worsening following sun exposure. A history of a reaction to sunscreens is a further indication. Grounds may be extended to testing anyone with an exposed-site distribution of dermatitis. Some patients have coexisting photosensitive disorders, causing practical problems in performing and interpreting the investigation.

Method. A British Photodermatology Group (BPG) workshop has achieved a consensus on the protocol for photopatch testing in the UK and Ireland [32], but the technique may vary slightly in other parts of the world. The BPG stated that photopatch testing is an evolving technique with a need for more research.

A UVA source is required, which in most centres will be the UVA lamps used for PUVA therapy, commonly in a hand/foot treatment unit. In photobiology centres, the more sophisticated irradiation monochromator may be used as an alternative. Other UVA sources include UVA blacklights and filtered metal halide and xenon arc lamps. In all cases irradiance should be measured with a calibrated UVA meter. The energy source must be monitored regularly as the tubes deteriorate with time.

Historically, administered dosages of UVA to the photopatch test site have generally ranged from 5 to 10 J/cm². However, the higher doses have the disadvantage of being more likely to induce false positive phototoxic responses without an increased detection of photoallergic subjects, and therefore a dose of 5 J/cm² is recommended. Modification of the dose may be necessary in UVA-photosensitive individuals, in which case 50% of the UVA minimal erythema dose is suggested. However, UVA phototesting to establish the minimal erythema dose is not always feasible or practicable, but is nevertheless advised before photopatch testing known photosensitive individuals. Application of the allergens is performed in an identical

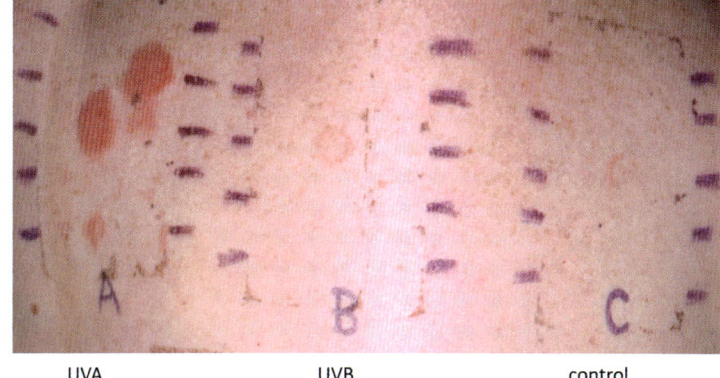

Figure 127.38 Phototesting demonstrating photo allergy after irradiation with UVA (A) but no response to the control (C) or after irradiation with UVB (B).

fashion to conventional patch tests, except that they must be applied in duplicate – one set is irradiated and the other (the control) is not. Usually, the two sets of tests are applied on either side of the vertebral column at the same level. It is suggested that the patient's back is positioned 15 cm from the front panel of the lamps. Steps must be taken to avoid any incidental irradiation by natural light of both the irradiated and the control set of allergens. The control site and the rest of the skin must be covered with opaque material during irradiation of the photopatch test site. Three protocols have been used and these are described in Table 127.11. There is evidence to show that a 48 h application is superior to a 24 h one [33], and one study failed to show an improved return with UVB irradiation (Figure 127.38) or with a 7-day reading [34].

Test materials. The principle of a baseline series also applies to photopatch tests. The EMCPPTS Taskforce has recommended such a series based on a recent European study (Table 127.12) [4,35]. However, for some centres more UV filters and other materials may be advisable as new exposures and photoallergens are identified.

Readings. A positive reaction on the irradiated side only is an indication of photoallergy. There are occasional difficulties distinguishing a false positive phototoxic reaction from photoallergy, but this is less likely with a dose of 5 J/cm². Readings are scored identically to conventional patch tests, but the positive symbol is preceded by the prefix Ph, for example Ph++ is a strong positive photoallergic reaction. If the same allergen provokes an equally strong reaction on both sides, it is an indication of contact allergy alone; if it is significantly

Table 127.12 Photopatch test baseline series.

Type of agent	Name of agent (INCI name for UV absorbers)	Concentration and vehicle	Comment
'Older' organic UV absorbers	Butyl methoxydibenzoylmethane	10% pet.	Among UV absorbers, the third highest cause of PPT reactions in the EMCPPTS. A commonly used UVA absorber
	Benzophenone-3	10% pet.	Among UV absorbers, the second highest cause of PPT reactions in the EMCPPTS. Many published reports of PACD over time
	Benzophenone-4	2% pet.	Permitted in sunscreens but mainly used in other cosmetics to prevent photodegradation. Few PPT reactions in the EMCPPTS
	Octocrylene	10% pet.	The UV absorber most frequently leading to PPT reactions in the EMCPPTS. Seems to have potential for cross-reacting with ketoprofen and benzophenone-3
	4-Methylbenzylidene camphor	10% pet.	These agents led to relatively few PPT reactions in the EMCPPTS, and continue to be used in sunscreens
	Ethylhexyl methoxycinnamate	10% pet.	
	Isoamyl-p-methoxycinnamate	10% pet.	
	PABA	10% pet.	Sunscreens in Europe are mostly PABA-free but this classic photoallergen may still be found in sunscreens bought elsewhere
'Newer' organic UV absorbers	Methylene bis-benzotriazolyl tetramethylbutylphenol	10% pet.	The agent most frequently leading to positive patch test reactions in the EMCPPTS. The role of the added surfactant decyl glucoside requires further elucidation
	Bis-ethylhexyloxyphenol methoxyphenyl triazine	10% pet.	These agents led to few PPT reactions in the EMCPPTS. However, owing to the relatively short time for which they have been present in the marketplace, further useful information on their photoallergenic potential will be gained by their inclusion in this European baseline photopatch test series
	Drometrizole trisiloxane	10% pet.	
	Terephthalylidene dicamphor sulfonic acid	10% aqua	
	Diethylamino hydroxybenzoyl hexyl benzoate	10% pet.	
	Ethylhexyl triazone	10% pet.	
	Diethylhexyl butamido triazone	10% pet.	
Topical NSAIDs	Ketoprofen	1% pet.	The agent most frequently leading to PPT reactions in the EMCPPTS, as well as in other studies in several countries
	Etofenamate	2% pet.	The second highest cause of PPT reactions in the EMCPPTS, often with unknown relevance
	Piroxicam	1% pet.	An NSAID class of its own responsible for PACD and systemic photosensitivity
	Benzydamine	2% pet.	Frequently responsible for PACD presenting as lip or hand dermatitis in Portugal and Spain. Also used in other European countries
Topical antihistamine	Promethazine	0.1% pet.	Widely used in several southern European countries as a topical antihistamine

Adapted from Gonçalo *et al.* 2013 [35] with permission of John Wiley & Sons.
EMCPPTS, European Multicentre Photopatch Test Study; INCI, International Nomenclature of Cosmetic Ingredients; NSAID, non-steroidal anti-inflammatory drug; PABA, *p*-aminobenzoic acid; PACD, photoallergic contact dermatitis; pet., petrolatum; PPT, photopatch test; UV, ultraviolet.

stronger on the irradiated side, then combined allergy and photocontact allergy may be occurring. Doubtful and slight amplification of photoallergic reactions may be the result of phototoxicity.

Management

Photoallergy to UV filters should be straightforward to eliminate. Once photoallergy has been demonstrated to a UV filter, the patient should be informed of the INCI name and synonyms of the material to which they are sensitive. UV filters relying totally on opaque/reflectant micronised titanium dioxide and zinc oxide should be free of chemical UV-filtering agents, and can be used for coexistent photodermatoses in those allergic to chemical UV filters. Where topical NSAIDs are commonly used, once the photoallergy has been confirmed, avoidance should be straightforward.

Allergic contact urticaria

Definition and nomenclature

The term contact urticaria was introduced by Fisher in 1973 [1] to describe a weal and flare reaction following contact with an external substance, usually appearing within 30 min and resolving within hours, without residual signs [2].

> **Synonyms and inclusions**
> - Immunological contact urticaria
> - Contact urticaria syndrome
> - Protein contact dermatitis

Introduction and general description

Contact urticaria (CU) falls into two types, immune (ICU) and non-immune (NICU). NICU is much more common, does not require prior sensitisation and is an irritant-type reaction occurring in many exposed individuals. NICU is typically triggered by low-molecular-weight chemicals such as benzoic acid, sorbic acid and cinnamic aldehyde, found in foods, personal care products and pharmaceuticals. ICU in contrast, requires prior sensitisation via a specific IgE-mediated response. It is mainly triggered by contact with proteins and is more common in atopic individuals. More rarely, low-molecular-weight chemicals can act as haptens and combine with cutaneous proteins to cause allergic CU.

CU can be part of the contact urticaria syndrome where local cutaneous reactions progress to become generalised and involve organs other than the skin including the respiratory, gastrointestinal and vascular systems, sometimes leading to anaphylaxis.

Protein contact dermatitis (PCD) is a separate condition where cutaneous contact with proteins, typically in handled foodstuffs, causes an eczematous eruption. This can be non-allergic or caused by an allergic type I hypersensitivity.

Epidemiology
Incidence and prevalence

Non-immune CU is caused by a wide variety of very common agents such as animals (e.g. ants, caterpillars, coral), foods (e.g. pepper, mustard), fragrance (e.g. cinnamic aldehyde), medicaments (e.g. menthol, witch hazel), plants (e.g. nettles) and preservatives (e.g. benzoic acid) [3]. Most of the reactions are mild and are not reported.

Most of the epidemiological data concerning CU come from occupational-based studies. The most recent report from the Finnish Register of Occupational Disease (2019) lists a combination of CU and PCD as the third most common cause of dermatology-related occupational disease, after allergic and irritant contact dermatitis, occurring in 11% of the 5265 reported cases. The mean age of the occupational CU/PCD cases was 39 years and the majority were female (64%) [4]. The most common causes of CU in the Finnish occupational data were cow dander, natural rubber latex and flour/grains/feed. In decreasing order of frequency, the most affected occupations were bakers, preparers of processed food and dental assistants [5].

A retrospective Australian study carried out in a tertiary-level occupational dermatology clinic identified a CU prevalence of 8.3%. Atopy was a significant risk factor for ICU induced by natural rubber latex, foodstuffs and ammonium persulphate. In this study, the three most common occupations associated with CU were health care workers, food handlers and hairdressers [6].

Changes in practice have resulted in a reduced incidence of latex CU in health care workers. In an occupational setting, CU most frequently develops in those who are exposed to animals such as agricultural workers, fish processors and slaughterhouse workers or those involved in food production such as bakers and chefs [7].

Gimenez-Arnau et al. have compiled a comprehensive list of CU causative substances aptly entitled 'a never ending story' [8]. The number of reported proteins and low-molecular-weight chemicals able to cause CU is vast, will continue to increase and is too long to list. The six main groups of substances reported to cause ICU are foods (e.g. seafood, meat, fruit, vegetables, dairy), cosmetic chemicals (e.g. fragrances, ammonium persulphate, hair dyes), topical medicaments (e.g. antibiotics, local anaesthetics), animal proteins (e.g. saliva, dander, placenta, hair), plants (e.g. latex, Compositae, ivy, yucca) and enzymes (e.g. amylase, papain).

Pathophysiology

Non-immune CU is thought to be secondary to the release of vasogenic mediators without the involvement of immunological processes. Urticating chemicals may have a direct effect on dermal vessel walls or cause a release of vasoactive substances such as histamine, slow-reacting substance A or bradykinin. NSAIDs such as aspirin are noted to inhibit NICU reactions, suggesting that prostaglandins play a role [2]. The clinical reaction is often redness without oedema rather than a true weal and flare response.

The pathogenesis of ICU involves the classic type I hypersensitivity reaction mediated by specific IgE in a presensitised individual. IgE binding to mast cells, their subsequent degranulation and release of histamine and other vasoactive mediators is described in detail in Chapter 9.

A third category of uncertain mechanisms also exists where the clinical symptoms resemble an immunological contact urticarial reaction yet no specific IgE can be demonstrated in the patient's serum or in the affected tissues, and passive transfer tests are negative. An example of this includes reactions to ammonium persulphate.

Predisposing factors

In addition to atopy, the presence of any pre-existing dermatitis predisposes to the development of ICU due to the presence of 'danger signals' that promote sensitisation. It has been reported that in patients with atopic eczema and raised IgE levels, the IgE may attach to the high-affinity IgE receptors on the surface of Langerhans cells or other antigen-presenting cells. This in turn may present protein allergens to Th2 cells, inducing a delayed-type hypersensitivity reaction resulting in eczematous lesions. This does not occur in atopic individuals with normal IgE levels or non-atopic controls and may explain why patients with atopic eczema have delayed hypersensitivity on patch testing to aeroallergens and develop a vesicular response to handling food proteins (PCD) [9,10].

Pathology

The histology of CU is identical to that of urticaria from other causes and is not further discussed here.

Genetics

There is a strong association of ICU with inherited atopic disease of all forms. There is also a reported association between the development of immediate-type hypersensitivity reactions, specifically to peanut, in individuals with filaggrin mutations [11].

Environmental factors

Changes in the exposure to an allergen in the environment will influence the development of contact allergy. This has been demonstrated by the reduced incidence of type I latex allergy by environmental measures and the use of low protein powder-free gloves [12].

Table 127.13 Examples of cross-reactions between foods, foods and pollens and foods and latex that may also cause contact urticaria.

	Risk (%), if known	Cross-reaction	Other cross-reacting allergens
Food type			
Fin fish, e.g. cod	5	Other fish, e.g. haddock, salmon	
Crustacea	75	Other crustacea	
Grain, e.g. wheat	20	Other grains, e.g. barley, rye	Grass pollens
Apple	55	Other Rosaceae fruit, e.g. peach, pear, cherry, plum	Birch tree pollen
Peanuts		Other legumes	Tree nuts, grass pollen
Cow's milk	92	Goat's milk	
Latex (latex–food syndrome)	35	Banana, avocado, kiwi, chestnut, potato, papaya	
Pollen type			
Birch		Raw apple, raw carrot, cherry, pear, peach, plum, fennel, walnut, potato, spinach, wheat, peanut, kiwi, hazelnut, fennel, coriander, cumin	
Mugwort		Celery, carrot, melon, watermelon, hazelnut	
Grass		Potato, melon, tomato, watermelon, orange, cherry, peanut	
Ragweed		Melon, chamomile, banana	

Adapted from Sicherer 2001 [26].

Clinical features

Presentation

The symptoms of ICU usually occur within 1 h and fade by 3 h. The spectrum of associated symptoms is wide. Local symptoms include itching and burning, and the development of redness and the characteristic weal and flare reaction. Early symptoms are commonly missed by physicians although well recognised by patients. In 'invisible' CU, only subjective symptoms (e.g. itching, tingling, burning) occur without any objective change or only mild redness. These reactions are often seen from cosmetics, fruits or vegetables.

Exposure to allergens in those who are highly sensitised, topically or via the oral or respiratory route, may result in widespread urticaria and swelling of the mucous membranes, resulting in conjunctivitis, rhinitis, oro-pharyngeal swelling, bronchoconstriction and rarely anaphylaxis.

Contact urticaria to foodstuffs. The most common causes of CU are foodstuffs, which can provoke oro-pharyngeal symptoms (the oral allergy syndrome) following ingestion, or cutaneous hand symptoms in food handlers. The oral allergy syndrome (pollen–food allergy syndrome) results from individuals already sensitised to plant pollens eating raw/uncooked/unprocessed fruits, vegetables and nuts that share antigens with the pollen. Symptoms are usually localised mucosal surface irritation or tingling. Clinical signs are usually confined to localised mucosal swelling, although anaphylaxis is rarely reported.

In the birch-rich areas of northern and central Europe almost all birch pollen-allergic patients are sensitised to Bet v1, the major allergen component of pollen from *Betula verrucosa*. Fifty to 90% of birch pollen-allergic patients have been reported to have some pollen-related food allergy – in particular to the Bet v1 homologous proteins (PR-10 proteins) in the *Rosaceae* family such as apple, peach and cherry [13]. Other clinically important food allergies commonly associated with Bet v1 are reactions to the *Apiaceae* family (e.g. celery, carrot) and/or the *Fabaceae* family (e.g. peanut, soybean). The Bet v1 homologous proteins in the *Rosaceae* family are very sensitive to heat and proteases. Clinical reactions therefore usually only occur with raw foods and do not occur when eating cooked or tinned fruit.

The most important molecular basis of the latex–fruit syndrome is the homology between the hevein (Hev b 6.02) of the latex with the hevein-like N-terminal domain of the class I chitinases of plants. This immunological phenomenon of cross-reactivity has consequences for the diagnosis and treatment of certain food allergies (Table 127.13) [14]. It is important to determine the clinical relevance of these cross-reactions and whether they represent sensitisation only or actual clinical reactivity (allergy). The dermatologist may be called upon to determine the risk of reactions to related foods and a variety of other plant-derived foods that may share proteins with pollens, latex and each other.

Clinical evaluation requires a careful history, skin prick tests and IgE-mediated blood tests. The pitfalls in evaluation are interpreting the clinical relevance of a positive skin prick test or specific IgE test and deciding when it is a false positive result. The use of component-resolved diagnostics that detects IgE antibodies to single allergen components can be used to help in this process.

Contact urticaria to natural rubber latex. Allergy to natural rubber latex was first recognised by Nutter in 1979 [15]. The allergens are present in the water-soluble protein moiety of the sap collected from the rubber-bearing tree *Hevea braziliensis*, harvested mainly in Malaysia and South-East Asia. The problem has been associated primarily with dipped rubber items, including gloves (Figure 127.39), condoms, balloons, catheters and medical tubing. These items are vulcanised at a lower temperature than solid rubber products such as tyres, seals and gaskets. With the advent of the acquired immune deficiency syndrome (AIDS) and the huge increase in the use of latex examination gloves among health care personnel, the production of inexpensive, disposable, natural rubber latex gloves escalated. During the production process, the natural rubber latex was not left to stand in holding tanks as long, the process was shortened by lower vulcanisation temperatures and there was less thorough washing of the final product [16]. All these measures led to an increase in the protein content of the gloves and this, coupled with their increasing use, resulted in an increase in the incidence of allergy to natural rubber latex.

Anaphylaxis can occur in any sensitised patient and seems to be particularly prevalent when challenge is via the mucosal surfaces,

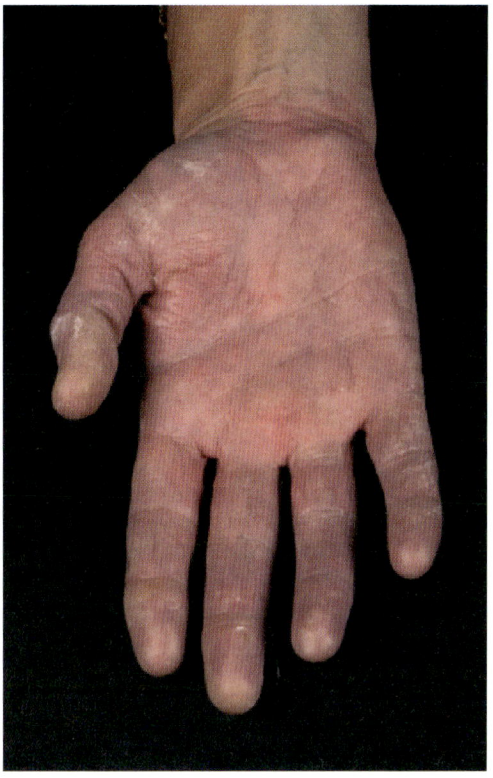
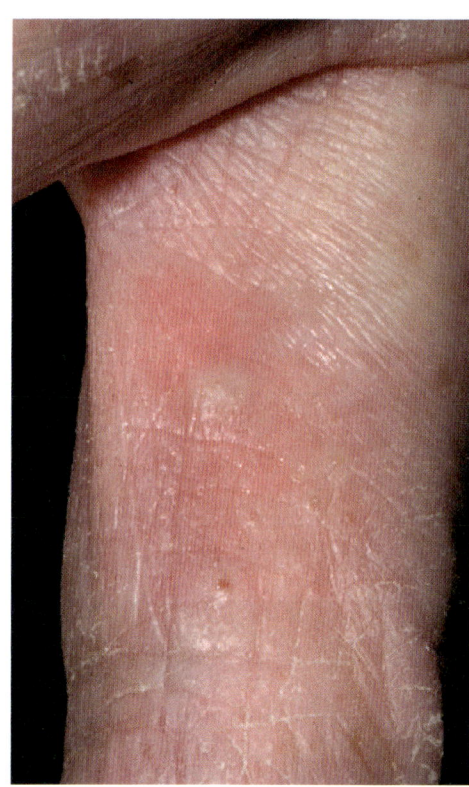

Figure 127.39 Allergic contact urticarial weals developing within 20 min following a powdered latex glove challenge in a natural rubber latex-allergic patient. Courtesy of Dr D. Orton.

as in dental and vaginal examinations, intraperitoneal operations, catheter changing (especially in spina bifida patients who have frequent surgery and catheter changes) and barium enemas. The allergenic proteins are multiple. Many of the allergenic peptides in natural rubber latex cross-react with those found in other plants [17], such as banana, lychees, chestnuts and avocado.

Due to several interventional measures including an increased use of powder-free latex gloves, low-protein latex gloves and non-latex gloves and medical equipment, the frequency of natural rubber latex allergy in health care workers seems to be reducing [12].

Protein contact dermatitis. Hjorth and Roed-Peterson defined this as an immediate dermatitis induced by contact with proteins. They described 33 caterers suffering from itch within 10–30 min following contact with meat, fish and vegetables, which was followed by redness and vesicle formation. Application of the relevant food to the affected skin resulted in either urticaria or eczema [18]. Patients who have repeated exposure of the hands, especially the fingertips, to contact urticants such as food proteins may develop PCD. Characteristically, the condition involves skin sites that have been affected previously by dermatitis. Damaged skin probably facilitates penetration of the allergens, and inflammatory cells already present in the dermis may explain the accelerated clinical response. An association between atopy and PCD occurs in approximately 50% of cases. It is common in dairy workers, veterinarians, slaughterhouse workers, chefs and sandwich makers, who become sensitised to the proteins they touch during work [7].

Differential diagnosis

The differential diagnosis of allergic CU is that of other forms of urticaria and is discussed in Chapter 42. In the identification of an exogenous cause, consideration of its possibility and referral for specialist investigation is essential. Localised symptomatic dermographism is a relatively common cause of urticaria to gloves in the absence of latex allergy [19], CU to rubber chemicals being extremely rare [20].

Classification of severity

The following staging system for the contact urticaria syndrome has been described by Amin and Maibach [21].
- Stage 1: localised urticaria (redness and swelling), dermatitis (eczema) and non-specific symptoms (e.g. itching, tingling, burning sensation).
- Stage 2: generalised urticaria.
- Stage 3: bronchial asthma (wheezing), rhinitis, conjunctivitis (e.g. runny nose, watery eyes), oro-laryngeal symptoms (e.g. lip swelling, hoarseness, difficulty in swallowing) and gastrointestinal symptoms (e.g. nausea, vomiting, diarrhoea, cramps).
- Stage 4: anaphylactoid reactions (shock).

Disease course and prognosis

Provided the allergen is identified and eliminated, even though sensitisation may persist, symptoms will resolve.

Investigations

The diagnosis of CU is based on a full medical history and skin testing with suspected substances. In particular, the study of chronic hand eczema in professional food handlers should include both immediate and delayed tests. A detailed history concerning the occurrence of immediate symptoms – whether confined to the skin or not – and their association, particularly with occupational exposure, should always be considered. With an unknown allergen,

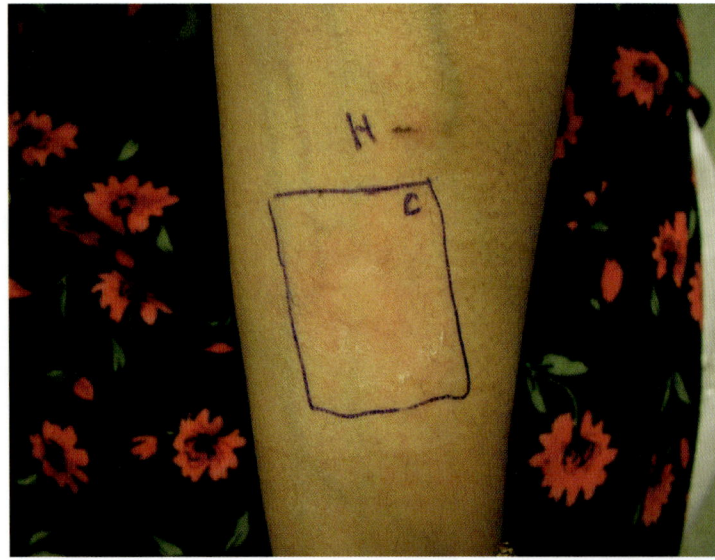

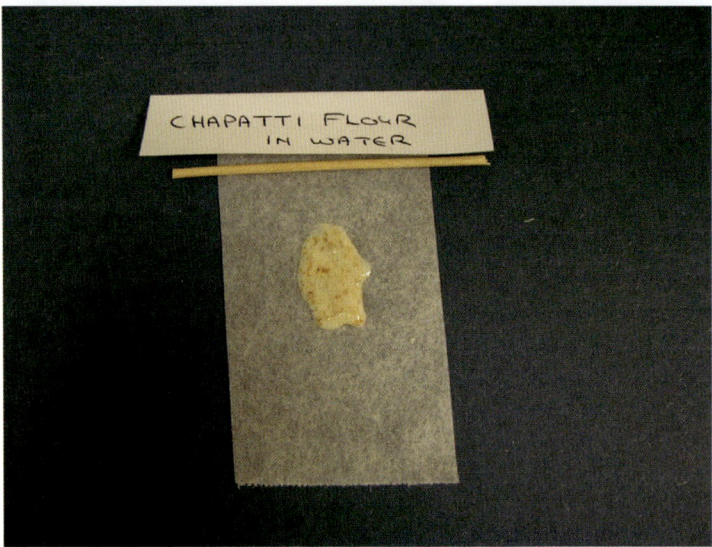

Figure 127.40 Open testing to a solution of chapatti flour causing an immune allergic contact urticarial response within 15 min. C, chapatti flour; H, histamine. Reproduced from Davies and Orton 2009 [25] with permission of John Wiley & Sons.

exposure should be graded with an initial application test (open and subsequently occluded) followed by a prick test and, if appropriate, an intradermal test. NSAIDs, antihistamines and exposure to UV light may all cause false negative results.

Von Krogh and Maibach produced guidelines for evaluating immediate types of cutaneous response [22]. The most simple test for CU is the open test, whereby 0.1 mL of the suspected causative agent is rubbed firstly on a 3 × 3 cm area of normal skin (upper back or flexor aspect of upper arm or forearm) (Figure 127.40). If this is negative, the test is then repeated on slightly affected skin or previously affected skin. The use of alcohol vehicles or the addition of propylene glycol to the vehicle enhances the sensitivity of the test [23]. A positive result occurs when oedema and/or redness is observed, usually within 15 min. The test sites are usually read at 20, 40 and 60 min to see the maximal response. ICU reactions typically appear within 15–20 min, whereas NICU reactions can be delayed up to 45–60 min following application. When performing tests with 'whole' foods at least six control subjects should also be tested.

When the open test is negative, prick testing of suspected agents with appropriate histamine and saline controls should be used. Although commercial allergen extracts are available, it should be remembered that unless standardised they may not contain the relevant protein allergens. The gold standard should always be to test and challenge with a sample of fresh material. Skin tests should only be performed where resuscitation facilities are available.

If the patient has experienced an anaphylactic reaction a specific IgE test should be performed initially, instead of a prick test, if available.

Scratch tests and scratch patch tests (contact with a small aluminium chamber for 15 min) are less standardised tests that should also be performed with appropriate controls. A small piece of the substance is applied on a closed patch test (Finn chamber, Epitest; Hyryla, Finland) to an area of skin. The skin may be lightly scarified with a needle or degreased with 96% alcohol prior to application [24]. After 20 min the area is examined for redness or weal and flare. Occasionally, there is no reaction on normal skin and the substance has to be applied to previously affected skin, for example the fingertips. The scratch patch test is particularly useful if testing non-standardised materials when a delayed reading is mandatory.

Management

Management is achieved by avoiding the causative substance or the use of appropriate personal protective equipment (e.g. gloves made of an appropriate material), since desensitisation for the majority of relevant allergens is not available. The general management of the symptoms of urticaria and its complications is discussed in Chapter 42. Treatment of the acute episode includes the use of systemic antihistamines and adrenaline in rare cases of anaphylaxis.

Key references

The full list of references can be found in the online version at https://www.wiley.com/rooksdermatology10e

Introduction
Aberer W, Andersen KE, White IR. Should patch testing be restricted to dermatologists only. *Contact Dermatitis* 1993;28:1–2.

Allergic contact dermatitis
Epidemiology
Incidence and prevalence
8 Diepgen TL, Ofenloch RF, Bruze M et al. Prevalence of contact allergy in the general population in different European regions. *Br J Dermatol* 2016;174:319–29.

Age
6 Lynch MD, McFadden JP, White JM et al. Age-specific profiling of cutaneous allergy at high temporal resolution suuggests age-related alterations in regulatory immune function. *J Allergy Clin Immunol* 2017;140:1451–3.

Impact of drugs on patch test reactions
2 Feuerman E, Levy A. A study of the effect of prednisolone and an antihistamine on patch test reactions. *Br J Dermatol* 1972;86:68–71.

Pathophysiology
1 Leonard A, Guttman-Yassky E. The unique molecular signatures of contact dermatitis and implications for treatment. *Clin Rev Allerg Immunol* 2019;56:1–8.

Sensitisation and elicitation
11 Dhingra N, Shemer A, Correa da Rosa J *et al*. Molecular profiling of contact dermatitis skin identifies allergen-dependent differences in immune response. *J Allergy Clin Immunol* 2014;362–72.

Predisposing factors
5 McFadden JP, Basketter DA. Contact allergy, irritancy and 'danger'. *Contact Dermatitis* 2000;42:123–7.
20 Friedmann PS. The relationships between exposure dose and response in induction and elicitation of contact hypersensitivity in humans. *Br J Dermatol* 2007;157:1093–102.

Genetics
1 Schnuch A, Westphal G, Mossner R, Uter W, Reich K. Genetic factors in contact allergy – review and future goals. *Contact Dermatitis* 2011;64:2–23.
24 Teo Y, McFadden JP, White IR *et al*. Allergic contact dermatitis in atopic individuals: results of a 30-year retrospective study. *Contact Dermatitis* 2019;81:409–16.

Clinical features
Presentation
Primary patterns
4 Hjorth N, Roed-Petersen J. Occupational protein contact in food handlers dermatitis. *Contact Dermatitis* 1976;2:28–42.

Clinical variants
Systemically reactivated contact dermatitis
11 Jensen CS, Menné T, Johansen JD. Systemic contact dermatitis after oral exposure to nickel: a review with a modified meta-analysis. *Contact Dermatitis* 2006;56:79–86.
23 Svedman C, Ekqvist S, Möller H *et al*. A correlation found between contact allergy to stent material and restenosis of the coronary arteries. *Contact Dermatitis* 2009;60:158–64.
24 Schalock PC, Menné T, Johansen JD *et al*. Hypersensitivity reactions to metallic implants – diagnostic algorithm and suggested patch test series for clinical use. *Contact Dermatitis* 2012;66:4–19.

Disease course and prognosis
1 Cahill J, Keegel T, Nixon R. The prognosis of occupational contact dermatitis in 2004. *Contact Dermatitis* 2004;51:219–26.
3 Kadyk DL, Hall S, Belsito DV. Quality of life of patients with allergic contact dermatitis: an exploratory analysis by gender, ethnicity, age, and occupation. *Dermatitis* 2004;15:117–24.
15 Sajjachareonpong P, Cahill J, Keegel T. Persistent post-occupational dermatitis. *Contact Dermatitis* 2004;51:278–83.

Investigations: patch tests
1 Johansen JD, Aalto-Korte K, Agner T *et al*. European Society of Contact Dermatitis guideline for diagnostic patch testing – recommendations on best practice. *Contact Dermatitis* 2015;73:195–221.
4 Rajagopalan R, Anderson RT, Sarma S *et al*. An economic evaluation of patch testing in the diagnosis and management of allergic contact dermatitis. *Am J Contact Dermatitis* 1998;9:149–54.
5 Thomson KF, Wilkinson SM, Sommer S *et al*. Eczema: quality of life by body site and the effect of patch testing. *Br J Dermatol* 2002;146:627–30.
16 Bruze M, Isaksson M, Gruvberger B, Frick-Engfeldt M. Recommendation of appropriate amounts of petrolatum preparation to be applied at patch testing. *Contact Dermatitis* 2007;56:281–5.
17 Goon AT, Bruze M, Zimerson E *et al*. Variation in allergen content over time of acrylates/methacrylates in patch test preparations. *Br J Dermatol* 2011;164:116–24.
18 Mowitz M, Zimerson E, Svedman C, Bruze M. Stability of fragrance patch test preparations in test chambers. *Br J Dermatol* 2012;167:822–7.
25 Svedman C, Isaksson M, Björk J, Mowitz M, Bruze M. 'Calibration' of our patch test reading technique is necessary. *Contact Dermatitis* 2012;66:180–7.
41 Wilkinson M, Gonçalo M, Aerts O *et al*. The European baseline series and recommended additions: 2019. *Contact Dermatitis* 2019;80:1–4.
44 Bruze M, Frick M, Persson L. Patch testing with thin-layer chromatograms. *Contact Dermatitis* 2003;48:278–9.

Investigations: other tests
4 Johansen JD, Bruze M, Andersen KE *et al*. The repeated open application test: suggestions for a scale of evaluation. *Contact Dermatitis* 1998;39:95–6.

Management
2 Noiesen E, Larsen K, Agner T. Compliance in contact allergy with focus on cosmetic labelling: a qualitative research project. *Contact Dermatitis* 2004;51:189–95.
16 Scheman A, Cha C, Jacob SE, Nedorost S. Food avoidance diets for systemic lip and oral contact allergy. *Dermatitis* 2013;23:248–47.
21 Thyssen JP, Johansen JD, Menné T. Contact allergy epidemics and their control. *Contact Dermatitis* 2007;56:185–95.
29 Jowsey IR. Proactive surveillance of contact allergies: an important component of the risk management strategy for skin sensitizers. *Contact Dermatitis* 2007;56:305–10.

Specific allergens
Fragrances, balsams, flavouring agents and spices
1 Johansen JD. Contact allergy to fragrances. Clinical and experimental investigations of the fragrance mix and its ingredients. *Contact Dermatitis* 2002;46:1–31.
8 Diepgen TL, Ofenloch R, Bruze M *et al*. Prevalence of fragrance contact allergy in the general population of five European countries: a cross-sectional study. *Br J Dermatol* 2015;173:1411–19.
14 Webber L, Keith D, Walker-Smith P, Buckley DA. Fragrance exposure in the UK: has there been a change in the last decade? *Br J Dermatol* 2018;179:1199–200.
51 Bennike NH, Zachariae C, Johansen JD. Non-mix fragrances are top sensitizers in consecutive dermatitis patients – a cross-sectional study of the 26 EU-labelled fragrance allergens. *Contact Dermatitis* 2017;77:270–9.
52 Paulsen E, Andersen F. Fragrant and sticky allergens from the pinewood: cohabiting and coreacting. *Contact Dermatitis* 2019;81:374–7.

Applied medicaments
2 Gilissen L, Goossens A. Frequency and trends of contact allergy to and iatrogenic contact dermatitis caused by topical drugs over a 25-year period. *Contact Dermatitis* 2016;75:290–302.

Cosmetics
4 Wilkinson M, Orton D. Acrylate allergy: time to intervene. *Contact Dermatitis* 2017;77:353–5.
16 Horton E, Uter W, Geier J *et al*. Developing a cosmetic series: results from the ESSCA network, 2009–2018. *Contact Dermatitis* 2021;84:82–94.

Antimicrobial agents and preservatives
Formaldehyde-releasing preservatives/biocides
5 Fasth IM, Ulrich NH, Johansen JD. Ten-year trends in contact allergy to formaldehyde and formaldehyde-releasers. *Contact Dermatitis* 2018;79:263–9.

Other cosmetic preservatives
Isothiazolinones
8 Goncalo M, Goossens A. Whilst Rome burns: the epidemic of contact allergy to methylisothiazolinone. *Contact Dermatitis* 2013;68:257–8.
21 Lundov MD, Opstrup MS, Johansen JD. Methylisothiazolinone contact allergy – a growing epidemic. *Contact Dermatitis* 2013;69:271–5.
22 Johnston GA; contributing members of the British Society for Cutaneous Allergy (BSCA). The rise in prevalence of contact allergy to methylisothiazolinone in the British Isles. *Contact Dermatitis* 2014;70:238–40.

Vehicles and other cosmetic excipients
Lanolin
5 Kligman AM. The myth of lanolin allergy. *Contact Dermatitis* 1998;39:103–7.
14 Wolf R. The lanolin paradox. *Dermatology* 1996;192:198–202.

Other excipients
4 Bhoyrul B, Solman L, Kirk S *et al*. Patch testing with alkyl glucosides: Concomitant reactions are common but not ubiquitous. *Contact Dermatitis* 2019;80:286–90.

p-Phenylenediamine and related dyes
4 Diepgen TL, Naldi L, Bruze M *et al*. Prevalence of contact allergy to p-phenylenediamine in the European general population. *J Invest Dermatol* 2016;136:409–15.

Methacrylate nail systems
1 Wilkinson M, Orton D. Acrylate allergy: time to intervene. *Contact Dermatitis* 2017;77:353–5.

Rubber
19 Warburton, KL, Uter W. Geier J *et al.* Patch testing with rubber series in Europe: a critical review and recommendation. *Contact Dermatitis* 2017;76:195–203.
21 Crepy M-N, Lecuen J, Ratour-Bigot C *et al.* Accelerator-free gloves as alternatives in cases of glove allergy in healthcare workers. *Contact Dermatitis* 2018;78:28–32.

Shoes
1 Nardelli A, Taveirne M, Drieghe J *et al.* The relation between the localization of foot dermatitis and the causative allergens in shoes: a 13-year retrospective study. *Contact Dermatitis* 2005;53:201–6.
5 Landeck L, Uter W, John SM. Patch test characteristics of patients referred for suspected contact allergy of the feet – retrospective 10-year cross-sectional study of the IVDK data. *Contact Dermatitis* 2012;66:271–8.

Resins and plastics
Epoxy resins
1 Aalto-Korte K, Pesonen M, Suuronen K. Occupational allergic contact dermatitis caused by epoxy chemicals: occupations, sensitizing products, and diagnosis. *Contact Dermatitis* 2015;73:336–42.

Acrylate resins
7 Goon AT, Bruze M, Zimerson E *et al.* Contact allergy to acrylates/methacrylates in the acrylate and nail acrylics series in southern Sweden: simultaneous positive patch test reaction patterns and possible screening allergens. *Contact Dermatitis* 2007;57:21–7.

Formaldehyde resins
2 Owen CM, Beck MH. Occupational allergic contact dermatitis from phenol-formaldehyde resins. *Contact Dermatitis* 2001;45:294–5.

Other plastics
1 Quartier S, Garmyn M, Becart S, Goossens A. Allergic contact dermatitis to copolymers in cosmetics – case report and review of the literature. *Contact Dermatitis* 2006;55:257–67.

Plants
1 Mitchell JC, Rook A. *Botanical Dermatology*. Philadelphia: Lea and Febiger, 1979.
2 Schmidt RJ, ed. *The Botanical Dermatology Database.* http://www.botanical-dermatology-database.info/ (last accessed July 2023).
3 Lovell CR. *Plants and the Skin*. Oxford: Blackwell Scientific Publications, 1993.
5 Paulsen E, Christensen LP, Andersen KE. Dermatitis from common ivy (*Hedera helix* L. subsp. *helix*) in Europe: past, present and future. *Contact Dermatitis* 2010;62:201–9.

Woods, colophony, turpentine and propolis
3 Woods B, Calnan CD. Toxic woods. *Br J Dermatol* 1976;94(Suppl. 13):1–97.
4 Pesonen M, Suuronen K, Suomela S, Aalto-Korte K. Occupational allergic contact dermatitis caused by colophonium. *Contact Dermatitis* 2019;80:9–17.
24 De Groot AC. Propolis: a review of properties, applications, chemical composition, contact allergy and other adverse effects. *Dermatitis* 2013;24:263–82.

Photoallergic contact dermatitis
4 European Multicentre Photopatch Test Study (EMCPPTS) Taskforce. A European photopatch test study. *Br J Dermatol* 2012;166:1002–9.
32 British Photodermatology Group. Photopatch testing: methods and indications. *Br J Dermatol* 1997;136:371–6.
35 Gonçalo M, Ferguson J, Bonevalle A *et al.* Photopatch testing: recommendations for a European photopatch test baseline series. *Contact Dermatitis* 2013;68:239–43.

Allergic contact urticaria
4 Aalto-Korte K, Koskela K, Pesonen M. 12-year data on dermatologic cases in the Finnish Register of Occupational Diseases I: distribution of different diagnoses and main causes of allergic contact dermatitis. *Contact Dermatitis* 2020;82:337–42.
8 Gimenez-Arnau A, Maurer M *et al.* Immediate contact skin reactions, an update of contact urticaria, contact urticaria syndrome and protein contact dermatitis – "a never ending story". *Eur J Dermatol* 2010;20:552–62.

---

10 Schubert S, Lessmann H, Schnuch A *et al.* Factors associated with p-phenylenediamine sensitization: data from the Information Network of Departments of Dermatology, 2008–2013. *Contact Dermatitis* 2018;78:199–207.
14 De Groot AC. Side-effects of henna and semi-permanent 'black henna' tattoos: a full review. *Contact Dermatitis* 2013;69:1–25.

CHAPTER 128

Irritant Contact Dermatitis

Jonathan M. L. White

Department of Dermatology, Hôpital Erasme, Brussels; Ecole de Santé Publique, Université libre de Bruxelles, Brussels, Belgium

Irritant contact dermatitis, 128.1	Phototoxic contact dermatitis, 128.9	Chemical burns, 128.11
Non-immune contact urticaria, 128.8	Subjective sensory irritation, 128.10	Key references, 128.12

Irritant contact dermatitis

Definition and nomenclature

Irritant contact dermatitis is the cutaneous response to the physical/toxic effects of a wide range of environmental exposures. This may be an acute (toxic) irritant contact dermatitis or a cumulative irritant/insult dermatitis.

Synonyms and inclusions
- 'Wear-and-tear' dermatitis
- Traumiterative dermatitis
- Contact dermatitis

Introduction and general description

Reversible cellular injury may cause contact urticaria or dermatitis dependent on the nature of the insult. Where there is no apparent cellular injury, various sensory symptoms such as stinging, smarting and burning may occur. The following types of irritant contact reaction may be distinguished:
1. Burns.
2. Irritant contact dermatitis:
   - Acute (toxic) irritant contact dermatitis.
   - Cumulative irritant/insult contact dermatitis.
3. Transient or immediate-type, non-immune, contact urticaria.
4. Symptomatic (subjective) irritant responses.
5. Other: pigmentary and granulomatous responses and those localised to appendageal structures (Table 128.1).

There is considerable variability in responses between individuals, as well as within the same patient due to various endogenous and exogenous variables (Table 128.2). Various chemicals have irritant properties, including plants (Boxes 128.1 and 128.2).

Table 128.1 Other irritant contact responses of the skin and their causes.

Contact reaction	Irritant
Folliculitis	Tar and oils, arsenic trioxide, fibreglass, occlusion
Acne	Halogenated aromatic hydrocarbons, oils, occlusion
Miliaria	Aluminium chloride, occlusion
Pigmentary:	
Hyperpigmentation	Phototoxic agents, metals (arsenic, silver, gold, mercury, bismuth)
Hypopigmentation	Substituted phenols and catechols
Granulomatous	Silica, talc, beryllium
Alopecia	Borax, chloroprene dimers

Table 128.2 Factors influencing irritancy potential of substances on human skin.

Exogenous	Endogenous	Cofactors
Chemical characteristics	*Individual susceptibility*	Mechanical
Molecular structure	Atopy	Thermal
pH	Ethnicity/skin colour/phenotype	Climatic
pK_a	Age	
Hydrophobicity (log P)	Hormonal	
Inherent toxicity	Barrier function	
Concentration/dose	Repair capacity	
Penetration characteristics	Eczema elsewhere	
Vehicle	Other skin diseases	
Solubility	Other unknown	
Duration of contact	Site of exposure	
Type of contact		

Epidemiology

Incidence and prevalence

Many studies on the epidemiology of irritant contact dermatitis are diagnostically vague or open to considerable selection bias.

A questionnaire study of 20 000 persons in an industrial town in the south of Sweden revealed a point prevalence of hand eczema of

---

Rook's Textbook of Dermatology, Tenth Edition. Edited by Christopher Griffiths, Jonathan Barker, Tanya Bleiker, Walayat Hussain and Rosalind Simpson.
© 2024 John Wiley & Sons Ltd. Published 2024 by John Wiley & Sons Ltd.

> **Box 128.1 Common irritants**
>
> - Water and wet work: sweating under occlusion
> - Household cleaners: detergent, soap, shampoo, disinfectant
> - Industrial cleaning agents, including solvents and abrasives
> - Alkalis, including cement
> - Acids
> - Cutting oils
> - Organic solvents
> - Oxidising agents, including sodium hypochlorite
> - Reducing agents, including phenols, hydrazine, aldehydes, thiophosphates
> - Certain plants, e.g. spurge, Boracinaceae, Ranunculaceae
> - Pesticides
> - Raw food, animal enzymes, secretions
> - Desiccant powders, dust, soil
> - Miscellaneous chemicals

> **Box 128.2 Irritating plants**
>
> - Ranunculaceae:
>   - *Ranunculus* (many species of buttercup)
>   - *Anemone*
>   - *Clematis*
>   - *Helleborus*
> - Araceae:
>   - *Dieffenbachia* (ornamental plant in tropics and house plant in Europe)
> - Euphorbiaceae (spurge; the milky latex of many species is intensely irritating):
>   - *Hippomane manchinella* (the manzanillo tree of the Caribbean contains a powerful irritant)
> - Cruciferae:
>   - *Brassica nigra* and other 'mustards'
> - Compositae:
>   - *Achillea* (milfoil and related species)
>   - *Anthemis* (mayweeds)
>   - *Matricaria*

> **Box 128.3 Occupations associated with irritant contact dermatitis**
>
> - Hairdressing
> - Medical, dental, veterinary
> - Cleaning
> - Agriculture, horticulture, forestry
> - Food preparation and catering
> - Printing and painting
> - Metal work
> - Mechanical engineering
> - Construction
> - Fishing

5.4% (with a 1-year period prevalence of 11%), and in 35% the hand eczema was thought to be irritant in nature. Atopic hand eczema accounted for 22% of cases, the presence of childhood eczema increasing the prevalence of hand dermatitis threefold compared with non-atopic individuals. Allergic contact dermatitis accounted for 19%. The most frequent sources of exposure were 'unspecified' chemicals, water, detergents, dust and dirt [1]. Occupationally, soaps (22.0% of cases), wet work (19.8%), petroleum products (8.7%) and cutting oils and coolants (7.8%) are the most frequently cited causes. Individuals involved in mining/manufacturing, hairdressing, agriculture and medical and nursing occupations had the highest frequency of dermatitis (Box 128.3) [2]. In one large study of adverse reactions to cosmetics [3], 16% were thought to be irritant. A study of 68 000 patch test subjects showed 13% had a diagnosis of irritant contact dermatitis (without concomitant allergic contact dermatitis) [4].

Sex
Females may be twice as commonly affected as males [1].

Ethnicity
In North America, there has been shown to be no ethnic difference in the prevalence of sensitive skin, although there are racial differences in how it is perceived. White Americans experience greater reactivity to wind and less to cosmetics; African Americans have reduced reactivity to most environmental factors; Asians have greater reactivity to spices, change in temperature and wind, and itch more frequently; Hispanics react less to alcohol. Overall, however, there were more similarities than differences [5]. This was confirmed by a study on populations from South Asia with differing skin pigmentation [6].

Associated diseases
These include allergic contact dermatitis and atopic eczema.

Pathophysiology
Certain chemicals have intrinsic irritant properties to varying degrees, but external factors may also influence this, including temperature (of the chemical, environment or individual), air flow (chapping), low humidity (by itself responsible for the common condition 'low humidity occupational dermatosis', which generally affects the face) and occlusion. Skin barrier dysfunction is a key reason for irritation.

The skin provides the first and most important line of defence against exogenous noxious agents, and this is one of its primary physiological functions [7]. This defence is far from perfect, as many substances penetrate readily into and through the epidermis, even when it is intact.

The principal epidermal barrier resides almost entirely in the stratum corneum. This is normally renewed every 17–27 days, but barrier function can be largely restored (depending on the site; for example, the barrier function of the sole of the foot takes a long time to heal) in 2–5 days following stripping or superficial injury. The stratum corneum appears to function as a homogeneous unit, the largest amount of penetrant always being found in the outermost layers. Damage to the stratum corneum is normally followed by an increase in percutaneous absorption and in transepidermal water loss (TEWL), with the increase in TEWL proportional to the decrease in thickness of the stratum corneum.

Solvent extraction studies indicate that epidermal lipid is a main contributor to the barrier, consisting of ceramides (45–50%), cholesterol (25%), free fatty acids (10–15%) and other lipids including cholesterol sulphate. The lipids are arranged as stacked membrane sheets in the intercellular space and are produced from lamellar granules in the cells of the granular cell layer of the epidermis. It follows that inherited abnormalities of the pathway might result in impaired barrier function usually associated with ichthyosis.

In addition to the lipid barrier, tight junctions between epidermal cells have also been shown to provide a block to water loss. Claudin-1 (an essential protein of tight junctions) knock-out mice developed wrinkly skin and greatly increased TEWL. They died within 1 day of birth [8].

For certain materials, there may be a second barrier at, or near, the dermal–epidermal junction or basement membrane [9] but, for most substances, the horny layer remains the principal barrier.

Emerging data suggest that filaggrin mutations may predispose to irritant contact dermatitis [10].

Mechanism of action of irritants

An irritant is any agent, physical or chemical, that is capable of producing cellular perturbation if applied for sufficient time and in sufficient concentration. Immunological memory is not involved and dermatitis occurs without prior sensitisation. Many chemicals penetrate the skin, and many substances will alter or damage skin cells. Dermatitis arises when the defence or repair capacity of the skin is exhausted, or when the penetration of chemicals excites an inflammatory response. Strong irritants will induce a clinical reaction in almost all individuals, whereas with less potent irritants the response may be subclinical, with dermatitis developing only in the most susceptible or in situations where there is repeated contact with irritants [11].

The relationship between physicochemical structure and cytotoxic activity remains to be fully elucidated, but it would appear that hydrophobicity (log P) and the dissociation constant (pK_a) are among the factors that contribute to irritation potential [12,13] (Table 128.2). For sodium lauryl sulphate, concentration has been shown to be a more important determinant of subsequent dermatitis than exposure time [14]. The nature of the response is in part determined by the irritant [15].

In the laboratory, barrier disruption has been shown to induce rapid interleukin 1α (IL-1α) release from a preformed pool in mouse epidermis [16] and upregulation of tumour necrosis factor α (TNF-α) and granulocyte–macrophage colony-stimulating factor (GM-CSF). There is then a rise in Langerhans cell-derived IL-1α stimulated by GM-CSF and IL-1α production. Concurrently, the loss of the normal extracellular calcium gradient stimulates lamellar body secretion and barrier repair [17]. Oxidative stress also contributes to the development of inflammation with various irritants [18].

Detergents at lower levels of exposure predominantly affect the horny layer, causing dryness and scaling by destroying lysosomal enzymes in the horny layer [19], whereas at higher concentrations they will dissolve cell membranes and damage lysosomes [20]. With repeated exposure, there will be signs of chronic inflammation, with increased DNA synthesis, acanthosis and changes in cellular metabolism over days to months.

Detergents and other irritants such as croton oil and phenol esters are chemotactic for polymorphonuclear leukocytes at non-toxic concentrations [21], and may cause pustular reactions. Organic solvents such as methanol or chloroform will damage blood vessels, causing hyperaemia [22], and dimethyl sulfoxide (DMSO) is a very effective degranulator of mast cells [23].

Irritants affect everyone, although individual susceptibility with regard to the development of dermatitis varies greatly. The body's immune response is important in generating dermatitis, and this has been shown in the attenuated response to irritants in CD4-deficient mice [24].

Whereas allergic contact dermatitis reactions are histologically almost always eczematous and rather monomorphic, those elicited by irritants show much greater variability. Histological changes vary according to the chemical nature and concentration of the irritant, the type and duration of exposure, the severity of the response and the time of sampling. Some irritant reactions may be histologically indistinguishable from allergic contact dermatitis, whereas others may possess morphological features characteristic of a certain type of chemical. More than one pattern of response may be induced by the same irritant.

Clinical features
History and presentation

Irritants produce a wide range of responses on the skin that are not necessarily eczematous. These may range from purely subjective sensations, such as stinging, smarting, burning or sensations of dryness and tightness, through delayed stinging or transient urticarial reactions to more persistent irritant reactions or irritant contact dermatitis. Irritant contact dermatitis has a spectrum of clinical features, ranging from a little dryness, redness or chapping through various types of eczematous dermatitis to an acute caustic burn. Irritants may also penetrate the skin via appendageal structures and cause folliculitis and other types of reaction (Table 128.1).

The same chemical may cause different irritant reactions depending on concentration; DMSO, for instance, is able to induce both conventional irritant dermatitis and immediate, non-immunological, contact urticarial reactions. The response may also vary according to the site and mode of application, the vehicle and the environmental conditions (mechanical, thermal, climatic) (Figure 128.1), and there is considerable variability between individuals (Table 128.2).

Irritant contact dermatitis frequently presents on the hand. However, constitutional, irritant and allergic factors frequently coexist. Although hand eczema is more common in women [25], this seems to be the result of increased irritant exposure rather than an inherent susceptibility [26]. Allergy can never be completely excluded on purely clinical grounds, nor is any pattern of hand dermatitis pathognomonic for a single causation. In spite of this, there are certain types of hand dermatitis that are at least suggestive of irritant contact dermatitis. These include a patchy 'housework'-type eczema affecting principally the dorsa, sides and webs of the fingers, or a 'ring' eczema – both are patterns associated with wet work and exposure to detergent. What may start as dryness can develop into patchy or diffuse redness with scaling, fissuring and even vesiculation.

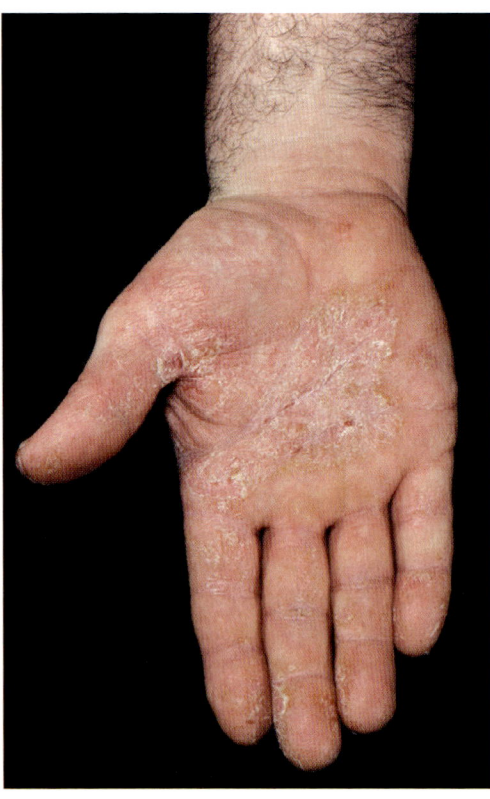

Figure 128.1 Mechanical irritation causing a psoriasiform irritant contact dermatitis of the palmar surface. Courtesy of St John's Institute of Dermatology, London, UK.

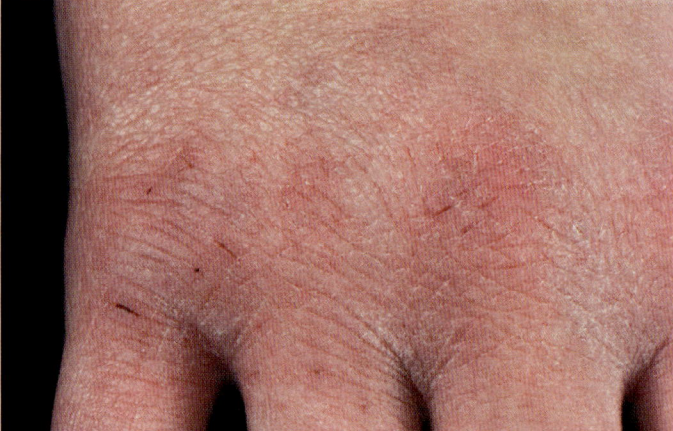

Figure 128.2 Fissuring on the dorsum occurs most commonly as a result of frequent hand washing and outdoor exposure. Courtesy of St John's Institute of Dermatology, London, UK.

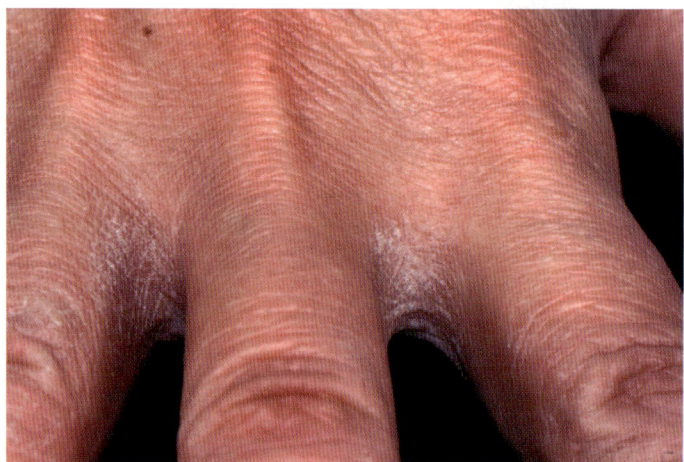

Figure 128.3 Interdigital irritant contact dermatitis is frequently caused by inadequate drying of the hand after washing. It is commonly seen in hairdressers on the non-dominant hand. Courtesy of St John's Institute of Dermatology, London, UK.

However, vesicles are less commonly seen in irritant than in allergic or constitutional eczema, and the principal clinical features are usually dryness or chapping. The wrists and distal arms may also be affected. With increased mechanisation in the house and at work, and with more widespread use of protective gloves and hand creams, this pattern of hand eczema is less common than previously.

Another common pattern of irritant hand eczema is the 'apron' or extended fingertip eczema, with dryness, redness and fissuring affecting principally the palmar aspects of the fingers and distal palm (Figures 128.2 and 128.3). This pattern of dermatitis commonly occurs in those who frequently hold wet cloths containing detergent or household chemicals in the unprotected hand. Friction, irritants and repetitive wetting/desiccation all play a part (Figures 128.4 and 128.5). A similar pattern may be seen in occupations where employees are repeatedly exposed to solvents, friction or irritating food components. Discoid or nummular hand eczema is another rarer pattern of irritant contact dermatitis, affecting especially the dorsa of the hands or fingers.

Clinical variants

Cosmetic dermatitis. Cosmetics, toiletries and skincare products, including sunscreens, quite frequently cause adverse irritant reactions [27]. In most cases, these are only mild or transient, and most consumers simply change to an alternative product. In a minority, reactions may be more severe, with redness, oedema, dryness and scaling. The eyelids are particularly susceptible to irritants [28], as are atopic individuals and those with very fair, rosaceous or seborrhoeic skins. It is of interest that irritant reactions are commoner in younger (premenopausal) women. Those using many products are at risk of 'cosmetic exhaustion', a form of cumulative cosmetic irritant contact dermatitis. Allergy is excluded only by comprehensive patch testing including both products and ingredients. Caution should be exercised when testing the patient's own cosmetics under occlusion. Some items (such as eye make-up) should be allowed to evaporate before being covered to prevent false positive reactions.

Volatile/airborne irritant contact dermatitis. Irritants, as well as allergens, may cause volatile contact dermatitis [29]. Volatile irritants are a not infrequent cause of eyelid dermatitis. In any exposed-site dermatitis, one should consider the possibility of irritant volatile fumes or airborne particles. The fumes can be from acids, alkalis, solvents, resins or any other irritant chemical, such as ammonia or formaldehyde. Irritant dusts include those of some (mostly tropical) woods, cement, fibreglass or rockwool, some metals and metal salts and powdered chemicals.

Cheilitis. Cheilitis is a common problem, often of multifactorial aetiology. Atopic eczema frequently predisposes to its

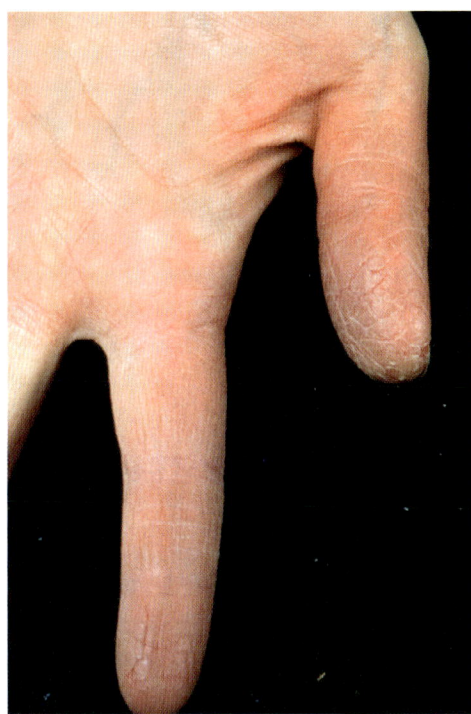

Figure 128.4 Pulpitis is usually caused by wet work. Courtesy of St John's Institute of Dermatology, London, UK.

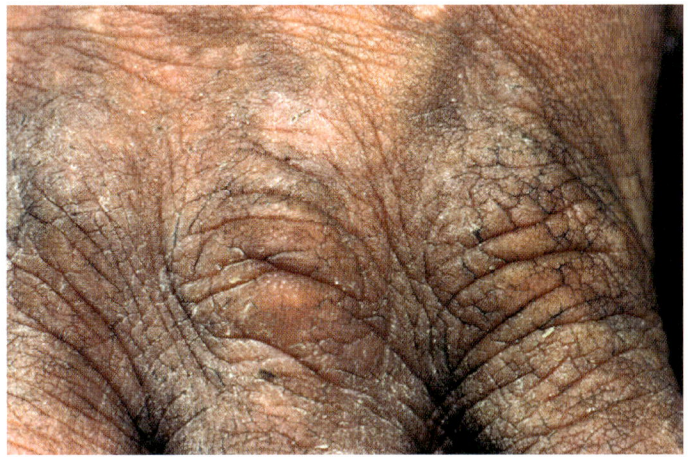

Figure 128.5 Lichenification from chronic irritation. Redness of the skin is less visible in darker skin types. Courtesy of St John's Institute of Dermatology, London, UK.

development [30]. The most common identifiable causes of cheilitis are irritant dermatitis, due to lip licking, cosmetics and medication, and allergic contact dermatitis, of many different causes.

Napkin (diaper/nappy), peristomal and perianal dermatitis. Irritant dermatitis will develop in situations of prolonged or too frequent contact with degraded urine or faeces/faecal residues [31]. Sweat, occlusion, irritant cleansers, secondary infection and secondary medicament allergy are all additional complicating factors. It occurs most frequently in the very young, or in elderly individuals in situations of urinary or faecal incontinence, although current disposable napkins reduce the risk of an irritant contact dermatitis as they are so absorbent. Measures to improve continence in the elderly and frequent changes of absorbent napkins [32] in infants are important, as are mild cleansers and protective pastes or silicone-based creams. Any dermatitis or secondary infection should be controlled with appropriate-strength topical steroids or steroid–antimicrobial combinations. In napkin dermatitis, secondary candidal infection is sufficiently common that routine treatment with an imidazole antifungal is frequently of benefit [33].

A similar situation appertains to perianal dermatitis, where mucus or faecal leakage may occur in association with haemorrhoids and/or poor sphincter function. A bidet or 'wet' cleansing routine using aqueous cream or equivalent is of benefit. Wet wipes and overzealous cleaning with detergents frequently aggravate the problem.

With peristomal dermatitis, there is the additional complication of the need to maintain a protective seal between the stoma bag and skin. The use of corticosteroid-containing lotions, either aqueous or alcoholic, has been shown to be effective without interfering with stoma bag adhesion [34] (Chapter 112). Dermatitis, as well as being caused by leakage, may also be due to continuous occlusion and repeated stripping of the skin. Where there is erosive disease, the use of topical sucralfate has been shown to promote healing in peristomal disease but not erosions from other causes [35]. The sucralfate acts as both a physical barrier and, it is suggested, by binding to basic fibroblast growth factor preventing its degradation, as a stimulus to healing.

Differential diagnosis

Other diagnoses including allergic contact dermatitis, pyoderma gangrenosum, infections, skin cancers, etc. should be considered in intractable cases or where response to treatment is unexpectedly poor. These include:
- Atopic eczema.
- Allergic contact dermatitis.
- Contact urticaria.
- Thermal injury.
- Non-accidental injury in children.

The differential diagnosis of hand dermatitis includes fungal infection, which may cause a unilateral palmar dermatitis resembling eczema on the dorsum of the hand. Skin scrapings are important to exclude tinea as the cause of a hard to treat 'dermatitis'. Psoriasis frequently affects the palms, resulting in a hyperkeratotic appearance. This can be difficult to distinguish from dermatitis when there are no lesions elsewhere. Furthermore, there may be a history of exacerbation when the disease leads to the Koebner phenomenon on the hands as a result of manual work. The presence of red scaling over the interphalangeal joints is often a helpful clue to the diagnosis. Scabies in the interdigital spaces can simulate an irritant dermatitis. Rarely, the presence of milia may suggest a diagnosis of porphyria cutanea tarda.

Classification of severity

In clinical practice, there are no objective ways of quantifying severity of irritant contact dermatitis. However, severity may be subjectively assessed by the degree of redness and surface change. Non-specific assessment tools such as the Physician Global Assessment or symptom-driven patient tools such as the Dermatology Life Quality Index (DLQI) may be used. A number of research tools exist that may quantify the irritant response by measuring redness,

TEWL, hydration and skin thickness. The optimal method to be used varies with the nature of the irritant [36].

Redness (erythema). Among the most overt clinical features of irritant reactions is redness, which may be quantified using a number of different approaches. Laser Doppler flowmetry (LDF) provides a measure of superficial blood flow by transmitting monochromatic light from a helium–neon laser through optical fibres to the skin surface. The light is Doppler-shifted by moving blood cells in the upper dermis, remaining unchanged in the surrounding stationary tissue. By means of a differential signal detector and signal processing arrangement, the back-scattered or reflected light is interpreted. The final output, which is linearly related to the product of the number of blood cells and their average velocity in the measured volume, is expressed in relative and dimensionless units. Studies by a number of investigators have shown that LDF generally correlates well with visually assessed redness, and is capable of discriminating between negative and weakly positive irritant reactions [37].

Alternative methods for objectively quantifying redness rely upon the generalised increase in red blood cells resulting from both increased blood flow and blood vessel dilatation. Those which are based upon remittance spectroscopy emit red and green light from a tungsten halogen lamp or light-emitting diode (LED) source. Oxyhaemoglobin in the blood vessels absorbs a proportion of the green light, and largely reflects the red light. Changes in the quantity of oxyhaemoglobin significantly alter the amount of green light absorbed, but have very little influence on the red light. An erythema index can therefore be calculated from the ratio between the reflected green and red light, such that the greater the redness, the higher the value of the erythema index [38].

Redness may also be quantified using tristimulus colorimeters, virtually all of which employ a system for colour definition known as the Commission Internationale de l'Eclairage (CIE) L*a*b* colour system. This provides a three-dimensional coordinate system where L* represents an axis for brightness, a* represents a green–red axis and b* represents a yellow–blue axis. Redness is more difficult to see and measure in those with darker skin types and in the context of postinflammatory hyperpigmentation. In real-life settings this can result in lower eczema severity scores which do not reflect the true disease burden [39].

Transepidermal water loss. In addition to inducing redness, irritants commonly affect barrier function, leading to alterations in TEWL. Measuring instruments employ open chambers, through which, when applied to the surface of the skin, water vapour evaporates, creating a water pressure gradient from which the evaporative TEWL (expressed in $g/m^2/h$) is calculated. Many variables influence TEWL measurements. Some relate to the environment and to instrument operation, necessitating a careful adherence to 'good laboratory practice', as outlined in a report from the Standardization Group of the European Society of Contact Dermatitis [40]. Others relate directly to the individual; age and anatomical site are among the most important variables. Measurements of TEWL have proved valuable in predicting susceptibility to skin irritation, assessing the protective effects of barrier creams and evaluating the irritancy potential of different chemicals, but it remains a research tool.

Hydration. Changes in the hydration state of the skin also commonly occur in irritant contact dermatitis and, again, this parameter may be objectively measured. Several different devices are available, based on differing biophysical approaches. Using the principle of capacitance, hydration of the stratum corneum can be measured to a depth of approximately 0.1 mm. In contrast, skin conductance has also been used as a measure of hydration. Studies suggest that capacitance may be more effective in the assessment of dry skin, whereas conductance is better suited for studies of water accumulation in the stratum corneum [41]. A third method uses the principle of impedance-based capacitance to assess hydration levels.

Skin thickness. Although not extensively applied, high-frequency ultrasound has also proved valuable for the assessment of another aspect of the irritant response, namely changes in skin thickness [42]. Line-field confocal optical coherence tomography and other similar techniques may yield even more precise detail.

Investigations

Irritant contact dermatitis is a clinical diagnosis based on knowledge of the chemical(s) involved and exposure factors. However, some chemicals may have both irritant and allergic potential, or the patient may be exposed to several chemicals with irritant or allergic potential. Consequently, patch testing should be undertaken to exclude an allergic component to the skin rash. Patch testing should never be undertaken with unknown chemicals supplied by the patient, and the testing clinician should either avoid testing known irritants, or carefully test with serial dilutions and be vigilant for false positive reactions.

Management

The successful management of irritant contact dermatitis requires both prevention and subsequently treatment if dermatitis develops [43]. The most important aspect of treatment is avoidance of the cause (Box 128.4). In an occupational setting, automation of the production process may avoid exposure but can be expensive. A cost-effective compromise is the use of personal protective equipment and/or substitution of a chemical. It should be remembered that natural rubber latex gloves provide protection against water-miscible substances but may be inappropriate for other exposures (Table 128.3). With organic solvents and chemicals, the choice of glove material may vary [44]; advice can be found on the material safety data sheet of each product.

Where present, dermatitis requires palliation of symptoms with topical steroids and emollients after irritant avoidance has been achieved. The efficacy of topical corticosteroids in irritant contact dermatitis has been questioned [45,46], although another study has shown benefit [47]. Retinoids and vitamin D analogues are not of any value [45].

Experimentally, an emollient alone has been shown to improve barrier repair. The choice of emollient may be important, with lipid-rich preparations being more effective. Studies have shown that barrier repair may be impaired or accelerated according to the constituents of a physiological lipid mixture [48]. For conditions like radiation dermatitis, sunburn, irritant dermatitis due to some surfactants and retinoids, or when treating premature infants under 33 weeks' gestation (where the lamellar body secretory system is

Box 128.4 Advice to patients with hand eczema

To speed healing and prevent your dermatitis from returning, you must now take great care of your hands and allow your skin to heal and recover its natural resilience/strength (this may take many months, even though the skin may look normal before then):

1. Use a moisturising hand cream frequently so that the skin does not become dry
2. Use the steroid creams/ointments as prescribed by the doctor
3. Hand washing. Use lukewarm water and soap substitute (e.g. aqueous cream). If soap is used, find a soap with no fragrance, tar or sulphur; use it sparingly; rinse thoroughly and then dry thoroughly (especially finger webs and wrists)
4. If wet work cannot be avoided, wear gloves; use plastic rather than rubber, preferably with a cotton lining. Consider the following:
   - Avoid contact with detergents and other cleaning agents. Always dilute them according to manufacturers' instructions. Keep the outside of the container clean or you will contaminate your hands with the neat product
   - When washing up, use running water and a pot brush rather than a cloth/sponge
   - Washing machines and dishwashers are a great help, but avoid contact with detergent powder or liquid – use a measure with a handle
   - Water softeners are helpful, but too expensive unless you are not contemplating moving house for a long time. Try adding water softener (e.g. Calgon) to dish water, washing water, baths, etc.; less soap/detergent is then required
   - Avoid contact with polish, e.g. metal, shoe, floor, car, furniture, window and wax polishes. NB: Spray polish carries a long way
   - Avoid contact with shampoo. Either use plastic gloves or get someone else to wash your own and your children's hair
   - Do not apply hair products with bare hands, e.g. setting mousse/gel/lotions, colourants, creams, brilliantine. Some of these are irritant, but the friction of running hands through hair is considerable
   - Avoid contact with solvents, e.g. white spirit and brush cleaners, petrol, trichlorethylene, xylene, carbon tetrachloride (e.g. dry cleaning and stain-removal agents). Solvents pass through rubber gloves. Buy vinyl for these jobs
   - Do not peel citrus fruits with bare hands, e.g. oranges, lemons, satsumas
5. Wear gloves when outdoors in cold weather
6. If the skin becomes inflamed and throbs, it is likely to be infected. Visit your doctor, who may take a skin swab and prescribe antibiotic treatment:
   - Individuals with hand eczema are at increased risk of contracting infection through damaged skin and should wear gloves when in contact with blood or potentially infectious biological secretions, e.g. when handling soiled linen, cleaning lavatories, etc.
   - Patients with hand eczema should not be involved in commercial food preparation because the bacteria that cause infection may also cause food poisoning

Your hand eczema should improve if you follow all these suggestions. Once the skin appears to have healed, you should always continue to take care of your hands

---

in napkin/diaper dermatitis), a mixture of cholesterol : ceramides : free fatty acids, in a 3 : 1 : 1 ratio, should be used to achieve a rapid return to normal barrier function [49].

In severe cases, phototherapy or systemic drugs such as corticosteroids, azathioprine and ciclosporin may be required. It is, as yet, unknown if dupilumab or other targeted treatments may influence irritant contact dermatitis. Where there is secondary infection, topical or systemic antimicrobial agents may be necessary. Regulation of occupational practice is essential in primary prevention (Box 128.5), and this is especially important as some patients may have persistent skin problems even after exposure has ceased [50] (Chapter 129).

Box 128.5 Recommended occupational skin protection programme

Washing
- Wash in lukewarm water – the damage caused by detergent is temperature dependent
- Rinse and dry thoroughly – dermatitis often develops in web spaces and other areas frequently missed
- Do not wear rings – soap and other irritants accumulate underneath

Disinfection
- Do not use unless a job requirement – disinfectants are more irritant than ordinary washing
- Alcohol gels may be preferable even if they sting – detergent-based disinfectants are more irritant [11]

Gloves
- Wear gloves – unprotected wet work is a major cause of irritant dermatitis
- Wear gloves for as short a time as possible – prolonged usage impairs barrier function
- Wear with a cotton liner – prevents the irritation induced by glove occlusion
- Change them frequently – occlusion enhances the effect of irritants that are contaminating or penetrate gloves

Emollients
- Apply during and after work – to prevent and treat dermatitis if it develops
- Apply to all of the hand – areas are often missed
- Use a lipid-rich product – more effective than the alternatives

At home
- Follow the same measures – domestic exposures are additive
- Wear warm gloves in winter – the skin is more susceptible to irritants in winter

Adapted from Holness and Nethercott 1991 [51].

Treatment ladder for irritant contact dermatitis

First line
- Irritant avoidance

---

impaired or immature), non-physiological lipids (e.g. petrolatum) should be considered for treatment. In most other causes of irritant dermatitis (where lipid metabolism has not been deranged such as

Table 128.3 Recommended glove materials for chemical protection.

Glove materials	Nitrile	Butyl	Neoprene	Fluorocarbon	PVC	PVA	Notes
Aliphatic hydrocarbons	+			+		+*	Except cyclohexane*
Aromatic hydrocarbons	+			+		+*	Except ethylbenzene*
Halogenated hydrocarbons			+		+*		Except methyl chloride* and halothane*
Aldehydes, amines, amides	+*						Except butylamine* and triethylamine*
Esters			+*			+†	Except butylacrylate* and octylphthalate†
Alkalis		+		+		+	
Organic acids	+*	+	+†				Except acrylic*†, methacrylic*† and acetic* acids
Inorganic acids	+*		+†		+‡		Except chromic†, hydrofluoric*, nitric*‡ and sulphuric*‡ acids

From Berardinelli 1988 [44].
*†‡, These gloves do not provide adequate protection with the listed chemical.
PVA, polyvinyl alcohol; PVC, polyvinyl chloride.

> **Second line**
> - Irritant substitution/personal protective equipment (e.g. appropriate gloves as listed in Table 128.3, protective clothing, etc.)
>
> **Third line**
> - Barrier creams, topical corticosteroids, systemic immunosuppressives

Non-immune contact urticaria

Definition and nomenclature
A localised redness or weal and flare reaction caused by contact with a substance where there is no substance-specific immune response.

> **Synonyms and inclusions**
> - Non-allergic contact urticaria

Introduction and general description
Immediate contact reactions may be either allergic or toxic. They are transient, developing within minutes, and fade quickly (usually within hours). They may appear on both normal and damaged/eczematous skin, and may present as only a transient, symptomatic redness or as a contact urticaria (Chapter 42). For some agents that cause immediate-type reactions, it is still unclear as to whether or not the mechanism is immunological. Non-immunological, immediate contact reactions occur without prior sensitisation. The reactions remain localised and may present as a transient redness or as an urticarial weal and flare, depending on concentration, area of contact, mode of exposure and agent involved [1,2]. Substances reported to cause non-immune contact urticaria are listed in Box 128.6. The most potent of these, such as benzoic acid, sorbic acid, cinnamic acid, cinnamal and nicotine acid esters, may induce a local reaction within 45 min in more than 50% of those tested. Reactions may occur at concentrations as low as 0.1% for benzoic acid, sorbic acid and sodium benzoate, and as low as 0.01% for cinnamal. Reactions are not enhanced by occlusion, but may affect mucosal surfaces; low concentrations of cinnamal are sometimes added to toothpaste and mouthwashes to impart a sensation of 'freshness'. Studies on an unselected population have shown that reactions to urticants are not predictable; an individual who reacted strongly to one urticant did not necessarily react to another. In addition, there was no significant correlation between age or sex and urticant response [3].

Epidemiology
Incidence and prevalence
These are unknown, but many patients with mild disease will not seek medical advice, hence there is likely to be considerable under-reporting.

Pathophysiology
The mechanism of action of non-immunological contact reactions is not known, but is presumed to be via direct release of inflammatory mediators, including prostaglandins and leukotrienes [4]; the reaction is blocked by non-steroidal anti-inflammatory drugs (NSAIDs) and ultraviolet (UV) light, or by pretreatment with capsaicin, but not by antihistamines [5–7].

Clinical features
Differential diagnosis
- Immunological contact urticaria (type I hypersensitivity).
- Chronic ordinary urticaria.

Investigations
Twenty-minute patch tests or skin prick tests may confirm the diagnosis but will not necessarily differentiate this from immunological contact urticaria. Control subjects may also be positive on testing.

Management

> **Treatment ladder for non-immune contact urticaria**
>
> **First line**
> - Urticant avoidance or substitution
>
> **Second line**
> - Personal protective equipment (e.g. gloves)
>
> **Third line**
> - Expectant therapy

Box 128.6 Agents reported to cause non-immune contact reactions

Animals
- Arthropods
- Caterpillars
- Coral
- Jellyfish
- Moths
- Sea anemones

Foods
- Cayenne pepper
- Fish
- Mustard

Fragrances and flavourings
- Benzaldehyde
- Cinnamic acid
- Cinnamal
- Cinnamon oil
- Myroxylon pereirae (balsam of Peru)
- Thyme

Medicaments
- Alcohols
- Benzocaine
- Camphor
- Cantharidin
- Capsaicin
- Chloroform
- Dimethyl sulfoxide
- Friars' balsam (compound benzoin tincture)

Plants
- Nettles
- Seaweed

Preservatives
- Benzoic acid
- Chlorocresol
- Formaldehyde
- Sodium benzoate
- Sorbic acid

Miscellaneous
- Butyric acid
- Cobalt
- Dimethyl fumarate
- Histamine
- Pine oil
- Pyridine carbo-aldehyde

Reproduced from Lahti and Basketter 2006 [2] with permission of Springer Nature.

Phototoxic contact dermatitis

Definition and nomenclature
Phototoxic contact dermatitis occurs when light is absorbed by a chemical which then is modified and becomes an irritant stimulus.

Synonyms and inclusions
- Photo-irritation

Introduction and general description
Chemicals applied either topically or systemically may absorb photons and be chemically modified to cause irritation. Clinically, the reaction resembles a sunburn and only occurs in sun-exposed areas of skin. Primary prevention is critical. An initial screen of potential phototoxic chemicals involves the measurement of its absorption spectrum. If this indicates the chemical may be photoreactive then the 3T3 neutral red uptake phototoxicity test (3T3 NRU PT) can be performed, which has been validated and accepted into legislation. This test compares the cytotoxicity of a chemical when tested with and without exposure to a non-cytotoxic dose of simulated solar light (UVA/visible spectrum). Mouse 3T3 fibroblasts are incubated with the chemical and the concentration-dependent reduction of the uptake of the vital dye neutral red is measured 24 h after treatment. Substances identified are likely to be phototoxic following systemic administration and distribution to the skin or following topical application. The test has been found to detect photoallergens in addition to irritants, and the use of further photobinding studies to human albumin may distinguish between the two. In general, photoallergy requires protein binding as a prelude to antigen presentation.

The use of ethical tests in human volunteers may be considered where testing *in vivo* is considered essential [1]. Strong irritants may cause dermatitis on first exposure, whereas weak irritants may be detected only by repeated application [2]. Internal standards are necessary to allow comparison with other established irritants [3].

Clinical features
History and presentation
Tetracycline-related antibiotics may cause phototoxicity, as can psoralens, porphyrins, amiodarone, phenothiazines and NSAIDs. Plant sap (e.g. from the giant hogweed) may cause a phototoxic reaction known as phytophotodermatitis. Such reactions can be flagellate or show linear vesicles. They often resolve with persistent hyperpigmentation.

Differential diagnosis
- Photoallergy.
- Allergic contact dermatitis.
- (Non-photo) irritant contact dermatitis.

Investigations
Photopatch testing is important to exclude a photoallergy in some cases; otherwise the diagnosis is clinical.

Management

Treatment ladder for phototoxic contact dermatitis

First line
- Primary prevention

Second line
- Phototoxin avoidance or substitution

Third line
- Emollients and topical corticosteroids for acute flares with sun avoidance

Subjective sensory irritation

Definition and nomenclature

Subjective sensory irritation is a subjective feeling of skin discomfort when in contact with a substance in the absence of any visible skin change.

Synonyms and inclusions
- Sensitive skin
- Subjective irritant response

Introduction and general description

With some irritants, there is little or nothing to see, but individuals complain of a subjective sensation of stinging, burning or smarting. These sensations most commonly affect the head and neck, may present as one form of cosmetic intolerance and are frequently termed 'sensitive skin' [1]. Although stinging potential is often assessed by the application of lactic acid to the naso-labial fold, the results do not necessarily correlate with the sensation perceived at other facial sites [2]. With soaps and detergents, the perceived sensory symptoms correlate with, and predict the development of, clinical signs of irritant dermatitis [3]. However, more typically the sensation does not correlate with a predisposition to irritant dermatitis or non-immune contact urticaria. Little is known of the mechanisms involved in subjective irritant reactions [1]. It is presumed that penetration of the irritant is primarily via sweat ducts and hair follicles, is not related to pH and that the reaction involves stimulation of sensory nerve endings. The reaction is substantially reduced in the absence of sweating and is commoner in the summer. Factors thought to predispose to sensitive skin include female sex and hormonal status, young age, fair skin, susceptibility to blushing/flushing, thin stratum corneum, increased number of sweat glands and innervation and impairment of epidermal barrier function. The presence of sensitive skin also affects quality of life scores, with affected individuals having an impaired psychological component, although there was no significant relationship to depressive symptoms [4]. Triggers are not necessarily chemical, and include environmental factors such as wind. Sensory irritation from woollen garments is also well known among patients with atopic eczema. Experimental studies have shown this to be due to stimulation of nerve fibres which transmit pain. It required a 100 mg force on the end of a 40 μm diameter textile fibre to trigger the nerve receptor. Thus, garments that induce the sensation will have protruding fibre ends that can withstand 100 mg pressure without buckling. Prickle was not experienced if the fabric was rubbed over the skin, if the skin was cold or if the area of contact was less than 1 cm^2. Moisture increased the severity of the sensation [5].

Individuals can be screened to ascertain whether they are 'stingers' or not by the application of 5% aqueous lactic acid to the naso-labial fold after the induction of sweating. Preparations can be screened for stinging potential by testing a predetermined panel of 'stingers and smarters'.

Immediate-type stinging. Some chemicals will cause painful sensations within seconds of contact [6]. These include acids, where the stinging may be a prodrome to the development of more severe cutaneous damage. Other chemicals, however, will cause stinging without any significant cutaneous damage. The best known of these are chloroform and methanol (1 : 1), and 95% ethanol. Responses vary according to site and individual susceptibility, and probably relate indirectly to stratum corneum thickness. The sensation abates quickly following removal of the irritant substance.

Delayed-type stinging. Delayed-type stinging may occur following contact with a number of substances (Box 128.7) [6]. Typically, there is no immediate stinging, but discomfort develops within 1–2 min, reaches a maximum in 5–10 min and fades slowly over the next half

Box 128.7 Substances known to cause delayed stinging or burning

Weak reaction
- Aluminium chloride 30% aq.
- Benzene 1% alc.
- Phenol 1% alc.
- Phosphoric acid 1% aq.
- Resorcinol 5% aq.
- Salicylic acid 5% alc.
- Zirconium hydroxychloride 30% aq.

Moderate reaction
- Benzoyl peroxide 5% aq.
- Diethyl toluamide 50% alc.
- Dimethyl acetamide 100%
- Dimethyl formamide 100%
- Dimethyl phthalate 50% alc.
- Dimethyl sulfoxide 100%
- 2-Ethyl-1,3-hexanediol 50% alc.
- Propylene carbonate 100%
- Propylene glycol 100%
- Propylene glycol diacetate 100%
- Sodium carbonate 15% aq.
- Trisodium phosphate 5% aq.

Severe reaction
- Amyldimethyl-*p*-aminobenzoic acid (Escalol 506) 5% alc.
- 2-Ethoxyethyl-*p*-methoxy-cinnamate (Giv-Tan FR) 2% alc.
- Hydrochloric acid 1.2% aq.
- Lactic acid 5% aq.
- Phosphoric acid 3.3% aq.
- Sodium hydroxide 1.3% aq.

Adapted from Frosch and John 2006 [6].

hour. The reaction normally affects only the face, especially in association with heat and humidity or sweating. The sensation is not alleviated by washing off the offending chemical. It is an idiosyncratic response, and only a proportion of the population will be affected.

Epidemiology
Incidence and prevalence
'Sensitive skin' might be considered a marker of a form of skin irritancy. In a questionnaire-based study of 3300 women and 500 men, 51.4% of women and 38.2% of men considered that they were susceptible [7]. Moreover, 57% of women and 31.4% of men had had an adverse reaction to a personal care product during their lives. Among women, symptoms of subjective skin irritation (burning, stinging, etc.) occurred more frequently in those who considered that they had a sensitive skin (53%) than in those who did not (17%). Dry skin and a predisposition to blushing/flushing were factors associated with a sensitive skin. An atopic background was a predictive factor for the presence of sensitive skin, as the incidence of atopy was higher among those with sensitive skin (49%) than among those in the non-sensitive group (27%). However, equal numbers of atopics and non-atopics constituted the sensitive skin group, indicating that other variables were involved.

Clinical features
Differential diagnosis
- Irritant contact dermatitis.
- Allergic contact dermatitis.
- Atopic eczema.
- Psychological illness.

Investigations
Sometimes patch testing can be helpful to eliminate other differential diagnoses.

Management
Treatment is largely that of avoidance, although strontium salts have been shown experimentally to inhibit the sensation [8]. Currently, this seems of little clinical value.

Chemical burns

Definition
A chemical burn results when tissue is exposed to a corrosive chemical, such as a strong acid or alkali. Irreversible cell damage and necrosis occurs (Chapter 125).

Introduction and general description
There is usually rapid onset of painful redness, often within minutes, at the site of exposure, followed by blistering and the development of necrotic ulcers. Weals may also be seen. Symptoms coincide with the exposure, but with some chemicals, including phenols and weak hydrofluoric acid, the onset may be delayed. Damage continues to occur until all of the agent has chemically reacted or has been neutralised as a result of treatment. Occupational settings are still common for chemical burns but the frequency of these burns in domestic settings is increasing [1]. The burn is classified according to depth (1 – superficial to 4 – extending deep to the skin).

Epidemiology
Incidence and prevalence
Scanty data exist but some studies suggest an incidence of 2–10% [1]. Chemical burns are relatively common, with an American survey showing that 119 hospitals treated 11 759 patients during a 1-year period. The majority of chemical burns involved the upper limb, with most occurring in young adults and infants. Occupational chemical burns are also relatively common, with 29% of chemical burns requiring admission being work related, with a rate of 26.4/10 000 employees. In women, chemical burns of the wrist and hand were most frequent, whereas in men eye involvement was more common. Welders, labourers, cooks and mechanics were most at risk [2].

Age
Limited data suggest that those of working age suffer most from chemical burns [1].

Sex
Men are more frequently affected than women (6 : 1 in some series [1]).

Associated diseases
Sometimes scars following burns may lead to functional disability, such as joint contractures.

Clinical features
History and presentation
Pain and redness are usually present within minutes of exposure, but presentation may be delayed. Most acids (e.g. sulphuric, nitric, hydrochloric, chromic) coagulate skin proteins, and as a result form a barrier that impedes further penetration. Some acids can discolour (e.g. nitric acid turns the skin yellow). Hydrofluoric acid [3] differs in that it causes a liquefactive necrosis, and penetration can continue for several days after exposure, even down to bone. Pain, which can last several days, is typical of burns due to hydrofluoric acid and other fluorides. It is related to the ability of the fluoride ion to bind calcium and disrupt neural function. If more than 1% of the body surface area is affected, systemic toxicity can develop.

Alkalis (e.g. sodium, calcium, potassium hydroxides; wet concrete [4]; sodium and potassium cyanides) degrade lipids, and saponification of the resulting fatty acids forms soaps which aid penetration deeper into the skin. As a consequence, damage is more severe than with most acids, and pain is also a feature. The dead skin turns brown and later black, usually without blistering, and forms a hard eschar. Phenols [5] and unhardened phenolic resins penetrate the skin easily and rarely can cause nerve damage in the absence of visible skin change. Vasoconstriction may contribute to the necrosis that develops, and in the case of systemic absorption can lead to shock and renal damage.

Differential diagnosis
- Irritant contact dermatitis.
- Allergic contact dermatitis.
- Contact urticaria.
- Thermal injury.
- Non-accidental injury in children.

Classification of severity

Burns are classified according to the depth of cutaneous involvement:

1. Superficial partial-thickness burns extend to the level of the dermal papillae. As the papillary blood vessels remain intact, the skin blanches on pressure and vasodilatation of the vessels results in the skin appearing shiny pink to red and wet as a result of capillary leakage. Blisters may be present, and sensation is preserved. The burn typically heals within 10–14 days without scarring.
2. Deep partial-thickness burns extend into the dermis but the appendages are spared. The burn appears white or pale pink and oedematous. Some sensation may be retained but often only that of deep pressure. Re-epithelialisation begins from the residual adnexal structures, taking up to 6 weeks to occur, with scarring.
3. Full-thickness burns extend into the subcutaneous tissue. The burn appears brown/black or pale white, with a leathery eschar. Sensation is completely lost and healing occurs slowly from the margins. Healing occurs with scarring and a risk of contracture.
4. Fourth-degree burns extend into the tendon, muscle, bone or joint.

Management

Knowledge of the chemical causing the burn is vital as decontamination or other specific neutralisation may be required. Initial treatment of chemical burns [6,7] requires irrigation with large volumes of lukewarm water and the removal of contaminated clothing. Where the chemical is insoluble in water, a soap solution or solvent may be used instead. High pressures should not be used to avoid splashing other areas of the body or bystanders with the corrosive material.

Although neutralising solutions offer an alternative to irrigation, theoretically an exothermic reaction and potential delay in obtaining the treatment might result in increased tissue damage, and they are not generally recommended [8]. Specific antidotes that have been suggested include the use of milk or egg whites for oxidising agents such as chromic acid and potassium permanganate. Reducing agents such as hydrochloric and nitric acids can be neutralised with soap or sodium and magnesium hydroxides.

Consideration should be given to referral to a burns unit in the following circumstances:

1. Partial-thickness burns with >10% surface area involvement.
2. Burns of the face, hands, feet, genitalia or over joints where contractures may affect function.
3. Full-thickness burns.
4. Chemical and inhalational injury where there is a risk of systemic involvement.
5. Burns in individuals with co-morbidities that may complicate management.

On arrival in hospital, initial assessment involves providing systemic support and fluid replacement. The fluid requirement varies depending on body weight and surface area involved. Jewellery should be removed to prevent it acting as a tourniquet as oedema develops. Tetanus status should be reviewed.

For some chemicals, such as hydrofluoric acid, specific antidotes should be used subsequently, for example 2.5% calcium gluconate gel. Application should be repeated 4-hourly and the disappearance of pain is a sign of successful treatment [9]. If the pain fails to resolve, infiltration or regional infusion has been used. If treatment is delayed, the fluoride ion disassociates and complexes with calcium and magnesium forming insoluble salts in the tissues, with the destruction of soft and bony tissue. Hypocalcaemia leads to cardiac arrhythmia. When there is a risk of toxicity from systemic absorption, as with chromic acid [10], early debridement of the necrotic areas reduces blood levels, and consideration should be given to the use of dialysis to remove circulating chromium. Ulcerated areas should be managed with antibacterial creams to prevent secondary infection while re-epithelialisation occurs. If there is a surrounding inflammatory reaction, a moderately potent topical corticosteroid can be applied. Vapour-permeable dressings are recommended in view of the role of TEWL in stimulating barrier repair [11].

Frequent review is required because the ulcers can progress over several days. Subsequent management with excision/debridement and/or grafting may speed up the healing process. Where the ulcer extends into the dermis, healing frequently results in a scar, and pigmentary change is common. Several chemicals (e.g. hydrofluoric acid, phenolic compounds, chromic acid, gasoline) carry a significant risk of systemic toxicity even when cutaneous involvement is small (c.1%). In these instances, regular monitoring of blood, liver and kidney function, with appropriate supportive treatment, is required [12].

When the chemical is a sensitiser, allergic contact dermatitis may subsequently occur on re-exposure to non-irritant concentrations, as burns and irritant dermatitis appear to promote sensitisation [13].

Treatment ladder for chemical burns

First line
- Thorough wound toilet
- Physiological dressings
- Topical antibiotics and topical corticosteroids

Second line
- Consider skin grafting/debridement for deep wounds

Third line
- Surgical correction of scarring if the scars cause functional impairment

---

Key references

The full list of references can be found in the online version at https://www.wiley.com/rooksdermatology10e

Irritant contact dermatitis

14 Aramaki J, Loffler C, Kawana S et al. Irritant patch testing with sodium lauryl sulphate: interrelation between concentration and exposure time. Br J Dermatol 2001;145:704–8.

36 Fluhr JW, Kuss O, Diepgen T et al. Testing for irritation with a multifactorial approach: comparison of eight non-invasive measuring techniques on five different irritation types. Br J Dermatol 2001;145:696–703.

43 Saary J, Qureshi R, Palda V et al. A systematic review of contact dermatitis treatment and prevention. *J Am Acad Dermatol* 2005;53:845–55.
44 Berardinelli SP. Prevention of occupational skin disease through use of chemical protective gloves. *Dermatol Clin* 1988;6:115–19.
50 Nicholson PJ, Llewellyn D, English JS. Evidence-based guidelines for the prevention, identification and management of occupational contact dermatitis and urticaria. *Contact Dermatitis* 2010;63:177–86.
51 Holness DL, Nethercott JR. Is a worker's understanding of their diagnosis an important determinant of outcome in occupational contact dermatitis? *Contact Dermatitis* 1991;25:296–301.

Non-immune contact urticaria
1 Wakelin SH. Contact urticaria. *Clin Exp Dermatol* 2000;26:132–6.

Phototoxic contact dermatitis
1 Cooper K, Marriott M, Peters L, Basketter DA. Stinging and irritating substances: their identification and assessment. In: Lóden M, Maibach HI, eds. *Dry Skin and Moisturisers*, 2nd edn. Boca Raton, FL: CRC Taylor & Francis, 2005:501–14.

Subjective sensory irritation
1 Farage M, Katsarou A, Maibach HI. Sensory, clinical and physiological factors in sensitive skin: a review. *Contact Dermatitis* 2006;55:1–14.

Chemical burns
1 Hardwicke J, Hunter T, Staruch R, Moiemen N. Chemical burns. An historical comparison and review of the literature. *Burns* 2012;38:383–7.

CHAPTER 129

Occupational Dermatology

Jonathan M. L. White

Department of Dermatology, Hôpital Erasme, Brussels; Ecole de Santé Publique, Université libre de Bruxelles, Brussels, Belgium

Occupational irritant contact dermatitis, 129.1	Occupational dyspigmentation, 129.13	Key references, 129.16
Occupational allergic contact dermatitis, 129.5	Occupationally induced skin tumours, 129.14	
Acne of chemical origin, 129.7	Vibration white finger, 129.15	

Occupational irritant contact dermatitis

Definition and nomenclature

Occupational irritant contact dermatitis is the cutaneous response to the physical/toxic effects of a wide range of environmental exposures in the workplace. This may be an acute (toxic) irritant contact dermatitis or a cumulative irritant/insult dermatitis (Chapter 128).

Synonyms and inclusions
- 'Wear-and-tear' dermatitis
- Traumiterative dermatitis
- Contact dermatitis

Introduction and general description

The principles of irritant contact dermatitis are described in Chapter 128. Occupational irritant contact dermatitis is the commonest form of occupational skin disease.

Dermatitis from the type of metal-working fluid or coolant most commonly known in the UK as 'soluble oil' is a prime example of occupational contact dermatitis that is usually primarily, and frequently totally, of cumulative irritant rather than allergic causation [1,2–6]. Soluble oils are oil-in-water emulsions used to cool and lubricate metal-working and certain other industrial manufacturing operations [7]. Synthetic coolants are aqueous chemical solutions and can have similar effects on the skin. Both types of product contain numerous additives, some of which are potential sensitisers (especially biocides [8,9]), but it is the substantial content of surface-active agents as emulsifiers or wetting agents in coolants that appears to underlie their potential for skin irritation [7,10]. Synthetic coolants also contain traces of nitrosamines, formed by triethanolamine or diethanolamine reacting with nitrites. Although currently under evaluation as carcinogens, there is no evidence that nitrosamines in coolants are irritant or sensitising to the skin.

Soluble oil dermatitis is typical of occupational irritant contact dermatitis in that it is cumulative and has a multifactorial aetiology [3,4]. The degree of skin contact [11], individual susceptibility, machine type and control method [12], and biocide additions [13] are all important factors, in addition to the specification and condition of the metal-working fluid itself. Clinically, the dorsa of the hands, finger webs, wrists and forearms are predominantly affected [14] and the dermatitis can have a patchy distribution that mimics nummular eczema (Figure 129.1) [4]. This is also true of several other forms of occupational contact dermatitis, including cement dermatitis [15] and dermatitis from machine oil in hosiery workers [16]. There are two reports [17,18] of soluble oil dermatitis presenting as 'dyshidrotic' eczema; a similar pattern has been described from mechanical irritancy [19]. The prognosis is highly variable but may eventually be good even without a change of work [20].

The skin can react in a variety of ways to excessive friction and microtrauma to produce a physical irritant contact dermatitis [21,22]. The reaction depends upon constitutional factors, such as a tendency to develop psoriasis (Figure 129.2), or the type of trauma [23]. Various types of reactions can occur: calluses, fissuring, lichenification, blistering, Koebner phenomenon aggravating psoriasis and granulomas.

Fibreglass dermatitis is a well-known example of a physical irritant contact dermatitis and was first described in 1942 [24]. Fibreglass consists of sharp glass spicules which are capable of penetrating the superficial part of the horny layer of the skin to cause immediate skin irritation. The acute irritation reaction results in a pruriginous dermatitis; as clothing may trap the fibreglass, this may occur on covered parts of the body, yet despite being very symptomatic, the clinical signs may be minimal.

Epidemiology
Incidence and prevalence
These vary considerably according to the irritant and profession involved (Table 129.1; Chapter 128). The annual population incidence of occupational contact dermatitis has been estimated to be in the range of 5.7–101 cases per 100 000 workers per year (with the

---

Rook's Textbook of Dermatology, Tenth Edition. Edited by Christopher Griffiths, Jonathan Barker, Tanya Bleiker, Walayat Hussain and Rosalind Simpson.
© 2024 John Wiley & Sons Ltd. Published 2024 by John Wiley & Sons Ltd.

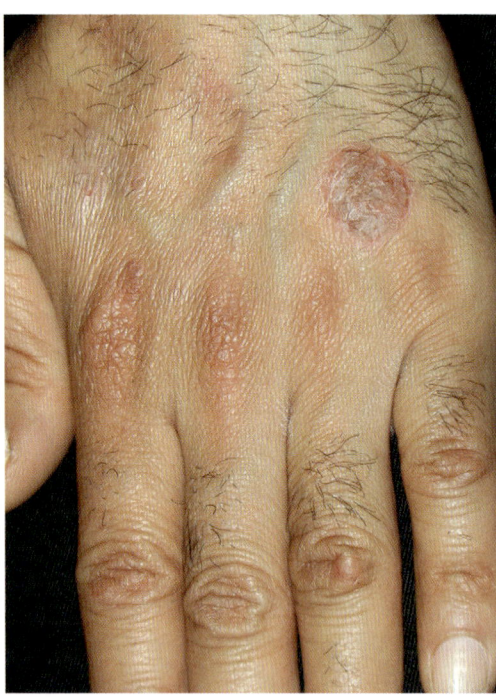

Figure 129.1 Discoid pattern of irritant contact dermatitis from soluble oil.

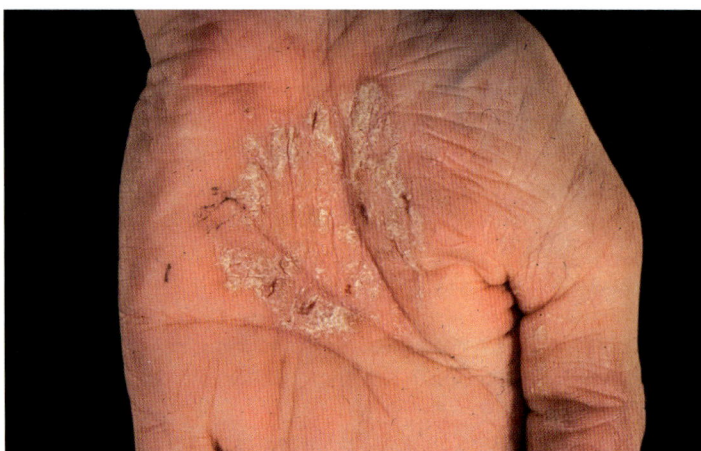

Figure 129.2 Psoriasis of the palm caused by frictional forces from repeated use of a screwdriver.

Table 129.1 Occupations with the highest risk of developing occupational irritant contact dermatitis (rate/100 000 employed/year), using labour force survey data as the denominator and cases reported to the UK EPIDERM survey as the numerator.

Occupation	Rate/100 000/year
Hairdressers	120
Printers	71
Machine tool operators	56
Chemical, gas and petroleum plant operatives	45
Car assemblers	35
Machine tool setters	34

majority of these being of irritant, not allergic, origin) [25]. Nearly 50% of all irritant contact dermatitis seen in patch test clinics may have an occupational cause [26].

Most available incidence statistics are unsuitable for comparison. Some do not distinguish between occupational accidents and illnesses; others fail to separate dermatitis from other skin conditions. Few give information on short periods of absence from work or on dermatitis without disability, and most are based on compensation paid. However, the ongoing experience of the British dermatologists (UK EPIDERM) and the Berufskrankheiten-Verordnung Saarland (BKH-S) surveillance schemes are addressing the epidemiology of occupational contact skin reactions [27,28]. Dermatitis was the predominant cutaneous reaction (73.5%), compared with urticaria (3.3%), infective conditions (21.7%) and neoplasia (18.0%) [27]. Recent findings show that skin diseases rank second (29%) to musculoskeletal conditions (57%) as causes of occupational disease [27]. The frequency of work-related skin reactions has been looked at in various occupational groups (Table 129.1).

The introduction of new chemicals may have increased the incidence of industrial dermatitis, but such a trend is counteracted by preventative and educational measures. The total number affected has increased as the number of persons employed in industry has risen. In a population sample from an industrial city, the overall 1-year period prevalence of hand eczema was 11.8% [29]. Hand eczema was significantly more common among those reporting potentially harmful skin exposures, cleaners for example having a corresponding prevalence rate of 21.3%.

In a joint European study of consecutive clinic patients with dermatitis, 30% of the men and 12% of the women had occupational dermatitis [30].

Of all occupational diseases, dermatoses comprise from 20% to 70% in different countries, and of the dermatoses between 20% and 90% are contact dermatitis. The relative proportions are determined by the extent and type of industrialisation in an area, and certainly also by the skill and interest of dermatologists in contact dermatitis [30].

The Covid-19 pandemic resulted in increased hand washing and sanitising hand gel use in all workplaces from 2020, with a corresponding increase in occupational skin disease. This was predominantly due to irritant contact dermatitis, but other skin diseases such as acne/rosacea due to personal protective equipment (e.g. face masks), infections, allergy and folliculitis as an occlusive effect were reported [31].

Age

Occupational dermatitis may occur at any age. The average age of onset varies from one occupation to another [32]. In some studies [33] two peaks appear, one at each end of working life. The young age group includes many patients with irritant and atopic eczema of the hands. Others find that the risk increases progressively with age [34]. Under reporting and bias (e.g. healthy worker effect) are likely to mean that occupational skin disease is more common than thought.

Pathophysiology

See Chapter 9.

Predisposing factors

Occupations. Certain industries and occupational groups contribute the majority of cases: in England and Germany, hairdressers [27,35], and in Italy, bricklayers [36]. Agriculture, manufacturing and construction consistently head the list in the USA [37,38]. If the number of persons exposed is taken into account, certain subgroups or departments of large industries have a particularly high risk of dermatitis [1]. A high chromium content in local cement may place building workers at the top of the list. Among 1071 building workers, 6% had occupational cement dermatitis and half of them were sensitised to chromium [39].

Certain high-risk groups may not be identified because the number employed is low. Thus, tilers were found to have a much higher risk than bricklayers when the number of cases seen was correlated with the number employed. Self-employed persons are rarely compensated and are therefore not registered. A high risk of dermatitis among veterinary surgeons thus escaped notice. The most common occupational contact dermatitis is probably housework dermatitis. In a Swedish public health examination, this affected approximately 1% of adult women; 38% of these had allergic contact dermatitis [40].

Period of exposure. Bakers get their dermatitis early, bricklayers later in life, which may in part be due to allergen potency and coexposure to irritants [32]. In one study, chromium in primers caused dermatitis after an average exposure of 5–7 months [41]. Hairdressers generally develop dermatitis early in their career [32], but the number who leave hairdressing before the age of 30 years is considerable and many leave for reasons other than dermatitis [42].

No comprehensive statistics have analysed the sum total of factors determining occupational risks. Wagner and Wezel [43] have suggested an approach. They base their calculations of occupational risk on three factors:
- The number of cases related to the number employed.
- The average age of onset of occupational dermatitis.
- The average period of work before onset.

Ideally, the number employed should be divided into age groups. All three factors vary independently. Many workers start a job late in life (e.g. unskilled labour in manufacturing industries) and develop their dermatitis rapidly. In others, dermatitis occurs after decades of work.

Genetics
On the background of atopy, filaggrin mutations seem to worsen severity of occupational irritant dermatitis [**44**]. Undoubtedly, other mutations will play a role in the interindividual variability in irritant responses.

Clinical features
History
Occupational contact dermatitis has the same morphology as any other contact dermatitis: cumulative irritant, allergic and photocontact dermatitis. The regional distribution, however, differs considerably because occupational contact dermatitis is mainly on exposed parts. The hands are affected, alone or together with other sites, in 80–90% of all cases of occupational contact dermatitis [25,45]. Irritant contact dermatitis started under finger rings in 12% of women and 2% of men [46]. The arms are also involved, especially if not covered by sleeves. Dusts and vapours affect the face and neck. Cement workers and miners often have dermatitis on the lower legs and feet. Those wearing rubber boots may have dermatitis from footwear.

Differential diagnosis
- Allergic contact dermatitis.
- Atopic eczema.
- Non-occupational irritant/allergic contact dermatitis.
- Fungal infection.

Classification of severity
There are no specific tools for occupational disease, but where the hands are affected, serial score of the hand eczema severity index (HECSI) can be clinically helpful [47].

Complications and co-morbidities
Fissured dermatitis commonly becomes infected and prolonged ill health and absence from work (with possible financial implications) may cause psychological disease such as anxiety and depression.

Disease course and prognosis
The disease course may be protracted, even after avoidance of known irritants. The most important aspect of prognosis in occupational dermatoses is that neither irritant nor allergic contact dermatitis may be as beneficially affected by change of work as some believe [**1**,32,48–51]. This has a profound influence on the management of the established case, as well as underlining the importance of primary prevention.

Investigations
Chemical investigations
There is an array of qualitative chemical spot tests [52,53], of which four are likely to be of particular use in the investigation of occupational cases. These are the dimethylglyoxime test for the presence of nickel [54], the diphenylcarbazide test for chromium [52], the lutidine test for formaldehyde [55] and the filter-paper test for epoxy resin [56]. These are all tests that can be carried out simply and reliably with minimum time and bench space.

Quantitative microanalysis of allergens and physicochemical techniques for the isolation of allergens [57] are likely to be beyond the scope of most dermatologists outside specialist departments, although they may be available within neighbouring departments. Thin-layer chromatography does, however, offer opportunities for relatively simple separation and identification, such as the detection of the sensitising low-molecular-weight oligomers of epoxy resin [53,56].

Liquid and gas chromatography, which may be linked to mass spectrometry, colorimetric spectrophotometry and atomic absorption and emission spectrophotometry all play important parts in current investigations [53].

Workplace visits
The diagnostic advantage to the dermatologist of seeing the way in which a patient carries out their work cannot be overestimated. Some general guidance is available [58,59,**60**,61,62], but it is the experience of making such visits that is the best instructor.

The main types of information that are worth establishing during such visits, and recording subsequently, are as follows:

- *Organisational.* Name, address (including postcode) and telephone number of the workplace; names and status of all medical, nursing, employer and employee representatives met.
- *Demographic.* Numbers employed overall and in the patient's work area; current expansion, contraction and turnover; shift system and pay scheme.
- *Technological.* Broad concept of production as a whole; detailed understanding of work carried out by the patient and in the patient's work area, including all potential irritants and allergens observed and their degree and extent of skin contact; names and addresses of suppliers of materials requiring further identification.
- *Preventative.* Broad impression of working conditions (e.g. space, lighting, ventilation); more detailed review of protective installations, protective clothing, skincare products and education; assessment of actual uptake and practical effectiveness of preventative methods.
- *Miscellaneous.* Industrial relations; psychological, sociological or economic factors; any similar problem in sister factory, etc.
- *Clinical.* Skin complaints in employees other than the patient, their clinical assessment and subdivision into occupational and non-occupational (often provisional).
- *Epidemiological.* Prevalence of skin complaints as a proportion of the total exposed; estimate of the prevalence of occupational dermatoses.
- *Aetiological.* Opinions of others, with attribution as to source and estimate of reliability; own opinion, with grounds for it (may be inconclusive).
- *Operational.* Summary of findings; recommendations for future investigation, management and review; follow-up.

Factory (or other workplace) visits can provide many major benefits [61] as follows:

- Detection of relevance of previously unexplained positive standard patch test reactions.
- Detection of missed allergen.
- Substantiation of diagnosis of irritant contact dermatitis.
- Diagnosis of mild or unfamiliar occupational dermatoses by their occurrence in several members of a workforce.
- Substantiation that various non-occupational skin conditions have been grouped together as a pseudo-occupational dermatosis [63], and why.
- Recognition of phenomenon of visible dermatoses, whether occupational or not, causing anxiety and subconsciously imitative symptoms in fellow employees [64].
- Initiation of research on new occupational dermatoses.
- Incidental effects, including improved dermatologist–occupational physician [65] and dermatologist–patient relationships.
- Progressive increase in dermatologist's overall knowledge of the working contactants of their patients.

A second-best alternative that can still provide useful information if a factory visit is impossible is to communicate with medical, nursing, employer or employee representatives by letter or telephone.

Management

Prevention [1,58,66,67]

Secondary preventative measures can reduce the risk of dermatitis in an established case, although success can be obtained only by close collaboration between the management of the factory and the dermatologist. Changes in the process, when practicable, are always likely to be more successful than personal protection [68]. Some preventative measures that are desirable from a dermatological point of view may be unsafe or impractical in an industrial environment. The wearing of gloves is often ruled out because of these strictures [69].

Materials selected for protective clothing may in practice allow many contactants to penetrate. Various sources provide practical guidance as to the choice of protective material [1,66–74]. There are now multilayered materials that show much greater resistance to allergens such as methyl-methacrylate [75] and irritants such as organic solvents [70]. Even when protective clothing is practicable and competent to protect, the way in which it is taken off and put on again may lead to contamination of inside surfaces. Because occlusion increases penetration, wearing a glove that has been contaminated on the inside can be more harmful than wearing no glove at all [67]. Correct procedures must therefore be instituted and maintained. *Personal protective equipment is only effective when selected carefully, removed safely and replaced/maintained regularly* [25]. Cotton-lined gloves can reduce the potential for irritant contact dermatitis [25].

Automated processes are often far from free of skin contact. Fregert [76] has listed many possible sources of skin contamination. Service engineers are particularly at risk [77].

Allergen replacement [58,77,78] is a useful concept. Extreme care must be taken to ensure as far as possible that the replacement is genuinely safer in all respects.

Some skincare creams ('barrier' and moisturising creams) have been demonstrated by various test methods [1,79–82] to have a protective effect against certain irritants. Their effectiveness in actual use remains less securely established and their use remains unproven [1,25]. Topical binding agents may have a role in the prevention of nickel dermatitis [83].

The basic principle of prevention of occupational contact dermatitis continues to be that of reduction of contact, or preferably avoidance. If chemicals remain on the skin for 24 h instead of 8 h, sensitisation and irritation occur more readily [67]. Evidence-based skincare recommendations have been published [84] (summarised in Box 129.1). If improvements are made to the working conditions by intensified preventative measures, then this is likely to lead to a reduction in cases of occupational contact dermatitis [85,86].

Box 129.1 Basic workplace skincare principles

- Lukewarm water for washing
- Use correct gloves before exposure for the shortest time
- Remove rings
- Cotton liners underneath protective gloves
- Avoid disinfectant hand cleansers
- Apply emollient hand creams
- Protect hands at home
- Workforce education

Management of the established case [1,58]
As most workers naturally prefer to continue their work, a detailed analysis of causative factors is required. Minor changes of procedure may be helpful once guided by a precise diagnosis. A change of job may be considered in first-year apprentices, in those with uncomplicated allergic contact dermatitis from readily avoidable substances or in atopics who have unavoidable contact with irritants. This should only be decided after full dermatological investigation. In the majority of cases, continuation in the same occupation should be made possible [32,58,87,88].

Assessment of dermatitic potential
The potential of chemicals to act as contact irritants [89,90], contact allergens [91–95], photoirritants [96] and photoallergens [95,97,98] can be assessed by test methods in laboratory animals and, to a lesser extent, in human volunteer subjects. These methods assess potential; they do not in themselves predict the incidence of dermatitis. Actual risk depends not only on dermatitic potential but also on other factors, the most important of which concern the conditions of exposure (i.e. concentration, frequency and duration) and the normality of skin. Also useful is background knowledge of the structure–activity relationships of chemical groups [99].

Modifications of widely accepted test procedures such as the guinea-pig maximisation test [94] tend to occur with experience of their use [100–102], and sufficiently different tests have been developed to justify separate names [95,103–105]. Standardisation of test procedures greatly reduces inter- and intralaboratory variation in results – but, as this is never likely to cease to be a problem to some degree [106], the development of new tests that may offer greater ease of standardisation (and economy) continues [107]. The use of mouse models and even *in silico* models for the prediction of sensitising potential is now well established [108,109]. Case reports of human exposure will continue to be important to alert fellow clinicians of the risk of individual chemicals.

Alkali tests
The usefulness of alkali resistance and alkali neutralisation tests as predictors of susceptibility to irritants remains controversial. Neither test is sufficiently simple and reliable to achieve widespread clinical use [110,111,112], and their diagnostic value has been overestimated.

More sophisticated tests with panels of irritants have been used to identify a 14% proportion of the general population with 'hyper-irritable skin' [110]. Susceptibility to one irritant, however, does not necessarily imply susceptibility to another irritant in the same individual [110,113]. Skin irritation thresholds have been correlated with the development of dermatitis in hairdressers [114].

Transepidermal water loss
Measurement of the baseline transepidermal water loss (TEWL) may be a useful indicator of reactivity to irritants, although there is variation between studies [110].

Measurement of skin contamination
Methods of quantifying the degree of skin contamination by substances include skin wiping [115], skin rinsing [116], exposure pads [117,118] and the use of natural fluorescence (oils and tars) [119] or fluorescent tracers [120].

> **Treatment ladder of occupational irritant contact dermatitis**
>
> **First line**
> - Prevention
>
> **Second line**
> - Irritant avoidance by minor changes in procedure or personal protective equipment
>
> **Third line**
> - Change of occupation and consideration of systemic immunosuppressive treatment if appropriate

Occupational allergic contact dermatitis

Definition and nomenclature
Occupational allergic contact dermatitis is a specific type IV hypersensitivity reaction to an allergen present in the workplace. It is eczematous in character and may be provoked by exposure to the allergen in the home/recreational environment as well as at least partly at work.

> **Synonyms and inclusions**
> - Work-related contact dermatitis
> - Occupational allergic dermatitis

Introduction and general description
Although less common than occupational irritant contact dermatitis, occupational allergic contact dermatitis [1,2–4] still tends to be underdiagnosed [5]. Better history taking [3], more extensive patch testing, workplace visiting and greater use of chemical investigations [3] significantly increase the proportion of patients found to have contact sensitisation relevant to their occupation. Allergic contact dermatitis also frequently complicates irritant contact dermatitis in occupational cases. A prime example of occupational allergic contact dermatitis is that from chromium [6,7] (Chapter 127).

Epidemiology
Incidence and prevalence
The annual population incidence of occupational contact dermatitis has been estimated to be in the range of 5.7–101 cases per 100 000 workers per year (but the majority of these will be due to irritant, not allergic, dermatitis) [8]. The most common allergens are acrylates, cobalt, chromium, cosmetics, fragrances, epoxy resin, nickel, plants, preservatives, resins and thiurams [8,9].

Pathophysiology (Chapter 127)
Atopy appears to be an independent risk factor for the development of occupational allergic contact dermatitis [8]. The overall role of filaggrin mutations has not yet been conclusively elucidated in occupational allergic contact dermatitis [10]. The effect of filaggrin

mutations on work-related sensitisation/elicitation reactions is likely to be allergen-specific. For example, nickel penetrates the skin more effectively in filaggrin null carriers than with wild-type filaggrin individuals [11].

Clinical features

The diagnostic approach to a suspected occupational dermatosis needs to be systematic. Most diagnostic difficulties arise from eczematous dermatoses [12]. Great care must be taken in the accurate distinction between contact dermatitis and endogenous eczema, and between irritant and allergic contact dermatitis (although there can be considerable overlap). Skill is needed in taking an occupational history [13,14] and in obtaining as detailed a picture as possible of what the patient actually does at work [1].

The clinical distinction on the hands, forearms or face between endogenous eczema, irritant contact dermatitis and allergic contact dermatitis is beset with pitfalls. Differences in the distribution and morphology are useful guides, but this can be misleading. There is a tendency for irritant contact dermatitis to affect the dorsa of the hands (see Figure 129.1) and fingers (Figure 129.3) and the finger webs, rather than the palms, and to be relatively devoid of vesicles. There is a tendency for vesicular eczema of the palms and sides of the fingers to be endogenous. However, certain irritants and allergens (Figure 129.4) can produce a vesicular eczema of the palmar aspects of the hands and fingers, and both allergic contact dermatitis and endogenous eczema frequently involve the dorsal aspects of the hands, fingers and webs. Discs of eczema on the dorsa of the hands and forearms are frequently endogenous, but allergic contact dermatitis from chromium and cumulative irritant contact dermatitis can present with a very similar distribution (see Figure 129.1). Gross eyelid swelling usually indicates allergic contact dermatitis, but degrees of eyelid swelling can occur in both irritant contact dermatitis and endogenous eczema.

It is difficult to overemphasise the importance of a sound working knowledge of occupational irritants, as well as allergens, and of

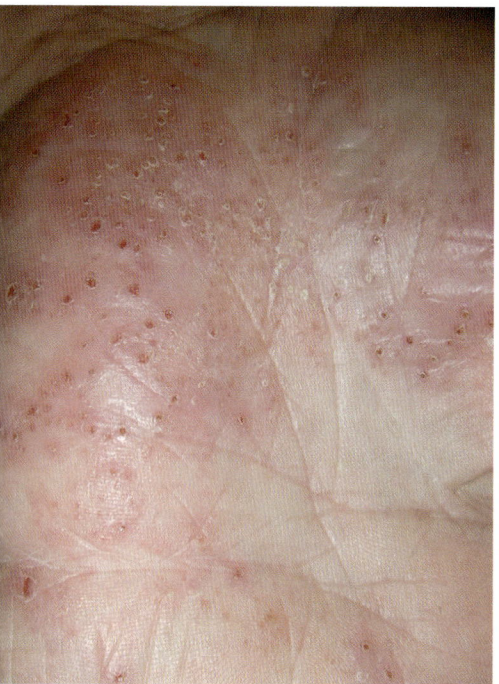

Figure 129.4 Allergic contact dermatitis from Compositae plants in a florist.

patch testing in overcoming these difficulties in clinical differentiation. It should be appreciated that hand eczemas, in particular, are often the joint outcome of endogenous, irritant, allergic and even general climatic factors, and may be partly occupational as well as wholly occupational or non-occupational. In identifying the primary and/or major cause of a contact dermatitis, antecedent and aggravating causes should not be neglected. The diagnosis of secondary bacterial infection in occupational contact dermatitis, for example, may allow significant improvement to be obtained with antibiotic therapy. Guidelines on patch testing and the management of contact dermatitis have been formulated by various bodies including the European Society of Contact Dermatitis [15] and the British Association of Dermatologists [16].

Differential diagnosis
- Non-occupational allergic contact dermatitis.
- Occupational irritant contact dermatitis.
- Non-occupational irritant contact dermatitis.
- Atopic eczema.

Classification of severity
See the section on classification of severity for occupational irritant contact dermatitis earlier in this chapter.

Disease course and prognosis
As seen in occupational irritant contact dermatitis, reactions can persist for months or years despite allergen avoidance (e.g. chromate). Prognosis is highly variable [8]. Up to 50% of patients experience significant adverse effects of quality of life, day-to-day activities and home relationships [8].

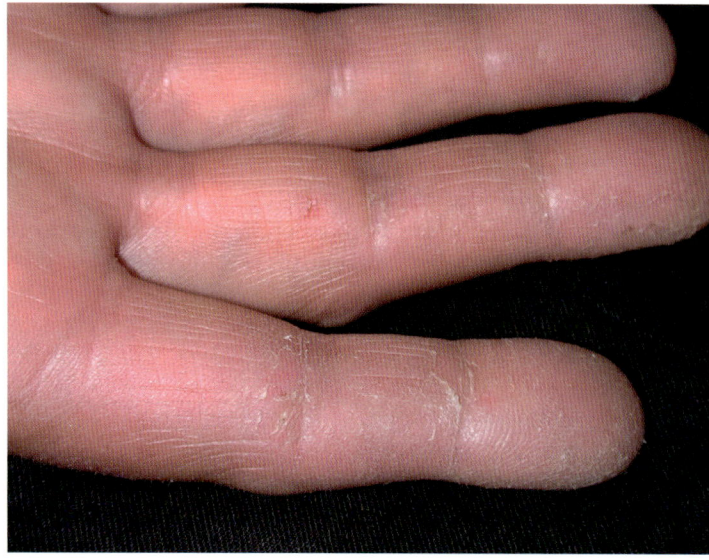

Figure 129.3 Irritant contact dermatitis of the fingers in a printer.

Investigations

Skin prick test/specific immunoglobulin E

Although testing for immediate hypersensitivity is not always a part of the assessment of contact dermatitis, it can be important, particularly in hand dermatitis when type 1 hypersensitivity to natural rubber latex (NRL) is suspected [17]. The two tests in common use are the skin prick test and the estimation of specific immunoglobulin E (IgE) in the blood (e.g. the radioallergosorbent test (RAST)). The glove usage or challenge test requires a highly allergenic brand of glove and is potentially dangerous – emergency treatment facilities for the management of anaphylaxis are needed [18].

Skin prick testing involves an intradermal puncture through a drop of allergen or glove. A positive reaction consists of an urticarial weal, which is usually apparent after 15 min, although it may take as long as 45 min to develop. A positive control test of histamine should also be performed to exclude a false negative reaction due to, for example, oral antihistamine ingestion. A negative control prick test with, for example, saline should also be performed to check if the patient is dermographic. There are occasional reports of anaphylaxis following prick testing with NRL extract [19] and appropriate consent from the patient should be obtained prior to testing. With the advent of standardised, commercially available NRL extracts, this risk is greatly reduced.

Some clinicians may prefer to perform specific IgE testing for NRL allergy, as they may not have adequate facilities or training to deal with anaphylaxis; however, the sensitivity and specificity may be less accurate compared with prick testing. Skin prick tests and use tests (where test substances are applied to the skin in ways close to real-life use/exposure and are then observed) are also useful when investigating protein contact dermatitis in occupations at risk, such as chefs or veterinarians [20].

Patch testing [21–25]

This standardised test is described in detail elsewhere (Chapter 127). Four general problems of patch testing are particularly relevant when testing in suspected occupational dermatitis:
- False positive reactions.
- False negative reactions.
- Unexplained positive reactions.
- Missed allergens.

False positive reactions are commonly obtained if industrial chemicals are applied undiluted as patch tests [23]. Such reactions can be shown to be false positive irritant reactions if testing in control subjects also demonstrates positive reactions; applying serial dilutions of the chemical to the original patient will often demonstrate an abrupt loss of the reaction. The uncritical use of undiluted chemical samples as patch tests also increases the risk of active sensitisation and other complications of patch testing (Chapter 127). When testing an unknown substance, extreme caution is required and where the test is unavoidable, a preliminary open test is advisable [24].

False negative reactions can also be obtained with samples acquired from the patient's workplace. This is because the concentration of an allergen in a sample (e.g. rubber) may be too low to elicit a positive patch test reaction. This problem also arises when allergens are found in irritant products such as cutting fluids, solvents and soaps. Dilution of these to avoid a false positive reaction from the irritancy of the sample may overdilute an allergen initially present in only low concentration (Chapter 127).

Unexplained positive reactions found on standard patch testing in suspected occupational cases should always be pursued for explanation [24,26]. This is particularly so when the allergens concerned are known to have a multiplicity of industrial uses, such as chromium, cobalt and colophonium. A factory visit can be invaluable in the detection of previously unsuspected sources of allergens [1,27,28].

When clinical assessment points strongly towards an occupational allergic contact dermatitis, the occurrence of negative patch test results should always raise the possibility of the responsible allergen having been inadvertently omitted from testing [25,26]. Another major function of a factory visit is to detect such *missed allergens*. Routine pre-employment testing with potential sensitisers to be used in the future job should not be carried out [22], mainly because of a risk of sensitising employees.

For chemical testing and the principles of a site visit, see the section on occupational irritant contact dermatitis earlier in this chapter.

Management

Primary prevention is key. Specific occupational hazards (both allergic and irritant) [1,3,29,30] are given in Box 129.2.

Treatment ladder for occupational allergic contact dermatitis

First line
- Primary prevention

Second line
- Allergen substitution or avoidance, including personal protective equipment

Third line
- Redeployment, topical or systemic immunosuppressive treatment

---

Acne of chemical origin

Definition and nomenclature

Acne of external or chemical origin is an acneform eruption caused by exposure to chemicals or physical irritation.

Synonyms and inclusions
- Chloracne

Introduction and general description

Various chemicals possess, to some degree, the capacity to induce acne by external contact [1]. Many are occupational hazards, but some may be encountered in the home. The occupational chloracnes are of outstanding medical importance because their development provides a valuable indicator of exposure to a toxic hazard. Many of the substances inducing chloracne are also hepatotoxic.

Box 129.2 Allergic and irritant occupational hazards

Agriculture [31–41]
Irritants. Artificial fertilisers, disinfectants and cleansers for milking utensils, petrol, diesel oil.
Sensitisers. Rubber (boots, gloves, milking machines), cement, local remedies for veterinary use, wood preservatives, plants, pesticides, antibiotics in animal feeds, penicillin for mastitis, nickel and cobalt in fertilisers, cobalt and vitamin K_3 in animal feeds, ethoxyquin (preservative) in feed, quinoxaline and derivatives (growth factor), dinitolmide (anticoccidiosis), phenothiazine sedatives, soil disinfectants.
Contact urticaria. Animal hair and dander.

Artists [42,43]
Irritants. Solvents, clay, plaster.
Sensitisers. Turpentine, cobalt–nickel pigments and chromium pigments, azo and phthalocyanine dyes, colophonium, epoxy, acrylic and formaldehyde resins.

Automobile, aerospace industries and aircrew [44–46]
Irritants. Solvents, oils, cutting oils, paints, glass fibre, carbon fibre, hand cleansers, low humidity, kerosene.
Sensitisers. Chromate (primers, anticorrosives, oils and cutting oils), nickel, beryllium, cobalt, rubber, epoxy and acrylic resins, dipentene in thinners.

Baking and pastry making [47–51]
Irritants. Flour, detergents.
Sensitisers. Citrus fruits, flour improvers, thiamine, spices (cinnamon, cardamom), essential oils, azo dyes, fat preservatives (lauryl gallate), sodium carboxymethyl cellulose.
Contact urticaria. Flour, spices, essential oils, α-amylase.

Bartenders [52–54]
Irritants. Detergents, citrus fruits, general wet work.
Sensitisers. Flavouring agents, citrus fruits, antibacterials in detergents, nickel.

Bathing attendants [55,56]
Irritants. Detergents, free or combined chlorine/bromine.
Sensitisers. Antimicrobial agents, sodium hypochlorite, formaldehyde, essential oils.
Contact urticaria. Sodium hypochlorite.

Bookbinders [57,58]
Irritants. Glues, solvents, paper.
Sensitisers. Glues, formaldehyde, plastic monomers, size (colophonium, maleopimaric acid).

Building trade [59–62]
Irritants. Cement, chalk, fly ash, hydrochloric and hydrofluoric acids, glass wool, wood preservatives (also phototoxic), organic tin compounds.
Sensitisers. Cement and fly ash (chromate, cobalt), rubber and leather gloves, additives in shale oils, glues (phenol- or urea-formaldehyde resins), wood preservatives, teak, glass wool impregnated with phenol-formaldehyde resin, epoxy resin, polyurethanes, rubber strip seals, jointing materials.

Butchers [50,63–66]
Irritants. Detergents, meat, entrails.
Sensitisers. Nickel, colophonium (sawdust), antiseptics, hardwood knife handles, meat.
Contact urticaria. Meat, blood.

Canning industry
Irritants. Brine, syrup, prawns and shrimps.
Sensitisers. Asparagus, carrots, preservatives (hexamethylene-tetramine in fish canning), rubber gloves.
Contact urticaria. Fruit, vegetables, prawns, shrimps.

Carpenters, cabinet makers [67–71]
Irritants. French polish, solvents, glues, cleansers, wood preservatives (also phototoxic), glass fibre.
Sensitisers. Exotic woods (teak, mahogany, rosewood, etc.), glues, polishes, turpentine, nickel, rubber (handles), plastics, colophonium, epoxy, acrylic, formaldehyde and isocyanate resins.

Chemical and pharmaceutical industry [72–76]
Irritants and sensitisers are numerous and specific for each workplace. Halogenated chemical intermediates are frequent sensitisers.

Cleaning work [77,78]
Irritants. Detergents, solvents.
Sensitisers. Rubber gloves, nickel, formaldehyde, perfumes.
Contact urticaria. Rubber gloves, perfumes, alcohols.

Coal miners [79–82]
Irritants. Stone dust, coal dust, oil, grease, hydraulic fluid, wood preservatives, cement, powdered limestone, anhydrous calcium sulphate.
Sensitisers. Rubber (boots), facemasks, explosives, chromate and cobalt in cement.

Cooks, catering industry [1,50,83–87]
Irritants. Detergents, dressings, vinegar, fish, meat, fruit and vegetable juices.
Sensitisers. Fruit and vegetables (onions, garlic, lemons, lettuce, artichokes), hardwood knife handles, spices, formaldehyde, rubber gloves.
Contact urticaria. Meat, fish, fruit, vegetables.

Dentists and dental technicians [77,88–90]
Irritants. Soap, detergents, plaster of Paris, acrylic monomer, fluxes.
Sensitisers. Local anaesthetics (tetracaine, procaine), mercury, rubber, ultraviolet-curing acrylates, aromatic epoxy acrylates, aliphatic acrylates, melamine-formaldehyde resin, BAC-ester chloride, disinfectants and sterilants (formaldehyde, glutaraldehyde, eugenol), nickel, epoxy resin (filling), periodontal dressing (*Myroxylon pereirae*, colophonium, eugenol), catalysts (methyl-*p*-toluenesulphonate and methyl-1,4-dichlorbenzenesulphonate) in impression and sealant materials.
Contact urticaria. Saliva, rubber gloves.

Dyers [3,60,91–94]
Irritants. Solvents, oxidising and reducing agents, hypochlorite, hair removers.
Sensitisers. Dyes, chromate, formaldehyde.

Electricians [29,95]
Irritants. Soldering flux.
Sensitisers. Soldering flux, insulating tape (rubber, colophonium, tar), rubber, nickel, bitumen, epoxy resins, glues (phenol-formaldehyde), polyurethanes.

Electronics industry [96–98]
Irritants. Soldering flux, organic solvents, hydrofluoric acid, fibreglass, antistatic agents.
Allergens. Soldering flux, chromate, cobalt, nickel, epoxy resins, anaerobic acrylic sealants.
Contact urticaria. Soldering flux.

Enamel workers [99]
Irritants. Enamel powder.
Sensitisers. Chromate, nickel, cobalt.

Fishing [83,100–104]
Irritants. Wet work, friction, oils, petrol, red feed from mackerel, fish juice (polypeptides).
Sensitisers. Tars, organic dyes in nets, rubber boots, rubber gloves, marine organisms (Dogger Bank itch) and plants.
Contact urticaria. Fish, marine organisms and plants.

Floor layers [29,105]
Irritants. Solvents, detergents, cement (can be ulcerative).
Sensitisers. Chromate (cement), epoxy resin, glues (phenol- and urea-formaldehyde), exotic woods, acrylates, varnish (urea-formaldehyde), polyurethanes.

Florists, gardeners and plant growers [106–110]
Irritants. Manure, bulbs, sap, fertilisers, pesticides, wet work.
Sensitisers. Plants (*Primula obconica*, chrysanthemum, Asteraceae (Compositae), weeds, tulips, narcissus, daffodils, *Alstroemeria*), formaldehyde, pesticides, lichens.

Food industry [50,51,83,85,87]
Irritants. Detergents, vegetables.
Sensitisers. Rubber gloves, spices, vegetables, fruits, preservatives.
Contact urticaria. Vegetables, fruits, meats, fish.

Foundry work [29,60,111]
Irritants. Oils, phenol-formaldehyde resins.
Sensitisers. Phenol- and urea-formaldehyde resins, furan and epoxy resins, chromate (cement, gloves, bricks).

Glaziers [29]
Sensitisers. Rubber, epoxy resin, hardwoods.

Hairdressers and barbers [1,77,112–114,**115**,116]
Irritants. Shampoos, soaps, permanent-wave liquids, bleaching agents.

Sensitisers. Hair dyes, rubber, nickel, perfumes, lanolin, thioglycolates, cocamidopropyl betaine, methylisothiazolinone.
Contact urticaria. Ammonium persulphate, henna, rubber gloves.

Histology technicians [29,117,118]
Irritants. Solvents, formaldehyde.
Sensitisers. Formaldehyde, glutaraldehyde, organic dyes, epoxy resin, acrylates, D-limonene.

Hospital workers [77,78,119–122]
Irritants. Disinfectants, quaternary ammonium compounds, hand creams, soaps, detergents.
Sensitisers. Rubber gloves, formaldehyde, chloroxylenol, penicillin, cephalosporins, streptomycin, neomycin, piperazine, phenothiazines, hand creams, nickel, glutaraldehyde, acrylic monomer, nitrogen mustard, local anaesthetics, propacetamol.
Contact urticaria. Rubber gloves, cisplatin.

Housework [85,87,123]
Irritants. Detergents, solvents, polishes, wet work, vegetables.
Sensitisers. Rubber (gloves), nickel, chromate, flowers and plants, hand creams and lotions, handles of knives and irons, oranges, balsams, spices, pyrethrum, methylisothiazolinone.
Contact urticaria. Vegetables, fruits, meats, fish, spices, rubber gloves.

Jewellers [29,124,125]
Irritants. Solvents, fluxes.
Sensitisers. Nickel, epoxy resins, enamels (chromate, nickel, cobalt), precious metals.

Masons [59,126]
Irritants. Cement, chalk, bricks, acids.
Sensitisers. Chromate and cobalt in cement, rubber and leather gloves, epoxy resin, hardwoods.

Mechanics [29,44,127,128]
Irritants. Solvents, detergents, degreasers, lubricants, oils, cooling system fluids, battery acid, soldering flux.
Sensitisers. Rubber, chromate, nickel, epoxy resin, polyester resin, D-limonene.

Metal workers [29,60,129,130]
Irritants. Cutting and drilling oils, hand cleansers, solvents.
Sensitisers. Nickel, chromate (antirust agents and dyes, welding fumes), cobalt, colophonium (tall oil), antibacterial agents and antioxidants in cutting oils, chromate, cobalt and nickel in used cutting oils.

Office workers [29,131–135]
Irritants. Photocopy paper, fibreglass, indoor climate, low humidity.
Sensitisers. Rubber (erasing rubber, mats, cords, finger stalls), nickel (clips, scissors, typewriters), copying papers, glue, felt-tip pen dyes.

Painters and maintenance workers [29,125,136–140]
Irritants. Solvents, turpentine, thinner, emulsion paints, wallpaper adhesive, organic tin compounds.
Sensitisers. Turpentine, dipentene, D-limonene, cobalt (dyes, driers), chromate (green, yellow), polyurethane, epoxy and acrylic resins, triglycidyl isocyanurate, glues (urea- and phenol-formaldehyde), varnish (colophonium, urea-formaldehyde), preservatives in water-based paints and glues (methylol-chloracetamide, chloracetamide, methyisothiazolinone), polyester paint pigments.

Performing artists [141–144]
Irritants. Mechanical, sweating.
Sensitisers. Cosmetics, colophonium, nickel, hardwoods.

Photography [29,145,146]
Irritants. Alkalis, reducing and oxidising agents, solvents.
Sensitisers. Metol (p-aminophenol), colour developers (azo compounds), chromate, formaldehyde, persulphate bleach accelerator-1 (PBA-1).

Plastics industry [147,148]
Irritants. Solvents, styrene, oxidising agents, acids.
Sensitisers. Low-molecular-weight raw materials, hardeners, additives, dyes, styrene.

Plating–electroplating (and electroforming) [29,60,149–153]
Irritants. Metal cleaners, alkalis, acids, detergents, heat, dust from metal blasting.
Sensitisers. Nickel, chromate, cobalt, mercury, gold, rhodium, rubber gloves.

Plumbers [29,154,155]
Irritants. Oils, soldering flux, hand cleansers.

Sensitisers. Rubber (gloves, packing, hoses), nickel, chromate (cement, antirust paint), epoxy resin, hydrazine, epichlorhydrin (solvent cement).

Printers [29,60,156,157]
Irritants. Solvents, acrylates in radiation-curing printing inks and lacquers.
Sensitisers. Nickel, chromate, cobalt, formaldehyde, isothiazolinones, colophonium, paper finishes, glues, turpentine, azo dyes, acrylates, etc., in radiation-curing printing inks, lacquers and printing plates, rubber gloves.

Radio and television repair [29,60]
Irritants. Soldering flux, solvents.
Sensitisers. Soldering flux (hydrazine, colophonium), epoxy resin, nickel, chromate.

Restaurant personnel [85,87]
Irritants. Detergents, vegetables, citrus fruits, shrimps, herring.
Sensitisers. Nickel, spices, vegetables, hardwoods (knife handles).
Contact urticaria. Vegetables, fruit, meat, fish.

Road workers [29]
Irritants. Sand–oil mix, asphalt (phototoxic), hand cleansers.
Sensitisers. Cement, gloves (leather, rubber), epoxy resin, tar, chromate in antirust paint.

Rubber workers [158–161]
Irritants. Talc, zinc stearate, solvents.
Sensitisers. Rubber chemicals, organic dyes, tars, colophonium, chromate, cobalt, phenol-formaldehyde resin.

Sheet metal workers [60,162,163]
Irritants. Solvents, paints.
Sensitisers. Chromium in paints and on zinc-galvanised sheets, glues.

Shoemakers [29,164–166]
Irritants. Solvents.
Sensitisers. Glues (*para*-tertiary butyl phenol-formaldehyde resin), leather (formaldehyde, chloroacetamide, chromate, dyes), turpentine, rubber, colophonium, bisphenol A.

Shop assistants [167]
Irritants. Detergents, vegetables, fruit, meats, fish.
Sensitisers. Nickel, colophonium (price labels).
Contact urticaria. Vegetables, fruit.

Tanners [29,60,168–170]
Irritants. Acids, alkalis, reducing and oxidising agents.
Sensitisers. Chromium, formaldehyde, glutaraldehyde, vegetable tanning agents, finishes, antimildew agents, dyes, resins.
Contact urticaria. Formaldehyde.

Textile workers [29,93,169,171,172]
Irritants. Solvents, bleaching agents, fibres, formaldehyde.
Sensitisers. Finishes (formaldehyde resins), dyes, mordants, caprolactam, nickel, diazo paper.
Contact urticaria. Formaldehyde.

Veterinarians [77,173–176]
Irritants. Hypochlorite, quaternary ammonium compounds, cresol, rectal and vaginal examinations of cattle.
Sensitisers. Rubber gloves, antibiotics (penicillin, streptomycin, neomycin, tylosin tartrate, virginiamycin), antimycotic agents, mercaptobenzothiazole (MBT) in medicaments, glutaraldehyde, preservatives in rectal lubricants.
Contact urticaria. Animal hair and dander, obstetric fluids, animal tissues, rubber gloves.

Welders [29,60]
Irritants. Oil.
Sensitisers. Chromium (welding fumes, gloves), nickel, cobalt.

Woodworkers [67–69,177–180]
Irritants. Woods, wood preservatives, solvents, detergents, fibreboard (urea-formaldehyde resin).
Sensitisers. Woods, wood preservatives, colophonium, turpentine, balsams, tars, lacquers, glues (urea, phenol- and *para*-tertiary butyl phenol-formaldehyde resins), *Frullania*, lichens.
Contact urticaria. Woods.

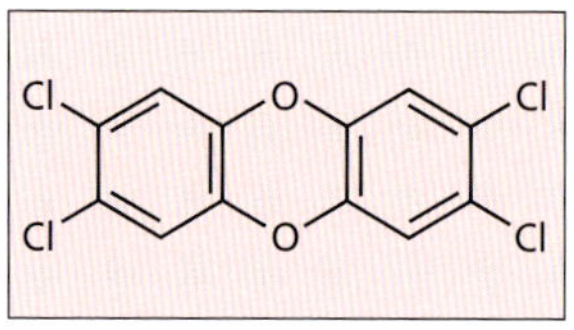

Figure 129.5 2,3,7,8-Tetrachlorodibenzo-*p*-dioxin – a halogenated aromatic compound – is highly toxic and causes chloracne.

Table 129.2 Clinical features of acne vulgaris versus halogen acne.

Clinical features	Acne vulgaris	Halogen acne
Usual age	Teenage	Any
Comedones	Present	>3 (if absent, it is not chloracne)
Straw-coloured cysts	Rare	Pathognomonic
Temporal comedones	Rare	Diagnostic
Inflammatory papules and cysts	≥3	Present
Retroauricular involvement	Uncommon	Common
Nose involvement	Often spared	Often spared
Associated systemic findings	Rare	Common

Halogenated aromatic hydrocarbons [2,3,4,5,6,7] are the most potent acnegenic agents. The chloronaphthalenes, chlorobiphenyls [8] and chlorobiphenyl oxides are used as dielectrics in conductors and insulators. Exposure occurs in those manufacturing these substances or making or handling cables [9,10]. A naphthalene wax used to 'feather proof' a counterpane caused acne on the face and arms of a child [11]. These substances will induce acne at any site [12] and at any age, usually after 1 or 2 months of exposure. The chlorophenols are used as insecticides, fungicides, herbicides and wood preservatives [13]. Their capacity to cause chloracne depends on the degree to which they are contaminated with chlorinated dioxins and the precise chemical structure of the latter, for example 2,3,7,8-tetrachlorodibenzo-*p*-dioxin (TCDD) (Figure 129.5) is the most powerful chloracnegenic agent known [14–18]. Similarly, the toxicity of the polychlorinated biphenyls (PCBs) is largely due to contamination with polychlorinated dibenzofurans (PCDFs). Chloracne has been caused by a weedkiller containing 2,4-dichlorophenoxyacetic acid and 2,4,5-trichlorophenoxyacetic acid [19], by sodium tetrachlorophenate used as a wood preservative [2], by the herbicide 2,6-dichlorobenzonitrile [20], by a trifluoromethylpyrazole derivative being developed as an antirheumatic drug [21] and by an intermediate product found in the manufacture of tetrachloroazobenzene [4].

As a consequence of industrial or other accidents, large numbers of individuals may be heavily exposed to such chemicals [22]. In such circumstances, TCDD caused serious systemic symptoms and severe chloracne [23]. After another industrial accident, the same chemical caused chloracne in members of the families of affected workers [24]. Following the Seveso accident in Italy, TCDD-induced chloracne, mainly in children, cleared well within a decade and systemic effects were absent [25].

The induction of chloracne by the ingestion of PCBs has occurred in two large epidemics caused by the contamination of cooking oil [2,26]: the chloracnegen was shown to have caused transplacental as well as direct toxicity [27]. Polybrominated biphenyls became widely distributed in the state of Michigan, USA, following a labelling error that resulted in their introduction into cattle feed [22].

Neat (insoluble) cutting oils, which are impure paraffin–oil mixtures, are the commonest chemical cause of acne because they are so widely used in the engineering industry, but their acnegenic capacity is inconstant and not necessarily high. Men are more readily affected than women, and those with acne vulgaris are particularly susceptible. The use of moulding oil in the manufacture of precast concrete can cause oil acne [28]. Brilliantines containing impure paraffins may have a similar effect [29]. Comedones and cysts behind the ears have been attributed to paraffin products in shaving soap inadequately rinsed from this region [30].

Crude petroleum is acnegenic in oilfield and refinery workers [7]. Diesel oil can cause acne in motor mechanics [31].

Heavy coal-tar distillates, especially pitch and creosote, are also to some extent acnegenic. Conduit makers and road workers are affected. Under experimental conditions the lesions induced by crude coal tar are more inflammatory in white people than in black people [32].

Cosmetics [33]: mild comedonal acne with occasional papulopustules occurs in one-third of adult women in the USA. Of 25 facial cosmetic creams tested in rabbits, 50% were comedogenic; so were lanolin, petrolatum and some vegetable oils [34]. Pomades had an even more marked effect in African Americans [29]. Also acnegenic were indigenous vegetable oils in India [35]. The salts of fatty acids in conventional soaps are comedogenic if used excessively [36]. Fatty acid esters, especially isopropyl linoleate, acetylated lanolin alcohol and grape seed and sweet almond oils, have been found to be particularly comedogenic in rabbits [37].

A large percentage of workers in a hardboard factory in Germany developed acne which was attributed to *asbestos* [38].

The continued application of *topical corticosteroids* under occlusive dressings may also induce comedo formation. It does not occur under the age of 10 years and is difficult to induce experimentally in subjects over 50 years of age [39].

A predominantly perioral acne can appear during *psoralen and ultraviolet A (PUVA) therapy* [1].

Epidemiology
Sporadic cases are reported in the literature, but there are no good estimates of population incidence or prevalence.

Clinical features
There are important clinical differences between acne vulgaris and acne of chemical origin, as listed in Table 129.2. Straw-coloured cysts, temporal comedones and retroauricular involvement are all important clues to a diagnosis of chloracne; however, it should be noted that those already with a tendency towards acne vulgaris may be more prone to acne of chemical origin.

Differential diagnosis (Table 129.3)
- Acne vulgaris
- Folliculitis

Disease course and prognosis
Improvement or resolution may occur on withdrawal of the offending item. However, the disease may take many years to resolve, or may persist nevertheless with potential scarring.

Table 129.3 Differential diagnosis of various forms of occupational acne.

Differential diagnosis	Aetiology	Location	Lesion
Chloracne	Halogenated aromatics	Malar, retroauricular, mandibular	Comedones, straw-coloured cysts (0.1–1.0 cm)
Oil folliculitis	Oil	Arms, thighs, buttocks	Red papules, pustules
Pitch acne	Tar/pitch	Exposed facial areas, especially malar	Open comedones
Tropical acne	Heat/humidity	Back, neck, buttocks, proximal extremities	Nodules, cysts

Management

If lesions persist despite acnegen avoidance, standard acne treatments can be employed (Chapter 88) such as oral antibiotics and oral isotretinoin.

> **Treatment ladder for acne of chemical origin**
>
> **First line**
> - Acnegen avoidance and/or occupational redeployment
>
> **Second line**
> - Oral antibiotics
>
> **Third line**
> - Oral isotretinoin

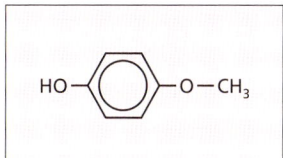

Figure 129.6 Monomethylether of hydroquinone (4-hydroxyanisole or 4-methoxyphenol) is an intermediate in the manufacture of several chemicals.

> **Box 129.3 Chemicals capable of causing occupational leukoderma**
>
> - Hydroquinone
> - Mercaptoamines, e.g. N-2-mercaptoethyl-dimethylamine hydrochloride (MEDA)
> - Monobenzylether of hydroquinone
> - Monoethylether of hydroquinone (p-ethoxyphenol)
> - Monomethylether of hydroquinone (p-methoxyphenol)
> - N,N′,N″-triethylenethiophosphoramide (thio-TEPA)
> - p-cresol
> - p-isopropylcatechol
> - p-methylcatechol
> - p-nonylphenol
> - p-octylphenol
> - p-phenylphenol
> - p-tert-amylphenol
> - p-tertiary-butylcatechol
> - p-tertiary-butylphenol
> - Physostigmine

Occupational dyspigmentation

Definition and nomenclature

Occupational dyspigmentation is a colour change on the skin partially, or entirely, due to work-related factors. More specifically, occupational leukoderma is defined as depigmentation or hypopigmentation of the skin due to industrial exposure to a chemical or chemicals known to have a destructive effect on epidermal melanocytes [1].

> **Synonyms and inclusions**
> - Occupational leukoderma

Introduction and general description

Certain chemicals, particularly the substituted phenols, are destructive to functional melanocytes [2]. Many of these compounds cause permanent depigmentation of the skin, resembling vitiligo. The most commonly implicated chemicals are para-tertiary butyl phenol, para-tertiary butyl catechol, monobenzyl ether of hydroquinone (Figure 129.6), hydroquinone and related compounds [1,2]. A list of chemicals known to cause occupational leukoderma is shown in Box 129.3.

Epidemiology

There are no convincing data on the incidence or prevalence of occupational leukoderma. Although it is more cosmetically obvious in a darker skin type, there is no evidence to suggest that ethnicity plays a role in the pathogenesis.

Pathophysiology

Agents associated with leukoderma usually cause apoptosis of melanocytes; however, the mechanisms effecting this may be very different [3].

Clinical features

The patient presents with asymptomatic hypopigmented macules in exposed areas (Figure 129.7), especially on the dorsa of the hands. Frequently, the individual will associate this with work exposure to chemicals. The diagnosis of occupational leukoderma should be suspected if a worker who potentially has been exposed to depigmenting chemicals develops localised or generalised hypopigmentation [4]. There should be particular suspicion if more than one worker is involved.

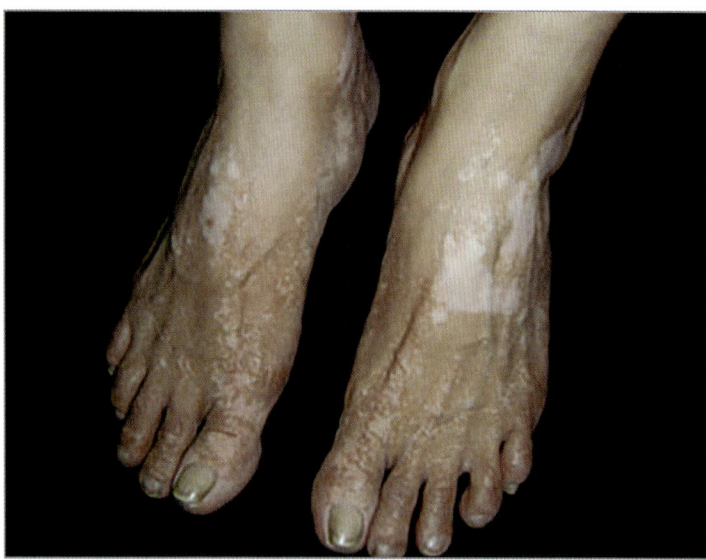

Figure 129.7 Numerous acquired confetti or pea-sized macules seen along with larger depigmented patches in chemical leukoderma. Reproduced from Ghosh and Mukhopadhyay 2009 [5].

Differential diagnosis
- Vitiligo.
- Postinflammatory hypopigmentation (e.g. from seborrhoeic dermatitis or irritant contact dermatitis).

Complications and co-morbidities
Psychological problems may be seen as a result of the cosmetic impact of this disease in severe cases.

Disease course and prognosis
Removal of the offending chemical may result in partial repigmentation, but this process may take years and may not occur at all.

Investigations
The chemicals to which the worker is exposed should be identified and investigation made to see if it or they are known to cause depigmentation. Chemicals that are prone to causing depigmentation at work are listed in Box 129.4. Patch testing may help to exclude leukoderma caused by an allergic contact dermatitis. Occasionally, a skin biopsy may help to exclude other differential diagnoses.

> **Box 129.4 Chemicals prone to causing depigmentation at work**
>
> - Insecticides, paints, plastics and rubber
> - Lubricating and motor oils
> - Photographic chemicals
> - Antimicrobials and disinfectants
> - Detergents and deodorants
> - Inks

Management
There is no specific treatment for occupational leukoderma. Treatment should be aimed at preventing further exposure. Camouflage cosmetics may be used and the depigmented skin should be protected from UV irradiation by sunscreens.

> **Treatment ladder for occupational dyspigmentation**
>
> **First line**
> - Primary prevention
>
> **Second line**
> - Personal protective equipment
>
> **Third line**
> - Topical sunscreens

Occupationally induced skin tumours

Definition
Occupational skin cancers are defined as those where a person's occupation has played a major role in the aetiology of the tumour. Multiple aetiological factors contribute to the development of skin cancer. There have previously been epidemics of skin cancer due to occupational exposures. The major occupational carcinogens recognised are polycyclic hydrocarbons, ionising radiation and arsenic; UV radiation is now the most important carcinogen in occupational skin cancer.

Introduction and general description
Sun exposure from outdoor work is the most common cause of occupational skin cancers, with other work-related exposure to chemicals, ionising radiation or other carcinogens being rare. Sunlight may easily be overlooked as an occupational carcinogen [1], although it is difficult to estimate how much UV radiation comes from work compared with non-occupational exposure [2]. There may also be differences in the carcinogenic potential of artificial UV sources compared with natural sunlight [3]. There is sometimes a long interval between exposure and development of the skin cancer.

In 1775, the first cancer of any type to be linked with occupational exposure was scrotal squamous carcinoma in British chimney sweeps, reported by Sir Percivall Pott [4]. In the rest of Europe, the disease was unknown because of wearing protective clothing and the reduced carcinogenicity of wood soot as opposed to coal soot from the coal predominantly burnt in Britain. Soot formed by burning wood has much lower levels of the polycyclic hydrocarbon, benzo(a)pyrene (Figure 129.8), implicated in the aetiology of skin cancer, compared with coal soot. Skin cancer was still reported in chimney sweeps in Britain in the 1950s. By 1945 in Britain, almost 50% of industrial skin cancer was attributable to exposure to pitch and tar in occupations such as cotton mule spinners, jute workers and the engineering industry [4–7]. Various skin tumours are still seen in the tar refining industry [8].

Epidemiology
There are no good population estimates of incidence and prevalence of occupational skin cancer.

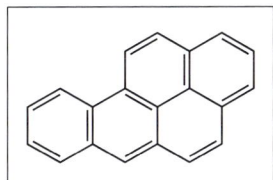

Figure 129.8 Benzo(a)pyrene.

Pathophysiology
See Box 129.5 and Table 129.4 for common causative agents and jobs associated with occupational skin tumours. Polycyclic hydrocarbons are produced by incomplete combustion and distillation of coal, natural gas and oil shale. These chemicals are contained in tar, fuel oils, lubricating oils and greases, oil shale and bitumen. The mechanisms of sun-induced skin cancers are discussed elsewhere (Chapter 10).

> **Box 129.5 Causative agents in occupational skin cancer**
>
> - Polycyclic hydrocarbons:
>   - Soot
>   - Tar
>   - Pitch
>   - Mineral oil
>   - Shale oil
>   - Crude paraffin
>   - Asphalt
> - Ionising radiation
> - Arsenic
> - UV light

Clinical features
The diagnosis of skin cancer is similar to that of non-occupational skin cancers. Generally, the exposed sites are involved. Previously, the scrotum was involved frequently because of continuous exposure to carcinogens and the increased likelihood of skin absorption in that site. There may be coexisting signs of exposure prior to or in addition to evidence of skin cancer. These may include oil folliculitis and hyperkeratoses, described in people working with mineral oil, and pitch or tar warts. Oil hyperkeratoses are flat, white, circular, hyperkeratotic smooth plaques, small in diameter and often clustered. In addition, there are verrucose, pigmented, round or oval, irregular, raised 'warts'. Tar 'warts' are pigmented small papules, often seen around the face on the eyes, eyelids, cheek, forearms and back of the hands.

Differential diagnosis
The differential diagnosis is skin cancer that is entirely coincidental with the current or previous occupation.

Investigations
Appropriate investigation of skin cancers is discussed elsewhere. A site visit may be required if there is doubt about exposure to potential carcinogens in the workplace.

Management
Prevention of the development of skin cancers is most important. Those at high risk of skin cancer (very pale skin types, renal transplant recipients, etc.) should be advised against outdoor work in sunny environments. In the workplace, it is important to consider substitution of carcinogens where possible; an example is the declining exposure to polycyclic hydrocarbons in recent decades. Protection of the skin, either with protective clothing or with engineering controls such as machine guarding, is important. Daily washing is essential. Since most of the skin cancers are associated with a very long latency period, it is important to have continued surveillance of older or retired workers. Finally, the skin cancers need to be treated as appropriate.

> **Treatment ladder for occupationally induced skin tumours**
>
> **First line**
> - Primary prevention
>
> **Second line**
> - Personal protective equipment (sun-protective clothing, topical sunscreens, etc.)
>
> **Third line**
> - Regular skin cancer surveillance for those at high risk

Table 129.4 Occupations with potential exposure to causative agents in occupational skin cancer.

Causative agent	Occupation
Polycyclic hydrocarbons	Tar distilling
	Coal gas manufacturing
	Briquettes manufacturing
	Shale oil workers
	Refinery workers
UV light	Outdoor workers
	Welders
	Laser exposure
	Printers
Ionising radiation	Nuclear power plant workers
	X-ray technicians
	Uranium mining

Vibration white finger

Definition and nomenclature
Vibration white finger is the episodic appearance of white finger skin patches (Raynaud phenomenon [1]) in response to vibrational tools (especially at 50–150 Hz) or environmental cold and is accompanied by secondary loss of sensation caused by vascular ischaemia (Chapter 122). It can be part of, but is not synonymous with, the hand–arm vibration syndrome [2].

> **Synonyms and inclusions**
> - Occupational Raynaud phenomenon

Introduction and general description

The pathogenesis of vibration white finger is poorly understood. Chronic vibration exposure may damage endothelial vasoregulatory mechanisms by disturbing the endothelial-derived relaxing factor-mediated vasodilatory function [3].

Epidemiology

There are no good population studies in this area and the prevalence and incidence are unknown. Black Africans may be more prone to vibration white finger than white people [4]. Sirtuin 1 single nucleotide polymorphism may be a diagnostic marker for this disease [5].

Pathophysiology

See Chapter 122.

Clinical features

Operatives using vibrating tools, such as lumberjacks, coal miners and road and construction workers, are at risk of developing vibration white finger. Affected individuals develop symptoms of Raynaud phenomenon on exposure to cold or vibration, usually after many years of working with vibrating tools [2]. Episodic numbness, tingling, colour change and loss of manual dexterity are typical.

Differential diagnosis

- Raynaud phenomenon of non-occupational origin.

Disease course and prognosis

Symptoms may be severe and compromise the ability to work.

Investigations

The diagnosis is usually made by the history alone. Ice provocation tests are not always reliable in precipitating attacks of vibration white finger [2].

Management

Widespread knowledge of its causes, controls over duration of use of relevant machinery and improved personal protective equipment have led to a reduction in the incidence of vibration white finger [2]. The treatment is the same as for the Raynaud phenomenon. It is generally believed that symptoms of vibration white finger regress some time after the cessation of exposure [2].

Treatment ladder for vibration white finger

First line
- Primary prevention: antivibration gloves

Second line
- Redeployment

Third line
- Standard treatments for Raynaud phenomenon such as keeping warm, stopping smoking, nifedipine, etc.

Resources

Further information

British Occupational Health Research Foundation (website is now only available for reference): www.bohrf.org.uk.

Patient resources

Canadian Centre for Occupational Health and Safety, resources for patients with occupational skin disease: www.ccohs.ca.
(Both last accessed March 2023.)

Key references

The full list of references can be found in the online version at https://www.wiley.com/rooksdermatology10e

Occupational irritant contact dermatitis

1 Rycroft RJG. Occupational contact dermatitis. In: Rycroft RJG, Menné T, Frosch PJ, Lepoittevin J-P, eds. *Textbook of Contact Dermatitis*, 3rd edn. Berlin: Springer, 2001:555–80.
14 Wilkinson DS, Budden MG, Hambly EM. A 10-year review of an industrial dermatitis clinic. *Contact Dermatitis* 1980;6:11–17.
21 Freeman S. Repeated low-grade frictional trauma. In: Kanerva L, Elsner P, Wahlberg JE, Maibach HI, eds. *Handbook of Occupational Dermatology*. Berlin: Springer, 2000:111–14.
26 Loman L, Uter W, Armario-Hita JC et al.; ESCC Working Group. European Surveillance System on Contact Allergies (ESSCA): characteristics of patients patch tested and diagnosed with irritant contact dermatitis. *Contact Dermatitis* 2021;85:185–97.
31 O'Neill H, Narang I, Buckley DA et al. Occupational dermatoses during the COVID-19 pandemic: a multicentre audit in the UK and Ireland. *Br J Dermatol* 2021;184:575–7.
44 Landeck L, Visser M, Skudlik C et al. Clinical course of occupational irritant contact dermatitis of the hands in relation to filaggrin genotype status and atopy. *Br J Dermatol* 2012;167:1302–9.
47 Held E, Skoet R, Johansen JD et al. The hand eczema severity index (HECSI): a scoring system for clinical assessment of hand eczema. A study of inter- and intra-observer reliability. *Br J Dermatol* 2005;152:302–7.
60 Carmichael AJ, Foulds IS. Performing a factory visit. *Clin Exp Dermatol* 1993;18:208–10.
84 Agner T, Held E. Skin protection programmes. *Contact Dermatitis* 2002;47:253–6.
85 Dickel H, Kuss O, Schmidt A, Diepgen TI. Impact of preventative strategies on trend of occupational skin disease in hairdressers: population based register study. *BMJ* 2002;324:1422–3.
110 Frosch PJ. Cutaneous irritation. In: Rycroft RJG, Menné T, Frosch PJ, eds. *Textbook of Contact Dermatitis*, 2nd edn. Berlin: Springer, 1995:28–61.
114 Smith HR, Armstrong DK, Holloway D et al. Skin irritation thresholds in hairdressers: implications for the development of hand dermatitis. *Br J Dermatol* 2002;146:849–52.

Occupational allergic contact dermatitis

2 Veien NK. Allergic contact dermatitis: immunological aspects and common occupational causes. In: English JSC, ed. *A Colour Handbook of Occupational Dermatology*. London: Manson, 1998:31–52.
3 Foussereau J, Benezra C, Maibach HI. *Occupational Contact Dermatitis*. Copenhagen: Munksgaard, 1982.
4 Dickel H. Kuss O, Schmidt A et al. Occupational relevance of positive standard patch-test results in employed persons with an initial report of an occupational skin disease. *Int Arch Occup Environ Health* 2002;75:423–34.
8 Nicholson PJ, Llewellyn D, English JS et al. Evidence based guidelines for the prevention, identification and management of occupational contact dermatitis and urticaria. *Contact Dermatitis* 2010;63:177–86.

9 DeKoven JG, DeKoven BM, Warshaw EM *et al*. Occupational allergic contact dermatitis: retrospective analysis of North American Contact Dermatitis Group Data 2001–2016. *J Am Acad Dermatol* 2022;86:782–90.

10 Brans R, Wilke A, Rodríguez E *et al*. Effectiveness of secondary prevention in metalworkers with work-related skin diseases and comparison with participants of a tertiary prevention program: a prospective cohort study. *Contact Dermatitis* 2020;83:497–506.

11 Julander A, Liljedahl ER, Korres de Paula H *et al*. Nickel penetration into stratum corneum in FLG null carriers – a human experimental study. *Contact Dermatitis* 2022;87:154–61.

12 Freeman S. Diagnosis and differential diagnosis. In: Adams RM, ed. *Occupational Skin Disease*, 3rd edn. Philadelphia: Saunders, 1999:189–207.

14 Lee WR, McCallum RI. The occupational history. In: Raffle PAB, Lee WR, McCallum RI, Murray R, eds. *Hunter's Diseases of Occupations*. London: Hodder & Stoughton, 1987:229–36.

15 Johansen JD, Aalto-Korte K, Agner T *et al*. European Society of Contact Dermatitis guideline for diagnostic patch testing – recommendations on best practice. *Contact Dermatitis* 2015;73:195–221.

16 Bourke J, Coulson I, English J. Guidelines for the management of contact dermatitis: an update. *Br J Dermatol* 2009;160:946–54.

20 Ale SI, Maibach HI. Occupational contact urticaria. In: Kanerva L, Elsner P, Wahlberg JE, Maibach HI, eds. *Handbook of Occupational Dermatology*. Berlin: Springer, 2000:201.

115 Cronin E, Kullavanijaya P. Hand dermatitis in hairdressers. *Acta Derm Venereol Suppl (Stockh)* 1979;85:47–50.

Acne of chemical origin

2 Crow KD. Chloracne: a critical review including a comparison of two series of cases of acne from chlornaphthalene and pitch fumes. *Trans St Johns Hosp Dermatol Soc* 1970;56:79–99.

5 Tindall JP. Chloracne and chloracnegens. *J Am Acad Dermatol* 1985;13:539–58.

7 Zugerman C. Chloracne, chloracnegens, and other forms of environmental acne. In: Adams RM, ed. *Occupational Skin Disease*, 2nd edn. Philadelphia: Saunders, 1990:127–35.

13 Coenraads PJ, Brouwer A, Olie K *et al*. Chloracne: some recent issues. *Dermatol Clin* 1994;12:569–76.

34 Kligman AM, Mills OH. Acne cosmetica. *Arch Dermatol* 1972;106:843–50.

Occupational dyspigmentation

1 Wattanakrai P, Miyamoto L, Taylor JS. Occupational pigmentary disorders. In: Kanerva L, Elsner P, Wahlberg JE, Maibach HI, eds. *Handbook of Occupational Dermatology*. Berlin: Springer, 2000:280–94.

Occupationally induced skin tumours

1 Gawkrodger DJ. Occupational skin cancers. *Occup Med (Lond)* 2004;54:458–63.

3 Surdu S, Fitzgerald EF, Bloom MS *et al*. Occupational exposure to ultraviolet radiation and risk of non-melanoma skin cancer in multinational European study. *PLOS One* 2013;8:e62359.

Vibration white finger

1 Raynaud M. *De l'asphyxie locale et la gangrène symétrique des extrémités* [Thesis]. Paris: Rignoux, 1862.

CHAPTER 130

Stings and Bites

Alfredo Siller Jr[1], Austinn C. Miller[1] and Stephen K. Tyring[2]

[1]Center for Clinical Studies, Houston, TX, USA
[2]University of Texas Health Science Center, Houston, TX, USA

STINGS, 130.1	Mollusca stings, 130.4	Snake bites, 130.5
Jellyfish, sea anemones and coral stings, 130.1	Venomous fish stings, 130.4	Dog and cat bites, 130.6
Sponge stings, 130.3		Human bites, 130.6
Sea urchin stings, 130.3	BITES, 130.5	
Sea mat stings, 130.4	Rodent bites, 130.5	Key references, 130.7

STINGS

Jellyfish, sea anemones and coral stings

Introduction and general description

Cnidaria is a phylum of over 9000 diverse species which includes jellyfish, sea anemones and corals [1,2,3]. All are aquatic and the majority are marine. Four of the five classes of Cnidaria have a medusa or 'jellyfish' stage in their life cycle and all have tentacles bearing batteries of stinging cells (nematocysts) that are used for defense and capturing prey. Within each nematocyst is a spirally coiled thread that can be everted, uncoiled and forcibly ejected. In contact with prey, or with human skin, the nematocysts are discharged and the threads inject venom. The nature and toxic effects of the venom vary by species; however, many species inflict at least some discomfort on humans, while others are potentially dangerous [3,4–7].

Pathophysiology
Pathology

Histopathology of an acute eruption following a cnidarian sting demonstrates intracellular oedema of the keratinocytes, many of which have pyknotic nuclei and a lymphocytic infiltrate in an oedematous superficial dermis [8]. Nematocysts were visible penetrating the epidermis in a 5-year-old child who suffered fatal envenomation from *Chironex fleckeri* [9].

The histology of recurrent reactions shows a spongiotic vesicular dermatitis with a dense, perivascular, lymphohistiocytic infiltrate, often containing large numbers of eosinophils [10,11]. There is oedema of the papillary dermis. Immunohistochemical studies suggest that Langerhans cells and helper T lymphocytes play a central role and that type IV delayed hypersensitivity is involved in the pathogenesis of the lesions [11]. Epithelioid granulomas and large CD30+ lymphocytes were present in a delayed reaction to a fire coral [12].

Causative organisms

Class Hydrozoa. This class includes the fire corals and free-floating members of the subclass Siphonophora. The Siphonophora are colonial organisms in which a number of individuals, specialised for different functions, are structurally associated. Perhaps the best known siphonophoran is *Physalia*, the Portuguese man-of-war, also known as the 'bluebottle' in Australia. It has an air-filled float, which acts as a sail, and trailing tentacles. The nematocysts occur in 'batteries' or 'sting buttons' along the tentacles and contact with them results in the extrusion of numerous nematocysts and the inoculation of venom.

Class Cubozoa. Often referred to as box jellyfish, several species are dangerous to humans [3]. The most notorious is *Chironex fleckeri* (the sea wasp), which has been responsible for a number of deaths in Australian waters. Other dangerous species include *Carybdea rastoni* (the jimble), *Carukia barnesi* (the Irukandji) [13], the 'Morbakka' (fire jelly or Moreton Bay stinger) [14] and the Hawaiian box jellyfish, *Alatina moseri*.

Class Scyphozoa. In this class, the medusa is the dominant form of the life cycle. These jellyfish are distributed worldwide. For example, *Pelagia noctiluca* (the mauve stinger) is well known in the Mediterranean and Adriatic but also has a wide distribution in the oceans of the world.

Class Anthozoa. This class contains several thousand species, including the sea anemones, the soft corals and the stony or true corals. Several species of sea anemone are known to inflict painful stings [2,3,15]. The reef-forming corals may cause injury to the skin with their nematocysts or with their calcareous outer skeletons [16].

Class Staurozoa. Staurozoa is a class of stalked jellyfish composed of over 50 species organised into 11 genera, 6 families and 2 suborders. It is the least known and least studied class of Cnidaria, but has been described to concentrate at mid-latitudes in intertidal and shallow subtidal regions [17].

Clinical features

Contact with *Physalia* tentacles usually results in a linear red eruption accompanied by severe local pain [3,18–20]. Because of the arrangement of the 'sting buttons' of nematocysts there is a beaded pattern of local, small weals. In humans, pain and skin lesions comprise the majority of reported toxicity, but occasionally more severe reactions may occur [21]. Haemolysis and acute renal failure in a 4-year-old girl [22] and fatalities have been reported [23,24].

The local effects of the box jellyfish's tentacle contact are immediate, severe pain and linear weals with a white, ischaemic centre. Larger weals may have a typical 'cross-hatched' or 'frosted/rope-ladder' pattern corresponding to the architecture of the tentacles (Figure 130.1). In mild cases, these cutaneous symptoms usually subside within 24 h [25]. Partial- or full-thickness skin necrosis may result. Box jellyfish may be responsible not only for localised lesions but also for severe systemic effects including nausea, vomiting and shock-like symptoms which may result in death [3,4,8,26–29]. The length of weals left on the skin can be used to predict prognosis of posioning: if the total length is greater than 2–4 m in children or 6 m in adults, there is increased risk of death [25].

In addition to acute skin lesions, which are regarded as toxic in nature, there may be delayed, persistent or recurrent eruptions at the original sites of cnidarian envenomation [10,30–36]. Recurrent episodes may be single or multiple and may take the form of red, urticarial lesions, papules or plaques. A delayed hypersensitivity response to jellyfish antigens has been demonstrated by a positive patch test reaction to a nematocyst preparation from *Olindias sambaquiensis* [37]. Other reported sequelae of jellyfish stings include erythema nodosum [38], cold urticaria [39] and Mondor disease [40].

Seabather's eruption is another reaction caused by jellyfish. It is an itchy, red dermatosis of papules and weals occurring predominantly under swimwear; lesions are usually concentrated in tight-fitting areas (Figure 130.2) [41–46]. Trapped underneath the

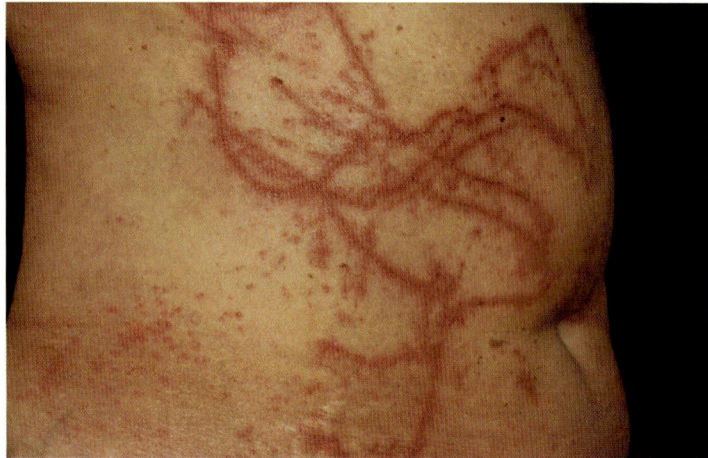

Figure 130.1 Serpiginous, red, papular/urticarial skin lesions on the abdomen 8 days after a jellyfish sting. From Neumann *et al.* 2020 [57].

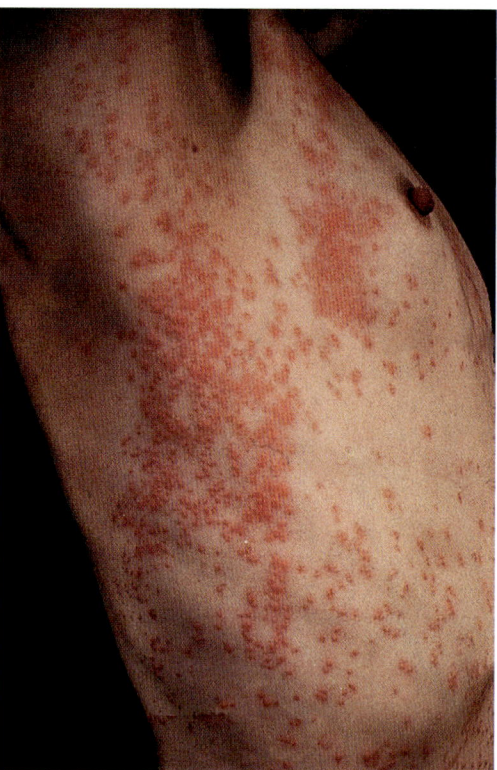

Figure 130.2 Seabather's eruption. Courtesy of Dr. R. MacSween, Kingston, Ontario, Canada.

bathing costume, the causative organisms become triggered and discharge their nematocysts. It is probable that a similar clinical picture can be produced by different coelenterates in different waters. In Florida, the Gulf of Mexico and the Caribbean, *Linuche unguiculata* (the thimble jellyfish) appears to be responsible, and evidence has recently been presented that all three free-swimming stages of this jellyfish can cause seabather's eruption [47]. Specific immunoglobulin G (IgG) antibodies against *L. unguiculata* antigen have been demonstrated by enzyme-linked immunosorbent assay (ELISA) in patients with seabather's eruption [48]. Cases in the Long Island region of New York have been attributed to larvae of the sea anemone *Edwardsiella lineata* [43].

It should be noted that seabather's eruption as described is completely distinct from 'swimmer's itch' or 'clam digger's itch', an eruption due to cercarial organisms that mainly affect uncovered skin, although both can occur in saltwater and the terms are sometimes loosely applied.

Envenomation by fire corals usually produces immediate burning or stinging pain, followed by urticarial lesions at the site of contact. These may in turn be followed by a localised vesiculobullous eruption and subsequently chronic granulomatous and lichenoid lesions [49–51]. Stinging of an aquarium shopworker by a stony coral, *Euphyllia picteti*, has been reported [52].

Management

An important aspect of first aid for cnidarian stings is the prevention of further discharge by nematocysts [3,20,53,54]. Vinegar has been shown to inhibit activation of the nematocyst spring mechanism of box jellyfish and should be poured over the affected area of skin as soon as possible. This should be done before attempting to remove any adhering tentacles to decrease risk of discharge. However, in other jellyfish such as *Physalia physalis*, nematocyst discharge is not inhibited and may be provoked by vinegar. In general, avoid using cold water or alcohol to treat stings as these cause immediate discharge worsening the skin reaction and poisoning [25].

The application of cold packs provides relief of mild to moderate pain resulting from stings by *Physalia* and a number of species of jellyfish, but heat has been demonstrated to be even more effective in pain relief, likely due to toxin inactivation. This observation may have wider therapeutic implications in the management of jellyfish envenomation [55,56]. For most jellyfish stings, tentacle removal and pain management is the primary therapy.

An antivenom is available for use in *Chironex fleckeri* envenomation. In Australia, containers of vinegar are avaliable on many beaches and protective clothing, in the form of Lycra 'stinger suits', is extremely useful in the prevention of jellyfish envenomation.

Sponge stings

Introduction and general description
Contact with certain sponges can induce a dermatitic eruption that is caused by spicules becoming lodged in the skin. Other skin signs may also follow contact with a noxious sponge and sometimes systemic symptoms occur as well. The syndrome typically occurs in divers and those who collect sponges, especially off the coasts of Australia and New Zealand [1].

Clinical features
Tedania ignis (the fire sponge) is capable of producing a severe dermatitis and has also been reported as inducing erythema multiforme-like lesions of the face, palms and soles 10 days after contact [2,3,4]. Dermatitis can also be caused by other sponges, including *Neofibularia nolitangere* (the poison bun sponge) and *Microciona prolifera* (the red sponge). Initial pruritus and burning may progress to redness with papules, vesicles or bullae. Although rare, patients may also complain of systemic symptoms such as nausea and vomiting.

Management
Treatment consists of wound irrigation with normal saline or sea water. Soaking the affected area in vinegar can also be helpful. Adhesive tape may be used in the removal of spicules. Topical corticosteroids can be prescribed for symptomatic relief. Pain, which may last for several weeks, is responsive to non-steroidal anti-inflammatory drugs (NSAIDs).

Sea urchin stings

Introduction and general description
The Echinoidea, or sea urchins, form part of the phylum Echinodermata, which also includes the starfishes and sea cucumbers [1,2,3]. Sea urchins are usually spherical or ovoid, enclosed in a shell of closely fitting plates supplied with numerous moveable spines and are found exclusively in saltwater bodies. The spines are formed by calcification of a cylindrical projection of subepidermal connective tissue. Situated between the spines are three-jawed pedicellariae, some of which are venomous. They are used to seize prey and are also used in defense. In some species of sea urchins, the spines are venomous.

Clinical features
Those who frequent saltwater ecosytems are most susceptible to sea urchin injuries (SUIs). SUIs occur on the feet in about 80% of cases, 15% involve the hands and the remaining 5% are distributed throughout the rest of the body [4]. Non-venomous spines generally produce mild inflammation and tenderness overlying the injury [4]. Envenomation by sea urchin spines or pedicellariae induces immediate burning pain, which may be intense and can persist for several hours [**1**,3,5,6]. The degree of local swelling can be variable, but is sometimes severe. In the absence of secondary infection, the puncture wounds heal within a week or two. Broken spine fragments result in dark punctae at the site of injury.

The development of secondary epidermoid cysts from implantation of fragmented epithelium driven into the wounds by the spines is recognised. Delayed granulomatous reactions usually develop several months after the original injury and take the form of bluish papules or nodules at the sites of penetration of the spines. Granulomatous inflammation is of a foreign body or sarcoidal type. It has been suggested that *Mycobacterium marinum* may play a pathogenic role in some cases of sea urchin granuloma [7,8].

On the digits, there may be diffuse fusiform swelling and limitation of movement. These lesions are persistent if not treated. Synovitis and joint damage may occur if the spines penetrate joint cavities [9]. Occasionally, systemic symptoms can accompany localised lesions.

A patient with a pruritic red eruption on the knees and ankles following injury by a sea urchin produced a positive patch test reaction to an extract of sea urchin spines [10].

Management
Timely and appropriate management can prevent long-term morbidity despite the deceptively innocuous appearance of these injuries [4]. Treatment should consist of quick and careful removal of spines and pedicellariae; however the fragile spines (made of calcium carbonate) break easily and may be difficult to extract. Immersion of the affected area in hot water (43–46°C) for 30–90 min will provide pain relief and may inactivate possible thermolabile toxins [11]. Local inhabitants, in certain areas where sea urchin injuries are common, apply hot candle wax to the area [12]. The spines often release pigment into the skin – if there is still a colour change 48 h after the initial puncture wound, it is likely that a spine remains lodged in the skin. Imaging with plain radiograph or ultrasound is warranted to help identify the remaining spines. Embedded spines are difficult to remove surgically, but erbium:yttrium-aluminium-garnet (Er:YAG) laser ablation has proved effective [13]. If the spines have penetrated a joint, surgical exploration is advisable. Granulomatous lesions may be treated with an intralesional steroid.

Sea mat stings

Introduction and general description
The Bryozoa are small, sedentary, colonial animals, which tend to form mat-like encrustations (hence the name sea mats) on rocks, seaweeds or other surfaces. Severe occupational dermatitis resulting from contact with *Alcyonidium diaphanum* (sea chervil) was originally described in North Sea fishermen, and was named 'Dogger Bank itch' because of its association with the Dogger Bank fishing grounds. However, *A. diaphanum* is widely distributed in waters around the British Isles and mainland Europe [1,2]. The eruption is an allergic contact dermatitis (rather than a physical dermatosis or sting) and occurs during the summer months, principally because the organism, which becomes detached in winter storms, proliferates in the spring and summer and is therefore encountered in greater numbers by fishermen.

Clinical features
The dermatosis caused by *A. diaphanum* is an acute, papular, occasionally bullous, contact dermatitis on the hands, arms and face [3–6], which may have a photoallergic component [5]. The allergen is the (2-hydroxyethyl)-dimethylsulphoxonium ion, a metabolite produced by the bryozoan [7,8]. Hypersensitivity to another bryozoan, *Electra pilosa*, has also been described [5,6].

Management
Topical therapy with a potent corticosteroid ointment is usually necessary, in combination with emollient.

Mollusca stings

Introduction and general description
The only important venomous univalve molluscs are the cone shells of the genus *Conus* [1,2,3]. All the species of this genus possess a venom apparatus and several species have caused human injury. The very small, floating mollusc *Creseis acicula* (Rang 1828) has been identified as a cause of stings in bathers in Florida [4]. The sting of some species, particularly the cone snail *Conus geographus*, may be fatal [2,5]. The tiny blue-ringed octopus (*Hapalochlaena maculosa*), a member of the Cephalopoda class of molluscs and found mainly in Australian and New Guinea coastal waters, has been called the world's most deadly octopus as its venom contains tetrodotoxin, one of the most deadly toxins in the world [6]. These creatures have been reported to bite humans when severely agitated. Their blue rings become very prominent when provoked.

Clinical features
Stings by molluscs cause painful puncture wounds, with local ischaemia, cyanosis and numbness. The numbness quickly spreads to involve the entire body. The bite of the blue-ringed octopus contains salivary conotoxins that may induce severe systemic symptoms culminating in death, usually from respiratory failure [6–8]. Cutaneous reactions following *H. maculosa* bites include intense pruritus and urticaria [3,7,9]. Redness, oedema and a burning sensation can follow the bite of *Octopus apollyon*, succeeded by a persistent red plaque and lymphoedema [10]. Overall envenomation-associated mortality with molluscs is up to 20%.

Management
The treatment of mollusca stings is largely supportive as there is no antivenom for conotoxins. The only therapeutic option for a patient stung by a cone snail, particularly in cases with respiratory arrest, is urgent intubation and admission of the patient to a critical care setting [6]. *H. maculosa* bites are treated in the same way, with the addition of pressure immobilisation used to reduce systemic venom spread.

Venomous fish stings

Introduction and general description
Numerous species of fish are capable of inflicting painful or even dangerous stings by means of dorsal or caudal spines provided with complex venom glands [1,2,3]. Most injuries caused by venomous fish result from contact with stingrays (class Chondrichthyes) or catfish and scorpionfish (class Osteichthyes). Venomous species are not confined to tropical waters. The lesser weeverfish (*Echiichthys vipera*) [4,5], the spiny dogfish (*Squalus acanthias*) and several species of stingray inhabit Atlantic coasts and can inflict serious stings. In warmer waters, species of stingray, scorpionfish, catfish [6], rabbitfish, stonefish [7], the aptly named 'bearded ghoul', stargazers and toadfish are potentially dangerous.

In many cases, envenomation results from victims inadvertently stepping on the fish in shallow water. The tail of the stingray carries serrated spines containing venom glands surrounded by an integumentary sheath. Treading on the fish results in a reflex 'whip' of the tail, which drives the spines into the skin, usually on the leg [8]. Several of these venomous species bury themselves in the sand in shallow waters, with their spines protruding, and are therefore a hazard to bathers.

Clinical features
Injuries commonly occur on the feet or legs as a result of the victim stepping on the fish. Fish stings are usually immediately painful. They present as painful lacerations or puncture wounds. Intense pain may continue for several hours; swelling and redness around the wounds may simulate an infective cellulitis. With some species, systemic symptoms may occur. The Raynaud phenomenon affecting individual digits penetrated by weeverfish spines has been reported [9,10]. Stingray spines may cause lacerations, or may be driven into the skin and break off. If the integumentary sheath ruptures, envenomation occurs. In severe stingray wounds, the affected area appears dusky or cyanotic and later becomes red or mottled, with necrosis of underlying fat and muscle [11].

The inflammatory infiltrate in one case of stingray envenomation contained numerous mononuclear cells, many of which were T-cell-restricted intracellular antigen 1 (TIA) positive, suggesting that an immunological reaction might contribute to the delayed healing commonly seen after stingray injury [12].

Fatalities have been attributed to venomous fish envenomation. These cases are poorly reported and may be more likely due to septicaemia from secondary bacterial infection.

Management
The venom of the weeverfish, like that of the stingray, stonefish and other venomous fish, is an unstable protein that is heat labile. Hot water is very effective in treating these types of stings [3,13–15]. The injured part should be immersed in hot water (someone other than the victim should gauge the temperature), and this will diminish the pain. An antivenom is available for stonefish stings. Tetanus prophylaxis should also be administered. Plain radiographs to ensure the removal of all spines should be performed [16]. Antibiotic prophylaxis may be warranted depending on the severity of the trauma and underlying co-morbidities of the victim [16].

BITES

Rodent bites

Introduction and general description
Approximately 20 000 rodent bites occur in the USA annually [**1**]. Although the risk of infection is low, there is concern for the transmission of zoonotic infection, particularly from rats, if the rodent is a carrier. Rat-bite fever (also known as Haverhill fever) is a febrile systemic illness caused by the bite or a scratch from an infected rat. Other risk factors for rat-bite fever are handling an infected rat, or contact with infected rat faeces. The disease is also probably transmitted by other rodents [2,3]. In one report approximately 30% of patients with rat-bite fever did not report having been bitten or scratched by a rat [4].

Pathophysiology
Causative organisms
The causative bacteria of rat-bite fever are *Streptobacillus moniliformis* and *Spirillum minus* (see Chapter 26).

Clinical features
The prodromal phase of the disease starts 2–10 days following exposure and is characterised by fever, myalgia and arthralgia, nausea, vomiting and headache. A rash on the extremities, and sometimes palms and soles, often ensues. It is typically described as maculopapular but can also be petechial, purpuric or pustular. A polyarthritis in up to 50% of patients can develop after the rash [5,6]. Some patients are left with persistent fevers and chills. These symptoms are typically relapsing or intermittent. The infection can be fatal in both children and adults, with a case fatality rate of up to 25% in untreated patients [7–9]. There are two reported cases of death secondary to sepsis in previously healthy adults [2].

Management
Preventative therapy is warranted in patients following a rat bite, even in the absence of clinical symptoms or signs of disease. The wound should be cleaned using appropriate wound management. The first line treatment is intravenous penicillin G (200 000 units every 4 h) for 5–7 days in adults. The second line treatment is tetracycline 500 mg PO four times a day for 7 days, or doxycycline 100 mg PO or IV twice a day for 7 days (adults).

Snake bites

Introduction and general description
The World Health Organization (WHO) has classfied snake bites as a neglected tropical disease, leading to underestimation of its public health importance and less effort in data collection. The highest incidences of snake bites recorded are in South America, West Africa, the Indian subcontinent and South-East Asia [1,2,**3**]. In India there are an estimated 46 900 deaths annually, and in Bangladesh snake bites cause about 6000 deaths per year [4]. Globally, there are an estimated 4–5 million snake bites each year which account for approximately 81 000–138 000 deaths [4]. Most deaths occur in areas that lack conventional medical treatment centres.

When venomous snakes bite, compressor muscles squeeze venom stored in glands behind the eyes through ducts that lead to the fangs. Depending on the venomous species, between 10% and 80% of bitten patients experience 'dry bites' without being envenomed. Symptoms of envenomed victims vary according to the composition of the venom. For example, bites of the spitting cobra (*Naja nigricollis*) produce local swelling and necrosis, haematological abnormalities and complement depletion [5]; the venom of the Malayan krait (*Bungarus candidus*) contains a toxin (bungarotoxin) that interferes with transmission at the neuromuscular junction [6]; and marked coagulation disturbances occur after envenomation by the Australian brown snakes (genus *Pseudonaja*) [7].

Clinical features
The first signs and symptoms of a venomous snake bite are often local pain, swelling, tenderness and bruising around the bite. Other non-specific signs that may suggest systemic envenoming include general malaise, headache, nausea and vomiting. Following envenomation, several syndromes must be distinguished: neurotoxicity, systemic toxicity, coagulopathy, rhabdomyolysis and renal failure. Local tissue necrosis is varied. Fang marks can be easily missed in most snake bites in Australia; in contrast bites from vipers and cobras may cause extensive tissue destruction.

Management [3,8]
The majority of snake bites do not result in envenomation. To determine if envenomation has occurred, patients should be closely monitored for signs and symptoms of envenomation before discharge from medical care. Antivenom is used when there are definite signs of systemic envenomation or massive local swelling and tissue destruction. Patients who do not receive antivenom should be instructed to seek medical care for worsening of symptoms, signs of coagulopathy or pain. Antibiotics should be prescribed to patients with signs of infection at the site of the bite.

Dog and cat bites

Introduction and general description
Dog bites are the most common animal bite [1]. The highest incidence of dog bites occurs in school-aged children. Most infections that develop from dog and cat bites are polymicrobial.

Pathophysiology
Causative organisms
Infections induced by dog and cat bites are often the result of multiple organisms, including aerobic bacteria (*Staphylococcus* species, *Streptococcus* species and *Corynebacterium* species) and anaerobic bacteria (*Bacteroides fragilis*, *Prevotella*, *Porphyromonas*, *Peptostreptococcus*, *Fusobacterium* species and *Veillonella parvula*) (Table 130.1) [2]. Cat scratch disease, caused by *Bartonella henselae*, can follow a bite from a cat (Chapter 26).

Capnocytophaga canimorsus is part of the normal oral flora of healthy dogs, cats and a number of other animals [3–7]. Approximately 80% of infections with *Capnocytophaga* follow dog bites or exposure to dogs. Previous splenectomy and alcoholism are important predisposing factors, but infection may occur in perfectly healthy persons. Confirmation of infection depends upon identifying Gram-negative rods within polymorphs on peripheral blood films, and isolation from blood and tissue cultures. The organism is sensitive to penicillin and ciprofloxacin.

Pasteurella multocida, an aerobic Gram-negative coccobacillus, is a normal component of the oral flora of dogs and cats and is frequently isolated from infected bites [3,4]. It is a virulent pathogen that provokes an intense inflammatory response and is likely to cause metastatic infection. Infective tenosynovitis can be a serious consequence of *P. multocida* infection, particularly in bites involving the hands.

Clinical features
Dog bites
Dog bites cause a range of injuries from minor scratches and abrasions to deep open lacerations and deep puncture wounds [8]. The extremities are the most frequent site of injury. The spectrum of illness from *Capnocytophaga* infection ranges from wound infection to fulminant septicaemia. Skin lesions include a localised eschar at the site of the bite, cellulitis, non-specific macular or maculopapular lesions, erythema multiforme [9], petechiae, purpura fulminans and symmetrical peripheral gangrene. The more severe changes occur as a consequence of septicaemia and disseminated intravascular coagulation [5–7].

Cat bites
Deep puncture wounds are of great concern with cats as they have long, sharp teeth [10]. Although less common than dog bites, cat bites are much more likely to become infected [1]. When bites occur in the hand, osteomyelitis or septic arthritis can occur due to bacteria being inoculated below the periosteum or into a joint [11].

Investigations
Wound culture should be obtained if the wound appears to be infected. Radiographs are warranted if the wound seems to have disrupted the underlying bones or joints. Soft-tissue injury, subcutaneous gas and osteomyelitis can all be detected.

Management
Standard wound care should be implemented for all dog and cat bites [1]. Wounds should be explored to exclude the possibility of a foreign body. The closure of bite wounds remains controversial. In general, primary closure can be undertaken with simple dog lacerations. In contrast, most cat wounds should be left open to heal by secondary intention. Prophylactic antibiotics should always be used with cat bites. Amoxicillin-clavulanate is considered first line therapy and effectively reduces the rate of animal bite infections [12]. Antibiotics lacking activity against *Pasteurella multocida* should be avoided. Clindamycin plus a fluoroquinolone or doxycycline are recommended as second line agents.

The patient's tetanus immunisation status should be determined for any bite that breaks the skin [13]. Certain patients may require a tetanus toxoid-containing vaccine. Patients with dirty wounds and less than three doses of tetanus toxoid, or if the vaccine status is unknown, should receive the human tetanus immune globulin. Patients should also be evaluated for the need of rabies post-exposure immunoprophylaxis.

Table 130.1 Predominant bacteria isolated from patients with animal and human bite wounds.

Bacteria	Animal bite	Human bite
Aerobic and facultative isolates		
Streptococcus spp.	+	+
Enterococcus spp.	+	+
Staphylococcus aureus	+	+
Staphylococcus epidermidis	+	+
Neisseria spp.	+	+
Corynebacterium spp.	+	+
Pasteurella multocida	+	
Eikenella corrodens	+	+
Acinetobacter spp.	+	
Weeksella zoohelcum	+	
Haemophilus spp.	+	+
Moraxella spp.	+	
Capnocytophaga spp	+	
Anaerobic isolates		
Peptostreptococcus spp.	+	+
Veillonella spp.	+	+
Bifidobacterium spp.		+
Eubacterium spp.		+
Fusobacterium spp.	+	+
Bacteroides spp.	+	+
Prevotella spp.	+	+

Adapted from Brook 2005 [14].

Human bites

Introduction and general description
Human bites are quite common; it is estimated that 250 000 human bites occur each year in the USA [1]. Clenched fist injuries ('fight

bites') are the most prevalent, and may introduce dangerous bacterial infection [2]. Necrotising fasciitis caused by group A streptococci has been reported in a human bite on the calf [3]. Transmission of herpesvirus types 1 and 2 and hepatitis B and C has also been documented. An epidemic of hepatitis B was traced to a carrier in a mental health residential institution who regularly bit his fellow residents [4]. Biting is also a possible transmission mode for human immunodeficiency virus (HIV) infection [5].

Pathophysiology
Causative organisms
Human bite wounds generally contain polymicrobial flora that reflects the aerobic and anaerobic microbiology of the oral flora of the biter, the skin of the victim and the environment (Table 130.1) [6]. Aerobic Gram-positive cocci are most commonly isolated from human bites, predominantly *Staphylococcus* species, *Streptococcus* species and *Eikenella spieces* [2].

Clinical features
Depending on the extent of the bite, a semicircular or oval area of redness or bruising will appear; the skin itself may or may not be intact.

Management
Standard wound care should be used in the management of human bites. Most wounds should be left open to heal by secondary intention. Some lesions may be closed due to cosmetic concerns, but this should only be implemented if the wound is clinically uninfected, less than 12 h old and not located on the hand or foot. Wounds on the hand typically have the highest rate of infection. Antibiotic prophylaxis should be given to patients who have bites that extend through the dermis. Amoxicillin-clavulanate is considered first line therapy; doxycycline is recommended as second line treatment (although not in children).

Key references

The full list of references can be found in the online version at https://www.wiley.com/rooksdermatology10e

Stings
Jellyfish, sea anemones and coral stings
3 Williamson JA, Fenner PJ, Burnett JW, Rifkin JF, eds. *Venomous and Poisonous Marine Animals*. Sydney: University of New South Wales Press, 1996.

Sponge stings
4 Burnett JW, Calton GJ, Morgan RJ. Dermatitis due to stinging sponges. *Cutis* 1987;39:476.

Sea urchin stings
1 Halstead BW. Class osteichthyes: venomous scorpion fishes. In: *Poisonous and Venomous Marine Animals of the World*, 2nd edn. Princeton, NJ: Darwin Press, 1978.

Sea mat stings
1 Porter JS, Ellis JR, Hayward PJ *et al*. Geographic variation in abundance and morphology of the bryozoan Alcyonidium diaphanum (Ctenostomata: Alcyonidiidae) in UK coastal waters. *J Mar Biol Assoc UK* 2002;82:529–35.

Mollusca stings
3 McGoldrick J, Marx JA. Marine envenomations part 2: invertebrates. *J Emerg Med* 1992;10:71–7.

Venomous fish stings
1 Halstead BW. *Poisonous and Venomous Marine Animals of the World*, 2nd edn. Princeton, NJ: Darwin Press, 1988.

Bites
Rodent bites
1 Hurt JB, Maday KR. Management and treatment of animal bites. *J Am Acad Physician Assist* 2018;31:27–31.

Snake bites
3 Warrell DA. Venomous bites, stings, and poisoning: an update. *Infect Dis Clin North Am* 2019;33:17–38.

Dog and cat bites
1 Hurt JB, Maday KR. Management and treatment of animal bites. *J Am Acad Physician Assist* 2018;31:27–31.

Human bites
1 Bula-Rudas FJ, Olcott JL. Human and animal bites. *Pediatr Rev* 2018;39:490–500.

PART 12
Neoplastic, Proliferative and Infiltrative Disorders Affecting the Skin

CHAPTER 131

Benign Melanocytic Proliferations and Melanocytic Naevi

Irene Stefanaki, Dimitris Sgouros and Alexander Stratigos

1st Department of Dermatology and Venereology, School of Medicine, National and Kapodistrian University of Athens, Andreas Sygros Hospital, Athens, Greece

---

Freckle or ephelis, 131.1

LENTIGINES, 131.3
Definition, 131.3
Introduction and general description, 131.3
Simple lentigo, 131.3
Solar or actinic lentigo, 131.5
Photochemotherapy (PUVA) lentigo, 131.7
Ink-spot lentigo, 131.8

MUCOSAL MELANOTIC LESIONS, 131.9
Pigmented melanotic macules, 131.9
Labial melanotic macules, 131.11

DERMAL MELANOCYTIC LESIONS, 131.12
Introduction and general description, 131.12
Mongolian spot, 131.12

Naevus of Ota, 131.12
Naevus of Ito, 131.14

CONGENITAL MELANOCYTIC NAEVI, 131.15
Speckled lentiginous naevus, 131.15

COMMON ACQUIRED NAEVI, 131.17
Acquired melanocytic naevi, 131.17

NAEVI IN UNUSUAL SITES, 131.21
Definition, 131.21
Introduction and general description, 131.22
Melanocytic naevi of the genital area, 131.22
Melanocytic naevi of the breast, 131.22
Melanocytic naevi of the scalp, 131.22
Acral naevi, 131.23
Conjunctival naevi, 131.24

Naevi of the nail matrix or nail bed, 131.24

NAEVI WITH UNUSUAL MORPHOLOGY, 131.24
Introduction and general description, 131.24
Combined melanocytic naevi, 131.24
Recurrent melanocytic naevi, 131.26
Halo naevus, 131.27
Meyerson naevus, 131.28
Cockade naevus, 131.30
Targetoid haemosiderotic naevus, 131.30

OTHER NAEVI, 131.32
Spitz naevus, 131.32
Blue naevus and variants, 131.38
Clinically atypical naevi, 131.40

Key references, 131.46

Freckle or ephelis

Definition
A freckle is a small reddish or pale to dark brown macule with a poorly defined border, on sun-exposed areas of the skin (Table 131.1). Freckles appear or darken during periods of UV exposure.

Epidemiology
Age
Freckles are common during childhood and often diminish with age.

Ethnicity
Freckles appear in all races but are more frequently seen in individuals with light skin complexion, red hair and blue eyes.

Pathophysiology
Exposure to UV radiation leads to overproduction of melanin by melanocytes, which is subsequently transferred through melanosomes to neighbouring keratinocytes. Freckles could be considered a hyperplastic and hyperactive response of melanocytes to UV radiation in predisposed individuals [1].

Table 131.1 Basic terminology and definitions used in benign melanocytic neoplasms.

Term	Description
Freckle (ephelis)	A pigmented macule on sun-exposed areas consisting of increased melanin pigmentation
Lentigo	A poorly demarcated area of uniform pigmentation consisting of increased melanin pigmentation, epidermal proliferation and replacement of basal cell keratinocytes by melanocytes
Café-au-lait macule	A well-circumscribed, uniformly light to dark brown macule or patch that spares mucous membranes and consists of increased melanin content in the basal cell layer
Nests of melanocytes	A group of melanocytes in contact with the basal layer of the epidermis but projecting downwards into the dermis
Junctional naevus	A pigmented melanocytic naevus in which the main histological feature is the presence of nests of melanocytes at the dermal–epidermal junction
Compound naevus	A pigmented melanocytic naevus in which the histological features include both junctional nests and the presence of naevus cells in the dermis
Intradermal/dermal naevus	A melanocytic lesion with naevus cells in the dermis. Melanin pigmentation is often absent and there is little or no abnormality of melanocytes in the epidermis. The deepest dermal cells tend to neural or fibroblastic differentiation

---

Rook's Textbook of Dermatology, Tenth Edition. Edited by Christopher Griffiths, Jonathan Barker, Tanya Bleiker, Walayat Hussain and Rosalind Simpson.
© 2024 John Wiley & Sons Ltd. Published 2024 by John Wiley & Sons Ltd.

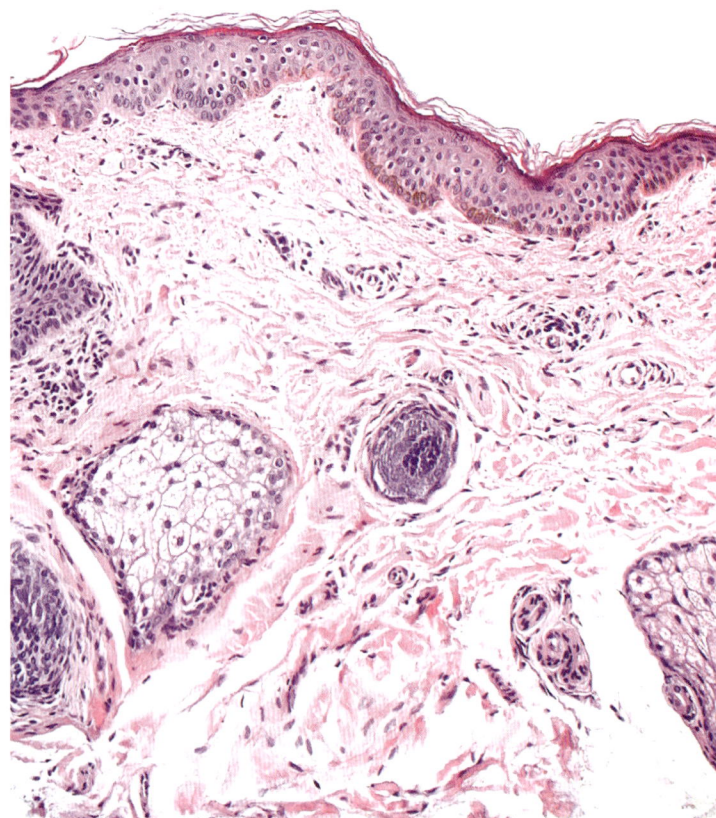

Figure 131.1 Epidermis of a freckle showing a hyperpigmented basal cell layer without elongated rete ridges or melanocytic hyperplasia. Magnification 20× (H&E). Courtesy of Dr K. Frangia, HBD HistoBio Diagnosis, Athens, Greece.

Pathology

The basal cell layer appears hyperpigmented, without alteration of the epidermal architecture (Figure 131.1). In contrast to lentigines, the number of melanocytes is normal.

Genetics

The melanocortin 1 receptor gene (*MCR1*) has been characterised as the major freckle gene [2]. Variants of *MC1R* have been associated with freckling, possibly through the induction of phaeomelaninogenesis (compared with eumelaninogenesis), although other mechanisms may exist. Other pigmentation genes (*TYR, IRF4, ASIP, BNC2*) have also been implicated [3,**4**].

Environmental factors

UV exposure is responsible for the exacerbated pigment production by melanocytes that results in the development of freckles.

Clinical features
Presentation

Freckles typically appear after excessive sun exposure (either chronic or intermittent) in light-skinned red- or fair-haired individuals. They present as areas of macular hyperpigmentation with a round or oval shape and ill-defined borders (Figure 131.2). In winter months freckles tend to lighten or even disappear.

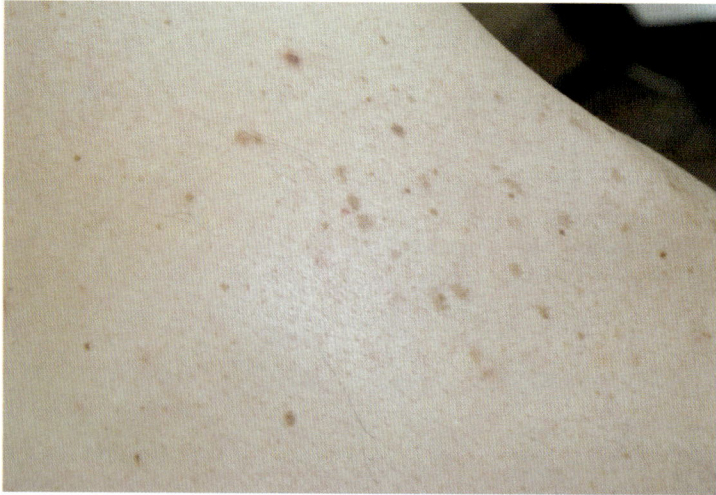

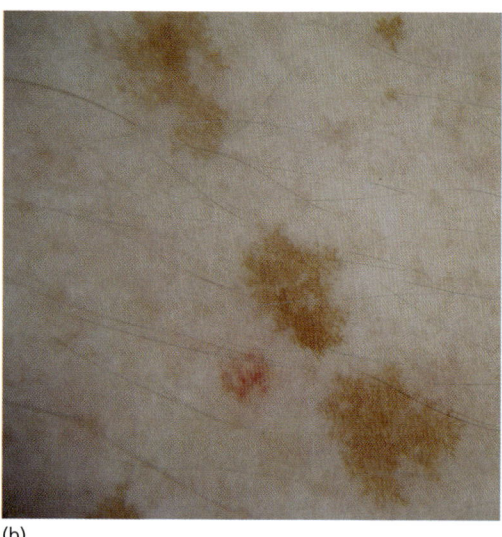

Figure 131.2 (a) Freckles. (b) Dermoscopic image showing hyperpigmented lesions with reticular pattern and moth-eaten edges.

Differential diagnosis

Freckles and solar lentigines are often grouped together in most studies, even though they are different. They are generally viewed as a response to sun exposure – solar lentigines to a greater extent – and both confer an increased risk for melanoma and epithelial skin cancers. They are distinguished from each other by the fact that lentigines persist even without UV exposure, they are usually larger, and tend to appear more frequently in older ages. In addition, lentigines are histologically characterised by an increased number of melanocytes at the dermal–epidermal junction. Freckling can occur in neurofibromatosis type 1 in which it is more commonly located in non-exposed areas (trunk and axilla), while other manifestations of neurofibromatosis are present.

Complications and co-morbidities

Freckles are considered risk factors for melanoma. The estimated relative risk of melanoma based on the presence of freckling in a

Table 131.2 Familial lentiginosis syndromes.

Disorder	Clinical manifestations	Inheritance	Related gene (chromosomal locus)
Peutz–Jeghers syndrome	Lentigines (lips, oral and bowel mucosa, palms, soles, eyes, nares, perianal region), hamartomatous GI polyps, neoplasms (GI tract, pancreas, breast, ovary, uterus, testis)	Autosomal dominant	LKB1/STK11 (19p13.3)
PTEN hamartomatous syndromes	Macrocephaly, lipomatosis, pigmentation of the glans penis, mental retardation, multiple hamartomas, neoplasms (breast cancer, follicular thyroid cancer, endometrial carcinoma)	Autosomal dominant	PTEN (10q23.31)
Carney complex	Lentigines (lips, conjunctiva, inner or outer canthi, genital mucosa), primary pigmented nodular adrenal cortical disease (PPNAD), cardiac and skin myxomas, schwannomas, acromegaly, breast and testicular tumours	Autosomal dominant	PRKAR1A (17q22–24)
Lentiginoses	Lentigines (centrofacial palmoplantar, trunk)	Autosomal dominant	Unknown
	Lentigines (centrofacial palmoplantar, trunk) plus mental retardation	Autosomal dominant/sporadic	Unknown
LEOPARD syndrome	Lentigines (mainly on face and upper trunk; rarely on oral mucosa, extremities, genitalia, conjunctiva), cardiac conduction abnormalities, aneurysms, pulmonic stenosis, cephalofacial dysmorphism, short stature, sensorineural deafness, mental retardation, skeletal abnormalities	Autosomal dominant Autosomal dominant	PTPN11 (12q24.1) – same as in Noonan syndrome RAF1 (3p25)

Adapted from Guerrero [6].
GI, gastrointestinal; LEOPARD, lentigines, electrocardiogram anomalies, ocular anomalies, pulmonary stenosis, abnormal genitalia, retardation of growth and deafness; PTEN, phosphate and tensin homologue.

meta-analysis was 1.99, with a population-attributable fraction of 0.23 [5].

Disease course and prognosis
Freckles are benign lesions and often fade with age.

Investigations
In dermoscopy freckles present with a uniform pigmentation and a moth-eaten edge (Figure 131.2b).

Management
No treatment is required. Chemical peels, lasers, topical depigmenting (more accurately termed 'pigment correcting') drugs and dermocosmetic products can be used for aesthetic reasons [6,7]. Since they are induced by UV exposure, photoprotection measures are indicated.

LENTIGINES

Definition

Lentigines are hyperpigmented macules that do not fade away in the absence of UV exposure. On microscopy they show increased melanin on the basal cell layer and increased numbers of singly arranged melanocytes, compared with the adjacent non-involved skin.

Introduction and general description

Lentigines are usually seen in light-skinned people and represent proliferative responses of melanocytes to natural or artificial UV radiation. The different subtypes discussed below are mainly artificial distinctions based on the history of UV radiation exposure, anatomical location and the specific morphological characteristics of the lesion. The subtypes include simple lentigo, actinic (or solar) lentigo, psoralen and UVA (PUVA) lentigo and ink-spot lentigo.

Rarely, lentigines arise in the setting of potentially serious hereditary multisystem syndromes related to malignancies. These familial lentiginosis syndromes are characterised by autosomal dominant inheritance and include the Peutz–Jeghers syndrome, the PTEN (phosphate and tensin homologue) hamartomatous syndromes (Ruvalcaba–Myhre–Smith or Bannayan–Zonnana syndromes and Cowden disease), the Carney complex (and the closely related NAME (naevi, atrial myxoma, myxoid neurofibroma and ephelides) and LAMB (lentigines, atrial myxomas, mucocutaneous myxomas and blue naevi) syndromes and the LEOPARD/Noonan syndrome (lentigines, electrocardiogram anomalies, ocular anomalies, pulmonary stenosis, abnormal genitalia, retardation of growth and deafness) (Table 131.2) (Chapter 68). Most of these syndromes are caused by mutations in the rat sarcoma–mitogen-actived protein (RAS-MAP) kinase and the mammalian target of rapamycin (mTOR) signalling pathway [8].

Lentiginosis profusa is a rare condition, with innumerable lentigines present at birth or arising early in life, without systemic abnormalities or mucosal involvement. The disorder has an autosomal dominant inheritance, but its exact genetic background is unknown. *Agminated or segmental lentiginosis* manifests as a circumscribed group of lentigines arranged in a segmental pattern that develop during childhood. They are presumed to represent mosaicism of an unidentified gene [9] and should be differentiated from neurofibromatosis type 1. Melanoma may occur in patients with segmental or generalised lentiginosis.

Simple lentigo

Definition and nomenclature
This is a light- to dark-brown or black macule that does not fade away once it appears, and is characterised histologically by increased melanocytes at the dermal–epidermal junction.

Synonyms and inclusions
- Lentigo simplex

Epidemiology

Incidence and prevalence
Simple lentigos are very common, particularly in those with red hair and fair skin.

Age
They usually appear during childhood and increase in number until the age of 40. The majority of lentigines remain unchanged in adult life.

Associated diseases
Generalised lentiginosis has been rarely associated with the development of melanoma. There has been a single case report of a patient with lentiginoses and gastrointestinal stromal tumours harbouring a *c-kit* gene mutation [9].

Pathophysiology

Predisposing factors
There have been reports of lentigines developing after topical immunotherapy with tacrolimus, squaric acid dibutylester and diphencyprone [10,11].

Pathology
There is a slight increase in the number of melanocytes along the dermal–epidermal junction, without nesting. Melanin hyperpigmentation is noted in melanocytes, adjacent keratinocytes and melanophages in the papillary dermis (Figure 131.3). The epidermal rete ridges are usually elongated and there might be a mild inflammatory infiltrate in the upper dermis.

Genetics
Multiple lentigines arising early in life on both exposed and non-exposed areas are usually a manifestation of inherited syndromes

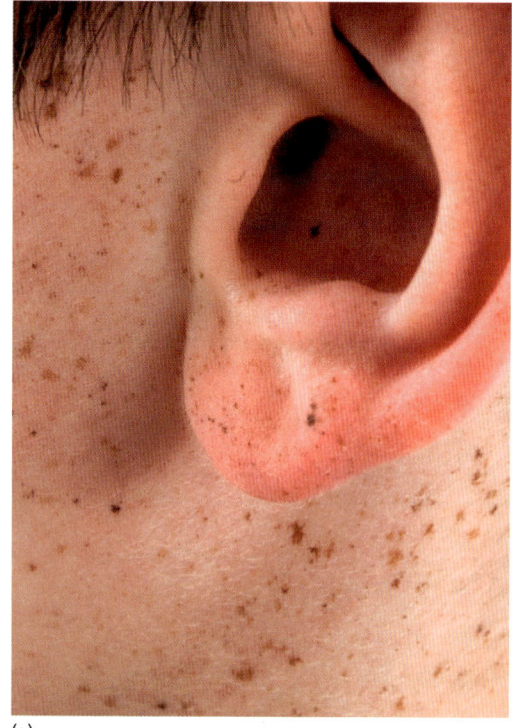

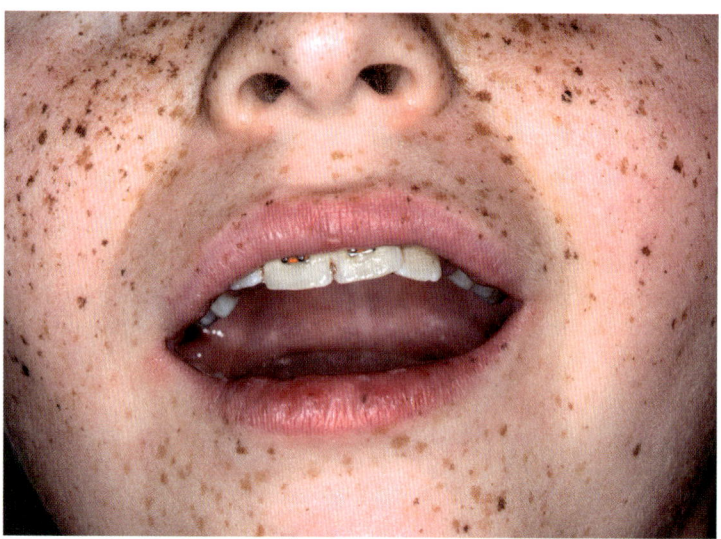

Figure 131.4 (a, b) Multiple lentigines in a patient with the Carney complex and a PRKAR1A mutation. Only about a third of patients with the complex have this classic pigmentation. Courtesy of Dr Constantine A. Stratakis, National Institutes of Health, Bethesda, MD, USA.

characterised by hyperplasias, hamartomas and neoplasia (Figure 131.4). Most of these syndromes are caused by mutations in the RAS-MAP kinase and the mTOR pathways.

Simple lentigos, solar lentigines and melanocytic naevi have been compared for mutations in the *BRAF* (common in melanocytic naevi), *FGFR3* and *PIK3CA* genes (common in solar lentigines and seborrhoeic keratoses). Simple lentigos did not show mutations in any of these genes and thus are genetically differentiated from melanocytic naevi and solar lentigines [12]. The *BRAF* mutations in

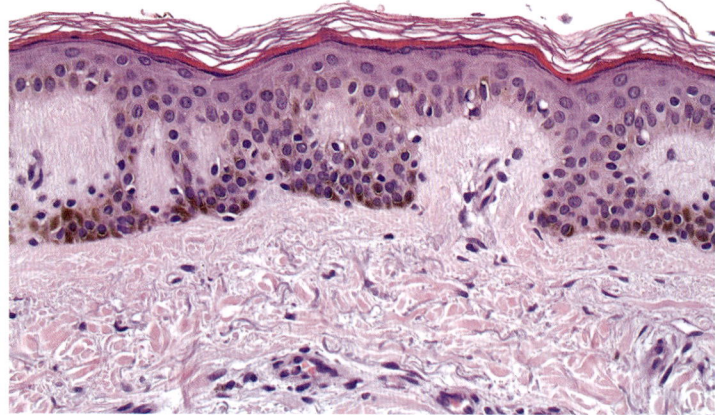

Figure 131.3 Lentigo simplex: hyperpigmentation is evident in the basal and squamous epidermal cells. There is a slight increase of non-atypical melanocytes between the epidermal basal cells. Magnification 40× (H&E). Courtesy of Dr K. Frangia, HBD HistoBio Diagnosis, Athens, Greece.

simple lentigos contradict the proposed lentigo–naevus sequence of evolution, but do not exclude it.

Environmental factors
Sunlight is the most important environmental factor.

Clinical features
Presentation
Lentigines are poorly circumscribed, uniformly pigmented macules, with a round or oval shape and a diameter of up to 5 mm (Figure 131.5). There may be slight scaling of the surface and several neighbouring lesions may coalesce. Their colour is pale to deep brown, depending on the skin colour of the individual. They are primarily located on photo-exposed areas as they are part of the spectrum of lesions (ephelides, simple lentigos, solar lentigos) resulting from excessive UV exposure.

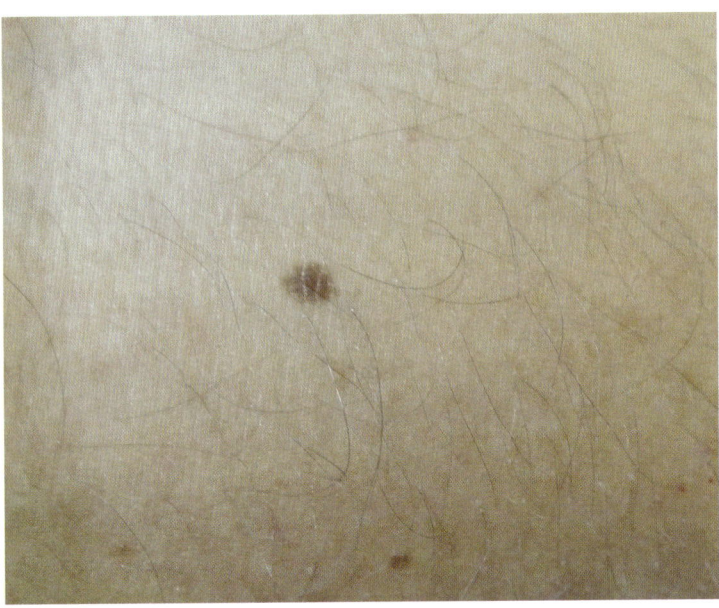
(a)

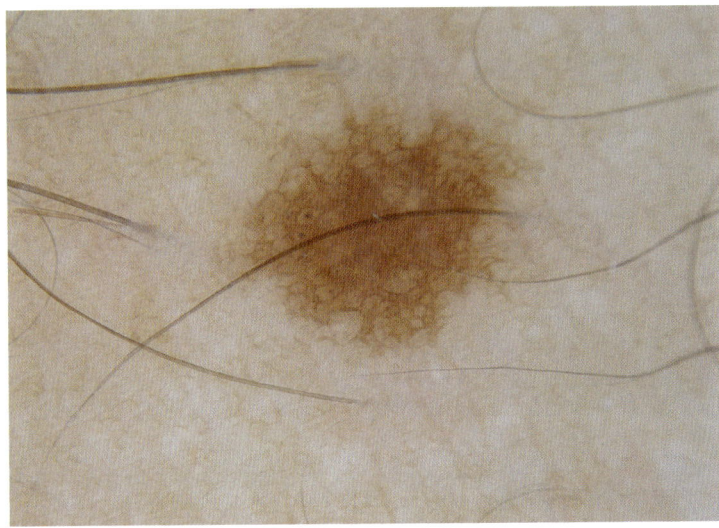
(b)

Figure 131.5 (a) Simple lentigo. (b) Dermoscopic image of simple lentigo.

Differential diagnosis
The differential diagnosis of lentigines from freckles is made clinically by their comparatively darker colour, more scattered distribution and by their unchanged status in relation to sunlight exposure. In contrast to freckles, lentigines present histologically with an increased number of melanocytes.

The differentiation of lentigines from small junctional naevi is often impossible on clinical grounds. On histology, naevi show nests of naevus cells, while, in lentigines, melanocytes are separated from one another and do not typically form nests. However, there are cases of larger lesions that clinically appear as lentigines but have small nests of naevus cells along the dermal–epidermal junction. This pattern is often referred to as the 'jentigo' pattern, meaning that the corresponding lesion combines features of both lentigo and junctional naevus. These transitional lesions may be regarded as precursors of future melanocytic naevi [1].

Lentigines may sometimes overlap clinically, or even histologically, with flat seborrhoeic keratoses (termed 'liver spots' when located at the dorsal hands). This overlap is clinically insignificant, as both are markers of light skin complexion, excessive sun exposure and a certain risk of skin cancer (Chapter 142).

Distinction from lentigo maligna is made by dermoscopy or pathology.

Disease course and prognosis
These are benign, relatively static lesions.

Investigations
With dermoscopy, lentigines show scalloped borders, a faint irregular network or pseudo-network and structureless areas (Figure 131.5b).

Management
There is no need for treatment. As the majority arise in sun-exposed areas, photoprotection could decrease the rate of new lesions developing. For cosmetic reasons, a variety of depigmenting topical agents and dermatological procedures such as chemical peels, lasers and photodynamic therapy reduces their pigmentation (Chapters 160 and 161) [13]. In patients with multiple lentigines arising early in life on non-sun-exposed sites, the possibility of a hereditary multisystem syndrome (Table 131.2) should be considered. In the very rare cases of generalised lentiginoses, individuals may be at increased risk for melanoma, and thus should be educated on avoidance of sunburn and self skin examination.

Solar or actinic lentigo

Definition and nomenclature
A solar lentigo is a brown macule appearing after excessive sun exposure.

Synonyms and inclusions
- Senile freckle
- Lentigo senilis
- Old age spot

Epidemiology
Age
The number of solar lentigines increases with ageing.

Pathophysiology
The pathogenetic mechanism leading to the development of solar lentigines remains unclear. UVB stimulates keratinocytes to produce interleukin 1α (IL-1α), leading to secretion of keratinocyte growth factor (KGF). KGF has been found to increase pigment production in both pigmented epidermal equivalents and human skin grafts, suggesting a possible involvement of KGF in the molecular pathogenesis of solar lentigo [14]. Another scenario favours the role of fibroblasts, which – after UV exposure – release melanogenic growth factors (hepatocyte growth factor, KGF and stem cell factor) that subsequently act through keratinocytes and contribute to the hyperpigmentation of solar lentigines [15].

Predisposing factors
A history of occupational radon exposure, as well as recreational sun exposure, has been implicated in the development of multiple lentigines in a single case report [16].

Pathology
The histological features of solar lentigo are the same as for simple lentigo. Solar elastosis of the dermis and photoactivation features of melanocytes are usually present.

Genetics
Mutations in *FGFR3* and *PIK3CA*, as well as in *IRF4*, *MC1R*, *RALY/ASIP* and *BNC2*, have been observed in both solar lentigo and seborrhoeic keratosis, suggesting a common genetic basis [12,17].

Environmental factors
Solar lentigines are associated with both intermittent and chronic sun exposure [3]. Solar lentigines on the back have also been associated with a history of sunburns before the age of 20 years, while facial solar lentigines have been associated with cutaneous signs of photodamage [3].

Clinical features
Presentation
In younger patients, solar lentigines are most commonly seen on sun-exposed sites, such as the face in both sexes and the shoulders in males. They are macular, tan coloured and may be very large, with a striking irregular border. There is frequently a history of acute sunburn, followed by the sudden appearance of large numbers of these irregular macular lesions [18,19]. In the UK, they are rare before the age of 12 years but in sunnier countries they may appear at a very young age.

Solar lentigines are also seen on older patients who have had excessive sun exposure (Figure 131.6) [19]. The backs of the hands and the face are common sites. Once again the lesions are large and macular, have an irregular edge and are usually a uniform shade of brown. They are situated in an area of clinically evident sun-damaged epidermis and often manifest a clinical and pathological overlap with flat seborrhoeic keratoses.

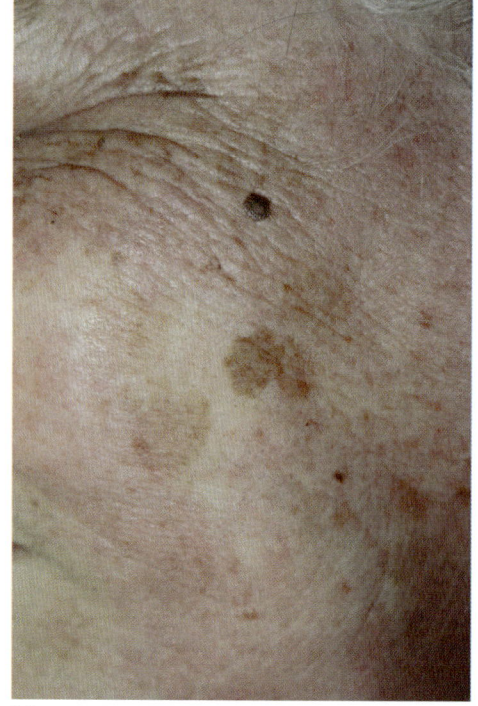
(a)

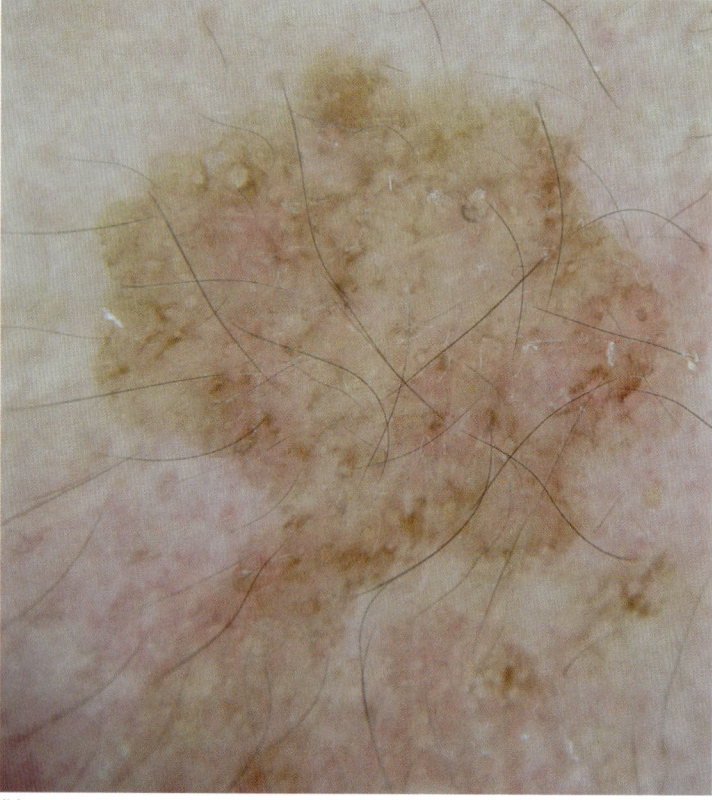
(b)

Figure 131.6 (a) Solar lentigo in the middle of the left cheek. (b) Dermoscopic image of solar lentigo showing a uniform structureless macule with sharply demarcated borders.

Differential diagnosis
Differential diagnosis includes simple lentigo, seborrhoeic keratosis and, in some cases, lentigo maligna and melanoma *in situ*.

Disease course and prognosis
It has been proposed that solar lentigo may sometimes evolve into seborrhoeic keratosis.

Investigations
Dermoscopy is the same as in simple lentigo, while adjacent skin may show features of photodamage. Solar lentigo should be differentiated from seborrhoeic keratosis exhibiting milia-like cysts, cerebriform patterns and sharply demarcated borders. Pigmented actinic keratoses show a prominent pigmented pseudo-network and a background red with a red pseudo-network ('strawberry pattern'). Lentigo maligna presents with specific dermoscopic features, such as asymmetrical follicular openings, 'annular–granular' pattern, pigmented rhomboidal structures and obliterated hair follicles that are absent in solar lentigines.

In some cases, the distinction between solar lentigo and lentigo maligna or melanoma *in situ* is very difficult when classic pathology is used. In such instances, immunohistochemistry is a valuable diagnostic tool. Several stains have been used, and microphthalmia-associated transcription factor (MiTF) seems to be superior in the differential diagnosis of solar lentigo from melanoma *in situ* [20,21].

Management
Patients often request treatment for these pigmented lesions located in visible body areas such as the face and back of hands.

Rigorous photoprotection with sun avoidance, use of a broad spectrum and high sun-protection-factor sunscreen, and appropriate clothing lowers the possibility of further lesions emerging in the future, and may also result in some degree of spontaneous resolution. General consensus supports the use of cryotherapy as first line therapy, with topical therapy (e.g. topical retinoids) as an alternative or used for maintenance. There is, however, an extensive literature on the cosmetic treatment of lentigines using a variety of other treatments such as intense pulsed light and pigment-specific (Q-switched) laser systems (Chapter 161).

Solar lentigines are benign lesions, but any pigmented lesion needs careful evaluation prior to treatment. There have been reports of cases that were referred for laser therapy or had already received treatment as solar lentigines, and were actually melanomas [22,23]. Furthermore, non-invasive confocal imaging has revealed remaining melanocytes at the site of solar lentigines of all subjects after Q-switched ruby laser treatment, even though there was hardly any observable skin pigmentation on clinical examination [24].

Photochemotherapy (PUVA) lentigo

Definition
Lentigines can arise after long-term use of PUVA therapy.

Epidemiology
Incidence and prevalence
PUVA lentigines usually occur in patients who have received a high cumulative dose of PUVA treatment. They have been reported in 20% of 198 patients with a mean cumulative dose of UVA of 169.5 J/cm^2 [25]. PUVA lentigines of any degree (slight, moderate or extensive) were also noted on the buttocks of 53% of 1380 psoriatic patients an average of 5.7 years after initiating PUVA therapy [26].

Pathophysiology
Predisposing factors
Fair-skinned individuals and patients who have received a greater number of PUVA treatments are at greater risk [27]. Lentigines appearing after narrow-band ultraviolet B (NB-UVB) radiation have also been reported [28].

Pathology
There are features resembling those of ephelides or lentigines. Melanocytes are increased in number and may have nuclear atypia. Ultrastructural studies have shown melanocytes with longer and more numerous dendrites as well as more active melanogenesis in PUVA lentigines, compared with solar lentigines and unexposed normal skin [29].

Clinical features
Presentation
PUVA lentigines are relatively large, pigmented macules that develop on the skin of patients receiving photochemotherapy (Figure 131.7).

Differential diagnosis
As in solar lentigo. There are also some reports that voriconazole-associated lentigines resemble PUVA lentigines.

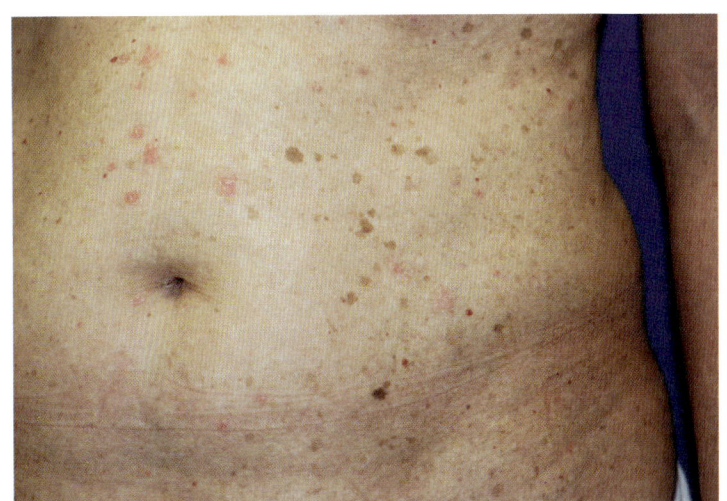

Figure 131.7 PUVA-induced lentigines in a patient with psoriasis.

Complications and co-morbidities
Follow-up of patients who had received PUVA in the USA revealed that PUVA lentigines are a marker of patients at increased risk of non-melanoma skin cancer [30]. An association with melanoma has not been firmly established. An increased risk was observed in a US study [26], but was not confirmed in a study from Scandinavia [31].

Disease course and prognosis
Some of the lesions persist for several months after completion of PUVA therapy.

Investigations
Dermoscopy helps to establish the diagnosis, revealing similar findings to solar lentigines.

Management
PUVA lentigines do not require treatment. Since they are considered potential markers for the development of non-melanoma skin cancer, patients with PUVA lentigines may benefit from regular follow-up.

Ink-spot lentigo

Definition and nomenclature
An ink-spot lentigo is a small, densely black macule resembling an ink spot displaying a markedly irregular outline, with a distribution similar to solar lentigo.

Synonyms and inclusions
- Reticulated black solar lentigo

Pathophysiology
Pathology
There is lentiginous hyperplasia of the epidermis and prominent hyperpigmentation of the basal cells, with 'skip' areas involving the rete ridges (Figure 131.8). A minimal increase in the number of melanocytes is reported [32].

Clinical features
Presentation
Ink-spot lentigines are sharply demarcated macules with a jet-black colour and irregular shape (Figure 131.9) [32]. They usually arise on exposed areas, such as the upper back, and although the same patient may have multiple solar lentigines, ink-spot lentigines are commonly solitary lesions.

Differential diagnosis
Due to their black colour, the differential diagnosis mainly includes lentigo maligna and melanoma *in situ*.

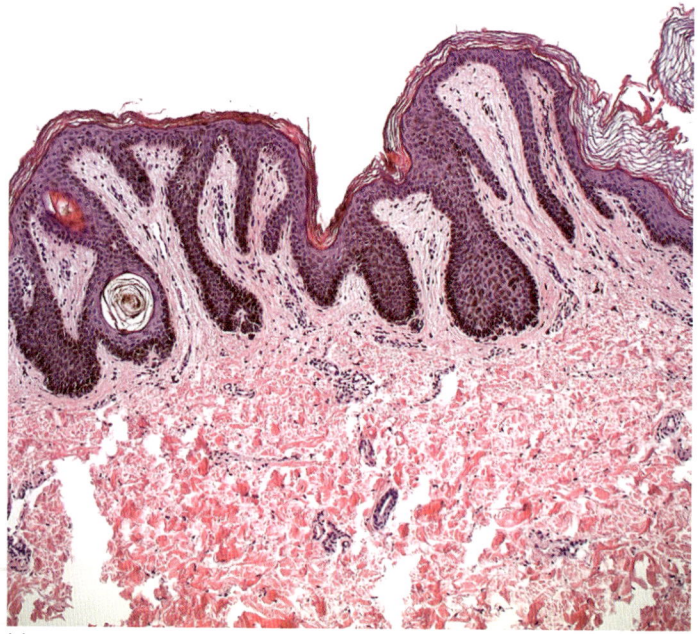

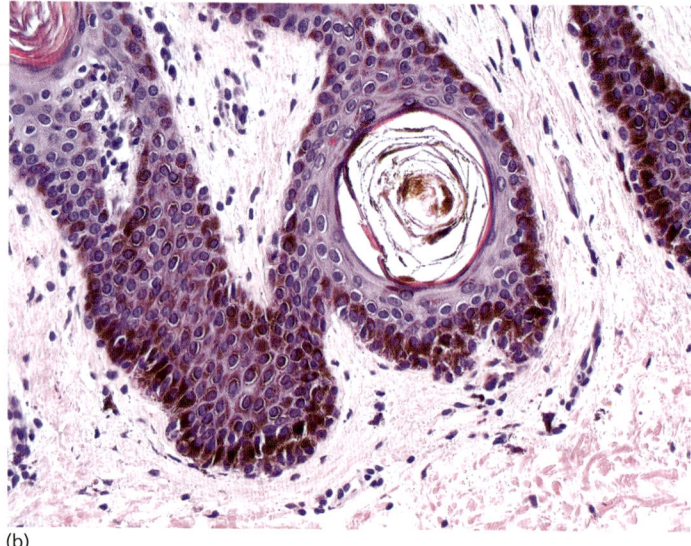

Figure 131.8 Ink-spot lentigo. (a) Epidermis with lentiginous hyperplasia and intensely hyperpigmented basal cells. Foci of less or no pigmentation are usually observed over the dermal papillae. Magnification 10× (H&E). (b) Hyperpigmentation is prominent to the lateral borders and the tips of the rete. There is a slight increase of melanocytes between the epidermal basal cells, and melanophages in the papillary dermis can be seen. Magnification 40× (H&E). Courtesy of Dr K. Frangia, HBD HistoBio Diagnosis, Athens, Greece.

Investigations
Dermoscopic features include a prominent black network with thin and/or thick lines.

Management
No treatment is required.

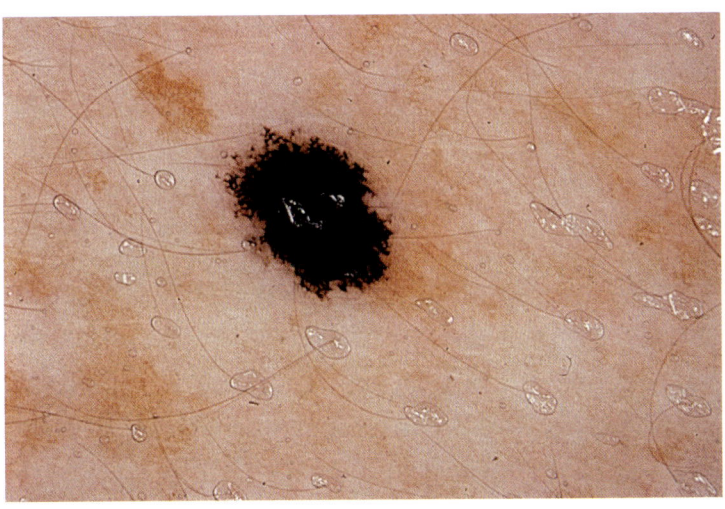

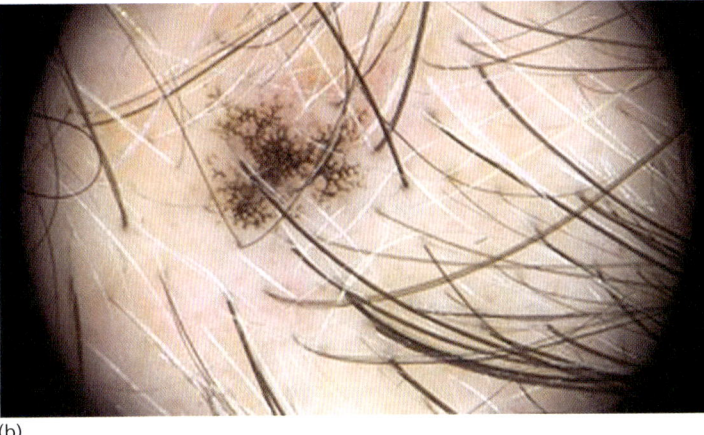

Figure 131.9 (a) Ink-spot lentigo. Courtesy of Dr S. Puig, Hospital Clinic Barcelona, IDIBAPS, Barcelona, Spain. (b) Dermoscopic image of an ink-spot lentigo showing a bizarre-looking black pigment network.

MUCOSAL MELANOTIC LESIONS

Pigmented melanotic macules

Definition and nomenclature
Mucosal melanotic macules (or lentigines) are benign pigmented patches of the mucosa. Although they occasionally have an alarming clinical appearance, histologically they are characterised by hyperpigmentation of basal keratinocytes and a normal or slightly increased number of melanocytes without atypical features or confluent proliferation.

Synonyms and inclusions
- Mucosal melanosis/genital lentiginosis (these terms have been used interchangeably)

Introduction and general description
Some degree of macular pigmentation of the mucosa in the mouth or on the genitalia is normal. More discrete, deeply pigmented macules are also common on the vulva and sometimes on the glans penis, where they are usually referred to as genital melanotic macules or mucosal melanosis. These macules result from local excessive pigment production with normal numbers of melanocytes [33]. Rarely, these melanotic macules may expand to several centimetres in size and be patchy in distribution. They may develop irregular deep pigmentation, which resembles melanoma and causes concern. Since melanoma in the genital area may begin with a protracted *in situ* phase that clinically resembles a mucosal melanotic macule, a biopsy is often performed to exclude this possibility.

Epidemiology
Incidence and prevalence
The exact incidence is not known. However, they are the most common solitary pigmented melanocytic lesions found in the oral mucosa (representing 86% of solitary melanocytic lesions of the mouth) [34] or the genitalia.

Age
These macules involve a wide variety of ages, from childhood to old age. Congenital cases have rarely been reported.

Sex
There is a 2:1 female predilection.

Ethnicity
Pigmented melanotic macules occur in all races, but are more common in individuals with darker skin complexion. Macules of the buccal mucosa may be more frequent in black people [35].

Associated diseases
Pigmented macules in the female genitalia have been occasionally associated with lichen sclerosus [36]. Histological examination of these lesions reveals features of atypical melanocytic naevi.

Pathophysiology
Predisposing factors
In oral lesions, pigmentation is more pronounced at sites of trauma. Smoking may also result in melanosis. Post-inflammatory pigmentation can be observed, for example following oral lichen planus. Familial lentiginosis manifests as multiple lentigines in a familial context. Some patients with HIV present with oral macules, but it is unclear if these are induced by the virus or by the treatment [37]. The pathogenesis of genital macules remains unclear.

Pathology
A mild acanthosis of the epidermis, hyperpigmentation of basal layer keratinocytes and a slight increase in the number of melanocytes without nesting is observed (Figures 131.10 and 131.11). Scattered melanophages are seen in the upper dermis as a result of melanin incontinence.

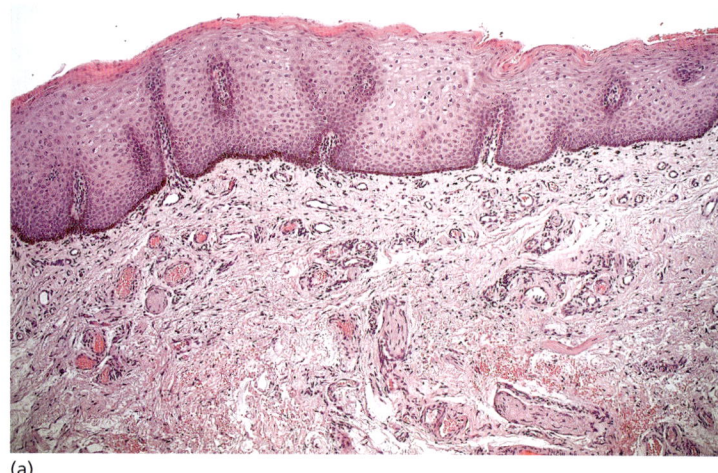

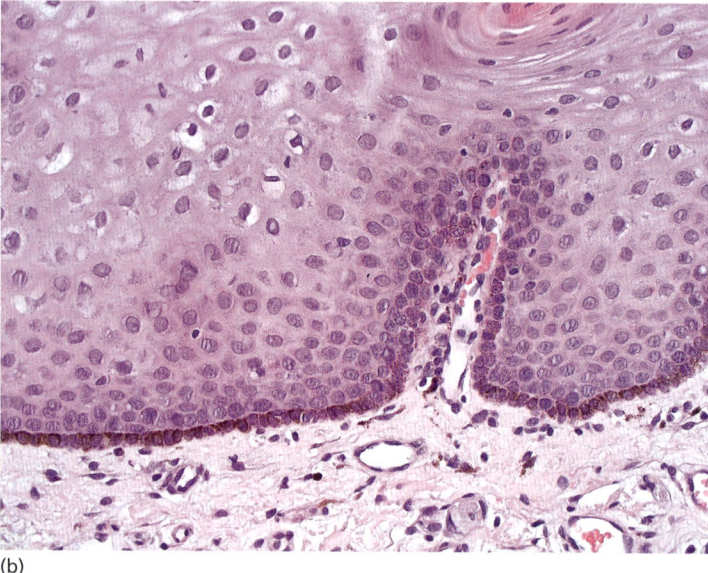

Figure 131.10 Mucosal melanosis. (a) Squamous epithelium of the oral cavity with hyperpigmentation of the basal cells. Magnification 10× (H&E). (b) Hyperpigmentation of the basal layer without melanocytic hyperplasia. Magnification 40× (H&E). Courtesy of Dr K. Frangia, HBD HistoBio Diagnosis, Athens, Greece.

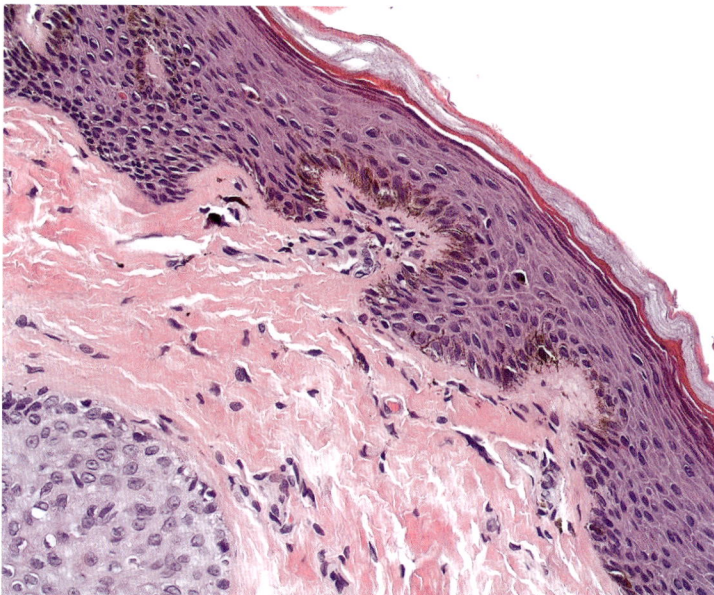

Figure 131.11 Penile lentiginosis: prominent melanocytic dendrites among the hyperpigmented basal layer cells. Magnification 40× (H&E). Courtesy of Dr K. Frangia, HBD HistoBio Diagnosis, Athens, Greece.

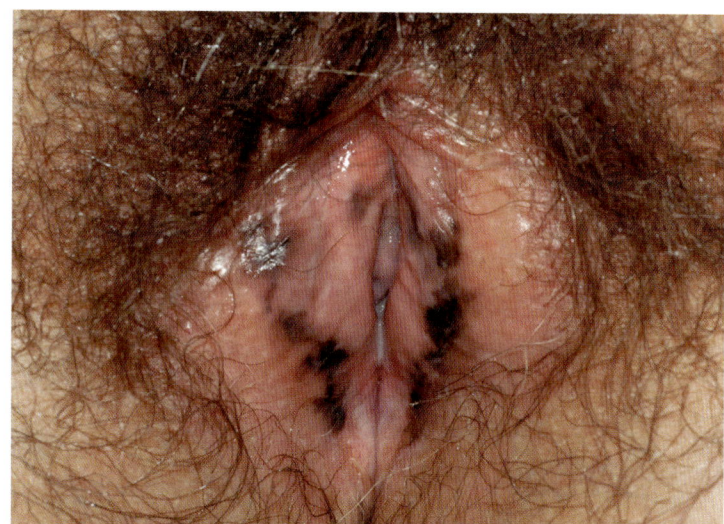

Figure 131.12 Genital melanosis.

Clinical features

Presentation
These are macules of uniform brown, black or grey pigmentation arising in the oral cavity (primarily on the lips and gingiva, followed by the palate and buccal mucosa) or the genitalia (mainly in the vulva, but also the penis or perineum) (Figure 131.12). Their diameter is relatively large, expanding slowly over time. They are usually single lesions, although multiple macules may arise occasionally. When located in the vulva, they are often asymmetrical with irregular borders and blue-black colour, simulating *in situ* melanoma.

Differential diagnosis
Oral melanotic macules should be distinguished from other solitary pigmented melanocytic lesions, including oral melanocytic naevi, blue naevi, oral melanoacanthomas and oral melanomas. Oral melanoma is quite rare, occurring usually on the palate and accounting for fewer than 1% of oral malignancies [38,39]. Exogenous pigmentation (e.g. amalgam tattoo), inflammatory hypermelanosis and smoker's melanosis should also be ruled out. Genital lentiginosis should be differentiated from lentigines, melanocytic naevi, clinically atypical naevi and *in situ* melanomas.

Disease course and prognosis
There are no reports of malignant transformation.

Investigations
Dermoscopic patterns of melanotic macules demonstrate a parallel, reticular, structureless pattern or globular pattern. A ring-like pattern, characterised by multiple white to tan structures with dark brown, well-defined regular borders, has been described in vulvar melanosis [40].

Management

If in clinical doubt, an incisional biopsy of an appropriately representative area is necessary to exclude melanoma. No treatment is needed if histology rules out malignancy. It is reasonable to follow up lesions with atypical clinical appearance in order to detect changes suggestive of melanoma.

If biopsy reveals significant melanocytic proliferation resembling lentigo maligna, then the lesion should be excised in its entirety and the tissue examined histologically. Topical imiquimod 5% followed by a new biopsy at the end of treatment may be considered in cases where surgical excision is technically difficult [41], although patients may suffer severe topical irritation.

Labial melanotic macules

Definition and nomenclature
A labial melanotic macule is a benign, hyperpigmented macule of the lip, quite similar to a freckle or simple lentigo.

Synonyms and inclusions
- Labial lentigo

Epidemiology
Incidence and prevalence
Such macules are encountered in approximately 3% of the general population.

Age
Labial melanotic macules usually appear around the age of 40, although in darker pigmented individuals it can present during adolescence [42].

Sex
They are more frequent in females.

Pathophysiology
Pathology
There is a linear increase in melanin pigment in the basal layer of the epidermis, with normal or slightly increased numbers of melanocytes, located singly between basal keratinocytes.

Environmental factors
Due to its common location in the middle of the lower lip, a UV-induced mechanism has been suggested.

Clinical features
Presentation
Such macules are brown to black and measure less than 6–7 mm (Figure 131.13). The most common location is the lower lip, especially the central third. It is usually a solitary lesion, developing rather rapidly in a young adult [42].

Differential diagnosis
Labial melanotic macules are differentiated from melanoacanthoma of the lip by the histological presence of intraepithelial dendritic

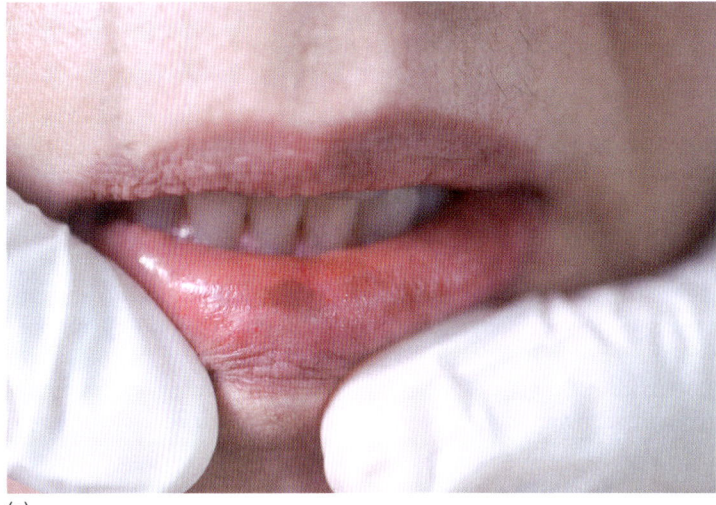

(a)

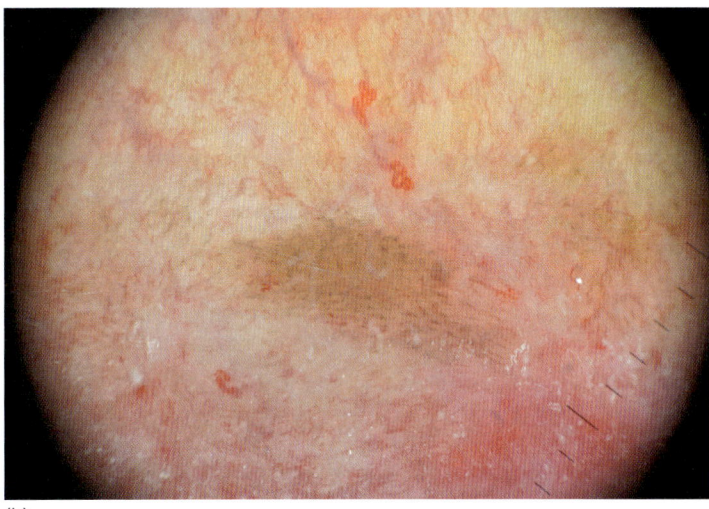

(b)

Figure 131.13 (a) Labial melanotic macule. (b) Dermoscopic image of a labial melanotic macule reveals a combination of grey-brown dots arranged in parallel lines and a background of light brownish homogeneous pigmentation.

melanocytes in the latter. The banal histological features of a labial melanotic macule are easily distinguished from melanoma.

Disease course and prognosis
Malignant transformation has not been reported in these lesions. In a study with a mean follow-up of approximately 6 years, no alarming change, indicative of malignancy, was observed [43].

Investigations
Dermoscopy confirms that this is a benign lesion, revealing a uniform brown colour with parallel lines ('fingerprint' pattern) (Figure 131.13b).

Management
Patients should be reassured about the benign nature of labial melanocytic macules. Removal for cosmetic purposes can be achieved using a variety of methods including cryotherapy, infrared coagulation or laser therapy [44]. In the case of a newly formed

lesion, or of changes in colour or size in a pre-existing lesion, a prompt evaluation of the patient is necessary.

DERMAL MELANOCYTIC LESIONS

Introduction and general description

Normally, during fetal life, melanocytes migrate from the neural crest to the dermal–epidermal junction. However, migrating melanocytes may occasionally remain entrapped in the dermis, not reaching their destination in the epidermis, and giving rise to dermal melanocytic lesions. These lesions have a bluish colour owing to the Tyndall effect.

Mongolian spot

Definition
Mongolian spots are congenital macular areas of blue-grey pigmentation of varying size and shape located on the sacral area in normal infants.

Epidemiology
Incidence and prevalence
Incidence varies among populations according to skin colour.

Age
The lesion develops *in utero*, increases in depth for a period during infancy and then diminishes.

Ethnicity
The Mongolian spot is uncommon in white people. In Europe it is more commonly observed in the Mediterranean region, while the highest incidence worldwide is documented in newborns with descent from the Far East. It has been observed in 13–26% of Turkish infants [45,46] and 11–71% of Iranian newborns [47,48]. Apart from genetic reasons, incidence differences among ethnicities could also be attributed to the amount of pigment produced in dermal melanocytes in darker individuals.

Associated diseases
There have been reports of association with Down syndrome, segmental café au lait macules and congenital haemangioma [49–51]. Extensive Mongolian spots have been associated with phakomatosis pigmentovascularis, congenital metabolic diseases, Hurler syndrome, GM1 gangliosidosis type 1 and mucolipidosis II [52–56], as well as with bilateral naevus of Ota [57].

Pathophysiology
Pathology
Elongated dendritic melanocytes are present around neurovascular bundles, and in a ribbon-like pattern between collagen fibres of the middle and lower dermis distributed in parallel levels to the skin surface. No fibrosis or dermal melanophages are present, distinguishing a Mongolian spot from a blue naevus.

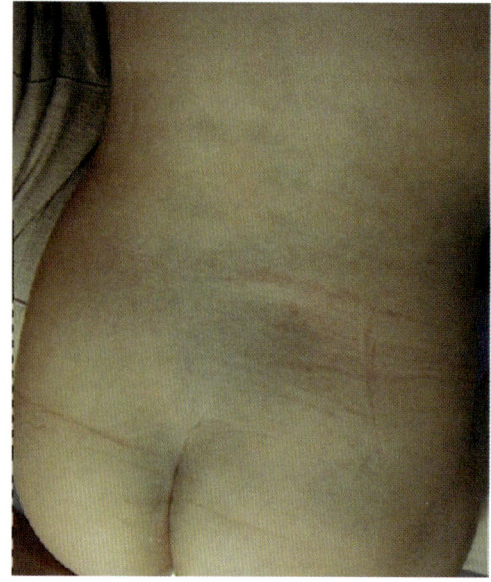

Figure 131.14 Mongolian spot in the lumbosacral area. Courtesy of Professor A. Katsarou-Katsari, Pediatric Dermatology Unit, Andreas Sygros Hospital, Athens, Greece.

Genetics
Extensive dermal melanocytosis and phakomatosis pigmentovascularis have been associated with activating mutations in *GNA11* and *GNAQ* [58].

Clinical features
Presentation
The lesion is a diffuse macule with rather uniform, relatively faint blue to grey colour. It has a round or oval shape, with a diameter of a few – usually up to 10 – centimetres. Normally it presents as a single lesion, but multiple Mongolian spots may occasionally occur (Figure 131.14). The most common location is the lumbosacral region. In the case of generalised lesions, the buttocks, flanks or even shoulders and lower legs may be affected.

Differential diagnosis
Mongolian spots can be clinically differentiated from congenital naevi, which are also macular and present at birth, by their grey-blue colour. Histologically, Mongolian spots resemble blue naevi.

Disease course and prognosis
Mongolian spots typically resolve during childhood, but may occasionally persist into adult life.

Management
No treatment is required. Q-switched lasers, intense pulsed light and bleaching creams have been used in persistent cases [59–61]. Adults usually have a less favourable outcome [59,60].

Naevus of Ota

Definition and nomenclature
A naevus of Ota is an extensive, bluish, patchy, dermal melanocytosis that affects the sclera and the skin adjacent to the eye, distributed

Associated diseases
It is rarely associated with naevus of Ito. Bilateral cases of naevus of Ota are sometimes associated with extensive Mongolian spots. Sturge–Weber and Klippel–Trenaunay syndromes have been infrequently associated with naevus of Ota.

Pathophysiology
Pathology
Elongated dendritic melanocytes are scattered among collagen bundles mainly of the superficial dermis and in larger numbers compared with Mongolian spots (Figure 131.16). Occasionally they may extend deeper in the dermis or subcutaneous tissue. Melanophages are seldom present.

Genetics
GNAQ mutations have been reported in 6% of naevi of Ota, suggesting *GNAQ* is a genetic link between naevus of Ota and uveal melanoma [63].

Clinical features
History
The condition is named after Masao Ota, who in 1939 used the term 'fuscocaeruleus ophthalmomaxillaris'.

Presentation
The lesion is often speckled, and is composed of blue and brown components that do not always coincide. This phenomenon can be better observed in the proximal eye, where the sclera appears blue and the conjunctiva brown. Brown pigmentation is patchy and superficial, following a reticular or geographical pattern; blue pigmentation is more diffuse and deeper.

Naevus of Ota is generally distributed along the ophthalmic and maxillary divisions of the trigeminal nerve. It presents in the periorbital region, involving the bulbar and palpebral conjunctiva and the sclera, as well as the temple, forehead, scalp, nose, ears, palate and malar area. It is usually unilateral, but bilateral lesions also exist.

Clinical variants
There have been several classifications based on clinical or histological features [64–66].

Differential diagnosis
Acquired bilateral naevus of Ota-like macules (Hori naevus) present as bilateral, blue-grey or brown, small, facial macules that are located in the same skin areas as naevus of Ota, but do not show mucous involvement [67]. They appear between the ages of 15 and 40 years in Asian women causing aesthetic problems. Their aetiopathogenesis is not clear [68], but oestrogens and UV radiation have been implicated.

Complications and co-morbidities
Meningeal melanocytomas of the brain, which are benign neoplasms, may complicate naevus of Ota [69]. Glaucoma and ipsilateral deafness have been associated with naevus of Ota [70–73]. The majority of melanomas associated with naevus of Ota occur in the meninges or in the choroid, iris or orbit [74–78]. There have been rare reports of cutaneous melanoma developing in a naevus of Ota.

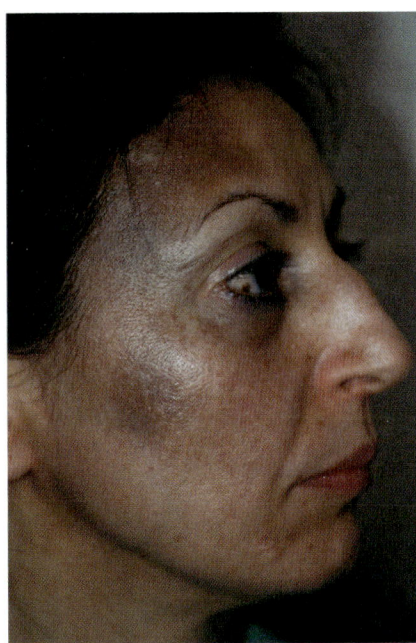

Figure 131.15 Naevus of Ota.

along the first and the second branches of the trigeminal nerve. Extracutaneous lesions may also present in the uveal tract, dura, nasopharynx, tympanum and palate.

Synonyms and inclusions
- Naevus fuscoceruleus ophthalmomaxillaris
- Congenital melanosis bulbi
- Oculodermal melanocytosis
- Oculomucodermal melanocytosis
- Melanosis bulborum
- Aberrant dermal melanocytosis

Epidemiology
Incidence and prevalence
Naevus of Ota usually presents in Asians, with an incidence between 0.014% and 0.034% [62]. It is very rare in other populations.

Age
Most lesions are present at birth or develop during the first year of life, increasing in size and number in subsequent years (Figure 131.15). A second peak of onset has been described in a minority of cases around puberty.

Sex
Lesions are more common in females.

Ethnicity
Naevus of Ota occurs more commonly in darkly pigmented individuals, particularly Asian and black people, although white people may also be affected. It is especially common in the Japanese (0.4–0.8% of dermatological patients).

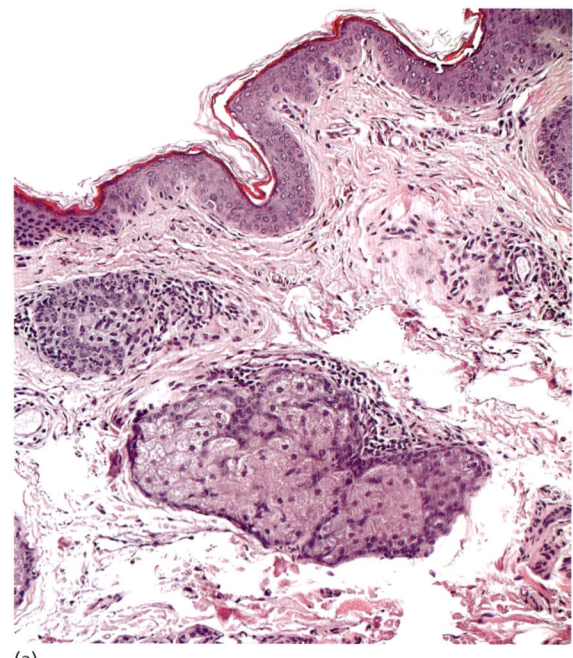

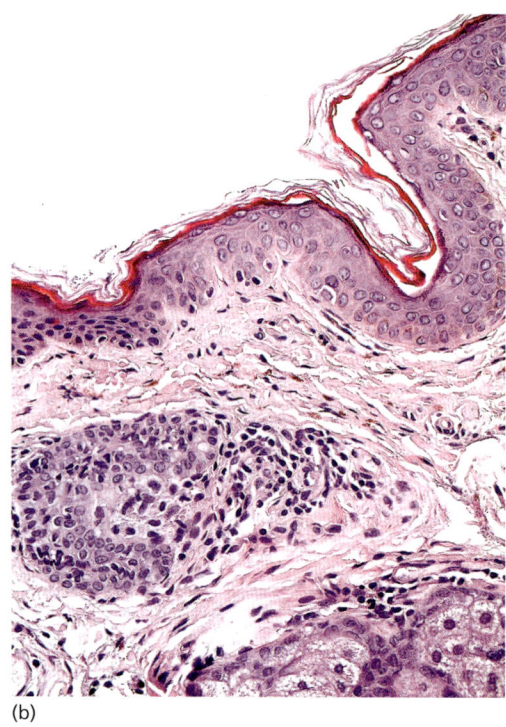

Figure 131.16 Naevus of Ota. (a) Skin with sparse dendritic melanocytes in the upper dermis and no melanocytic hyperplasia in the overlying epidermis. Magnification 20× (H&E). (b) Isolated dendritic melanocytes distributed among collagen bundles of the upper reticular dermis. Magnification 40× (H&E). Courtesy of Dr K. Frangia, HBD HistoBio Diagnosis, Athens, Greece.

Disease course and prognosis
Unlike Mongolian spots, it does not disappear with time.

Management
Q-switched lasers are the first line treatment, achieving a high rate of pigment clearing, depending on the age of the patient, the colour and histological depth of the lesion [79]. Post-treatment hypo- or hyperpigmentation, scarring and recurrence of the lesion can occur [62,80–82]. Cosmetic camouflage can also be used.

Despite the rare occurrence of malignant transformation in naevus of Ota, close ophthalmological monitoring is essential in cases where the eye is involved. Any new subcutaneous nodule arising on a naevus of Ota should be further investigated histologically to exclude the possibility of melanoma.

Naevus of Ito

Definition and nomenclature
Naevus of Ito is a dermal melanocytosis involving the acromioclavicular region and the upper chest.

Synonyms and inclusions
- Naevus fusocoeruleus acromiodeltoideus

Epidemiology
Incidence and prevalence
Naevus of Ito is a rare disorder, presenting more commonly in Asians. It is less frequent than naevus of Ota.

Ethnicity
This naevus primarily occurs in Chinese and Japanese people.

Pathophysiology
Pathology
Histological features are identical to those of naevus of Ota.

Clinical features
History
This naevus was originally described by Minor Ito in 1954.

Presentation
Naevus of Ito presents as a unilateral, blue-greyish macular discoloration. It is distinguished from naevus of Ota by its location in the area innervated by the posterior supraclavicular and lateral cutaneous brachial nerves (Figure 131.17). Bilateral distribution has been reported occasionally [83–86].

Differential diagnosis
A Becker naevus is a large, pigmented, often hairy, patch on the shoulder, chest or back of young males (Chapter 73). Histologically it shows hyperpigmentation of the basal layer, mild acanthosis, elongation of the rete ridges and numerous melanophages in the upper dermis.

Complications and co-morbidities
Naevus of Ito is a benign lesion. There are only three cases of transformation to melanoma reported in the literature [87–89].

Disease course and prognosis
This is the same as in naevus of Ota.

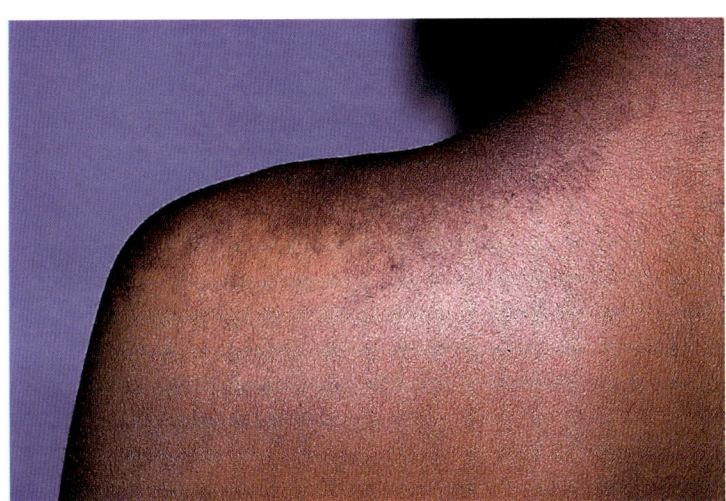

Figure 131.17 Naevus of Ito, showing a typical distribution over the shoulder area.

Management
Pigment targeting Q-switched laser systems are the treatment of choice.

CONGENITAL MELANOCYTIC NAEVI

See Chapter 73 and Table 131.3.

Speckled lentiginous naevus

Definition and nomenclature
Speckled lentiginous naevus (SLN) is a congenital melanocytic naevus presenting as a lentiginous macule early in life, and subsequently developing multiple darkly pigmented macules or papules in a speckled distribution (Table 131.3).

Synonyms and inclusions
- Naevus spilus
- Speckled naevus spilus
- Speckled lentiginous spilus
- Zosteriform lentiginus naevus

Epidemiology
Incidence and prevalence
The estimated prevalence is about 1–2%.

Age
The naevus may be present at birth or appear during childhood.

Sex
There is no sex predilection.

Associated diseases
Speckled lentiginous naevi are occasionally part of complex disorders such as speckled lentiginous naevus syndrome (SLN syndrome), phakomatosis pigmentovascularis (PPV) or phakomatosis pigmentokeratotica (PPK) [90–92]. SLN syndrome (or papular naevus spilus syndrome as recently proposed) is characterised by a papular SLN associated with ipsilateral neuromuscular, peripheral nerve and/or central nervous system defects [93]. Phakomatosis spilorosea, which according to the new classification by Happle in 2005 is a type of PPV corresponding to previous types IIIa and IIIb, is characterised by the coexistence of a macular SLN with a pale pink telangiectatic naevus [94]. PPK is characterised by the presence of a sebaceous naevus and a papular SLN, with or without skeletal and neurological disturbances.

Pathophysiology
Pathology
The background macule shows a subtle increase in melanocytes, whereas darkly pigmented speckles present a 'jentigo' pattern. Papular lesions correspond to superimposed dermal or compound melanocytic naevi.

Genetics
Phakomatosis pigmentovascularis was considered to be a didymosis with early postzygotic recombination [95]. However, Groesser and co-workers proposed that both naevi (sebaceous naevus and SLN) in PPK are caused by a postzygotic *HRAS* mutation in a multipotent progenitor cell and should therefore be viewed as a mosaic RASopathy [96].

Clinical features
Presentation
An SLN comprises a flat macule on a tan background, often faintly appearing, and more darkly pigmented lentigo-like lesions or naevi (Figure 131.18). Other types of naevi, such as blue naevi, Spitz naevi or rarely congenital melanocytic naevi, can occur within the lesion. The sites more commonly involved are the trunk and the upper and lower extremities. Naevi present in various sizes and occasionally show zosteriform or segmental distributions.

Clinical variants
Vidaurri de la Cruz *et al.* performed an extensive review of case reports on SLN and proposed two distinct subtypes of naevus spilus: macular (naevus spilus maculosus) and papular (naevus spilus papulosus) [97]. Macular SLN is characterised by a light brown macule with darker flat speckles, resembling a polka-dot pattern. In papular SLN, the light brown macule is superimposed with multiple papules or nodules with uneven distribution, reminiscent of a star map, while dark macules may also be present. Macular SLN is related to the phakomatosis spilorosea type of PPV, whereas papular SLN is present in PKK and SLN syndrome.

Differential diagnosis
Speckled lentiginous naevi can be confused with café-au-lait spot, congenital melanocytic naevus, Becker naevus, agminated naevomelanocytic naevus and segmental lentiginosis.

Disease course and prognosis
There have been a few reports of melanoma arising within SLNs of various sizes, but the relative risk is unknown. Considering the

Table 131.3 Basic clinical, pathological and dermoscopic patterns of acquired and congenital melanocytic naevi (Chapter 73).

Type of naevus	Subtype	Clinical presentation	Pathological characteristics	Dermoscopic presentation
Congenital naevi	Small (<1.5 cm) Medium (1.5–20 cm) Giant (>20 cm)	Light to dark brown colour, flat or elevated, with smooth to mammillated to verrucous surface and well-defined borders; may acquire coarse hair	Deeper naevus cells exhibit a tendency to extend deeply in relation to skin appendages	Reticular, globular or mixed pattern; milia-like cysts, perifollicular hypo-/hyperpigmentation, black or brown dots/globules and hypertrichosis may be present
	Speckled lentiginous naevus	Multiple darkly pigmented macules or papules (representing junctional and compound naevi) arising on a lentiginous macule	Banal naevi arising in a macular lentigo with a subtle increase in melanocyte number	Globular, reticular, structureless brown and mixed patterns on a faint network
Common acquired naevi	Junctional naevus	Uniformly pigmented brown macule, with a diameter of 2–1 mm	Benign proliferations of melanocytes in the epidermis	Globular, reticular, structureless brown and mixed patterns
	Compound naevus	Slightly raised, oval or round papule with symmetrical shape; pigmented with variable shades of brown	Benign proliferations of melanocytes in the epidermis, showing evidence of migration of cells into the dermis and 'maturation' of those cells within the deeper dermis	Globular, reticular, structureless, brown, multicomponent and mixed patterns
	Intradermal/dermal naevus	Flesh-coloured, dome-shaped, exophytic papule or nodule	Benign tumours of melanocytes in which there is no longer epidermal proliferation; the naevus cells have migrated into the dermis and matured there	Symmetrical homogeneous pattern; may have a slight pigmented globular pattern or black dots. Comedo-like openings, crypts and comma vessels may be present
Naevi in unusual sites	Naevus of the genital area	Usually hyperpigmented and larger in size compared with common acquired naevi	Atypical junctional proliferation of melanocytes may be present (large nests, discohesion of melanocytes)	Asymmetrical in colour and structure, often with irregular dots/globules or grayish-black blotches
	Naevus of the scalp	Often asymmetric and poorly circumscribed in younger ages, presenting as dermal naevus later in life	Large pleomorphic dyscohesive nests; lentiginous growth	Globular and combination of globular and reticular patterns
	Acral naevus	Macular or slightly elevated, uniformly pigmented lesion with irregular and sharp borders	Atypical junctional proliferation of melanocytes may be present	Parallel furrow, lattice-like or fibrillar pattern
	Nail-associated naevus	Longitudinal parallel and homogeneous light to dark brown to black pigmentation of the nail plate	Junctional or compound naevus with prominent hyperpigmentation and nuclear hyperchromasia	Brown, longitudinal parallel lines with regular spacing and thickness
Naevi with unusual morphology	Combined melanocytic naevus	Bluish macule or papule surrounded by a macular brown area	Two different types of naevi (one of which is usually a blue naevus) within the same lesion	Usually a brownish reticular and/or globular pattern with central or eccentric structureless blue pigmentation
	Recurrent melanocytic naevus	Macular area with hyper- or hypopigmentation, linear streaks and mottled pigmentation arising within a scar	Intraepidermal presence of melanocytes with abundant melanin and occasionally atypia, above the level of a scar	Irregular prominent network, globules and heterogeneous pigmentation, usually within the borders of the scar
	Halo naevus	A melanocytic naevus surrounded by a depigmented halo	Dense lymphocytic infiltrate in the early phase and subsequent elimination of naevus cells	Central naevus exhibits the globular and/or homogeneous patterns, surrounded by a white rim
	Meyerson naevus	A melanocytic naevus that develops a red-squamous halo	Benign naevus with overlying spongiosis of the epidermis	Pattern of the involved naevus is often blurred by an overlying yellowish superficial crust
	Cockade naevus	A naevus with a target-like appearance	Central junctional or compound component, while the periphery consists of junctional nests	Darker central globular or homogeneous pattern, surrounded by a structureless inner ring and a more peripheral darker reticular ring
	Targetoid haemosiderotic naevus	Brown or red-brown or violaceous papule surrounded by a thin pale area and a peripheral ecchymotic ring	Naevus cells mingled with extravasated blood vessels	Red to purple colour haemorrhage surrounding a naevus
Spitz naevus	Classic Spitz naevus	Solitary, firm, symmetrical, sharply demarcated, round or dome-shaped pink to red to reddish brown nodule (≤5–6 mm in diameter)	Symmetrical naevus of orderly architecture; consists of epithelioid/spindle cells arranged in nests showing zonation and maturation at the depth of lesion; intact epidermis, Kamino bodies, few superficial mitoses	Dotted vascular pattern with intersecting white lines (classic non-pigmented type); a 'starburst' pattern, aglobular pattern (blue-grey pigmentation surrounded by a rim of pigmented globules) or a multicomponent atypical pattern is seen in pigmented variants
	Reed naevus	Solitary, densely pigmented, irregularly shaped, dark-brown or black papule or nodule	Similar to classic Spitz naevi; junctional melanocytic activity with large quantities of melanin pigment	'Starburst' pattern (diffuse blue-black pigmentation with radial streaks in the periphery)

Table 131.3 (continued)

Type of naevus	Subtype	Clinical presentation	Pathological characteristics	Dermoscopic presentation
Blue naevus	Common blue naevus	Blue-black or deep blue dome-shaped papule, with a diameter <1–2 cm	Spindle or dendritic melanocytes within the dermis, containing pigment, even deeply in the dermis	Structureless, homogeneous, diffuse blue, blue-grey to steel blue pattern
	Cellular blue naevus	Same as common blue naevus; usually larger diameter	Dermal naevus cells are more numerous and extend into the deep reticular dermis or to subcutaneous fat	Similar to blue naevus; may have pale or yellowish periphery
	Deep penetrating naevus	Larger than common blue naevus, may show diffuse and irregular lateral margin	Extension of naevus cells deep into the dermis with a wedge shape	Negative globular pattern with blue-brown homogeneous pigmentation
Clinically atypical naevus		Larger than 5 mm with irregular borders and pigmentation; may contain a reddish hue. A central papular component is often surrounded by a macular periphery	Characteristic architectural and cytological atypia (see Table 131.5)	Multiple patterns; a common dermoscopic pattern shows central homogeneity and reticulated network or dots at the periphery

limited number of reported malignant transformation and the estimated 1–2% prevalence of SLN in the population, it is likely that this risk is quite low.

Management

There is no standardised management algorithm for SLN. Although they are not considered a major risk factor for melanoma or true melanoma precursors, patients should be instructed to monitor their naevi. Baseline photos and subsequent documenting of clinical changes could be useful. For patients with large naevi covering extensive body surface areas that are difficult for the patient to self-examine, clinical surveillance and sequential dermoscopic examination should be offered. Prophylactic excision is not justified, but suspicious lesions should be biopsied.

Excision, ablative and non-ablative lasers and dermabrasion for cosmetic reasons have been used with varying results [98–101].

COMMON ACQUIRED NAEVI

Acquired melanocytic naevi

Definition and nomenclature

These are common benign proliferations of uniform melanocytes that are located initially at the dermal–epidermal junction, and over time tend to migrate into the dermis and regress with subsequent morphological changes.

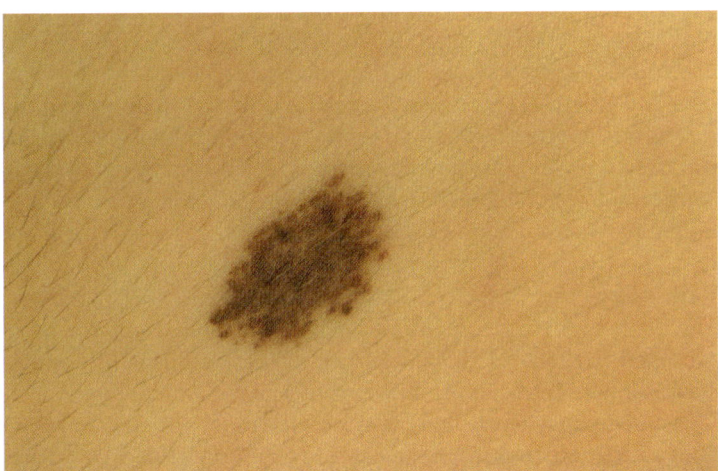
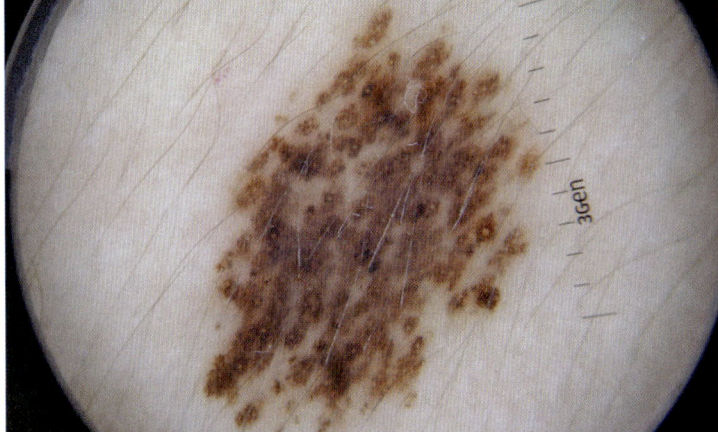

Figure 131.18 (a) Speckled lentiginous naevi. Numerous darker macules and papules (representing junctional and compound naevi) can be seen on a faintly visible tan macular background. (b) Dermoscopic image showing patchy diffuse distribution of brown reticular spots with regular network over a light brownish background. Follicular openings can also be observed.

Synonyms and inclusions
- Cellular naevus
- Naevocytic naevus
- Mole

Introduction and general description

Acquired melanocytic naevi are benign neoplasms of melanocytic naevus cells that begin to proliferate at the dermal–epidermal junction (junctional naevus) and over time tend to migrate into the dermis while a component remains in contact with the basal layer (compound naevus) (Table 131.3). At the end stage of this process, all the naevus cells are completely detached from the overlying epidermis (intradermal naevus). The typical life cycle of a common melanocytic naevus follows the stages of initiation, promotion, senescence and involution.

Epidemiology

Incidence and prevalence

Acquired melanocytic naevi are the most common neoplasms among white people and are usually multiple. Higher naevi counts have been associated with fair skin and freckling [102,103].

Age

The number of acquired melanocytic naevi increases from childhood to midlife and decreases progressively thereafter. The occurrence of a new melanocytic lesion in a young individual is a common event, while the same phenomenon in a patient older than 60 years should raise concern of melanoma.

Sex

There is no sex predilection.

Ethnicity

These naevi present in all races, but their incidence and number are higher in white people.

Associated diseases

The presence of multiple acquired melanocytic naevi is a risk factor for melanoma. Patients with more than 100 naevi have a sevenfold increase in melanoma risk [104]. The risk of malignant transformation of an acquired melanocytic naevus is extremely low, ranging on an annual basis from one in 200 000 for men and women younger than 40 years, to one in 33 000 for men older than 60 years [105].

Pathophysiology

The exact mechanism of melanocytic naevus development is unknown, but probably involves an interplay of genetic and environmental factors. A common scenario proposes that naevi originate from a single precursor melanocyte of unknown nature.

Predisposing factors

Variations in naevus numbers have been observed among different groups of patients. Sun exposure and sun-protection habits during childhood may modify naevus count [106,107]. Chemotherapy administered for leukaemia in childhood [108] or after renal transplantation [109] has been associated with increased naevus count. Local trauma may trigger the development of eruptive naevi in predisposed patients [110]. Hormonal factors in females may also play a role in naevogenesis, as postmenarche status [106], and the use of oral contraceptives or hormone replacement therapy have been linked with higher naevi count [111]. Individuals with Turner syndrome have increased numbers of melanocytic naevi [112]. Children with atopic dermatitis present fewer naevi compared with control subjects, suggesting that the pro-inflammatory cytokine milieu in the atopic skin might inhibit naevogenesis [113,114].

Pathology

The pathology of acquired naevi consists of naevomelanocytes arranged partially in clusters or nests. They are usually round or cuboidal with intracytoplasmic granules of melanin pigment.

In junctional naevus, along the dermal–epidermal junction, single naevus cells are present in the basal layer. Nests of naevus cells are distributed mainly at the tips or, less commonly, between the rete ridges (Figure 131.19).

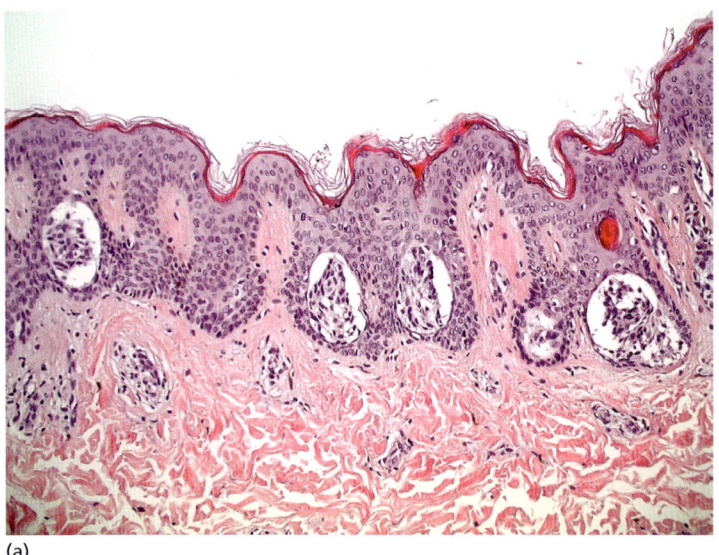
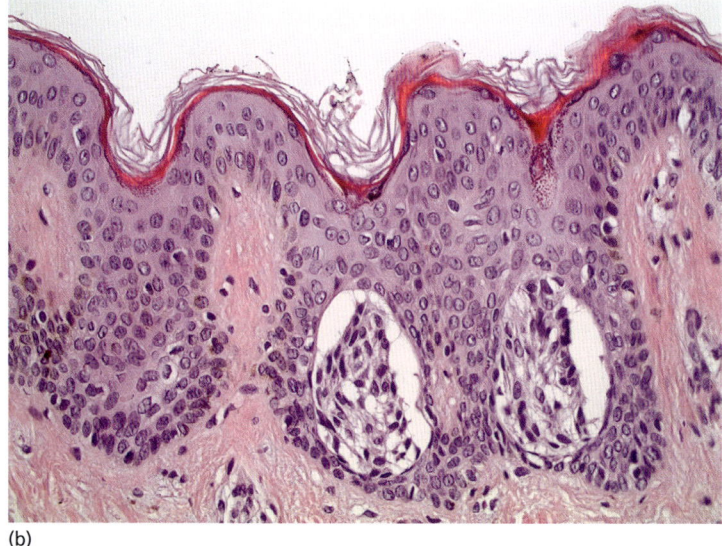

Figure 131.19 Junctional naevus. (a) Aggregates of naevomelanocytic cells in the rete ridges of a hyperplastic epidermis. There is no dermal component. Magnification 10× (H&E). (b) Naevomelanocytic nests are usually located in the tips and basilar area of the rete ridges and are often separated from the adjacent squamous cells by a clear space. Magnification 40× (H&E). Courtesy of Dr K. Frangia, HBD HistoBio Diagnosis, Athens, Greece.

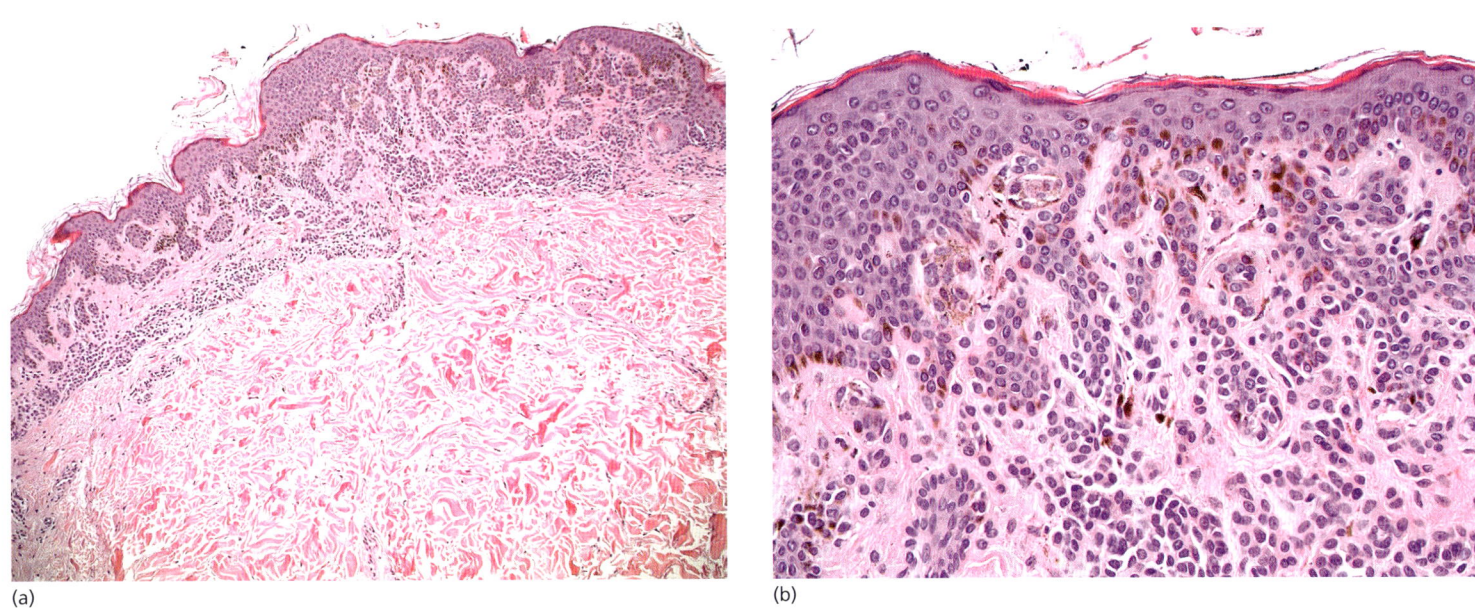

Figure 131.20 Acquired compound naevus. (a) Naevomelanocytic proliferation in the junctional area and the dermis. The dermal component extends beyond the boundaries of the junctional component. Magnification 10× (H&E). (b) Naevus cells type A (epithelioid) or type B (without significant atypia) present in the dermal–epidermal junction and in the dermis, in an isolated or nesting pattern of development. Melanin pigment is more pronounced in the upper portion of the lesion. Magnification 40× (H&E). Courtesy of Dr K. Frangia, HBD HistoBio Diagnosis, Athens, Greece.

A compound naevus has a junctional and an intradermal component with a variety of morphological types of naevomelanocytes (A, B and C cells) arranged in nests, cords or single units in the dermis (Figure 131.20a). Type A or epithelioid cells with intracytoplasmic melanin pigment in an abundant cytoplasm are typically found in the upper dermis. Type B or naevic cells are smaller than type A, contain less melanin and lie in cords deeper in the dermis (Figure 131.20b). Type C or spindle cells rarely contain melanin and have a neurotised, schwannian morphology. They are located in the lower dermis, often in strands or in loose, fibrillar aggregates, called naevic corpuscles. Multinucleated cells may also be present at the upper dermis.

An intradermal naevus has identical features to the dermal component of a compound naevus, with melanocytes gradually losing their ability to produce melanin as they progress from the upper to the deeper dermis (Figure 131.21). When the spindle-shaped type C cells prevail, the lesion mimics a neurofibroma and the term neural naevus is used for the variant without a type A or B cell component. The presence of fat cells between the naevus cells and of atypical senescence of naevomelanocytes are considered to indicate ageing of the lesion. The overlying epidermis may be hyperplastic, with hyperkeratosis and papillomatosis.

In general, melanocytes gradually lose their ability to produce pigment as they progress from the epidermis to the dermis and 'senesce'. These stages are not necessarily followed by every naevus. Additionally, naevi seem to retain the ability to respond physiologically to certain conditions, such as pregnancy or exposure to UV radiation, including increasing proliferative rates, while maintaining their benign nature [**115**].

The balloon cell naevus is a histological subtype of compound naevi. It consists of characteristic cells with swollen, vacuolated cytoplasm, containing none or a few small melanin granules, which are sometimes multinucleated. Regular melanocytes can be found at the periphery of the naevus. The biological significance of balloon cells is unknown, and they are not precursors to balloon cell melanoma. It is speculated that 'ballooning' is an intrinsic cellular degenerative process due to an arrest in the biosynthesis of melanin in melanosomes [116]. Rare cases of balloon cell naevi in the upper aerodigestive tract mucosa and conjunctiva have been reported [117,118].

Genetics

Somatic *BRAF* mutations (most commonly BRAF p.V600E) are present in the majority (c. 80%) of acquired melanocytic naevi (especially in those with a dermal component) [119] and *NRAS* are encountered less often, implicating activation of the RAS/MAPK kinase pathway in the pathogenesis of naevi. *BRAF* mutations are an early initiating event in naevogenesis, leading to melanocytic proliferation and the formation of neoplastic clones [**115**,120]. In the absence of other genetic alterations these clones enter cell cycle arrest and senescence through the induction of p16INK4a and acidic β-galactosidase [121]. Genomewide association studies have identified several genetic loci on chromosomes 9p21 and 22q13 that are potentially associated with naevus counts and melanoma development [122,123].

Environmental factors

Although the prevalence of common naevi has not always been associated with UV exposure [124], international comparative studies have documented increased numbers of naevi in children living in sunnier climates compared with children of similar ethnicity residing in northern countries [125,126]. Several studies have demonstrated that ambient sunlight and sunburn is associated with increased naevus counts in children [106,127–129].

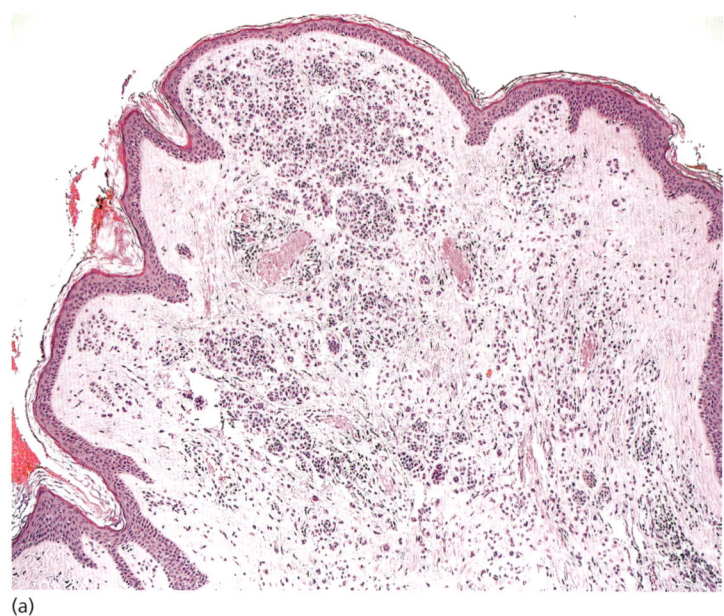
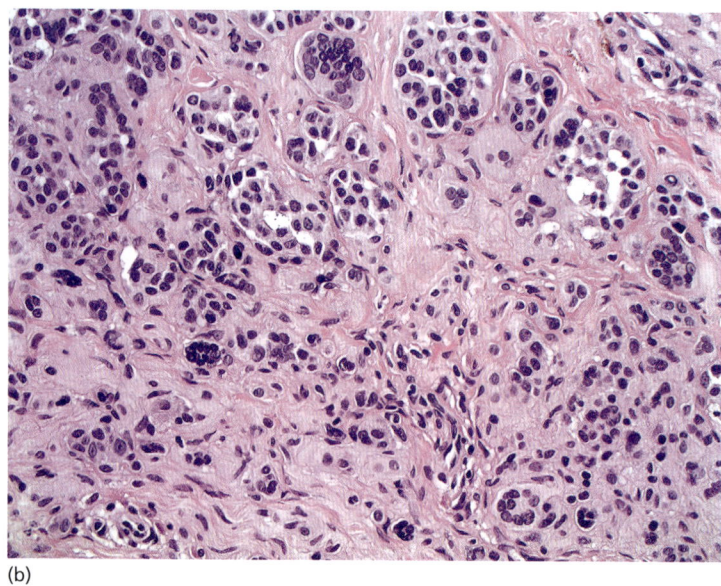

Figure 131.21 Acquired dermal naevus. (a) Nested pattern of development in the upper portion of the lesion. There is no junctional component. Magnification 10× (H&E). (b) All types of naevic cells (A, B, C and giant cells) are present in an isolated or nested pattern. Magnification 40× (H&E). Courtesy of Dr K. Frangia, HBD HistoBio Diagnosis, Athens, Greece.

Clinical features

Presentation

A newly formed melanocytic naevus is a junctional naevus, presenting as a uniformly pigmented brown macule, with a diameter of 2–10 mm (Figure 131.22). Naevus pigmentation is related to individual skin colour, with lighter phototypes typically presenting paler naevi. It is also associated with UV exposure, gaining a darker shade after exposure to sunlight (e.g. after a summer vacation) or artificial UV sources. It can be located anywhere in the body, but it is found more commonly on the trunk and the extremities.

A compound naevus is a slightly raised, oval or round papule with symmetrical shape (Figure 131.23). This naevus is also pigmented, with shades of brown according to the patient's skin colour.

Intradermal (or dermal) naevi are flesh-coloured, dome-shaped nodules that can be larger than junctional naevi (Figure 131.24). Their surface is usually smooth but can also appear papillomatous. They are located primarily on the head, neck and shoulders. One or a few hair shafts may project from the naevus surface. Acute inflammation of intradermal naevi, presenting as painful red-coloured swelling can occur due to mechanical friction or bacterial infection of the hair follicles inside the naevus and should not cause concern of malignant transformation.

Clinical variants

Agminated and eruptive melanocytic naevi can occasionally occur (Chapter 147).

Differential diagnosis

The distinction between very small congenital and common acquired melanocytic naevi during the first years of life may be very difficult both clinically and dermoscopically.

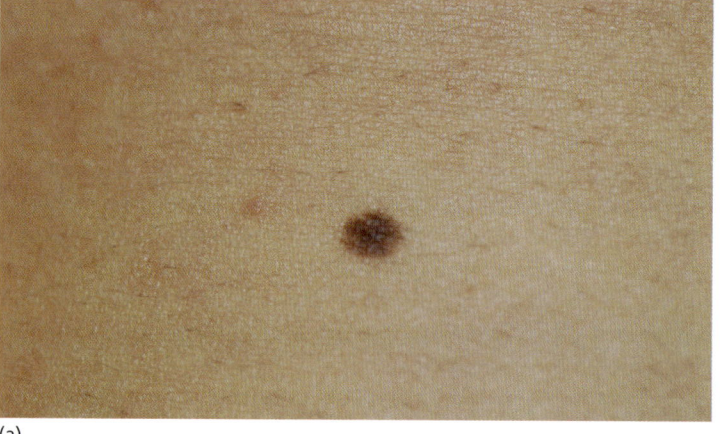
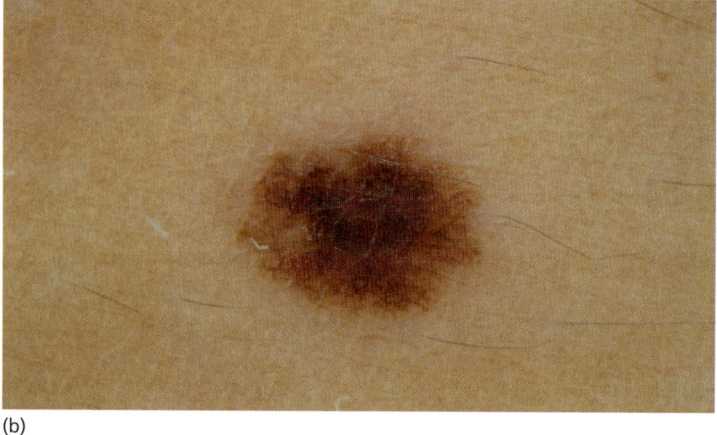

Figure 131.22 (a) Junctional naevus. (b) Dermoscopic image of a junctional naevus showing a reticular pattern with a smooth ending at the periphery.

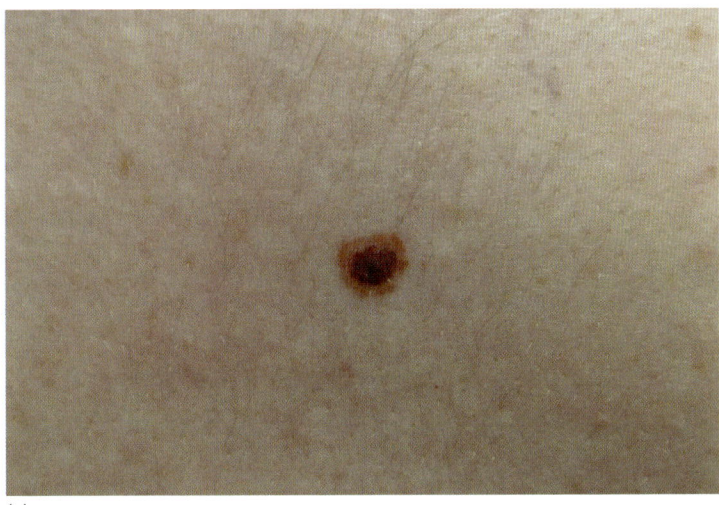

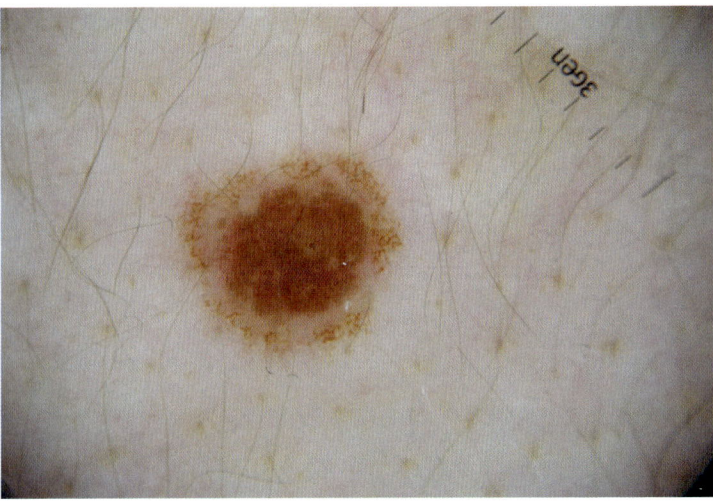

Figure 131.23 Compound naevus. (a) Hyperpigmented papule surrounded by symmetrical, lighter brown, macular area. (b) Dermoscopic image showing a structureless brown centre with reticulated periphery.

Disease course and prognosis

Although 25–30% of melanomas arise in association with pre-existing naevi, malignant transformation of naevi is a very rare event.

Investigations

Upon dermoscopy (Figures 131.21b, 131.22b and 131.23b), common acquired melanocytic naevi can be classified into globular, reticular, structureless brown and mixed patterns, which correlate to different histopathological features. Dermoscopic patterns are also related to the patient's age and skin pigmentation, as well as anatomical location [130].

Management

No treatment is required. Surgical removal is performed only for aesthetic purposes, but has the potential risk of scarring. Superficial removal techniques, like curettage, dermabrasion, shave excision, electrosurgery and lasers, do not destroy all naevus cells, so the naevus can recur with an atypical presentation ('pseudo-melanoma').

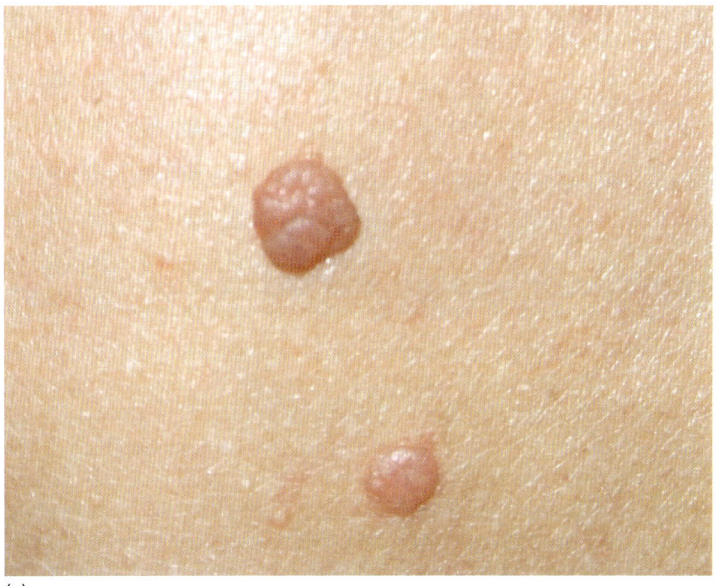

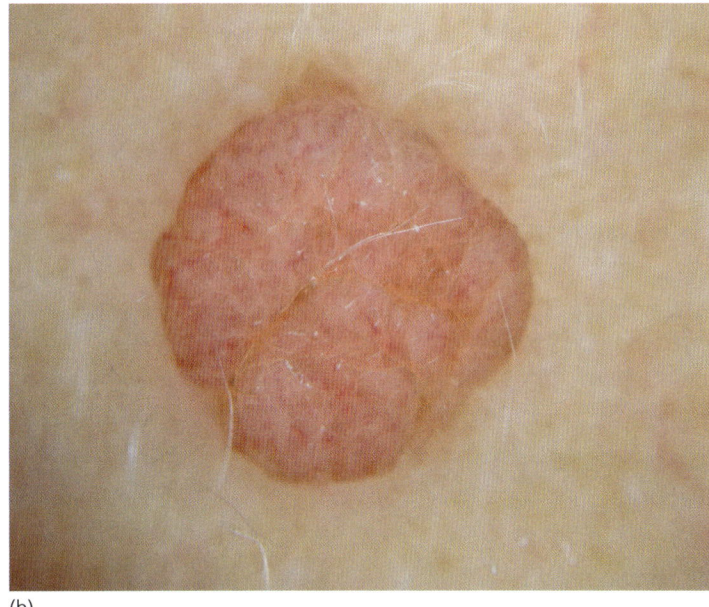

Figure 131.24 (a) Dermal naevi. (b) Dermoscopic image showing a symmetrical, flesh-coloured, homogeneous pattern with comma-shaped vessels.

Scarring, inflammation, neovascularisation and postinflammatory hyper- or hypopigmentation are also frequent sequelae associated with these methods.

NAEVI IN UNUSUAL SITES

Definition

Naevi in certain locations include a group of benign melanocytic naevi with histological features resembling clinically atypical naevi or melanoma [131]. They are located in distinct anatomical areas such as the scalp, ear, embryonic milkline, flexural sites, breast, genitalia and acral sites but comprise only a subset of naevi that present on these sites (see Table 131.3).

Synonyms and inclusions
- Melanocytic naevi of special sites
- Naevi with site-related atypia

Introduction and general description

Although not broadly accepted as a unique entity, these lesions have a different morphological pattern from banal melanocytic naevi. This is partially due to anatomical factors, hormonal influences, trauma, UV exposure and epidermal thickness [132]. These naevi are clinically more atypical, presenting with a larger size and colour variegation. They exhibit distinct histological patterns such as pagetoid speading (acral naevi) [133], enlarged junctional nests with discohesion of melanocytes (flexural and genital naevi) [134] or large nests with bizarre shapes that extend down to the follicular epithelium (scalp) [135]. They can also present with atypical nesting patterns, stromal fibrosis and atypical dermal cytology [136]. Their course is benign and, just as in naevi on other sites, they should be monitored clinically. Inspection of all these usually 'hidden' areas should be included in total body examination.

Melanocytic naevi of the genital area

Epidemiology
Incidence and prevalence
These hamartomas are uncommon, found in 2.3% of patients undergoing routine gynaecological examinations [137].

Pathophysiology
Pathology
Most are compound naevi characterised by a florid junctional melanocytic proliferation, cellular dyscohesion and atypical cytology [138]. Melanocytic naevi arising within lichen sclerosus may demonstrate additional features mimicking melanoma [139].

Clinical features
Presentation
These naevi are predominantly located in the vulva, but also occur in the perineum, mons pubis, penis and scrotum. A small subset of genital naevi (5%), termed atypical melanocytic naevi of the genital type, occurs mainly in young premenopausal women and is characterised by marked architectural and atypical cytology [140]. Clinically, these lesions are often hyperpigmented and larger in size compared with common acquired naevi.

Differential diagnosis
Despite their benign course, these lesions are often difficult to differentiate from vulval melanoma, which is seen primarily in postmenopausal women [141]. Atypical genital naevi and genital melanomas have also distinct and non-overlapping somatic mutational patterns [142].

Melanocytic naevi of the breast

Epidemiology
Incidence and prevalence
They occur in both males and females [**131**,136].

Pathophysiology
Pathology
They tend to exhibit more atypical characteristics than naevi from other sites, with nesting irregularities, melanocytes with atypia in the papillary dermis and maturation in the deep dermis, and dermal fibroplasia [136,**139**].

Clinical features
Presentation
They can be located anywhere in the breast, including the nipple, and are often larger than 6 mm with irregular borders (Figure 131.25) [**139**,143].

Melanocytic naevi of the scalp

Epidemiology
Incidence and prevalence
Atypical melanocytic naevi of the scalp are more prevalent in younger ages [135].

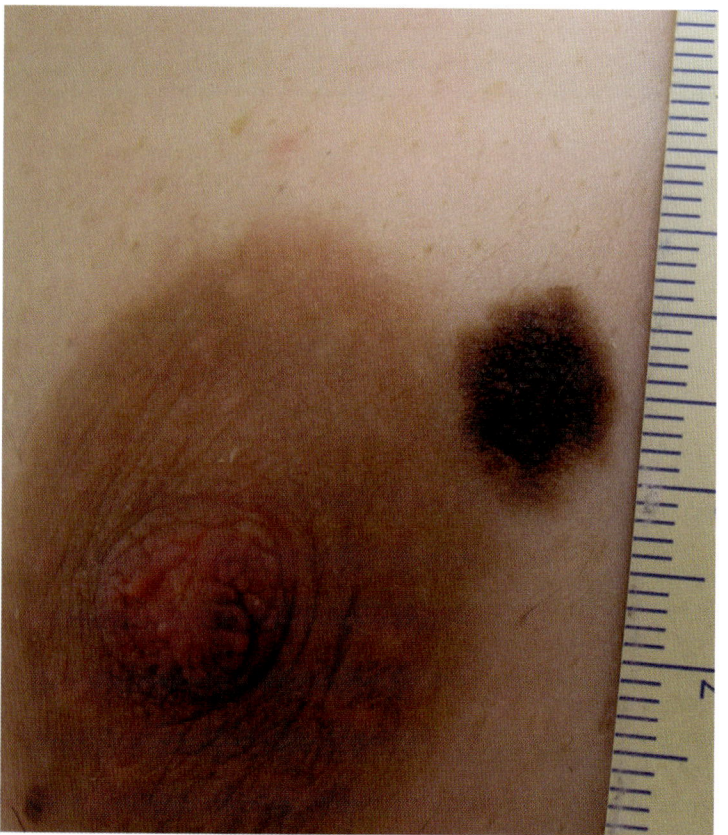

Figure 131.25 Breast naevus with irregular borders.

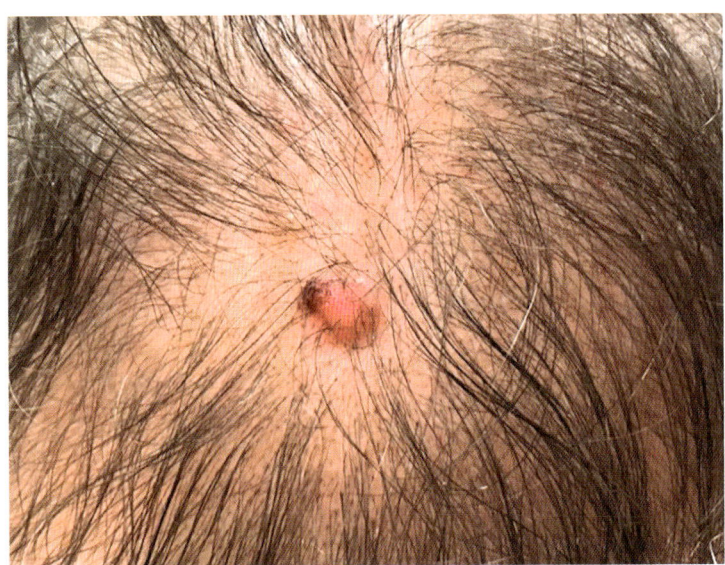

Figure 131.26 Naevus of the scalp.

Pathophysiology
Pathology
Scalp naevi often show large pleomorphic dyscohesive nests, lentiginous growth, melanocytes with large nuclei, follicular involvement and superficial fibroplasia [131].

Clinical features
Presentation
These naevi tend to be asymmetric and poorly circumscribed, especially in children, adolescents and young adults. In older patients they usually become raised with a smooth or papillomatous surface, and less pigmented or flesh-coloured (Figure 131.26) [143]. Blue naevi and their variants are frequent on the scalp [143].

Investigations
Globular and a combination of globular and reticular patterns, as well as perifollicular hypopigmentation, and central hypopigmentation (eclipse naevus), are frequent dermoscopic features in children and adolescents [143].

Acral naevi

Synonyms and inclusions
- Melanocytic naevus of the acral skin
- Melanocytic acral naevus with intraepidermal ascent of cells

Pathophysiology
Pathology
Histologically, these naevi share the same features with common acquired naevi in other locations, although they are usually more cellular. They can be junctional, compound or intraepidermal (Figure 131.27a) [144,145]. Lentiginous melanocytic proliferation and some degree of upward migration of naevus cells are seen

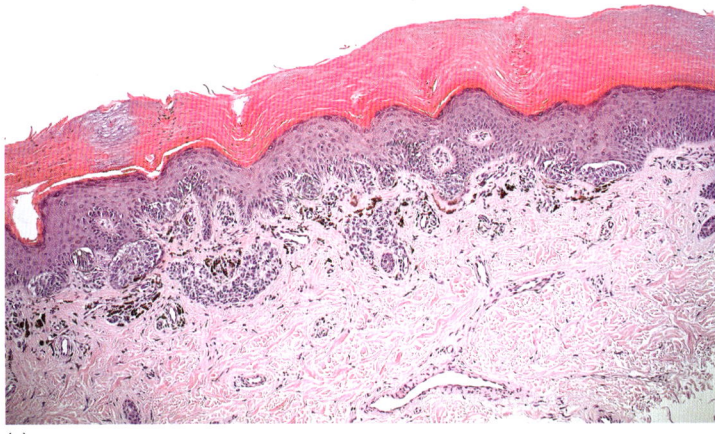

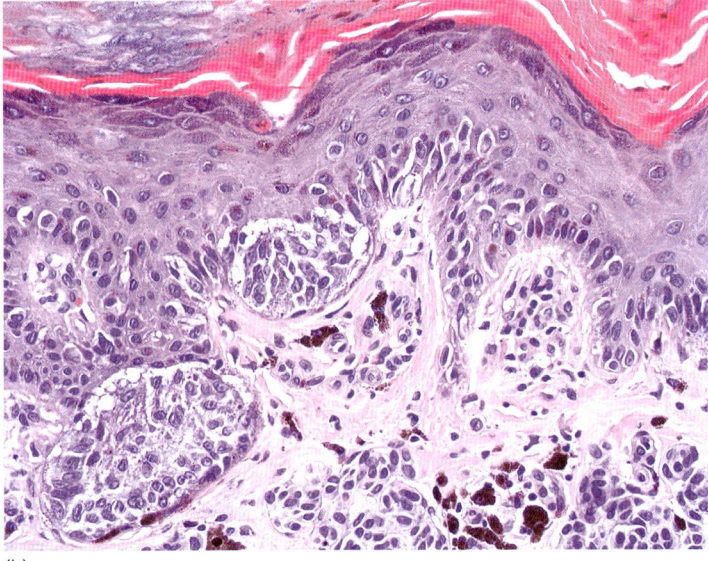

Figure 131.27 Compound acral naevus. (a) The junctional component predominates, with variable sized and shaped nests located mainly to the tips of the rete ridges. A dermal component is also present. Magnification 10× (H&E). (b) Single melanocytes present in the epidermis in a pagetoid spreading pattern may lead a pathologist to the erroneous diagnosis of melanoma. Magnification 40× (H&E). Courtesy of Dr K. Frangia, HBD HistoBio Diagnosis, Athens, Greece.

(Figure 131.27b), the latter due to a transepidermal elimination effect from frequent trauma and friction on these sites. The dermal component of acral naevi shows maturation, bland cytology and lack of mitoses. A prominent inflammatory infiltrate should raise concern for malignancy [131].

Clinical features
Presentation
Acral naevi are usually macular or slightly elevated, uniformly pigmented lesions with irregular and sharp borders [144]. Their colour can range from brown to dark brown and they often present with a striated appearance, distributed along the parallel furrows of acral skin (Figure 131.28), in contrast to melanomas that are situated along the ridges of the palms and soles. Acral naevi of the soles are usually located on non-weight-bearing areas, in contrast to melanomas [146].

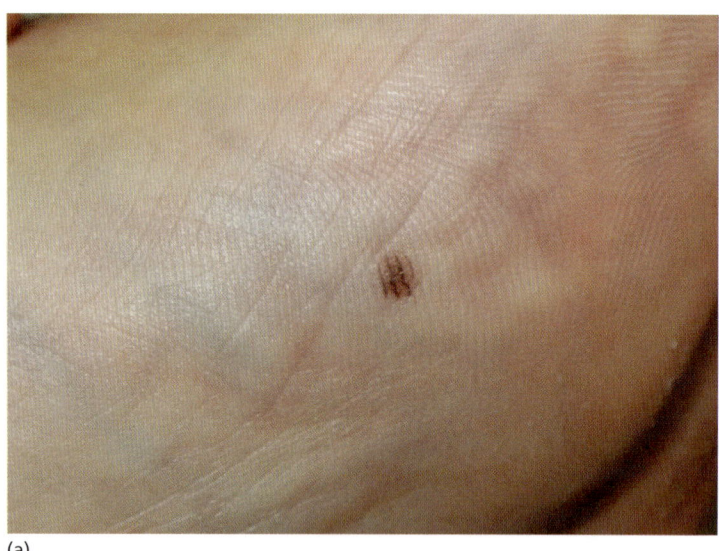

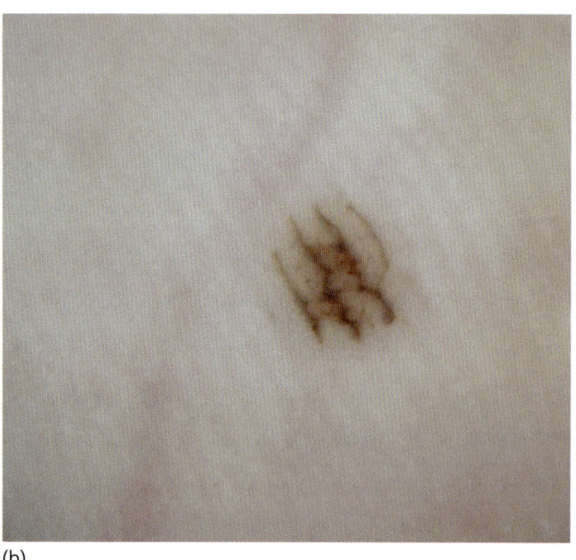

Figure 131.28 (a) Naevus on the sole of a foot. (b) Dermoscopic image of acral naevus showing a parallel furrow pattern.

Investigations
The most common dermoscopic pattern of acral naevi is the parallel furrow pattern (Figure 131.28b), followed by the lattice-like and fibrillar patterns [147].

Management
Despite their slightly atypical histology, the majority of acral naevi are clinically and histologically indistinguishable from benign naevi in other sites and should be managed similarly.

Conjunctival naevi

Epidemiology
Incidence and prevalence
Conjunctival naevi are the most common tumours of the conjunctiva and can be of the acquired or congenital type [148].

Pathophysiology
Pathology
Histologically, the compound type predominates although all histological variants have been reported, including a rapidly growing and often concerning lesion in children and adolescents [149]. The characteristic feature of conjunctival naevi is the histological presence of intralesional cysts (Figure 131.29).

Clinical features
Presentation
These naevi are similar to those occurring in the skin and present as circumscribed, flat or slightly raised macules or papules, occurring most commonly on the bulbar conjunctiva [150] (Figure 131.30). They are often amelanotic (30% of cases), particularly in children in whom they often acquire pigmentation after puberty.

Disease course and prognosis
The prognosis is excellent. There are no specific clinical signs that predict the transformation of a conjunctival naevus to melanoma (presumed to occur in fewer than 1% of naevi). Attachment to the sclera, extension into the cornea and development of 'feeder' vessels upon slit lamp examination represent worrisome changes [151,152].

Naevi of the nail matrix or nail bed

Melanonychia is covered in Chapter 93.

NAEVI WITH UNUSUAL MORPHOLOGY

Introduction and general description
There is a distinct group of naevi that exhibit unusual clinicopathological and dermoscopic features. These naevi, designated as 'special' naevi, include those with clinically atypical presentation that simulate melanoma (e.g. combined and recurrent naevi) and those with targetoid morphology (e.g. halo, Mayerson, cockade and targetoid haemosiderotic naevi) (see Table 131.3).

Combined melanocytic naevi

Definition
Combined naevi present as two different types of benign melanocytic proliferations within the same naevus [153]. The most frequent combination is that of a blue naevus associated with a congenital, acquired or Spitz naevus.

Epidemiology
Incidence and prevalence
Combined naevi correspond to approximately 1% of excised naevi [154].

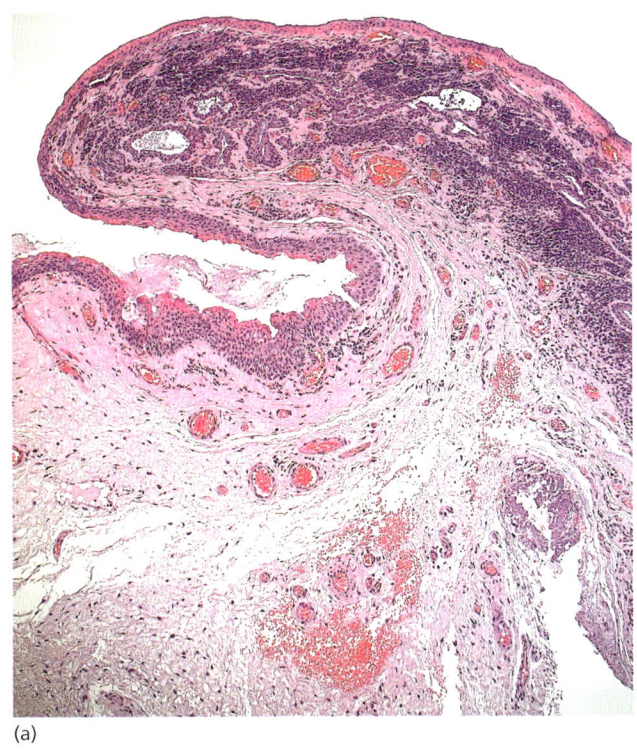

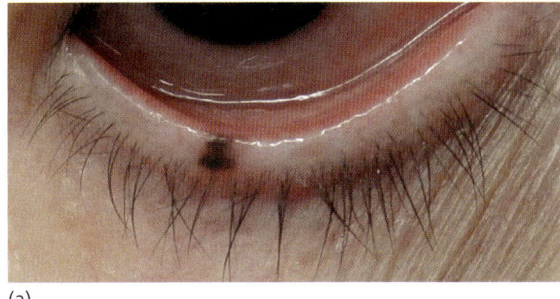

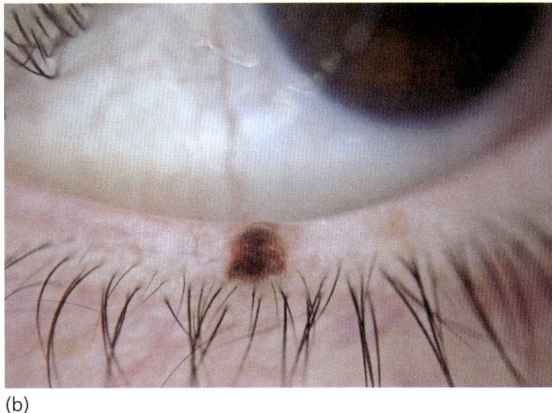

Figure 131.30 Conjunctival naevus. (a) A well-circumscribed papule of various shades of brown. (b) Dermoscopic image showing homogeneous brown-greyish pigmentation with a reddish hue. Courtesy of Dr D. Sgouros, Andreas Sygros Hospital, Athens, Greece.

Pathophysiology
It is unclear whether pathogenetically they represent a mere coexistence of two different naevi populations or if they derive from a single cell proliferation differentiating into two different types of naevi.

Clinical features
Presentation
The clinical presentation of this naevus depends on the combination and distribution of its cellular components [131]. Combined naevi containing a blue naevus often present as a bluish macule or papule (representing a blue naevus) surrounded by a macular brown area (representing a compound naevus) (Figure 131.31) [155]. The back is a frequent location.

Genetics
The genetic profile of these naevi varies. A subset of combined naevi with a spitzoid component shows inactivation of *BAP1* (combined *BAP1*-inactivated naevus) [156,157]. Germline mutations of *BAP1* lead to multiple combined *BAP1*-inactivated naevi and melanocytomas [131,158,159].

Differential diagnosis
Due to the presence of two different naevi components, combined naevi are characterised by colour variegations that raise the suspicion of melanoma. For this reason, excision and histopathological analysis of these lesions is generally recommended.

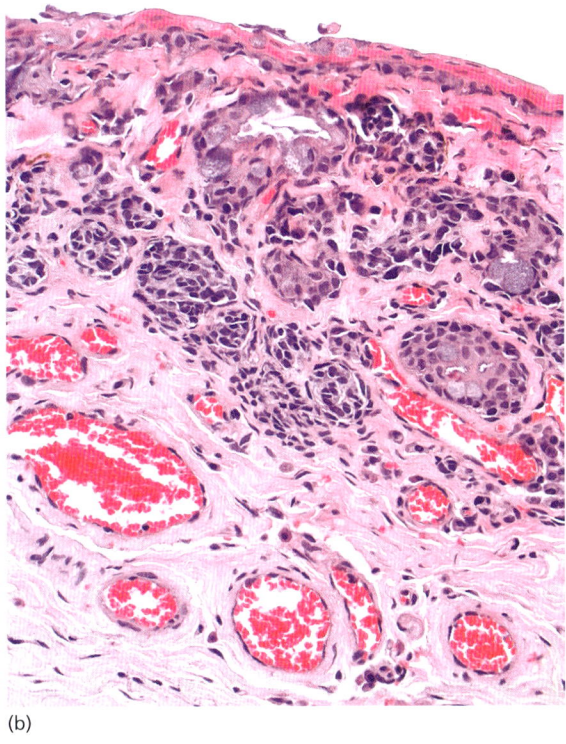

Figure 131.29 Compound conjunctival naevus. (a) Naevic aggregates are observed mainly beneath the conjunctival epithelium, in the substantia propria and partially around cystic epithelial inclusions. Magnification 10× (H&E). (b) Nests of fairly uniform naevomelanocytes showing a partial relationship to the epithelium of local cystic epithelial inclusions. There is also a small naevic component at the base of the surface epithelium. Magnification 40× (H&E). Courtesy of Dr K. Frangia, HBD HistoBio Diagnosis, Athens, Greece.

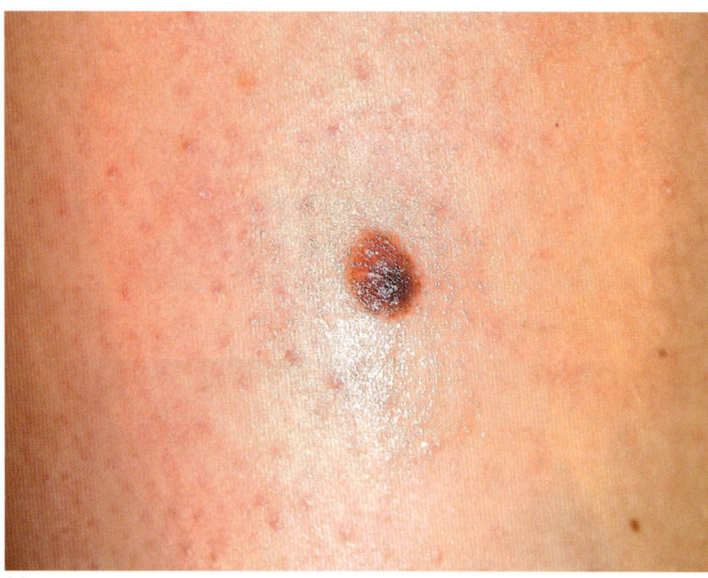

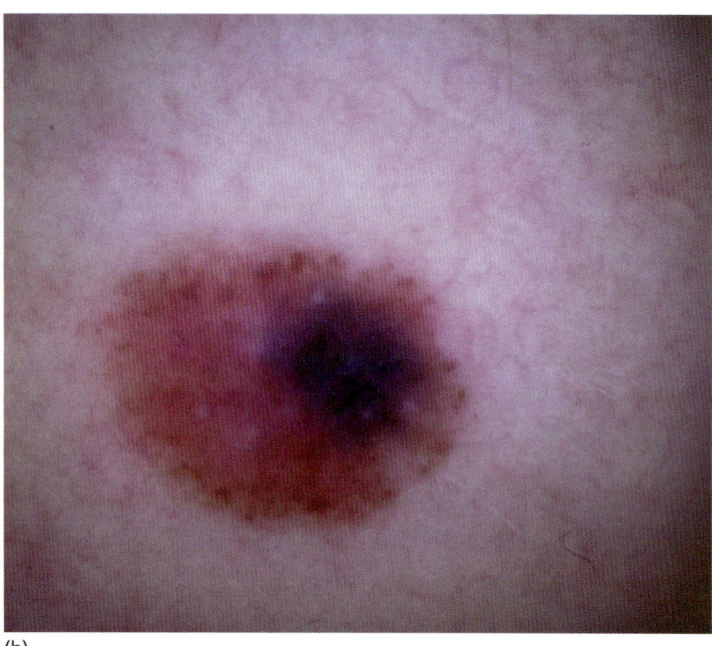

Figure 131.31 (a) Combined naevus. (b) Combined naevus with eccentric, structureless, bluish area and peripheral, brown, globular pattern. Courtesy of Dr D. Sgouros, Andreas Sygros Hospital, Athens, Greece.

Investigations

Dermoscopically, the most frequent pattern is a typical brownish reticular and/or globular pattern with central or eccentric structureless blue pigmentation (Figure 131.31b) [160,161].

Recurrent melanocytic naevi

Definition and nomenclature

Recurrent melanocytic naevi are benign melanocytic naevi that recur after incomplete surgical excision or trauma.

Synonyms and inclusions
- Persistent naevus
- Pseudomelanoma

Epidemiology
Incidence and prevalence
They occur more frequently in women aged 20–30 years of age.

Pathophysiology
Various theories have been proposed such as regrowth from a residual dermal naevus, repopulation from seeded melanocytes after initial removal or from adnexal structures, and junctional stimulation from remaining hair roots or from the periphery of the lesion [153].

Pathology
Histopathologically, recurrent naevi have an intraepidermal presence of melanocytes above the level of a scar. Effacement of rete ridges and a lentiginous or nested proliferation of naevus cells is also seen. The naevomelanocytes have abundant melanin and uniform nucleoli, although low grade atypical cytology can be observed occasionally.

Clinical features
History
Recurrent naevi usually originate from acquired ordinary melanocytic naevi removed by shave biopsy for cosmetic reasons. Recurrences after incomplete removal of blue naevi, Spitz naevi and clinically atypical or dysplastic naevi have been also reported [162]. Recurrences typically arise in the centre of the scar, usually within a time frame from 6 weeks to 6 months after removal of the initial naevus [163].

Presentation
Clinically, they appear as a macular area with hyper- or hypopigmentation, linear streaks and mottled pigmentation (halo, stippled or diffuse) measuring 2–5 mm in diameter (Figure 131.32) [164]. Due to their atypical clinical and histopathological presentation, they are viewed as simulators of melanoma, hence the term 'pseudo-melanoma'. Their most common location is the trunk (back), followed by the face and extremities [163].

Differential diagnosis
The differential diagnosis of recurrent naevi is often difficult to make from recurrent melanoma and reactive pigmentation of scars. The history of occurrence after the removal of a pre-existing naevus, the distribution of pigmentation within the scar and specific dermoscopic findings are important parameters in setting the correct diagnosis. Their presentation within 6 months of excision and their confinement within the boundaries of the scar point more towards a recurrent naevus [165]. In contrast, a recurrent melanoma arises more slowly and tends to grow beyond the borders of the scar into the adjacent normal skin.

Investigations
Dermoscopy of recurrent naevi reveals an irregular prominent network, the presence of globules and a heterogeneous pigmentation

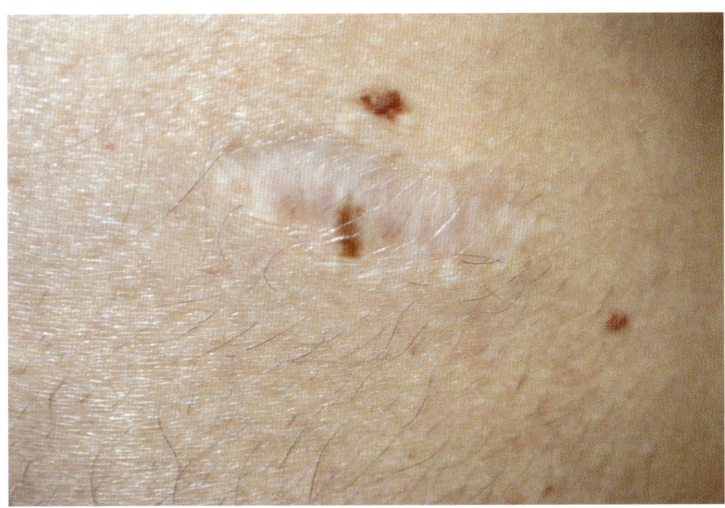

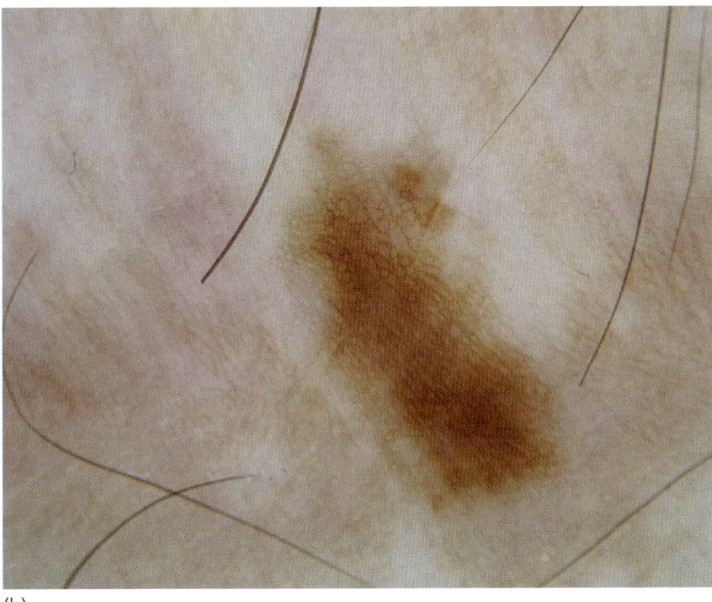

Figure 131.32 Recurrent naevus. (a) Macule developing within the scar of a previously excised melanocytic naevus. (b) Dermoscopic image showing a slightly asymmetrical macule consisting of a smooth reticular network of fine lines and brownish colour on a whitish scar. Courtesy of Dr D. Sgouros, Andreas Sygros Hospital, Athens, Greece.

(Figure 131.32b) [166]. According to a study examining the dermoscopic features of recurrent naevi versus recurrent melanomas, there is a more symmetrical and centrifugal growth confined within the area of the scar in recurrent naevi compared with the chaotic, often eccentric and non-continuous pigmentation of recurrent melanoma extending beyond the scar's edge [167].

Management

The management of these lesions is often not straightforward. Factors such as the patient's age, the anatomical site, the time from removal, the type of removal (surgical versus destructive modality) and the growth pattern are important clues, but the most important is the histopathology of the first excision. If the diagnosis of the primary lesion was that of a banal naevus then no further treatment is warranted. If there is a previous report of an atypical naevus or if the histopathology of the primary lesion is not available, then a thorough excision of the recurrent lesion and a histopathological evaluation is necessary.

Halo naevus

Definition and nomenclature
A halo naevus is a melanocytic naevus surrounded by a depigmented area resembling a halo.

Synonyms and inclusions
- Sutton naevus
- Leukoderma acquisitum centrifugum
- Perinaevoid vitiligo

Epidemiology
Incidence and prevalence
Halo naevi are relatively common, presenting in approximately 1% of the population. They may present as solitary or multiple lesions.

Age
These naevi are more commonly seen in children, adolescents and young adults.

Sex
There is no sex predilection.

Associated diseases
Halo naevi can be associated with autoimmune disorders like vitiligo, Hashimoto thyroiditis, alopecia areata and atopic eczema.

Pathophysiology
The exact pathophysiology of halo naevi is unknown. They are considered an autoimmune response against naevus cells. There is some laboratory evidence of local and circulating immunological T-cell activation in patients with unexcised halo naevi [168].

Predisposing factors
Stress and puberty are considered to be triggering factors [153]. Familial cases have been reported [169]. Regression of several melanocytic naevi in patients with metastatic melanoma receiving ipilimumab has been observed [170,171]. Halo naevi have also been observed in relation with imatinib [172] and tocilizumab treatment [173,174].

Pathology
Halo naevi are usually compound melanocytic naevi, although junctional or dermal naevi are occasionally noted. At the time of the halo appearing, they demonstrate a heavy, lichenoid, lymphocytic infiltrate within the dermis, with naevus cells arranged in nests or singly among the inflammatory cells (Figure 131.33). In

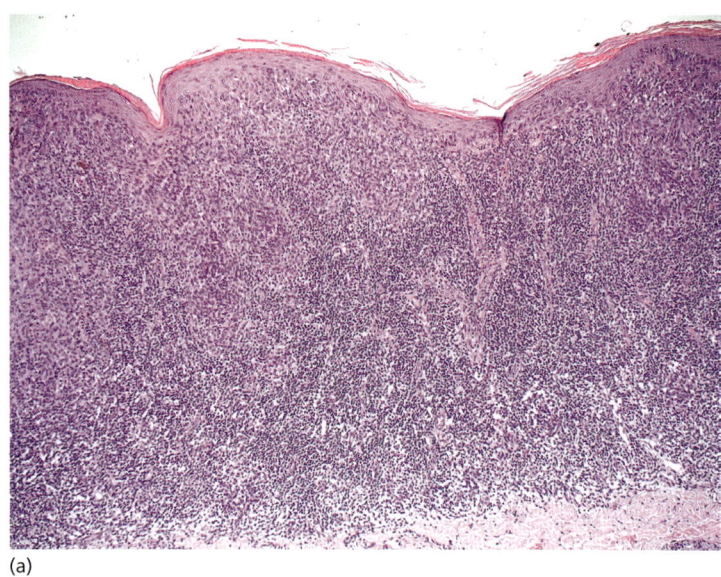
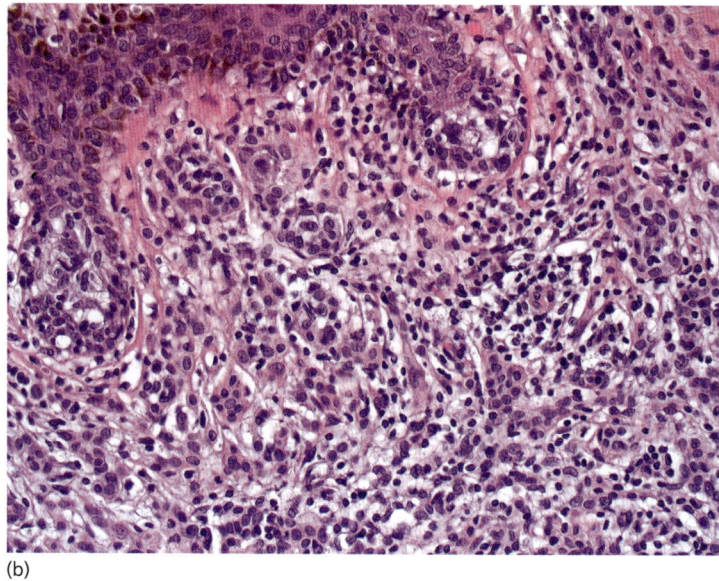

Figure 131.33 Halo naevus. (a) Dense lymphocytic infiltrate with disruption of the naevomelanocytic aggregates, especially in the mid and deep portion of the dermal component of the naevus. Magnification 10× (H&E). (b) Small lymphocytes disrupt the naevic aggregates and intermingle with single naevomelanocytes in the dermal component of the naevus. Lymphocytes are also distributed between the basal cells of the overlying epidermis and the naevic cells of junctional nests. Magnification 40× (H&E). Courtesy of Dr K. Frangia, HBD HistoBio Diagnosis, Athens, Greece.

the intraepidermal component single lymphocytes are distributed among the naevomelanocytes, in a linear pattern, extending beyond the boundaries of the dermal component in cases of compound naevi. Dihydroxy-phenylalanine staining reveals a loss of epidermal melanocytes in the depigmented area.

Environmental factors
Halo naevi sometimes appear after intense sun exposure [175].

Clinical features
Presentation
Initially, a rim of depigmentation appears around a pre-existing melanocytic naevus (Figure 131.34). This white halo is particularly visible during the summer months when the unaffected adjacent skin acquires a tan. During the following months the naevus may gradually shrink or even disappear completely, leaving a white macule. Approximately half of halo naevi undergo total clinical and histological regression.

Halo naevi are located primarily in the back. Multiple halo naevi may develop, while other adjacent naevi remain unchanged.

Differential diagnosis
In older patients presenting a single lesion, the possibility of a melanoma in regression should be excluded. In a case of melanoma, both the central pigmented area and the surrounding halo appear irregular, while the centre of the lesion presents dermoscopic features that are suggestive of melanoma. In suspicious cases, excisional biopsy should be performed.

Disease course and prognosis
The depigmented area usually persists for a decade or longer. A subgroup may progress through stages of involution with a return to normal colour, but even these lesions usually persist for several years (average of 7.8 years) [176].

Investigations
In dermoscopy, the central naevus exhibits the globular and/or homogeneous patterns characteristic of melanocytic naevi in young ages, surrounded by a rim of white regression-like depigmentation with a variable diameter (Figure 131.34b) [**153**,177].

Management
No treatment is required. Patients should be reassured, particularly in case of multiple lesions, and UV protection measures to avoid sunburn of the depigmented skin area is advised. A halo naevus presenting in an older patient should raise concern, especially in the absence of vitiligo and no history of halo naevi in the past. In such cases, a thorough skin and lymph node examination is recommended to exclude melanoma elsewhere.

Meyerson naevus

Definition and nomenclature
This is a melanocytic naevus that develops an eczematous-like inflammatory reaction.

Synonyms and inclusions
- Halo eczema naevus
- Halo dermatitis naevus

Epidemiology
Incidence and prevalence
A Meyerson naevus is an unusual type of naevus.

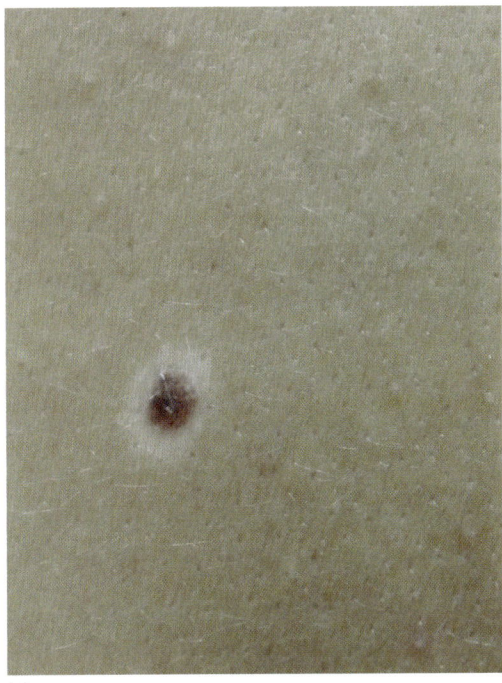

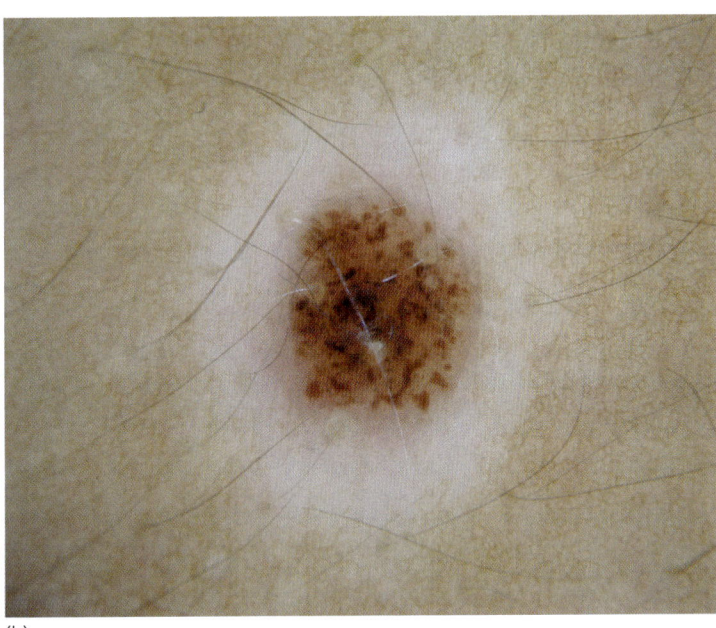

Figure 131.34 (a) Halo naevus. (b) Dermoscopic image of a halo naevus showing a symmetrical compound naevus (globular pattern) surrounded by a whitish halo.

Age
It usually presents in young individuals.

Associated diseases
Meyerson naevi have been associated with atopic eczema.

Pathophysiology
The aetiopathogenesis of this naevus remains unclear. Theories proposing an atypical pityriasis rosea-like reaction, subacute allergic dermatitis or a hypersensitivity reaction have not been confirmed [178–181].

Predisposing factors
Treatment with interferon α has been reported prior to the development of Meyerson naevi [182,183].

Pathology
Histology reveals a common, usually compound, melanocytic naevus with associated spongiotic dermatitis of the overlying epidermis. Also seen is a dense, perivascular infiltrate in the upper dermis composed mainly of CD4+ lymphocytes and occasionally eosinophils.

Environmental factors
Severe sunburn has been implicated [184].

Clinical features
Presentation
Meyerson naevus, originally described by Meyerson in 1971, presents as a melanocytic naevus that develops a red-coloured halo with overlying scales (Figure 131.35). The lesion resembles a naevus with superimposed discoid eczema and it may be slightly pruritic. It usually arises on the trunk and proximal extremities. Multiple lesions can occur.

Halo dermatitis has been reported around various benign skin lesions (e.g. common acquired and congenital naevi, Sutton naevi, Spitz naevi, clinically atypical naevi, sebaceous naevus, keloids, insect bites, seborrhoeic keratoses, dermatofibromas) and malignant skin lesions (e.g. melanoma, basal and squamous cell carcinomas) [185].

Differential diagnosis
Single lesions could occasionally be confused with melanoma or halo naevus. In multiple Meyerson naevi, the differential diagnosis includes pityriasis rosea and roseola of secondary syphilis [153].

Disease course and prognosis
The eczematoid changes usually resolve spontaneously after a few months, leaving the involved naevus intact, although some degree of hypopigmentation or even complete resolution of the naevus has been described [186]. Meyerson naevus is a similar lesion to halo naevus and may coexist with this entity in the same patient. Occasionally, a Meyerson naevus can progress to a halo naevus or vice versa [187,188].

Investigations
Dermoscopy reveals the benign pattern of the involved melanocytic naevus, often blurred by a yellowish, overlying, superficial serocrust (Figure 131.35b) [153].

Management
Normally, the eczematous reaction subsides after 1–2 weeks of treatment with a moderately potent topical steroid. Clinical re-evaluation and dermoscopic examination will confirm that the underlying naevus is benign.

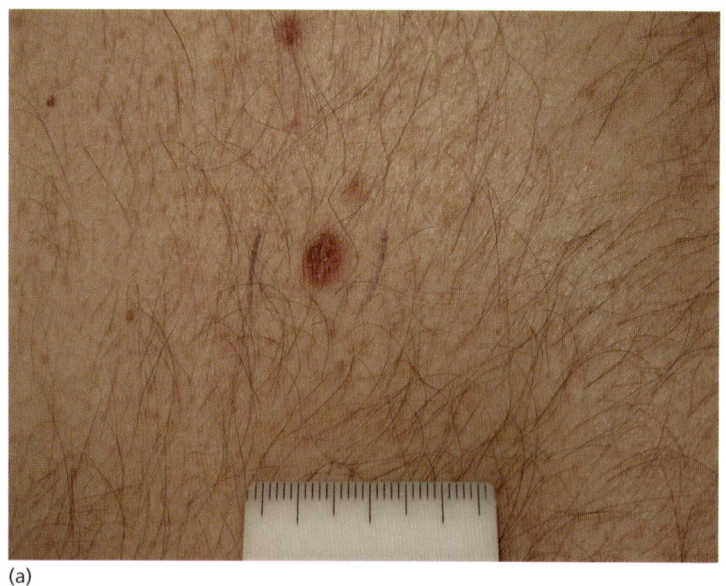
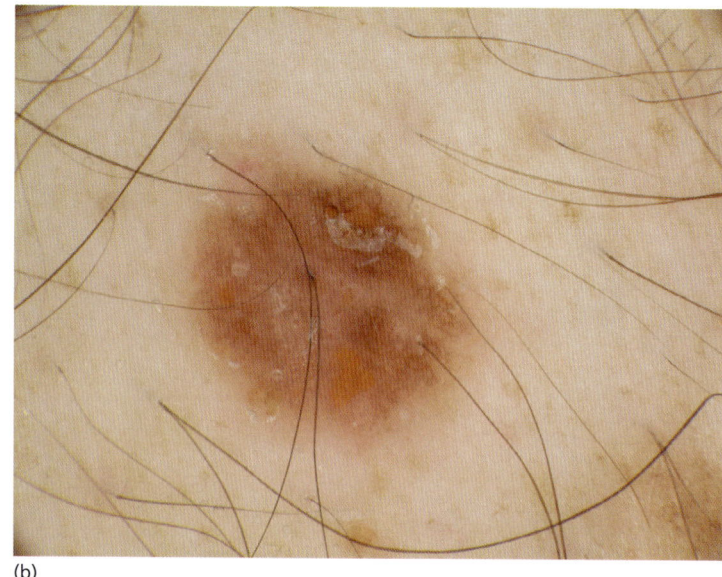

Figure 131.35 Meyerson naevus. (a) A small-sized naevus with an eczematous component. (b) Dermoscopic image showing yellowish crusts covering a naevus with a faint brownish network. Courtesy of Dr I. Zalaudek, Skin Cancer Unit Arcispedale Santa Maria Nuova – IRCCS Reggio Emilia, Italy.

Cockade naevus

Definition and nomenclature
A cockade naevus is a benign melanocytic lesion with a target-like appearance resembling a rosette.

Synonyms and inclusions
- Target-like naevus
- Kokarden naevus
- Naevus en cocarde

Epidemiology
Incidence and prevalence
A cockade naevus is an uncommon type of naevus.

Age
It usually presents in children and adolescents.

Pathophysiology
It has been proposed that naevus cells in the central and peripheral areas produce melanin more actively [189], or that there is a lack of melanin synthesis involving the melanocytes of the non-pigmented rim [190].

Pathology
The central component of the naevus is that of a junctional or compound type, while the periphery of the lesion is composed of junctional nests and may present increased pigment in the dermis [191].

Clinical features
Presentation
The central component of the naevus is a dark, often papular area, which is surrounded by a non-pigmented circular zone and an outer pigmented ring (Figure 131.36). Lesions are usually multiple and located on the trunk, or on the scalp in young patients.

Differential diagnosis
A target-like appearance has also been reported in association with blue naevi [192] and melanoma [193].

Investigations
Dermoscopy reveals a naevus with a darker, central globular or homogeneous pattern, surrounded by a structureless inner ring and a more peripheral darker reticular ring (Figure 131.36b) [194,195].

Management
A cockade naevus is a benign lesion, thus no treatment is required.

Targetoid haemosiderotic naevus

Definition
A targetoid haemosiderotic naevus derives from mechanical trauma of a melanocytic naevus, which is usually elevated or exophytic.

Epidemiology
Incidence and prevalence
It is common in children and young adults. The upper chest is the most common location [196,197].

Naevi with unusual morphology

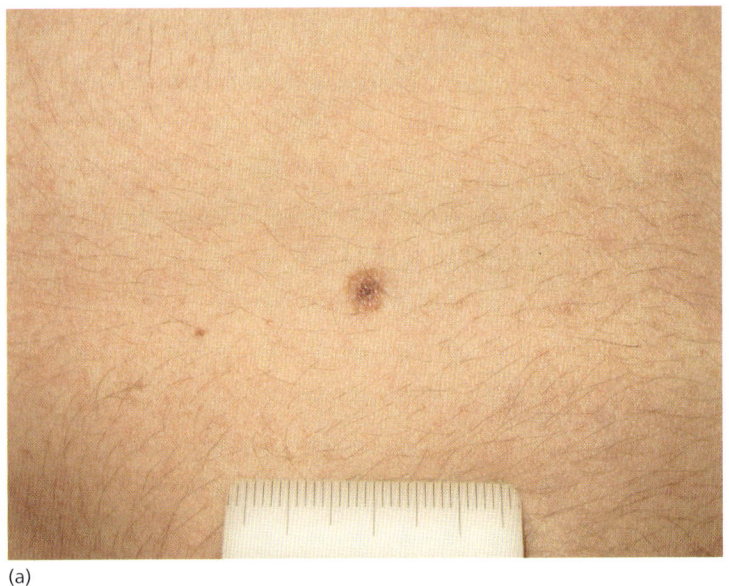
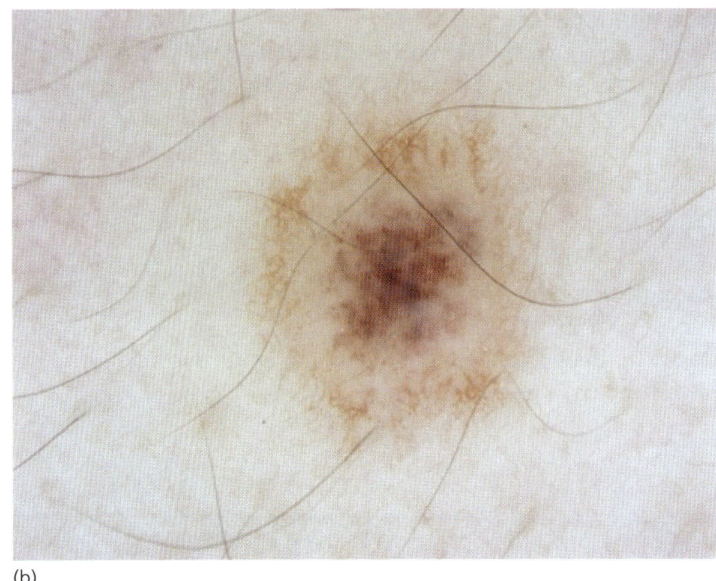

Figure 131.36 (a) Cockade naevus. (b) Dermoscropic image of a cockade naevus showing a darker, central homogeneous pattern, a lighter inner ring and a peripheral brown reticular ring. Courtesy of Dr I. Zalaudek, Skin Cancer Unit Arcispedale Santa Maria Nuova – IRCCS Reggio Emilia, Italy.

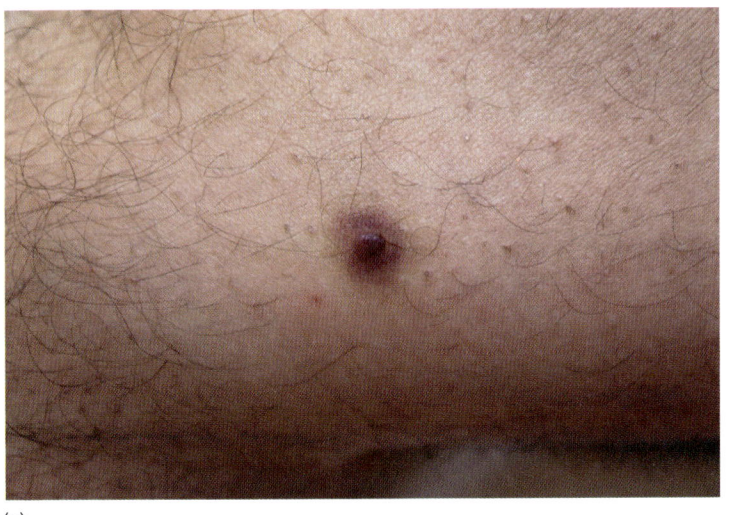
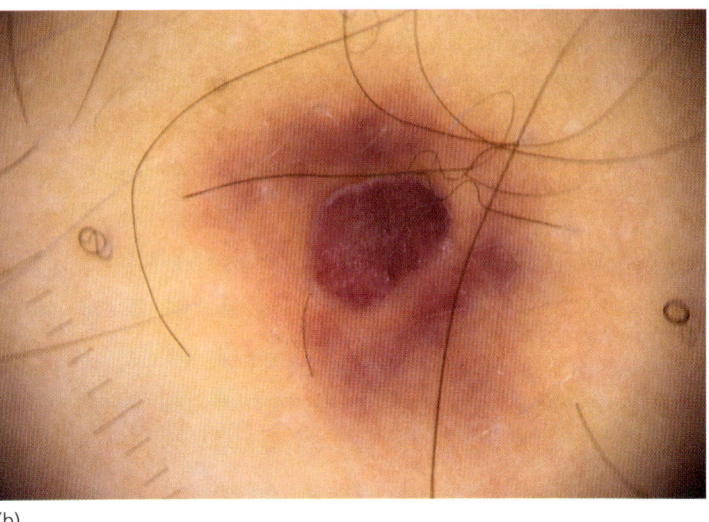

Figure 131.37 Targetoid haemosiderotic naevus. (a) Naevus acutely presenting with a haemorrhagic halo. (b) Dermoscopic image showing a peripheral, structureless, purple rim around a central pre-existing naevus.

Pathophysiology
Pathology
Histopathologically, targetoid haemosiderotic naevus consists of naevus cells mingled with extravasated blood vessels and an increased number of irregular, ectatic, vascular channels. The peripheral halo demonstrates extensive haemorrhage with haemosiderin and fibrin deposits combined with slit-shaped vascular channels that dissect in between collagen bundles. A mild, inflammatory, primarily eosinophilic infiltrate is also seen.

Clinical features
History
Targetoid haemosiderotic naevus usually appears as a sudden change of pigmentation in a pre-existing naevus following mechanical irritation, usually from clothing, shaving or scratching [196,197]. A history of trauma or irritation is not always apparent to the patient. Symptoms indicating trauma such as pain, tenderness or pruritus are common.

Presentation
Clinically, the lesion presents as a brown, red-brown or violaceous papule surrounded by a thin pale area and a peripheral ecchymotic area that tends to expand, become fainter and resolve while the central papule persists (Figure 131.37).

Differential diagnosis
The differential diagnosis includes targetoid haemosiderotic haemangioma, cockade naevus, traumatised angiokeratoma and melanoma.

Investigations
Dermoscopy reveals haemorrhagic changes with a red to purple colour, surrounding a naevus with a usually globular pattern (Figure 131.37b) [198]. Jet-black areas with irregular shape and size as well as comma-shaped vessels are also seen. The periphery of the lesion representing the ecchymotic halo shows an ill-defined, pale area surrounded by a reddish zone with jagged edges.

Management
Management includes reassurance of the patient and the use of a topical antibiotic or steroid preparation until the inflammatory/haemorrhagic changes have resolved.

OTHER NAEVI

Spitz naevus

Definition and nomenclature
A Spitz naevus is a melanocytic lesion characterised by spindled and/or epitheloid naevomelanocytes.

Synonyms and inclusions
- Spindle and epithelioid cell naevus
- Spitz tumour
- Benign juvenile melanoma

Introduction and general description
Spitz naevus was initially described by Sophie Spitz as an unusual type of melanocytic proliferation in children, with features histologically indistinguishable from melanoma (hence the original term of 'juvenile melanoma'), but with a favourable prognosis [199]. Currently the entity of Spitz naevi remains a subject of controversy due to their clinical and histological variability, their overlapping histological characteristics with melanoma and the uncertainty of their biological behaviour in certain cases. Refinement of the various clinical and histological subtypes of Spitz naevi has resulted in a highly complex morphological classification of these tumours [200,**201**]. At one end of the spectrum is the common or classic Spitz naevus (see Table 131.3), a benign proliferation frequently occurring in children; at the other end are lesions with extensive pleomorphic features sufficient for the diagnosis of melanoma ('malignant Spitz tumours' or 'Spitz melanoma'). In between lies a heterogeneous group of lesions with varying features and unknown malignant potential termed 'atypical Spitz tumours' or 'Spitzoid lesions of uncertain malignant potential (STUMP)' [202–205]. These and other borderline lesions, such as atypical blue naevi and deep penetrating naevi, are included in 'melanocytic tumours of uncertain malignant potential (MELTUMP)', a term used for atypical melanocytic proliferations in the dermis that are tumourigenic, but lack the specific criteria needed to distinguish between benign and malignant lesions [131].

Epidemiology
Incidence and prevalence
Spitz naevi account for 1% of excised naevi in children [206].

Age
Spitz naevi are more commonly seen in younger ages. Approximately 40% of lesions occur in patients under the age of 15 years and 77% before the age of 30 [207].

Sex
Both sexes are equally affected, although age-dependent variations may be observed [207–210].

Ethnicity
Spitz naevi occur predominantly in white populations, but they have also been described in black, Hispanic and Asian groups [211,212].

Associated diseases
Disseminated, eruptive Spitz naevi have been reported to occur with Addison disease, HIV infection, chemotherapy, puberty and pregnancy [213,214].

Pathophysiology
Most lesions are acquired, but up to 7% of Spitz naevi can occur congenitally [215].

Pathology
The 'classic' Spitz naevus typically is a symmetrical and well-defined compound naevus. Intraepidermal and intradermal forms have been also reported [216]. There is a degree of epidermal hyperplasia overlying the naevus, without evidence of malignant intraepidermal pagetoid spreading of naevic cells (Figure 131.38a). Naevomelanocytic nests are neatly located between keratinocytes, unlike their disorderly arrangement in melanoma. The naevomelanocytic nests at the dermal–epidermal junction are often separated from the surrounding keratinocytes by a cleft caused by a retraction artefact. The naevus cells may be either spindle shaped, streaming into the dermis in interlacing bundles, or epithelioid, arranged in clusters, with giant and multinucleated naevus cells seen among them.

Kamino bodies (i.e. amorphous eosinophilic globules containing periodic acid–Schiff-positive basement membrane constituents) are noted intraepidermally and at the dermal–epidermal junction (Figure 131.38b) [217,218]. Their presence is neither sensitive nor specific for Spitz naevi as they may also be present in early melanoma.

In classic Spitz naevi, dermal naevomelanocytic nests and fascicles exhibit a zonation phenomenon with depth, for example uniformity in size, shape and spacing along horizontal planes. Typical mitoses may occur, especially in the upper and mid-portion of the lesion. They usually do not exceed a rate of $2/mm^2$. Dermal vessels are dilated, and the stroma is oedematous and infiltrated by lymphocytes [210].

Several histological features have been considered to indicate a more aggressive behaviour. A Spitz naevus thicker than 1 mm in

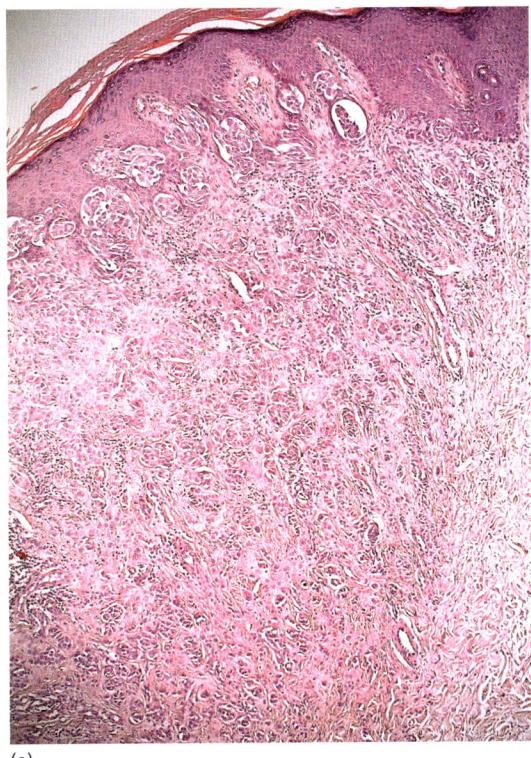

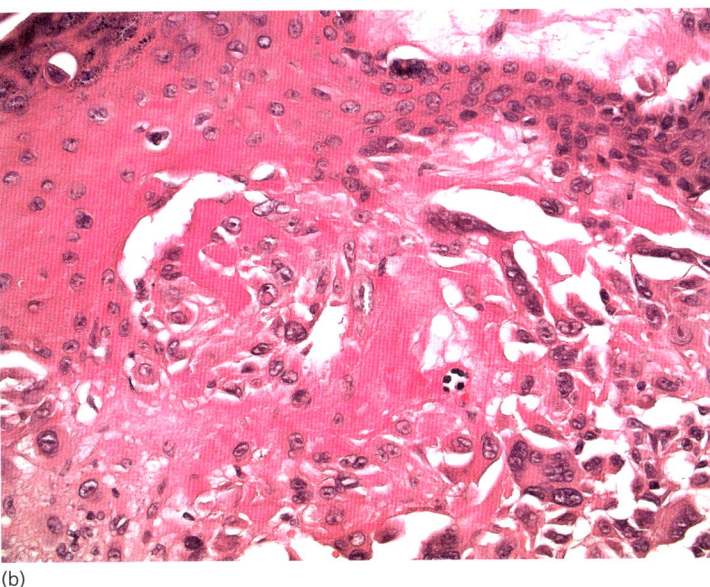

Figure 131.38 Compound naevus of Spitz. (a) Sparsely demarcated naevomelanocytic proliferation at the junctional area and mainly in the dermis. The dermal component has prominent cellular pleomorphism and evidence of maturation in the deeper portion of the lesion. Magnification 10× (H&E). (b) Epithelioid cells with eosinophilic cytoplasm and nuclear pleomorphism with prominent nucleoli. Multinucleated giant cells are common. Eosinophilic, partially coalescent, Kamino bodies are present in the junctional area and upper papillary dermis. Magnification 40× (H&E). Courtesy of Dr K. Frangia, HBD HistoBio Diagnosis, Athens, Greece.

depth, with asymmetry, poor circumscription, deeper extension and ulceration is considered to have increased metastatic potential [219]. In addition, single cell pagetoid spread beyond the epidermal nests, lack of zonation with depth and persistent expansile deep nests with more deeply seated mitotic activity, are considered to be atypical histological features. Cellular heterogeneity and atypical cytology (higher nuclear to cytoplasmic ratios, hyperchromatism and abnormal nuclear borders) are additional findings supportive of an atypical lesion [220].

Reed naevi, widely considered to be a pigmented subtype of Spitz naevi, presents with an organised symmetrical and uniform architecture, similar to classic Spitz naevi. A well-demarcated junctional melanocytic activity with large quantities of melanin pigment is noted (Figure 131.39a). Spindle-shaped melanocytes proliferate downwards towards the papillary dermis but rarely involve the reticular dermis (Figure 131.39b) [221].

Desmoplastic Spitz naevi are predominantly intradermal lesions, characterised by a relatively small number of mainly isolated large and bizarre cells with copious cytoplasm distributed among thick collagen fibres. Mitotic figures are rare [222].

Immunohistochemistry can be used to differentiate Spitz naevi from melanoma. MIB-1, which stains the proliferative marker Ki-67, has a lower expression in Spitz naevi compared with melanoma [223], while HMB-45 is more superficially expressed with diminished staining in the deeper dermal component [224]. S100 and Mart-1 are more weakly stained in Spitz naevi [225], whereas the S100A6 subtype shows more intense and diffuse expression in Spitz naevi compared with its weak and patchy staining in melanoma [226]. p16 reactivity is stained more intensely in desmoplastic Spitz naevi, while it is largely absent in melanomas [227].

Genetics

The very rare incidence of *NRAS* and *BRAF* mutations in Spitz naevi compared with other melanocytic lesions, and the presence of *HRAS* mutations in a subgroup of Spitz naevi (c. 20%), suggests a distinct activation of the RAS pathway components in different melanocytic neoplasms [228–230]. A number of copy number aberrations have been described in atypical Spitz tumours, including isolated loss at 3p21 (in *BAP1*-associated Spitz tumours), 6q23 and 9p21 [231,232]. The majority (c. 55%) of Spitz naevi and atypical Spitz tumours have mutually exclusive kinase fusions as primary initiating genomic events [131,233]. Genomic rearrangements activate oncogenic signalling pathways and involve the kinases *ALK*, *ROS1*, *NTRK1*, *NTRK3*, *BRAF*, *RET* and *MET* [131,234–237].

In contrast to tumours with heterozygous 9p21 deletions on FISH, atypical Spitz tumours with homozygous 9p21 deletions have been associated with a considerably worse prognosis [232].

Multiple cutaneous, spitzoid, melanocytic tumours can occur in the context of a familial autosomal dominant syndrome caused by inactivating mutations of the *BAP1* gene. Skin-coloured papules and nodules (Figure 131.40) characterised histologically by a naevoid silhouette with large epithelioid melanocytes and an immunohistochemical loss of *BAP1* (termed naevoid melanoma-like melanocytic proliferations, BAPomas, or *BAP1*-inactivated naevi) are typical features of this syndrome, along with a predisposition to cutaneous and uveal melanoma [156,238].

Clinical features
History
Spitz naevi usually develop rapidly over a period of 3–6 months, reaching sizes of 1–2 cm. Following this rapid growth period, the lesions remain stable in size. Reports of spontaneous involution over

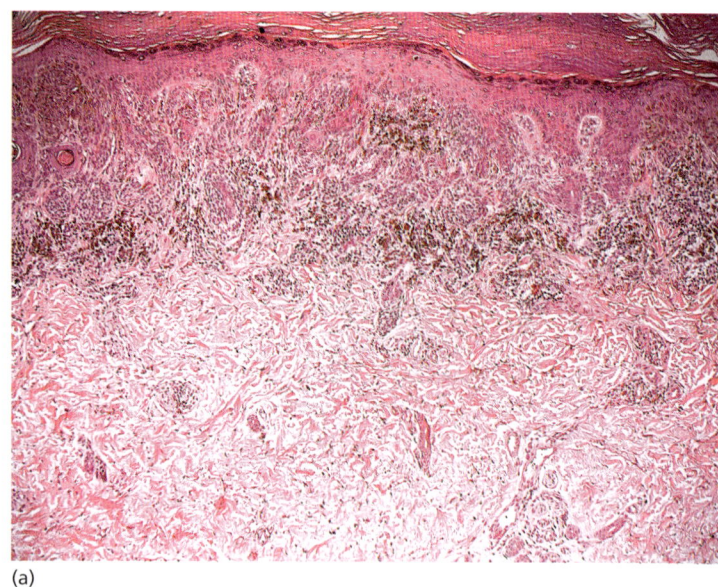
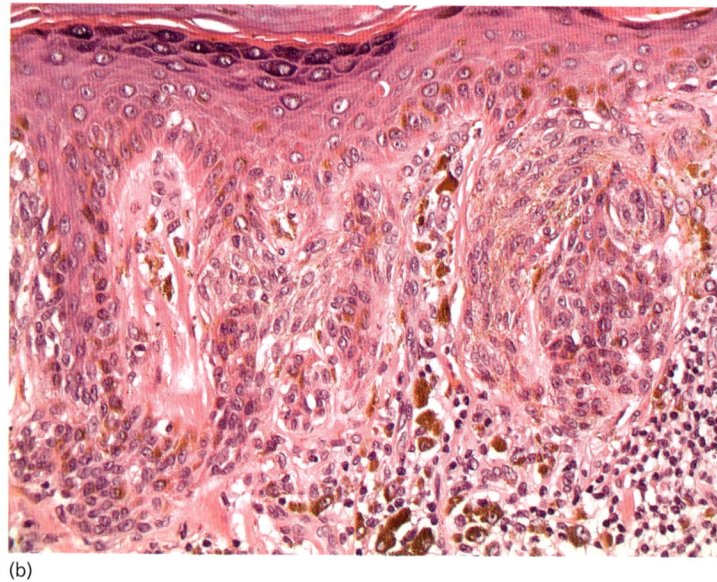

Figure 131.39 Pigmented spindle cell naevus of Reed. (a) An almost exclusively intraepidermal naevomelanocytic lesion with heavily pigmented spindle cells arranged in fascicles. There are aggregates of melanophages in the dermis beneath the lesion. Magnification 10× (H&E). (b) Epithelioid cells arranged in fascicles, often orientated vertically to the surface of the skin. A chronic inflammatory component with melanophages is prominent beneath the lesion. Magnification 40× (H&E). Courtesy of Dr K. Frangia, HBD HistoBio Diagnosis, Athens, Greece.

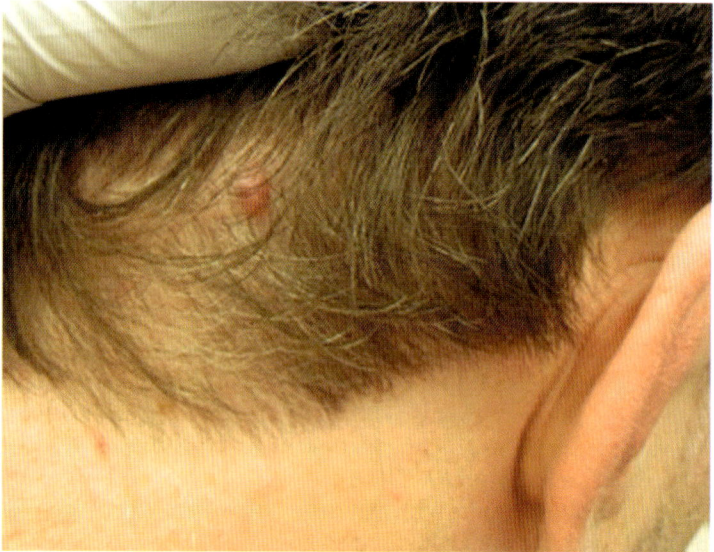

Figure 131.40 *BAP1*-inactivated naevus of the scalp. Courtesy of Dr H. Tsao, MGH Melanoma and Pigmented Lesion Center, Dermatology, Massachusetts General Hospital, MA, USA.

time or conversion to more common types of melanocytic naevi have been reported [239].

Presentation

The classic Spitz naevus usually appears as a solitary, firm, symmetrical, sharply demarcated, round or dome-shaped nodule of equal or less than 5–6 mm diameter on average. The colour of the lesion is pink to red to reddish brown (Figure 131.41). Firm pressure or diascopy reveals the degree of melanin pigmentation. Ten per cent of Spitz naevi are pigmented lesions with colours that range from tan to brown to black (Figure 131.42). The surface of the lesion is smooth, with a thin, fragile epidermis, often causing bleeding and crusting after minor injury. The commonest sites for Spitz naevi are the head and neck area (37%), particularly the face and cheek in children, and the lower extremities (28%) in young adults [240,241]. Atypical Spitz tumours tend to be larger, more asymmetrical or ulcerated with irregular pigmentation and border outline (Table 131.4; Figure 131.43).

Clinical variants

A more deeply pigmented variant of Spitz naevus, called the spindle cell naevus of Reed, and initially described in 1975 [243], occurs mainly in young females and is most commonly seen on the thighs. It usually presents as solitary, densely pigmented, irregularly shaped, dark-brown or black nodule (Figure 131.44) [241].

Rare accounts of multiple eruptive or disseminated Spitz naevi involving the entire cutaneous surface have been reported [244–246]. In agminated Spitz naevi, multiple Spitz naevi can also occur in a grouped fashion, resembling a speckled congenital naevus.

Desmoplastic Spitz naevus is a rare subtype of the Spitz naevus encountered most commonly in adults [208]. These lesions are usually pink or red, firm, raised nodules with little or no clinically visible melanocytic pigmentation. A desmoplastic Spitz is often the presenting type of a recurrent Spitz naevus following incomplete removal [247,248].

Differential diagnosis

The differential diagnosis of Spitz naevi includes acquired, dysplastic and congenital variants of melanocytic naevi and melanoma. A number of non-melanocytic entities should also be considered such as dermatofibroma, molluscum contagiosum, pyogenic granuloma, haemangioma, mastocytoma, juvenile and adult xanthogranuloma, angiofibroma, histiocytoma and granuloma.

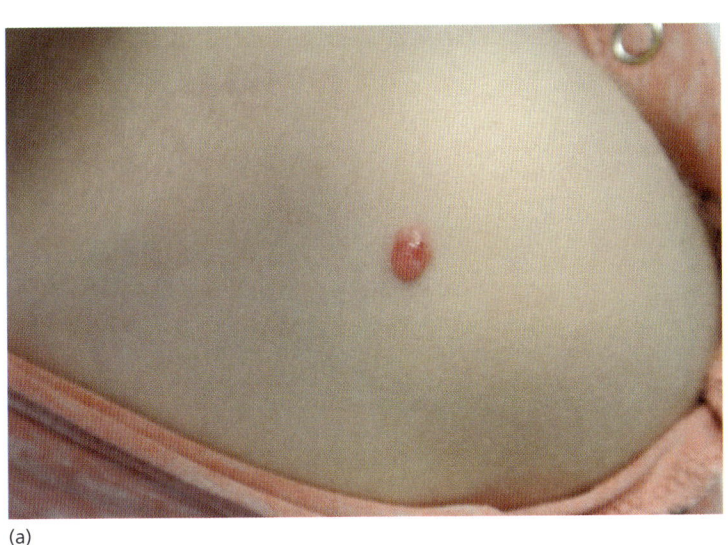
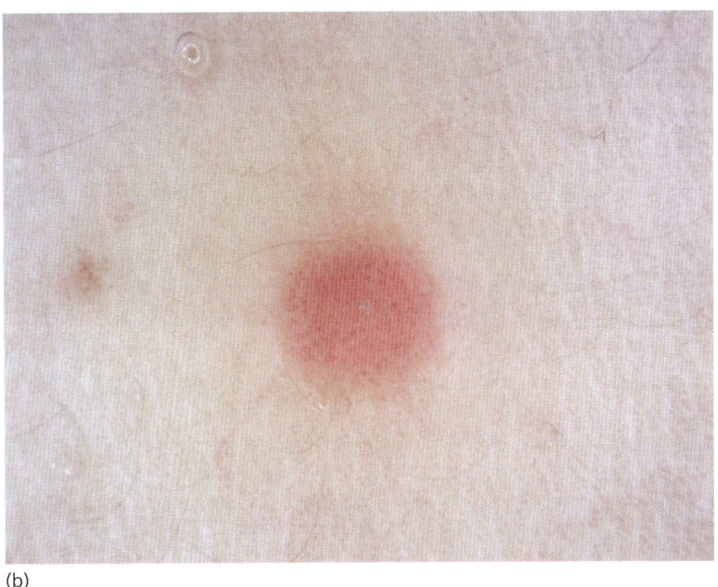

Figure 131.41 Classic Spitz naevus. (a) A well-circumscribed pink nodule. (b) A round, symmetrical lesion with dotted vessels and lack of pigmentation.

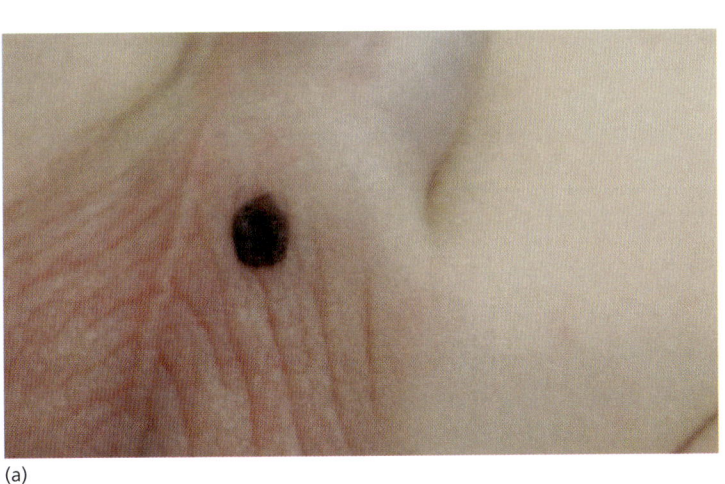
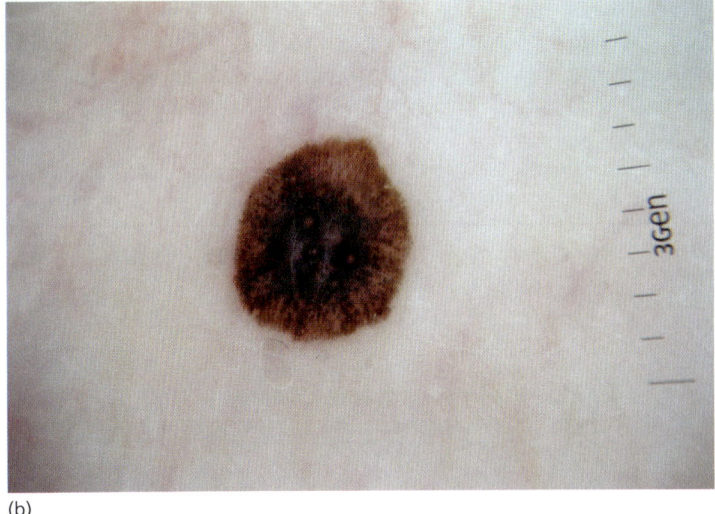

Figure 131.42 (a) Pigmented Spitz naevus. (b) Dermoscopic image of a pigmented Spitz naevus showing a well-circumscribed symmetrical nodule with a papillomatous surface and various shades of brown pigmentation.

Disease course and prognosis

Even though the metastatic behaviour of atypical Spitz tumours is well established, their malignant potential is debated since they only rarely result in a fatal outcome [249,250]. The use of sentinel lymph node biopsy in atypical Spitz tumours has clarified the rate of lymph node positivity (average of 39%) [251–256]. Only 19% of sentinel lymph node biopsy positive cases resulted in positive nodes after complete lymphadenectomy and very few led to death in the immediate follow-up period [256]. Risk stratification schemes using pathological criteria have attempted to classify Spitz tumours based on their metastatic potential. One study identified abnormal mitoses, mitotic counts of over $2/mm^2$ and deep mitoses as suggestive of spitzoid melanoma [257]. Spatz *et al.* have identified age over 10 years, diameter over 10 mm, ulceration, invasion to subcutaneous fat and mitotic activity of over $6/mm^2$ as suggestive of spitzoid melanoma rather than Spitz naevi [219]. Interobserver variations, even between expert pathologists, for spitzoid lesions are significant [200].

Investigations

Upon dermoscopy, Spitz naevi can demonstrate a diversity of patterns [258]. The classic, less pigmented variant (pink colour) shows a predominantly dotted vascular pattern with reticular depigmentation (see Figure 131.41b). Pigmented Spitz naevi or Reed naevi exhibit a 'starburst' pattern, a globular pattern or a multicomponent atypical pattern (see Figures 131.42b and 131.44b) [259]. Although there are no reliable dermoscopic features that characterise atypical Spitz tumours [260], these lesions often exhibit

Table 131.4 Clinical, histological, immunohistochemical and molecular features of classic and atypical Spitz naevi.

	Classic Spitz naevi	Atypical Spitz tumours
Clinical features		
Age	<10 years	>10 years
Location	Face, neck, extremities (thighs)	Trunk (back in men)
Diameter	<10 mm (usually 5–6 mm)	>10 mm
Symmetry	Usually symmetrical	Increasing asymmetry
Border	Well defined	Irregular
Surface	Smooth	Possibly ulcerated
Colour	Pink/red	Irregular
Histology features		
Architecture	Symmetrical, sharply demarcated, dome shaped, non-disruptive, orderly dispersion and regular spacing of nests and cells	Asymmetrical, poorly demarcated, infiltrating, irregular spacing and disorderly arrangement of nests and cells
Epidermal changes	Intact epidermis	Ulceration
Pagetoid spread	Limited pagetoid spread in lower epidermis	Single-cell pagetoid spread, beyond epidermal nests
Clefting	Presence of junctional clefting	Lack of junctional clefting
Kamino bodies	Aggregates of Kamino bodies	Absent or few Kamino bodeis
Zonation	Uniformity of cytological features across horizontal planes	Lack of zonation
Maturation	Maturation (smaller nests with depth), lack of deep involvement	Persistent expansile nests, subcutaneous involvement
Cell type	Spindle or epithelioid cell type	Heterogeneous cell types
Mitoses	Mitoses <2 mm^2, superficial, usually not atypical	Mitoses >2–6 mm^2, deeply located, atypical
Cytology	Low nuclear to cytoplasmic ratio	High nuclear to cytoplasmic ratio
	Ground glass or opaque cytoplasm	Granular or 'dusty' cytoplasm in epithelioid cells, scant in spindle cells
Nuclear changes	Uniform nucleoli, delicate, dispersed chomatin	Large, eosinophilic nucleoli, hyperchromatism
Immunohistochemistry features		
Immunohistochemistry	Weaker stain for S100 and Ki-67; low Ki-67 proliferation index (<5%); superficial expression of HMB45	Stronger expression of S100 and Ki-67; low to intermediate Ki-67 proliferation index (5–15%); deeper stain for HMB45
Molecular features		
Cytogenetic techniques (CGH, FISH) and mutational profile	Array CGH: isolated gains of 7p, 11q; *HRAS* mutations; kinase fusions	Array CGH: often ≥1 chromosomal abnormality; kinase fusions; *PTEN* mutations; heterozygous or homozygous loss of 9p21

CGH, comparative genomic hybridisation; FISH, fluorescent *in situ* hybridisation. Adapted from Elder *et al.* 2018 [**131**]; Luo *et al.* 2011 [**201**]; Spatz *et al.* 1999 [**219**]; Barnhill 2006 [**242**].

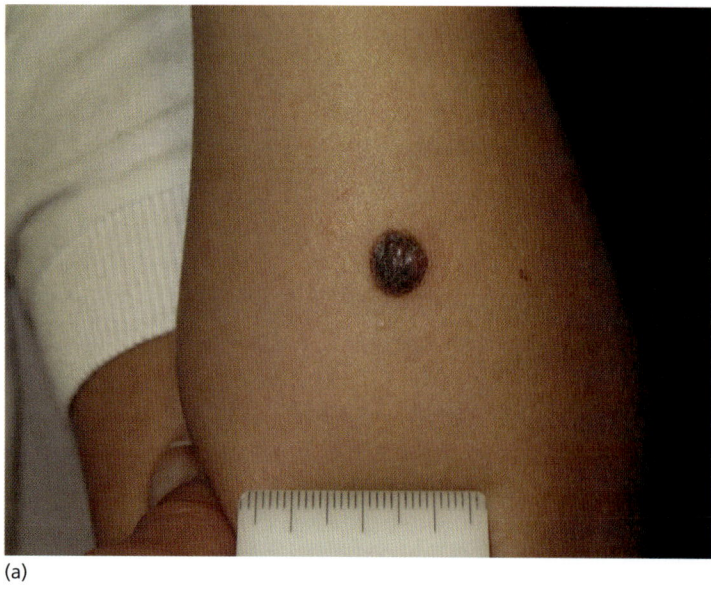

(a)

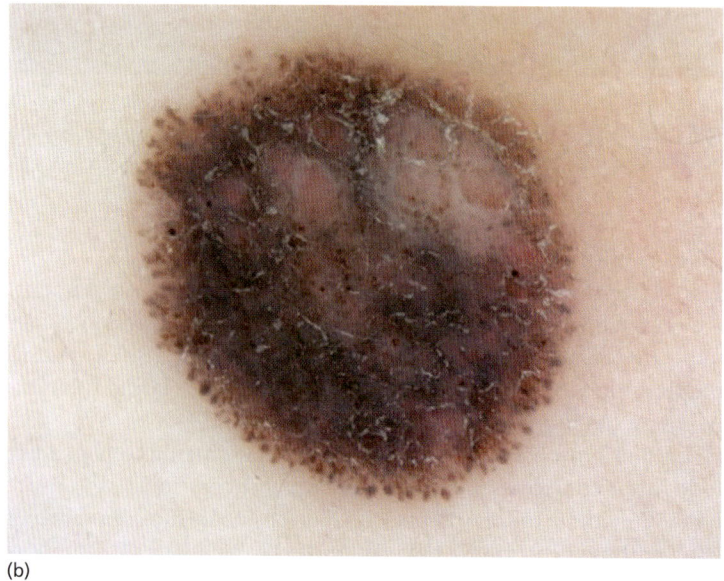

(b)

Figure 131.43 Atypical Spitz tumour. (a) Asymmetrical nodule with heterogeneous pigmentation. (b) Dermoscopic image of the symmetrical, peripheral distribution of pigmented streaks and heterogeneous pigmentation with bluish/black and whitish hue. Courtesy of Dr I. Zalaudek, Skin Cancer Unit Arcispedale Santa Maria Nuova – IRCCS Reggio Emilia, Italy.

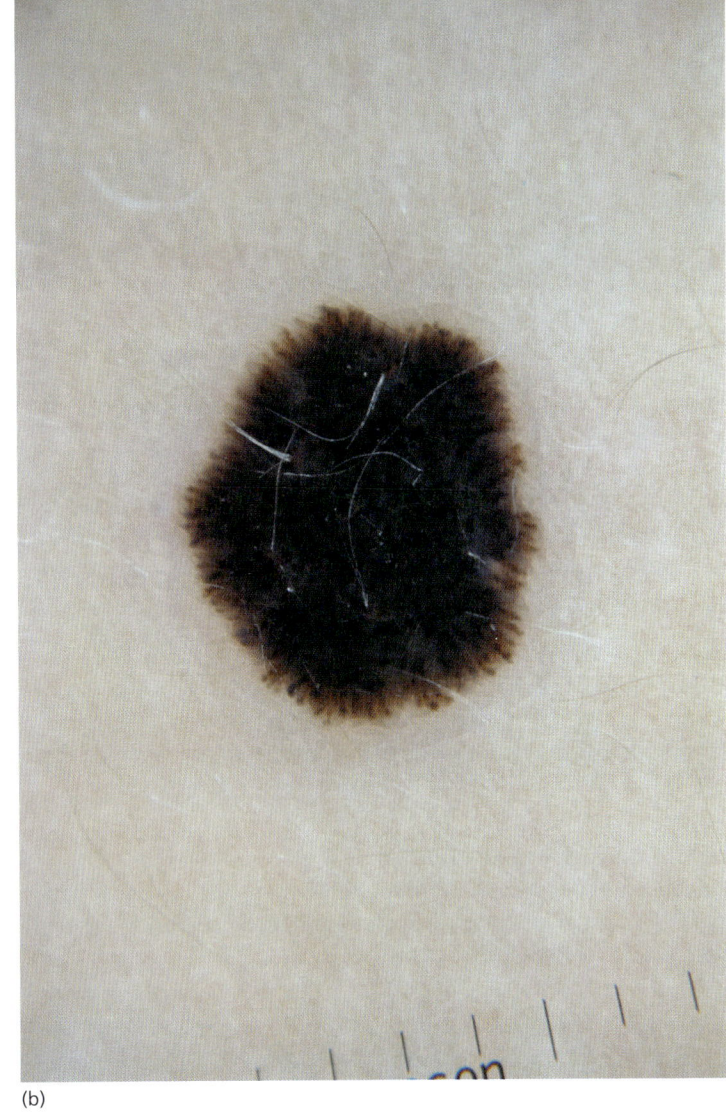

Figure 131.44 Reed naevus. (a) Darkly pigmented symmetrical macule. (b) Dermoscopic image showing a 'starburst' pattern with diffuse blue-black pigmentation and symmetrically distributed radial streaks in the periphery.

nodularity, asymmetrical peripheral distribution of pigmented streaks, heterogeneous pigmentation with bluish-black and whitish hue and white lines (see Figure 131.43b). *In vivo* reflectance confocal microscopy can offer further assistance in differentiating Spitz naevi from melanomas for lesions showing starburst and globular patterns on dermoscopy [261].

Management

There is a lack of consensus regarding management. Because of the clinical and histological overlap between Spitz naevi and melanoma some authors suggest that all spitzoid lesions should be surgically removed and examined histologically. Local excision of the lesion with a margin of 1–3 mm is usually sufficient to confirm the diagnosis [262]. Since local recurrences have been reported at a rate of 7–16% [263], often presenting with a more atypical histology and increased desmoplasia, incompletely removed tumours should be re-excised [206]. Due to the benign nature of typical or classic Spitz naevi in childhood, some experts suggest close monitoring of dermoscopically symmetric, flat spitzoid-looking lesions in children younger than 12 years, as an alternative to surgical excision [264,265]. Taking no further action in this specific setting of lesions and age group has also been proposed [266]. The histological diagnosis of an atypical Spitz tumour should be approached more aggressively and treated with a wide margin resection following the guidelines of melanoma resection. Patients can be reassured that the lesion may in fact be benign.

The significance of sentinel lymph node biopsy positivity and how to manage the presence of nodal disease further is questionable [249]. Given the low fatality rate of atypical Spitz tumours, the limited evidence of a survival benefit from selective lymphadenectomy in sentinel lymph node biopsy positive cases and the potential morbidity associated with lymphadenectomy, a more judicious case-by-case use of sentinel lymph node biopsy has been recommended [267]. Results of a systematic review analysis did not show any prognostic benefit of sentinel lymph node biopsy for patients with atypical Spitz tumours [256].

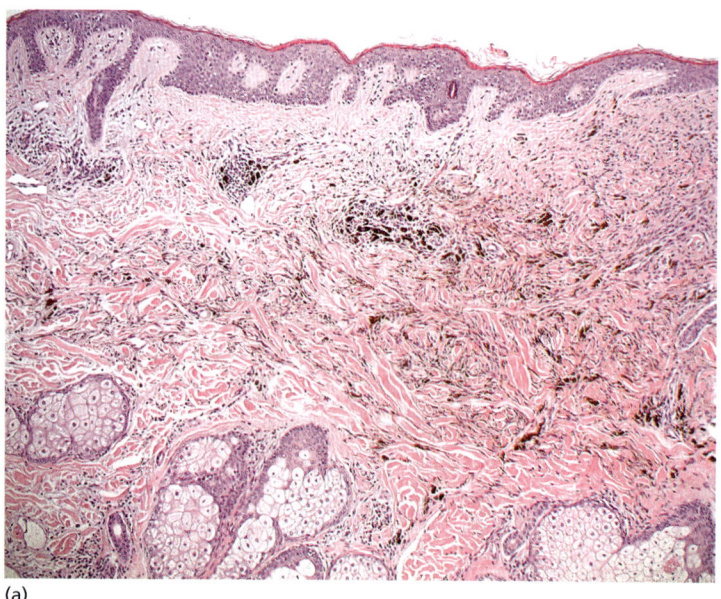
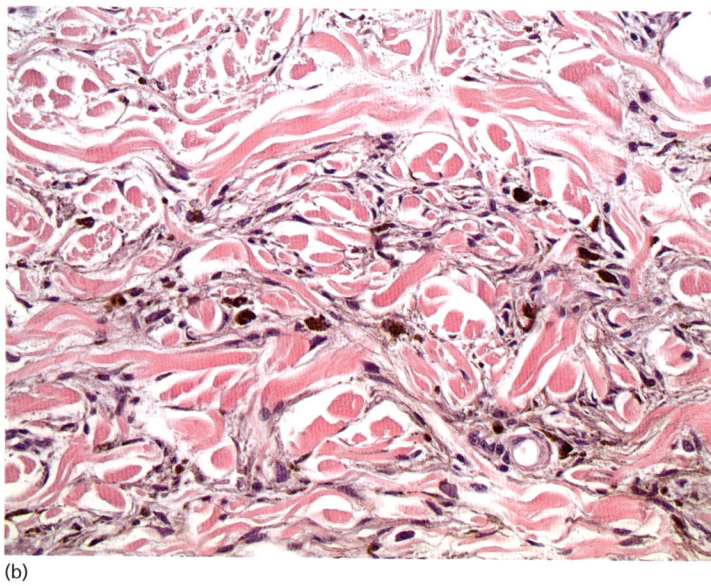

Figure 131.45 Common blue naevus. (a) Poorly circumscribed area of elongated, pigmented melanocytes in the dermis. The dendritic melanocytes are located between the collagen bundles of the reticular dermis. The overlying epidermis may be slightly hyperplastic. Magnification 10× (H&E). (b) A proliferation of elongated, dendritic melanocytes without atypia or mitoses and with finely distributed intracytoplasmic melanin can be seen among the collagen bundles of the reticular dermis. Round melanophages with heavily pigmented cytoplasm and coarse melanin intermingle with the melanocytes. Magnification × (H&E). Courtesy of Dr K. Frangia, HBD HistoBio Diagnosis, Athens, Greece.

Blue naevus and variants

Definition and nomenclature
This is a relatively common blue, blue-grey or blue-black benign melanocytic naevus comprised of dermal melanocytes, with several clinical and histological variants (see Table 131.3).

> **Synonyms and inclusions**
> - Blue naevus of Jadassohn–Tièche
> - Blue neuronaevus

Epidemiology
Incidence and prevalence
Their estimated prevalence in white populations is 0.5–4%.

Age
Blue naevi usually present during childhood, puberty or early adulthood, but can occur at all ages.

Sex
They are more common in females.

Associated diseases
Multiple epithelioid blue naevi may be associated with the LAMB (*l*entigines, *a*trial and *m*ucocutaneous myxomas and multiple *b*lue naevi) syndrome.

Pathophysiology
The aetiopathogenesis is unclear. The most favoured hypothesis proposes that blue naevi originate from latent dermal dendritic melanocytes, which are remnants of the melanocyte migration from the neural crest to the epidermis during gestation.

Pathology
Common blue naevi consist of spindle-shaped, dendritic melanocytes admixed with ovoid or fusiform, elongated melanocytes, located in the dermis in an inverted wedge shape (Figure 131.45a). Naevus cells can extend into the lower dermis along appendages or in the perivascular and perineural areas. The dendritic melanocytes do not show significant mitotic activity or atypical cytology and stain positively for S100, HMB-45 and MART-1 (Figure 131.45b). An admixture of melanophages with intracytoplasmic coarse melanin granules is often seen. With the exception of combined blue naevi, in which a blue naevus coexists with a congenital, acquired or Spitz naevus, blue naevi have no junctional component. A varying degree of stromal fibroplasia is also noted.

The cellular blue naevus has a characteristic architecture related to a 'dumb-bell'-shaped extension of the lesion to the deep reticular dermis or the subcutaneous fat (Figure 131.46). In common blue naevi there are nodules or fascicles of larger, oval to spindle naevomelanocytes with clear vacuolated, less pigmented cytoplasm. These cells stain positively for S100, HMB-4 and MART-1, and show rare mitotic activity or cytological atypia [268]. Variable numbers of melanophages with coarse melanin pigment are also present.

Cellular blue naevi with increased atypia and mitoses (3–4 mitoses/mm^2) have been designated as atypical cellular blue naevi, a term used to denote a biological behaviour intermediate between cellular blue naevus and malignant blue naevus.

Epithelioid blue naevus (or pigmented epithelioid melanocytoma) can occur sporadically or in association with the Carney complex. The histological features that distinguish it from common

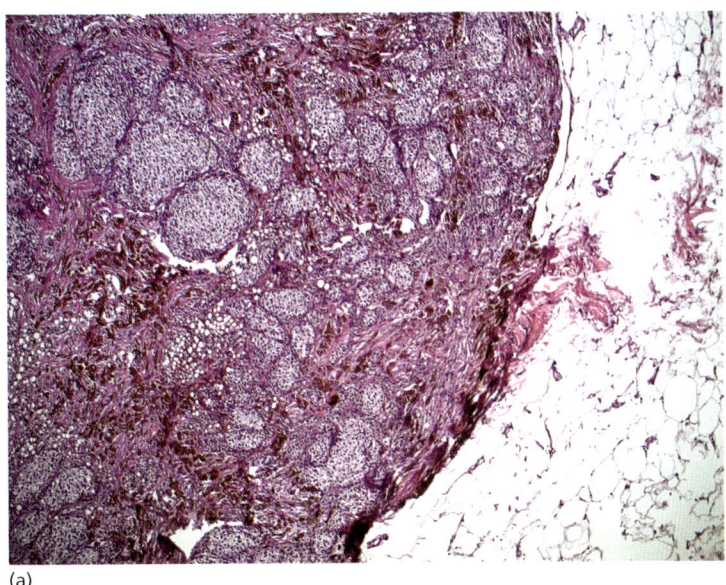
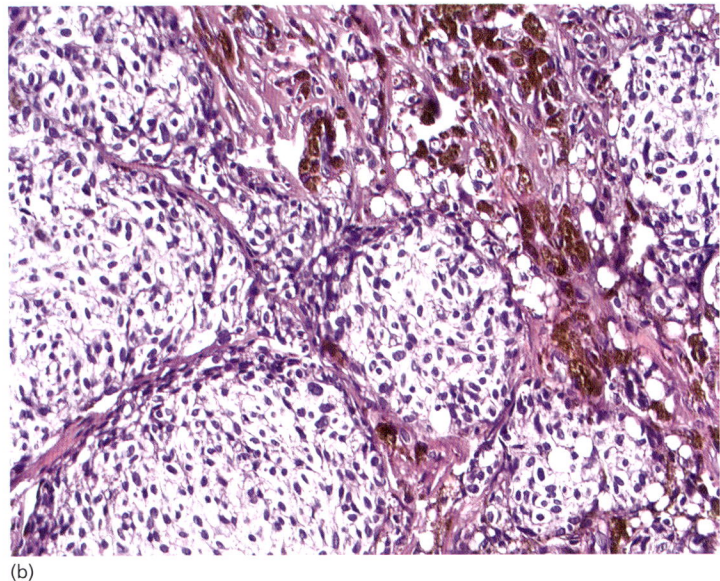

Figure 131.46 Cellular blue naevus. (a) Multiple amelanotic nodules of naevomelanocytes are characteristic. The cellular component of blue naevus extends deep to the reticular dermis of the skin and often projects into the adjacent subcutaneous fat. There is no necrosis. Magnification 10× (H&E). (b) The cellular nodules consist of almost uniform melanocytes with light eosinophilic or even clear cytoplasm. There is focal, finely distributed, intracytoplasmic melanin pigment. Between the cellular nodules there are aggregates of heavily pigmented dendritic melanocytes. Magnification 40× (H&E). Courtesy of Dr K. Frangia, HBD HistoBio Diagnosis, Athens, Greece.

blue naevi include vesicular rather than hyperchromatic nuclei of the dendritic cells and the presence of pigmented, polygonal and – more characteristically – large epithelioid cells.

A deep penetrating naevus is characterised by loosely organised nests of pleomorphic, pigmented epithelioid cells that penetrate in an inverted wedge configuration deep into the dermis or subcutaneous fat [269]. Unlike the majority of blue naevi, the deep penetrating naevus does not harbour mutations in Gnaq and Gna11 proteins. The identification of *HRAS* mutations in these naevi suggest that they may be considered variants of Spitz rather than blue naevi [270]. The majority of deep penetrating naevi harbour activating mutations in the β-catenin and the MAP-kinase pathways and could be seen as an intermediate stage in a step-wise progression from naevus to melanoma [271].

Sclerosing (or desmoplastic) blue naevi show marked dermal fibrosis and hyaline sclerosis and should be differentiated from desmoplastic melanoma.

Occasionally, blue naevi can be amelanotic or hypomelanotic. Due to the lack of pigment, a diagnosis of blue naevus is based on the presence of dermal spindle cells that are HMB-45 positive on immunohistochemistry.

Genetics
Blue naevi do not show oncogenic mutations in the signalling components of the MAP kinase pathway (such as *BRAF* or *NRAS*) which are common in other types of melanocytic naevi as well as melanomas. Somatic mutations of the *GNAQ* gene (codon 209), a member of the G-protein α subunit, converting it into a dominant-acting oncogene are present in 46–83% of blue naevi, 50% of malignant blue naevi and 46% of ocular melanoma of the uvea [63]. A smaller proportion of blue naevi (7–16%) have mutations in the *Gna11* gene, also a membrane bound guanosine triphosphatase (GTPase), *PLCB4* and *CYSLTR2* [272,273].

Clinical features
Presentation
Blue naevi typically present as single, blue-black or deep blue, dome-shaped papules, with a diameter of less than 1–2 cm. Large or giant lesions, ulceration or the development of subcutaneous nodules can also be observed but are rare events. The blue colour is caused by the 'Tyndall effect': dermal pigment absorbs the longer wavelengths of light and scatters blue light. Locations more commonly involved are the face and scalp, the dorsal area of the distal extremities (Figure 131.47) and the buttocks.

Blue naevi can incidentally arise in the prostate, female genital tract, lymph nodes, conjunctiva, nasal and oral mucosa and lungs.

Clinical variants
A variety of clinical variants have been described, such as the large congenital blue naevus, large plaque blue naevus with subcutaneous cellular nodules, and agminate, eruptive and target blue naevi.

Some of the histological variants of blue naevi may also present with distinct clinical features. The combined blue naevus may have an unusual appearance, causing concern. A cellular blue naevus (Figure 131.48) may develop before birth, but frequently becomes apparent around puberty. The deep penetrating naevus is more commonly observed on the head and neck, presenting with a diffuse, irregular lateral margin.

Differential diagnosis
The most important distinction is between the blue naevus and melanoma. Blue naevi have distinct dermoscopic features and are relatively static lesions. The histology of each is characteristic and can easily help separate the two entities. Immunohistochemistry and FISH assay may be useful in distinguishing challenging cases.

Satellite lesions of blue naevi resembling cutaneous metastases of melanoma have been reported [274].

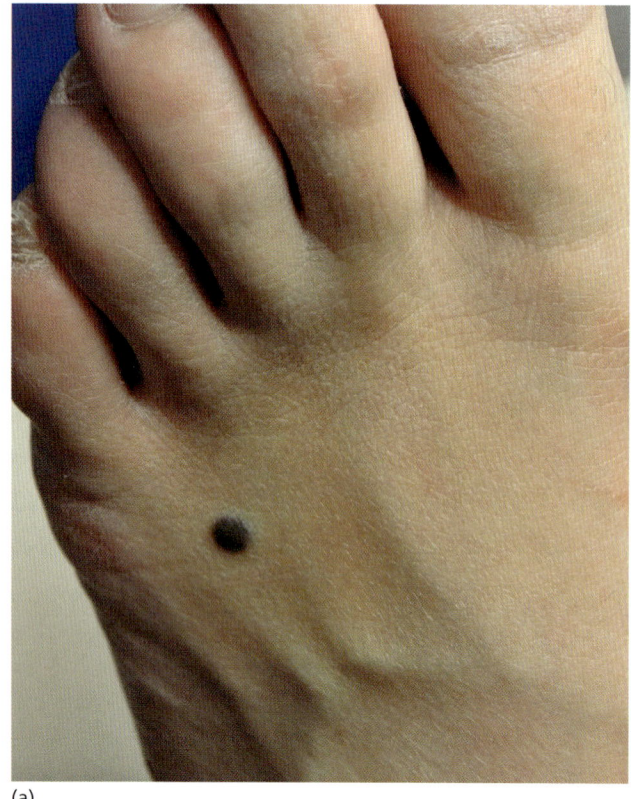

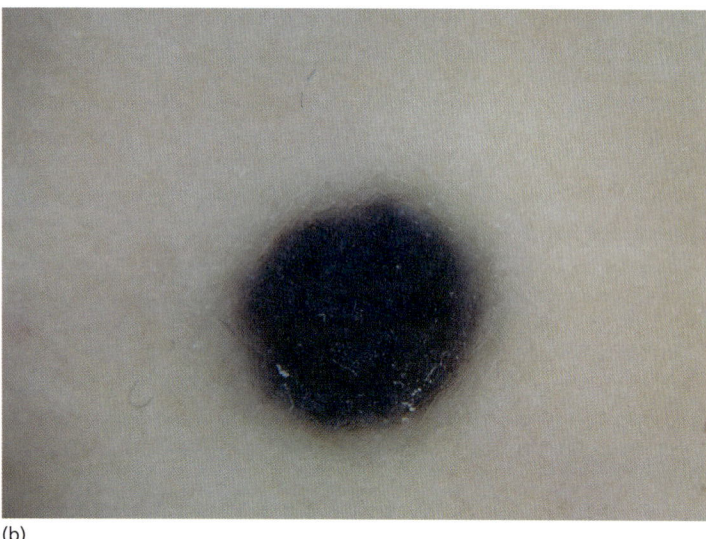

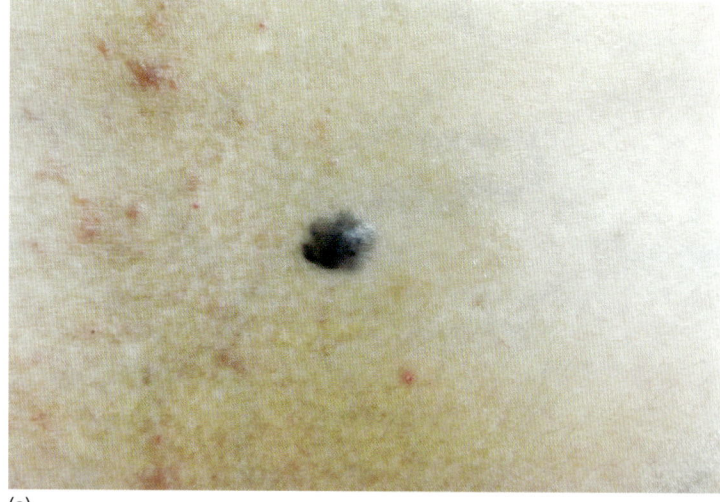

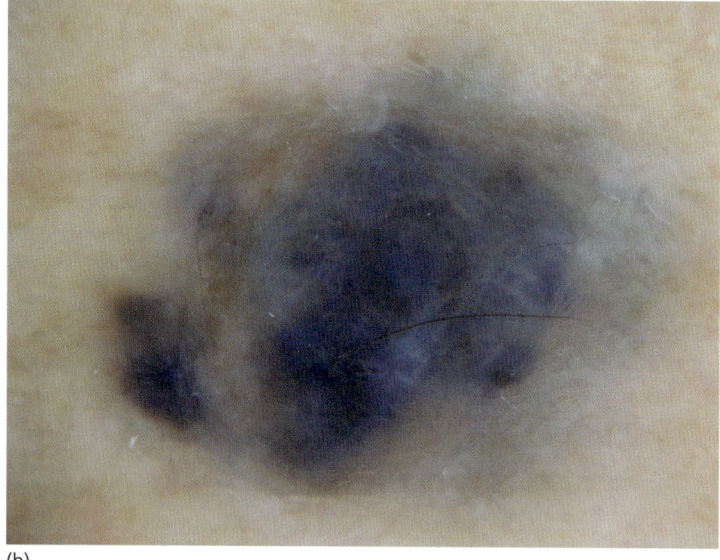

Figure 131.47 (a) Blue naevus. (b) Dermoscopic image of a blue naevus showing a homogeneous blue pattern.

Figure 131.48 (a) Cellular blue naevus. (b) Dermoscopic image of a cellular blue naevus showing a well-circumscribed, protuberant nodule with homogeneous dark blue pigmentation and randomly distributed whitish zones corresponding histopathologically to fibrosis.

Disease course and prognosis
Blue naevi are generally non-progressive proliferations. Enlargement of the lesion may raise concern of malignant transformation.

Investigations
Dermatoscopically, blue naevi lack the pigmented network of other melanocytic lesions and show a distinct homogeneous, structureless, blue, blue-grey, blue-brown or blue-black colour (Figure 131.47b). However, the dermoscopy of blue naevi may vary and lesions with polychromatic pigmentation and local dermoscopic criteria (dots/globules, whitish, scar-like areas, peripheral streaks and vessels) are not uncommon, making their distinction from melanoma difficult (Figure 131.48b) [275].

Management
Blue naevi do not require treatment, except for cosmetic reasons (e.g. facial location). When in clinical doubt, an excisional biopsy should be performed to rule out melanoma.

Clinically atypical naevi

Definition and nomenclature
These are melanocytic naevi, 5 mm or larger in diameter, with a macular component, irregular and poorly defined borders, asymmetrical outline and variable pigmentation (see Table 131.3).

> **Synonyms and inclusions**
> - Dysplastic naevus
> - Clark naevus
> - B-K naevus
> - Naevus with architectural disorder and cytological atypia of melanocytes
> - Familial atypical multiple mole melanoma syndrome (FAMMM)
> - Dysplastic naevus syndrome (DNS)
> - Atypical naevus syndrome (ANS)
> - B-K mole syndrome

Introduction and general description

In 1978 Clark *et al.* described members of melanoma-prone families who had a personal history of melanoma and who exhibited high numbers of naevi with distinct clinical and histological characteristics [276]. These naevi were named B-K moles and the syndrome B-K mole syndrome after the initials of two probands. Their malignant potential was considered analogous to cervical dysplasia. During the same year, Lynch *et al.* used the term familial atypical multiple mole melanoma (FAMMM) syndrome in the same context [277]. In 1980, Elder *et al.* introduced the term dysplastic naevus syndrome (DNS) with familial and sporadic variants, stating that these naevi were precursors of melanoma due to their histological features [278]. The term dysplastic naevus was also proposed during the same year by Greene *et al.* as a distinction from banal naevi and an intermediate naevus phenotype in the spectrum of melanoma development [279]. Ever since, the confusion and controversy caused by differences in terminology, definitions and criteria (clinical and histological) used has not ceased [280].

Clinically atypical naevi are currently considered a distinct subgroup of naevi. Although they are benign lesions, they exhibit clinicopathological characteristics that may resemble early radial growth phase melanomas. They are also risk factors of melanoma and, to a much lesser extent, potential precursors of melanoma.

For the purposes of this chapter, the term 'atypical naevus' is used as a clinical description, while 'dysplastic naevus' is used as a histological one.

Epidemiology
Incidence and prevalence
The prevalence of atypical naevi varies considerably among different studies, ranging from 2% up to 50% [281]. Their frequency among melanoma patients is higher, ranging from 34% to 59% [282]. They are less frequent than banal naevi in the general population, their prevalence increasing in 'high risk' individuals with a personal or family history of melanoma [283].

Age
They are more prevalent in younger ages (less than 30–40 years of age), probably because some of them regress later in life. Typically, they appear during childhood and they become more prominent in puberty. Atypical naevi occur in older ages at a lower rate and should be cautiously examined to rule out melanoma.

Sex
There is no sex predilection.

Ethnicity
Their prevalence among different ethnicities is variable.

Associated diseases
Clinically, atypical naevi have consistently been associated with melanoma risk in relevant studies. This risk seems to depend on the number of atypical naevi, as well as on the personal and family history of melanoma. In sporadic atypical naevi, the presence of one naevus confers a relevant risk of 1.45, rising up to 6.36 for five atypical naevi [104]. In the study by Tucker *et al.* [284], 10 or more atypical moles conferred a 12-fold risk of melanoma. Atypical naevi are also associated with a higher risk of multiple primary melanomas [285–289]. In the setting of melanoma kindreds with increased numbers of atypical naevi and multiple common naevi (FAMMM, DMS, AMS), the relative risk for melanoma is even greater, reaching 85-fold in melanoma-prone family members with dysplastic naevi (Figure 131.49) [290].

Pathophysiology
Predisposing factors
Similar to common naevi, atypical naevi are also considered to be genetically determined, based on evidence from twin studies [291]. The role of environmental exposures is unknown although sunburn may be important [292].

Pathology
The main histological features of clinically atypical or dysplastic naevi include characteristic architectural and cytological features,

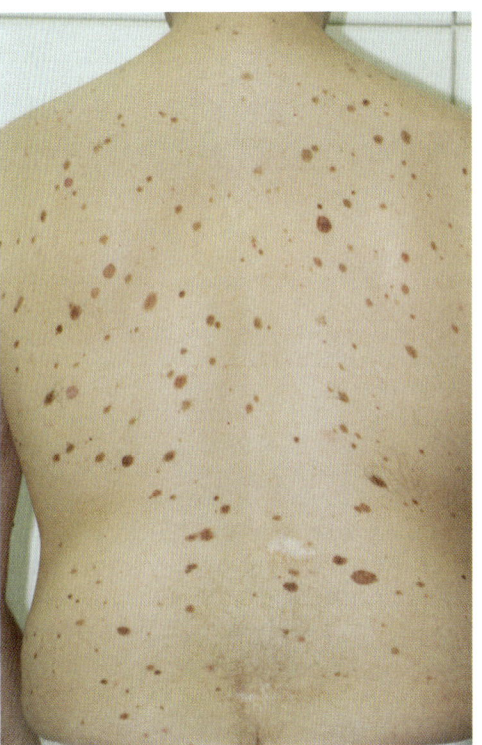

Figure 131.49 Dysplastic naevus syndrome: multiple clinically atypical naevi on the back. The lower surgical scar on the sacral area corresponds to a previously removed superficial spreading melanoma. The patient also had a second primary melanoma on the scalp.

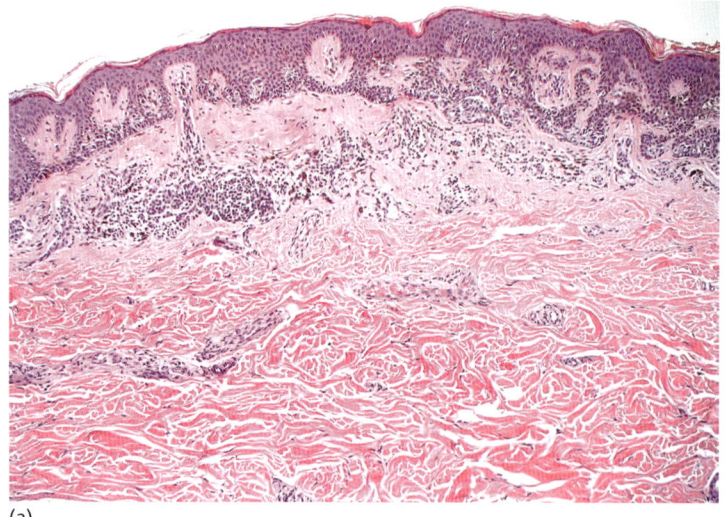

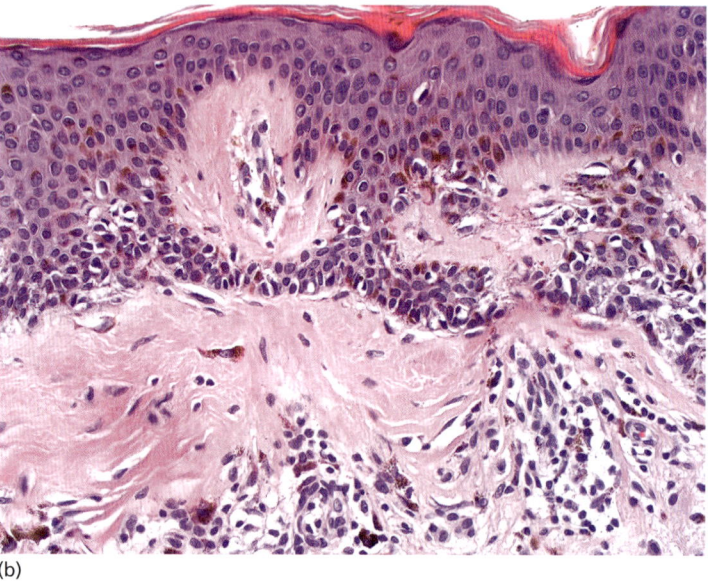

Figure 131.50 Compound dysplastic naevus. (a) Hyperplastic epidermis with bridging of the adjacent rete ridges. Nests of melanocytes, of variable sizes and shapes, can be seen in the junctional area as well as lamellar fibrosis of the dermis beneath the rete ridges. There is focal lymphocytic infiltrate of the dermis. Magnification 10× (H&E). (b) There are atypical or multinucleated giant melanocytes in the junctional portion of the naevus. Magnification 40× (H&E). Courtesy of Dr K. Frangia, HBD HistoBio Diagnosis, Athens, Greece.

as well as a fibrotic and inflammatory host response (Figure 131.50). These features were originally thought to be specific; however, there is a significant overlap with other types of naevi (e.g. acquired naevi smaller than 5 mm, some congenital naevi, atypical lentiginous naevi, naevi of special sites) [293] as well as with lentigo maligna and radial growth phase melanomas. Diagnostic criteria for dysplastic naevi have been proposed by several groups [294–298] and are presented in Table 131.5. The National Institutes of Health has proposed that the term dysplastic naevus be abandoned and replaced by the term 'naevus with architectural disorder' accompanied by a statement describing the presence and degree of melanocyte atypia [299].

Although a clinically atypical naevus usually exhibits histological dysplasia, and vice versa, this is not always the case. This discordance between clinical and histological diagnosis may not pose a real problem since the true value of the histological examination of a melanocytic lesion with clinically atypical features lies in the exclusion of melanoma.

Genetics

At a molecular level, at least a subset of atypical naevi exhibit features that place them in an intermediate position on a spectrum ranging from common naevi to overt melanoma [300–302]. CGH analysis and exome sequencing have revealed that melanocytic naevi differ from melanoma as they show no chromosomal aberrations or have a restricted set of alterations with basically no overlap with melanoma [303,304]. The *BRAF* V600E mutation rate is high in both common (~80%) and dysplastic (~60%) naevi [305]. However, dysplastic naevi can also harbour *BRAF* non-V600E, *NRAS* and, in a subset of dysplastic naevi adjacent to melanomas, *TERT* promoter mutations [301]. Although studies have not always been in accordance with each other, the most common molecular findings in atypical naevi include mutation/deletion of the *p16* gene, altered expression of p53, increased microsatellite instability, alterations of pigmentation pathways, mismatch repair gene expression, upregulation of genes involved in proliferation, cell adhesion and migration, and increased expression of follicular keratinocyte and inflammation-related genes [306–311].

Environmental factors

Episodes of painful sunburn before the age of 20 years have been associated with an increased risk for the development of melanocytic naevi (odds ratio (OR) 1.5; confidence interval (CI) 1.1–2.0) and atypical naevi (OR 1.4; CI 0.88–2.3) [312].

Clinical features
Presentation
Clinically, atypical naevi are larger than 5 mm with irregular borders and pigmentation (Figure 131.51). They sometimes present with a reddish hue that corresponds to a degree of inflammation. A central papular component is often surrounded by a macular periphery, so that the naevus resembles a 'fried egg' appearance. The well-known ABCDE rule of melanoma also applies to these naevi, albeit to a less pronounced extent.

Differential diagnosis
The critical distinction is between an atypical naevus and an *in situ* or early radial growth phase melanoma [313]. While the early detection of melanoma is of paramount importance in terms of prognosis, excessive prophylactic excision of benign naevi that are quite common in the general population is unjustified. Congenital melanocytic naevi and compound blue naevi sometimes can also exhibit atypical clinical features.

Classification of severity
Several studies have attempted to relate the grade of histological atypia (mild/moderate/severe or low-grade/high-grade) of these lesions to the risk of developing malignant melanoma

Table 131.5 Published histological criteria of the definition of dysplastic melanocytic naevi.

Parameters	Clark's histological criteria [294]	International Melanoma Pathology Study Group (IMPSG) criteria [131][a]	EORTC criteria [295][b]	Duke University criteria/grading system [296][c]
Architecture	Nests bridge rete ridges Nests at the side of rete ridges Single cells between nests Lentiginous elongation of rete ridges Anastomosis of rete ridges Little or no pagetoid spread	Both of the following: • Irregular (i.e. horizontaly orientated, bridging adjacent rete, and/or varying in shape and size) and/or dyscohesive nests of intraepidermal melanocytes • Increased density of non-nested junctional melanocytes (e.g. more melanocytes than keratinocytes in an area ≥ 1 mm^2)	Marked junctional proliferation Irregular naevus nests	Junctional component nested at both edges Overall symmetry >5% of nests cohesive Suprabasal spread (prominent or at edge) >50% confluence of proliferation Single cell proliferation absent or focal
Cytological atypia	Variable slight to moderate atypia Few (if any) mitoses Scattered epithelioid naevus cells and cells with finely granular melanin	Presence of cytological atypia, which is graded on the basis of the highest degree of cytological atypia present in more than a few melanocytes (WHO classification 2018 [131])	Large nuclei	Nuclei round or oval and euchromatic Nuclei larger than those of basal keratinocytes Nucleoli prominent Cell diameter twice that of basal keratinocytes
Host response	Patchy lymphocytic infiltrate Eosinophilic fibroplasia Lamellar fibroplasia		Lymphohistiocytic infiltrate	

Adapted from Elder et al. 2018 [131]; Elder et al. 1982 [294]; de Wit et al. 1993 [295]; Shea et al. 1999 [296].
[a] Also requires width >4 mm in fixed sections (>5 mm clinically). Reproduced from: Shors et al. [297] and Xiong et al. [298].
[b] Three or more of the listed features are required for the diagnosis of dysplastic naevus.
[c] For each group (architectural disorder/cytology) a grading score is assigned as follows: mild, 0–1 criteria; moderate, 2 criteria; severe, 3–4 criteria.

[131,283,294,314]. Although patients with more severe histologically atypical naevi seem to have a higher risk of developing melanoma, the prognostic value of this classification is still limited due to a lack of uniform and objective criteria. It has been reported that the diameter (>4.40 mm) of a dysplastic naevus may be a stronger predictor of melanoma than the degree of histological dysplasia [298].

Disease course and prognosis
The usual natural history of acquired benign melanocytic naevi is that of a progression from junctional to compound and finally to dermal naevi, with subsequent termination of naevomelanocytic proliferation. Atypical naevi retain their ability to proliferate for an extended period before their maturation, resulting in a larger size and irregular shape and pigmentation compared with common naevi. Although the vast majority of naevi follow this course, there are some cases of both common and atypical naevi that evolve into radial growth phase melanomas. Histological examination of melanomas reveals that approximately one-quarter to one-third develop on pre-existing naevi. However, the rate of malignant transformation of naevi into melanomas is very low [105]. There are no data to support the notion that atypical naevi are more likely to progress to melanomas than common naevi and the prevalence of naevus-associated melanoma does not seem to depend on whether the naevus was dysplastic or non-dysplastic [315]. Therefore, atypical naevi should mainly be viewed as risk markers – and occasionally simulants – for melanomas rather than true precursor lesions.

Investigations
Dermoscopy is always useful in assessing a melanocytic lesion with clinically atypical features. Different methods of analysis, such as qualitative pattern analysis, the ABCD rule and the seven-point checklist, yield different percentages of diagnostic accuracy for melanoma, yet they all add to the clinical differential diagnosis between atypical naevi and melanomas. Dermoscopic features that can be seen in atypical naevi vary [316–322]. It is usual to note an atypical or irregular pigmentation network, irregularly distributed and shaped brown globules and dots, as well as areas of regression (Figure 131.51, right hand images). *In vivo* confocal microscopy (Figure 131.52) and other non-invasive imaging techniques increase diagnostic accuracy when combined with dermoscopy in equivocal cases, yet their use is currently limited due to the high cost and limited availability.

Artificial intelligence-based tools are continuously being developed and their role in assisting skin lesion classification is expected to grow.

Management
Since atypical naevi are risk markers rather than melanoma precursors, there is no need to excise for prophylactic reasons. The risk of melanoma conferred by the presence of atypical naevi remains even after their excision, since the genetic susceptibility of an individual cannot be altered. Additionally, the majority of melanomas develop *de novo*, and there are currently no molecular markers for the identification of lesions at higher risk for transformation [311]. 'Prophylactic' excision is therefore unlikely to truly protect against future melanoma development, while it involves the patient with the additional cost and morbidity of the procedure, and possibly a false sense of safety. Patients with atypical naevi, especially those with high numbers of atypical and common naevi and/or a personal or family history of melanoma, are at high risk for melanoma development. These patients should be taught to self-examine their existing naevi as well as the rest of their skin

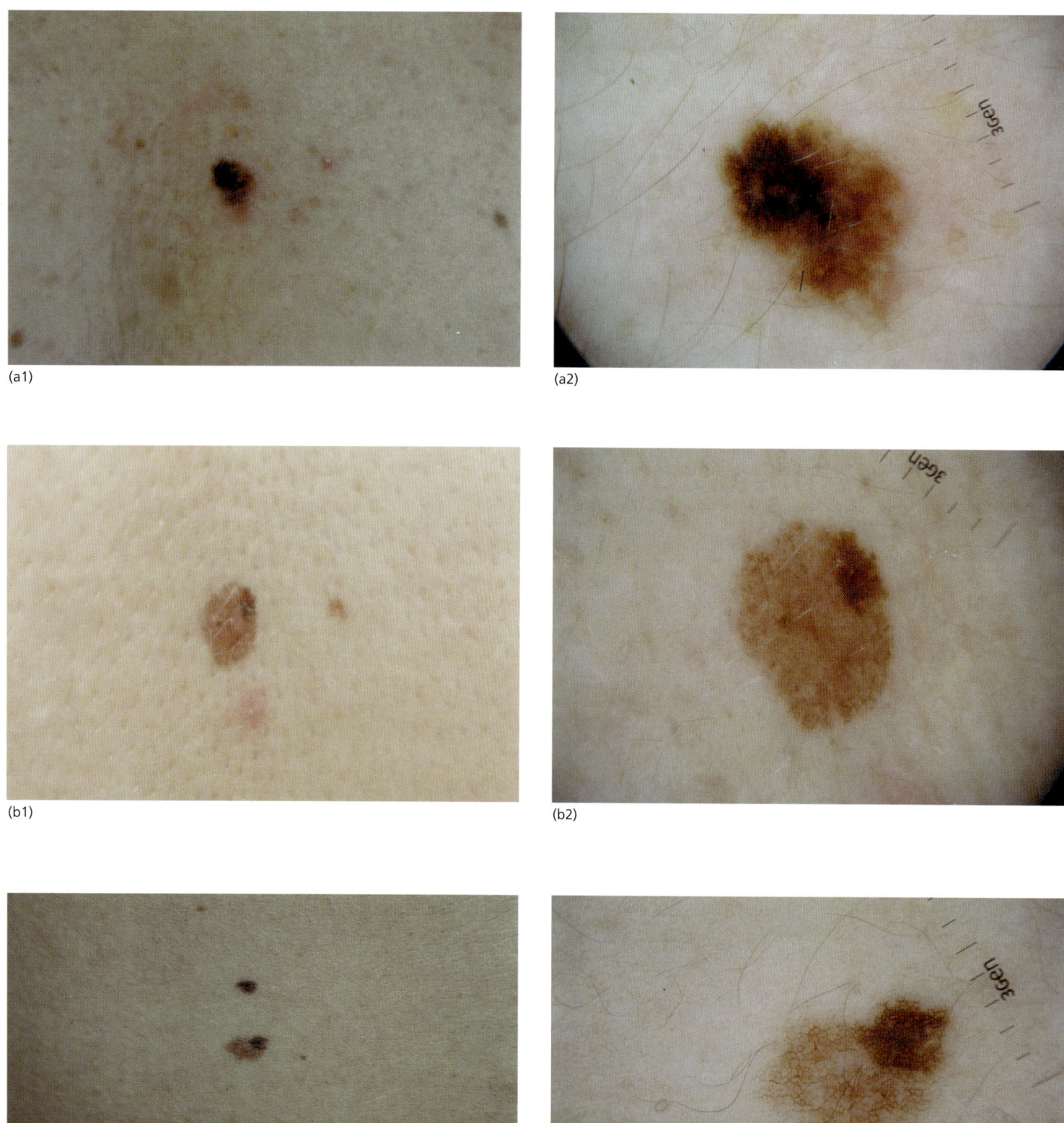

Figure 131.51 (a–e) Clinically atypical naevi of variable shapes, sizes and pigmentary patterns (on the left) and their corresponding dermoscopic images (on the right). Parts c and e courtesy of Dr D. Sgouros, Andreas Sygros Hospital, Athens, Greece.

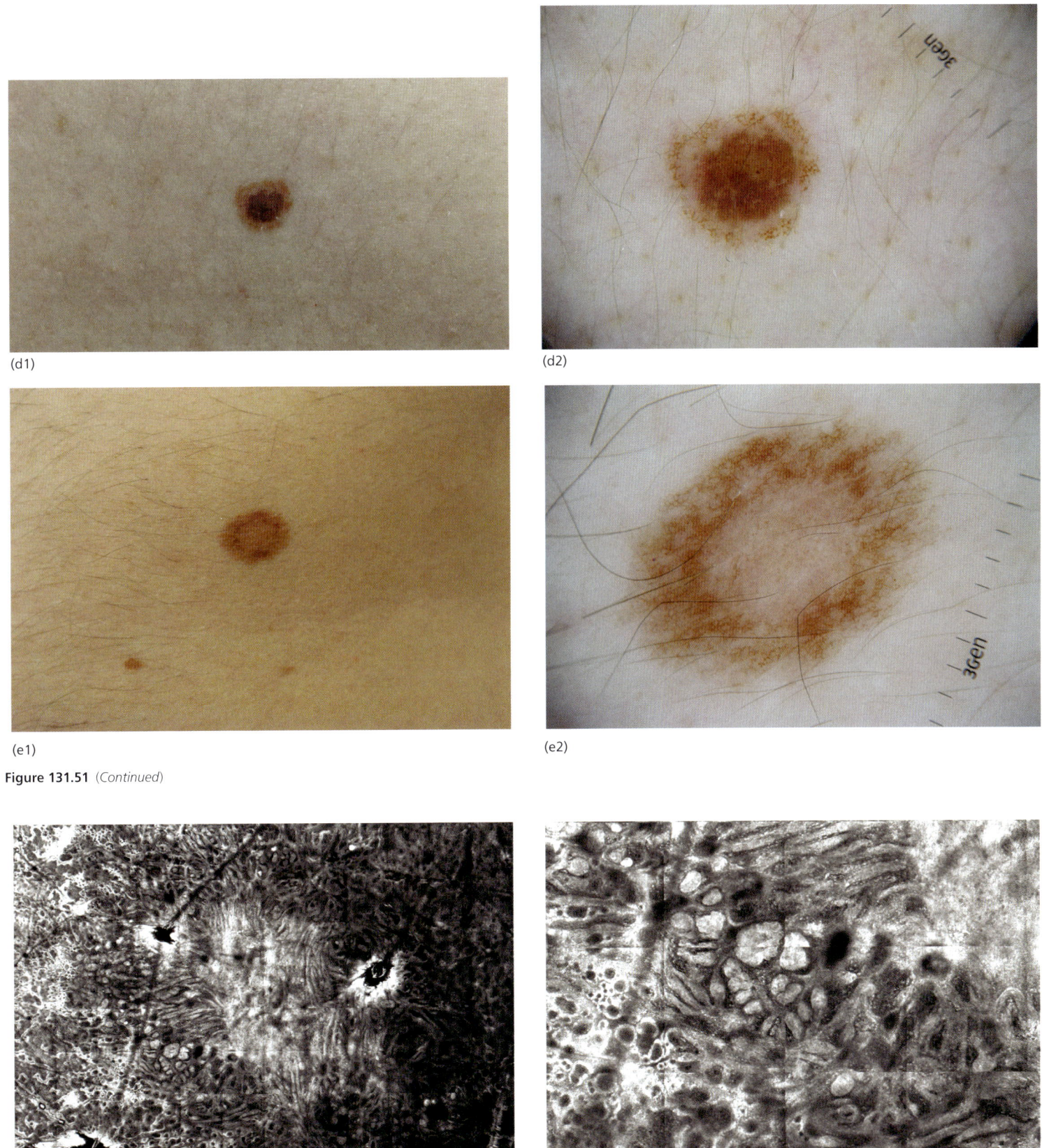

Figure 131.51 (Continued)

Figure 131.52 (a) Dysplastic naevus (4.2 × 6 mm) by reflectance confocal microscopy showing a more disarranged pattern with elongated junctional nests in the centre and some nests bulging from the side of the cristae. (b) Detail (1.4 × 2 mm) at a higher magnification where a few large (>40 μm) bright nucleated cells are also visible within the nests, corresponding to atypical melanocytes. Courtesy of Dr Giovanni Pellacani, Department of Dermatology, University of Modena and Reggio Emilia, Italy.

for potentially suspicious lesions. They should also be counselled about sun protection strategies. Apart from a full skin examination, dermoscopy and photographic recording (ideally by digital dermoscopic imaging and/or total body photography) should be used in patients with atypical naevi. There is no consensus on the frequency of follow-up visits or on the overall time period of surveillance for individual lesions. In the case of particularly atypical lesions, complete surgical excision with a 2–3 mm clinical margin and subsequent histological examination to rule out melanoma *in situ* or early melanoma should be performed [323,324].

Resources

Patient resources

American Academy of Dermatology. Moles: who gets and types. https://www.aad.org/public/diseases/a-z/moles-overview (last accessed July 2023).
https://www.cancer.gov/types/skin/moles-fact-sheet (last accessed July 2023).

Key references

The full list of references can be found in the online version at https://www.wiley.com/rooksdermatology10e

4 Praetorius C, Sturm RA, Steingrimsson E. Sun-induced freckling: ephelides and solar lentigines. *Pigment Cell Melanoma Res* 2014;27:339–50.

105 Tsao H, Bevona C, Goggins W, Quinn T. The transformation rate of moles (melanocytic nevi) into cutaneous melanoma: a population-based estimate. *Arch Dermatol* 2003;139:282–8.

115 Damsky WE, Bosenberg M. Melanocytic nevi and melanoma: unraveling a complex relationship. *Oncogene* 2017;36:5771–92.

131 Elder DE, Massi D, Scolyer RA *et al.*, eds. *WHO Classification of Skin Tumors*, 4th edn. IARC: Lyon, 2018.

139 Ahn CS, Guerra A, Sangüeza OP. Melanocytic nevi of special sites. *Am J Dermatopathol* 2016;38:867–81.

153 Larre Borges A, Zalaudek I, Longo C *et al*. Melanocytic nevi with special features: clinical-dermoscopic and reflectance confocal microscopic-findings. *J Eur Acad Dermatol Venereol* 2014;28:833–45.

201 Luo S, Sepehr A, Tsao H. Spitz nevi and other Spitzoid lesions part I. Background and diagnoses. *J Am Acad Dermatol* 2011;65:1073–84.

278 Elder DE, Goldman LI, Goldman SC *et al*. Dysplastic nevus syndrome: a phenotypic association of sporadic cutaneous melanoma. *Cancer* 1980;46:1787–94.

283 Duffy K, Grossman D. The dysplastic nevus: from historical perspective to management in the modern era: part I. Historical, histologic, and clinical aspects. *J Am Acad Dermatol* 2012;67:e1–16; quiz 7–8.

CHAPTER 132

Benign Keratinocytic Acanthomas and Proliferations

Edward Seaton[1] and Vishal Madan[2]

[1]OneWelbeck Skin Health and Allergy, London, UK
[2]Dermatology Centre, Salford Royal NHS Foundation Trust, Salford, UK

BENIGN KERATINOCYTIC ACANTHOMAS, 132.1	Dermatosis papulosa nigra, 132.4	OTHER BENIGN PROLIFERATIONS, 132.8
Seborrhoeic keratosis, 132.1	Warty dyskeratoma, 132.5	Skin tags, 132.8
Stucco keratosis, 132.4	Clear cell acanthoma, 132.6	Pseudoepitheliomatous hyperplasia, 132.9
Inverted follicular keratosis, 132.4	Lichenoid keratosis, 132.7	Key references, 132.10

BENIGN KERATINOCYTIC ACANTHOMAS

Acanthomas are benign proliferations of keratinocytes. Acanthomas show varied histological features including acanthosis, hyperkeratosis, dyskeratosis and acantholysis.

Seborrhoeic keratosis

Definition and nomenclature
Seborrhoeic keratoses (SK) are very common benign tumours of epidermal keratinocytes. SK typically appear in mid-life, the lesions increase in number gradually and affect the majority of older adults. Dermatosis papulosa nigra and stucco keratosis are considered as variants of SK.

Synonyms and inclusions
- Seborrhoeic wart
- Senile wart
- Senile keratosis
- Basal cell papilloma

Introduction and general description
SK are discrete and often multiple, well-demarcated, raised lesions, with a wart-like surface and a rough texture. They are typically hyperpigmented. However, pigmentation is variable and may be absent, so that lesions can be brown, black, yellow, flesh-coloured or red. They are typically asymptomatic but may be mildly pruritic or inflamed.

Epidemiology
Age
SK are the most prevalent benign skin tumours and increase markedly with age. They are rare in young adults, common in late middle age and affect the majority of older people. In adults aged over 50 years, 90% had SK in Korea and 100% in Australia [1,2]. SKs were present in 56% of Berlin elderly care home residents, and in 45% of people in northern Finland aged 46 [3,4]. In a study of 90 880 industrial workers in Germany, prevalence was 1.4% between ages 16 and 20 years, 24% between ages 41 and 50 and 67% between 61 and 70 [5].

Sex
The distribution is equal between the sexes [5].

Ethnicity
Lighter skin types seem more prone to the development of SK, perhaps reflecting the influence of sun exposure in their pathogenesis. They are commoner in white and Asian skin types than in black skin. In contrast, the dermatosis papulosa nigra variant occurs predominantly in black and pigmented skin [6].

Associated diseases
The eruptive development of multiple SK or a sudden increase in size of existing lesions has been described in relationship to several types of underlying malignancy, particularly gastric, colonic and rectal adenocarcinoma as well as several other solid tumours. This is sometimes described as the sign of Leser–Trélat and is certainly rare. A true association is controversial: SK are almost ubiquitous in older adults, and the sign does not fulfil the Curth postulates, a set of clinical criteria that evaluate the temporal relationship between skin signs and underlying cancer [7]. However, it is suggested that the coexistent presence of eruptive SK with pruritus or acanthosis nigricans should heighten the suspicion of malignancy [8]. The release of growth factors and cytokines by the tumour is thought to be responsible, particularly epidermal growth factor α (EGF-α) and overexpression of EGF receptor. If suspected, a thorough history and review of systems should be undertaken. Referral for upper and lower gastrointestinal endoscopy may be considered, along with

Rook's Textbook of Dermatology, Tenth Edition. Edited by Christopher Griffiths, Jonathan Barker, Tanya Bleiker, Walayat Hussain and Rosalind Simpson.
© 2024 John Wiley & Sons Ltd. Published 2024 by John Wiley & Sons Ltd.

mammography, chest X-ray and prostate-specific antigen testing as appropriate. Eruptive SK has also been reported in pregnancy, erythroderma, human immunodeficiency virus (HIV) infection and transplant recipients.

Pathophysiology

SK are thought to result from the clonal expansion of proliferating keratinocytes as a result of somatic mutations. Patients with large numbers of SKs often have a family history, but a clear demonstration of the mechanisms of genetic susceptibility is lacking. Previous sun exposure is a key factor in their development. SKs occur more commonly on sun-exposed sites such as the temples, neck, trunk, hands and forearms, appear earlier in photo-exposed skin and are also more numerous, larger and more often flat at these sites [9]. Under the age of 40, more Australians than British people have SK, including 12% of Australians aged 15–25 years [10]. Four-fifths of SKs exhibit typical ultraviolet-induced mutations. In fact, the frequency of dypyrimidine mutations C>T and CC>TT in SK is actually higher than basal and squamous cell carcinoma [11].

SKs have been found to harbour multiple somatic mutations, but despite this are genetically stable, and not premalignant. The keratinocytes proliferate upwards, respecting the integrity of the basement membrane. The commonest mutations are FGFR3 in approximately half of lesions, PIC3CA in one-third and TERT promotor, OXNAD1 and DPH3 in a quarter each. Increased FGFR3 in SK has been correlated with increased FOXN1 transcription factor levels, production of which might stall malignant transformation [11,12].

Pathology

Keratinocyte proliferation results in acanthosis (thickening of the entire epidermis) and papillomatosis. Other common histological features are hyperkeratosis (thickening of the stratum corneum), horny invaginations, which appear cross-sectionally as pseudo-horn cysts, and true horn cysts (areas of keratinisation surrounded by a thin granular layer) (Figure 132.1).

Six histological subtypes are recognised: acanthotic, hyperkeratotic, melanoacanthoma, adenoid, clonal and irritated [13]. More than three-quarters of SK are acanthotic, hyperkeratotic or a mixture of these two variants. Acanthotic SK have a markedly thickened epidermis and horny invaginations which appear as pseudo-horn cysts. Adenoid SK have numerous thin tracts of epidermal cells extending from the epidermis and branching and weaving through the dermis, often containing only a double row of basaloid cells.

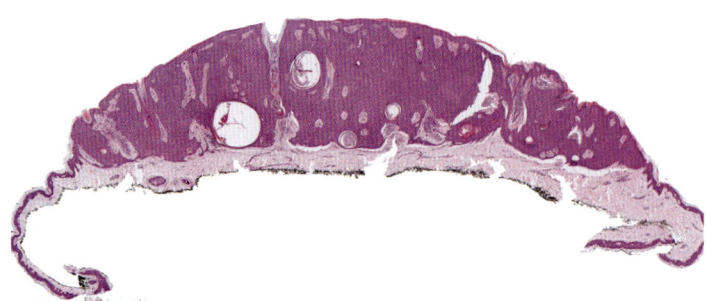

Figure 132.1 Histopathological features of seborrhoeic keratosis showing skin with hyperkeratosis, irregular acanthosis, keratin-filled invaginations and small pseudocysts.

Melanoacanthoma is often described as a rare variant, but it has been found to comprise 8–9% of SK in some pathology series. Melanoacanthomas have hyperpigmentation throughout all layers of the thickened epidermis and melanocytes with pronounced dendrites throughout the epidermis [14]. Clonal SK are a rare variant with well-demarcated interepithelial nests of pale or basaloid cells occurring within the epidermis. This intraepidermal proliferation is described as the Borst–Jadassohn phenomenon, which is also seen in hidroacanthoma simplex and Bowen disease.

Clinical features

SK usually appear slowly over months and years. They are mostly asymptomatic, unless they become inflamed, for example after trauma or rubbing, or when there is coexistent xerosis. Typically, they are noticed incidentally on examination, but patients with SK are often referred to dermatologists to exclude the possibility of skin cancer. They are usually multiple.

SK can appear at any site other than mucosal surfaces, most commonly on the temples, chest, back, neck, scalp, dorsal hands and forearms. They may appear grouped, for example in flexural sites, such as in the inframammary folds. They typically range between 2 and 20 mm in size but may reach several centimetres across. SK are often oval in shape but may be irregular. Hyperpigmentation is the norm, varying from light brown to black; however some patients may have multiple lesions that are flesh-coloured, yellow or slightly red.

Typical SK are flat-topped with a warty, greasy-looking, non-reflective, irregular surface and a characteristic stuck-on appearance (Figure 132.2). Black comedo-like openings, or white cysts each 1–2 mm in size, may be visible in the surface. In hair-bearing areas, hair density is often reduced over the keratosis itself. Flat SK are well demarcated and may have a faintly perceptible rough surface to touch. Verrucous or pedunculated SKs often occur in areas of skin folding, such as the inguinal region, inframammary folds or axillae. SK may become inflamed, red or crusted. Markedly hyperkeratotic SK may present as a keratin horn, with a steeple-shaped, firmly adherent scale.

Clinical variants

The following are considered to be clinical variants of SK:
- Stucco keratosis.
- Inverted follicular keratosis (Chapter 137).
- Dermatosis papulosa nigra.

Differential diagnosis

Diagnosis of SK is often straightforward, with important exceptions. Flat SKs, commonly seen on the face, may mimic solar lentigos, lentigo maligna or melanoma. Hyperkeratotic, red SKs may mimic hyperkeratotic actinic keratosis, squamous cell carcinoma or viral warts. Malignant melanoma may mimic SK. A melanoma should be suspected if there is a history of change in a pigmented or red lesion, with an absence of clearly identifiable diagnostic features of SK or other benign lesions, especially if it appears solitary or different from other lesions.

Investigations

Dermoscopy is a very useful means of distinguishing SK from melanocytic lesions and skin cancer (Figure 132.3). The presence of

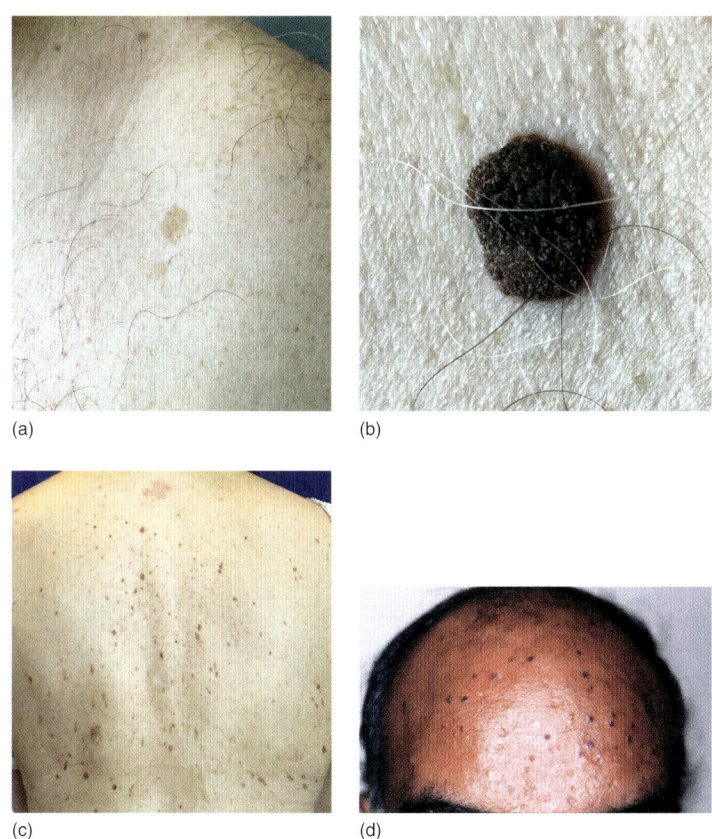

Figure 132.2 (a) Flat seborrhoeic keratosis (SK). A lightly hyperpigmented lesion with a 'stuck-on' appearance. (b) SK with a verrucous, non-reflective surface, dark hyperpigmentation and a well-demarcated, 'stuck-on' appearance. (c) Multiple SKs on the trunk. A family history of SK and excessive sun exposure is common in such patients. (d) SK occurs in all skin types and increases markedly with age. (d) Reproduced from Inamada and Palit 2003 [40] with permission of John Wiley & Sons.

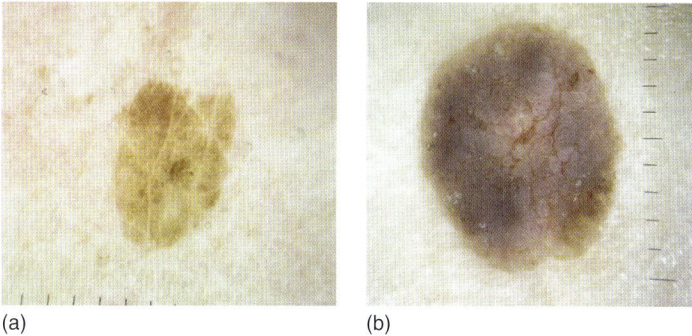

Figure 132.3 Dermoscopy of seborrhoeic keratosis (SK). (a) A well-demarcated border around the whole periphery and a fingerprint-like appearance typical of a flat SK. The absence of a pigment network is an important feature in distinguishing from melanocytic lesions. (b) A well-demarcated border around the whole periphery and a central cerebriform appearance, resembling the surface of a brain. Peripherally, comedo-like openings are seen as darker circles and milia-like cysts as white circles. No pigment network is seen.

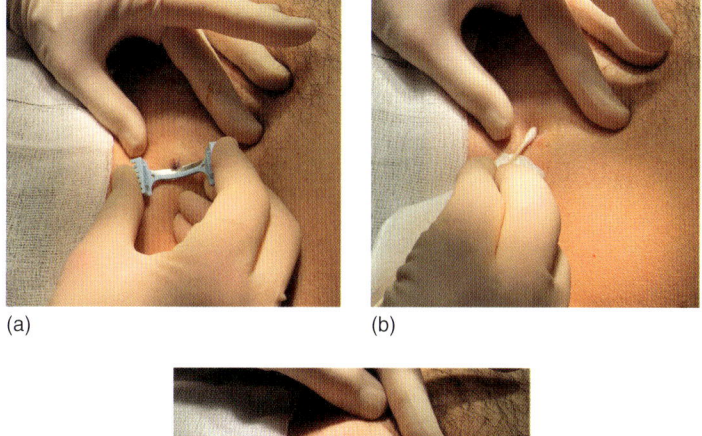

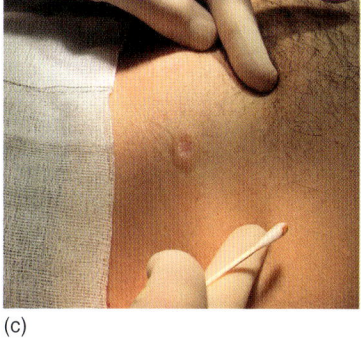

Figure 132.4 (a) Surgical removal of a seborrheic keratosis under local anaesthetic. The lesion is removed with a flat blade, flush with the surrounding skin and at the level of the superficial dermis. (b) Haemostasis is obtained by using 20% aluminium chloride hexahydrate applied with gentle pressure using a cotton tip. (c) Appearance of the surgical wound prior to the application of a dressing.

a reticulated pigment network is not a typical feature of SK and is more likely to indicate a melanocytic lesion [15].

The six dermoscopic features of SK are:
- Sharply demarcated border around the whole periphery.
- Black comedo-like openings.
- White milia-like structures.
- Cerebriform surface (with ridges and fissures resembling the sulci and gyri of a brain).
- Fingerprint-like appearance (often in flat SK).
- Fine hairpin-like vessels with a white halo.

Management

SK are benign and does not require treatment unless symptomatic or done for cosmetic reasons.

Carefully directed liquid nitrogen cryotherapy is an effective treatment. The duration of treatment varies from 10 to 30 seconds depends on the body site and the thickness of the keratosis. Treated lesions become crusted or black and fall off the skin within 2 weeks. Thicker lesions may require a second treatment. Side effects include redness, which may last a few weeks, and hypopigmentation, which is usually faint but can be permanent, particularly with longer treatment durations. For this reason, cryotherapy should be avoided or used very cautiously in patients with darkly pigmented skin. Lesions over 15 mm in size are harder to treat evenly with cryotherapy and surgical treatment is often preferable.

Surgical treatment under local anaesthetic is effective, including shave excision using a flat blade, or curettage, in each case aiming to remove the lesion flush with the surrounding skin just at the level of the superficial dermis, indicated by pinpoint bleeding (Figure 132.4). Bleeding can be stopped by the application of 20% aluminium chloride hexahydrate solution or by gentle electrocautery. Electrocautery should be used cautiously as it may produce scarring.

For patients with multiple SK, topical treatment by lesional application of trichloracetic acid solution (50–75%) is effective [16]. Post-treatment redness and hyperpigmentation may last a few months. Treatment with 40% hydrogen peroxide solution has shown some efficacy in a randomised study [17].

Ablative laser therapy including erbium:yttrium-aluminium-garnet (Er:YAG) and carbon dioxide devices, and more recently nanosecond pulsed electrical field treatment, have been used to treat SK. Post-treatment hyperpigmentation and hypopigmentation may occur [18,19].

Stucco keratosis

Definition and nomenclature
Stucco keratosis (StK) is considered to be a variant of seborrhoeic keratosis and typically presents as multiple small, non-pigmented, white keratotic plaques that are seen on the distal limbs of elderly people.

Synonyms and inclusions
- Keratosis alba

Epidemiology
StK is thought to be four times commoner in males than females and tends to appear after the age of 40. Prevalence is reported to be 7–20%. It is commoner in lightly pigmented skin types [20,21].

Pathophysiology
Pathology
Typical features are epidermal papillomatosis resembling a church spire or sawtooth and orthohyperkeratosis. Horn cysts and pseudocysts are not a feature. StKs are similar histologically to hyperkeratotic SK. StKs are stable with no malignant potential (Figure 132.5).

Genetics
StK has been found to harbour PIKC3A mutations [22].

Environmental factors
The cutaneous distribution suggests lifetime cumulative sun exposure is important in pathogenesis, although lesions do not occur on the face.

Clinical features
Presentation
Stucco keratoses are asymptomatic. They are typically white or white-grey scaly papules a few millimetres in diameter that appear in older adults on the extensor surfaces of the forearms and lower legs, especially near the ankles and dorsal surfaces of the hands and feet. They are often multiple, numbering over a hundred.

Differential diagnosis
Diagnosis is usually straightforward. Non-pigmented SK, hypertrophic actinic keratosis and viral warts may look similar.

Management
Treatment is not required. Emollients may improve the appearance, particularly those containing keratolytics such as urea or salicylic acid. Cryotherapy or surgical treatment may be done but are not usually undertaken because of the large number of lesions. There is no consistently effective topical or systemic drug treatment.

Inverted follicular keratosis

See Chapter 137.

Dermatosis papulosa nigra

Definition
Dermatosis papulosa nigra (DPN) is considered to be a variant of seborrhoeic keratosis in which multiple, small, pigmented papules develop on the face and neck. It is much commoner in black and Asian skin.

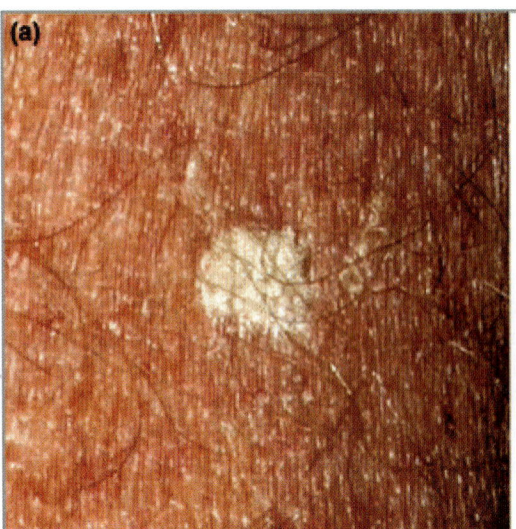
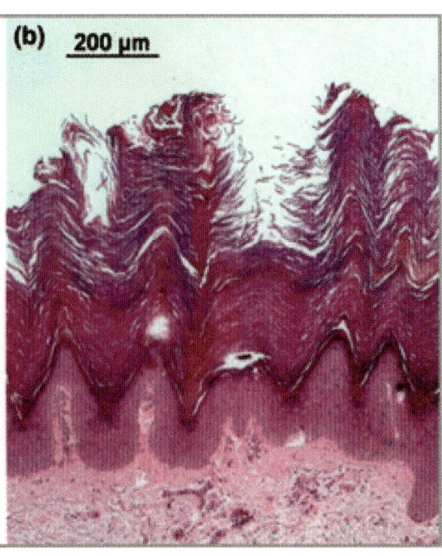

Figure 132.5 (a) Stucco keratosis is a white or white-grey papule a few millimetres in diameter, typically seen on the limbs of older adults. They are usually multiple. (b) Histopathological appearance of stucco keratosis with epidermal papillomatosis resembling a church spire or sawtooth with orthohyperkeratosis. Reproduced from Hafner et al. 2009 [22] with permission of John Wiley & Sons.

Epidemiology

Age
DPN often appears in early adult life at an earlier age than SK. The papules increase in number gradually and become multiple. They are not usually seen in children.

Ethnicity
Prevalence in black people is reported at between 10% and 30%. One study found a prevalence of 77% in black patients [6,23,24]. It is also commonly seen in India, China and Mexico [25,26]. It occurs much more rarely in white skin.

Sex
DPN is commoner in females with a gender ratio of 2 : 1.

Pathophysiology

Pathology
Histologically, DPN demonstrates acanthosis, papillomatosis and hyperpigmentation. It resembles the acanthotic variant of SK, although horn cysts and pseudocysts are less common. It is stable with no malignant potential.

Genetics
A family history of DPN present in four-fifths of cases. DPN lesions have been found to harbour FGFR3 mutations [22].

Clinical features

Presentation
Lesions are typically black or dark brown, shallow, dome-shaped papules measuring 1–5 mm in diameter (Figure 132.6). The cheeks, forehead and neck are most commonly affected, but lesions can also occur on the limbs or trunk.

Management
Treatment is usually done for cosmetic reasons. Electrodesiccation and curettage under local anaesthetic is effective. It may be prudent to undertake a test patch and allow time for healing to ensure satisfaction with outcome before treating a large number of lesions, especially in patients with pigmented skin. Electrodesiccation energies should be kept low and desiccated lesions curetted gently and shallowly.

Laser treatment can also be effective. Successful treatment is reported for carbon dioxide, neodymium (Nd):YAG, pulsed dye and potassium titanyl phosphate (KTP) laser devices [27,28].

> **Treatment ladder for dermatosis papulosa nigra**
>
> **First line**
> - Electrodesiccation and curettage
>
> **Second line**
> - Ablative laser

Warty dyskeratoma

Definition and nomenclature
Warty dyskeratoma (WD) is a benign epidermal tumour typically presenting as a discrete, wart-like, cup-shaped nodule with a keratotic plug. Dyskeratosis and acantholysis are characteristic histological features.

> **Synonyms and inclusions**
> - Focal acantholytic dyskeratoma
> - Isolated dyskeratosis follicularis

Epidemiology
WD is rare and usually occurs in older people.

Pathophysiology
The cause of WD is unknown but is probably multifactorial. Ultraviolet light, smoking, viral infection, chemical carcinogens and a reaction to inflammation have been proposed as aetiological factors. WDs have been observed during vemurafenib treatment [29]. Smoking is thought to be the main cause of oral lesions [30]. It has been suggested that WD may represent a sporadic localised error in epithelial maturation and cohesiveness. WDs can occur within or adjacent to other epithelial, fibrohistiocytic and melanocytic lesions and in inflammatory dermatoses.

Pathology
Histology of WD reveals a cup-shaped invagination surrounding a plug of epidermal hyperparakeratosis, with suprabasal acantholysis, multiple upward-pointing villus-like structures, dyskeratotic cells and corps ronds (Figure 132.7). Origination from a hair follicle has been proposed, because of the frequent proximity or connection to pilosebaceous units and the results of immunohistochemical studies [31,32].

Clinical features
WD usually presents in older adults on sun-exposed skin of the scalp, face or neck. It also occurs on oral and vulval mucosa. Multiple WDs have been reported. At non-mucosal sites, a pruritic

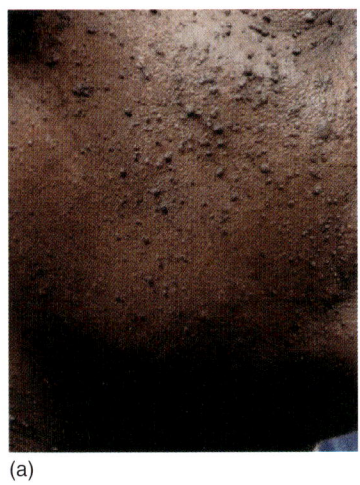
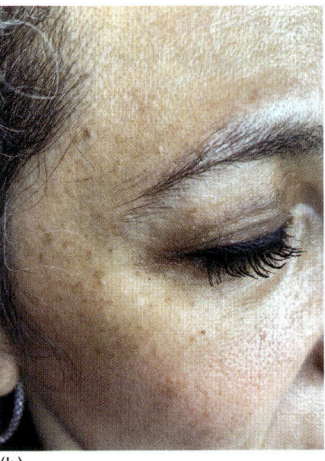

(a) (b)

Figure 132.6 (a) Dome-shaped papules of dermatosis papulosa nigra with a characteristic upper facial distribution. It is commonest in Fitzpatrick skin types IV–VI. (b) Dermatosis papulosa nigra can also occur in fairer skin.

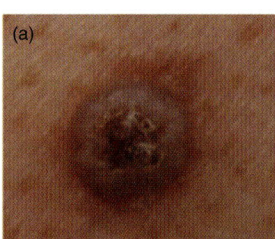
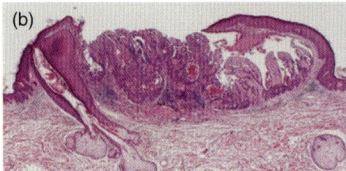
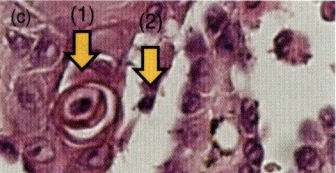

Figure 132.7 Warty dyskeratoma. (a) A solitary cup-shaped lesion with a central keratotic plug. (b) A cup-shaped invagination surrounding a plug of epidermal hyperparakeratosis with multiple upward-pointing villus-like structures and acantholysis. (c) Corps ronds (arrow 1) and grains (arrow 2) are visible at higher power. Reproduced from Nakagawa et al. 2018 [41] with permission of John Wiley & Sons.

solitary lesion is seen with a central keratotic plug. Other symptoms may include recurrent foul-smelling cheese-like discharge or bleeding with trauma.

Differential diagnosis
WD may be mistaken clinically for basal cell carcinoma, actinic or seborrhoeic keratosis, sebaceous hyperplasia, epidermoid cyst, keratoacanthoma, squamous cell carcinoma, Bowenoid papulosis, adnexal tumour or a viral wart. Histologically, focal acantholytic dyskeratosis can be seen in acantholytic squamous cell carcinoma, actinic keratosis, Darier disease, Grover disease, Hailey–Hailey disease and pemphigus vulgaris.

Management

> **Treatment ladder for warty dyskeratoma**
>
> **First line**
> - Surgical excision
>
> **Second line**
> - Shave excision
> - Curettage and cautery

Clear cell acanthoma

Definition and nomenclature
Clear cell acanthoma (CCA) is an asymptomatic benign lesion that typically presents as a red, dome-shaped papule on a lower limb. The epidermis contains clear glycogen-containing cells.

> **Synonyms and inclusions**
> - Degos acanthoma
> - Pale acanthoma
> - Acanthome cellules claires of Degos and Civatte

Epidemiology
Clear cell acanthoma is usually seen in mid-life, with a peak at age 50–60 years, with an equal sex incidence and no clear racial predilection. It is not seen in children [33,34,**35**].

Pathophysiology
The cause of CCA is unknown. On one hand it has been proposed to be a benign neoplasm, of epidermal, sweat gland or pilar origin, possibly a variant of seborrhoeic keratosis with abundant keratinocyte glycogen production. On the other it has been suggested as a reactive inflammatory process, because cytokeratin production is similar to that seen in some inflammatory dermatoses, such as psoriasis, and because CCA has been noted on psoriatic plaques, as well as in association with venous stasis eczema, varicose veins, SK, bacterial or viral infections and insect bites [36].

Pathology
Histological examination reveals acanthosis, psoriasiform hyperplasia and a characteristic pale epidermis that is sharply demarcated from the darker normal epidermis immediately adjacent (Figure 132.8). There may be intercellular oedema and an infiltrate containing many polymorphonuclear leukocytes forming parakeratotic microabscesses. The papillary dermis is oedematous with increased blood vessels. The cytoplasm of the clear cells contains glycogen, which stains with periodic acid–Schiff with diastase sensitivity. Phosphorylase enzyme necessary for the degradation of glycogen has been found to be absent in CCA keratinocytes. Electron microscopy reveals the displacement of tonofibrils with glycogen.

Clinical features
CCA usually presents as a red or red-brown asymptomatic dome-shaped papule or nodule with a 'stuck-on' appearance. The surface may look moist or crusted, and bleeding can occur with trauma. A collarette of fine peripheral scale is occasionally present (Figure 132.9). The lesions enlarge slowly over years and range from a few millimetres to a couple of centimetres in size. The lower limb is the commonest area affected, but lesions have been observed at multiple other sites.

Clinical variants
Giant, polypoid/pedunculated, atypical, cystic and pigmented patterns may be seen. Rarely eruptive multiple lesions are noted, tending to appear over a few months.

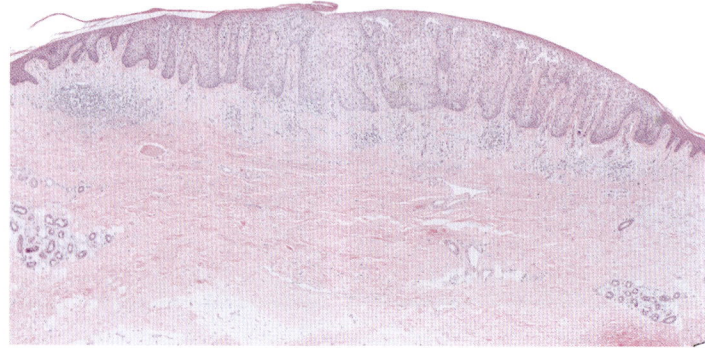

Figure 132.8 Histopathological features of clear cell acanthoma with a papulonodular lesion showing a well-demarcated area of epidermal hyperplasia (acanthosis). The lesional cells show keratinocytic pallor due to the accumulation of glycogen.

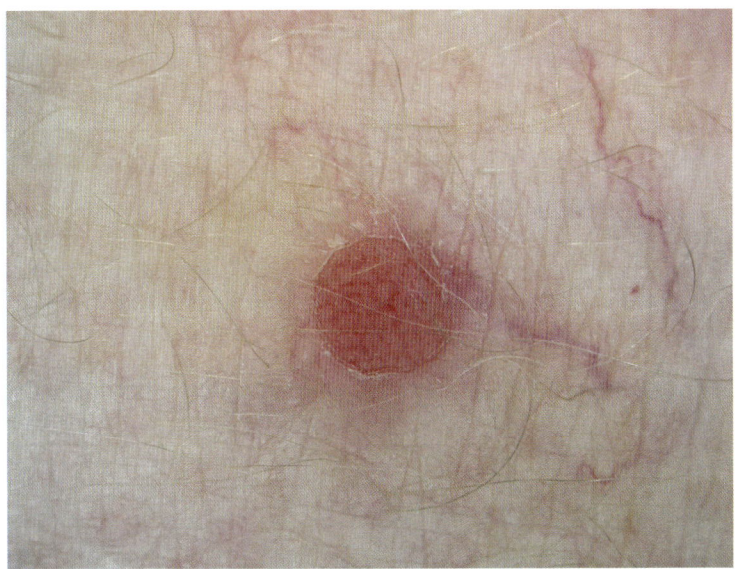

Figure 132.9 Clear cell acanthoma. Reproduced from Bowling 2022 [42] with permission of John Wiley & Sons.

Differential diagnosis

Differential diagnosis includes pyogenic granuloma, actinic keratosis, Bowen disease, basal cell carcinoma, squamous cell carcinoma, eccrine poroma, clear cell hidradenoma, amelanotic melanoma and cutaneous metastatic carcinoma.

Investigations

Dermoscopy shows an abundance of striking glomerular blood vessels with pin-point capillary loops in a streaky, curvilinear, reticulated pattern. This vascular pattern of dotted and coiled vessels in a serpiginous arrangement gives it a characteristic 'string of pearls' appearance (Figure 132.10).

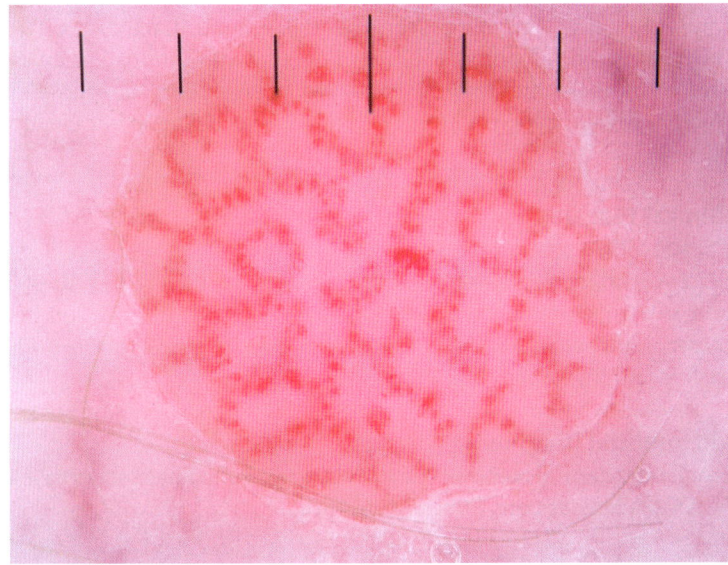

Figure 132.10 Dermoscopy of clear cell acanthoma. Striking glomerular blood vessels with pin-point capillary loops in a streaky, curvilinear, reticulated pattern can be seen: a 'string of pearls' appearance. Reproduced from Bowling 2022 [42] with permission of John Wiley & Sons.

Management

> **Treatment ladder for clear cell acanthoma**
>
> **First line**
> - Treatment is not always required but shave biopsy may be prudent to exclude malignancy in view of the possible differential diagnoses
>
> **Second line**
> - Curettage and cautery or shave excision to dermis
>
> **Third line**
> - Cryotherapy or carbon dioxide or other ablative therapy may be appropriate for multiple lesions

Lichenoid keratosis

Definition and nomenclature

Lichenoid keratosis (LK) is a solitary pink to red-brown plaque most commonly seen on the trunk or lower limbs, often with a preceding history of a pigmented macule or plaque.

> **Synonyms and inclusions**
> - Lichen planus-like keratosis
> - Solitary lichen planus
> - Involuting lichenoid plaque

Epidemiology

LK is common. The mean age of presentation is 60–65 years. Lesions are unusual below the age of 35. There is an increased prevalence among white people and women [37].

Pathophysiology

LKs are thought develop as a chronic inflammatory involution of a pre-existing skin lesion, most commonly a solar lentigo, actinic keratosis or seborrhoeic keratosis. The inflammatory stimulus is unknown.

Pathology

Rete ridges are typically flattened in LK and the dermal–epidermal junction is obscured by a band-like lichenoid lymphocytic infiltrate. Variable numbers of neutrophils, plasma cells and eosinophils are identified as well as epidermal parakeratosis, features that distinguish LK from typical lichen planus. Epidermal acanthosis is common in the classic variant; several other variants are described. A bullous subtype of LK has intraepidermal or subepidermal bullous cavities with necrotic basal keratinocytes. Atypical-type LK demonstrates enlarged CD3 and CD30+ lymphocytes with large hyperchromatic nuclei. The early interphase type has single lymphocytes along the dermal–epidermal junction, without acanthosis. The regressed or atrophic LK variant shows epidermal atrophy, papillary scarring and melanin incontinence, which can be

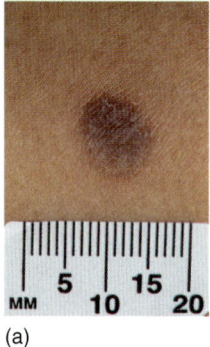
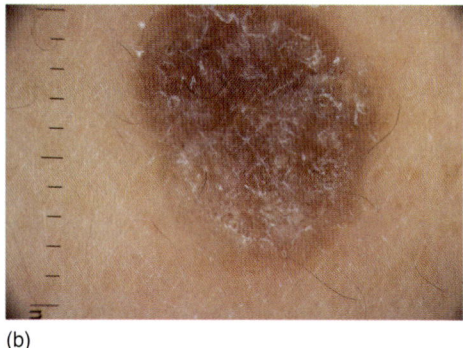

Figure 132.11 Lichenoid keratosis. (a) A solitary hyperpigmented papule without specific diagnostic features. (b) Dermoscopic appearance of the same lesion.

difficult to distinguish from the appearance of regressing melanoma *in situ* [37].

Clinical features
Presentation
LKs are usually solitary. Histologically, classic, bullous and atypical LKs typically present as a pink papule or plaque. The early interphase type often presents as a red or hyperpigmented macule (Figure 132.11). The regressed or atrophic variant is typically a violaceous plaque. Three-quarters of LKs occur on the trunk. The extremities are another common site. Less than one-tenth develop on the head and neck.

Differential diagnosis
It is difficult to make a confident clinical diagnosis of an LK even with experience. Clinicians suspect basal cell carcinoma in half of cases biopsied [38,39]. Other common differential diagnoses are seborrhoeic keratosis, actinic keratosis, solar keratosis, squamous cell carcinoma, Bowen disease, psoriasis and melanoma.

Investigations
LKs show a mixture of dermoscopic features, but none are pathognomonic or typically diagnostic. These include diffuse or localised granular patterns of pigmentation, blood vessels and blue-white structures. Similar features can be seen in regressing melanoma.

Management

> **Treatment ladder for lichenoid keratosis**
>
> **First line**
> - Excision with narrow margins should be undertaken if there is any question of melanoma
> - Shave excision
> - Curettage and cautery
>
> **Second line**
> - Cryotherapy
> - Carbon dioxide laser or erbium:YAG laser ablation

OTHER BENIGN PROLIFERATIONS

Skin tags

Definition and nomenclature
A skin tag is a benign lesion occurring mainly on the neck and major skin flexures as a small soft pedunculated protrusion. They are typically multiple.

> **Synonyms and inclusions**
> - Soft fibromas
> - Acrochordon
> - Fibroepithelial polyp

Epidemiology
Age
Skin tags are very common in middle-aged and older adults.

Associated diseases
Skin tags are commoner in obesity, dyslipidaemia, hypertension and insulin resistance and may therefore indicate a predisposition to atherosclerosis and cardiovascular disease [1]. They may appear in pregnancy. A combination of skin tags with multiple fibrofolliculomas is seen in Birt–Hogg–Dubé syndrome, an autosomal dominant condition with increased risk of colon and kidney cancer, pulmonary cysts and spontaneous pneumothorax.

Pathophysiology
Pathology
Skin tags are polypoid lesions with a core of loosely arranged collagen fibres and blood vessels (Figure 132.12). The epidermis may either be flattened, especially in larger lesions, or may be hyperplastic, resembling a seborrhoeic keratosis. Larger skin tags may have central adipose tissue. Pagetoid dyskeratosis may be seen as an incidental finding. Ischaemic necrosis may be seen after torsion. Melanocytic proliferation and naevus cells are not usually seen.

Clinical features
Presentation
Skin tags are pedunculated and are typically 1–5 mm in size. Round and soft tags are easy to diagnose. They may be skin coloured or hyperpigmented. The most common sites are the sides of the neck, axillae and inguinal folds.

Differential diagnosis
Small intradermal melanocytic naevi and pedunculated seborrhoeic keratoses may appear clinically identical.

Complications and co-morbidities
A skin tag may twist on its pedicle and become inflamed.

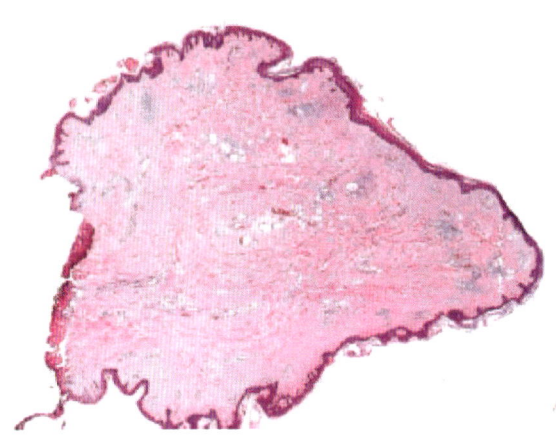

Figure 132.12 Histology of a skin tag: polypoid skin covered by mildly hyperkeratotic epidermis, containing thin- and thick-walled blood vessels in the dermal stroma.

Management

> **Treatment ladder for skin tags**
>
> **First line**
> - Snip excision, which may be done without anaesthetic for small lesions. Application of aluminium chloride hexahydrate with a cotton tip is useful to obtain haemostasis
> - Standard cryotherapy, taking care to avoid overtreatment to the surrounding normal skin. The use of metal forceps dipped in liquid nitrogen and held to the base of the tag for 20–30 seconds is also effective

Pseudoepitheliomatous hyperplasia

Definition and nomenclature
A benign, reactive proliferation of the epidermis that occurs secondary to a variety of inflammatory and neoplastic conditions. It mimics squamous cell carcinoma both clinically and histologically.

> **Synonyms and inclusions**
> - Pseudocarcinomatous hyperplasia
> - Invasive acanthosis
> - Verrucoid epidermal hyperplasia
> - Carcinomatoid hyperplasia

Pathophysiology
Predisposing factors
Conditions associated with pseudoepitheliomatous hyperplasia (PSE) can be grouped into three major categories:
1. Dermatoses causing chronic inflammation or irritation.
2. Infections.
3. Neoplasia.

Inflammatory causes include lichen simplex chronicus, prurigo nodularis or hypertrophic lichen planus, which are all fairly common conditions. Hypertrophic cutaneous lupus erythematosus may cause PSE and be misdiagnosed as multiple recurrent squamous cell carcinomas. Other inflammatory causes include vulval lichen sclerosis, chronic leg ulcers, burns, pemphigoid vegetans and halogenodermas, which are cutaneous reactions to ingested bromides or iodides or topical fluoride gels applied to the oral mucosa.

Infectious causes include cutaneous tuberculosis, deep fungal infections and as a complication of ulcers overlying chronic osteomyelitis.

Neoplastic causes include granular cell tumours, cutaneous lymphoma, especially nasal natural killer/T-cell lymphoma, and CD30+ lymphoproliferative diseases. PSE may also occur overlying melanocytic lesions, such as Spitz naevi and melanoma [2].

It is well reported that PSE can occur after tattoos, most commonly with red or purple pigment. A verrucous or fungating growth typically appears days or months after the procedure.

Pathology
Elongated, thick, downward projections of acanthotic epidermis occur, often with jagged borders and a sharply pointed base. Hypergranulosis, orthokeratosis and parakeratosis are common and abnormal areas of keratinisation, known as 'keratin pearls', may be seen. Slight keratinocyte atypia occurs, usually at the stratum basale, but keratinocyte necrosis is usually absent, and mitotic figures are not numerous or atypical. The general appearance is of an invasive proliferation of the epithelium, but with individual cells not showing the typical features suggestive of malignancy (Figure 132.13). Nevertheless, histological distinction from squamous cell carcinoma can be difficult.

A systematic histological approach to assessment may be helpful, dividing PSE into categories with or without a main pathological process in the dermis [2]. In simple ulcers and inflammatory lesions, by far the commonest causes, there is disturbance of the upper part of the dermis, often with young fibroblasts and a rather myxomatous connective tissue stroma replacing the normal dermal collagen. If there is significant dermal inflammation, infection should be ruled out, especially if histiocytes and multinucleated giant cells are present. In these cases special stains for mycobacteria and fungi

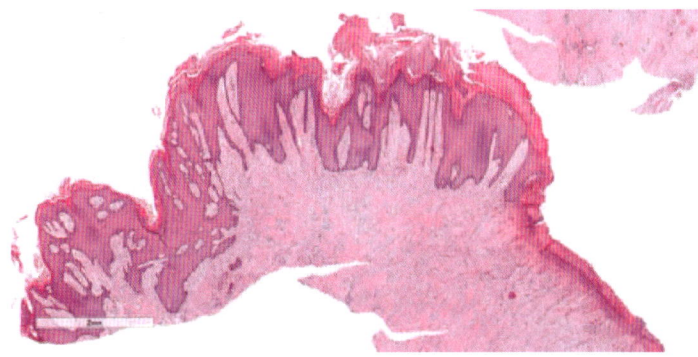

Figure 132.13 Histological features of pseudoepitheliomatous hyperplasia showing compact hyperkeratosis with uneven prominent epidermal downgrowths and dermal fibrosis. Vertically orientated capillaries are seen in the papillary dermis.

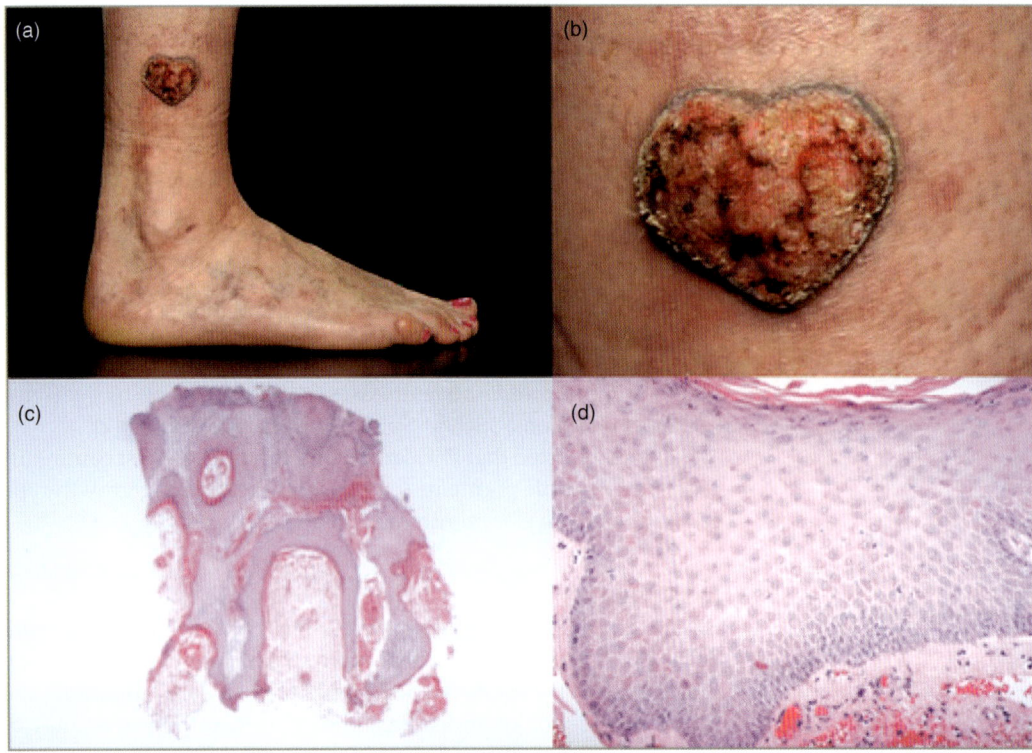

Figure 132.14 (a, b) Pseudoepitheliomatous hyperplasia secondary to a red tattoo and presenting as a fungating exophytic plaque with a verrucous surface, mimicking squamous cell carcinoma. (c, d) Histology revealed no cellular atypia. Reproduced from Kiss et al. [4] with permission of John Wiley & Sons.

should be done, and re-biopsy with fresh tissue culture for these organisms be considered. Some reports have identified immunohistochemical differences between PSE and squamous cell carcinoma at certain sites, however the usefulness and reproducibility of these not yet been established in clinical practice.

Clinical features
Presentation
PSE typically presents as a reddish well-demarcated plaque or nodule with variable degrees of scale, crust and verrucous change (Figure 132.14). Ulceration may occur. Features of the underlying process can often be observed. When caused by a chronic ulcer, colostomy site or burn scar, the margin may be heaped up in PSE, often giving the appearance of a rolled border, which improves and resolves as the ulcer is successfully treated. Pigmentation may be seen when PSE overlies melanoma. In deep fungal infection such as blastomycosis, PSE may present as a large plaque with central scarring and an active or serpiginous border. A palpable deep dermal nodule in association with PSE should raise the possibility of lymphoma.

Differential diagnosis
Differentiation from squamous cell carcinoma is important but can be difficult. Careful correlation of clinical and histopathology findings is required.

Investigations
DNA microarray studies show a distinct gene expression pattern that distinguishes squamous cell carcinoma from PSE. Gene *C15orf48* has a higher expression than *KRT9* in squamous cell carcinoma, but lower expression than *KRT9* in PSE [3].

Management
Skin biopsy should be undertaken to rule out squamous cell carcinoma. Treatment is directed at the underlying disorder.

Key references

The full list of references can be found in the online version at https://www.wiley.com/rooksdermatology10e

Benign keratinocytic acanthomas
6 Del Bino S, Duval C, Bernerd F. Clinical and biological characterization of skin pigmentation diversity and its consequences on UV impact. *Int J Mol Sci* 2018;19:2668.
9 Bernett CN, Schmieder GJ. Leser Trelat sign (updated 2020). In: *StatPearls [Internet]*. Treasure Island, FL: StatPearls Publishing, 2021.
11 Heidenreich B, Denisova E, Rachakonda S et al. Genetic alterations in seborrheic keratoses. *Oncotarget* 2017;8:36639–49.
13 Roh NK, Hahn HJ, Lee YW, Choe YB, Ahn KJ. Clinical and histopathological investigation of seborrheic keratosis. *Ann Dermatol* 2016;28:152–8.
22 Hafner C, Landthaler M, Mentzel T, Vogt T. FGFR3 and PIK3CA mutations in stucco keratosis and dermatosis papulosa nigra. *Br J Dermatol* 2010;162:508–12.
31 Kaddu S, Dong H, Mayer G, Kerl H, Cerroni L. Warty dyskeratoma – "follicular dyskeratoma": analysis of clinicopathologic features of a distinctive follicular adnexal neoplasm. *J Am Acad Dermatol* 2002;4:423–8.
35 Usmani A, Qasim S. Clear cell acanthoma: a review of clinical and histologic variants. *Dermatopathol (Basel)* 2020;7:26–37.
37 Morgan MB, Stevens GL, Switlyk S. Benign lichenoid keratosis: a clinical and pathologic reappraisal of 1040 cases. *Am J Dermatopathol* 2005;27:387–92.
39 Gori A, Oranges T, Janowska A et al. Clinical and dermoscopic features of lichenoid keratosis: a retrospective case study. *J Cutan Med Surg* 2018;22:561–6.

Other benign proliferations
2 Zayour M, Lazova R. Pseudoepitheliomatous hyperplasia: a review. *Am J Dermatopathol* 2011;33:112–22, quiz 123–6.

CHAPTER 133

Cutaneous Cysts

Vishal Madan[1] *and Edward Seaton*[2]

[1] Dermatology Centre, Salford Royal NHS Foundation Trust, Salford, UK
[2] OneWelbeck Skin Health and Allergy, London, UK

Introduction and general description, 133.1	Milia, 133.4	Steatocystoma multiplex, 133.6
Classification of cutaneous adnexal cysts, 133.1	Vellus hair cysts, 133.4	Cutaneous keratocysts, 133.6
CYSTS WITH INFUNDIBULAR EPITHELIAL WALL, 133.1	CYSTS WITH ISTHMIC EPITHELIAL WALL, 133.4	Key references, 133.7
Epidermoid cysts, 133.1	Trichilemmal cysts, 133.4	
Comedones, 133.3	CYSTS WITH SEBACEOUS DUCT EPITHELIAL WALL, 133.6	

Introduction and general description

The common terms used to describe cutaneous cysts are *sebaceous*, *epidermoid* and *trichilemmal*.

Classification of cutaneous adnexal cysts

While clinical differentiation of cysts can be difficult, their histology is distinct and characteristic. Classification is based on the pathogenesis, the nature of cyst contents and their wall lining (Table 133.1). Kaya and Saurat have classified cysts by examining the lining of the cystic structures [1]. Epidermal or epidermoid cysts have an epithelial wall containing a granular layer with lamellar keratinisation, indicating an origin from the follicular infundibulum (Figure 133.1). Tricholemmal or trichilemmal cysts have an undulating epithelial wall with no granular layer and a compact keratinisation as seen in the outer root sheath of hair follicles, signifying origin from follicular isthmus. In steatocystoma multiplex, dermoid cyst and folliculosebaceous hamartoma, the epithelial lining shows a crenulated appearance as seen in the sebaceous duct, hence these are the true sebaceous cysts [1].

Hidrocystoma shows the characteristic cuboidal epithelial lining of sweat glands with decapitation secretion in its apocrine forms. The hair matrix cyst wall is composed of basaloid cells maturing to squamoid cells, as seen in the normal hair matrix and shadow cells in the lumen. Metabolising acquired dioxin-induced skin hamartoma (MADISH) is a cystic lesion with lamellar keratinisation, and no sebaceous glands [1].

CYSTS WITH INFUNDIBULAR EPITHELIAL WALL

Epidermoid cysts

Definition and nomenclature
Cysts containing keratin and its breakdown products, which are surrounded by an epidermoid wall.

Synonyms and inclusions
- Epithelial cyst
- Epidermoid inclusion cyst
- Infundibular cyst
- Epidermal inclusion cyst

Epidemiology
Incidence and prevalence
These are the commonest cutaneous cysts. They are sometimes described incorrectly as sebaceous cysts.

Age
They are most frequently seen in young and middle-aged adults.

Sex
No predilection for either sex.

Table 133.1 Kaya and Saurat's classification of cutaneous adnexal cysts. Reproduced from [1].

Cysts with infundibular epithelial wall
    Epidermal (infundibular) cyst
    Comedon
    Milia
    Vellus hair cyst
Cysts with isthmic epithelial wall
    Tricholemmal cyst
Cysts with sebaceous duct epithelial wall
    Steatocystoma
    Cutaneous keratocyst
Cysts with glandular epithelial wall
    Eccrine/apocrine hidrocystoma
Cysts with hair matrix epithelial wall
    Hair matrix (pilomatrical) cyst
Hamartomatous cysts
    Dermoid cyst
    Folliculosebaceous hamartoma
    MADISH (metabolizing acquired dioxin-induced skin hamartoma)

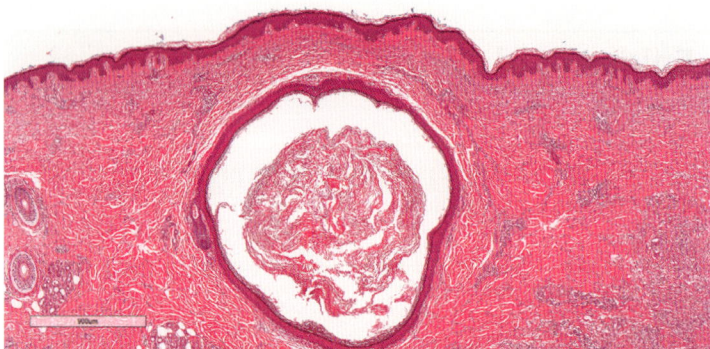

Figure 133.1 Histopathology of an epidermoid cyst.

Associated diseases
Epidermoid cysts are seen in Gardner syndrome (see Chapter 78) which is a variant of familial adenomatous polyposis and naevoid basal cell carcinoma syndrome (NBCCS) (see Chapter 140) [1,2].

Pathophysiology
The common epidermoid cyst is the result of squamous metaplasia in a damaged sebaceous gland. Many are the result of inflammation around a pilosebaceous follicle. Multiple cysts can therefore be seen in patients with more severe lesions of acne vulgaris. Some may result from deep implantation of a fragment of epidermis by a blunt penetrating injury (inclusion cysts). Those that occur as a part of Gardner syndrome and of the NBCCS are probably caused by a developmental defect.

Clinical features
History
Epidermoid cysts are most commonly seen on the face and upper trunk (Figure 133.2). They are situated in the dermis and push the epidermis upwards, appearing as a skin-coloured, white or slightly yellow, firm, spherical, smooth papule or nodule that is mobile over the deeper structures. They are tethered to the epidermis and may have a central keratin-filled punctum that is visible to the naked eye or by using a dermatoscope. The size varies from a few millimetres to more than 5 cm in diameter and the lesions may be solitary but are commonly multiple. They typically enlarge slowly and are stable, but may become acutely inflamed, increasing significantly in size with pain and tenderness.

Traumatic inclusion cysts usually occur on the palmar or plantar surfaces, buttock or knee. A history of penetrating injury may not always be obtained.

Differential diagnosis
Trichilemmal cysts are usually situated on the scalp and do not have a punctum. Lipomas are soft in their consistency. Other benign and rounded dermal tumours (Figures 133.3 and 133.4) may be mistaken for epidermoid cysts and inflammatory granulomas such as cutaneous leishmaniasis may mimic an inflamed cyst. On rare occasions, metastatic cancers to the subcutaneous or dermal compartments may simulate a cyst.

Complications and co-morbidities
Suppuration may occur which may lead to an offensive smelling discharge. Rupture of the cyst wall can give rise to acute and intense inflammation. Epidermoid cysts occurring secondary to acne and subject to recurrent inflammation may be scarred and difficult to remove completely. Calcification of the contents of epidermoid cysts cannot usually be detected clinically; when it occurs in multiple cysts of the upper part of the trunk it may be noted on chest X-ray and cause some diagnostic confusion. Dystrophic calcification of scrotal cysts is common. Malignant degeneration of epidermoid cysts has been reported rarely [3].

Disease course and prognosis
Prognosis is usually excellent.

Investigations
Diagnosis is usually clinical and can be confirmed on excision biopsy. On ultrasound, the appearance is that of an avascular mass located in the subcutaneous tissue with dorsal acoustic amplification and lateral shadowing. On magnetic resonance imaging, they have slightly hypointense signal intensity on T1-weighted images and intermediate to high signal on T2-weighted images [4].

Management
Uncomplicated cysts may not require any treatment, although patients should be advised of the possibility of slow enlargement or acute inflammation.

Surgical excision is effective. Removal of the entire cyst lining is important to reduce the risk of recurrence. Excision of an intact cyst can be undertaken via a narrow elliptical incision, which should be designed to include any visible punctum. Injection of anaesthetic around and not into the cyst itself is important. The cyst lining can usually be identified by making the initial scalpel incisions angled away from the centre of the ellipse and parallel to the cyst walls to avoid immediate puncture of the sac. Forceps can be used to securely hold the cyst via the ellipse of skin at its surface. The cyst walls may then be dissected away from the surrounding tissues, and once reached, the underside of the cyst can be freed using scissors.

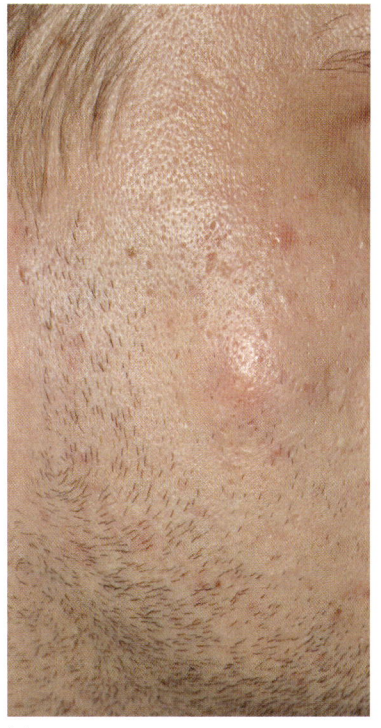
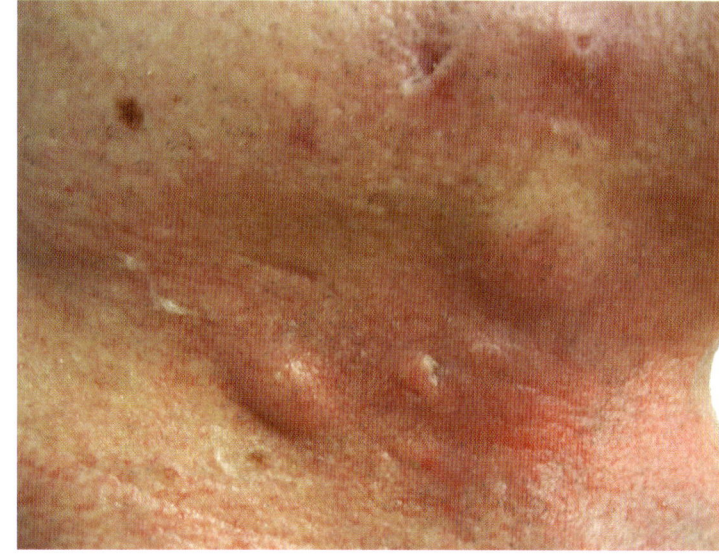

Figure 133.2 An epidermoid cyst on the (a) cheek and (b) neck.

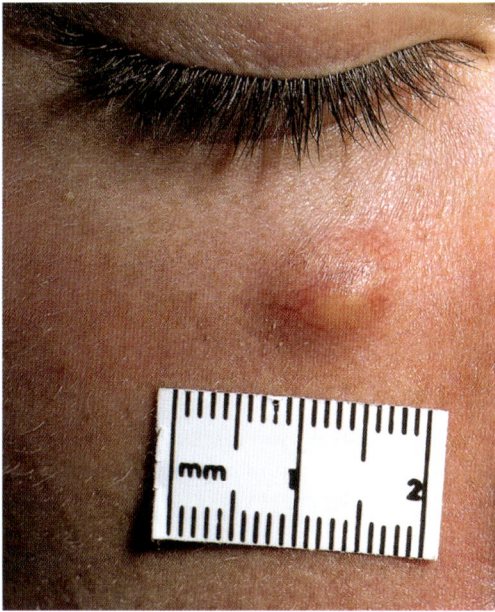

Figure 133.3 Calcified cyst just below the eyelid margin.

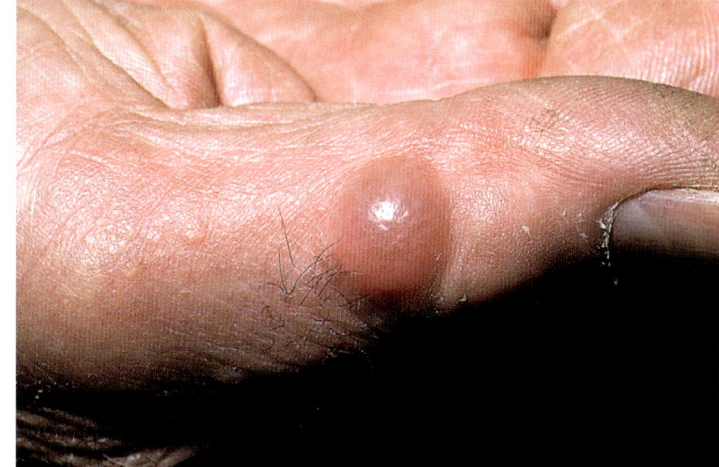

Figure 133.4 Inclusion cyst following trauma to the thumb.

An alternative procedure is punch extrusion: the cyst is directly punctured using a punch biopsy blade, including the punctum if it is visible. The keratinous contents are extruded by compression. The cyst wall is then identified and removed. Use of haemostatic forceps (e.g. mosquito) is helpful to grasp and apply gentle traction of the wall as the cyst is dissected out gradually using fine scissors. Punch extrusion produces a shorter scar than elliptical excision and may be helpful in areas where cosmetic outcome is important, such as on the face. Elliptical excision may be more appropriate for larger cysts or those that are recurrent or scarred. An acutely inflamed cyst may require incision and drainage to relieve symptoms of pain, after which it is allowed to heal by secondary intention, perhaps with packing of the defect. Alternatively, acutely inflamed cysts can be injected with triamcinolone to reduce inflammation and encourage shrinkage before excision that is delayed by a few weeks. Oral antibiotics are often given for acutely inflamed cysts, although the lesions are often not actually infected, and evidence of benefit is lacking. Inflamed acne cysts may respond to a small amount of intralesional triamcinolone given at low dose, thus obviating the need for excision.

Comedones

For detailed information please see Chapter 88.

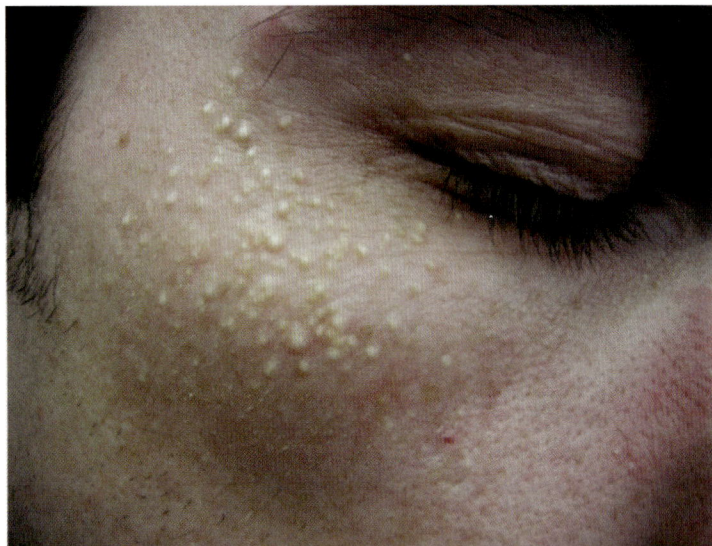

Figure 133.5 Milia on the periorbital area.

Milia

Definition
These are small subepidermal keratin cysts.

Introduction and general description
Milia are isolated or grouped small uniform spherical white papules with a smooth non-umbilicated top.

Epidemiology
Incidence and prevalence
Milia are quite common at all ages.

Associated diseases
Rombo and Bazex syndromes.

Pathophysiology
Predisposing factors
Second-degree burns, epidermolysis bullosa, porphyria cutanea tarda, bullous lichen planus, following dermabrasion, in areas of chronic topical corticosteroid-induced atrophy and radiotherapy.

Pathology
Simple common milia of the face are found within the undifferentiated sebaceous collar that encircles many vellus hair follicles. The milial cyst has a stratified squamous epithelial lining with a granular layer. The white milium body is composed of lamellated keratin. Milia that follow blistering can often be traced to eccrine sweat ducts in serial sections. Those at the margin of an irradiated area are usually situated in the distorted remnant of the pilosebaceous duct.

Clinical features
Presentation
Milia are firm, white or yellowish, rarely more than 1 or 2 mm in diameter and appear to be immediately beneath the epidermis. They are usually noticed only on the face and occur in the areas of vellus hair follicles, on the cheeks and eyelids particularly (Figure 133.5).

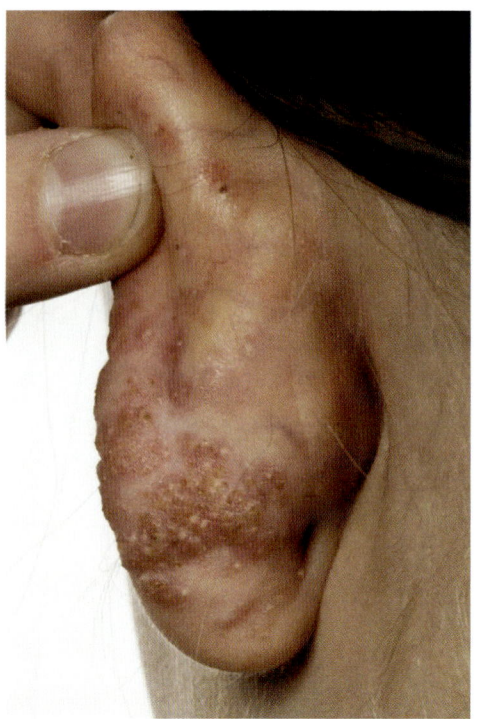

Figure 133.6 Milia en plaque on pinna.

Clinical variants
Milia en plaque appear as a cluster of white papules on a red, oedematous base. These are most commonly seen in the postauricular area (Figure 133.6).

Management
First line
Incision of the overlying epidermis and expressing the contents is curative. Recurrence is uncommon. Spontaneous disappearance occurs in many milia in infants.

Second line
Laser ablation or puncturing the milia or electrodessication can be very effective. Topical tretinoin may be effective.

Vellus hair cysts

For detailed information please see Chapter 137.

CYSTS WITH ISTHMIC EPITHELIAL WALL

Trichilemmal cysts

Definition and nomenclature
Trichilemmal cysts contain keratin and its breakdown products. They are usually situated on the scalp and their wall resembles external hair root sheath, hence the name.

Synonyms and inclusions
- Pilar cyst
- Tricholemmal cyst

Introduction and general description
Trichilemmal cysts may resemble epidermoid cysts but are not as common.

Epidemiology
Incidence and prevalence
They account for about 5–10% of keratinous cysts seen by surgical pathology services [1] but in a recent study they were felt to be more common [2].

Age
They are more common in middle age.

Sex
They are more common in women.

Pathophysiology
Pathology
Trichilemmal cysts are lined by stratified squamous epithelium (Figure 133.7). There are no distinct intercellular bridges visible among the epithelial cells and they show a distinct peripheral palisading [2]. Individual cells become larger towards the lumen. The keratinisation is abrupt with no intervening granular layer. The cyst contents are homogeneous and eosinophilic. Cholesterol clefts are common in the keratinous material which on immunohistochemistry is positive for keratins K10 and K17. Calcification of cyst contents can occur in some cases. Rupture of the cyst can lead to foreign body giant cell reaction and significant inflammation, making complete excision of the cyst difficult. Proliferating trichilemmal cysts may show gross epithelial hyperplasia of the cyst lining with minimally cystic areas mimicking clinically and histologically a squamous cell carcinoma [3]. True malignant transformation in scalp cysts is very rare.

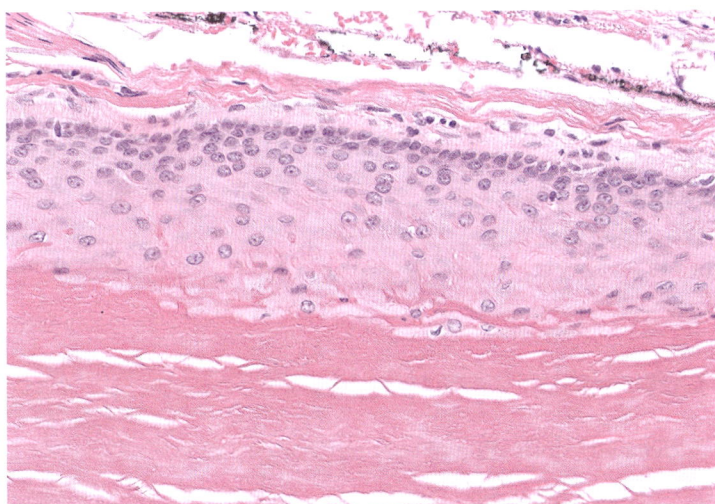

Figure 133.7 Pilar cyst showing typical pathological features (see text). Courtesy of Eduardo Calonje.

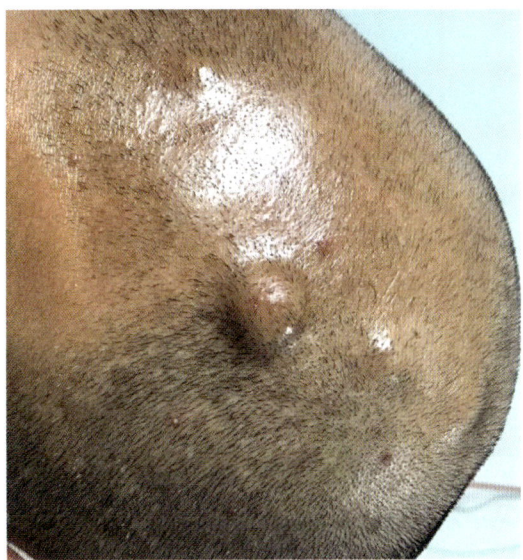

Figure 133.8 Clinical illustration of typical pilar cysts on the scalp.

Genetics
They may be inherited as an autosomal dominant disorder [3].

Clinical features
Presentation
These are usually multiple and occur mainly on the scalp and present as smooth, mobile, firm and rounded nodules (Figure 133.8). Unlike epidermoid cysts, there is usually no punctum.

Inflamed cysts may become tender and the cyst wall can rupture following an infection. The cyst wall may fuse with the epidermis to form a crypt (marsupialised cyst), which can occasionally terminate by discharging its contents and healing spontaneously. In contrast, the contents may protrude above the surface to form a soft cutaneous horn.

Clinical variants
Proliferating trichilemmal tumours are uncommon solitary, multilobular, large, exophytic masses with a predilection for the scalp in elderly females. Malignant transformation to trichilemmal carcinoma is very uncommon.

Differential diagnosis
Epidermoid cyst and proliferating trichilemmal cyst.

Investigations
Excisional biopsy.

Management
Uncomplicated cysts can be extirpated with relative ease and usually with an intact cyst wall. A simple linear incision or narrow ellipse is often sufficient. The cyst wall should be fully removed, which is often achieved easily using pressure applied to the skin on either side of the incision, with gentle blunt dissection around the sac if necessary (Figure 133.9). Proliferating cysts need to be excised with a margin because they will recur if tissue is left behind.

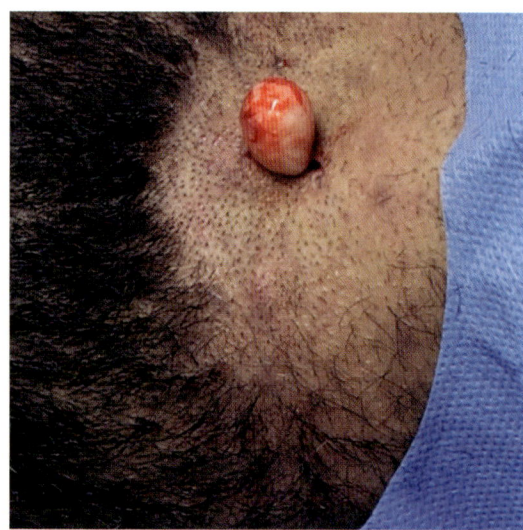

Figure 133.9 An intact pilar cyst excised from scalp.

Pathology
The cyst is situated in the mid-dermis. The cyst wall is thin and composed of keratinising epithelium with an absent granular layer (Figure 133.10). In some sections, lobules of sebaceous glands can be seen to form part of the wall or to empty into the cyst via ducts. The contents are oily and composed of unsplit esters (precursors) of sebum. They may contain hairs. Hair roots and, occasionally, sweat glands may be found connected with the cyst, and the whole complex is joined to the epidermis by a short strand of undifferentiated cells.

Genetics
Keratin 17 mutations have been implicated [1].

Clinical features
History
Multiple, smooth, skin-coloured to yellow, compressible dermal papules and nodules are present. Size varies from a few millimetres to 20 mm or more (Figure 133.11). The trunk and proximal part of the limbs are most commonly involved, particularly the pre-sternal area. Lesions may also appear on the face and acral sites [2]. No punctum is usually apparent over the cyst, but there may be multiple comedones. In these cases, differentiation from acne can be difficult. If pricked, an oily fluid can be expressed. There is an association with eruptive vellus hair cysts and pachyonychia congenita type 2.

Presentation
Presentation is usually in adulthood with lesions appearing around puberty [3].

Differential diagnosis
Nodular acne, vellus hair cysts.

Complications and co-morbidities
They are usually asymptomatic. Some lesions become inflamed, suppurate and heal with scarring.

Management
First line
Excision is often impractical because of the large number of cysts. Oral isotretinoin may reduce the size of pre-existing cysts or reduce the rate of development of new lesions [4].

Second line
Carbon dioxide or erbium:YAG laser perforation and extirpation of the cysts appears to be effective [5].

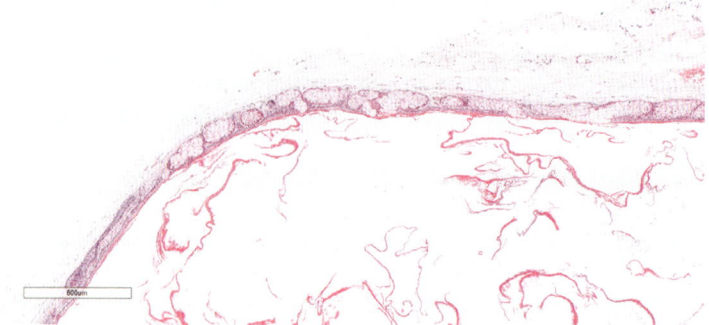

Figure 133.10 Histopathology of steatocytoma multiplex. A cyst lined by epithelium resembling the sebaceous duct. Mature sebaceous glands are present in the wall.

CYSTS WITH SEBACEOUS DUCT EPITHELIAL WALL

Steatocystoma multiplex

Definition and nomenclature
Steatocystoma multiplex is an uncommon autosomal dominant condition, which presents as multiple dermal cysts composed of sebaceous gland lobules in their wall and containing sebum. These can be regarded as true sebaceous cysts.

> **Synonyms and inclusions**
> - Sebocystomatosis
> - Hereditary epidermal polycystic disease

Pathophysiology
Steatocystoma multiplex is most likely to be a genetically determined failure of canalisation between the sebaceous lobules and the follicular pore.

Cutaneous keratocysts

For detailed information please see Chapter 140.

See Chapter 137 for discussion of:
- Cysts with glandular epithelial wall (eccrine/apocrine hidrocystoma)

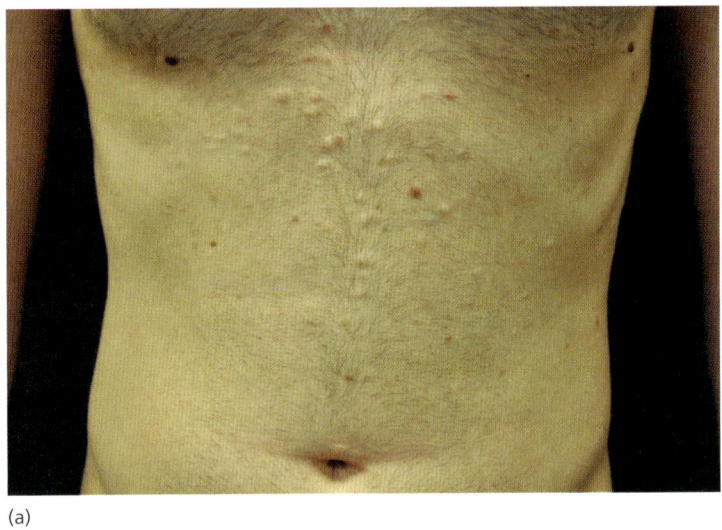 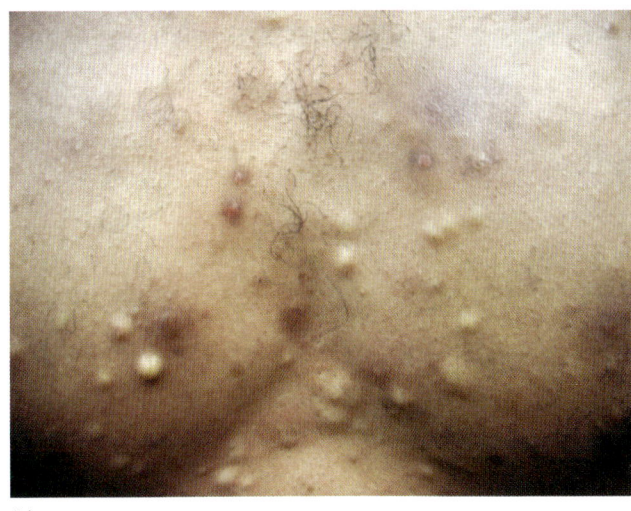

(a) (b)

Figure 133.11 (a, b) Multiple skin-coloured cysts of steatocystoma multiplex.

- Cysts with hair matrix epithelial wall (hair matrix (pilomatrical)) cyst
- Folliculosebaceous hamartoma

See Chapter 116 for discussion of:
- Dermoid cysts

See Chapters 88 and 129 for discussion of:
- MADISH (metabolising acquired dioxin-induced skin hamartoma) – chloracne

Key references

The full list of references can be found in the online version at https://www.wiley.com/rooksdermatology10e

Epidermoid cysts

1 Juhn E, Khachemoune A. Gardner syndrome: skin manifestations, differential diagnosis and management. *Am J Clin Dermatol* 2010;11:117–22.
2 Gorlin RJ. Nevoid basal cell carcinoma syndrome. *Dermatol Clin* 1995;13:113–25.
3 Morritt AN, Tiffin N, Brotherston TM. Squamous cell carcinoma arising in epidermoid cysts: report of four cases and review of the literature. *J Plast Reconstr Aesthet Surg* 2012;65:1267–9.

Trichilemmal cysts

1 Ramaswamy AS, Manjunatha HK, Sunilkumar B, Arunkumar SP. Morphological spectrum of pilar cysts. *N Am J Med Sci* 2013;5:124–8.
2 Kamyab K, Kianfar N, Dasdar S, Salehpour Z, Nasimi M. Cutaneous cysts: a clinicopathologic analysis of 2,438 cases. *Int J Dermatol* 2020;59:457–62.
3 Leppard BJ, Sanderson KV. The natural history of trichilemmal cysts. *Br J Dermatol* 1976;94:379–90.

Steatocystoma multiplex

1 Covello SP, Smith FJ, Sillevis Smitt JH *et al*. Keratin 17 mutations cause either steatocystoma multiplex or pachyonychia congenita type 2. *Br J Dermatol* 1998;139:475–80.
2 Rollins T, Levin RM, Heymann WR. Acral steatocystoma multiplex. *J Am Acad Dermatol* 2000;43:396–9.
3 Cho S, Chang SE, Choi JH, Sung KJ, Moon KC, Koh JK. Clinical and histologic features of 64 cases of steatocystoma multiplex. *J Dermatol* 2002;29:152–6.
4 Statham BN, Cunliffe WJ. The treatment of steatocystoma multiplex suppurativum with isotretinoin. *Br J Dermatol* 1984;111:246.
5 Bakkour W, Madan V. Carbon dioxide laser perforation and extirpation of steatocystoma multiplex. *Dermatol Surg* 2014;40:658–62.

CHAPTER 134

Lymphocytic Infiltrates

Fiona Child[1] and Sean J. Whittaker[1,2]

[1] St John's Institute of Dermatology, Guy's and St Thomas' NHS Foundation Trust, London, UK
[2] Division of Genetics and Molecular Medicine, King's College London, London, UK

Pseudolymphoma, 134.1	Small plaque parapsoriasis, 134.6	Jessner lymphocytic infiltrate, 134.10
Pityriasis lichenoides, 134.3	Large plaque parapsoriasis, 134.7	Key references, 134.11
Parapsoriasis, 134.6	Lymphocytoma cutis, 134.8	

Pseudolymphoma

Definition and nomenclature
Pseudolymphoma is not a specific disease but encompasses a group of benign lymphoid proliferations in the dermis, which may be difficult to distinguish from low-grade malignant lymphoma and possibly may rarely transform to a lymphoma in some cases [1–3]. The term cutaneous lymphoid hyperplasia has been suggested and both terms are more commonly used to describe a pathological rather than a clinical appearance [4]. Pseudolymphomas may be of T-cell or B-cell origin. B-cell pseudolymphoma is also called lymphocytoma cutis. T-cell pseudolymphoma may be idiopathic but may also include lymphomatoid drug eruptions, lymphomatoid contact dermatitis and actinic reticuloid. Confusion between pseudolymphoma and lymphoma can easily arise if a biopsy is submitted to the pathologist without an adequate history of recent events such as drug ingestion or scabies infestation.

> **Synonyms and inclusions**
> - Cutaneous lymphoid hyperplasia
> - Lymphocytoma cutis (B-cell pseudolymphoma)

Epidemiology
Incidence and prevalence
These are not established.

Age
It is more common in patients younger than 40 years of age.

Sex
Localised pseudolymphoma (B-cell pattern) has a female to male ratio of 2:1.

Ethnicity
No link with ethnicity has been established.

Pathophysiology
Predisposing factors
Both B- and T-cell pseudolymphomas may occur in tattoos as a reaction to certain pigments [5,6], after vaccination [7], trauma, acupuncture [8] or in association with infections. T-cell pseudolymphomas may arise as a form of adverse drug reaction. The range of causative drugs is wide but includes anticonvulsants, angiotensin-converting enzyme inhibitors, β-blockers, calcium channel blockers, cytotoxics, antirheumatics, antihistamines, antidepressants and various biologic agents [9–13,**14**]. T-cell pseudolymphoma may also occur in the context of persistent contact dermatitis [15,16].

Pathology [17–22]
In order to help distinguish between pseudolymphoma and lymphoma, it is vital to give the pathologist a good clinical history, as the pathological, phenotypic and molecular differentiation is not absolute. A T- or B-cell lymphoid proliferation is present, which is usually nodular in B-cell and nodular or band-like in T-cell proliferations (Figure 134.1). There may be a few mitotic figures but there is minimal atypical cytology. In B-cell proliferations germinal centres may or may not be present, but typically reactive germinal centres have tingible body macrophages. T-cell pseudolymphomas do not usually show significant epidermotropism. Rarely, the lymphoid cells may be very bizarre and resemble mitogen-stimulated lymphocytes seen *in vitro* during the lymphocyte transformation test [23].

Immunophenotypic studies show a normal T-cell phenotype and a mixed κ/λ expression. When germinal centres are present, Bcl-2 is not expressed in B-cell pseudolymphomas [24]. CD68 highlights tingible body macrophages. T-cell receptor (TCR)

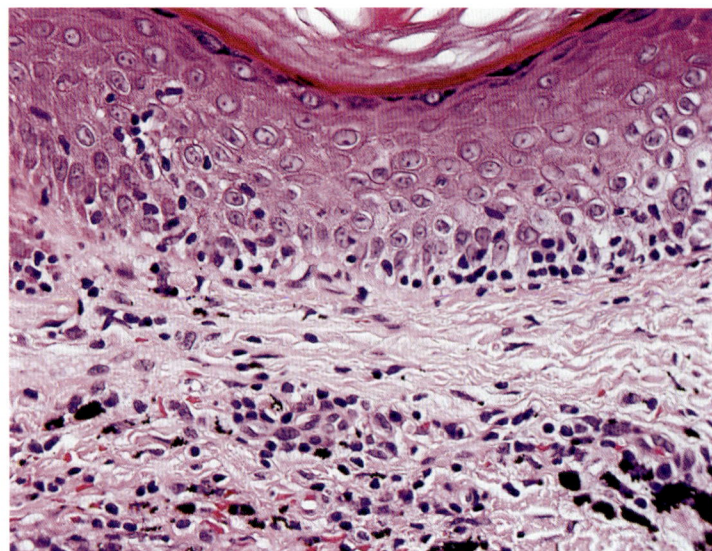

Figure 134.1 H&E-stained section of skin from a patient with a pseudolymphoma with conspicuous tagging of lymphocytes along the basal epidermis, resembling lichenoid mycosis fungoides; tattoo pigment is present in the dermis. Original magnification 400×. Courtesy of Dr Alistair Robson.

and immunoglobulin gene analysis usually shows a polyclonal pattern, but rarely a monoclonal pattern may be detected, suggesting a neoplastic proliferation. However, the significance of this finding remains unclear [25–28,29].

Causative organisms

Persistent nodular scabies and arthropod bites may cause a T-cell pseudolymphomatous histology [30–32], possibly caused by retained foreign material stimulating a persistent antigenic reaction. B-cell pseudolymphomas may be associated with *Borrelia burgdorferi* [33,34,35], *Leishmania* [36], molluscum contagiosum [37] and herpes zoster [38,39] infections. Borrelia species can also induce T-cell-rich pseudolymphomatous infiltrates [40].

Clinical features

Presentation and clinical variants

B-cell pseudolymphomas usually present as solitary or multiple, itchy or asymptomatic, smooth surfaced or excoriated, dermal papules and nodules, which may also be subcutaneous. T-cell pseudolymphomas present with solitary or scattered papules, nodules and plaques (Figure 134.2), but can also present as persistent red or purple discoloration, which may develop into an exfoliative erythroderma [41], particularly when caused by drug reactions or contact dermatitis; there may also be persistent lymphadenopathy, low-grade fever and other symptoms including headache, malaise and arthralgia.

Differential diagnosis

The most important differential diagnosis is of cutaneous B- and T-cell lymphoma. Careful clinicopathological correlation is vital in order to distinguish between them. Primary cutaneous CD4+, small/medium-sized pleomorphic T-cell lymphoproliferative disorder is an increasingly recognised entity that may have very similar clinical and histological features to pseudolymphoma and has an indolent behaviour [42,43].

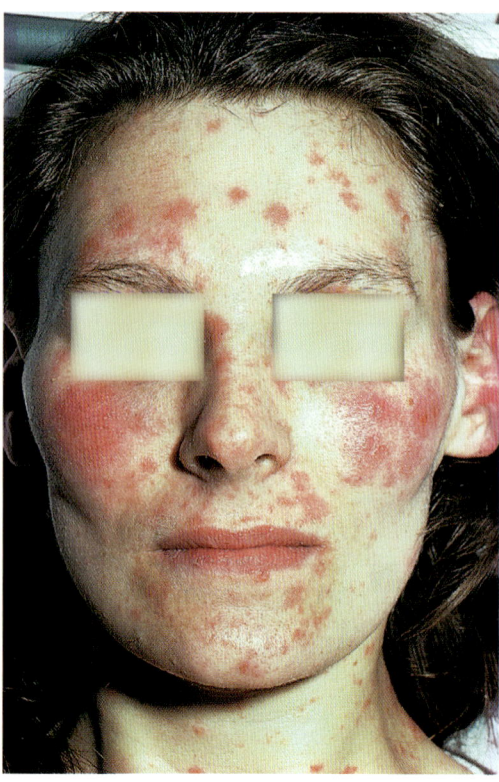

Figure 134.2 Multiple nodules and plaques of T-cell pseudolymphoma affecting the face due to a drug eruption induced by co-trimoxazole.

Complications and co-morbidities

Reports suggest cases have evolved to lymphoma; however, many of these cases may have been subtle low-grade lymphoma initially.

Disease course and prognosis

If a potential cause is identified it should be removed as soon as possible, but it may take weeks or months for the cutaneous reaction to subside. In the absence of an identifiable cause, pseudolymphomas may be persistent. The diagnosis and prognosis of pseudolymphoma should be guarded, as in a number of cases clear progression from apparent pseudolymphoma to malignant lymphoma has been recorded [1–3,25,44]. This appears to confirm the concept that chronic, initially benign, reactive inflammatory conditions may very rarely progress to frank lymphoma or that these conditions may be low-grade lymphomas initially, which then transform and adopt a more obvious malignant cellular cytology/morphology.

Investigations

A skin biopsy is needed for histology and TCR/immunoglobulin gene rearrangement analysis. *Borrelia burgdorferi* serology should be checked. Patch testing may be indicated if lymphomatoid contact dermatitis is suspected. In severe cases of drug-induced T-cell pseudolymphoma, full blood count (FBC) and liver function tests should be checked as eosinophilia and hepatitis may occur.

Management

The suspected cause should be removed. This is easiest in the case of an adverse drug reaction, but it may take weeks or even months for the cutaneous reaction to subside. Drug-induced pseudolymphomas may also present many months or even years after the therapy has been started. There are no randomised clinical trials; all treatments are based on anecdotal reports and small studies. Topical steroids may be given for symptomatic relief of itch and intralesional steroids can be injected into solitary small nodules. Hydroxychloroquine may be used for generalised disease. Treatments for lymphocytoma cutis are discussed later in the chapter.

Patients with extensive cutaneous involvement and systemic symptoms, usually when a causal drug is suspected, may require admission for supportive measures.

Pityriasis lichenoides

Definition and nomenclature

The cause of pityriasis lichenoides is unknown. Clinically, pityriasis lichenoides is divided into two main conditions: pityriasis lichenoides chronica (PLC) and pityriasis lichenoides et varioliformis acuta (PLEVA). The distinction between PLC and PLEVA is based on clinical morphology and histology rather than disease course and there may be considerable overlap between the two entities. A third, much more rare and aggressive form, febrile ulceronecrotic Mucha–Habermann disease (FUMHD), also occurs [1,2,3,4]. Pityriasis lichenoides has been considered to be a variant of parapsoriasis and may also show overlap with lymphomatoid papulosis (Chapter 139) [1,5].

> **Synonyms and inclusions**
> - Mucha–Habermann disease

Epidemiology
Incidence and prevalence
The incidence is not known, although PLC is the most common type. Both PLEVA and PLC last on average 18 months with an episodic course.

Age
It occurs most frequently in children and young adults. One large study suggested that PLEVA is the most common pattern in younger children (57% compared with 37% PLC and 6% mixed pattern) [6]. All types are rare in infancy and old age, but PLEVA has been reported at birth [7]. Most cases of FUMHD occur in the second or third decade of life [3].

Sex
In children with PLC there is a male predominance [8] but in adults there is an approximately equal sex incidence [3,8]. There is a strong male predominance in FUMH (approximately 75%) [3].

Ethnicity
Pityriasis lichenoides has been reported mainly from Europe and America, but there is no specific geographic variation in incidence or racial predisposition.

Associated diseases
PLC-like lesions have been described in patients with typical features of mycosis fungoides, and identical T-cell clones have been identified in both types of cutaneous lesions from the same patients [9]. Evidence of T-cell clonality has been detected in most cases of PLEVA and some cases of isolated PLC [8,10,11], and in FUMHD [12,13]. PLEVA has also been reported with an associated lymphoma [14]. These findings suggest that at least some cases represent a cytotoxic CD8$^+$ T-cell lymphoproliferative disease, which may coexist with other primary cutaneous T-cell lymphomas. The term 'atypical pityriasis lichenoides' has been suggested for patients with a clinicopathological presentation of pityriasis lichenoides but with an aberrant immunophenotype. These patients should be monitored in order to detect possible evolution to mycosis fungoides [15].

Pathophysiology
Predisposing factors
The aetiology is unknown. Reported triggers include medications, such as chemotherapeutic agents, oral contraceptives and vaccinations [16], in addition to infective (mainly viral) triggers. Aetiological hypotheses include an inflammatory reaction triggered by an infection or drug, an inflammatory response to a T-cell dyscrasia or an immune complex hypersensitivity vasculitis.

Pathology [3,17,18]
The histology varies with the stage, intensity and extent of the reaction; changes are more severe in PLEVA than in PLC. In early lesions, an infiltrate of predominantly small lymphocytes surrounds and involves the walls of dilated dermal capillaries, which show endothelial proliferation (Figure 134.3). In PLEVA, the infiltrate may be deep, dense and wedge-shaped rather than predominantly perivascular. The epidermis is oedematous, with an interface dermatitis composed mainly of CD8$^+$ lymphocytes. Some necrotic keratinocytes are often present, especially in PLEVA. Intraepidermal and perivascular extravasation of erythrocytes is typical. Later, over the centre of the lesion, a parakeratotic scale forms, containing lymphocytic pseudo-Munro abscesses, and there is prominent exocytosis of lymphocytes. Mild cytological atypia can be present. If the reaction is still more intense, as occurs in FUMHD, frank necrosis occurs and the lesion may be difficult to distinguish from other forms of acute necrosis of the skin on histology. In FUMHD there may be marked fibrinoid necrosis of deep vessels with luminal thrombi, partial necrosis of follicles and complete necrosis of eccrine glands.

Immunofluorescence studies variably demonstrate IgM, C3 and fibrin in the vessel walls of fresh lesions [16]. Macrophages are increased in number and Langerhans cells are decreased. HLA-DR is expressed by the lymphocytic infiltrate and the overlying epidermis.

There is a histological resemblance to many other conditions, including common inflammatory conditions such as psoriasis and resolving eczema. The most important is the distinction from parapsoriasis and particularly (as they may also be clinically similar) differentiation between PLEVA and lymphomatoid papulosis. The most useful distinction from lymphomatoid papulosis is that the latter shows a more pronounced collection of papulonodular

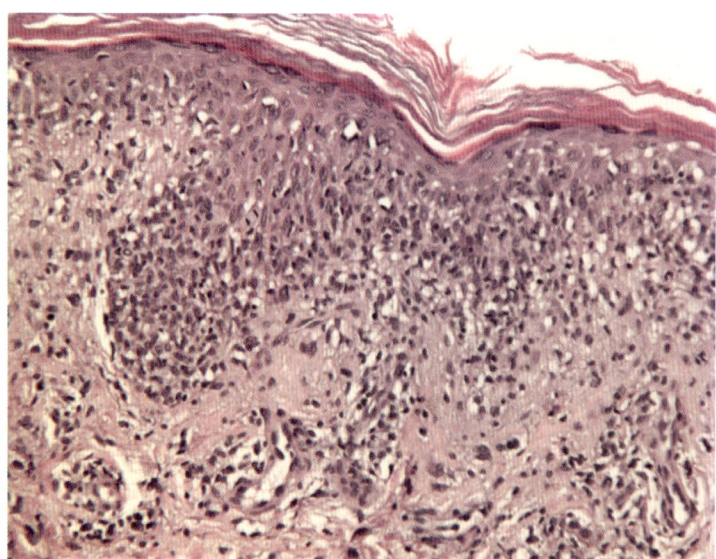

Figure 134.3 H&E-stained section of skin illustrating a florid lymphocytic infiltrate obscuring the dermal–epidermal junction. There is no cytological atypia. Original magnification 400×. Courtesy of Dr Alistair Robson.

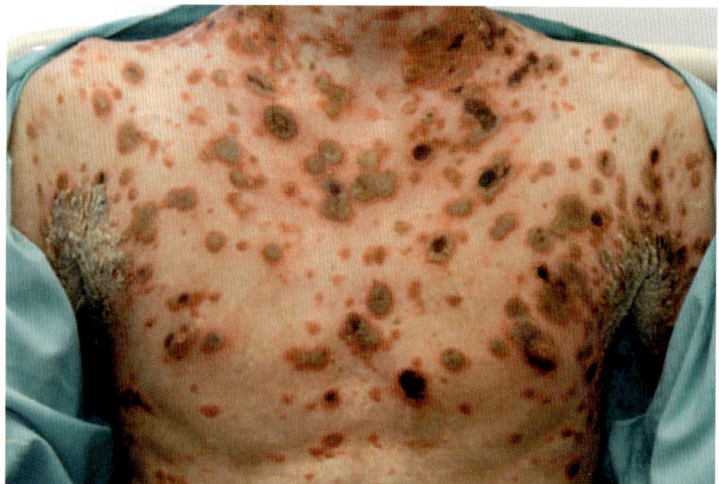

Figure 134.4 Crusted necrotic and ulcerative plaques in a young man with febrile ulceronecrotic Mucha–Habermann disease.

lesions with a predominant population of large atypical CD30+ cells (usually CD4+ but occasionally CD8+) whereas atypical CD30+ cells in pityriasis lichenoides are usually few and invariably CD8+ [9]. Cutaneous lymphocyte-associated antigen (CLA) and T-cell intercellular antigen 1 (TIA-1) are expressed in both conditions and indicate a proliferation of cytotoxic T cells [19].

Causative organisms

Histological features of an underlying vasculitis in PLEVA suggest an immune complex-mediated pathogenesis. In support of this hypothesis there are many documented cases of infective triggers. Seasonal peaks of onset in autumn and winter [6], and rare familial outbreaks [20], suggest the possibility of an infectious trigger. Numerous potential infectious triggers have been summarised in reviews [3,18], and include toxoplasmosis [21,22], cytomegalovirus [23], parvovirus B19 [24,**25**,26], adenovirus [27], Epstein–Barr virus (EBV) [28,29], herpes simplex [30], varicella-zoster virus [31,32], HIV [33], measles, MMR and human papillomavirus vaccines [16,34,35], streptococci [36], staphylococci and *Mycoplasma* infections. In many such reports, there is evidence of seroconversion at the time of onset or of resolution of pityriasis lichenoides when the infective trigger was treated, supporting a causal relationship. Parvovirus B19 genomic DNA was identified in lesional skin in 30% of patients with PLEVA [37]. A therapeutic response of PLC to tonsillectomy in the setting of chronic tonsillitis has been reported [38], as well as responses to antibiotics such as erythromycin [1,39,40] or tetracycline [41]. Resolution has also followed pegylated interferon and ribavirin in a patient with hepatitis C infection [42]. In one study, human herpesvirus 8 DNA in lesional skin was discovered in 11 (21%) patients with pityriasis lichenoides, but in none of the controls [43].

Clinical features

History and presentation [1,2,3,4,5,39,43–46]

Pityriasis lichenoides et varioliformis acuta. The eruption develops in crops and consequently appears polymorphic. Constitutional symptoms such as fever, headache, malaise and arthralgia may precede or accompany the onset of lesions. The initial lesion is an oedematous pink papule that undergoes central vesiculation and haemorrhagic necrosis. In the vesicular forms the vesicles may be small or so large that the eruption appears frankly bullous [44]. The rate of progression of individual lesions varies greatly, as do the frequency and extent. New lesions may cause irritation or a burning sensation as they appear, but are often asymptomatic. The trunk, thighs and upper arms, especially the flexor aspects, are most frequently affected, but the eruption may be generalised. Lesions on the palms and soles are less common, and the face and scalp are often spared; red or necrotic lesions affecting the mucous membranes may be present. Lesions heal with scarring, which may be varioliform. PLEVA in pregnancy carries a potential risk of premature labour if there are mucosal lesions in the region of the cervical os [45].

Febrile ulceronecrotic Mucha–Habermann disease. In the acute ulceronecrotic form there is high fever and large necrotic lesions (Figure 134.4); new crops may continue to develop over many months. About 50–75% of cases occur in adults, with a fulminating course that may even be fatal [1,2,46,47]. General malaise, weakness, myalgia, neuropsychiatric symptoms and lymphadenopathy occur, with non-specific serological markers of inflammation such as raised erythrocyte sedimentation rate (ESR) and C-reactive protein; there may be serological evidence of associated viral infection.

Pityriasis lichenoides chronica. The characteristic lesion is a small, firm, lichenoid papule 3–10 mm in diameter, and reddish brown in colour (Figure 134.5). An adherent 'mica-like' scale can be detached by gentle scraping to reveal a shining brown surface – a distinctive diagnostic feature. Over the course of 3 or 4 weeks, the papule flattens and the scale separates spontaneously to leave a pigmented macule, which gradually fades. Postinflammatory hypopigmentation may occur, and is occasionally persistent, but scarring is unusual in PLC. The body site distribution is the same as for PLEVA but an isolated acral form may occur [48–50] and segmental forms have been reported [51].

Differential diagnosis
The acute vesicular form must be distinguished from varicella; acute necrotic lesions may suggest other necrotic skin infections, vasculitis or pyoderma gangrenosum. Lymphomatoid papulosis is a particularly difficult differential diagnosis in patients with necrotic lesions in view of its histological similarity, although lymphomatoid papulosis is usually characterised by less vesicular and more necrotic papulonodular lesions than those of PLEVA.

PLC must be differentiated from guttate psoriasis and lichen planus. The acral form of PLC in particular may mimic psoriasis, and secondary syphilis needs to be excluded, especially if the palms and soles are involved or if there are mucosal lesions. The single, detachable 'mica-like' scale on the red-brown papule is a characteristic sign of PLC. Gianotti–Crosti syndrome is less likely to be confused with pityriasis lichenoides, but insect bites and drug eruptions should be included in the differential diagnosis.

Complications and co-morbidities
In FUMH and PLEVA, ulcerated lesions may become secondarily infected.

Disease course and prognosis
The course of pityriasis lichenoides varies. If the onset is acute, new crops may cease to develop after a few weeks, and many cases are clear within 6 months. However, acute recurrences may occur over a period of years, or may become chronic. In some cases, all lesions are of the chronic scaling type from the onset, and new crops of similar lesions may develop from time to time over the years. Uncommonly, acute attacks occur after chronic lesions have been present for months or years. In general, the immediate prognosis is said to be better when the onset is acute and the lesions that occur in successive crops are also of the acute type. However, one large study of 124 children showed only a small difference in clearance times between PLEVA (mean 18 months) and PLC (mean 20 months) [6]. A smaller study comparing adults and children found that the disease tended to run a longer course in children, with a greater extent of lesions, more pigmentation and a poor response to conventional treatments [52].

Investigations
A skin biopsy is needed for histology, immunohistochemistry and TCR gene rearrangement analysis. In cases of FUMH, a causative infectious agent may be implicated and investigations should be tailored to each patient's presentation. They may include antistreptolysin (ASO) titre, throat swab, hepatitis, EBV and HIV serology, monospot and investigations for *Toxoplasma* infection.

Management
Management of both PLC and PLEVA is similar and, in the small number of controlled trials that have been conducted, both conditions are included. Topical corticosteroids may improve symptoms and healing of lesions but do not alter the course of the disease. There are also reports of disease clearance with the application of topical tacrolimus ointment [53,54]. In adults, phototherapy [3] is usually the first line treatment of choice, and includes natural sunlight, UVB [55], narrow-band UVB [56–58], UVA-1 [59] and psoralen and UVA (PUVA) [60]. Responses are also reported with the addition of acitretin to PUVA in refractory disease [61].

A randomised trial comparing narrow-band UVB with PUVA showed no significant difference in response rate between the two therapies [57]. In children, treatment options include antibiotics such as tetracyclines [62] or erythromycin [6,40,52] (preferred in young children because of the dental pigmentation side effects of tetracycline). In more aggressive or refractory disease of PLEVA or FUMHD pattern, and less commonly in PLC, various immunosuppressive agents including methotrexate [63], ciclosporin and dapsone [3] and intravenous immunoglobulin [64] may prove successful. Elevated levels of serum tumour necrosis factor α (TNF-α) in a patient with FUMHD [65] have resulted in the successful use of anti-TNF-α inhibitors in a small number of patients [66,67]. However, there are also reports of infliximab, adalimumab and etanercept causing pityriasis lichenoides [68–71].

Treatment ladder

Pityriasis lichenoides chronica

First line
- Topical steroids/immunomodulators

Second line: adults
- Phototherapy (broad-/narrow-band UVB, PUVA)
- Antibiotics (tetracycline, erythromycin)

Second line: children
- Antibiotics (erythromycin)

Third line: adults
- Acitretin (acitretin plus PUVA)
- Methotrexate, ciclosporin, dapsone, UVA-1

Third line: children
- Methotrexate, ciclosporin, dapsone

Pityriasis lichenoides et varioliformis acuta

First line
- Oral antibiotics (erythromycin)

Second line: adults
- Phototherapy (broad-/narrow-band UVB, PUVA)
- Acitretin plus PUVA

Second line: children
- Phototherapy (broad-/narrow-band UVB)

Third line: adults
- Systemic corticosteroids, methotrexate, ciclosporin, dapsone, UVA-1

Third line: children
- Systemic corticosteroids, methotrexate, ciclosporin, dapsone

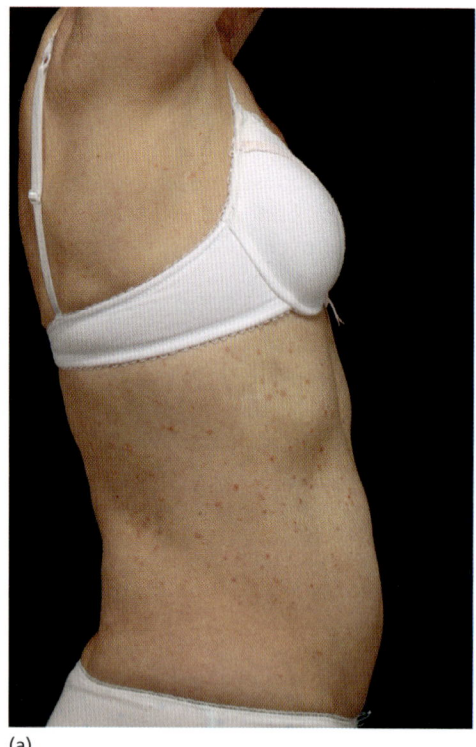 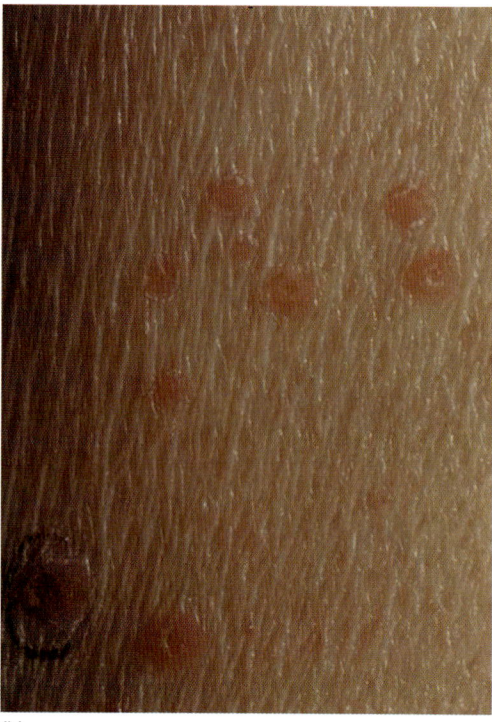

Figure 134.5 (a) Scattered scaly papules on the trunk in a patient with pityriasis lichenoides chronica (PLC). (b) Close-up of individual lesions of PLC showing the mica-like scale.

Parapsoriasis

This term has caused confusion since its introduction in 1902 because of the lack of a universally agreed definition of the clinical entities to be included. For this reason, many dermatologists prefer not to use the term at all, and to substitute one of the many synonyms for clinical conditions that might be included in one of the parapsoriasis groups. There is unresolved controversy as to whether two of the parapsoriasis variants are either precursors of cutaneous T-cell lymphoma, mycosis fungoides (MF) variant (so-called premycotic eruptions) or established, but early, MF from the outset. There is a broad division of parapsoriasis into small and large plaque variants, each with a number of synonyms. The evidence that the majority of cases of small plaque parapsoriasis (SPP) are a chronic, benign condition is reasonable. In contrast, a large series of patients with large plaque parapsoriasis (LPP) recorded the development of definite MF in 11% of cases but whether these cases were MF from the outset remains unclear [1]. However, a more recent retrospective study of both SPP and LPP showed that 10% of patients with SPP and 35% of those with LPP evolved into MF over a median period of 10 and 6 years, respectively [2]. Unfortunately, TCR gene rearrangement studies have been inconclusive, although the proportion of cases with evidence of monoclonality is lower in SPP [3–6]. Long-term follow-up of these cases is required.

Small plaque parapsoriasis

Definition and nomenclature

This is a chronic asymptomatic condition, characterised by the presence of persistent, small, scaly plaques, mainly on the trunk [1,2,3].

Synonyms and inclusions
- Chronic superficial scaly dermatitis
- Persistent superficial dermatitis
- Digitate dermatosis
- Xanthoerythroderma perstans

Epidemiology
Incidence
The incidence of SPP is not known and may be underreported as it is usually asymptomatic.

Age
It normally presents in middle age with a peak incidence in the fifth decade.

Sex
It is more common in males, with a 3 : 1 male to female incidence.

Pathophysiology
Pathology
This is non-specific. There are small focal areas of hyperkeratosis and parakeratosis, and in the underlying dermis there are small aggregates of morphologically normal CD4$^+$ T cells, mainly around the vasculature. There is no epidermotropism and no Pautrier microabscesses (Figure 134.6).

Immunophenotypic studies reveal a normal mature T-cell phenotype. Reports have identified 'dominant T-cell clones' in some cases of SPP using polymerase chain reaction (PCR) analysis [3,4]. The significance of this observation in terms of its relationship to MF and disease progression is not yet clear. There is also a report of a

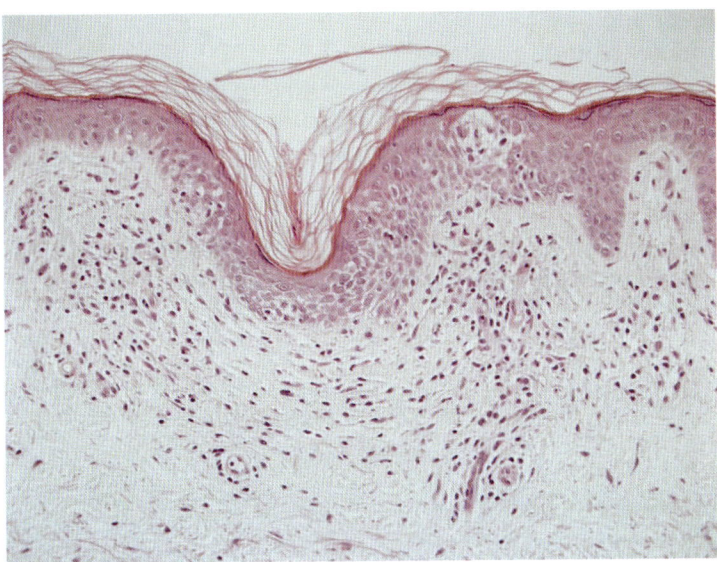

Figure 134.6 H&E-stained section of skin illustrating spongiosis, light lymphocytic dermal inflammation and exocytosis – features commonly seen in chronic superficial scaly dermatitis. Original magnification 100×. Courtesy of Dr Alistair Robson.

higher frequency of clonal T cells in the peripheral blood of patients with SPP [6] with no evidence of clonality in the skin, although the significance of this finding is questionable because non-pathological T-cell clones can be found in the peripheral blood of patients with benign cutaneous infiltrates and normal, healthy volunteers [7,8].

Clinical features
Presentation
The lesions usually appear insidiously and asymptomatically on the trunk and, to a lesser extent, on the limbs of young adults. Individual lesions are monomorphic, round or oval red/purple/dusky patches, 2.5–5 cm in diameter, with slight scaling (Figure 134.7). Some have a slightly yellow, waxy tinge. The digitate dermatosis is a distinctive form, which consists of finger-like projections following dermatomes on the lateral aspects of the chest and abdomen. The lesions persist for years or even decades and may be more obvious during the winter. There is sparing of the pelvic girdle area and the striking polymorphic appearance of individual patches seen in MF is lacking.

Differential diagnosis
This includes other inflammatory dermatoses that may present with scaly, red/purple/dusky patches and includes discoid eczema, guttate psoriasis, pityriasis versicolor and allergic contact dermatitis. Early-stage cutaneous T-cell lymphoma should also be considered.

Disease course and prognosis
It may persist for many years and subsequently resolve spontaneously. There are reports of progression to MF in a minority of cases [1,2,9].

Investigations
The diagnosis is usually made clinically as histology is non-specific. However, a skin biopsy should be taken for histology and TCR gene rearrangement studies if there is any suspicion of MF.

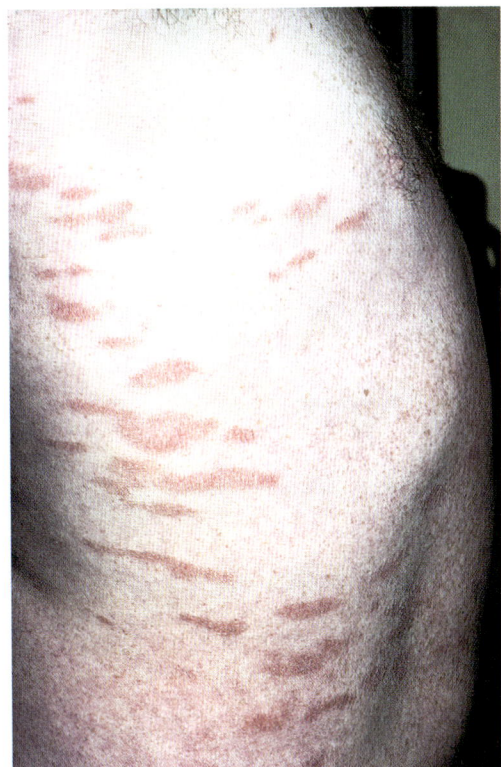

Figure 134.7 Typical pattern of chronic, superficial, scaly dermatosis showing finger-like projections on the sides of the torso.

Management
Often, little treatment is needed. Emollients may help control the scaling. There are no randomised clinical trials, but retrospective and prospective studies have shown that both PUVA and narrow-band UVB phototherapy may result in temporary clearance of the lesions [10–12,13]. Both complete and partial responses have also been reported with topical nitrogen mustard [14].

Large plaque parapsoriasis

Definition and nomenclature
This is a chronic condition characterised by the presence of fixed, large, atrophic, red/purple/dusky plaques, usually on the trunk and occasionally on the limbs.

Synonyms and inclusions
- Parakeratosis variegata
- Retiform parapsoriasis
- Atrophic parapsoriasis
- Poikilodermatous parapsoriasis

Epidemiology
Sex
There is a slight male predominance.

Associated diseases
It may progress to MF [2] although it may be early-stage MF from the outset.

Pathophysiology
Pathology [15,16]
There is frequently epidermal atrophy and a lichenoid or interface reaction may also be seen at the dermal–epidermal junction. There is a band-like lymphocytic infiltrate in the papillary dermis and there may also be free red cells present. The histology is not diagnostic for MF and most biopsies only show a mild dermatitis. Immunophenotypic studies reveal a normal T-cell phenotype. In one study TCR gene rearrangement studies identified a clonal T-cell population in the skin in 6 of 12 patients, but progression to overt cutaneous T-cell lymphoma was only noted in 1 of the 12 patients [17].

Clinical features
Patients present with persistent, large, yellow-orange atrophic patches and thin plaques on the trunk and limbs. The involvement of covered skin on the breast and buttock areas suggests MF and in these cases patches and plaques may show striking polymorphism and poikiloderma with slow progression [18].

Investigations
A skin biopsy is needed for histology, immunohistochemistry and TCR gene rearrangement analysis.

Management
Topical emollients, UVB and PUVA are all helpful in offering symptomatic relief [19,20]. Topical nitrogen mustard can also lead to clearance of disease [21]. There is one report of the successful use of the excimer laser (308 nm) with long-term benefit [22]. Topical steroids should be used with caution because of the atrophic nature of the condition. In view of the risk of progression to cutaneous T-cell lymphoma, patients should be offered intermittent dermatology review.

Lymphocytoma cutis

Definition and nomenclature
Lymphocytoma cutis is a benign, cutaneous, B-cell lymphoproliferative disorder that is included as a subtype of pseudolymphoma. It encompasses a spectrum of benign B-cell lymphoproliferative diseases that share clinical and histopathological features. It occurs as a response to known or unknown antigenic stimuli that result in the accumulation of lymphocytes and other inflammatory cells in a localised region on the skin.

Synonyms and inclusions
- Spiegler–Fendt sarcoid
- Lymphadenosis benigna cutis of Bafverstedt
- Reactive cutaneous lymphoid hyperplasia

Epidemiology
Incidence and prevalence
Not known, although in Europe lymphocytoma cutis associated with *Borrelia burgdorferi* infection occurs primarily in areas where the *Ixodes ricinus* tick is endemic [1].

Age
It can occur at any age but is most commonly seen in early adulthood. Borrelial lymphocytoma is more common in children than adults [2].

Sex
There is a female preponderance, with a female to male ratio of approximately 2 : 1 [3].

Ethnicity
There is no racial predilection.

Pathophysiology
Pathology [3,4,5,6]
The epidermis is usually unaffected and is often separated by a relatively acellular grenz zone from the dermis, which is replaced by a nodular, dense infiltrate extending through the full thickness of the dermis but without cellular atypia (Figure 134.8). In classic cases, lymphocytes and histiocytes form a follicular arrangement (germinal centre) resembling the appearance of a lymph node (Figure 134.9). Mitotic figures may be visible in the cells of the follicles and occasional eosinophils may also be present. Appendages and blood vessels are spared. Some cases lack well-defined lymphoid follicles, although the histological appearance with normal lymphocytes and histiocytes is otherwise similar. The majority of lymphocytes in the dermis are B cells. In cases with well-formed germinal centres, a cuff of reactive T cells may be seen around the periphery of the main B-cell aggregate. The germinal centres also retain cells that express CD10 and Bcl-6 but expression of Bcl-2 by germinal centre cells is not seen. There is polytypic expression of κ and λ light chains. The histological differential diagnosis includes primary cutaneous lymphoma, particularly of marginal zone origin.

Causative organisms
Infectious stimuli include *Borrelia burgdorferi* [1,2], molluscum contagiosum and *Leishmania donovani* [7]. Lymphocytoma cutis may also present in scars from previous herpes zoster virus infections [8].

Environmental factors
Other reported stimuli causing lymphocytoma cutis include trauma, vaccinations [9], allergy hyposensitisation injections [10], drug ingestion, arthropod bites, acupuncture, metallic pierced earrings [11] and treatment with leeches [12].

Clinical features
Presentation
Most patients show solitary or grouped, asymptomatic, red or plum-coloured papules, nodules or plaques, most commonly on

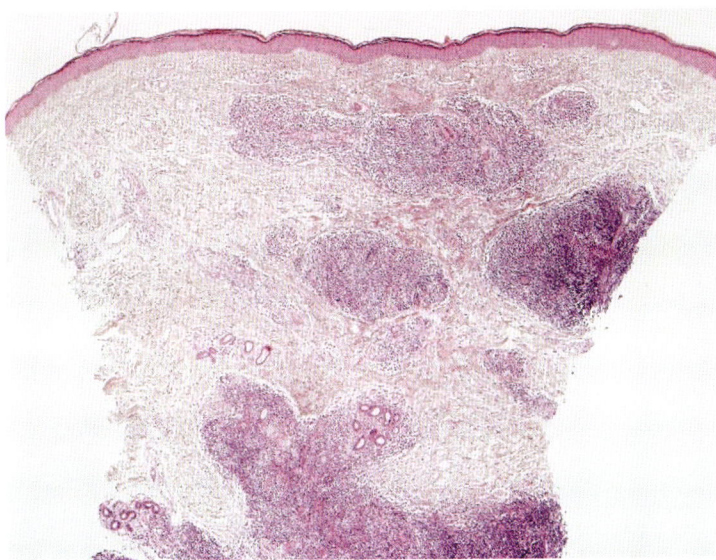

Figure 134.8 H&E-stained section of skin illustrating a dense, nodular infiltrate in the dermis. There is a grenz zone and a normal epidermis. Original magnification 20×. Courtesy of Dr Alistair Robson.

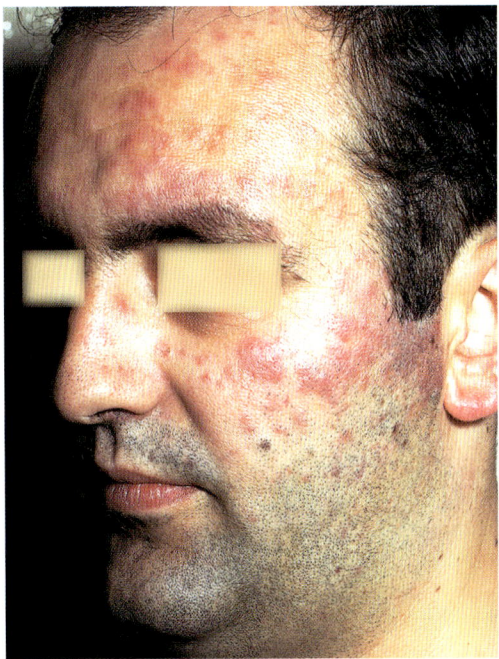

Figure 134.10 Extensive dermal nodules of lymphocytoma cutis on the face.

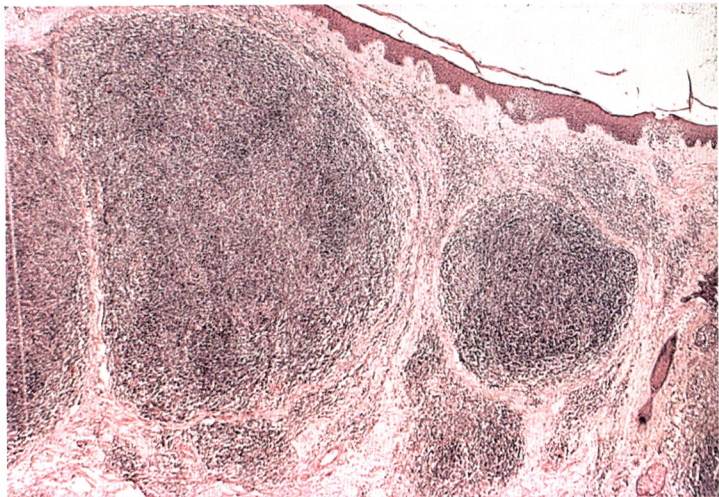

Figure 134.9 H&E-stained section demonstrating the large reactive lymphoid follicles that can be seen in lymphocytoma cutis.

the face, chest and upper extremities (Figure 134.10). Occasionally, they may have a translucent appearance. They are usually asymptomatic but can occasionally be itchy or tender. They enlarge slowly and may reach a diameter of 3–5 cm. Associated sunlight sensitivity has been reported in some patients [13]. Bafverstedt [14] has described an unusual form of lymphocytoma that presented as a solitary tumour of the scrotal skin. Disseminated or miliary lymphocytoma cutis is also reported [15–17]. Lymphocytoma cutis secondary to *Borrelia* infection is most frequently seen at sites with low skin temperature such as the earlobes, nipples, nose and scrotum [1].

Differential diagnosis
Histological examination should distinguish lymphocytoma cutis from granulomatous disorders including sarcoidosis, granuloma faciale and rosacea. Distinction from primary cutaneous B-cell marginal zone lymphoma (MZL) is difficult, although the presence of atypical lymphoid cells, immunoglobulin light chain restriction and detection of a clonal immunoglobulin gene rearrangement by molecular analysis would suggest a primary cutaneous MZL. Insect bite reactions may also be impossible to distinguish from lymphocytoma cutis.

Jessner benign lymphocytic infiltration, tumid discoid lupus erythematosus and polymorphic light eruption can also cause difficulties. However, in Jessner lymphocytic infiltrate, which characteristically waxes and wanes in severity, the dermal lymphocytic infiltrate is dominated by T cells. The presence of basal cell liquefaction degeneration and positive direct immunofluorescence helps distinguish lupus erythematosus.

Disease course and prognosis
The course of disease varies but is often chronic and indolent. If the cause is identified, the lesions may resolve once the cause is removed. Some lesions resolve spontaneously. Long-term follow-up of these patients suggests that a small proportion progress to or begin as a primary cutaneous B-cell lymphoma (MZL) [5,18,19].

Investigations
A skin biopsy is needed for histology, immunohistochemistry and immunoglobulin gene analysis. Serology is required to test for *Borrelia burgdorferi*. Patch testing may be requested if a possible contact allergen is suspected.

Management
There is no treatment of proven value for lymphocytoma cutis, with only anecdotal reports and small case series, and no clinical trials. If a causal agent is identified, it should be removed if possible.

First line therapies for localised disease include excision, topical or intralesional corticosteroids and oral antibiotics if the *Borrelia* serology is positive. In generalised disease, hydroxychloroquine [20] may be of benefit. Second line therapies for localised disease with reported success include superficial radiotherapy [21], intralesional interferon α (IFN-α) [22,23], cryotherapy, intralesional rituximab [24], topical 0.1% tacrolimus ointment [25] and topical photodynamic therapy [26–28]. Subcutaneous IFN-α [29,**30**], thalidomide [16,31,32] and methotrexate [33] have also shown benefit in generalised disease.

Jessner lymphocytic infiltrate

Definition
This is a chronic, benign, inflammatory condition, usually affecting photo-exposed skin. First described in 1953 by Jessner and Kanof [1], it remains poorly understood. It has many similarities with lupus erythematosus tumidus, both clinically and histologically [2,**3**,**4**].

Epidemiology
Incidence and prevalence
The incidence and prevalence are not known but it is uncommon.

Age
It mainly occurs in adults below the age of 50 years. It may occur in children [5] and familial cases have also been reported [6,7].

Sex
There are conflicting reports of male and female predominance.

Ethnicity
There is no known racial predilection.

Associated diseases
Recent literature suggests that it may be a variant of lupus erythematosus.

Pathophysiology
It is not well understood. Its relationship to lupus erythematosus and other benign cutaneous lymphocytic infiltrates is not clear.

Pathology [2,8–10]
The epidermis is usually normal with no atrophy, follicular plugging or basement membrane thickening. There is a moderately dense superficial and deep perivascular dermal lymphocytic infiltrate. It may also be perifollicular and extend to the subcutis (Figure 134.11). The infiltrate contains small mature lymphocytes, with occasional large lymphoid cells, plasmacytoid and plasma cells. Copious dermal mucin is not seen. Immunohistochemistry confirms a mixed lymphocytic infiltrate with a dominant population of CD8+ cells. Direct immunofluorescence is negative. Both T-cell and B-cell populations are polyclonal on molecular analysis.

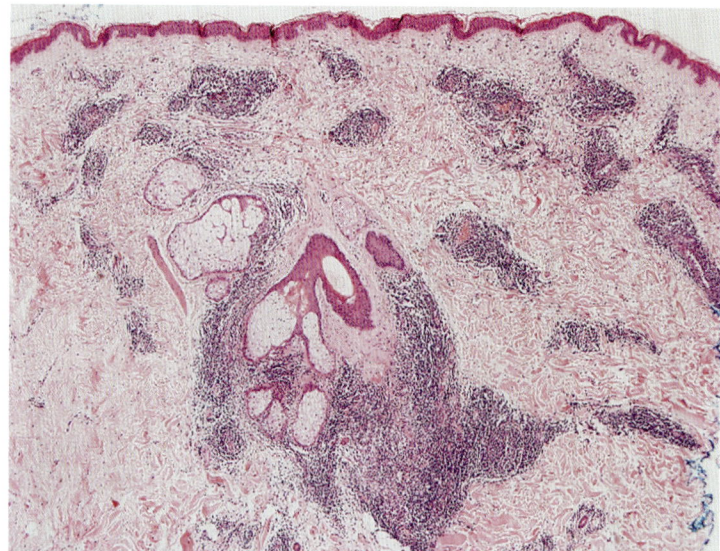

Figure 134.11 H&E-stained section of skin from a patient with Jessner lymphocytic infiltrate showing a moderately dense superficial and deep perivascular dermal lymphocytic infiltrate. Original magnification 40×.

Clinical features
Presentation
It presents with asymptomatic, non-scaly, red/purple/dusky papules and plaques, mainly affecting the face, neck and upper chest. There may be one, a few or numerous lesions and central clearing of lesions may occur, giving them an annular appearance (Figure 134.12). There is no atrophy or follicular plugging. There may or may not be a history of onset following sun exposure. The lesions may last months or years and often resolve spontaneously but can recur, either at the same or a different site.

Differential diagnosis
Polymorphic light eruption can usually be excluded from the history and short duration of lesions. Lupus erythematosus and lymphocytoma cutis can be excluded histologically. Lesions of CD4+ small/medium T-cell pleomorphic lymphoproliferative disorder are usually solitary and although histological features are similar, the follicular T-cell immunophenotype can help distinguish it from Jessner lymphocytic infiltrate [11].

Disease course and prognosis
Prognosis is good as it is benign in nature and may resolve spontaneously; there is no increase in mortality.

Investigations
A skin biopsy is needed for histology, direct immunofluorescence and molecular gene rearrangement studies. Serology testing for systemic lupus erythematosus should be considered, including antinuclear antibodies, ESR, anti-Ro and anti-La antibodies, FBC and urinalysis. Phototesting may be useful in those patients with a history of photosensitivity.

Management
Treatments are often unsatisfactory and based on case reports. It may require no treatment if it is asymptomatic. Cosmetic camouflage,

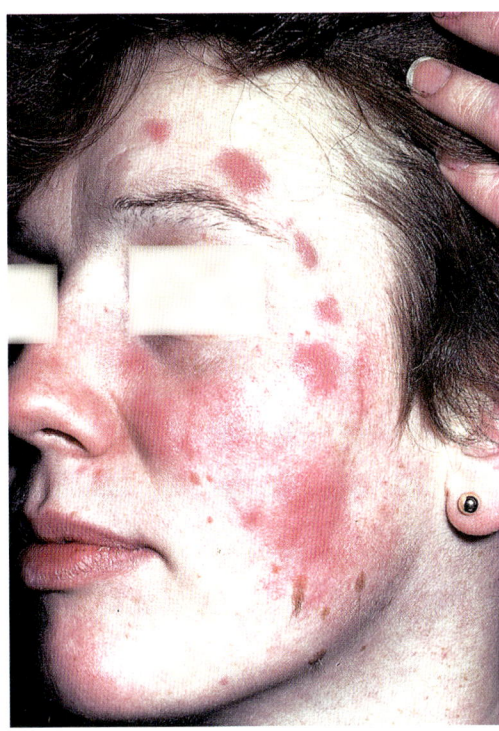

Figure 134.12 Non-scaly red plaques on the face of a young woman with Jessner lymphocytic infiltrate.

excision of small lesions, photoprotection and topical [2] or intralesional [5] steroids may provide benefit. Hydroxychloroquine [2], systemic steroids and cryotherapy have been used with success. There are reports of benefit with methotrexate [12], retinoids [13] and oral auranofin [14]. There is one randomised double blind cross-over study comparing thalidomide with placebo in 27 patients; 59% remained in complete remission 1 month after stopping treatment [15]. Clearing of lesions has also been reported with pulsed dye laser [16] and methyl aminolevulinate photodynamic therapy [17].

Key references

The full list of references can be found in the online version at https://www.wiley.com/rooksdermatology10e

Pseudolymphoma

14 Magro CM, Daniels BH, Crowson AN. Drug induced pseudolymphoma. *Seminars in Diagnostic Pathol* 2018;35:247–59.
29 Wood GS. Analysis of clonality in cutaneous T-cell lymphoma and associated diseases. *Ann NY Acad Sci* 2001;941:26–30.
34 Colli C, Leinweber B, Mulleegger R, Chott A, Kerl H, Cerroni L. Borrelia burgdorfori-associated lymphocytoma cutis: clinicopathological, immunophenotypic and molecular study of 106 cases. *J Cutan Pathol* 2004;31:232–40.

42 Beltraminelli H, Leinweber B, Kerl H, Cerroni L. Primary cutaneous CD4+ small-/medium-sized pleomorphic T-cell lymphoma: a cutaneous nodular proliferation of pleomorphic T lymphocytes of undetermined significance? A study of 136 cases. *Am J Dermatopathol* 2009;31:317–22.

Pityriasis lichenoides

3 Bowers S, Warshaw EM. Pityriasis lichenoides and its subtypes. *J Am Acad Dermatol* 2006;55:557–72.
6 Ersoy-Evans S, Greco F, Mancini AJ et al. Pityriasis lichenoides in childhood. A retrospective review of 124 patients. *J Am Acad Dermatol* 2007;56:205–10.
15 Borra T, Custrin A, Saggini A et al. Pityriasis lichenoides, atypical pityriasis lichenoides, and related conditions: a study of 66 cases. *Am J Surg Pathol* 2018;42:1101–12.
25 Kempf W, Kazakov DV, Palmedo G, Fraitag S, Schaerer L, Kutzner H. Pityriasis lichenoides et varioliformis acuta with numerous CD30(+) cells: a variant mimicking lymphomatoid papulosis and other cutaneous lymphomas. A clinicopathologic, immunohistochemical, and molecular biological study of 13 cases. *Am J Surg Pathol* 2012;36:1021–9.

Parapsoriasis

2 Vakeva L, Sama S, Vaalati A, Pukkala E, Kariniemi AL, Ranki A. A retrospective study of the evolution of parapsoriasis en plaques into mycosis fungoides. *Acta Derm Venereol* 2005;85:318–23.
3 Klemke CD, Dippel E, Dembinski A et al. Clonal T cell receptor gamma-chain rearrangement by PCR-based GeneScan analysis in the skin and blood of patients with parapsoriasis and early-stage mycosis fungoides. *J Pathol* 2002;197:348–54.
13 Aydogan K, Karadogan SK, Tunali S, Adim SB, Ozcelik T. Narrowband UVB phototherapy for small plaque parapsoriasis. *J Eur Acad Dermatol Venereol* 2006;20:573–7.
14 Lindahl LM, Fenger-Gron M, Iversen L. Topical nitrogen mustard therapy in patients with mycosis fungoides or parapsoriasis. *J Eur Acad Dermatol Venereol* 2013;27:163–8.

Lymphocytoma cutis

1 Colli C, Leinweber B, Mullegger R, Chott A, Kerl H, Cerroni L. Borrelia burgdorferi-associated lymphocytoma cutis: clinicopathologic, immunophenotypic, and molecular study of 106 cases. *J Cutan Pathol* 2004;31:232–40.
4 Sarantopoulos GP, Palla B, Said J et al. Mimics of cutaneous lymphoma. Report of the 2011 Society for Haematopathology/European Association for Haematopathology Workshop. *Am J Clin Pathol* 2013;139:536–51.
6 Bergman R, Khamaysi K, Khamaysi Z, Ben Arie Y. A study of histologic and immunophenotypical staining patterns in cutaneous lymphoid hyperplasia. *J Am Acad Dermatol* 2011;65:112–24.
30 Singletary HL, Selim MA, Olsen E. Subcutaneous interferon alfa for the treatment of cutaneous pseudolymphoma. *Arch Dermatol* 2012;148:572–4.

Jessner lymphocytic infiltrate

1 Jessner M, Kanof NB. Lymphocytic infiltration of the skin. *Arch Dermatol* 1953;68:447–9.
3 Lipsker D, Mitschler A, Grosshans E, Cribier B. Could Jessner's lymphocytic infiltration of the skin be a dermal variant of lupus erythematosus? An analysis of 210 cases. *Dermatology* 2006;213:15–22.
4 Rémy-Leroux V, Léonard F, Lambert D et al. Comparison of histopathologic-clinical characteristics of Jessner's lymphocytic infiltration of the skin and lupus erythematosus tumidus: multicenter study of 46 cases. *J Am Acad Dermatol* 2008;58:217–23.

CHAPTER 135

Cutaneous Histiocytoses

Thai Hoa Tran[1], Elena Pope[2] and Sheila Weitzman[2]

[1] CHU Sainte-Justine, Montreal, Quebec, Canada
[2] Hospital for Sick Children, Toronto, Ontario, Canada

Introduction, 135.1
Ontogeny of histiocytes, 135.1
Function of histiocytes, 135.1
Langerhans cell histiocytosis, 135.2
Haemophagocytic lymphohistiocytosis, 135.11

NON-LANGERHANS CELL HISTIOCYTOSES, 135.14

DISORDERS WITH MAINLY SKIN INVOLVEMENT WITH/WITHOUT A SYSTEMIC COMPONENT, 135.14

Juvenile xanthogranuloma, 135.14
Benign cephalic histiocytosis, 135.17
Generalised eruptive histiocytosis, 135.18
Papular xanthoma, 135.18

Progressive nodular histiocytosis, 135.19
Xanthoma disseminatum, 135.19

DISORDERS IN WHICH SKIN MAY BE INVOLVED BUT SYSTEMIC COMPONENT PREDOMINATES, 135.21

Erdheim–Chester disease, 135.21

DISORDERS WITH MAINLY SKIN INVOLVEMENT WITH/WITHOUT A SYSTEMIC COMPONENT, 135.22

Reticulohistiocytoma, 135.22
Familial sea-blue histiocytosis, 135.22
Hereditary progressive mucinous histiocytosis, 135.23
Malakoplakia, 135.23

Necrobiotic xanthogranuloma, 135.24

DISORDERS IN WHICH SKIN MAY BE INVOLVED BUT THE SYSTEMIC COMPONENT PREDOMINATES, 135.25

Multicentric reticulohistiocytosis, 135.25
Sinus histiocytosis with massive lymphadenopathy, 135.27

MALIGNANT HISTIOCYTOSES, 135.29

Malignant histiocytosis, 135.29
True histiocytic lymphoma, 135.30
Histiocytic sarcoma, 135.31

Key references, 135.32

Introduction

Skin involvement is common in all forms of histiocytic disorders and is seen at all ages. In general, for convenience, the histiocytoses were divided into those involving dendritic cells (DC disorders) and those involving the macrophage–monocyte lineage (or non-DC disorders). Recent molecular insights, however, led to a new World Health Organization (WHO) classification system in 2016 in which disorders that commonly harbour mutations in the MAPK pathway are classified together as the L group, while disorders that mainly involve skin and mucosa form the C group, the various forms of Rosai–Dorfman disease constitute the R group, the malignant histiocytoses represent the M group, and finally the family of haemophagocytic lymphohistiocytoses comprises the H group [1]. The C group is further subdivided into those with predominant skin and mucosa involvement and those cutaneous histiocytoses that have a major systemic component [2]. This chapter will provide an overview of the histiocytic disorders including a brief discussion of possible pathogenetic mechanisms, followed by an in-depth discussion of the skin manifestations, pathology and therapy of the histiocytic disorders. The similarities and differences between childhood and adult forms of the diseases will be highlighted.

Ontogeny of histiocytes

Histiocytes represent the cells of the mononuclear phagocyte system. They all share a common bone marrow progenitor cell, the neutrophil–macrophage colony-forming unit (NM-CFU). Histiocytes can be broadly divided into two functionally distinct cell populations: the 'professional' phagocyte and the antigen-presenting cell (APC) of which the Langerhans cell (LC) is the primary example. In contrast to all other dendritic cell populations, LCs do not arise from adult bone marrow-derived myeloid progenitor cells but originate from fetal liver-derived monocyte precursors that populate the skin prior to birth [1]. Postnatally, they repopulate directly from other skin LC cells during steady-state conditions, but when major inflammation occurs, they can be replaced by circulating monocytes [2]. Monocytes arise from NM-CFUs and following their release into the circulation migrate to various tissues, where they differentiate into macrophages and other histiocytic lines.

Function of histiocytes

The phagocytes include the majority of resident tissue and immature macrophages. Macrophages are specialised in particle uptake and degradation by phagocytosis. Phagocytosis starts with recognition of the foreign material via surface receptors, in particular the carbohydrate and lectin receptors, followed by endocytosis [1]. This mechanism is involved in the phagocytosis of bacteria and possibly tumour cells. Phagocytes also express the specific complement component receptors CR1 and CR3, which bind to C3b and C3bi, respectively, and Fc fragment of immunoglobulin receptors, which bind to the Fc fragment of IgG. These receptors are important in the phagocytosis of material that has bound IgG and complement, which act as opsonins and augment phagocytosis. Although limited, phagocytes also possess some antigen-presenting capacity. They generally present antigen to sensitised T cells but not to naive or 'memory' T cells.

APCs are histiocytic cells, or in some instances other cell types, that have specialised functional activity in presenting antigen to T cells. These cells are represented in humans by the blood dendritic cell, epidermal LC, interdigitating reticulum cell of the lymph node paracortex and veil cell of the efferent lymph. These cells have no phagocytic activity and, unlike 'professional' phagocytes, are unable to adhere to surfaces. They are able to internalise antigen by endocytosis, process it by lysosomal digestion and re-express the antigen on their surface in association with major histocompatibility complex (MHC) molecules (class II for external antigens and class I for internal antigens). These cells are potent antigen-presenting cells and are able to present antigen not only to sensitised T cells but also to memory and naive T cells [2].

Langerhans cell histiocytosis

Definition and nomenclature
Langerhans cell histiocytosis (LCH) is a proliferative disease characterised by excess accumulation of CD1a+ LCs in various sites, leading to tissue damage. It is the commonest of the histiocytic disorders and the commonest 'L' group disorder.

Synonyms and inclusions
- Histiocytosis X
- Eosinophilic granuloma
- Letterer–Siwe disease
- Hand–Schüller–Christian syndrome
- Hashimoto–Pritzker syndrome
- Self-healing histiocytosis
- Pure cutaneous histiocytosis
- Langerhans cell granulomatosis
- Type II histiocytosis
- Non-lipid reticuloendotheliosis

Epidemiology
Incidence and prevalence
LCH is a rare disease affecting 2–5 children per million per year with an estimated prevalence of 1:50 000 in children under 15 years of age [1]. A study from Sweden reported a higher incidence of 8.9 children per million per year [2]. However, the true incidence may be underestimated due to disease heterogeneity, especially in those with localised bone or skin LCH who may remain undiagnosed or undergo spontaneous resolution.

Age
LCH can present at any age, from the neonatal period until old age, but the disease is most common in the 0–4-year age group. The median age at diagnosis is 30.2 months as reported by the French LCH Study Group, which included 348 patients younger than 15 years of age [1]. Single system (SS) disease accounts for 70% of paediatric LCH, with bone being the most commonly affected organ and skin being seen in around 10% of SS-LCH patients [3]. Unifocal bone disease occurs in 50% of children with SS bone LCH over the age of 5, while multifocal bone disease is found in children aged between 2 and 5 years of age [1]. Multisystem (MS) LCH usually occurs in children younger than 2 years of age.

In adults, the mean age at diagnosis is 35 years, with 10% being older than 55 years. Sixty-nine percent of adults with LCH from the Histiocyte Society Adult Registry had MS disease with skin and lung involvement in 51% and 62%, respectively [4]. Of the 31% of adult patients with SS disease, the lung was involved in 51%, most of whom were smokers, followed by bone and skin in 38% and 14%, respectively.

Sex
Most studies consistently report a slight male to female predominance, although some series have reported a male predominance as high as 2:1 [1].

Pathophysiology
Pathology
The LC is a unique APC found within the epidermis, bronchi and mucosa. LCs are characterised phenotypically by low levels of MCH-II, intermediate CD11c and high expression of Langerin (CD207) [5]. Langerin is associated with the formation of tennis-racket-shaped intracellular organelles known as Birbeck granules, which represent the structural hallmark of LCs [6]. The Langerin immunostain (anti-CD207) has replaced electron microscopic analysis as a diagnostic marker for LC and LCH cells. Human LCs express myeloid markers CD13 and CD33; the leukocyte marker CD45; adhesion molecules such as CD40, CD44 and E-cadherin; and CD1a, an MCH class I-like protein that has the function of presenting lipid antigen to T cells [7].

The origins of LCs have been the matter of intense debate – whether LCs are blood-borne or derived from *in situ* localised epidermal LC precursors. However, recent evidence suggests a dual origin of the LC network. During steady state, LCs may originate from a localised LC precursor in the epidermis that maintains LC renewal, while LCs could source from a blood-borne precursor during inflammation [6,8–10].

The clinical heterogeneity of LCH is surprisingly unified by the histopathology of one abnormal population of LCH cells. They represent pathological cells with the same immunophenotype as LCs, including a surface rim of CD1a and a granular cytoplasmic and surface staining for Langerin (Figure 135.1). Moreover, S100 immunostain will give a nuclear and cytoplasmic blush to the cells. Fascin is demonstrable in low to moderate amounts in only a few cells. HLA-II (LN3 antibody) and CD68 (KP-1) display punctate

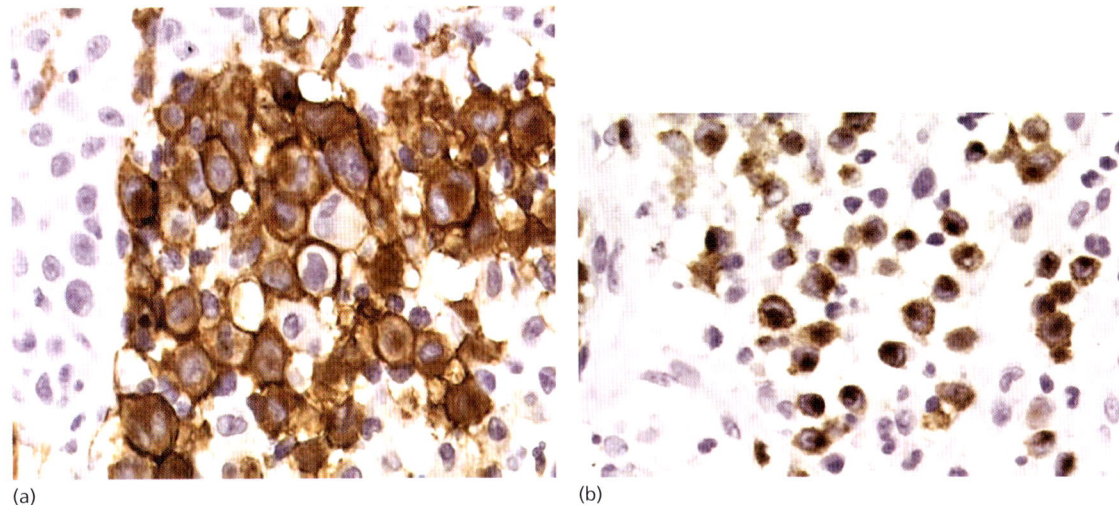

Figure 135.1 Langerhans cell histiocytosis (LCH) lesion in the skin showing (a) characteristic CD1a-positive staining of LCH cells and (b) skin LCH cells showing cytoplasmic and surface staining for langerin.

paranuclear Golgi-like intracytoplasmic staining [11]. Morphologically, LCH cells are round to oval in shape, measuring 15–25 µm in size (2–3 times as large as lymphocytes), most commonly found in aggregates and lacking the 'dendritic' morphology, which helps to distinguish them from inflammatory CD1a+ dendritic cells characterised by a branching morphology [12]. Their nucleus is lobulated, coffee bean or boat shaped, but the most typical LCH nuclei have complex angular and elaborate folds. The cytoplasm is generous and homogeneously pink. A prototypical LCH lesion usually displays LCH cells interspersed with inflammatory cells, mainly eosinophils and lymphocytes. Macrophages, both phagocytic and giant cell forms, can be found in many sites. Osteoclast-like giant cells predominate in any lesion involving bone [11].

Genetics

The aetiology of LCH is unknown, but recent advances in molecular genetics have provided important insights into the pathophysiology of LCH and have deepened our understanding of the disease. For a prolonged period, immune dysregulation and abnormal cytokine expression have been stipulated as potential pathogenic mechanisms in LCH, given the immune and inflammatory nature of LCs and based on the observation of regulatory T-cell expansion in LCH [13–15]. However, no specific immune dysfunction has been demonstrated and patients do not have an increased risk of infection. More recently, advances in molecular and genomic technologies have supported the concept of LCH as a myeloid neoplastic disease. The clonality of pathological LCH cells identified in non-pulmonary LCH provided the first argument supporting the idea of LCH as a neoplasm [16,17]. The identification of the *BRAF* V600E mutation in 57% of LCH cases tested in addition to the demonstration of RAS pathway activation in all of the cases, even those without the *BRAF* mutation, suggest a common mechanism of activation of the signal transduction pathway and give strong support to the designation of LCH as a neoplasm, although not necessarily a malignancy [18,19]. The *BRAF* V600E mutation was found in all risk groups and had no impact on overall survival, although its presence conferred a twofold increased risk of reactivation ($P = 0.04$) [19]. Given the universal RAS-MAPK pathway activation in LCH, alterations in other MAPK pathway genes were suspected because only 50–65% of LCH cases harboured the *BRAF* V600E mutations.

Whole-exome sequencing of 41 LCH cases revealed activating *MAP2K1* mutations in 33% of wild-type *BRAF* LCH cases, which were mutually exclusive from those harbouring *BRAF* mutations [20]. In the remaining LCH cases without *BRAF* V600E or *MAP2K1* mutations, *BRAF* exon 12 in-frame deletions and the *FAM73A-BRAF* gene fusion were detected in 29% of cases, both alterations shown to activate *ERK* in LCH model systems [21]. In summary, genomic and functional studies identified MAPK pathway gene mutations in over 90% of LCH cases and highlighted the central role of *ERK* in LCH pathogenesis.

Clinical features

Despite the identical histopathological appearance of various forms of LCH, the disease encompasses a heterogeneous clinical profile and affects many organs. The classification of LCH is based on the number of organ systems involved, with an initial subdivision into SS and MS disease. SS-LCH is further subdivided into unifocal and multifocal disease, while MS-LCH is divided into 'low-risk' disease and 'risk' disease, where risk represents the risk of death. For clarity, the latter group will be referred to as 'high risk' in this chapter.

Presentation

SS bone LCH is the most common form of LCH, except in the first year of life when MS-LCH predominates [22]. The skull vault is the most frequent site of disease; however, any bone can be involved except for the hands and feet. SS skin LCH (skin-only LCH) is the second most common site (Table 135.1). MS-LCH refers to the involvement of any organ, although gonads and kidneys are usually spared. The 'risk' designation is limited to involvement

Table 135.1 Distribution of Langerhans cell histiocytosis in 170 children with single system-Langerhans cell histiocytosis treated in the DAL-HX studies.

Sites	Patients (%)
Unifocal bone	68
Multifocal bone	19
Isolated skin	11
Isolated lymph node	2

Reproduced from Titgemeyer et al. 2001 [23] with permission of John Wiley & Sons.

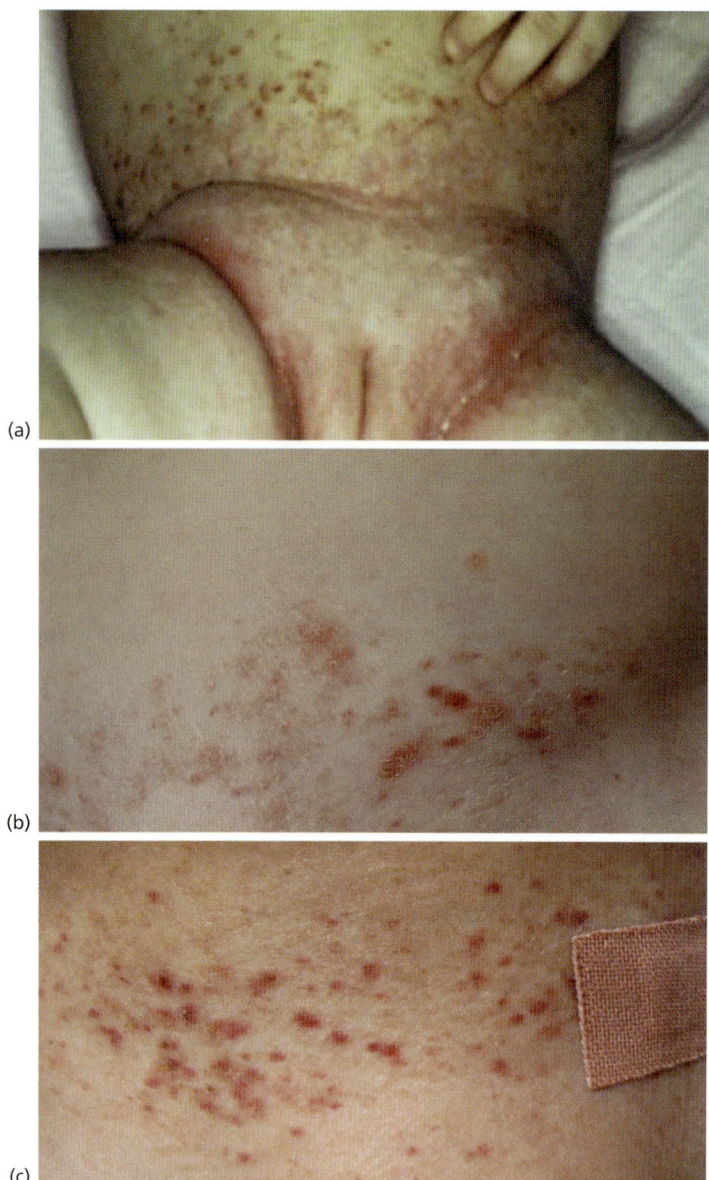

Figure 135.2 (a) Langerhans cell histiocytosis (LCH) showing a polymorphic eruption of papules, vesicles, crusts and telangiectasias affecting the nappy area, including the folds, in an infant. (b) Groin rash in LCH: polymorphic eruption with greasy papules, crusting and petechiae. (c) Groin rash in LCH: hemorrhagic papules, crusting, purpura on the groin.

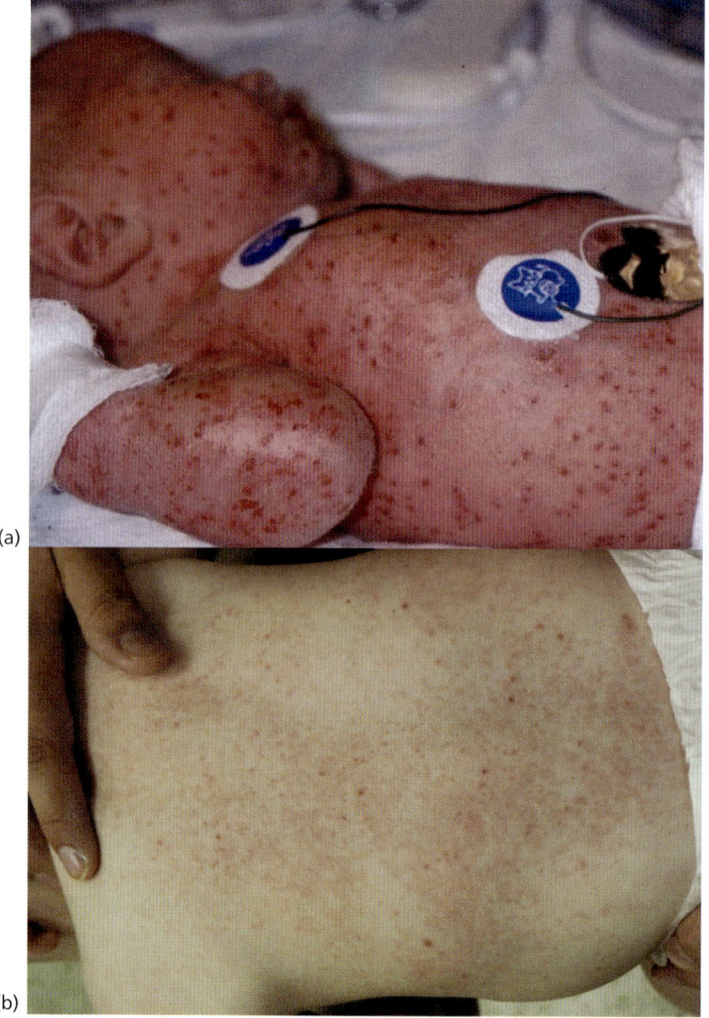

Figure 135.3 Generalised rash in Langerhans cell histiocytosis. (a) Polymorphic eruption with haemorrhagic crusts, petechiae and papules. (b) Diffuse papular eruption with petechiae.

of the haematopoietic system, liver and spleen. In contrast to the adult smokers' lung LCH, isolated paediatric lung LCH is no longer thought to give a major risk of death [24]. In this chapter, only skin LCH and its variants will be discussed in detail.

Skin is the second most commonly involved organ, reported in 30–60% of paediatric cases, with skin being the only affected site in 10% (skin-only LCH) [25]. Skin LCH can occur at any age. The appearance of the skin lesions is very variable and includes macules, papules, plaques, scales, vesicles, pustules, crusts, bullae and ulcerative lesions (Figures 135.2 and 135.3). The most characteristic cutaneous lesion of LCH in children consists of papulosquamous lesions with greasy scales, affecting the scalp, resembling seborrhoeic dermatitis (Figure 135.4). Other sites include skin folds such as the gluteal cleft and midline of the trunk, but any area can be involved including the nails. Persistent eruption on the scalp and in skin flexures outside of infancy should raise the suspicion of LCH even in the absence of other signs and symptoms. However, unusual persistence of 'cradle cap' or 'nappy rash' even in infancy should suggest the possibility of LCH and warrants a biopsy. Petechiae or areas of purpura can accompany skin lesions when the platelet count is reduced. Involvement of the external ear canal is usually considered part of skin LCH and may be associated with secondary infection with *Pseudomonas aeruginosa*. By contrast, LCH of the middle and inner ear is often associated with temporal bone disease. The mucous membranes of the mouth and genital tract may also be involved, the latter being seen more commonly in adult patients [24].

Clinical variants

Skin LCH in adults. The International Histiocyte Society compiled a registry of adult patients with LCH and found that 14.3% of adults with SS-LCH and 62% with MS-LCH have skin involvement [4]. Skin lesions are often the presenting feature of the disease. Adult

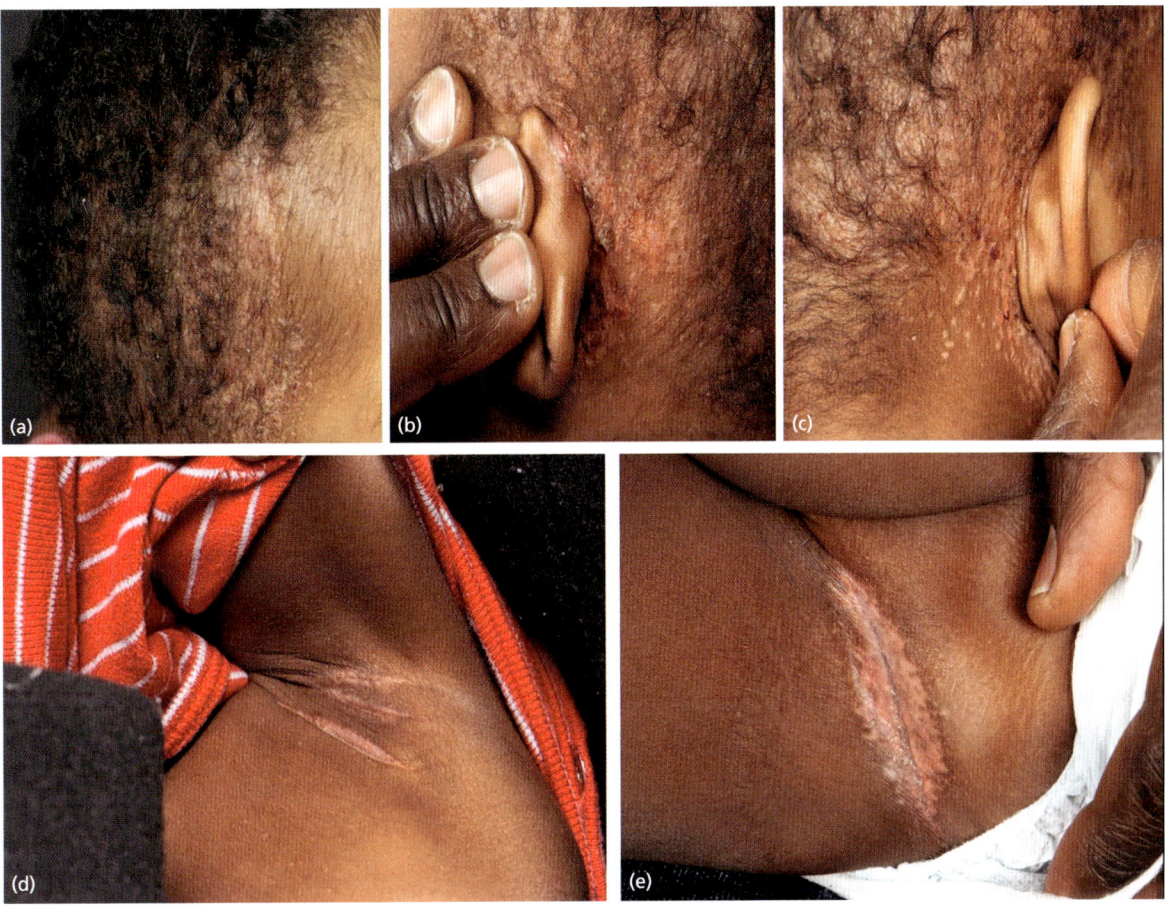

Figure 135.4 Langerhans cell histiocytosis showing crusted and petechial papules in a seborrheic dermatitis distribution in a child (a, b, c) and ulcerated erythematous plaques in the axillary (d) and groin areas (e). Courtesy of Dr Afshin Hatami.

skin LCH can mimic many common dermatoses including eczema, guttate psoriasis, candida infections, prurigo nodularis, lichen planus or lichenoid dermatitis, and a skin biopsy is often needed to confirm or exclude skin LCH [26].

The areas of involvement are similar to those seen in children but ulceration of the flexures, groin, perianal or vulvar area is common. Inframammary involvement may also occur. As with children, lesions may be papular, pustular, nodular, erythematous, poikilodermatous-like, xanthomatous, polypoid and peduncular. They may involve the nails and mucosa, including the genital mucosa. They may be asymptomatic or may be pruritic or burning [25,27,28]. Pure varicella-like vesicular eruptions are rarely observed in adults, whereas pruritic ulcerative lesions in the ano-genital area are a common presentation of adult LCH [26].

Skin-only LCH. LCH localised to the skin occurs in approximately 10% of children and adults with SS-LCH. Skin-only LCH in children is seen in the very young child and may undergo spontaneous regression within weeks to many months (Figure 135.5). Alternatively, in a proportion of cases, the disease may progress to high-risk MS-LCH, which can be fatal. This can be seen in young infants despite the improvement in the skin lesions (Figure 135.6). Of 12 skin-only infants in a series from the Hospital for Sick Children, Toronto [29], 10 were observed without therapy; 4 of the 10 progressed to MS disease 5 weeks to 5 months after diagnosis, resulting in two deaths. Additionally, one patient developed a single bone lesion almost 4 years after diagnosis with skin-only LCH. In infants from birth to 4 weeks of age, skin-only LCH is sometimes called Hashimoto–Pritzker disease or the congenital self-healing reticulohistiocytosis (CSHRH) variant (Figure 135.7). Skin-only LCH and CSHRH share the same pathology and immunostaining. Although some dermatologists claim to be able to distinguish CSHRH from skin-only LCH clinically, the literature does not support that unless myelin-dense bodies, thought to represent senescent mitochondria, are seen on electron microscopy. Battistella *et al.* described a series of 31 patients, 21 'self-regressive' and 10 'non-self-regressive', and found that monolesional forms, necrotic lesions and hypopigmented macules at presentation, in addition to distal extremity involvement, were seen only in patients with self-regressive cutaneous LCH [30]. Since both skin-only LCH and CSHRH require initial investigations to exclude systemic disease and both forms can be observed without therapy if limited to the skin, it is felt that the distinction is without real value. We emphasise that all young children with skin-only disease should be carefully observed and the diagnosis of spontaneously regressing disease should only be made retrospectively [29].

No prospective studies have looked at whether patients with skin-only LCH have a risk of long-term complications such as diabetes insipidus (DI). In two small published retrospective series,

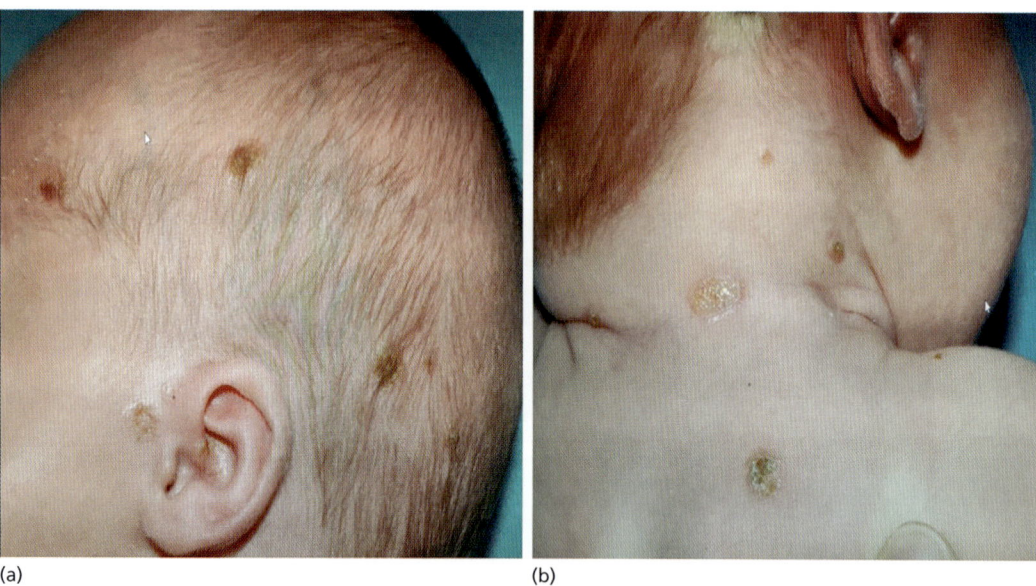

Figure 135.5 Ulcerated lesions of self-healing histiocytosis in an infant. Courtesy of Dr Antonio Torrelo.

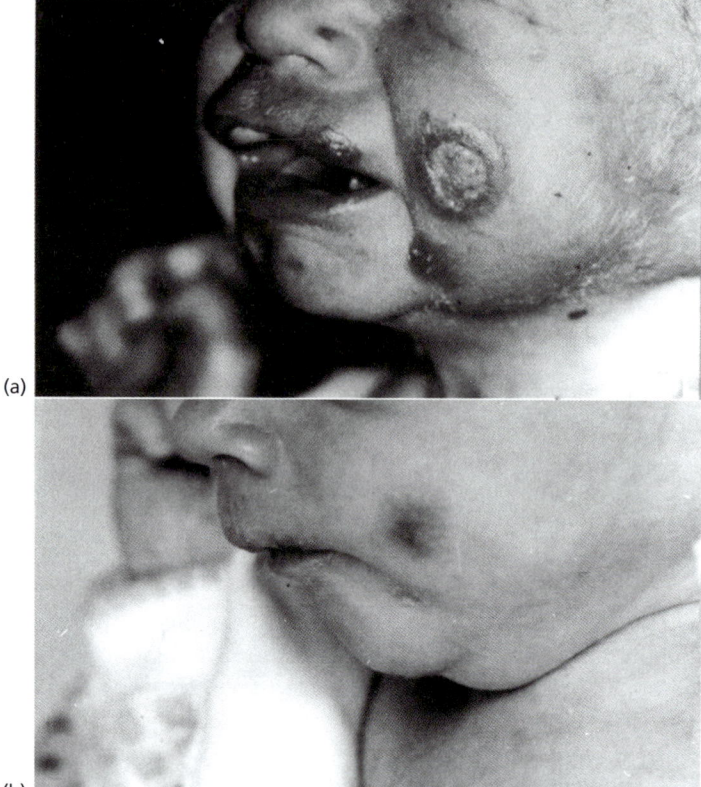

Figure 135.6 (a) A neonate presenting with multiple ulcerative lesions in the face and (b) at 6 weeks of age. Healing of the skin lesions is seen at the same time as high-risk multisystem Langerhans cell histiocytosis was found.

one consisting of 25 infants [31] and the other of 19 infants [32] with skin-only LCH, one patient in each series eventually developed DI. Prolonged follow-up is, therefore, recommended but in view of the generally good prognosis, radiological investigations should be limited and based on clinical suspicion.

Skin LCH as part of low-risk multisystem disease. This skin LCH clinical variant was formerly known as Hand–Schüller–Christian syndrome. This entity is a chronic, multifocal form of LCH. It is characterised by the presence of lytic bone lesions, exophthalmos, DI and skin lesions, although all these features are not required for diagnosis. The age of onset is usually later than the onset of skin-only LCH, typically between 2 and 6 years. Cutaneous manifestations include nodules and tumours that are yellow-brown in colour or with a seborrhoea-like picture, but any skin picture may be seen. Oral mucosa may be involved with gingival ulceration and haemorrhage. Premature tooth eruption may be the first manifestation of this variant [28].

Skin involvement as part of disseminated disease. This variant was previously known as Letterer–Siwe disease and represents the most extensive and severe form of LCH. It occurs in fewer than 15% of paediatric cases and is usually seen under the age of 2 years, often in the neonatal period. The skin is involved in 75–100% of cases, manifesting as a typical seborrhoea-like pattern in the scalp and diaper area; however, any part of the body may be affected. Extensive ulceration, superinfection, petechia and purpura may accompany skin lesions. Multiple organs are involved including the bones, liver, spleen, lungs, central nervous system (CNS) and haematopoietic system. This form carries the worst prognosis, is the least likely to resolve spontaneously and always requires systemic therapy [22].

Differential diagnosis

Nodular lesions of LCH should be differentiated from non-LCH lesions such as xanthogranulomas, mastocytosis or scabies as well as malignant lesions such as neuroblastoma, leukaemia and lymphoma. If the lesions are vesicular, herpes simplex and zoster infections, acropustulosis of infancy and bacterial infections should be ruled out. TORCH infections and syphilis should be considered in cases where skin lesions accompany multisystem involvement. The polymorphic characteristics of the rash and the 'seborrheic

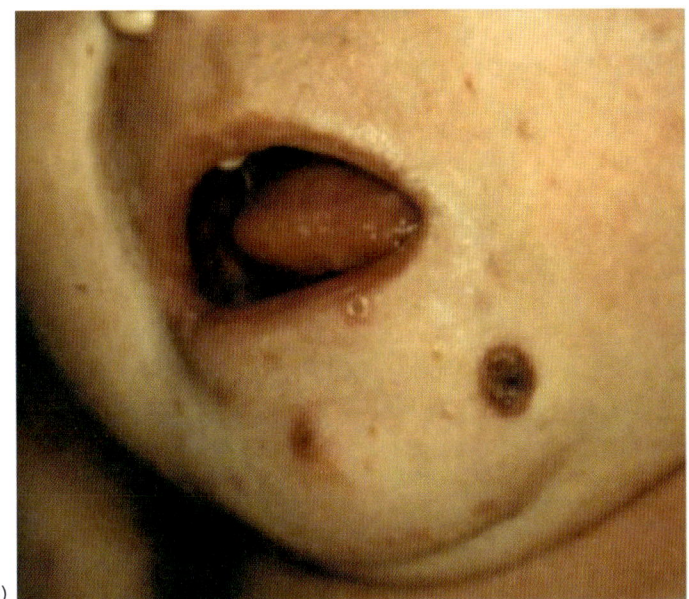

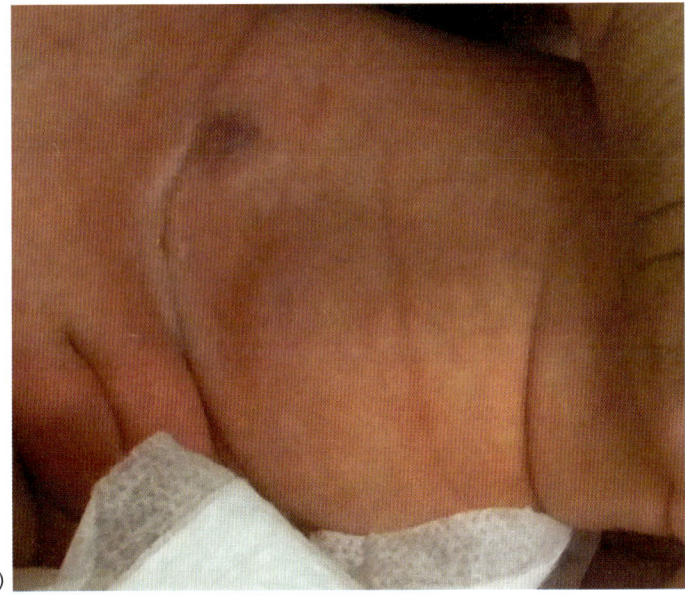

Figure 135.7 Congenital self-healing reticulohistiocytosis (Hashimoto–Pritzker disease) showing (a) ulcerated nodules in an infant, and (b) a single nodule, violaceous, firm to palpation in the groin area of a newborn.

for the development of significant long-term sequelae, of which DI is the commonest and CNS disease the most serious.

Patients with SS disease tend to undergo spontaneous regression or respond well to limited therapy. In an earlier series from the Hospital for Sick Children, Toronto, consisting of 180 patients with bone LCH, 12% of SS unifocal bone reactivated and there were no cases of DI. Of those with SS multifocal bone, 25% reactivated and the risk of DI was 12%; while in bone as part of low-risk MS disease, the reactivation rate was 50% and more than 25% developed DI [3]. In very young children with high-risk organ involvement, the mortality rate decreased to 10% with the advent of the most recent therapy protocols [33]. Historically, of those high-risk MS-LCH children who respond well to therapy, 50% reactivate in low-risk organs such as bone; these patients had a similar risk of long-term sequelae such as DI and CNS disease as the low-risk MS group. In the recently published LCH-III study, therapy was prolonged to 12 months for all high-risk MS patients, and the low-risk MS patients were randomised to receive 6 months versus 12 months of therapy. In both subgroups, extension of therapy to 12 months resulted in a reduction of the reactivation rate from 50% to about 30%, but it has not yet been proven whether that also results in reduction in late sequelae [33]. The open LCH-IV study is randomising patients to either 12 or 24 months of therapy to see if the reactivation rate can be further reduced and is following patients long-term to evaluate the effect on serious late complications.

The natural history of LCH in adults is less clear but it is thought that spontaneous regression, even in SS disease, is less likely to occur and that they typically require some form of therapy depending on the extent of organ involvement. In adult LCH, survival rates of patients with SS disease approach 100% [4]. The survival of adult patients with MS disease including skin is better than that seen in children due to the lower number of organs involved [28,34].

In this molecular era, LCH genotype may have clinical implications and confer prognostic significance. In a retrospective study of 41 LCH cases with available genotype and clinical data, there were no significant differences in sex, age, presence of risk organ or number of LCH lesions between patients with *BRAF* V600E ($n = 20$), *MAP2K1* mutation ($n = 7$) or neither mutation ($n = 14$) [20]. While overall survival (OS) was similar in the three genotypes ($P = 0.6653$), *BRAF*-mutated patients were almost three times as likely to have a recurrence compared with those without *BRAF*, even after adjusting for age and sex (hazard ratio (HR): 2.9; $P = 0.015$; 95% confidence interval (CI) 1.2–6.8) [35]. In a large French cohort of 315 LCH cases, the presence of *BRAF* V600E was associated with high-risk disease, permanent injury and poor response to chemotherapy. Compared with wild-type *BRAF* patients, those with *BRAF* V600E mutation had a higher 5-year reactivation rate (42.8% vs 28.1%; $P = 0.006$) and had more permanent, long-term consequences from disease or treatment (27.9% vs 12.6%; $P = 0.001$) [36]. Although limited by the small number, heterogeneous patient population and retrospective data, patients with *MAP2K1* mutations had a decreased risk in disease progression compared with those with *BRAF* V600E ($P = 0.0360$) [20]. Large-scale prospective studies of uniformly treated patients are needed for validation of these preliminary observations.

dermatitis' distribution (diaper area and retroauricular involvement) help to narrow the diagnostic possibilities. In adults, other conditions such as hidradenitis suppurativa, Paget disease, keratosis follicularis and sexually transmitted diseases may have to be considered.

Disease course and prognosis

The natural history of paediatric LCH varies from spontaneous regression to a low-grade chronic disease with multiple reactivations and the possibility of significant long-term consequences, to a 'high-risk' disease that can be fatal. Its course also varies with different subgroups and depending on the extent of disease. The mortality from SS and low-risk MS-LCH is extremely low. The problem for these subgroups is the propensity for reactivations and

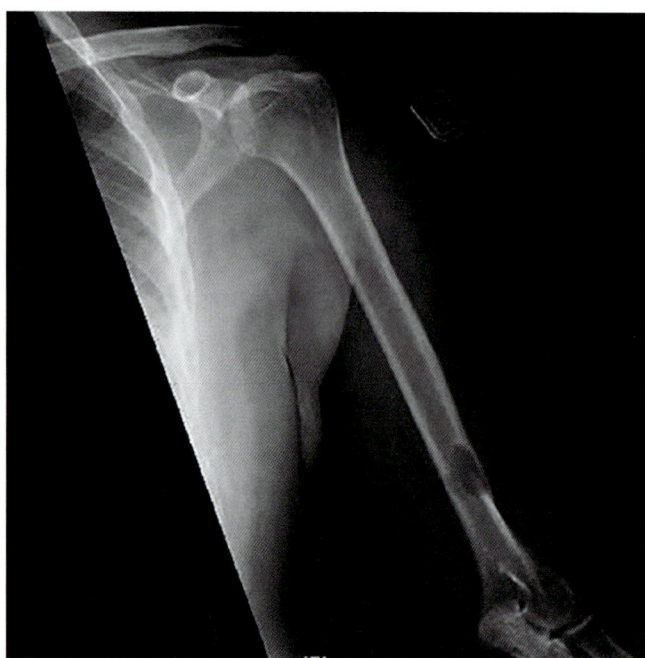

Figure 135.8 Radiograph of a humerus showing a typical punched-out lytic lesion of bone Langerhans cell histiocytosis.

Investigations

Diagnosis

LCH is diagnosed by the characteristic histology and immunostaining made on biopsy. Because LCs are normally found in the skin, nodes and lung, it is important to differentiate LCH from reactive LCs in these areas (see Figure 135.1). Thus, LCH is a *clinicopathological* diagnosis, confirmation requiring the typical histology and immunostaining in the *appropriate clinical setting* (R. Jaffe, personal communication).

Evaluation

The aim of evaluation is to assess disease extent to guide treatment planning and follow-up. Patients may present with skin, bone, lymph node, pituitary, lung or liver disease as the primary site, but need to be fully investigated before a diagnosis of SS disease can be made. Plain radiography, as part of the skeletal survey, is usually the first modality to assess bone involvement (Figure 135.8). Guidelines for diagnosis, work-up and treatment of paediatric LCH have been published [37]. Box 135.1 details the investigations that should be conducted on all suspected LCH cases and the indication for more specialised investigations in some patients.

Management

The modern treatment approach utilises a risk stratification strategy based on the extent and severity of disease, which represent the main determinants of outcome. Paediatric patients with SS-LCH generally have a benign course with a high chance of spontaneous remission over a period of months to years, and a favourable outcome with no or limited treatment [23].

In unifocal bone disease, simple curettage or even biopsy can be curative. Intralesional corticosteroids (75–150 mg of methylprednisolone) have been shown to be an effective and safe treatment

> **Box 135.1 Investigating patients with Langerhans cell histiocytosis**
>
> **Investigations on all patients**
> - Full blood count
> - Electrolytes, urea, creatinine, liver function tests, coagulation studies, erythrocyte sedimentation rate and C-reactive protein
> - Skeletal survey
> - Chest X-ray
> - Biopsy of site(s) of involvement
> - BRAF immunohistochemistry or *BRAF* mutation analysis or RAS-MAPK pathway mutations by molecular tests (optional)
>
> **Tests indicated in some patients**
> - Magnetic resonance imaging of the brain if lytic skull lesions, diabetes insipidus, symptoms suggestive of central nervous system involvement
> - Water deprivation test if polyuria, polydipsia
> - High-resolution computed tomography (CT) of the chest if adult smoker or patients with respiratory symptoms
> - Lung function tests if lung involvement
> - Abdominal ultrasound, liver biopsy if abnormal liver function tests
> - Fluorodeoxyglucose positron emission tomography (FDG PET)/CT scan appears to be the most sensitive test for detection of LCH lesions as well as assessment of response to therapy. However, the radiation dose needs to be taken into account when this modality is being considered.

modality, typically for symptomatic bone lesions [38]. Due to concerns of long-term sequelae and secondary malignancy, radiation at low dose (6–10 Gy) should be reserved only for emergency circumstances when vital structures such as the optic nerve and/or spinal cord are compromised [38].

Systemic therapy is reserved for MS-LCH, multifocal bone disease and for disease defined as 'risk' bone disease. 'Risk' bones include those bones thought to be associated with increased risk of DI as well as vertebral body LCH with a soft tissue mass which may result in spinal cord compression. Many drugs have been used, from non-steroidal anti-inflammatory drugs and steroids to cytotoxic chemotherapy such as vincristine, vinblastine, etoposide, 6-mercaptopurine (6-MP), methotrexate, cytarabine, cladribine and clofarabine, in addition to the immune-modulating agents (interferon α, anti-tumour necrosis factor α (anti-TNF-α), ciclosporin A, thalidomide, etc.) [7,39,40]. Most recently, BRAF/MEK inhibitors are being increasingly used.

In the last 20 years, three large-scale, international, prospective, therapeutic trials conducted by the Histiocyte Society (LCH-I, LCH-II, LCH-III) yielded important insights into the management of MS-LCH [33,41,42]. Firstly, the most frequently used regimen consisting of vinblastine with a corticosteroid is a safe and effective regimen. The addition of either etoposide or methotrexate to the vinblastine–steroid–6-MP backbone did not improve outcomes of patients with MS-LCH or with high-risk organ involvement [33,43]. In patients with MS-LCH, a 12-month maintenance period reduces the rate of reactivation compared with a 6-month maintenance period [33]. The combination of vincristine, steroid and cytarabine, as reported by the Japanese cooperative group, represents an equivalent therapeutic alternative [44]. For refractory low-risk MS disease, cladribine monotherapy has been shown to be an effective therapeutic option [45]; while for refractory high-risk MS-LCH, salvage therapy with cladribine in combination with cytarabine has proven to be effective [46,47]. Another useful salvage therapy option is single-agent clofarabine [48]. Haematopoietic stem cell transplantation (HSCT) can also be considered in patients with high-risk organ involvement who are refractory to salvage therapy [49]. A recent article comparing outcomes using reduced-intensity conditioning (RIC) to myeloablative conditioning (MAC) for refractory LCH found that the 3-year projected OS was 77% after MAC and 71% after RIC. Relapse rates were 28% after RIC and 8% after MAC regimens. The investigators concluded that MAC transplant was better in centres with good supportive care [50]. However, in the molecular era, patients failing salvage chemotherapy are more likely to be treated with targeted therapy, if available.

Targeted therapies

The recent discovery that the majority of LCH cells carry the *BRAF* V600E mutation and that all have activation of the RAS-MAPK pathway raises the possibility of BRAF and other MAPK pathway inhibitors as promising novel therapies in LCH. A dramatic efficacy of vemurafenib, an approved BRAF inhibitor for metastatic melanoma, has been shown in patients with multisystemic and refractory Erdheim–Chester disease (ECD) and LCH harbouring the *BRAF* V600E mutation [51]. The follow-up report including four patients with mixed LCH and ECD with *BRAF* V600E confirmed sustained response to vemurafenib with a median follow-up duration of 10.5 (range: 6–16) months [52]. An international observational study of off-label use of vemurafenib in 54 children with refractory *BRAF* V600E-positive MS-LCH reported a complete response in 38 (70%) patients and a partial response in 16 (30%) patients at 8 weeks of vemurafenib. However, reactivations occurred rapidly upon discontinuation of vemurafenib with a 12-month reactivation rate of 84% (95% CI 68–95%) [53]. Disease recurrence was associated with the detection of circulating *BRAF* V600E-positive cells in the blood which persist even after HSCT [53]. The results of the phase 2, open-label, non-randomised, histology-agnostic study in patients with *BRAF* V600E mutation, the VE-BASKET trial, confirmed the objective response rate (ORR) of 61.5% (95% CI 40.6–79.8), the 2-year progression-free survival (PFS) and OS of 86% and 96%, respectively, for the entire cohort [54]. Based on these results, vemurafenib has been approved by the Food and Drug Administration (FDA) in 2017 for patients with *BRAF* V600-mutant ECD and defines a new standard of care for these patients. Clinical trials of other BRAF inhibitors such as dabrafenib as monotherapy or in combination with a MEK inhibitor (trametinib) are underway. Rapid and excellent responses of refractory skin LCH have been seen with compassionate use of dabrafenib in young LCH patients with MS-LCH in which all organs except the skin responded to salvage therapy (S. Weitzman, personal communication). The problem that remains is that the length of therapy is unknown in view of the fact that to date, the majority of LCH patients treated on targeted kinase inhibitor therapy relapse when the drug is stopped. Whether longer use or combination of dual targeted therapies (BRAF and MEK inhibitors) or combination of targeted therapy and conventional chemotherapy may allow inhibitors to be safely discontinued remains to be determined.

Management of skin LCH

Paediatrics. With skin-only LCH, these young patients can be observed and therapy given only if there is pain, bleeding and/or ulceration. Physicians should avoid treating for cosmetic reasons alone. If treatment is required, topical therapy such as topical corticosteroids should be tried first. Other topical therapies that have been described, but that are not commonly used, include topical imiquimod, topical pimecrolimus or tacrolimus, narrow-band UVB and psoralen–UVA (PUVA) [28,39]. If topical tacrolimus is used over a large percentage of the skin surface area, tacrolimus levels should be monitored to prevent systemic complications.

For skin involvement as part of MS-LCH, management usually consists of systemic chemotherapy. The most commonly used protocol is the combination of vinblastine and prednisolone as per the standard arm of the LCH-II and LCH-III protocols of the Histiocyte Society [33,41] with or without topical therapy (usually consisting of medium- to high-potency corticosteroids). Other possibilities are intravenous cytarabine alone or with vincristine and prednisolone. For patients refractory to these therapies, salvage chemotherapy, targeted kinase inhibitor therapy or HSCT could be tried as discussed previously.

Treatment ladder for skin LCH in children

Skin-only LCH
- First line: observation (unless there is pain, ulceration or bleeding)
- Second line: topical mid-potency corticosteroid
- Third line: UVB therapy/PUVA or topical tacrolimus (for paediatric patients >2 years of age with serum tacrolimus levels) or systemic therapy if severe

Skin as part of low-risk MS-LCH
- First line: vinblastine/prednisolone (as per arm A of the LCH-III study)
- Second line: vincristine/cytarabine with or without prednisolone
- Third line: cladribine monotherapy or BRAF/MEK inhibitors if evidence of RAS-MAPK pathway gene mutations

Skin as part of high-risk MS-LCH
- First line: vinblastine/prednisolone (as per arm A of the LCH-III study)
- Second line: cladribine in combination with other agents (e.g. cytarabine) or single-agent clofarabine
- Third line: BRAF/MEK inhibitors if evidence of RAS-MAPK pathway gene mutations. Recent clinical experience suggests that these targeted inhibitors work rapidly and well to control refractory skin disease but are not utilised as first or second line therapy because of uncertainty whether they can ever be safely stopped. In very ill young infants who fail first line therapy, anecdotal experience suggests that BRAF inhibitors work quickly and with less immediate toxicity than salvage chemotherapy.
- Fourth line: haematopoietic stem cell transplantation

Adults. In contrast to the young child, adult patients with skin-only LCH usually require some form of therapy. In general, prospective trials have been limited to paediatric MS disease and most of the published reports on therapy in adult LCH consist of single case reports or small series. The adult LCH study group of the Histiocyte Society recently published guidelines for the management of adult LCH [55] and these guidelines continue to be refined. Possible therapies for skin LCH in adults include surgery, topical, ultraviolet light, radiation or systemic therapy.

- *Surgery.* Surgical excision is a good option for limited skin lesions, but mutilating surgery such as vulvectomy or hemivulvectomy should not be performed.
- *Topical therapy.* First line topical therapy usually consists of high-potency corticosteroids or intralesional steroids. Other options include topical tacrolimus, which has been successful in anecdotal reports, but systemic toxicity limits its use, especially for a large treatment area or ulcerated lesions. If utilised, tacrolimus levels should be measured. Topical imiquimod for 5 days/week for 2 months was used successfully in one adult patient with disease refractory to other therapy [56].
- *Ultraviolet light therapy.* Whole body UVB and PUVA have been utilised successfully in adult patients with skin LCH [57]. In addition, a recent report described the successful use of narrowband UVB delivered locally by means of an Excimer laser [58]. However, response of scalp and intertriginous lesions is limited [26].
- *Radiation therapy.* Localised radiation therapy and electron beam radiation therapy have been used but would not be the first choice of treatment [59].
- *Systemic therapy.* Adults do not tolerate or respond as well as their paediatric counterparts to vinblastine and prednisolone therapy. Nonetheless, a vinblastine and steroid combination remains the first line systemic therapy for adult LCH in many centres, particularly in Europe, including for skin LCH requiring systemic therapy. Other centres prefer to avoid these drugs and suggest starting with single-agent cytarabine given for 5 days every month. Other systemic therapy utilised in adult LCH patients and summarised by Girschikofsky *et al.* [55] includes weekly oral methotrexate [60], daily oral etoposide [29] and oral chlorambucil (A. Chu, personal communication). Daily oral etoposide has been demonstrated to be less myelosuppressive and to carry much less risk of causing secondary acute myeloblastic leukaemia than the intravenous form of the drug. Biweekly pegylated interferon-α has been successful in some refractory cases [27,61], similar to oral thalidomide (100 mg PO daily) [62], as well as oral lenalidomide [63] and oral isotretinoin [57]. The combination of interferon-α and thalidomide proved successful in patients with skin disease refractory to either agent alone [64]. Other therapies successful in adult skin LCH are azathioprine and 6-mercaptopurine as well as oral methotrexate as single agent or in combination with a thiopurine.
- *Targeted therapies.* BRAF/MEK inhibitors emerge as promising therapeutic options for patients with skin involvement as part of high-risk MS-LCH or relapsed/refractory low-risk MS-LCH with evidence of RAS-MAPK pathway gene mutations, as previously described.

With all forms of therapy, a relapse of skin LCH following the discontinuation of therapy is common, but the disease often responds again to reinstitution of the same therapy for a prolonged period and a slow taper may be required.

Treatment ladder for skin LCH in adults

Skin-only LCH
- Topical therapy
- Topical or intralesional corticosteroids
- Topical imiquimod (one case report)
- Topical nitrogen mustard (reported in children)
- Topical tacrolimus/sirolimus (with blood levels)
- Ultraviolet light therapy
- UVB/PUVA
- Surgical excision for localised disease (mutilating surgery such as hemivulvectomy is contraindicated)
- Radiation therapy
- Systemic therapy

Skin-only LCH unresponsive to topical therapy or as part of low-risk MS-LCH
First line options include
- Methotrexate 20 mg PO/SC per week
- Azathioprine 2 mg/kg PO per day or 6-mercaptopurine
- Thalidomide 100 mg PO (prolonged therapy) or lenalidomide
- Interferon-α 6 mega units once daily or pegylated interferon-α biweekly (prolonged therapy)
- Combination of interferon-α and thalidomide
- Etoposide PO

Additionally in multifocal bone LCH
- Zoledronic acid 4 mg IV every 1–6 months (depending on extent and response)

Second line options
- Cytarabine 100 mg/m^2 IV days 1–5 every 4 weeks
- Etoposide 100 mg/m^2 IV days 1–5 every 4 weeks
- Vinblastine/prednisolone (as in paediatric studies)
- BRAF/MEK inhibitors if evidence of RAS-MAPK pathway mutations

Skin as part of high-risk MS-LCH
- First line: cladribine 6 mg/m^2 SC/IV days 1–5 every 4 weeks (2–6 courses) *or* vinblastine/prednisolone (institutional choice) (LCH-A1 protocol)
- Second line: clofarabine 20–40 mg/m^2/day for 5 days every 4 weeks (2–6 courses) (risk of cumulative cytopenia may be additive to cladribine)
- Third line: BRAF/MEK inhibitors if evidence of RAS-MAPK pathway mutations

Adapted from Girschikofsky *et al.* 2013 [55] and Girschikofsky and Tazi 2018 [26]

Resources

Further information
Euro-Histio-Net: www.eurohistio.net (last accessed June 2023).
Histiocyte Society: www.histiocytesociety.org (last accessed June 2023).

National Cancer Institute at the National Institutes of Health. *Langerhans Cell Histiocytosis Treatment.* http://www.cancer.gov/cancertopics/pdq/treatment/lchistio/HealthProfessional (last accessed June 2023).

Haemophagocytic lymphohistiocytosis

Definition and nomenclature
Haemophagocytic lymphohistiocytosis (HLH) is a hyperinflammatory condition resulting from uncontrolled ineffective immune response.

Introduction and general description
HLH is a rare histiocytosis characterised by widespread infiltration of multiple organs by lymphocytes and mature histiocytes showing prominent phagocytosis. HLH with an underlying genetic defect is regarded as 'primary HLH', while all other forms are reactive, such as macrophage activation syndrome (MAS), thus grouped as 'secondary HLH' [1]. Primary HLH can be divided into those inherited cases where HLH is the only clinical manifestation (e.g. familial haemophagocytic lymphohistiocytosis (FHL)), and those with other manifestations including oculocutaneous albinism where HLH is an important part of the clinical picture. In both subtypes, HLH is often due to gene mutations underlying a deficiency in the triggering of apoptosis. In secondary forms of HLH, haemophagocytosis occurs as a result of macrophage activation by a known stimulus, which can be infectious, malignant, autoimmune or physical. A number of infections, Epstein–Barr virus (EBV) being the commonest, have been shown to be associated with secondary HLH. Despite different aetiologies, the common pathway involves a production of high levels of pro-inflammatory cytokines by T-helper cells (interferon-γ, tumour necrosis factor, IL-1, IL-2, IL-6, IL-10, IL-12, IL-18 and granulocyte macrophage-colony stimulating factor), and excessive activation of monocytes and macrophages leading to phagocytosis of blood cells [2,3].

Epidemiology
Incidence and prevalence
The estimated incidence of FHL is 1 in 50 000 live births [4], but this figure will almost certainly increase as more genetic defects are being discovered.

Age
The majority of FHL patients present before the age of 1 year, while most adult cases are due to secondary HLH. However, primary HLH can occur at any age including in adults.

Sex
The male to female ratio is 1:1 [4], although some studies demonstrate a slight male preponderance [5].

Ethnicity
There is an increased incidence in ethnic groups with higher rates of consanguinity [6].

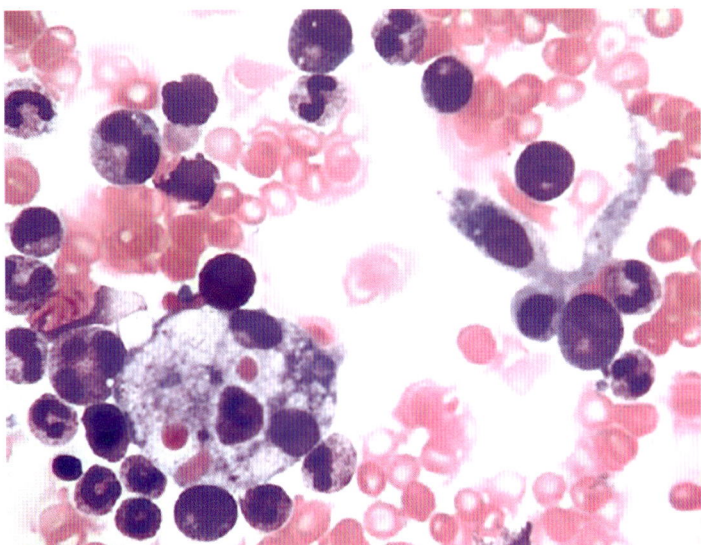

Figure 135.9 Haemophagocytosis in haemophagocytic lymphohistiocytosis.

Associated diseases
The association of secondary HLH and EBV infection has been well described, with more than 50% of patients coming from the Far East from Japan, China or Taiwan [7]. EBV may also trigger HLH in patients with primary HLH. More than half of EBV-associated HLH cases occur in children younger than 3 years of age [7]. Infections and lymphomas are the most common causes of adult-onset secondary HLH [8].

Pathophysiology
Pathology
Histologically, involved tissues show a diffuse infiltrate with lymphocytes and mature histiocytes. The histiocytes exhibit active phagocytosis, especially of erythrocytes but also of leukocytes and occasionally platelets (Figure 135.9). The histiocytes stain positively for acid phosphatase, non-specific esterase, lysozyme and α-antichymotrypsin. A striking histological finding is lymphocyte depletion of the lymph nodes, spleen and thymus [9]. Biopsy of the associated rash usually has non-specific findings with dermal perivascular infiltrates. Although haemophagocytosis is not usually found in the skin, one of the authors' patients had HLH confirmed by haemophagocytosis within an infiltrative skin nodule (S. Weitzman, personal communication).

Genetics
The pathophysiology of HLH is characterised by hypercytokinaemia and a concomitant defect in effector lymphocytes, namely cytotoxic T lymphocytes (CTLs) and natural killer (NK) cells [6,10,11]. FHL is an autosomal recessive disease but certain X-linked conditions, such as both forms of the X-linked lymphoproliferative syndrome (XLP) as well as X-linked severe combined immunodeficiency (SCID) and X-linked hypogammaglobulinaemia, also result in the HLH phenotype [12], as do increasing numbers of primary immunodeficiency syndromes [2]. Recent genetic studies have revealed that perforin gene mutations account for 20–40% of FHL cases [13]. Another 20–25% cases of FHL harbour mutations in MUNC13-4 [13]. Perforin is an apoptosis-triggering agent required

for CTLs and NK cells to induce apoptosis in target cells [14] and MUNC13-4 mediates the exocytosis of the perforin-containing granules from effector lymphocytes [15]. Most of the genetic HLH cases are due to mutations of important genes in the same pathway. These underlying genetic defects provide a plausible explanation for the defect in cytotoxicity observed in HLH [16].

Clinical features
Presentation
The cardinal clinical features are prolonged high fever, hepatosplenomegaly and cytopenias. Fever is usually the first sign of the disease, with symptoms of an upper respiratory tract or gastrointestinal infection. Pallor, anorexia, vomiting, irritability and hepatosplenomegaly are usually present at presentation. Around half of patients develop a transient, non-specific, maculopapular rash, which is often seen at times of high fever [17]. About 20% of patients have neurological symptoms, presenting with seizures or other signs of meningeal irritation.

The initial clinical picture of HLH often resembles a harmless viral illness; however, progression of clinical symptoms and worsening of laboratory values such as rising inflammatory markers or progressive cytopenias in a sick child should alert the physician to the possibility of HLH. Patients may improve initially with supportive care such as transfusions or antibiotics, but responses are usually short lived and the disease can rapidly be fatal.

Investigations
Diagnosis
The diagnosis of HLH is made by compiling a number of clinical and laboratory features that raise the possibility of HLH (Box 135.2). Laboratory tests should include a complete blood count that usually reveals cytopenia, initially with anaemia or thrombocytopenia. Up to 28% have leukocytosis, with either neutrophilia or lymphocytosis [17]. Neutropenia affects most children eventually and progressive pancytopenia is seen in untreated patients. Transaminitis is almost universal, sometimes associated with hyperbilirubinaemia. Some patients exhibit a consumptive coagulation picture with hypofibrinogenaemia, and D-dimers are elevated in most patients. Hypertriglyceridaemia is present in most children and may reach levels >10 mmol/L. Hyperferritinaemia >500 μg/mL is found in the majority of patients, but serum ferritin levels above 10 000 μg/mL are more suggestive of HLH [12]. Isolated hyperferritinaemia is not diagnostic of HLH whatever the level found. In adult patients, the highest ferritin levels were seen in autoimmune haemolytic anaemia [18]. A positive Coombs' test and platelet antibodies are present in some patients. Immunological testing shows abnormalities of both humoral and cellular components of the immune system. CTL and NK cell activity is markedly reduced or absent in affected patients. Elevated levels of the α-chain of the soluble interleukin 2 receptor (sCD25) and of the soluble FAS (CD178) ligand reflect stimulation of histiocytes and T cells, while elevated soluble CD163 (sCD163) reflects activation of the alternative pathway of macrophage activation.

Many centres do not have the ability to measure NK cell activity or sCD25. Furthermore, in many centres the NK cell activity by the chromium release assay has been replaced by the CD107a degranulation assay, which has been shown to be a reliable screening test for defects in the perforin/granzyme release pathway. This test does not diagnose perforin deficiency, however, since the killer cells will still degranulate and the presence of perforin protein should be assessed by flow cytometry prior to the degranulation assay. In addition, what is missing from the diagnostic criteria is assessment of organ damage which is necessary for the diagnosis of HLH. Accordingly, finding of high transaminases, hypoalbuminaemia, hyponatraemia, coagulopathy and CNS involvement (brain magnetic resonance imaging (MRI) and cerebrospinal fluid) support the diagnosis [2]. Furthermore, studies have shown that these criteria are not useful in secondary HLH associated with systemic juvenile idiopathic arthritis. A group of international experts have published diagnostic criteria for MAS in the setting of systemic juvenile idiopathic arthritis [19]. It is as yet unclear whether these criteria are useful in diagnosing MAS in other rheumatological diseases such as systemic lupus erythematosus (SLE) and Kawasaki disease.

Evaluation
A bone marrow examination is mandatory to exclude underlying malignancy, but only a minority of people show haemophagocytosis at presentation. Haemophagocytosis alone does not make the diagnosis of HLH without the other clinical manifestations and laboratory criteria. A lumbar puncture and brain MRI should also be performed, as more than 50% of patients will have asymptomatic neurological pathological abnormalities. Molecular genetic studies are now available to establish the diagnosis of a number of FHLs but not all the genes have as yet been identified (Table 135.2). However, these studies take weeks to complete so that they are not helpful in making the necessary early diagnosis. Flow cytometric studies available within a few days such as the CD107a degranulation assay, perforin protein assay, SAP and XIAP protein in males (XLP) and measurement of cytokines such as sCD25 and sCD163 are more useful. It is important to perform a thorough history and diagnostic

---

Box 135.2 Diagnostic criteria for the HLH-2004 treatment protocol

The diagnosis of haemophagocytic lymphohistiocytosis (HLH) can be established if one of either 1 or 2 below is fulfilled:
1 A molecular diagnosis consistent with HLH
2 Diagnostic criteria for HLH are fulfilled (i.e. five of the following eight criteria are fulfilled):
- Fever
- Splenomegaly
- Cytopenias (affecting ≥2 or 3 lineages in the peripheral blood: haemoglobin <90 g/L (in infants <4 weeks: haemoglobin <100 g/L), platelets <100 × 10^9/L or neutrophils <1.0 × 10^9/L
- Hypertriglyceridaemia and/or hypofibrinogenaemia: fasting triglycerides >3.0 mmol/L (e.g. ≥265 mg/dL) or fibrinogen ≤1.5 g/L
- Haemophagocytosis in bone marrow or spleen or lymph nodes
- Low or absent natural killer cell activity (according to local laboratory references)
- Ferritin ≥500 μg/L
- Soluble CD25 (i.e. IL-2 receptor) ≥2400 units/mL

From Gupta and Weitzman 2010 [12].

Table 135.2 Genetic defects leading to haemophagocytic lymphohistiocytosis (HLH).

Disease	Gene[a]
FHL1	Unknown
FHL2	PRF1
FHL3	MUNC13.4
FHL4	STX11
FHL5	STXBP2
Chediak–Higashi	LYST
Griscelli II	RAB27a
Hermansky–Pudlak II	AP3B1
XLP1	SH2D1A (SAP)
XLP2	BIRC4 (XIAP)

Adapted from Weitzman 2011 [20].
Diseases: FHL1–5, familial haemophagocytic lymphohistiocytosis 1 to 5; XLP1–2, X-linked lymphoproliferative disease type 1 and 2. Genes: *PRF1*, perforin; *STX11*, syntaxin 11; *STXBP2*, syntaxin-binding protein 2; *LYST*, lysosomal trafficking regulator; *RAB27A*, RAS-associated protein 27A; *AP3B1*, adaptor 3 B1 subunit; *SH2D1A*, signalling lymphocyte activation molecule-associated protein; *BIRC4*, baculoviral IAP repeat-containing 4.

work-up to rule out the variety of underlying conditions leading to the same hyperinflammatory phenotype. Infections, systemic inflammatory rheumatic disorders, malignancies, inherited genetic defects and inborn errors of metabolism have been associated with the HLH phenotype.

Except for XLP and the primary immunodeficiencies, all known genetic HLH is caused by mutations in genes important in the cytolytic secretory pathway that causes perforin and granzymes to induce apoptosis in target cells. Primary immunodeficiencies associated with HLH (other than those already mentioned these include chronic granulomatous disease, SCID, Wiskott–Aldrich syndrome, X-men syndrome, interleukin-2 inducible T-cell kinase deficiency and others) [2]. Inherited metabolic defects such as lysinuric protein intolerance and Wolman disease may also present with the HLH phenotype and should be considered when investigating young infants [21].

Management

Principles of therapy include the following:
1 Suppression of the cytokine storm.
2 HSCT to replace the defective gene is necessary in all patients with primary HLH.
3 Treatment of the underlying condition in secondary HLH. However, many patients will require HLH-type therapy concomitantly to allow patients to survive long enough for the disease-specific therapy to work.

FHL is rapidly fatal if left untreated, with a reported median survival of fewer than 2 months from diagnosis, with 96% of patients dying within 12 months. Diagnosis can be challenging when there is no family history or no evidence of a molecular defect. Therefore, sometimes treatment must begin on a strong clinical suspicion even when diagnostic criteria are not completely fulfilled. Major improvements in survival were only observed when the combination of etoposide with corticosteroids was introduced into HLH therapy [22]. The HLH-94 treatment protocol consists of an induction phase with etoposide and corticosteroids for 8 weeks, followed by the addition of ciclosporin in the continuation phase. The 3-year probability of survival for the 113 eligible patients was 55% and the 3-year probability of survival for those who underwent HSCT was 62% [5]. All surviving HSCT patients are free of disease. The HLH-2004 treatment protocol investigated the upfront incorporation of ciclosporin to the 8-week dexamethasone/etoposide-based initial therapy and the addition of prednisolone to intrathecal therapy in 369 patients, the largest prospective HLH study to date. Although the projected 5-year survival of HLH-2004 was 61%, the pre-HSCT mortality rates between HLH-94 and HLH-2004 treatment protocols were not statistically significant; HLH-94 thus remains the standard of care treatment [23]. It has been suggested that etoposide dosing should be lowered in adolescents and adult patients by giving the drug once a week and using lower doses such as 50–100 mg/m^2 instead of the 150 mg/m^2 of the HLH-94 protocol, depending on the severity of symptoms and response [24]. Treatment of milder forms of HLH, as in secondary HLH, can be initiated with corticosteroids alone or in combination with intravenous immunoglobulin. If they fail to respond or progress, immunosuppressive agents such as etoposide should be added early (within days).

Allogeneic HSCT remains the only cure to date for primary HLH. Primary HLH patients slated for transplant should remain on maintenance therapy until transplant occurs. HSCT should be carried out as early as possible to prevent early deaths. Transplant is best performed in patients who have responded to chemoimmunotherapy but a 3-year survival of 54% was achieved following HSCT in patients with persisting HLH [25]. Experience in HLH HSCT is necessary for centres undertaking these difficult transplants. Alemtuzumab is an integral part of the RIC regimen which has successfully reduced the high transplant-related mortality associated with HLH transplants, although primary graft rejection is common and donor lymphocyte infusions are often necessary [26]. This has led to the successful implementation at some centres of reduced toxicity rather than reduced intensity protocols (D. Wall, personal communication).

Salvage therapy

For patients who failed induction on the HLH-94 protocol, some responded to increased doses of the same drugs, in particular a higher dose of dexamethasone. If that strategy fails, therapy with the anti-CD52 antibody alemtuzumab has proven to be the best salvage therapy at present [27].

Based on the presence of hypercytokinaemia in HLH, cytokine targeting has been another therapeutic avenue to dampen the hyperinflammatory state in HLH. Emapalumab, a fully human anti-interferon-γ monoclonal antibody, was investigated in a phase 2/3 study for previously treated and untreated children with primary HLH as interferon-γ is thought to play a central role in HLH pathogenesis. Among 34 patients who received emapalumab, 65% had a response at 8 weeks, of which 21% had a complete response, 32% had a partial response and 12% had improvement in measures of HLH [28]. Twenty-two (65%) patients proceeded to HSCT and the estimated 1-year OS was 69.3% in the emapalumab group [28]. Ten patients who received emapalumab died, but none of the deaths was attributed to emapalumab. Therefore, emapalumab was found to be effective with an acceptable toxicity profile in the treatment of primary HLH. Investigators from the

Histiocyte Society HLH committee, however, pointed out that emapalumab inhibits only interferon-γ and that when used as front-line therapy, no one reached no active disease status, in contrast to current standard therapy with dexamethasone and etoposide which attack the cells producing the cytokines. Their conclusion was that we need to learn how best to utilise anti-interferon-γ and other cytokine-directed agents in the treatment of primary HLH, either as stand-alone therapies or in conjunction with dexamethasone and etoposide [29].

Other agents blocking individual cytokines such as anakinra, a recombinant IL-1 receptor antagonist, and tocilizumab, an anti-IL-6 receptor antibody, have been shown to induce responses in retrospective case series of secondary HLH [30–32]. Furthermore, key cytokines in HLH such as interferon-γ, IL-2 and IL-6 bind to receptors that mediate downstream JAK-STAT signalling activation, suggesting that JAK inhibition may decrease the cytokine-driven hyperinflammation in HLH [33,34] and overcome cytokine-mediated resistance of CD8+ T cells to dexamethasone in preclinical models [35]. Several reports of ruxolitinib, a JAK1/2 inhibitor, exhibiting prompt clinical improvement and short-term HLH disease control in relapsed/refractory HLH [36] and more recently in the frontline setting [37,38] have since emerged. Nevertheless, prospective randomised clinical trials of ruxolitinib versus standard of care using standardised definitions of disease activity and response are urgently needed. Combination of anti-cytokine agents or combination with chemotherapy may prove to be the optimal way to utilise these and other emerging therapies.

Treatment ladder for HLH

Primary HLH

First line
- High-dose dexamethasone, etoposide as per HLH-94 and intrathecal therapy followed by haematopoetic stem cell transplant (HSCT) (as early as possible). Maintenance therapy with dexamethasone should be continued until HSCT. Supportive care with pneumocystis and antifungal prophylaxis. In adults, the addition of intravenous immunoglobulin and viral prophylaxis has been suggested

Salvage therapy
- High-dose pulse corticosteroids and/or alemtuzumab
- DEP chemotherapy (doxorubicin, etoposide and methylprednisolone)
- Emapalumab
- Other anti-cytokine agents (tocilizumab, infliximab)
- Ruxolitinib (remains experimental at this time)

Secondary HLH

First line
- Corticosteroids alone with careful observation. Etoposide added early for patients failing to respond to single-agent steroids
- For systemic juvenile idiopathic arthritis-MAS: anakinra ± corticosteroids ± intravenous immunoglobulin given as first line therapy
- For adolescents and adult patients with presumed secondary HLH, the etoposide administration can be modified to once weekly plus lower doses (50–100 mg/m^2) depending on severity of disease and response
- CNS HLH is commoner in primary HLH but intrathecal therapy may be necessary for some patients with secondary HLH
- Supportive care as outlined under primary HLH

Second line
- Rituximab should be added early in Epstein–Barr virus-associated HLH
- Consider addition of tumour necrosis factor-inhibiting agents, IL-1 inhibitors or anti-IL-6 antibodies in macrophage activation syndrome
- Ruxolitinib and emapalumab remain experimental in this setting

NON-LANGERHANS CELL HISTIOCYTOSES

The non-Langerhans cell histiocytoses (non-LCHs) are a diverse group of disorders defined by the accumulation of histiocytes that do not meet the phenotypical criteria for the diagnosis of LCH. The non-LCHs are generally benign proliferative disorders. Clinically, they can be further stratified into two major groups: (i) those that predominantly affect the skin but may have a systemic component (e.g. juvenile xanthogranuloma, reticulohistiocytoma); and (ii) those such as ECD and sinus histiocytosis with massive lymphadenopathy (Rosai–Dorfman disease) that are primarily systemic diseases where skin may be involved.

DISORDERS WITH MAINLY SKIN INVOLVEMENT WITH/WITHOUT A SYSTEMIC COMPONENT

Juvenile xanthogranuloma

Definition and nomenclature

Juvenile xanthogramuloma (JXG) is a proliferative disorder of histiocytes occurring in early infancy and childhood that spontaneously regresses in most cases. A small percentage of cases present with isolated extracutaneous disease with no skin involvement or it may present with disseminated disease with a poor prognosis. On occasion, JXG and LCH can occur in the same patient simultaneously or one may precede the other. In this setting, 'true' JXG needs to be differentiated from LCH of the skin which may heal leaving behind a xanthomatous scar.

Epidemiology

Incidence and prevalence
JXG is the commonest of the non-LCH, non-HLH histiocytic disorders. The incidence of JXG is unknown and is likely underestimated due to its natural history of spontaneous involution.

Age
JXG occurs predominantly during infancy with median ages at onset ranging from 5 months to 1 year as reported in two large series [1,2]. Lesions may occur at birth and very rarely in adults [3].

Sex
There is no sex predilection, although male preponderance was much higher (male:female 12:1) in children with multiple skin lesions [4].

Ethnicity
There is a racial predilection, being 10 times more common in white than in black children.

Associated diseases
JXG has been associated with neurofibromatosis type 1 (NF1) and juvenile myelomonocytic leukaemia (JMML) [5]. Patients with JXG and NF1 have a significantly higher risk of developing myeloid leukaemia than normal [6].

Pathophysiology

Pathology
JXG is characterised by a dense infiltrate of small histiocytes in the dermis, which stain positively for factor XIIIa, CD68, CD163, CD14 and fascin (Figure 135.10a,b). Stains for S100 and CD1a are negative. Touton giant cells, seen in 85% of JXG cases, can be distinguished by the characteristic wreath of nuclei around a homogeneous eosinophilic centre and prominent xanthomatisation in the periphery (Figure 135.10c) [1]. In extracutaneous JXG lesions, Touton cells are absent or reduced in numbers. In young infants younger than 6 months old, JXG can present with mainly vacuolated histiocytes, without foamy histiocytes or giant cells. Most of the cutaneous non-LCH disorders share an identical immunophenotype with JXG and are collectively known as the JXG family. These disorders include benign cephalic histiocytosis, generalised eruptive histiocytosis, xanthoma disseminatum and progressive nodular histiocytosis. The JXG family also includes the non-cutaneous disorder Erdheim–Chester disease.

The pathogenesis of JXG remains unclear. Lipid abnormalities do not play any role in JXG. It is suggested that dermal dendrocytes are the precursor cells of most non-LCHs, including JXG [4,5,7]. An origin from dermal dendrocytes was postulated based on the positive immunostaining for factor XIIIa, but derivation from an earlier circulating precursor cell has been suggested recently as being able to better explain the occurrence of extracutaneous JXG [6].

Genetics
Since neurofibromin, the protein product of the gene involved in NF1, negatively regulates the *RAS* oncogene, the association of JXG with NF1 and JMML has led to the speculation that the

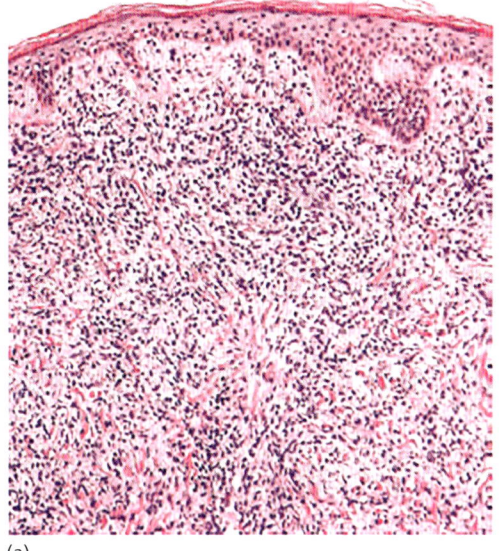

(a)

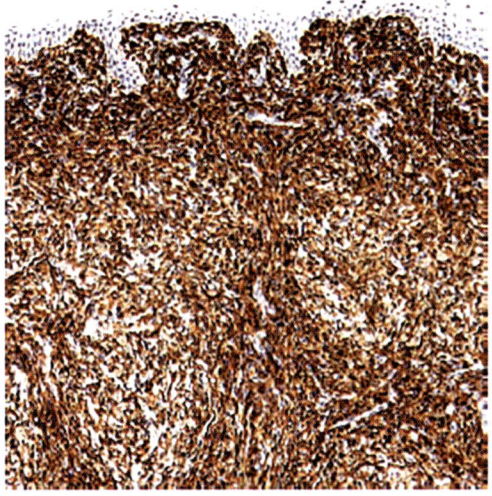

(b)

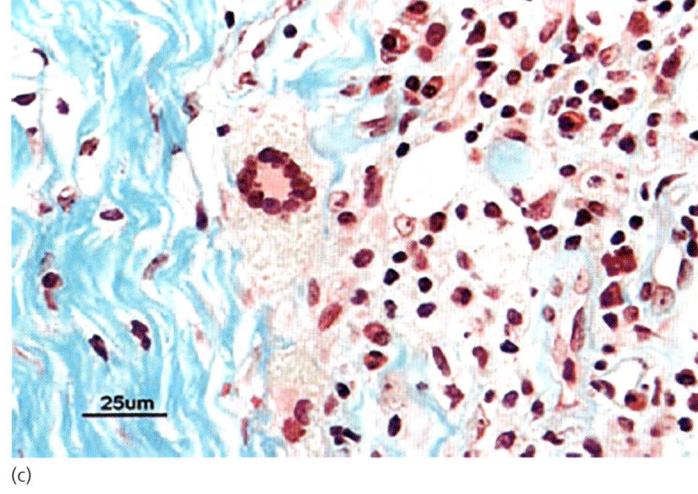

(c)

Figure 135.10 Juvenile xanthogranuloma. (a) Small, slightly spindled histiocytes permeate the dermis, splaying collagen fibres. Touton cells are not represented. Magnification 200× (H&E). (b) This lesion has a high content of factor XIIIa. Magnification 200× (diaminobenzidine). (c) Touton giant cells with CD68-positive immunoreactivity. Courtesy of Dr R. Jaffe, Children's Hospital of Pittsburgh, Pittsburgh, USA.

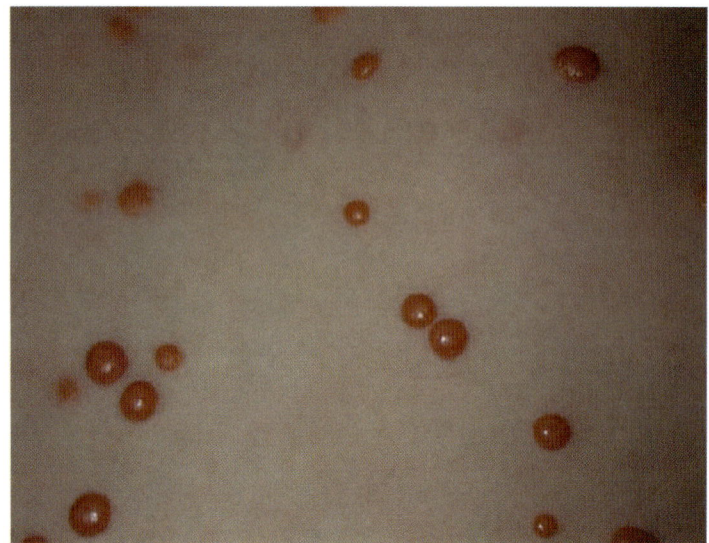

Figure 135.11 Juvenile xanthogranuloma showing multiple, disseminated, yellow papules.

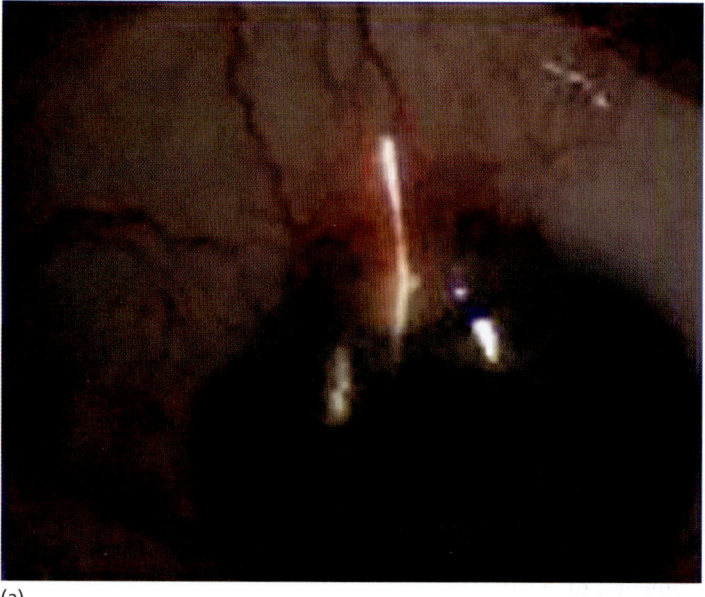
(a)

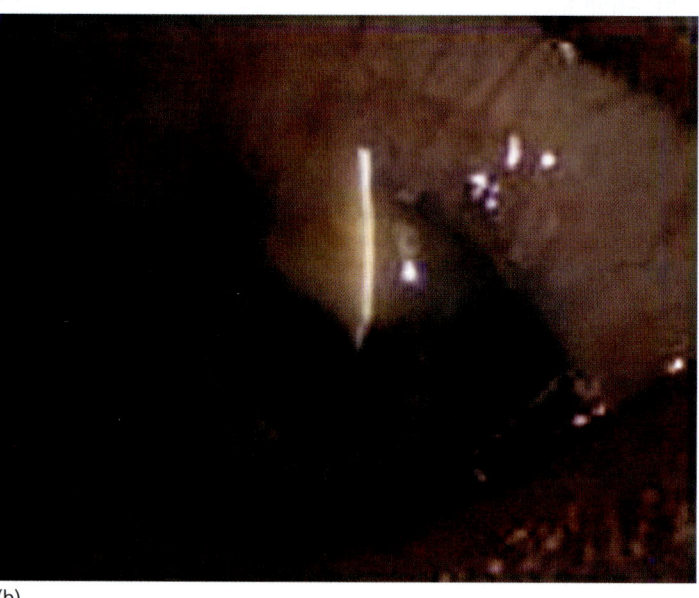
(b)

Figure 135.12 Juvenile xanthogranuloma of the iris. (a) Right eye, November 2001. (b) Right eye, July 2003. Courtesy of Dr J. Donadieu, Trousseau.

dysregulation of apoptosis via dysfunction of the *RAS* oncogene may lead to both leukaemia and JXG [6]. Interestingly, the *BRAF* V600E mutation in LCH [7] and ECD [8] has not been identified in JXG thus far [9], except for two cases from Texas Children's Hospital with features of both LCH and JXG that harbour the *BRAF* V600E mutation [10]. This is despite many published case reports of JXG and LCH occurring in the same patient [11–13], either simultaneously or with LCH first and then JXG. Because it appears that some LCH lesions may become xanthomatous when inactive, this needs to be distinguished from true active JXG that can be seen with or following LCH. More recently, DNA-based and RNA-based next-generation sequencing of 55 cases of JXG identified several kinase-activating alterations: *MAP2K1* ($n = 6$); *CSF1R* ($n = 5$); *KRAS* ($n = 4$); *NRAS* ($n = 3$); *KIT* ($n = 3$); *JAK3* ($n = 2$); *ALK* ($n = 2$); *MET* ($n = 1$); *CSF3R* ($n = 1$); *NTRK1* fusions ($n = 6$); *BRAF* fusions ($n = 4$); *RET* fusions ($n = 2$); and *ALK* fusion ($n = 1$) [14]. Activating *CSF1R* mutations and *NTRK1* fusions are specifically enriched in JXG, constituting 10% and 12% of cases, respectively [14]. These findings suggest that some JXG lesions may be targetable with the relevant kinase inhibitors.

Clinical features
Presentation
Clinically, cutaneous lesions are the most common presentation of JXG, which presents with single to multiple papules or nodules with a predilection for the face, head and neck, followed by the upper torso and upper and lower extremities. Single lesions (unifocal JXG) are the most common, but multiple lesions, ranging from a few to hundreds, may occur, particularly in young male infants. They usually start as reddish yellow macules/papules, which may enlarge and evolve into yellow-brown patches/plaques with surface telangiectasias (Figure 135.11). The consistency is generally firm and rubbery. Giant JXG, defined as a lesion greater than 2 cm in diameter, has been reported. It usually occurs in females younger than 14 months of age, on the proximal extremity or upper back, and may be misdiagnosed as haemangioma, particularly as it can be preceded by a congenital precursor lesion [15].

Clinical variants
Systemic involvement occurs in 4% of children, mostly during infancy with a median age of 0.3 years [5]. Systemic JXG has an overall mortality of 5–10%, mainly associated with involvement of liver or brain. Almost half of the patients have no skin lesions. The most common site is a solitary mass in the deep soft tissues (deep JXG) followed by the liver, spleen, lung and CNS. Most systemic lesions undergo spontaneous resolution; however, ocular and CNS involvement leads to significant complications.

Ocular JXG occurs in up to 10% of cases, but in fewer than 1% of children with coexisting cutaneous JXG [16]. Eye involvement is usually, but not always, unilateral and commonly presents with redness, irritation and photophobia, which may lead to acute hyphaema, glaucoma and blindness [17] (Figure 135.12). Thus, recognition of eye JXG is important for the prevention of vision loss.

Liver involvement presents clinically with jaundice, hepatosplenomegaly and transaminitis, while lung involvement is usually associated with multiple nodules. Rarely JXG may involve the bone marrow, resulting in cytopenias.

Disease course and prognosis
JXG, either cutaneous or systemic, usually follows a benign course with spontaneous resolution of lesions within 1–5 years. Large lesions may leave anetoderma (loose, stretched skin) and pigmentary changes. Long-term sequelae are rarely reported. However, CNS involvement may result in significant morbidity with seizures, ataxia, increased intracranial pressure, subdural effusions, developmental delay, diabetes insipidus and other neurological deficits [18]. Fatalities have been reported in cases of progressive CNS JXG [18,19] and neonates with hepatic involvement [20].

Investigations
The diagnosis of JXG is made on immunohistochemistry. Extensive work-up should be reserved for those with clinical suspicion of systemic involvement.

Management
The management of JXG depends upon the site(s) of involvement. For patients with single and accessible lesions, surgical excision appears to be curative, although most childhood lesions will resolve spontaneously. As a result, cutaneous JXG does not require treatment, although parents need to be warned that occasionally resolution may result in a scar. For ocular JXG, therapy includes topical, intralesional and subconjunctival corticosteroids; surgery may be required to treat complications such as hyphaema and glaucoma; and systemic corticosteroids, chemotherapy or low-dose 'non-cataractogenic' radiation therapy (300–400 cGy) may be required for non-responders [21]. Ophthalmological surveillance is recommended for high-risk patients younger than 2 years of age, who should undergo screening at diagnosis and every 3–6 months until age 2 [21]. For systemic JXG, there is currently no established standard chemotherapeutic regimen. A variety of regimens have been tried with variable results; most of these regimens incorporate LCH-based agents such as vinblastine, prednisolone and/or methotrexate [22], but response to chemotherapy is unpredictable. Supportive care should be strongly emphasised due to the potential toxicity in these young infants. Multiagent chemotherapy, including cytarabine, methotrexate, vincristine and prednisolone, is reserved for life-threatening or progressive disease [23]. CNS involvement has been successfully treated with cladribine [24], but the disease does not always respond. Thalidomide and clofarabine have been reported to have activity in heavily pretreated, refractory patients [25,26]. Targeted tyrosine kinase inhibitors may be considered for those with kinase-activating alterations. For instance, a patient with disseminated JXG skin lesions harbouring the *NCOA4-RET* fusion exhibited a meaningful clinical response following 12 weeks of selpercatinib, a RET inhibitor [14].

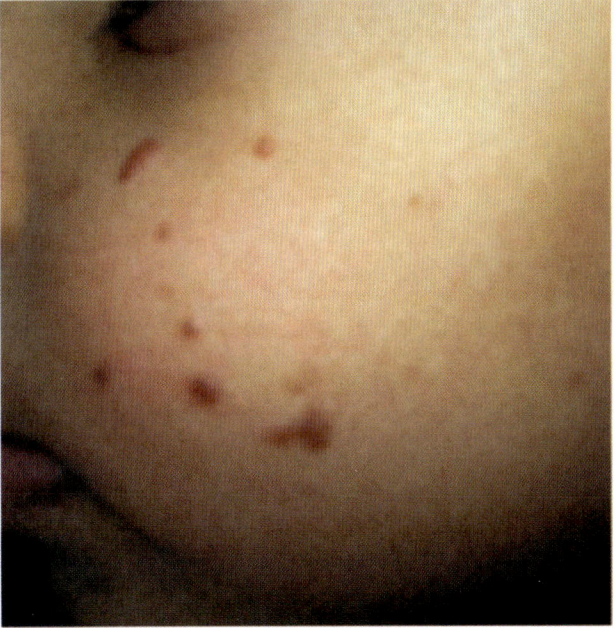

Figure 135.13 Benign cephalic histiocytosis showing multiple, asymptomatic, red/brown papules on the face of a toddler.

Benign cephalic histiocytosis

Definition and nomenclature
Benign cephalic histiocytosis (BCH) is a rare, self-limiting histiocytic disorder. Many consider BCH as a clinical variant or a milder form of juvenile xanthogranuloma without systemic involvement [1,2].

> **Synonyms and inclusions**
> - Papular histiocytosis of the head

Pathophysiology
Pathology
Immunohistochemically, BCH cells are identical to JXG. On electron microscopy, they may show 'worm-like' cytoplasmic inclusions.

Clinical features
Patients are typically young children with a mean age of onset of 15 months (range 2–66 months) [3]. Asymptomatic, red to brown macules/papules/nodules develop on the cheeks and spread to the forehead, earlobes and neck (Figure 135.13). Extension onto the trunk, upper limbs and rarely buttocks may be seen. There is no mucosal involvement.

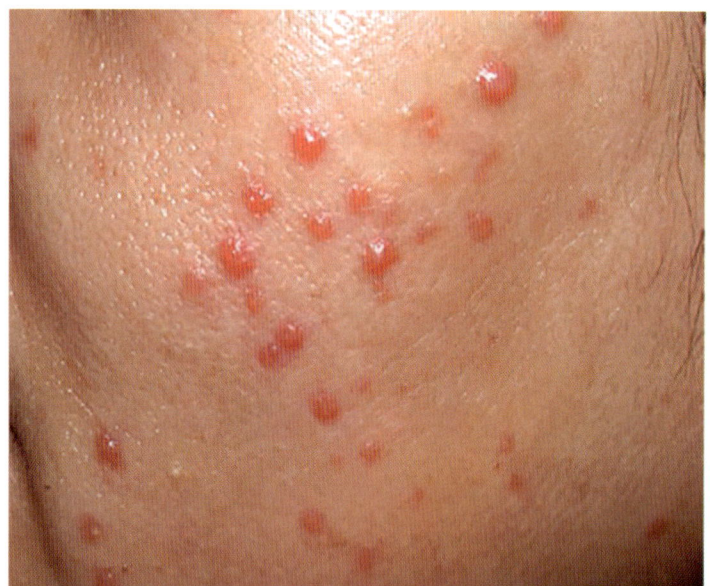

Figure 135.14 Generalised eruptive histiocytosis showing multiple, small, symmetrical, red-brown papules in an adult. Courtesy of Dr S. Walsh, Sunnybrook Hospital, Toronto, Canada.

Management
Given the self-limiting course of the disease, no therapy is required.

Generalised eruptive histiocytosis

Introduction and general description
Generalised eruptive histiocytosis (GEH) is a rare cutaneous histiocytosis that mainly affects adults, although paediatric cases have been reported [1,2]. It is characterised by asymptomatic, symmetrical papules on the face, trunk and arms, usually sparing the flexures. GEH must be distinguished from the eruptive histiocytomas associated with hyperlipidemia. The course is usually benign and self-limited, but a few cases have been reported that were associated with various forms of leukaemia [3].

Pathophysiology
Pathology
Histology shows a proliferation of monomorphic histiocytic cells in the upper and mid dermis. No giant cells or foam cells are present. Scattered lymphocytes may be present. Immunohistochemically, the cells are identical to JXG with positivity for CD68, Mac-387, lysozyme and factor XIIIa and negative for S100 and CD1a.

Clinical features
Presentation
The disease presents as multiple, symmetrical, small, red-brown papules on the face, trunk and arms, usually sparing the flexures (Figure 135.14). The lesions are asymptomatic and variable in number. The characteristic feature of GEH is the rapid appearance of a crop of lesions, which resolve spontaneously or leave a macular area of hyperpigmentation. Mucosal involvement is rare.

Management
The evolution of GEH to other non-LCHs has been reported. Patients need to be re-biopsied if lesions become xanthomatoid or flexural or if systemic symptoms develop [2]. The disease is generally self-limiting and often does not require treatment. One paediatric case demonstrated healing in sun-exposed areas, suggesting the value of ultraviolet light as a therapeutic option [4]. Twenty treatments with systemic PUVA were subsequently shown to be effective in a 32-year-old woman with widespread disease with no evidence of recurrence [5]. One patient treated for cosmetic and psychological reasons responded well to chloroquine, thalidomide and glucocorticoid therapy [6]. One patient with GEH harbouring the *FIP1L1-PDGFRA* fusion and chronic eosinophilic leukaemia responded to imatinib [7].

Papular xanthoma

Introduction and general description
This is a rare histiocytic disorder that was first described in adults and subsequently reported in children [1]. Whether it represents a separate clinicopathological entity or a variant of other xanthogranulomatous conditions is debatable.

Pathology
Histologically, there is an upper and mid dermal infiltrate of foamy histiocytes and giant cells. Few inflammatory cells are present. Histiocytic cells are positive for CD68 and factor XIIIa and negative for S100 and CD1a [1,2]. More recent studies, however, have shown that the foamy cells in this disease are factor XIIIa negative [3,4]. In such a rare condition, further studies are needed to confirm the dermal dendrocyte origin of the lesional cells. Electron microscopy shows similar changes to those seen in mature juvenile xanthogranuloma, with myeloid bodies filling the cytoplasm of the histiocytes with associated lysosomal inclusions, laminate bodies and lipid droplets.

Clinical features
Presentation
Clinically, it can resemble JXG, but has not been associated with systemic involvement or café-au-lait spots, and may resemble xanthoma disseminatum, but papules do not coalesce and there is no predilection for flexures. It is characterised by 2–15 mm yellow or reddish yellow papules/plaques affecting both the skin and mucous membranes. The back and head are the most common locations. Clinical presentation in adults is different from children. Mucosal involvement and risk for disease progression are features of adult presentation. In contrast, spontaneous resolution is the norm in children, with involution starting after weeks or months and being complete in 1–5 years, often leaving anetoderma-like scarring [2].

Management
No treatment is needed in children, while none has been shown to be effective in adults.

Progressive nodular histiocytosis

Definition and nomenclature
Progressive nodular histiocytosis (PNH) is a rare benign histiocytic disorder of unknown aetiology. It is characterised clinically by the development of multiple superficial skin-coloured or reddish orange papules and deep nodules distributed at random over the body.

Synonyms and inclusions
- Progressive nodular histiocytoma
- Spindle cell xanthogranuloma

Introduction and general description
PNH is a rare variant of non-LCH disorders that affects skin and mucosa. The skin manifestations consist of two types of lesions: superficial papules and deeper subcutaneous nodules, mainly consisting of spindle-shaped histiocytes [1]. The disease occurs most commonly in adults, although PNH in childhood has been occasionally reported [2,3].

Pathology
Histologically, this is a dermal disease with neither epidermal involvement nor epidermotropism. Early lesions show an accumulation of xanthomatised and scalloped histiocytes with some infiltrating lymphocytes. In older lesions, the histiocytes are spindle shaped and arranged in a storiform pattern. Occasional giant cells may be present. Mitotic figures are absent. Cells are positive for CD68 and factor XIIIa. Stains for S100 and CD1a are negative [4].

Clinical features
Presentation
The disease is characterised by the progressive appearance of asymptomatic cutaneous lesions and can result in severe disfigurement with time (Figure 135.15). Superficial papules are 2–10 mm in diameter and yellow-orange, while deep subcutaneous nodules are 1–5 cm in diameter and may be skin coloured or reddish orange due to overlying telangiectasia [5]. Both types of lesions can reach hundreds in number. Distribution is random with no predilection for the flexures. About 40–50% of the patients have mucosal lesions, including oral, nasopharyngeal, respiratory, anal or conjunctiva. About 50% of patients are complicated with diabetes insipidus; the clinical manifestations of polydipsia and polyuria are mild and mostly temporary, and can be relieved with the disappearance of skin lesions [3].

Management
PNH is not generally associated with systemic involvement or other disorders. No treatment has yet been demonstrated to be effective in reducing the size of skin lesions or in inducing remission [6]. However, Chu *et al.* suggest that the early stages of PNH may be more sensitive to chemotherapy and radiation therapy [7], but these modalities have generally not been shown to be useful. Large or painful lesions are usually excised surgically or by carbon dioxide laser. One patient was reported to respond well to intermediate dose cytarabine both clinically and on PET/CT imaging; further investigation of this drug is needed [8].

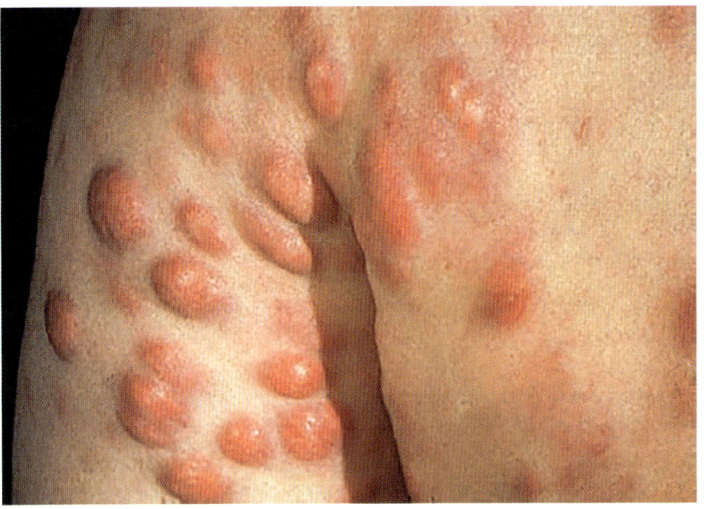

Figure 135.15 Progressive nodular histiocytosis in a 48-year-old man with nodular lesions in the posterior axillary fold. Courtesy of Professor J. M. Naeyaert, University Hospital, Ghent, Belgium.

Xanthoma disseminatum

Definition and nomenclature
Xanthoma disseminatum (XD) is a rare non-familial disease, characterised by proliferation of histiocytic cells in which lipid deposition is a secondary event.

Synonyms and inclusions
- Disseminated xanthosiderohistiocytosis
- Montgomery disease

Introduction and general description
XD is characterised by proliferation of histiocytic cells in which lipid deposition is a secondary event, with involvement of the skin, mucous membranes of eyes, upper respiratory tract and meninges. Rarely, other organs may be affected, including the liver, spleen and bone marrow [1].

Epidemiology
The disease predominantly affects male children and young adults but can occur at any age and in either sex. Fifty per cent of lesions appear before the age of 25 and 36% of patients are children [2].

Pathophysiology
XD is thought to be a reactive rather than a neoplastic process with a pathological immune response induced by unknown inflammatory triggers. The lesional cell appears to be an inflammatory lipid-laden macrophage with a characteristic foamy appearance which could represent increased uptake, synthesis or decreased efflux of lipids [3].

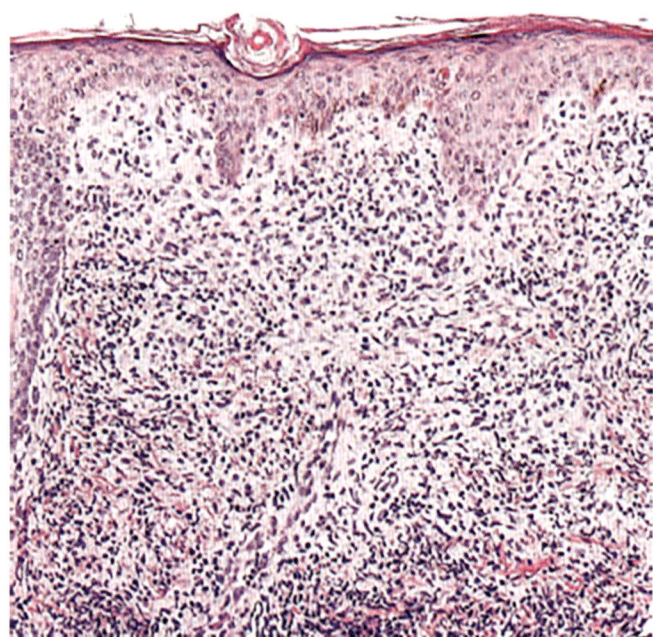

Figure 135.16 Xanthoma disseminatum: similar histological picture to juvenile xanthogranuloma consisting of dermal infiltrate of small spindled histiocytes (H&E). Courtesy of Dr R. Jaffe, Children's Hospital of Pittsburgh, Pittsburgh, USA.

Pathology

Histologically, XD is a dermal disease, characterised by early infiltration of the dermis with spindle-shaped mononuclear cells, foamy histiocytes, giant cells, lymphocytes, polymorphs and eosinophils (Figure 135.16). Lesional cells in XD have irregular scalloped borders with extensive cytoplasm and ovoid vesicular nuclei. Cells label strongly with factor XIIIa, CD68 and Ki-M1p and are negative for S100 and CD1a. Iron and lipid can be detected in the histiocytes. In older lesions, more foamy histiocytes are evident and Touton giant cells may be observed. At the ultrastructural level, histiocytic cells contain myeloid bodies and membrane-bound fat droplets.

The various members of the factor XIIIa-positive xanthogranuloma family, XD, PNH and GEH, may be indistinguishable from one another on histopathology and the diagnosis may depend on the clinical presentation. Some described differences in morphology of the cells, such as foamy xanthoma cells versus oncolytic or epithelioid cells, may be a function of when the biopsy was done in the course of evolution of the disease rather than a difference in diagnosis [4].

Clinical features

Presentation

The clinical lesions of XD are reddish or yellow-brown papules and nodules, which are symmetrically distributed on the trunk, scalp, face and proximal extremities. The lesions become confluent, especially in flexures, to form xanthomatous plaques, which may become verrucous (Figure 135.17). In 39–60% of patients, the mucous membranes are affected, with particular involvement of the lips, pharynx, larynx, conjunctivae and bronchus. XD also has the tendency to involve the upper respiratory tract (trachea, larynx) rather than lower respiratory tract, leading to stridor or respiratory

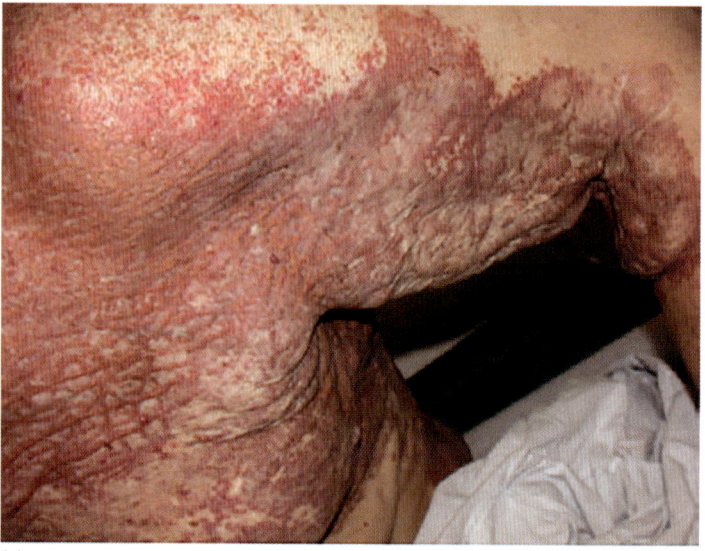
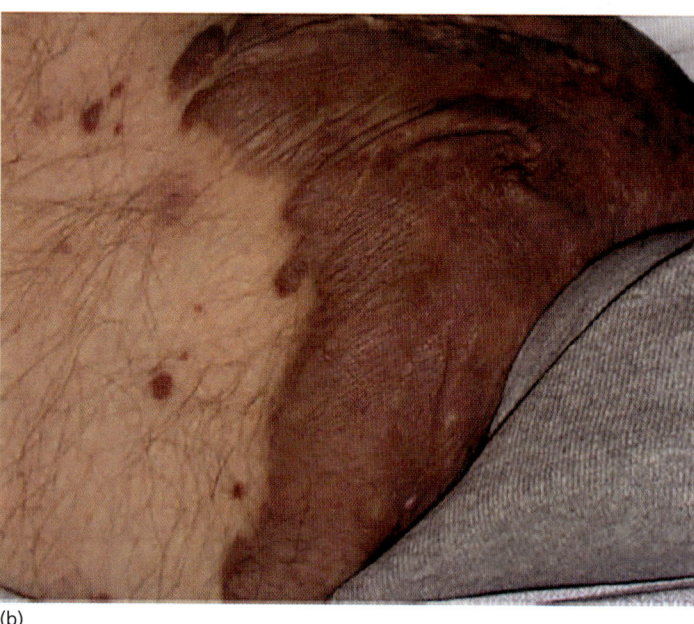

Figure 135.17 (a, b) Xanthoma disseminatum showing large, yellow-brown plaques affecting the skin folds. Courtesy of Dr S. Walsh, Sunnybrook Hospital, Toronto, Canada.

compromise [5,6]. Meningeal involvement is common, with infiltration at the base of the brain leading to diabetes insipidus in up to 40% of cases, which may, however, be transient. Other manifestations of meningeal involvement are seizures and growth retardation. Intracranial involvement presenting as a discrete mass simulating glioma has been reported [7] and progressive intracranial disease may be fatal in as many as 63% of patients [8]. Hepatic and bone involvement have been reported but represent rare complications of the disease.

Disease course and prognosis

XD is a self-limiting disease but may be locally destructive and persist for years. Three clinical patterns have been identified: a rare self-healing form, a chronic, often progressive form and a progressive multiorgan form, which may be fatal.

Management

Skin lesions of XD are disfiguring and patients often request treatment. A carbon dioxide laser has been used with good results [9]. Other forms of surgical removal, excision, dermabrasion and electrocoagulation have been used with moderate effect [2,9]. Localised conjunctival involvement can be treated with surgery. Surgery has also been used in CNS disease but recurrences may occur and not all CNS lesions are amenable to resection. Systemic involvement with lung, liver or CNS involvement requires active treatment but the response to therapy is not predictable and may not be long lasting. Glucocorticoids, chlorambucil, azathioprine and cyclophosphamide have been effective in some patients with cutaneous disease [3,10]. Recently, cladribine was found to be useful in two small case series [11,12]. One recent patient was successfully treated with imatinib [13] and another with anakinra [14]. Interestingly, one patient had a partial response to a combination of three lipid-lowering agents, rosiglitazone, simvastatin and the niacin analogue acipimox [3], and a second patient had a dramatic response after 5 months of simvastatin alone [15]. Anti-inflammatory and lipid-lowering drugs such as the statins need further evaluation in refractory XD patients, keeping in mind the possibility of spontaneous resolution, which may make assessment of response to therapy more difficult.

Treatment ladder for xanthoma disseminatum

Cutaneous xanthoma disseminatum

First line
- Carbon dioxide laser

Second line
- Surgical excision or dermabrasion or electrocoagulation

Systemic xanthoma disseminatum (lung, liver, CNS)

First line
- Chemotherapy (e.g. corticosteroids, chlorambucil, azathioprine, cyclophosphamide)

Second line
- Cladribine or anti-inflammatory and lipid-lowering agents (e.g. statins) have been used in small case series

Third line
- Anakinra or imatinib – successfully treated refractory XD in one case each.

DISORDERS IN WHICH SKIN MAY BE INVOLVED BUT SYSTEMIC COMPONENT PREDOMINATES

Erdheim–Chester disease

Definition and nomenclature
This disease is characterised by infiltration of viscera, bones, retroperitoneum and skin.

Synonyms and inclusions
- Uber lipoid granulomatose

Introduction and general description
Erdheim–Chester disease (ECD) is a rare lipoid granulomatosis characterised by infiltration of the viscera, bones, retroperitoneum and skin. ECD may represent a variant of JXG with mostly osseous and visceral involvement, which can be distinguished from JXG clinically and radiographically [1,2]. With the 2016 WHO revision of the histiocytoses classification, ECD now belongs to the 'L' group, along with LCH [3].

Epidemiology
This is predominantly a disease of adults, with a mean age of 53 years (range 7–84 years) [4]. The male to female ratio was reported as 33:26 [4].

Pathophysiology
Pathology
Morphologically and immunohistochemically, ECD histiocytes are identical to those of JXG. They are positive for CD68 and factor XIIIa, but negative for CD1a and S100. Histological examination shows a xanthogranulomatous infiltration by lipid-laden histiocytes within a mesh and surrounded by fibrosis. Factor XIIIa-positive histiocytes are known to stimulate fibroblast proliferation, resulting in fibrosis, which is common in this disorder [5]. Touton giant cells and eosinophils may be prominent.

Genetics
The pathogenesis of ECD is poorly understood. Recent identification of the *BRAF* V600E mutation in more than half of ECD patients suggests involvement of the RAS signalling pathway and has important therapeutic implications [6,7]. Furthermore, comprehensive genomic analysis of ECD cases with whole-exome and whole-transcriptome sequencing unravelled recurrent activating mutations in *MAP2K1* (30%), *NRAS* or *KRAS* (27%), *PIK3CA* (11%), *ARAF* and kinase fusions involving *BRAF*, *ALK* and *NTRK1*. Activating *CSF1R* mutations have been identified in 6% of ECD cases without MAPK pathway gene mutations [8].

Clinical features
Presentation
The clinical presentation can range from asymptomatic to fulminant organ failure. Bone pain in the knees and ankles is the most common presenting symptom. Constitutional symptoms such as weakness, weight loss and fever are frequent. Bilateral symmetrical long bone involvement is nearly always present [2,3]. Diagnosis is made on the basis of radiological features of osteosclerosis in addition to the classic histology.

Complications and co-morbidities
In Veyssier-Belot's series of 59 patients, 86% of reported cases have involvement of the long bones, with the distal femur, proximal fibula and tibia being most commonly affected [4]. Up to 30% of patients show lytic lesions in the flat bones, which can be difficult

to distinguish from LCH. Unlike JXG, skin involvement is less common in ECD, affecting approximately 20% of patients and presenting as xanthoma-like lesions despite normal plasma lipid levels, usually on the eyelids but occasionally on the trunk and submammary area [9]. Pulmonary involvement is seen in 25–50% of patients [10], and although mostly asymptomatic, the presence of cough and progressive dyspnoea carries a poor prognosis. However, pulmonary involvement was not found to be an independent predictor of decreased survival in one large series [11]. Cardiac involvement is relatively common in ECD, with periaortic fibrosis in 55.6%, pericardial involvement in 44.4% and myocardial involvement in 30.6% among 72 patients with ECD and cardiovascular involvement [12]. CNS involvement is seen in 15% of patients, presenting with ataxia, paraparesis, hemiparesis or change in mental state [13]. Neurological imaging can reveal thickening of the dura or more rarely intracerebral masses that can resemble meningioma-like tumours [13].

Disease course and prognosis
ECD appears to have a significantly worse prognosis compared with other histiocytoses, with an overall mortality of around 60% in one series [4], mainly from cardiorespiratory failure from lung fibrosis or renal failure from retroperitoneal fibrosis.

Management
Not all patients with ECD require treatment at the time of diagnosis. Active treatment is typically reserved for symptomatic patients. However, treatment for patients with asymptomatic CNS involvement is recommended since it represents an independent predictor of a worse outcome [14]. A variety of therapeutic options are available with varying degrees of success. These include surgical debulking, high-dose corticosteroids, ciclosporin, interferon-α, systemic chemotherapy and radiation therapy [4,15]. The commonest chemotherapy drugs utilised have been vinca alkaloids, anthracyclines and cyclophosphamide [16]. Interferon-α was recommended as first line therapy because of the durable response seen in three patients with advanced disease initially, followed by large case series subsequently [3,17,18]. In May 2019, the 5-year survival of 261 patients with ECD treated with interferon-α was 79% [2,17]. Nevertheless, half of patients experienced depression and fatigue with interferon-α treatment [18]. Several case reports have also shown activity of imatinib in ECD [19,20]. Although the exact role of imatinib in the treatment paradigm remains undefined, it offers an alternative therapeutic option for patients who fail to respond or are intolerant to interferon-α. A growing body of literature on the successful use of BRAF (vemurafenib, dabrafenib) or MEK inhibitors (trametinib, cobimetinib) in refractory ECD patients harbouring MAPK pathway mutations paves the way for molecularly targeted therapies in ECD [21–23]. Vemurafenib was approved for *BRAF* V600-mutant ECD by the FDA in November 2017 based on the results of the phase 2 VE-BASKET trial which showed a response rate of 43%, a 12-month PFS of 91% and OS of 100% in the ECD/LCH cohort [24]. In addition, for patients without the *BRAF* V600E mutation, the phase 2 study of cobimetinib (NCT01953926) which enrolled 18 patients with various histiocytic neoplasms (12 ECD, 2 LCH, 2 RDD and 2 mixed histiocytosis) reported an ORR of 89% with 72% having a complete response [25].

DISORDERS WITH MAINLY SKIN INVOLVEMENT WITH/WITHOUT A SYSTEMIC COMPONENT

Reticulohistiocytoma

Definition and nomenclature
Reticulohistiocytoma is an uncommon, incompletely characterised histiocytic tumour of the skin and soft tissues.

> **Synonyms and inclusions**
> - Solitary epithelioid histiocytoma
> - Solitary histiocytoma

Introduction and general description
Reticulohistiocytoma is the localised variant of multicentric reticulohistiocytosis. This uncommon tumour is generally solitary and asymptomatic. Lesions are less than 1 cm in diameter and present as papules or dome-shaped nodules. They may occur anywhere on the body including the genitalia. Oral mucosal lesions have been reported [1]. They are thought to represent a non-neoplastic reactive process.

Epidemiology
Reticulohistiocytoma tends to occur in young adult males. Rarely, it may appear in the newborn period.

Pathology
Histology shows nodules of large epithelioid histiocytes with abundant, glassy, eosinophilic cytoplasm extending from the papillary dermis to the mid dermis associated with lymphoid cells and occasionally neutrophils. Cells may have a lacuna space-like clearing at the periphery and scalloped cytoplasm. Cells are CD68 and CD163 positive and generally CD1a and S100 negative. The presence of factor XIIIa is variable. In a study of five cases of solitary reticulohistiocytoma, factor XIIIa was found to be positive [1,2].

Management
Treatment is surgical excision. Follow-up in 12 patients, with a median follow-up of 13 years, showed no recurrence after primary excision.

Familial sea-blue histiocytosis

Introduction and general description
This is a rare inherited abnormality of lipid metabolism in which characteristic histiocytic cells are found in the bone marrow and other tissues. The histiocytes are identified by the May–Gruenwald stain, which colours the cytoplasmic granules a deep azure blue, hence the name 'sea-blue histiocytosis'. Secondary sea-blue histiocytes have been described in a variety of disorders of lipid metabolism such as Niemann–Pick disease, in patients with

prolonged use of intravenous fat emulsions, and in cases of partial sphingomyelinase deficiency, myelodysplastic syndromes, lymphomas, chronic myeloid leukaemia, idiopathic thrombocytopenic purpura, autoimmune neutropenia, total parenteral nutrition and β-thalassemia major [1].

Epidemiology
It usually presents in young adulthood with hepatosplenomegaly and thrombocytopenia, although the age at presentation ranges from 1 to 83 years [1].

Pathophysiology
The biological abnormality is poorly understood, but the condition probably represents a storage disease in which glycolipid, phospholipid or both accumulate in histiocytic cells in various organs including the bone marrow, liver and spleen.

Pathology
Histologically, it is characterised by micronodular infiltrates of large monomorphous histiocytes with cytoplasmic vacuoles and granules. The granules appear yellow-brown with H&E, dark blue with Giemsa and 'sea-blue' with May–Gruenwald staining [2].

Genetics
It is one of a group of related lipid disorders caused by changes in the *APOE* gene. The genetic change associated with this condition is inherited in an autosomal dominant manner [3].

Clinical features
The skin, lungs, gastrointestinal tract, eye and nervous system may be involved. Skin manifestations are common in more than 80% of cases and may cause disfigurement. They present as patchy and irregular brownish grey pigmentation or subcutaneous nodules. Affected sites are face, upper chest and shoulders. In the eye, white stippled deposits may be observed at the margins of the fovea or macula, with discoloration of the macular region. Neurological symptoms occur early, with ataxia, epilepsy and dementia. Sea-blue histiocytosis is usually benign, but it may disseminate and lead to death from heart, liver or lung involvement.

Management
There is no specific treatment for sea-blue histiocytosis. Specific treatment of the associated disorder of lipid metabolism may induce resolution of the disease. Nevertheless, it has been suggested that splenectomy may worsen the condition.

Hereditary progressive mucinous histiocytosis

Definition
Hereditary progressive mucinous histiocytosis is a rare autosomal dominant genodermatosis consisting of lesions affecting the nose, hands, forearms and thighs.

Epidemiology
This is a rare autosomal dominant genodermatosis, which was first described in 1988. All case reports to date have been in women, thus suggesting a link to hormones [1].

Pathophysiology
Histologically, the epidermis is normal but within the dermis there are small collections of epithelioid histiocytes with telangiectatic vessels in the upper dermis in early lesions. As tumours develop, the infiltrate changes to nodular mid dermal aggregates of tightly packed, spindle-shaped cells. In both early and established lesions, there is moderate to extensive mucin production by the epithelioid histiocytes and spindle-shaped cells. On electron microscopy, the spindle-shaped cells are shown to be dendritic histiocytes with abundant lysosomal storage organelles, myelin bodies and zebra bodies. Immunohistochemically, these cells stain with CD68 and MS1 [2].

Clinical features
Skin lesions appear in the first decade of life and gradually increase throughout life. Lesions consist of skin-coloured to red-brown papules that characteristically affect the nose, hands, forearms and thighs.

Management
The condition is progressive, with a gradual increase in the numbers of tumours throughout life. These patients show no evidence of spontaneous resolution. No systemic involvement has been described and no treatment seems to have any impact on the disease [3,4].

Malakoplakia

Definition
Malakoplakia is an immunodeficiency disease in which macrophages fail to phagocytose and digest bacteria adequately. The term 'malakoplakia', which means soft plaque, was adopted as a descriptive term.

Pathophysiology
Pathology
Histologically, sheets of large histiocytic cells with abundant cytoplasm are present in the skin, affecting any level from the epidermis to the subcutaneous fat. The cells have fine eosinophilic granules in their cytoplasm and are referred to as Hansemann cells. They also contain one or more round basophilic inclusion bodies (Michaelis–Gutmann bodies). Michaelis–Gutmann bodies are 5–15 μm in diameter and stain positively with periodic acid–Schiff stain (PAS), von Kossa stain (for calcium) and Perls ferrocyanide reaction (for ferric iron). They are considered pathognomonic for this disease and are thought to represent abnormal degradation of bacteria, with calcium and iron deposited on the remaining glycolipid [1].

Causative organisms

The aetiology of malakoplakia is still unclear. However, chronic infection has been suggested to play a role in the pathogenesis of the disease [2]. Common associated organisms include *Escherichia coli*, *Proteus species*, *Mycobacterium tuberculosis* and *Staphylococcus aureus* [2].

Clinical features
Presentation

Malakoplakia can affect many organs but most commonly affects the urinary and gastrointestinal tracts [3,4]. Cutaneous lesions are rare, non-specific and variable. Draining abscesses, sinuses, ulcers, fluctuant masses, isolated tender nodules and grouped papules have been reported [5,6]. Mucous membranes may be affected, including the tongue and cervix.

Disease course and prognosis

The disease generally runs a benign self-limiting course, but fatal cases have been reported [6].

Management

Management includes different combinations between surgical excision and/or use of antibiotics for the associated infections. Some case reports suggest higher cure rates with surgical excision when compared with antibiotic therapy [7]. In addition, when comparing antibiotics, quinolones seem to be superior [7].

Necrobiotic xanthogranuloma

Definition

Necrobiotic xanthogranuloma (NXG) is a rare, multisystem histiocytic disease in which widespread infiltrated xanthomatous nodules and plaques are strongly associated with haematological malignant conditions.

Epidemiology

Only about 100 cases have been reported in the literature since it was first recognised as a distinct dermatosis in 1980 [1].

Pathophysiology

The pathogenesis of NXG is unknown. Some believe that paraproteins function as autoantibodies leading to fibroblast proliferation and the deposition of dermal macrophages [2], while others suggest that the abnormal paraprotein becomes complexed with lipid and deposits in the skin, where it produces a foreign body giant cell granulomatous reaction [3]. However, this does not explain NXG cases without paraproteinaemia. The possibility of an infectious aetiology was raised by the finding of *Borrelia* species in some skin biopsy specimens [4]. Approximately 80–90% of patients have an underlying monoclonal gammopathy [5], among whom IgG-κ is the most frequent monoclonal gammopathy of unknown significance (MGUS) (65%), followed by IgG-λ (35%) and, much less commonly, IgA [1]. When a gammopathy is present, the underlying haematological condition is MGUS in half of the cases and myeloma in the other half [6], which can manifest years after the development of

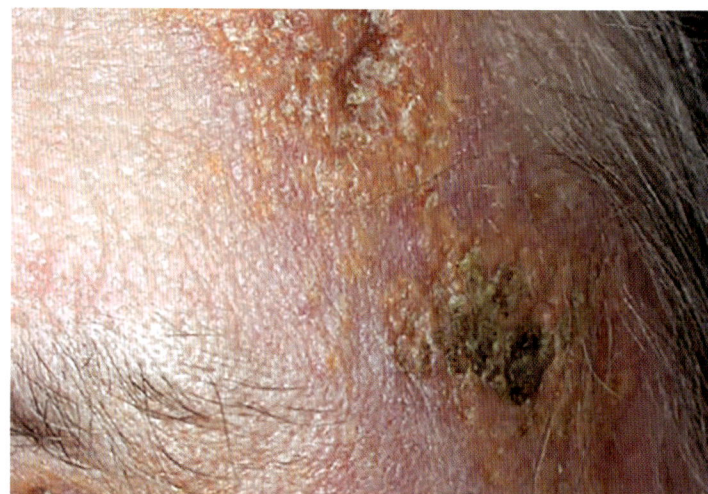

Figure 135.18 Necrobiotic xanthogranuloma showing a reddish yellow, infiltrative plaque with evidence of necrosis. Courtesy of Dr S. Walsh, Sunnybrook Hospital, Toronto, Canada.

skin lesions. Because of the prolonged gap between the onset of the skin disease and these malignancies, their role in pathogenesis remains uncertain.

Pathology

Histologically, confluent granulomatous masses are present as either sheets or nodules, replacing much of the dermis and extending into the subcutaneous tissue. Hyaline areas of necrobiosis separate individual nodules. Numerous giant cells are present, with Touton cells and bizarre, angulated giant cells [7]. Cholesterol clefts, lymphoid nodules (some of which develop germinal centres) and perivascular aggregates of plasma cells are frequent features. Less common, but characteristic when present, are palisading cholesterol cleft granulomas and xanthogranulomatous panniculitis [8]. Granulomatous invasion of blood vessels with thrombosis has been described.

Clinical features
Presentation

The clinical picture of NXG consists of slowly progressive, reddish yellow, xanthomatous plaques/nodules that are infiltrative and destructive (Figure 135.18) [9]. More than 80% of the lesions are periorbital but may occur on the trunk and limbs where subcutaneous nodules and xanthomatous plaques are present with atrophy and ulceration. The eyes are often affected with conjunctivitis, keratitis, uveitis, iritis and proptosis. Blindness has been reported in two affected patients [10].

Complications and co-morbidities

Association with haematological and lymphoproliferative malignant disorders such as myeloma, non-Hodgkin lymphoma and chronic lymphocytic leukaemia has been well described and typically occurs approximately 2 years from the onset of skin manifestations [1,5]. The diagnosis of NXG should prompt a thorough evaluation to rule out these conditions. Only one case report of a patient with typical cutaneous lesions and cerebral involvement presenting as tonic–clonic seizures has been published [11]. Systemic symptoms have been reported, including nausea, vomiting, fatigue, epistaxis, back pain and the Raynaud phenomenon. Atypical forms of NXG have been reported, including solitary tumours of the skin [12].

Management
Due to the rarity of the condition, there is no consensus regarding the optimal therapy. Treatment is generally directed to the associated paraproteinaemia. Alkylating agents such as melphalan, with or without prednisolone, have resulted in temporary clearing of the skin [9]. Other therapies included intralesional corticosteroids, high-dose systemic steroids, chlorambucil, interferon-α, cyclophosphamide, methotrexate, hydroxychloroquine and azathioprine [9]. A recent review of reported cases treated with chlorambucil supported its use as a frontline agent in selected cases [13]. In one patient where cytotoxic drugs had failed, plasmapheresis reduced the level of the circulating monoclonal IgG and resulted in clearing of the skin [10]. Radiotherapy was successful in one case involving the eye [12]. Cutaneous disease has also been successfully treated with carbon dioxide laser with no evidence of relapse after 12 months [14]. Two patients were successfully treated with intravenous immunoglobulin [2]. A single case report described one patient achieving long-term remission following the combination of thalidomide for 2 years and pulse dexamethasone for 9 months [9]. These authors felt that this combination should be tried as first line in patients who need systemic therapy but that high-dose and prolonged treatment is necessary.

DISORDERS IN WHICH SKIN MAY BE INVOLVED BUT THE SYSTEMIC COMPONENT PREDOMINATES

Multicentric reticulohistiocytosis

Definition and nomenclature
Multicentric reticulohistiocytosis (MRH) is a rare non-LCH disorder characterised by the association of specific nodular skin lesions and destructive arthritis. It is classified as a Group C histiocytosis (cutaneous and mucocutaneous).

Introduction and general description
This is a rare multisystem disorder characterised by papulonodular cutaneous and mucosal involvement in addition to a destructive arthropathy that can also affect other organs including lungs and heart. The arthropathy usually precedes nodular skin involvement and mucosal infiltration. About 28% of patients have an associated internal malignancy. This must be differentiated from solitary or multiple reticulohistiocytomas that are restricted to skin with neither associated arthropathy nor internal malignancy. Moreover, differentiation from fibroblastic rheumatism (FR), which can also present with a destructive polyarthritis and skin lesions, is important as it differs both in prognosis and therapy. FR was originally classified as a class IIB histiocytic disorder, but recent studies have suggested that FR more properly belongs to the fibroblastic disorders [1].

Epidemiology
MRH is a disease of middle-aged adults, predominantly female [2], although rare paediatric cases have been reported [2–4]. The female to male ratio is 3:1, and 85% of reported adults were white [2].

Pathophysiology
Pathogenesis is unknown. The disease was generally considered to be a reactive histiocytosis. Inflammatory cytokines such as TNF-α, IL-1 and IL-6 have been found to be highly expressed in MRH nodules [5]. IL-6 may also result in the osteoclastogenesis, accounting for the multinucleated giant cells seen in the lesions.

Recent genetic analysis using whole exome sequencing (WES) and RNA sequencing of two patients with MRH in Japan suggested that MRH is not an autoimmune or inflammatory disease, but a neoplastic disease which may involve aberrant activation of the RAS-MAPK pathway or a tyrosine kinase pathway. Both genetic alterations detected (*KIF5B-FGFR1* fusion in patient 1 and *MAP2K1* deletion in patient 2) are potentially druggable, suggesting that targeted therapy using FGFR or MEK inhibitors may be effective treatment for MRH [6].

Pathology
The characteristic pathological picture in the skin and mucous membranes is infiltration by mono- and multinucleated giant cells with voluminous ground-glass cytoplasm (Figure 135.19). In early lesions, the predominant infiltrating cells are histiocytes, lymphocytes and eosinophils, with few giant cells, but the giant cell infiltrate quickly follows. The giant cells are large (100 μm diameter) with 1–20 nuclei, which may be distributed randomly at the periphery or in the centre. The cells are PAS positive, contain diastase-resistant material and variable amounts of lipid and free or esterified cholesterol. In older lesions, fibrosis usually signals regression of the lesions, with a reduction in the inflammatory cell infiltrate. Ultrastructural studies have shown type IV collagen inclusions in MRH. These inclusions were both intracytoplasmic and extracytoplasmic. Such inclusions are usually found in lymphohistiocytic neoplasms, suggesting that MRH is a proliferative rather than an inflammatory disorder [7]. Immunocytochemical studies show a histiocytic phenotype of the cells, which are positive for acid phosphatase, adenosine triphosphatase, lysozyme and α_1-antitrypsin. The cells are also positive for vimentin, CD45, CD68, CD11b and HAM56, but negative for CD1, S100, CD34 and factor XIIIa [8]. CD14 is usually positive in osteoclast-like macrophages and negative in true osteoclasts [9].

Causative organisms
No infective agent has been implicated, but in one study 33% of patients had evidence of tuberculosis exposure and 5% had active tuberculosis on examination [10].

Clinical features
Presentation
The disease is often limited to the skin, mucosa and joints but systemic involvement of the heart and other organs has been described. Two-thirds of patients present with symmetrical polyarthritis, followed by the appearance of skin lesions. The arthropathy typically affects the hands, but other joints may be involved as well, including the knees, shoulders, wrists, hips, ankles, feet, elbows, spine and

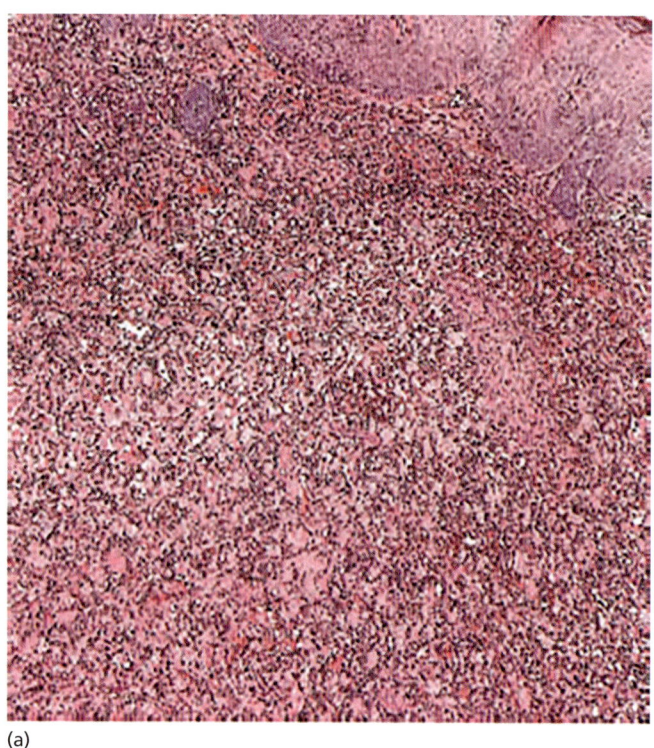

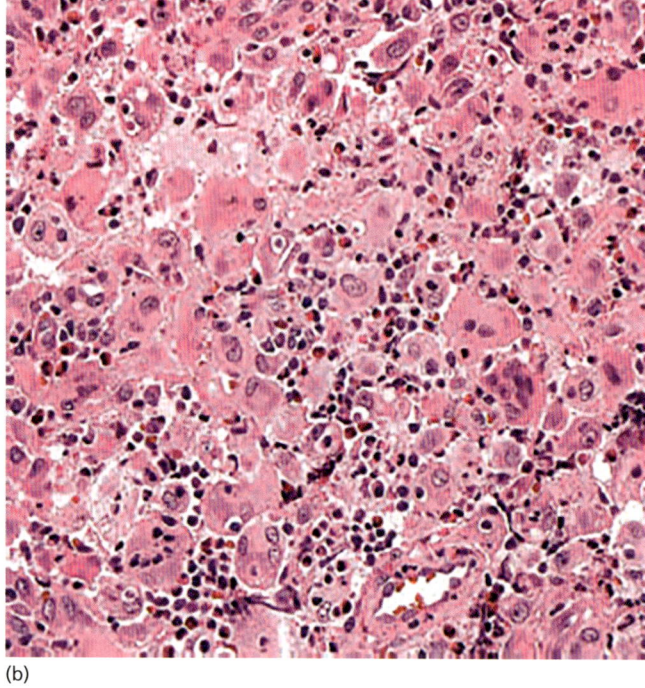

Figure 135.19 Reticulohistiocytoma/multicentric reticulohistiocytosis. (a) The dermis contains an infiltrate of large, eosinophilic, cytoplasm-rich histiocytes with an interspersed inflammatory cell component. Magnification 100× (H&E). (b) The large eosinophilic histiocytes generally have a single nucleus or two nuclei. Interspersed lymphocytes and eosinophils are prominent in this example. Some emperipolesis is noted. Magnification 400× (H&E). Courtesy of Dr R. Jaffe, Children's Hospital of Pittsburgh, Pittsburgh, USA.

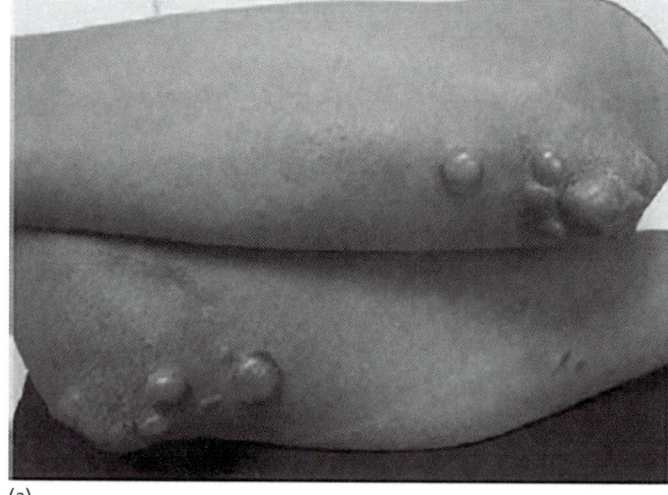

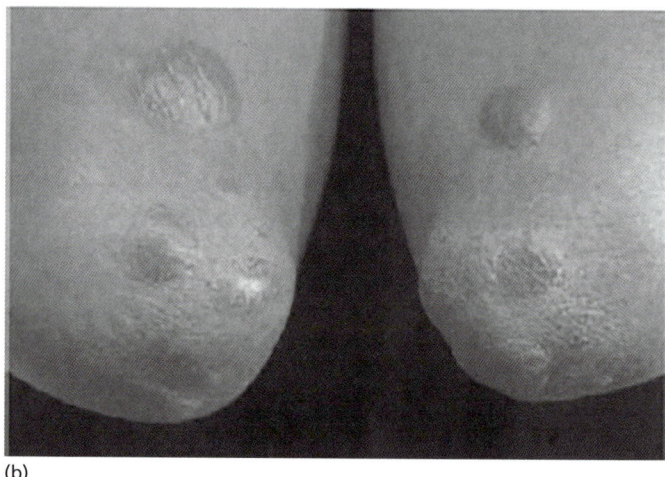

Figure 135.20 Multicentric reticulohistiocytosis nodules over the elbows (a) that shrank after an infusion of zoledronic acid (photograph taken 43 days after infusion) (b). From Codriansky et al. 2008 [12]. Reproduced with permission from John Wiley & Sons.

temporo-mandibular joints. Although it often remits spontaneously, 15–50% of cases progress to mutilating osteoarthropathy with disabling deformities [3,11]. In 20% of cases, skin nodules appear first while simultaneous skin and joint lesions emerge in the remainder [12]. The classic skin lesions are firm brown or yellow papules and plaques, which predominantly affect extensor surfaces, particularly on the hands and forearms (Figure 135.20). The face, scalp, hands and ears are often affected but involvement of the lower trunk and legs is rare. Coral bead-like lesions may occur around the nail folds, which may result in nail dystrophy. Skin lesions are of variable size and rarely ulcerate. Large nodular lesions in proximity to the affected joints and cystic swellings of the tendon sheaths may occur. About 25% of patients complain of pruritus associated with skin lesions. One-third of patients have symptoms of fever, weight loss and malaise. More than 50% of patients have mucosal involvement, characteristically of the lips and tongue, but it can also affect the mouth, gingiva, pharynx, larynx and sclera.

Complications and co-morbidities

Around 15% of patients have an associated autoimmune disease such as SLE, diabetes or Sjögren syndrome, while 20% of patients have been found to have an associated internal malignancy. The commonest tumours are gastric, ovarian [13], breast and uterine carcinomas [14], myeloma, melanoma [15] and lymphomas. The diagnosis of MRH precedes that of the neoplasm in most cases, and the disease may relapse with recurrence of the neoplasm.

Disease course and prognosis
The prognosis is good, with the disease becoming quiescent in 7–8 years if there is no systemic malignancy. Fatal cardiac involvement may occur with widespread systemic involvement [16]. MRH may, however, leave considerable morbidity, with a crippling arthropathy and scarred skin [17].

Management
Treatment of the underlying disease is important, although it does not usually influence the disease course. Resolution of MRH was seen in a patient with renal cell carcinoma following nephrectomy. Most children have a self-limiting disease with non-deforming arthritis. However, this is not true for adults, in whom therapy is usually indicated. Gold, tamoxifen and d-penicillamine failed in all cases [18]. Several reports suggest that methotrexate alone or in combination may be effective [2–4,19]. Cyclophosphamide alone induced complete remission in three cases [19]. Other immunosuppressive agents such as ciclosporin, leflunomide [20], prednisolone and azathioprine [21] have resulted in complete remission in single case reports. Successful therapy with bisphosphonates alone or in combination with prednisolone and methotrexate has also been reported [22,23]. Anti-TNF agents such as etanercept, infliximab and adalimumab have been reported to be beneficial [17,21], as has the anti-IL-6 receptor antibody tocilizumab, in patients resistant to methotrexate and prednisolone [5].

A reasonable approach in the past was to begin therapy with a combination of corticosteroid and low-dose methotrexate, and to add cyclophosphamide for poor responders. Consideration could be given to combining methotrexate with or without corticosteroid with one of these newer targeted agents as frontline therapy in severely affected or resistant patients. As with all of the non-LCH disorders, different patients may respond differently and a switch from one agent to another may be needed in individual patients. The recent finding of activated kinase signalling pathways in two patients with MRH suggests that druggable targets may be present and that WES and RNA sequencing should be performed in patients with MRH, particularly in patients resistant to the therapies discussed here.

Sinus histiocytosis with massive lymphadenopathy

Definition and nomenclature
Sinus histiocytosis with massive lymphadenopathy (SHML) is a rare, non-neoplastic disorder of unknown aetiology that is usually self-limiting. It is characterised by abundant histiocytes in the lymph nodes throughout the body. It was first described by a French pathologist, Pierre Paul Louis Lucien Destombes, in 1965. It is now known as Rosai–Dorfman–Destombes disease (RDD) as Juan Rosai and Ronald Dorfman analysed 34 cases of SHML in 1969 [1].

Synonyms and inclusions
- Rosai–Dorfman–Destombes disease

Epidemiology
Most patients are young adults (mean age 20.6 years), but with a wide age distribution from birth to 74 years [2]. Patients presenting with isolated intracranial disease appear to be older (mean age 37.5 years) [3]. The disease is slightly more common in males (58%) and in black people [4].

Pathophysiology
Predisposing factors
The aetiology of SHML is unknown. It is postulated that an infectious or malignant process may result in aberrant activation of the macrophage system with excessive cytokine release by the macrophages and T cells. An increased incidence of autoimmune disorders such as autoimmune haemolytic anaemia and various rheumatological disorders has been reported [5].

Pathology
Histologically, involved lymph nodes show massive sinus infiltration of large histiocytes admixed with lymphocytes and plasma cells (Figure 135.21). Immunohistochemicallly, SHML cells are positive for S100, CD68, CD163, HAM-56, α_1-antichymotrypsin and α_1-antitrypsin, but negative for CD1a [2]. SHML lesions show strong expression of IL-1 and TNF-α and moderate expression of IL-6 [6]. The latter may be related to the observed polyclonal plasmacytosis and hypergammaglobulinaemia. A hallmark of SHML is the presence of emperipolesis (phagocytosis of intact leukocytes, particularly lymphocytes) in histiocytes that express S100. In the skin, a dense, upper dermal, histiocytic infiltration with scattered multinucleate giant cells and plasma cells is seen [7]. Emperipolesis is less prominent in the skin than in the nodes.

Genetics
In contrast to LCH and ECD, the *BRAF* V600E mutation is rarely found in RDD [8]. Recent studies have identified other MAPK pathway mutations (*KRAS, NRAS, ARAF, MAP2K1*) and *CSF1R* mutations in patients with RDD [9].

Clinical features
Presentation
Clinically, about 80% of patients present with bilateral, painless, cervical adenopathy, which may be associated with fever, malaise, night sweats, weight loss, leukocytosis and hypergammaglobulinaemia. Other nodal groups, such as axillary, mediastinal and inguinal, can also be involved. The lymph node enlargement can reach massive proportions. Extranodal involvement is described in 43% of patients and skin represents the most common extranodal site [10].

Clinical variants
Skin is the most common extranodal site and is found in isolation in 50% of patients (Figure 135.22) [7]. Skin lesions are usually yellow

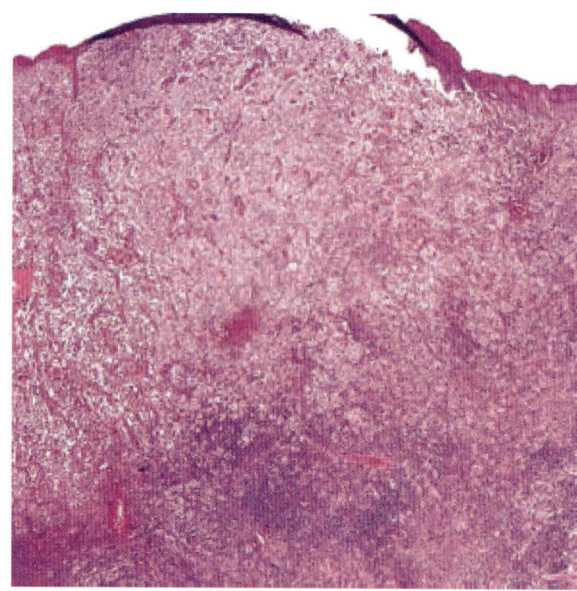

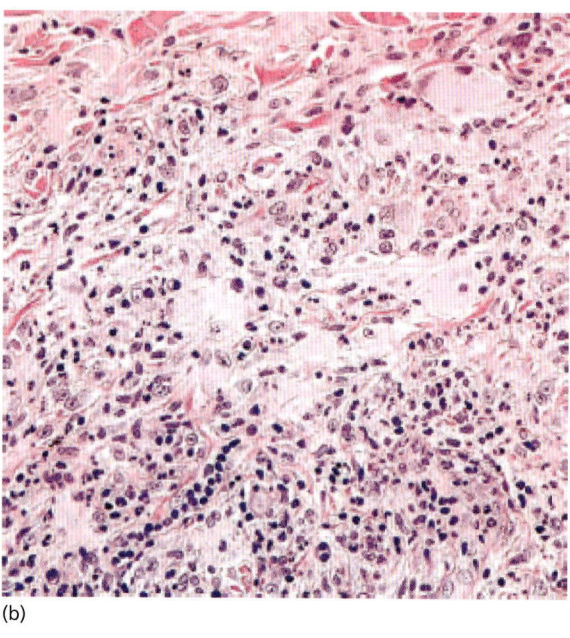

Figure 135.21 Rosai–Dorfman disease. (a) The 'lymph node-in-skin' appearance is highlighted at a low-power magnification of 20× (H&E). (b) Rosai–Dorfman histiocytes have very abundant water-clear cytoplasm and one or two large hypochromatic nuclei. Emperipolesis of intact lymphocytes is notable in the cytoplasm. Magnification 400× (H&E). Courtesy of Dr R. Jaffe, Children's Hospital of Pittsburgh, Pittsburgh, USA.

but may be violaceous or purple. Red macules, papules, nodules or infiltrated plaques have been reported. Scaling is often present and telangiectasias may be observed. Skin lesions may occur anywhere and there is no predilection for any site [11].

Complications and co-morbidities

Other reported extranodal sites include the lung, uro-genital tract, breast, gastrointestinal tract, liver and pancreas. Head and neck involvement occurs in 22% of patients [10], with the nasal cavity and parotid gland as the commonest sites. Isolated intracranial disease can occur in SHML without extracranial lymphadenopathy, which makes the diagnosis challenging. Most intracranial lesions

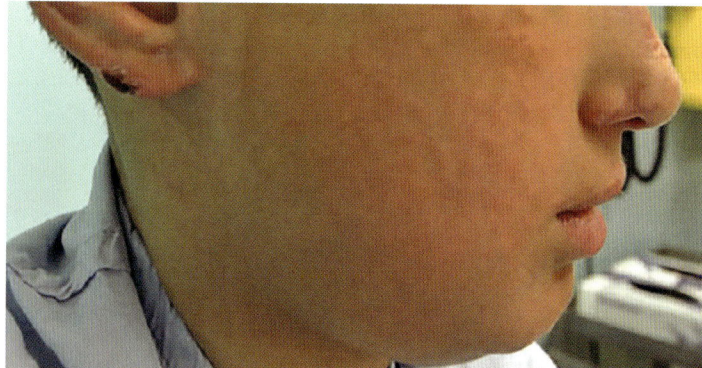

Figure 135.22 Rosai–Dorfman disease showing multiple nodules/tumours with superficial crusting and old scars on the nose.

are attached to the dura and patients present with headaches, seizures, numbness or paraplegia [12].

Disease course and prognosis

The clinical course of SHML is unpredictable, with episodes of exacerbation and remission that may extend over many years. The outcome is usually good and the disease is often self-limiting. Nonetheless, about 5–11% of patients die from the disease. Patients with underlying immunological abnormalities at or prior to onset have a worse prognosis with more widespread nodal disease and higher fatality rate [10,13].

Investigations

Laboratory investigations usually show a mild normochromic normocytic anaemia or hypochromic microcytic anaemia with an elevation of the erythrocyte sedimentation rate. Serum proteins are often abnormal, with a low serum albumin and polyclonal gammopathy. Serum lipids are normal. Chest computed tomography or head imaging should be considered depending on clinical symptomatology.

Management

There is no defined treatment approach for RDD and treatment is tailored to the patient's clinical presentation. Treatment is only necessary when a vital organ is being compromised or nodal enlargement leads to significant problems such as airway obstruction [14]. For intracranial dural-based lesions, surgical excision alone is successful in most cases [3]. There is currently no consensus on guidelines for systemic treatment when indicated. Antibiotics are not useful. Surgical debulking of resectable lesions achieved complete remission in eight of nine patients [14]. Systemic corticosteroids are useful in decreasing size and symptoms, but regrowth often occurs within a short period of discontinuation. Chemotherapy is generally unsuccessful. Variable response has been observed with vinblastine, anti-metabolite chemotherapy (methotrexate or mercaptopurine) could be used as maintenance therapy, and complete remission has been achieved in 7 out of 11 patients with severe, disseminated or refractory RDD treated with cladribine [1,15–17]. Complete remissions achieved with interferon-α plus chemotherapy [18,19], thalidomide or acyclovir have been reported in case reports [20]. Sirolimus has been effective in the treatment of severe autoimmune cytopenia in the context of RDD [21].

Rituximab, a chimeric anti-CD20 antibody, has been successful in recent anecdotal reports including three patients treated by the author (S. Weitzman, personal communication), one of whom had severe liver involvement. Relapse after discontinuation of rituximab was seen in another anecdotal case. Retreatment and prolongation of therapy, similar to cases of follicular lymphoma, may be indicated in these refractory patients, but this approach is obviously experimental. A recent study of the efficacy of MEK1/MEK2 inhibition with cobimetinib in 18 adult patients with various histiocytic disorders included 2 patients with RDD. Although the response by disease type was not given, it is notable that the overall response rate was 89% with 72% achieving CR, 17% PR and 6% stable disease. Median duration of response and median PFS had not been reached after a median follow-up of 11.9 months. No responding patient had progressed by the time of reporting, 56% required dose reduction for toxicity, but all patients maintained their responses at the lower dose [22]. Further investigation is indicated but targeted therapy with a MEK inhibitor could be considered in RDD patients failing standard approaches.

MALIGNANT HISTIOCYTOSES

Malignant histiocytoses are malignancies of the monocyte/macrophage series of cells. These diseases are separated into monocytic leukaemia, malignant histiocytosis, true histiocytic lymphoma and histiocytic sarcoma based on clinical criteria, but there is an enormous overlap and it may not always be possible to differentiate them.

Malignant histiocytosis

Definition and nomenclature
Malignant histiocytosis (MH) is a widespread neoplastic proliferation of histiocytic cells that typically involves liver, spleen, lymph nodes and bone marrow.

Synonyms and inclusions
- Malignant reticulohistiocytosis
- Malignant reticulosis
- Histiocytic medullary reticulosis
- Sinusoidal haematolymphoid malignancy
- Malignant astrocytosis
- Aleukaemic reticulosis
- Histiocytic reticulosis

Introduction and general description
The widespread increase in histiocytic cells in MH typically involves the liver, spleen, lymph nodes and bone marrow. The cells usually arise from sinusoidal histiocytes, although very rare cases of malignant histiocytosis of LC phenotype have been reported. In addition, many cases previously reported as MH were eventually shown to be T- and B-cell lymphomas including anaplastic large cell lymphoma [1].

Epidemiology
Sex
MH is a rare disease with a male to female ratio of 3.5:1. It has been reported in all age groups, with a median age of 35 years [2]. Childhood disease is uncommon with few reported series [3]. The disease tends to occur earlier in women (second to third decades) than in men (third to fourth decades) [4].

Ethnicity
Reports have suggested an increased incidence of this disease in parts of tropical Africa, with reports from Malawi and Uganda [5,6]. A recent review of deaths from 'histiocytosis' in the USA between 1979 and 2006 showed that LCH was significantly more common as a cause of death in people younger than 5 years of age irrespective of sex (P value <0.0001), whereas death rates from MH were significantly greater in ages >54 years (P value <0.00001) [7]. There were more MH deaths among males than females.

Pathophysiology
MH is a neoplastic proliferation of cells of the mononuclear phagocyte system.

Pathology
The histological picture in the skin and lymph nodes is similar and the diagnosis can be established in either site. Characteristically, there is an infiltrate of histiocytic cells showing varying degrees of atypia that are typically non-cohesive. Cells are large (up to 50 μm in diameter) with abundant cytoplasm and distinct cytoplasmic membranes. The histiocytic cells are heterogeneous. Some show more marked histiocytic differentiation, with pale cytoplasm, prominent vacuolation or even foamy cytoplasm, and exhibit phagocytosis of erythrocytes, leukocytes and cellular debris. Other cells are more 'primitive', with deeply eosinophilic or amorphous cytoplasm. Nuclei are usually lobulated, with finely granular or reticulated chromatin and prominent or bizarre nucleoli. Nuclear membranes tend to be thickened. Mitoses are common.

Immunohistochemistry showing a histiocytic origin and negative for myeloid, dendritic or other lymphoid markers is essential for the diagnosis of all the histiocytic malignancies. Cytochemical and immunohistochemical studies have shown that the cells in MH are negative for chloracetate esterase, Sudan black B, alkaline phosphatase and β-glucuronidase [8]. The presence of non-specific esterase, acid phosphatase and lysozyme is variable, with the better differentiated cells showing these enzymes [9]. The more differentiated phagocytosing cells usually stain for factor XIIIa and the antimonocyte monoclonal antibody MOI [10]. In some cases, epithelial membrane antigen (EMA), HLA-DR, CD25, CD30, CD68 and CD71 have been detected. In rare cases, CD1a or CD21/35 may be found. In lymph nodes, the architecture is disarranged but not effaced by the malignant cells.

In the skin, there is extensive perivascular and periappendageal infiltration of the dermis, with extension into the subcutaneous fat. In advanced lesions, fat necrosis may occur. The epidermis and papillary dermis are characteristically spared, but in the more tumid lesions epidermal ulceration may be present.

Causative organisms
There is no evidence of a viral aetiology in this disease and no reported familial incidence.

Genetics
There have been reports of a characteristic chromosomal translocation t(5;6)(q35;p21) in MH [11,12], but it is unclear whether those cases would be called MH by current criteria.

Clinical features
Presentation
Malignant histiocytosis is usually of acute onset, with fever, sweats, wasting, generalised painful lymphadenopathy and hepatosplenomegaly. As the disease progresses, jaundice, purpura, anaemia and leukopenia occur. In 50% of patients, extranodal extension of the disease is seen, most commonly affecting the skin, bone and gastrointestinal tract [13]. Cutaneous involvement occurs in 10–15% of cases, manifesting with single or multiple skin-coloured to violaceous papulonodular lesions [14]. These lesions tend to have a predilection for the lower extremities and buttocks but may occur anywhere. Large lesions may ulcerate. A widespread, papulonodular eruption similar to that in acute monocytic leukaemia may also be seen. In the bone, the lesions are focal, destructive, lytic and may become widespread with associated hypercalcaemia. Gastrointestinal involvement is usually observed late in the disease. The small and large bowel may be involved, with infiltration of the lamina propria and local intraluminal masses. This presents with obstruction or haemorrhage or both. A rare presentation with multiple lesions is with malabsorption.

This disease was invariably lethal in the past, with death occurring within weeks to months of diagnosis. However, with aggressive management (radiotherapy or radiotherapy and chemotherapy) complete remission has been reported in up to 50% of cases, with a mean duration of complete remission of over 12 months [2]. Microscopic evidence of vascular invasion carries a poor prognosis [13].

Differential diagnosis
The major differential diagnosis is with large cell anaplastic lymphomas, in which the clinical and histological features may be similar. Other diseases that may be confused with malignant histiocytosis are familial haemophagocytic lymphohistiocytosis, virus-associated haemophagocytic syndrome, Hodgkin disease and SHML.

Investigations
Diagnosis can usually be established on clinicopathological features of the disease, although special stains may be needed to exclude large cell anaplastic lymphoma.

Management
MH is sensitive to both radiotherapy and chemotherapy but treatment must be started early, as many patients die before therapy can be started [3]. A review of the treatment of MH has been published [15], but similar to the other malignant histiocytic disorders, there are no recent large studies to inform therapy decisions. Conventional chemotherapy and radiotherapy remain the mainstays of treatment. In a study of 27 children with MH, complete remission was achieved in 22 children using a regimen of vincristine, cyclophosphamide, doxorubicin and prednisolone, with a 5-year survival of 81% [16]. There are anecdotal reports of success with LCH-type salvage therapy, such as cladribine and cytosine arabinoside as per the LCH-S-2005 protocol, as well as T-cell acute lymphoblastic leukaemia therapy. In patients who relapse after conventional chemotherapy, bone marrow transplantation has successfully achieved long-term remission [15]. Large skin tumours or ulcerated tumours, non-responsive to chemotherapy, can be treated with local radiotherapy.

True histiocytic lymphoma

Definition and nomenclature
True histiocytic lymphoma is a malignant histiocytic neoplasm that may disseminate.

Synonyms and inclusions
- Reticulum cell sarcoma
- Histiosarcoma
- Monocytic sarcoma

Introduction and general description
The disease represents a malignant proliferation of non-LC histiocytes or more rarely of LCs. Differentiation from malignant histiocytosis may be difficult. Many early cases of 'histiocytic lymphoma' have been reclassified as other lymphomas, including primary cutaneous B-cell lymphoma, and it has been recently suggested that histiocytic lymphomas should be classified and treated as histiocytic sarcomas [1].

Pathophysiology
The aetiology is unknown. True histiocytic lymphoma exhibits many of the features described in malignant histiocytosis, with infiltrating cells being predominantly dermal and non-cohesive. Nemes and Thomazy suggest that the cells in true histiocytic lymphoma are more differentiated than those in malignant histiocytosis and that the cell population is more homogeneous, showing phagocytosis and labelling for factor XIIIa [2]. These cells stain with macrophage markers CD11c and CD68 and are negative for T- and B-cell markers [3]. A rare spindle cell variant has been described that expressed CD163, CD68, CD45, lysozyme and neuron-specific enolase (NSE) [4].

Clinical features
This is a localised tumour of malignant histiocytes that may be nodal or extranodal. In 40% of patients, presentation is with the painless enlargement of one or more groups of superficial lymph nodes. Constitutional symptoms of malaise, anorexia, sweating and fever may be present. Extranodal presentation may be with bone, gastrointestinal tract or skin lesions. Bone and gastrointestinal tract lesions are as described in malignant histiocytosis. Skin lesions are localised bluish red tumours that can attain a large size. An isolated skin tumour of true histiocytic lymphoma in a 79-year-old patient

has been described that reached 20 cm in diameter at presentation [5]. Hepatosplenomegaly occurs in only a minority of patients with true histiocytic lymphoma and peripheral blood involvement is rare. In one case report, a 44-year-old man with true histiocytic lymphoma was treated with autologous bone marrow transplantation and subsequently developed histiocytic leukaemia classified as M5c monocytic leukaemia [6]. True histiocytic lymphoma is treatable and the prognosis is probably better than in malignant histiocytosis.

Management
Review of the literature reveals no recent advances in therapy except for the testing of many new agents against a 'histiocytic lymphoma' cell line U937. From the earlier literature, it appears that true histiocytic lymphoma is both radiosensitive and chemosensitive. Complete remission has been achieved in localised skin disease using electron beam therapy [5]. Reports of therapeutic responses are difficult to evaluate because of doubt over the diagnosis in older series.

Histiocytic sarcoma

Definition
Histiocytic sarcoma (HS) is an extremely rare, non-LCH disorder of unknown cause that most commonly presents with symptoms due to unifocal or multifocal extranodal tumours that can involve the intestinal tract, skin, soft tissues, bone marrow, CNS and spleen. It is an aggressive tumour that responds poorly to standard therapies. A small number of patients have resectable tumours with a much more favourable outcome following surgical resection [1].

Epidemiology
It mainly occurs in adults, but paediatric cases have been reported. HS can occur at any age (range 3 months to 89 years) without sex predilection [2].

Pathophysiology
Pathology
HS is composed of cells that morphologically and immunohistochemically resemble mature tissue histiocytes. Histological examination demonstrates widespread infiltration of large, epithelioid cells with round to oval nuclei, large distinct nucleoli, finely to moderately dispersed chromatin, and abundant cytoplasm that is acidophilic with H&E and greyish with Giemsa staining [3]. Binucleated cells are common and multinucleated giant tumour cells can be found occasionally. The Ki67 index ranged from 5% to 40% with a mean of 18.8% in one analysis [4]. Tissue necrosis is not prominent. The immunohistochemical profile includes reactivity for CD45, CD68, lysozyme and CD163 with a variable expression of S100. LC–dendritic cell markers such as CD1a, CD21 and CD35 should be negative.

Genetics
The pathogenesis of HS is unknown. Whole exome and targeted DNA/RNA sequencing of six cases of HS revealed alterations in *MAP2K1* ($n = 2$), *BRAF* V600E ($n = 1$), *KRAS* ($n = 2$), *CSF1R* ($n = 1$) and *BRAF* fusion ($n = 1$) [5]. Several studies have described cases of HS as well as other histiocytic disorders arising from lymphoid haematological malignancies, most commonly acute lymphoblastic leukaemias [6,7] and lymphomas [7–11]. These histiocytic sarcomas share the same molecular or cytogenetic abnormality as the primary malignancy, suggesting a clonal relationship between the two entities. Next-generation sequencing technologies have been able to show that some mutations are not shared between the two tumours, supporting the hypothesis that a common lymphoid precursor accumulates genetic alterations leading to two different malignancies with different prognoses [12]. HS has also been found in association with germ cell tumours and teratomas [13].

Clinical features
Presentation
The clinical presentation of HS varies depending on the site of involvement – most commonly affecting the intestinal tract, skin and soft tissues. In the largest series of HS, consisting of 18 cases [4], the three paediatric cases presented with multiple, isolated skin lesions, multiple lymph node involvement and disseminated disease, respectively. Among adults, sites of involvement can be diverse and have been reported in the thyroid gland, gastrointestinal tract, kidney, spleen, testes and CNS [4,14]. The median age at presentation was 46 years.

Disease course and prognosis
HS is usually aggressive. Among the 12 patients with available follow-up, 6 had no response to treatment and died of progressive disease; 3 of the 5 patients who went into remission experienced relapse within 3–5 years; only one survived but with a chemoresistant tumour [4]. Due to the rarity of the disease, prognostic factors remain unclear. However, sites of involvement, localised disease and tumour size may impact prognosis, with small, localised, low-grade tumours that are amenable to surgical resection having better outcomes [15]. For cases of HS arising with/after lymphoid malignancies, the prognosis is usually poor, with three of four patients dying despite therapy in a review [6]. Cases are being described, however, in which a targetable mutation is found in the HS allowing the use of targeted therapy with an improved prognosis.

Management
HS is a rare but highly aggressive disease. It generally shows poor response to treatment consisting of a combination of surgery, chemotherapy and radiotherapy. Chemotherapy is usually derived from non-Hodgkin lymphoma protocols such as ICE (ifosfamide/carboplatin/etoposide) or CHOP (cyclophosphamide/doxorubicin/vincristine/prednisolone) regimens, while surgery and radiotherapy are reserved for localised disease [16]. Optimal therapy in the refractory or relapsed setting is unknown. Single case reports have suggested efficacy for high-dose chemotherapy and autologous/allogeneic stem cell transplantation [17]. The anti-CD52 antibody alemtuzumab was successful in a refractory HS patient [18] and prolonged use of thalidomide appears to have been effective in four patients who did not respond to multiple other therapies [19,20]. Recent identification of druggable targets in four cases of HS with an expression of platelet-derived growth factor

receptor, vascular endothelial growth factor receptor and epidermal growth factor receptor [21], and a few cases of *BRAF* V600E [13,22], suggest that novel targeted therapies will improve the outlook for these patients in the future.

Key references

The full list of references can be found in the online version at https://www.wiley.com/rooksdermatology10e

Introduction
1 Emile JF, Abla O, Fraitag S et al. Revised classification of histiocytoses and neoplasms of the macrophage-dendritic cell lineages. *Blood* 2016;127:2672–81.

Langerhans cell histiocytosis
21 Chakraborty R, Burke TM, Hampton OA et al. Alternative genetic mechanisms of BRAF activation in Langerhans cell histiocytosis. *Blood* 2016;128:2533–7.
33 Gadner H, Minkov M, Grois N et al. Therapy prolongation improves outcome in multisystem Langerhans cell histiocytosis. *Blood* 2013;121:5006–14.
41 Gadner H, Grois N, Potschger U et al. Improved outcome in multisystem Langerhans cell histiocytosis is associated with therapy intensification. *Blood* 2008;111:2556–62.
54 Diamond EL, Subbiah V, Lockhart AC et al. Vemurafenib for BRAF V600-mutant Erdheim-Chester disease and Langerhans cell histiocytosis: analysis of data from the histology-independent, phase 2, open-label VE-BASKET study. *Bone Marrow Transplant* 2018;4:384–8.

Haemophagocytic lymphohistiocytosis
28 Locatelli F, Jordan MB, Allen C et al. Emapalumab in children with primary hemophagocytic lymphohistiocytosis. *N Engl J Med* 2020;382:1811–22.
33 Das R, Guan P, Sprague L et al. Janus kinase inhibition lessens inflammation and ameliorates disease in murine models of hemophagocytic lymphohistiocytosis. *Blood* 2016;127:1666–75.

Juvenile xanthogranuloma
14 Durham BH, Lopez Rodrigo E, Picarsic J et al. Activating mutations in CSF1R and additional receptor tyrosine kinases in histiocytic neoplasms. *Nat Med* 2019;25:1839–42.

Erdheim–Chester disease
3 Goyal G, Heaney ML, Collin M et al. Erdheim-Chester disease: consensus recommendations for evaluation, diagnosis, and treatment in the molecular era. *Blood* 2020;135:1929–45.

Sinus histiocytosis with massive lymphadenopathy
1 Abla O, Jacobsen E, Picarsic J et al. Consensus recommendations for the diagnosis and clinical management of Rosai-Dorfman-Destombes disease. *Blood* 2018;131:2877–90.

CHAPTER 136

Soft-tissue Tumours and Tumour-like Conditions

Eduardo Calonje[1] *and Zlatko Marušić*[2]

[1] St John's Institute of Dermatology, Guy's and St Thomas' NHS Foundation Trust, London, UK
[2] Clinical Department of Pathology and Cytology, University Hospital Center Zagreb, Zagreb, Croatia

Introduction and general description, 136.2

FIBROUS AND MYOFIBROBLASTIC TUMOURS, 136.2
Fibrous papule of the face, 136.2
Storiform collagenoma, 136.3
Pleomorphic fibroma, 136.4
Acquired digital fibrokeratoma, 136.4
EWSR1-SMAD3-rearranged fibroblastic tumour, 136.4
Nodular fasciitis, 136.5
Fibro-osseous pseudotumour of the digits, 136.6
Ischaemic fasciitis, 136.6
Fibrous hamartoma of infancy, 136.6
Calcifying fibrous tumour/pseudotumour, 136.7
Calcifying aponeurotic fibroma, 136.7
Dermatomyofibroma, 136.8
Plaque-like CD34-positive dermal fibroma, 136.8
Angiomyofibroblastoma, 136.9
Cellular angiofibroma, 136.9
Elastofibroma, 136.10
Inclusion body (digital) fibromatosis, 136.10
Fibroma of tendon sheath, 136.11
Desmoplastic fibroblastoma, 136.11
Nuchal-type fibroma, 136.12
Palmar and plantar fibromatosis (superficial fibromatoses), 136.12
Penile fibromatosis, 136.13
Lipofibromatosis, 136.13
Dermatofibrosarcoma protuberans, 136.14
Giant cell fibroblastoma, 136.15
CD34-positive superficial fibroblastic tumour, 136.16
Myxoinflammatory fibroblastic sarcoma, 136.17
Undifferentiated sarcoma, 136.17
Myxofibrosarcoma, 136.18
Low-grade fibromyxoid sarcoma, 136.18

FIBROHISTIOCYTIC TUMOURS, 136.19
Tenosynovial giant cell tumour, 136.19
Fibrous histiocytoma (dermatofibroma), 136.19
Plexiform fibrohistiocytic tumour, 136.22

Atypical fibroxanthoma/pleomorphic dermal sarcoma, 136.22

VASCULAR TUMOURS, 136.23
REACTIVE VASCULAR LESIONS, 136.23
Intravascular papillary endothelial hyperplasia, 136.23
Reactive angioendotheliomatosis, 136.24
Glomeruloid haemangioma, 136.25
BENIGN VASCULAR TUMOURS, 136.25
Papillary haemangioma, 136.25
Lobular capillary haemangioma (pyogenic granuloma), 136.25
Cirsoid aneurysm, 136.27
Epithelioid haemangioma, 136.27
Cutaneous epithelioid angiomatous nodule, 136.28
Acquired elastotic haemangioma, 136.29
Hobnail haemangioma, 136.29
Microvenular haemangioma, 136.30
Sinusoidal haemangioma, 136.30
Spindle cell haemangioma, 136.31
Symplastic haemangioma, 136.31
Poikilodermatous plaque-like haemangioma, 136.32
VASCULAR TUMOURS OF INTERMEDIATE MALIGNANCY, 136.32
Retiform haemangioendothelioma, 136.32
Papillary intralymphatic angioendothelioma, 136.33
Composite haemangioendothelioma, 136.33
Pseudomyogenic haemangioendothelioma, 136.34
MALIGNANT VASCULAR TUMOURS, 136.34
Angiosarcoma, 136.34
Epithelioid haemangioendothelioma, 136.36
Epithelioid angiosarcoma, 136.37

LYMPHATIC TUMOURS, 136.37
Acquired progressive lymphangioma, 136.38
Atypical vascular proliferation after radiotherapy, 136.38
Diffuse lymphangiomatosis, 136.39

TUMOURS OF PERIVASCULAR CELLS, 136.39
Infantile myofibromatosis and adult myofibroma, 136.39
Myopericytoma, 136.40
Glomus tumour, 136.41

PERIPHERAL NEUROECTODERMAL TUMOURS, 136.42
Neuromuscular hamartoma, 136.42
Dermal hyperneury, 136.42
Multiple mucosal neuromas, 136.43
Amputation stump neuroma, 136.43
Morton neuroma, 136.43
Solitary circumscribed neuroma, 136.43
Schwannoma, 136.44
Solitary neurofibroma, 136.45
Plexiform neurofibroma, 136.46
Diffuse neurofibroma, 136.46
Perineurioma, 136.47
Dermal nerve sheath myxoma, 136.47
Cellular neurothekeoma, 136.48
Granular cell tumour, 136.48
Meningothelial heterotopias, 136.49
Glial heterotopic nodules, 136.50
Epithelial sheath neuroma, 136.50
Pigmented neuroectodermal tumour of infancy, 136.50
Malignant peripheral nerve sheath tumour, 136.51
Cutaneous Ewing sarcoma, 136.51
CIC-rearranged sarcoma, 136.52

TUMOURS OF MUSCLE, 136.52
Smooth muscle hamartoma, 136.52
Leiomyoma, 136.53
Leiomyosarcoma/atypical smooth muscle tumour (dermal and subcutaneous), 136.54

SKELETAL MUSCLE TUMOURS, 136.55
Rhabdomyomatous congenital hamartoma, 136.55
Rhabdomyoma, 136.55
Cutaneous rhabdomyosarcoma, 136.55

TUMOURS OF FAT CELLS, 136.56	Liposarcoma, 136.59	Perivascular epithelioid cell tumour ('PEComa'), 136.61
Angiolipoma, 136.56	TUMOURS OF UNCERTAIN HISTOGENESIS, 136.59	Deep ('aggressive') angiomyxoma, 136.62
Lipoma, 136.56		Angiomatoid fibrous histiocytoma, 136.62
Hibernoma, 136.57	Acral fibromyxoma, 136.59	Epithelioid sarcoma, 136.63
Lipoblastoma and lipoblastomatosis, 136.57	Superficial angiomyxoma, 136.59	Clear cell sarcoma, 136.64
Spindle cell and pleomorphic lipoma, 136.58	Digital mucous cyst, 136.60	
Atypical lipomatous tumour, 136.58	Dermal non-neural granular cell tumour, 136.60	Key references, 136.64
	Haemosiderotic fibrolipomatous tumour, 136.60	

Introduction and general description

For many clinical dermatologists, soft-tissue tumours arising in the dermis, subcutis or deeper soft tissues are a confusing group of lesions. This is probably partly explained by the facts that there is a very long list of soft-tissue tumours and that a large majority of these can arise in the skin or affect it secondarily. Most of these tumours have no characteristic clinical appearance and present as non-specific, dermal or deep-seated nodules. However, it is necessary for all clinical dermatologists to have an understanding of the range of tumours that may arise in the dermis and also of the likely biological behaviour of individual lesions. Although cutaneous malignant soft-tissue tumours are rare, many benign lesions may be histologically confused with a malignancy. Furthermore, there is a group of soft-tissue tumours that have low-grade malignant potential (intermediate malignancy) with frequent local recurrences but little or no potential for metastatic spread (e.g. dermatofibrosarcoma protuberans (DFSP)). These tumours may cause important morbidity, and their recognition is therefore essential for the planning of treatment and follow-up. Recognising a wide range of soft-tissue tumours is also important as a number of these lesions – particularly when multiple – may be markers of genetic syndromes (e.g. multiple neurofibromas and plexiform neurofibroma in neurofibromatosis type 1).

A broad division can be made between tumours according to the morphological lines of differentiation. The latter include fibroblastic, myofibroblastic, neural, vascular, muscular and adipocytic types. While there is a significant number of tumours with an unclear line of differentiation, as a normal cell of origin cannot be identified (e.g. epithelioid sarcoma), in recent years some progress has been made in this group, namely in the classification of clinically and genetically distinct undifferentiated round cell sarcomas previously considered subtypes of Ewing sarcoma. In a still larger group of tumours, their origin is descriptively ascribed to fibrohistiocytic cells, but with mounting evidence that many of these lesions have fibroblast and/or myofibroblastic differentiation and almost none display true histiocytic differentiation. The list of tumours discussed in this chapter is not all-inclusive. For a full account of the very wide range of these tumours, the reader is referred to the standard major works in this field [1,2]. True histiocytic tumours (Chapter 135), keloids and hypertrophic scars (Chapter 94) and metastatic malignant tumours (Chapter 148) are covered elsewhere.

The most useful biological triage is into totally benign lesions; lesions that may recur locally but never or almost never metastasise; and those that are truly malignant and may metastasise. The great majority of dermal or superficial soft-tissue tumours come into the first two categories, while truly malignant soft-tissue tumours much more frequently arise below the deep fascia. In the case of these rare malignant tumours, there is a relationship between bulk and prognosis, smaller lesions carrying a better prognosis. More superficially situated lesions tend to carry a better prognosis than those deeply situated. Mitoses (particularly abnormal mitotic figures) and necrosis both tend to be associated with malignant rather than benign lesions.

The usual clinical presentation of many of the tumours described in this chapter is of a non-specific lump or nodule. An incisional biopsy should be arranged, and it must be adequately deep so that the nature of the lesion at its deepest margin can be determined. Once the pathologist has established the nature of the tumour, appropriate definitive surgery can be planned. Prior consultation with the pathologist is strongly recommended, as samples may be needed for immunohistochemistry or cytogenetics. All of these may be helpful in arriving at an accurate diagnosis.

FIBROUS AND MYOFIBROBLASTIC TUMOURS

Fibrous papule of the face [1]

Definition and nomenclature
A small facial papule with a distinctive fibrovascular component on histological examination.

Synonyms and inclusions
- Fibrous papule of the nose

Epidemiology
Incidence and prevalence
Lesions are very common [2,3,4].

Age
Most patients are middle-aged adults.

Sex
Both sexes are equally affected.

Pathophysiology
It has been suggested that the condition may be a variant of a melanocytic naevus [2,4], but others disagree [3]. S100 protein is never present in lesional cells, giving further support to the theory of a non-melanocytic proliferation.

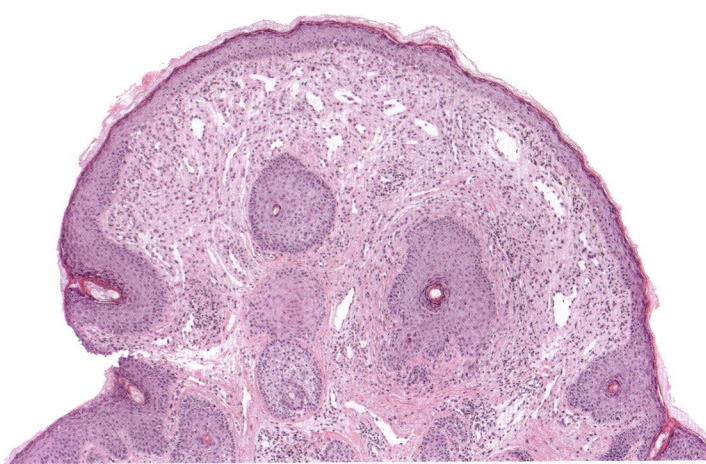

Figure 136.1 Fibrous papule with hyalinised collagen bundles and increased dilated vascular channels.

Pathology [2,3,4]

The epidermis appears normal, although there may be an increased number of clear cells overlying the lesion. In the dermis, there is increased collagen with a hyalinised appearance and scattered, somewhat dilated, vascular channels (Figure 136.1). In the background, there is increased cellularity with mono- and multinucleated cells with a histiocyte-like appearance. In some lesions, epithelioid or clear cells and exceptionally granular cells may predominate [5–8]. There are prominent dilated capillaries.

Clinical features [2,3,4]
History and presentation
The lesions usually occur singly on the nose. Occasionally, they may occur on the forehead, cheeks, chin or neck, and they may rarely be multiple. The papule develops slowly as a dome-shaped, skin-coloured or slightly red or pigmented lesion, which is usually sessile. Most are asymptomatic, but about one-third bleed on minor trauma.

Differential diagnosis
The main clinical consideration is that of an intradermal melanocytic naevus and, less commonly, a basal cell carcinoma.

Management
The lesion is benign, but it may easily be excised usually by shave biopsy for cosmetic reasons.

Storiform collagenoma [1,2]

Definition and nomenclature
Storiform collagenoma is a fibrous hypocellular cutaneous lesion which, when multiple, may be associated with Cowden disease or phosphatase and tensin homologue (PTEN) hamartoma syndrome (multiple hamartoma and neoplasia syndrome; see Chapter 148) [3].

Synonyms and inclusions
- Sclerotic fibroma

Epidemiology
Incidence and prevalence
It is relatively rare.

Age
There is a wide age range with a predilection for adults [2,3].

Sex
No sex predilection.

Pathophysiology
The aetiology of sporadic cases is unknown. In the setting of Cowden syndrome, the development of multiple lesions is associated with loss-of-function mutations in PTEN, leading to hyperactivity of the mTOR pathway.

Pathology
Storiform collagenoma typically consists of a fairly well-circumscribed dermal nodule with prominent hypocellular hyalinised collagen bundles in a storiform pattern (Figure 136.2). Bland spindle-shaped cells are rare. A similar histological pattern may be seen in the late stages of lesions as diverse as pleomorphic fibroma, fibrous histiocytoma (FH) and myofibroma and it has been proposed that it does not represent a distinctive entity but a reaction pattern [4,5].

A more cellular variant containing multinucleated bizarre cells has been described as giant cell collagenoma [6]. The latter is a potential link between pleomorphic fibroma (see later) and sclerotic fibroma as it has been proposed that both entities are part of the same spectrum [7].

Clinical features
History and presentation
Storiform collagenoma usually presents as a small, solitary, asymptomatic papule, with wide anatomical distribution. Segmental presentation has been described in association with the PTEN hamartoma tumour syndrome [8].

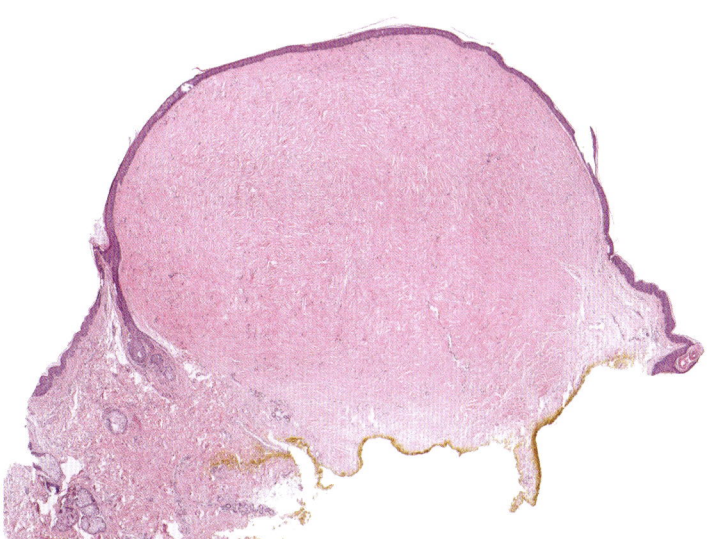

Figure 136.2 Storiform collagenoma. Poorly cellular stroma composed of hyalinised collagen in a characteristic 'plywood' pattern.

Management
Excision is curative.

Pleomorphic fibroma

Definition [1]
Pleomorphic fibroma is a relatively rare lesion with features very similar to those of a fibroepithelial polyp (skin tag), but characterised histologically by bizarre mono- or multinucleated stromal cells.

Epidemiology
Incidence and prevalence
Pleomorphic fibroma is relatively rare.

Age
Mainly in adults.

Sex
No sex predilection.

Pathophysiology
The aetiology is unknown.

Pathology
Normal or mildly acanthotic epidermis surrounds a collagenous and vascular stroma containing scattered bizarre mono- or multi-nucleated cells with hyperchromatic and pleomorphic nuclei. Mitotic figures are rare.

Clinical features
History and presentation
Presentation is in the form of a lesion with clinical findings of a fibroepithelial polyp with wide anatomical distribution with some predilection for perianal skin and the face.

Management
Simple excision is curative, and there is no tendency for local recurrence.

Acquired digital fibrokeratoma [1]

Definition
A benign lesion, possibly a reaction to trauma, which occurs on the fingers and toes [2] (Figure 136.3), although the palms and the soles have occasionally been involved.

Epidemiology
Incidence and prevalence
The incidence is low.

Age
Adults are usually affected.

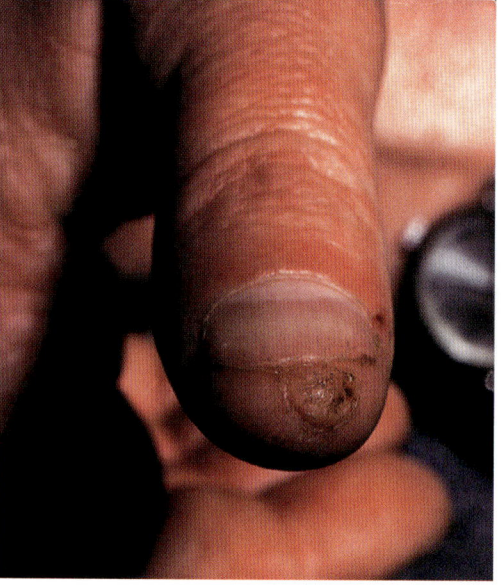

Figure 136.3 Clinical appearance of an acquired digital fibrokeratoma.

Sex
There is no sex predilection.

Pathophysiology
Pathology
The histology shows thick collagen bundles, thin elastic fibres and increased vascularity. Occasionally, there is an obvious increase in fibroblasts, and rarely the collagen bundles may be separated by oedema [3]. The epidermis is relatively normal, but acanthosis and hyperkeratosis may occur.

Clinical features
History and presentation
The lesion usually occurs as a solitary dome-shaped lesion, with a collarette of slightly raised skin at its base. Occasionally, it may be elongated or pedunculated. Giant lesions may occasionally occur [4]. The surface may appear to be slightly warty.

Differential diagnosis
There is a wide clinical differential diagnosis, which includes dermatofibroma, viral wart, supernumerary digit and cutaneous horn. Histologically, the lesion is extremely similar to the Koenen tumour [5], the periungual fibrous lesion that arises from the nail fold in tuberous sclerosis.

Management
Excision is curative.

EWSR1-SMAD3-rearranged fibroblastic tumour [1,2]

This is an emerging benign entity typically presenting as a small and superficial acral nodule, composed of intersecting cellular fascicles of bland spindled fibroblasts with an occasional acellular centre, showing diffuse nuclear ERG expression and negative CD34.

Nodular fasciitis [1,2,3,4,5]

Definition and nomenclature
A rapidly enlarging subcutaneous neoplasm due to a proliferation of myofibroblasts and fibroblasts and that histologically resembles a sarcoma.

Synonyms and inclusions
- Pseudosarcomatous fasciitis
- Pseudosarcomatous fibromatosis

Epidemiology
Incidence and prevalence
It is relatively common. The intravascular and cranial variants of fasciitis are rare [6,7].

Age
It is more common in young adults but can occur at any age. Intravascular fasciitis is more common in young adults and cranial fasciitis tends to occur in children younger than 2 years of age [6,7].

Sex
There is no predilection for either sex except for cranial fasciitis that is more common in males [7].

Pathophysiology
Predisposing factors
There is no clear evidence that trauma initiates the lesions although trauma may play a role in cranial fasciitis [8].

Pathology [1,2,3,4,5]
These lesions may look extremely worrying in view of the high mitotic rate and rapid growth (see later). The tumour is only focally circumscribed and it is composed of bundles of fairly uniform fibroblasts and myofibroblasts with pink cytoplasm, vesicular nuclei and a single small nucleolus. Myxoid change and mucin deposition is often prominent, resulting in a typical tissue culture-like appearance (Figure 136.4). In the background, there are numerous small delicate blood vessels, extravasated red blood cells and scattered mononuclear inflammatory cells. Multinucleated giant cells may be seen, and they resemble osteoclasts. Mitoses are usually numerous, but there are no abnormal forms. Hyalinised collagen bundles are often present and may display a keloidal appearance. At the periphery, compact bundles of fibroblasts and capillaries probe the fascial planes and may infiltrate fat or skeletal muscle. It is not surprising that this histological picture is relatively often confused with that of a malignant tumour. Variants of nodular fasciitis include: those with metaplastic bone (ossifying fasciitis); a variant that involves the periosteum (periosteal fasciitis); a variant that involves the scalp and tends to occur in children (cranial fasciitis) [6]; and a variant within the lumen of a blood vessel (intravascular fasciitis) [7,9]. A rare variant of intradermal nodular fasciitis has also been described [10,11]. Intra-articular location may also be seen [12]. Tumour cells are variably positive for smooth muscle actin and calponin [13] and usually negative for

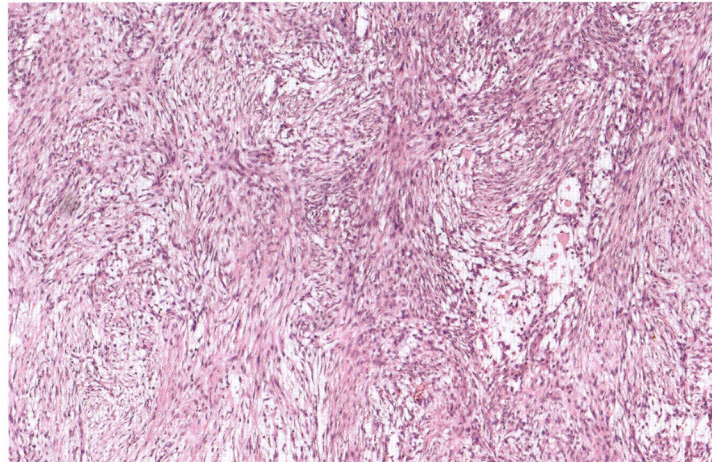

Figure 136.4 Typical tissue culture-like appearance of nodular fasciitis with prominent myxoid background.

smooth muscle markers including desmin and h-caldesmon [14]. The histological diagnosis may be very difficult, especially in small biopsies. Confusion with a sarcoma or with fibromatosis are major pitfalls, with obvious detrimental consequences.

Immunohistochemistry may be useful in the distinction between fibromatosis and nodular fasciitis. The former tends to display nuclear β-catenin positivity, while the latter are usually negative or display cytoplasmic positivity only [15]. However, some fibromatoses, especially those superficially located, are negative for this marker and the diagnosis should be based on careful clinicopathological correlation.

Genetics
The *MYH9-USP6* fusion gene has consistently been identified in lesions confirming the neoplastic nature of this tumour [16]. Lesions like this with a self-limited life and a distinctive clonal genetic translocation have been referred to as transient neoplasms [16]. Subsequently, multiple *USP6* fusion partner genes have been described in nodular fasciitis [17].

Clinical features [1,2,3,4]
History and presentation
The majority of tumours appear as tender rapidly growing masses beneath the skin. The average size is 1–3 cm in diameter. The commonest situation is the upper extremities, particularly the forearm, but the lesion can occur anywhere, including the orbit and the mouth [9]. Lesions on the head and neck often present in children. In nearly half the patients, the tumour has been noticed for only 2 weeks or fewer when they come for advice.

Differential diagnosis
The rapid growth of the lesion may suggest a clinical diagnosis of malignancy.

Disease course and prognosis
Resolution usually follows incomplete surgical removal. Local recurrence is exceptional.

Management
Excision is therefore an adequate treatment.

Fibro-osseous pseudotumour of the digits [1,2,3,4]

Definition
This is a *USP6*-driven myofibroblastic proliferation with bone formation, which occurs exclusively on the digits.

Epidemiology
Incidence and prevalence
It is rare.

Age
It presents predominantly in young adults although presentation can be at any age.

Sex
Males are more often affected than females.

Pathophysiology
Predisposing factors
Trauma appears to be an important factor in the development of the tumour.

Pathology
The tumour is ill-defined and similar to nodular fasciitis, except for the fact that there is formation of osteoid and mature bone. Oedematous stroma, vascular proliferation and bundles of spindle-shaped myofibroblast-like cells are seen intermixed with osteoid and mature bone. Mitotic figures are found and their number depends on the age of the lesion.

Genetics
COL1A1-USP6 gene rearrangement has been identified as a consistent genetic alteration in these lesions [4].

Clinical features
History and presentation
The lesion grows rapidly and it is not attached to bone. The fingers are more commonly affected than the toes.

Disease course and prognosis
Local recurrence is rare.

Management
Simple excision is the treatment of choice.

Ischaemic fasciitis [1–3,4,5]

Definition and nomenclature
Ischaemic fasciitis is a reactive pseudosarcomatous fibroblastic/myofibroblastic proliferation that often occurs as a result of alterations in local circulation and sustained pressure in immobilised patients.

Synonyms and inclusions
- Atypical decubitus fibroplasia

Epidemiology
Incidence and prevalence
Ischaemic fasciitis is relatively rare.

Age
Most patients are elderly, usually between the seventh and ninth decades of life.

Sex
There is a slight predilection for males.

Pathophysiology
Predisposing factors
Persistent ischaemia and trauma to the affected area in immobilised patients is an important factor in the development of the lesion. However, in many cases there is no association with immobility or debilitation [4].

Pathology
The lesion is poorly circumscribed and contains areas of fibrosis, vascular proliferation, necrosis and focal myxoid change. Thrombosed blood vessels with recanalisation and areas of fibrinoid necrosis, focal haemorrhage and mononuclear inflammatory cells are additional features. In the background, there are variable numbers of spindle-shaped myofibroblasts/fibroblasts with vesicular or hyperchromatic nuclei and a prominent nucleolus. Mitotic figures may be seen but are not prominent.

Clinical features
The lesion presents as an asymptomatic subcutaneous mass, predominantly over bony prominences that may extend to deeper soft tissues and to the overlying dermis.

Management
Excision of the lesion is an adequate treatment.

Fibrous hamartoma of infancy [1–5]

Definition
This is a benign, fibroblastic/myofibroblastic, deep dermal and subcutaneous tumour presenting in children and characterised by three distinctive pathological components, as described below.

Epidemiology
Incidence and prevalence
This is a rare tumour.

Age
The majority of cases present in children under the age of 2. A quarter of the cases present at birth.

Sex
Males are more affected than females.

Pathophysiology
Pathology
The tumour is composed of three components:
1 Bundles of interlacing, elongated, bland, wavy spindle-shaped cells in a variable collagenous background.
2 Nests of more immature round cells with focal myxoid change.
3 Mature adipose tissue.

In a number of cases a focal pseudoangiomatous component is seen [6]. A focal resemblance to a neurofibroma may be seen when the first component predominates, but tumour cells are actin positive and S100 negative [7].

In the dermis overlying the tumour, eccrine glands may show secondary changes including hyperplasia, papillary projections and squamous syringometaplasia [8].

Genetics
EGFR exon 20 insertion/duplication mutations have been identified as the driving genetic event in these lesions [9].

Clinical features
History and presentation
Most cases present as an asymptomatic, solitary, skin-coloured plaque/nodule only a few centimetres in diameter. Exceptional tumours are very large and multifocal [10]. Rarely, pigmentary changes and/or hypertrichosis may be seen [11]. The tumour grows rapidly and has a predilection for the axillae, arm and shoulder girdle [1–3]. Rare cases occur on the head and neck [6]. A familial association has not been reported.

Disease course and prognosis
Local recurrence is exceptional.

Management
Simple excision is the treatment of choice [5]; recurrences are exceptional.

Calcifying fibrous tumour/pseudotumour [1,2,3]

Definition
This is a rare, benign, hypocellular tumour characterised by dense collagen bundles, areas of calcification and a patchy mononuclear cell infiltrate. This lesion has no relation with inflammatory myofibroblastic tumour as was originally suggested [3].

Epidemiology
Incidence and prevalence
This is very rare.

Age
Most lesions occur in children but rare cases may present in young adults.

Sex
There is no sex predilection.

Pathophysiology
Pathology
The tumour typically consists of haphazardly arranged collagen bundles with scattered bland fibroblasts, focal small calcifications and focal aggregates of lymphocytes and plasma cells. Tumour cells are positive for CD34 and may be focally positive for smooth muscle actin and more rarely for desmin [3].

Clinical features
History and presentation
Lesions present as a fairly large subcutaneous or deeper asymptomatic mass with a wide anatomical distribution. Cases may also occur in internal organs [3].

Disease course and prognosis
Local recurrence is rare.

Management
The treatment of choice is simple excision.

Calcifying aponeurotic fibroma [1,2,3,4,5]

Definition
This is a rare fibroblastic tumour characterised by a nodular proliferation of bland spindle-shaped cells surrounding nodules at different stages of calcification. Cartilage and, less commonly, bone formation may be seen.

Epidemiology
Incidence and prevalence
Tumours are very rare.

Age
Most cases present in children.

Sex
There is no sex predilection.

Pathophysiology
Pathology
The growth pattern is multinodular. Tumour cells are elongated, with scanty pink cytoplasm, vesicular nuclei and very rare mitotic figures. Tumour nodules frequently contain areas of calcification, which are surrounded by tumour cells in a pattern reminiscent of palisading.

Genetics
The *FN1-EGF* fusion is the main driver mutation in calcifying aponeurotic fibroma.

Clinical features
History and presentation
Lesions have a predilection for the hands and, less commonly, the feet. Occurrence at other sites is rare but tumours may present in

places as diverse as the knee, back and thigh [2,3]. Tumours are small, slowly growing and usually asymptomatic. Multiple lesions are exceptional [4].

Disease course and prognosis
Local recurrence is observed in 50% of cases but malignant transformation is exceptional [5].

Management
Simple excision is the treatment of choice.

Dermatomyofibroma

Definition and nomenclature [1–4]
Dermatomyofibroma presents as a benign, dermal and superficial subcutaneous myofibroblastic proliferation microscopically mimicking a fibromatosis. The tumour, however, has no potential for local recurrence and lacks an infiltrative growth pattern.

Synonyms and inclusions
- Dermal plaque-like fibromatosis

Epidemiology
Incidence and prevalence
Dermatomyofibroma is relatively rare.

Age
Most patients are young adults with children only exceptionally affected [5–7].

Sex
There is predilection for females.

Pathophysiology
Pathology
Low-power examination reveals a plaque-like proliferation of fascicles of myofibroblast-like cells with an almost parallel orientation to the epidermis. Tumour cells are bland and mitotic figures are very rare. The tumour does not destroy adnexal structures but may extend focally into the subcutaneous tissue. Rare cases with haemorrhage may mimic plaque-stage Kaposi sarcoma (Chapter 138) [8]. The latter, however, is always positive for human herpes virus 8 (HHV8). Tumour cells are variably positive for smooth muscle actin and calponin. The latter two markers, however, may be negative or minimally positive in some cases. CD34 is focally positive in around 20% of cases [7].

Clinical features
History and presentation
Dermatomyofibroma presents as a solitary, asymptomatic, skin-coloured or hypopigmented plaque measuring less than 4 cm in diameter. Multiple lesions are rarely seen and an exceptional case has presented with a linear pattern [9].

Disease course and prognosis
Local recurrence is almost never seen.

Management
Simple excision is curative.

Plaque-like CD34-positive dermal fibroma [1,2,3]

Definition and nomenclature
This is a very rare lesion characterised by a superficial dermal plaque-like proliferation of fibroblasts and not of dermal dendrocytes as originally reported [1].

Synonyms and inclusions
- Medallion-like dermal dendrocytic hamartoma

Epidemiology
Incidence and prevalence
Tumours are very rare.

Age
The age range is wide. Earlier reports were mainly in children but tumours also present in adults. Rare lesions are congenital.

Sex
Females are more frequently affected than males.

Pathophysiology
Pathology
The epidermis appears unremarkable or slightly flattened and in the dermis there is a fairly monotonous proliferation of spindle-shaped bland cells in a plaque-like distribution. These cells are positive for CD34 and negative for S100. Only a few scattered cells in the background are positive for factor XIIIa (FXIIIa). The appearance may resemble early DFSP and distinction between the two conditions is very important. Plaque-like CD34-positive dermal fibroma hardly ever extends only focally into the subcutis and does not do it in a lace-like pattern. Furthermore, this tumour does not show the t17;22 translocation typically found in DFSP [3].

Clinical features
History and presentation
There is predilection for the trunk and limbs. Lesions are sometimes round or oval and have an atrophic appearance and a yellow-red colour. More often, however, clinical features are non-distinctive.

Disease course and prognosis
Lesions are benign.

Management
Simple excision is the treatment of choice.

Angiomyofibroblastoma [1,2–4]

Definition
Angiomyofibroblastoma is a distinctive benign neoplasia that occurs almost always in the pelvis and perineum, particularly affecting the vulva. There is some overlap with another tumour that presents in the pelvis and perineum (cellular angiofibroma, see later) and also with aggressive angiomyxoma [5].

Epidemiology
Incidence and prevalence
It is rare.

Age
Young to middle-aged females and very rarely in elderly females.

Sex
Predominantly in females. Exceptional cases in males.

Pathophysiology
Pathology
Lesions are well circumscribed and consist of a mixture of round and spindle-shaped bland cells in a myxoid or oedematous stroma with numerous small dilated blood vessels. There is a tendency for tumour cells to surround the vascular channels. Mitotic activity is not usually present. In a number of cases, there are collections of mature adipocytes [4].

Cytological atypia secondary to degeneration is sometimes seen. Tumour cells are positive for desmin and for oestrogen and progesterone receptors. They are only focally positive for smooth muscle actin and muscle-specific actin. Some tumours are variably positive for CD34.

Clinical features
History and presentation
Tumours present mainly in the vulva and in males usually affect the scrotum. Lesions are subcutaneous, asymptomatic and measure less than 5 cm in diameter. Occasional larger pedunculated lesions have been reported [6].

Disease course and prognosis
Tumours are benign with no tendency for local recurrence. Only one malignant tumour has been reported [7].

Management
The treatment is simple excision.

Cellular angiofibroma [1–4]

Definition and nomenclature
Cellular angiofibroma is a distinctive benign neoplasm that occurs almost exclusively in the vulva and less commonly in the scrotum and inguinal soft tissues of men. Some cases overlap histologically with angiomyofibroblastoma and a relationship with spindle cell lipoma and mammary-type myofibroblastoma has been suggested [2]. The latter is based on histological overlap and also on the presence of a distinctive cytogenetic abnormality (see later).

> **Synonyms and inclusions**
> - Male angiomyofibroblastoma-like tumour

Epidemiology
Incidence and prevalence
It is relatively rare.

Age
Predominantly in young adults.

Sex
Most tumours occur in females.

Pathophysiology
Pathology
Tumours are sharply circumscribed but not encapsulated and are characterised by short, usually bland, spindle-shaped cells with scanty ill-defined pale pink cytoplasm. These cells are arranged in bundles and the degree of cellularity varies. In the background, there are thin collagen bundles and numerous small to medium-sized blood vessels. Mitotic figures are rare and cytological atypia may be occasionally seen in some cases. Scattered mononuclear inflammatory cells, mainly lymphocytes, and degenerative changes are often identified. The latter consist of haemorrhage, thrombosis, hyalinisation and haemosiderin deposition. In myxoid areas, mast cells are present and many tumours contain variable numbers of mature adipocytes. The most consistent immunohistochemical finding is the presence of diffuse positivity for CD34 in many cases. Muscular markers including actin and desmin tend to be negative but positivity has been reported in male tumours. In a few cases, there is focal positivity for oestrogen and progesterone receptors.

Genetics
A monoallelic deletion of RB1 located on chromosome 13q14 is often found [5].

Clinical features
History and presentation
Tumours presenting as a small, well-circumscribed, asymptomatic, subcutaneous nodule. In males, lesions tend to be larger and may be related to a hydrocoele or a hernia [2].

Disease course and prognosis
Lesions are benign with little or no tendency for local recurrence. Histologically, exceptional tumours with atypia or sarcomatous transformation have been described but they have not behaved in an aggressive manner, although follow-up was limited [5,6].

Management
Simple excision is the treatment of choice.

Elastofibroma [1,2,3]

Definition and nomenclature
Elastofibroma is a reactive, probably degenerative, process of the elastic fibres of deep soft tissues that occurs almost exclusively around the shoulder. Although the lesion is regarded as degenerative, the finding of chromosomal alterations (see later), and of clonality in some cases, has led to the suggestion that it represents a neoplastic process [4].

Synonyms and inclusions
- Elastofibroma dorsi

Epidemiology
Incidence and prevalence
Unknown. However, computed tomography (CT) scans detected incidental lesions in 2% of persons more than 60 years of age and in 16% of adult autopsies in persons older than 55 [5,6].

Age
Most lesions occur in old-aged individuals.

Sex
No sex predilection.

Pathophysiology
Predisposing factors
Although elastofibroma has been regarded as the result of a degenerative process involving elastic fibres and in association with trauma, the presence of cytogenetic abnormalities in some tumours suggest that it is more likely to be neoplastic (see later).

Genetics
Comparative genomic hybridisation in a series of elastofibromas has found chromosomal alterations in a percentage of cases. The most common alteration consists of gains at chromosome Xq12-q22 [7].

Pathology
The mass is poorly circumscribed, and the appearances are characteristic. Abundant hypocellular hyalinised collagen containing numerous large thick eosinophilic elastic fibres is the most distinctive feature. Sometimes the fibres are beaded and fragmented. Staining for elastic tissue nicely highlights the changes.

Clinical features
History and presentation
It presents as an asymptomatic slowly growing mass on the posterior upper trunk. Pain is very rare. Lesions in other locations, including internal organs, are exceptional. Multiple lesions are usually bilateral and may be symmetrical [8].

Disease course and prognosis
There is no tendency for local recurrence.

Management
Simple excision is the treatment of choice.

Inclusion body (digital) fibromatosis [1–3,4]

Definition and nomenclature
Inclusion body fibromatosis is a fibro/myofibroblastic proliferation that almost only occurs on the fingers and toes. It is characterised by bright, round, intracytoplasmic, eosinophilic inclusions.

Synonyms and inclusions
- Infantile digital fibromatosis
- Recurring digital fibrous tumour of childhood

Epidemiology
Incidence and prevalence
Lesions are rare, representing 2% of fibroblastic tumours in childhood [5].

Age
Most lesions present either at birth or during the first year of life. Presentation in adults is exceptional [6].

Sex
Males and females are equally affected.

Pathophysiology
Pathology
Monomorphic bundles of bland myofibroblast-like cells are seen in the dermis (Figure 136.5a) and often the subcutis. Tumour cells have vesicular nuclei, an inconspicuous nucleolus and pink cytoplasm. Some mitotic figures may be seen. A distinctive feature is the presence of variable numbers of small round eosinophilic intracytoplasmic inclusions in tumour cells (Figure 136.5b). These are periodic acid–Schiff (PAS) negative, but stain red with Masson trichrome. They also stain for smooth muscle actin.

Clinical features
History and presentation
Lesions present as small multiple nodules with a predilection for the dorsal or dorsolateral aspect of the third, fourth and fifth digits. Involvement of the first digits (thumb and hallux) does not occur. Simultaneous involvement of fingers and toes is very rare. New lesions often develop over a long period of time. Only rare cases have been described at other sites including the leg, arm and breast [4,7].

Disease course and prognosis
Spontaneous regression is sometimes seen [8]. Local recurrence may be seen in up to 25% of cases. Aggressive behaviour has not been described.

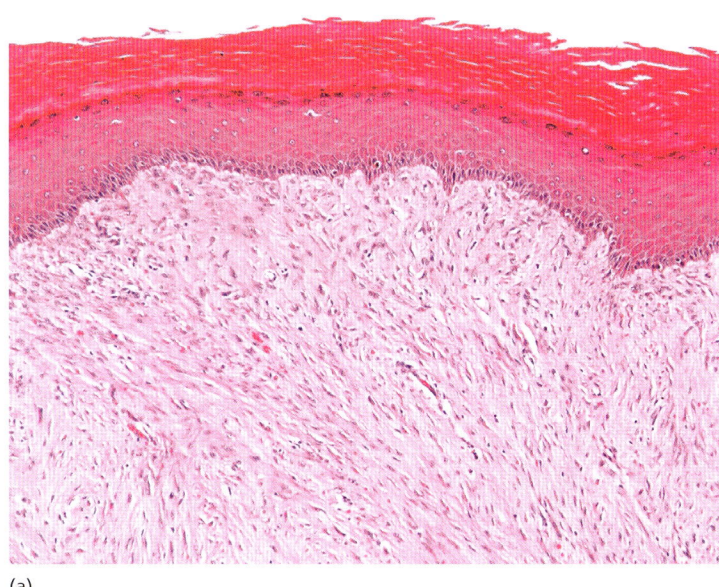
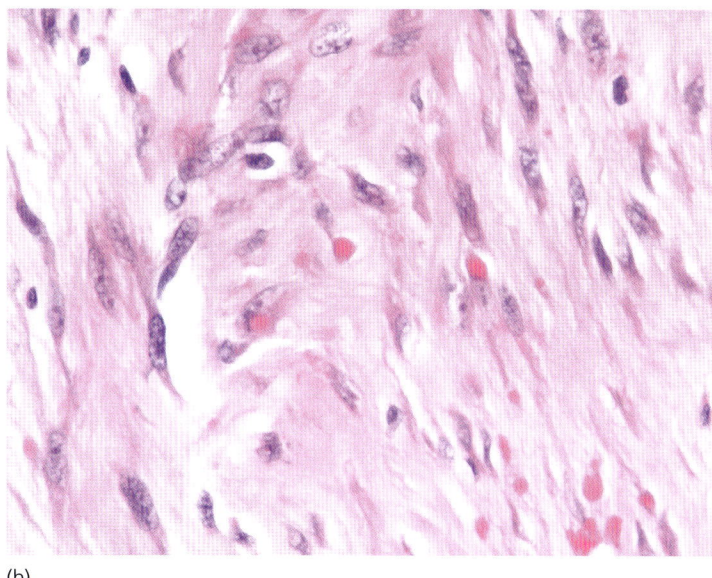

Figure 136.5 (a) Bundles of bland myofibroblast-like cells in the dermis in a case of inclusion body fibromatosis. (b) Numerous typical eosinophilic intracytoplasmic eosinophilic inclusions.

Management
Simple excision may be required for lesions that interfere with function, but simple observation of histologically confirmed lesions may be all that is necessary.

Fibroma of tendon sheath [1,2]

Definition and nomenclature
This is a distinctive well-circumscribed fibroblastic tumour, presenting almost exclusively on the distal extremities.

Synonyms and inclusions
- Tenosynovial fibroma

Epidemiology
Incidence and prevalence
Tumours are rare.

Age
Fibroma of tendon sheath presents mainly in young to middle-aged adults and exceptionally in children.

Sex
Males and females are equally affected.

Pathophysiology
Pathology [1,2,3]
The neoplasm is multilobular and well circumscribed, and consists of cellular or poorly cellular areas on a background of variably hyalinised stroma. Stromal clefting is usually prominent. Tumour cells are spindle shaped, with scanty cytoplasm and vesicular nuclei. Cytological atypia tend to be absent, and the mitotic count is low. Degenerative changes are seen in some cases and consist of cystic degeneration, myxoid change and bony metaplasia. Rare giant cells are sometimes identified.

Genetics
USP6 translocations with various partner genes have been demonstrated in a large proportion of tendon sheath fibromas (cellular variant) [4].

Clinical features [1,2,3]
History and presentation
It is a small slowly growing asymptomatic tumour, with a marked predilection for the distal upper limb, particularly the hand and fingers (1st, 2nd and 3rd). Rare lesions may present with carpal tunnel syndrome [5]. Tumours on the foot are much less common.

Disease course and prognosis
About 20% of cases recur locally but the growth is not destructive.

Management
Simple excision is the treatment of choice.

Desmoplastic fibroblastoma [1,2]

Definition and nomenclature
Desmoplastic fibroblastoma represents a distinctive subcutaneous fibroblastic tumour consisting of a prominent collagenous stroma.

Synonyms and inclusions
- Collagenous fibroma

Epidemiology

Incidence and prevalence
Tumours are relatively common.

Age
Presentation is in middle-aged to old adults.

Sex
Males are twice as frequently affected as females.

Pathophysiology

Pathology
This is a well-circumscribed tumour composed of bland elongated or stellate cells, with a background collagenous stroma and focal myxoid change. Mitotic figures are very rare.

Genetics
A translocation t(2;11)(q31;q12) is characteristically found in this tumour [3]. The rearrangement of the 11q12 chromosome results in the deregulated expression of FOSL1 [3,4]. Desmoplastic fibroblastomas show strong and diffuse FOSL1 nuclear immunoreactivity [5].

Clinical features

History and presentation
Lesions present as an asymptomatic nodule, a few centimetres in diameter, at any body site with a predilection for the back and limbs.

Disease course and prognosis
There is no tendency for local recurrence.

Management
Simple excision is the treatment of choice.

Nuchal-type fibroma [1,2]

Definition and nomenclature
Nuchal fibroma is a dermal or subcutaneous tumour consisting of hypocellular dense collagen.

Synonyms and inclusions
- Collagenosis nuchae

Epidemiology

Incidence and prevalence
Occurrence is rare.

Age
Most cases present in adults between the third and fifth decades of life.

Sex
Males are much more commonly affected than females.

Pathophysiology

Predisposing factors
Patients often have type 2 diabetes.

Pathology
Dense aggregates of collagen with very few cells and entrapment of adipose tissue. Inflammation is minimal and consists of a few scattered lymphocytes. In some cases, focal proliferation of nerves is seen mimicking a traumatic neuroma.

Clinical features

History and presentation
The great majority of cases present by far on the nape of the neck. Tumours can also present on the upper back, limbs and face [3]. Coexistence with scleroedema is possible, probably reflecting the association with diabetes, and lesions identical to nuchal fibroma are recognised to occur in Gardner syndrome (Chapter 78) and are known as Gardner-associated fibromas [3,4]. The latter may be multiple, present in various locations and may recur. These lesions may be the first clue as to the existence of Gardner syndrome.

Disease course and prognosis
Local recurrence is common but lesions do not behave aggressively.

Management
Simple excision is the treatment of choice.

Palmar and plantar fibromatosis (superficial fibromatoses) [1,2]

Definition and nomenclature
Palmar and plantar fibromatoses are superficial neoplastic proliferations of fibroblasts and myofibroblasts that have a tendency for local recurrence, but do not metastasise.

Synonyms and inclusions

Plantar fibromatosis
- Ledderhose disease

Palmar fibromatosis
- Dupuytren disease
- Dupuytren contracture

Epidemiology

Incidence and prevalence
Palmar fibromatosis is fairly common and more common than plantar fibromatosis. The incidence of both conditions, but particularly the former, increases with age.

Age
Both conditions affect middle-aged to elderly patients and are uncommon in younger individuals. However, children may rarely be affected, particularly by plantar fibromatosis [3].

Sex
Both lesions are more common in men, but the sex difference is more marked in palmar lesions.

Ethnicity
Affected patients are mainly of northern European origin; non-whites are rarely affected.

Pathophysiology
Predisposing factors
Genetic predisposition, as well as trauma, is thought to play an important role in the pathogenesis of these conditions. Associations with diabetes, alcoholic liver disease and epilepsy have also been described.

Pathology
Early lesions are fairly cellular and consist of bundles of bland fibroblasts with some collagen deposition. The latter increases considerably in older lesions. Interestingly, although superficial fibromatoses are very similar histologically to deep fibromatosis (abdominal, extra-abdominal and mesenteric fibromatosis), the behaviour of superficial fibromatosis is not usually aggressive. This may be due to the fact that deep fibromatosis often display mutations of the APC gene or somatic mutations of the gene encoding β-catenin, while these mutations are absent in superficial fibromatosis. Intriguingly however, although deep fibromatoses often display nuclear expression of β-catenin, this is also seen in a smaller percentage of superficial fibromatoses without gene mutations [4].

Coexistence between the two variants of fibromatoses and desmoid tumours, penile fibromatosis (Peyronie disease) and knuckle pads, may be seen.

Clinical features
History and presentation
Palmar fibromatosis presents as indurated nodules or as an ill-defined area of thickening, bilateral in about 50% of cases that may result in contracture. Plantar fibromatosis usually consists of a single nodule.

Disease course and prognosis
Functional limitation is common. Lesions are prone to local recurrence.

Management
Complete excision is desirable. Another, non-surgical option is treatment with *Clostridium histolyticum* injectable collagenase [5].

Penile fibromatosis [1,2,3]

Definition and nomenclature
Although usually regarded as a variant of superficial fibromatosis, it is more likely that this disease represents a reactive fibrotic disorder of unknown aetiology.

Synonyms and inclusions
- Peyronie disease

Epidemiology
Incidence and prevalence
The condition is rare.

Age
Most patients are middle-aged.

Pathophysiology
Predisposing factors
There is an association with type 2 diabetes.

Pathology
In early lesions, there is a patchy chronic mononuclear inflammatory cell infiltrate and focal vasculitic changes. These changes lead to dense bands of hyalinised collagen in late stages.

Clinical features
History and presentation
It presents as a solitary nodule or multiple nodules close to the corpus cavernosum on the dorsal surface of the shaft and in most the lesion is small. Pain and curvature of the penis on erection are frequent complaints. The presence of diabetes increases the severity of the disease [4].

Disease course and prognosis
The condition results in penile deformity and sexual dysfunction.

Management
Surgery is the treatment of choice but in recent years less invasive therapies have been attempted. The latter include intralesional injections of interferon α-2b or of *Clostridium histolyticum* collagenase [5].

Lipofibromatosis [1]

Definition and nomenclature
Lipofibromatosis is a locally aggressive childhood tumour composed of variable amounts of mature adipose and fibroblastic elements.

Synonyms and inclusions
- Infantile/juvenile fibromatosis variant (non-desmoid type)

Epidemiology
Incidence and prevalence
The condition is very rare.

Age
Tumours occur in infants and children; the majority of cases presenting in the first decade of life.

Sex
There is male predominance (around 60% of cases).

Pathophysiology
Pathology
Tumours are infiltrative and consist of lobules of mature adipose tissue intermixed with bundles of fibroblast-like cells with no cytological atypia and low mitotic activity. By immunohistochemistry, tumour cells are focally positive for S100 protein, CD34, bcl-2, actin, epithelial membrane antigen (EMA) and CD99. The lesion closely resembles a fibrous hamartoma of infancy but has more prominent adipose tissue and lacks the third cellular component seen in the latter, which consists of round primitive-looking cells in a myxoid background.

Genetics
Many of the cases show fusions involving various tyrosine kinase receptor genes [2].

Clinical features
History and presentation
Some tumours are congenital. There is a male predominance. The classical presentation is of a slowly growing ill-defined mass. There is a predilection for the hands and feet, but other sites in the limbs, and less commonly on the trunk, may be affected. The rate of local recurrence is high.

Disease course and prognosis
The tumour is locally aggressive with no metastatic potential. There is high tendency for local recurrence.

Management
Complete excision (with a free margin) is desirable, as the lesions are infiltrative.

Dermatofibrosarcoma protuberans [1–3]

Definition
DFSP is a locally invasive, low grade malignant tumour arising in the dermis and showing fibroblastic differentiation.

Epidemiology [1–3]
Incidence and prevalence
DFSP is uncommon but represents one of the most common dermal sarcomas. The incidence in the USA has been estimated as 4.2 cases per million [4].

Age
Tumours more commonly develop during the third and fifth decades of life. However, presentation during childhood and late life is not particularly rare [5–7]. Congenital cases have been described [7,8].

Sex
There is a slight female predilection.

Ethnicity
It is more common in black than in white patients [4].

Pathophysiology
Predisposing factors
Some cases develop at the site of previous trauma and reports have included a burn scar [9] and the site of vaccination. Exceptional cases have been associated with previous radiotherapy to the area [10]. There is an association between DFSP and children with adenosine deaminase deficient severe combined immunodeficiency [11]. Patients affected by the latter have a higher incidence of tumours presenting at early age and often multicentric.

Pathology [1–3]
The tumour is usually a solitary multinodular mass. The dermis and subcutaneous tissue are replaced by bundles of uniform spindle-shaped cells with little cytoplasm and elongated hyperchromatic, but not pleomorphic, nuclei. Usually there is little mitotic activity. Deeper involvement may be seen in some cases. Laterally, the tumour cells infiltrate widely between collagen bundles of the deeper dermis and blend into the normal dermis, forming quite definite bands, which interweave or radiate like the spokes of a wheel; this is described as a 'storiform' pattern (Figure 136.6). The interstitial tissue contains collagen fibres, except in the most cellular parts of the tumour. The subcutaneous tissue is extensively infiltrated and replaced in a typical lace-like pattern. Myxoid change may be focal or, rarely, prominent; in the latter setting, the histological diagnosis is difficult [12,13]. Some tumours are colonised by scattered deeply pigmented melanocytes, a variant known as pigmented DFSP (Bednar tumour) [14,15]. A further variant consists of myoid nodules and is thought to represent myofibroblastic differentiation [16]. Rare cases show focal granular cell change.

Fibrosarcomatous DFSP [17,**18**,19,20] is an important variant of this tumour, which is recognised by the focal presence of areas with long sweeping fascicles of tumour cells intersecting at acute angles in a typical 'herring-bone' pattern, almost identical to that seen in fibrosarcoma. In these areas, mitoses are increased and there is more nuclear hyperchromatism. P53 expression is increased in fibrosarcomatous areas [20]. Identification of the presence of

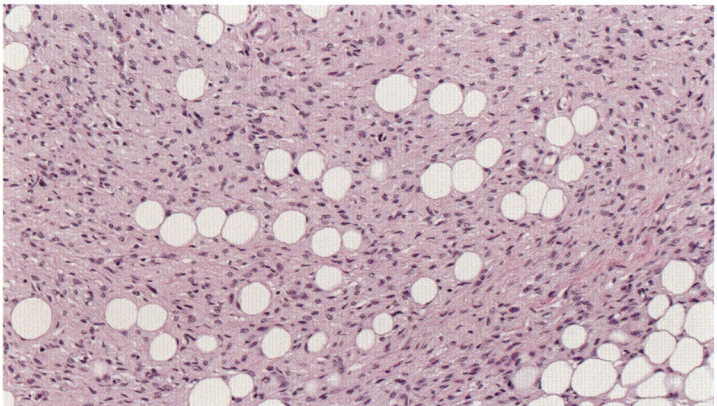

Figure 136.6 Pathological appearance of dermatofibrosarcoma protuberans showing the diffuse distribution of fairly uniform, spindle-shaped tumour cells with characteristic 'honeycomb' fat infiltration.

this pattern, and its quantity, is very important, as it is related to metastatic potential. Fibrosarcomatous areas are more common in recurrent tumours. Very rare variants of DFSP may show areas of high-grade sarcoma either in the primary tumour or in a recurrence [21]. DFSP may show areas of giant cell fibroblastoma (see later) and either tumour may recur, displaying features of the other tumour [22].

The majority of the lesions are positive on staining with the antibody CD34, although this is not specific for DFSP [23]. Other markers are usually negative, but in some cases focal positivity for epithelial membrane antigen may be seen. Fibrosarcomatous areas often show decreased staining with CD34 [19].

Genetics
Cytogenetic studies are helpful, as ring chromosomes indicative of a 17;22 translocation are invariably found [22]. However, it is important to highlight that some cases demonstrate a variant ring chromosome with cryptic rearrangements of chromosomes 17 and 22 [24]. This chromosomal translocation involves the collagen type I α1 (*COL1A1*) gene on chromosome 17 and the platelet-derived growth factor B (*PDGFB*) gene on chromosome 22. The abnormal fusion transcripts resulting from this translocation leads to autocrine stimulation of PDGFB and platelet-derived growth factor receptor β (*PDGFRB*) and cell proliferation. The fusion transcript is found in almost all examples of the tumour by polymerase chain reaction (PCR) and fluorescence *in situ* hybridisation (FISH) [23]. The same cytogenetic abnormality is found in giant cell fibroblastoma, confirming that both tumours are part of the same spectrum. The progression of DFSP to fibrosarcomatous DFSP involves activation of Akt-mTOR pathway proteins and PDGFR [25].

Clinical features
History and presentation
The tumour is more often situated on the trunk (up to half of the cases), particularly in the flexural regions, than on the extremities or the head [1,2]. Involvement of the limbs is usually proximal. Presentation on the hands and feet, particularly on the digits, is very rare. It may begin in early adult life with one or more small, firm, painless, flesh-coloured or red dermal nodules (Figure 136.7).

The tumour starts as a plaque, which may occasionally be atrophic [6,26]. Progression is usually very slow and may occur over many years; a significant proportion of tumours only become protuberant after a long period of time [27]. Eventually, nodules develop, coalesce and extend, becoming redder or bluish as they enlarge to form irregular protuberant swellings. At this stage, the base of the lesion is a hard indurated plaque of irregular outline. In the later stages, a proportion of lesions become painful and there may be rapid growth, ulceration and discharge.

Differential diagnosis
In the early stages, it may be impossible to distinguish this tumour from a histiocytoma or a keloid. Some lesions may also be confused with morphoea profunda. The slow progression, deep red or bluish-red colour and the characteristic irregular contour and extended plaque-like base are strongly suggestive of DFSP.

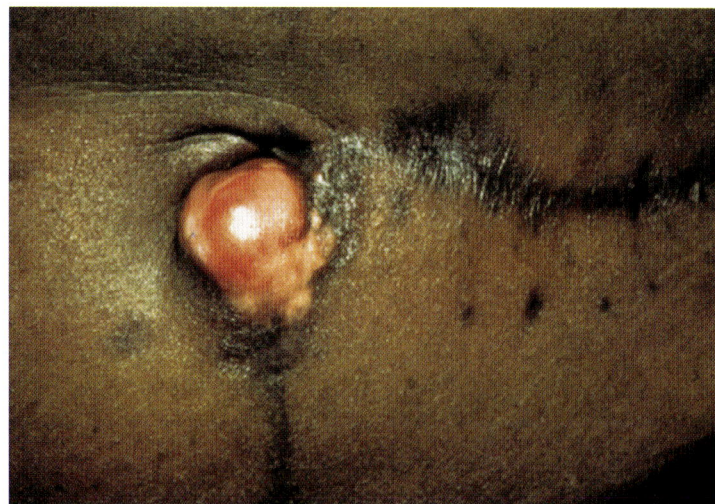

Figure 136.7 Recurrent abdominal dermatofibrosarcoma protuberans.

Disease course and prognosis
Local recurrence of ordinary DFSP is reported to vary from 15% to up to 60% [3,28,29]. The fibrosarcomatous variant has a similar rate of local recurrence but a higher rate of metastatic spread [20,21,30,31,32]. Metastases to lymph nodes and internal organs tend to be extremely rare in pure DFSP [20,33,34] but occur in up to 13% of cases with fibrosarcomatous transformation [20,21,22,31,32].

Management
The tumour should be excised completely, with a generous margin of healthy tissue [35]. The best chance of achieving a complete cure with no recurrence is early detection of small tumours. Local recurrence invariably follows inadequate removal; the clearance necessary to cure the tumour is often underestimated [36]. A margin of between 2 and 4 cm has been recommended [29,37]. Mohs micrographic surgery has been reported as effective in reducing the rate of local recurrence and it has become the recommended standard treatment where available [38,39]. If this type of treatment is used it should be performed using formalin-fixed paraffin-embedded sections rather than frozen sections, and evaluation should be by an individual experienced in interpreting cutaneous neoplasms, ideally a pathologist, dermatopathologist or a dermatologist (the qualifications of medical specialties in histopathological examination vary between different parts of the world). Although Mohs surgery clearly reduces the rate of local recurrences, the latter still occur and sometimes this happens more than 5 years after surgery [40]. Postsurgical radiotherapy has been advocated to reduce the rate of local recurrence [41] but this type of treatment has not been assessed in large series of patients. In recent years, it has been demonstrated that imatinib mesylate, a potent inhibitor of a number of protein kinases including the PDGFR, results in good clinical response in patients with large unresectable or metastatic tumours [42–46].

Giant cell fibroblastoma [1–3,4]

Definition
This is a locally recurrent fibroblastic tumour, closely related to DFSP. It is characterised by spindle-shaped, oval or stellate, mono

or multinucleated cells in a fibromyxoid stroma with irregular pseudovascular spaces lined by tumour cells.

Epidemiology
Incidence and prevalence
Tumours are rare.

Age
Most cases present in children. Rare cases are seen in young adults and only exceptionally in older adults.

Sex
About 60% of patients are male.

Pathophysiology
Pathology
Solid fibromyxoid areas with variable collagen deposition contain stellate and spindle-shaped mono- and multinucleated tumour cells with hyperchromatic nuclei. Dilated irregularly branching pseudovascular spaces are commonly seen scattered throughout the lesion. These spaces are lined by tumour cells, which often appear multinucleated (Figure 136.8). Mitotic figures are exceptional. Aggregates of perivascular lymphocytes in an onion-ring pattern and focal haemorrhage are often seen [4]. Focal areas identical to DFSP may be seen and can occupy a substantial part of the tumour. Excised lesions can recur as a pure giant cell fibroblastoma, as a tumour with focal DFSP, or as pure DFSP [4,5–7]. All types of tumour cells are positive for CD34.

Genetics
Ring chromosomes with sequences of chromosomes 17 and 22, identical to those found in DFSP, have been described in this tumour, confirming their close histogenetic relationship [8,9].

Clinical features [1–3,4]
History and presentation
The large majority of cases present as a subcutaneous ill-defined mass but rare tumours are polypoid. It is rare in young adults and more exceptional in older adults. The trunk, axilla and groin are much more commonly involved than the proximal limbs. Head and neck tumours are rare. Lesions typically measure a few centimetres in diameter and tend to be asymptomatic.

Disease course and prognosis
Recurrence may be seen in about half of the cases, but metastasis has not been reported.

Management
Complete surgical excision with adequate margins is the treatment of choice.

CD34-positive superficial fibroblastic tumour [1,2]

Definition
This is a distinctive low-grade cutaneous/subcutaneous tumour, composed of spindled cells with copious, eosinophilic, glassy or granular cytoplasm and marked nuclear pleomorphism, growing in sheets or fascicles.

> **Synonyms and inclusions**
> - PRDM10-rearranged soft tissue tumour

Epidemiology
Incidence and prevalence
Tumours are rare.

Age
Most patients are middle-aged adults.

Sex
There is a slight male predilection.

Pathophysiology
Pathology
The tumours are relatively circumscribed, but at least partially infiltrative. The cells are spindled to epithelioid, grow in sheets or fascicles and show abundant granular or glassy eosinophilic cytoplasm. Occasional lipidisation of cells may be present. Nuclear pleomorphism is moderate to marked. The nuclei may exhibit bizarre shapes, pseudoinclusions, hyperchromatic nuclei and prominent nucleoli. However, mitotic activity is very low and necrosis is infrequent. All cases show strong, diffuse CD34 positivity, while focal cytokeratin expression is noted in 70% of cases [1].

Genetics
PRDM10 rearrangement has been shown in three cases [2].

Clinical features
History and presentation
The tumour most frequently occurs in the superficial soft tissues of the lower extremities, especially the thigh, with a mean diameter of 4.1 cm.

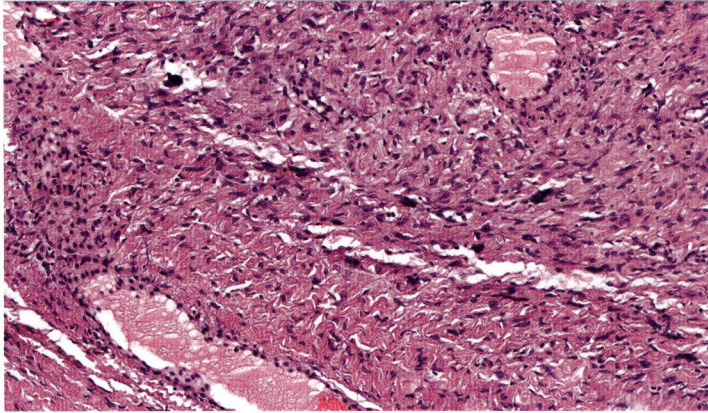

Figure 136.8 Typical pseudovascular spaces focally lined by multinucleated cells in a case of giant cell fibroblastoma.

Disease course and prognosis
There have been no local recurrences reported, and only one regional lymph node metastasis 7 years after an incomplete excision.

Management
The treatment of choice is local excision with free margins.

Myxoinflammatory fibroblastic sarcoma [1–3,4]

Definition and nomenclature
Myxoinflammatory fibroblastic sarcoma is a distinctive, neoplastic process with marked predilection for acral sites, and with histological features closely mimicking an inflammatory process due to the presence of prominent inflammation and virocyte-like inclusions in the nuclei of tumour cells. The latter features were initially thought to indicate an infectious aetiology. A relationship with haemosiderotic fibrolipomatous tumour is likely (see later). Both tumours share a similar translocation (see later). Hybrid tumours or metachronous evolution of the former to myxoinflammatory fibroblastic sarcoma have been documented, with adverse outcomes in some cases [5,6].

Synonyms and inclusions
- Inflammatory myxohyaline tumour of the distal extremities with virocyte or Reed–Sternberg-like cells
- Acral myxoinflammatory fibroblastic sarcoma

Epidemiology
Incidence and prevalence
Tumours are rare.

Age
Most patients are middle-aged adults. Presentation in children [6] and elderly patients is very rare.

Sex
There is a slight female predilection.

Pathophysiology
Pathology
Lesions are lobulated and poorly circumscribed and involve the subcutaneous fat and often extend to the dermis and deeper tissues, sparing bone. Low-power examination is misleading and the initial impression is that of an inflammatory process. Lobules of hyalinised and myxoid tissue containing variable numbers of inflammatory cells are seen. The latter include lymphocytes, histiocytes, neutrophils and less commonly eosinophils and plasma cells. Closer examination reveals variable numbers of neoplastic cells that vary from round to spindle shaped. Some of these cells may be multinucleated. Round cells mimic ganglion cells with nucleoli resembling viral inclusions. Less commonly, vacuolated tumour cells resembling lipoblasts are seen. Mitotic activity is very low. Lesions displaying one or more of the following histological features appear to have a higher rate of local recurrence: areas with complex sarcoma-like vasculature, hypercellular areas and increased mitotic activity or the presence of atypical mitotic figures [4]. Immunohistochemistry shows that tumour cells are variably positive for bcl-1 (94.5%), FXIIIa (89%), CD10 (80%), D2-40 (56-86%), CD34 (50%), keratins (33%), actin (26%), CD68 (27%) and very rarely for desmin, S100 and EMA [4,7].

Genetics
FISH and array comparative genomic hybridisation performed in a substantial number of cases show *BRAF* alterations or the t(1;10) involving *TGFBR3* and *OGA* in around 5% of cases, respectively, while amplification of *VGLL3* on chromosome 3 can be found in approximately 40%. Currently there is no sufficiently robust genetic or immunohistochemical diagnostic signature and the diagnosis rests mainly on clinicopathological features [8].

Clinical features
History and presentation
Characteristically, tumours are longstanding, asymptomatic and slowly growing, multinodular and usually measure no more than 4 cm. The great majority occur on acral sites, particularly the dorsal aspect of the hands and wrists, followed by the feet. However, lesions may rarely present elsewhere on the limbs (the arm, forearm and thigh) [4,6,9,10] and exceptionally elsewhere in the body, including the head and neck [4,5,9]. Most cases are clinically diagnosed as a ganglion cyst or as a giant cell tumour of tendon sheath.

Disease course and prognosis
The rate of local recurrence is high, varying from 11% to 67% in different series [1,2,4]. The absence of clear surgical margins correlates with higher recurrence rate. Distal metastases are exceptional and are mainly to regional lymph nodes.

Management
The treatment of choice is wide local excision and this often implies amputation.

Undifferentiated sarcoma [1–4]

In pertinent classifications, undifferentiated soft tissue sarcoma (USTS) has replaced 'malignant fibrous histiocytoma' which was an umbrella term historically encompassing a heterogeneous group of neoplasms that included five different clinicopathological subtypes: pleomorphic, myxoid, giant cell, inflammatory and angiomatoid. There was little relation between these five morphological types; the angiomatoid variant was reclassified in the group of fibrohistiocytic tumours and the name changed to 'angiomatoid FH'. What was formerly known as myxoid variant of malignant FH is now known as 'myxofibrosarcoma', and it is likely to show fibroblastic differentiation; this tumour often involves the skin because of its frequent origin in the subcutis and it will therefore be discussed in more detail later. Angiomatoid FH has been described under fibrohistiocytic tumours. Currently, USTS may be roughly divided into pleomorphic, spindle cell, round cell and epithelioid subsets by morphology, but these have no specific defining features other than their common denominator – lack of identifiable differentiation. If cases classified as USTS are extensively studied with ancillary studies including immunohistochemistry, electron microscopy and cytogenetics [5,6], a certain percentage may be reclassified as pleomorphic variants of other soft-tissue tumours, including liposarcoma, rhabdomyosarcoma and leiomyosarcoma.

Myxofibrosarcoma [1–3,4]

Definition and nomenclature

Myxofibrosarcoma (MFS) is a neoplasm of the subcutis and deeper soft tissues with variable cellularity, myxoid change and cells with pleomorphic nuclei. The cellular end of the spectrum is identical to undifferentiated sarcoma and the diagnosis is made based on the presence of myxoid areas with less cellularity and a lobular pattern. The myxoid change should be seen in 10% or more of the tumour before a lesion is classified as myxofibrosarcoma.

Synonyms and inclusions
- Myxoid malignant fibrous histiocytoma

Epidemiology
Incidence and prevalence

Age
Presentation is mainly in middle-aged to old adults.

Sex
There is a slight male predilection.

Pathophysiology
Pathology [4]
These tumours have a lobular growth pattern. They are classified according to the degree of cellularity and pleomorphism into low, medium and high grade. Low-grade tumours are paucicellular and consist of round or elongated bland and pleomorphic cells in a prominent myxoid stroma. The atypical cells have irregular hyperchromatic nuclei and mitotic figures are relatively frequent. In the background, a fairly prominent number of thin-walled vascular channels with a typical curvilinear pattern are seen. Vacuolated, Alcian blue positive cells, focally mimicking lipoblasts, are relatively frequent. In some tumours, hypocellular areas blend with more cellular areas containing cells with increased pleomorphism; such tumours are classified as intermediate grade. Tumours with high cellularity (high grade) are indistinguishable from undifferentiated sarcoma and may have necrosis. Grading of lesions is important, because the rate of local recurrence and metastasis varies (see later). Some tumours, particularly high-grade lesions, may have epithelioid morphology [5]. Focal SMA and/or CD34 reactivity may be encountered.

Genetics
Myxofibrosarcomas show complex karyotypes, with a large number of driver genes, some of them potentionally actionable. Methylation-based analysis groups MFS into three clusters, associated with particular driver mutations, different clinical outcomes and immune cell compositions [6].

Clinical features
History and presentation
This tumour mainly presents in the extremities, particularly the lower limbs followed by the upper limbs and less commonly the trunk, head and neck [4]. Typically, an asymptomatic mass, measuring several centimetres in diameter, is found in the subcutis or deeper soft tissues. This is one of the sarcomas that more often involves the dermis as a result of extension from the subcutis or deeper soft tissues, rather than having a dermal origin. About 50% of cases arise in the subcutaneous tissue and involve the overlying dermis [5]. Exceptional cases have been reported in association with a burn scar [7].

Disease course and prognosis
High-grade lesions have a higher tendency for local recurrence and for metastatic spread to regional lymph nodes. The overall 5-year survival is between 60% and 70% [4,5,7]. Tumours with epithelioid morphology appear to have a more aggressive behaviour [8].

Management [4]
Excision with clear margins is essential.

Low-grade fibromyxoid sarcoma [1–3]

Definition and nomenclature
This distinctive neoplasm is regarded as a low-grade variant of fibrosarcoma. It is characterised by deceptive, bland, spindle-shaped cells in a stroma with curvilinear blood vessels and either collagenous or myxoid background.

Synonyms and inclusions
- Hyalinising spindle cell tumour with giant rosettes

Epidemiology
Incidence and prevalence
Tumours are rare.

Age
It is seen mainly in young to middle-aged adults.

Sex
There is no sex predilection.

Pathophysiology
Pathology [1–3]

The tumour consists of a proliferation of wavy, bland, spindle-shaped cells arranged in short fascicles and surrounded by a collagenous or myxoid stroma. Cellularity varies and tumour cells are usually bland with very rare mitotic figures. Frequent, elongated, thin-walled blood vessels are seen throughout the tumour. Only a small number of cases display some degree of cytological atypia. As a result of the deceiving histological appearances, the tumour is often diagnosed as benign. In a proportion of cases there are focal areas with hyalinised collagen surrounded by epithelioid tumour cells forming rosettes. This variant of the tumour was originally described as hyalinising spindle cell tumour with giant rosettes [4]. The presence of rosettes does not influence the behaviour of the neoplasm. Diffuse and intense cytoplasmic MUC4 staining is a highly sensitive and specific marker for low-grade fibromyxoid sarcoma [5].

Genetics
The majority of tumours are characterised by a t(7;16)(q33;p11) translocation, leading to fusion of the *FUS* and *CREB3L2* genes [6]. Small numbers harbour a FUS-CREB3L1 fusion resulting from t(11;16)(p11;p11), while rare cases harbour the EWSR1-CREB3L1 fusion [7] resulting from t(11;22)(p11;q12). These findings are useful for confirmation of the diagnosis by FISH.

Clinical features
History and presentation

The tumour usually presents as a slowly growing lesion in young to middle-aged adults, with an equal sex incidence; it has a predilection for the proximal extremities, followed by the trunk. Tumours tend to be longstanding and asymptomatic and present as a mass, measuring several centimetres in diameter, and located in the subcutis or deeper soft tissues. Subcutaneous lesions are often clinically diagnosed as a lipoma.

Disease course and prognosis
In the largest series of cases reported so far it has been shown that local recurrence occurs in 9% of cases, metastases in 9% and mortality in 2% [7]. It seems that areas with higher grade morphology do not confer a more aggressive behaviour. However, this needs to be confirmed in further studies. Metastatic spread may occur many years after the original diagnosis and therefore long-term follow-up is indicated.

Management
Excision with clear margins is essential.

FIBROHISTIOCYTIC TUMOURS

Tenosynovial giant cell tumour [1,2,3,4]

Definition
This is a benign tumour that in its localised variant occurs mainly on the hands and consists of a nodular proliferation of histiocyte-like cells with scattered multinucleated giant cells and variable numbers of mononuclear inflammatory cells. The diffuse variant of this tumour that involves joints is not discussed further in this chapter.

Epidemiology
Incidence and prevalence

Tumours are relatively rare.

Age

Young to middle-aged adults.

Sex

There is a predilection for females.

Pathophysiology
Pathology

It is a multinodular lesion composed of sheets of histiocyte-like cells with bland vesicular nuclei, intermixed with multinucleated giant cells, foamy cells, siderophages and scattered mononuclear inflammatory cells. Hyalinisation, haemosiderin deposition and cholesterol clefts are often seen. No histological features predict lesions that recur locally [3].

Genetics
The tumours are characterised by rearrangements of CSF1 (macrophage colony-stimulating factor) [4].

Clinical features
History and presentation

Tumours present mainly on the hands with a predilection for the fingers. They are typically between 1 and 3 cm in diameter and asymptomatic, although they may interfere with function. Multiple tumours are very rare [5].

Disease course and prognosis
The rate of local recurrence varies from 5% to 15% [3,6].

Management
Excision is the treatment of choice.

Fibrous histiocytoma (dermatofibroma) [1–4]

Definition and nomenclature
Fibrous histiocytoma (FH) is a benign dermal and often superficial subcutaneous proliferation of oval cells resembling histiocytes, and spindle-shaped cells resembling fibroblasts and myofibroblasts. Their line of differentiation remains uncertain, but these lesions are descriptively classified as fibrohistiocytic tumours because of the microscopic appearance of the tumour cells. Evidence of clonality in FH was confirmed by cytogenetic studies in the 1990s [5], and more recently gene fusions involving protein kinase C genes were found in a proportion of FHs [6]. The neoplastic nature of FH is

also confirmed by their clinical persistence and by the frequency of local recurrence of some variants (cellular, aneurysmal and atypical; see later) as well as the exceptional metastases (rarely leading to death as a result of disseminated disease) of some tumours (cellular, aneurysmal and atypical and, more exceptionally, epithelioid and even ordinary types) [7–9,10,11,12].

> **Synonyms and inclusions**
> - Histiocytoma cutis
> - Subepidermal nodular fibrosis
> - Sclerosing angioma

Epidemiology
Incidence and prevalence
Ordinary FH is probably the most common cutaneous soft-tissue tumour. Important clinicopathological variants (cellular, atypical and aneurysmal) are much more uncommon. Cellular FH represents fewer than 5% of all FHs [12]. Aneurysmal and atypical FHs are less common than the latter.

Age
Most FHs occur in young to middle-aged adults. Cellular, atypical and epithelioid FHs are more common in young adults.

Sex
Ordinary FH is more common in females. Cellular and atypical FHs are more common in males. The other variants are more common in females.

Pathophysiology
Pathology
The overlying epidermis frequently shows a degree of epidermal hyperplasia [13] (Figure 136.9). The latter displays different patterns including changes mimicking a squamous papilloma, a seborrhoeic keratosis and lichen simplex chronicus. Occasionally, the epidermal proliferation is associated with immature follicular structures, which are often confused with a basal cell carcinoma. In the dermis, there is a localised proliferation of histiocyte-like cells and fibroblast-like cells, associated with variable numbers of mononuclear inflammatory cells. Foamy macrophages, siderophages and multinucleated giant cells are also variably present. A focal storiform pattern is often seen. The tumour blends with the surrounding dermis. Collagen bundles at the periphery of the lesion are surrounded by scattered tumour cells and appear somewhat hyalinised. Focal myofibroblastic differentiation is often suggested, particularly in the cellular variant. Older lesions show focal proliferation of small blood vessels in association with haemosiderin deposition and fibrosis, hence the older name of 'sclerosing haemangioma'.

Cellular FH [12] also shows epidermal hyperplasia, but the lesions are more cellular, less polymorphic and consist of bundles of spindle-shaped cells with pink cytoplasm and a focal storiform pattern (Figure 136.10). The mitotic rate varies and necrosis may be found in up to 12% of cases. Extension into the subcutaneous tissue is more prominent than that seen in ordinary FH. However, the pattern of infiltration is mainly along the septae and only focally into the subcutaneous lobule in a lace-like pattern. The cellularity and growth pattern often make distinction from DFSP difficult, particularly in small biopsies. DFSP is, however, more monomorphic, tends to infiltrate the subcutaneous tissue diffusely and is generally uniformly positive for CD34. Cellular FH may be focally positive for CD34, but this is predominantly seen at the periphery of the tumour. Staining for FXIIIa is positive in a percentage of background cells in FH and negative in DFSP. Furthermore, cellular FH is often focally positive for smooth muscle actin, whereas this marker is negative in DFSP.

Aneurysmal FH [14,15] shows extensive haemorrhage, with prominent cavernous-like pseudovascular spaces (Figure 136.11), which are not lined by endothelial cells. The mitotic rate varies but may be prominent. The background is that of an ordinary FH.

Atypical FH [16,17] shows variable numbers of mono- or multinucleated, pleomorphic, spindle-shaped or histiocyte-like cells on a background of an ordinary FH. These cells may be very prominent, making the histological diagnosis difficult. Mitotic figures, including atypical forms, may be seen. These lesions used to be classified as 'atypical fibroxanthoma (AFX) occurring in non-sun-exposed skin of young patients'.

Epithelioid FH [18,19,20] contains a predominant population of cells with abundant pink cytoplasm and vesicular nuclei, and there is often myxoid change and a prominent vascular component. Most

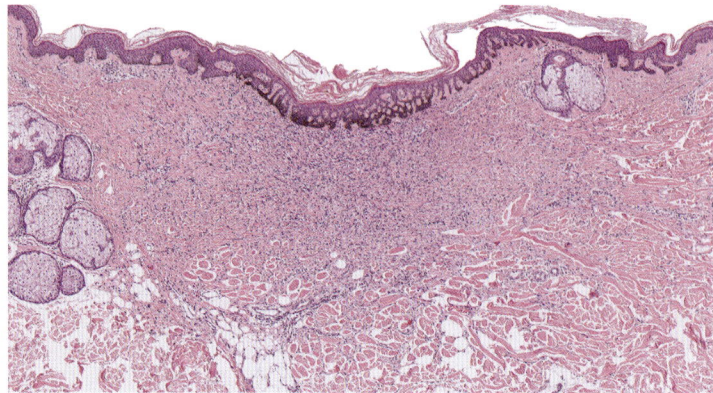

Figure 136.9 Histological appearance of dermatofibroma, showing epidermal hyperplasia and pigmentation overlying the dermal sclerotic component.

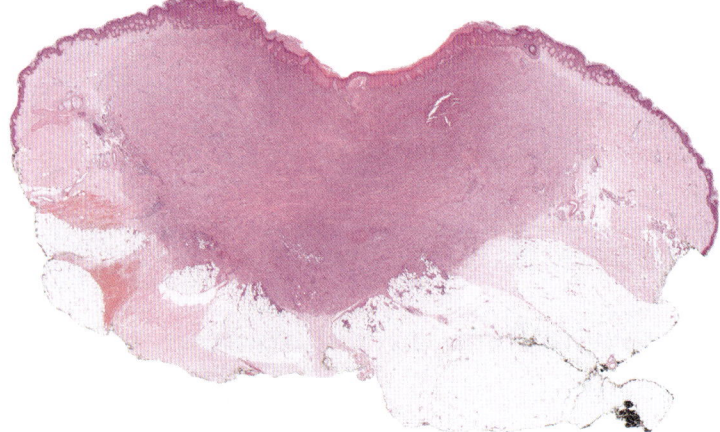

Figure 136.10 Cellular fibrous histiocytoma. Note the increased cellularity, fascicular appearance and focal extension into the subcutis.

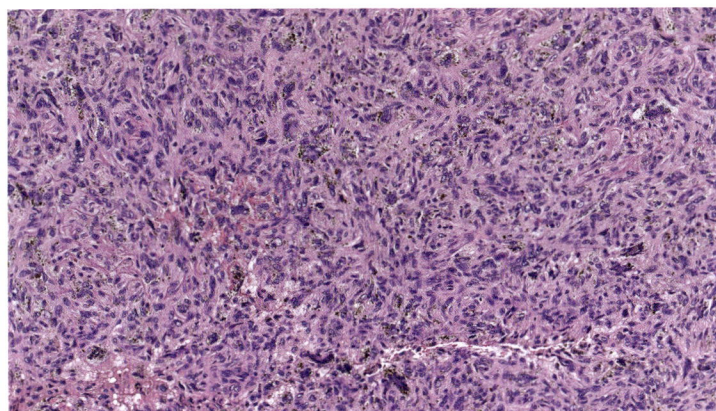

Figure 136.11 Aneurysmal fibrous histiocytoma. Prominent haemorrhage and haemosiderin deposition within a typical fibrous histiocytoma background.

epithelioid FH harbour *ALK* rearrangement and show ALK overexpression by immunohistochemistry. Distinction from a Spitz naevus may be difficult on histological grounds alone, but in epithelioid FH there is no junctional component, tumour cells are not nested, they are negative for S100 and usually ALK positive.

Many histological variants of FH have been described; recognising these variants is important to avoid misdiagnosis. They include lesions with palisading granular cell change [21], abundant lipid (ankle-type) [22], clear cell change [23], balloon cell change [24] and keloidal change [25]. The presence of lipid within lesions of FH is not usually associated with systemic lipid abnormalities [26].

Clinical features
History and presentation
FH is commonest on the limbs and appears as a firm papule which is frequently yellow-brown in colour and slightly scaly (Figure 136.12). If the overlying epidermis is squeezed, the 'dimple sign' will be seen, indicating tethering of the overlying epidermis to the underlying lesion. Giant lesions (>5 cm in diameter) are occasionally seen [27] and large tumours are more often encountered in some of the variants (see later). Multiple lesions may develop and eruptive variants have been described. The latter may be familial [28], or may be associated with immunosuppression (e.g. HIV) [29], with systemic disease, including autoimmune diseases such as lupus erythematosus and neoplasia, particularly haematological malignancies [30–34], and even with highly active antiretroviral therapy (HAART) [35].

A number of clinicopathological variants of FH mentioned before has been described, which should be recognised by clinicians and pathologists in order to avoid a misdiagnosis of malignancy. These variants include: cellular FH [12], aneurysmal FH [14,15], atypical FH (pseudosarcomatous FH, dermatofibroma with monster cells) [16,17] and epithelioid FH [18,19,20]. A further variant, described as 'atrophic' [36], may mimic a scar and does not usually pose a problem in differential diagnosis. Rare cases may be ulcerated, erosive or lichenoid [37].

Cellular FH, like ordinary FH, has predilection for the limbs. However, the distribution of age and site is wide; cellular FH is not infrequent in children, and on sites such as the head, neck, fingers and toes. The size of these lesions is also larger than that of ordinary FH. Most cellular FHs are less than 2 cm in diameter, but lesions measuring more than 5 cm may occur. Recognition of this variant is important, because it has a local recurrence rate of 25%, and metastases have been reported anecdotally in a small number of cases [7,8,**10**,11].

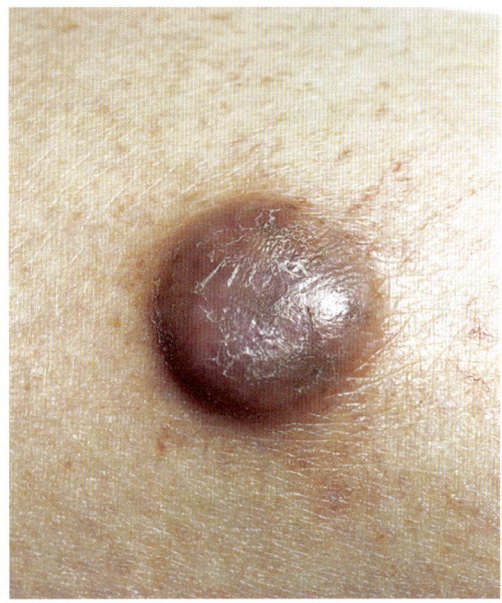

Figure 136.12 Clinical appearance of a fibrous histiocytoma or dermatofibroma.

Aneurysmal FH is usually rapidly growing and may attain a very large size. They clinically mimic a vascular tumour. Exceptional tumours are multiple [38]. The rate of local recurrence is 19% [**15**].

Atypical FH presents as a papule, nodule or plaque, usually less than 1.5 cm in diameter. The rate of local recurrence is around 14%, and exceptional metastases have been reported [17].

Epithelioid FH [18,19,**20**] presents on the limbs of young patients, with a predilection for females. The typical clinical appearance is that of a polypoid, often vascular, lesion resembling a non-ulcerated pyogenic granuloma.

Disease course and prognosis
Ordinary and epithelioid FHs hardly ever recur locally. Cellular FH recurs in 25% of cases, aneurysmal FH recurs in 19% of cases and atypical FH recurs in 14% of cases. Exceptional metastases have been reported in all clinicopathological variants including ordinary and epithelioid FH. This phenomenon, although exceptional, is more common in cellular, aneurysmal and atypical FHs [7–9,**10**,11]. In one case of cellular FH, transformation to a pleomorphic sarcoma has been reported [11]. Morphological features do not allow prediction of tumours that will behave in a more aggressive manner [**10**]. Metastatic tumours are more often associated with chromosomal abnormalities as demonstrated by array comparative genomic hybridisation [11,39]. Fatal tumours are associated with the highest number of chromosomal abnormalities [39].

Management
Most FHs are no more than a cosmetic nuisance and no treatment is necessary. However, cellular, atypical and aneurysmal variants should be completely removed conservatively, because of the risk of local recurrence and the occurrence of occasional distant metastases.

Plexiform fibrohistiocytic tumour [1–4,5]

Definition and nomenclature
Plexiform FH is a distinctive predominantly subcutaneous tumour with two distinctive components:
1 A fibro/myofibroblastic fascicular component.
2 A nodular histiocytic-like component, which also includes giant cells.

Despite its new name, it does not represent a plexiform variant of an ordinary FH (dermatofibroma). An association with cellular neurothekeoma, a tumour that occurs primarily in the dermis, has been suggested based on morphological similarities [5,6].

> **Synonyms and inclusions**
> - Plexiform fibrous histiocytoma

Epidemiology
Incidence and prevalence

Age
It mainly occurs in children and young adults. An exceptional case has been congenital [7].

Sex
It is most common in females.

Pathophysiology
Pathology [1–4,5]
Low-power examination reveals a predominantly subcutaneous tumour with focal involvement of the dermis and a distinctive plexiform growth pattern. Purely dermal lesions are occasionally seen [8]. Two components are usually identified and consist of fascicles of bland spindle-shaped fibro/myofibroblast-like cells and nodules of histiocyte-like cells with scattered giant cells, focal haemorrhage and haemosiderin deposition. In some tumours, one of the components may predominate. The spindle-shaped cells stain focally for smooth muscle actin and the cells in the nodules are focally positive for CD68.

Clinical features [1–4,5]
History and presentation
Tumours have a predilection for the upper limbs. The tumour is solitary, measures no more than a few centimetres in diameter and is asymptomatic.

Disease course and prognosis
Local recurrences are observed in up to 30% of cases. Metastases to regional lymph nodes or to the lungs have been reported [1,3,9].

Management
Complete surgical excision and follow-up are indicated. Histological features do not predict cases with more aggressive behaviour.

Atypical fibroxanthoma/pleomorphic dermal sarcoma [1,2,3,4]

Definition
Atypical fibroxanthoma (AFX), by definition, arises in the sun-damaged skin of elderly people. It is a paradoxical tumour with histological features of a highly malignant neoplasm and low-grade clinical behaviour. Tumours with more aggressive histological features should be diagnosed as dermal pleomorphic sarcoma (see later) [5].

Epidemiology
Age
Most patients are elderly in the seventh to eighth decades of life. Tumours in younger patients occur very rarely in the setting of xeroderma pigmentosum [6].

Sex
Tumours are much more frequent in males than in females.

Ethnicity
It is a tumour almost exclusively restricted to white people.

Pathophysiology
Predisposing factors
UV radiation-induced *p53* mutations have been observed in these lesions, confirming the association with sun-damaged skin [7]. More recently, telomerase reverse transcriptase (TERT) promoter mutations with UV signature have been identified in AFXs giving further support to the relationship to sun exposure [8].

Pathology
The tumours are exophytic, fairly well circumscribed and surrounded by an epidermal collarette. The remarkable and paradoxical feature of AFX is its histological resemblance to a highly malignant soft-tissue sarcoma (Figure 136.13) [9–11]. It arises in the dermis and may extend very focally into the fat, but the edge is pushing rather than infiltrative. It is composed of large

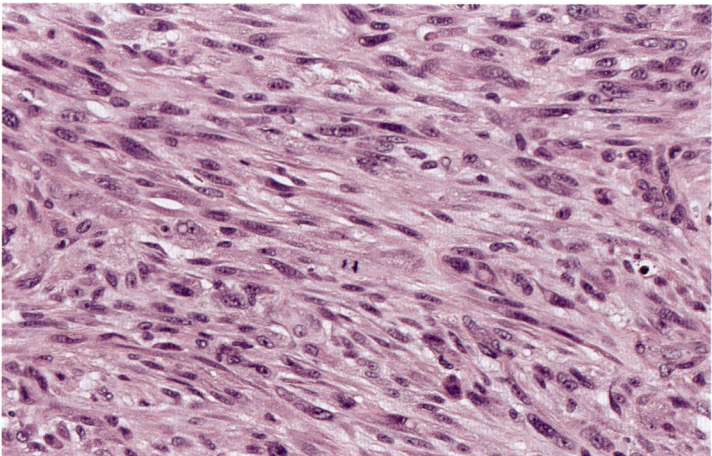

Figure 136.13 Prominent cellular pleomorphism in a case of atypical fibroxanthoma.

spindle-shaped and histiocyte-like pleomorphic cells, many of which appear multinucleated. The cells are arranged in a haphazard fashion and mitotic figures, including atypical forms, are frequent. The histiocytic cells may contain lipid or haemosiderin [12,13]. A series of a less pleomorphic spindle cell variant, which may cause considerable problems in differential diagnosis, has been described [14]. Rare cases display prominent sclerosis [15], and partial or total regression may rarely be seen [16]. In some tumours, there is focal or prominent clear or granular cell change, keloid-like areas, prominent myxoid change, osteoclast-like giant cells and pseudoangiomatous areas [17–19,20]. Tumours with an infiltrative growth pattern, involvement of deeper tissues (including the subcutis), tumour necrosis, lymphovascular invasion and perineural invasion should be classified as pleomorphic dermal sarcomas (PDS) as they have a more aggressive behaviour than conventional AFXs (see later) [5]. The diagnosis of AFX is a diagnosis of exclusion. An immunohistochemical panel to rule out melanoma (S100), sarcomatoid squamous cell carcinoma (pankeratin, mainly MNF 116 and AE1/AE3, as the low molecular weight keratin Cam 5.2 is usually negative in sarcomatoid squamous cell carcinoma of the skin) and even leiomyosarcoma (desmin, h-caldesmon) should be performed in all cases. The basic panel should be enough to accurately diagnose most cases of AFX. Other markers have been described that are often positive in AFX and tend to be negative in other tumours that enter the differential diagnosis. These include CD99, CD10 and pro-collagen 1 [21–23]. CD31 is often focally positive in tumour cells as is EMA and very rare focal positivity for melan-A has been reported [20,24]. Since the advent of immunohistochemistry, reports of metastatic tumours have been very rare. This suggests that many lesions reported in the past as metastatic AFX, which were diagnosed by examination of haematoxylin and eosin stained slides alone, probably represented other tumours, such as spindle cell melanomas or sarcomatoid squamous cell carcinoma. Tumours described in younger patients in non-sun-damaged skin represent examples of atypical FH.

Genetics
AFX and pleomorphic dermal sarcoma (PDS) have unspecific molecular traits, but show similar mutational and DNA methylation profiles, as well as copy number alterations, that do not overlap significantly with other cutaneous tumours in the differential diagnosis [25,**26**].

Clinical features
History and presentation
The lesions occur most frequently on the ears, bald scalp and cheeks (Figure 136.14). The lesions are often ulcerated and have a red fleshy appearance; they rarely exceed 30 mm in diameter and are usually of less than 6 months' duration. Exceptional cases occur as a result of immunosuppression in cardiac transplant [27]. Multiple lesions have been reported [28].

Disease course and prognosis
Local recurrence may be seen in about 10% of cases and metastases to lymph nodes and internal organs are occasionally reported [29,30]. The latter, however, may be examples of tumours that are classified as PDS. The latter have a local recurrence rate of around 28% and metastatic rate of 10% [5].

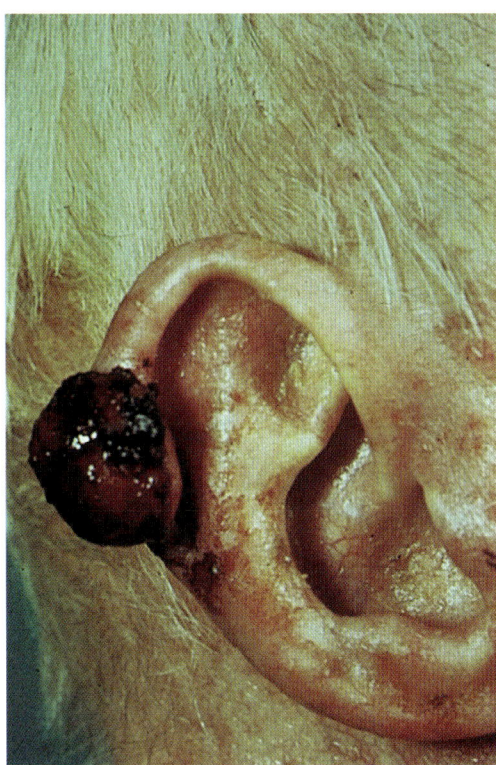

Figure 136.14 Typical clinical appearance of an atypical fibroxanthoma with a polypoid architecture.

Management
The benign behaviour of the tumour enables it to be treated by limited local removal. Although rare cases are treated by Mohs micrographic surgery [31], tumours are usually relatively well circumscribed and the former treatment is rarely needed to achieve good clearance. Radiotherapy is not usually recommended.

VASCULAR TUMOURS

Reviews of vascular tumours may be found in [1,2]. The vascular ectasias (Chapter 101), verrucovenous malformation (verrucous haemangioma), cavernous and capillary haemangiomas, congenital haemangiomas, tufted angioma and kaposiform haemangioendothelioma (Chapter 116) are described elsewhere.

REACTIVE VASCULAR LESIONS

Intravascular papillary endothelial hyperplasia [1,2,3,4]

Definition and nomenclature
Intravascular papillary endothelial hyperplasia is regarded as a form of organising thrombus in which endothelial cells line hyalinised papillae. It usually presents as a primary phenomenon within a thrombosed blood vessel, usually a vein [2,**3**,4]. The

secondary variant is commonly seen as an incidental finding within other vascular tumours, or in lesions such as haemorrhoids. Exceptionally, the same phenomenon is seen within a haematoma [4].

Synonyms and inclusions
- Masson pseudoangiosarcoma
- Masson vegetant intravascular haemangioendothelioma

Epidemiology
Incidence and prevalence
A relatively common lesion.

Age
In general, this presents with a wide age range, although the primary form of the disease is more common in young adults.

Sex
The primary form is slightly more common in females.

Pathophysiology
All forms of the condition are the result of reactive proliferation of endothelial cells as a result of an organising thrombus most often but not always secondary to trauma.

Pathology
The pathology is that of a widely dilated vascular channel in the dermis or subcutis, containing an organising thrombus and prominent papillary projections with a hyalinised collagenous core. The latter are usually lined by a single layer of bland endothelial cells. Mitotic figures are rare. The presence of hyalinised collagen lined by endothelial cells produces an appearance similar to the 'dissection of collagen bundles' described in angiosarcoma. Distinction from angiosarcoma, however, is easy, as the latter is only exceptionally purely intravascular; it also displays cytological atypia, multilayering and mitotic figures. In secondary forms of Masson tumour, the changes are seen within one or several vascular channels of a vascular tumour, usually a cavernous haemangioma or a vascular malformation.

Clinical features
History and presentation
The primary form presents as a slowly growing solitary asymptomatic or slightly painful bluish nodule less than 20 mm in diameter. The site of predilection is the head and neck, followed by the hand (particularly the fingers). Multiple lesions are exceptional [5].

Disease course and prognosis
Behaviour is benign and there is no tendency for local recurrence.

Differential diagnosis
Clinical presentation is that of a vascular tumour.

Management
Simple excision is usually curative.

Reactive angioendotheliomatosis [1–3]

Definition
A reactive vascular proliferation is usually multifocal and is associated with a number of systemic diseases. In the past, it was divided into a reactive and a malignant form. With the advent of immunohistochemistry, it became apparent that the malignant form is a variant of aggressive intravascular lymphoma (Chapter 139).

Epidemiology
Incidence and prevalence
The condition is rare.

Age
The age range is wide although most cases occur in adults.

Sex
No sex predilection.

Pathophysiology
Predisposing factors
It has been described in association with systemic diseases, including bacterial endocarditis, peripheral vascular atherosclerotic disease, cryoglobulinaemia [2], liver and renal disease, antiphospholipid syndrome [4], amyloidosis [5] and sarcoidosis [6]. It is not clear how systemic diseases induce the vascular proliferation.

Pathology [7]
The dermis and, in some cases, the subcutis show a multifocal proliferation of clusters of capillaries lined by plump endothelial cells with little or no cytological atypia. A layer of pericytes surrounds each capillary. In some areas, dilated capillaries appear to contain smaller vascular channels within their lumina. Patients with cryoglobulinaemia show thrombosis of capillaries by hyaline eosinophilic globules.

Clinical features
History and presentation
Most patients present with multiple red and/or haemorrhagic macules, papules and plaques located on the trunk and limbs. Patients with fewer, more localised, lesions may also be seen. In the latter cases, the association with systemic disease is not usually present. In patients with antiphospholipid syndrome or cryoglobulinaemia, ulcerated lesions may be present.

Disease course and prognosis
The condition is self-limited and usually resolves spontaneously within weeks.

Differential diagnosis
Not infrequently patients present with a livedo-like pattern in an unusual location (proximal rather than acral). Distinction from a vasculitic process may be difficult but ulceration is rare except in the very rare cases associated with the antiphospholipid syndrome or with cryoglulinaemia.

Management
There is no treatment available, but the condition is usually self-limited and resolves spontaneously within a few weeks.

Glomeruloid haemangioma [1,2]

Definition
This is a distinctive multifocal vascular proliferation that occurs in association with POEMS syndrome (*p*olyneuropathy, *o*rganomegaly, *e*ndocrinopathy, *M* protein and *s*kin changes; Chapter 149) or with multicentric Castleman disease. This condition is best considered as a form of reactive angioendotheliomatosis in the setting of POEMS syndrome. Exceptional cases with no clinical features of POEMS syndrome have been reported [3,4].

Epidemiology
Incidence and prevalence
This is a rare disease that presents almost exclusively in the context of POEMS syndrome and multicentric Castleman disease.

Age
It presents in adults.

Sex
There is no sex predilection.

Pathophysiology
Pathology
The histological appearances in a typical case are striking, consisting of a multifocal dermal proliferation of clusters of closely packed dilated capillaries with a striking similarity to renal glomeruli. A layer of pericytes surrounds each capillary. Vacuolated cells are focally present and, in some cases, there are eosinophilic hyaline globules within the lumina of capillaries. These globules represent deposits of protein.

Clinical features
History and presentation
Patients present with multiple vascular papules on the trunk and limbs. Only a minority of these vascular lesions have the histological appearance of glomeruloid haemangioma; most have the histological appearance of cherry angiomas.

Management
The lesions do not tend to regress spontaneously. Individual lesions can be removed surgically, but because of their numbers this is not generally a practical option.

BENIGN VASCULAR TUMOURS

Papillary haemangioma [1]

Definition
A distinctive dermal tumour characterised by vascular channels with papillary projections.

Epidemiology
Incidence and prevalence
Lesions are very rare.

Age
It presents in adults.

Sex
There is predilection for males.

Pathophysiology
Pathology
Tumours are relatively well circumscribed and consist of multiple dilated thin-walled vascular channels lined by bland endothelial cells and associated with papillary projections containing endothelial cells and pericytes and thick basement membrane-like material. A distinctive feature is the presence of intracytoplasmic eosinophilic globules within the endothelial cells.

Clinical features
History and presentation
Most lesions occur on the head and neck as a single asymptomatic papule.

Disease course and prognosis
Lesions are benign.

Management
Simple excision is the treatment of choice.

Lobular capillary haemangioma (pyogenic granuloma) [1,2]

Definition and nomenclature
A vascular nodule that develops rapidly, often at the site of a recent injury, and which is composed of a lobular proliferation of capillaries in an oedematous stroma.

Synonyms and inclusions
- Granuloma telangiectaticum

Epidemiology
Incidence and prevalence
Lesions are very common.

Age
The age range is wide but there is a peak in the second decade of life [3].

Sex
There is predilection for males except in lesions presenting in the oral cavity which are more common in females [4].

Pathophysiology
Predisposing factors
In a minority of cases, a minor injury, usually of a penetrating kind, has occurred a few weeks before the nodule appears. Lesions may also occur at the sites of burns [5].

Granuloma gravidarum is a variant of pyogenic granuloma that presents in the oral cavity during pregnancy.

Pathology
There is a lobular proliferation of small blood vessels, which erupt through a breach in the epidermis to produce a globular pedunculated tumour. The epidermis forms a collarette at the base of the lesion and covers part, or all, of the tumour in a thin layer. The proliferating vessels are set in a myxoid stroma, lacking in collagen in the earlier stages and relatively rich in mucin. The endothelial cells are plump, as in new granulation tissue, lining the vessels in a single layer. They are surrounded by a mixed cell population of fibroblasts, mast cells, lymphocytes, plasma cells and, where the surface is eroded, polymorphonuclear leukocytes (Figure 136.15). Mitotic figures may be prominent. Older lesions tend to organise and partly fibrose and may show focal bone formation. Late lesions can display focal degenerative atypia, raising the possibility of malignancy. In rare instances, particularly in children, and sometimes following treatment, satellite lesions, which have a similar pathology to the primary lesion, may develop around a pyogenic granuloma. These respond to simple destructive measures, thus ruling out malignancy [6]. In exceptional cases, extramedullary haemopoiesis may be seen [7]. Bacillary angiomatosis shows an almost identical histology to that of pyogenic granuloma [8]. However, in bacillary angiomatosis, pale epithelioid endothelial cells are prominent, neutrophils and nuclear dust are seen throughout the lesion and violaceous amorphous aggregates of bacilli which are positive with either Giemsa or Warthin–Starry stains are easily identified. The causative organism may also be identified by PCR.

Genetics
BRAF mutations have been reported in a large proportion of secondary pyogenic granulomas occurring within port-wine stains, and less frequently in sporadic cases [9].

Clinical features
History and presentation
The tumour is vascular, bright red to brownish-red or blue-black in colour. It is partially compressible but cannot be completely blanched and does not show pulsation. The surface of early bright-red lesions is usually thin intact epidermis. Older and darker lesions are frequently eroded and crusted and may bleed very easily. Occasionally, the surface is raspberry-like or even verrucous. The size is commonly between 5 and 10 mm, but may reach 50 mm. The outline is rounded. The base is often pedunculated and surrounded by a collar of acanthotic epidermis; the lesion may be sessile. The common sites are the hands, especially the fingers (Figure 136.16), the feet, lips, head and upper trunk, and the mucosal surfaces of the mouth and perianal area. The initial evolution is rapid, but growth ceases after a few weeks. Spontaneous disappearance is rare. Lesions are not painful; patients mainly complain of the appearance or of recurrent bleeding. Rarely, pyogenic granulomas may occur within a port-wine stain [10]. There are reported cases of multiple pyogenic granulomas developing after exfoliative dermatitis [11] and, in a periungual location, after HAART [12]. Lesions mimicking pyogenic granuloma may occur during therapy with gefitinib [13], systemic 5-fluorouracil [14] and capecitabine [15]. Eruptive forms of this tumour have rarely been reported [16]. In this setting, distinction from bacillary angiomatosis is crucial because the latter often presents with multiple lesions that can be clinically and histologically difficult to distinguish from pyogenic granuloma. Multiple lesions closely resembling pyogenic granulomas have been reported after systemic [17] and topical [18] treatment with retinoids. Subcutaneous [19,20] and intravascular [21] variants are rarely seen and do not have distinctive clinical features. Interestingly, two cases of subcutaneous lesions have been described in patients with antiphospholipid antibodies [22].

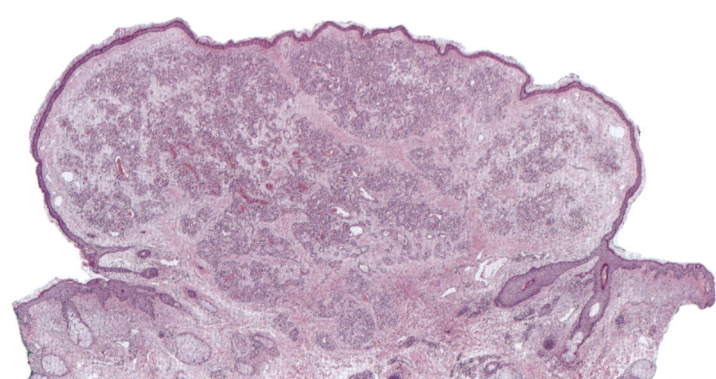

Figure 136.15 Typical lobular proliferation of capillaries in a case of pyogenic granuloma.

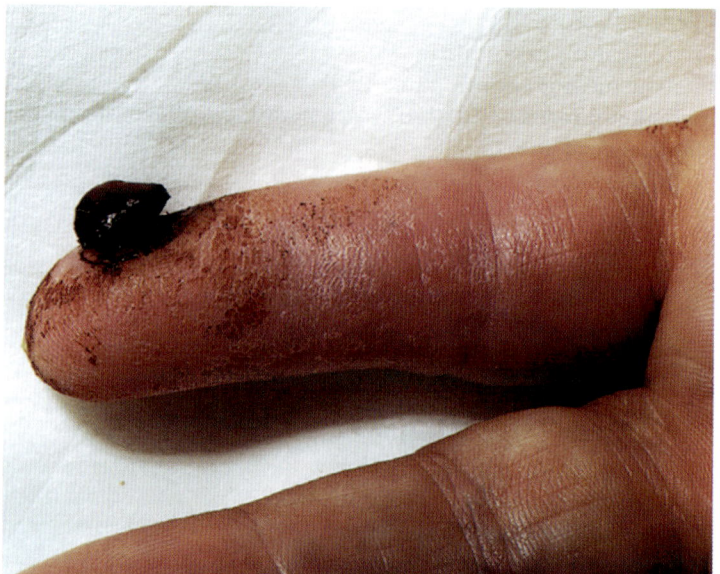

Figure 136.16 Clinical appearance of a thrombosed pyogenic granuloma on a typical site at the tip of the finger.

Differential diagnosis
In most cases, the history and clinical appearance leave little doubt about the diagnosis, and microscopic confirmation is straightforward. In 38% of one case series, the clinical diagnosis of pyogenic granuloma proved to be wrong [23]. The errors included keratoacanthoma and other epithelial neoplasms, inflamed seborrhoeic keratoses, melanocytic naevi, melanoma and Spitz naevi, viral warts, molluscum contagiosum, angioma, glomus tumour, eccrine poroma, Kaposi sarcoma and metastatic carcinoma.

Disease course and prognosis
Simple excision is the treatment of choice, as lesions do not regress spontaneously. Local recurrence may be seen after incomplete excision.

Management
The pedunculated lesions are easy to treat by curettage with cauterisation or diathermy coagulation of the base. A considerable proportion of pyogenic granulomas recur after such treatment because the proliferating vessels in the base extend in a conical manner into the deeper dermis. In some areas – for instance in the nail fold or on the palmar aspect of a finger – it may be reasonable to carry out curettage and adopt an expectant approach thereafter. Wherever possible, it is desirable to excise a narrow, but deep, ellipse of skin beneath the lesion – such a wound may be repaired primarily or allowed to heal by second intention. A small number of lesions have been treated with topical imiquimod 5% cream both in children and adults with complete resolution [24,25]. Other treatment modalities that have been used include Nd:YAG laser [26], cryosurgery [27], intralesional steroids, flash lamp pulsed dye laser, sclerotherapy with sodium tetra decyl sulphate [28] and even injection of absolute ethanol [29].

Cirsoid aneurysm [1,2,3,4]

Definition and nomenclature
Cirsoid aneurysm is a small vascular proliferation characterised by small- to medium-sized channels with features of arteries and veins. As opposed to deeper tumours showing similar features, shunting is absent.

> **Synonyms and inclusions**
> - Cutaneous arteriovenous haemangioma
> - Acral arteriovenous tumour

Epidemiology
Incidence and prevalence
Lesions are relatively common.

Age
Most patients are young adults.

Sex
There is no sex predilection.

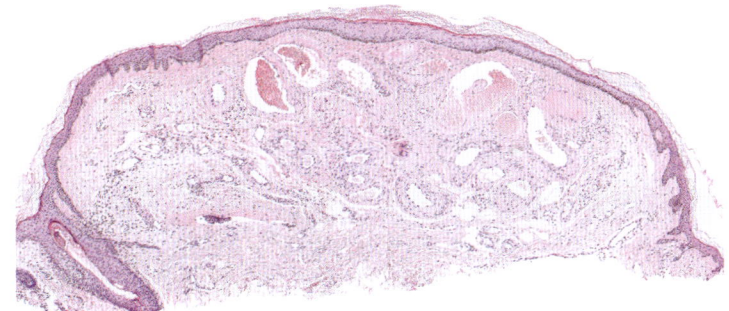

Figure 136.17 A dermal collection of thick- and thin-walled blood vessels in a typical case of cirsoid aneurysm.

Pathophysiology
Pathology
The dermis contains a mixture of scattered blood vessels with thick walls and features of veins and arteries (Figure 136.17).

Clinical features
History and presentation
Most lesions present on the head and neck region of young adults, with no sex predilection, as a small blue-red asymptomatic papule.

Management
As there is no associated shunting or deep component, simple excision is the treatment of choice.

Epithelioid haemangioma [1,2]

Definition and nomenclature
A benign locally proliferating lesion composed of vascular channels lined by endothelial cells with abundant pink cytoplasm and vesicular nuclei. There has, on occasion, been a difficulty with nomenclature such that the term Kimura disease has been applied but this condition is now viewed as distinct. In Kimura disease, the lesions occur in younger patients, are deeper seated, are associated with lymphadenopathy, have no initial overlying skin lesions and do not contain epithelioid endothelial cells [3,4]. Furthermore, peripheral blood eosinophilia is much more common in Kimura disease. Exceptionally, epithelioid haemangioma may coexist with Kimura disease [5].

> **Synonyms and inclusions**
> - Angiolymphoid hyperplasia with eosinophilia (ALHE)
> - Pseudopyogenic granuloma
> - Histiocytoid haemangioma

Epidemiology
Incidence and prevalence
These lesions have now been reported from many parts of the world. In a proportion of cases the findings suggest a reactive process [6], while other cases show consistent gene rearrangements [7].

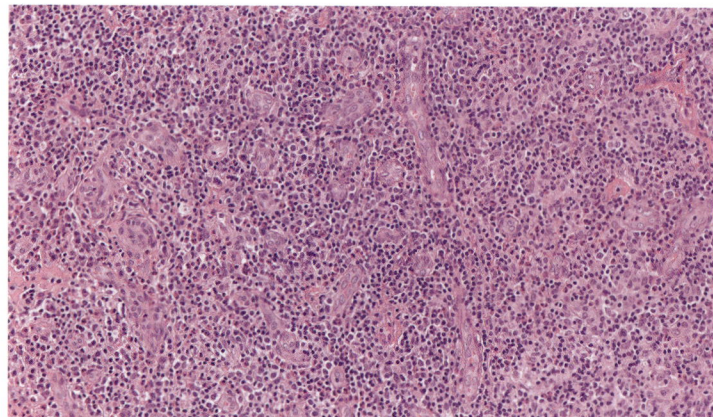

Figure 136.18 Vascular channels lined by epithelioid endothelial cells surrounded by numerous eosinophils in a case of epithelioid haemangioma.

Age
The age range is wide but lesions most commonly occur in young adults.

Sex
Both sexes are equally affected.

Pathophysiology
Pathology [2,8]
A poorly circumscribed lobular lesion is seen. It is composed of clusters of proliferating capillaries and often thicker blood vessels lined by plump epithelioid endothelial cells (Figure 136.18) with little cytological atypia and rare mitotic figures. Around the blood vessels there is a cellular inflammatory infiltrate composed mainly of lymphocytes and large numbers of eosinophils. However, only less than half of cases contain a prominent infiltrate. Older lesions show sclerosis of the stroma and the epithelioid endothelial cells become more prominent. A frequent finding, particularly in larger lesions, is the involvement of larger blood vessels. Rare cases are entirely intravascular [9,10]. The endothelial cells stain for vascular markers including CD34, CD31 and ERG (avian v-ets erythroblastosis virus E26 oncogene homologue). In cutaneous cases, the epithelioid endothelial cells are usually negative for keratins. They also consistently stain for the FOSB antigen [11], a finding that would not be expected from the proportion of cutaneous cases that harbour *FOS* gene rearrangements.

Genetics [7,12,13]
FOS gene rearrangements occur in a substantial proportion of EH with deep (bone, soft tissue) involvement, while they are rare in intravascular and more superficial (ALHE-type) cutaneous cases. Recently, novel *GATA6-FOXO1* fusions have been found in a number of cases.

Clinical features [14–17] (Figure 136.19)
History and presentation
Affected individuals present with a cluster of small translucent nodules on the head and neck, particularly around the ear or the hairline [18]. The lesions may also involve the oral mucosa [19]. Less

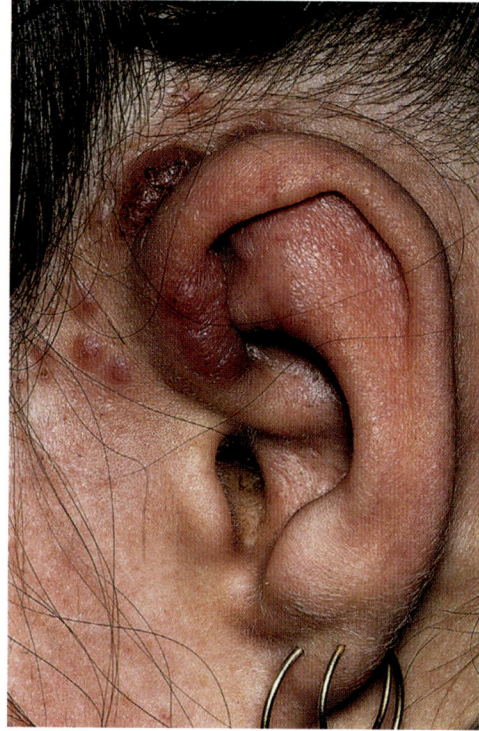

Figure 136.19 Epithelioid haemangioma. Courtesy of and copyright of Dr R. H. Champion, Addenbrooke's Hospital, Cambridge, UK.

frequently, lesions can involve the trunk and extremities. Involvement of deeper soft tissues and internal organs, including bone, can be seen. Individual nodules rarely exceed 2–3 cm in diameter, but occasionally deeper extension and larger subcutaneous lesions occur. Peripheral blood eosinophilia may be present but only in fewer than 10% of patients.

Disease course and prognosis
Spontaneous regression is seen in some cases after a variable period of time.

Management
Both surgery and radiotherapy are effective, but local recurrences are common. Treatment with Nd:YAG laser has been effective [20] and there is an anecdotal report of response to imiquimod cream [21].

Cutaneous epithelioid angiomatous nodule

Definition
This is tumour within the spectrum of vascular lesions characterised by epithelioid endothelial cells [1,2,3]. It is regarded by some as part of the spectrum of epithelioid haemangioma.

Epidemiology
Incidence and prevalence
Lesions are rare.

Age
Presentation is usually in adults.

Sex
There is no sex predilection.

Pathophysiology
Pathology
The majority of lesions are superficial, well circumscribed and surrounded by an epithelial collarette. Occasional deeper tumours may be observed. It is composed of sheets of epithelioid endothelial cells with abundant pink cytoplasm, vesicular nuclei and a single small nucleolus. Cytological atypia is mild or absent and mitotic figures are variable. There is little tendency for formation of vascular channels but individual endothelial cells often contain intracytoplasmic vacuoles. In the background, scattered mononuclear inflammatory cells and eosinophils may be seen.

Clinical features
History and presentation
Lesions consist of a papule or nodule presenting in an adult, with a predilection for the trunk and limbs and, less commonly, involving the face. Multiple lesions are exceptional [1,4,5]. A lesion arising in a capillary malformation has been reported [6]. Immunosuppression may play a role in a subset of cases [7].

Disease course and prognosis
There is no tendency for recurrence after surgical treatment.

Management
Simple excision is the treatment of choice.

Acquired elastotic haemangioma [1,2]

Definition
This is a distinctive vascular lesion that develops in sun-exposed skin in association with solar elastosis.

Epidemiology
Incidence and prevalence
This is a rare lesion.

Age
Middle-aged to elderly people.

Sex
Predilection for females.

Ethnicity
Patients have fair skin.

Pathophysiology
Predisposing factors
The development of the lesion is clearly associated with sun exposure.

Pathology
Lesions are well circumscribed and consist of a superficial band-like proliferation of capillaries in the background of solar elastosis. Each capillary is surrounded by a layer of pericytes.

Clinical features
History and presentation
Lesions present mainly on the forearms or neck as a small red or blue circumscribed and asymptomatic plaque.

Disease course and prognosis
Lesions are benign and there is no tendency for local recurrence after excision.

Management
Simple excision is the treatment of choice and there is no tendency to local recurrence.

Hobnail haemangioma [1,2,3,4]

Definition and nomenclature
This is a benign vascular dermal proliferation characterised by small channels lined by endothelial cells with little cytoplasm and a prominent dark nucleus (hobnail cells). Formation of small papillae is also often seen. The original name proposed for this condition (targetoid haemangioma) was based on a distinctive targetoid clinical appearance produced by bleeding and haemosiderin deposition. However, only a minority of lesions present with this typical appearance and therefore the alternative name of hobnail haemangioma has been proposed. The denomination of superficial haemosiderotic lymphovascular malformation has been proposed and has been used synonymously [5–7].

Synonyms and inclusions
- Targetoid haemosiderotic haemangioma
- Superficial haemosiderotic lymphovascular malformation

Epidemiology
Incidence and prevalence
It is relatively uncommon.

Age
It has a predilection for young to middle-aged adults. Some lesions occur in children.

Sex
There is a slight predilection for males.

Pathophysiology
Predisposing factors
Trauma may play a part in its pathogenesis [4]. Occasionally, lesions vary according to the timing within the menstrual cycle [8].

Pathology
Pathological examination shows dilated vascular channels in the papillary and high reticular dermis, with a single layer of endothelial cells lining intraluminal papillary projections. These cells have a hobnail ('matchstick') appearance. They may occasionally be more numerous and appear to fill the lumen of the vessel. The vascular channels tend to disappear in the mid and lower reticular dermis, and the endothelial cells become less prominent and lose the hobnail appearance. Haemosiderin deposition is prominent and can be highlighted with a Perl stain. The endothelial cells stain for the lymphatic marker podoplanin (D2-40), suggesting that these lesions represent lymphangiomas rather than haemangiomas [9]. This has led to the suggestion that lesions represent a form of lymphatic malformation [5]. This is based on the usually negative staining of the endothelial cells in the proliferation for the endothelial cell marker Wilm tumour 1 (*WT1*) gene [6,7]. The pathological appearance may resemble Kaposi sarcoma, but this differential diagnosis can usually be resolved by clinicopathological correlation, as hobnail haemangioma is a solitary entity whereas Kaposi sarcoma is usually composed of multiple lesions. Histological distinction can be made if attention is paid to the symmetry of the lesion, the presence of hobnail endothelial cells with papillary projections and the absence of inflammation in hobnail haemangioma. Furthermore, hobnail haemangioma is not associated with HHV8 while all cases of Kaposi sarcoma are associated with this virus.

Clinical features
History and presentation
This entity presents as a rapidly developing asymptomatic solitary red or brown lesion, which in some cases has a central raised violaceous papule and is surrounded by a paler brown halo (targetoid appearance) [1]. Lesions with a clinical targetoid appearance are easy to diagnose. The anatomical distribution is wide, but it has a predilection for the lower limbs and trunk. The oral mucosa may also be affected [3].

Disease course and prognosis
Lesions are benign and there is no tendency for local recurrence.

Management
Simple surgical excision is the treatment of choice; there is no tendency for recurrence.

Microvenular haemangioma [1,2,3]

Definition
This is a benign dermal vascular lesion characterised by proliferation of small vascular channels with features suggestive of venules.

Epidemiology
Incidence and prevalence
It is relatively rare.

Age
It presents mainly in young adults. Presentation in children is rare [4].

Sex
There is no sex predilection.

Pathophysiology
Pathology
There is a superficial and deep dermal proliferation of angulated thin-walled vascular channels, all of which are surrounded by a single layer of pericytes. These channels look like venules, are lined by flat bland endothelial cells and are surrounded by somewhat hyalinised collagen. A frequent finding is the infiltration of arrector pili muscles by vascular channels. Inflammation is not usually a feature. These lesions are negative for HHV8 [5].

Clinical features
History and presentation
It presents as a solitary red-brown or bluish papule, nodule or plaque with a predilection for the limbs. Most lesions are less than 10 mm in diameter. Multiple lesions are rarely described [6].

Disease course and prognosis
Lesions are benign and there is no tendency for local recurrence.

Management
Simple surgical excision is the treatment of choice.

Sinusoidal haemangioma [1]

Definition
This is a benign dermal and/or subcutaneous variant of cavernous haemangioma composed of thin-walled dilated vascular spaces in a typical sieve-like distribution.

Epidemiology
Incidence and prevalence
Lesions are rare.

Age
It usually presents in adults.

Sex
There is a slight predilection for females.

Pathophysiology
Pathology
The lesion is usually well circumscribed, but several lobules of subcutaneous tissue may be focally affected by the tumour. A striking feature is the presence of back-to-back, dilated and congested thin-walled vascular channels. These channels are interconnected, and transverse sectioning is, in part, responsible for the distinctive sinusoidal appearance. Pseudopapillary projections are focally present and thrombosis with dystrophic calcification may also be seen. Focal cytological atypia secondary to degenerative changes may be seen. Distinction from angiosarcoma, particularly in tumours presenting in the breast, is based on the fact that the latter occurs in the breast parenchyma and only invades the dermis and subcutis secondarily. Tumour cells in angiosarcoma also display cytological atypia, multilayering and mitotic figures.

Clinical features
History and presentation
Sinusoidal haemangioma presents as a solitary blue asymptomatic nodule, particularly on the trunk or upper limbs. The dermis and subcutaneous tissue overlying the breast is not uncommonly involved and may suggest a diagnosis of angiosarcoma (differentiating features are discussed below).

Disease course and prognosis
Lesions are benign with no tendency for local recurrence.

Management
Simple surgical excision is the treatment of choice.

Spindle cell haemangioma [1–5]

Definition and nomenclature
This is a benign vascular neoplasm. Although initially described as a low-grade malignant lesion with a high tendency for local recurrence and minimal potential for metastasis, further studies demonstrated that it is a benign multifocal process [3–5]. Confirmation of its benign nature has led to change of the name 'haemangioendothelioma' for 'haemangioma', as the former implies malignant potential [6].

Synonyms and inclusions
- Spindle cell haemangioendothelioma

Epidemiology
Incidence and prevalence
Spindle cell haemangioma is relatively rare.

Age
The age range is wide but lesions often present in childhood or adulthood.

Sex
Males and females are affected equally.

Pathophysiology
Pathology
Low-power magnification reveals single or multiple fairly well-circumscribed haemorrhagic nodules. Origin from a pre-existing blood vessel is often seen, and individual lesions may be entirely intravascular. Dilated, thin-walled, congested, cavernous-like vascular spaces are intermixed with more cellular areas composed of bland short spindle-shaped cells with the formation of slit-like spaces. Scattered, more epithelioid cells, with pink cytoplasm and prominent vacuolation, are also seen. The spindle-shaped cells are a mixture of endothelial cells, pericytes and fibroblasts. Focal degenerative cytological atypia may be present. Immunohistochemistry reveals staining for CD31 and CD34 and focal staining for smooth muscle actin.

Genetics
R132C *IDH1* and *IDH2* heterozygous mutations identical to those found in the enchondromas of Maffucci and Ollier syndrome have been found in most cases, with improved consistency using novel molecular techniques [7,8].

Clinical features
History and presentation
The process is often associated with lymphoedema, Maffucci syndrome (multiple enchondromas) [9], early-onset varicose veins or Klippel–Trenaunay syndrome. The majority of cases present in the distal limbs, particularly the hands and feet, as multiple cutaneous or subcutaneous, red or bluish nodules. Deeper tumours are rare. Presentation at other sites including the neck and oral cavity is very rare [10,11]. Lesions continue to appear over many years, indicating multifocality rather than true recurrences. Most nodules are less than a few centimetres in diameter; they may occasionally be painful.

Disease course and prognosis
Behaviour is benign but new lesions appear over time.

Management
Single lesions are easily treated with simple excision. Treatment is more difficult in the presence of multiple lesions.

Symplastic haemangioma

Definition
This is not a distinctive variant of haemangioma but represents extensive degenerative changes in a pre-existing haemangioma, closely mimicking malignancy [1,2,3]. Only a handful of cases have been reported. From personal experience with a small number of cases, the pre-existing vascular lesion is often either not identifiable or it represents a cirsoid aneurysm.

Epidemiology
Incidence and prevalence
Lesions are rare.

Age
It presents in adults.

Sex
There is no sex predilection.

Pathophysiology
Pathology
These tumours are often polypoid and well circumscribed, and do not tend to be ulcerated. The typical histological picture consists of dilated and congested, thin- to thick-walled vascular spaces surrounded by a variable cellular stroma with frequent myxoid change and haemorrhage. Stromal cells and smooth muscle cells

within the vessel walls show variable cytological atypia, consisting of nuclear enlargement and hyperchromatism. The endothelial cells lining the vascular spaces may be plump but do not display cytological atypia, multilayering or mitotic activity, allowing distinction from an angiosarcoma. Often cells have a bizarre appearance and multinucleated cells are common. Mitotic figures may be found but tend to be rare. Very occasional atypical mitotic figures may also be seen.

Clinical features

History and presentation
These are not distinctive. However, the patient is usually an adult, and the description is usually of a longstanding lesion that has rapidly increased in size.

Disease course and prognosis
Lesions are benign.

Management
Simple excision is the treatment of choice.

Poikilodermatous plaque-like haemangioma

Definition
This is a newly described entity that most likely represents a true haemangioma [1,2] with an indolent course. It clinically resembles poikilodermatous mycosis fungoides, but has a different histological appearance, emphasising the need for clinicopathological distinction from mycosis fungoides.

Epidemiology

Incidence and prevalence
Lesions are rare.

Age
It presents in the elderly.

Sex
There is a marked male predilection.

Pathophysiology

Pathology
There is a diffuse band-like vascular proliferation of thin-walled vascular channels in the papillary and superficial reticular dermis. The vessels have features of post-capillary venules and are lined by a single layer of cytologically bland endothelial cells without mitoses. Only focal lobular arrangement of vessels is noted. The endothelial cells are positive for CD31 and ERG. Dilated surrounding D2-40 positive lymphatic vessels may be present. The overlying epidermis is usually somewhat acanthotic, and there is often a background of dermal oedema and fibrosis, with diminished elastic fibres within the proliferation.

Clinical features

History and presentation
It presents as a slowly growing and asymptomatic, solitary (rarely multiple), large, red or violaceous atrophic plaque, predominantly in elderly males on the lower extremities and pelvic girdle.

Disease course and prognosis
Lesions are benign.

Management
The majority of patients receive no treatment because the lesions are stationary. Early distinction from mycosis fungoides is important to prevent unnecessary investigation and treatment.

VASCULAR TUMOURS OF INTERMEDIATE MALIGNANCY

Retiform haemangioendothelioma
[1,2,3]

Definition and nomenclature
Retiform haemangioendothelioma is a rare variant of low-grade angiosarcoma with a tendency for local aggressive behaviour. It is characterised by arborising vascular channels lined by endothelial cells with hobnail morphology.

Synonyms and inclusions
- Hobnail haemangioendothelioma

Epidemiology

Incidence and prevalence
Tumours are rare.

Age
Presentation is mainly in young adults.

Sex
There is no sex predilection.

Pathophysiology
Pathology
Scanning magnification is distinctive and reveals an infiltrative tumour composed of arborising, thin-walled, narrow, vascular channels with a striking resemblance to the rete testis. Vascular spaces are lined by bland hobnail endothelial cells with prominent nuclei and scanty cytoplasm. Intravascular papillae with collagenous cores, similar to those seen in papillary endolymphatic angioendothelioma, are sometimes seen. The surrounding stroma often appears hyalinised; a prominent mononuclear inflammatory cell infiltrate is common. The endothelial cells stain for vascular markers. The lineage is likely to be lymphatic but positivity for lymphatic endothelial cell markers such as podoplanin is not consistently demonstrated [4]. There is no relationship to HHV8.

Genetics
Recurrent *YAP1* and *MAML2* gene rearrangements have been found in retiform haemangioendothelioma [5].

Clinical features [1,2,3,6]
History and presentation
Retiform haemangioendothelioma presents as a slowly growing asymptomatic dermal and subcutaneous plaque or nodule. Lesions rarely present as a bruise [7]. Presentation with multiple lesions is exceptional [8]. Rarely, there is an association with lymphoedema or radiotherapy and in one case the tumour arose in the setting of a cystic lymphangioma [9].

Disease course and prognosis
Local recurrence occurs in up to 60% of cases. At the time of writing there has only been one report of a tumour metastasising to a regional lymph node, and a further lesion has spread locally to soft tissues [10]. No tumour-related deaths have been reported.

Management
Wide local excision is the treatment of choice.

Papillary intralymphatic angioendothelioma [1]

Definition and nomenclature
Defining this entity is difficult because since its original description in 1969, few further convincing cases have been described [1–4]. Furthermore, the original series included some examples of what is now known as retiform haemangioendothelioma. Recently, the tumour has been better characterised under the preferred name of 'papillary intralymphatic angioendothelioma' (PILA) [5]. It belongs to the family of tumours with hobnail endothelial cells and it is characterised by dilated cavernous-like lymphatic spaces with frequent papillary projections.

> **Synonyms and inclusions**
> - Endovascular lymphatic angioendothelioma
> - Dabska tumour

Epidemiology
Incidence and prevalence
Tumours are very rare.

Age
It presents mainly in infants and children, with 25% of the cases occurring in adults.

Sex
There is no sex predilection.

Pathophysiology
Pathology
This tumour is composed of dilated thin-walled channels simulating a cavernous lymphangioma. These channels are lined by bland hobnail endothelial cells with very rare mitotic figures. A striking feature is the formation of intraluminal papillary tufts with hyaline cores. Aggregates of mononuclear inflammatory cells may be seen around the vascular channels.

Clinical features
History and presentation
Presentation is as a slowly growing asymptomatic plaque or nodule with a predilection for the limbs.

Disease course and prognosis
In the original series of six cases, a tendency for local recurrence and metastasis to regional lymph nodes was reported [1], but in a series of 12 cases, none of the eight cases with follow-up recurred locally or metastasised [5]. It therefore seems likely that the behaviour of this tumour is benign. Further studies are needed to confirm whether it deserves to be kept in the group of tumours of intermediate behaviour.

Management
Until the issue regarding the biological behaviour of this tumour is resolved, complete excision is recommended.

Composite haemangioendothelioma [1,2,3–5]

Definition
This is a tumour defined as a vascular neoplasm made of a mixture of varying proportions of different histological patterns including benign, low grade and/or malignant.

Epidemiology
Incidence and prevalence
Tumours are very rare.

Age
Most tumours present in adults although cases in children have been described exceptionally.

Sex
There is no sex predilection.

Pathophysiology
Pathology
Tumours are infiltrative and occupy the dermis and subcutaneous tissue. There is presence of at least two morphologically distinct vascular tumour elements that most often resemble retiform haemangioendothelioma and epithelioid haemangioendothelioma but may include spindle cell haemangioma, lymphangioma circumscriptum, papillary intralymphatic angioendothelioma haemangioendothelioma. Cases with a component resembling conventional angiosarcoma are exceedingly rare and should be diagnosed only after true angiosarcoma has been ruled out. There is a distinctive subset with neuroendocrine differentiation that has a predilection for deep locations and displays more aggressive behaviour [2].

Genetics
Recurrent *YAP1* and *MAML2* gene rearrangements have been found in composite haemangioendothelioma, with *PTBP1-MAML2* fusion reported more frequently in the few analysed cases with neuroendocrine differentiation [3].

Clinical features
History and presentation
The tumours present predominantly on the limbs, with a predilection for the hands and feet, as longstanding nodules or plaques, red or blue in colour, and often haemorrhagic. Most lesions are several centimetres in diameter and lymphoedema is a common occurrence. Rare patients have associated Maffucci syndrome [4].

Disease course and prognosis
It is possibly determined by the tumour with the highest histological grade. There is an increased tendency for local recurrence and lymph node metastases have been documented [5], and the neuroendocrine variant has been associated with systemic spread and lethal outcome.

Management
Complete excision is the treatment of choice.

Pseudomyogenic haemangioendothelioma [1,2,3,4–6]

Definition and nomenclature
A low-grade, rarely metastasising malignant vascular. It is often multifocal, lacking histological vasoformative features and displaying features that mimic epithelioid sarcoma or a myogenic tumour [1,2,3].

Synonyms and inclusions
- Fibroma-like epithelioid sarcoma
- Epithelioid sarcoma-like haemangioendothelioma

Epidemiology
Incidence and prevalence
Tumours are rare.

Age
It has a predilection for young adults but a smaller number of tumours develop in older individuals.

Sex
There is marked predilection for males.

Pathophysiology
Pathology
Tumours are infiltrative and consist of sheets of cells many of which have abundant pink cytoplasm simulating rhabdomyoblasts. A smaller percentage of cells are spindle shaped or purely epithelioid. Nuclei are vesicular and a small nucleolus is often seen. Cytological atypia that can be pronounced is observed in a small percentage of cases. Mitotic activity is low and up to half of the tumours contain abundant neutrophils [3]. Tumour cells are usually positive for the pankeratin marker AE1/AE3 and also for vascular endothelial cell markers mainly FLI1 and ERG. CD31 is only positive in 50% of cases. Other keratins, mainly MNF116, are usually negative. Nuclear staining for FOSB is a consistent finding [6].

Genetics
Recurrent translocations resulting in a *SERPINE-FOSB* and *ACTB-FOSB* fusion genes have been described [7,8].

Clinical features
History and presentation
The evolution of the tumours is usually short, frequently less than 2 years. Almost 70% of patients present with multiple discontinuous nodules that affect the dermis and subcutis, and often deeper soft tissues including skeletal muscle (up to half of patients). Bone involvement is seen in 20% of cases [3]. Most tumours present on lower limbs, less commonly on the trunk and upper limbs and very rarely on the head and neck. Pain is a frequent symptom and tumours are usually less than 3 cm in diameter.

Disease course and prognosis
About 60% of patients develop local recurrence or development of similar lesions in the same area. Regional lymph node metastasis was reported in one case and only two patients have died of the disease [1,3].

Management
Complete surgical excision is the treatment of choice.

MALIGNANT VASCULAR TUMOURS

Angiosarcoma [1,2–4]

Definition and nomenclature
This is a malignant vascular tumour arising from both vascular and lymphatic endothelium. Except for the pure epithelioid variant of angiosarcoma (see later), cutaneous angiosarcoma almost exclusively occurs in three settings: idiopathic angiosarcoma of the face, scalp and neck [2–4], angiosarcoma associated with chronic lymphoedema (Stewart–Treves syndrome) [5–9] and post-irradiation angiosarcoma [10–12]. In this chapter, the terms 'angiosarcoma' and 'lymphangiosarcoma' are used interchangeably.

Synonyms and inclusions
- Malignant haemangioendothelioma
- Haemangiosarcoma
- Lymphangiosarcoma

Epidemiology
Incidence and prevalence
Angiosarcoma of the scalp and face of the elderly is very rare.

Stewart–Treves syndrome occurs in 0.5% of patients who survive mastectomy for more than 5 years and the mean interval between mastectomy and the appearance of the tumour is 10.5 years [9]. Not all patients have received radiotherapy in association with the mastectomy and not all have had axillary nodes removed. Lymphoedema is not invariably present, or it may be late in appearing and antedate the tumour by only a short time. The incidence and cause of postmastectomy lymphoedema have been reviewed [13]. In the majority of cases, the clinical course and autopsy findings have shown that the treatment of the breast carcinoma was successful and that patients have had less frequent involvement of the axillary nodes than usual [9]. A small number of cases have arisen in lymphoedema of the lower limb, or in the upper limb without breast cancer and mastectomy [14]. Most of these patients were women. Multiple primary malignancies have occurred in 8% of cases of Stewart–Treves syndrome [6] and a systemically acting carcinogen has been suggested [8,9]. There is no evidence to support this.

Post-irradiation angiosarcoma is rare and most cases arise in the skin after radiotherapy for breast or, less commonly, internal cancer [10–12].

Angiosarcoma occurring in other settings is very rare. Angiosarcoma may also exceptionally occur in association with vascular grafts and orthopaedic prostheses [15], benign vascular tumours including vascular malformations [16], in a large blood vessel [17], in association with a plexiform neurofibroma in neurofibromatosis [18], in a schwannoma [19], in a malignant peripheral nerve sheath tumour [20,21], in xeroderma pigmentosum [22], in a gouty tophus [23], in association with vinyl chloride exposure [24], in association with immunosuppression in organ transplantation [25] and as the mesenchymal component in a metaplastic carcinoma [26]. An exceptional case of an angiosarcoma producing granulocyte colony-stimulating factor and inducing a leukaemoid reaction has been described [27].

Age

- Angiosarcoma of the scalp and face of the elderly by definition affects patients in the seventh to ninth decades of life and only rarely patients in the sixth decade of life.
- Stewart–Treves syndrome: the mean age at appearance of the angiosarcoma is 62 years.
- Post-irradiation angiosarcoma: occurs mainly in adults, predominantly old-aged patients.
- Angiosarcoma occurring in other settings: mainly adults. Presentation in children is extremely rare [28].

Sex

- Angiosarcoma of the scalp and face of the elderly affects mainly males.
- Stewart–Treves syndrome and post-irradiation angiosarcoma affects mainly women. Two cases of Stewart–Treves syndrome have been reported in men following mastectomy [29].
- Angiosarcoma occurring in other settings: there is no sex predilection.

Pathophysiology
Pathology [4,30–32]
In the well-differentiated tumour, vascular channels infiltrate the normal structures in a disorganised fashion, as if trying to line every available tissue space with a layer of endothelial cells. The collagen is characteristically lined by tumour cells in a pattern that has been described as 'dissection of collagen' (Figure 136.20). Tumour cells may be plumper than normal, double-layered in places and form solid intravascular buds. The pattern of growth is more suggestive of lymphatic vessels than blood vessels, but both are probably involved. Haemorrhage is often prominent. Less well-differentiated tumours show more atypical pleomorphic endothelial cells, often with spindle cell morphology, which may be heaped into several layers or become syncytial. Advancing malignancy may be associated with loss of vascular pattern and proliferation of cell masses. Rare cases are composed of granular cells [33]. In exceptional cases, tumours may be extensively infiltrated by lymphocytes or macrophages. In these cases, distinction from a lymphoma may be difficult [34,35].

Immunohistochemical studies have indicated that membranous staining for CD31 and nuclear staining for ERG are the most reliable markers for routine use, compared with antibodies against CD34 and von Willebrand factor (now rarely used) [7,36]. However, a panel of antibodies including three markers is recommended in difficult cases as positivity to the different markers varies. An antibody against the carboxy terminal of the FLI-1 protein, a nuclear transcription factor member of the ETS family of DNA-binding transcription factors, has been shown to be a fairly specific marker of endothelial cells [37].

Genetics
Most analysed cases have shown complex karyotypes, without recurrent chromosomal abnormalities [38]. Angiogenesis-related and vascular-specific receptor tyrosine kinase genes are usually upregulated. A subset of cases in younger patients exhibiting epithelioid morphology and poorer survival are associated with *CIC* gene abnormalities [39]. *MYC* gene amplification and overexpression by immunohistochemistry has been demonstrated mainly in post-irradiation angiosarcomas [40]. However, it may also occur in other types of cutaneous angiosarcomas [41].

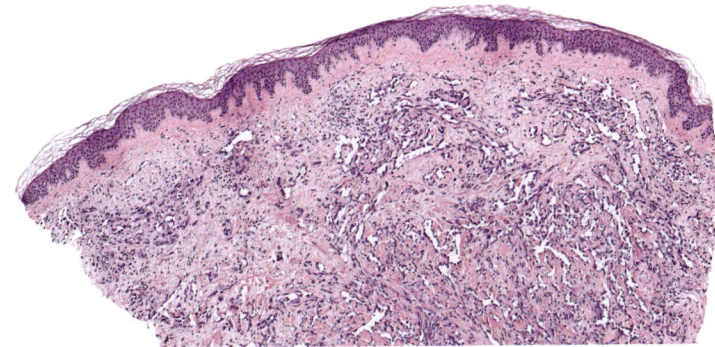

Figure 136.20 Well-differentiated angiosarcoma, with thin-walled irregular vascular channels lined by atypical endothelial cells. Note the dissection of collagen pattern.

Clinical features

History and presentation [3,4,42,43]

In all types of angiosarcoma, the first sign may be an area of bruising, often thought by the patient to be traumatic (Figure 136.21). Dusky blue or red nodules develop and grow rapidly, and fresh discrete nodules appear nearby. In some cases, haemorrhagic blisters are a prominent feature. As the tumours grow, the oedema may increase and older lesions may ulcerate. Multifocality is a very frequent finding; this makes surgical excision very difficult, particularly in those cases occurring on the face and scalp. Dissemination occurs early, with the first visceral deposits usually being in the lung and pleural cavity.

Disease course and prognosis

Most studies reporting outcomes have confined their attention to idiopathic angiosarcoma of the face, neck and scalp, in which the reported 5-year survival is low, at between 12% and 33% [3,44]. Angiosarcomas arising in the setting of chronic lymphoedema and after radiotherapy appear to be equally aggressive. Combined series of idiopathic angiosarcoma of the face and scalp, other cutaneous angiosarcomas and angiosarcomas occurring in internal organs report 5-year survival rates varying between 24% and 34% [1,45,46,47]. Features found to affect prognosis vary between different studies. Tumour size and completeness of excision appear to be more reliable factors to predict outcome [27]. It has been suggested that a high mitotic count correlates with poor prognosis and that a heavy mononuclear inflammatory cell infiltrate correlates with good prognosis [3,5,27]. A recent study of cutaneous sporadic angiosarcomas, excluding those associated with radiotherapy or with chronic lymphoedema, has found by univariate analysis that factors associated with higher mortality include older age, lesions on the trunk and limbs compared with those on the head and neck, necrosis and epithelioid cell morphology [48]. Tumours with necrosis and epithelioid morphology were classified as high risk and confirmed by multivariate analysis to be associated with higher mortality. The depth of invasion correlated with higher risk of local recurrence. The caveat with this study is that it combines traditional head and neck angiosarcomas with those showing a purer epithelioid cell morphology that usually occurs elsewhere and are usually classified under a different category.

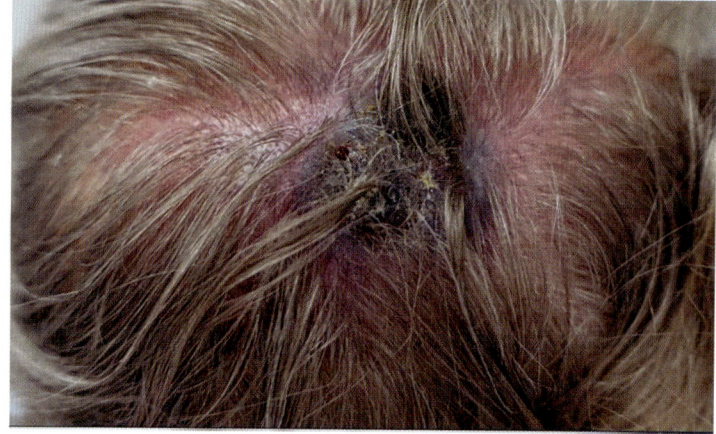

Figure 136.21 Typical haemorrhagic appearance of an angiosarcoma.

Management [3]

All angiosarcomas, regardless of the setting in which they occur, have a bad prognosis. In the less malignant types, wide excision and grafting has controlled some cases. The response to radiotherapy alone is disappointing and is usually only palliative. In the early stages of angiosarcoma of a limb, radical amputation may offer a hope of cure. In idiopathic angiosarcoma of the head and neck, a very small percentage of patients with smaller lesions (usually less than between 5 and 10 cm in diameter at presentation) can be successfully treated with radical wide-field radiotherapy and surgery [1,45,46,47]. The best chance of survival in these patients resides in wide surgical excision followed by radiotherapy [49]. A combination of radiotherapy and taxanes (paclitaxel and docetaxel), the latter used for induction and maintenance therapy, has been shown to improve the overall survival of patients with cutaneous angiosarcoma compared with those treated with surgery and radiotherapy [50]. Combination of taxanes and anthracyclines has also been described to have some effect in the control of disease [51]. As in other types of sarcoma, anti-angiogenic therapy in the treatment of angiosarcoma has not yet produced the expected promising results [52]. The best approach to the management of these tumours is by individualising cases in a multidisciplinary setting.

Epithelioid haemangioendothelioma [1,2,3]

Definition

Epithelioid haemangioendothelioma is a distinctive tumour characterised by epithelioid endothelial cells arranged in strands or as individual units, in a myxoid or hyalinised stroma. It was initially described as a low-grade malignant tumour, but was subsequently classified as a fully malignant neoplasm, in view of the associated morbidity and mortality [3]. However, small primary cutaneous lesions appear to have an indolent behaviour.

Epidemiology

Incidence and prevalence

This tumour may occur in many internal organs, and it is more commonly seen in deeper soft tissues. Involvement of the skin may occur primarily or as a result of direct extension from a deep-seated primary. Fewer than 10% of cases occur primarily in the skin [4].

Age

There is predilection for middle-aged adults.

Sex

Males are equally affected than females.

Pathophysiology

The neoplasm is infiltrative and is composed of strands, cords and nests of endothelial cells in a hyaline or myxoid stroma. Dermal lesions often consist of a fairly well-defined nodule. The tumour cells have epithelioid morphology and consist of pink cytoplasm, vesicular nuclei and inconspicuous nucleoli. Angiocentricity is commonly seen and tumours often arise from a medium-sized vein or even an artery. Formation of vascular channels is not readily apparent but a common finding is the presence of intracytoplasmic vacuoles with or without red blood cells. A small number of cases display cytological atypia, which may be prominent, and a high mitotic count. There is no clear correlation between cytological grade and behaviour. Occasional tumours overlap with epithelioid angiosarcoma. Staining for endothelial cell markers, including ERG and CD31, is usually positive, and 20–30% of cases are focally positive for keratin [3,5]. Podoplanin (D2-40) is also frequently positive in tumour cells.

Genetics
Most tumours show a translocation t(1;3) (p36.3;q25) that results in fusion of the WWTR1 and CAMTA1 genes [6–9]. In a group of tumours, a novel fusion, involving genes YAP1 and TFE3 on chromosomes 11 and X, respectively, has been demonstrated.

Clinical features [1,2,3]
History and presentation
Cutaneous tumours are usually small, but deeper lesions are often several centimetres in diameter. Pain is a frequent complaint, probably due to angiocentricity. Involvement of other organs, including the lung, liver and bone, may be seen in some cases, and it is not clear whether this represents multicentricity or metastatic spread.

Disease course and prognosis
Purely cutaneous tumours appear to have a benign behaviour, but there is some tendency for local recurrence. Deeper tumours have a recurrence rate of up to 15% and a mortality rate of 20% [1,2,3].

Management
Complete excision with clear margins is essential.

Epithelioid angiosarcoma [1–3,4]

Definition
A distinctive variant of angiosarcoma composed almost exclusively of endothelial cells with an epithelioid morphology, often mimicking a carcinoma. This tumour represents the malignant end of the spectrum of tumours with epithelioid cell morphology.

Epidemiology
Incidence and prevalence
This is a rare tumour that mainly occurs in deep soft tissue but that may present primarily in the skin or other organs.

Age
There is a predilection for young to middle-aged adults.

Sex
Males are more frequently affected.

Pathophysiology
Pathology [1–3,4]
Sheets of atypical epithelioid cells with abundant pink cytoplasm, vesicular nuclei and a single eosinophilic nucleolus occupy the dermis and/or subcutis. Haemorrhage and haemosiderin deposition is often seen. Formation of vascular channels is not readily apparent and the main feature is the presence of intracytoplasmic vacuoles with or without red blood cells in variable numbers of tumour cells. Mitotic figures are common. Tumour cells are variably positive for vascular markers including ERG, CD31, CD34, FLI-1 and von Willebrand factor. In 50% of cases, there is positivity for cytokeratin. Focal positivity for epithelial membrane antigen is also seen in 25% of cases [4]. Ordinary angiosarcomas such as those occurring on the head of elderly patients, those associated with radiotherapy and those associated with chronic lymphoedema may display focal areas with epithelioid endothelial cells. These tumours should not be classified as epithelioid angiosarcomas.

Genetics
CIC gene abnormalities were shown to occur in angiosarcomas with epithelioid morphology affecting younger patients, with an inferior disease-free survival [5].

Clinical features [1–3,4]
History and presentation
Cutaneous tumours present in young to middle-aged adults, with a predilection for the extremities. The typical presentation is that of solitary, or more rarely multiple, asymptomatic papules or nodules which are often haemorrhagic. It is not clear whether multiple lesions represent multifocality or metastatic disease. Occasional cases have been reported in association with a foreign body [6], radiotherapy [1] or an arteriovenous fistula [7]. Epithelioid angiosarcoma arising in another organ may present with cutaneous metastases [8].

Disease course and prognosis
Although it was initially suggested that cutaneous epithelioid angiosarcoma has a relatively good prognosis, this was based on only very few cases with limited follow-up [2]. Overall, the behaviour of these tumours appears to be aggressive with a mortality rate of more than 55% after 3 years [4].

Management
Complete excision and close follow-up are indicated.

LYMPHATIC TUMOURS

Kenneth Y. Tsai
Departments of Dermatology & Immunology, University of Texas MD Anderson Cancer Center, Houston, TX, USA

Cavernous lymphangioma, cystic hygroma and lymphangioma circumscriptum are described in Chapter 103.

Acquired progressive lymphangioma

Definition and nomenclature
This is a benign dermal tumour composed of irregular lymphatic channels dissecting between collagen bundles.

Synonyms and inclusions
- Benign lymphangioendothelioma

Epidemiology
Incidence and prevalence
Tumours are very rare.

Age
There is a predilection for middle-aged adults but children may be affected.

Sex
Males are slightly more affected than females.

Pathology [1–3,4]
Low-power examination reveals an ill-defined often pan-dermal proliferation of irregular thin-walled lymphatic channels dissecting between collagen bundles. These channels tend to be orientated parallel to the epidermis and are lined by a single layer of bland endothelial cells. Involvement of the subcutaneous tissue is rare. Distinction from the lymphangiomatous variant of Kaposi sarcoma is often very difficult, but in the former there are aggregates of inflammatory cells including plasma cells and the cells lining the vascular channels are usually positive for HHV8. Distinction from a well-differentiated angiosarcoma is based on the absence of cytological atypia and mitotic figures.

Clinical features [1–3,4]
Lesions typically present as slow-growing nondescript solitary vascular or pigmented, 0.3–10 cm macules or papules on the head and neck, and less frequently on the oral mucosa, extremities and trunk [4]. Multiple lesions are exceptional [3].

Management
Excision is all that is required; there is no tendency for local recurrence [1,4,5]. Recently, pulsed dye laser has been successfully used [6].

Atypical vascular proliferation after radiotherapy [1–3,4,5–7]

Definition and nomenclature
Atypical vascular proliferation after radiotherapy (AVPR) defines a group of vascular lesions that occur months or years after radiotherapy – mainly, but not exclusively, after breast cancer. Lesions may also present after radiotherapy for ovarian and endometrial carcinoma.

Synonyms and inclusions
- Atypical post-radiation vascular lesion

Epidemiology
Incidence and prevalence
These lesions are rare.

Age
Most patients are middle-aged to elderly.

Sex
Almost all cases affect females.

Associated diseases
AVPRs have been described almost exclusively in the context of prior radiation therapy for breast cancer, particularly breast-conserving therapy with adjuvant radiation therapy, although cases related to radiation therapy for multiple myeloma, cervical carcinoma, Hodgkin disease, ovarian cancer, endometrial carcinoma and melanoma have been reported [4].

Pathophysiology
MYC gene amplification and overexpression by immunohistochemistry has been demonstrated in post-irradiation angiosarcomas but not in AVPRs and this is an important aid in differential diagnosis [8].

There is a clear aetiological link with radiotherapy [1–3,4,5–7]. The demonstration of staining of the endothelial cells for lymphatic markers suggests a lymphatic line of differentiation. Although the relationship between AVPR and post-radiation angiosarcoma has been controversial, the more commonly accepted view is that AVPR represents part of a spectrum of lesions with post-radiation angiosarcomas [4]. Most AVPR are banal but occasionally progression from AVPR to angiosarcoma is seen.

Pathology (Figure 136.22)
Irregular lymphatic-like vascular channels, lined by a single layer of endothelial cells, are seen in the dermis and may be multifocal. The endothelial cells are flat or have a hobnail appearance, and papillary projections can also be found. Careful examination of multiple sections is recommended.

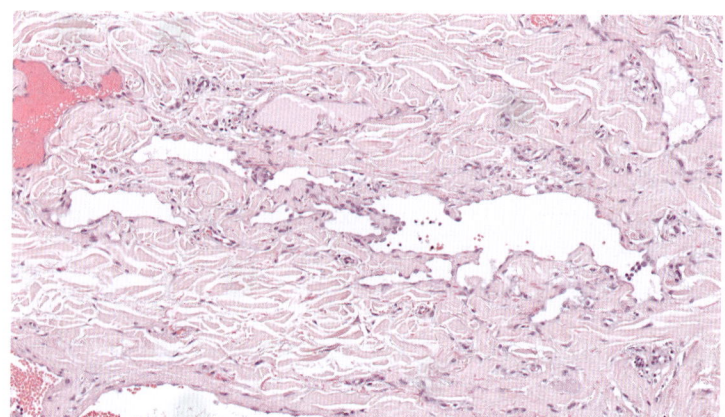

Figure 136.22 Histopathology of atypical vascular proliferation after radiotherapy.

Clinical features
History
AVPR presents a few years or months after radiotherapy for breast cancer (by comparison, post-irradiation angiosarcomas usually but not always tend to present many years after radiotherapy) [1–3]. As acute and chronic radiation dermatitis typically stabilises within 3 years, changes noted after this period should prompt suspicion of AVPR. The median latency period following radiation exposure is 5–6 years [4,6,7,9].

Presentation
Characteristic lesions are solitary or grouped red to violaceous macules, papules, nodules or vesicles. These may range in size from 0.3 to 20 cm, with surrounding ecchymoses, induration or telangiectasia [1,4,6,9].

Disease course
Although usually benign in clinical course [1,7], the ultimate outcome is somewhat indeterminate as a result of recurrence, development of new AVPRs, angiosarcoma present upon re-excision (5/11 in one series) and transition from AVPR to angiosarcoma within 2 years in a handful of cases [2,4,9,7].

Prognosis
Most lesions behave in a benign fashion. However, as mentioned before, it is controversial whether these lesions are uniformly benign or whether they overlap with radiation-induced angiosarcoma.

Management
There is no standardised management algorithm and practices differ widely. Given that there have been several reports of AVPR being reclassified as angiosarcoma upon re-excision [6] and transition to angiosarcoma as early as within 2 years [4,9], wide excision and close clinical follow-up are appropriate, although even in instances where margins were reported to be clear, recurrence was common.

Diffuse lymphangiomatosis

Definition and nomenclature
A rare condition characterised by extensive and variable involvement of the viscera (particularly the lung), bone, soft tissue and occasionally the skin by lymphatic malformations.

> **Synonyms and inclusions**
> - When involving bone, it is sometimes referred to as Gorham syndrome, Gorham–Stout disease or disappearing/vanishing/phantom bone disease

Introduction and general description
Diffuse lymphangiomatosis can involve the bone, lungs, spleen, liver, soft tissue and skin, as well as other structures in the thorax [1]. Though histologically benign, the space-occupying nature of the lesions, with the generation of effusions, can severely compromise organ function leading to death. The disease is thought to be congenital, with most clinical presentations in childhood. There is no strong sex predominance or pattern of inheritance [2–7].

Pathophysiology
Pathology
The histological findings are similar to those of acquired progressive lymphangioma except that they are not confined to the dermis, often penetrating into the subcutis, involving soft tissue, fascia, muscle and organ parenchyma [8,9]. Involvement of the skin is relatively uncommon in Gorham–Stout syndrome [6,7,**10**], though it can be extensive over affected bone [9]. Haemangiomata are also reported, involving bone, soft tissue and overlying skin [8]. The endothelial cells lining the dilated vascular spaces express CD31, factor VIII, UEA-1, LYVE-1, VEGF-R3, VEGF-C and podoplanin, consistent with lymphatic origin [1,8,9,11].

Clinical features
The clinical features reflect the degree and site of involvement. Pulmonary involvement manifests as cough or dyspnoea, and bone involvement with pain, pathological fracture and osteolytic lesions. Any part of the skeleton may be involved. Diffuse pulmonary disease has a poor prognosis complicated by chylothorax, pleural and pericardial effusions, and infection. Skin involvement is typified by overlying haemangiomata or lymphangiomata [1–3,5–7], and lymphangiomatosis should be considered if accompanied by symptoms of bone or pulmonary involvement.

Management
Generally, treatment is supportive including the draining of effusions, placement of shunts and sclerotherapy. Radiation therapy and surgical correction of skeletal defects can be successful early in the clinical course [1,**10**,12]. Responses to interferon α-2b and bisphosphonates have been reported for bone involvement [3,13]. Anecdotal successes have been reported with sirolimus [14], bevacizumab [15] and propranolol [16].

TUMOURS OF PERIVASCULAR CELLS

Infantile myofibromatosis and adult myofibroma [1–6]

Definition and nomenclature
This tumour is composed of cells showing differentiation towards perivascular contractile cells and has been described in the past as infantile haemangiopericytoma [7]. Infantile myofibromatosis and adult myofibroma/myofibromatosis are best regarded as part of the spectrum of lesions described more recently as myopericytomas (see later) [8,9].

> **Synonyms and inclusions**
> - Congenital generalised fibromatosis
> - Infantile haemangiopericytoma

Epidemiology

Incidence and prevalence
Solitary lesions both in children and adults are relatively rare. Multiple lesions are uncommon.

Age
Most cases of infantile myofibromatosis, present before the age of 2 years, with slight male predominance. Congenital tumours occur in up to a third of the cases. Solitary myofibroma tends to occur in adults, with the same anatomical distribution as that of cutaneous and soft-tissue lesions presenting in infantile myofibromatosis [5,6]; multiple superficial tumours are rarely seen in adults. Intraoral lesions tend to be more common in young adults [10,11].

Sex
Tumours are more common in males.

Pathophysiology

Predisposing factors
Rare myopericytomas but not classic myofibromas are associated with Epstein–Barr virus and have been reported in patients with HIV/AIDS [12] (see Chapter 31).

Pathology [1,2,5,6,7,8]
Tumours have a distinctive biphasic growth pattern:
- Areas composed of bundles of mature spindle-shaped myofibroblasts with pink cytoplasm and vesicular nuclei.
- Areas composed of immature round cells, with scanty cytoplasm arranged around small blood vessels, often displaying a haemangiopericytoma-like pattern ('staghorn-like').

Protrusion of tumour cells into vascular lumina is frequent, often mimicking vascular invasion. Old lesions often undergo hyalinisation of the more mature areas. Mitotic figures and necrosis are relatively common. Tumour cells, particularly in the mature areas, are focally positive for actin.

Genetics
A germline mutation in *PDGFRB* is encountered in familial infantile myofibromatosis cases [13]. Recurrent somatic *PDGFRB* mutations have also been demonstrated in sporadic infantile/solitary adult myofibromas [14].

Clinical features [1–3]

History and presentation
Presentation is usually as single or solitary nodules that may be skin coloured or blue/red. Multiple lesions are present in 25% of patients. The preferred sites are the head and neck, followed by the trunk. Familial cases are rare. Involvement of other organs, including the gastrointestinal tract, lungs and bone, is seen in some cases. Multicentric involvement may be associated with mortality. Multiple lesions in the skin and soft tissues behave in a benign fashion and may regress spontaneously. Exceptionally, associated thrombocytopenia has been reported [15].

Disease course and prognosis
Lesions tend to regress spontaneously, but it is important to remember that patients with visceral tumours may die from the disease. Solitary lesions do not tend to recur locally.

Management
Simple excision is the treatment of choice for solitary lesions.

Myopericytoma

Definition
For many years, tumours thought to differentiate towards pericytes (perivascular myoid cells) were divided into two main categories: infantile haemangiopericytoma and adult haemangiopericytoma. Both variants, however, appear to have very little in common except for the histological presence of a pericytomatous pattern characterised by elongated branching thin-walled vascular spaces with a stag-horn pattern. With the combination of immunohistochemistry and electron microscopy, most tumours previously classified as adult haemangiopericytoma on light microscopy represent other tumours, including synovial sarcoma, mesenchymal chondrosarcoma and solitary fibrous tumour [1]. In very few cases the line of differentiation remains obscure, and these represent the 'true' adult haemangiopericytomas. They are more likely to arise from an undifferentiated mesenchymal cell than from a pericyte. 'True' adult haemangiopericytomas do not usually occur in the skin and will not be discussed further here.

The concept of myopericytoma was introduced to describe a group of lesions characterised by short oval to spindle-shaped myofibroblasts and a characteristic concentric perivascular growth [2]. Tumours tend to be mainly deep dermal and subcutaneous, and include lesions classified in the past as glomangiopericytoma, myopericytoma, myofibroma and myofibromatosis in adults. Infantile haemangiopericytoma and infantile myofibromatosis represent identical conditions and the former term has been abandoned.

Infantile myofibroma/myofibromatosis has already been described in the section on myofibroblastic tumours.

Epidemiology

Incidence and prevalence
Tumours are relatively rare.

Age
Most lesions present in middle-aged adults.

Sex
There is no sex predilection.

Pathophysiology

Pathology
The histological spectrum of myopericytoma is wide and varies from lesions that are very similar to myofibromatosis, to tumours that closely resemble glomus tumours and even to angioleiomyoma. Tumours in all the latter categories are regarded as belonging within the same spectrum. Lesions are well circumscribed and composed of a mixture of solid cellular areas intermixed with variable numbers of vascular channels. The latter are often elongated and display prominent branching, resulting in a stag-horn appearance (haemangiopericytoma-like). The cells in the solid areas are bland, round or short and spindle shaped with eosinophilic

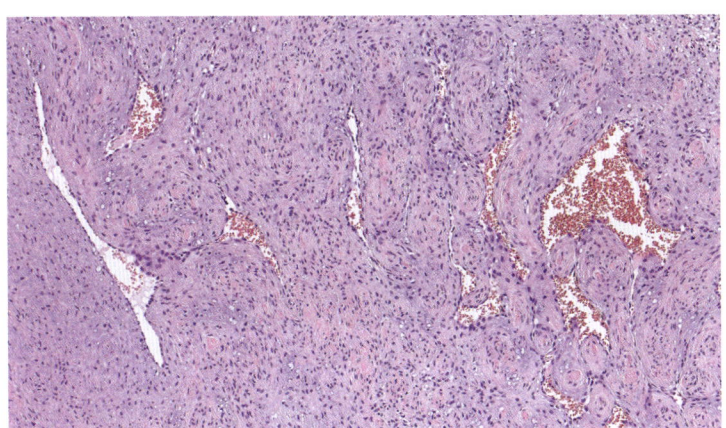

Figure 136.23 Numerous vascular channels surrounded by layers of pericytes in a case of myopericytoma.

or amphophilic cytoplasm and vesicular nuclei. Mitotic figures are exceptional. A common feature is the presence of concentric layers of tumour cells around vascular channels resulting in a typical onion-ring appearance (Figure 136.23). Myxoid change may be focally prominent. Occasional findings include hyalinisation, cystic degeneration and bone formation. Nodules of tumour cells may protrude into the lumina of vascular channels. Rare examples are entirely intravascular [3]. In some cases, tumour cells closely resemble glomus cells and are characterised by round punched-out central nuclei and pale eosinophilic cytoplasm. These cases are referred to as glomangiopericytomas. Tumour cells are positive for smooth muscle actin and in most cases negative for desmin.

Genetics
PDGFRB alterations have been demonstrated in myopericytoma [4].

Clinical features
History and presentation
Myopericytoma is relatively rare and presents mainly in middle-aged adults with a predilection for the limbs, especially the distal lower limb. Lesions are small (no more than 2 cm in diameter), longstanding, usually asymptomatic and may be solitary or, rarely, multiple [2,5,6]. Exceptionally, they are painful. In the setting of multiple myopericytomas, these often develop simultaneously with a predilection for a single anatomical site.

Disease course and prognosis
Behaviour is benign even in cases with an intravascular location. Very rarely, malignant examples of myopericytoma have been reported [7].

Management
Simple excision is the treatment of choice.

Glomus tumour [1–3]

Definition and nomenclature
A tumour of the myoarterial glomus, composed of vascular channels surrounded by proliferating glomus cells. The tumours have variable quantities of glomus cells, blood vessels and smooth muscle. According to this finding, they are classified as either solid glomus tumour, glomangioma or glomangiomyoma.

> **Synonyms and inclusions**
> - Glomangioma
> - Glomangiomyoma

Epidemiology
Incidence and prevalence
Glomus tumours are comparatively uncommon.

Age
Some are present at birth; they rarely appear during infancy, but from the age of 7 years onwards the incidence increases gradually. Multiple tumours are 10 times more frequent in children than in adults [3,4]. Tumours in adults present mainly during the third or fourth decades of life.

Sex
There is no sex predilection.

Pathophysiology
Pathology
The tumour is lobulated, well circumscribed and situated in the dermis. The proportion of glomus cells to vascular spaces varies. The smaller painful lesions tend to be mainly cellular. The larger, multiple and often painless lesions are angiomatous, with only a band of cells around the dilated vascular channels. The glomus cell is cuboidal, with a well-marked cell membrane and a round central nucleus. The cells align themselves in rows around the single layer of endothelial cells of the vascular spaces and in a somewhat less orderly fashion further out. More than 50% of tumours can be classified as glomangiomas and a minority (fewer than 15%) are classified as glomangiomyomas (Figure 136.24). Electron microscopy [5–7] suggests that glomus cells are transversely cut smooth muscle cells and that there are many mast cells around the tumour, but that nerve fibres are not associated with the glomus cells. Tumour cells are

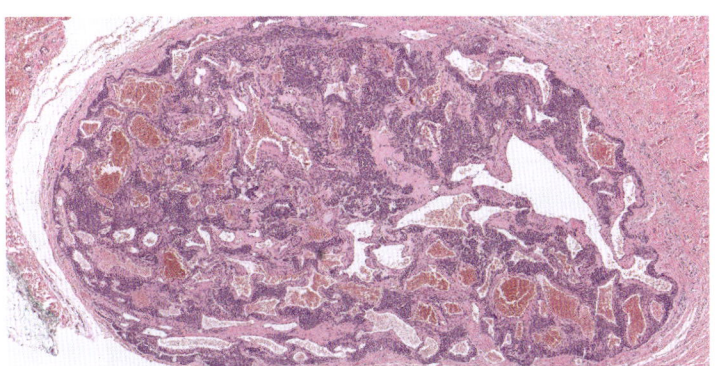

Figure 136.24 A typical case of glomangiomyoma displaying vascular channels, smooth muscle and thin layers of glomus cells.

universally positive for smooth muscle actin and are usually negative for desmin. Positivity for CD34 may be seen [8]. An oncocytic variant has been described [9], and also variants developing within a cutaneous nerve [10] and within a vein [11]. Malignant glomus tumour (glomangiosarcoma) is exceedingly rare. Even cutaneous tumours that are histologically malignant rarely metastasise, but they have a potential for local recurrence [12,13].

Genetics
NOTCH gene fusions have been demonstrated in a number of benign and malignant glomus tumours [14].

Clinical features
History and presentation
A solitary glomus tumour is a pink or purple nodule varying in size from 1 to 20 mm; it is conspicuously painful (Figure 136.25). Pain may be provoked by direct pressure or a change in skin temperature, or may be spontaneous. The commonest site is the hands, particularly the fingers, followed by other sites on the extremities including the head, neck and penis [15]. Tumours beneath the nail are particularly painful, and patients present for treatment while the lesions are still very small. The affected nail has a bluish-red flush. An association between subungual glomus tumour and neurofibromatosis type 1 has been reported [16,17]. Glomus tumours may also involve internal organs.

Multiple glomus tumours are larger and usually dark blue in colour, and are situated deep in the dermis. They are less restricted to the extremities, may be widely scattered and are not usually painful [18–21]. In some cases, grouped multiple tumours may be painful, and pain, intermittent discoloration and sweating of a limb may precede the development of a palpable tumour.

Differential diagnosis
The solitary tumour is to be distinguished from other painful tumours such as leiomyoma and eccrine spiradenoma. Distinction is usually only possible on histological examination. The multiple glomangioma may be indistinguishable clinically from a cavernous haemangioma and is possibly identical to 'blue rubber bleb' naevus [5].

Disease course and prognosis
Local recurrence is very rare and occurs mainly after incomplete excision. Most recurrences are seen in deeper lesions with an infiltrative growth pattern [21]. These lesions have been described as infiltrating glomus tumours [22].

Management
Surgical excision is usually curative.

PERIPHERAL NEUROECTODERMAL TUMOURS

Neural tumours are reviewed in [1,2].

Neuromuscular hamartoma [1,2]

These lesions appear to be combined hamartomas of both muscular and neural tissue. The clinical appearance is of a subcutaneous mass. Multinodular masses of skeletal muscle are mixed with both myelinated and unmyelinated nerve fibres. Malignant triton tumours, composed of a mixture of schwannoma-like material and rhabdomyosarcoma, are very much commoner than the benign variety of triton tumour. Surgical excision is required.

Synonyms and inclusions
- Triton tumour

Dermal hyperneury [1,2,3]

Increase in the amount of dermal nerve fibres has been noted in normal skin of patients with multiple endocrine neoplasia type 2b [1]. Rarely, dermal hyperneury can manifest in other familial cancer syndromes, such as Cowden syndrome. Solitary and multiple presentation has been described outside the syndromic setting as well [2,3]. The clinical appearance in those cases is that of pink or skin-coloured papules. On histology, well-formed and conspicuous nerves, unusually large for the level of cutis, are present within the lesions.

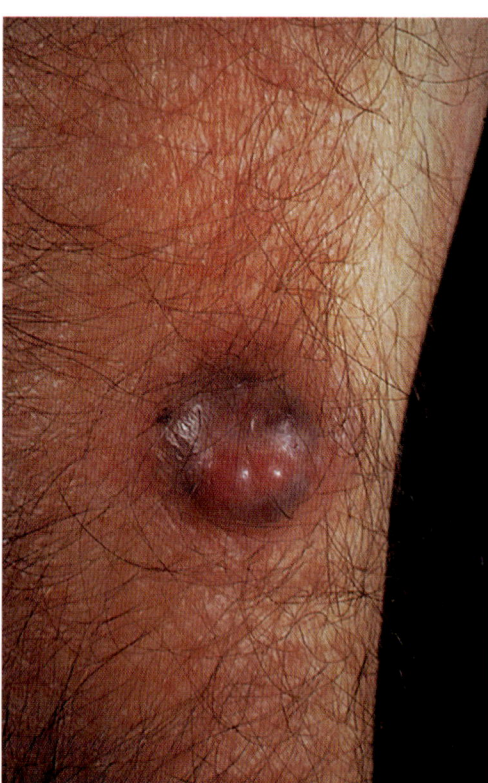

Figure 136.25 Clinical appearance of a glomus tumour.

Morton neuroma [1,2]

Definition and nomenclature
This is the result of damage to the plantar digital nerve, followed by fibrosis. The condition has been associated with the use of high-heeled footwear.

Synonyms and inclusions
- Morton metatarsalgia

Epidemiology
Incidence and prevalence
It is rare.

Age
Adults.

Sex
Most common in females.

Pathophysiology
Pathology
On pathological examination, there is very prominent perineurial, endoneurial and epineurial fibrosis. Perivascular fibrosis and intimal thickening are also seen.

Clinical features
History and presentation
Patients complain of severe pain, usually between the third and fourth metatarsals, especially when walking.

Management
Excision is the recommended therapy and is curative.

Solitary circumscribed neuroma

Definition and nomenclature
This is a distinctive variant of cutaneous neuroma composed of variable proportions of the normal components of nerve tissue.

Synonyms and inclusions
- Palisaded encapsulated neuroma

Epidemiology
Incidence and prevalence
Lesions are relatively common.

Age
Most cases present in adults.

Sex
There is equal sex incidence.

Synonyms and inclusions
- Multiple cutaneous neuromas

Multiple mucosal neuromas [1]

Multiple neuromas of the oral mucosa are a feature of Sipple syndrome (multiple endocrine neoplasia type 2) and may be associated with phaeochromocytoma, parafollicular thyroid cysts secreting calcitonin, medullary thyroid carcinoma and opaque nerve fibres on the cornea (Chapter 148).

Synonyms and inclusions
- Sipple syndrome
- Multiple endocrine neoplasia type 2

Amputation stump neuroma [1]

Definition and nomenclature
This is a benign response of nerve tissue to injury.

Synonyms and inclusions
- Traumatic neuroma

Pathophysiology
Pathology
Foci of proliferating nerve tissue surrounded by scar tissue are typically seen (Figure 136.26). Accessory digits may show a very similar pattern of tissue involvement.

Clinical features
History and presentation
A small tender nodule is found in a scar site.

Management
Surgical excision is usually required. The problem can be prevented by apposing the ends of nerves at the sites of injury.

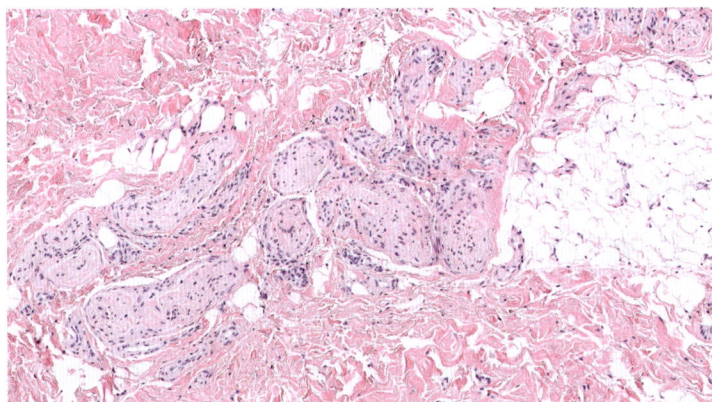

Figure 136.26 Histological appearance of an amputation neuroma. Small nerves proliferate in the dermis in a background of fibrosis.

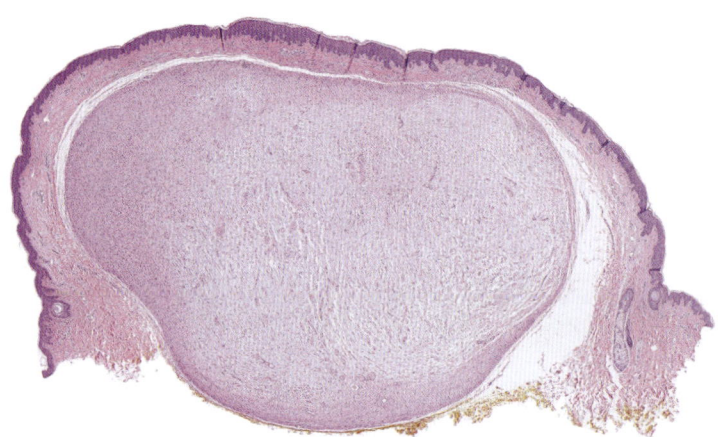

Figure 136.27 Sharply demarcated dermal nodule in a case of solitary circumscribed neuroma.

Pathophysiology
Pathology [1,2,3]
Examination reveals a well-circumscribed partially encapsulated dermal nodule (Figure 136.27), often associated with a nerve in the deep dermis. It is composed of uniform cells with pink cytoplasm in a collagenous background and with artefactual clefting between bundles. The capsule displays epithelial membrane antigen-positive perineurial cells. Most of the cells within the nodule are S100 protein positive and special stains may demonstrate axons.

Clinical features [1,2,3]
History and presentation
It is fairly common and presents mainly on the face of adults as a small asymptomatic papule, which may resemble a naevus.

Disease course and prognosis
Lesions are benign.

Management
Simple excision is curative.

Schwannoma

Definition and nomenclature
A tumour of nerve sheaths composed of Schwann cells.

Synonyms and inclusions
- Neurilemmoma

Epidemiology
Incidence and prevalence
The tumour is relatively rare in the skin and relatively uncommon in other sites including soft tissues.

Age
It may occur at any age but is most common in the fourth and fifth decades.

Sex
Females are affected more often than males [1].

Pathophysiology
Pathology [2,3]
The tumour is rounded, circumscribed and encapsulated. It is situated in the course of a nerve, usually in the subcutaneous fat. The cells are spindle shaped with poorly defined cytoplasm and elongated wavy basophilic nuclei. Variable amounts of collagen are seen in the background. Cells are arranged in bands, which stream and interweave. The nuclei display palisading and are arranged in parallel rows with intervening eosinophilic cytoplasm in a typical appearance known as Verocay bodies (Figure 136.28). Cellular areas known as Antoni A areas are intermixed with areas showing prominent myxoid change known as Antoni B areas [4]. The latter areas are likely to be the result of degeneration. In some tumours, there is mucous secretion, producing a vacuolated stroma. Scattered mononuclear inflammatory cells are often seen. In some cases, the nerve of origin may be found associated with the capsule. Electron microscopy shows that tumour cells have typical features of Schwann cells [5]. S100 protein staining is strong and uniform [6]. For many years, it was thought that schwannomas lack axons and this was regarded as a useful way of distinguishing these tumours from neurofibromas, which contain variable numbers of axons. The presence of the latter is demonstrated by immunostaining for neurofilaments. This view, however, has been challenged as both hereditary and sporadic schwannomas may contain axons, suggesting that both entities may in fact be more closely related than previously thought [7]. This explains the rare occurrence of hybrid lesions combining features of neurofibroma and schwannoma [8].

There are several variants of schwannoma, some of which may be confused histologically with other benign or malignant tumours:
1. *Hybrid schwannoma/perineuriomas* are tumours that have two clearly defined populations of cells, Schwann cells and perineural cells positive for S100 protein and EMA, respectively [9].
2. *Ancient schwannoma* [10] often occurs in a deep location and is characterised by prominent degenerative changes, which often result in cytological atypia. Ectatic blood vessels, haemorrhage,

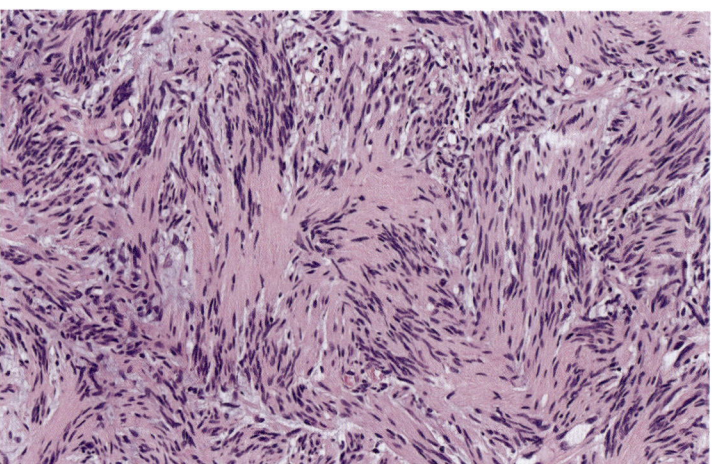

Figure 136.28 Typical Verocay body in a case of schwannoma.

haemosiderin deposition and focal inflammation consisting of lymphocytes are often seen. There is loss of Antoni A areas, which makes histological diagnosis difficult.

3 *Cellular schwannoma* [11] also tends to have a predilection for deep soft tissues. It is characterised by high cellularity, with almost complete absence of Antoni B areas. This, coupled with the presence of mitotic figures, often leads to a misdiagnosis of malignancy [12]. A multinodular plexiform variant may occur in children and some examples are congenital.
4 *Plexiform schwannoma* [13,14] tends to occur in younger patients, may be painful and has a predilection for the dermis. Multiple cellular nodules composed of bland Schwann cells are seen in the dermis. Distinction from plexiform neurofibroma is important, as these tumours are not usually associated with neurofibromatosis type 1. Multiple cutaneous plexiform schwannomas, however, are associated with neurofibromatosis type 2 [1,15].
5 *Malignant melanotic schwannian tumour (previously known as melanotic schwannoma)* [16] only exceptionally occurs in the skin; it has a predilection for spinal nerve roots. Tumour cells are epithelioid and melanin pigment is prominent. The importance of this variant is that these tumours previously regarded as benign have now been classified as malignant and may be a marker of Carney complex (Chapter 148) [17]. These neoplasms are characterised by *PRKAR1A* inactivating mutations [18].
6 *Pacinian schwannoma* is a rare variant composed of structures closely resembling the Pacinian corpuscles.
7 *Neuroblastoma-like schwannoma* is very rare and characterised histologically by areas composed of round blue small Schwann cells which may form perivascular rosettes or rosettes with collagenous cores [19]. The tumour in other areas has the typical appearance of a schwannoma and the immunohistochemical profile is typical of the latter.
8 *Epithelioid schwannoma* is an infrequent type of schwannoma composed predominantly of cells with epithelioid morphology [20]. However, although these tumours are positive for S100 protein, they lack palisading, are composed of uniform tumour cells and contain a population of CD34-positive cells. It has therefore been proposed that these lesions do not represent classical examples of schwannomas [21].
9 *Glandular schwannoma* [22,23] represents in most cases an ordinary schwannoma with entrapment of normal sweat glands.

Genetics
Inactivation of the *NF2* gene has been demonstrated as the main genetic event in sporadic schwannomas, as well as in schwannomatosis [24].

Clinical features [25]
History and presentation
It arises most frequently from the acoustic nerve. Bilateral acoustic schwannomas are characteristic of neurofibromatosis type 2. A further manifestation of the latter is the occurrence of multiple cutaneous plexiform schwannomas. There is no association with neurofibromatosis type 1. In the peripheral nervous system, it is usually found in association with one of the main nerves of the limbs, usually on the flexor aspect near the elbow, wrist or knee, the hands or the head and neck [25]. It may be seen on the tongue. Other sites include the wall of the gastrointestinal tract and the posterior mediastinum. They are rounded or ovoid circumscribed nodules varying in size up to 5 cm, usually firm (but sometimes soft and cystic) in consistency and sometimes painful. The colour is pink-grey or yellowish. Small lesions may be intradermal, but larger ones are subcutaneous. They usually grow slowly.

Disease course and prognosis
Most tumours are benign. Malignant transformation of a schwannoma is exceedingly rare and may contain areas of epithelioid angiosarcoma [26,27,28].

Management
Simple excision is curative. Wider margins should be obtained for malignant melanotic schwannian tumour.

Solitary neurofibroma [1,2,3,4]

Definition
An isolated lesion probably arising from the endoneurium and composed of a mixture of Schwann cells, fibroblasts and perineurial fibroblasts. It is not related to neurofibromatosis type 1. Although it was regarded as hamartomatous in nature, the demonstration of clonality suggests a neoplastic origin [5].

Epidemiology
Incidence and prevalence
Lesions are relatively common.

Age
Tumours are more common in adults.

Sex
There is no sex predilection.

Pathophysiology
It has been suggested that cutaneous neurofibromas develop as a result of precursor cells that are pluripotent, probably arise from the hair roots and have a NF1 (+/−) genotype [6].

Genetics
Biallelic genetic inactivation of the *NF1* tumour suppressor gene in the Schwann cell population is the sole recurrent somatic event detectable in neurofibroma. RAS/RAF/MEK/ERK and PI3K/AKT/mTOR pathways are involved in *NF1* tumour pathogenesis [7].

Pathology
These lesions differ from schwannomas in that they do not have a capsule, they are only focally positive for S100 protein and they do not have Antoni A and Antoni B areas. Instead, they are composed of bland spindle-shaped cells with wavy nuclei in a myxoid or collagenous stroma. Mast cells are usually prominent. Degenerative changes are sometimes seen but mitotic activity is absent. Tumours

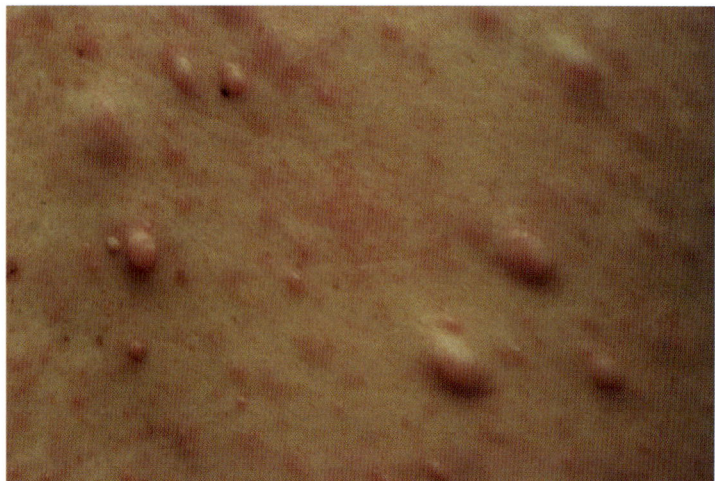

Figure 136.29 Multiple soft papules, typical of neurofibroma in a patient with neurofibromatosis type 1.

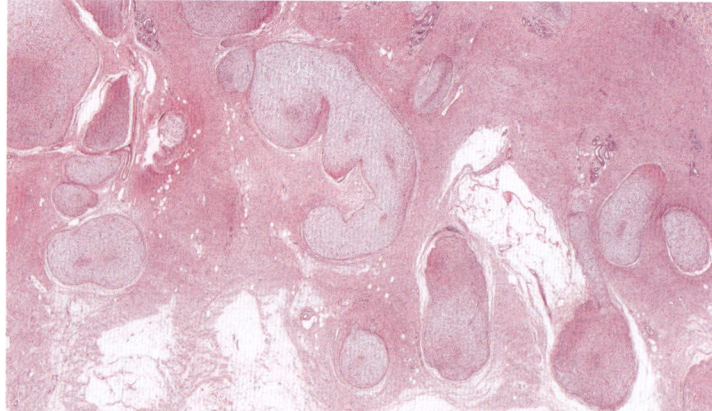

Figure 136.30 Numerous plexiform neural fascicles within plexiform neurofibroma.

with scattered atypical cells (nuclear enlargement and hyperchromatism) are classified as atypical but they are not associated with aggressive behaviour [8]. Fewer than 50% of the cells in these lesions are S100 positive. There is also focal positivity for CD34 and EMA.

Several histological variants of neurofibroma have been described, including epithelioid neurofibroma, granular cell neurofibroma, pigmented neurofibroma [11] and a variant with dendritic cells and pseudorosettes [3,10].

Clinical features
History and presentation
Any body site may be affected. It usually appears as a slow-growing small polypoid lesion. Multiple neurofibromas are rare outside the setting of neurofibromatosis type 1 (Figure 136.29).

Disease course and prognosis
Malignant change is said not to occur outside the setting of neurofibromatosis type 1.

Management
Simple excision is curative.

Plexiform neurofibroma

This tumour is considered to be pathognomonic of neurofibromatosis type 1 (Chapter 78). However, it has been contested whether the presence of a single plexiform neurofibroma in the absence of other signs of neurofibroma can be regarded as pathognomonic of neurofibromatosis type 1 [1,2]. Interestingly, cytogenetic analysis of a sporadic plexiform neurofibroma has shown biallelic inactivation of NF1 [3]. It presents in children and young adults of either sex, with a predilection for the lower limbs and the head and neck. Tumours are large and located in the dermis, subcutis and even deeper soft tissues. The overlying skin is folded and hyperpigmented and the lesion is described as having an appearance and feeling on palpation of a 'bag of worms' (Figure 136.30). This

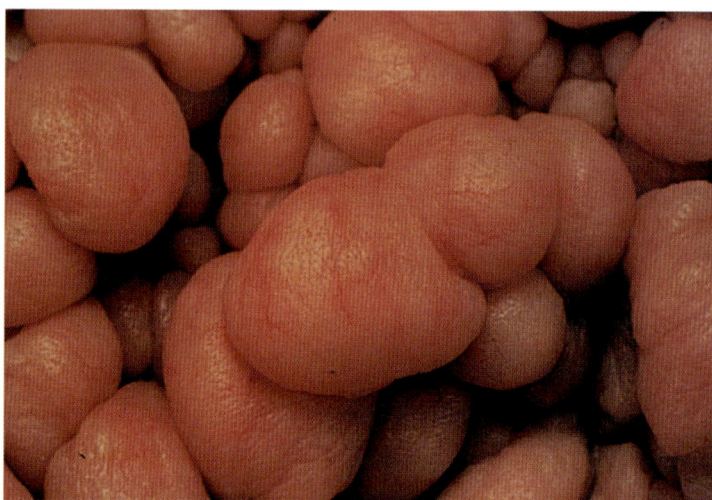

Figure 136.31 Clinical appearance of a plexiform neurofibroma.

reflects the typical histological appearance of nerve trunks of different sizes randomly distributed throughout the involved tissues (Figure 136.31). Careful histological examination of these lesions is necessary because the presence of mitotic activity usually indicates malignant transformation.

Surgical removal of these lesions is usually very difficult because of the extensive involvement. MEK inhibition has been shown to exhibit efficacy in *NF1*-related tumours [4] and the use of MEK inhibitors is likely to increase substantially in NF1 [5]. When planning the surgical removal of these tumours, surgeons should remember that there is a tendency for haemorrhage within the tumour that may lead to morbidity or mortality.

Diffuse neurofibroma

This lesion presents as a diffuse poorly defined induration or plaque-like lesion of the skin and subcutaneous tissue in children or young adults, with a predilection for the trunk and head and neck area. A number of cases are associated with neurofibromatosis type 1. The histological features are identical to those of a solitary neurofibroma except for the fact that there is diffuse replacement of involved tissue by the tumour. Local recurrence is frequent unless the lesion is widely excised. Very rare sporadic tumours recur repeatedly and show a tendency for malignant transformation [1].

Perineurioma [1,2,3,4]

Definition and nomenclature
Perineurioma is a tumour originally described in soft tissues. It is relatively common in the skin and it is composed of cells showing differentiation towards perineural fibroblasts.

Synonyms and inclusions
- Storiform perineural fibroma

Epidemiology
Incidence and prevalence
Lesions are rare.

Age
Most tumours present in young adults.

Sex
There is predilection for females.

Pathophysiology
Pathology
Tumours are well circumscribed and composed of bipolar and slender bland thin spindle-shaped cells with scanty cytoplasm and wavy nuclei. They are often arranged in concentric whorls (Figure 136.32) or in a storiform pattern. Cellularity varies and is low in the sclerosing variant where hyalinised collagen predominates. The architecture may be plexiform in some cases [4]. Tumour cells are distinctively positive for EMA. They are also positive for a tight junction associated protein, claudin-1 [5]. Focal positivity for CD34 may also be seen. Rare cutaneous tumours may be intraneural [6].

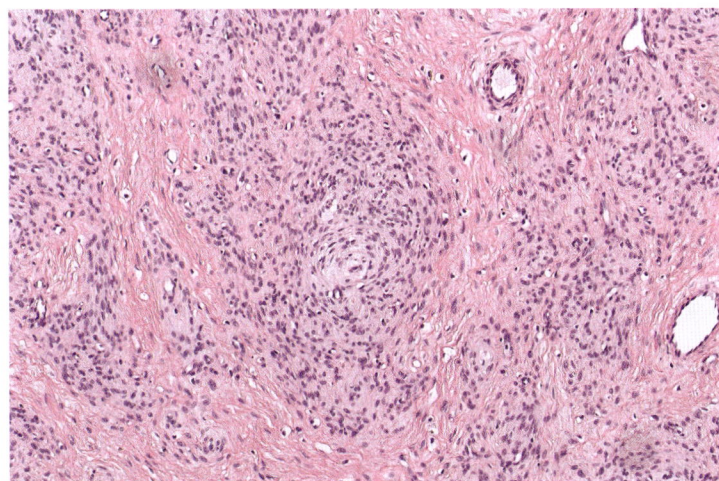

Figure 136.32 Typical whorling appearance and some degree of sclerosis in a case of perineurioma.

Clinical features
History and presentation
The lesion has a predilection for the lower limbs of young females. Tumours are small and asymptomatic. Multiple lesions are exceptional [7]. A distinctive sclerosing variant has been described, affecting most commonly, but not always, the hands [8,9].

Disease course and prognosis
Lesions are entirely benign.

Management
Simple excision is the treatment of choice.

Dermal nerve sheath myxoma [1–3,4]

Definition and nomenclature
This is a myxoid tumour that is thought to display nerve sheath differentiation.

Synonyms and inclusions
- Neurothekeoma

Epidemiology
Incidence and prevalence
Tumours are rare.

Age
Young adults.

Sex
There is predilection for males.

Pathophysiology
Pathology [1–3]
The dermis shows a well-defined tumour composed of lobules that vary in size and shape and are separated by fibrocollagenous stroma. Each lobule is composed of slender stellate or spindle-shaped Schwann cells with bland nuclei and indistinct cytoplasm margins in the background of prominent myxoid change. Mitotic figures are very rare. Tumour cells are uniformly positive for S100. They are also positive for glial fibrillary acid protein and CD57 [4]. EMA-positive cells are seen in the periphery of tumour lobules. These tumours have no relationship with the so-called cellular neurothekeoma [5].

Clinical features [1,2,4]
History and presentation
This presents most commonly on the upper limbs (particularly the fingers and hands) and lower limbs (mainly the knees, shins or feet). The trunk and head and neck are rarely affected. Lesions are longstanding, small, usually less than 1 cm, skin coloured and asymptomatic.

Disease course and prognosis
Tumours are benign but there is some tendency for local recurrence [4].

Management
Simple excision is the treatment of choice.

Cellular neurothekeoma [1–4]

Definition
Despite its name, this tumour is not related to dermal nerve sheath myxoma, and its line of differentiation has not been established. Gene expression profiles of this tumour has suggested that they may be related to fibrous histiocytoma [5]. The tumour should not be confused with ordinary nerve sheath myxomas showing focal cellular areas [1–3].

Epidemiology
Incidence and prevalence
Tumours are relatively common.

Age
The age range is wide but most cases occur in children and young adults.

Sex
It is more common in females.

Pathophysiology
Pathology
In the dermis and frequently extending into the subcutis [6], there is an ill-defined tumour composed of nests and fascicles of epithelioid or spindle-shaped cells (Figure 136.33) with vesicular nuclei and a single small eosinophilic nucleolus. Lesions presenting in the face may extend into the underlying skeletal muscle. Mitotic figures are relatively common and scattered multinucleated cells may be seen. Myxoid change is present in some lesions and it may be extensive [7]. Tumour cells resemble melanocytes and this often leads to the lesion being confused with a melanoma. However, there is no junctional activity, and cells are invariably negative for S100 protein, HMB45 and melan-A. Rare tumours display perineural extension [7,8]. Some tumours are larger in size, have more cytological atypia and increased mitotic count, and these tumours have been classified as atypical cellular neurothekeoma [4,6,8]. However, this does not seem to be related to a more aggressive behaviour. Tumour cells are often positive for smooth muscle actin (in about 57% of cases), NKI-C3, neuron-specific enolase, PGP 9.5 and microphthalmia transcription factor [6,9]. The tumours are negative for Sox10, which is useful in the distinction from melanocytic and nerve sheath tumours [10]. A rare plexiform tumour with hybrid features of perineurioma and cellular neurothekeoma and predilection for the lips has been described [11].

Clinical features
History and presentation
The tumour presents as a small asymptomatic papule with a predilection for the upper limbs and face and neck [4,6]. Multiple lesions are exceptional [12].

Disease course and prognosis
There is very little tendency for local recurrence even in cases classified histologically as atypical.

Management
Simple excision is curative.

Granular cell tumour [1,2,3]

Definition and nomenclature
A tumour composed of cells with characteristic granular cytoplasm. The histogenesis of the classic granular cell tumour seems to be neural [4,5]. However, it is worth remembering that many tumours of different histogenesis may show granular cell change, due to the cytoplasmic accumulation of secondary lysosomes.

> **Synonyms and inclusions**
> - Abrikossoff tumour
> - Granular cell myoblastoma

Epidemiology
Incidence and prevalence
Tumours are rare.

Age
It is usually seen between the fourth to sixth decades of life. It can occur in childhood.

Sex
It is more common in males than females.

Pathophysiology
Pathology
Large polyhedral cells arranged in sheets, which infiltrate the dermal connective tissue and subcutaneous fat, form the tumour. The cytoplasm is pale and contains brightly acidophilic granules.

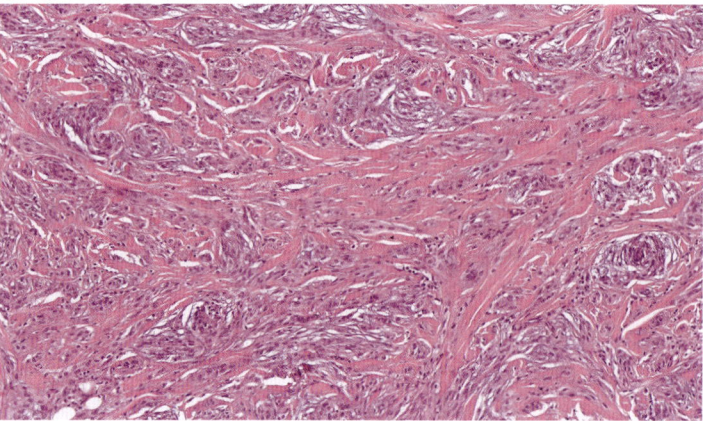

Figure 136.33 Cellular neurothekeoma. Nests of epithelioid cells in the background of a hyalinised stroma. In cases with cytological atypia and mitotic activity, confusion with a melanoma is more likely.

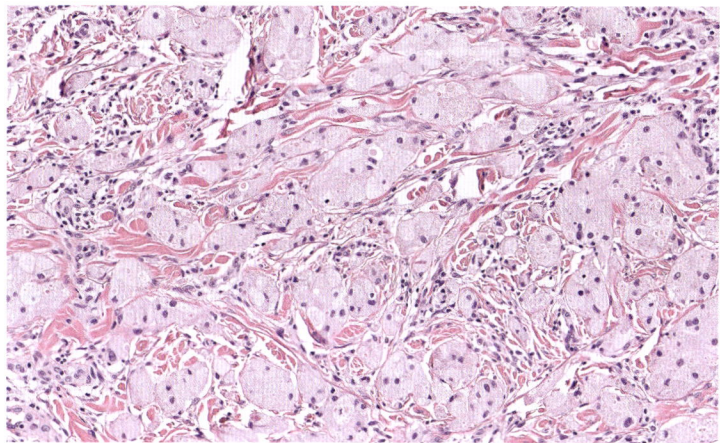

Figure 136.34 Abundant eosinophilic and granular cytoplasm in a case of granular cell tumour.

Tumour cells often display large eosinophilic granules surrounded by a clear halo and known as pustulo-ovoid bodies of Milian [6]. The nuclei are relatively small and round, and tend to be vesicular. Clear cell change may occasionally be prominent [7]. The epithelium over the area may show pseudoepitheliomatous hyperplasia and in small biopsies this may be confused with a squamous cell carcinoma (Figure 136.34). Perineural extension is often seen. Vascular invasion may be seen occasionally and this does not seem to have any bearing on behaviour [8]. Occasionally, tumour cells involve the epidermis and distinction from melanoma may be difficult [9]. However, although S100 positivity is seen in both tumours, HMB45 is usually negative in granular cell tumour. It is important, however, to take into account that rare granular cell tumours may show focal positivity for melan-A and that microphthalmia transcription factor is positive in a percentage of tumours [10]. The original suggestion that the cells are myoblasts probably arose from the examination of tumours of the tongue in which infiltration between the striated muscle bundles gave the impression of origin from the muscle. The general belief now is that the cells are of neural or nerve sheath origin.

Genetics

Loss-of-function mutations in the endosomal pH regulators *ATP6AP1* and *ATP6AP2* are found in granular cell tumours and result in the characteristic accumulation of intracytoplasmic granules [11].

Clinical features

History and presentation

The tumour is usually solitary, situated in the skin, beneath the epithelium of the tongue or in deeper soft tissues or internal organs (mainly the gastrointestinal tract) [2,3]. It is firm and rounded but with rather indefinite margins, sessile or pedunculated, and between 5 and 20 mm in diameter, although larger tumours may be seen. A warty appearance may be seen due to epidermal hyperplasia. The colour may vary from flesh colour to pink or greyish-brown. Rare tumours are painful. Multiple tumours may occur both in adults and in children [3]. Multiple lesions have also been reported in Noonan syndrome [12]. The tumour grows slowly. Malignant tumours are very rare.

Disease course and prognosis

Local recurrence is sometimes seen after incomplete excision.

Management

Simple excision is the treatment of choice.

Meningothelial heterotopias [1–3,4,5–8]

Definition and nomenclature

Meningeal heterotopias are defined as lesions with meningothelial elements presenting in the skin and soft tissue and can be the result of heterotopias or secondary extension from a primary central nervous system tumour (see later).

> **Synonyms and inclusions**
> - Cutaneous meningioma

Epidemiology

Incidence and prevalence

All types of meningothelial heterotopias are very rare.

Age

See later.

Sex

There is no sex predilection.

Pathophysiology

Pathology [6–8]

Low-power examination often reveals a lesion with a striking resemblance to a lymphangioma. Irregular dilated spaces are seen dissecting between collagen bundles. The spaces are partially lined by plump epithelioid cells, which are also seen in clusters in the surrounding stroma. Focal formation of psammoma bodies may be present. The dermal collagen and blood vessels also appear to be increased. Some lesions contain more solid areas. The presence of meningothelial cells can be demonstrated by positive staining for EMA. These cells are also positive for p63 but negative for keratins and S100 protein [9].

Clinical features

History and presentation

Meningeal heterotopias were divided into three groups by Lopez *et al*. [4]. The first two groups of lesions represent meningothelial heterotopias or hamartomas (ectopic meningothelial hamartoma). The main difference between both groups is that affected patients are children in the first group and adults in the second group. The third group consists of intracranial meningiomas that extend secondarily into the skin or soft tissues. This group will not be discussed in more detail here.

A small number of cases of meningothelial heterotopias have been associated with von Recklinghausen disease [1]. The tumour occurs over the scalp or in the paraspinous region of the trunk of children and young adults. Occasionally, it appears to be familial [6]. In the scalp, the area is often bald. The skin is adherent to the mass, which is dermal or subcutaneous, and there may be a central depression with epidermal atrophy or ulceration. A connection with the cranial cavity is not usually demonstrated. The size ranges from 2 to 10 cm.

Management
Simple excision is the treatment of choice.

Glial heterotopic nodules [1,2]

Definition and nomenclature
This represents the presence of heterotopic mature glial tissue in the dermis or subcutis, predominantly on the central face. It may be considered to be a developmental defect in the closure of the neural tube. However, rare cases occur away from the midline, suggesting a different unexplained mechanism for its occurrence [3].

Synonyms and inclusions
- Nasal glioma

Epidemiology
Incidence and prevalence
Lesions are very rare.

Age
Most lesions present in infants and children. Presentation in adults is exceptional.

Sex
There is no sex predilection.

Pathophysiology
Pathology
Nodules of astrocytes in a neurofibrillar background are characteristic. Less commonly, oligodendrocytes are seen; neuronal elements are exceptional.

Clinical features
History and presentation
Most lesions present as a subcutaneous mass on the bridge of the nose. Communication with the cranial cavity is present in up to 20% of cases.

Management
Excision is curative, but it is very important to make sure that an underlying communication with the cranial cavity is ruled out, as failure to do so may result in complications such as meningitis or cerebrospinal fluid leakage.

Epithelial sheath neuroma [1]

Definition
This is a relatively novel, rare and intriguing dermal lesion that combines a neural and an epithelial component. Although some features suggest that this may be a hamartoma, the fact that it has only been described in adults makes this possibility unlikely. A further theory is that the lesions may represent a variant of nerve hyperplasia with epidermal origin [2].

Epidemiology
Incidence and prevalence
Lesions are very rare.

Age
It presents in adults.

Sex
There is no sex predilection.

Pathophysiology
Pathology
Histologically there are scattered prominent nerves in the superficial dermis, encased by mature non-dysplastic squamous epithelium with focal keratinisation and dyskeratotic cells. Immunohistochemistry displays the normal staining of nerves and epidermis, respectively.

Clinical features
History and presentation
In view of the fact that so few cases have been described, very little can be said about the clinical features. The clinical presentation is not distinctive and lesions appear to have a predilection for the back.

Management
Simple excision is the treatment of choice.

Pigmented neuroectodermal tumour of infancy [1,2]

Definition and nomenclature
A pigmented tumour of childhood, combining neural and melanocytic elements. It is thought to recapitulate the early stages of development of the retinal epithelium although the finding of raised urinary excretion of vanillylmandelic acid in some cases, suggest a neural crest derivation [3–6].

Synonyms and inclusions
- Melanotic progonoma
- Retinal anlage tumour
- Melanotic neuroectodermal tumour

Epidemiology
Incidence and prevalence
Tumours are very rare.

Age
Most cases present in infants between 3 and 6 months old. Occurrence in adults is exceptional.

Sex
There is no sex predilection.

Pathophysiology [7,8]
Pathology
A mass of irregular alveolar spaces surrounded by fibrous stroma is seen. Two types of cells are easily recognised: small round blue cells with scanty cytoplasm in a fibrillary matrix, and large epithelioid cells with pink cytoplasm and vesicular nuclei. These cells often contain melanin. Both types of tumour cells stain for synaptophysin and neuron-specific enolase, and are negative for S100 protein. The large cells are positive for cytokeratin and HMB45.

Clinical features
This tumour occurs most frequently in the anterior part of the maxilla and often presents as a pigmented oral mass [9]. It has been reported also in the anterior fontanelle, shoulder, epididymis, femur, mediastinum and even the foot. It may cause a high urinary excretion of vanillylmandelic acid [3]. This tumour has been mistaken for malignant melanoma and could also be confused with a cellular blue naevus. The clinical appearance is that of a rapidly expanding nodule in the jaw, which may affect dentition.

Disease course and prognosis
Although classified as benign, the lesions may cause considerable local destruction, and around 5% of cases may metastasise and prove fatal [10].

Management
Complete surgical excision is the treatment of choice.

Malignant peripheral nerve sheath tumour [1,2]

Definition and nomenclature
A malignant tumour arising from the nerve sheath.

Synonyms and inclusions
- Neurofibrosarcoma
- Malignant schwannoma

Epidemiology
Incidence and prevalence
Tumours are very rare.

Age
Young adults are more commonly affected in the setting of neurofibromatosis type 1. Sporadic cases occur in older individuals.

Sex
Cutaneous tumours usually arise from a plexiform neurofibroma in patients with NF1 [3]. Rare cutaneous lesions may arise within ordinary neurofibromas or *de novo* [4]. Deep-seated lesions arise *de novo* or in association with NF1. Patients with this disease develop malignancy in 30–50% of cases.

Pathophysiology
Pathology
The basic pattern is that of fascicles of tumour cells, often with a herringbone pattern and resembling a fibrosarcoma. Tumour cells tend to concentrate around blood vessels and myxoid change is common. The degree of pleomorphism and the number of mitotic figures varies. S100 is only focally positive and often entirely negative. H3K27me3 loss is a sensitive and specific marker for high grade MPNSTs, particularly outside the NF1 setting [5]. The rare epithelioid variant of the neoplasm consists of sheets of epithelioid cells often mimicking melanoma and tumour cells are usually diffusely positive for S100 but negative for other melanocytic markers, with loss of SMARCB1 on immunohistochemistry in approximately 50% of cases [6].

Genetics
MPNSTs harbour complex karyotypes and usually show inactivating mutations in the *NF1, p16* or *PRCA2* pathways [7], while about a half of epithelioid MPNSTs show *SMARCB1* inactivation.

Clinical features [8]
The diagnosis should be suspected when a previously static tumour in a patient with NF1 begins to enlarge or becomes painful. The pain may become radicular as the lesion progresses but the tumours are not always associated with nerve trunks. The commoner sites are the flexor aspects of the limbs. A minority of cases occur as a complication of radiotherapy.

Disease course and prognosis
Tumours behave in an aggressive manner. Systemic metastases particularly to the lungs are common. The prognosis is worse in cases occurring after previous radiotherapy.

Management
Wide local excision or amputation is necessary.

Cutaneous Ewing sarcoma [1–4,5]

Definition and nomenclature
An undifferentiated small round cell tumour displaying a spectrum of neuroectodermal differentiation.

Synonyms and inclusions
- Peripheral primitive neuroectodermal tumour

Epidemiology
Incidence and prevalence
Tumours are very rare.

Age
Most tumours present in children but presentation is at a later age than conventional Ewing sarcoma [5].

Sex
There is slight predilection for females.

Pathophysiology
Pathology
Tumours are composed of sheets of small blue round cells that are fairly homogeneous, with scanty pale cytoplasm and fine chromatin. Mitotic figures are common. Tumour cells are diffusely positive for CD99 (in a cytoplasmic membrane pattern) and focally positive for FLI-1. NKX2-2 is a sensitive but imperfectly specific marker for cutaneous PNET. Keratin is positive in up to a third of cases.

Genetics
This tumour usually presents a reciprocal chromosome translocation t(11;22)(q24;q12) that is an important aid in diagnosis and can be demonstrated by FISH.

Clinical features
History and presentation
The tumour presents in children and has no distinctive clinical features, although it is often confused with a vascular tumour.

Differential diagnosis
This tumour should be distinguished from undifferentiated round cell sarcomas with *CIC* rearrangement, as the latter show a poor prognosis.

Disease course and prognosis
Cutaneous tumours appear to have a better prognosis than those presenting in deeper soft tissues [4].

Management
Surgical followed by chemotherapy and in some cases also radiotherapy [4].

CIC-rearranged sarcoma [1,2–5]

Definition and nomenclature
A high grade round cell sarcoma with poor prognosis. Other members of the undifferentiated round cell sarcoma group apart from Ewing sarcoma typically involve bones or deeper soft tissue and will not be discussed further.

> **Synonyms and inclusions**
> - *CIC-DUX4* sarcoma

Epidemiology
Incidence and prevalence
Tumours are very rare.

Age
The age range is wide, but there is a striking predilection for young adults.

Sex
There is slight predilection for males.

Pathophysiology
Pathology
The architecture is typically nodular or sheet-like, composed of round cells with necrosis and haemorrhage separated by dense hyaline bands. The cells are characterised by vesicular chromatin, prominent nucleoli and frequent mitotic figures. Spindling and epithelioid/rhabdoid phenotype may be present, and focal myxoid stromal changes are frequent. On immunohistochemistry, the tumours are positive for CD99 and DUX4. Nuclear expression of WT1 and ETV4 is very frequent [2]. ERG and calretinin may be positive.

Genetics
A *CIC* gene rearrangement, most frequently a *CIC-DUX4* translocation, is the defining genetic feature. A significant minority of cases can be missed by FISH testing alone.

Clinical features
History and presentation
Rapid growth within the deep soft tissue with predominant affection of the trunk and limbs. Presentation at various anatomical sites (genital, visceral, other) has been documented. Superficial cases are rare and most represent involvement from deeper soft tissue [5].

Differential diagnosis
The most important distinction is from cutaneous Ewing sarcoma, as the latter shows a much better prognosis.

Disease course and prognosis
Prognosis is poor, with most cases showing rapid metastatic spread and death from disease within 2 years. Based on few anecdotal reports, the rare tumours limited to the dermis appear to have a better prognosis than those presenting in deeper soft tissues.

Management
Surgical followed by chemotherapy and in some cases also radiotherapy.

TUMOURS OF MUSCLE

Smooth muscle hamartoma

Definition and nomenclature [1]
Smooth muscle hamartoma is a proliferation of smooth muscle within the dermis.

> **Synonyms and inclusions**
> - Arrector pili hamartoma
> - Congenital pilar and smooth muscle naevus
> - Congenital smooth muscle naevus

Epidemiology [1,2,3,4]
Incidence and prevalence
It is a rare tumour.

Age
Usually it is congenital. Acquired lesions with onset in puberty or adulthood have been reported.

Sex
There is a slight male predominance.

Pathophysiology
Genetics [5–10]
Familial cases have been reported [5,6]. An association with Xp microdeletion syndrome [7] or with familial paracentric inversion of chromosome 7q and Michelin tyre syndrome has been suggested [8–10].

Pathology [1,2,3,4,5,11–13]
Microscopically, within the dermis or the subcutis, variably orientated bundles of smooth muscle are seen. The overlying epidermis may be acanthotic and hyperpigmented. Follicles may be prominent but are not increased in numbers. Becker naevus may show similar histology; it has been suggested that both lesions may be a part of the same spectrum [14]. Associations with other skin lesions, such as naevus flammeus and blue naevi, have been reported [11,12].

Clinical features [1,2,3,4–15]
History and presentation
The typical presentation is that of a solitary macule or plaque of variable size, which may be associated with hyperpigmentation, hypertrichosis or both. The lumbosacral area, trunk and proximal extremities are the sites of predilection. However, unusual sites such as the head and neck, including the oral cavity, scrotum and conjunctiva have been reported. Sometimes lesions may be atrophic or linear. Another unusual presentation is folding of the skin including Michelin tyre syndrome. Pseudo-Darier sign has been described [16].

Prognosis
It is an entirely benign lesion.

Management
Complete excision is curative in almost every case. This is mainly done for cosmetic reasons.

Leiomyoma

Definition
A benign tumour of smooth muscle derived from the arrector pili muscle (pilar leiomyoma), from the media of blood vessels (angioleiomyoma) or from smooth muscle of the scrotum, labia majora or nipples (genital leiomyoma) [1,2–4,5,6–8].

Epidemiology [1,2–4,5,6–8]
Incidence and prevalence
Tumours in the three types are relatively uncommon. Pilar leiomyoma is the most common. Genital leiomyoma is the least common followed by angioleiomyoma. The cutaneous variety in general is about six times more frequent than the genital type [2].

Age
Pilar leiomyoma (leiomyoma cutis) can occur at any age from birth onwards, but appears usually in early adult life. Genital leiomyoma (dartoic myoma) can occur at any age. Angioleiomyoma is seen mainly in middle-aged adults.

Sex
Pilar and genital leiomyomas present equally in both sexes. Angioleiomyoma is more frequent in females.

Pathophysiology
Pathology [1,2–4,5,6–9]
The smooth muscle cells proliferate to produce interweaving bundles of spindle-shaped cells, which are strongly eosinophilic (Figure 136.35). The nuclei are long and thin, and the general appearance of the mass in ordinary sections may suggest a hypertrophic fibrous reaction. The smooth muscle cells can be distinguished from collagen by their different reaction with trichrome stains, and by the presence of myofibrils, which stain with phosphotungstic acid haematoxylin, and by their blunt-ended nuclei. Tumour cells are positive for actin and desmin. Loss of fumarate hydratase immunohistochemical expression in cutaneous leiomyomas can be helpful in the screening for hereditary leiomyomatosis and renal cancer (HLRCC) [2].

The tumour of pilomotor origin (leiomyoma cutis, multiple cutaneous leiomyomas) is usually composed of numerous dermal nodules with vague margins where the cells penetrate the surrounding collagen bundles and an upper border that approaches

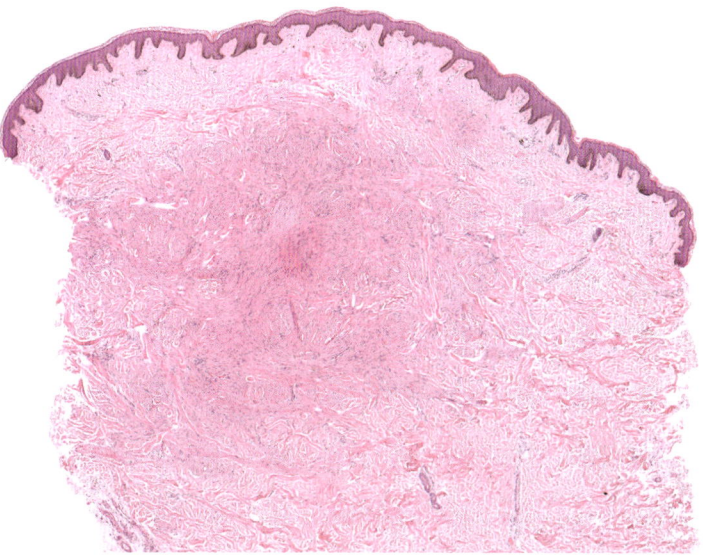

Figure 136.35 Pathology of leiomyoma, showing spindle-shaped cells with eosinophilic cytoplasm arranged in bundles closely resembling the arrector pili muscle.

the papillary body. Associated epidermal hyperplasia is common. Focal nuclear atypia likely to be degenerative in origin and very low mitotic activity (up to one per 10 high-power fields) may be seen without this being indicative of malignant degeneration [1]. Genital leiomyomas are nodular tumours with a similar appearance. Scrotal tumours are less circumscribed and more cellular than those developing in the vulva. The angioleiomyomas are related to veins in the subcutaneous tissue, and are rounded and well circumscribed [4,5]. Vessels of variable thickness are intermixed with bundles of mature smooth muscle. Focal degenerative cytological atypia may be seen, but mitotic figures are absent. Calcification, hyalinisation and thrombosis of vessels are often seen.

Genetics

The gene that predisposes to multiple pilar leiomyomas has been mapped to chromosome 1q 42.3-q43 [10]. It also predisposes to uterine leiomyomas (multiple cutaneous and uterine leiomyomatosis, Reed syndrome (MCUL)) and to renal cancer (mainly papillary renal cell carcinoma) [11–14]. This is as a result of mutations in the gene encoding the enzyme fumarate hydratase. In patients with associated renal cancer, the syndrome is known as hereditary leiomyomatosis and renal cancer (HLRCC).

Clinical features [1,3]

Pilar leiomyoma has been reported in identical twins, in siblings and in several generations of a family. The cases with a familial background have all had multiple tumours and are associated with MCUL and renal cancer syndrome. It generally presents as a collection of pink, red or dusky brown, firm dermal nodules of varying size but usually less than 15 mm diameter (Figure 136.36). The nodules are often subject to episodes of pain and may be tender. The pain can be provoked by touching or chilling the skin, or by emotional disturbance, and is often worse in winter. Some lesions contract and become paler when painful. The condition usually begins with the appearance of one small nodule, which gradually increases in size, and further similar lesions appear nearby or at some other area. Adjacent tumours may coalesce to form a plaque. The areas most commonly affected are the extremities, with the proximal and extensor aspects somewhat favoured. The trunk is involved more often than the head and neck. Multiple lesions may be regional and unilateral, or more than one region can be affected. Solitary lesions may occur, apart from the dartoic type.

Genital leiomyoma is a solitary dermal nodule occurring most commonly in the scrotum, but also appearing on the penis, labia majora and nipple area [6–9]. Scrotal tumours are often large. Pain is less frequent than with pilar leiomyoma. Contraction in response to stimulation by touch or cold can occur.

Angioleiomyoma is usually a solitary, flesh-coloured, rounded, subcutaneous or deep dermal tumour up to 40 mm in diameter [4,5]. It is more frequent on the lower limb than the upper and may appear on the trunk or face. About half the reported cases have been painful. Lesions are longstanding and present between the fourth and sixth decades of life. Pain may be triggered by changes in temperature, pregnancy or menses.

Differential diagnosis

The multiple type should cause little difficulty and even without pain it is fairly distinctive. The solitary painful lesion may be mistaken for a glomus tumour or an eccrine spiradenoma, and a history of contraction is helpful.

Disease course and prognosis

The behaviour is benign and local recurrences are exceptional.

Management

Surgical excision cures the solitary tumour. The severity of the pain may make the patient demand treatment and extensive lesions require plastic surgery. Medical treatments that may relieve pain include calcium-channel blockers and gabapentin. However, the effect is not long-lasting.

Leiomyosarcoma/atypical smooth muscle tumour (dermal and subcutaneous) [1–4]

Definition and nomenclature

A histologically malignant tumour displaying smooth muscle differentiation. Tumours are divided into those occurring in the subcutaneous tissue and those arising in the dermis. Pure dermal lesions have a very different behaviour from those arising in the subcutis and it is therefore important to separate them. Due to the benign behaviour of dermal tumours, it has recently been proposed that they should be renamed as atypical intradermal smooth muscle neoplasms [5].

> **Synonyms and inclusions**
> - Atypical intradermal smooth muscle neoplasm

Epidemiology

Incidence and prevalence

Both variants (dermal and subcutaneous) are rare. There does not seem to be an association with fumarate hydratase germline mutations.

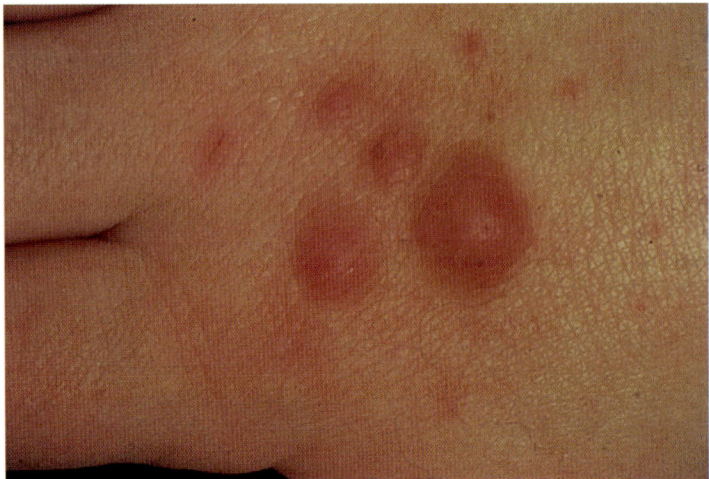

Figure 136.36 Clinical appearance of multiple leiomyomas.

Age
Atypical intradermal smooth muscle neoplasm (dermal leiomyosarcoma) is more common in middle-aged adults. Subcutaneous leiomyosarcoma affects middle-aged to elderly patients.

Sex
Both dermal lesions and subcutaneous leiomyosarcomas have predilection for males.

Pathophysiology
Pathology [3,6–10]
The lesion is distinguished from other dermal malignant tumours composed of spindle-shaped cells by the presence of fascicles of eosinophilic spindle-shaped cells with vesicular cigar-shaped nuclei. The degree of differentiation varies and necrosis tends to be present in deeper tumours, and it is rare in those arising primarily in the dermis. Mitotic figures are common in both variants. Most tumours are actin, calponin, desmin and h-caldesmon-positive, but staining may be lost in poorly differentiated variants. Dermal variants tend to be consistently positive for all markers. Rare cases have a desmoplastic stroma making histological diagnosis difficult [11,12]. About 45% of leiomyosarcomas are immunohistochemically positive for keratin and this is usually focal.

Clinical features [5,6,13,14]
History and presentation
Both types of tumours are more common in the trunk and lower extremities. Dermal lesions usually present as a skin-coloured or red papule or nodule. The latter is usually larger than a leiomyoma and may be painful. Subcutaneous tumours present as nodular tumours, ulcerated plaques [15] or diffuse swellings [16]. They may invade underlying muscle fascia. Rare subcutaneous tumours may arise from the penis [17] or vulva. An exceptional tumour has been reported arising in a naevus sebaceous [18].

Disease course and prognosis
Atypical intradermal smooth muscle neoplasms have a 5% recurrence rate, but they almost never metastasise [5,6]. Subcutaneous tumours metastasise in up to 50% of cases and they are associated with a mortality of about 30% [9].

Management
Wide surgical excision is necessary, as local recurrence follows inadequate excision [5].

SKELETAL MUSCLE TUMOURS

Rhabdomyomatous congenital hamartoma [1,2,3,4–9]

Definition and nomenclature [1,2,3]
Rhabdomyomatous mesenchymal hamartoma is a dermal lesion with a prominent component of skeletal muscle.

Synonyms and inclusions
- Striated muscle hamartoma
- Congenital midline hamartoma
- Hamartoma of cutaneous adnexa and mesenchyme

Epidemiology [1,2,3,4]
Incidence and prevalence
It is a very rare tumour.

Age
Typically it is congenital. Exceptional cases in adults have been reported [4,5].

Sex
A female predominance is noticed.

Pathophysiology
Genetics [3,4]
Aberrant embryonic migration of mesodermally derived tissues, or a genetic defect predisposing to the formation of hamartomas, has been suggested as possible aetiological factors.

Pathology [1,2,3,4–7]
Microscopically intersecting bundles of mature skeletal muscle orientated perpendicular to the epidermis are admixed with varying amounts of mature fat, collagen and adnexal structures.

Clinical features [1,2,3,4–9]
History and presentation
The majority of lesions present as papules or polyps, resembling skin tags. The head and neck (especially the central face) is the site of predilection. An association with other congenital abnormalities as well as Delleman syndrome has been reported.

Prognosis
The tumour is benign. Spontaneous regression may rarely occur.

Management
Complete excision is curative.

Rhabdomyoma

Rhabdomyomas are divided into adult, fetal and genital types. They mainly occur in soft tissues, vulva or vagina, upper respiratory tract and internal organs. Presentation in the skin is almost never seen and they will not be discussed further in this chapter.

Cutaneous rhabdomyosarcoma

Malignant tumours with skeletal-muscle differentiation are classified into two large groups, the embryonal and alveolar types. Although rhabdomyosarcomas represent up to 8% of tumours in children, primary involvement of the skin by this tumour is very rare [1]. Much more common is involvement of the skin by direct extension from deeper soft tissues. A relatively small number of primary cutaneous rhabdomyosarcomas have been reported in the literature so far, showing bimodal age distribution and male predominance, similar to rhabdomyosarcoma in deep soft tissue [2,3,4]. The most common subtype occurring in the skin is the alveolar variant. The majority of cases have presented on the face. The prognosis is difficult to estimate because of the rarity of these cases and the limited follow-up available.

TUMOURS OF FAT CELLS

Angiolipoma [1–11]

Definition
Angiolipoma is a benign tumour composed of mature white adipose tissue admixed with a variable amount of thin-walled vessels. By definition, some of the vessels should contain fibrin microthrombi.

Epidemiology [1–3]
Incidence and prevalence
It is a relatively common tumour.

Age
Lesions usually occur in young adults. They are rare in children, the middle aged and the elderly.

Sex
A male predominance is observed.

Pathophysiology
Pathology [1–4]
Angiolipomas are encapsulated. They consist of mature adipose tissue intermingled with a prominent vascular component usually more prominent in the periphery of tumour lobules. Some of the blood vessels contain fibrin thrombi. Cases with a prominent vascular component obscuring the adipocytic component have been termed 'cellular angiolipomas' [4].

Genetics [5,6]
Cytogenetic studies have consistently shown no karyotypic abnormality. This is a unique finding in adipocytic tumours, which has given rise to arguments regarding its pathogenesis. It has been proposed that the lesion is primarily a vascular tumour and that it should be named lipoangioma.

Clinical features [1–3,7–11]
History and presentation
Typically, angiolipomas are multiple variably painful subcutaneous nodules. They are usually small and well circumscribed. A predilection for the upper limbs is observed, followed by the trunk and lower limbs. Intraosseous cases have been reported [7].

Familial incidence is well documented in a subset of angiolipomas [8–12].

Prognosis
The tumour is benign. Local recurrence and malignant transformation does not occur.

Management
Complete excision is curative.

Lipoma [1–20]

Definition
Lipoma is a benign tumour composed of variable amounts of mature white adipose tissue.

Epidemiology [1–3]
Incidence and prevalence
It is the most common human mesenchymal neoplasm. It is more frequent in the obese.

Age
Tumours occur in adults (40–60 years old). They are rare in children. Congenital lesions have been reported.

Sex
It is more common in females.

Pathophysiology
Genetics [4–10]
Chromosome aberrations have been found in more than half of the cases examined. Three types of chromosomal abnormalities have been described: tumours with a 12q13-15 rearrangement affecting the *HMGA2* gene (the most common), tumours with a 6p21-23 rearrangement and lesions with deletion of 13q.

Pathology [1–3,11–16]
Tumours are usually encapsulated and consist of lobules of mature adipose tissue divided by delicate fibrous septa. Adipocytes are uniform in size and shape. Nuclear atypia is not a feature. There is no mitotic activity. Degenerative changes frequently occur, usually in the form of fat necrosis. Myxoid change is not uncommon.

Some lipomas may contain fibrous tissue in variable amounts. Metaplastic bone, cartilage or muscle tissue may be observed.

Clinical features [1–3,11–21]
History and presentation
The typical presentation is of a slowly growing and painless subcutaneous mass. There is a predilection for the trunk, abdomen and neck. Other sites, such as the proximal extremities, face, scalp and less commonly the hands and feet, may be affected. Spinal cord and pancreatic lipomas have been reported [19,20].

Lipomas are usually solitary but multiple lesions have been described, some of them in a setting of an autosomal dominant disorder.

Size is variable and large lesions may occur. They are most often well-circumscribed but deep-seated variants, such as intramuscular lipomas, may be ill defined.

Dermal examples may resemble fibroepithelial polyps.

Prognosis
The tumour is benign. Local recurrence is not a frequent feature. Progression to liposarcoma is exceptional.

Management
Complete excision is curative in almost every case.

Hibernoma [1–9]

Definition [1,2]
Hibernoma is a benign tumour composed of brown granular multivacuolated cells (resembling normal brown fat) admixed with a variable amount of mature white adipose tissue.

Epidemiology [3]
Incidence and prevalence
It is a rare tumour.

Age
It predominantly occurs in young adults (third and fourth decades). Approximately 5% of the tumours occur in children and 7% in elderly individuals.

Sex
A female predominance is noticed.

Pathophysiology
Pathology [3–7]
Hibernomas are usually encapsulated and lobulated. Typical cases consist of adipocytes with an eosinophilic granular multivacuolated cytoplasm and a centrally located nucleus. Mature white adipose tissue is present in a variable proportion. Variants include the lipoma-like, myxoid and spindle cell hibernoma.

By immunohistochemistry, the adipocytes are positive for S100 protein. UCP1 is highly expressed in brown adipose tissue, including hibernomas, and can distinguish hibernomas from other adipocytic and most non-adipocytic soft tissue tumours.

Genetics [8,9]
Cytogenetic studies, in most cases, have shown aberrations of the 11q13-21 region, and in fewer cases of 10q22. Concomitant deletions of the *MEN1* and *AIP* tumour suppressor genes are essential for the pathogenesis.

Clinical features [3–5]
History and presentation
Hibernoma presents as painless subcutaneous mass of long duration. The site of predilection is the thigh. This is followed by the trunk, upper limbs and head and neck. Deep-seated lesions can occur. Visceral locations, such as the retroperitoneum, have been described.

Prognosis
The tumour is benign. Local recurrence is not a feature.

Management
Local excision is curative.

Lipoblastoma and lipoblastomatosis
[1,2,3]

Definition
Lipoblastoma is a tumour that occurs almost exclusively in infants and children. It is characterised by a proliferation of immature fat cells in a myxoid stroma (that may mimic myxoid liposarcoma) and intermixed with mature adipocytes [1]. Lipoblastoma is a well-circumscribed subcutaneous tumour; lipoblastomatosis refers to a deeper lesion or those that have an infiltrative growth pattern.

Epidemiology
Incidence and prevalence
Tumours are rare.

Age
Most cases present during the first few years of life.

Sex
There is predilection for males.

Pathophysiology
Pathology [1,2,3]
Tumours have a characteristic lobular appearance. Each tumour lobule is separated by fibrous septae and consists of a mixture of small, univacuolated, signet-ring cells, spindle-shaped or stellate cells and scattered mature adipocytes. In the background, there are prominent myxoid changes and numerous small vessels in a typical 'crow's feet' distribution, mimicking a myxoid liposarcoma. Distinction from the latter may be very difficult, especially in small biopsies. The clinical information is therefore crucial, as myxoid liposarcoma is vanishingly rare in children and almost never occurs before the age of 10 years [4]. Furthermore, lipoblastoma tends to be less cellular than myxoid liposarcoma and has a lobular architecture. Over time, maturation occurs, and in some cases most of the tumour is composed of mature fat cells.

Genetics
Cytogenetic studies in lipoblastoma have shown rearrangements of the *PLAG1* and *HMGA2* genes [5,6].

Clinical features [1,2,3]
The majority of tumours occur on the limbs and trunk as an asymptomatic mass no more than a few centimetres in diameter. Lipoblastoma is much more common than lipoblastomatosis.

Disease course and prognosis
Tumours behave in a benign fashion but deep-seated lesions may recur locally usually as a result of incomplete excision.

Management
The tumour is benign and simple excision is the treatment of choice.

Spindle cell and pleomorphic lipoma
[1–12,13]

Definition
Spindle cell lipoma is composed of mature adipocytes and variable numbers of short bland spindle-shaped cells with indistinct cytoplasm. Pleomorphic lipoma is composed of mature adipocytes, cells with hyperchromatic nuclei and frequent multinucleation, and collagen bundles. Both types of tumour may overlap and they are therefore considered to be part of the same spectrum.

Epidemiology
Incidence and prevalence
Lesions are relatively rare.

Age
There is predilection for middle-aged to old patients with a median of 55 years.

Sex
Tumours have a strong predilection for males.

Pathophysiology
Pathology [1,2,4–7,9]
Spindle cell lipoma presents as a well-circumscribed tumour composed of mature adipocytes intermixed with short spindle-shaped cells with wavy nuclei. Hyalinised collagen bundles and focal myxoid change are prominent. Pseudovascular spaces are prominent in some cases. The spindle-shaped cells stain for CD34 and the adipocytes are positive for S100 protein. Loss of nuclear Rb expression is found in spindle cell and pleomorphic lipoma [6]. Pleomorphic lipoma is also well circumscribed and composed of mature adipocytes intermixed with uninucleated or multinucleated cells with hyperchromatic nuclei. The nuclei in the multinucleated cells are often arranged in a circle (floret cell). The histological diagnosis may be quite difficult in cases with few or no mature fat cells [7]. Rare variants contain real prominent vascular spaces [9].

Genetics
Cytogenetic studies of both tumours have shown variable abnormalities, most commonly in chromosome 16q and rarely in chromosomes 13q and 6p [10–12].

Clinical features [1,2,4,5]
History and presentation
Spindle cell/pleomorphic lipoma usually presents as a small subcutaneous nodule on the upper back or nape of the neck. Purely dermal examples are rare [13], but more frequent in females, as are atypical locations including the face and extremities [8]. Multiple lesions and familial cases occur rarely [3].

Disease course and prognosis
Local recurrence after excision is very rare.

Management
Simple excision is the treatment of choice.

Atypical lipomatous tumour [1–4]

Definition and nomenclature
This is a lesion composed of lobules of mature adipose cells with scattered larger cells with variation in nuclear size and hyperchromatism. The term 'atypical lipomatous tumour' is usually used for neoplasms occurring in the subcutis or within skeletal muscle. Similar tumours occurring in the abdominal cavity are regarded as well-differentiated liposarcomas in view of the fact that they have a potential to cause death as a result of extensive growth. Only subcutaneous skin lesions will be discussed here.

Synonyms and inclusions
- Well-differentiated liposarcoma

Epidemiology
Incidence and prevalence
Tumours are relatively frequent in the subcutaneous tissue and exceptional in the dermis.

Age
Middle-aged to old adults.

Sex
There is no sex predilection.

Pathophysiology
Pathology
Typically, lobules of mature adipose tissue, with or without fibrous tissue and myxoid change, are seen. Focal variation in the size and shape of adipocytes is seen and this is associated with nuclear enlargement and hyperchromatism. Vacuolated cells may also be found. Atypical cells are often present in the fibrous tissue. Some tumours are classified as cellular based on the presence of non-lipogenic areas of increased cellularity with low-mitotic activity [5]. De-differentiated tumours are lesions that develop a high-grade sarcomatous component that is associated with poor prognosis [6]. This change does not usually develop in tumours that are superficially located.

Genetics
Cytogenetic studies of these neoplasms have found chromosomal abnormalities in most cases. About a third of cases show supernumerary ring chromosomes affecting chromosome 12q.13-15 [4]. This results in amplification of *MDM2* and *CDK4* genes [7]. Expression of these genes can be detected by FISH, real-time PCR and immunohistochemistry, making it a useful diagnostic aid. Of these methods,

FISH and real-time PCR, but particularly the former, are more sensitive than immunohistochemistry for detection of these amplifications [8].

Clinical features [1–3]
History and presentation
Tumours may be large, are asymptomatic and have the same clinical appearance as a lipoma. Dermal tumours may be identical to a fibroepithelial polyp [9].

Disease course and prognosis
There is a tendency for local recurrence, but metastases are not seen unless the tumour undergoes dedifferentiation, which does not tend to happen in superficially located tumours, particularly those in the subcutaneous tissue [6].

Management
Complete surgical excision is indicated.

Liposarcoma [1]

Myxoid and round cell liposarcoma and pleomorphic liposarcoma are vanishingly rare in the skin. Only a few cases of primary cutaneous liposarcoma have been described. Follow-up is limited, but the behaviour seems to be better than that of their deeper counterparts, probably reflecting early detection and treatment and the easy accessibility to the skin. Additional information on this tumour can be found in other texts.

TUMOURS OF UNCERTAIN HISTOGENESIS

Acral fibromyxoma [1–3,4,5]

Definition and nomenclature
Acral fibromyxoma is a distinctive benign dermal and/or subcutaneous, fibroblastic tumour with a strong predilection for digits of both the hands and feet.

> **Synonyms and inclusions**
> - Digital fibromyxoma
> - Cellular digital fibroma

Epidemiology
Incidence and prevalence
It is relatively frequent.

Age
The age range is wide but most patients are middle aged.

Sex
There is predilection for males.

Pathophysiology
Pathology
Lesions are circumscribed and consist of bland stellate and spindle-shaped cells in a variably prominent myxoid and collagenous stroma and with small blood vessels in the background. Some lesions are more cellular and have been described in the literature under the rubric of cellular fibroma of the digits [2,5]. In myxoid areas, mast cells are often seen. Scattered multinucleated cells may be seen in some cases. Mitotic figures are very rare. Tumour cells are diffusely positive for CD34 and may be focally positive for EMA, CD99 and smooth muscle actin. *RB1* loss/deletion is frequent in acral fibromyxoma and loss of Rb expression is found in 90% of tumours [6].

In the past, it is likely that these tumours were classified as neurofibromas because of the cytomorphology of tumour cells and the myxoid background, with fairly frequent mast cells. However, neurofibroma is rare in acral sites, tumour cells are positive for S100 protein, only focally positive for CD34 and there is no loss of Rb expression.

Clinical features
History and presentation
Most cases present as a longstanding, solitary mass measuring between 1 and 2 cm, on the hands and feet (overwhelmingly involving the digits, often in a subungual location) [1–3,4].

Disease course and prognosis
Local recurrence is exceptional and is usually associated with incomplete excision.

Management
Simple local excision is the treatment of choice.

Superficial angiomyxoma [1,2]

Definition
Superficial angiomyxoma is a dermal or subcutaneous tumour composed of a mixture of small blood vessels and sparse spindle-shaped cells in a prominent myxoid stroma.

Epidemiology
Incidence and prevalence
Lesions are rare.

Age
Most patients are adults.

Sex
There is no sex predilection.

Pathophysiology
Pathology
Tumours are multilobulated, with copious myxoid stroma, numerous delicate small blood vessels and spindle-shaped or stellated

bland cells, probably representing fibroblasts. Aggregates of inflammatory cells, mainly neutrophils, are frequent. In up to 30% of cases epithelial structures, probably representing hyperplastic trapped adnexal structures (particularly hair follicles), are identified.

Clinical features [1,2]
Most cases present as an asymptomatic solitary papule or nodule. Lesions are usually less than 3 cm and have a wide anatomical distribution with a predilection for the trunk, head and neck and genital skin. In patients with multiple lesions, the possibility of Carney complex should be considered (Chapter 148) [3].

Disease course and prognosis
The behaviour is benign. Local recurrence after surgical treatment is seen in up to 30% of cases [1,2].

Management
Excision is the treatment of choice.

Digital mucous cyst [1]

Digital mucous cyst presents mainly on the fingers as a small solitary painful nodule. Females are much more commonly affected than males and there is a tendency for local recurrence. Lesions are poorly circumscribed and consist of abundant myxoid stroma with only scattered bland spindle-shaped cells (Chapter 57).

Synonyms and inclusions
- Cutaneous myxoid cyst

Dermal non-neural granular cell tumour

Definition and nomenclature
This is a distinctive dermal tumour with no specific line of differentiation, initially described as primitive polypoid granular cell tumour in 1991 [1]. Tumours are not related to neural granular cell tumours, which are uniformly S100 positive. They occur both in the dermis and in subcutaneous tissue.

Synonyms and inclusions
- Primitive polypoid granular cell tumour
- Primitive non-neural granular cell tumour

Epidemiology
Incidence and prevalence
Tumours are rare.

Age
There is a wide age range but most patients are adults.

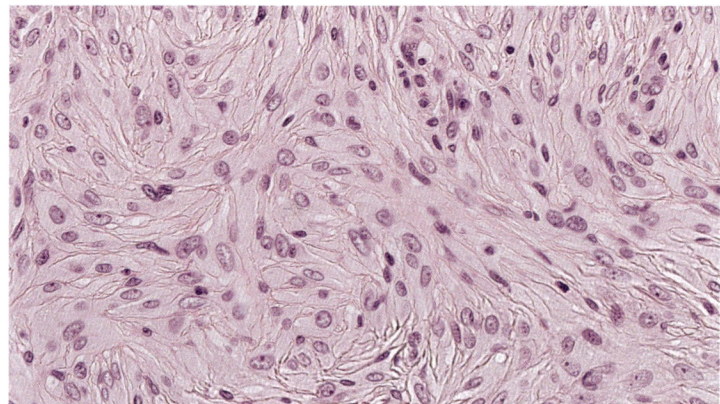

Figure 136.37 Large cells with prominent granular cell change in a case of dermal non-neural granular cell tumour.

Sex
There is no sex predilection.

Pathophysiology
Pathology
Histologically, lesions show rounded or spindle-shaped cells with prominent granular cell change (Figure 136.37). Polypoid tumours have an epithelial collarette. Nuclear pleomorphism varies but does not tend to be prominent. Mitotic figures may be prominent. Multinucleated cells are sometimes seen. There is diffuse positivity for NKI-C3, which is a non-specific marker for lysosomes, and focal positivity for CD68 and neuron-specific enolase (NSE). Tumour cells do not stain for keratin, EMA, actin, desmin, h-caldesmon or S100 [2,3].

Genetics
Recurrent *ALK* gene fusions have recently been demonstrated in 60% of the cases tested [5].

Clinical features
History and presentation
This tumour usually presents as an exophytic small lesion with a wide anatomical distribution, wide age range and no sex predilection. Not all tumours are polypoid. Clinical behaviour is usually benign with only rare local recurrences [2,3,4]. However, a single case of metastasis to a regional lymph node has been reported [2].

Management
Complete conservative excision is the treatment of choice.

Haemosiderotic fibrolipomatous tumour [1,2]

Definition and nomenclature
This is a distinctive rare lesion that occurs almost exclusively on the foot, particularly the ankle, and was initially thought to represent a reactive process [1]. A relationship with impaired circulation, particularly stasis, has been suggested [3]. However, it is now believed that

lesions are neoplastic. A relation to pleomorphic hyalinising angiectatic tumour [4] and myxoinflammatory fibroblastic sarcoma has been suggested [5]. The association with the latter is not only based on the coexistence of both tumours in some cases but also on cytogenetic analysis (see later).

Synonyms and inclusions
- Haemosiderotic fibrohistiocytic lipomatous lesion

Epidemiology
Incidence and prevalence
Tumours are rare.

Age
There is predilection for middle-aged to elderly adults.

Sex
Females are more frequently affected than males.

Pathophysiology
Pathology
The tumour is fairly circumscribed and it is composed of lobules of mature adipose tissue with scattered areas containing variable numbers of spindle-shaped cells, which may be slightly hyperchromatic and often contain abundant intracytoplasmic haemosiderin. Histiocyte-like cells may also be seen. These cells are bland and only rarely slightly atypical. In the background, there may be a few mononuclear inflammatory cells, mainly lymphocytes. Mitotic figures are exceptional. Spindle cells are positive for calponin and CD34 and may be positive for CD68 but negative for other markers, including desmin and h-caldesmon.

Genetics
These tumours frequently show a t(1;10) translocation with rearrangements of *TGFBR3* and *MGEA5* [5], confirming their close and complex relationship with myxoinflammatory fibroblastic sarcoma (MIFS). However, the translocation is much more frequent in hybrid HFLT/MIFS than in classic MIFS, indicating that hybrid HFLT/MIFS may represent HFLTs with sarcomatous progression rather than tumours closely related to classic MIFS [6].

Clinical features
History and presentation
Lesions present as a slowly growing fairly well-defined subcutaneous tumour, which tends to be asymptomatic. Size is variable and may be several centimetres in diameter.

Disease course and prognosis
Behaviour is usually benign with occasional local recurrences. However, a tumour that recurred as a myxoinflammatory fibroblastic sarcoma metastasised resulting in the demise of the patient [7].

Management
The treatment of choice is complete surgical excision.

Perivascular epithelioid cell tumour ('PEComa')

Definition
Perivascular epithelioid cell tumour is part of a spectrum of neoplasms that includes clear cell 'sugar' tumour of the lung, angiomyolipoma, lymphangioleiomyomatosis and clear cell myomelanocytic tumour of the falciform ligament [1,2,3]. Occurrence in the skin and soft tissue is rare but it is likely that the lesion is underrecognised. Although tumour cells are usually positive for melanocytic markers such as HMB45 and Melan-A, the cell of origin has not been identified.

Epidemiology
Incidence and prevalence
Cutaneous tumours are rare [4].

Age
Most patients are young adults.

Sex
There is predilection for females.

Pathophysiology
Pathology [3,4]
Histology is distinctive and consists of bland epithelioid cells, typically arranged radially around thin-walled vascular channels. A smaller population of spindle cells is often seen. Tumour cells have pale pink cytoplasm and vesicular nuclei. Malignant examples may be seen but have not been reported in the skin. The immunophenotype is distinctive, as the tumour cells stain for melanocytic markers including HMB45, MITF-1, Melan-A and tyrosinase and for muscular markers including SMA, desmin and calponin. They are usually negative for S100 and keratin.

Genetics
Recurrent chromosomal alterations leading to inactivation of the *TSC1* or *TSC2* genes or rearrangements of *TFE3* have been demonstrated in visceral PEComas. However, the latter rearrangement does not seem to occur in cutaneous tumours [5]. Recently, *MITF* translocations have been described in tumours with clear cell myo-melanocytic differentiation [6,7].

Clinical features
History and presentation
Tumours present as a small nondescript lesion, more frequently on the lower extremities.

Disease course and prognosis
Behaviour is benign. Malignant tumours are very rare.

Management
Simple excision is the treatment of choice.

Deep ('aggressive') angiomyxoma
[1,2,3]

Definition
Deep 'aggressive' angiomyxoma is a distinctive tumour occurring in the genital region and pelvis, predominantly in females. It is characterised by bland spindle-shaped cells in the background of a prominent myxoid stroma and frequent thick-walled blood vessels.

Epidemiology
Incidence and prevalence
Tumours are rare.

Age
Most cases present during the reproductive years particularly during the fourth decade of life [3]. Presentation after the menopause and in children is rare [4].

Sex
It occurs almost exclusively in females although rare lesions have been described in males [5].

Pathophysiology
Pathology
The lesion is infiltrative and is composed of spindle- or stellate-shaped bland cells with scanty cytoplasm, surrounded by prominent myxoid stroma. Small to medium-sized thick-walled blood vessels are seen throughout the tumour. Mitotic figures are very rare. Rare cases contain multinucleated giant cells [6]. Interestingly, tumour cells are positive for actin and desmin. Tumour cells are often positive for oestrogen and/or progesterone receptors [7]. Immunohistochemistry for HMGA2 protein is a useful aid in the diagnosis of this neoplasm as it is positive in most aggressive angiomyxomas and negative or minimally positive in other mimics [8], while it can also be used for the assessment of resection margins. However, the staining is not entirely specific and may be encountered in other tumours in the vulvovaginal region, such as smooth muscle tumours and fibroepithelial polyps [9].

Genetics
Cytogenetics demonstrate a translocation involving the chromosomal region 12q14-15, involving a rearrangement of *HMGA2* (an architectural transcription factor) [10].

Clinical features
History and presentation
Cases in children may involve the spermatic cord [4]. Tumours are slowly growing, and by the time of presentation they are large and ill-defined, often measuring 10 cm or more. The most commonly affected sites are the vulva and perineum. Extension into deeper soft tissues is often found.

Disease course and prognosis
Local recurrence is observed in up to a third of cases. Exceptional metastases have been reported [11,12].

Management
Complete surgical excision is the treatment of choice but it is usually difficult because of the infiltration of surrounding tissue. However, recurrences are not usually destructive, and radical surgical procedures are therefore not indicated [13]. Furthermore, the outcome of patients with resection positive margins does not seem to be very different compared with those with resection negative margins [2]. An alternative to surgical management may be the use of gonadotrophin-releasing hormone agonists, a treatment that was shown to be promising in isolated case reports [14,15]. It was subsequently confirmed to have a potential of disease control in larger trials, establishing a role in treatment in combination with surgery [16].

Angiomatoid fibrous histiocytoma
[1,2,3–5]

Definition and nomenclature
Angiomatoid fibrous histiocytoma (FH) was initially described as a variant of malignant FH [1]. It has recently been reclassified as a neoplasm with low-grade malignant behaviour, unrelated to malignant FH. Although it is considered to be 'fibrohistiocytic' due to the cytological resemblance of tumour cells to histiocytes, focal positivity of these cells to desmin raises the possibility of muscular differentiation. However, the lesion is now regarded as of uncertain histiogenesis.

> **Synonyms and inclusions**
> - Previously known as angiomatoid malignant fibrous histiocytoma

Epidemiology
Incidence and prevalence
Represents a rare tumour.

Age
It presents in children and young adults and rarely in older patients.

Sex
There is no sex predilection.

Pathophysiology
Pathology [1,2,3–8]
Low-power examination reveals haemorrhagic, pseudovascular, cavernous-like, cystic spaces filled with red blood cells. Mononuclear inflammatory cells are prominent (including lymphocytes, histiocytes and plasma cells) and germinal centres and sclerosis are present in some cases [6]. Eosinophils may be seen. Tumour cells are arranged in sheets and consist of short spindle-shaped and round cells with pink cytoplasm and vesicular nuclei. Myxoid variants have been described [7]. Cytological atypia is sometimes present, and the mitotic count tends to be low. Up to 85% of angiomatoid FH cases are positive for ALK with certain antibody clones without a demonstrable *ALK* rearrangement, which represents a potential pitfall [8]. Tumour cells are focally positive to desmin in about half of the cases [3,4]. Positivity for other markers including EMA, muscle-specific actin, calponin, CD99 and CD68 may be seen.

Genetics
Initial cytogenetic studies demonstrated a translocation between chromosomes 16p11 involving the *FUS* (*TLS*) gene and chromosome 12q13 involving the *ATF1* gene. The resultant protein (FUS/ATF1) is similar to the protein present in clear cell sarcoma (EWS/ATF1) involving t(12;22)(q13;q12) [9]. However, other cases show a different fusion gene, *EWSR1-CREB1*, which seems to be the most common fusion gene in these tumours [10].

Clinical features
History and presentation
It presents as an asymptomatic blue or skin-coloured subcutaneous or deeper mass. Primary dermal tumours are exceptional. Most cases occur on the limbs and patients may present with systemic symptoms including fever, anaemia and weight loss. Generalised lymphadenopathy may also be seen.

Disease course and prognosis
Local recurrence is observed in about 15% of patients and, exceptionally, metastasis to neighbouring soft tissues or regional lymph nodes may occur. Complete excision and follow-up are therefore indicated. Local recurrence is more likely with deep tumours, those with an infiltrative growth pattern and those that are incompletely removed [2].

Management
Most cases are cured after adequate excision.

Epithelioid sarcoma [1,2,3,4]

Definition
A distinctive, malignant mesenchymal tumour composed of cells with epithelial differentiation. It is divided into two clinicopathological subtypes: conventional (classic) involving mainly acral sites (granuloma-like) and proximal-type involving the trunk and proximal limbs (solid growth) [5,6].

Epidemiology
Incidence and prevalence
It is an uncommon tumour representing fewer than 1% of all soft-tissue sarcomas [7]. The proximal type variant is much less common than the conventional variant.

Age
Conventional tumours are more common in early adult life. The proximal type variant is more common in older patients. Both variants can present in any age group.

Sex
Males are more often affected than females in both variants.

Pathophysiology
The tumour is composed of firm nodules, 5–50 mm or larger in diameter, surrounded by fibrous tissue and fat. It is often closely associated with fascia, periosteum, tendon or nerve sheaths. The cut surface is greyish-white and flecked or mottled with yellow or brown, reflecting the presence of areas of necrosis. Microscopically, there are masses of large round polygonal or spindle cells with acidophilic cytoplasm. Spindle cells are often present and may predominate. The larger nodules have necrotic centres and show so-called 'geographical necrosis', which may be mistaken on scanning power microscopy for a granuloma. Mitotic figures are common and binucleate cells occur. Variable cytological atypia is always present and may be prominent. Intercellular hyalinised collagen increases the acidophilia, while calcification, with osteoid or bone formation (in about 20% of cases), may take place in the necrotic areas. The tumour spreads along dense fibrous structures and may ulcerate in areas with little subcutaneous fat. Local recurrence after excision is common and metastasis, principally to lymph nodes, lung and pleura, may occur. Tumour cells show clear histological, ultrastructural and immunohistochemical evidence of epithelial differentiation.

The proximal type of epithelioid sarcoma shows a similar multi-nodular growth pattern but tumour cells are larger and with a more rhabdoid appearance consisting of abundant cytoplasm and large nuclei with or without a prominent eosinophilic nucleolus [5,6].

Immunohistochemically, tumour cells in both variants of epithelioid sarcoma have the same profile. They are positive for vimentin, keratin and EMA, and 50% of cases are positive for CD34 [8]. Most examples of both variants of the tumour show loss of nuclear expression of INI1 [9].

Genetics
Tumours often display complex chromosomal abnormalities involving chromosome 22q11 [10,11]. Some of these changes involve deletions or mutations of the tumour suppressor gene *SMARCB1* (*INI1*, *hSNF5*). Loss of nuclear expression of the latter can be demonstrated by immunohistochemistry and this is a very useful aid in the differential diagnosis of these tumours [9] (see later).

Clinical features [1,2,3,4,8,12]
History and presentation
The presenting sign can be a dermal nodule that grows outwards and may ulcerate early, a nodule or lobular subcutaneous tumour that is painless and grows slowly, or a tumour attached to deeper structures that is rather poorly defined and causes pain, paraesthesiae or muscular wasting when growing along a large trunk nerve. As a result of prominent perineurial and perivascular extension of tumour cells, multiple nodules in a sporotrichoid distribution may be seen. The distal extremities are the usual situation for the tumour, particularly the flexor aspect of the finger and the palm. It may grow at a deceptively slow rate.

The proximal-type epithelioid sarcoma presents as a large, often deep-seated, mass on the proximal limbs, genitalia, buttocks, trunk (mainly axilla) or head and neck [5,6].

Disease course and prognosis
Local recurrence and metastasis may occur years after the original diagnosis. The survival rate has been estimated at between 60% and 80% at 5 years and between 42% and 62% at 10 years [8,13–18]. The proximal-type variant has a worse prognosis.

Features associated with poorer prognosis include male sex, older age at diagnosis, proximal location, deep involvement, rhabdoid phenotype, tumour size, mitotic rate, necrosis, vascular invasion, local recurrence and lymph node metastasis [3,13–18].

Management
Complete removal by surgical excision is essential if local recurrence and eventual metastasis are to be avoided, and the earlier this is done the less likely is the process to spread along fascial planes. Surgical excision followed by radiotherapy is often recommended. Involvement of regional lymph nodes is associated with distant metastasis (mainly to the lungs) and death [18].

Clear cell sarcoma [1–4,5]

Definition and nomenclature
Clear cell sarcoma is a distinctive, malignant soft-tissue tumour that displays melanocytic differentiation.

Synonyms and inclusions
- Melanoma of soft parts

Epidemiology
Incidence and prevalence
Tumours are rare. Primary dermal clear cell sarcomas are exceptional [6,7].

Age
The tumour is more common in young adults.

Sex
There is predilection for females.

Pathophysiology
Pathology
The lesion has a lobular growth pattern. Tumour cells are fairly homogeneous and contain clear or pale pink cytoplasm and a prominent eosinophilic nucleolus. Mitotic figures are not prominent, but multinucleated giant cells with a wreath-like arrangement of the nuclei are often identified. Loose thin bands of collagen surround tumour cells. Secondary involvement of the dermis is relatively common. Necrosis is sometimes seen. Melanin is sometimes identified, and S100, HMB45 and Melan-A are usually positive. Exceptional cases of clear cell sarcoma may display a junctional component [8,9]. This may lead to a misdiagnosis of Spitz naevus. Electron-microscopic examination of tumour cells reveals the presence of melanosomes.

Genetics
Cytogenetic analysis often reveals a translocation t(12;22)(q13;q12); this translocation is not found in melanoma, which often has mutations in the *BRAF* gene (a feature exceptional in clear cell sarcoma) [10–12]. The clear cell sarcoma translocation results in an *EWSR1-ATF1* fusion gene. Rare cases of clear cell sarcoma may also show *KIT* mutations [13]. In recent years, a subset of clear cell tumours with melanocytic differentiation and what seems to be a more indolent prognosis have been linked to translocations involving *CRTC1-TRIM11* or *MITF* genes, thus expanding the differential diagnosis of clear cell sarcoma [14–16].

Clinical features
Most cases occur on the lower limbs, with a predilection for the foot. The upper limb is affected in about 25% of cases. Tumours tend to grow around tendons, are usually less than 3 cm in diameter and are often painful.

Disease course and prognosis
About 50% of patients develop metastatic disease, often many years after the initial diagnosis. Prognosis is associated with mitotic index, size of the tumour and presence of necrosis [17,**18**]. The 5- and 10-year survival rates are 52% and 25%, respectively [**18**]. Tumour size appears to be associated with worse prognosis [19]. It is not clear whether purely dermal tumours have a better prognosis than those deeply located.

Management [1–4,17,**18**,19]
Wide excision is the treatment of choice. Chemotherapy does not seem to be effective in the treatment of disseminated disease.

Key references

The full list of references can be found in the online version at https://www.wiley.com/rooksdermatology10e

Introduction
1. Goldblum JR, Weiss SW, Folpe A. *Enzinger and Weiss's Soft Tissue Tumors*, 7th edn. St Louis: Elsevier, 2019.
2. WHO Classification of Tumours Editorial Board. *Soft Tissue and Bone Tumours*, 5th edn. Lyon, France: WHO, 2020.

Fibrous and myofibroblastic tumours
4. de Cambourg G, Cribier B. Fibrous papules of the face: a retrospective anatomo-clinical study of 238 cases. *Ann Dermatol Venereol* 2013;140:763–70.

Storiform collagenoma
2. Metcalf JS, Maize JC, LeBoit PE. Circumscribed storiform collagenoma (sclerosing fibroma). *Am J Dermatopathol* 1991;13:122–9.

Pleomorphic fibroma
1. Kamino H, Lee JY, Berke A. Pleomorphic fibroma of the skin: a benign neoplasm with cytologic atypia – a clinicopathologic study of eight cases. *Am J Surg Pathol* 1989;13:107–13.

Acquired digital fibrokeratoma
3. Kint A, Baran R, de Keyser H. Acquired (digital) fibrokeratoma. *J Am Acad Dermatol* 1985;12:816–21.

EWSR1-SMAD3 rearranged fibroblastic tumour
2. Habeeb O, Korty KE, Azzato EM *et al*. EWSR1-SMAD3 rearranged fibroblastic tumor: case series and review. *J Cutan Pathol* 2021;48:255–62.

Nodular fasciitis
3 Shimizu S, Hashimoto H, Enjoji M. Nodular fasciitis: an analysis of 250 patients. *Pathology* 1984;16:161–6.

Fibro-osseous pseudotumour of the digits
3 Chaudhry IH, Kazakov DV, Michal M et al. Fibro-osseus pseudotumor of the digit: a clinicopathological study of 17 cases. *J Cutan Pathol* 2010;37:323–9.

4 Švajdler M, Michal M, Martínek P et al. Fibro-osseous pseudotumor of digits and myositis ossificans show consistent COL1A1-USP6 rearrangement: a clinicopathological and genetic study of 27 cases. *Hum Pathol* 2019;88:39–47.

Ischaemic fasciitis
4 Liegl B, Fletcher CD. Ischemic fasciitis: analysis of 44 cases indicating an inconsistent association with immobility or debilitation. *Am J Surg Pathol* 2008;32:1546–52.

Fibrous hamartoma of infancy
6 Saab ST, McClain CM, Coffin CM. Fibrous hamartoma of infancy: a clinicopathologic analysis of 60 cases. *Am J Surg Pathol* 2014;38:394–401.

9 Park JY, Cohen C, Lopez D et al. EGFR exon 20 insertion/duplication mutations characterize fibrous hamartoma of infancy. *Am J Surg Pathol* 2016;40:1713–18.

Calcifying fibrous tumour/pseudotumour
3 Nascimento AF, Ruiz R, Hornick JL et al. Calcifying fibrous 'pseudotumor': clinicopathologic study of 15 cases and analysis of its relationship to inflammatory myofibroblastic tumor. *Int J Surg Pathol* 2002;10:189–96.

Calcifying aponeurotic fibroma
1 Puls F, Hofvander J, Magnusson L et al. FN1-EGF gene fusions are recurrent in calcifying aponeurotic fibroma. *J Pathol* 2016;238:502–7.

3 Fetsch JF, Miettinen M. Calcifying aponeurotic fibroma: a clinicopathologic study of 22 cases arising in uncommon sites. *Hum Pathol* 1998;29:1504–10.

Dermatomyofibroma
7 Mentzel T, Kutzner H. Dermatomyofibroma: clinicopathologic and immunohistochemical analysis of 56 cases and reappraisal of a rare and distinct cutaneous entity. *Am J Dermatopathol* 2009;31:44–9.

Plaque-like CD34-positive dermal fibroma
3 Kutzner H, Mentzel T, Palmedo G et al. Plaque-like CD34-positive dermal fibroma ('medallion-like dermal dendrocyte hamartoma'). Clinicopathologic, immunohistochemical, and molecular analysis of 5 cases emphasizing its distinction from superficial, plaque-like dermatofibrosarcoma protuberans. *Am J Surg Pathol* 2010;34:190–201.

Angiomyofibroblastoma
1 Fletcher CD, Tsang WY, Fisher C et al. Angiomyofibroblastoma of the vulva. A benign neoplasm distinct from aggressive angiomyxoma. *Am J Surg Pathol* 1992;16:373–82.

Cellular angiofibroma
5 Flucke U, van Krieken JHJM, Mentzel T. Cellular angiofibroma: analysis of 25 cases emphasizing its relationship to spindle cell lipoma and mammary-type myofibroblastoma. *Mod Pathol* 2011;24:82–9.

Elastofibroma
2 Nagamine N, Nohara Y, Ito E. Elastofibroma in Okinawa: a clinicopathologic study of 170 cases. *Cancer* 1982;50:1794–805.

Inclusion body (digital) fibromatosis
4 Laskin WB, Miettinen M, Fetsch JF. Infantile digital fibromatosis: a clinicopathological and immunohistochemical study of 69 tumors from 57 patients with long-term follow-up. *Am J Surg Pathol* 2009;33:1–13.

Fibroma of tendon sheath
2 Pulitzer DR, Martin PC, Reed RJ. Fibroma of tendon sheath: a clinicopathologic study of 32 cases. *Am J Surg Pathol* 1989;13:472–9.

Desmoplastic fibroblastoma
2 Miettinen M, Fetsch JF. Collagenous fibroma (desmoplastic fibroblastoma): a clinicopathological analysis of 63 cases of a distinctive soft tissue lesion with stellate-shaped fibroblasts. *Hum Pathol* 1998;29:676–82.

Nuchal-type fibroma
2 Michal M, Fetsch JF, Hes O et al. Nuchal-type fibroma: a clinicopathologic study of 52 cases. *Cancer* 1999;85:156–63.

Palmar and plantar fibromatosis (superficial fibromatoses)
1 Allen PW. The fibromatoses: a clinicopathologic classification based on 140 cases. *Am J Surg Pathol* 1977;1:255–70.

Penile fibromatosis
1 Smith BH. Peyronie's disease. *Am J Clin Pathol* 1966;85:670–8.

Lipofibromatosis
1 Fetsch JF, Miettinen M, Laskin WB et al. A clinicopathologic study of 45 soft tissue tumors with an admixture of adipose tissue and fibroblastic elements, and a proposal for classification as lipofibromatosis. *Am J Surg Pathol* 2000;24:1491–500.

2 Al-Ibraheemi A, Folpe AL, Perez-Atayde AR et al. Aberrant receptor tyrosine kinase signaling in lipofibromatosis: a clinicopathological and molecular genetic study of 20 cases. *Mod Pathol* 2019;32:423–34.

Dermatofibrosarcoma protuberans
18 Conelly JH, Evans HL. Dermatofibrosarcoma protuberans: a clinicopathologic review with emphasis on fibrosarcomatous areas. *Am J Surg Pathol* 1992;16:921–5.

22 Rubin B, Fletcher J, Fletcher CD. The histologic, genetic and biological relationships between dermatofibrosarcoma protuberans and giant cell fibroblastoma: an unexpected story. *Adv Anat Pathol* 1997;4:336–41.

31 Llombart B, Monteagudo C, Sanmartin O et al. Dermatofibrosarcoma protuberans: a clinicopathological, immunohistochemical, genetic (COL1A1-PDGFB), and therapeutic study of low-grade versus high-grade (fibrosarcomatous) tumors. *J Am Acad Dermatol* 2011;65:564–75.

32 Voth H, Landsberg J, Hinz T et al. Management of dermatofibrosarcoma protuberans with fibrosarcomatous transformation; an evidence-based review of the literature. *J Eur Acad Dermatol Venereol* 2011;25:1385–91.

40 Snow SN, Gordon EM, Larson PO et al. Dermatofibrosarcoma protuberans: a report on 29 cases treated by Mohs micrographic surgery with long-term follow-up and review of the literature. *Cancer* 2004;101:28–38.

Giant cell fibroblastoma
4 Jha P, Moosavi C, Fanburg-Smith JC. Giant cell fibroblastoma: an update and addition of 86 cases from the Armed Forces Institute of Pathology, in honor of Dr. Franz M. Enzinger. *Ann Diagn Pathol* 2007;11:81–8.

CD34-positive superficial fibroblastic tumour
1 Carter JM, Weiss SW, Linos K et al. Superficial CD34-positive fibroblastic tumor: report of 18 cases of a distinctive low-grade mesenchymal neoplasm of intermediate (borderline) malignancy. *Mod Pathol* 2014;27:294–302.

Myxoinflammatory fibroblastic sarcoma
4 Laskin WB, Fetsch JF, Miettinen M. Myxoinflammatory fibroblastic sarcoma: a clinicopathologic analysis of 104 cases with emphasis on predictors of outcome. *Am J Surg Pathol* 2014;38:1–12.

8 Suster D, Michal M, Huang H et al. Myxoinflammatory fibroblastic sarcoma: an immunohistochemical and molecular genetic study of 73 cases. *Mod Pathol* 2020;33:2520–33.

Undifferentiated sarcoma
5 Fletcher CD. Pleomorphic malignant fibrous histiocytoma: fact or fiction? A critical reappraisal based on 159 tumors diagnosed as pleomorphic sarcoma. *Am J Surg Pathol* 1992;16:213–28.

Myxofibrosarcoma
4 Mentzel T, Calonje E, Wadden C et al. Myxofibrosarcoma: clinicopathologic analysis of 75 cases with emphasis on the low-grade variant. *Am J Surg Pathol* 1996;20:391–405.

Low-grade fibromyxoid sarcoma
7 Lau PP, Lui PC, Lau GT et al. EWSR1-CREB3L1 gene fusion: a novel alternative molecular aberration of low-grade fibromyxoid sarcoma. *Am J Surg Pathol* 2013;37:734–8.

Fibrohistiocytic tumours
Tenosynovial giant cell tumour
2 Ushjima M, Hashimoto H, Tsuneyoshi M et al. Giant cell tumor of the tendon sheath (nodular tenosynovitis): a study of 207 cases to compare the large joint group with the common digit group. *Cancer* 1986;57:875–84.

Fibrous histiocytoma (dermatofibroma)
10 Doyle LA, Fletcher CD. Metastasizing "benign" cutaneous fibrous histiocytoma: a clinicopathologic analysis of 16 cases. *Am J Surg Pathol* 2013;37:484–95.
12 Calonje E, Mentzel T, Fletcher CDM. Cellular benign fibrous histiocytoma: clinicopathologic analysis of 74 cases of a distinctive variant of cutaneous fibrous histiocytoma with frequent recurrence. *Am J Surg Pathol* 1994;18:668–76.
15 Calonje E, Fletcher CDM. Aneurysmal benign cutaneous fibrous histiocytoma: clinicopathologic analysis of a tumor frequently misdiagnosed as a vascular lesion. *Histopathology* 1995;26:323–31.
17 Kaddu S, McMenamin M, Fletcher CD. Atypical fibrous histiocytoma of the skin: clinicopathologic analysis of 59 cases with evidence of infrequent metastasis. *Am J Surg Pathol* 2002;26:35–46.
20 Dickson BC, Swanson D, Charames GS et al. Epithelioid fibrous histiocytoma: molecular characterization of ALK fusion partners in 23 cases. *Mod Pathol* 2018;31:753–62.

Plexiform fibrohistiocytic tumour
5 Moosavi C, Jha P, Fanburg-Smith JC. An update on plexiform fibrohistiocytic tumor and addition of 66 new cases from the Armed Forces Institute of Pathology, in honor of Franz M. Enzinger, MD. *Ann Diagn Pathol* 2007;11:313–19.

Atypical fibroxanthoma/pleomorphic dermal sarcoma
1 Beer TW, Drury P, Heenan PJ. Atypical fibroxanthoma: a histological and immunohistochemical review of 171 cases. *Am J Dermatopathol* 2010;32:533–40.
2 Fretzin DF, Helwig EB. Atypical fibroxanthoma of the skin: a clinicopathological study of 140 cases. *Cancer* 1973;31:1541–52.
20 Luzar B, Calonje E. Morphological and immunohistochemical characteristics of atypical fibroxanthoma with a special emphasis on potential diagnostic pitfalls: a review. *J Cutan Pathol* 2010;37:301–9.
26 Griewank KG, Wiesner T, Murali R et al. Atypical fibroxanthoma and pleomorphic dermal sarcoma harbor frequent NOTCH1/2 and FAT1 mutations and similar DNA copy number alteration profiles. *Mod Pathol* 2018;31:418–28.

Vascular tumours
Reactive vascular lesions
Intravascular papillary endothelial hyperplasia
3 Hashimoto H, Daimaru Y, Enjoji M. Intravascular papillary endothelial hyperplasia: a clinicopathologic study of 91 cases. *Am J Dermatopathol* 1983;5:539–45.

Reactive angioendotheliomatosis
7 McMenamin ME, Fletcher CD. Reactive angioendotheliomatosis: a study of 15 cases demonstrating a wide clinicopathologic spectrum. *Am J Surg Pathol* 2002;26:685–97.

Glomeruloid haemangioma
1 Chan JKC, Fletcher CDM, Hicklin GA et al. Glomeruloid hemangioma: a distinctive cutaneous lesion of multicentric Castleman's disease associated with POEMS syndrome. *Am J Surg Pathol* 1990;14:1036–46.

Benign vascular tumours
Papillary haemangioma
1 Suurmeijer AJ, Fletcher CD. Papillary haemangioma. A distinctive cutaneous haemangioma of the head and neck area containing eosinophilic hyaline globules. *Histopathology* 2007;51:638–48.

Lobular capillary haemangioma (pyogenic granuloma)
3 Harris MN, Desai R, Chuang TY et al. Lobular capillary hemangioma: an epidemiologic report, with emphasis on cutaneous lesions. *J Am Acad Dermatol* 2000;42:1012–16.

Cirsoid aneurysm
2 Connelly MG, Winkelmann RK. Acral arteriovenous tumor: a clinicopathologic review. *Am J Surg Pathol* 1985;9:15–21.

Epithelioid haemangioma
1 Olsen TG, Helwig EB. Angiolymphoid hyperplasia with eosinophilia. *J Am Acad Dermatol* 1985;12:781–96.
7 Huang SC, Zhang L, Sung YS et al. Frequent FOS gene rearrangements in epithelioid hemangioma: a molecular study of 58 cases with morphologic reappraisal. *Am J Surg Pathol* 2015;39:1313–21.

Cutaneous epithelioid angiomatous nodule
1 Brenn T, Fletcher CDM. Cutaneous epithelioid angiomatous nodule: a distinct lesion in the morphologic spectrum of epithelioid vascular tumors. *Am J Dermatopathol* 2004;26:14–21.

Acquired elastotic haemangioma
1 Requena L, Kutzner H, Mentzel T. Acquired elastotic hemangioma: a clinicopathologic variant of hemangioma. *J Am Acad Dermatol* 2002;47:371–6.

Hobnail haemangioma
3 Guillou L, Calonje E, Speight P et al. Hobnail hemangioma: a pseudomalignant vascular lesion with a reappraisal of targetoid hemosiderotic hemangioma. *Am J Surg Pathol* 1999;23:97–105.

Microvenular haemangioma
1 Hunt SJ, Santa Cruz DJ, Barr RJ. Microvenular hemangioma. *J Cutan Pathol* 1991;18:235–40.

Sinusoidal haemangioma
1 Calonje E, Fletcher CDM. Sinusoidal hemangioma. *Am J Surg Pathol* 1991;15:1130–5.

Spindle cell haemangioma
6 Perkins P, Weiss SW. Spindle cell hemangioendothelioma: an analysis of 78 cases with reassessment of its pathogenesis and biologic behavior. *Am J Surg Pathol* 1996;20:1196–204.

Symplastic haemangioma
3 Goh N, Dayrit J, Calonje E. Symplastic hemangioma. Report of two cases. *J Cutan Pathol* 2006;33:735–40.

Poikilodermatous plaque-like haemangioma
1 Semkova K, Carr R, Grainger M et al. Poikilodermatous plaque-like hemangioma: case series of a newly defined entity. *J Am Acad Dermatol* 2019;81:1257–70.

Vascular tumours of intermediate malignancy
Retiform haemangioendothelioma
1 Calonje E, Fletcher CD, Wilson Jones E et al. Retiform hemangioendothelioma: a distinctive form of low-grade angiosarcoma delineated in a series of 15 cases. *Am J Surg Pathol* 1994;18:115–25.

Papillary intralymphatic angioendothelioma
5 Fanburgh-Smith JC, Michal M et al. Papillary intralymphatic angioendothelioma (PILA): a report of twelve cases of a distinctive vascular tumor with phenotypic features of lymphatic vessels. *Am J Surg Pathol* 1999;23:1004–10.

Composite haemangioendothelioma
1 Nayler SJ, Rubin BP, Calonje E et al. Composite hemangioendothelioma: a complex, low-grade vascular lesion mimicking angiosarcoma. *Am J Surg Pathol* 2000;24:352–61.

2 Perry KD, Al-Ibraheemi A, Rubin BP et al. Composite hemangioendothelioma with neuroendocrine marker expression: an aggressive variant. Mod Pathol 2017;30:1589–602.

Pseudomyogenic haemangioendothelioma
3 Hornick JL, Fletcher CD. Pseudomyogenic hemangioendothelioma: a distinctive, often multicentric tumor with indolent behavior. Am J Surg Pathol 2011;35:190–201.

Malignant vascular tumours
Angiosarcoma
1 Mark RJ, Poen JC, Tran LM et al. Angiosarcoma: a review of 67 patients and review of the literature. Cancer 1996;77:2400–6.
46 Abraham JA, Hamicek FJ, Kaufman AM et al. Treatment and outcome of 82 patients with angiosarcoma. Ann Surg Oncol 2007;14:1953–67.
48 Deyrup AT, McKenney JK, Tighiouart M et al. Sporadic cutaneous angiosarcomas: a proposal for risk stratification based on 69 cases. Am J Surg Pathol 2008;32:72–7.

Epithelioid haemangioendothelioma
3 Mentzel T, Beham A, Calonje E et al. Epithelioid hemangioendothelioma of skin and soft tissues: clinicopathologic and immunohistochemical study of 30 cases. Am J Surg Pathol 1997;21:363–74.

Epithelioid angiosarcoma
4 Suchak R, Thway K, Zelger B et al. Primary cutaneous epithelioid angiosarcoma: a clinicopathologic study of 13 cases of a rare neoplasm occurring outside the setting of conventional angiosarcomas and with predilection for the limbs. Am J Surg Pathol 2011;35:60–9.

Lymphatic tumours
Acquired progressive lymphangioma
4 Guillou L, Flecher CDM. Benign lymphangioendothelioma (acquired progressive lymphangioma), a lesion not to be confused with well-differentiated angiosarcoma and patch stage Kaposi's sarcoma: clinicopathologic analysis of a series. Am J Surg Pathol 2000;24:1047–57.

Atypical vascular proliferation after radiotherapy
4 Brenn T, Fletcher CD. Radiation-induced cutaneous atypical vascular lesions and angiosarcoma: clinicopathologic analysis of 42 cases. Am J Surg Pathol 2005;29:983–96.

Diffuse lymphangiomatosis
10 Bruch-Gerharz D, Gerharz CD, Stege H et al. Cutaneous lymphatic malformations in disappearing bone (Gorham-Stout) disease: a novel clue to the pathogenesis of a rare syndrome. J Am Acad Dermatol 2007;56(Suppl.):S21–5.

Tumours of perivascular cells
Infantile myofibromatosis and adult myofibroma
7 Mentzel T, Calonje E, Nascimento AG et al. Infantile hemangiopericytoma versus infantile myofibromatosis: study of a series suggesting a continuous spectrum of infantile myofibroblastic lesions. Am J Surg Pathol 1994;18:922–30.
13 Cheung YH, Gayden T, Campeau PM et al. A recurrent PDGFRB mutation causes familial infantile myofibromatosis. Am J Hum Genet 2013;92:996–1000.

Myopericytoma
6 Mentzel T, Dei Tos AP, Sapi Z et al. Myopericytoma of skin and soft tissues: clinicopathologic and immunohistochemical study of 54 cases. Am J Surg Pathol 2006;30:104–13.

Glomus tumour
13 Folpe AL, Fanburgh-Smith JC, Miettinen M et al. Atypical glomus tumors: analysis of 52 cases, with a proposal for the reclassification of glomus tumors. Am J Surg Pathol 2001;25:1–12.
15 Schiefer TK, Parker WL, Anakwenze OA et al. Extradigital glomus tumors: a 20-year experience. Mayo Clin Proc 2006;81:1337–44.

Peripheral neuroectodermal tumours
1 Rodriguez-Peralto JL, Riveiro-Falkenbach E, Carrillo R. Benign cutaneous neural tumors. Semin Diagn Pathol 2013;30:45–57.

Neuromuscular hamartoma
2 Markel SF, Enzinger FM. Neuromuscular hamartoma: a benign 'triton tumor' composed of mature neural and striated muscle elements. Cancer 1982;49:140–4.

Dermal hyperneury
1 Winkelmann RK, Carney JA. Cutaneous neuropathology in multiple endocrine neoplasia, type 2b. J Invest Dermatol 1982;79:307–12.
2 Ieremia E, Marušić Z, Mudaliar V et al. Expanding the clinical spectrum of dermal hyperneury: report of nine new cases and a review of the literature. Histopathology 2019;75:738–45.

Multiple mucosal neuromas
1 Gorlin RJ, Sedano HO, Vickers RA et al. Multiple mucosal neuromas, pheochromocytoma and medullary carcinoma of the thyroid: a syndrome. Cancer 1968;22:293–9.

Amputation stump neuroma
1 Cieslak AK, Stout AP. Traumatic and amputation neuromas. Arch Surg 1946;53:646–51.

Morton neuroma
1 Lassmann G, Lassmann H, Stockinger L. Morton's metatarsalgia: light and electron microscopic observations and their relation to entrapment neuropathies. Virchows Arch (A) 1976;370:307–21.

Solitary circumscribed neuroma
2 Fletcher CDM. Solitary circumscribed neuroma of the skin (so-called palisaded, encapsulated neuroma): a clinicopathologic and immunohistochemical study. Am J Surg Pathol 1989;13:574–80.

Schwannoma
11 White WM, Shiu MH, Rosenblum MK et al. Cellular schwannoma: a clinicopathologic study of 57 patients and 58 tumors. Cancer 1990;66:1266–75.
21 Laskin WB, Fetsch JF, Lasota J et al. Benign epithelioid peripheral nerve sheath tumors of the soft tissues: clinicopathologic spectrum of 33 cases. Am J Surg Pathol 2005;29:39–51.
24 Agnihotri S, Jalali S, Wilson MR et al. The genomic landscape of schwannoma. Nat Genet 2016;48:1339–48.
26 Woodruff JM, Selig AM, Crowley K et al. Schwannoma (neurilemmoma) with malignant transformation: a rare, distinctive peripheral nerve tumor. Am J Surg Pathol 1994;18:882–95.

Solitary neurofibroma
3 Megahed M. Histopathological variants of neurofibroma: a study of 114 lesions. Am J Dermatopathol 1994;16:486–95.

Plexiform neurofibroma
3 Beert E, Brems H, Renard M et al. Biallelic inactivation of NF1 in a sporadic plexiform neurofibroma. Genes Chromosomes Cancer 2012;51:852–7.

Perineurioma
3 Fetsch JF, Miettinen M. Sclerosing perineurioma: a clinicopathological study of 15 cases of a distinctive soft tissue lesion with a predilection for the fingers and palms of young adults. Am J Surg Pathol 1997;21:1433–42.

Dermal nerve sheath myxoma
4 Fetsch JF, Laskin WB, Miettinen M. Nerve sheath myxoma: a clinicopathologic and immunohistochemical analysis of 57 morphologically distinctive, S-100 protein and GFAP positive myxoid peripheral nerve sheath tumors with a predilection for the extremities and a high local recurrence rate. Am J Surg Pathol 2005;29:1615–24.

Cellular neurothekeoma
6 Hornick JL, Fletcher CD. Cellular neurothekeoma: detailed characterization in a series of 133 cases. Am J Surg Pathol 2007;31:329–40.

Granular cell tumour
2 Lack EE, Worsham GF, Calliham MD et al. Granular cell tumor: a clinicopathologic study of 100 patients. *J Surg Oncol* 1980;13:301–9.

Meningothelial heterotopias
4 Lopez DA, Silvers DN, Helwig EB. Cutaneous meningiomas: a clinico-pathologic study. *Cancer* 1974;34:728–44.

Glial heterotopic nodules
1 Fletcher CDM, Carpenter G, McKee PH. Nasal glioma: a rarity. *Am J Dermatopathol* 1986;8:341–6.

Epithelial sheath neuroma
1 Requena L, Grosshans E, Kutzner H et al. Epithelial sheath neuroma: a new entity. *Am J Surg Pathol* 2000;24:190–6.

Pigmented neuroectodermal tumour of infancy
7 Johnson RE, Scheithauer BW, Dahlin DC. Melanotic neuroectodermal tumor of infancy: a review of seven cases. *Cancer* 1983;52:661–6.

Malignant peripheral nerve sheath tumour
4 Allison KH, Patel RM, Goldblum JR et al. Superficial malignant peripheral nerve sheath tumor: a rare and challenging diagnosis. *Am J Clin Pathol* 2005;124:685–92.

Cutaneous Ewing sarcoma
5 Delaplace M, Lhommet C, de Pinieux G et al. Primary cutaneous Ewing sarcoma: a systematic review focused on treatment and outcome. *Br J Dermatol* 2012;166:721–6.

CIC-rearranged sarcoma
1 Antonescu CR, Owosho AA, Zhang L et al. Sarcomas with CIC-rearrangements are a distinct pathologic entity with aggressive outcome: a clinicopathologic and molecular study of 115 cases. *Am J Surg Pathol* 2017;41:941–9.

Tumours of muscle
Smooth muscle hamartoma
3 González IA, Dehner LP. Smooth muscle hamartoma and striated muscle hamartoma: clinicopathologic characterization of two rare entities and literature review. *J Cutan Pathol* 2021;48:237–46.

Leiomyoma
1 Raj S, Calonje E, Kraus M et al. Cutaneous pilar leiomyoma: clinicopathologic analysis of 53 lesions in 45 patients. *Am J Dermatopathol* 1997;19:2–9.
5 Hachisuga T, Hashimoto H, Enjoji M. Angioleiomyoma: a clinical reappraisal of 562 cases. *Cancer* 1984;54:126–30.
10 Alam NA, Bevan S, Churchman M et al. Localization of a gene (MCUL1) for multiple cutaneous leiomyomata and uterine fibroids to chromosome 1q,42.3–q43. *Am J Hum Genet* 2001;68:1264–9.

Leiomyosarcoma/atypical smooth muscle tumour (dermal and subcutaneous)
5 Kraft S, Fletcher CD. Atypical intradermal smooth muscle neoplasms: clinicopathologic analysis of 84 cases and a reappraisal of cutaneous "leiomyosarcoma". *Am J Surg Pathol* 2011;35:599–607.

Skeletal muscle tumours
Rhabdomyomatous congenital hamartoma
3 Rosenberg AS, Kirk J, Morgan MB. Rhabdomyomatous mesenchymal hamartoma: an unusual dermal entity with a report of two cases and review of the literature. *J Cutan Pathol* 2002;29:238–43.

Cutaneous rhabdomyosarcoma
3 Marburger TB, Gardner JM, Prieto VG et al. Primary cutaneous rhabdomyosarcoma: a clinicopathologic review of 11 cases. *J Cutan Pathol* 2012;39:987–95.

Tumours of fat cells
Lipoblastoma and lipoblastomatosis
3 Collins MH, Chatten J. Lipoblastoma/lipoblastomatosis: a clinicopathologic study of 25 tumors. *Am J Surg Pathol* 1997;21:1131–7.

Spindle cell and pleomorphic lipoma
13 Mentzel T. Cutaneous lipomatous neoplasms. *Semin Diagn Pathol* 2001;18:250–7.

Atypical lipomatous tumour
5 Evans HL. Atypical lipomatous tumour, its variants, and its combined forms: a study of 61 cases, with a minimum follow-up of 10 years. *Am J Surg Pathol* 2007;31:1–14.

Liposarcoma
1 Dei Tos AP, Mentzel T, Fletcher CD. Primary liposarcoma of the skin: a rare neoplasm with unusual high-grade features. *Am J Dermatopathol* 1998;20:332–8.

Tumours of uncertain histogenesis
Acral fibromyxoma
4 Hollmann TJ, Bovee JVMG, Fletcher CDM. Digital fibromyxoma (superficial acral fibromyxoma): a detailed characterization of 124 cases. *Am J Surg Pathol* 2012;36:789–98.

Superficial angiomyxoma
2 Calonje E, Guerin D, McCormick D et al. Superficial angiomyxoma: clinicopathologic analysis of a series of distinctive but poorly recognized cutaneous tumors with a tendency for recurrence. *Am J Surg Pathol* 1999;23:910–17.

Digital mucous cyst
1 Johnson WC, Graham JH, Helwig EB. Cutaneous myxoid cyst: a clinicopathologic and histochemical study. *JAMA* 1965;191:15–20.

Dermal non-neural granular cell tumour
2 Lazar AJ, Fletcher CD. Primitive nonneural granular cell tumors of the skin: clinicopathologic analysis of 13 cases. *Am J Surg Pathol* 2005;29:927–34.

Haemosiderotic fibrolipomatous tumour
2 Browne TJ, Fletcher CD. Haemosiderotic fibrolipomatous tumour (so-called haemosiderotic fibrohistiocytic lipomatous tumour): analysis of 13 new cases in support of a distinct entity. *Histopathology* 2006;48:453–61.

Perivascular epithelioid cell tumour ('PEComa')
3 Hornick JL, Fletcher CD. PEComa: what do we know so far? *Histopathology* 2006;48:75–82.

Deep ('aggressive') angiomyxoma
2 Fetsch JF, Laskin WB, Lefkowitz M et al. Aggressive angiomyxoma: a clinicopathologic study of 29 female patients. *Cancer* 1996;78:79–90.

Angiomatoid fibrous histiocytoma
2 Costa MJ, Weiss SW. Angiomatoid malignant fibrous histiocytoma: a follow-up study of 108 cases with evaluation of possible predictors of outcome. *Am J Surg Pathol* 1990;14:1126–32.

Epithelioid sarcoma
3 Fisher C. Epithelioid sarcoma of Enzinger. *Adv Anat Pathol* 2006;13:114–21.
5 Guillou L, Wadden C, Coindre JM et al. Proximal-type epithelioid sarcoma, a distinctive aggressive neoplasm showing rhabdoid features: clinicopathologic, immunohistochemical, and ultrastructural study of a series. *Am J Surg Pathol* 1997;21:130–46.

Clear cell sarcoma
5 Meis-Kindblom JM. Clear cell sarcoma of tendon and aponeuroses: a historical perspective and tribute to the man behind the entity. *Adv Anat Pathol* 2006;13:286–92.
18 Coindre JM, Hostein I, Terrier P et al. Diagnosis of clear cell sarcoma by real-time reverse transcriptase-polymerase chain reaction analysis of paraffin embedded tissues: clinicopathological and molecular analysis of 44 patients from the French sarcoma group. *Cancer* 2005;107:1055–64.

CHAPTER 137
Tumours of Skin Appendages

Eduardo Calonje[1] and Zlatko Marušić[2]

[1] St John's Institute of Dermatology, Guy's and St Thomas' NHS Foundation Trust, London, UK
[2] Clinical Department of Pathology and Cytology, University Hospital Center Zagreb, Zagreb, Croatia

---

Introduction, 137.1

HAIR FOLLICLE TUMOURS, 137.2
Inverted follicular keratosis, 137.2
Dilated pore, 137.3
Tumour of the follicular infundibulum, 137.3
Pilar sheath acanthoma, 137.4
Trichoadenoma, 137.4
Comedo naevus, 137.4

EXTERNAL ROOT SHEATH TUMOURS, 137.5
Trichilemmal cyst, 137.5
Proliferating trichilemmal tumour, 137.5
Trichilemmoma, 137.6
Trichilemmal carcinoma, 137.6

HAMARTOMAS AND HAIR GERM TUMOURS AND CYSTS, 137.7
Hair follicle naevus, 137.7
Eruptive vellus hair cyst, 137.7
Trichofolliculoma, 137.8
Trichoepithelioma, 137.9
Desmoplastic trichoepithelioma, 137.10
Trichoblastoma, 137.10
Adamantinoid trichoblastoma, 137.11
Basaloid follicular hamartoma, 137.12

HAIR MATRIX TUMOURS, 137.12
Pilomatricoma, 137.12
Pilomatrical carcinoma, 137.14

LESIONS OF HAIR FOLLICLE MESENCHYME, 137.14
Trichodiscoma, 137.14
Perifollicular fibroma, 137.15
Fibrofolliculoma, 137.15

SEBACEOUS GLAND TUMOURS, 137.15
Sebaceous adenomas and sebaceomas, 137.16
Sebaceous carcinoma, 137.17

APOCRINE GLAND TUMOURS, 137.18
Apocrine hidrocystoma, 137.18
Syringocystadenoma papilliferum, 137.19
Hidradenoma papilliferum, 137.20
Nipple adenoma, 137.20
Apocrine tubular adenoma, 137.21
Apocrine carcinoma, 137.21

ECCRINE GLAND HAMARTOMAS AND TUMOURS, 137.22
Eccrine angiomatous hamartoma, 137.22
Eccrine hidrocystoma, 137.23
Hidroacanthoma simplex, 137.23
Eccrine dermal duct tumour, 137.24
Eccrine poroma, 137.24
Eccrine syringofibroadenoma, 137.25
Syringoma, 137.26
Tubular adenoma, 137.27

ECCRINE OR APOCRINE/FOLLICULAR TUMOURS, 137.27
Hidradenoma, 137.28

Cylindroma, 137.28
Spiradenoma, 137.29
Mixed tumour of the skin, 137.31
Cutaneous myoepithelioma, 137.32

SWEAT GLAND CARCINOMAS, INCLUDING DUCTAL APOCRINE/FOLLICULAR CARCINOMAS, 137.32
Eccrine gland carcinomas, 137.32
Malignant eccrine poroma, 137.32
Squamoid eccrine ductal carcinoma, 137.33
Digital papillary adenocarcinoma, 137.33
Eccrine or apocrine/follicular carcinomas, 137.34
Malignant cylindroma, 137.34
Hidradenocarcinoma, 137.34
Spiradenocarcinoma, 137.35
Microcystic adnexal carcinoma, 137.35
Adnexal carcinoma NOS, 137.36
Mucinous carcinoma, 137.37
Endocrine mucin-producing sweat gland carcinoma, 137.37
Adenoid cystic carcinoma, 137.38
Secretory carcinoma, 137.38

MISCELLANEOUS TUMOURS, 137.39
Tumours of ano-genital mammary-like glands, 137.39
Paget disease of the nipple, 137.39
Extramammary Paget disease, 137.41
Lymphoepithelioma-like carcinoma, 137.42

Key references, 137.43

Introduction

The anatomical relationships of the epidermis and dermis are fully discussed in Chapter 3. The skin appendages are of particular interest in this respect, in that they clearly show a morphological and, in some instances, functional interrelationship. The appendageal tumours discussed in this chapter either differentiate towards or arise from the pilosebaceous apparatus (including the apocrine gland) and eccrine sweat gland [1–5,6,7].

The pilosebaceous apparatus can be divided into the hair follicle, the adjacent sebaceous gland and, in some body sites, the apocrine glands. Small strips of smooth muscle, the arrector pili muscle, are also found in association with these structures.

The pilosebaceous apparatus is concentrated in the head and neck area, with the pilar element predominant on the scalp and the sebaceous element on the face, chest and upper back. Thus, tumours arising from these structures are found predominantly at these anatomical sites.

Rook's Textbook of Dermatology, Tenth Edition. Edited by Christopher Griffiths, Jonathan Barker, Tanya Bleiker, Walayat Hussain and Rosalind Simpson.
© 2024 John Wiley & Sons Ltd. Published 2024 by John Wiley & Sons Ltd.

The eccrine sweat glands are, in contrast, found on all body sites and comprise a double-layered, deeply situated secretory structure and a more superficial excretory duct winding through the dermis and spiralling through the epidermis to reach the surface of the skin.

The excretory (ductal) portions of the eccrine and apocrine glands are identical and cannot be differentiated on morphological grounds unless the apocrine duct can be identified entering the hair follicle. To complicate matters further, the apocrine duct rarely opens directly into the epidermis, and there are no histochemical or immunohistochemical stains that allow distinction between eccrine and apocrine tumours. From this, it can be inferred that adnexal tumours showing ductal differentiation may be either eccrine or apocrine, and distinction is not possible unless there is concomitant follicular differentiation. It has therefore been proposed that the classification of adnexal tumours should follow a more logical approach that takes this into consideration [6]. It has become apparent that tumours traditionally considered to be of eccrine differentiation, such as cylindroma, spiradenoma and mixed tumour (so-called chondroid syringoma) may show either line of differentiation and this is probably most often apocrine. Even a classical eccrine tumour such as poroma has been described occasionally as differentiating towards the apocrine duct [7].

A wide range of cells make up the secretory and excretory components of the appendage ducts, the hair follicles and the sebaceous glands. As each cell type capable of dividing can give rise to a tumour as a result of inappropriate transfer of genetic material and cell division, it follows that an equal number of tumours are theoretically possible. The great majority of these appendage-derived tumours are benign, while behaviour and prognosis for most tumours with malignant potential is no worse than the one seen in basal cell carcinoma. Thus, although local recurrence is well recorded, metastases are rare, with the exception of the malignant eccrine and apocrine gland-derived tumours and ocular sebaceous carcinoma. It is important to take into account that malignant adnexal tumours with metastasis are overreported in the literature and that this has led to overestimation of their biological behaviour.

Appendage tumours are relatively rare and their clinical appearance is commonly non-specific. The great majority are not diagnosed as such until after excision and pathological study. Classification systems for these lesions tend to be controversial, but in general the system groups lesions according to their morphological similarity to normal appendage structures.

HAIR FOLLICLE TUMOURS

A large number of tumours are theoretically capable of arising from the hair follicle and matrix, depending on the exact type of cell and its situation within the dermis. A representative selection of these tumours is described here. For a comprehensive list, the reader is referred to specialised publications [1,2]. Studies on the role of the sonic hedgehog gene and related proteins in basal cell carcinoma (Chapter 140) have been extended to hair follicle tumours [3]. The *PTCH* gene is located on chromosome 9q22.3, and loss of heterozygosity has been identified in sporadic trichoepitheliomas [4]. Overexpression of Gli-1, which is integral to this pathway, has been observed in trichoepitheliomas in mice [5]. Multiple familial trichoepitheliomas exhibit mutations in the *CYLD* gene [6]. Trichilemmal carcinomas have been shown to harbour *TP53* mutations and fusions previously encountered in melanoma [7].

β-Catenin plays a key role in signal transduction and subsequent tissue modelling, and mutations in the β-catenin gene have been recorded in pilomatricomas [8,9].

Inverted follicular keratosis [1–3,4]

Definition and nomenclature
A localised area of hyperkeratosis found in association with the pilosebaceous orifice, considered as a variant of seborrheic keratosis (Chapter 132).

Synonyms and inclusions
- Endophytic seborrheic keratosis

Epidemiology
Age
Middle aged and elderly.

Sex
Men are affected much more frequently than women.

Pathophysiology
A number of these lesions arise as a result of infection of the infundibulum of the hair follicle by human papillomavirus (HPV). It is likely that a majority of these lesions may be regarded as the most superficial tumour of the follicular infundibulum (see later), arising as the result of irritation.

Pathology
The pathological features show an endophytic lesion connected to the infundibulum of the hair follicle. Irritated keratinocytes form whorls of cells, so-called 'squamous eddies', and keratin cysts. All of these features may give rise to problems with the differential diagnosis of squamous cell carcinoma, especially on small biopsies. This can be relatively easily distinguished on low-power examination, as there is no individual cell invasion into the dermis. At higher power, mitotic figures may be seen, but they are not abnormal mitoses. The appearances are identical to an irritated seborrhoeic keratosis, but the latter is exophytic.

Clinical features
History and presentation
In common with many of the lesions described in this chapter, this lesion presents as a solitary papule on the head and neck area. It may reach a considerable size, and be inflamed and pruritic. Recently, an attempt to establish dermoscopic features has been made [5].

Disease course and prognosis
Occasionally, the lesions recur [3].

Management
Local surgical excision is generally not needed once diagnostic shave biopsy excludes other entities requiring excision.

Dilated pore [1,2]

Definition and nomenclature
An area of expanded follicular infundibulum with a dilated poral opening extending down to subcutaneous fat [2].

Synonyms and inclusions
- Pore of Winer
- Infundibuloma

Epidemiology
Incidence and prevalence
Relatively common.

Age
Adults in the fourth to sixth decade.

Sex
There is male predilection.

Pathophysiology
Pathology
There is a wide, crater-like cavity from which acanthotic areas of follicular epithelium radiate. The follicle is lined by outer root sheath epithelium and there is little evidence of a sebaceous gland or a well-formed emerging hair. Rare lesions may be associated with trichoblastoma [3] and exceptionally with either basal cell carcinoma [4] or squamous cell carcinoma [5].

Clinical features
History and presentation
The pore is a comedo-like lesion found mainly on the head and neck area. Dermoscopy features have been described [6]. One case with multiple lesions has been described [7].

Disease course and prognosis
The lesion is benign.

Management
No treatment is necessary except when lesions become persistently inflamed or for cosmetic reasons. Treatment options include cosmetic strips and topical application of retinoids. Mechanical evacuation can be used as well, but refilling of the lesion is common. Laser therapy or surgical excision may be used on more resistant cases.

Tumour of the follicular infundibulum [1]

Definition and nomenclature
This lesion may be considered the hair follicle equivalent of the eccrine dermal duct tumour (see later). It is a tumour that shows differentiation towards the follicular infundibulum or isthmus.

Synonyms and inclusions
- Isthmicoma
- Infundibuloma
- Infundibulomatosis (eruptive form)

Epidemiology [2]
Incidence and prevalence
The tumour is rare.

Age
It is more common in elderly people (median age: 66 years). The rare eruptive form tends to occur in younger patients.

Sex
It shows a slight female predilection.

Pathophysiology
Pathology [3–5]
The pathology is that of a large horizontally orientated plate of small dark cells situated in the superficial dermis, usually with multiple connections to the overlying epidermis. The cellular detail is focally similar to that seen in the trichilemmoma, with large numbers of small polygonal cells with clear cytoplasm contained within a palisaded border. Basaloid cells are often seen. The resemblance to basal cell carcinoma is striking, but the stromal element is lacking. Occasionally, sebaceous differentiation may be seen [6]. These lesions with sebaceous differentiation have been termed superficial epithelioma with sebaceous differentiation [7] and acanthomatous, superficial, sebaceous hamartoma [8].

Clinical features
History and presentation
These lesions are usually found on facial skin and may be relatively large irregular nodules. They are usually biopsied or excised to obtain a diagnosis because the clinical appearance is not specific. It has been suggested that they can be divided into four main groups: solitary lesions; those in association with Cowden disease; multiple eruptive tumours [9]; and follicular infundibulum-like changes in the epidermis [1]. An association with other skin tumours may be seen [10] especially with basal cell and squamous cell carcinoma [11,12]. In some cases, changes identical to those seen in the tumour are identified incidentally [10,13]. Dermoscopy features have been described [14].

Disease course and prognosis
The lesion is benign.

Management
For solitary tumours surgical excision is curative. Eruptive variants are difficult to treat due to the number of lesions.

Pilar sheath acanthoma [1]

Definition and nomenclature
A follicular tumour with differentiation towards the infundibulum and the isthmus.

Synonyms and inclusions
- Infundibulo-isthmicoma

Epidemiology [2,3]
Incidence and prevalence
Lesions are very rare.

Age
Middle aged to elderly.

Sex
There is no sex preference.

Pathophysiology
Pathology
The pathology is that of an expanded area of the outer root sheath epithelium within an irregularly branched cystic cavity, with large lobules of epithelial cells radiating outwards from this cavity area. A plaque-like architectural pattern may be seen [4].

Clinical features
History and presentation
These lesions, described in 1978 [1], are most commonly seen on the upper lip area [2]. A few cases have been described at other locations such as the lower lip and cheeks and postauricular area [3]. Presentation is a solitary asymptomatic skin-coloured nodule with a central pore-like opening measuring 3–5 mm. Biopsy is usually required to obtain a definite diagnosis.

Disease course and prognosis
Lesions have a benign behaviour.

Management
Usually the lesion is completely removed to obtain a definite diagnosis.

Trichoadenoma [1,2]

Definition
A rare benign tumour with multiple cystic structures closely resembling the infundibular portion of the hair follicle. The keratin profile expression supports the theory that this tumour differentiates towards the follicular infundibulum and the follicular bulge region [3]. It has been shown on cell lines that tumours with trichoadenoma histology arise from a specific compartment within the stem cell population [4].

Epidemiology [5]
Incidence and prevalence
The lesion is rare.

Age
It is more common in adults. Congenital lesion or occurrence in childhood is rarely seen.

Sex
There is no sex predilection.

Pathophysiology
Pathology
The lesions are in the upper dermis, and on light microscope scanning power give the impression of a cluster of cysts. On higher power, these cyst-like structures have an appearance similar to the infundibular portion of the hair follicle but turned through 90°; no recognisable hair shafts are seen. By immunohistochemistry, trichadenomas retain the CK20-positive Merkel cells [6].

Clinical features
History and presentation
This lesion presents as a non-specific nodule, usually on the face, although there are some reports of lesions on the buttocks. It may occur within a naevus sebaceous [7] or coexist with an intradermal naevus [8]. Dermoscopy features have been described [9].

Disease course and prognosis
The lesion is benign.

Management
Usually complete surgical excision is required to obtain a definite diagnosis.

Comedo naevus [1,2,3]

Definition and nomenclature
A rare abnormality of the follicular infundibulum presenting as a group of comedo-like lesions. It is suggested that it is a rare type of epidermal naevus. It is part of the naevus comedonicus syndrome [2].

Synonyms and inclusions
- Naevus comedonicus
- Naevus acneiformis unilateralis
- Naevus a comedons
- Naevus follicularis keratosus
- Naevus zoniforme

Epidemiology
Incidence and prevalence
The prevalence has been estimated to be from 1 in 45 000 to 1 in 100 000 [2].

Age
They may be present at birth or develop throughout adult life.

Sex
It shows no gender predilection.

Pathophysiology
Pathology
A rudimentary pilosebaceous follicle is present, with a large overlying keratin-filled crater. The surface of the keratinous material oxidises to give the comedone-like appearance. Rarely, lesions develop trichilemmal cysts [4].

Genetics
Somatic mutations in NEK9 cause comedo naevus [2].

Clinical features
History and presentation
These lesions are rare and are seen mainly on the head and neck area. Cases may also occur at other sites including the palm and wrist [5]. The palm is not an area that contains hair follicles and the unusual presentation of naevus comedonicus in this location has led to the suggestion that these lesions may really represent variants of sweat duct naevus [6,7]. They appear as a cluster of comedones or as a single giant lesion [3]. NC syndrome is mainly associated with ocular, skeletal and neural abnormalities, most typically ipsilateral congenital cataract and malformations of fingers and toes [8,9].

Disease course and prognosis
Lesions are benign.

Management
Treatment options, for cosmetic reasons or in complicated cases, include topical retinoid therapy (adapalene), laser and surgery [2].

EXTERNAL ROOT SHEATH TUMOURS

Trichilemmal cyst

See Chapter 133.

Proliferating trichilemmal tumour [1,2]

Definition and nomenclature
A tumour of external root sheath derivation usually arising in a pre-existent pilar cyst.

Synonyms and inclusions
- Proliferating trichilemmal cyst
- Pilar tumour of the scalp

Epidemiology [1,2,3,4,5]
Incidence and prevalence
These lesions are uncommon.

Age
It occurs mainly in the elderly.

Sex
It shows a marked predilection for females (6/1).

Pathophysiology
Pathology
These lesions may arise from pre-existing trichilemmal cysts and remnants of a classic trichilemmal cyst may be present [1,2,3,4]. The architecture is lobular and expansile, without an infiltrative growth pattern. Tumour lobules are cystic and composed of pale squamous cells with mild atypia. However, tumour cells in the periphery of the lobules may display more prominent cytological atypia and mitotic activity. This is particularly true in early lesions that are actively growing. The surrounding stroma may be fibrotic with inflammation consisting of lymphocytes and plasma cells and a foreign-body granulomatous reaction may be seen in areas where cystic structures have ruptured. Cholesterol clefts and areas of calcification may also be seen. Rarely sebaceous, apocrine and matrical differentiation may be present [5,6].

Exceptionally, a malignant spindle cell component has been described [7,8]. If there is frank invasion into adjacent structures in association with tumour necrosis, cytological atypia and increased mitotic activity, the diagnosis of a malignant proliferating trichilemmal tumour should be made [9,10,11,12]. Such tumours are often characterised clinically by rapid growth and large size [11]. The diagnosis is often very difficult in small samples of tissue and ideally the whole tumour should be submitted for histological examination to avoid confusion with a squamous cell carcinoma. The increased expression of p53 by tumour cells similar to that seen in ordinary squamous cell carcinoma but much lower than that seen in trichilemmal cysts suggests that all these lesions may represent low-grade malignancies [13].

Clinical features
History and presentation
The tumour presents as a rapidly growing large nodule, commonly on the head (scalp and less commonly the face) and neck area followed by the trunk [1,3]. Exceptionally, an association with a naevus sebaceous is seen. Some lesions are very large and may be more than 10 cm in diameter. The history of rapid expansion frequently gives rise to concern about malignancy. Malignant change has been rarely reported in these lesions (see later). Occasionally, tumours may develop within a pre-existing naevus sebaceous [14]. Multiple lesions are exceptional [15].

Disease course and prognosis
Local recurrence takes place. In malignant proliferating trichilemmal tumour metastases may occur, leading to death.

Management
Complete excision is necessary. Radiotherapy and or chemotherapy may be used in malignant tumours. Clinical follow-up is advisable because histology may not correlate with clinical behaviour [3].

Trichilemmoma [1,2,3]

Definition and nomenclature
This lesion is classically considered to be a proliferation of the external root sheath of the hair follicle [4,5]. However, immunohistochemical studies with different molecular weight keratins normally expressed by different components of the hair follicle have not only confirmed the latter but suggest that the lesion also displays infundibular keratinisation [6].

> **Synonyms and inclusions**
> - Tricholemmoma

Epidemiology [7,8,9,10,11,12,14]
Incidence and prevalence
Solitary trichilemmoma is a relatively common lesion. Patients with Cowden syndrome (Chapter 78) or multiple hamartoma and neoplasia syndrome [7,8,9,10,11,12,14] – which is associated with a very high incidence of breast, thyroid and gastrointestinal carcinomas – have large numbers of trichilemmomas. The incidence of this condition is estimated to be 1:200 000 [15].

Age
Lesions usually present in young and middle-aged adults.

Sex
The solitary variant shows no sex predilection but lesions in patients with Cowden syndrome show a slight female predominance.

Pathophysiology
Pathology
These lesions are well-circumscribed lobular tumours extending down from the epidermis and often connected to a hair follicle. Tumour cells display prominent clear cytoplasm secondary to the deposition of glycogen. The presence of glycogen can be confirmed with a positive periodic acid–Schiff (PAS) stain, which becomes negative after treatment with diastase. There is an irregular enclosing PAS-positive diastase-resistant membrane. In a number of cases, there is prominent hyperplasia of the surface epithelium, with hypergranulosis, clumping of keratohyalin granules and hyperkeratosis. This suggests induction of some lesions by HPV. A viral association has been confirmed by demonstration of HPV DNA by polymerase chain reaction in some [16] but not in all cases of the tumour [17]. Trichilemmomas are often found within a naevus sebaceous.

A variant of trichilemmoma, described as desmoplastic trichilemmoma, is more rarely seen [18]. The periphery of this lesion has histological features identical to those of ordinary trichilemmoma, but towards the centre there are strands of squamous cells embedded in a desmoplastic stroma. This stroma appears to contain type I collagen and tenascin but not laminin or type IV collagen [19]. This results in an infiltrative appearance that may be confused with a squamous cell carcinoma, particularly in small biopsy samples.

Genetics
Mutations of the *PTEN* tumour suppressor gene on chromosome 10q23 are found in Cowden syndrome [14,20]. The number of mutations identified is large and continues to increase [21]. It seems that the benign lesions in Cowden syndrome occur without loss of the second *PTEN* allele while the malignant tumours require inactivation of both alleles and additional somatic mutations [22]. Trichilemmomas show a high frequency of HRAS activating mutations [23]. While many of the Cowden syndrome-associated trichilemmomas show loss of *PTEN* expression, it is noted only rarely in sporadic trichilemmomas [24,25].

Clinical features [14–17]
History and presentation
Clinically, these lesions are small non-specific papules on facial skin; the diagnosis of multiple trichilemmomas should stimulate a search for other evidence of Cowden syndrome. This includes a characteristic 'cobblestone' appearance of the oral epithelium, multiple skin tags, squamous papillomas and sclerotic fibromas (storiform collagenomas).

Disease course and prognosis
The lesion although benign can recur if treated by shave biopsy.

Management
Few treatment options are available, ranging from surgical excision to carbon dioxide laser tissue ablation for multiple cases.

Trichilemmal carcinoma [1,2,3,4]

Definition
A rare tumour, probably underdiagnosed, with low metastatic potential, usually arising in sun-exposed skin of the elderly. Most cases are likely to be diagnosed as squamous cell carcinomas without further qualification.

Epidemiology
Incidence and prevalence
Relatively uncommon.

Age
Elderly.

Sex
It is more common in women.

Pathophysiology
Pathology
These lesions are not uncommonly *in situ* involving predominantly the epidermis and neighbouring hair follicles. Due to the lobular and deep involvement of the latter, tumours are often diagnosed erroneously as invasive. Tumour cells are squamoid and lobules may have a surrounding PAS-positive membrane, and there is central trichilemmal (abrupt) keratinisation. There is a high mitotic rate, with abnormal mitoses present. The diagnosis of trichilemmal carcinoma should only be made in the presence of clear evidence of trichilemmal differentiation. The presence of clear-cell change is not enough to make this diagnosis. Most malignant cutaneous tumours with clear-cell change are squamous cell carcinomas and often show at least focal evidence of keratinisation. An exceptional case of trichilemmal carcinoma with neuroendocrine differentiation has been reported [5]. Immunohistochemical studies in a single case of trichilemmal carcinoma, suggest that the tumour shows differentiation towards the follicular infundibulum rather than towards the outer root sheath as ordinary trichilemmomas usually do [6]. However, the latter also show infundibular follicular differentiation and it is possible that malignant counterparts lose the expression of markers of outer sheath differentiation.

Genetics
Trichilemmal carcinomas exhibit some generic genetic alterations similar to other cutaneous tumours, such as *TP53* mutations [7].

Clinical features
History and presentation
This lesion presents as a solitary expanding often ulcerating lesion on the face. Clinically, it may be misdiagnosed as a basal cell carcinoma. Exceptionally, multiple tumours have been described [8]. Trichilemmal carcinoma may arise from a trichoblastoma and in the context of a naevus sebaceous [9]. It has also been described in the setting of solid-organ transplantation [10,11].

Disease course and prognosis
These lesions represent low-grade carcinomas with rare recurrence and extremely low metastatic potential [12]. Spontaneous regression has exceptionally been reported [13].

Management
Surgical excision with clear margins is the treatment of choice. Mohs surgery approach may show excellent results [14].

HAMARTOMAS AND HAIR GERM TUMOURS AND CYSTS

Hair follicle naevus [1,2,3,4]

Definition and nomenclature
Hair follicle naevus is a rare hamartoma composed of vellus hair follicles [3]. The lesion is now considered a distinct entity and not a variant of trichofolliculoma although they represent two closely related follicular hamartomas [2,4].

> **Synonyms and inclusions**
> - Congenital vellus hamartoma

Epidemiology
Incidence and prevalence
Lesions are very rare.

Age
They present in children and may be congenital. Few cases occurring in adults have been described.

Sex
There is no gender predilection.

Pathophysiology
Pathology
The pathology of this entity consists of a group of normal vellus hair follicles clustered together. A case associated with sebaceous hyperplasia has been reported [5].

Clinical features
History and presentation
These are recognised as plaque-like lesions with small tufts of hairs. The so-called 'faun tail naevus' is a hair follicle naevus on the sacral skin. Rare cases occur following Blaschko lines [6]. A rare association with frontonasal dysplasia has been reported [7]. It is not clear whether some hair follicle naevi are variants of accessory tragi [8–10]. An exceptional lesion on abdominal skin has been reported [11].

Disease course and prognosis
The lesion is benign.

Management
No treatment is necessary other than for cosmetic reasons.

Eruptive vellus hair cyst

Definition and nomenclature
Occlusion and cystic dilatation of vellus hair follicles.

> **Synonyms and inclusions**
> - Vellus hair cyst

Epidemiology
Incidence and prevalence
Relatively rare. They are more frequent than expected in patients with pachyonychia congenita [1,2].

Age
Mainly seen in the second decade of life [3]. In familial cases, lesions present at birth or early infancy [4]. A case occurring after 3% minoxidil application has been described [5].

Sex
There is no sex predilection.

Pathophysiology
Pathology
Cysts are located in the mid-dermis and are lined by squamous epithelium. They contain vellus hair and keratin debris. Biopsies from some lesions show features indistinguishable from steatocystoma, with absence of vellus hairs. This finding shows that there is an overlap with steatocystoma multiplex [6,7].

Clinical features
History and presentation
These present as small red or brown papules on the chest [3]. They are usually multiple and family clusters have been reported with some lesions showing features of eruptive vellus hair cysts, other lesions showing features of steatocystoma and some displaying hybrid features [8,9,**10**]. Lesions may rarely be unilateral [11] or even generalised [12] and have been reported in chronic renal failure [13]. An association with Lowe syndrome, with attention deficit hyperactivity disorder and with syringomas has been described [14–16]. Rarely, lesions present on the vulva or may be acneform or even resemble a naevus of Ota [17–20]. Dermoscopy may be useful in reaching a diagnosis, as lesions display a red maroon halo with occasional irregular radiating capillaries at the periphery and the vellus hairs can be identified opening onto the epidermis [21,22].

Disease course and prognosis
The lesion is benign. Spontaneous resolution has been reported in 25% of lesions [4].

Management
If treatment is requested, the lesions may clear after application of topical retinoids [20]. Curettage and laser therapy may also be effective, but it is easy to cause scarring. Pulsed carbon dioxide laser is useful for facial lesions but this treatment may induce hypertrophic scarring if used for truncal lesions. Success has been reported at the latter site with an erbium:YAG laser [23]. However, when this treatment is used on facial lesions, although initial results are good, there is a tendency for local recurrence. This is due to the fact that the depth of ablation of facial lesions is superficial to avoid scarring and atrophy [**24**].

Trichofolliculoma [1]

Definition
This lesion is regarded as a hamartoma of the pilosebaceous follicle, which results in several hairs being formed within the follicular opening and all protruding onto the epidermal surface from a pilosebaceous orifice [2–6].

Epidemiology
Incidence and prevalence
It is a rare lesion.

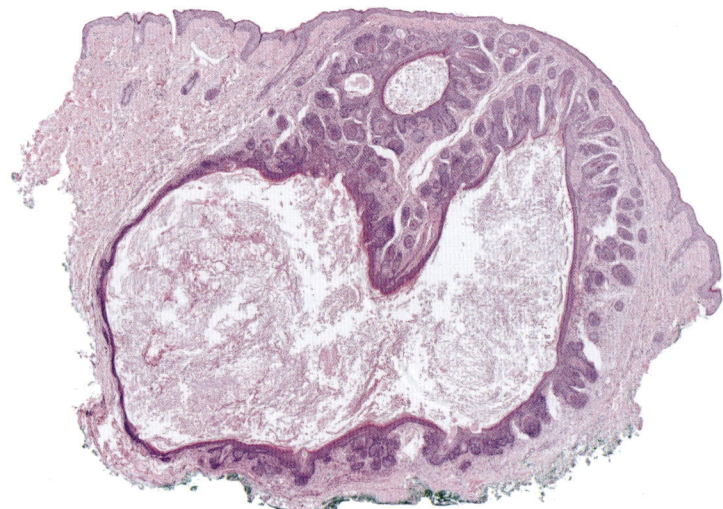

Figure 137.1 Trichofolliculoma. A large central follicular structure from which immature follicular structures radiate.

Age
Most cases occur in young adults [7].

Sex
There seems to be a slight male predilection [7].

Pathophysiology
Pathology
The pathological appearance is that of a dilated and abnormally large pilosebaceous canal containing numerous poorly formed hairs, with several pilosebaceous-like structures opening into the canal (Figure 137.1). The components of the lesion undergo evolutionary changes similar to those of the normal hair follicle [8]. Malignant change has been suggested in a single case with perineural invasion [9]. The so-called folliculosebaceous cystic hamartoma is considered by some authors to be a variant of trichofolliculoma in a late stage of development [10,11]. This theory, however, is not agreed upon by other authors [12,13].

Genetics
It has been suggested that inhibition of bone morphogenetic protein (BMP) signalling in P-cadherin positive hair progenitor cells may play a role in the pathogenesis of trichofolliculoma [**14**,15].

Clinical features
History and presentation
Trichofolliculoma shows a predilection for the head and neck, particularly the face [**16**]. Occasionally, tumours present in the vulva [17] or other unusual sites including the upper extremities, external ear, penis and scrotum [18]. Clinically, lesions can be recognised as small raised nodules with two or three hairs protruding together in a small tuft (Figure 137.2).

Disease course and prognosis
The lesion is benign. Recurrence may occur in exceptional cases.

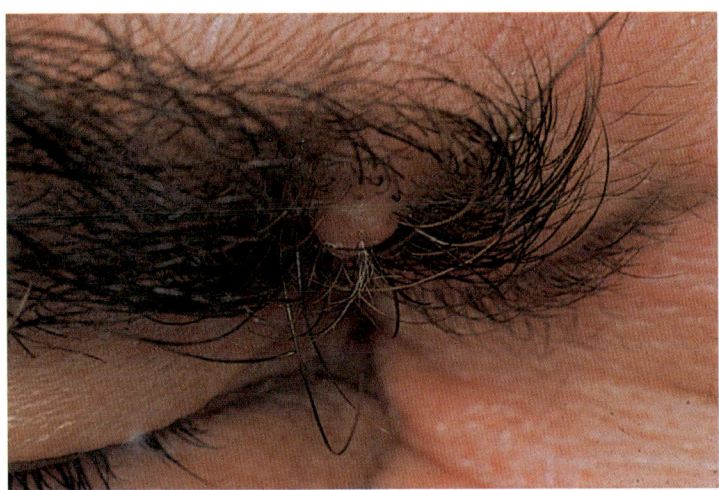

Figure 137.2 Typical example of a trichofolliculoma with a small tuft of hairs in the centre.

Management

Simple surgical excision is the treatment of choice.

Trichoepithelioma [1]

Definition and nomenclature

A hamartoma of the hair germ composed of immature islands of basaloid cells with focal primitive follicular differentiation and induction of a cellular stroma. Trichoepithelioma is now regarded as part of the spectrum of trichoblastoma and it is increasingly described under the same heading in some textbooks.

Synonyms and inclusions
- Epithelioma adenoides cysticum
- Brooke's tumour

Epidemiology

Age
Most affected patients are young adults.

Sex
There is female predilection.

Pathophysiology

Pathology [2,3]
The pathology is identical for solitary or multiple lesions and consists of lobules of small dark basaloid cells, often with a degree of peripheral palisading surrounding a central area of eosinophilic amorphous material (Figure 137.3). Occasionally, hair shaft-like structures can be seen in these central areas. A fibrous cellular stroma is seen around the cellular lobules. There is frequently a strong resemblance to basal cell carcinoma and at times differentiating between the two can be very difficult. However, the stroma in trichoepithelioma is distinctive in that it contains clefts, with an absence of retraction artefact between tumour cells and the surrounding stroma.

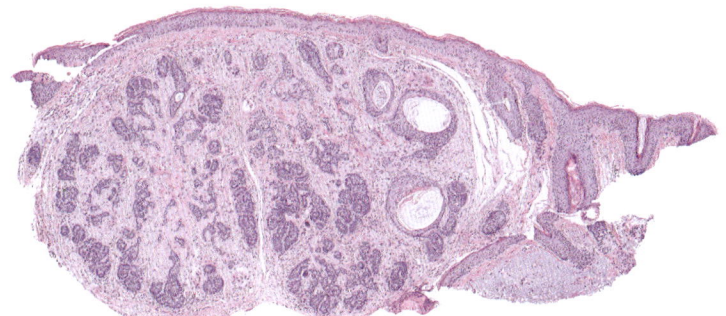

Figure 137.3 Trichoepithelioma. A lobular basaloid tumour with induction of stroma and immature follicular differentiation.

Genetics

The gene for multiple trichoepitheliomas has been mapped to a locus on chromosome 9p21 [4]. The commoner sporadic cases of trichoepithelioma have, in a proportion of cases, deletions at chromosome 9q22.3, the site of the human homologue of the *Drosophila patched* gene [5]. Familial basal cell carcinomas and some cases of sporadic basal cell carcinomas also show this deletion. It has been proposed that in multiple trichoepitheliomas, tumours develop from undifferentiated germinative cells of the pilosebaceous–apocrine unit [6]. This explains why in some cases tumours have features of spiradenoma and/or cylindroma, particularly in the Brooke–Spiegler syndrome. The Brooke–Spiegler syndrome inherited by autosomal dominant transmission consists of multiple trichoepitheliomas, cylindromas and spiradenomas and the gene for this syndrome has been mapped to chromosome 16q12–13 [7–9]. Mutations in *CYLD* and *PTCH* tumour suppressor genes are responsible for the manifestations of the disease, although *CYLD* and *PTCH* mutation-negative cases have been described [10].

Clinical features

History and presentation
The presentation of a solitary lesion is that of a smooth nodule, usually on the face, which clinically resembles a non-ulcerated basal cell carcinoma. Multiple lesions, which are inherited by autosomal dominant transmission, are seen as multiple small pearly lesions, mainly on centrofacial skin (Figure 137.4). In multiple lesions [11–14], larger lesions may be yellow, pink or sometimes bluish from pigmentation, and there may be dilated blood vessels over the surface. Individual tumours reach a limiting size, but the numbers may increase over the years. Multiple trichoepitheliomas have been described in combination with epidermoid cysts of the vulva [15].

Disease course and prognosis

The lesion is benign although it can recur. Malignant transformation is extremely rare [16,17].

Management

Any suspicion of malignant change calls for adequate excision and histological examination. The only other reason for treatment is cosmetic. Partial destruction is usually followed by regrowth. Many treatment modalities may be used including surgical excision, curettage, cryotherapy and dermabrasion. High-energy pulsed carbon

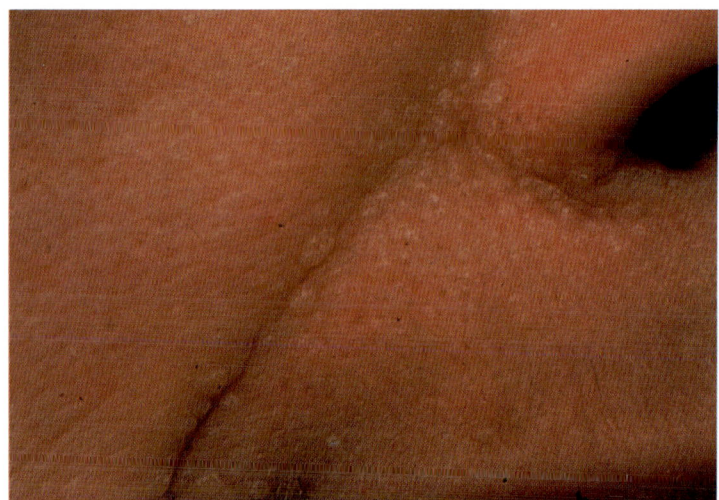

Figure 137.4 Multiple trichoepitheliomas on the central face.

dioxide laser and monopolar microneedle radiofrequency ablation has also been advocated as a useful treatment [18,19,20]. Oral vismodegib for metastatic basal cell carcinoma in one patient with concurrent multiple trichoepitheliomas has shown a serendipitous regressive effect on multiple familial trichoepitheliomas [21].

Desmoplastic trichoepithelioma [1,2]

Definition and nomenclature
A slowly expanding plaque containing structures differentiating towards the superficial part of the hair follicle and regarded as a hamartoma.

> **Synonyms and inclusions**
> - Sclerosing epithelial hamartoma

Epidemiology

Age
It occurs mainly in young persons but also in middle-aged adults [3].

Sex
There is predilection for females.

Pathophysiology
Pathology
Tumours are symmetrical on scanning magnification. The three features that characterise this lesion are large numbers of small keratin-filled cysts, strands and ribbons of small dark epithelioid cells, and a dense fibrous stroma surrounding the first two structures. Perineural extension and pseudocarcinomatous hyperplasia may be a feature [4,5]. The striking palisading of the basal cell carcinoma is absent. There is, however, a considerable similarity to the sclerosing (morphoeic) variant of basal cell carcinoma, although the number of cysts is very much greater in the desmoplastic trichoepithelioma. Distinction from microcystic adnexal carcinoma may be impossible in a small and superficial biopsy. The latter, however, shows a diffuse infiltrative pattern, with prominent perineural invasion. Merkel cells are present in desmoplastic trichoepithelioma and absent in microcystic adnexal carcinoma and in most cases of morphoeic basal cell carcinoma [6]. Immunostaining with cytokeratin 20, to identify Merkel cells, is therefore useful in the differential diagnosis of these neoplasms. MYB staining has been reported to discriminate between desmoplastic trichoepithelioma and basal cell carcinoma [7]. An electron microscopic and immunohistochemical study with different types of keratins has suggested that this tumour derives from basal cells in the outer root sheath of the hair follicle which can differentiate into various components of the folliculosebaceous and apocrine unit [8]. Occasional desmoplastic trichoepitheliomas are combined with a benign melanocytic naevus and even blue naevus [9].

Clinical features
History and presentation
These two terms were introduced almost simultaneously: the US group of Brownstein and Shapiro used the term 'desmoplastic trichoepithelioma' [1], while MacDonald, Wilson Jones and Marks in the UK suggested the term 'sclerosing epithelial hamartoma' [2]. Lesions are found mainly on the face and have a depressed centre and a raised rolled edge in many cases, causing clinical confusion with basal cell carcinoma. Exceptionally, lesions may be familial [10] and a congenital case has been described [11]. Dermoscopic features have been described in a case and consist of a well-defined ivory-white lesion with marked arborising telangiectasia [12].

Disease course and prognosis
The lesion is benign.

Management
Local excision is effective in the majority of cases. Alternative methods include curettage and electrodissection.

Trichoblastoma [1,2,3,4]

Definition and nomenclature
Tumours of the hair germ composed of follicular germinative cells.

> **Synonyms and inclusions**
> - Trichogenic fibroma
> - Trichoblastic fibroma

Epidemiology [5,6]
Incidence and prevalence
It is a rare lesion.

Age
It is more common in the fifth to seventh decade but any age group can be affected. Occurrence in children is exceptional.

Sex
Both sexes are affected equally.

Pathophysiology
Pathology
Nests of basophilic basaloid cells with a lobular architecture and prominent induction of stroma are seen in the dermis and/or subcutaneous tissue. Focal evidence of follicular differentiation is seen, but this usually consists of less mature structures than those seen in trichoepithelioma. Characteristically, condensation of cellular stroma is seen around aggregates of basaloid cells but true follicular papillae are not usually formed, as the stroma does not invaginate into the epithelial component. Mitotic figures vary and may be frequent. Usually, the tumour is not connected to the epidermis. According to the degree of follicular differentiation and the amount of stroma induced, lesions have been subclassified into different categories, including trichogenic and trichoblastic fibromas. However, all tumours in this category are best classified as variants of trichoblastoma. Some tumours display sebaceous and even ductal (apocrine) differentiation confirming the theory that they differentiate towards the folliculosebaceous and apocrine germ [7,8]. Melanin deposition is often seen, may be prominent and is not uncommonly associated with the presence of melanocytes [9] within the tumour as seen in normal hair follicles. In some cases, rows of tumours cells are arranged parallel to each other in a pattern that has been described as rippled trichoblastoma [10]. Occasional neoplasms consist mainly of clear cells, a change that indicates trichilemmal differentiation [11]. Histological overlap with trichoepithelioma is often seen and there is a tendency to regard all these tumours as part of the same spectrum. Distinction between nodular trichoblastoma and follicular basal cell carcinoma may be very difficult, particularly in small biopsies. Distinction is usually based on the presence of a deep infiltrative pattern in the latter [12]. The presence of Merkel cells in trichoblastoma identified by immunohistochemical markers (cytokeratin 20, chromogranin) is useful in the differentiation from basal cell carcinoma, which lacks these cells [13]. However, deep-seated tumours often have few or no Merkel cells. Based on clinicopathological features and the presence of Merkel cells in the neoplasm, it has been proposed that fibroepithelioma of Pinkus is a variant of trichoblastoma rather than a variant of basal cell carcinoma [14]. A further aid in the differential diagnosis between basal cell carcinoma and trichoblastoma is the immunohistochemical expression of androgen receptor. It is purported that the latter is usually positive in basal cell carcinoma and negative in benign follicular neoplasms [15].

Clinical features
History and presentation
These are deeply or superficially situated dermal and/or subcutaneous nodules [16], found – as is common with follicular tumours – on the head and neck. A variant presenting with multiple facial plaques has been described [17]. Rare occurrence in the vulva has been reported [18]. Often lesions are found within naevus sebaceous [19] and trichoblastoma is regarded as the most common neoplasm occurring in this hamartoma [20,21]. Association with melanocytic tumours including naevi and melanoma is uncommon [22,23]. Tumours may be induced by low-dose X-ray depilatory treatment such as was previously used to treat ringworm and acne [24].

Disease course and prognosis
Behaviour is usually benign but malignant transformation of the epithelial or even the mesenchymal component (trichoblastic carcinoma/sarcoma) may occasionally occur [25,26]. Loss of p53 and alterations in the *AKT* signalling pathway have been suggested to play a role in malignant transformation [27]. The tumours with malignant alteration appear to be less aggressive than previously thought, despite concerning histological characteristics [28].

Management
Complete excision is often desirable as exclusion of a basal cell carcinoma may be difficult in small biopsies.

Adamantinoid trichoblastoma [1,2,3,4,5–8]

Definition and nomenclature
This entity was first described in 1991 [**1**]. Follicular, sebaceous and ductal differentiation has been demonstrated and therefore this tumour is regarded as a variant of trichoblastoma, a neoplasm differentiating towards the folliculosebaceous and apocrine germ [**4**,**8**].

Synonyms and inclusions
- Cutaneous lymphadenoma

Epidemiology
Incidence and prevalence
It is relatively rare.

Age
Usually occurs in young adults although the age range is broad. Congenital cases have been described [9,10].

Sex
Both sexes are affected equally.

Pathophysiology
Pathology
The tumour consists of nests and lobules of basaloid cells in the reticular dermis, with no connection to the epidermis. These aggregates of cells are embedded in a fibrous stroma. Tumour cells are bland and display focal peripheral palisading. A striking feature is the presence of prominent infiltration of tumour lobules and nests by T lymphocytes and histiocytes (Figure 137.5). These inflammatory cells are mainly located in the centre of the tumour lobules. No cellular atypia is seen and mitotic figures are rare. Focal areas of keratinisation are seen in some cases. The pattern of cytokeratin 17 expression is patchy and peripheral in cutaneous lymphadenoma, as opposed to diffuse expression in basal cell carcinoma [11].

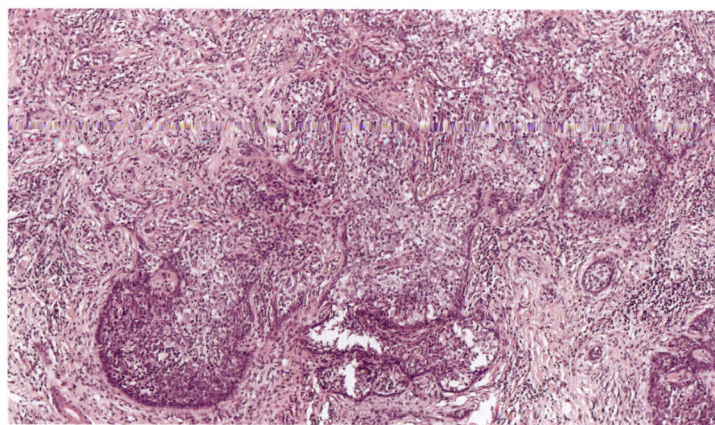

Figure 137.5 Lymphadenoma. Nests and lobules of epithelial cells with peripheral palisading and prominent infiltration by lymphocytes.

Clinical features
History and presentation
Cutaneous lymphadenoma was first described in 1991 by Santa Cruz et al. [1]. The lesions are seen mainly on the head and neck area, and present as non-specific papules or nodules. The preoperative clinical diagnosis is frequently either basal cell carcinoma or intradermal naevus.

Disease course and prognosis
The behaviour is entirely benign. A case with malignant transformation has been reported [12].

Management
Local excision is recommended. Mohs micrographic surgery has been suggested as an option but is hard to justify for a benign lesion that has no infiltrative growth pattern [13,14].

Basaloid follicular hamartoma [1,2,3,4]

Definition
A hamartoma consisting of a proliferation of basaloid cells, with frequent involvement of hair follicles. Induction of immature hair follicles is often seen.

Epidemiology [2]
Incidence and prevalence
The lesion is very rare.

Age
It may be congenital or acquired. The range is broad but it seems to be more common in middle-aged and elderly individuals.

Sex
There is a slight predilection for women.

Pathophysiology
Pathology
A multifocal proliferation of cords, strands and nests of basaloid cells is seen, with frequent connections to the epidermis. Basaloid cells focally replace neighbouring hair follicles. In addition, immature follicular bulbs may also be seen.

Genetics
It is associated with deregulation of the *PTCH* pathway; in fact, basaloid follicular hamartoma syndrome may genetically and clinically fall within the spectrum of naevoid basal cell carcinoma syndrome [5].

Clinical features
History and presentation
These lesions are usually small multiple papules that may become confluent to form a plaque. Involvement of the face is common but lesions may also present on the trunk. Presentation may be generalised or localised and the latter may be linear [4,6]. They may be present in isolation or inherited as an autosomal dominant trait [7,8,9]. Association with autoimmune diseases and alopecia has been described particularly in the generalised variant [10]. The autoimmune diseases include lupus erythematosus [11] and myasthenia gravis [7]. Other rare associations include cystic fibrosis [12], milia and hypohidrosis [13].

Disease course and prognosis
The lesion is benign. In exceptional cases, basal cell carcinomas may develop within the lesions [14].

Management
May be excised for cosmetic reasons or if a basal cell carcinoma is suspected.

HAIR MATRIX TUMOURS

Pilomatricoma [1,2–4]

Definition and nomenclature
A benign tumour considered to be a hamartoma of the hair matrix composed of cells resembling those of the hair matrix and cortex and inner root sheath. The cells usually undergo 'mummification', i.e. a particular form of degeneration with retained cellular outlines.

Synonyms and inclusions
- Benign calcifying epithelioma of Malherbe
- Trichomatricoma
- Pilomatrixoma

Epidemiology
Incidence and prevalence
This lesion makes up around 20% of all hair follicle-related tumours in most series and is therefore the commonest hair follicle tumour [5]. A number of familial cases are recorded [6]. Association with myotonic dystrophy [6], Turner syndrome [7,8], Rubinstein–Taybi syndrome [9] and Kabuki syndrome [10] have been described. MYH-associated polyposis is an autosomal recessive variant of familial adenomatous polyposis with susceptibility to colorectal

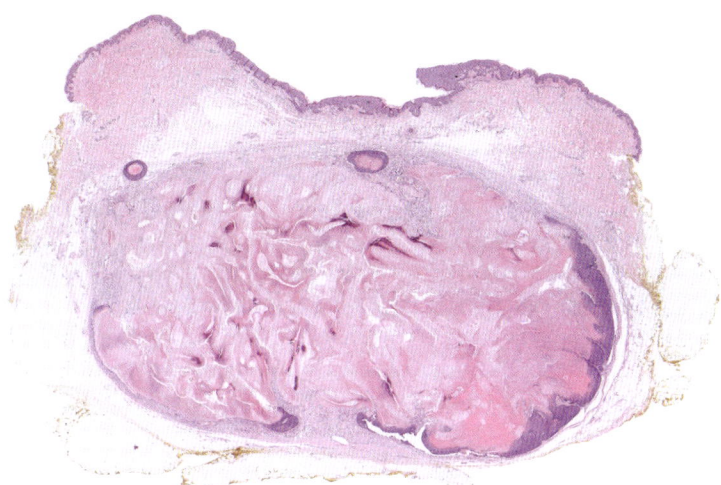

Figure 137.6 A dermal/subcutaneous tumour with central pale pink area containing ghost cells focally surrounded by a thin peripheral rim of basaloid cells.

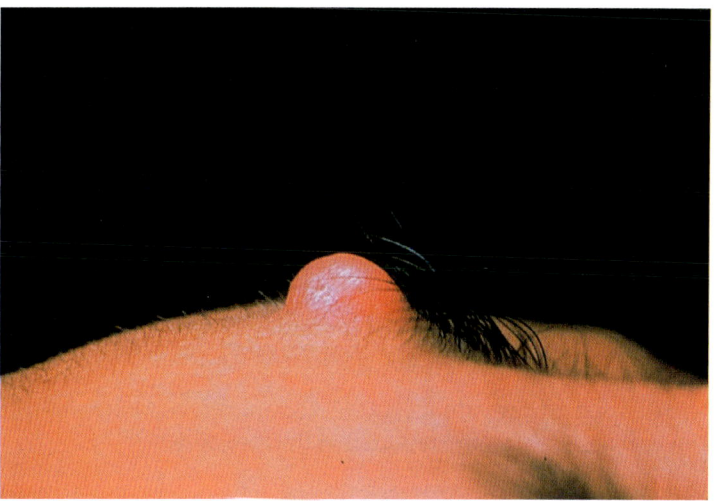

Figure 137.7 Pilomatricoma. Small red firm papule.

carcinoma and association in some affected individuals with multiple pilomatricomas [11].

Age
It may occur at any age from infancy and is frequently seen in children [5,12]. The majority of patients are under 20 years of age.

Sex
Females are affected more often than males.

Pathophysiology
Pathology [13,14,15–18]
The tumour is situated in the dermis and is composed of well-circumscribed rounded islands giving a lobulated contour. The outer cells are small and their rounded nuclei crowded together make this region deeply basophilic. Normal mitotic figures can usually be seen and are often numerous. The cytoplasm is scanty and the cell margins indistinct, but intercellular connections can be seen. Towards the centre of the mass, the cytoplasm becomes more abundant and eosinophilic. The nuclear outline persists, but the chromatin is sparse and clumped in dark granules; when all basophilic material disappears, a mummified 'ghost cell' remains (Figure 137.6). The ultrastructural and histochemical characteristics of these cells mark them as hair matrix cells maturing towards the cortex or root sheath [3,19,20]. The central areas often calcify and calcium can be demonstrated in the basophilic areas of the tumour. In older lesions, the basophilic cells may be greatly reduced or disappear entirely. Melanin may be present and dendritic melanocytes have been found between the tumour cells. The stroma that encapsulates the masses usually contains inflammatory and foreign-body giant cells, and occasionally ossifies. A rare variant of superficial pilomatricoma presenting clinically as a cutaneous horn and with an intraepidermal location has been reported [21]. A bullous appearance may occur consequent on lymphangiectasia [22], and anetoderma can occur in the dermis surrounding the tumour [23]. Occasional hybrid cysts may show areas of pilomatrical differentiation identical to pilomatricoma [24]. Melanocytic matricoma is a rare tumour consisting of islands and nodules of matrical cells associated with colonisation by prominently pigmented dendritic melanocytes [19,20].

Genetics
Studies have shown that 75% of pilomatricomas possess activating mutations of the β-catenin gene [25,26,27,28]. The sites of β-catenin expression within pilomatricomas suggest that this may affect cell–cell adhesion [28]. More recently, mutations of various fibroblast growth factor receptors have been reported [29,30].

Clinical features
History and presentation [31,32,33]
The lesion is usually a solitary, deep, dermal or subcutaneous tumour 3–30 mm in diameter situated on the head, neck or upper extremities (Figure 137.7). Very large tumours occur occasionally [34]. The skin over the tumour is normal and the lesion has a firm to stone-hard consistency and a lobular shape on palpation. In adult life, there may be quite a short history [4] and there is usually no evidence of a preceding cyst. It may be subject to periodic inflammation and can present as a granulomatous swelling. Rarely, ulcerated lesions may show transepithelial elimination [35]. An unusual case associated with hypercalcaemia and high levels of parathyroid hormone has been described [36]. Malignant change is very rare (see later). The diagnosis can be suspected if a subcutaneous nodule feels hard and lobular. The presence of calcium salts may be apparent on radiographs, but these can also be deposited in other cysts and tumours of the skin.

Disease course and prognosis
The lesion is benign but there is a tendency for local recurrence. Malignant change is recorded in several cases and appears to arise chiefly in large pilomatricomas that have been present for many years (see later) [37].

Management
Local excision is sufficient for benign lesions. Wider excision will be needed if malignancy is suspected.

Pilomatrical carcinoma [1–4]

Definition and nomenclature
The malignant counterpart of the pilomatricoma, possessing metastatic potential.

Synonyms and inclusions
- Pilomatrix carcinoma

Epidemiology [5,6,7]
Incidence and prevalence
Fewer than 150 cases are reported in the literature.

Age
The average age of the patients is 70 years.

Sex
Males are more often affected than females.

Pathophysiology
Pathology
Definition of malignancy is usually very difficult on histological grounds. Malignant tumours usually have a very large predominant basaloid component, an infiltrative growth pattern and extensive necrosis. In addition, there are numerous mitotic figures, and both lymphatic and vascular invasion may be seen.

Genetics
As in pilomatricoma, mutations in β-catenin have been demonstrated in pilomatricarcinomas suggesting the activation of a common cellular pathway in both types of neoplasms despite the difference in clinical behaviour [8,9]. More recently, a novel oncogenic mutation in FGFR4 has been demonstrated by whole exome sequencing in a case of pilomatrical carcinoma [10].

Clinical features
History and presentation
The lesion presents as a rapidly expanding firm nodule. Most tumours develop on the head and neck followed much less frequently by the trunk [5]. It can present *de novo* or on a longstanding benign pilomatricoma.

Disease course and prognosis
Pilomatrical carcinomas are locally aggressive with a tendency to recur [11]. There may be metastases to distant organs such as the lungs, bone and lymph nodes [12,13–17]. At least two cases have proved fatal.

Management
Wide local excision is usually curative, but follow-up is required because of the possibility of metastatic spread. There are no specific recommendations for follow-up, but a follow-up schedule similar to high-risk squamous cell carcinoma is applicable.

LESIONS OF HAIR FOLLICLE MESENCHYME

According to the World Health Organization (WHO) trichodiscoma and fibrofolliculoma are now considered to represent the late and early stage, respectively, of the same appendageal tumour, which differentiates towards the mantle of the hair follicle. Trichodiscoma was described by Pinkus as a hamartomatous proliferation of the mesodermal component of the Haarscheibe. The Haarscheibe is considered to be a slowly reacting mechano-receptor associated with the hair follicle (hair disc). Neurofollicular hamartoma is considered the same as trichodiscoma. The term fibrofolliculoma has been used to refer to perifollicular fibroma and the term mantleoma has been used to refer to both fibrofolliculoma and trichodiscoma.

Trichodiscoma [1]

Epidemiology
Incidence and prevalence
It is a rare lesion.

Age
It occurs in young to middle-aged individuals (third to fourth decade).

Sex
There is no sex predilection.

Pathophysiology
Pathology
A discrete but non-encapsulated area of myxoid, poorly cellular stroma with focal collagen deposition is seen in the dermis, associated with a proliferation of blood vessels, some of which are thick-walled. The proliferating cells are CD34 positive [2]. A variant with a cellular spindle-cell component has been described [3] which may represent what is called neurofollicular hamartoma. Pilosebaceous units are often seen on both sides of the myxoid stroma. Trichodiscomas and trichofolliculomas usually show histological overlap. Interestingly, the acrochordon-like lesions in Birt–Hogg–Dubé syndrome display the histological features of either trichodiscomas or trichofolliculomas [4].

Genetics
Multiple trichodiscomas, trichofolliculomas and acrochordon-like lesions as well as perifollicular fibromas have been described as part of the Birt–Hogg–Dubé syndrome [5]. This syndrome is an autosomal dominant genodermatosis also associated with lung cysts, spontaneous pneumothorax and renal neoplasms (chromophobe renal carcinoma and oncocytoma) [6]. The causative gene, FLCN, has been mapped to chromosome 17p12q11. A case of multiple trichodiscomas negative for FLCN mutation has been reported in association with multiple endocrine neoplasia type I (MEN1) syndrome [7].

Clinical features

History and presentation
The clinical appearance of the trichodiscoma is that of multiple discrete flat-topped papules 2–3 mm in diameter. They occur mainly in the central area of the face. Familial cases are recorded [8,9].

Disease course and prognosis
The lesion is benign.

Management
It is excised for cosmetic reasons. In Birt–Hogg–Dubé syndrome skin lesions may be the first manifestation of the disease [10] therefore screening and follow-up is advisable as the risk for developing renal tumours increases with age.

Perifollicular fibroma [1–4]

Definition
A cutaneous hamartoma of unknown aetiology that shows differentiation in the connective tissue sheath of the hair follicle.

Epidemiology

Incidence and prevalence
It is a very rare lesion.

Age
The lesion may be single (congenital or acquired) or multiple (late onset).

Sex
There is no sex predilection.

Pathophysiology

Pathology
The pathology is that of a striking concentric fibrous proliferation around a relatively normal pilosebaceous apparatus.

Genetics [5]
See under trichodiscoma.

Clinical features

History and presentation [1–4,5,6–8,9]
The clinical appearance of these lesions has not been well described and is not distinctive. Mostly it consists of small firm papules/papule either flesh coloured or pink usually on the face and neck. Other sites may be exceptionally affected. Association with colonic polyps has been described and it is known as Hornstein–Knickenberg syndrome [7]. It seems that Birt–Hogg–Dubé syndrome, which was described later, represents the same entity [8,9].

Disease course and prognosis
The lesion is benign but multiple perifollicular fibromas are associated with Birt–Hogg–Dubé syndrome [5].

Management
See under trichodiscoma.

Fibrofolliculoma

Definition
A fibrous lesion of perifollicular connective tissue [1]. See also Lesions of hair follicle mesenchyme, earlier.

Epidemiology

Incidence and prevalence
It is rare.

Age
These lesions usually first appear in middle age (third to fourth decade) [2].

Sex
There is no sex predilection.

Pathophysiology

Pathology
Histology shows multiple small poorly formed pilosebaceous follicles set in a very striking fibrous stroma. There is also an obvious proliferation of the outer root sheath similar to that seen in the perifollicular fibroma.

Genetics
Multiple lesions are seen in the Birt–Hogg–Dubé syndrome, which is an autosomal dominant condition mapped to chromosome 17p11.2 [3–6].

Clinical features

History and presentation
It can rarely present as a solitary lesion or more often as multiple lesions either isolated or as a part of Birt–Hogg–Dubé syndrome [2]. It can also be associated with other conditions such as thyroid carcinoma [3] and tuberous sclerosis (Chapter 78) [7]. They tend to affect the upper part of the body.

Disease course and prognosis
The lesion is benign. In the Birt–Hogg–Dubé syndrome, fibrofolliculomas are seen in association with trichodiscomas, acrochordon-like lesions, renal tumours most commonly chromophobe carcinoma and spontaneous pneumothorax [8,9].

Management
See under trichodiscoma.

SEBACEOUS GLAND TUMOURS

The following tumours or tumour-like conditions of the sebaceous glands are considered elsewhere:
1 Naevus sebaceous (Chapter 35).

2 Senile sebaceous hyperplasia (Chapter 91).
3 Steatocystoma multiplex (Chapter 133).

The two main conditions discussed in this section are sebaceous adenomas and sebaceomas, and sebaceous carcinoma. The old term 'sebaceous epithelioma' is no longer used, as it causes confusion with the exceptionally rare basal cell carcinoma with sebaceous differentiation.

Sebaceous adenomas and sebaceomas [1–6]

Definition
Benign tumours composed of incompletely differentiated sebaceous cells of varying degrees of maturity. Sebaceous adenoma and sebaceoma are described together, as they do not have distinctive clinical features and, although histological separation is possible in most cases, there is also some degree of overlap.

Epidemiology
Incidence and prevalence
These are relatively rare tumours [4].

Age
Most cases of solitary type occur in the elderly.

Sex
The solitary type may occur in either sex.

Pathophysiology
Pathology [3,6–8]
The tumours are multilobular and usually connected to the epidermis. The lobules are well defined, composed of variable numbers of small basophilic sebaceous matrix cells peripherally and larger cells – mature sebaceous cells – containing cytoplasmic fat globules. The proportion of immature, transitional and mature sebaceous cells may vary widely from one area to another. In sebaceous adenoma, mature sebaceous cells predominate in the centre of the lobules (Figure 137.8) while in sebaceoma immature basaloid sebaceous cells predominate, occupying large areas of the lobules. In both tumours, there may also be cystic spaces lined by a thin layer of eosinophilic material similar to the intraglandular sebaceous ducts. The outline of the tumour is less regular than normal sebaceous glands and may be irregular. However, some sebaceous adenomas closely mimic the normal sebaceous gland, except for an increase in the number of immature sebaceous cells. Mitotic figures are frequent in the immature sebaceous cells, and this feature should not be regarded as evidence of malignancy. Larger and deeper tumours with cystic degeneration usually represent sebaceomas, but adenomas may also be seen. Some of these tumours have atypical histological features [9]. The cystic space contains abundant holocrine (sebaceous) material. It has been suggested that these cystic sebaceous tumours are a marker for the mismatch, repair-deficient subtype of Muir–Torre syndrome, which has a high risk of internal malignancies [9]. However, a more recent study, although demonstrating that sebaceous keratoacanthomas are often associated with the syndrome, failed to show the same correlation with cystic sebaceous neoplasms [10]. Glandular apocrine differentiation may occur rarely in some sebaceous neoplasms [11].

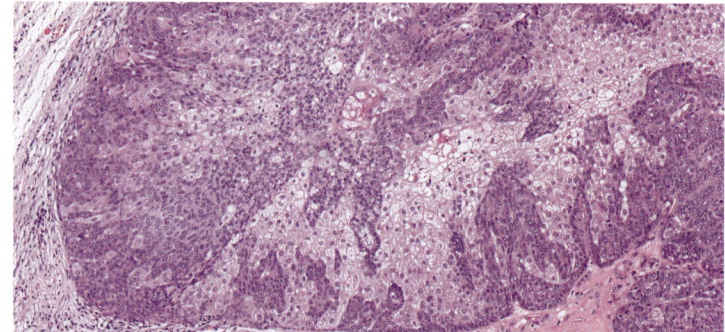

Figure 137.8 Sebaceous adenoma. Lobular lesion with prominent maturation in the centre and immature cells in the periphery.

Genetics
Patients with multiple benign sebaceous tumours (other than sebaceous hyperplasia) should be suspected of having the Muir–Torre syndrome (Chapter 141), associated with multiple visceral malignancies [7,12–18,**19**,**20**,21,22]. It is important to note, however, that a single sebaceous neoplasm and more uncommonly a sebaceous carcinoma particularly in an extraocular location may represent a marker of the syndrome [23]. It has also been suggested that a single sebaceous tumour outside the head and trunk is a strong indicator of the syndrome [**10**]. Muir–Torre syndrome is a rare subset of the hereditary non-polyposis colorectal carcinoma (Lynch syndrome), representing 1–2% of cases of the latter [24,25]. It is characterised by cutaneous sebaceous tumours, gastrointestinal malignancies, especially colonic and, more rarely, renal, uterine and breast neoplasms [5]. The internal malignancies tend to be fairly low grade, and often patients develop them earlier in life than the equivalent neoplasm in the general population. Sebaceous neoplasms tend to develop later in life. Patients with Muir–Torre syndrome may also develop sebaceous keratoacanthomas [**10**] and ordinary keratoacanthomas. Microsatellite instability has been reported in the Muir–Torre syndrome [26,**27**], which results in the loss of a number of mismatch repair proteins particularly MLH1 and MSH2 and less commonly PMS2 and MSH6. The protein most commonly lost is MSH2, which was lost 10 times more frequently than MLH1 in Muir–Torre syndrome [24]. The loss of expression of MLH1, MSH2, PMS2 and MSH6 may be demonstrated by immunohistochemical methods [28,29]. While loss of expression should not be regarded as a diagnostic test for Muir–Torre syndrome, it could be useful as an initial screening tool for Muir–Torre syndrome [30]. The finding should be used in combination with personal and family history and germ line genetic testing to confirm the diagnosis [**31**]. The Mayo Clinic has proposed a clinical scoring system based on a number of parameters including age at presentation at which the first sebaceous neoplasm occurs, number of sebaceous neoplasms, and family and personal history of related neoplasms to help identify patients at risk [**32**].

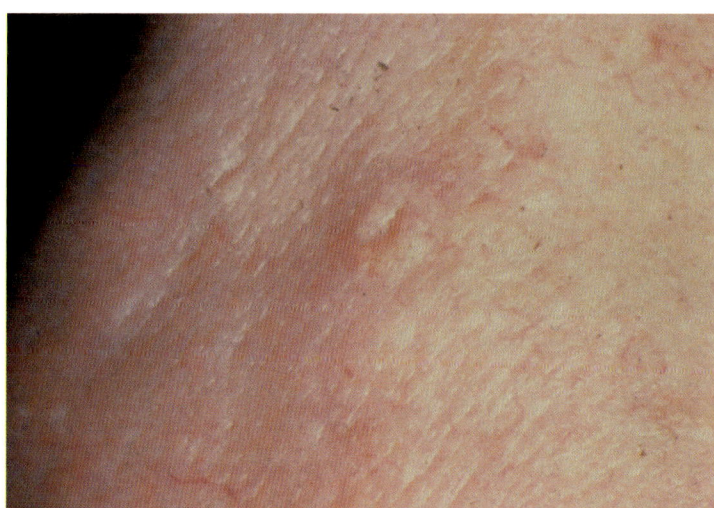

Figure 137.9 Sebaceous adenoma. Small yellowish papule.

Clinical features

History and presentation

Tumours are usually rounded, raised and either sessile or somewhat pedunculated (Figure 137.9). They are normally less than 10 mm in diameter, but older lesions may form plaques or ulcerate. Occasional tumours are more deeply located and appear cystic. The colour is fleshy or of a waxy yellowish hue and the surface may be papilliferous. The common situation is the face or scalp and it may occur on the eyelid. It usually grows slowly, but a sudden increase in growth rate can occur. A yellow-tinged facial nodule may be suggestive, but clinical differentiation from other epithelial tumours, especially basal cell carcinoma, may be impossible. The microscopic diagnosis is more certain. They may be associated with a cutaneous horn [6]. There is no evidence that actinic radiation or other recognised carcinogens are to blame.

Disease course and prognosis

The lesion is benign. The risk of local recurrence is low.

Management

Surgical excision is the treatment of choice.

Sebaceous carcinoma [1,2,3]

Definition

A malignant tumour composed of cells showing differentiation toward sebaceous epithelium.

Epidemiology

Incidence and prevalence

The variable incidence reported for this tumour reflects the differing diagnostic criteria of different workers. It is, however, rare, comprising fewer than 1% of all skin malignancies. The tumour has been reported following radiodermatitis [4] and in a patient with multiple arsenical skin cancers. Lesions may rarely occur in naevus sebaceous [5]. It is likely that a number of sebaceomas with high mitotic activity have been reported in the past as sebaceous carcinomas.

Age

Most lesions occur in middle-aged and particularly old individuals [6–14]. Exceptional cases have been reported in children [15].

Sex

There is a slight predilection for males.

Pathophysiology

Pathology

The same problem of terminology exists with sebaceous carcinoma as with the adenomas. Basal cell carcinoma with sebaceous differentiation is not included in the description of sebaceous carcinoma. The essential feature is cytological evidence of sebaceous differentiation. The proportion of cells showing fat globules and the degree of cytoplasmic vacuolation are variable. The undifferentiated cells are of moderate size, with round centrally placed nuclei and rather basophilic cytoplasm, and they tend to group themselves in masses of a multilobular configuration. The differentiating cells tend to be more central. There are, in addition, cytological features of malignancy and evidence of an infiltrative growth pattern. Mitotic figures including atypical forms are frequent. Pagetoid infiltration of the epidermis is frequent, particularly in tumours arising around the eye [6]. Demonstration of sebaceous differentiation by histochemistry is possible by the use of oil red O but it requires frozen sections and these are usually not available. By immunohistochemistry, sebaceous differentiation can be demonstrated by epithelial membrane antigen (EMA) but only in cells with good differentiation. Adipophilin and peripilin are more recently added immunohistochemical stains useful in demonstrating sebaceous differentiation [16,17]. Peripilin seems to be more specific than adipophilin except in cases of carcinoma *in situ* with clear-cell change in which tumour cells are often positive for the former marker [17].

Genetics

Sebaceous carcinoma may rarely be associated with the Muir–Torre syndrome (Chapter 141) [18,19]. The latter association is mainly seen with extraocular carcinomas and those tumours occurring outside the head and neck area [20]. Studies have shown activation of *PI3K* signalling pathways [21] and *TERT* promoter mutations [22] in sebaceous carcinomas.

Clinical features

History and presentation

The tumour is solitary, firm, sometimes translucent and covered with normal or slightly verrucose epidermis. The colour may be yellow or orange. The face and scalp [23] are the commonest sites, especially the eyelid (Figure 137.10). The evolution may be very slow, and a size of 5 cm or more may be reached after many years without metastasis. Some tumours grow rapidly and invade early, but metastasis is uncommon [24,25]. Clinical features are not distinctive and eyelid lesions may be confused with a

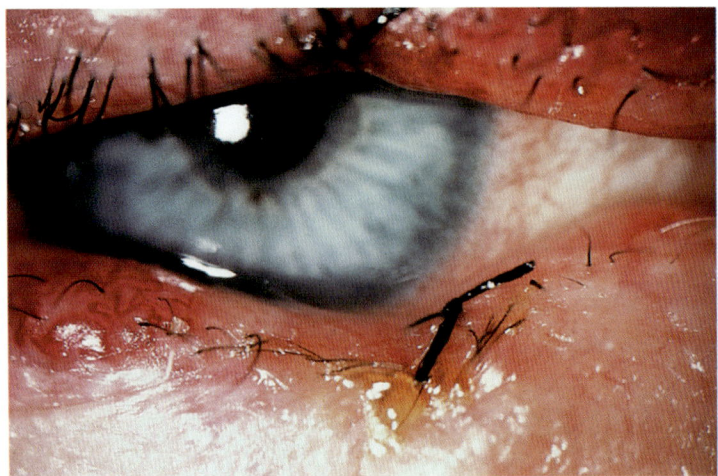

Figure 137.10 Sebaceous carcinoma. Ulcerated yellowish lesion of the eyelid.

chalazion. Sebaceous carcinomas may occur in immunosuppressed organ transplant patients, and these tumours are associated with microsatellite instability [18].

Disease course and prognosis
It is uncommon for the lesion to be aggressively invasive on the skin, although it frequently is when situated on the eyelid [6–10,**26**]. There are, however, individual case reports of extraocular aggressive lesions with occasional metastatic spread [27,28].

Management
Complete surgical excision is required [12,29]. Reports of excellent results with Mohs surgery suggest that this may be the treatment of choice [**30**].

APOCRINE GLAND TUMOURS [1]

Apocrine hidrocystoma [2]

Definition and nomenclature
A lesion produced by cystic dilatation of apocrine secretory glands. Although the terms apocrine hidrocystoma and cystadenoma have been used as synonyms, and the clinical features of both lesions are identical, there are a number of histological findings that set them apart (see later).

Synonyms and inclusions
- Apocrine cystadenoma

Epidemiology
Incidence and prevalence
The lesion is not uncommon, but is most often seen in ophthalmological, surgical and dermatology clinics.

Age
It occurs in adult life, in no particular age group.

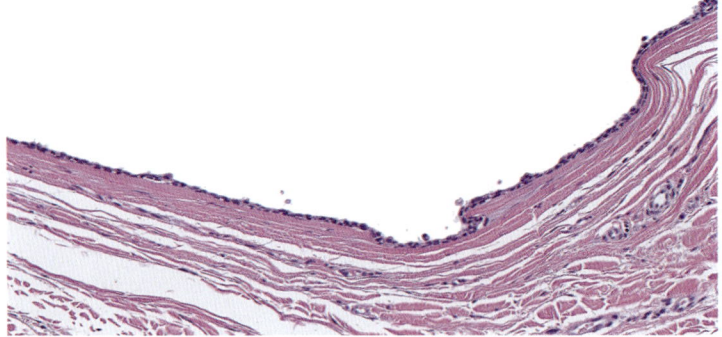

Figure 137.11 Apocrine hidrocystoma. Cystic cavity lined by an outer layer of myoepithelial cells surrounding an inner layer of flattened cuboidal cells with pink cytoplasm.

Sex
Males and females are equally affected.

Pathophysiology
Pathology [3–5]
Large cystic cavities are found in the dermis if the lesion has been carefully dissected out. Commonly, the cyst is punctured and has collapsed before fixation. The cavities are lined by cuboidal or high-columnar apocrine secretory cells with decapitation secretion and a peripheral layer of myoepithelial cells (Figure 137.11). Papillary projections or solid buds of secretory cells may break the smooth contour of the cyst lining. The secretory cells may contain pigment [6,7], which is neither melanin nor haemosiderin. Polarisable calcium oxalate crystals may be found within the lumina [8]. The secretions in the cysts may be coagulated and stained using the PAS technique. There is a well-organised fibrous stroma. Electron microscopy confirms the apocrine nature of the secretory epithelium [9]. Lesions designated as apocrine cystadenoma are regarded as proliferative lesions with true papillary projections (containing a fibrous core). These tumours may display focal cytological atypia and mitotic activity. Based on these atypical features in cystadenoma, complete excision is suggested for tumours classified as such [**10**].

Clinical features
History and presentation [6,7,11,12]
The lesions are solitary or occasionally multiple, well-defined, dome-shaped, translucent nodules [13]. The surface is smooth and the colour varies from a skin colour to greyish or blue-black; pigmentation may affect only part of the cyst [14]. The commonest site is around the eye, particularly lateral to the outer canthus (Figure 137.12). It has also been reported on the penis [1], vulva [15], lip [16], fingers [17] and multiple lesions bilaterally in both axillae [18]. There are no symptoms. The cyst increases slowly in size and may become 10 mm or more in diameter. Multiple lesions may be seen in Schöpf–Schulz–Passarge syndrome (a form of ectodermal dysplasia syndrome characterised by hypotrichosis, hypodontia, nail dystrophy, palmoplantar keratoderma and periocular apocrine hidrocystomas) [19]. The lesion must be differentiated from basal cell carcinoma, which is usually of a firmer consistency, less regular in its surface contour and has surface telangiectases. The cystic nature of the lesion, which can often be shown by transillumination,

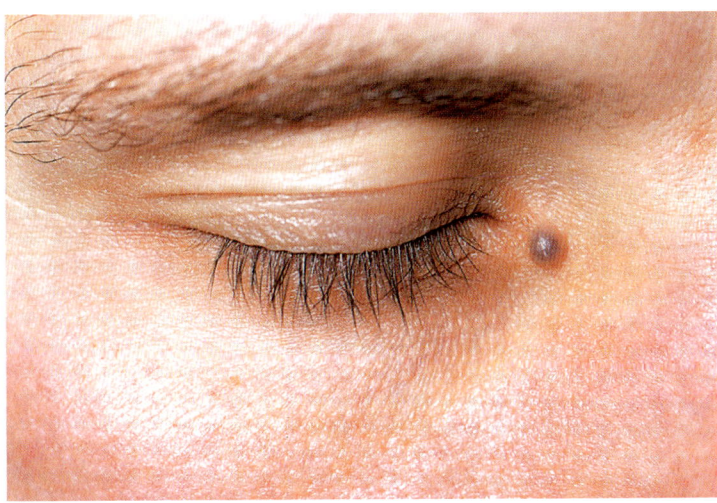

Figure 137.12 Apocrine hidrocystoma. Cystic translucent papule on the right inner canthus.

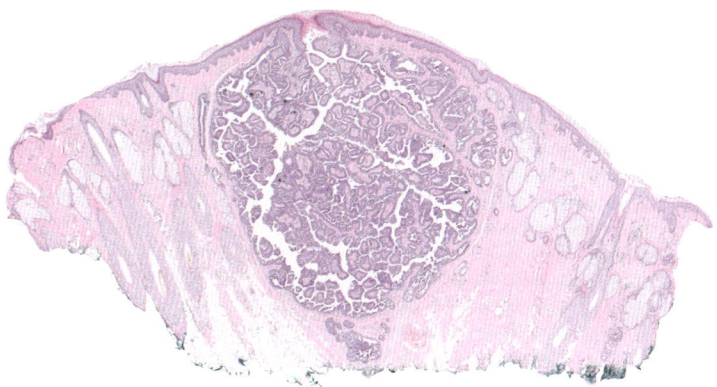

Figure 137.13 Syringocystadenoma papilliferum. Papillary projections with a fibrovascular stroma.

separates it from blue naevi and malignant melanoma when pigment is present.

Disease course and prognosis
The lesion is benign.

Management
The tumour is cured by surgical removal, which is commonly also needed for diagnosis. Other treatment modalities are the same as those used for eccrine hidrocystomas (see later). Multiple lesions have been treated successfully with trichloroacetic acid [20].

Syringocystadenoma papilliferum [1,2]

Definition and nomenclature
An exuberant proliferating lesion, commonly seen on the scalp in association with an organoid naevus (naevus sebaceous), and showing differentiation in an apocrine pattern [3].

> **Synonyms and inclusions**
> - Naevus syringadenomatosus papilliferus

Epidemiology [4–6]
Incidence and prevalence
It is not an uncommon lesion.

Age
These lesions may be present at birth or in childhood [5], but the majority are seen on the face and scalp of young adults.

Sex
There is no sex predilection.

Pathophysiology
Pathology [7–9]
The epidermal surface shows papillomatous expansion and from these areas cystic invaginations are seen. The cystic structures are lined by papillae that have a lining of a double layer of columnar epithelium, which shows an apocrine pattern of secretion (Figure 137.13). The underlying stroma is rich in plasma cells [10]. Sebaceous differentiation may occasionally be seen [11]. Superficial lesions with features of apocrine tubular adenoma (see later) may overlap histologically with those of syringocystadenoma papilliferum [12].

Genetics
Molecular biological studies have identified loss of heterozygosity at chromosome 9q22, the locus of the *patched* gene [13], as well as *RAS* mutations [14] and *BRAF* V600E mutation [15].

Clinical features
History and presentation
There is frequently a history of papillomatous expansion of a small pre-existing lesion at or around puberty and lesions often occur in a pre-existing organoid naevus. The lesion is composed of multiple warty papules, some of which are translucent and pigmented (Figure 137.14). Tumours may be seen in other locations [16] including the vulva [17], external ear [18], lower leg [19], scrotum [20] and the nipple [21].

Disease course and prognosis
The lesion is benign. Occasionally, basal cell carcinoma, a squamous cell carcinoma (including verrucous carcinoma) [22] or a ductal carcinoma [23] develops on a pre-existing syringocystadenoma papilliferum. *In situ* carcinoma [24] and invasive apocrine carcinoma are exceptional [25,26].

Management
Surgical excision is recommended, both to confirm the diagnosis and for cosmetic reasons.

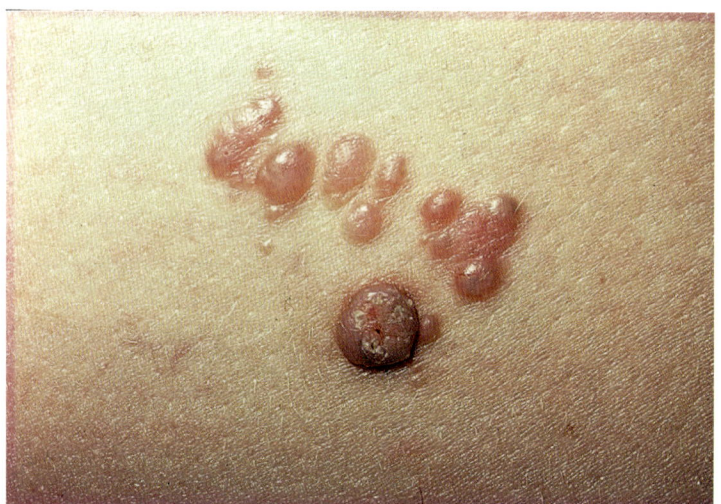

Figure 137.14 Syringocystadenoma papilliferum. Papular lesion with superficial erosion.

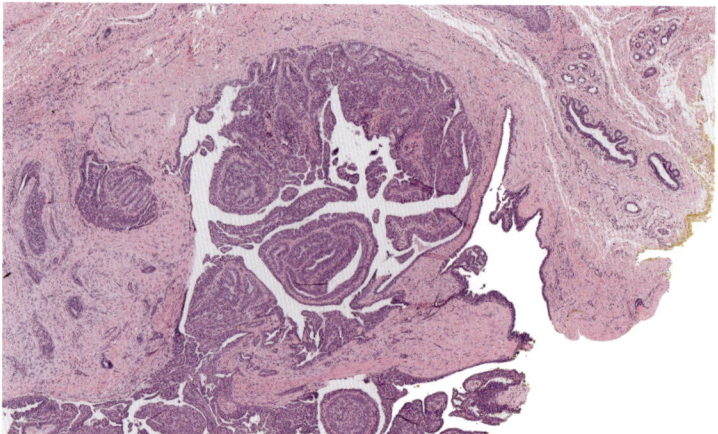

Figure 137.15 Hidradenoma papilliferum. Well-circumscribed tumour with glands and papillary projections.

Hidradenoma papilliferum

Definition and nomenclature
A skin tumour of the ano-genital area of adult females composed of frond-like papillae lined by apocrine epithelium. It most likely arises from ano-genital mammary-like glands [1,2].

> **Synonyms and inclusions**
> - Papillary hidradenoma
> - Mammary-like gland adenoma of the vulva [3]

Epidemiology
Incidence and prevalence
This is an uncommon tumour although it is the most frequent benign adnexal vulvar tumour [4]. In one large series, the subjects were exclusively white, and 75% were between the ages of 25 and 40 years. It occurs four times as commonly on the vulva as in the perianal area [5].

Age
More frequent in middle-aged adults.

Sex
It occurs predominantly in women.

Pathophysiology
Pathology
The tumour is well circumscribed and located just below the skin surface. It is usually spherical in shape and enclosed by compressed connective tissue stroma. Lesions are composed partly of slender fronds of connective tissue lined by one or two layers of epithelial cells and partly of glandular structures (Figure 137.15). The epithelial cells have histochemical characteristics in keeping with an apocrine origin [6,7]. The tumour originates from the ano-genital mammary-like glands [1–3,8]. Sebaceous differentiation is seen occasionally [9]. Mitotic figures vary and may be frequent. In the absence of other features indicative of malignancy, the mitotic count does not imply malignant behaviour [10]. Rare cases have a component connected to the epidermis and overlap with syringocystadenoma papilliferum [11].

Genetics
Molecular biological studies have identified recurrent mutations in *PIK3CA* and *AKT1* in a majority of cases [12].

Clinical features
History and presentation [13–15]
The patients usually seek advice for a lump in the vulval or perianal area, which may be symptomless or, less frequently, may be tender or liable to bleed. The tumour is rounded, freely mobile, often elevated and may feel firm, soft or even cystic. It may range in size from 1 to 40 mm. The commonest site is the labium majus, but it may occur elsewhere on the vulva or perianal area and, exceptionally, in other sites such as the eyelid [9,15], nose [16], arm [17] and chest [18]. Coexistence with a naevus comedonicus has been described [19]. Occasionally, the epithelial surface will ulcerate and the tumour becomes everted to form a reddish-brown papillary mass, which may be suspected of being malignant [5]. The tumour is usually mistaken for a cyst, polyp, angioma or haemorrhoid. A prolonged history and a firm spherical form make the last three diagnoses unlikely.

Disease course and prognosis
The lesion is benign. Malignant transformation is exceptional [18,19].

Management
Excision is curative.

Nipple adenoma [1,2–4,5]

Definition and nomenclature
A complex benign tumour arising from the lactiferous ducts of the nipple.

Synonyms and inclusions
- Benign papillomatosis of the nipple
- Florid papillomatosis of the nipple ducts
- Erosive adenomatosis of the nipple
- Subareolar duct papillomatosis
- Superficial papillary adenomatosis

Epidemiology
This is an uncommon tumour, which occurs mainly in middle-aged women, but it can occur at any age [6], and occasionally in males [7–9]. In one case, the lesion developed 10 years after treatment for carcinoma of the prostate by bilateral orchidectomy and diethylstilboestrol [10].

Pathophysiology
Pathology [1,4,11–14]
The lesion consists of tubules, with an inner layer of columnar cells and an outer layer of cuboidal myoepithelial cells. A major feature is the presence of superficial keratocysts lined by both squamous and columnar epithelium, and filled with keratin flakes and an eosinophilic material, apparently secreted by the columnar cells. The cysts seem to reproduce the terminal portion of the nipple duct system. Within some of the superficial cysts or ducts, foreign-body giant cells may be seen.

Some degree of intraluminal growth (intraductal papillomatosis) is present in many cases. This ranges from small papillary epithelial tufts to almost complete occlusion of the lumina by solid epithelial plugs, and there may be evidence of apocrine decapitation secretion. The overlying epidermis may show acanthosis and hyperkeratosis. The major histopathological diagnostic pitfall is confusing erosive adenomatosis with sweat gland tumours and as it may also be difficult to differentiate from papillary breast carcinoma. Immunohistological techniques are of value in demonstrating the layer of myoepithelial cells [12,13].

Genetics
Mutations in *PIK3CA* and *BRAF V600E* are frequently found in nipple adenomas [14].

Clinical features
These are variable. The condition may start with a blood-stained or serous discharge, and the nipple may be enlarged, eroded, crusted or eczematous. There may be a small nodule on the nipple and the symptoms may be worse in the premenstrual phase. The condition is commonly misdiagnosed as Paget disease or eczema [15]. It is usually unilateral, but bilateral involvement has been reported [16,17], and it has been described in an accessory nipple [18]. Dermoscopy can be useful in distinguishing nipple adenoma from eczema or psoriasis [19].

Management
Excision is curative – either simple local excision, or partial or complete resection of the nipple, depending on the size of the tumour [20]. There are reports of successful treatment by cryosurgery [21] and Mohs surgery [22].

Apocrine tubular adenoma [1,2,3]

Definition
A tumour usually arising on the scalp.

Epidemiology
Incidence and prevalence
It is a rare lesion.

Age
Presentation is usually in middle-aged adults.

Sex
There is slight female predilection.

Pathophysiology
Pathology
Clusters of tubular structures are seen in the dermis, with a lining of cells showing decapitation secretion. There is no surrounding inflammatory response. Cytological atypia and an infiltrative margin are absent. As with many adnexal tumours, often one finds histological overlap between tubular apocrine adenoma and papillary eccrine adenoma [3,4]. Overlapping features with syringocystadenoma papilliferum are also seen, especially in superficial tumours [5]. Sometimes they coexist [6].

Genetics
Apocrine tubular adenomas frequently harbour *BRAF V600E* mutations [7].

Clinical features
History and presentation
These are usually large slowly expanding lesions on the scalp. Other locations such as the nose and the vulva have been reported [8,9]. The lesion often arises in association with a naevus sebaceous.

Disease course and prognosis
Tumours are benign.

Management
Simple surgical excision is the treatment of choice.

Apocrine carcinoma [1–3]

Definition
A malignant adnexal carcinoma showing clear evidence of apocrine differentiation: large cells with abundant pink cytoplasm and decapitation secretion.

Epidemiology
Incidence and prevalence
This is a rare entity.

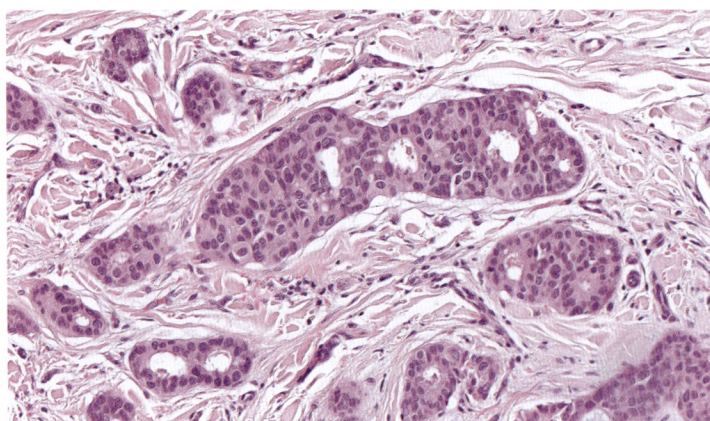

Figure 137.16 Apocrine carcinoma. Prominent glands with decapitation secretion.

Age
Patients are middle aged or elderly.

Sex
There is a slight predilection for females.

Pathophysiology
Pathology
Three histological patterns may be seen: tubular, tubulopapillary and solid (Figure 137.16). The degree of differentiation varies and the diagnosis is often difficult in poorly differentiated tumours. Mitotic figures, local invasion and nuclear pleomorphism all suggest a malignant lesion. The most specific pathological feature is the presence of decapitation secretion [1]. Some cases are associated with prominent pagetoid spread, particularly those presenting on genital skin [4]. Tumour cells are positive for gross cystic disease fluid protein-15 (GCDFP-15) [5] and they show positivity for oestrogen, progesterone and androgen receptors in up to a third of cases [6]. Recently, it has been suggested that an immunohistochemical panel of adipophilin, ER, PR, HER2, cytokeratin 5/6 and mammaglobin may be helpful in distinguishing cutaneous apocrine carcinoma from mammary apocrine carcinoma as the former is positive for these markers while the latter tends to be negative [7]. A histologically distinctive variant of apocrine carcinoma has been described as cribiform apocrine carcinoma [8]. The designation as malignant is surprising as this tumour shows little cytological atypia, low mitotic activity, does not tend to recur and no metastases have been reported.

Clinical features
History and presentation
Lesions have been reported mainly from the head and neck area, including the eyelid and external ear, ano-genital skin and also the axilla [9]. It is not possible on morphological grounds or with the help of immunohistochemistry to separate a cutaneous axillary apocrine carcinoma from an apocrine breast carcinoma spreading or invading the skin by direct extension. Breast imaging is advisable to rule out a primary breast tumour. Some tumours arise within a naevus sebaceous [6,10]. The tumour presents as a nodule, usually measuring more than 1 cm in diameter. Rare cases may be bilateral [11].

Genetics
Apocrine carcinomas have been shown to exhibit polysomy or trisomy of *EGFR*, as well as mutations of *AKT-1*, *PIK3CA* and *TP53* [12].

Disease course and prognosis
It has been found that grading tumours according to the modified Bloom–Richardson method of grading breast carcinoma is very useful in establishing prognosis [6]. Patients with grade 3 tumours have a poor prognosis [6]. Metastatic spread to regional lymph nodes and internal organs occurs in between 20% and 30% of the cases [6,13].

Management
Wide excision and close follow-up are required. Based on the similarities between breast and apocrine carcinoma, breast carcinoma adjuvant therapy regimens may be considered in high grade tumours [6].

ECCRINE GLAND HAMARTOMAS AND TUMOURS

Eccrine gland-derived lesions make up a large and relatively common group of appendage tumours. Hidroacanthoma simplex, dermal duct tumour and eccrine poromas form a fairly homogeneous family derived from eccrine duct and pore. However, there are clear examples of apocrine poroma. Eccrine syringofibroadenoma probably also belongs in this subsection. Eccrine hidradenoma, although closely related, has features suggesting both secretory and ductal differentiation, which makes the term 'acrospiroma' misleading, and thus is perhaps best kept in a separate category.

Malignant tumours of sweat glands are relatively rare, but important to recognise. Their morphology and behaviour are variable.

Eccrine angiomatous hamartoma
[1,**2**,3–8]

Definition and nomenclature
Eccrine angiomatous hamartoma is a rare condition most commonly found in acral skin. It is characterised histologically by numerous eccrine structures and capillary channels.

Synonyms and inclusions
- Sudoriparous angioma

Epidemiology
These lesions appear at birth or during childhood in most cases and there is a slight male predilection [9].

Pathophysiology
Pathology
Histologically, lesions show nests of large but otherwise normal eccrine glands [2,3], enmeshed in loose fibrous tissue, which contains numerous thin-walled blood vessels and lymphatics [4]. There may be a very intimate association between the glandular and vascular elements [5,6]. The overlying epidermis may be mildly acanthotic. Other components, particularly hair follicles, may also be closely associated with the eccrine angiomatous complexes [7,8]. Some have shown fat [9,10,11] or mucin deposition [3,12]. Immunohistochemical findings are similar to normal eccrine glands [9].

Clinical features
Mostly solitary, they take the form of a nodule or plaque, flesh-coloured or with a bluish colour and angiomatous appearance. Eighty per cent occur on the extremities [13], particularly the palm and sole, but also on other parts of the feet, on the face, neck and on the trunk. Occasionally, there are multiple lesions [1,9,13–17]. Most are painful on pressure [4,9,18]. Nail destruction with underlying osteolysis has been reported [14]. Some demonstrate hypertrichosis [15] and/or hyperhidrosis [3], but not all [19]. Generally, they enlarge very gradually; more rapid growth has been described during pregnancy and adolescence [20]. One atypical case presented at the age of 73 years on the buttock and was verrucous [21]. They are usually unassociated with other anomalies but accompanied Cowden syndrome in one case [22] and neurofibromatosis in another [23]. A familial occurrence was noted in one report [17].

Management
Painful lesions may require removal, particularly those on the palm or sole; this has been successfully achieved by deep excision with full-thickness grafting [4]. There have been (fortunately rare) cases where pain control and lack of function required amputation [20]. Pulsed dye laser was helpful in only one of two patients [24]. Spontaneous regression has been reported [25].

Eccrine hidrocystoma [1,2–7]

Definition
A tumour produced by mature deformed eccrine sweat units, whose secretions dilate the ducts. Lesions are usually situated on the face and are often multiple.

Epidemiology
Incidence and prevalence
This is a rare tumour. It was formerly reported as being more common in those who had to work exposed to heat, such as cooks. A report indicating that the lesion is usually solitary and situated close to the eyelid underlines the problem of differentiating eccrine from apocrine hidrocystomas [1]. Eccrine hidrocystoma is currently classified into two types according to the number of lesions: the Smith type, which is the most prevalent and presents with a solitary lesion, and the rare Robinson type consisting of multiple lesions [1,2].

Age
Middle-aged individuals are typically affected. It can exceptionally occur in children [3].

Sex
It occurs mainly in women.

Pathophysiology
Pathology [4–6]
The general features are those of a dermal cystic lesion uni- or multilocular lined by two layers of cells. The inner layer of cells is columnar and the outer layer consists of elongated myoepithelial cells. In cases with prominent dilatation, the epithelium appears flattened. Distinction from apocrine hidrocystoma is based on the presence of decapitation secretion in the cells of the inner layer.

Clinical features
History and presentation [1]
The lesions are largely confined to the cheeks and eyelids. They are cystic, often blue in colour and there is frequently a history of enlargement when the skin is exposed to heat and flattening of the lesion when the skin is exposed to cold. Administration of atropine also induces disappearance of the cyst [7]. The lesions may be multiple and pigmented [8]. Exceptionally, multiple eccrine hidrocystomas have been reported in Graves disease with resolution after treatment of the condition [9].

Disease course and prognosis
The lesion is benign.

Management
Treatment may consist of topical atropine or scopolamine but this is usually discontinued due to side effects [10]. Oral oxybutinin is an anticholinergic agent that has been successfully used in the treatment of multiple hidrocystomas [11]. Electrodesiccation, carbon dioxide laser, pulse dye laser and botulinum toxin (with temporary effect) have been used with good results [12,13,14]. Excision produces satisfactory results.

Hidroacanthoma simplex [1,2,3,4,5,6]

Definition
An intraepidermal tumour derived from the eccrine duct epithelium, which could be considered an intradermal eccrine poroma [2,3].

Epidemiology
Incidence and prevalence
It is a rare tumour.

Age
Mainly occurs in elderly individuals.

Sex
There is no sex predilection.

Pathophysiology
Pathology
Nests of clearly discrete small rounded cells are seen within the normal epidermal cells. They are smaller and more cuboidal than surrounding keratinocytes and are rich in glycogen and the glycolytic enzymes. These lesions may be confused with intraepidermal or clonal seborrhoeic keratoses, demonstrating what has in the past been called the 'Borst–Jadassohn phenomenon' [7]. The individual cells in these lesions are larger and less rich in glycogen. However, for the diagnosis to be made, ductal differentiation should be demonstrated. In a histogenetic study of classic poroma, hidroacanthoma simplex, dermal duct tumour and poroid hidradenoma, a common histogenesis was demonstrated for these neoplasms; they seem to derive from the basal keratinocytes of the sweat duct ridge and the lower acrosyringium as the majority of the poroid cells in these tumours expressed K14, islands of K10-positive and K77-negative large cells. K77 expression was limited to luminal cells of intact ductal structures within the tumours [3].

Clinical features
History and presentation
Hidroacanthoma simplex is a verrucous plaque or ring with a hyperkeratotic usually brown surface. It often mimics a flat seborrhoeic keratosis. Ulceration or elevation of the lesion suggests a dermal component. From the few reports available, it appears that the limbs are more likely to be involved than the head or trunk.

Disease course and prognosis
The lesion is benign. Malignant change has been reported in hidroacanthoma simplex including pigmented and clear cell variants [8–12].

Management
Excision is recommended both to confirm the diagnosis and for management. If malignant change occurs, wider excision and follow-up is advisable.

Eccrine dermal duct tumour [1,2]

Definition
A benign proliferation of the eccrine dermal duct located in the dermis.

Epidemiology
Incidence and prevalence
It is a very rare tumour.

Age
Usually occurs in the elderly.

Sex
There is female predilection.

Pathophysiology
Pathology
The pathology is similar to that of the hidroacanthoma simplex, but the nests of tumour cells making up the lesion are located in the dermis. The cells are small, cuboidal, regular and stain strongly with PAS. Ductal structures are often seen. An intraepidermal component may be seen in some cases, confirming that this lesion is part of the spectrum of eccrine poroma. In some cases, there is prominent clear-cell change [3]. Poroid hidradenoma is regarded as a variant of poroma with overlapping features of hidradenoma (dermal solid and cystic nests) and poroma (poroid cells and ductal differentiation) [4]. This lesion more likely represents part of the spectrum of dermal duct tumour. As with all poroid tumours, dermal ductal tumour can display apocrine and sebaceous differentiation.

Clinical features
History and presentation
The clinical picture is that of a nondescript dermal nodule, occasionally with verrucous change overlying it.

Disease course and prognosis
The lesion is benign.

Management
Excision is required for diagnostic and therapeutic purposes.

Eccrine poroma [1,2]

Definition
A tumour deriving from the intraepidermal eccrine duct (acrosyringium). Traditionally, all poromas have been regarded as eccrine. However, a number of lesions may show apocrine differentiation.

Epidemiology
Incidence and prevalence
Tumours are relatively common.

Age
Most patients are adults, tumours rarely presenting in children [3].

Sex
There is no sex predilection.

Pathophysiology
Pathology [4–6]
These lesions are relatively easy to diagnose, with a clear margin between adjacent normal epidermal keratinocytes and a population of smaller cuboidal cells, usually with darker nuclei protruding down into the underlying dermis (Figure 137.17). The cells are similar to those seen in the dermal duct tumour [7]. Reports, however, have stressed the fact that some poromas may show either sebaceous or apocrine differentiation [8,9,**10**] highlighting the fact that adnexal tumours with ductal differentiation may be either eccrine or apocrine, as the ducts of both structures are identical. YAP1-fused tumours seem to harbour reproducible histopathological features, such as broad and bulbous architecture,

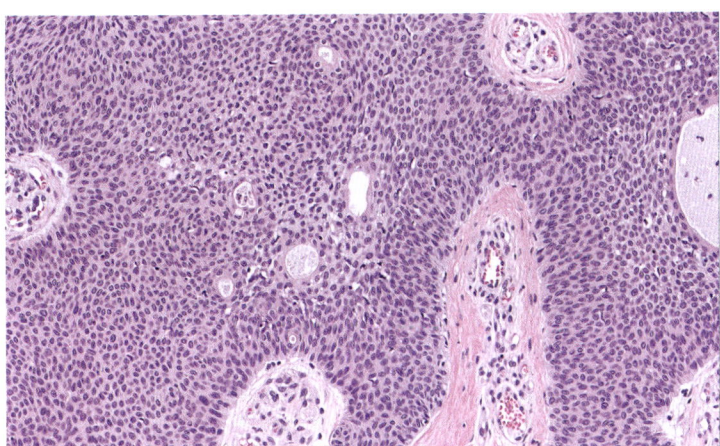

Figure 137.17 Poroma. Cuboidal cells and ductular differentiation.

squamatised cuticles and ductules, nuclear grooves and pseudonuclear inclusions [11]. Recently, NUT expression and loss of YAP1 by immunohistochemistry have been demonstrated in eccrine poromas [12,13].

Genetics
Eccrine poromas are characterised by highly recurrent YAP1-MAML2 and YAP1-NUTM1 fusions [14].

Clinical features
History and presentation [1,2,3–23,24,26]
This lesion is one of the easiest of the appendage tumours to recognise in the clinic. The great majority of these lesions are found on the palms and soles (Figure 137.18), in contrast to other skin appendage tumours, which tend to be concentrated around the head and neck area. The anatomical distribution is, however, wide and it has been demonstrated that the head, neck and trunk regions represent common sites. They are moist exophytic lesions, pink or red in colour, and may reach 1–2 cm in diameter. Occasional lesions are pigmented and look similar to pigmented basal cell carcinoma under dermoscopy [24,25]. Exceptional examples of poroma have been reported in a naevus sebaceous [26], with rapid growth during pregnancy [27], after electron beam therapy for mycosis fungoides [22], after radiotherapy [22] and at the site of a burn [28]. Multiple poromas (poromatosis) have been reported in a case of hidrotic ectodermal dysplasia as well as in patients with a history of lymphoproliferative disorders [29,30], after radiotherapy and during pregnancy [31,32].

Disease course and prognosis
The lesion is benign. Malignant change has been recorded in up to 18% of cases (see under porocarcinoma).

Management
Benign eccrine poromas are treated by surgical excision.

Eccrine syringofibroadenoma [1]

Definition and nomenclature
It is an uncommon tumour with eccrine ductal differentiation.

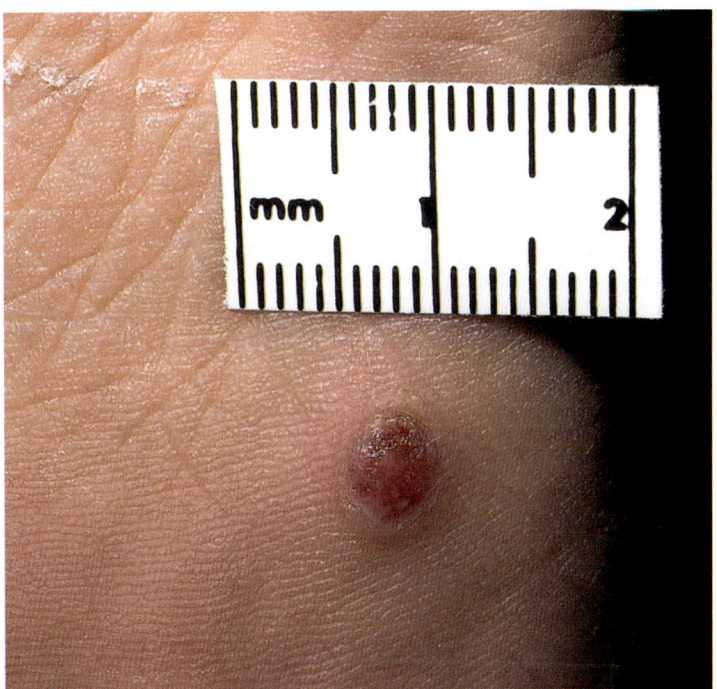

Figure 137.18 Poroma. Note the red shiny surface, which often leads to misdiagnosis of a pyogenic granuloma.

Synonyms and inclusions
- Acrosyringeal naevus

Epidemiology
Incidence and prevalence
This is a very rare entity. Fewer than 100 have been reported in the English literature to date [2].

Age
Although the age of onset varies depending on the clinical subtype, in most cases it presents in elderly individuals.

Sex
There is no sex predilection.

Pathophysiology
Pathology
It is still unclear whether the lesion is hyperplastic, hamartomatous or neoplastic in nature. It is possible that the lesion represents a spectrum of clinical findings, rather than being separate in nature [3]. Histologically, a network of epithelial cells extends down from the epidermis, forming a mesh-like structure in the underlying epidermis. These cords are composed of smaller cells than in the overlying epidermis and may contain ductal structures. This mesh is surrounded by a fibrovascular stroma. Unlike basal cell carcinoma, there is no palisading [4,5]. Clear cells may occasionally predominate [6].

Clinical features
History and presentation
Five clinical subtypes have been described:
- Type I: multiple – associated with ectodermal dysplasia.
- Type II: multiple without other cutaneous features.
- Type III: unilateral linear (naevoid).
- Type IV: solitary neoplastic [7].
- Type V: reactive [8].

It may present as a solitary, often warty nodule on the arms or legs, especially on distal sites. The lesion may be reactive, representing hyperplasia as a result of diverse stimuli, or may be neoplastic usually presenting as a single lesion. Unusual presentations including plaques and multiple lesions [9], occasionally with a linear distribution, may be seen [7]. Coexistence with a squamous cell carcinoma and porocarcinoma has rarely been described [10,11] and lesions may rarely present within naevus sebaceous [12]. Syringofibroadenomatous hyperplasia of the sweat ducts is seen in the background of other tumours, a healing ulcer, stasis, a reparative process after bullous diseases, in skin affected by leprosy, in peristomal skin, in burn scars and in association with ectodermal dysplasia [13,14,**15**,16–19]. In small biopsies, this type of hyperplasia may be confused with a syringofibroadenoma.

Disease course and prognosis
The lesion is benign. Malignant transformation has exceptionally been described [4,20].

Management
Excision is the treatment of choice.

Syringoma [1,2,3]

Definition and nomenclature
A benign skin tumour composed of sweat ducts that is usually multiple.

> **Synonyms and inclusions**
> - Hidradénomes eruptifs
> - Syringocystadenoma
> - Syringocystoma

Epidemiology
Incidence and prevalence
It is a relatively common lesion.

Age
It is most likely to appear at adolescence, and further lesions may develop during adult life. It does not appear to be hereditary.

Sex
It occurs more commonly in females.

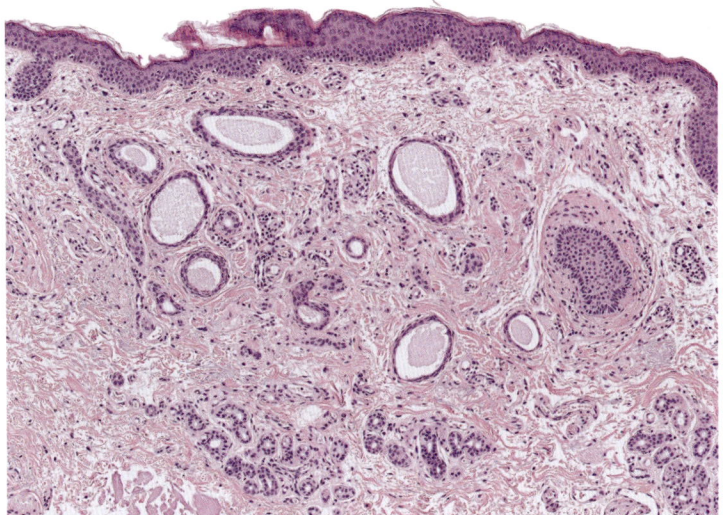

Figure 137.19 Syringoma. Typical ductal structures with a tadpole appearance.

Pathophysiology
Pathology [4,5]
The lesion has a characteristic architectural pattern on light microscope scanning power. Collections of convoluted and cystic ducts are seen in the upper half of the dermis. Most are lined by a double layer of cells similar to, but flatter than, those that line normal eccrine ducts. The lumina contain amorphous debris. A characteristic feature is the tail-like strand of cells projecting from one side of the duct into the stroma, giving a resemblance to a tadpole or comma (Figure 137.19). Occasional cases show cells with prominent clear-cell change [6,7]. The ducts may be enclosed in a fibrous stroma similar to the hair follicle hamartomas, but in most cases it is narrower and less cellular.

Clinical features
History and presentation
The individual small dermal papules are skin coloured, yellowish or mauve, but sometimes appear translucent and cystic. The surface may be rounded or flat-topped and the outline sometimes angular. Rarely, injury to the surface will allow a drop of clear watery fluid to escape. They vary in size from 1 to 5 mm, but most are less than 3 mm. Rare cases present in a linear naevoid distribution [8] and exceptionally lesions are associated with alopecia [9]. Some cases resemble milia and in these cases the histology reveals a number of cystically dilated structures [10,11]. In most cases, there are multiple tumours, and they tend to have a bilateral symmetry in distribution. The front of the chest, face and neck are the chief areas affected. A few lesions are usually found on the eyelids when the cheeks are involved (Figure 137.20). Eruptive syringomas have a predilection for the neck, chest, abdomen, pubic area and more rarely on the buttocks [12,13]. Eruptive vulval and less commonly penile syringomas may also have been described [14–17]. Syringomas are seen more often than expected in patients with Down syndrome [**18**,19] and may erupt dramatically (Figure 137.21). Familial cases rarely occur [20]. A case of multiple syringomas probably sun induced and in an acral location has been described [21]. Multiple syringomas have also been reported during radiotherapy for breast cancer [22]. The lesions regressed after cessation of radiotherapy. Syringoma is most likely to be confused with trichoepithelioma on

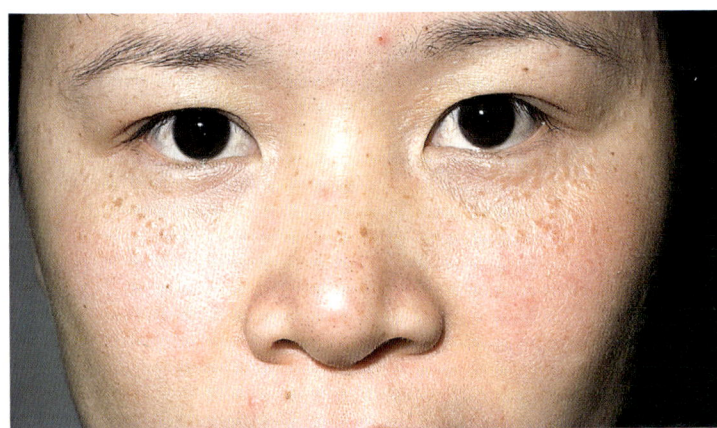

Figure 137.20 Multiple syringomas on the upper cheek area.

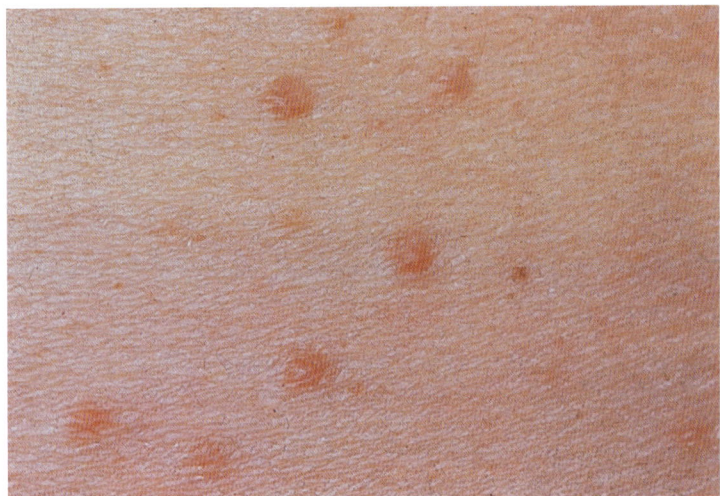

Figure 137.21 Eruptive syringomas. Multiple tiny brownish or red lesions are often seen on the trunk and limbs.

the face. The syringomas tend to be smaller, rather less superficial, more flat-topped and disposed more evenly over the cheeks and eyelids, rather than favouring the naso-labial creases. There is no family history. Lesions on the lids may be mistaken for xanthelasma but lack the orange colour. Those erupting on the trunk may be mistaken for disseminated granuloma annulare.

Disease course and prognosis
The lesion is benign.

Management
The main reason for treatment is cosmetic. Careful destruction with diathermy can produce good cosmetic results. Lesions treated with carbon dioxide laser may recur. Botulinum toxin has also been used in combination with laser or as monotherapy (temporary effect) in the treatment of localised syringomas [23].

Tubular adenoma [1,2,3,4]

Definition and nomenclature
It is not entirely settled whether papillary eccrine adenoma represents the same entity as tubular apocrine adenoma [2]. It is likely that most tumours are probably apocrine [3], while true eccrine lesions are unusual and arise in areas where no apocrine glands are present normally, such as the limbs [4]. However, current classifications unify this entity under the name of tubular adenoma [5].

Synonyms and inclusions
- Papillary eccrine adenoma
- Tubular apocrine adenoma

Epidemiology [1]
Incidence and prevalence
It is a rare lesion. Fewer than 50 cases have been described.

Age
There is a wide age range.

Sex
There is a predilection for females.

Pathophysiology
Pathology
The lesion is in the mid–lower dermis and consists of ductal structures with papillary projections. These ductal structures may display either eccrine or apocrine differentiation (decapitation secretion). Dilated ducts form a complex honeycomb-like structure. The lumina are filled with an eosinophilic amorphous material, which is diastase resistant, PAS positive and Alcian blue positive. The most important differential diagnosis is from aggressive digital papillary adenocarcinoma, which has a more infiltrative growth pattern, and displays nuclear and cytoplasmic pleomorphism and numerous mitotic figures.

Clinical features
History and presentation
This rare lesion was first described in 1977 [1]. It presents in a non-diagnostic manner as a slowly growing solitary nodule usually on the limbs of darker skinned individuals [6].

Disease course and prognosis
The lesion is benign. Recurrence is exceptional [1].

Management
Excision is the treatment of choice.

ECCRINE OR APOCRINE/FOLLICULAR TUMOURS

In recent years, it has become apparent that a number of adnexal tumours that were regarded as exclusively showing eccrine ductal differentiation often display ductal apocrine differentiation. Because of the close relationship between the apocrine and the pilosebaceous unit, these tumours may also show evidence of focal follicular and even sebaceous differentiation [1,2]. The list of tumours with potential to display apocrine ductal differentiation continues to expand and even includes rare examples of poromas showing apocrine differentiation.

Hidradenoma [1]

Definition and nomenclature
A relatively rare tumour of sweat gland origin. Although traditionally regarded as displaying eccrine differentiation, it is now accepted that tumours can show either eccrine or apocrine differentiation [2]. In fact, it is now believed that apocrine hidradenomas are more common [3].

> **Synonyms and inclusions**
> - Nodulocystic hidradenoma
> - Clear-cell hidradenoma
> - Acrospiroma

Epidemiology
Incidence and prevalence [4]
This is a relatively uncommon tumour.

Age
It is found mainly in adults. Lesions in children are very rare [5].

Sex
It is excised more commonly in women than in men.

Pathophysiology
Pathology [6–9]
The tumour may connect with the epidermis. It forms lobulated circumscribed masses and is composed of two cell types – polygonal cells, whose glycogen content may give the cytoplasm a clear appearance; and elongated, darker and smaller cells, which may occur at the periphery. Often, tumours do not contain cells with clear cytoplasm, and the name 'clear-cell hidradenoma' is therefore misleading. Cuboidal or columnar cells are seen lining duct-like spaces and clefts. In cases with a connection to the epidermis, the superficial component displays poromatous features. Focal squamous differentiation may be seen [10] and occasional mucinous cells are also present. The latter is often seen in lesions with apocrine differentiation. A small number of tumours have features that are worrying but do not fulfil the criteria for malignancy. These lesions are regarded as atypical hidradenomas [11]. Malignant transformation is very rare, and the diagnosis relies on identification of the pre-existing benign component [12–15]. Such tumours are characterised by deep extension, infiltrative growth pattern, necrosis, substantial cytological atypia and increased mitotic activity [11].

Genetics
Approximately one half of hidradenomas contain a CRTC1-MALM2 fusion [16].

Clinical features
History and presentation
The tumours are firm dermal nodules, 5–30 mm in size, and may be attached to the overlying epidermis, which can be either thickened or ulcerated (Figure 137.22). Growth is slow and there may be a history of serous discharge. The lesions are usually solitary and are most likely to be found on the scalp, face, anterior trunk and proximal limbs. When the tumour is attached to the epidermis, the diagnosis may be suspected on clinical grounds, especially if there is a history of discharge. Ulcerated lesions may resemble basal cell carcinoma. Dermal nodules are non-diagnostic by clinical inspection.

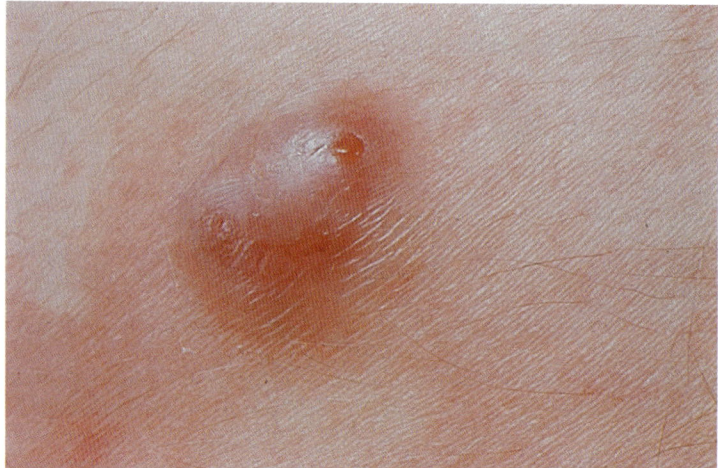

Figure 137.22 Hidradenoma. Red-brown irregular papule.

Disease course and prognosis
The lesion is benign. Local recurrences are rare [17]. Lymphatic invasion and regional lymph node metastasis have been reported in tumours that are histologically entirely benign. This finding does not seem to alter prognosis but the number of cases reported is too low and follow-up is limited to be certain of this [18]. Atypical hidradenomas appear to have some tendency for local recurrence but no metastatic potential [11]. Malignant eccrine hidradenoma may metastasise.

Management
Surgical excision will cure benign lesions. Long follow-up is suggested for histologically benign lesions that display lymphatic invasion or lymph node metastasis [18]. In patients with the latter finding, staging should also be performed.

Cylindroma [1,2,3]

Definition and nomenclature
A skin tumour traditionally regarded as showing sweat gland lineage with a characteristic histology (see later) that usually manifests as nodules or tumours of the scalp.

> **Synonyms and inclusions**
> - Turban tumour
> - Spiegler's tumour

Epidemiology
Incidence and prevalence
This is an uncommon tumour. It is frequently familial and an autosomal dominant gene determines its inheritance [4,5]. It has been reported to follow radiotherapy epilation of the scalp.

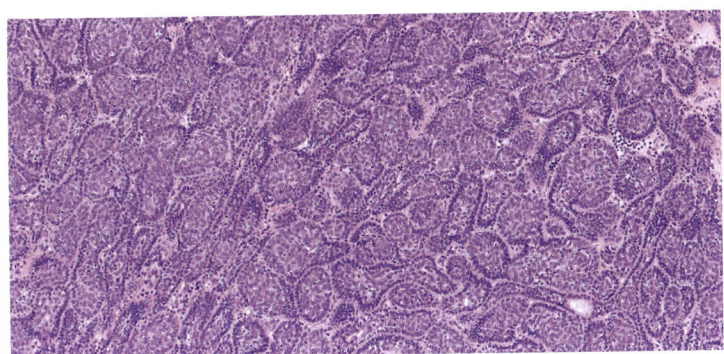

Figure 137.23 Cylindroma. Classical jigsaw-puzzle architecture with basaloid tumour lobules.

Age
The onset is usually in early adult life but may be in childhood or adolescence.

Sex
It involves females more frequently than males.

Pathophysiology
Pathology [6,7,8,9–11]
The tumours have a rounded outline and are composed of closely set mosaic-like masses ('jigsaw-puzzle' appearance) and columns of cells that are invested by a hyaline basal membrane of variable thickness. Thin bands of stroma (Figure 137.23) separate tumour lobules from one another. The cells are of two types: one large, with a moderate amount of cytoplasm and a vesicular nucleus; and the other small, with little cytoplasm and a compact nucleus. The small cells tend to be peripheral; they also surround duct-like spaces or masses of hyaline material within the tumour lobule. There are strong immunohistochemical similarities between cylindromas and spiradenomas, and they may coexist in the same individual [12–14]. Malignant transformation is very rare and a sarcomatous component may exceptionally be seen [15,16,17].

Genetics
The lesions may be familial and a suppressor gene (cylindromatosis gene, *CYLD*) has been identified on chromosome 16q12–13, loss of which is associated with cylindroma development [18–20]. Somatic mutations have also been identified in sporadic cases. The loss of this gene causes activation of necrosis factor β (NF-β), which is a transcription factor with antiapoptotic activity [19]. Based on genetic studies and the identification of mutations in the same gene in the Brooke–Spiegler syndrome, multiple familial trichoepitheliomas and familial cylindromatosis, it is suggested that the three diseases have the same genetic basis and are phenotypic expressions of the same disease [21]. It has been demonstrated that benign sporadic dermal cylindromas express the *MYB-NFIB* gene fusion [22], which is also expressed in adenoid cystic carcinomas of the breast, head and neck. Transition from cylindroma to spiradenoma in *CYLD* defective tumours associated with reduced *DKK2* expression has been reported [23]. MYB expression is increased in cylindromas of Brooke–Spiegler syndrome in the absence of *MYB-NFIB* fusion, which suggests that MYB is one of the key players in the development of inherited cylindromas [24]. Mutations in *DNMT3A* and *BCOR* have been demonstrated in a proportion of cylindromas, both in syndromic and sporadic settings [25,26].

Clinical features
History and presentation
The tumours are frequently multiple, smooth, firm, pink to red in colour and often somewhat pedunculated (Figure 137.24). The rate of growth of cylindroma is slow and often seems to cease when a certain size has been reached. Some tumours become 5 cm or more in diameter, but most are smaller. Pain is an occasional symptom. The commonest site is the scalp and adjacent skin. Tumours on the scalp may be almost hairless when pedunculated, but the smaller lesions form dermal nodules with little loss of overlying hair. Multiple tumours have attracted much attention in the literature, but solitary lesions are not uncommonly seen by surgical pathology services. A proportion of lesions occur on the face and neck away from the scalp margin; in fewer than 10% of cases, they are situated on the trunk and limbs. Rare lesions may occur in the breast sporadically or in association with Brooke–Spiegler syndrome. When the lesions are multiple, new tumours arise over the years. In some patients, there may be an admixture with trichoepithelioma, either in separate tumours or sometimes in the same tumour. This is a clear confirmation of what can be inferred from the syndromes associated with cylindromas and follicular neoplasms, which is that cylindromas are more likely to be related to the apocrine gland than to the eccrine gland. The multiple type on the scalp is most likely to be confused with tricholemmal cyst, which is, however, usually smoother, firmer and more mobile. Small tumours are difficult to diagnose, and must be distinguished from trichoepithelioma, steatocystoma or basal cell carcinoma if solitary. Large, pedunculated and lobular tumours are almost unmistakable.

Disease course and prognosis
Lesions behave in a benign fashion. Malignant transformation is very rare.

Management
Surgery is the treatment of choice. Extensive involvement of the scalp may require wide excision and skin graft reconstruction. Topical salicylic acid has been used with some success in patients with multiple cylindromas [27].

Spiradenoma [1,2]

Definition and nomenclature
A benign tumour of sweat gland lineage, which is usually solitary and is distinguished by its histology (see later).

Synonyms and inclusions
- Eccrine spiradenoma

Epidemiology
Incidence and prevalence
It is relatively uncommon and is rarely familial (see under cylindroma).

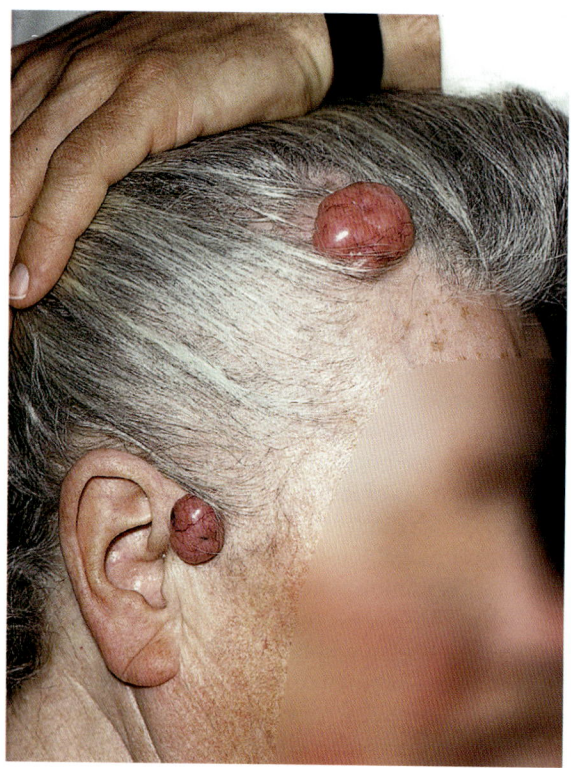

Figure 137.24 Cylindroma. Two large tumours on the head of an elderly woman.

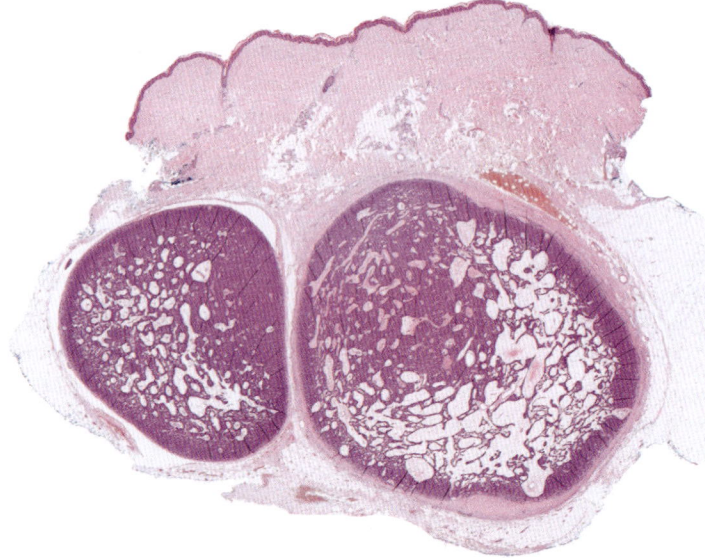

Figure 137.25 Eccrine spiradenoma. Well-circumscribed subcutaneous bluish tumour nodules (so-called 'blue balls').

Age
It appears mainly in young adults.

Sex
Both sexes are equally affected.

Pathophysiology
Pathology [3,4]
The tumour is lobular (Figure 137.25), with two cell types in the islands. Larger paler cells may be grouped around lumina and smaller darker cells form the periphery. Small tubular structures or cystic spaces may occur and large thin-walled dilated vascular channels are also present [5,6]. The lobules are surrounded by condensed connective tissue, which may encroach on the islands as hyaline droplets. Degenerative changes in old tumours are often prominent. Haemorrhage and ischaemic necrosis as a result of degeneration often obscure the histological features, and only focal areas display the typical features of a spiradenoma (Figure 137.26). Old tumours with degenerative changes tend to be very large. Malignant transformation may occur and usually presents in long-standing tumours [7–12]; lesions may have features of cylindroma and spiradenoma [13]. The diagnosis of a malignant spiradenoma is often only made after a residual benign component is identified. Rare tumours have a sarcomatous component [14]. Four general patterns have been described [15] in malignant neoplasms arising from pre-existing benign spiradenomas/cylindromas. A high rate of p53 expression has been reported but its utility is limited as it can be negative in clearly malignant neoplasms [16].

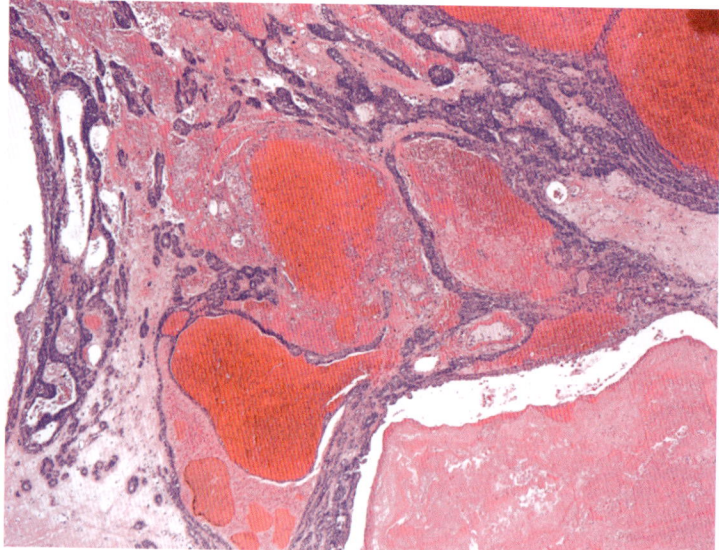

Figure 137.26 Eccrine spiradenoma. Extensive haemorrhage with or without ischaemic necrosis may result in rapid clinical growth. Only small areas of residual spiradenoma remain.

Genetics
Lesions with features of spiradenoma may be part of the Brooke–Spiegler syndrome [3]. Spiradenoma often overlaps with cylindroma and this gives support to the theory that they are part of the same spectrum (see Cylindroma) [17]. A recurrent missense mutation in the kinase domain of the *ALPK1* gene that can activate the NF-κB pathway and is mutually exclusive with *CYLD* mutations has been demonstrated in spiradenomas and spiradenocarcinomas [18].

Clinical features
History and presentation [19,20]
The lesion is usually solitary and painful and consists of a firm rounded bluish dermal nodule 3–50 mm in diameter [19]. The usual site is on the front of the trunk and proximal limbs. Rare sites include the vulva, breast and external ear. Congenital tumours are

exceptional and in one case lesions followed Blaschko lines on the face [21]. Multiple neoplasms in a linear or zosteriform distribution may also be seen [22,23] and tumours may rarely be seen in a naevus sebaceous [24]. Furthermore, the coexistence of spiradenoma with follicular tumours confirms an apocrine line of differentiation at least in a percentage of these tumours. Clinical differentiation from other dermal tumours and cysts may be made if the tumour is firm, dark blue and domed.

Disease course and prognosis
The lesion is benign but may rarely recur locally. Malignant tumours may metastasise but it is difficult to be certain of how aggressive these neoplasms are because of their rarity and the bias to report mainly cases with aggressive behaviour. It seems that tumours with low grade malignant transformation exhibit a good prognosis in general [25].

Management
Surgical excision should be complete, as there may be recurrence.

Mixed tumour of the skin [1]

Definition and nomenclature
Although traditionally regarded as a tumour showing eccrine derivation, it has been demonstrated that a majority of lesions are folliculosebaceous–apocrine and only rare tumours are truly eccrine [2].

Synonyms and inclusions
- Chondroid syringoma

Epidemiology
Age
It occurs most commonly in middle-aged males. Lesions in children are rare [3].

Sex
There is no sex predilection.

Pathophysiology
Pathology [4]
This is usually a large multilobulated tumour located in the dermis and/or subcutaneous tissue. Tumour lobules are separated by fibrous septa. A myxoid, hyalinised or chondroid stroma is variably seen in all tumours. The epithelial component consists of nests and strands of cells with pink cytoplasm and vesicular nuclei with a single inconspicuous nucleolus. Cytological atypia is absent and mitotic figures are sometimes seen. Tubular structures and ductal differentiation are frequently seen. Epithelial cells may show various types of metaplasia and differentiation including squamous and mucinous metaplasia and clear-cell change and columnar and oxyphilic change [2]. Larger tumour cells with a plasmacytoid appearance are a frequent finding and suggest myoepithelial differentiation. Myoepithelial cells may also be spindle shaped or display

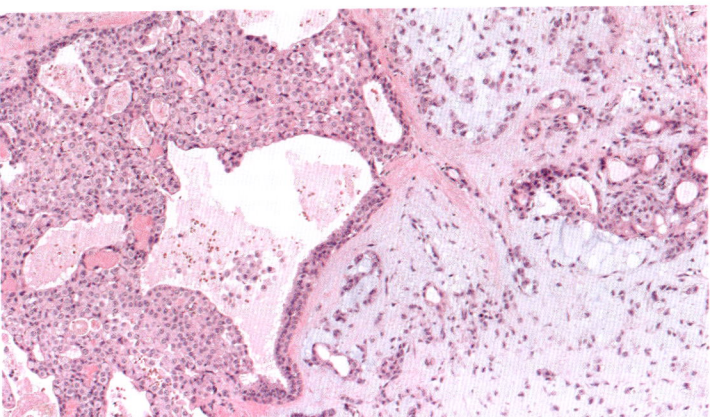

Figure 137.27 Apocrine mixed tumour. Notice the apocrine glands with a surrounding myxoid/hyalinised stroma.

hyaline or clear-cell change and collagenous spherulosis [2]. Ductal structures usually have a peripheral layer of flattened myoepithelial cells. Immunohistochemical studies reveal positivity for keratin and focal positivity for S100 and smooth muscle actin, confirming myoepithelial differentiation. Areas clearly indicative of apocrine (Figure 137.27) and follicular differentiation are often identified [5,6]. Tumours with follicular differentiation often show numerous keratocysts indicating infundibular differentiation. Staining with cytokeratin 20 may be helpful to identify Merkel cells which, when present, confirms follicular differentiation [7]. The stroma stains positively with Alcian blue, indicating the presence of chondroitin sulphate and hyaluronic acid. Focal calcification, mature fat and bone formation may also be seen [2,8]. From this description, it is clear that all the different cellular elements in mixed tumours including the epithelial, myoepithelial and stromal components may show a wide spectrum of differentiation and metaplastic changes that may make histological interpretation difficult and a potential source of pitfalls [2]. Tumours composed exclusively of myoepithelial cells are regarded as myoepitheliomas [9]. In some cases of mixed tumours, focal architectural and cytological atypia may be seen but this does not seem to imply a more aggressive behaviour [10].

Genetics
PLAG1 gene rearrangements have been shown in a subset of mixed tumours of the skin [11].

Clinical features
History and presentation [1]
This tumour is usually found on the head and neck, followed by the trunk and the extremities, as a solitary nodule. The lesions are frequently large and nodular, sometimes with a diameter of 5–10 cm.

Disease course and prognosis
The lesion is benign. Local recurrence is rarely seen. Malignant chondroid syringomas have been reported, including rare cases with metastasis [12–17,**18**,19,21].

Management
Local excision is recommended. If there is any suspicion of malignancy, wide excision and follow-up are required.

Cutaneous myoepithelioma

Definition and nomenclature
A tumour composed predominantly of myoepithelial cells. Myoepithelial tumours include mixed tumours of the skin, cutaneous myoepitheliomas and myoepithelial carcinomas.

> **Synonyms and inclusions**
> - Ectomesenchymal chondromyxoid tumour
> - Parachordoma

Epidemiology [1,2–4,5,6,7–9,10,11]
Incidence and prevalence
Myoepithelial tumours of the skin are uncommon.

Age
A wide age range is reported.

Sex
A male predominance is observed in cutaneous myoepitheliomas.

Pathophysiology
Pathology [1,2–4,5,6,7–9,10,11,12]
Cutaneous myoepitheliomas show a wide histological spectrum. Usually they are confined to the dermis. Overlying epidermal hyperplasia and/or a collarette can be observed. Syncytial cutaneous myoepithelioma, which is the most common variant, is a poorly circumscribed lesion composed of sheets of epithelioid or histiocytoid cells with bland nuclei and typically a small amount of intervening stroma. Focal areas of myxoid stroma or adipocytic differentiation may additionally be observed. Only a minority of cutaneous myoepitheliomas show the same appearances as their soft-tissue counterparts, with a lobulated architecture, a nested or trabecular pattern, a prominent myxoid stroma and a spindled, or plasmacytoid cytology. The presence of at least moderate to severe atypia is considered the only reliable criterion of malignancy. Cutaneous myoepitheliomas are immunoreactive for both S100 protein and EMA. Glial fibrillary acidic protein (GFAP) is also positive in the majority of cases. Calponin and smooth muscle antibody (SMA) may be positive. Keratin expression is usually absent although dot-like MNF116 positivity has been reported [12]. If positive, cutaneous tumours stain for AE1/AE3.

Genetics
A subset of cutaneous myoepitheliomas harbour an *EWSR1* gene rearrangement [10]. *PLAG1* gene rearrangement has also been reported recently in myoepitheliomas containing an important epithelial component [11].

Clinical features
History and presentation
Cutaneous myoepitheliomas usually present as a longstanding asymptomatic nodule in the extremities, although any site can be affected. Their size is usually small, ranging from 0.5 to 3 cm.

Disease course and prognosis
Local recurrence is observed in approximately 20% of cutaneous myoepitheliomas. Rarely, regional lymph node metastases have been reported but with no adverse clinical outcome. Conversely, carcinomas do show an aggressive clinical course with a high rate of metastatic disease and mortality.

Management
Complete excision is indicated.

SWEAT GLAND CARCINOMAS, INCLUDING DUCTAL APOCRINE/FOLLICULAR CARCINOMAS

These lesions can be divided into two broad groups. The first group represents the situation in which malignant change develops in a pre-existing, apparently benign lesion such as hidradenoma, mixed tumour, spiradenoma, cylindroma and eccrine poroma. The latter is the most commonly recorded example of such malignant progression [1,2]. In most adnexal tumours, with the exception of malignant eccrine poroma, the diagnosis usually requires identification of a benign component. Even when there is unmistakable cytological evidence of malignancy, the biological behaviour of malignant tumours of skin appendages is generally relatively benign, with local recurrence being much more common than cutaneous metastases.

The second group of carcinomas consists of lesions that develop as carcinomas *ab initio*. The primary eccrine carcinomas include microcystic adnexal carcinoma, adnexal carcinoma not otherwise specified (NOS), aggressive digital papillary adenocarcinoma, mucinous carcinoma and adenoid cystic carcinoma. Lymphoepithelioma-like carcinoma of the skin is also included in this group.

Eccrine gland carcinomas

Malignant eccrine poroma [1,2]

Definition and nomenclature
A malignant tumour arising from intraepidermal eccrine ducts. In up to 18% of cases, tumours arise from a pre-existing benign eccrine poroma [3].

> **Synonyms and inclusions**
> - Porocarcinoma

Epidemiology
Incidence and prevalence [4–7]
These are relatively common malignancies (0.01–0.005% of all cutaneous tumours).

Age
The lesion presents in older patients, with an average age at presentation of 73 years.

Sex
Females are more commonly affected than males.

Pathophysiology
Pathology [3,8,9,10]
Tumours show multiple connections to the epidermis, and a pre-existing benign eccrine poroma may be present. *In situ* lesions are seen occasionally [3,11]. The tumour infiltrates the dermis and the subcutaneous tissue in nests and lobules composed of relatively small cells that do not have a basaloid appearance. Peripheral palisading is absent. Ductal differentiation is necessary for the diagnosis to be made. This may be demonstrated by the use of immunohistochemical stains for carcinoembryonic antigen (CEA) and EMA. YAP1 loss and expression of NUT1 can be useful in the diagnosis of porocarcinoma [12]. A PAS stain may also be used, but this only highlights the ducts in very well-differentiated tumours forming ducts with a cuticle. Comedo necrosis is often present. Clear-cell change and squamous differentiation may be seen, and the latter may be prominent in some cases making it difficult to decide whether the tumour represents a squamous cell carcinoma with ductal differentiation or a porocarcinoma with squamous differentiation [13]. Sarcomatoid change may be seen in rare cases [14].

Poor prognostic factors are a large number of mitotic figures, lymphovascular invasion, tumour depth greater than 7 mm and an infiltrating rather than a pushing border [3].

Genetics
A large proportion of malignant poromas are characterised by YAP1-MAML2 and YAP1-NUTM1 fusions [15].

Clinical features
History and presentation
The lesion presents as an endoexophytic often ulcerated tumour, most often on the lower limbs (44% of cases). Tumours may attain a very large size and are frequently longstanding. A small number of patients present with multiple lesions and it is not clear whether this phenomenon represents epidermotropic metastasis or true multifocality [1,3,16]. An exceptional case has been reported arising in a scar [17], and a further metastatic lesion was associated with exposure to poison gas [18]. A neoplasm developed from a poroma in a child [19]. Pigmented variants may mimic melanoma [20].

Disease course and prognosis
Local recurrence is seen in 17% of cases. Regional lymph node metastases and systemic metastases occur in 19% and 11% of patients, respectively [3]. Two series, including a total of 93 cases, suggest that these lesions may have less metastatic capacity than thought previously [3,21]. In a smaller series of 12 cases, half displayed metastases to regional lymph nodes [22]. There is a mortality rate of 67% in patients with lymph node metastases. Distant metastases are rare [23].

Management
Wide excision and follow-up are required. Mohs micrographic surgery is useful in those cases with a prominent infiltrative growth pattern [24].

Squamoid eccrine ductal carcinoma [1,2,3]

Definition
A very malignant, rare but probably underreported neoplasm displaying dual differentiation, i.e. ductal eccrine and squamous.

Epidemiology
Incidence and prevalence
It is a rare neoplasm.

Age
Most patients are old.

Sex
There is predilection for males.

Pathophysiology
Pathology
Tumours are frequently connected to the epidermis and consist of nests and strands of variably atypical cells in a frequently desmoplastic stroma. Squamous differentiation is often seen in areas closer to the surface while ductal differentiation is more apparent in deep parts of the tumour. Mitotic activity is frequent and many tumours display perineural invasion.

Clinical features
Tumours present as a nodule or plaque.

Disease course and prognosis
Tumours have a tendency for local recurrence. Metastatic spread may be seen but appears to be low.

Management
Wide excision and follow-up are indicated.

Digital papillary adenocarcinoma

Definition and nomenclature
A rare tumour found on the hands and feet, with a high risk both of local recurrence and metastasis. Prior publications have described a benign, aggressive digital papillary adenoma and a carcinoma [1,2], but the lack of pathologically diagnostic or prognostic differentiating features suggests that all lesions in this category should be treated as carcinomas.

Synonyms and inclusions
- Aggressive digital papillary adenocarcinoma

Epidemiology
Incidence and prevalence
It is a rare tumour [3].

Age
The age range is wide with a mean age of 43 years. Few patients are less than 20 years old [3,4].

Sex
Both sexes are affected.

Pathophysiology
Pathology [1,2,5]
The lesions are obviously cystic on low-power microscopic examination and have papillary projections into the cystic cavities. Ductal and tubuloalveolar structures are also present. There may be focal necrosis and both nuclear hyperchromatism and a high mitotic count. In some cases, a tubular architecture tends to predominate and papillary projections may not be so prominent. Histological features do not allow accurate prediction of behaviour, as tumours with low-grade histology may metastasise [2]. Tumours may invade surrounding soft tissues and blood vessels and can destroy bone.

Genetics
Gene expression profiling studies point to *FGFR2* gene as a potential oncogenic driver [6].

Clinical features
History and presentation
The lesion presents as a non-diagnostic asymptomatic nodule on the fingers, toes, palms or soles. Delayed diagnosis is frequent [1,2,5,7]. Lesions may masquerade as either a fibrokeratoma [8] or paronychia [9].

Disease course and prognosis
There is a high recurrence rate, both locally and via metastatic spread [1,2,10,11]. Delayed occurrence of metastases and a protracted course despite metastatic disease has been noted in some patients [3].

Management
Wide local excision including amputation of the affected digit and long-term follow-up are recommended. It remains to be seen if Mohs surgery can play a successful role in the treatment of this tumour. Sentinel lymph node biopsy predicts systemic recurrence in digital papillary adenocarcinoma [11].

Eccrine or apocrine/follicular carcinomas

Malignant cylindroma [1,2,3,4,5]

Definition and nomenclature
A rare tumour which usually develops from a pre-existing benign dermal cylindroma.

Synonyms and inclusions
- Cylindroadenocarcinoma

Epidemiology
Incidence and prevalence
These are unusual tumours [6]. Fewer than 40 cases have been reported so far.

Age
It presents in the fifth to seventh decades [7].

Sex
No sex preference has been established although there seems to be a slight female predilection.

Pathophysiology

Genetics
Malignant cylindromas have been reported, mostly in familial cases of cylindromas [1,2,3,4] (see Cylindroma).

Pathology
These lesions have the characteristic architecture of a dermal cylindroma, with deeply basophilic small cells surrounded by an eosinophilic basement membrane [5,6,7,8]. In addition, however, there is marked nuclear atypia, irregularity of cell size and an infiltrative growth pattern. Mitotic figures, both normal and abnormal, are present. Exceptionally, a sarcomatous component may be seen [9].

Clinical features
History and presentation
These tumours develop as expanding nodules, usually on the scalp or very rarely in the external ear [10]. They may be suspected by expansion of a previously static dermal cylindroma or turban tumour.

Disease course and prognosis
It is locally aggressive and often metastasises [5].

Management
Wide local excision and follow-up are required.

Hidradenocarcinoma

Definition and nomenclature
A malignant tumour traditionally regarded as displaying eccrine differentiation and arising from a pre-existing hidradenoma.

Synonyms and inclusions
- Malignant hidradenoma
- Malignant acrospiroma

Epidemiology
Incidence and prevalence
It is very rare.

Age
They are commonest in older adults, but cases have been recorded in children [1–4].

Sex
No sex preference is established.

Pathophysiology
Pathology
Large clusters of glycogen-rich clear cells are present in some cases, but others may resemble basal cell carcinoma [5,6–9]. Focal necrosis may be present and the range of mitoses is highly variable. Squamous differentiation may be prominent [10]. Tumour cells are usually positive for EMA, CEA, S100, gross cystic disease fluid protein-15, the keratin cocktail AE1/AE3 and cytokeratin 5/6 [11]. Tumours may be eccrine or apocrine.

Genetics
Rarely hidradenocarcinomas show a t(11;19) translocation. More unusual is the amplification of the *Her2/neu* gene. There is also a low frequency of *TP53* mutations despite a high rate of p53 protein expression at the immunohistochemical level [11]. A single case of *MAML2* translocation similar to its benign counterpart has been described in hidradenocarcinoma [12].

Clinical features
History and presentation
These lesions are most often recorded as red ulcerated solitary nodules on the face, hands or feet.

Disease course and prognosis
The lesions may recur locally and/or metastasise. They may be very aggressive and pulmonary metastases have occurred. The prognosis is poor [13].

Management
Wide local excision is recommended. Mohs surgery has been used successfully for lesions on the foot [14]. Follow-up is essential [15]. Sentinel lymph node biopsy has been used exceptionally to demonstrate early metastatic disease [16]. In a case with lymph node metastases, amplification of the *Her2/neu* gene has been demonstrated [17]; based on this finding, the patient was treated with trastuzumab. The value of the adjuvant radiotherapy and chemotherapy has not been confirmed [18].

Spiradenocarcinoma [1]

Definition and nomenclature
A rare tumour, which usually arises in a pre-existing spiradenoma.

Synonyms and inclusions
- Malignant spiradenoma

Epidemiology
Incidence and prevalence
It is very rare.

Age
Presentation is usually in the seventh decade. An exceptional case in a child has been reported [2].

Sex
The sex distribution appears equal.

Pathophysiology

Genetics
TP53 mutations have been described, as well as mutations of the *ALPK1* kinase in a proportion of tumours [3,4].

Pathology [5,6,7]
These lesions usually show evidence of origin from a pre-existing benign spiradenoma. Necrosis, a high mitotic count, loss of the dual cell population, loss of infiltrating T lymphocytes and an infiltrative growth pattern are features that usually indicate malignant transformation.

Clinical features
History and presentation
Sudden expansion of a pre-existing nodule is the most likely presentation [1]. A study of 12 cases reports the commonest site as the trunk, with the limbs, head and neck less frequently involved [5].

Disease course and prognosis
Up to 20% of these tumours have been reported to metastasise [5,6–8]. However, tumours with low grade morphology seem to have an excellent prognosis [9].

Management
Excision and follow-up are required. There is little data on the effectiveness of Mohs surgery. Imaging for staging should be reserved for high grade tumours. Adjuvant chemoradiotherapy does not seem to alter survival [10].

Microcystic adnexal carcinoma

Synonyms and inclusions
- Sclerosing/syringomatous sweat duct carcinoma
- Malignant syringoma

Epidemiology [1,2,3,4]
Incidence and prevalence
This tumour is relatively rare.

Age
The age range is very wide, but young and middle-aged patients are more frequently affected.

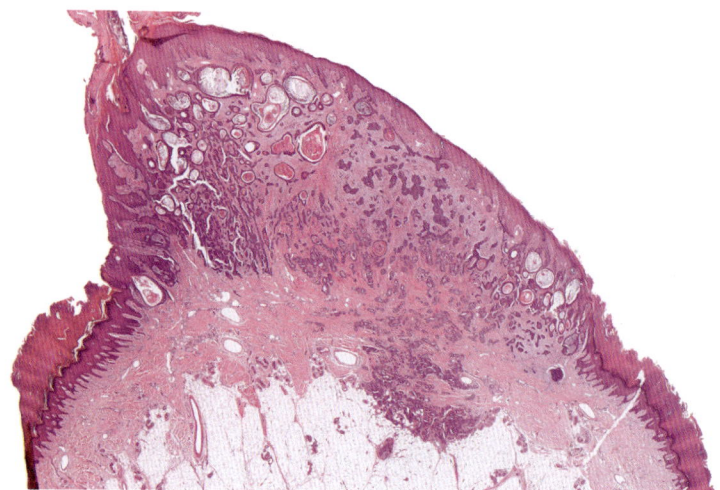

Figure 137.28 Microcystic adnexal carcinoma. Microcysts in the superficial part and nests/ductules with an infiltrative growth pattern in the deeper part of tumour.

Sex
It has an equal sex incidence.

Pathophysiology
Pathology [5,6]
The salient histological features are the presence of cords of cytologically banal epithelial cells with focal, variable ductal differentiation set in a very sclerotic desmoplastic stroma [2,3,4]. Horn cysts are seen in many cases, and pilar and sebaceous differentiation may also occur (Figure 137.28) [5,6–8]. Superficial areas show a resemblance to syringoma, desmoplastic trichoepithelioma and, in some cases, to infiltrative basal cell carcinoma. The diagnosis can therefore be impossible if only a small superficial biopsy is evaluated, as clues to the correct diagnosis reside in an infiltrative growth pattern and prominent perineural invasion. Even so, one should carefully examine the base of the specimen for any inconspicuous infiltrative growth in the form of small tubules or cords. Immunohistochemistry is of limited value as an aid in the histological diagnosis of microcystic adnexal carcinoma. Although it has been claimed that BerEP4 is consistently negative in microcystic adnexal carcinoma [9] and this may allow distinction from infiltrative basal cell carcinoma, which is consistently positive for this marker, this finding is contradicted by a more recent study in which 38% of microcystic adnexal carcinomas were positive for this marker [10]. In approximately 20% of cases that harbour *p53* mutations, expression of p53 protein is significantly higher than in syringomas and microcystic adnexal carcinomas unrelated to *p53* mutations [11]. Although desmoplastic trichoepithelioma and microcystic adnexal carcinoma may both show positivity for CK15 and BerEP4, it has been shown that CK15 tends to be negative in infiltrative basal cell carcinoma and this may be a useful marker in the histological differential diagnosis of both tumours [12].

Genetics
Next generation sequencing [11] has shown that microcystic adnexal carcinomas are molecularly heterogeneous tumours, with inactivated p53 or activated JAK/STAT signalling in a subset of cases (up to 40% in total).

Clinical features
History and presentation
The tumour has a predilection for the central area of the face, often as an inconspicuous, elevated or depressed sclerotic plaque or nodule in the upper lip area [1,2,3,4]. The trunk is also rarely involved. If the lesion is not promptly treated, or if local recurrence occurs, the lesions may present with pain or a burning sensation because of perineural spread. Cases have been reported both in patients with generalised immunosuppression and in sites of previous radiotherapy [13–15]. It has also rarely been reported arising within a naevus sebaceous [16]. Multiple tumours are exceptional [17].

Disease course and prognosis [18–20,21]
Morphologically high-grade transformation in microcytic adnexal carcinoma is a rare phenomenon that might not necessarily confer a risk for aggressive behavior. Metastatic spread is very rare, but extensive local recurrence can be a major problem. The rate of local recurrence is very high (up to 40%). Bone involvement is rarely seen. Tumours may rarely extend into the brain as a result of perineural invasion.

Management
The importance of this tumour is that perineural permeation is common, and for this reason microscopically controlled surgical excision is recommended. Mohs surgery or excision with complete circumferential peripheral and deep margin assessment has been recommended as the surgical approach of choice [22,23]. Radiotherapy can be considered as an adjuvant for microcystis adnexal carcinoma at high risk for recurrence, surgically unresectable tumours or patients who cannot have surgery for medical reasons [23].

Adnexal carcinoma NOS [1,2,3,4]

> **Synonyms and inclusions**
> - Sweat duct carcinoma
> - Syringoid eccrine carcinoma

Epidemiology
Incidence and prevalence
Freeman and Winkelmann, who considered it to be a basal cell tumour with eccrine differentiation [1,2], first described this rare tumour in 1969. However, the tumour does not represent a basal cell carcinoma with eccrine differentiation [3]. Some authors have proposed that it is part of the spectrum of microcystic adnexal carcinoma. Fewer than 50 cases [5] are currently reported in the world literature. The lesion has some resemblance to both benign syringoma and to dermal cylindroma. Syringoid eccrine carcinoma is the most accepted term in the literature.

Age
Most often affects the middle aged.

Sex
There is a female predilection.

Pathophysiology
Pathology
The tumour consists of cords and clusters of small dark-staining cuboidal basophilic cells set in a very dense stroma. The cells are cytologically abnormal with a high nuclear/cytoplasmic ratio and mitotic figures are seen. These features occur in the lower part of the dermis, extending into the subcutaneous fat. The islets of cells have a surrounding PAS-positive membrane. In addition to syringoma-like tadpole structures and glandular differentiation, these tumours can also exhibit squamoid and cribriform growth patterns [6]. The importance of adnexal carcinoma NOS lies in its similarity to adenocarcinoma metastatic to the skin.

Clinical features
History and presentation
Two-thirds of the cases so far reported have occurred on the scalp as large non-specific sometimes ulcerated nodules. They may be painful, due to their position in the deep dermis.

Disease course and prognosis
Adnexal adenocarcinoma NOS can recur and metastasise.

Management
Wide local excision is required. Follow-up is essential.

Mucinous carcinoma

Definition
A rare adnexal apocrine mucin-producing carcinoma arising on the head and neck area in more than 90% of the cases. This tumour is very similar to mucinous carcinoma of the breast [1].

Epidemiology [2–7]
Incidence and prevalence
This is a rare neoplasm.

Age
Most cases appear in the elderly. Occasional tumours develop in younger patients [7].

Sex
Males are affected more frequently than females.

Pathophysiology
Pathology
These lesions are relatively deeply situated and consist of clusters of cells with pink cytoplasm and some degree of cytological atypia. The central cells are paler and surrounded by darker staining cells arranged in a palisaded fashion. Broad fibrous septa run between these cytologically malignant cells and both cells and septae are separated by lakes of mucin (Figure 137.29) [8,9]. The mucin stains with diastase-resistant PAS, and acid Alcian blue (pH 2.5). Distinction from metastatic breast of gastrointestinal mucinous carcinoma is difficult. In many cases of primary cutaneous mucinous carcinoma, there is evidence of an *in situ* component in neighbouring glands and this confirms a tumour as primary arising in the skin [1,10]. Tumours presenting in the trunk often originate in the breast and those with dirty necrosis usually represent a metastasis from a gastrointestinal primary [1].

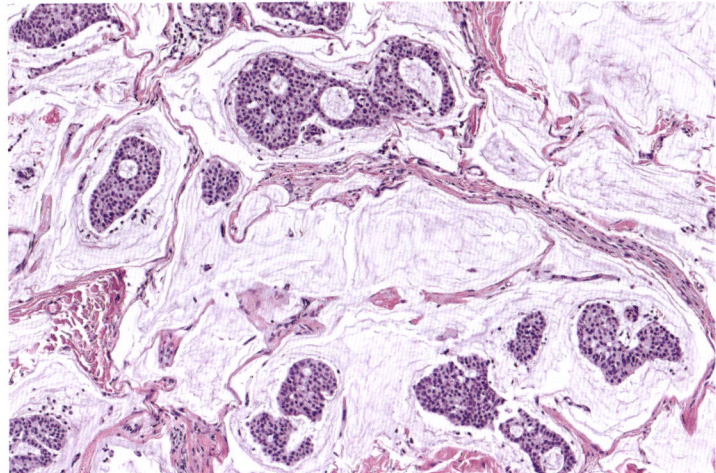

Figure 137.29 Mucinous carcinoma. Nests of tumour cells surrounded by pools of mucin.

Clinical features
History and presentation
The most frequently described clinical presentation is that of a grey nodule on the face often in the periorbital area [2–6]. Rarely tumours are bilateral [11]. An important clinical differential diagnosis is a cutaneous secondary deposit from a more common site for mucinous carcinoma such as the stomach and breast [12]. The distinction between a primary skin tumour and a metastasis is often very difficult and has to rely on some histological features (see later), clinicopathological correlation and additional studies to rule out an internal primary. In the case of a suspected metastatic mucinous breast carcinoma, staining for oestrogen and progesterone receptors is not useful, as primary cutaneous mucinous carcinomas are often positive for these markers [13].

Disease course and prognosis
Extensive metastatic spread and invasion of bone is very rare [14,15]. Local recurrence is often seen and the risk of metastatic spread to regional lymph nodes increases after a recurrence.

Management
Surgical excision, preferably with Mohs micrographic surgery, is recommended [16,17,18].

Endocrine mucin-producing sweat gland carcinoma
[1,2,3–6,7,8]

Definition
Endocrine mucin-producing sweat gland carcinoma is a rare low-grade sweat gland carcinoma that is believed to represent a precursor of mucinous carcinoma.

Epidemiology
Incidence and prevalence
It is rare. Up to date, around 150 cases have been described.

Age
More common in middle-age and elderly patients.

Sex
There is predilection for women.

Pathophysiology
Pathology [1,2,3–6,7,8]
Histologically, it is a well-circumscribed usually multinodular tumour with solid or cystic nodules which display more often papillary and sometimes cribriform structures composed of uniform small slightly atypical epithelial cells with lightly eosinophilic to bluish cytoplasm, stippled chromatin and inconspicuous nucleoli. Intracytoplasmic and extracellular mucin is usually present. Mitotic activity tends to be low. Immunohistochemically at least one neuroendocrine marker (synaptophysin or chromogranin) is expressed as well as other non-specific markers of neuroendocrine differentiation such as CD57 and neuron-specific enolase. The tumour is positive in epithelial markers such as low molecular cytokeratin, epithelial membrane antigen and cytokeratin 7 but usually negative for cytokeratin 20. There is expression of oestrogen and progesterone receptors. S100 protein is negative. Immunohistochemical stains for p63 or other myoepithelial markers may highlight areas of *in situ* carcinoma enabling the differential diagnosis from a metastatic tumour.

Clinical features
History and presentation
The tumour usually presents as a slowly growing cyst or nodule located on the lower and less often on the upper eyelid. Lesions on the cheek have exceptionally been reported [2]. Clinically, the lesion may mimic a cyst, a basal cell carcinoma or a chalazion.

Disease course and prognosis
It is a low-grade carcinoma with only rare local recurrences and no metastasis reported so far [9].

Management
Complete excision and close follow-up is recommended.

Adenoid cystic carcinoma [1–4]

Definition and nomenclature
This is a particularly rare variant of adnexal carcinoma, which has only been recognised as an entity since 1975. Adenoid cystic carcinomas arise relatively frequently from salivary glands and direct spread or even metastasis from this site should be ruled out before the diagnosis of primary cutaneous adenoid cystic carcinoma is made [4].

> **Synonyms and inclusions**
> - Primary cutaneous adenocystic carcinoma

Epidemiology [5,6,7,8,9]
Incidence and prevalence
The tumour is very rare.

Age
It usually appears in middle-aged to old individuals.

Sex
Males are equally affected than females.

Pathophysiology
Pathology [6,10–12]
The pathology is that of large masses of cells with mild or no cytological atypia, arranged in a distinct adenoid or cribriform pattern. The cystic spaces are occupied by mucin, which stains with Alcian blue (pH 2.5). The lesion usually involves the mid to deep dermis and may extend into the subcutaneous tissue. A more solid variant may be seen occasionally. Many of these tumours show at least focal evidence of myoepithelial differentiation. Perineural invasion is frequently seen but is less common than in primary adenoid cystic carcinomas presenting in salivary glands [6]. Diffuse expression of MYB is present in a majority of cases, regardless of *MYB* alterations [13].

Genetics
MYB translocations have been found in about half of cases, in both myoepithelial and ductoglandular cells [14].

Clinical features
History and presentation [1,2]
These lesions are non-specific sometimes painful nodules on the head and neck area. The pain is attributed to perineural spread although this symptom is rare. Rarely, tumours develop elsewhere in the skin including the scrotum [3]. Patients with adenoid cystic carcinoma have a higher risk of developing lymphohaematopoietic and thyroid cancers [9].

Disease course and prognosis
Five-year survival is up to 96% [9]. Local recurrence is common and metastasis to the lung and regional lymph nodes has rarely been reported [9,15–18]. Metastatic spread to the lungs has also been reported, rarely many years after removal of the primary cutaneous tumour [19]. Erosion of bone at the primary site has also been recorded.

Management
The management of these lesions is by wide local excision and Mohs surgery is a good treatment option [20].

Secretory carcinoma [1,2–5,6,7–9]

Definition and nomenclature
Cutaneous secretory carcinoma is the morphological and genetic analogue of secretory carcinoma encountered in the breast and the salivary glands.

Synonyms and inclusions
- Primary cutaneous mammary analogue secretory carcinoma
- Mammary-type secretory carcinoma of the skin

Epidemiology [6,7]
Incidence and prevalence
The tumour is very rare.

Age
It is encountered mostly in the young and in middle age, but there is a wide age span.

Sex
There is a slight female predominance.

Pathophysiology
Pathology [2,6,7]
The cutaneous tumours are characterised by low grade histology. They are typically well circumscribed but not surrounded by capsule. There are microcystic and tubular spaces with characteristic eosinophilic luminal secretions. The cells lining the lumina are oval, round or cuboidal, and bland in appearance. Solid areas, and focal pseudopapillary or mucinous foci can be seen.

Genetics
Similarly to its breast and salivary gland counterparts, most of secretory carcinomas are characterised by a t(12;15)(p13;q25) translocation, resulting in an *ETV6-NTRK3* fusion [3,6,7].

Clinical features
History and presentation [1,2,4,5]
The cases are typically encountered in locations rich with apocrine glands, such as the axillae, eyelids, head and neck and the vulva [5].

Disease course and prognosis
The cutaneous tumours reported so far have followed an indolent course, without recurrence or metastasis. A small proportion of breast tumours, however, have shown distant metastatic potential [8].

Management
The management of these lesions is by local excision with negative margins. Even though metastatic disease has not been reported in cutaneous tumours so far, an excellent response to NTRK inhibitor therapy has been described in a metastatic breast secretory carcinoma case [9].

MISCELLANEOUS TUMOURS

Tumours of ano-genital mammary-like glands

For many years, it was assumed that a number of female genital tumours with features identical to those arising in the breast

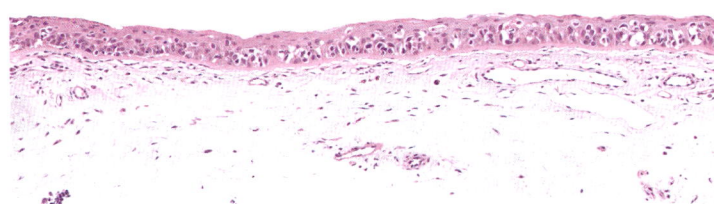

Figure 137.30 Pathology of Paget disease: note colonisation of the epidermis with large pleomorphic cells.

were derived from ectopic mammary gland tissue along the milk lines. Van der Putte, however, has proposed that this theory is not accurate as primordia of mammary glands do not extend beyond the axillary–pectoralis area [1]. His proposal is that there is a group of distinctive mammary-like genital glands that share features with true mammary glands and eccrine and apocrine glands and from which most genital glandular neoplasms arise [1,2]. The latter include hidrocystoma, hidradenoma papilliferum, extramammary Paget disease and tumours identical to those arising in breast tissue including fibroadenoma, cystosarcoma phylloides and adenocarcinoma [3–7].

Paget disease of the nipple [1]

Definition
A progressive, marginated, scaling or crusting of the nipple and areola due to invasion of the epidermis by malignant cells, which usually but not always originate from an intraductal carcinoma of the breast. There is a strong current view that Paget disease arises from apocrine duct-derived epithelial cells.

Epidemiology
Incidence and prevalence [2]
Paget disease of the nipple is an uncommon occurrence, considering the frequency of breast cancer [3,4]. In one series, it occurred in fewer than 3% of breast cancers. Published cases suggest that the disease is more common in Anglo-Saxon countries. Although the incidence of breast cancer is increasing, the incidence of Paget disease has decreased by 45% in the USA in the last decades [5]. Equally, the incidence of Paget disease associated with underlying invasive cancer of ductal carcinoma *in situ* has also decreased [5].

Age
It is rare before the fourth decade and is most frequent in the fifth and sixth.

Sex
It occurs chiefly in women, although rare cases have been recorded in men [6].

Pathophysiology
Pathology [7–9]
The epidermis is thickened, with papillomatosis, enlargement of the interpapillary ridges and hyperkeratosis or parakeratosis on the

surface (Figure 137.30). Within the epidermis, characteristic Paget cells are dispersed between the prickle cells. They vary in number and when profuse the Malpighian layers may be disrupted and the surface covered by a crust. There is a chronic inflammatory reaction in the upper dermis. In the later stages, the epidermis may be atrophic or eroded. On scanning microscopy, the differential diagnosis may include superficial spreading malignant melanoma. The Paget cells have a clear abundant cytoplasm and do not establish intercellular bridges with the adjacent normal keratinocytes. Both the cells and their nuclei are rounded; the nuclei are vesicular or hyperchromatic with a high nuclear/cytoplasmic ratio. The cytoplasm is PAS positive and diastase resistant, which indicates the presence of neutral polysaccharides and supports the glandular origin of the cells [10]. Staining with antibodies to CEA is also positive [11,12]. As many as 90% of cases are positive for HER2. Androgen receptor expression is present in most cases, while oestrogen and progesterone receptor expression is present in a much smaller contingent of cases (10–30%) [13]. The cells are distributed singly among the prickle cells, or in clusters in a pattern similar to that seen in superficial spreading melanoma. The Paget cells may also be seen in appendage ducts, so that it can be impossible to determine if these cells are migrating from these ducts to the epidermis or invading downwards into the ducts from the epidermis. An underlying breast carcinoma, if present, is not always seen on biopsy, as it may be deeply set. Careful examination of the underlying breast specimen may show an intraduct carcinoma, sometimes of quite small dimensions, usually situated most distally, but sometimes in the terminal ducts, and often appearing to spread between the two layers of epithelial cells of the duct. The cells may accumulate within and distend the ducts and spread in both directions. A number of ducts are usually involved. At a later stage, the carcinoma becomes invasive and behaves like classic breast carcinoma.

The main pathological challenge is to distinguish Paget disease from malignant melanoma, the latter exceptionally presenting in the nipple [14,15]. Paget disease cells will be CEA positive, EMA positive and Cam 5.2 positive, while those of melanoma will be positive for melanocytic markers [14,15]. Positivity to antibody to S100 protein is not useful, as although it is positive in the great majority of melanomas, this is also the case in a proportion of cases of Paget disease. The absence of melanophages and the presence of neutral mucopolysaccharides (PAS positive) in tumour cells are also helpful.

The histogenesis of Paget disease is still unclear. The current view is that the majority of cases of Paget disease arise from either invasive or *in situ* ductal carcinoma in the deeper breast tissue. In a minority of cases no underlying *in situ* or invasive carcinoma is found [16].

Genetics
NY-BR-1 expression or loss of *pRb* expression has been described in Paget disease. Overexpression of *ras* p21 has been demonstrated in mammary and extramammary Paget disease [17,18].

Clinical features
History and presentation [18,19]
The early changes may be minimal, with a small, crusted and intermittently moist area on the nipple giving a brownish stain on

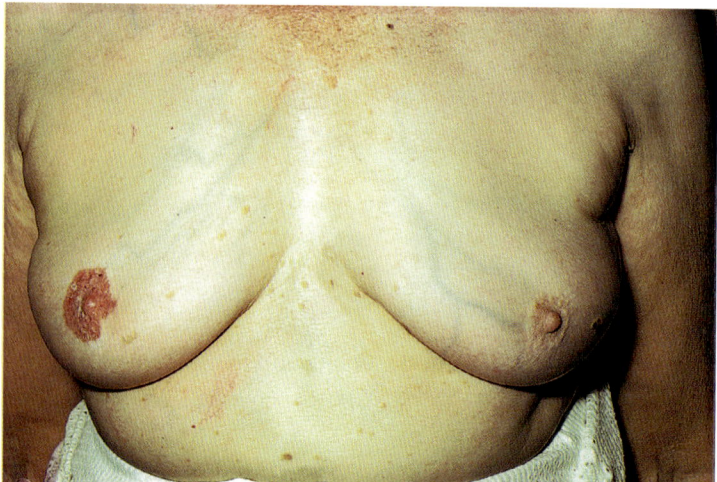

Figure 137.31 Paget disease of the nipple. Distant clinical view showing unilateral lesion.

clothing, or producing itching, pricking or burning sensations. Less often, there is a serous or blood-stained discharge from the nipple, or a lump may be noticed in the breast (Figure 137.31). The surface changes persist and gradually spread to produce an eczematous appearance. The nipple, areola and, at a later stage, skin of the breast are red and moist or crusted (Figure 137.32). The change is sharply marginated and may spare a segment of the areola. The edge is slightly raised and irregular in outline. If the crusts are removed, a red, glazed, moist or vegetating surface is revealed. Itching may be a prominent symptom and excoriations may be found in the established lesion. Some areas may be ulcerated. The nipple itself may be retracted, and a subjacent mass or a lump deeper in the breast may be felt. The regional glands should be examined; they are rarely enlarged when a mass cannot be felt but are enlarged in more than half the cases with a detectable tumour. It is exceptionally bilateral [20]. The change may occasionally involve not only the skin of the breast but also spread on to the chest wall. An exceptional case has been recorded in which the patient presented with ipsilateral eruptive seborrhoeic keratoses of the nipple and areola (Leser–Trélat sign) [21].

The principal differential diagnosis is eczema of the nipple. This is frequently bilateral and runs a more fluctuating course, improving in response to local treatment and spreading rapidly when irritated. Eczema lacks the sharp, raised and rounded margin and the superficial induration of Paget disease. In doubtful cases, biopsy will be required. Bowen disease and superficial basal cell carcinoma may also produce a similar clinical picture. They are both very uncommon on the nipple and can be differentiated histologically. Psoriasis and erosive adenomatosis of the nipple may also need to be considered in the clinical differential diagnosis, and again a biopsy to obtain pathology will clarify the situation.

Disease course and prognosis
The rate of spread of the skin changes is slow and patients often wait a year or more before seeking advice. Poor prognosis is associated with invasive disease and the presence of a palpable mass [22].

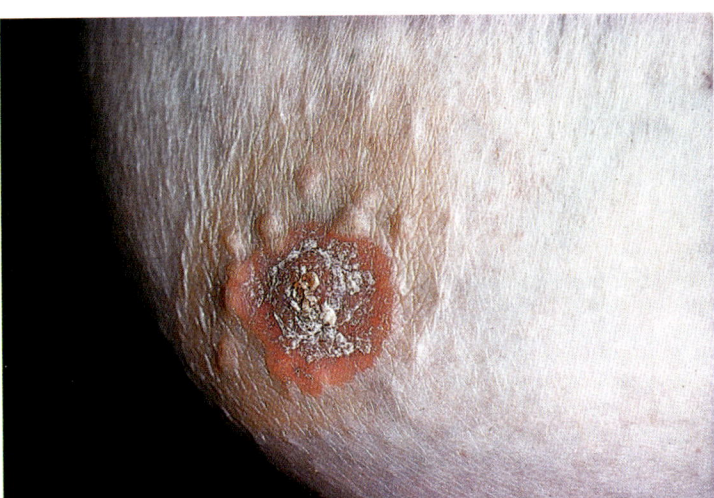

Figure 137.32 Paget disease of the nipple. Close-up view showing redness and well-marked lateral edge of the lesion.

Management [23]

All patients should have a mammogram or ultrasound to establish whether or not there is deeper pathology in the underlying breast, as this will help determine the extent of surgery required. Surgery should be carried out as for carcinoma of the breast. In patients with no evidence of an underlying breast carcinoma, conservation may be a realistic option [24,25]. Some studies have confirmed this, recommending breast conserving therapy with or without radiotherapy according to the presence or absence of an invasive component as the treatment of choice [26]. Sentinel lymph node biopsy is performed in cases with an invasive component [19]. Surgery should always include the whole of the nipple–areolar complex [19].

Extramammary Paget disease [1]

(Chapter 110)

Definition

A marginated plaque resembling Paget disease clinically and histologically, but occurring in sites rich in apocrine glands, such as the vulva, ano-genital region and axilla. There is currently controversy as to how often this condition arises on the background of an underlying carcinoma and how often it arises primarily in the epidermis or apocrine ductal tissue of the affected area. This has given rise to the concept of primary and secondary extramammary Paget disease (EMPD) [2].

Epidemiology

Incidence and prevalence

This is a rare disease. The current view is that in about 75% of cases, extramammary Paget disease arises as a primary intraepidermal neoplasm, possibly from apocrine gland ductal cells or from keratinocyte stem cells. It has also been suggested that the disease may originate from Toker cells [3], while some findings suggest that rare cases of primary EMPD may originate in ano-ngenital mammary-like glands [4]. In the remaining 25% of cases, an underlying primary adenocarcinoma is found. These cases are referred to as secondary Paget disease.

Age

It starts usually in the fifth decade or after.

Sex

It occurs more frequently in women.

Pathophysiology
Pathology

The changes in the epidermis are essentially similar to Paget disease. The cells stain positively for acid as well as neutral mucopolysaccharides. They may contain melanin granules. Immunohistochemistry shows cells positive for CEA and Cam-5.2 and other low-molecular-weight keratins such as CK7 and CK8/18 [5]. GCDFP-15 is a marker of apocrine epithelium [6] and is frequently strongly expressed in primary vulval or perianal Paget disease with no detectable underlying malignancy. Cytokeratin 20 is usually negative in primary cases and tends to be positive in lesions associated with an internal gastrointestinal tumour. Cases of intraepidermal vulval and penile and scrotal EMPD usually have a phenotype that is MUC1 positive, MUC2 negative and MUC5AC positive. In contrast, mammary Paget disease is usually negative for the latter marker and perianal lesions associated with underlying rectal adenocarcinoma are positive for MUC2 and only variably positive for MUC1 and MUC5AC. Vulval lesions with underlying apocrine carcinoma tend to be negative for MUC5AC.

Genetics

EMPD is characterised by alterations involving the *PI3K-AKT* pathway [7].

Clinical features
History and presentation

The lesion has many features in common with Paget disease of the nipple. The margin is sharp, rounded and slightly raised, and encloses an area that is pink or red. The surface may be scaly and small greyish crusts may cover erosions. Itching is a prominent feature and there may be excoriations or lichenification. Variable hyperpigmentation may be present, adding to the pathological confusion between EMPD and superficial spreading melanoma. In a proportion of cases, there may be leukoplakia.

The appearance varies somewhat according to the site. The commonest area involved is the vulva [8–10] (Figure 137.33), followed by the perianal area, which is more frequently affected in men than women, the scrotum, penis and axilla [11,12]. The first symptom, especially in vulval lesions, is itching and burning, which may be persistent and spread. Quite often it is regarded as eczema and may be irritated by topical therapy. The mucosal surfaces of the labia are frequently a rather more vivid red than the skin when both areas are involved and the change may spread to the thighs, mons pubis and into the vaginal introitus. There may occasionally be a papillomatous surface. Perianal lesions may extend up into the anal canal. Lesions on the scrotum spread to the thigh or onto the shaft of the penis. Very occasionally, EMPD may be present

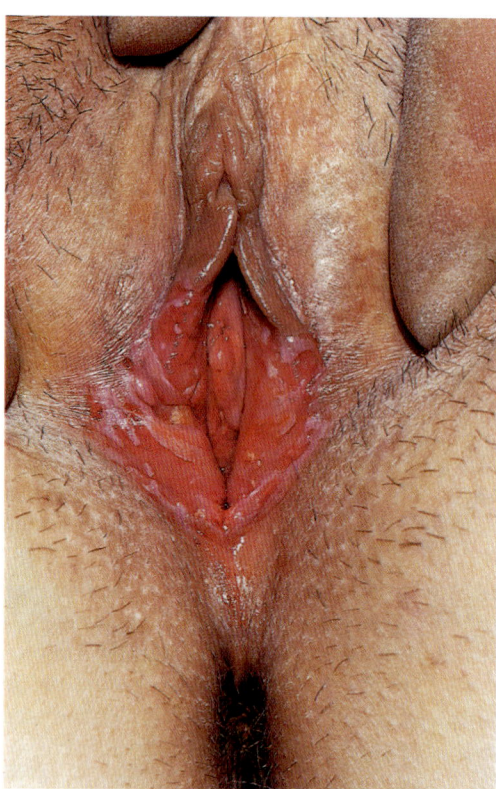

Figure 137.33 Extramammary Paget disease of the vulva showing inflamed eczematous presentation.

on the eyelids or ears. Characteristic clinical features include the relentless progression, despite all local applications, and the sharp margin. Eventually, one area may become thickened and ulcerated as evidence of invasion downwards. Lymph node or distant metastases can occur. Although most of the cases in which a primary carcinoma is found result from an underlying sweat gland adenocarcinoma, it is necessary to examine the patient for evidence of an adenocarcinoma elsewhere, particularly of the cervix and rectum. The differential diagnosis from eczema, intertrigo and pruritus vulvae is made by the steady spread, lack of response to topical anti-inflammatory agents and the sharp and extending margin. Bowen disease is usually more raised and verrucous, and superficial basal cell carcinoma has a thread-like margin. It may be difficult to differentiate leukoplakia or Bowen disease of the mucosal surfaces and a biopsy may be required. As with mammary Paget disease, superficial spreading melanoma is an important pathological differential diagnosis.

Disease course and prognosis

Local recurrence is common, even in cases with a wider excision [13]. Poor prognosis is associated with depth of invasion and with elevated serum levels of CEA [14].

Management

Adequate tissue sampling and other investigations are essential to establish whether or not there is an associated underlying malignancy requiring surgical excision. If an underlying malignancy is present, it should be excised together with all clinically abnormal epithelium. If no underlying malignancy is detected on careful examination, the entire affected area of epithelium should be excised. Mohs surgery with careful control of excision margins may be useful, because a common cause of recurrence is inadequate excision of the lesion [15,16,**17**].

Promising results are reported with photodynamic therapy, but larger series and longer periods of follow-up are required [18–20]. In cases with limited disease, the use of topical imiquimod has been advocated with good results [21,**22**]. Radiotherapy has been advocated either as an adjunct to surgical therapy [23] or as an alternative therapy for elderly patients in whom surgery may be difficult [24,**25**].

Lymphoepithelioma-like carcinoma

Definition

Lymphoepitheliomas are well-recognised tumours of the nasopharynx and an entity with similar histological features has also been observed in the skin [1]. However, the latter is not generally associated with Epstein–Barr virus (EBV) infection and its behaviour appears to be less aggressive than that of upper respiratory tract lesions [2,3]. Association with other viruses including HPV and simian virus 40 has not been found either [4].

Epidemiology [5]
Incidence and prevalence
It is a very rare tumour.

Age
It mainly affects older individuals.

Sex
There is an equal sex distribution.

Pathophysiology
Pathology
The pathological features are those of a very dense infiltrate of inflammatory mononuclear cells, including lymphocytes and histiocytes, with small strands and nests of atypical epithelial cells. Inflammatory cells extensively infiltrate nests and strands of tumour cells, and the epithelial nature of these cells is often not immediately apparent unless more or less intact nests of epithelial cells are found. Confusion with a lymphoma is therefore a possibility, and often immunostaining for keratin and lymphoid cells is necessary to distinguish the two populations of cells. A case associated with marginal zone lymphoma has been described [6]. Cytological atypia is usually present and mitotic figures are common. Focal evidence of adnexal differentiation and even neuroendocrine differentiation may be seen [7–12]. Some tumours appear to be arising from a squamous cell carcinoma. A sarcomatoid component may be seen [13]. It has therefore been suggested that this is not a distinctive entity but a morphological pattern in various cutaneous carcinomas [14]. It has been suggested that it represents a variant of poorly differentiated squamous cell carcinoma. A case associated with EBV has been documented [15].

Clinical features
History and presentation
The clinical appearance is of non-specific nodules on the head and neck area of older patients. Occasional cases present on the eyelid [16] and the trunk and vulva [17] are also rarely involved.

Disease course and prognosis
The lesion has a low malignant potential [18] but local recurrence and distant metastases, with one tumour-associated death, have been recorded [8,10,**19**].

Management
Surgery followed by radiotherapy is recommended. Some cases have been treated by Mohs surgery [**20**].

Key references

The full list of references can be found in the online version at https://www.wiley.com/rooksdermatology10e

Introduction
6 McCalmont TH. A call for logic in the classification of adnexal neoplasms. *Am J Dermatopathol* 1996;18:104–9.

Hair follicle tumours
1 Ackermann AB. *Neoplasms with Follicular Differentiation.* New York: Lea & Febiger, 1993.
8 Kajino Y, Yamaguchi A, Hashimoto N et al. Beta catenin gene mutation in human hair follicle related tumours. *Path Int* 2001;51:543–8.

Inverted follicular keratosis
4 Sim-Davis D, Marks R, Wilson Jones E. The inverted follicular keratosis: a surprising variant of seborrheic wart. *Acta Derm Venereol* 1976;56:337–44.
5 Armengot-Carbo M, Abrego A, Gonzalez T et al. Inverted follicular keratosis: dermoscopic and reflectance confocal microscopic features. *Dermatology* 2013;227:62–6.

Dilated pore
1 Winer L. The dilated pore, a trichoepithelioma. *J Invest Dermatol* 1954;23:181–8.
6 Moreira A, Menezes N, Guedes R et al. Dermoscopy of a dilated pore of Winer. *Eur J Dermatol* 2010;20:229.

Tumour of the follicular infundibulum
1 Cribier B, Grosshans E. Tumours of the follicular infundibulum: a clinicopathological study. *J Am Acad Dermatol* 1995;33:979–84.
6 Mahalingam M, Bhawan J, Finn R et al. Tumor of the follicular infundibulum with sebaceous differentiation. *J Cutan Pathol* 2001;28:314–17.

Pilar sheath acanthoma
1 Mehregan AH, Brownstein MH. Pilar sheath acanthoma. *Arch Dermatol* 1978;114:1495–7.

Trichoadenoma
1 Rahbari H, Mehregan AM, Pinkus H. Trichoadenoma of Nikolowski. *J Cutan Pathol* 1977;4:90–8.
6 Shimanovich I, Krahl D, Rose C. Trichoadenoma of Nikolowski is a distinct neoplasm within the spectrum of follicular tumors. *J Am Acad Dermatol* 2010;62:277–83.

Comedo naevus
2 Levinsohn JL, Sugarman JL; Yale Center for Mendelian Genomics et al. Somatic mutations in NEK9 cause nevus comedonicus. *Am J Hum Genet* 2016;98:1030–7.
8 Torchia D. Nevus comedonicus syndrome: a systematic review of the literature. *Pediatr Dermatol* 2021;38:359–63.

External root sheath tumours
Proliferating trichilemmal tumour
1 Wilson-Jones E. Proliferating epidermoid cysts. *Arch Dermatol* 1966;94:11–19.
3 Miyachi H, Togawa Y, Yamamoto Y et al. Proliferating trichilemmal tumour: a comparison of dermoscopic, ultrasonographic and histopathological features. *Eur J Dermatol* 2016;26:400–2.
11 Folpe AL, Reisenauer AK, Mentzel T et al. Proliferating trichilemmal tumors: clinicopathologic evaluation is a guide to biologic behavior. *J Cutan Pathol* 2003;30:492–8.

Trichilemmoma
1 Brownstein MH, Shapiro L. Trichilemmoma. *Arch Dermatol* 1973;107:866–9.
8 Brownstein MH, Mehregan AH, Bikowski B et al. The dermatopathology of Cowden's syndrome. *Br J Dermatol* 1979;100:667–73.
11 Starink TM, Hausman R. The cutaneous pathology of extrafacial lesions in Cowden's disease. *J Cutan Pathol* 1984;11:338–44.
18 Hunt SJ, Kilzer B, Santa Cruz DJ. Desmoplastic trichilemmoma: histologic variant resembling invasive carcinoma. *J Cutan Pathol* 1990;17:45–52.
20 Liew D, Marsh DJ, Li J et al. Germline mutations of the PTEN gene in Cowden's disease. *Nat Genet* 1997;16:64–7.
24 Al-Zaid T, Ditelberg JS, Prieto VG et al. Trichilemmomas show loss of PTEN in Cowden syndrome but only rarely in sporadic tumors. *J Cutan Pathol* 2012;39:493–9.

Trichilemmal carcinoma
2 Wong TY, Suster S. Tricholemmal carcinoma. *Am J Dermatopathol* 1994;16:463–73.
4 Reis JP, Tellechea O, Unha MF et al. Trichilemmal carcinoma: a study of seven cases. *J Cutan Pathol* 1993;20:44–9.

Hamartomas and hair germ tumours and cysts
Hair follicle naevus
2 Labandeira J, Peteiro C, Toribio J. Hair follicle naevus: case report and review. *Am J Dermatopathol* 1996;18:90–3.
3 Komura A, Tani M. Hair follicle nevus. *Dermatology* 1992;185:154–5.

Eruptive vellus hair cyst
1 Takeshita T, Takeshita H, Irie K. Eruptive vellus hair cyst and epidermoid cyst in a patient with pachonychia congenita. *J Dermatol* 2000;27:655–7.
7 Kiene P, Hauschild A, Christopher E. Eruptive vellus hair cysts and steatocystoma multiplex variants of one entity? *Dermatology* 1996;134:365–7.
10 Rodgers SA, Kitagawa K, Selim MA et al. Familial eruptive vellus hair cysts. *Pediatr Dermatol* 2012;29:367–9.
24 Coras B, Hohenleutner U, Landthaler M et al. Early recurrence of eruptive vellus cysts after Er:YAG laser therapy: case report and review of the literature. *Dermatol Surg* 2005;31:1741–4.

Trichofolliculoma
1 Gray HR, Helwig EB. Trichofolliculoma. *Arch Dermatol* 1962;86:619–25.
11 Wu YH. Folliculosebaceous cystic hamartoma or trichofolliculoma? A spectrum of hamartomatous changes inducted by perifollicular stroma in the follicular epithelium. *J Cutan Pathol* 2008;35:843–8.
14 Kan L, Liu Y, Kessler JA. Inhibition of BMP signaling in P-Cadherin positive hair progenitor cells leads to trichofolliculoma-like hair follicle neoplasias. *J Biomed Sci* 2011;18:92.
16 Romero-Pérez D, García-Bustinduy M, Cribier B. Clinicopathologic study of 90 cases of trichofolliculoma. *J Eur Acad Dermatol Venereol* 2017;31:e141–e142.

Trichoepithelioma
3 Bettencourt MS, Prieto VG, Shea R. Trichoepithelioma: a 19-year clinicopathologic re-evaluation. *J Cutan Pathol* 1999;26:398–404.
4 Harada H, Hashimoto K, Ko MS. The gene for multiple familial trichoepithelioma maps to chromosome 9p21. *J Invest Dermatol* 1996;107:41–3.
6 Clarke J, Ioffreda M, Helm KE. Multiple familial trichoepitheliomas: a folliculosebaceous-apocrine genodermatosis. *Am J Dermatopathol* 2002;24:402–5.

10 Ponti G, Nasti S, Losi L *et al.* Brooke–Spiegler syndrome: report of two cases not associated with a mutation in the CYLD and PTCH tumor-suppressor genes. *J Cutan Pathol* 2012;39:366–71.
20 Retamar RA, Stengel F, Saadi ME *et al.* Brooke–Spiegler syndrome – report of four families: treatment with CO_2 laser. *Int J Dermatol* 2007;46:583–6.
21 Baur V, Papadopoulos T, Kazakov DV *et al.* A case of multiple familial trichoepitheliomas responding to treatment with the Hedgehog signaling pathway inhibitor vismodegib. *Virchows Arch* 2018;473:241–6.

Desmoplastic trichoepithelioma
1 Brownstein MH, Shapiro L. Desmoplastic trichoepithelioma. *Cancer* 1977; 40:2979–86.
4 Jedrych J, Leffell D, McNiff JM. Desmoplastic trichoepithelioma with perineural involvement: a series of seven cases. *J Cutan Pathol* 2012;39:317–23.
12 Khelifa E, Masouyé I, Kaya G *et al.* Dermoscopy of desmoplastic trichoepithelioma reveals other criteria to distinguish it from basal cell carcinoma. *Dermatology* 2013;226:101–4.

Trichoblastoma
2 Wong TY, Reed JA, Suster S. Benign trichogenic tumours: a report of two cases supporting a simplified nomenclature. *Histopathology* 1993;22:575–80.
4 Altman DA, Mikhail GR, Johnson TM *et al.* Trichoblastic fibroma. *Arch Dermatol* 1995;131:198–201.
21 Idriss MH, Elston DM. Secondary neoplasms associated with nevus sebaceus of Jadassohn: a study of 707 cases. *J Am Acad Dermatol* 2014;70:332–7.

Adamantinoid trichoblastoma
1 Santa Cruz DJ, Barr RJ, Headington JT. Cutaneous lymphadenoma. *Am J Surg Pathol* 1991;15:101–10.
4 Díaz-Cascajo C, Borghi S, Rey López A *et al.* Cutaneous lymphadenoma: a peculiar variant of nodular trichoblastoma. *Am J Dermatopathol* 1996;18:186–92.

Basaloid follicular hamartoma
2 Brownstein MH. Basaloid follicular hamartoma: solitary and multiple types. *J Am Acad Dermatol* 1992;22:237–40.
3 Walsh N, Ackerman AB. Basaloid follicular hamartoma. *J Am Acad Dermatol* 1993;29:125–7.
8 Wheeler CE, Carroll MA, Groben PA *et al.* Autosomal dominantly inherited generalized basaloid follicular hamartoma syndrome: report of a new disease in a North Carolina family. *J Am Acad Dermatol* 2000;43:189–206.

Hair matrix tumours
Pilomatricoma
1 Forbis R Jr, Helwig EB. Pilomatrixoma (calcifying epithelioma). *Arch Dermatol* 1961;83:606–18.
6 Chiaramonti A, Gilgor RS. Pilomatricomas associated with myotonic dystrophy. *Arch Dermatol* 1978;114:1363–5.
8 Handler MZ, Derrick KM, Lutz RE *et al.* Prevalence of pilomatricoma in Turner syndrome: findings from a multicenter study. *JAMA Dermatol* 2013;149:559–64.
14 Kaddu S, Soyer HP, Hodl S *et al.* Morphological stages of pilomatricoma. *Am J Dermatopathol* 1996;18:333–8.
27 Durand M, Moles JP. Beta catenin mutations in a common skin cancer: pilomatricoma. *Bull Cancer* 1999;86:725–6.
28 Park SW, Suh KS, Wang HY *et al.* Beta catenin expression in the transitional zone of pilomatricoma. *Br J Dermatol* 2001;145:624–9.
33 Julian CG, Bowers PW. A clinical review of 209 pilomatricomas. *J Am Acad Dermatol* 1998;39:191–5.

Pilomatrical carcinoma
5 Hardisson D, Linares MD, Cuevas-Santos J *et al.* Pilomatrix carcinoma: a clinicopathologic study of six cases and review of the literature. *Am J Dermatopathol* 2001;23:394–401.
8 Lazar AJ, Calonje E, Grayson W *et al.* Pilomatrix carcinoma contain mutations in CTNNB1, the gene encoding beta-catenin. *J Cutan Pathol* 2005;32:148–57.
12 Cornejo KM, Deng A. Pilomatrix carcinoma: a case report and review of the literature. *Am J Dermatopathol* 2013;35:389–94.

Lesions of hair follicle mesenchyme
Trichodiscoma
1 Pinkus H, Cosket R, Burgess GH. Trichodiscoma. *J Invest Dermatol* 1974;63:212–18.
5 Schmidt L, Warren M, Nickerson M *et al.* Birt–Hogg–Dubé syndrome, a genodermatosis associated with spontaneous pneumothorax and kidney neoplasia, maps to chromosome 17p11.2. *Am J Hum Genet* 2002;69:876–82.
10 Menko FH, van Steensel MA, Giraud S *et al.* European BHD Consortium. Birt–Hogg–Dubé syndrome: diagnosis and management. *Lancet Oncol* 2009;10:1199–206.

Perifollicular fibroma
5 Shvartsbeyn M, Mason AR, Bosenberg MW *et al.* Perifollicular fibroma in Birt–Hogg–Dubé syndrome: an association revisited. *J Cutan Pathol* 2012;39:675–9.
9 Happle R. Hornstein–Birt–Hogg–Dubé syndrome: a renaming and reconsideration. *Am J Med Genet A* 2012;158A:1247–51.

Fibrofolliculoma
2 Foucar K, Rosen T, Foucar E *et al.* Fibrofolliculoma: a clinicopathologic study. *Cutis* 1981;28:429–32.
8 Zbar B, Alvord WG, Glenn G *et al.* Risk of renal and colonic neoplasms and spontaneous pneumothorax in the Birt–Hogg–Dubé syndrome. *Cancer Epidemiol Biomarkers Prev* 2002;11:393–400.

Sebaceous gland tumours
Sebaceous adenomas and sebaceomas
10 Singh RS, Grayson W, Redston M *et al.* Site and tumor type predicts DNA mismatch repair status in cutaneous sebaceous neoplasia. *Am J Surg Pathol* 2008;32:936–42.
19 Lynch HT, Fusaro RM, Roberts L *et al.* Muir–Torre syndrome in several members of a family with a variant of the cancer family syndrome. *Br J Dermatol* 1985;113:295–301.
20 Schwartz RA, Torre DP. The Muir–Torré syndrome: a 25-year retrospect. *J Am Acad Dermatol* 1995;33:90–104.
27 Southey MC, Young MA, Whitty J *et al.* Molecular pathologic analysis enhances diagnosis and management of the Muir–Torre syndrome and gives an insight into its underlying molecular pathogenesis. *Am J Surg Pathol* 2001;25:936–41.
31 Everett JN, Raymond VM, Dandapani M *et al.* Screening for germline mismatch repair mutations following diagnosis of sebaceous neoplasm. *JAMA Dermatol* 2014;150:1315–21.
32 Roberts ME, Riegert-Johnson DL, Thomas BC *et al.* A clinical scoring system to identify patients with sebaceous neoplasms at risk for the Muir–Torre variant of Lynch syndrome. *Genet Med* 2014;16:711–16.

Sebaceous carcinoma
1 Nelson BR, Hamlet KR, Gillard M *et al.* Sebaceous carcinoma. *J Am Acad Dermatol* 1995;33:1–15.
16 Ostler DA, Prieto VG, Reed JA *et al.* Adipophilin expression in sebaceous tumors and other cutaneous lesions with clear cell histology: an immunohistochemical study of 117 cases. *Mod Pathol* 2010;23:567–73.
26 Dasgupta T, Wilson LD, Yu JB. A retrospective review of 1349 cases of sebaceous carcinomas. *Cancer* 2009;115:158–65.
30 Spencer JM, Nossa R, Tse DT *et al.* Sebaceous carcinoma of the eyelid treated by Mohs micrographic surgery. *J Am Acad Dermatol* 2001;44:1004–9.

Apocrine gland tumours/Apocrine hidrocystoma
10 Sugiyama A, Sugiura M, Piris A *et al.* Apocrine cystadenoma and apocrine hidrocystoma: examination of 21 cases with emphasis on nomenclature according to proliferative features. *J Cutan Pathol* 2007;34:912–17.

Syringocystadenoma papilliferum
10 Kazakov DV, Bisceglia M, Calonje E *et al.* Tubular adenoma and syringocystadenoma papilliferum: a reappraisal of their relationship. An interobserver study of a series, by a panel of dermatopathologists. *Am J Dermatopathol* 2007;29:256–63.
16 Yap FB, Lee BR, Baba R. Syringocystadenoma papilliferum in an unusual location beyond the head and neck region: a case report and review of literature. *Dermatol Online J* 2010;16:4.

25 Kazakov DV, Requena L, Kutzner H et al. Morphologic diversity of syringocystadenocarcinoma papilliferum based on a clinicopathologic study of 6 cases and review of the literature. Am J Dermatopathol 2010;32:340–7.

Hidradenoma papilliferum

2 Konstantinova AM, Michal M, Kacerovska D et al. Hidradenoma papilliferum: a clinicopathologic study of 264 tumors from 261 patients, with emphasis on mammary-type alterations. Am J Dermatopathol 2016;38:598–607.

3 Scurry J, Van der Putte SC, Pyman J et al. Mammary-like gland adenoma of the vulva: review of 46 cases. Pathology 2009;41:372–8.

4 Baker GM, Selim MA, Hoang MP. Vulvar adnexal lesions: a 32-year, single-institution review from Massachusetts General Hospital. Arch Pathol Lab Med 2013;137:1237–46.

12 Pfarr N, Sinn HP, Klauschen F et al. Mutations in genes encoding PI3K-AKT and MAPK signaling define anogenital papillary hidradenoma. Genes Chromosomes Cancer 2016;55:113–19.

18 Pelosi G, Martignoni G, Bonetti F. Intraductal carcinoma of mammary-type apocrine epithelium arising within a papillary hidradenoma of the vulva. Report of a case and review of the literature. Arch Pathol Lab Med 1991;115:1249–54.

Nipple adenoma

1 Brownstein MH, Phelps RG, Magnin PH. Papillary adenoma of the nipple: analysis of fifteen new cases. J Am Acad Dermatol 1985;12:707–15.

5 Montemarano AD, Sau P, James WD. Superficial papillary adenomatosis of the nipple: a case report and review of the literature. J Am Acad Dermatol 1995;33:871–5.

13 Diaz NM, Palmer JO, Wick MR. Erosive adenomatosis of the nipple: histology, immunohistology and differential diagnosis. Mod Pathol 1992;5:179–84.

14 Liau JY, Lee YH, Tsai JH et al. Frequent PIK3CA activating mutations in nipple adenomas. Histopathology 2017;70:195–202.

Apocrine tubular adenoma

3 Fox SB, Cotton D. Tubular apocrine adenoma and papillary eccrine adenoma: entities or unity? Am J Dermatopathol 1992;14:149–54.

5 Kazakov DV, Bisceglia M, Calonje E et al. Tubular adenoma and syringocystadenoma papilliferum: a reappraisal of their relationship. An interobserver study of a series, by a panel of dermatopathologists. Am J Dermatopathol 2007;29:256–63.

7 Liau JY, Tsai JH, Huang WC et al. BRAF and KRAS mutations in tubular apocrine adenoma and papillary eccrine adenoma of the skin. Hum Pathol 2018;73:59–65.

Apocrine carcinoma

6 Robson A, Lazar AJF, Ben Nagi J et al. Primary cutaneous apocrine carcinoma. A clinico-pathologic analysis of 24 cases. Am J Surg Pathol 2008;32:682–90.

7 Piris A, Peng Y, Boussahmain C et al. Cutaneous and mammary apocrine carcinomas have different immunoprofiles. Hum Pathol 2014;45:320–6.

12 Le LP, Dias-Santagata D, Pawlak AC et al. Apocrine-eccrine carcinomas: molecular and immunohistochemical analyses. PLoS One 2012;7:e47290.

Eccrine gland hamartomas and tumours
Eccrine angiomatous hamartoma

2 Sulica RL, Kao GF, Sulica VI, Penneys NS. Eccrine angiomatous hamartoma (nevus): immunohistochemical findings and review of the literature. J Cutan Pathol 1994;21:71–5.

9 Patterson AT, Kumar MG, Bayliss SJ et al. Eccrine angiomatous hamartoma: a clinicopathologic review of 18 cases. Am J Dermatopathol 2016;38:413–17.

12 Smith VC, Montesinos E, Revert A et al. Eccrine angiomatous hamartoma: report of three patients. Pediatr Dermatol 1996;13:139–42.

Eccrine hidrocystoma

1 Smith JD, Chernosky ME. Hidrocystomas. Arch Dermatol 1973;108:676–9.

12 Sarabi K, Khachemoune A. Hidrocystoma – a brief review. Med Gen Med 2006;8:57.

Hidroacanthoma simplex

3 Battistella M, Langbein L, Peltre B et al. From hidroacanthoma simplex to poroid hidradenoma: clinicopathologic and immunohistochemic study of poroid neoplasms and reappraisal of their histogenesis. Am J Dermatopathol 2010;32:459–68.

6 Anzai S, Arakawa S, Fujiwara S et al. Hidroacanthoma simplex: a case report and analysis of 70 Japanese cases. Dermatology 2005;210:363–5.

Eccrine dermal duct tumour

1 Winkelmann RK, McLeod WA. The dermal duct tumour. Arch Dermatol 1966;94:50–5.

Eccrine poroma

2 Hyman AB, Brownstein MH. Eccrine poroma: an analysis of 45 new cases. Dermatologica 1969;138:29–38.

10 Kazakov DV, Kutzner H, Spagnolo DV et al. Sebaceous differentiation in poroid neoplasms: report of 11 cases, including a case of metaplastic carcinoma associated with apocrine poroma (sarcomatoid apocrine porocarcinoma). Am J Dermatopathol 2008;30:21–6.

12 Macagno N, Kervarrec T, Sohier P et al. NUT is a specific immunohistochemical marker for the diagnosis of YAP1-NUTM1-rearranged cutaneous poroid neoplasms. Am J Surg Pathol 2021;45:1221–7.

14 Sekine S, Kiyono T, Ryo E et al. Recurrent YAP1-MAML2 and YAP1-NUTM1 fusions in poroma and porocarcinoma. J Clin Invest 2019;129:3827–32.

23 Chen CC, Chang YT, Liu HN. Clinical and histological characteristics of poroid neoplasms: a study of 25 cases in Taiwan. Int J Dermatol 2006;45:722–7.

24 Kuo HW, Ohara K. Pigmented eccrine poroma: a report of two cases and study with dermatoscopy. Dermatol Surg 2003;29:1076–9.

30 Miura T, Yamamoto T, Navi D et al. Poromatosis: the occurrence of multiple eccrine poromas. Dermatol Online J 2008;14:3.

Eccrine syringofibroadenoma

5 Ohnishi T, Suzuki T, Watanabe S. Eccrine syringofibroadenoma. Br J Dermatol 1995;134:449–54.

7 Starink TM. Eccrine syringofibroadenoma multiple lesions representing a new cutaneous marker of the Schopf syndrome, and solitary nonhereditary tumors. J Am Acad Dermatol 1997;36:569–76.

15 Nomura K, Kogawa T, Hashimoto I et al. Eccrine syringofibroadenomatous hyperplasia in a patient with bullous pemphigoid: a case report and review of the literature. Dermatologica 1991;182:59–62.

Syringoma

3 Winkelmann RK, Muller SA. Sweat gland tumors. Arch Dermatol 1964;89:827–31.

12 Soler-Carrillo J, Estrach T, Mascaró JM. Eruptive syringoma: 27 new cases and review of the literature. J Eur Acad Dermatol Venereol 2001;15:242–6.

18 Urban CD, Cannon JR, Cole RD. Eruptive syringomas in Down's syndrome. Arch Dermatol 1985;117:374–9.

Tubular adenoma

1 Rulon DB, Helwig EB. Papillary eccrine adenoma. Arch Dermatol 1977;113:596–8.

4 Mizuoka H, Senzaki H, Shikata N et al. Papillary eccrine adenoma: immunohistochemical study and literature review. J Cutan Pathol 1998;25:59–64.

Eccrine or apocrine/follicular tumours

2 Wong TY, Suster S, Cheek RF, Mihm MC Jr. Benign cutaneous adnexal tumours with combined folliculosebaceous, apocrine, and eccrine differentiation: study of eight cases. Am J Dermatopathol 1996;18:124–36.

Hidradenoma

3 Nandeesh BN, Rajalakshmi T. A study of histopathologic spectrum of nodular hidradenoma. Am J Dermatopathol 2012;34:461–70.

11 Nazarian RM, Kapur P, Rakheja D et al. Atypical and malignant hidradenomas: a histologic and immunohistochemical study. Mod Pathol 2009;22:600–10.

16 Winnes M, Mölne L, Suurküla M et al. Frequent fusion of the CRTC1 and MAML2 genes in clear cell variants of cutaneous hidradenomas. Genes Chromosomes Cancer 2007;46:559–63.

18 Stefanato CM, Ferrara G, Chaudhry IH et al. Clear cell nodular hidradenoma involving the lymphatic system: a tumor of uncertain malignant potential or a novel example of "metastasizing" benign tumor? Am J Surg Pathol 2012;36:1835–40.

Cylindroma

1 Crain RC, Helwig EB. Dermal cylindroma (dermal eccrine cylindroma). *Am J Clin Pathol* 1961;35:504–15.
4 Biggs PJ, Chapman P, Lakhani SR *et al*. The cylindromatosis gene on chromosome 16q may be the only tumour suppressor gene involved in the development of cylindromas. *Oncogene* 1996;12:1375–7.
5 Takahashi M, Rapley E, Biggs PJ *et al*. Linkage and LOH studies in 19 cylindromatosis families show no evidence of genetic heterogeneity and refine the CYLD locus on chromosome 16q12-q13. *Hum Genet* 2000;106:58–65.
8 Gottschalk HR, Graham JH, Aston EEIV. Dermal eccrine cylindroma, epithelioma adenoides cysticum, and eccrine spiradenoma. *Arch Dermatol* 1974;110:473–4.
17 Durani BK, Kurzen H, Jaeckel A *et al*. Malignant transformation of multiple dermal cylindromas. *Br J Dermatol* 2001;145:653–6.

Spiradenoma

1 Castro C, Winkelmann RK. Spiradenoma: histochemical and electron microscopic study. *Arch Dermatol* 1974;109:40–8.
4 Hashimoto K, Lever WF. Histogenesis of skin appendage tumors. *Arch Dermatol* 1969;100:356–69.
13 Granter SR, Seeger K, Calonje E *et al*. Malignant eccrine spiradenoma (spiradenocarcinoma): a clinicopathologic study of 12 cases. *Am J Dermatopathol* 2000;22:97–103.
15 Kazakov DV, Zelger B, Rütten A *et al*. Morphologic diversity of malignant neoplasms arising in preexisting spiradenoma, cylindroma, and spiradenocylindroma based on the study of 24 cases, sporadic or occurring in the setting of Brooke–Spiegler syndrome. *Am J Surg Pathol* 2009;33:705–19.
18 Rashid M, van der Horst M, Mentzel T *et al*. ALPK1 hotspot mutation as a driver of human spiradenoma and spiradenocarcinoma. *Nat Commun* 2019;10:2213.

Mixed tumour of the skin

2 Kazakov DV, Belousova IE, Bisceglia M *et al*. Apocrine mixed tumor of the skin ('mixed tumor of the folliculosebaceous–apocrine complex'). Spectrum of differentiation and metaplastic changes in the epithelial, myoepithelial, and stromal components based on a histopathologic study of 244 cases. *J Am Acad Dermatol* 2007;57:467–83.
4 Headington JT. Mixed tumors of the skin: eccrine and apocrine types. *Arch Dermatol* 1961;84:989–96.
9 Mentzel T, Requena L, Kaddu S *et al*. Cutaneous myoepithelial neoplasms: clinicopathologic and immunohistochemical study of 20 cases suggesting a continuous spectrum ranging from benign mixed tumor of the skin to cutaneous myoepithelioma and myoepithelial carcinoma. *J Cutan Pathol* 2003;30:293–302.
10 Kazakov DV, Bisceglia M, Spagnolo DV *et al*. Apocrine mixed tumors of the skin with architectural and/or cytologic atypia: a retrospective clinicopathologic study of 18 cases. *Am J Surg Pathol* 2007;31:1094–102.
11 Bahrami A, Dalton JD, Krane JF *et al*. A subset of cutaneous and soft tissue mixed tumors are genetically linked to their salivary gland counterpart. *Genes Chromosomes Cancer* 2012;51:140–8.
18 Metzler G, Schaumburg-Lever G, Hornstein O *et al*. Malignant chondroid syringoma. *Am J Dermatopathol* 1996;18:83–9.

Cutaneous myoepithelioma

1 Kilpatrick SE, Hitchcock MG, Kraus MD *et al*. Mixed tumors and myoepitheliomas of soft tissue: a clinicopathologic study of 19 cases with a unifying concept. *Am J Surg Pathol* 1997;21:13–22.
5 Hornick JL, Fletcher CD. Myoepithelial tumors of soft tissue: a clinicopathologic and immunohistochemical study of 101 cases with evaluation of prognostic parameters. *Am J Surg Pathol* 2003;27:1183–96.
6 Hornick JL, Fletcher CD. Cutaneous myoepithelioma: a clinicopathologic and immunohistochemical study of 14 cases. *Hum Pathol* 2004;35:14–24.
10 Jo VY, Antonescu CR, Zhang L *et al*. Cutaneous syncytial myoepithelioma: clinicopathologic characterization in a series of 38 cases. *Am J Surg Pathol* 2013;37:710–18.

Sweat gland carcinomas, including ductal apocrine/follicular carcinomas

1 Urso C, Bondi R, Paglierani M *et al*. Carcinomas of sweat glands: report of 60 cases. *Arch Pathol Lab Med* 2001;125:498–505.

Eccrine gland carcinomas

Malignant eccrine poroma

3 Robson A, Greene J, Ansari N *et al*. Eccrine porocarcinoma: a clinicopathologic study of 69 cases. *Am J Surg Pathol* 2001;25:710–20.
10 Shaw M, McKee PH, Lowe D, Black MM. Malignant eccrine poroma: a study of 27 cases. *Br J Dermatol* 1982;107:675–80.
14 Mahomed F, Blok J, Grayson W. The squamous variant of eccrine porocarcinoma: a clinicopathological study of 21 cases. *J Clin Pathol* 2008;61:361–5.
15 Sekine S, Kiyono T, Ryo E *et al*. Recurrent YAP1-MAML2 and YAP1-NUTM1 fusions in poroma and porocarcinoma. *J Clin Invest* 2019;129:3827–32.
21 Goh SG, Dayrit JF, Calonje E. Sarcomatoid eccrine porocarcinoma: report of two cases and a review of the literature. *J Cutan Pathol* 2007;34:55–60.

Squamoid eccrine ductal carcinoma

3 van der Horst MP, Garcia-Herrera A, Markiewicz D *et al*. Squamoid eccrine ductal carcinoma: a clinicopathologic study of 30 cases. *Am J Surg Pathol* 2016;40:755–60.

Digital papillary adenocarcinoma

1 Kao GF, Helwig EB, Graham JH. Aggressive digital papillary adenoma and adenocarcinoma: a clinicopathological study of 57 cases. *J Cutan Pathol* 1987;14:129–46.
2 Duke WH, Sherod TT, Lupton GP. Aggressive digital papillary adenocarcinoma (aggressive digital papillary adenoma and adenocarcinoma revisited). *Am J Surg Pathol* 2000;24:775–84.
3 Suchak R, Wang WL, Prieto VG *et al*. Cutaneous digital papillary adenocarcinoma: a clinicopathologic study of 31 cases of a rare neoplasm with new observations. *Am J Surg Pathol* 2012;36:1883–91.
11 Bartelstein MK, Schwarzkopf E, Busam KJ *et al*. Sentinel lymph node biopsy predicts systemic recurrence in digital papillary adenocarcinoma. *J Surg Oncol* 2020;122:1323–7.

Eccrine or apocrine/follicular carcinomas

Malignant cylindroma

1 Pizinger K, Michal M. Malignant cylindroma in Brooke–Spiegler syndrome. *Dermatology* 2000;201:255–7.
3 Kazakov DV, Zelger B, Rütten A *et al*. Morphologic diversity of malignant neoplasms arising in preexisting spiradenoma, cylindroma, and spiradenocylindroma based on the study of 24 cases, sporadic or occurring in the setting of Brooke–Spiegler syndrome. *Am J Surg Pathol* 2009;33:705–19.
4 Kazakov DV, Grossmann P, Spagnolo DV *et al*. Expression of p53 and TP53 mutational analysis in malignant neoplasms arising in preexisting spiradenoma, cylindroma, and spiradenocylindroma, sporadic or associated with Brooke–Spiegler syndrome. *Am J Dermatopathol* 2010;32:215–21.
7 Iyer PV, Leong AS. Malignant dermal cylindromas: do they exist? A morphological and immunohistochemical study and review of the literature. *Pathology* 1989;21:269–74.

Hidradenocarcinoma

5 Mambo NC. The significance of atypical nuclear changes in benign eccrine acrospiromas: a clinical and pathological study of 18 cases. *J Cutan Pathol* 1984;11:35–44.
11 Kazakov DV, Ivan D, Kutzner H *et al*. Cutaneous hidradenocarcinoma: a clinicopathological, immunohistochemical, and molecular biologic study of 14 cases, including Her2/neu gene expression/amplification, TP53 gene mutation analysis, and t(11;19) translocation. *Am J Dermatopathol* 2009;31:236–47.
14 Souvatzidis P, Sbano P, Mandato F *et al*. Malignant nodular hidradenoma of the skin: report of seven cases. *J Eur Acad Dermatol Venereol* 2008;22:549–54.
18 Nash JW, Barrett TL, Kies M *et al*. Metastatic hidradenocarcinoma with demonstration of Her-2/neu gene amplification by fluorescence in-situ hybridization: potential treatment implications. *J Cutan Pathol* 2007;34:49–54.

Spiradenocarcinoma

3 Kazakov DV, Grossmann P, Spagnolo DV *et al*. Expression of p53 and TP53 mutational analysis in malignant neoplasms arising in preexisting spiradenoma, cylindroma, and spiradenocylindroma, sporadic or associated with Brooke–Spiegler syndrome. *Am J Dermatopathol* 2010;32:215–21.

5 Granter SR, Seeger K, Calonje E, Busam K, McKee PH. Malignant eccrine spiradenoma: a study of 12 cases. *Am J Dermatopathol* 2000;22:97–103.

Microcystic adnexal carcinoma
2 Chiller K, Passaro D, Scheuller M *et al*. Microcystic adnexal carcinoma: forty-eight cases, their treatment, and their outcome. *Arch Dermatol* 2000;136:1355–9.
5 Goldstein D, Barr R, Santa Cruz D. Microcystic adnexal carcinoma: a distinct clinicopathologic entity. *Cancer* 1982;50:566–72.
18 Nagatsuka H, Riveras RS, Gunduz M *et al*. Microcystic adnexal carcinoma with mandibular bone marrow involvement: a case report with immunohistochemistry. *Am J Dermatopathol* 2006;28:518–22.
19 Brenn T, Wiedemeyer K, Calonje E. Morphologically high-grade microcystic adnexal carcinoma: a report of two cases. *Histopathology* 2020;77:449–52.
20 Gabillot-Carré M, Weill F, Mamelle G *et al*. Microcystic adnexal carcinoma: report of seven cases including one with lung metastasis. *Dermatology* 2006;212:221–8.
23 Worley B, Owen JL, Barker CA *et al*. Evidence-based clinical practice guidelines for microcystic adnexal carcinoma: informed by a systematic review. *JAMA Dermatol* 2019;155:1059–68.

Adnexal carcinoma NOS
3 Urso C, Bondi R. Eccrine epithelioma: an enigma or a chimera? *Am J Dermatopathol* 1992;14:179–80.
6 Sidiropoulos M, Sade S, Al-Habeeb A *et al*. Syringoid eccrine carcinoma: a clinicopathological and immunohistochemical study of four cases. *J Clin Pathol* 2011;64:788–92.

Mucinous carcinoma
1 Kazakov DV, Suster S, LeBoit P *et al*. Mucinous carcinoma of the skin, primary and secondary: a clinicopathologic study of 63 cases with emphasis on the morphologic spectrum of primary cutaneous forms: homologies with mucinous lesions in the breast. *Am J Surg Pathol* 2005;29:764–82.
13 Hanby AM, McKee P, Jeffery M *et al*. Primary mucinous carcinomas of the skin express TFF1, TFF3, estrogen receptor and progesterone receptors. *Am J Surg Pathol* 1998;22:1125–31.
15 Marra DE, Schanbacher CF, Torres A. Mohs micrographic surgery of primary cutaneous mucinous carcinoma using immunohistochemistry for margin control. *Dermatol Surg* 2004;30:799–802.
18 Kamalpour L, Brindise RT, Nodzenski M *et al*. Primary cutaneous mucinous carcinoma: a systematic review and meta-analysis of outcomes after surgery. *JAMA Dermatol* 2014;150:380–4.

Endocrine mucin-producing sweat gland carcinoma
1 Flieder A, Koerner FC, Pilch BZ *et al*. Endocrine mucin-producing sweat gland carcinoma: a cutaneous neoplasm analogous to solid papillary carcinoma of breast. *Am J Surg Pathol* 1997;21:1501–6.
2 Zembowicz A, Garcia CF, Tannous ZS *et al*. Endocrine mucin-producing sweat gland carcinoma: twelve new cases suggest that it is a precursor of some invasive mucinous carcinomas. *Am J Surg Pathol* 2005:29;1330–9.
7 Dhaliwal CA, Torgersen A, Ross JJ *et al*. Endocrine mucin-producing sweat gland carcinoma: report of two cases of an under-recognized malignant neoplasm and review of the literature. *Am J Dermatopathol* 2013;3:117–24.

Adenoid cystic carcinoma
5 Rocas D, Asvesti C, Tsega A *et al*. Primary adenoid cystic carcinoma of the skin metastatic to the lymph nodes: immunohistochemical study of a new case and literature review. *Am J Dermatopathol* 2014;36:223–8.
6 Ramakrishnan R, Chaudhry IH, Ramdial P *et al*. Primary cutaneous adenoid cystic carcinoma: a clinicopathologic and immunohistochemical study of 27 cases. *Am J Surg Pathol* 2013;37:1603–11.
9 Dores GM, Huycke MM, Devesa SS *et al*. Primary cutaneous adenoid cystic carcinoma in the United States: incidence, survival, and associated cancers, 1976 to 2005. *J Am Acad Dermatol* 2010;63:71–8.
13 North JP, McCalmont TH, Fehr A *et al*. Detection of MYB alterations and other immunohistochemical markers in primary cutaneous adenoid cystic carcinoma. *Am J Surg Pathol* 2015;39:1347–56.

19 Pappo O, Gez E, Craciun I *et al*. Growth rate analysis of lung metastases appearing 18 years after resection of cutaneous adenoid cystic carcinoma: case report and review of the literature. *Arch Pathol Lab Med* 1992;116:76–9.
20 Krunic AL, Kim S, Medenica M *et al*. Recurrent adenoid cystic carcinoma of the scalp treated with Mohs micrographic surgery. *Dermatol Surg* 2003;29:647–9.

Secretory carcinoma
1 Brandt SM, Swistel AJ, Rosen PP. Secretory carcinoma in the axilla: probable origin from axillary skin appendage glands in a young girl. *Am J Surg Pathol* 2009;33:950–3.
6 Bishop JA, Taube JM, Su A *et al*. Secretory carcinoma of the skin harboring ETV6 gene fusions: a cutaneous analogue to secretory carcinomas of the breast and salivary glands. *Am J Surg Pathol* 2017;41:62–6.

Miscellaneous tumours
Tumours of ano-genital mammary-like glands
1 van der Putte SC. Mammary-like glands of the vulva and their disorders. *Int J Gynecol Pathol* 1994;13:150–60.
2 van der Putte SC, van Gorp LH. Adenocarcinoma of the mammary-like glands of the vulva: a concept unifying sweat gland carcinoma of the vulva, carcinoma of supranumerary mammary glands and extramammary Paget's disease. *J Cutan Pathol* 1994;21:157–63.

Paget disease of the nipple
1 Lloyd J, Flanagan AM. Mammary and extramammary Paget's disease. *J Clin Pathol* 2000;53:742–9.
2 Ordoñez NG, Awalt H, MacKay B. Mammary and extramammary Paget's disease. *Cancer* 1987;59:1173–83.
5 Chen CY, Sun LM, Anderson BO. Paget disease of the breast: changing patterns of incidence, clinical presentation, and treatment in the U.S. *Cancer* 2006;107:1448–58.
12 Reed W, Oppedal BR, Eeg Larsen T. Immunohistology is valuable in distinguishing between Paget's disease, Bowen's disease and superficial spreading melanoma. *Histopathology* 1990;16:583–8.

Extramammary Paget disease
5 Liegl B, Liegl S, Gogg-Kamerer M *et al*. Mammary and extramammary Paget's disease: an immunohistochemical study of 83 cases. *Histopathology* 2007;50:439–47.
13 Black D, Tornos C, Soslow RA *et al*. The outcomes of patients with positive margins after excision for intraepithelial Paget's disease of the vulva. *Gynecol Oncol* 2007;104:547–50.
14 Hatta N, Yamada M, Hirano T *et al*. Extramammary Paget's disease: treatment, prognostic factors and outcome in 76 patients. *Br J Dermatol* 2008;158:313–18.
17 Thomas CJ, Wood GC, Marks VJ. Mohs micrographic surgery in the treatment of rare aggressive cutaneous tumours: the Geisinger experience. *Dermatol Surg* 2007;33:333–9.
22 Sanderson P, Innamaa A, Palmer J *et al*. Imiquimod therapy for extramammary Paget's disease of the vulva: a viable non-surgical alternative. *J Obstet Gynaecol* 2013;33:479–83.
25 Hata M, Koike I, Wada H *et al*. Definitive radiation therapy for extramammary Paget's disease. *Anticancer Res* 2012;32:3315–20.

Lymphoepithelioma-like carcinoma
1 Swanson SA, Cooper PH, Mills SE *et al*. Lymphoepithelioma-like carcinoma of the skin. *Mod Pathol* 1988;1:359–65.
18 Welch PQ, Williams SB, Foss RD *et al*. Lymphoepithelioma-like carcinoma of head and neck skin: a systematic analysis of 11 cases and review of literature. *Oral Surg Oral Med Oral Pathol Oral Radiol Endod* 2011;111:78–86.
19 Hall G, Duncan A, Azurdia R *et al*. Lymphoepithelioma-like carcinoma of the skin: a case with lymph node metastasis at presentation. *Am J Dermatopathol* 2007;29:365–9.
20 Glaich AS, Behroozan DS, Cohen JL *et al*. Lymphoepithelioma-like carcinoma of the skin: a report of two cases treated with complete microscopic margin control and review of the literature. *Dermatol Surg* 2006;32:316–19.

CHAPTER 138

Kaposi Sarcoma

Kenneth Y. Tsai

Departments of Anatomic Pathology and Tumor Biology, H. Lee Moffitt Cancer Center and Research Institute, Tampa, FL, USA

Kaposi sarcoma, 138.1	Key references, 138.6

Kaposi sarcoma

Definition and nomenclature

Kaposi sarcoma (KS) is a multifocal, endothelial proliferation caused by human herpesvirus 8 (HHV-8), most often with cutaneous involvement and with or without visceral extension. There are five distinct clinicopathological subtypes: classic, endemic, iatrogenic, AIDS-associated and HIV-negative MSM (men who have sex with men).

Synonyms and inclusions
- Multiple haemorrhagic sarcoma
- Multiple pigment sarcoma

Classification links
- ICD-10: C46
- MIM: 148000

Introduction and general description

KS, first described by dermatologist Moritz Kaposi in 1872, is a multifocal endothelial proliferation of low-grade malignant potential. Debate remains as to whether this is a true neoplasm or a reactive process [1,2,3], although in its later stages there is evidence of monoclonality [4]. Its precise histogenesis has also been somewhat controversial, although recent evidence points towards a lymphatic origin [5]. A strong predisposition among immunocompromised individuals, such as in HIV-infected individuals or solid organ transplant recipients, reflects a dependence upon host immune status. The worldwide age-standardised incidence varies dramatically from fewer than 1 per 100 000 in most areas of western Europe and North America to over 22 per 100 000 in central Africa where the disease occurs in its endemic form and HIV infection is rampant [1].

Epidemiology

Epidemiological details are given in Table 138.1.

Pathophysiology

Predisposing factors

Although HHV-8 is considered the causative agent, it is likely insufficient to cause KS alone [1,40]. Multiple co-factors are required, the most powerful of which is HIV co-infection, which elevates the risk up to 20 000-fold [1,41,42]. A few weakly contributory genetic polymorphisms in immune-related genes have also been identified [1,3].

Pathology

The histopathological changes of KS typically parallel the clinical progression of patch, plaque and tumour stages and do not differ between the clinicopathological subtypes. Patch-stage KS (Figure 138.1) manifests as a mild increase in the number of vessels, which are classically arranged in a horizontal fashion, dissecting through collagen bundles, around adnexae and surrounding pre-existing vessels (promontory sign) (Figure 138.2). A chronic lymphoplasmacytic infiltrate may be present, with extravasated erythrocytes and haemosiderin deposition. The plaque stage has more obvious and extensive vessel expansion, lined by single-layered, plump endothelial cells. Surrounding them are more spindled cells with eosinophilic cytoplasm and hyperchromatic nuclei (Figure 138.3). The chronic inflammatory infiltrate remains. Finally, in tumour-stage or nodular KS, there is a circumscribed mass of spindled cells with unlined slit-like spaces with extravasated erythrocytes (Figure 138.4). Mitotic activity is readily appreciated, as are periodic acid–Schiff stain (PAS) positive, diastase-resistant, amorphous eosinophilic globules that are red on Mallory trichrome stain and probably represent degenerated erythrocytes [43].

Immunohistochemical studies demonstrate a strong expression of CD31, CD34, factor VIII-related antigen and podoplanin (D2-40) [44–47]. The latent nuclear antigen-1 of HHV-8 exhibits granular nuclear expression, which is highly specific for KS (Figure 138.5) [48,49].

Causative organisms

All forms of KS are associated with HHV-8 infection as the aetiological agent. Discovered in 1994 and originally termed Kaposi sarcoma herpesvirus [50], this γ-herpesvirus is easily transmitted through

---

Rook's Textbook of Dermatology, Tenth Edition. Edited by Christopher Griffiths, Jonathan Barker, Tanya Bleiker, Walayat Hussain and Rosalind Simpson.
© 2024 John Wiley & Sons Ltd. Published 2024 by John Wiley & Sons Ltd.

Table 138.1 Features of the five types of Kaposi sarcoma (KS).

Subtype	Incidence and prevalence	Age	Sex	Ethnicity	Associated conditions
Classic	0.47–8.8 per 100 000 per year in areas of Italy and Greece [6–12]; 0.2% of cancers in the USA [13]	Elderly, fifth to seventh decades, rarely children	Male predominance, over 10 : 1 ratio	Southern European (Italian, Greek); eastern European Jews	
Endemic	Up to 10% of cancers in central Africa [14–22]	Children, adults	Near unity in childhood; 15 : 1 male predominance by puberty	Equatorial Africa (Congo, Uganda, Zaire)	Epstein–Barr virus infection [23,24]
Iatrogenic	0.3–1.6% among transplant recipients in the USA and Europe [25–30]; up to 5.3% of renal transplant patients in Saudi Arabia [26,31]; 100–500-fold increased incidence over general population [32,33]	Adults, usually younger than classic or adult endemic	Male predominance; 1.5 : 1 in Saudi Arabia [34]	Increased risk is superimposed upon ethnogeographic predisposition seen in classic KS	Organ transplantation, post-treatment lymphoma, corticosteroid and ciclosporin use
AIDS-associated	Most common neoplasm in untreated HIV-infected individuals [35]; 30 per 1000 patient-years (pre-HAART) to 0.3 per 1000 patient-years (post-HAART) [36]; up to 40% of homosexual men with AIDS (pre-HAART) [37]	Young men, 20–40 years	Male predominance (particularly homosexuals), up to 7 : 1		HIV infection, drug abuse
HIV-negative MSM [38,39]		Young to middle-aged men			

AIDS, acquired immune deficiency syndrome; HAART, highly active antiretroviral therapy; HIV, human immunodeficiency virus; KS, Kaposi sarcoma; MSM, men who have sex with men.

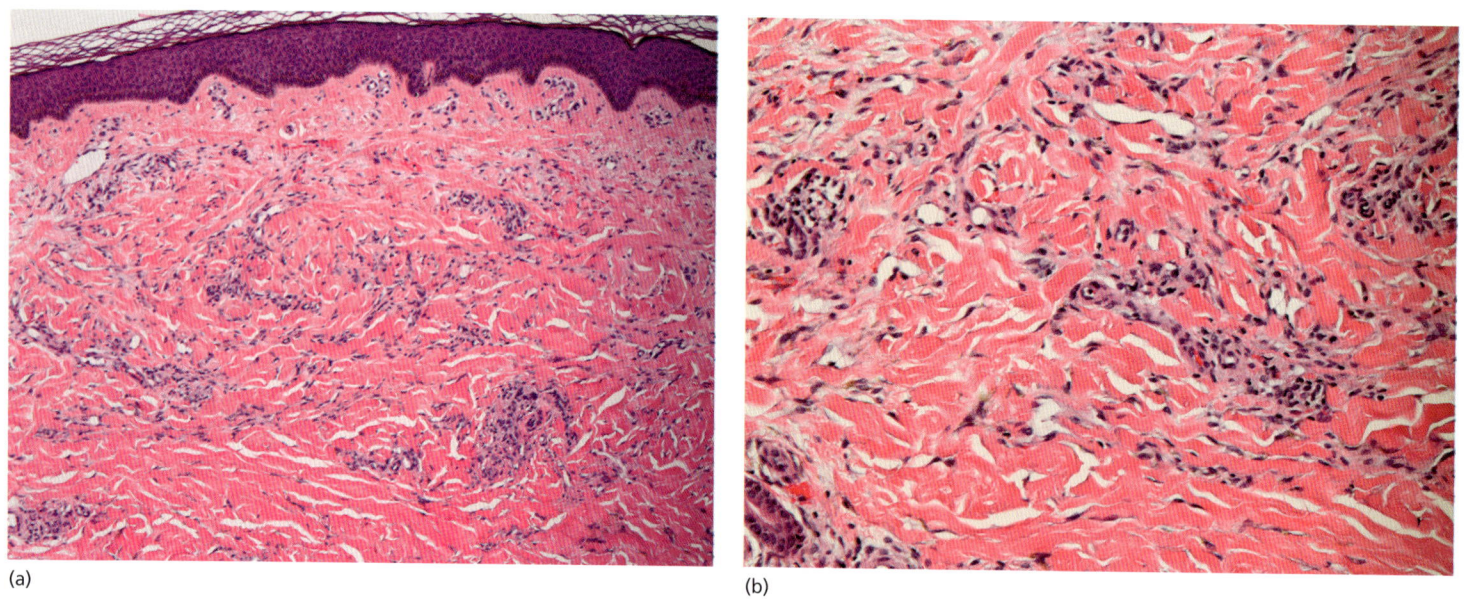

Figure 138.1 Patch-stage Kaposi sarcoma. (a) Lesions can be subtle and typically consist of horizontally arranged, irregular vessels that dissect through collagen and around adnexae. (b) Vessels are lined by endothelial cells that may be plump and hyperchromatic, with areas of erythrocyte extravasation and hemosiderin deposition.

saliva and blood products and infects endothelial cells, epithelial cells, B cells, monocytes, fibroblasts and dendritic cells [51–54]. Seroprevalence correlates highly with KS incidence [1] although HHV-8 seropositivity can be observed in a myriad of other non-KS conditions. The characteristic spindle cells of KS lesions are latently infected with HHV-8, and expression of latent-associated nuclear antigen, v-cyclin, viral FLIP and viral microRNAs suppresses apoptosis and drive proliferation [1,55–62]. Even in the lytic phase, in which cellular lysis occurs, it is thought that HHV-8 genes drive pro-tumourigenic cytokine production [1,63].

Many of these alterations, including those driven by vGPCR, converge upon cancer-related signalling pathways including canonical MAP-kinase (JNK, ERK), PI3K-AKT-mTOR, and NF-κB pathways [64–69]. Gene expression studies demonstrate that KS spindle cells

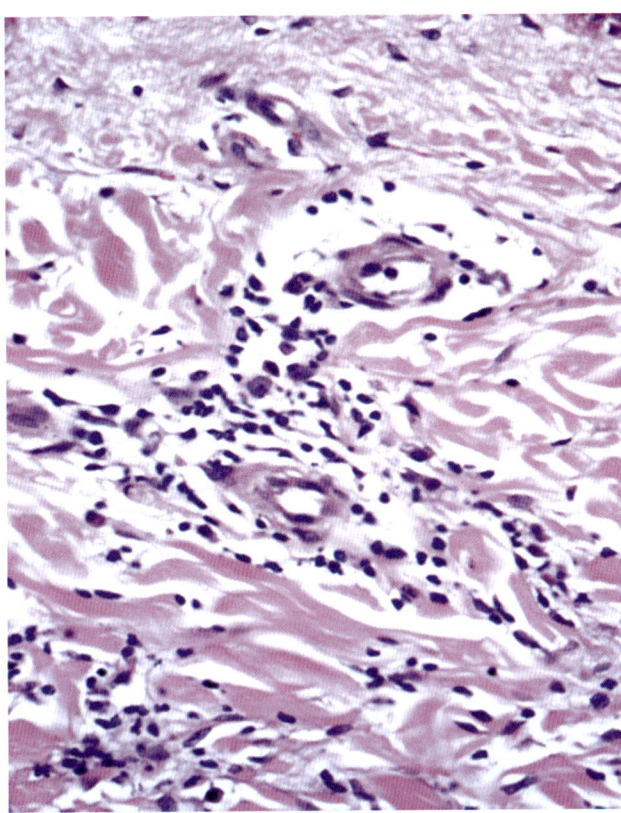

Figure 138.2 Promontory sign. This finding shows normal vessels or adnexae ensheathed within new abnormal vascular spaces.

have overlapping features of lymphatic and blood endothelial cells, but more strongly resemble the former [70]. In addition, HHV-8 drives aberrant differentiation of blood endothelial cells by inducing the expression of lymphatic markers including PROX1 and podoplanin [5,71–73].

Genetics and genomics
The genetic basis for the ethnogeographic predisposition of KS in the classic and endemic subtypes is unclear at present, although there are case reports of germline mutations causing early onset KS in childhood. There is one report of autosomal recessive OX40 deficiency causing classic KS in a child of consanguineous parents [74]. This loss of OX40 function resulted in decreased effector CD4+ T cell function. In another family with inherited susceptibility to KS, a *STAT4* mutation was implicated [75].

Transcriptomic analyses of KS have now been conducted and reflect a wide diversity of transcriptional profiles showing activation of interferon pathways and alterations in host cell glucose and lipid metabolism [76,77]. Interestingly, these studies have not identified significant intrinsic differences between endemic and AIDS-associated forms of KS [78].

Environmental factors
The contribution of additional exposures has been suggested but there is no clear mechanistic basis established for them at this time. These include exposure to quinine (used as an antimalarial and used to process heroin), nitrile inhalants (a common drug of abuse preceding the start of the AIDS epidemic), angiotensin-converting enzyme

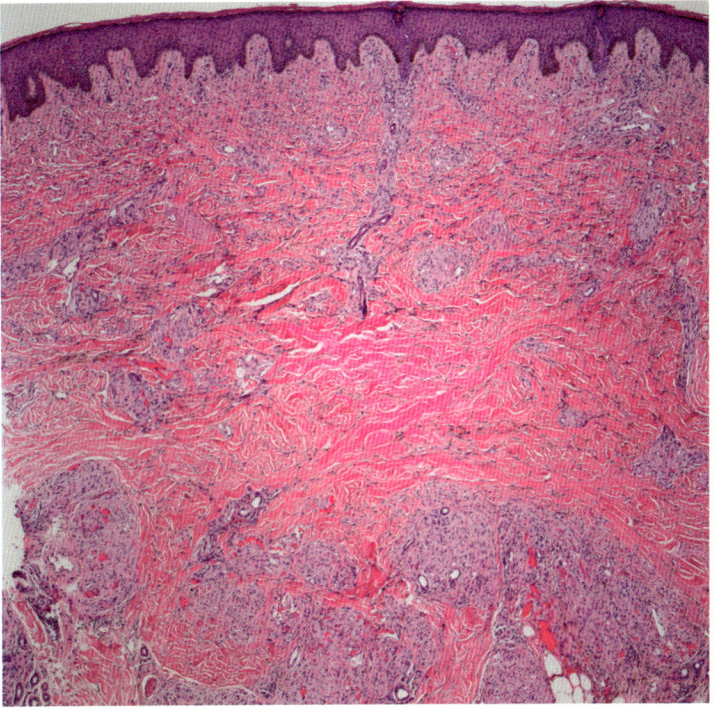

(a)

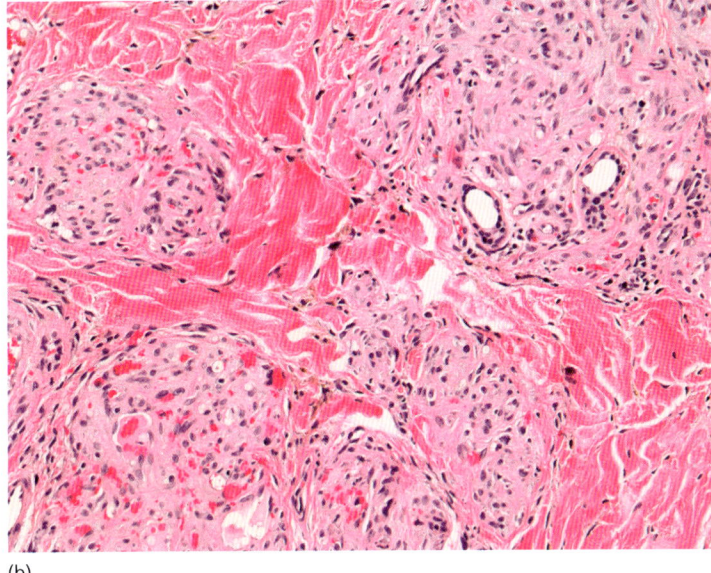

(b)

Figure 138.3 Plaque-stage Kaposi sarcoma. The histological findings (a) are more exaggerated than those of patch-stage KS, with deeper involvement, more prominent extension of spindled cells around vessels, erythrocyte extravasation and hemosiderin deposition (b).

(ACE) inhibitors and volcanic soil silicates (areas with endemic KS) [63,79,80].

Clinical features
Presentation
Cutaneous lesions commonly present in the extremities, most often on the feet and occasionally on the hands, ears or nose [40,81,82]. Lesions are typically dark blue or purple and may partially blanche when tumid (Figure 138.6). They are most often multifocal, fusing to

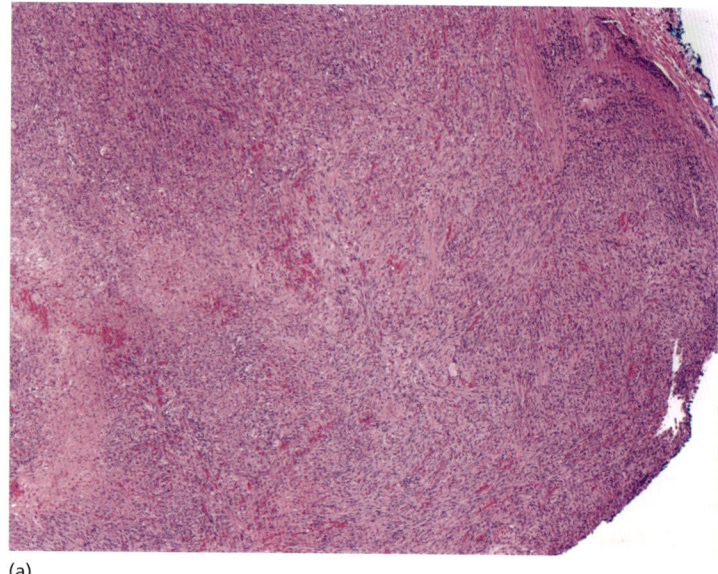

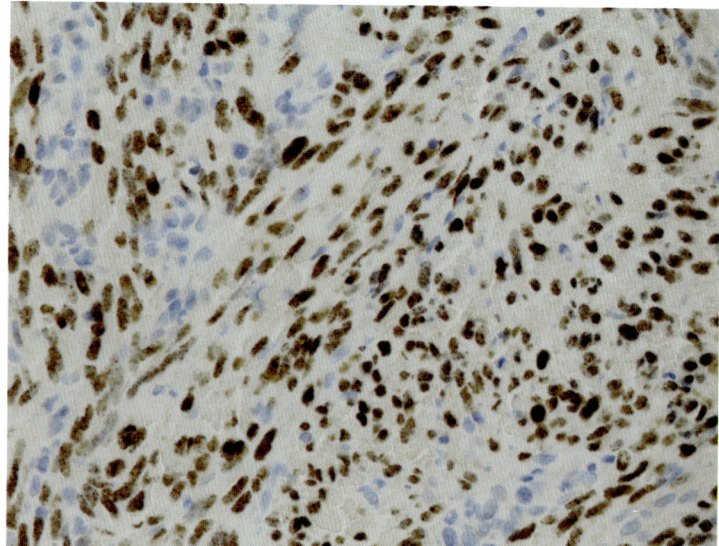

Figure 138.5 Human herpesvirus 8 (HHV-8) staining. Immunohistochemical staining for the latent nuclear antigen-1 of HHV-8 is specific for KS and demonstrates strong granular nuclear staining of the spindled cells.

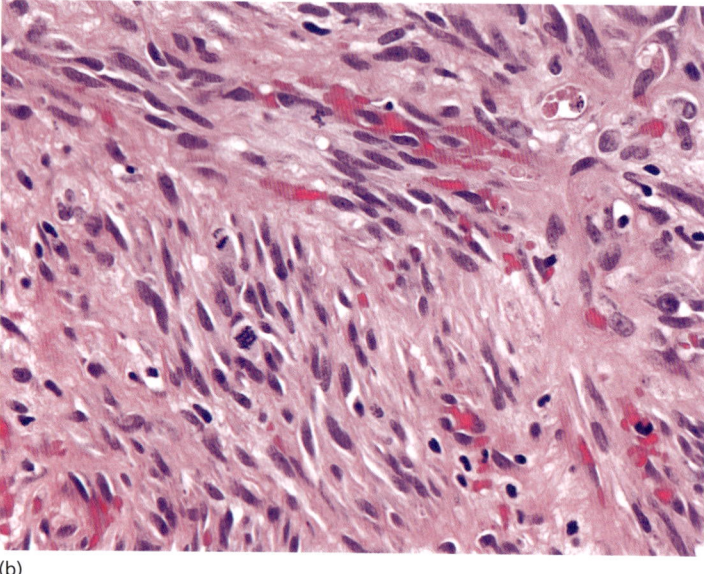

Figure 138.4 Nodular Kaposi sarcoma. (a) A circumscribed tumour nodule occupies the dermis with a dense, whorled arrangement of spindled cells. (b) Erythrocyte extravasation within slit-like spaces is prominent, with readily observed mitoses and eosinophilic globules.

eventually form plaques and tumours to a size of several centimetres (Figure 138.7) [83]. Oedema of the associated limb can follow, although it is sometimes the presenting finding, particularly in the endemic form in adults. Locally aggressive lesions can ulcerate, fungate or leave pigmented scars. Lymph nodes, mucosae and viscera may be involved as the disease progresses, although this can occur without skin involvement. The endemic form in children is classically lymphadenopathic [40,84]. Patients with KS in the context of immunosuppression may have subtle lesions that resemble bruises or trauma.

Clinical variants

The most distinguishing clinical features among the clinicopathological subtypes are the rate of progression and the degree of non-cutaneous involvement. Classic KS typically starts in the skin of the lower extremities and progresses very slowly. Iatrogenic KS resembles classic KS in presentation with a more varied site of presentation and more subtle lesions. In adults, the African endemic form can be locally aggressive in the skin but is rarely so systemically. The African endemic form in children is typically lymphadenopathic with or without cutaneous involvement and is often fatal within 2 years [85]. AIDS-associated KS can be rapidly progressive, often involving the head, neck, trunk and mucous membranes; fulminant disease with widespread nodal and visceral involvement is expected, particularly in the absence of highly active antiretroviral therapy (HAART) [40,86,87]. In this context, lesions can also arise during immune reconstitution inflammatory syndrome [88,89]. The newest subtype, arising in MSM without HIV infection and typically presents with indolent, localised disease [2,3].

Differential diagnosis

The differential diagnosis of cutaneous lesions is typically that of other vascular lesions, particularly haemangiomas as well as melanocytic proliferations. Acroangiodermatitis due to severe stasis changes has an overlapping site distribution with KS, and bacillary angiomatosis can coexist with KS, particularly in the context of immunosuppression [40].

Classification of severity

Staging of KS was originally developed in the context of AIDS by the AIDS Clinical Trial Group (ACTG) (Table 138.2) [90,91]. Originally, the CD4 T cell count was thought to be a critical prognostic indicator, but more recent refinements suggest that tumour stage and systemic disease status are more important [40,92]. Stratifying treatment of patients with T0 vs T1 status with combination antiretroviral therapy vs combination antiretroviral therapy and liposomal anthracycline therapy, respectively, improved outcomes by effectively treating T1 disease while sparing those with T01 disease from systemic anthracyclines [93].

Kaposi sarcoma 138.5

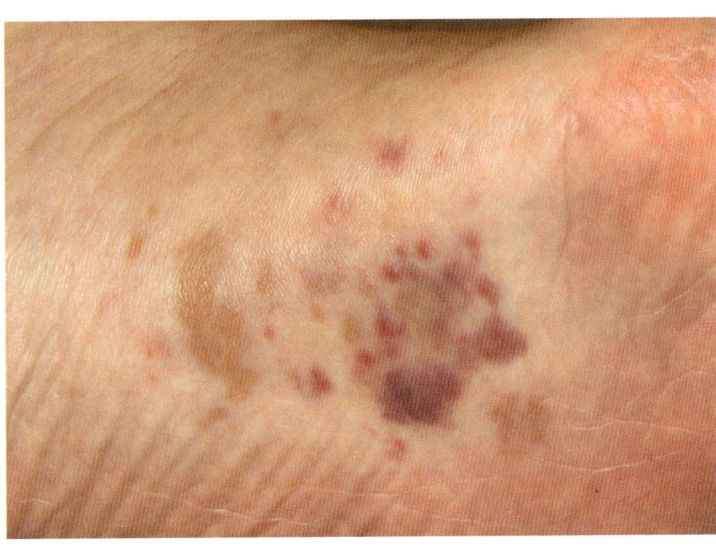

(a)

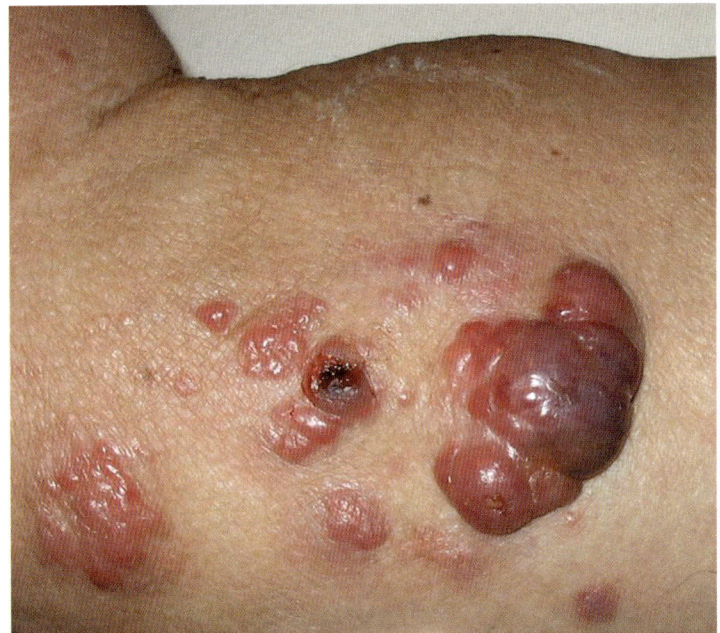

Figure 138.7 Nodular Kaposi sarcoma. Clinical lesions consist of well-demarcated, red-violaceous, firm nodules, often with accompanying lymphoedema.

Table 138.2 AIDS Clinical Trial Group staging system for Kaposi sarcoma (KS).

	0	1
Tumour (T)	Cutaneous or lymph node-only involvement with few oral macules	Oedema, ulceration, extensive oral KS with papules, extracutaneous and extranodal involvement
Immune (I)	CD4 T-cell count >150/mm^3	CD4 T-cell count <150/mm^3
Systemic (S)	No history of opportunistic infections or thrush; no B symptoms (unexplained fever, night sweats, unintentional weight loss of >10%, diarrhoea); Karnofsky performance status >70	History of opportunistic infections or thrush; one or more B symptoms; Karnofsky performance status <70; other HIV-related illness such as neurological involvement or lymphoma

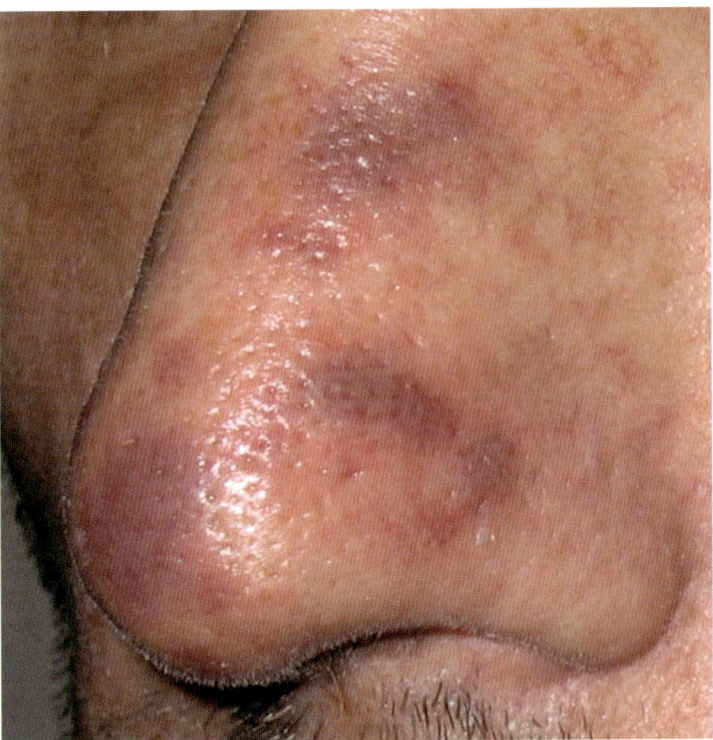

(b)

Figure 138.6 Patch-stage Kaposi sarcoma. Clinical lesions consist of violaceous to brown patches and plaques, most often involving the feet in classic KS (a) and often involving the face in AIDS-associated KS (b).

Other staging systems have been proposed as well that concentrate mostly on features of extent and rapidity of tissue involvement [94–97].

Complications and co-morbidities
KS has been associated with both Hodgkin and non-Hodgkin lymphomas [14,15,98–101] and HHV-8 has aetiological roles in multicentric Castleman disease and primary effusion lymphoma [102–104].

Disease course and prognosis
Disease outcome depends heavily upon tumour extent and systemic involvement. The ACTG T1S1 group has a 3-year survival of 53% versus over 80% for all other groups [92]. The gastrointestinal tract, particularly the small intestine, is the most common site of visceral involvement with massive haemorrhage as a serious potential complication. The lungs, heart and liver are most commonly involved but many organs may be involved [105–113]. Visceral involvement is particularly common in AIDS-associated KS with lungs, gastrointestinal tract and lymph nodes being the most common sites [105].

Investigations
Laboratory studies are typically normal in KS and direct testing for HHV-8 is not routinely used [40]. Testing for HIV status is important given the efficacy of HAART.

Management

Management depends on the clinical subtype, although no approach is definitively curative [114]. KS is highly radiosensitive with complete responses in up to 93% of patients [115]. In localised cutaneous disease, excision and cryotherapy can be used. Intralesional vinblastine, interferon-α2b and imiquimod are effective although recurrence is common [116–119]. For AIDS-associated KS, the institution of HAART to treat HIV infection often results in regression of KS, but up to 50% never achieve total remission [120]. Similarly, diminution or cessation of immunosuppression in iatrogenic KS can lead to the regression of lesions. In this setting, sirolimus has been reported mostly to induce the regression of KS [121–125]. Disseminated KS is responsive to therapy, although no definitive regimen is established given the lack of large, well-controlled clinical trials. However, response rates of over 70% are reported with liposomal doxorubicin, vinca alkaloids, etoposide and taxanes [114,126–137]. Liposomal doxorubicin and paclitaxel are approved by the US Food and Drug Administration as first line and second line treatments, respectively, for advanced KS. In resource-limited settings where AIDS-associated KS predominates and anthracyclines are not readily available, paclitaxel was superior to oral etoposide and the combination of bleomycin and vincristine, together with ART [**138**] with a 50% progression-free survival at 48 weeks. Pegylated doxorubicin achieved an 80% response rate in this setting [139]. Bortezomib has also demonstrated activity in the setting of AIDS [140]. There are also anecdotal reports of responses to imatinib and sorafenib [141–143].

Importantly, the advent of immunotherapy has also impacted KS and several reports detail therapeutic success using nivolumab or pembrolizumab (anti-PD1), including in the AIDS-associated setting [144,145,**146**], as well as with combined anti-CTLA4 (ipilimumab) and anti-PD1 (nivolumab) therapy [147].

Key references

The full list of references can be found in the online version at https://www.wiley.com/rooksdermatology10e

2 Dupin N. Update on oncogenesis and therapy for Kaposi sarcoma. *Curr Opin Oncol* 2020;32:122–8.

3 Cesarman E, Damania B, Krown SE, Martin J, Bower M, Whitby D. Kaposi sarcoma. *Nat Rev Dis Primers* 2019;5:9.

13 Dourmishev LA, Dourmishev AL, Palmeri D, Schwartz RA, Lukac DM. Molecular genetics of Kaposi's sarcoma-associated herpesvirus (human herpesvirus-8) epidemiology and pathogenesis. *Microbiol Mol Biol Rev* 2003;67:175–212.

50 Chang Y, Cesarman E, Pessin MS et al. Identification of herpesvirus-like DNA sequences in AIDS-associated Kaposi's sarcoma. *Science* 1994;266(5192):1865–9.

63 Ruocco E, Ruocco V, Tornesello ML, Gambardella A, Wolf R, Buonaguro FM. Kaposi's sarcoma: etiology and pathogenesis, inducing factors, causal associations, and treatments: facts and controversies. *Clin Dermatol* 2013;31:413–22.

90 Krown SE, Testa MA, Huang J. AIDS-related Kaposi's sarcoma: prospective validation of the AIDS Clinical Trials Group staging classification. AIDS Clinical Trials Group Oncology Committee. *J Clin Oncol* 1997;15:3085–92.

92 Nasti G, Talamini R, Antinori A et al. AIDS-related Kaposi's sarcoma: evaluation of potential new prognostic factors and assessment of the AIDS Clinical Trial Group Staging System in the Haart Era – the Italian Cooperative Group on AIDS and Tumors and the Italian Cohort of Patients Naive From Antiretrovirals. *J Clin Oncol* 2003;21:2876–82.

138 Krown SE, Moser CB, MacPhail P et al. Treatment of advanced AIDS-associated Kaposi sarcoma in resource-limited settings: a three-arm, open-label, randomised, non-inferiority trial. *Lancet* 2020;395(10231):1195–207.

146 Galanina N, Goodman AM, Cohen PR, Frampton GM, Kurzrock R. Successful treatment of HIV-associated Kaposi sarcoma with immune checkpoint blockade. *Cancer Immunol Res* 2018;6:1129–35.

CHAPTER 139

Cutaneous Lymphomas

Sean J. Whittaker

St John's Institute of Dermatology, Guy's and St Thomas' NHS Foundation Trust, London, UK; School of Basic and Medical Biosciences, Kings College London, London, UK

Introduction, 139.1

PRIMARY CUTANEOUS T-CELL LYMPHOMAS, 139.2
Introduction and general description, 139.2
Mycosis fungoides, 139.2
Follicular mucinosis, 139.14
Pagetoid reticulosis, 139.15
Granulomatous slack skin disease, 139.16
Sézary syndrome, 139.16
Molecular features of mycosis fungoides and Sézary syndrome, 139.19
Management of mycosis fungoides and Sézary syndrome, 139.20
Skin-directed therapy, 139.21
Systemic therapy, 139.22

PRIMARY CUTANEOUS CD30+ LYMPHOPROLIFERATIVE DISORDERS, 139.25
Introduction and general description, 139.25
Lymphomatoid papulosis, 139.26
Primary cutaneous anaplastic (CD30+) large-cell lymphoma, 139.28

PRIMARY CUTANEOUS T-CELL LYMPHOMA VARIANTS, 139.29
Introduction and general description, 139.29
Subcutaneous panniculitis-like T-cell lymphoma, 139.29
Primary cutaneous aggressive epidermotropic CD8+ T-cell lymphoma, 139.31
Primary cutaneous γδ T-cell lymphoma, 139.32
Primary cutaneous CD4+ small/medium pleomorphic T-cell lymphoproliferative disorder (provisional), 139.33
Primary cutaneous acral CD8+ T-cell lymphoma (provisional), 139.33
Adult T-cell leukaemia–lymphoma (HTLV-1 associated), 139.34
Extranodal NK/T-cell lymphoma (nasal type), 139.36

PRIMARY CUTANEOUS B-CELL LYMPHOMAS, 139.37
Introduction and general description, 139.37
Primary cutaneous marginal zone lymphoma, 139.38

Primary cutaneous follicle centre cell lymphoma, 139.40
Primary cutaneous diffuse large B-cell lymphoma, 139.41

SECONDARY CUTANEOUS B-CELL LYMPHOMAS, 139.43
Intravascular large B-cell lymphoma, 139.43
Lymphomatoid granulomatosis, 139.44

SECONDARY CUTANEOUS T-CELL LYMPHOMAS, 139.45
Angioimmunoblastic T-cell lymphoma, 139.45

OTHER DISORDERS, 139.45
Blastic plasmacytoid dendritic cell neoplasm (CD4+/CD56+ haematodermic neoplasm), 139.45
Post-transplant lymphoproliferative disorder, 139.47
Leukaemia cutis, 139.47
Cutaneous manifestations of Hodgkin disease, 139.48

Key references, 139.49

Introduction

Advances in the biology of lymphoid cells have greatly improved our classification and understanding of the pathogenesis of primary cutaneous lymphomas. Specifically, the 2018 World Health Organization (WHO) classification is based on clinical, pathological, immunopathological, molecular and cytogenetic findings [1]. It implicitly recognises that the site of origin of extranodal lymphomas and tumour morphology determines clinical behaviour, which in turn has a critical influence on prognosis and therapeutic approach.

In 1975, it was demonstrated that the majority of lymphoid infiltrates associated with the skin were of T-cell type and Edelson introduced the term cutaneous T-cell lymphoma (CTCL). In Europe, the Dutch Cutaneous Lymphoma Working Party (DCLWP) and the Austrian Graz group delineated different subsets of primary cutaneous T- and B-cell lymphomas, which led directly to the European Organization of Research and Treatment of Cancer (EORTC) proposal for the classification of primary cutaneous lymphomas (Table 139.1) [2] which is now reflected in the 2018 WHO classification of haematological malignancies [1].

Mycosis fungoides (MF) and its variants are the most common primary CTCL subset, but other subsets with clearly identifiable clinicopathological features and varying prognoses have also been described. A critical observation has been the realisation that lymphomas with a similar pathology arising in different organs have different prognoses and distinct pathogenesis: nodal CD30+ anaplastic large-cell lymphomas are usually anaplastic lymphoma kinase (ALK) positive but ALK-negative variants are associated with a poor prognosis, whereas primary cutaneous CD30+ anaplastic large-cell lymphomas are invariably ALK negative and have a good prognosis [2]. The majority of primary cutaneous B-cell lymphomas also have an excellent prognosis [2], and primary cutaneous follicle centre lymphomas are pathogenetically distinct from nodal follicular lymphomas. Furthermore, it is appreciated

Table 139.1 WHO–EORTC 2018 classification of primary cutaneous lymphomas (frequency and prognosis based on Dutch and Austrian clinical data, 2002–2017).

WHO–EORTC classification	Frequency (%)	Disease-specific 5-year survival (%)
Primary cutaneous T-cell lymphoma		
Indolent clinical behaviour:		
Mycosis fungoides	39	88
Folliculotropic mycosis fungoides	5	75
Pagetoid reticulosis	<1	100
Granulomatous slack skin disease	<1	100
Primary cutaneous anaplastic large cell lymphoma	8	95
Lymphomatoid papulosis	12	99
Subcutaneous panniculitis-like T-cell lymphoma	1	87
Primary cutaneous CD4+ small/medium pleomorphic T-cell lymphoproliferative disorder[a]	6	100
Primary cutaneous acral CD8+ T-cell lymphoma[a]	<1	100
Aggressive clinical behaviour:		
Sézary syndrome	2	36
Primary cutaneous NK/T-cell lymphoma, nasal type	<1	16
Primary cutaneous epidermotropic CD8+ T-cell lymphoma[a]	<1	31
Primary cutaneous γδ T-cell lymphoma	<1	11
Primary cutaneous peripheral T-cell lymphoma, (NOS)	2	15
Cutaneous B-cell lymphoma		
Indolent clinical behaviour		
Primary cutaneous marginal zone B-cell lymphoma	9	99
Primary cutaneous follicle centre cell lymphoma	12	95
EBV+ mucocutaneous ulcer[a]	<1	100
Intermediate clinical behaviour:		
Primary cutaneous diffuse large B-cell lymphoma, leg type	4	56
Primary cutaneous diffuse large B-cell lymphoma, other	<1	50
Primary cutaneous intravascular large B-cell lymphoma	<1	72

Adapted from Willemze *et al*. 2019 [2].
[a] Provisional entities.
EBV, Epstein–Barr virus; EORTC, European Organization of Research and Treatment of Cancer; NK, natural killer; NOS, not otherwise specified; NR, not reached; WHO, World Health Organization.

that cutaneous and systemic T-cell lymphomas are usually derived from specific tissue-resident T-cell subsets (Figure 139.1).

PRIMARY CUTANEOUS T-CELL LYMPHOMAS

Introduction and general description

The most common type of primary CTCL is MF, which is characterised by distinct clinicopathological features but is closely related to other subtypes of CTCL such as Sézary syndrome (SS). Indeed patients may have coexistent MF and lymphomatoid papulosis due to the same T-cell clone. In addition there are numerous clinical variants of MF that can make diagnosis challenging, and MF can clinically mimic other T-cell-mediated inflammatory dermatoses. However, there are a number of rare CTCL variants that must be distinguished from classic MF as their treatment and prognoses are different.

The concept of a subset of circulating lymphocytes with a special avidity or affinity for the skin has been supported by the identification of T cells expressing the cutaneous lymphocyte antigen (CLA), which binds to its ligand, E-selectin, on dermal endothelial cells [1]. These subsets of skin-trafficking T cells comprise the skin-associated lymphoid tissue, and contribute to skin immunity, in a similar manner to other mucosal sites such as gut mucosa-associated lymphoid tissue (MALT). The expression of the chemokine receptors CCR4 and CCR10 by tumour cells may also contribute to epidermotropism in CTCL, while the expression of the lymph node chemokine receptor CCR7 may contribute to tumour dissemination in SS [2]. There is now considerable evidence that mature T-cell malignancies are derived from specific subsets of mature tissue-resident T cells and accumulating evidence that MF is derived from skin-resident effector memory T cells, whereas SS is derived from central memory T cells (Figure 139.1) [3].

The completion of several large international randomised controlled trials in CTCL has been facilitated by consensus clinical end points and response criteria for MF and SS, which has led to regulatory approval of novel therapies [4].

Mycosis fungoides

Definition

This is the most common variant of primary CTCL; it is generally associated with an indolent clinical course and is characterised by well-defined clinicopathological features.

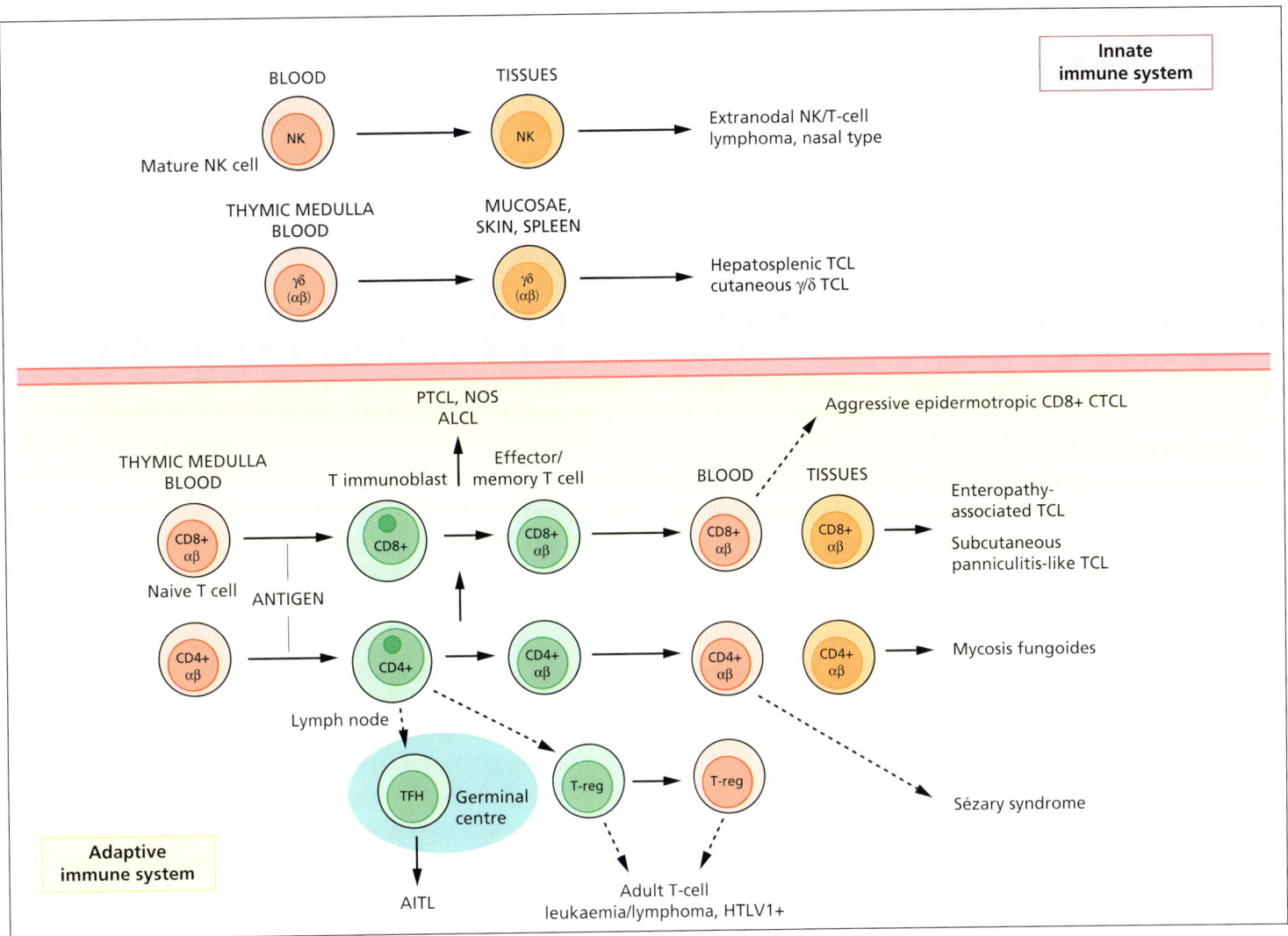

Figure 139.1 Cell of origin for mature T-cell leukaemia–lymphomas. AITL, angioimmunoblastic T-cell lymphoma; ALCL, anaplastic large-cell lymphoma; CTCL, cutaneous T-cell lymphoma; HTLV, human T-cell leukaemia virus; NK, natural killer; NOS, not otherwise specified; PTCL, peripheral T-cell lymphoma; TCL, T-cell lymphoma; TFH, T follicular helper.

Epidemiology

The incidence of MF (0.64/100 000) is increasing but the explanation for this is unclear. The rise could represent a combination of improved diagnosis and previous incorrect coding as well as a genuine increasing disease incidence, as seen for other non-Hodgkin lymphoma [1].

Pathophysiology
Predisposing factors

The human T-cell leukaemia virus 1 (HTLV-1) retrovirus was first isolated from a patient with CTCL but subsequently it was appreciated that this patient had a distinct lymphoma, namely adult T-cell leukaemia–lymphoma (ATLL). There are striking clinical and pathological similarities between MF and cutaneous involvement in ATLL, but studies have failed to identify HTLV-associated viruses in MF. A higher proportion of patients working in the petrochemical, textile, machine and metal industries has been reported in CTCL patients, and other case–control studies have suggested possible links with occupational exposure to glass, pottery and ceramics. A significantly higher incidence of allergies and skin infections compared with healthy controls and an increased incidence of atopic disease have also been reported in MF patients with reports of CTCL developing in patients with severe atopic eczema [1]. However, an association with atopic disease was not confirmed in one case–control study [2], and links to occupational or environmental exposure have also not been confirmed.

In contrast, studies have shown that CTCL is associated with an ultraviolet (UV) mutational signature identical to that seen in non-melanoma and melanoma skin cancers and distinct from other mature systemic T-cell lymphomas [3]. This finding confirms that UV is the major cause of mutations in CTCL and that this is not related to phototherapy. Previous studies suggested that CTCL occurs more commonly in workers exposed to solar radiation. In contrast a large epidemiological study of UV radiation exposure and incidence of non-Hodgkin lymphoma (NHL) concluded that the incidence of NHL, including CTCLs such as MF/SS, increases with distance from the equator suggesting that UV radiation has a protective effect. However, as CTCL is rare, the role of environmental UV exposure might reflect a specific susceptibility in a skin-resident T cell [3].

A large study of US Food and Drug Administration (FDA) adverse event reporting data on tumour necrosis factor α (TNF-α) inhibitors has concluded that there is an increased risk of T-cell NHL, specifically hepatosplenic and CTCL (MF/SS), in patients on TNF-α inhibitors in combination with thiopurines but not on TNF-α inhibitors alone [4]. Whether this reflects a drug effect, diagnostic issues or a specific effect of the underlying chronic inflammatory condition remains unclear.

Pathology

The histological features of MF vary according to the clinical stage [1,2]. The earliest pathological features of MF are the presence of a moderate lymphocytic infiltrate in the papillary dermis. Many of the small lymphoid cells may be hyperchromatic and show a tendency to 'line up' at the dermal–epidermal junction. Spongiosis is usually absent but can occur rarely. As the disease progresses with the development of thicker plaques, prominent epidermotropism develops (Figure 139.2), which is characterised by the selective colonisation of the epidermis by atypical T cells either by single-cell colonisation, often along the basal layer, or by clusters of atypical lymphocytes in the epidermis – so-called Pautrier microabscesses. The malignant T cells in the epidermis are often strikingly cerebriform (Figure 139.3), with a very irregular nuclear outline and heavy nuclear staining as well as a characteristic halo appearance to the cells. If these cells are examined either under high power or with thin sections, the cerebriform and irregular nature of the nuclei can be better appreciated. In early MF, the T-cell infiltrate may be associated with a number of other cell types including small numbers of plasma cells or eosinophils. However, with later stages of disease the infiltrate becomes denser, monotonous and monomorphic. Granulomatous features may be rarely present and a prominent histiocytic infiltrate can be seen, so-called interstitial MF. Whether granulomatous variants of MF have a worse prognosis is currently unclear [3] but some reports suggest such patients are more resistant to skin-directed therapies.

In more advanced stages of disease (IIB–III), the epidermotropic infiltrate may be lost, with scattered larger tumour cells showing marked cellular atypia. Large-cell transformation may also occur and is a poor prognostic feature on univariate analysis, although this does not appear to be independent of age and stage of disease on multivariate analysis [4]. Indeed large-cell transformation appears to be independently associated with an increased risk of disease progression but not overall survival on multivariate analysis [5] or when compared with those advanced disease patients without large-cell transformation. Large-cell transformation (Figure 139.4) is defined as the presence of more than 25–50% of large cells (either CD30 positive or negative) within the dermal infiltrate or the development of microscopic dermal nodules consisting of larger cells with pleomorphic and occasionally anaplastic or blastic morphology [4]. It is important to distinguish large histiocytic cells from large tumour cells with an anaplastic morphology; occasionally the presence of reactive germinal centres in MF can also cause histological confusion.

The diagnostic differentiation between large-cell transformation in MF and primary cutaneous CD30+ lymphoproliferative disorders with excellent prognoses, such as lymphomatoid papulosis or anaplastic large cell lymphoma, is crucial and based on a

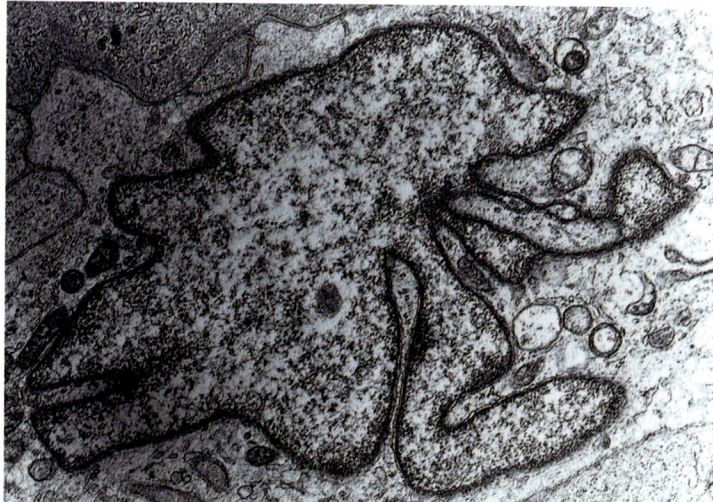

Figure 139.3 Electron micrograph of a T cell infiltrating the epidermis in mycosis fungoides, showing the striking cellular contours of the typical cell of Lutzner with a typical highly convoluted nucleus.

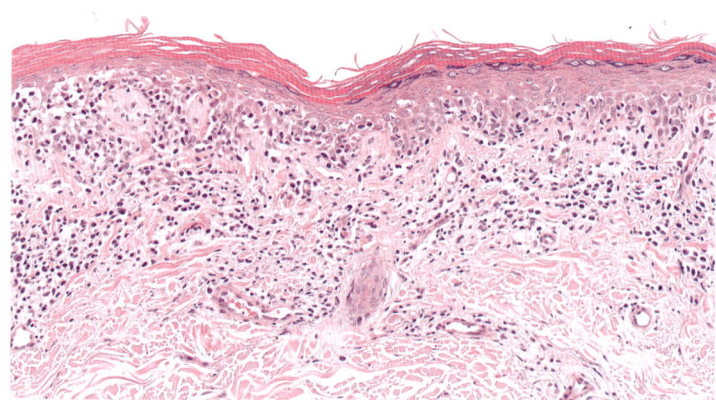

Figure 139.2 Histology of mycosis fungoides showing striking epidermotropism with the presence in the epidermis of cytologically atypical, small, dark cells proven to be CD4+ helper T lymphocytes. Courtesy of Eduardo Calonje.

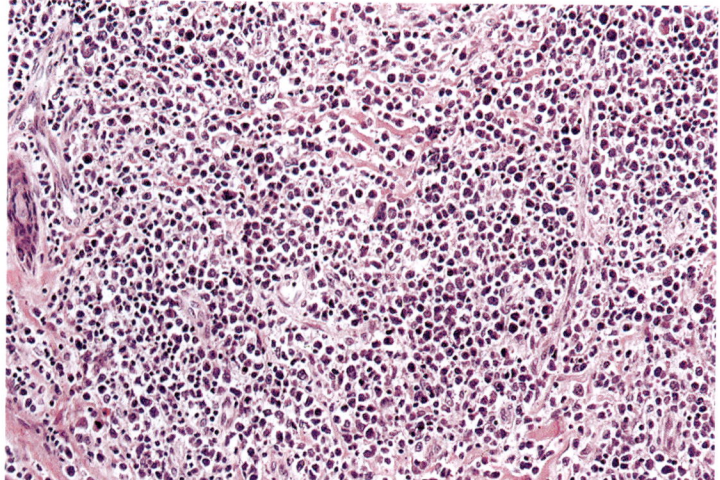

Figure 139.4 High-power view of large-cell transformation in mycosis fungoides. Courtesy of Eduardo Calonje.

careful clinical assessment of the patient. The development of large tumours in patients with typical polymorphic patches or plaques of MF would suggest large-cell transformation of MF. In contrast, the presence of more than 75% of CD30+ large cells in only one or a few isolated tumours developing in patients with no concurrent or previous clinical evidence of MF suggests that the patient has a primary cutaneous CD30+ lymphoproliferative disorder.

Immunopathology (Figure 139.5)

The tumour cells in MF are CD3+, CD4+, CD45RO+ and usually CD7− T cells. This is the phenotype of a mature helper T cell of memory subtype. The tumour cells are CLA+, CCR4+ and CCR10+, consistent with a skin homing T cell. In rare cases, the tumour cells are CD8+ rather than CD4+ but this does not appear to have any prognostic significance. Interestingly, CD8+ cases of MF are more common in childhood and in hypopigmented variants [1]. CD8+ MF must be distinguished from an epidermotropic cytotoxic variant of CTCL with a poor prognosis. Occasionally, there is a very prominent infiltrate of reactive tumour-infiltrating CD8+ T cells expressing cytotoxic proteins, which may indicate a good prognosis. The dermal infiltrate often consists of a prominent population of CD1a+ dendritic cells and CD68+ histiocytic cells. In advanced disease, tumour cells may express an aberrant phenotype with either the loss of T-cell surface antigen 'null cell phenotype' or the expression of the CD30 antigen either by scattered larger tumour cells or by prominent dermal nodules consisting of large pleomorphic or anaplastic tumour cells [2,3]. CD30 expression may or may not be associated with large-cell transformation but any prognostic significance remains unclear [3,4]. The tumour cells usually express the αβ T-cell receptor (TCR) and only rarely express cytotoxic proteins such as T-cell intracellular antigen 1 (TIA-1), perforin and granzyme. Cases of MF/SS have been reported with the immunophenotype of follicular helper T cells [5].

A subset of CD4+, CD25+ T cells has been defined with suppressive function. These regulatory T cells (T-regs) are cytotoxic T-lymphocyte antigen 4+ (CTLA4+) and express the transcription factor FoxP3. Studies in MF/SS have analysed the expression of FoxP3, as well as T-reg function, and have established that a proportion of the intraepidermal and dermal T cells in early stages of MF are FoxP3+ T cells but that this proportion decreases significantly with more advanced disease. This suggests that in MF the presence of T-regs may be a good prognostic factor and that T-regs may actually suppress the expansion of tumour cells. Whether tumour cells also function as T-regs remains to be established. CTLA4 is expressed by a proportion of Sézary cells, and Sézary cells with immunosuppressive T-reg function have only been described in a minority of SS patients.

Pathological differential diagnosis

In early MF, the main differential diagnosis includes a dermatitis reaction. The epidermotropic quality of the T-cell infiltrate in MF may be helpful, as may the cytology of the individual T cells, as in MF these intraepidermal lymphocytes tend to be larger than the surrounding keratinocytes and to have intensely stained nuclei with a very irregular outline. Spongiosis, if present in association with epidermotropic T cells or Pautrier microabscesses, is minimal, whereas this tends to be more striking in dermatitis. A useful clue may be the characteristic basal layer colonisation and the larger size of the intraepidermal T cells compared with the dermal mononuclear cells (Figure 139.6).

The pathological diagnosis of early MF can still, however, be extremely subjective and is best made in full collaboration with the clinician and only after careful correlation with the clinical features. It is often wise to take several elliptical biopsies from lesions that do not show secondary changes such as excoriation or impetiginisation, and if necessary to repeat biopsies as the clinical picture evolves over a period of months or even years. An algorithm for establishing an early clinical and histological diagnosis of MF has been proposed by the International Society for Cutaneous Lymphoma (ISCL) (Table 139.2) [1]; grading systems have also been proposed [2].

Immunophenotypic studies are usually of minimal value in differentiating early MF from other cutaneous lymphocytic infiltrates, as the majority of these cells will also be CD3+ and CD4+. However, a predominance of larger CD4+ cells within the epidermis compared with the mixed population of smaller cells within the dermis can sometimes be helpful.

The distinction of early MF from conditions such as arthropod bites and lymphomatous drug eruptions can also be difficult, and clinicopathological correlation is essential. In general, reactions to arthropod bites tend to show a higher proportion of eosinophils, and the disposition of the infiltrate in lymphomatous drug reactions will be perivascular rather than epidermotropic. In a proportion of cases, however, the diagnosis is suspected on clinical grounds but cannot confidently be made with certainty on histological examination. In these cases, sequential biopsies at 3–6-month intervals may be needed.

Pathology of extracutaneous disease

The usual pattern of extracutaneous spread is from the skin to the draining peripheral lymph nodes and rarely to visceral sites such

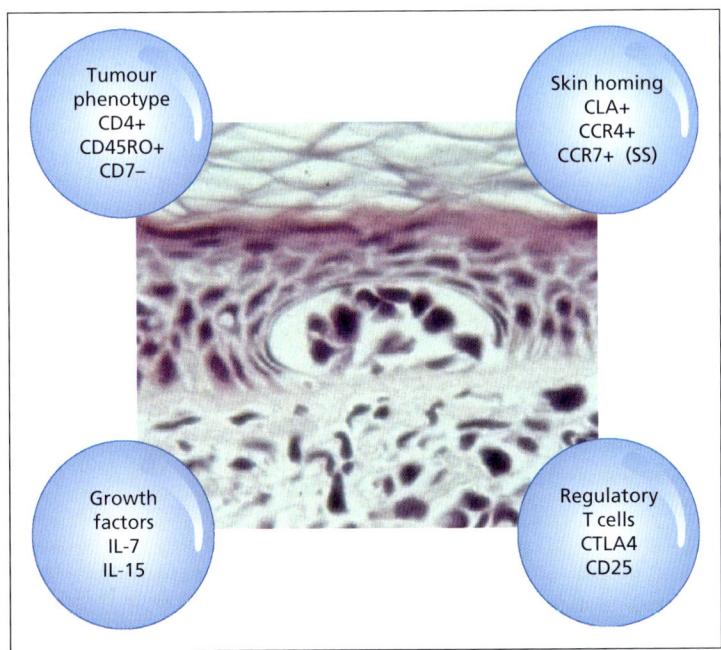

Figure 139.5 Immunopathology of mycosis fungoides/Sézary syndrome (SS). IL, interleukin.

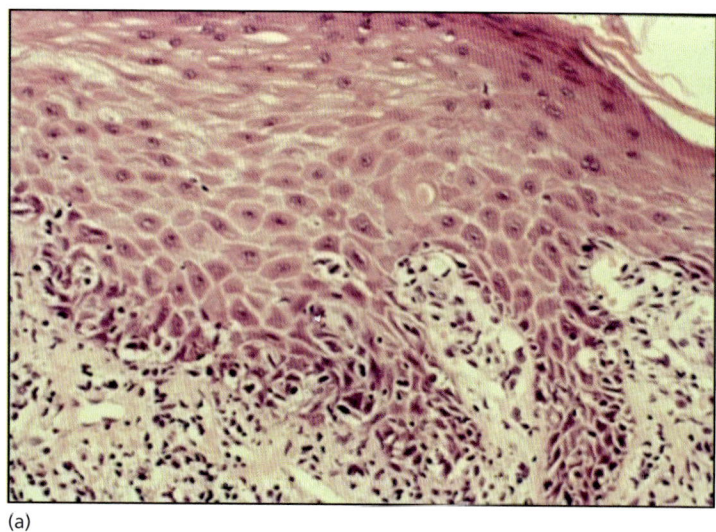

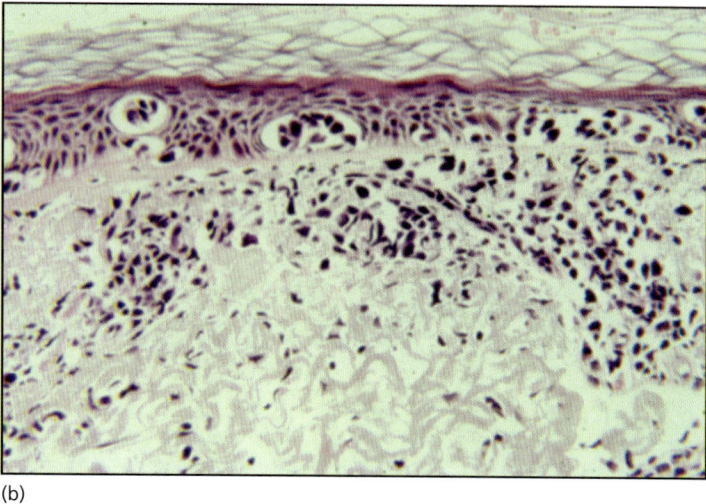

Figure 139.6 (a) Colonisation of basal layer by hyperchromatic lymphoid cells. (b) Pautrier microabscesses.

Table 139.2 International Society for Cutaneous Lymphoma diagnostic criteria for early mycosis fungoides (a total of 4 points is required for the diagnosis of MF).

Criteria	Major (2 points each)	Minor (1 point each)
Clinical Persistent and/or progressive patches and plaques **plus** 1 Non-sun-exposed location 2 Size/shape variation 3 Poikiloderma	Any 2	Any 1
Histopathological Superficial lymphoid infiltrate **plus** 1 Epidermotropism 2 Atypia	Both	Either
Molecular/biological Clonal TCR rearrangement		Present
Immunopathological 1 CD2, CD3, CD5 <50% 2 CD7 <10% 3 Epidermal discordance		Any 1

Adapted from Pimipinelli *et al.* 2005 [9].
TCR, T-cell receptor.

as pulmonary, naso-pharynx, skeletal and central nervous system (CNS) sites.

The National Cancer Institute (NCI) classification system [1] classified lymph node architecture as preserved in LN1–3 in which dermatopathic changes predominate. LN1 is characterised by single, infrequent, atypical cells; LN2 shows small clusters of atypical lymphocytes; and LN3 shows larger aggregates of atypical cells in paracortical areas. In contrast, LN4 is characterised by partial or complete effacement by atypical cells [1].

A further histological assessment of peripheral nodes was proposed by Scheffer *et al.* [2]. Those biopsies with no abnormalities are recorded as LN0 while those with dermatopathic changes are designated LN1 (dermatopathic lymphadenopathy). LN1 is characterised by enlargement of the paracortical area of the lymph node because of the presence of large numbers of macrophages and pale dendritic (interdigitating reticulum) cells (grade 1 = LN1–2). The macrophages contain aggregates both of melanin and lipid material, giving rise to the older term 'lipomelanic reticulosis'. Histological evidence of possible involvement (grade 2 = LN3) is characterised by the additional presence of small clusters of larger atypical mononuclear cells within the expanded paracortical areas (Figure 139.7). In contrast, partial (grade 3 = LN4) or complete (grade 4 = LN4) effacement of the lymph node architecture is consistent with definite lymphomatous involvement (Figure 139.7).

A comparison of these systems has shown that both have a poor prognosis for partial or totally effaced nodes, with non-effaced nodes showing no difference in survival [3]. In the WHO classification system, a modification of these classifications has been proposed whereby LN1 and LN2 have been grouped together as grade I (no histological involvement), with LN3 as grade II and LN4 as grade III, both representing definite histological involvement, although this system has not yet been validated [4]. However, there is a subtle difference in this system because in the WHO proposal, grade I can be characterised by scattered but not clusters of atypical cerebriform cells, whereas nodes showing clusters of atypical cerebriform cells are graded as II (LN3).

The ISCL–EORTC revised staging classification (Tables 139.3 and 139.4) suggests grouping lymph node biopsies N1 (with no definite histological involvement; grade 1/LN1–2), N2 (possible involvement; grade 2/LN3) and N3 (definite involvement; grade 3–4/LN4), with each group reflecting the results of TCR gene analysis as clone absent or present (a/b) [5].

T-cell receptor gene analysis

T-cell receptor gene analysis consists of analysis of DNA from tissue samples for the detection of clonal rearrangements of the TCR genes as a marker of a monoclonal T-cell population. A similar approach can be used to identify a B-cell clone using analysis of immunoglobulin genes. A clonal lymphoid population is usually synonymous with a neoplastic proliferation but this does not signify malignancy. In contrast, the malignant potential of a lymphoid clone is dependent on the underlying somatic mutations. Analysis of TCR genes in MF is now a standard approach that has diagnostic, prognostic and therapeutic implications. Most studies are based on

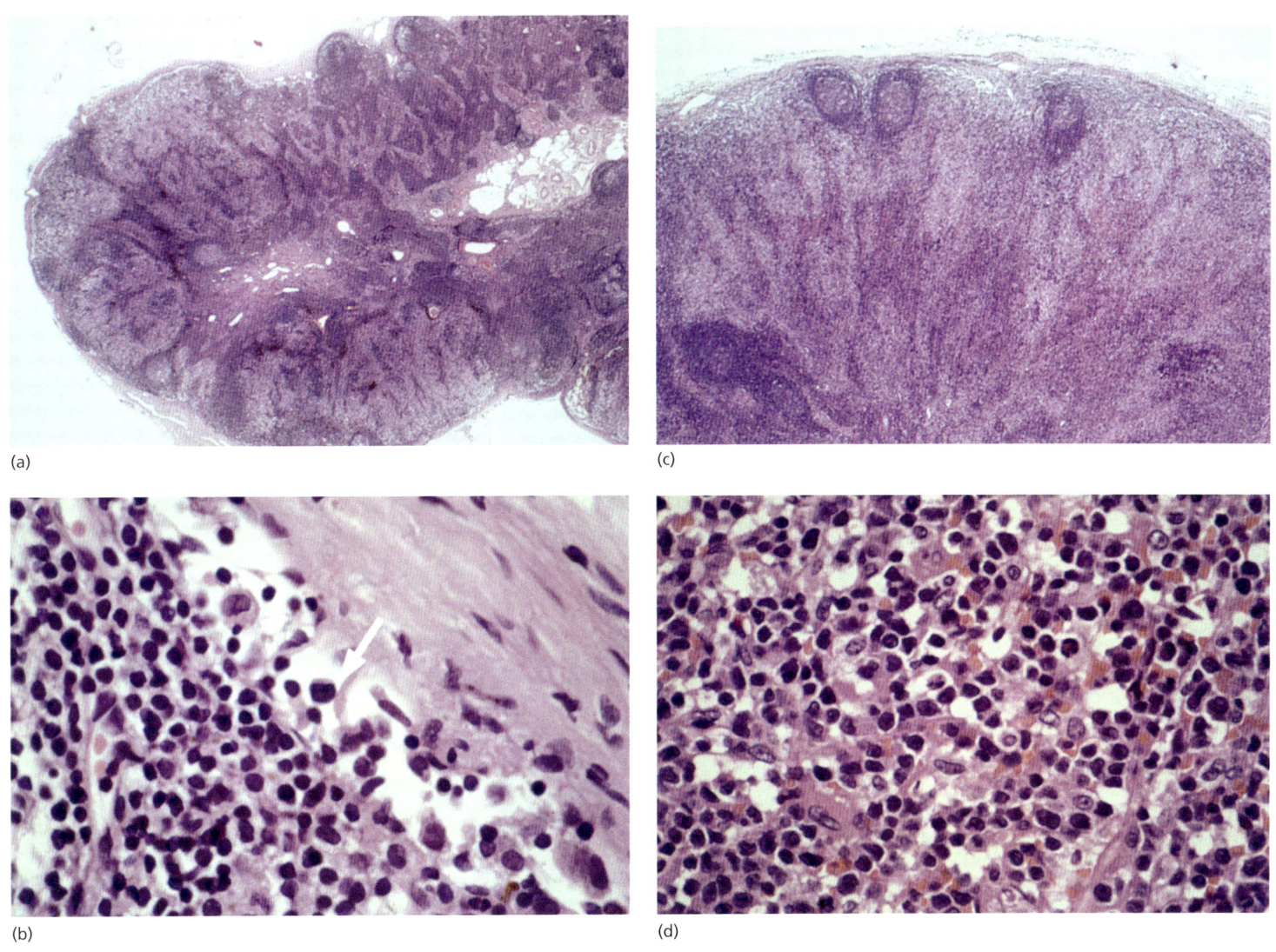

Figure 139.7 Photomicrographs showing features of dermatopathic lymphadenopathy. (a) LN1 is characterised by dermatopathic changes with melanin deposition and occasional atypical lymphocytes. (b) LN2 shows paracortical expansion of T-cell areas (arrow points at an atypical cell). (c, d) LN3–LN4 shows lymph node effacement by small- and medium-sized atypical convoluted cells ((d) high power view).

Table 139.3 Clinical staging system for mycosis fungoides related to the TNM classification.

Stage	T (tumour)	N (node)	M (metastasis)	B (blood)
IA	T1a/b	N0	M0	B0–1
IB	T2a/b	N0	M0	B0–1
IIA	T1–2	N1	M0	B0–1
IIB	T3	N0–2	M0	B0–1
IIIA	T4	N0–2	M0	B0
IIIB	T4	N0–2	M0	B1
IVA1	T1–4	N0-2	M0	B2
IVA2	T1–4	N3	M0	B0–2
IVB	T1–4	N0–3	M1	B0–2

Adapted from Olsen *et al.* 2007 [15].

sensitive polymerase chain reaction (PCR) techniques and several different platforms are employed including denaturing gradient gel electrophoresis (DGGE), temperature gradient gel electrophoresis (TGGE), single-strand conformational gel electrophoresis (SSCP) and Genescan analysis of the γ and β TCR genes [1,2]. These different methodologies have not been compared adequately for cutaneous lymphomas but most results are broadly consistent and standardisation has been partly achieved by the use of Biomed 2 primers for the γ and β TCR genes [3]. High-throughput sequencing platforms have also been applied to TCR and immunoglobulin (Ig) gene analysis, and are emerging as potential sensitive platforms especially for the detection of minimal residual disease [4].

T-cell clones can be detected in a proportion (*c.*70% overall) of skin biopsies from patients with early-stage disease and are almost invariable in patients with later stages of disease [1]. The lack of T-cell clones in all patients with early stages of disease almost certainly reflects a lack of sensitivity of the technique, although studies have shown that those early-stage patients without a T-cell clone achieve a higher complete remission rate with skin-directed therapy than those with a T-cell clone [5]. This suggests that the proportion of non-tumour cells in the infiltrate, possibly reflecting the host immune response, may also be critical. Identical T-cell clones can be detected in the peripheral blood of a proportion of patients with

Table 139.4 Revised American Joint Committee on Cancer staging classification for mycosis fungoides/Sézary syndrome.

TNMB stage	Description
Skin	
T1	Limited patches, papules and plaques covering <10% of the skin surface; may further stratify into T1a (patch only) versus T1b (plaque ± patch)
T2	Patches, papules and plaques covering ≥10% of the skin surface; may further stratify into T2a (patch only) versus T2b (plaque ± patch)
T3	One or more tumours (≥1 cm diameter)
T4	Confluence of erythroderma covering ≥80% body surface area
Node	
N0	No clinically abnormal peripheral lymph nodes; biopsy not required
N1	Clinically abnormal peripheral lymph nodes; histopathology Dutch grade 1 or NCI LN0–2
N1a	Clone negative
N1b	Clone positive
N2	Clinically abnormal peripheral lymph nodes; histopathology Dutch grade 2 or NCI LN3
N2a	Clone negative
N2b	Clone positive
N3	Clinically abnormal peripheral lymph nodes; histopathology Dutch grades 3–4 or NCI LN4; clone positive or negative
NX	Clinically abnormal peripheral lymph nodes; no histological conformation
Visceral	
M0	No visceral organ involvement
M1	Visceral involvement (must have pathology confirmation and organ involved should be specified)
Blood	
B0	Absence of significant blood involvement; ≤5% of peripheral blood lymphocytes are atypical (Sézary cells)
B0a	Clone negative
B0b	Clone positive (identical to skin T-cell clone)
B1	Low blood tumour burden; >5% of peripheral blood lymphocytes are atypical (Sézary cells) but does not meet the criteria of B2
B1a	Clone negative
B1b	Clone positive (identical to skin T-cell clone)
B2	High blood tumour burden; ≥1000/μL Sézary cells with positive clones

Reproduced from Olsen *et al.* 2007 [15] with permission of Elsevier.
NCI, National Cancer Institute.

all stages of disease and this has independent prognostic significance (stage B0b) [1,4,5]. In contrast, peripheral blood T-cell clones can also be detected that are not identical to the original tumour clone in the skin. Such peripheral blood T-cell clones may not be pathological, emphasising that results from all samples must be carefully compared. In patients with both MF and lymphomatoid papulosis, identical T-cell clones can be found, indicating a common pathogenesis but different phenotype. T-cell clones identical to those in the skin can also be detected in dermatopathic lymph nodes (LN1–LN2/N1b) and this might provide independent prognostic information, although larger studies are required to prove this conclusively [6]. The assessment of enlarged lymph nodes with fine-needle aspirate in CTCL has shown that T-cell clones cannot be detected with the same frequency compared with core biopsies or excised nodes, suggesting sampling error. Because of the sensitivity of these PCR-based techniques, T-cell clones or oligoclonal proliferations are rarely detected in non-neoplastic inflammatory disorders and therefore it is critical that the presence or absence of a clonal TCR gene rearrangement is always interpreted in conjunction with the clinical and pathological features. PCR-based studies have also detected clonal T-cell proliferations in some cases of pityriasis lichenoides acuta, small- and large-plaque parapsoriasis and pityriasis lichenoides chronica [7,8]. The clinical significance of these findings is unclear at present, although these results would support clinical impressions that large-plaque parapsoriasis probably represents early-stage MF. T-cell clones are detected rarely in small-plaque parapsoriasis, which is generally thought to be an inflammatory condition not related to MF, although patients require careful follow-up. The findings in pityriasis lichenoides acuta support previous suggestions that this represents part of a spectrum with lymphomatoid papulosis, and, intriguingly, lesions resembling pityriasis lichenoides chronica can be associated with MF [8].

Molecular features

The molecular features of MF and SS are discussed later in this chapter.

Clinical features

Presentation

Mycosis fungoides is specifically characterised by polymorphic patches and plaques usually involving limb/girdle sites, the breast and especially the buttock area. Only about 34% of patients progress from having limited patches and plaques to extensive plaques or tumours and even erythroderma, which is usually associated with severe pruritus [1]. MF is characterised by subtle and variable fine, scaly and often slightly atrophic (wrinkled) red patches (Figure 139.8), which may be associated with mild pruritus but patients are often asymptomatic. Plaques are more obvious, persistent, polymorphic, red lesions with a similar distribution (Figure 139.9). Individual plaques may become very large, and there may be some degree of regression, giving rise to unusual arcuate lesions that can show considerable variation in colour, degree of scaling and border definition. Striking psoriasiform scaling can sometimes be a feature. Once again, patients may complain of pruritus or be asymptomatic. Rarely, individual plaques may become eroded or ulcerated and painful, which is often associated with secondary bacterial infection and such patients may have a very poor quality of life and high morbidity despite having an early stage of disease. Tumours can show considerable variation in size (Figure 139.10). A *tumeur d'emblée* form of MF, in which patients rapidly develop large nodules and tumours without the prior presence of patches and plaques, has been described, but it is now appreciated that many of these patients have other CTCL variants, which should be excluded on the basis of a critical assessment of the histological and immunophenotypic features. Patients may also rarely present with erythroderma and the differential diagnosis for these patients includes inflammatory dermatoses and SS.

The development of peripheral lymphadenopathy in MF may be associated with typical 'B' symptoms such as drenching night sweats and weight loss. Histological involvement of the central lymph nodes and other organs is a very poor prognostic sign. Any systemic organ can be involved but the most common visceral sites

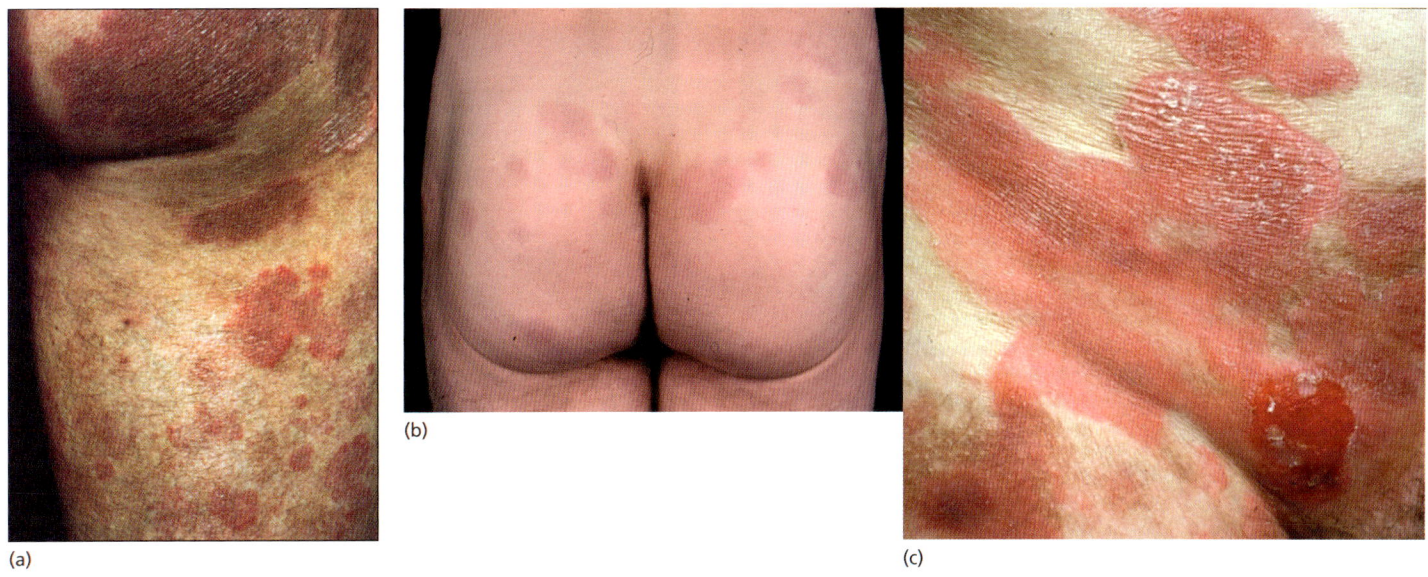

Figure 139.8 (a–c) Mycosis fungoides: patches and plaques showing typical morphology characterised by variable shape, colour, scale and thickness and distribution with involvement of the pelvic girdle area.

involved include the pulmonary, skeletal, naso-pharyngeal and central nervous system.

Clinical variants

There are a large number of clinical variants of MF (Box 139.1; Figure 139.11). Some plaques have a verrucous or hyperkeratotic appearance, and bullae may rarely develop from individual plaques. Rare ichthyosiform variants have been described. An important subset of patients have MF that appears to involve pilo-sebaceous follicles, giving rise to a follicular clinical pattern often with alopecia and occasionally boggy plaques with mucinorrhoea (pilotropic or folliculotropic MF). There is evidence that these patients may be resistant to treatment and have a poorer prognosis independent of their stage of disease [1]. Rarely, younger patients present with a purpuric eruption not unlike the pigmented purpuric dermatosis associated with capillaritis but with histological features of MF. Non-white, younger adult patients may also present with a hypopigmented variant of MF, characterised by striking hypopigmented scaly patches often involving the trunk and especially the pelvic girdle area rather than the limbs. Histologically in contrast to the subtle clinical features, these lesions tend to show marked epidermotropism and loss of melanocytes probably due to a direct cytotoxic effect of the CD8+ tumour cells [2]. In poikilodermatous MF, patients develop clinical lesions characterised by either widespread or isolated poikiloderma, which may or may not be associated with typical patches and plaques of MF. The trunk is usually involved and the breasts and pelvic girdle area may also be affected (Figure 139.12). The poikiloderma is typically characterised by atrophy, pigmentation and telangiectasia, and must be distinguished from poikiloderma resulting from other disorders by appropriate histology. Rarely, patients may have extensive poikiloderma as a feature of erythrodermic disease. These clinical variants do not have any prognostic significance with the exception of folliculotropic/pilotropic MF [1]. Solitary MF is a controversial entity in which patients may subsequently develop multiple characteristic polymorphic patches and plaques, but the prognosis is excellent.

> **Box 139.1 Clinical variants of mycosis fungoides**
>
> - Folliculotropic/pilotropic
> - Poikiloderma
> - Hypopigmented
> - Capillaritis-like
> - Verrucous/hyperkeratotic
> - Psoriasiform
> - Icthyosiform
> - Bullous

Differential diagnosis

In the early stages of MF, the clinical differential diagnosis may include such diverse conditions as allergic contact dermatitis, atopic eczema, pityriasis rosea, psoriasis and fungal infections. Any patient with persistent polymorphic patches and plaques, particularly involving the pelvic girdle area, should have a skin biopsy and histological confirmation of the disease. The diagnosis of MF must then be based on a combination of the clinical and pathological features. Clinicopathological criteria for the early diagnosis of MF have been published by the ISCL (see Table 139.2) [1].

Staging and classification

The revised ISCL and EORTC staging system for MF and SS [1] distinguishes patients with early stage IA/IB who only have patches, and stratifies peripheral blood and nodal status as well as molecular findings (see Tables 139.3 and 139.4) [1]. The prognostic value of this staging system has been validated (Figure 139.13) [2]. Patients with patches involving <10% of the skin surface area (IA) are distinguished from those with patches involving >10% of the skin surface area (IB), while those with patches only (T1a/T2a) are distinguished from those with patches and plaques (T1b/T2b) and this distinction has prognostic impact [2]. Early-stage patients may also have dermatopathic nodes (IIA). In contrast, advanced stage

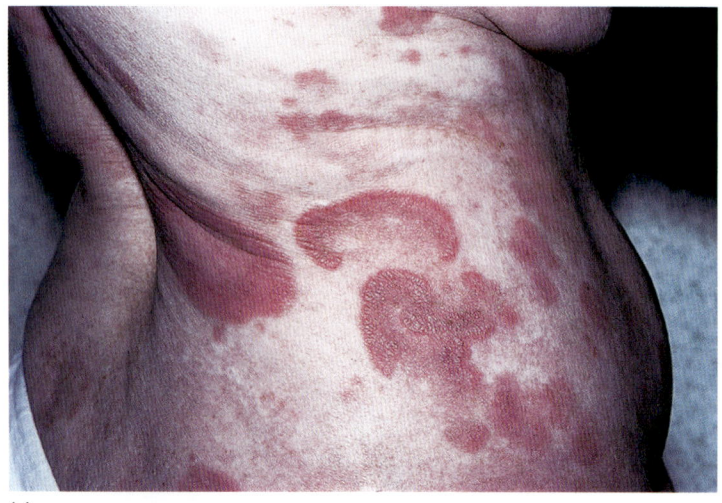

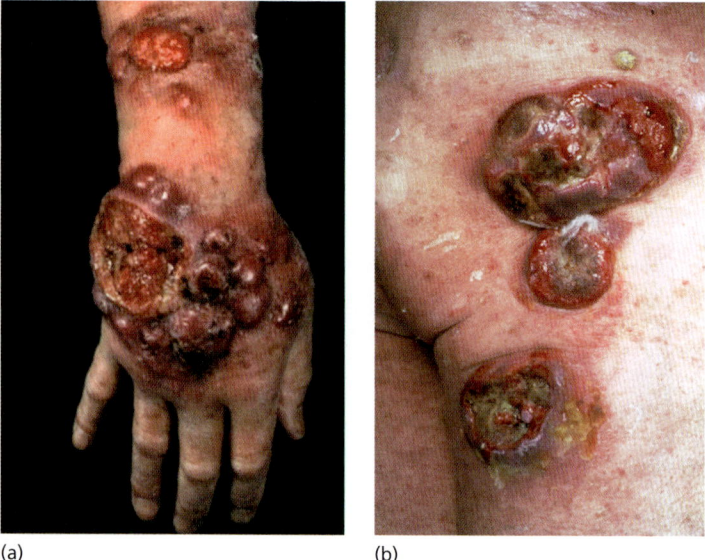

Figure 139.10 (a, b) Mycosis fungoides: extensive ulcerated skin tumours.

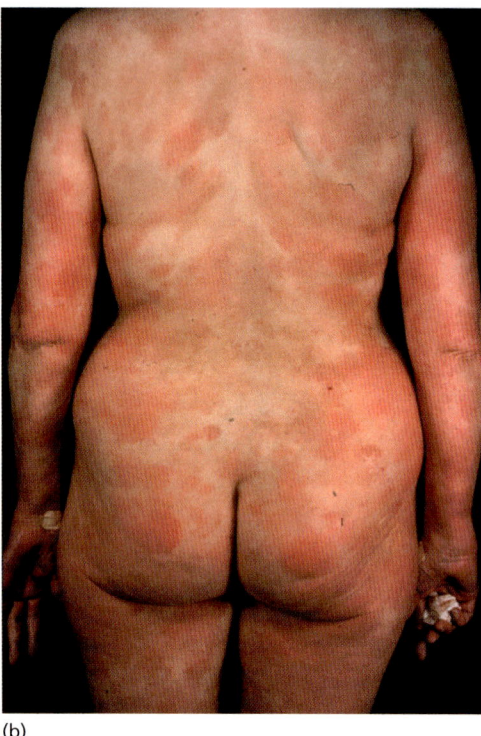

Figure 139.9 Mycosis fungoides. (a) Typical polycyclic plaques. (b) Extensive patches and thin plaques stage IB (T2b).

patients may have tumours (IIB) or erythroderma without peripheral blood involvement (IIIA) or with low-level peripheral blood involvement characterised by Sézary cells constituting >250/μL but <1000/μL on flow analysis (B1) (classified as stage IIIB). SS patients with high levels of peripheral blood (>1000/μL; B2) are also divided into those without (IVA1) or with (IVA2) nodal involvement, while those with visceral disease are classified as stage IVB.

Disease assessment

Several tools have been adopted to monitor disease response [1] including CAILS (cutaneous assessment individual lesions), which is used to assess a limited number of skin lesions based on assessment of different clinical features, and mSWAT (modified skin weighting assessment tool). The latter provides a means to assess the whole skin response based on the sum of the body surface area (BSA) of the patches, plaques and tumours (total mSWAT = patches ×1 + plaques ×2 + tumours ×4) and this approach has been adapted for erythrodermic patients. Global response criteria are now also in clinical use to combine mSWAT with assessment of nodal and blood responses. These approaches provide more rigorous assessment of disease response in randomised clinical trials [1] and are available free as a 'cutaneous lymphoma resource tools' app compatible with iOS and Android systems.

Disease course and prognosis

Age at onset (over 60 years), skin stage and the presence of nodal (IVA) or visceral (IVB) disease are independent prognostic factors in MF [1–3]. The overall survival (OS) rates at 5 and 10 years in MF are 68–80% and 53–57%, respectively, with disease-specific survival (DSS) rates of 81–89% and 75% at 5 and 10 years, respectively, and an overall risk of progression of 34% (Tables 139.5 and 139.6). In contrast, SS patients (T4, N1–3, M0, B2) have a poor prognosis, with an overall median survival of 32 months from diagnosis [1–4].

A wide variety of clinical (thick plaques), histological (granulomatous) and haematological (eosinophilia) features have been suggested to have prognostic significance in MF but generally these conclusions are based on small cohort studies that have lacked adequate statistical power [1–3]. Multivariate analysis has identified risk factors for progression and survival in a large cohort of 1502 MF/SS patients (Table 139.6; Figure 139.13) [4]. Specifically, male gender and age (>60 years) are key risk factors. The presence of plaques (T1b/T2b), histological evidence of folliculotropic disease and palpable or histologically confirmed dermatopathic peripheral nodes (N1/Nx) are also critical prognostic factors in early-stage MF [4]. Thus, while patients with early-stage IA MF are unlikely to die of their disease, patients with stage IB have a variable prognosis (84% overall 5-year survival), which is partly determined by age, gender, the presence or absence of folliculotropism, plaques and a peripheral blood T-cell clone identical to that in the skin (B0b) [4,5].

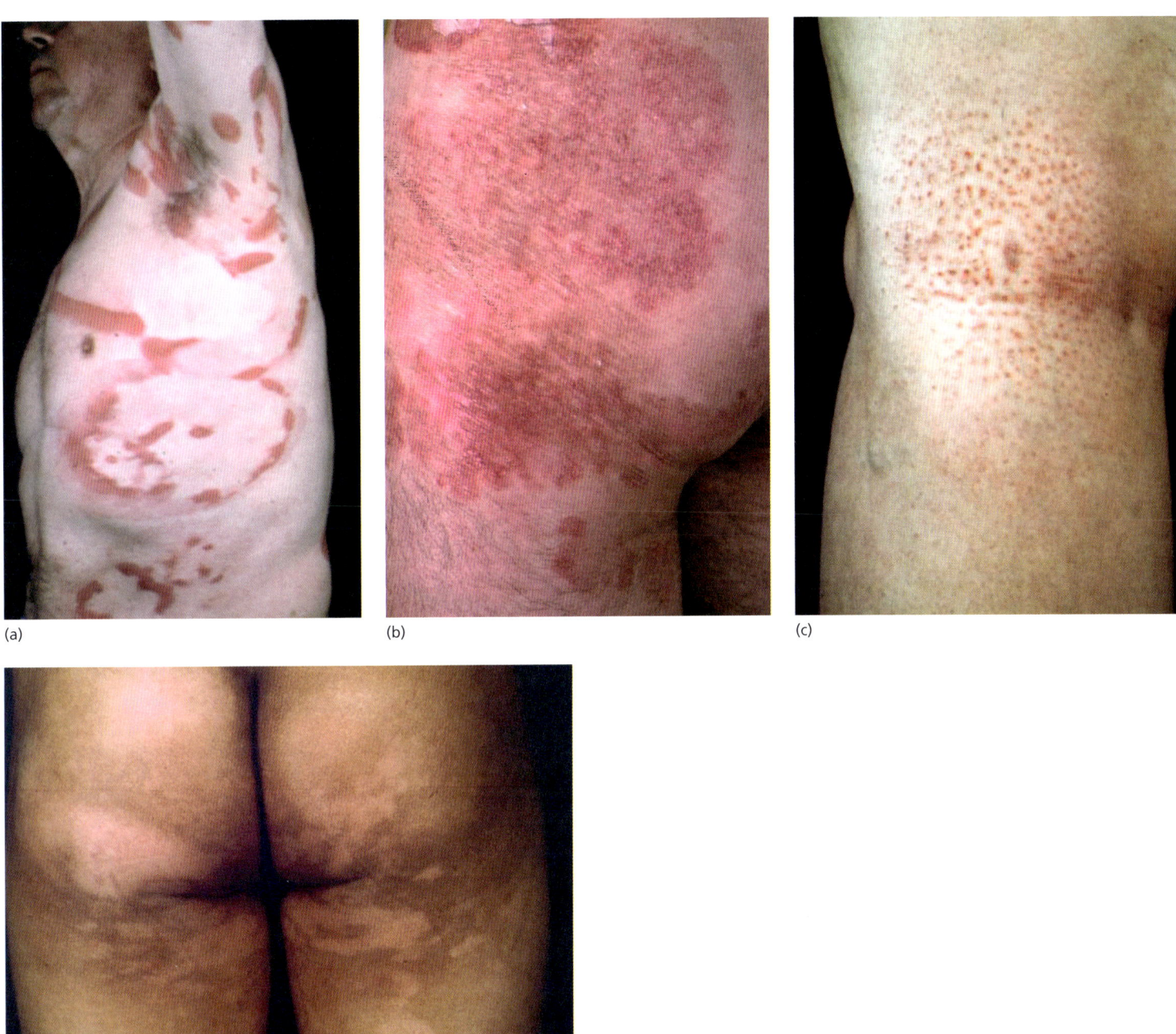

Figure 139.11 Clinical variants of mycosis fungoides: (a) annular/polycyclic; (b) poikilodermatous; (c) folliculotropic; (d) hypopigmented.

Patients with tumours (IIB) have a poor prognosis (40–65% 5-year survival) but the published data show marked variation, probably reflecting the heterogeneous nature of stage IIB MF both in terms of tumour burden and biology [1–4]. The 5-year survival for stage III erythrodermic MF patients (40–47%), without evidence of lymph node or peripheral blood involvement, is broadly similar to stage IIB MF. In contrast the prognosis for stage IV patients is poor (5-year OS 18–34%) depending on the presence of peripheral blood (IVA1), nodal disease (IVA2) or visceral disease (IVB) [1–6].

Recently, a cutaneous lymphoma prognostic index (CLIPi) has been proposed based on modelling these independent multivariate prognostic factors (Table 139.7). This defines separate models for early- and late-stage disease with five risk factors in each group defining significantly different prognostic groups (early-stage model: male gender, age, presence of plaques, folliculotropism, palpable or dermatopathic nodes; late-stage model: male gender, age, blood, nodal or visceral involvement). This now forms the basis for a prospective study (ProCLIPi) to define a prognostic index with which to stratify patients for future clinical trials and treatment decision (Figure 139.14).

A high incidence of second malignancies in MF patients is seen, notably non-melanoma skin cancer and pulmonary small cell lung cancer. A smaller incidence of melanoma also occurs. It is, however, unclear whether these malignancies are related to prior therapy [7].

Table 139.5 Published prognostic data for mycosis fungoides patients from diagnosis.

	Clinical stage										
	IA (%)	IB (%)	IIA (%)	IIB (%)	III (%)	IVA (%)	IVB (%)	Overall (%)	Reference	No. in study	Med FU (years)
OS at 5 years	99	86	49	65		40	0	80	Doorn et al. 2000 [2]	309	5.2
	100	84		52	57				Zackheim et al. 1999 [3]	489	4.7
	97	72		40	41	27	27	68	Kim et al. 2003 [1]	525	5.5
OS at 10 years	84	61	49	27		20	0	57	Doorn et al. 2000 [2]	309	5.2
	100	67		39	41				Zackheim et al. 1999 [3]	489	4.7
	88	55		26	24			53	Kim et al. 2003 [1]	525	5.5
DSS at 5 years	100	96	68	80		40	0	89	Doorn et al. 2000 [2]	309	5.2
	100	95	84	56	65	30	30	81	Kim et al. 2003 [1]	525	5.5
DSS at 10 years	97	83	68	42		20	0	75	Doorn et al. 2000 [2]	309	5.2
DSS at 15 years	98	85	71	32	49	14	14	74	Kim et al. 2003 [1]	525	5.5
Median survival	NR	12.1 years		3.3 years	4.0 years	1.2	0.7		Kim et al. 2003 [1]	556	9.8
Disease progression (5 years)	4	21	65	32		70	100		Doorn et al. 2000 [2]	309	5.2
	10	22		56	48				Kim et al. 2003 [1]	525	5.5
Disease progression (10 years)	10	39	65	60		70	100		Doorn et al. 2000 [2]	309	5.2
	13	32		72	57				Kim et al. 2003 [1]	525	5.5
Disease progression (20 years)	16	40		81	78				Kim et al. 2003 [1]	525	5.5

Comments:
1. All actuarial survival curves are calculated according to method of Kaplan–Meier and are based on stage at diagnosis.
2. In the study by Doorn et al. [2] (and in a subsequent publication: van Doorn et al. [9]), the presence of follicular mucinosis was an independent poor prognostic feature, possibly related to depth of infiltrate in patients with stage IB disease (DSS of 81% and 36% and OS of 75% and 21% at 5 and 10 years, respectively). A lack of a complete response to initial therapy was also associated with a poor outcome ($P < 0.001$) in a multivariate analysis as well as increasing clinical stage and the presence of extracutaneous disease. A different staging system was used in this study (based on Hamminga et al. [10]) but for the purposes of this table the staging has been altered to be consistent. Only three patients had stage IVB disease and only 18 patients each had stage IIA and IVA disease. Therefore the results for these stages must be interpreted cautiously.
3. In the study by Zackheim et al. [3], black patients had a relatively more advanced stage of disease than white patients. The TNM classification was used in this study. Lymph node stage had an unfavourable impact on survival but this trend did not reach significance for each individual T stage because of a lack of sufficient power (an estimated 1700 subjects required) and IIA/IVA patients were not designated separately. Similar considerations apply to peripheral blood involvement. Similar outcomes for patients with stage IIB (T3) and III (T4) disease is consistent with other studies but this might reflect a lack of lymph node staging data included in this study.
4. The study by Kim et al. [1] included data on 525 patients and showed that the majority presented with early-stage disease and that independent multivariate prognostic factors were age, skin stage and presence of extracutaneous disease at presentation. With the exception of stage IA, the relative risk for death is greater in MF than in a control population: 2.2 for stage IB/IIA; 3.9 for stage IIB/III; 12.8 for stage IV disease.

DSS, disease-specific survival; FU, follow-up; NR, not reached; OS, overall survival.

Table 139.6 Clinical outcomes for 1502 mycosis fungoides/Sézary syndrome patients from diagnosis.

Clinical stage	No. in study	%	Median survival (years)	OS (%)			DSS (%)			RDP (%)		
				5 years	10 years	20 years	5 years	10 years	20 years	5 years	10 years	20 years
IA	438	29.2	35.5	94	88	73	98	95	90	8	12	18
IB	583	38.8	21.5	84	70	52	89	77	67	21	38	47
IIA	40	2.7	15.8	78	52	47	89	67	60	17	33	41
IIB	167	11.1	4.7	47	34	21	56	42	29	48	58	71
IIIA	100	6.7	4.7	47	37	25	54	45	31	53	62	74
IIIB	56	3.7	3.4	40	25	NR	48	45	NR	82	73	NR
IVA1	67	4.5	3.8	37	18	15	41	20	17	62	83	86
IVA2	37	2.5	2.1	18	15	3	23	20	6	77	80	94
IVB	14	0.9	1.4	18	NR	NR	18	NR	NR	82	NR	NR

Reproduced from Agar et al. 2010 [4] with permission of Wolters Kluwer Health, Inc.
DSS, disease-specific survival; NR, not reached; OS, overall survival; RDP, risk of disease progression.

Other types of lymphoma–leukaemia and Hodgkin lymphoma have also been described in association with MF and SS [8].

Investigations (Box 139.2)

All patients with MF should have a full clinical examination and adequate diagnostic biopsies for histology as well as immunophenotypic and molecular TCR studies, as even stage IA disease studies suggest that patients with a detectable T-cell clone have a shorter duration of response and a higher rate of treatment failure. Often, multiple elliptical skin biopsies and the opinion of experienced dermatopathologists are required to make a diagnosis. Peripheral blood samples should be taken at diagnosis for routine haematology, biochemistry, serum lactate dehydrogenase (LDH), lymphocyte flow cytometry, HTLV-1 serology, TCR gene analysis

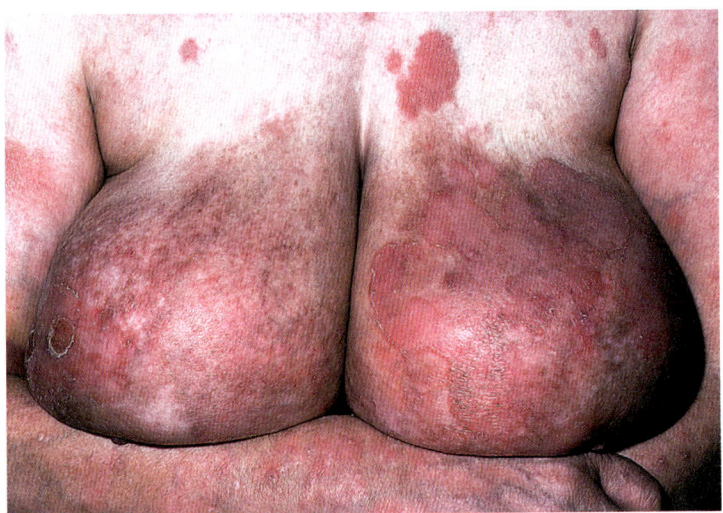

Figure 139.12 Poikilodermatous mycosis fungoides showing involvement of both breasts.

Table 139.7 Independent prognostic factors (CLIPi) for mycosis fungoides/Sézary syndrome patients (a) and overall survival at 5 and 10 years (b).

(a)

Stage	Adverse factors
Early IA–IIA	Male >60 years Plaques Folliculotropic N1/Nx
Late IIB–IVB	Male >60 years B1/B2 N2/N3 Visceral (M1)

(b)

	Risk group	No. of risk factors	N (%)	5-year OS (%)	10-year OS (%)
Early	I Low	0–1	482 (45.6)	96.0	90.3
	II Intermediate	2	330 (31.2)	87.6	76.2
	III High	3–5	245 (23.2)	73.5	48.9
Late	I Low	0–1	133 (29.9)	63.2	53.2
	II Intermediate	2	178 (40.0)	37.8	19.8
	III High	3–5	134 (30.1)	22.1	15.0

Adapted from Benton et al. 2013 [11].
CLIPi, cutaneous lymphoma prognostic index; OS, overall survival.

and a blood film for Sézary cells. These tests are necessary to distinguish patients with ATLL and those patients with peripheral blood T-cell clones identical to skin who may have a poor prognosis. Any palpable bulky peripheral nodes should be biopsied but the practice of 'blind' lymph node biopsy of non-palpable nodes is not essential, although histological evidence of lymphoma can rarely be detected in the absence of palpable lymphadenopathy. Fine-needle aspirates are not appropriate for histological assessment of lymph nodes in MF/SS. Core biopsies can yield relevant information in those patients with large bulky nodes but excision node biopsies are required to formally assess lymph node status in some situations. Staging computed tomography (CT) scans of the neck, chest, abdomen and pelvis are indicated in all those patients with stage IIA, IIB, III and IV MF, but not indicated for those with stage IA or IB MF. Peripheral nodes with a diameter greater than 1.5 cm in the short axis are considered to be abnormal in patients with cutaneous lymphomas, whereas for central nodes a diameter greater than 1 cm is considered to be the limit. Positron emission tomography (PET)/CT in MF can increase the detection rate of systemic disease with PET activity correlating to histological lymph node grade [1] and enabling the choice of the nodal basin for biopsy. Bone marrow aspirate and trephine biopsies are not indicated unless patients have unexplained peripheral blood abnormalities as the overall positive yield is low even in those with SS. The significance of bone marrow infiltration in MF/SS is currently unknown and is not incorporated into the revised staging system.

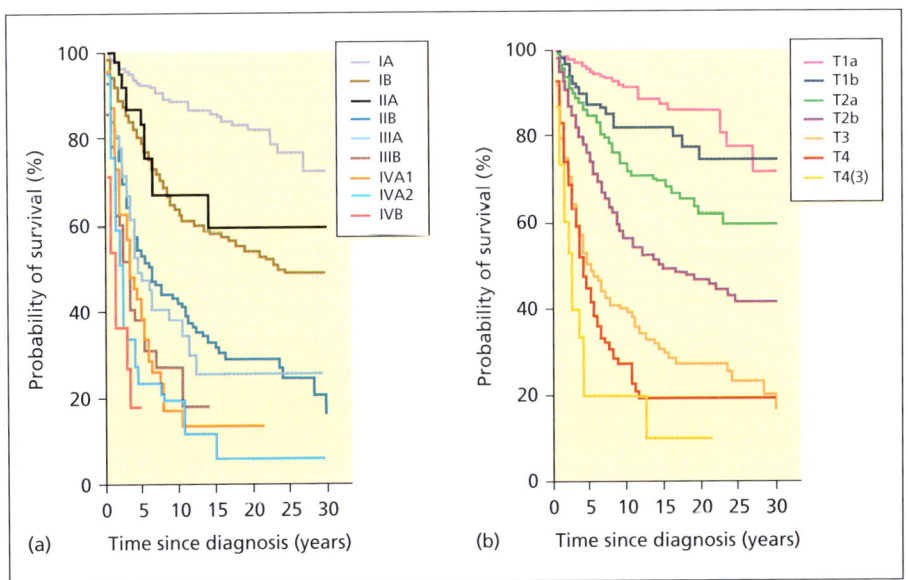

Figure 139.13 Disease-specific survival according to (a) clinical stage and (b) T classification at diagnosis. Reproduced from Agar et al. 2010 [4] with permission of Wolters Kluwer Health, Inc.

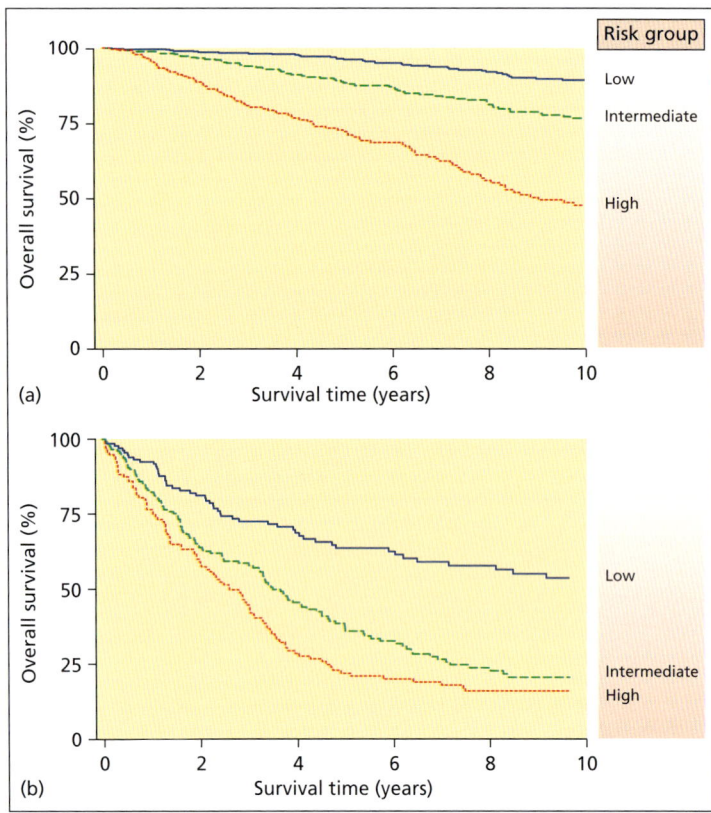

Figure 139.14 Overall survival according to prognostic group for mycosis fungoides/Sézary syndrome. (a) Early-stage group. (b) Late-stage group [11].

Box 139.2 Investigations for mycosis fungoides/Sézary syndrome

- Skin biopsies from representative patches/plaques/tumours (often multiple required, preferably incisional elliptical biopsies as opposed to small punch biopsies)
- Haematology; LDH; β_2 microglobulin; lymphocyte subsets (flow cytometry); Sézary cell count; HTLV-1 serology
- TCR gene analysis of skin, peripheral blood lymphocytes and any nodal tissue
- PET/CT scans for stages IIB–IV; lymph node excision/core biopsies for palpable peripheral nodes or those nodes >1.5 cm in short axis
- Bone marrow trephine biopsy if unexplained haematological findings

CT, computed tomography; HTLV, human T-cell leukaemia virus; LDH, lactate dehydrogenase; PET, positron emission tomography; TCR, T-cell receptor.

Management

See the separate section on the management of MF/SS later in this chapter.

Follicular mucinosis

Definition and nomenclature

This consists of boggy cutaneous plaques showing follicular prominence and histological evidence of mucinous degeneration of the hair follicles. It is often associated with an atypical pilotropic T-cell infiltrate and clinical features of MF (pilotropic or folliculotropic MF).

Synoyms and inclusions
- Alopecia mucinosa

Pathophysiology

Follicular mucinosis represents a follicular (pilotropic) variant of MF with mucinous degeneration of the hair follicle. This is supported by the presence of this clinical and histological pattern in patients with typical features of MF. The poor prognosis of folliculotropic variants may relate to the poorer efficacy of skin-directed therapies because of the depth of the associated T-cell infiltrate or a currently unknown biological difference.

Pathology

There is degeneration of the involved hair follicles, associated with a prominent pilotropic, atypical T-cell infiltrate in MF. There may also be associated interfollicular epidermotropism. Mucin stains such as Alcian blue show the presence of large quantities of mucin although the reason for mucin deposition is unknown (Figure 139.15). In MF, a pilotropic or folliculotropic infiltrate may also occur without mucinosis.

In contrast, the inflammatory form of follicular mucinosis does not show a prominent atypical pilotropic T-cell infiltrate, although repeated biopsies may be required to fully exclude MF [1]. It may be impossible to distinguish these two forms with confidence and there is an emerging consensus that most, if not all, patients with follicular mucinosis have a form of CTCL (pilotropic MF) [2]. However, histological features of follicular mucinosis, without atypia, can also occur as an incidental histological feature in the context of various inflammatory dermatoses.

Immunophenotype

The tumour cells in both follicular mucinosis and folliculotropic/pilotropic MF are usually CD3+, CD4+ and CD8–. Prominent CD30+/– blast cells may be a feature of large-cell transformation [2]. Clonal TCR gene rearrangements can be detected in both MF-associated follicular mucinosis and so-called benign forms of inflammatory follicular mucinosis, consistent with suggestions that both may represent MF variants [2].

Clinical features

There are two distinct forms of follicular mucinosis, one associated with MF and a separate, benign, inflammatory form of follicular mucinosis which is not associated with the development of MF. The clinical features of these two types of follicular mucinosis are identical: follicular papules and plaques often associated with severe pruritus and a predilection for the face and scalp although the trunk and limbs can be affected. In MF, classic polymorphic patches and plaques may also be present. A younger age group is affected by the inflammatory form but there are no satisfactory criteria for distinguishing this presumed inflammatory process from MF-associated follicular mucinosis [3]. Prominent giant comedones

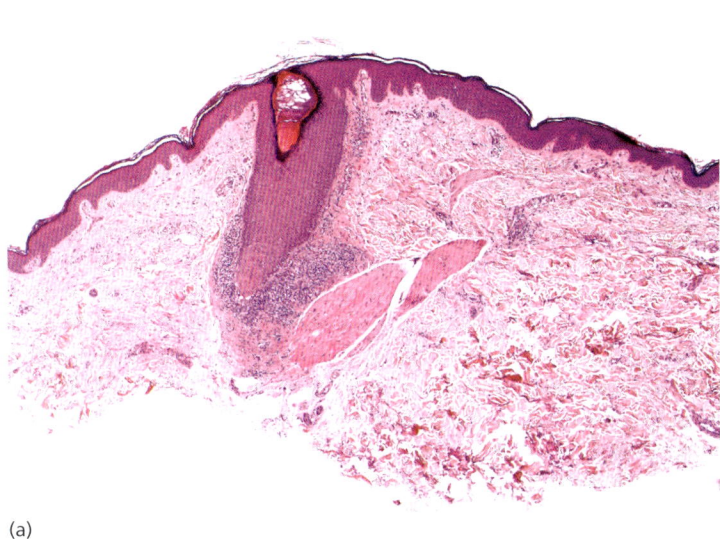

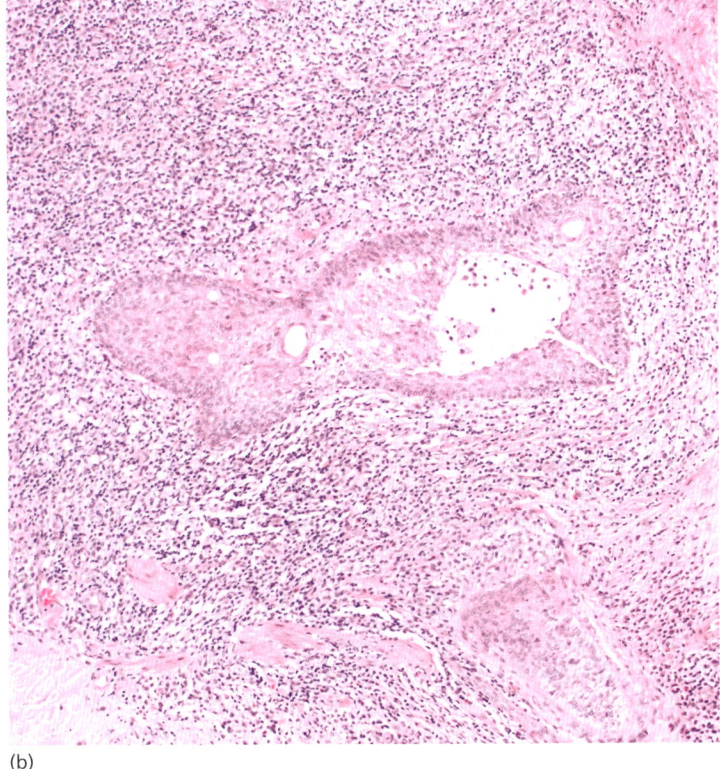

Figure 139.15 (a) Prominent perifollicular lymphoid infiltrate without epidermotropism or spongiosis and (b) high power view showing cytological atypia and striking mucinous deposition. (b) Courtesy of Eduardo Calonje.

are often a feature with acneiform lesions (Figure 139.16), and significant alopecia may be present, rarely with mucinorrhoea [1].

Disease course and prognosis

There is evidence that follicular variants of MF have a worse prognosis, with disease-specific survival rates of 81% at 5 years and 36% at 10 years [1,4,5].

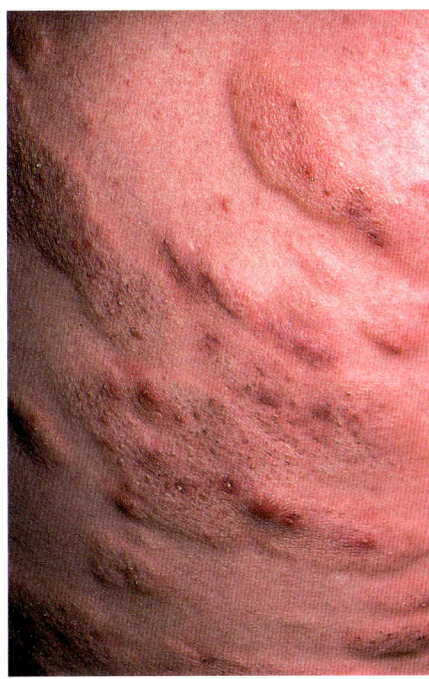

Figure 139.16 Clinical appearance of follicular mucinosis showing boggy mucin-secreting plaques on the trunk.

Management

Mycosis fungoides associated with follicular mucinosis is treated with skin-directed therapy as for the early stages of MF (see section on management of MF and SS later in this chapter), but patients may also require systemic treatment with interferon α (IFN-α) or rexinoids (bexarotene). Radiotherapy is ideal for isolated plaques of folliculotropic MF. Total skin electron beam therapy may be appropriate for resistant cases. Dapsone can be effective for inflammatory forms of follicular mucinosis. However, if the hair follicles have been destroyed, scarring alopecia will be present and hair loss is permanent. Evolution of folliculotropic MF to SS has been described [6].

Pagetoid reticulosis

Definition and nomenclature

This is a localised, solitary variant of CTCL, which histologically shows intense epidermotropism.

Synonyms and inclusions
- Woringer–Kolopp disease

Pathophysiology

This entity may either represent a localised epidermotropic variant of MF [1] or be closely related to the more recently described CD8+ epidermotropic CTCL [2].

Pathology

Biopsies show very striking colonisation of an acanthotic epidermis by atypical, large, pale, mononuclear cells, which usually either fail

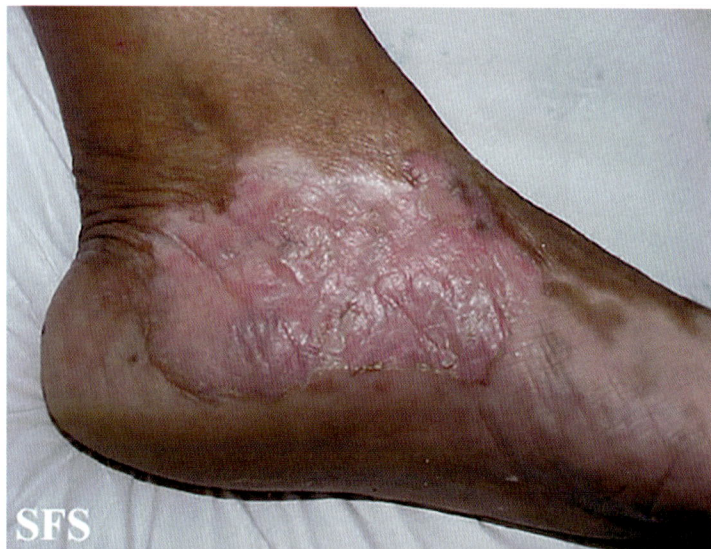

Figure 139.17 Pagetoid reticulosis at an acral site.

to express lymphoid markers or express an aberrant T-cell phenotype. However, the detection of an aberrant T-cell phenotype (CD4– and CD8–) in some cases and clonal TCR gene rearrangements defines this as a CTCL variant.

Clinical features
This entity was first described in 1939 [3] and is rare but appears to affect younger adults and is characterised by an isolated, persistent, scaly plaque, commonly involving an acral site (Figure 139.17). The lesion may be asymptomatic and slowly expands, but no further plaques develop on other body sites. The plaque may show psoriasiform or Bowenoid features. A more generalised variant with multiple plaques at other sites has also been described (Ketron–Goodman variant), but this almost certainly represents an epidermotropic variant of MF or the more recently described CD8+ epidermotropic CTCL variant [2].

Disease course and prognosis
The natural history of this lesion is of very slow local extension with an excellent prognosis.

Management
Successful durable remission has been reported with both surgical excision and low-dose superficial radiotherapy.

Granulomatous slack skin disease

Definition
This is a very rare disease characterised clinically by the slow development of pendulous folds of lax reddish skin often affecting flexural sites and histologically by dermal granulomas and elastolysis.

Pathophysiology
While some patients have only features of granulomatous slack skin, some patients show typical clinical features of MF, but whether this condition represents a granulomatous variant of MF or a CTCL variant is currently unclear [1,2], especially as a novel balanced translocation has recently been detected in granulomatous slack skin [3].

Pathology
Histology reveals a dense granulomatous dermal infiltrate (Figure 139.18) with the destruction of dermal elastic tissue (elastolysis) [4]. The destruction appears to be mediated by histiocytic giant cells [5]. Similar granulomas may occasionally be found in the spleen and lymph nodes. The lymphocytic infiltrate in the dermis shows some cytological atypia and may have an aberrant T-cell phenotype suggestive of lymphoma. TCR gene analysis confirms that T-cell clones are present, suggesting a CTCL variant in most cases [6].

Clinical features
The lesions develop slowly, usually in middle-aged adults, and then progress over several years [7]. The sites of skin involvement are typically flexures and consist of thickened, pendulous folds (Figure 139.19). This condition appears to be caused by cutaneous elastolysis associated with an underlying lymphoma. Several patients have died of Hodgkin disease or non-Hodgkin lymphoma, and the otherwise unaltered epidermis may show epidermotropism similar to that seen in MF. The condition must be distinguished from other forms of cutis laxa.

Disease course and prognosis
The prognosis is usually excellent.

Management
No definitive therapy has yet been identified but radiotherapy, IFN-α, retinoids and surgery can be effective [8–10].

Sézary syndrome [1,2]

Definition
This syndrome consists of a clinical triad of erythroderma, peripheral lymphadenopathy and atypical mononuclear cells (Sézary cells) comprising a total Sézary count of more than $1000 \times 10^9/\text{L}$ (1000/μL peripheral blood stage B2) and the presence of a peripheral blood T-cell clone identical to that detected in the skin/node on TCR gene analysis [3].

Epidemiology
The majority of SS patients are elderly males and may develop the syndrome either *ab initio* or rarely as progression from classic MF.

Pathophysiology
Pathology
Skin biopsies can show large numbers of atypical mononuclear cells in the dermis with epidermotropism, but non-diagnostic and lymphomatoid histology is frequently seen in proven cases of SS [4]. The presence of atypical (Sézary-like), cerebriform, mononuclear

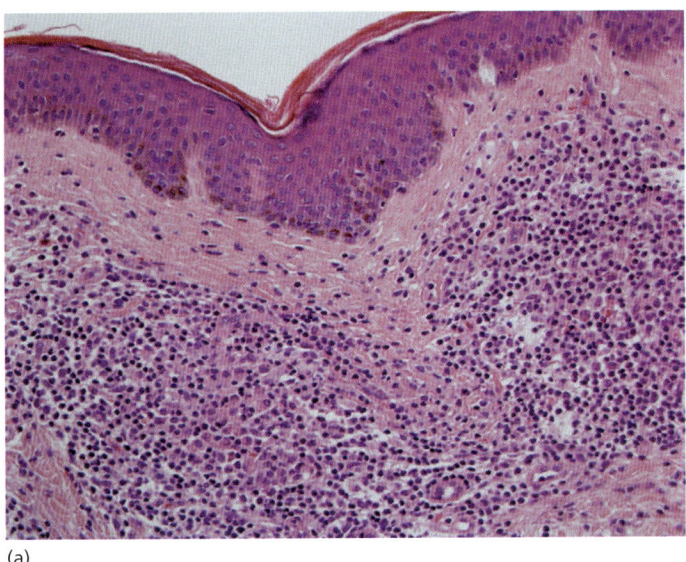

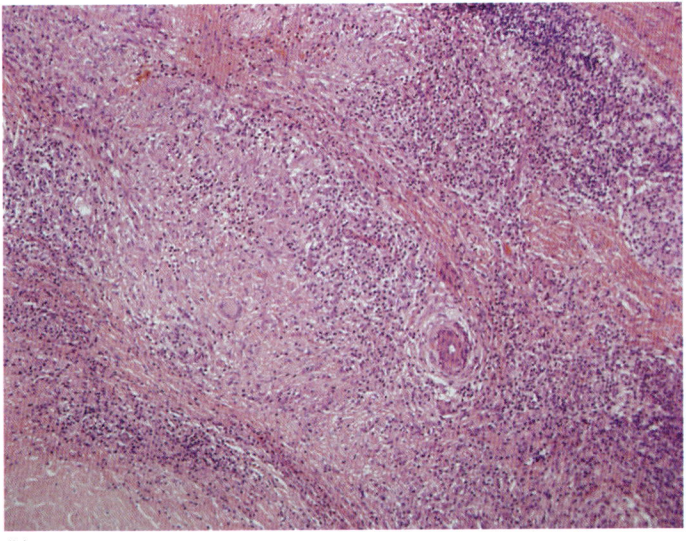

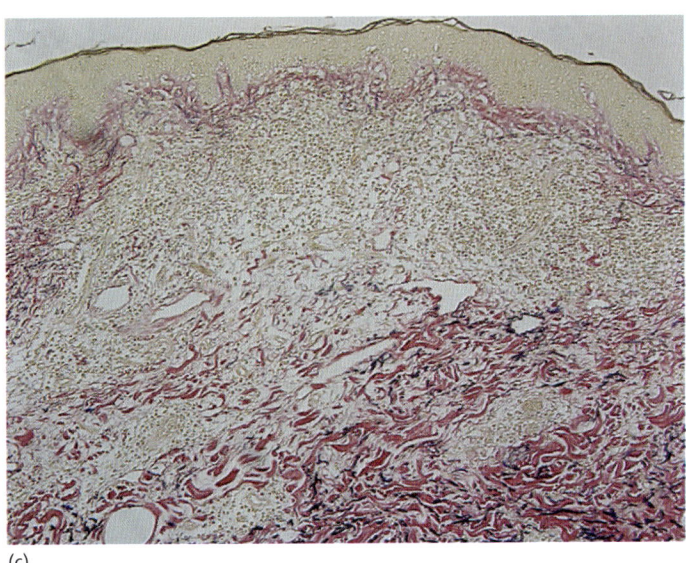

Figure 139.18 (a) Histology showing a prominent infiltrate of histiocytic cells and lymphoid cells with mild cytological atypia. (b) Giant cells are also present. (c) There is a marked loss of elastic tissue (elastolysis) in the upper dermis (elastic van Gieson stain).

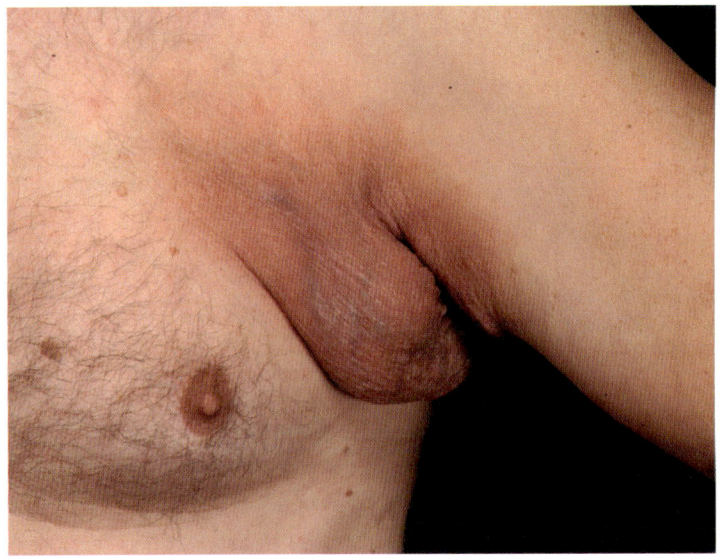

Figure 139.19 Granulomatous slack skin showing prominent, lax folds of markedly indurated axillary skin with superficial scaling and wrinkling.

cells has also been reported in the peripheral blood of patients with a variety of inflammatory conditions including actinic reticuloid, erythrodermic eczema, psoriasis and severe drug reactions (Figure 139.20). Usually the percentage of atypical cells in such conditions is lower (<250/ μL) than in SS. In addition, T cells with the morphological and ultrastructural features of Sézary cells can be identified in the peripheral blood of normal healthy individuals [5]. However, it is important to appreciate that the total lymphocyte count may not be raised for the diagnosis of SS to be made. Consequently, it can be difficult to conclusively distinguish cases of SS from inflammatory dermatoses. Large Sézary cell variants (>16 μm diameter) are easier to recognise but small Sézary cell variants (12–14 μm) are more common and difficult to distinguish morphologically from activated lymphocytes [2].

Immunophenotype

Sézary cells are usually CD3+, CD4+, CD7– and CD26– T cells but CD26+, CD7+ and CD8+ variants have been reported and CD26 loss can occur in control populations albeit at low levels. Absolute CD4 counts and CD4 : CD8 ratios are usually elevated. A peripheral blood CD4 : CD8 ratio greater than 10 distinguishes most cases of SS from an inflammatory dermatosis associated with Sézary cells but represents a large peripheral blood tumour burden. Consensus diagnostic criteria include the clinical triad of features plus the presence of peripheral blood Sézary cells based on flow cytometry showing >40% of lymphocytes with a CD4+/CD26– phenotype and/or >30% of lymphocytes with a CD4+/CD7– phenotype. Flow should also determine that the total CD4+/CD26– and/or CD4+/CD7– counts is >1000/ μL with a blood film showing Sézary cells and a peripheral blood T-cell clone identical to skin detected by TCR gene analysis [3]. Those patients without evidence of a T-cell clone may have a benign inflammatory dermatosis with an excellent prognosis. SS should also be distinguished from other T-cell malignancies such as T-prolymphocytic leukaemia, which can rarely present with cutaneous involvement including erythroderma. This diagnosis is usually apparent on the basis of clinicopathological

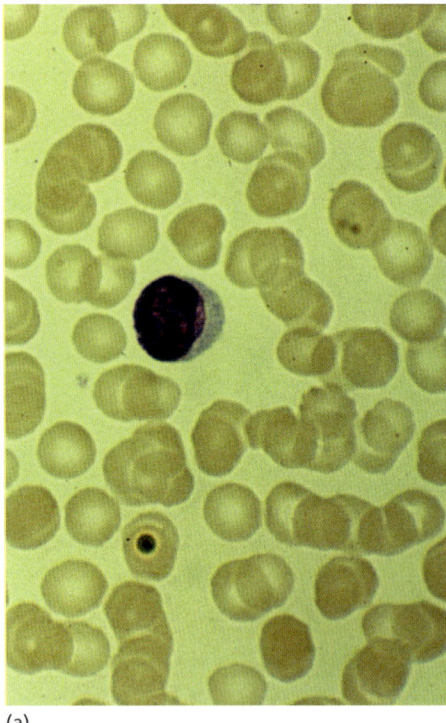

Molecular features
See later in this chapter for a separate discussion of the molecular features of MF and SS.

Clinical features
History
Many patients describe a prolonged history of 'dermatitis' but rarely patients may have a previous history of MF.

Presentation
Patients present with a generalised exfoliative erythroderma, and may have systemic problems because of shunting blood through grossly dilated cutaneous vasculature resulting in high-output cardiac failure. There may be associated ectropion, scalp alopecia, palmoplantar hyperkeratoses and fissuring and the nails often show gross subungual hyperkeratoses (Figure 139.21). Peripheral lymphadenopathy is often present. Rarely, patients may present

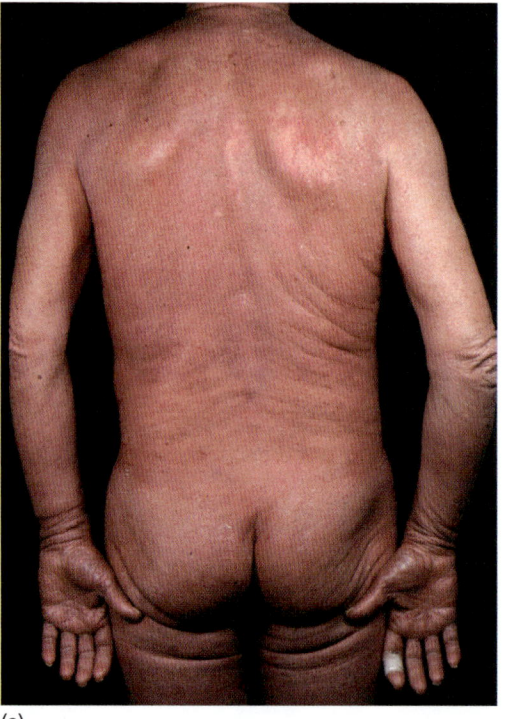

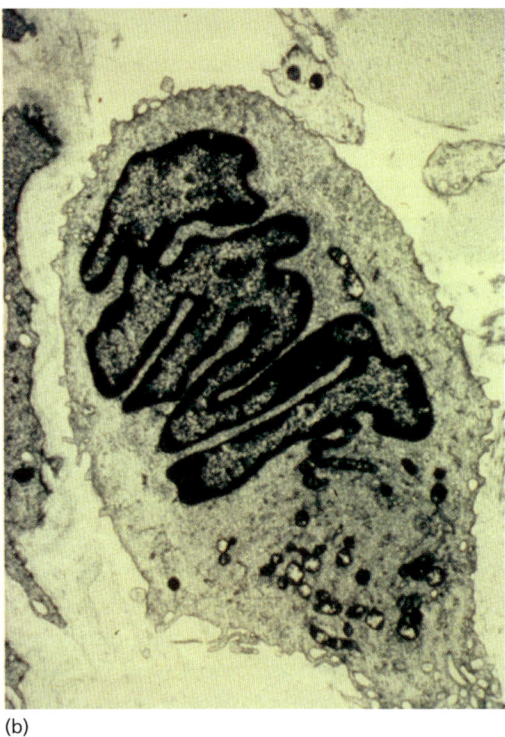

Figure 139.20 High-power views of Sézary cells in the peripheral blood showing (a) a large cell with a very large nucleus and minimal cytoplasm and (b) the ultrastructural features of a typical cerebriform nucleus.

and immunophenotypic features including a characteristic tumour cytology in the peripheral blood and bone marrow and an aberrant T-cell phenotype (CD4+/CD8+). Studies have suggested that SS is derived from central memory T cells while MF is derived from skin-resident, peripheral, memory T cells [6].

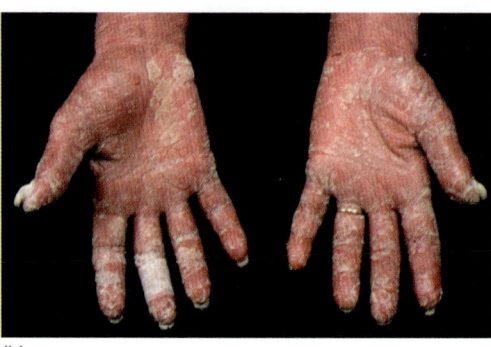

Figure 139.21 Sézary syndrome showing (a) erythroderma on the back with (b) palmoplantar hyperkeratoses and prominent nail dystrophy.

with limited skin involvement and a leukaemic phase with a high peripheral blood Sézary cell count.

Differential diagnosis

The distinction from erythrodermic MF is based on the degree of peripheral blood involvement. The historical definition of SS, as suggested in the original NCI staging system, comprised a Sézary count of 5% or more of peripheral blood lymphocytes on a buffy coat smear (peripheral blood stage B1). However, low numbers of Sézary cells can be detected in the peripheral blood of healthy individuals and patients with inflammatory dermatoses. In 1988, the NCI published a revised staging system, with over 20% Sézary cell count (per 100 lymphocytes) as the B1 rating [7], based on previous studies showing that this figure had prognostic significance in SS. An absolute Sézary cell count of over $1000/mm^3$ ($1000/\mu L$) as a criterion for the diagnosis of SS (peripheral blood stage B2) was subsequently included in the revised staging classification. However, patients with a lower tumour burden (Sézary cell count >5% of lymphocytes or CD4+/CD26– and/or CD4+/CD7– total count >250/μL but <1000/μL) are classified as erythrodermic MF (stage B1) as opposed to SS [4]. Distinction from inflammatory causes of erythroderma can be extremely challenging partly because: (i) skin biopsies in erythrodermic CTCL may be non-diagnostic; (ii) peripheral blood activated T cells may resemble Sézary cells; and (iii) accurate delineation of peripheral blood involvement using flow analysis is based on percentages of CD4+/CD7– and CD4+/CD26– T-cell populations that can fluctuate in the context of inflammatory dermatoses. This issue has been exemplified by a multicentre study of SS and erythrodermic inflammatory dermatoses which showed that: (i) loss of CD26 (>80% CD4+ T cells) and/or CD7 (>40% CD4+ T cells) gated on CD4+ T cells; and (ii) altered gene expression of *STAT4* (reduced), *TWIST1* and *DNM3* or *PLS3* (all increased) were more more specific and sensitive than existing criteria [8].

Disease course and prognosis

The prognosis in SS is poor with an 11% 5-year overall survival and median survival of 32 months from diagnosis [9]. The presence of lymph node disease is an independent prognostic factor, while the degree of peripheral blood involvement may have prognostic significance; age and gender are also key prognostic factors [9]. Most patients die of opportunistic infection. Spontaneous resolution of SS has been rarely described [10].

Management

For the management of MF and SS see later in this chapter.

Molecular features of mycosis fungoides and Sézary syndrome

Extensive studies have provided critical insights into the underlying molecular pathogenesis and have shown striking similarities between MF and SS (Figure 139.22). The availability of large whole exome/genome sequencing (WES/WGS) datasets of CTCL and systemic T-cell lymphomas (403 cases) has allowed analysis of the mutational spectrum [1,2–8]. All mature T-cell lymphomas exhibit signature 1 which is related to cellular age and is due to spontaneous deamination of methylated cytosine residues, therefore reflecting derivation from memory T cells. Intriguingly, MF and SS (137 cases) are associated with the UV signature 7 which contributes 52% of the mutational burden in MF and 23% in SS. Overall 41% of these patients were treatment naïve and the detection of a mutational signature is dependent on the presence of a clonal population, suggesting that the malignant T cell in CTCL accumulates UV-associated mutations before transformation and clonal expansion [1]. The UV signature was also detected in CD4+-enriched peripheral blood leukaemic cells from SS patients. In addition, analysis of WGS data from treatment-naïve patients with advanced stages of MF showed a UV signature 7 with a high frequency of CC>TT double substitutions at dipyrimidine sites and transcriptional strand bias, both characteristic of UV irradiation [1]. This confirms that for CTCL, in contrast to systemic T-cell lymphomas, the major causal factor is environmental UV irradiation of T cells either resident or circulating through the skin.

These high-throughput sequencing studies have also identified a heterogeneous pattern of genomic abnormalities with at least 55 potential driver gene mutations [9]. The most frequent recurrent gene variants affect TCR signalling pathways (*PLCG1*, *CARD11*, *CD28*, *RLTPR*) and selectively upregulate the nuclear factor κB (NFκB) pathway (Figure 139.23). Other pathways affected by driver

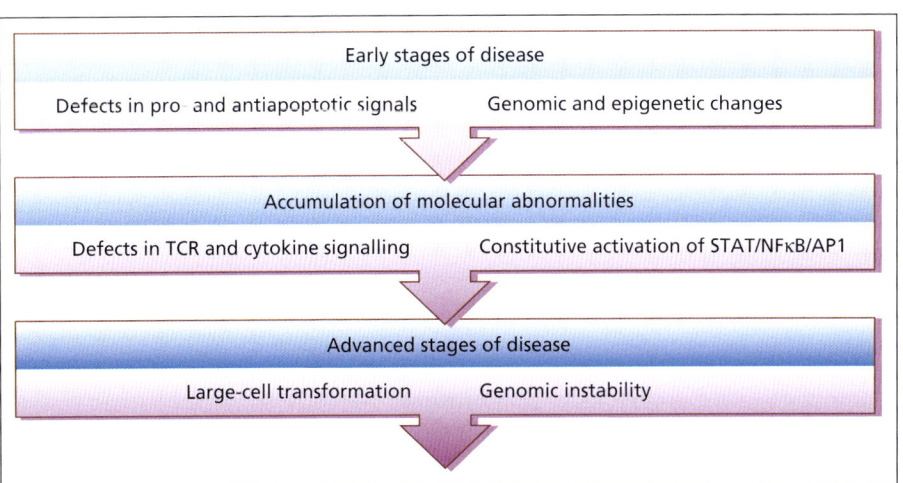

Figure 139.22 Molecular pathogenesis of mycosis fungoides/Sézary syndrome. NFκB, nuclear factor κB; TCR, T-cell receptor.

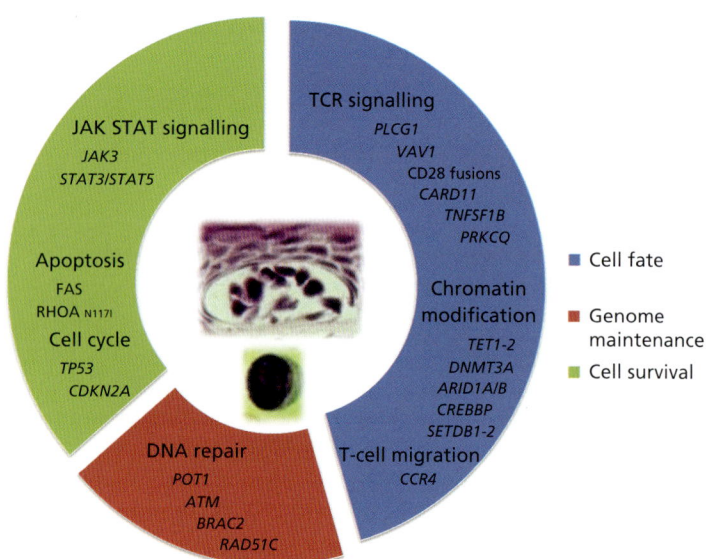

Figure 139.23 Genomic landscape of mutations in cutaneous T-cell lymphoma. JAK, Janus kinase; STAT, signal transducer and activator of transcription; TCR, T-cell receptor.

gene mutations (>10%) include DNA damage response pathways (*TP53, POT1, ATM, BRAC1-2*), chromatin modification (*ARID1A, TRRAP, DNMT3A, TET2*) and JAK (Janus kinase) STAT (signal transducer and activator of transcription) signalling (*STAT5B, JAK3*) (Figure 139.23). Critically these gene variants have been functionally validated, confirming that they are bona fide driver gene mutations with either gain or loss of function. Two of the most common CTCL gene mutations, *PLCG1* and *CARD11*, include recurrent variants, appear to be mutually exclusive and occur in almost 30% of SS cases. These *PLCG1* and *CARD11* gene variants are gain-of-function mutations that increase downstream T-cell signalling specifically through enhanced NFκB transcriptional activity and also NFAT (nuclear factor of activated T cells) and AP1 (activator protein 1) activity [10–12]. These transcription factors regulate the expression of genes involved in cell proliferation, survival and differentiation. Crucially, many of these variants induce downstream signalling *without T-cell stimulation* suggesting that these mutations lead to constitutive activation of T-cell signalling.

In addition, data from WGS studies mainly in advanced MF samples have shown a complex pattern of chromosomal rearrangements and translocations with no recurrent balanced translocations. However, specific gains (17q, 8q) and losses (10q, 17p) are seen frequently,

confirming previous studies using conventional cytogenetics, allelo-typing and metaphase and array comparative genomic hybridisation (CGH) techniques showing recurrent numerical and structural chromosomal abnormalities in all stages of MF and SS [13–16]. Minimal regions of deletion have been detected on 10q, suggesting a number of potential candidate genes [17]. Specifically, chromosomal abnormalities have been detected in early stages of MF, suggesting that chromosomal instability occurs early [18].

Extensive studies have also revealed that the silencing of specific tumour suppressor genes in CTCL due to promoter hypermethylation includes the genes involved in cell cycle regulation (*TP53, CDKN2A/2B*), DNA repair (*MLH1, MGMT*), apoptosis (*FAS*) and JAK-STAT signalling (*SHP-1*) [19–25]. This hypermethylation may reflect the high frequency of mutations affecting genes encoding DNA methyltransferases (*DNMT3A*), cytosine methylation (*TET2*) and chromatin modification (*ARID1A/1B*) in MF/SS [9].

MF and SS are characterised by UV-induced mutations of genes involved in: (i) TCR signalling facilitating activation of T cells without antigenic stimulation; (ii) downstream activation of the NFκB and JAK-STAT pathways; (iii) epigenetic modification enabling aberrant methylation and inactivation of genes involved in the cell cycle and apoptosis; and (iv) DNA damage response pathways contributing to genomic instability (Figure 139.24).

Management of mycosis fungoides and Sézary syndrome

The current treatment of MF and SS includes a range of options (Table 139.8) but few have been subjected to randomised controlled trials with rigorous disease assessment tools and appropriate end points. The choice of initial treatment for the MF patient depends on the clinical stage and performance status. A significant proportion of patients with MF are frail elderly and the patient's quality of life should always be considered. The current consensus is that patients with early-stage disease should receive skin-directed therapies in view of the low risk of progression [1,2,3]. Systemic therapies are reserved for those with either early-stage disease resistant to skin-directed therapy or advanced disease (Table 139.8) [2,3,4]. A randomised trial in MF reported on 103 patients who received either total skin electron beam therapy (TSEBT) (3000 cGy total skin electron beam) together with cyclophosphamide, daunorubicin, etoposide and vincristine (a rigorous 'treat to cure' regimen) or

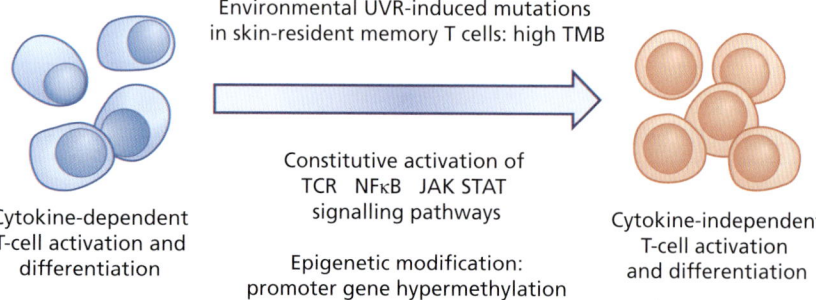

Figure 139.24 Driver gene mutations in cutaneous T-cell lymphoma. JAK, Janus kinase; NFκB, nuclear factor κB; STAT, signal transducer and activator of transcription; TCR, T-cell receptor; TMB, tumour mutational burden; UVR, ultraviolet radiation.

Table 139.8 Treatment algorithm for mycosis fungoides/Sézary syndrome.

Prognostic group (stage)	First line	Second line	Third line
Low risk (IA–IIA)	Expectant or SDT	SDT	Trials
Intermediate risk (IA–IIA) and stage IIB[a]	SDT	HDACi[c]; Onzar[c]	
	PUVA + maintenance IFN-α	Mogamulizumab[d]	
	PUVA + maintenance Bex	Brentuximab[d]	
	TSEBT	Trials	Trials
Erythrodermic (III)	MTX	Alemtuzumab	RicAlloSCT
	ECP/IFN-α/Bex combinations	Brentuximab[d]	Chemotherapy
		HDACi[c]; Ontak[c]	TSEBT
		Mogamulizumab*	
	Trials	Trials	Trials
High risk (IIB[b]/IV)	Radiotherapy (incl TSEBT)	HDACi[c]; Ontak[c]	
	Chemotherapy	Brentuximab[d]	
		RicAlloSCT	
		Mogamulizumab[d]	
	Trials	Trials	Trials

[a] Limited tumours.
[b] Extensive tumours.
[c] US Food and Drug Administration (FDA) and European Medicines Agency (EMA) approved.
[d] US FDA approved;
Bex, bexarotene; ECP, extracorporeal photopheresis; HDACi, histone deacetylase inhibitors (vorinostat/romidepsin); IFN-α, interferon α; MTX, methotrexate; Ontak, denileukin diftitox; PUVA, psoralen and ultraviolet A; RicAlloSCT, reduced-intensity conditioned allogeneic stem cell transplant; SDT, skin-directed therapy (topical therapy, phototherapy (TLO1/PUVA) or radiotherapy); TSEBT, total skin electron beam therapy.

sequential topical therapy consisting of nitrogen mustard, superficial radiotherapy and TSEBT, progressing to psoralen and UVA (PUVA) if required (a 'gentle palliative' regimen) [5]. After a median follow-up time of 75 months, there was no difference in disease-free or overall survival between the 52 patients who received TSEBT plus chemotherapy and the 51 who received sequential palliative topical therapy [5]. This study established a consensus that therapy in MF should be based on the stage of disease and aimed at disease palliation rather than an aggressive intent to cure and this is supported by more recent data showing that chemotherapy does not produce durable disease control [1]. Various therapies have been approved for CTCL by either the US FDA and/or the European Medicines Agency (EMA), including a rexinoid, bexarotene (FDA and EMA), that binds to the retinoid X receptor [6]; INF-α (EMA); a diphtheria interleukin 2 (IL-2) fusion toxin, denileukin diftitox (Onzar or Ontak, FDA) [7]; two histone deacetylase inhibitors (FDA), suberoylanilide hydroxamic acid (SAHA or vorinostat) [8] and depsipeptide (romidepsin) [9]; brentuximab (FDA and EMA) [10]; mogamulizumab (FDA and EMA) [11]; and topical mechlorethamine (FDA and EMA) [12]. Many of these trials have included disease response assessments of all tumour compartments and appropriate clinical end points based on consensus recommendations [13–15].

Skin-directed therapy
Topical steroids
For patients with limited early-stage MF, life expectancy may not be adversely affected and it is acceptable to simply use emollients with or without moderate potency topical steroids for symptomatic relief. Potent topical corticosteroids can produce a clinical response, although this is usually short lived [1].

Topical chemotherapy: mechlorethamine and carmustine
Topical mechlorethamine (nitrogen mustard) is effective for superficial disease with response rates of 51–80% for IA, 26–68% for IB and 61% for IIA disease [1,2]. Previous compounded products were difficult to use and associated with irritancy or allergic dermatitis in sensitised individuals (35–58%). A novel 0.02% gel formulation, compared with a compounded formulation, was approved after a successful non-inferiority trial with an overall response rate (ORR) of 47.7–58.5% depending on the use of different disease assessment tools [3], but both products showed similar rates of skin irritancy/allergic contact dermatitis. This product must not be used in pregnancy and there are rare reports of non-melanoma skin cancer in patients treated with topical mechlorethamine. There is no consensus as to whether mechlorethamine should be applied to individual lesions or to the whole skin, daily or twice weekly, or about the duration of topical therapy after a clinical remission has been produced. Responses can be sustained for prolonged periods.

Topical carmustine (BCNU) is an alternative but rarely used topical chemotherapeutic agent in MF, with similar efficacy to mechlorethamine as indicated by response rates of 86% in stage IA, 47% in stage IB and 55% in stage IIA patients. Alternate day or daily treatment with 10 mg carmustine in 60 mL dilute alcohol (95%) or 20–40% carmustine ointment can be used. Hypersensitivity reactions occur less often (5–10%) than with mechlorethamine. All patients treated topically with carmustine should have regular monitoring of their full blood counts and treatment is normally given for only 2–4 weeks to avoid myelosuppression; maintenance therapy is contraindicated.

Topical rexinoids
Targretin 1% (bexarotene) gel is approved by the US FDA for topical therapy in stage I MF patients who are resistant to, or intolerant of, other topical therapies [1]. In open uncontrolled studies, response rates of 63% with 21% complete response rates were reported in 67 patients with early-stage (IA–IIA) disease. Median time to and duration of response were 20 and 99 weeks, respectively.

Other topical therapies
There has only been one randomised, placebo-controlled trial of topical therapy in MF. Topical peldesine cream (BCX-34, an inhibitor of the purine nucleoside phosphorylase enzyme) showed no benefit, compared with vehicle, with response rates of 28% and 24%, respectively, emphasising the difficulties in interpretation of uncontrolled studies of topical therapy in early stages of MF [1]. Other topical therapies reported in small cohort studies to have efficacy in early-stage MF include imiquimod and 5-fluorouracil creams.

Phototherapy and photochemotherapy

Psoralen and UVA photochemotherapy may induce a complete response rate of 79–88% in stage IA and 52–59% in stage IB disease [1–3]. Flexural sites ('sanctuary sites') often fail to respond completely and the duration of response varies. There is no significant response in tumour (IIB) stage disease. One study showed that 56% of stage IA and 39% of stage IB complete PUVA responders had no recurrence of disease after 44 months follow-up without maintenance therapy [4]. A retrospective study on long-term outcome for MF patients treated with PUVA reported that 50% of patients with a higher cumulative UVA dose achieved a longer duration of response. However these patients also received maintenance therapy while those who relapsed early did not, making interpretation difficult. Furthermore, there was no difference in clinical outcome in terms of disease progression or survival in the two groups. Randomised controlled trails are rare but an EORTC study showed an ORR for PUVA of 75% with complete response rates of 25%, where only a minority of patients had a prolonged duration of response [5]. Maintenance therapy is rarely effective at preventing relapse and therefore should be avoided so as to limit the total cumulative dose, as patients will often require repeated courses over many years.

PUVA is an ideal therapy for patients with stage IB–IIA disease who are intolerant of, or fail to respond to, topical therapies such as mechlorethamine, although both therapies can be complementary for some patients. Treatment regimens have varied between two to four times weekly with different protocols for incremental dosage, but usually two to three times weekly treatment is acceptable until disease clearance or best partial response, usually over a minimum of 12–14 weeks. Patients with a high total cumulative UVA dosage will have increased risks of non-melanoma and rarely melanoma and Merkel cell carcinomas. Efforts should be made to restrict the total PUVA dosage to less than 200 treatment sessions or a total cumulative dose of 1200 J/cm^2. In some circumstances patients may receive a greater total dosage if clinically justified and with consent. PUVA remains one of the most effective therapies for patients with early-stage disease but there are surprisingly no data to establish if PUVA can improve overall survival or reduce rates of disease progression in stage IB. PUVA therapy is rarely tolerated in erythrodermic (stage III) disease but occasional patients will respond.

Broad- and narrow-band UVB and high-dose UVA-1 phototherapy have also been used in MF with success [6,7]. There have been no adequate comparative studies of different phototherapy regimens in CTCL but narrow-band UVB therapy may be an effective option for patients with only patches as opposed to plaques. Small cohort studies have suggested that patients with limited cutaneous disease may respond to photodynamic therapy and 308 nm excimer laser treatment.

Radiotherapy and total skin electron beam therapy

Mycosis fungoides and other CTCL variants are highly radiosensitive malignancies. Individual thick plaques or tumours can be treated successfully with low-dose superficial radiotherapy (ortho-voltage or electrons), often administered in several fractions (e.g. two or three fractions of 400 cGy at 80–120 kV). Large tumours may require a different energy source. Radiotherapy is very well tolerated and often used with other therapeutic modalities such as PUVA, and closely adjacent and overlapping fields can often be retreated because of the low doses used [1].

Whole body TSEBT has been evaluated extensively in CTCL [2]. Different field arrangements have been used in an attempt to treat the whole skin uniformly to a depth of 1 cm with various total dosages administered and additional radiotherapy to shielded areas. A meta-analysis of open uncontrolled and mostly retrospective studies of TSEBT as monotherapy in 952 patients with CTCL established that responses are stage dependent, with complete responses of 96% in stage IA, IB and IIA disease. However, disease relapse rates are high, indicating that this approach is not curative even in early-stage disease [3]. In stage IIB disease, complete responses are less common (36%), but erythrodermic (stage III) disease shows complete responses of 60%. Greater skin surface dose (32–36 Gy) and higher energy (4–6 MeV electrons) are associated with a higher rate of complete response, and 5-year relapse-free survivals of 10–23% were noted [3]. One study using mSWAT as a rigorous method for assessing disease response reported ORRs of 95% and complete responses of 51%, with a median time to relapse of 12 months and to disease progression of 44 months [4]. A retrospective study of erythrodermic disease has also shown 60% complete responses with 26% progression-free at 5 years. In this study, the overall median survival was 3.4 years with a median dose of 32 Gy given as 5-weekly fractions over 6–9 weeks. Patients with stage III disease did best compared with those erythrodermic patients with nodal or visceral (IVA–B) disease. The duration of response was also longer for those who received more than 20 Gy using 4–9 MeV. Comparative studies of TSEBT versus topical mechlorethamine in early-stage MF show similar response rates and duration of response, suggesting that TSEBT should be reserved for those who fail first and second line therapies [5,6]. Adverse effects of TSEBT include temporary alopecia, telangiectasia and skin malignancies, and the treatment is only available in a limited number of centres [7]. Although full-dose TSEBT is usually only given once in a lifetime, several reports have documented patients who have received two or three courses, where the total dosage tolerated and duration of response were lower with subsequent courses [8]. EORTC and international consensus guidelines have been produced for TSEBT [9,10]. Low-dose TSEBT regimens (10–30 Gy) have shown similar response rates although the duration of response is lower but these schedules (e.g. 12 Gy over eight sessions) have become the standard protocol for TSEBT as treatment is well tolerated and allows repeated palliative courses [11–13].

Systemic therapy
Immunotherapy

Different forms of immunotherapy have been evaluated in CTCL, with the intention of enhancing antitumour host immune responses by promoting the generation of cytotoxic T cells and Th1 cytokine responses. IFN-α shows ORRs of 45–74%, with complete responses of 10–27% [1,2]. Various regimens have been employed (from 3 MU three times weekly to 36 MU/day) and it appears that response rates are higher for larger dosage regimens (overall responses of 78% compared with 37% for the lower dosage regimen) [1]. ORRs are also higher in early (IB–IIA: 88%) compared with late (III–IV: 63%) stages of disease [1]. IFN-α availability is now limited but pegylated IFN-α is available and may be more effective and better tolerated [3] although response data are limited.

Pilot studies have shown that both IL-12 and IFN-γ can produce clinical responses in CTCL but their therapeutic value remains to be established and neither are approved. Ciclosporin has been used in erythrodermic MF/SS to relieve severe pruritus but there is evidence that treatment may cause rapid disease progression and its use in CTCL is not recommended with the exception of subcutaneous panniculitis-like T-cell lymphoma (SPTCL). CTCL frequently expresses PD-1 and phase II trials of nivolumab and pembrolizumab have shown efficacy in both MF and SS with ORRs as high as 38%, but these immune checkpoint inhibitors have not yet been approved for CTCL [4].

Retinoids and rexinoids

Oral retinoid therapy has been used both as a single agent and in combination with interferons and PUVA in the management of MF. A non-randomised small study comparing acitretin and isotretinoin in MF and SS showed no obvious differences, with complete responses of 21% in both groups.

Bexarotene, a rexinoid, is approved for MF/SS [1,2]. Bexarotene selectively binds and activates the rexinoid X receptor and promotes apoptosis and inhibits cell proliferation. It is relatively selective and therefore should have little effect on the retinoid acid receptor involved in cell differentiation. In phase II and III trials of 152 CTCL patients, response rates of 20–67% were reported [3,4]. The most effective tolerated oral dosage is 300 mg/m^2/day, although responses improve with higher dosage. Side effects are transient and generally mild but most patients while on therapy require treatment for hyperlipidaemia and central (hypothalamic) hypothyroidism according to an algorithm (Figure 139.25) [3,4]. At a dosage of 300 mg/m^2/day in early-stage disease (IA, IB, IIA), ORRs of 54% have been noted [1], while 45% of advanced MF patients (IIB–IVB) respond with a notable reduction in pruritus in stage III disease [2].

Combination therapy

Combined IFN-α and retinoid therapy produces similar response rates to IFN alone and is not recommended [1]. Studies comparing PUVA and IFN-α with IFN-α and acitretin in early-stage disease have shown complete response rates of 70% and 38%, respectively, but there are no data on duration of response [2]. Uncontrolled studies of combined PUVA and IFN-α (maximum tolerated dosage 12 MU/m^2 three times weekly) in MF and SS have shown ORRs of 100%, with 62% complete response rates [3]. This combination may also be useful for patients with resistant early-stage disease, such as those with thick plaques and folliculotropic disease. Open studies comparing PUVA with combined PUVA and acitretin have shown similar complete response rates (73% and 72%, respectively), although the cumulative dose to best response was lower in

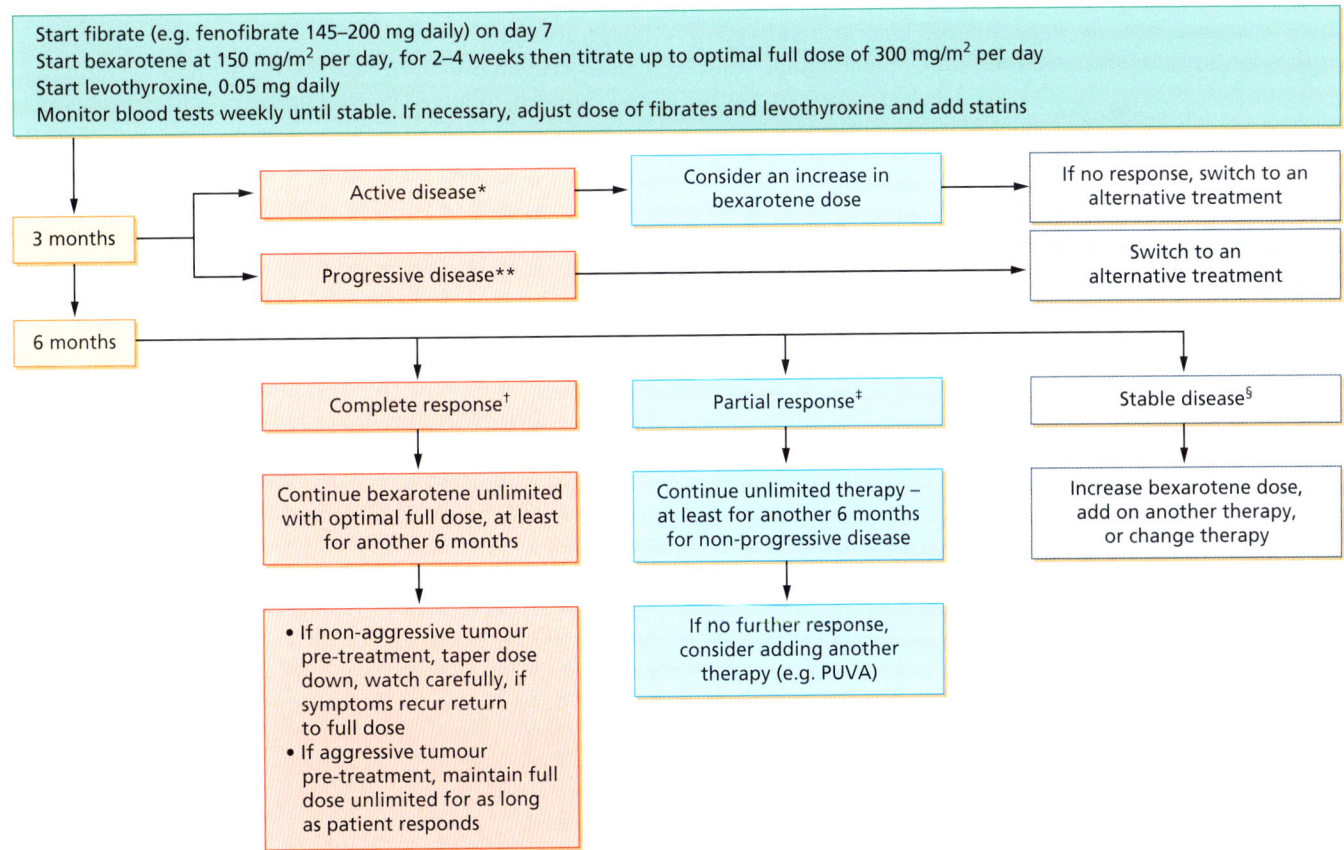

Figure 139.25 Suggested management algorithm for bexarotene in cutaneous T-cell lymphoma. PUVA, psoralen and ultraviolet A therapy. * Active disease = a slight increase in the extent of skin disease, e.g. <25%; ** progressive disease = increasing clinical stage or same stage, more tumours; † complete response = complete disappearance of all cutaneous disease; ‡ partial response = at least a 50% improvement compared with baseline; § stable disease = no new tumours, no stage progression, but no significant response. Reproduced from Gniadecki et al. 2007 [3] with permission of John Wiley & Sons.

patients receiving the combination therapy [4]. Bexarotene has been safely used in combination with PUVA [5,6] but a prospective randomised study in early-stage MF comparing PUVA with PUVA and bexarotene combined showed no difference in response rates [7]. At present there are few data on the impact on disease-free and overall survival.

Systemic chemotherapy

Mycosis fungoides and SS are relatively chemoresistant and responses are usually short lived [1]. This may partly reflect the low proliferative rate of tumour cells and a high prevalence of inactivating p53 mutations, which produce a relative resistance to tumour cell apoptosis. A systematic review of published data on different regimens has shown complete response (CR) rates of 33% in 526 patients treated with single-agent chemotherapy with a median duration of 3–22 months [2]. Combination chemotherapy regimens including cyclophosphamide, doxorubicin, vincristine and prednisolone (CHOP), in 331 patients, produced CR rates of 38%, with a median duration of 5–41 months [2]. CTCL patients are prone to infection and septicaemia is a common preterminal event.

Chemotherapy should not be used in patients with early-stage IA, IB or IIA disease. For patients with stage IIB–IVB disease, individual tumours and effaced peripheral lymph nodes will respond to superficial radiotherapy, and additional chemotherapy should be considered in patients with a good performance status (WHO 0–2). However, responses are likely to be short lived and patients should always be considered for clinical trials. Single-agent chemotherapy in stage IIB–IVB disease, and especially erythrodermic patients, includes oral chlorambucil (four to six cycles of 0.15–0.2 mg/kg/day for 2 weeks every 28 days), methotrexate and etoposide, and the intravenous purine analogues 2-deoxycoformycin, 2-chlorodeoxyadenosine and fludarabine [2].

Open studies of 2-deoxycoformycin in MF and SS have reported response rates of 35–71%, with CR rates of 10–33% [3]. Methotrexate has been reported in an uncontrolled study to produce a CR rate of 41% in 29 patients with erythrodermic (stage III/T4) disease, with a median survival of 8.4 years with single weekly doses of 5–125 mg [4]. In contrast, liposomal doxorubicin and gemcitabine have shown excellent responses in stage IIB and IVA non-erythrodermic MF with ORRs of 88% (44% CR) and 70–85% (10–22% CR), respectively. Once again, the duration of response is often short lived with a median duration of response of 10 months for CR patients treated with gemcitabine. In other studies, liposomal doxorubicin showed similar responses (56% ORR with 20% CR) in both transformed MF and erythrodermic SS patients, while an EORTC prospective study showed a lower response rate using a rigorous disease assessment tool [5]. Pralatrexate, a folate analogue, is well tolerated in MF and has shown moderate response rates [6]. Temozolomide is also effective in a minority of advanced stage MF/SS patients [7] and also for patients with CNS disease. A UK study of combination gemcitabine and bexarotene showed no additional benefit of this combination [8].

A phase III randomised controlled trial compared the anti-CD30 antibody–drug conjugate brentuximab with physician's choice of either methotrexate or bexarotene in CD30+ MF/anaplastic large-cell lymphoma (ALCL). This study showed a global ORR of 67%, CR of 16% and ORR lasting at least 4 months of 56.3% for brentuximab compared with a ORR of 20%, CR of 2% and ORR at 4 months of 12.5% for the physician's choice. These data led to FDA and EMA approval of brentuximab for CD30+ CTCL patients who are resistant to one systemic therapy [9].

Studies assessing the use of TSEBT and/or total body irradiation combined with high-dose conditioning chemotherapy prior to autologous stem cell transplantation in patients with stage IIB–IVA disease have shown good clinical responses [10] but high relapse rates. It does not appear that this approach affects disease-free or overall survival rates. Full allogeneic stem cell or bone marrow transplantation has only been used in a few patients, with encouraging results, but the associated mortality suggests that this approach is difficult to justify. However, reduced intensity allogeneic stem cell transplantation has shown promising results with clear evidence of a graft-versus-lymphoma effect and durable long-term complete remission in 50% of patients with advanced stages of CTCL [11–18]. At present there is no consensus regarding the most effective conditioning regimen but many reported series utilise a conditioning protocol consisting of TSEB, total lymphoid irradiation (TLI) and antithymocyte globulin (ATG) [18]. Specifically, the use of alemtuzumab (Campath) is not advised because of significant early relapses [13]. For patients with advanced disease and a good performance status, a reduced intensity conditioning allogeneic stem cell transplant is the most appropriate option producing a molecular complete remission in 43% with an overall survival of 56% at 5 years and non-relapse mortality of 14% [18].

Photopheresis

Extracorporeal photopheresis (ECP) involves the administration of oral psoralen, followed by the *ex vivo* collection of an enriched buffy coat preparation using a cell separator. These leukocytes are then passed through thin polythene tubing with exposure to UVA and the cells thereafter returned to the patient. This regimen is repeated on two successive days and the 2-day cycle repeated monthly or fortnightly in an accelerated regimen. There is evidence that a proportion of the UVA-exposed leukocytes, including some tumour lymphocytes, undergo apoptosis and that dendritic cells are activated during the *ex vivo* circulation with the induction of a host antitumour immune response after the treated cells are returned to the patient. Different models of autoimmune disease support this suggestion and the activation of dendritic cells during an expanded period of *ex vivo* incubation overnight (transimmunisation) has been shown.

ECP is FDA approved for the treatment of CTCL but there are no randomised studies to clarify whether ECP has an impact on overall survival. The original open study of ECP in 29 patients with erythrodermic CTCL reported a response rate of 73%, but response rates in patients with earlier stages of MF were much lower (38%) [1]. Subsequently, a median survival of 62 months was reported in the original cohort of 29 erythrodermic patients, which compares favourably with historical controls (30 months). A study of 33 patients with SS treated with ECP reported a median survival of 39 months, which was similar to historical controls from the same institution. Other studies have shown more prolonged median survival data [2]. An accelerated regimen consisting of nine collections rather than six for each cycle and an accelerated treatment schedule every 2 weeks has shown ORRs of 50%, with 18% CRs in erythrodermic disease. A systematic review of response rates in erythrodermic disease (stage III–IVA) with ECP reported overall responses of 35–71%, with CRs of 14–26%. Other studies are more difficult to interpret because they have either involved small numbers or patients with earlier stages of disease and in most studies many of the patients have been on concurrent therapies. Preliminary pilot studies suggest that the combination of IFN-α and ECP is more effective than ECP alone, but this has yet to be confirmed in randomised studies [3,4]. There are isolated case reports of combined ECP and IFN-α and/or bexarotene that have induced complete clinical and molecular responses [5]. There have also been claims that the CD8 count is critical in predicting whether patients will respond to ECP, although others have provided evidence that the total baseline Sézary cell count is the only predictor of response [6].

Toxin therapies

Denileukin diftitox, a DAB389–IL-2 fusion toxin (Onzar in Europe, Ontak in the USA), received FDA approval for the treatment of resistant or recurrent CTCL after the completion of several open label, phase II studies and a prospective randomised placebo-controlled study. Onzar is a recombinant fusion protein consisting of peptide sequences for the enzymatically active domain (389) of diphtheria toxin and the membrane translocation domain of IL-2 that is capable of inhibiting protein synthesis in tumour cells expressing high levels of the IL-2 receptor, resulting in cell death.

A study of 71 heavily pre-treated patients with stage IB–IVA disease, and more than 20% CD25+ T cells, showed an ORR of 30%, including 10% with complete responses [1]. The median duration of response was 6.9 months (range 2.7–46.1 months). The optimally tolerated intravenous regimen was 18 μg/kg/day for 5 days, repeated every 21 days for four to eight cycles. Adverse effects included fever, chills, myalgia, nausea and vomiting, and a mild increase in transaminase levels. Acute hypersensitivity reactions occurred in 60%, invariably within 24 h and during the initial infusion but this can be prevented with steroid pre-treatment [2]. A vascular leak syndrome characterised by hypotension, hypoalbuminaemia and oedema can be seen within the first 14 days of a given dose in 25% of patients. Myelosuppression is rare. Five per cent of adverse effects are severe or life threatening. The clinical relevance of antibody responses to denileukin diftitox is unclear. A prospective randomised phase III study comparing two different doses (9 and 18 μg/kg) with a placebo showed an ORR of 44% (higher with the 18 μg/kg dose) with 10% complete remission compared with a 16% ORR in patients receiving placebo [3]. Progression-free survival was significantly prolonged (median 2 years) for those patients on active treatment compared with placebo. Rare complete remissions noted in patients on the placebo arm emphasise that spontaneous remission can occur even in patients with advanced disease [3]. Current access to Onzar has been limited by purification challenges in the bacterial expression system, but a newer diphtheria toxin–IL-2 fusion protein is currently in clinical trials (E777, Eisai).

Monoclonal antibody therapy

The first antibody approach was a humanised chimeric anti-CD4 monoclonal antibody used to treat eight patients with CTCL, of whom seven showed a clinical response although this was of short duration. A radiolabelled anti-CD5 antibody has also been used in MF with some objective results and trials of a fully humanised anti-CD4 antibody (zanolimumab) for bexarotene-refractory MF/SS have shown an overall response of 56% and a median response duration of 81 weeks [1] but neither has been developed further for CTCL.

Campath (anti-CD52/alemtuzumab) for stage III patients has shown overall responses of 55–85% and a median response duration/time to treatment failure of 12 months [2]. A low-dose Campath regimen has also been reported with excellent response rates in SS [3–5] and remains a useful palliative option.

A phase III randomised controlled trial of mogamulizumab, a monoclonal antibody targeting a C–C chemokine receptor 4 (CCR-4) expressed in CTCL, compared with an FDA-approved oral histone deacetylase (HDAC) inhibitor, vorinostat, reported a significant improvement in progression-free survival (7.7 months) compared with vorinostat (3.1 months). This has led to FDA and EMA approval [6].

Histone deacetylase inhibitors

A novel class of drugs has been assessed in both MF and SS in a series of open label studies. These HDAC inhibitors affect gene expression by inhibiting deacetylation of histone proteins, which causes the chromatin structure to adopt an open configuration therefore allowing binding of transcription factors to promoter regions and gene transcription. While the effect of these drugs on histone proteins within chromatin is best understood, there are almost certainly widespread effects on non-histone proteins as well, which may be therapeutically important. There are four classes of HDAC inhibitors, and several including SAHA (vorinostat) and depsipeptide (romidepsin) are approved by the FDA for the second line treatment of both MF and SS [1–3]. Phase I/II studies of vorinostat have shown ORRs of 30% with a median time to progression of 5 months and romidepsin has shown overall global disease response rates of 34% with complete remission in 6% [1–3]. Side effects include lethargy, thrombocytopenia, gastrointestinal symptoms and prolongation of the QT interval. Whether HDAC inhibitors are best used as maintenance therapy or in combination for advanced disease remains unclear but dysregulation of STAT3 may confer resistance to HDAC inhibition in MF/SS [4].

PRIMARY CUTANEOUS CD30+ LYMPHOPROLIFERATIVE DISORDERS

Introduction and general description

Primary cutaneous CD30+ lymphoproliferative disorders consist of a spectrum of conditions. Lymphomatoid papulosis and CD30+ anaplastic large-cell lymphomas are defined on the basis of clinical and pathological features. Where a distinction cannot be made, patients are designated as 'borderline cases'. This group represents approximately 30% of all primary cutaneous lymphomas.

In the skin, CD30+ lymphoproliferative disorders are invariably of T-cell origin although nodal CD30+ lymphomas can be derived from B, T or null cells. By definition, primary cutaneous CD30+ disorders do not have any systemic or nodal involvement

Table 139.9 Treatment algorithm for cutaneous CD30+ lymphoproliferative disorders.

Disease	First line	Second line
Lymphomatoid papulosis	Expectant	MTX
	SDT	IFN-α
	Radiotherapy	
Anaplastic large-cell lymphoma	Surgical excision (solitary lesions)	CHOP
	Radiotherapy	Brentuximab[a]
	MTX	

[a] US Food and Drug Administration (FDA) and European Medicines Agency (EMA) approved.
CHOP, cyclophosphamide, doxorubicin, vincristine and prednisolone; IFN-α, interferon α; MTX, methotrexate; SDT, skin-directed therapy (topical therapy, phototherapy (TLO1/psoralen and ultraviolet A) or radiotherapy).

at diagnosis [1]. CD30 expression was originally identified on Reed–Sternberg cells in Hodgkin disease, but CD30 is also expressed on a proportion of activated T and B cells. Importantly primary cutaneous CD30+ lymphomas are associated with a good prognosis, in contrast to systemic nodal CD30+ lymphomas. A proportion of nodal systemic CD30+ lymphomas are associated with a disease-specific t(2;5) (p23;q35) translocation signified by expression of anaplastic lymphoma kinase (ALK), which is almost never found in primary cutaneous CD30+ lymphoproliferative disorders [2]. In MF, tumour cells may acquire CD30 expression but this should be distinguished from primary cutaneous CD30+ lymphoproliferative disorders by careful assessment of the associated clinical features. In MF, CD30 expression can be associated with large-cell transformation although this is not invariable. Patients with MF may also have concurrent skin lesions which have the classic clinical and pathological features of lymphomatoid papulosis.

Although the Epstein–Barr virus (EBV) genome can be detected in a proportion of CD30+ infiltrates in Hodgkin disease, EBV has not been found in patients with primary cutaneous CD30+ lymphoproliferative disorders. CD30 is a cell surface receptor for TNF-α-like cytokines, and it has been demonstrated that CD30 expression can be upregulated by EBV and in activated T cells.

The EORTC, ISCL and US Cutaneous Lymphoma Consortium (USCLC) consensus guidelines for the treatment of primary cutaneous CD30+ lymphoproliferative disorders have been published (Table 139.9) [3].

Lymphomatoid papulosis

Definition
This term was first used in 1968 by Macaulay to describe a 'self-healing rhythmical paradoxical papular eruption, histologically malignant but clinically benign' [1–3]. It is a chronic, recurrent, self-healing papulonecrotic or papulonodular eruption with the histological features of a CD30+ cutaneous lymphoma.

Pathophysiology
Mutations of *JAK1* and/or *STAT3* and *NPM1-TYK2* gene fusions have only been reported rarely in pcCD30+ ALCL and lymphomatoid papulosis [4]. Chromosomal rearrangements involving the 6p25.3 locus have only been identified in a minority (5%) of lymphomatoid papulosis cases [5]. This rearrangement involves the *DUSP22-IRF4* (MUM1) locus, and is associated with downregulation of DUSP22 encoding dual-specificity phosphatase-22, a tumour suppressor gene, which inhibits TCR signalling and promotes apoptosis. However, MUM1 expression is not specific for this rearrangement. This rearrangement has also been detected in a subset (25%) of systemic ALK-CD30+ ALCL cases; patients have a good prognosis [6]. In contrast, *TP63* rearrangements identified in aggressive variants of systemic ALK-CD30+ ALCL have not been detected in pcCD30+ lymphoproliferative disorders, which probably explains their excellent prognosis [7].

MUM1 is a transcription factor encoded by the *IRF4* gene and expressed in myeloma and lymphomas with plasmacytoid differentiation as well as activated T cells and Hodgkin lymphoma. It is expressed by the CD30+ cells in a majority of lymphomatoid papulosis but only rarely in primary cutaneous CD30+ ALCL [8]. Furthermore, *TRAF1*, expressed by activated T cells and in Hodgkin lymphoma, is also differentially expressed, being restricted mostly to lymphomatoid papulosis as opposed to primary cutaneous ALCL [9]. The functional significance of differential *MUM1* and *TRAF1* expression in lymphomatoid papulosis is unclear.

Clonal TCR gene rearrangements can be identified and are identical in different lesions from the same patient, but some biopsies may not show a clonal pattern because of a lack of sensitivity to detect a small clonal T-cell population [1,10]. Identical T-cell clones can be detected in skin biopsies from patients with both MF and lymphomatoid papulosis [10]. Studies using laser-captured CD30+ cells and sequencing of TCR genes have shown contradictory findings. One study suggested that the large CD30+ cells show clonal TCR gene rearrangements while other studies have shown that these large CD30+ cells are polyclonal and that the monoclonal population resides in the smaller population of CD30– cells [11]. The 6p25.3 rearrangement involving the *DUSP22-IRF4* locus is detected in a minority of cases (5%) [6]. In contrast, the t(2;5) translocation characteristic of nodal CD30+ lymphomas is not detected in lymphomatoid papulosis.

Pathology
The histological features consist of a relative lack of epidermotropism and Pautrier microabscesses, and the presence in the dermis of a mixed infiltrate composed of atypical lymphocytes with large nuclei and frequent abnormal mitoses, eosinophils, neutrophils, extravasated red cells and large histiocytic cells. Some of these cells may show marked cytological atypia (Figure 139.26). The epidermis may be ulcerated and the infiltrate may extend deeply into the reticular dermis. True vasculitis is rarely seen.

Lymphomatoid papulosis can be divided on histological grounds into types A, B, C, D and E subgroups [12–14]. In the A subgroup there appears to be a predominance of scattered, large, strikingly atypical CD30+ cells similar to those seen in Hodgkin disease [15]. In the B subgroup, smaller atypical T lymphocytes with convoluted nuclei similar to those seen in MF predominate and are CD3+ and CD4+ but CD30–. Group C lesions have large clusters of CD30+ cells and an overall pattern suggestive of an anaplastic CD30+ large-cell lymphoma [15]. In type D cases atypical CD30+ lymphoid cells express CD8 with a cytotoxic phenotype and in type E there

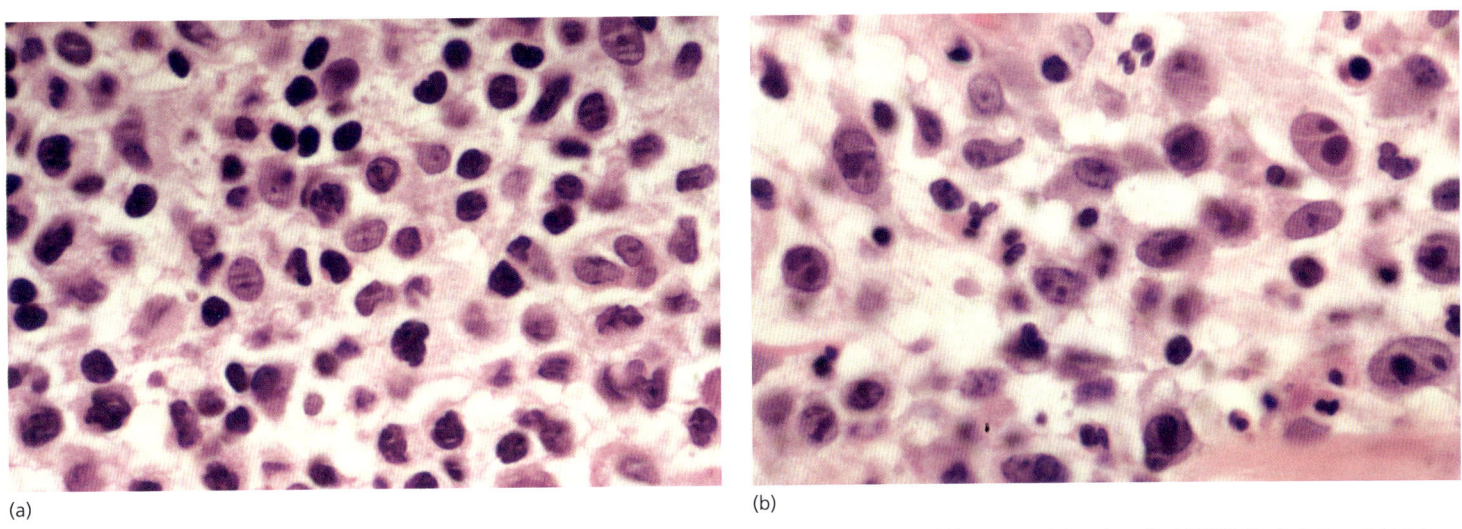

Figure 139.26 Composite high-power view of atypical cerebriform cells in (a) type B lymphomatoid papulosis and (b) large 'Reed–Sternberg-like' (CD30+) cells in type A histology.

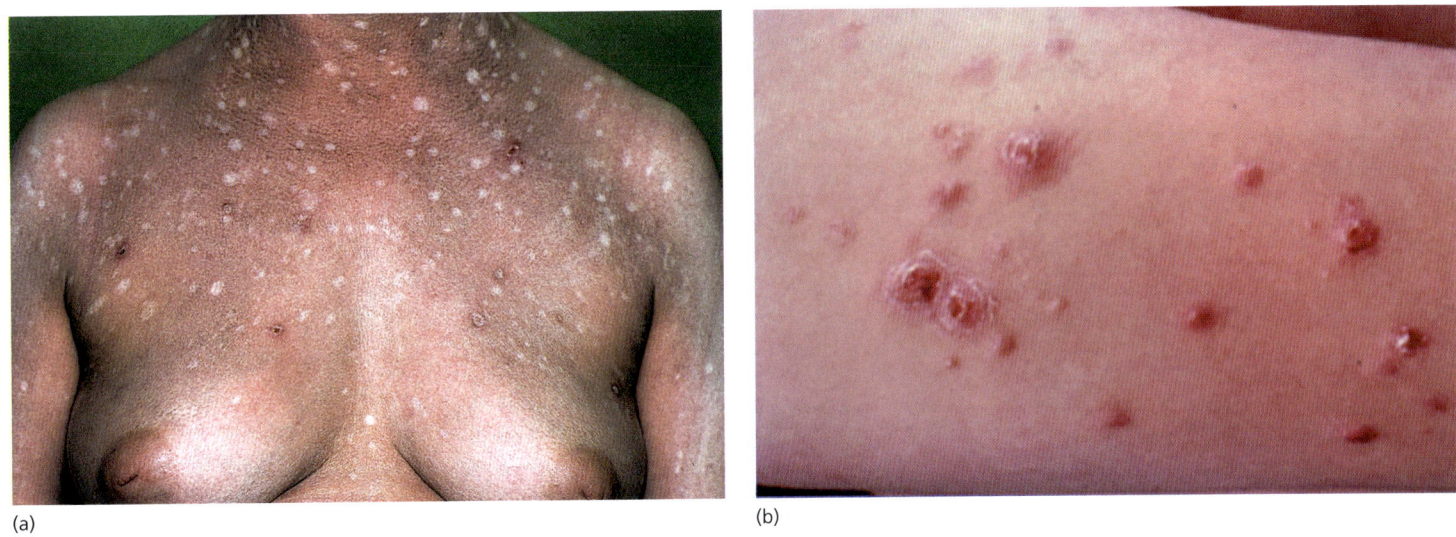

Figure 139.27 (a) Lymphomatoid papulosis. Note the multiple varioliform scars on the upper chest area of this patient, with a small number of fresh papular lesions. (b) Regional lymphomatoid papulosis.

is an angioinvasive pattern [13,14]. Many patients have multiple types of lesions coexisting simultaneously or a mixed pattern of A and B. Some patients with clinical lesions resembling pityriasis lichenoides et varioliformis acuta show a lymphomatoid histology and this probably represents a form of lymphomatoid papulosis (type B). These different pathological subtypes do not have any clinical or prognostic significance.

Clinical features

Patients have recurrent crops of papular or papulonecrotic or nodular lesions predominantly affecting the trunk, although any body site can be involved and localised regional variants may occur (Figure 139.27). These lesions grow rapidly over a few days and may develop ulcerated necrotic centres. Occasional patients develop isolated large necrotic tumours. Healing occurs slowly over 3–12 weeks, with fine atrophic circular or varioliform scars, but the cycle recurs every few months, with no obvious initiating factor. Critically for the diagnosis, every individual skin lesion resolves spontaneously and there may eventually be a persistent clinical remission. The lesions generally occur first in adult life and may recur in crops for up to 40 years. A small number of cases have been reported in children. Systemic symptoms at the time of disease flares are very rare.

The original description of lymphomatoid papulosis suggested a benign chronic and non-progressive disease, but there are well-documented rare cases of patients with lymphomatoid papulosis developing primary cutaneous or nodal CD30+ large-cell anaplastic T-cell lymphoma and Hodgkin disease. Similarly, some patients develop lymphomatoid papulosis-like lesions with a preceding history of Hodgkin disease. In contrast, patients more commonly have coexistent MF, and indeed patients with pre-existing MF may also subsequently develop lesions indistinguishable from those of lymphomatoid papulosis [15]. A follicular variant of the condition has been described and rarely lymphomatoid papulosis involving the subcutaneous tissues has been reported but these cases may represent other CTCL variants.

Disease course and prognosis

Long-term follow-up is necessary in all cases because of the risk of progression to a more aggressive lymphoma such as a primary cutaneous CD30+ anaplastic lymphoma, MF or Hodgkin disease in less than 5% of cases. The prognosis in patients with both MF and lymphomatoid papulosis appears to be excellent [16,17]. A review of 118 patients with lymphomatoid papulosis followed for many years suggested that only approximately 4% will develop extracutaneous disease within 10 years and that the 5-year overall survival is 100%. At present there are no proven prognostic indicators to identify those patients who might be more likely to develop associated lymphomas.

Management (Table 139.9)

There is no current treatment that alters the natural history of the disease but some therapies do reduce the frequency and severity of new lesions or prevent recurrent disease flares. Intensive combination chemotherapy is not recommended and is only associated with a short duration of response.

Low-dose radiotherapy may accelerate clearance of individual lesions and is especially useful for large necrotic lesions. Narrow-band UVB therapy and PUVA benefit individual patients for short periods of time. Low-dose once-weekly oral methotrexate is the most useful systemic therapy, and there are reports of a beneficial effect with oral dapsone [18,19].

Primary cutaneous anaplastic (CD30+) large-cell lymphoma

Definition

This is a primary cutaneous CD30+ anaplastic (or rarely pleomorphic or blastic) large-cell lymphoma in which the CD30+ tumour cells comprise the majority of the infiltrate. Clinical features of MF are absent and, unlike lymphomatoid papulosis, these tumours do not resolve spontaneously.

Pathophysiology

Primary cutaneous CD30+ ALCL expresses CCR3 and Th2 cytokines as well as CCR4 as in MF/SS. There is no evidence for the t(2;5) chromosomal translocation detected in systemic nodal CD30+ anaplastic lymphomas. This balanced translocation is found in ALK+ ALCL and usually involves the nucleophosmin (*NPM*) gene juxtaposed with the *ALK* gene although there are several other ALK partners identified in a minority of cases [1]. Mutations of *JAK1* and/or *STAT3* and kinase fusions such as the *NPM1-TYK2* gene fusion have been reported rarely in pcCD30+ ALCL and lead to constitutive activation of the JAK-STAT pathway [2]. Chromosomal rearrangements involving the 6p25.3 locus have been identified in pcCD30+ ALCL (25%). This rearrangement involves the *DUSP22-IRF4* (MUM1) locus and is associated with downregulation of DUSP22 encoding dual-specificity phosphatase-22, a tumour suppressor gene, which inhibits TCR signalling and promotes apoptosis [3]. Primary cutaneous CD30+ ALCL cases also have allelic loss at 9p21-22 [4].

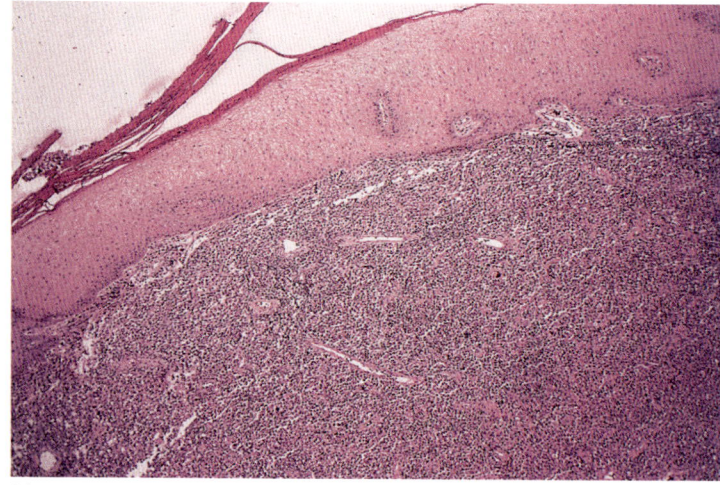

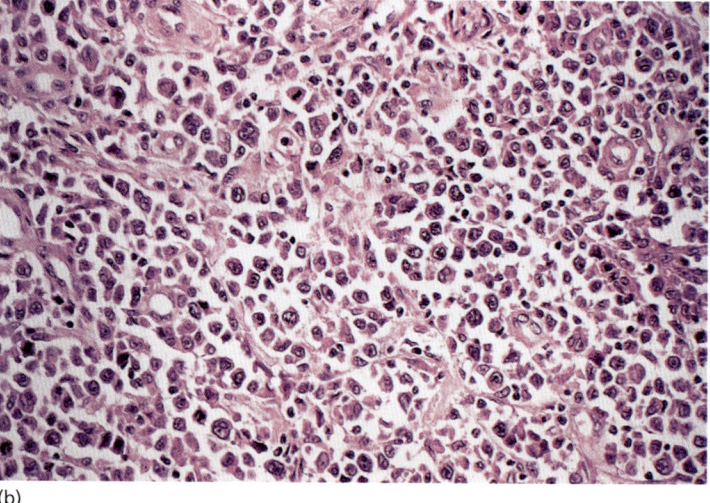

Figure 139.28 (a) Low-power view of CD30+ infiltrate showing a lack of epidermotropism but dense infiltrate in the underlying dermis. (b) CD30+ lymphocytic infiltrate showing striking large atypical cells.

Pathology

Biopsies show a dense lymphocytic infiltrate consisting of sheets of large atypical cells with an anaplastic morphology and mitoses, but usually there is no epidermotropism as seen in MF (Figure 139.28). The tumour cells variably express T-cell antigens and the vast majority will be CD30+. Some tumour cells show a pleomorphic or blast-like morphology [5]. Pseudoepitheliomatous hyperplasia may occur. Clonal TCR gene rearrangements are detected in almost all cases consistent with a T-cell origin.

Immunophenotype

The tumour cells are generally CD4+ and by definition CD30+ with expression of cytotoxic proteins such as perforin, granzyme B and TIA-1. There is variable loss of other T-cell antigens such as CD2, CD5 and CD3. Some cases are CD8+. Tumour cells are epithelial membrane antigen and CD15 negative. ALK is not expressed, in contrast to those systemic CD30+ lymphomas with secondary cutaneous involvement, but CD56 may be rarely expressed. The t(2;5) translocation is absent [1]. While the morphology and phenotype are similar in lymphomatoid papulosis [6], the key distinguishing feature is the presence of cohesive nodules and sheets of anaplastic cells in primary cutaneous ALCL, and in primary cutaneous ALCL the tumour cells generally do not express *MUM1* and *TRAF1* unlike in lymphomatoid papulosis [7].

Clinical features

These lymphomas are usually seen in adults and present as large solitary or multiple and often ulcerated nodules (Figure 139.29), most often on the trunk. There are no patches or plaques of MF elsewhere, and some individual lesions may partially but never completely regress. Some individuals develop disease localised to a limb, and others will show a clinical spectrum characterised by large persistent nodules of ALCL and coexistent lesions of lymphomatoid papulosis. Progression to extracutaneous sites is rare but has been recorded in approximately 10% of cases [5] and recent evidence suggests that patients with extensive regional disease may be at higher risk of disease progression.

Clinical variants

Flynn *et al.* described patients with large ulcerative nodules, often on the thighs and buttocks, which show variable rates of spontaneous resolution and were labelled as 'regressing atypical histiocytosis' [8]. These 'borderline cases' are now considered to be closely related to both lymphomatoid papulosis and primary cutaneous CD30+ large-cell lymphoma, with the detection of a T-cell phenotype and clonal rearrangements of the TCR gene confirming a T-cell origin.

A rare locoregional nodal variant has been described in which there are palpable and pathologically involved regional lymph nodes at presentation, but no evidence of lymphoma beyond the regional draining nodal basin [5]. The limited evidence to date on treatment and prognosis suggests that this lymphoma has a similar prognosis to primary cutaneous CD30+ ALCL.

Differential diagnosis

Careful staging consisting of bone marrow and PET/CT scans is required to exclude systemic CD30+ ALCL in which there is secondary cutaneous involvement.

Disease course and prognosis

Disease-related 5-year survival rates of 90% have been reported but they may be as low as 50% for those patients presenting with generalised tumours [5].

Management (Table 139.9)

Both excision and localised radiotherapy are acceptable methods of treating isolated lesions [9]. The recurrence rate on the treated site is low, but new lesions may develop elsewhere on the skin. Low-dose methotrexate may also be effective. Systemic chemotherapy, including CHOP, is effective but is only the treatment of choice for patients with widespread cutaneous disease. Rare variants with regional nodal disease have been successfully treated with radiotherapy and do not always require systemic chemotherapy. Brentuximab has shown a high rate of durable complete remissions in a pivotal phase III randomised controlled trial and is FDA/EMA approved for patients who are resistant/refractory to one prior systemic therapy [10].

PRIMARY CUTANEOUS T-CELL LYMPHOMA VARIANTS

Introduction and general description

Rare primary CTCL variants represent a heterogeneous group of T-cell malignancies, which are defined by distinct clinicopathological features. In all cases MF must be carefully excluded especially on the basis of the clinical features. Several subtypes are currently considered as provisional entities [1]. For patients who do not fulfil the characteristic features of these rare variants, the designation of primary cutaneous peripheral T-cell lymphoma (not otherwise specified –(NOS)) should be used. The prognosis may be poor with a high probability of systemic involvement. Full staging investigations are required for all patients to exclude a systemic nodal/extranodal peripheral T-cell lymphoma (NOS).

Subcutaneous panniculitis-like T-cell lymphoma

Definition

This is a rare, cytotoxic T-cell lymphoma, representing less than 1% of all non-Hodgkin lymphomas, which usually affects younger adults with an equal sex incidence [1]. Two subsets have been defined consisting of those cases derived from an αβ T cell, which have an indolent course, and those derived from a γδ T cell [2]. The term subcutaneous panniculitis-like T-cell lymphoma (SPTCL) is now restricted to those lymphomas derived from an αβ T cell [1].

Pathophysiology

The underlying molecular pathogenesis has been clarified. Two germline variants of the gene *HAVCR2* have been detected in SPTCL patients [3]. These founder variants are detected in a majority of patients [4]. *HAVCR2* encodes the checkpoint inhibitor TIM3

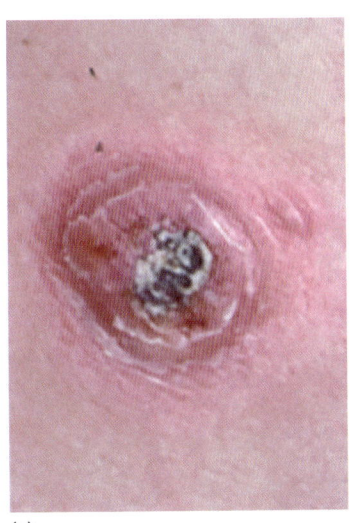
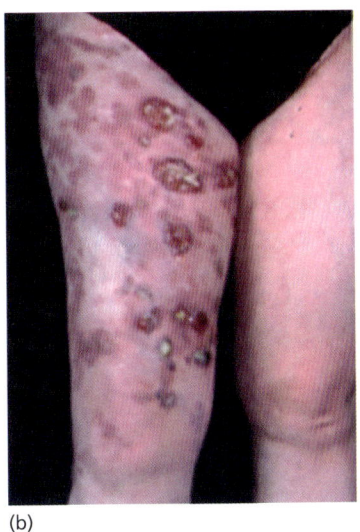

Figure 139.29 (a) Solitary primary cutaneous CD30+ anaplastic large-cell lymphoma (ALCL). (b) Multifocal pcCD30+ALCL.

and the germline homozygous variants cause loss of function leading to T-cell activation. Relatives with heterozygote mutations may be asymptomatic or develop lupus-like symptoms [4]. Somatic variants detected in *HAVCR2* mutant and wild-type SPTCL include *TET2*, *ARID1B* and other epigenetic modifiers as well as genes involved in the PI3K/AKT/mTOR (phosphatidylinositol 3-kinase/protein kinase B/mammalian target of rapamycin) pathways and the JAK-STAT pathway [4]. Studies have characterised a specific pattern of chromosomal abnormalities using CGH, loss of heterozygosity (LOH) and FISH techniques; these have shown losses of 10q, 17p and 19, with additional 5q and 13q gains, which appear to be distinct from findings in MF/SS [5].

Pathology

There is a diffuse infiltrate restricted to and extending throughout the subcutis without epidermotropism [1,2]. In contrast, primary cutaneous γδ T-cell lymphomas may show prominent involvement of the subcutis but there is invariably associated dermal and/or epidermal involvement [1]. The degree of cellular atypia can be minimal but medium-sized and occasionally large pleomorphic cells are usually present (Figure 139.30). Rimming of the tumour cells around fat cells is a characteristic feature, although not restricted to SPTCL. A prominent reactive inflammatory infiltrate is common and the tumour cells may show vascular invasion with angiocentricity. Necrosis and erythro-lymphophagocytosis may be present.

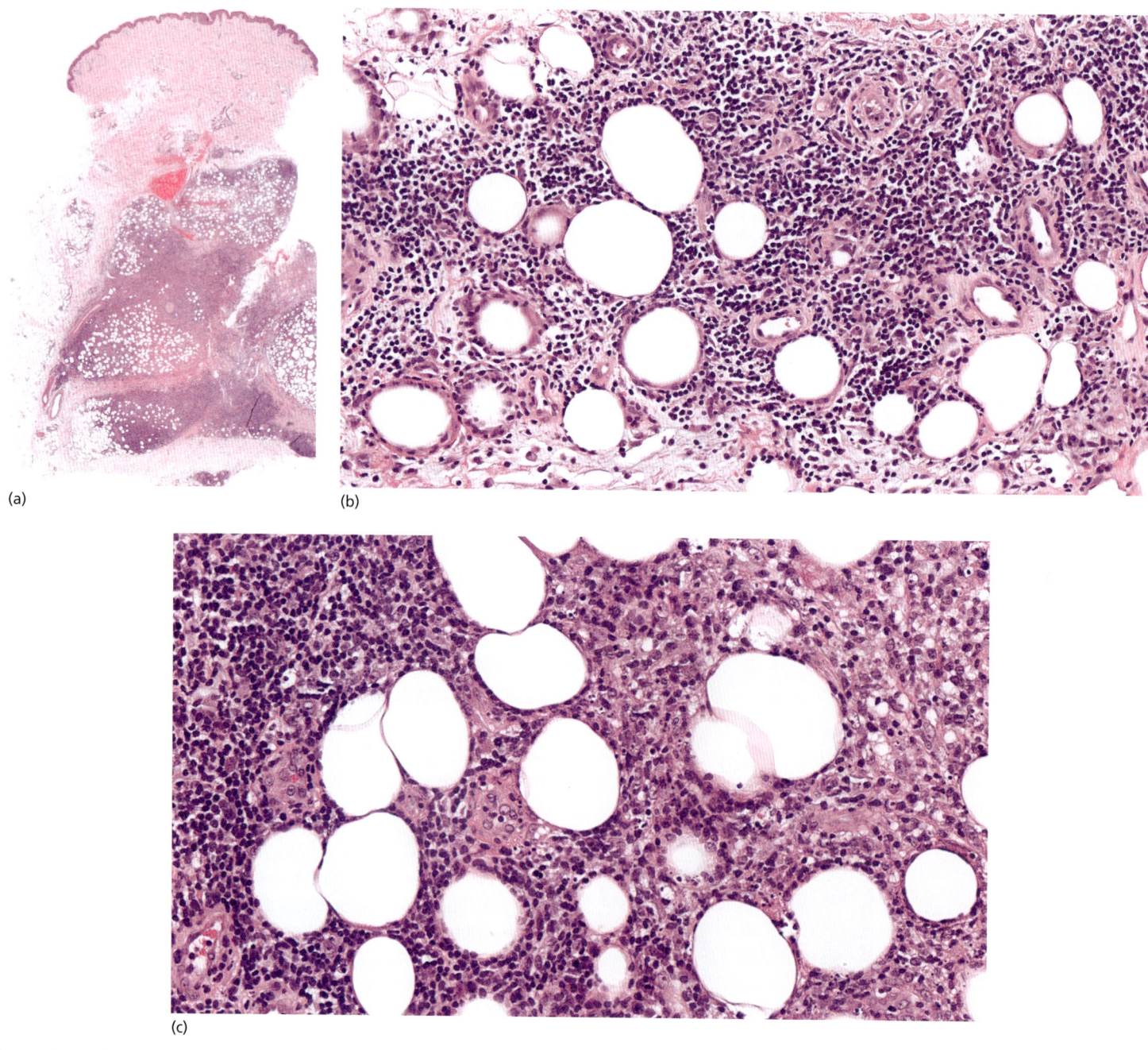

Figure 139.30 Subcutaneous panniculitis-like T-cell lymphoma. Low-power view of subcutaneous infiltrate (a), with high-power views showing rimming of fat cells by atypical mononuclear cells (b) and medium/large pleomorphic tumour cells (c). Courtesy of Eduardo Calonje.

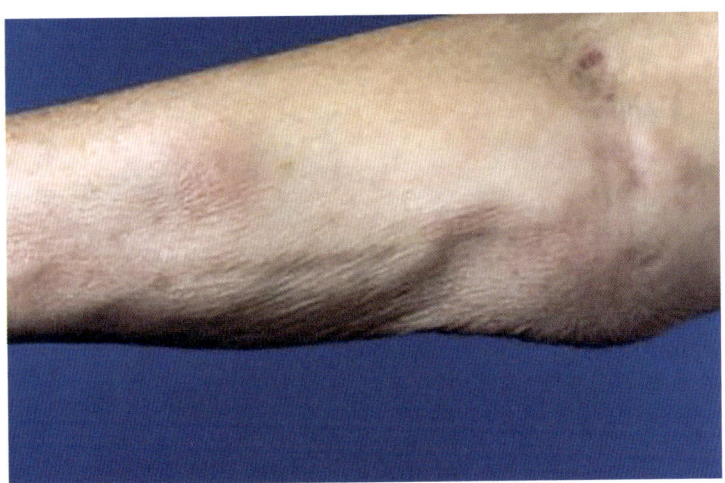

Figure 139.31 Subcutaneous panniculitis-like T-cell lymphoma. Subcutaneous indurated plaques with lipoatrophy.

Table 139.10 Treatment algorithm for cutaneous T-cell lymphoma variants.

Disease	First line	Second line
Subcutaneous panniculitis-like T-cell lymphoma	Prednisolone Radiotherapy Ciclosporin	CHOP
Epidermotropic CD8+ cutaneous T-cell lymphoma	Chemotherapy TSEBT	RicAlloSCT
Small/medium CD4+ T-cell lymphoproliferative disorder and acral CD8+ T-cell lymphoma	Surgical excision Radiotherapy	

CHOP, cyclophosphamide, doxorubicin, vincristine and prednisolone; RicAlloSCT, reduced-intensity conditioned allogeneic stem cell transplant; TSEBT, total skin electron beam therapy.

Indolent cases were previously diagnosed as benign cytophagic histiocytosis (Weber–Christian disease) [6,7].

Immunophenotype
Tumour cells have a mature T-cell phenotype and are usually βF1+, CD3+, CD8+ and CD4– [1,2]. CD30 and CD56 are generally negative. Tumour cells may express cytotoxic molecules including granzyme B, perforin and TIA-1. Clonal rearrangements of the TCR genes are present [2,8].

Clinical features
Patients present with indolent, slowly expanding, subcutaneous nodules or plaques usually involving the limbs, which may initially be misdiagnosed as panniculitis (Figure 139.31). Occasionally, patients present with more diffuse erythematous induration mimicking cellulitis. Ulceration is rare. Lymphadenopathy is usually absent at presentation and systemic progression is rare although nodal involvement can be characterised by tumour cells restricted to the perilymph node fatty tissue. There is often a prolonged indolent phase before the diagnosis is established. Systemic symptoms may occur, particularly in those patients who develop a haemophagocytic syndrome consisting of fever, pancytopenia and hepatosplenomegaly, although this is more common in those with a γδ T-cell lymphoma.

Differential diagnosis
Cases must be carefully distinguished from lupus panniculitis as both conditions share similar clinical and pathological features, which is likely to reflect the presence of germline *HAVCR2* mutations [9].

Disease course and prognosis
The prognosis is reasonable, with a 5-year survival of 80%. Dissemination to extracutaneous sites is rare in contrast to primary cutaneous γδ T-cell lymphomas, which have a poor prognosis [1].

Management (Table 139.10)
Patients with αβ SPTCL can be treated successfully with systemic steroids [10] and ciclosporin, which may be more effective in those patients with germline *HAVCR2* mutation [1,11]. Superficial radiotherapy can be used for individual lesions. Denileukin diftitox has been used successfully in SPTCL [12], as have bexarotene and romidepsin [13,14]. Combination chemotherapy can be associated with successful clinical responses and resolution of the haemophagocytic syndrome, although this is usually restricted to those with extracutaneous disease [1]. High-dose therapy and autologous/allogeneic stem cell transplantation have also been successful in patients with refractory and usually systemic disease [15–17].

Primary cutaneous aggressive epidermotropic CD8+ T-cell lymphoma

Definition
This is a primary cutaneous CD8+ T-cell lymphoma that expresses cytotoxic proteins and shows a prominent epidermotropic infiltrate [1,2]. Although rare, the distinctive pathological and immunophenotypic features and poor prognosis suggest that it represents a distinct subtype of CTCL [1,2].

Pathophysiology
This CTCL variant was previously designated as disseminated pagetoid reticuloses (Ketron–Goodman variant). Clonal TCR gene rearrangements are detected but the underlying pathogenesis has not yet been established. Although the number of cases reported is small, these cases should be distinguished from primary cutaneous γδ T-cell lymphomas (βF1–) that show clonal rearrangements of the γ TCR gene with the β TCR gene in a germline configuration [1]. WGS and RNA sequencing studies have identified gain-of-function *JAK2* fusions and mutations activating the JAK-STAT pathway as well as a complex pattern of large-scale chromosomal gains and losses including *CDKN2A/B* [3].

Pathology
These lymphomas show a striking epidermotropic band-like infiltrate (pagetoid) with nodular infiltrates of large or small to

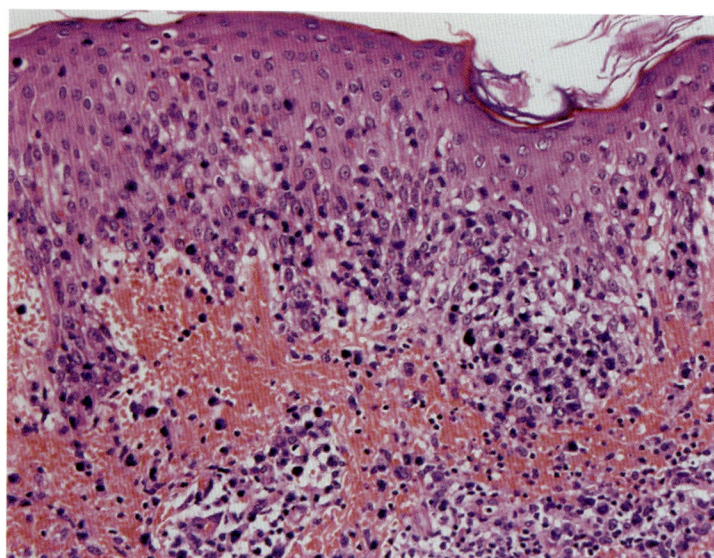

Figure 139.32 An epidermotropic infiltrate of large pleomorphic lymphoid cells and marked papillary dermal haemorrhage.

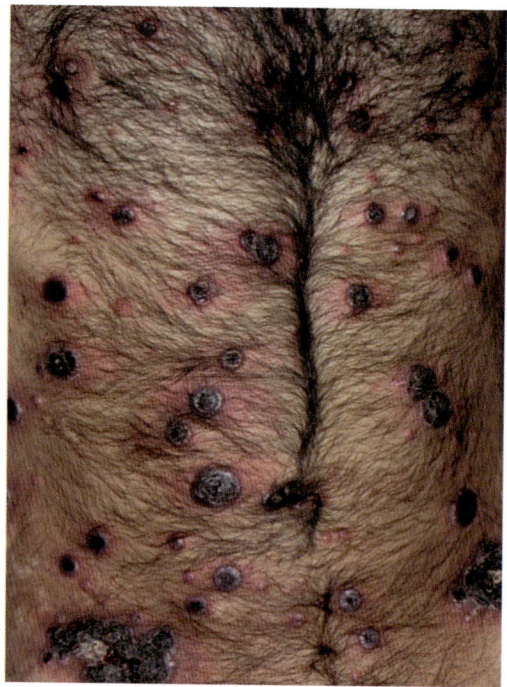

Figure 139.33 Primary cutaneous aggressive epidermotropic CD8+ cutaneous T-cell lymphoma showing necrotic haemorrhagic plaques.

medium-sized pleomorphic or blastic T cells, usually accompanied by haemorrhage in the upper dermis (Figure 139.32). Angiocentricity and invasion can be a feature. These cutaneous lymphomas must be distinguished from CD8+ MF variants, primary cutaneous γδ T-cell lymphomas [1,4], primary cutaneous CD30+ lymphoproliferative disorders with a CD8+ phenotype and rare indolent CD8+ cutaneous lymphomas characterised by solitary nodular lesions, often around the ear or acral sites [5–7].

Immunophenotype
The tumour cells are CD8+ and usually βF1+, CD45RA+ and CD3+ [1,2]. The tumour cells also express cytotoxic proteins such as TIA-1, granzyme B and perforin. CD4, CD45RO, CD56 and CD30 are negative. EBV is not detected, in contrast to nasal-type natural killer (NK)/T-cell lymphomas [1].

Clinical features
These patients rapidly develop generalised and monomorphic plaques, nodules and/or tumours (Figure 139.33), which often show ulceration, haemorrhage and necrosis [1,2]. Mucosal involvement may occur. There are no preceding characteristic clinical features of MF, namely polymorphic patches and plaques and involvement of the limb–girdle areas.

Disease course and prognosis
The prognosis is very poor, with a 5-year survival of 18% [1].

Management (Table 139.10)
These patients have a very poor prognosis and dissemination to visceral sites such as the CNS, testis and lung is more common than to nodal sites. Responses to radiotherapy and chemotherapy are limited and the treatment of choice may be a reduced-intensity allogeneic stem cell transplant for selected patients with a reasonable performance status who achieve a good clinical response.

Primary cutaneous γδ T-cell lymphoma

Definition
This is a CTCL consisting of γδ T cells with a cytotoxic phenotype, which presents primarily with skin involvement. A subgroup of patients with subcutaneous panniculitis-like T-cell lymphoma derived from γδ T cells are included in this category [1,2].

Pathophysiology
This variant must be distinguished from transformed MF, ATLL, primary cutaneous aggressive epidermotropic cytotoxic CD8+ CTCL, SPTCL derived from αβ T cells and blastic NK cell or extranodal NK/T-cell lymphomas (nasal type). Oncogenic mutations in the JAK-STAT, mitogen-activated protein kinase (MAPK), *MYC* and chromatin modification pathways have been identified but no mutations affecting the TCR signalling pathway, in contrast to MF/SS [3]. It has also been established that this CTCL variant is derived from Vδ1 γδ T cells although those subtypes that show additional subcutaneous involvement are derived from Vδ2 γδ T cells [3].

Pathology
Prominent nodular or diffuse infiltrates are characteristic with medium to large pleomorphic or blast-like T cells. Epidermotropism may occur but the infiltrate is often extensive with dermal and subcutaneous patterns. Angiocentricity and rimming of fat cells may occur.

Immunophenotype
The tumour cells are usually CD2+, CD3+, CD5−, CD7+/− and CD56+ but are negative for CD4, CD8 and βF1. EBV is negative and clonal TCR gene rearrangements are usually present.

Clinical features
The characteristic presentation is the sudden appearance of multiple cutaneous plaques, nodules or tumours, which may be ulcerated and with no preceding polymorphic plaques or patches typical of MF. The clinical presentation may be similar to primary cutaneous aggressive epidermotropic CD8+ lymphomas but some patients present with only subcutaneous involvement. Mucosal involvement and extranodal involvement is common. Some cases of disseminated pagetoid reticulosis (Ketron–Goodman variant) may have represented cutaneous γδ T-cell lymphomas [4–6]. A haemophagocytic syndrome may complicate some cases.

Disease course and prognosis
The prognosis is very poor [1,2].

Management
Superficial radiotherapy and multiagent chemotherapy are usually required but the overall prognosis is very poor and allogeneic stem cell transplantation may be appropriate for selected patients with a reasonable performance status who achieve a good clinical response.

Primary cutaneous CD4+ small/medium pleomorphic T-cell lymphoproliferative disorder (provisional)

Definition
This provisional entity is usually characterised by solitary skin lesions associated with a dermal infiltrate consisting of small to medium-sized pleomorphic tumour cells which are CD4+ [1].

Pathophysiology
Currently, little is known about the underlying aetiology and pathogenesis but the immunophenotype suggests a derivation from follicular helper T cells [2–4]. Cases must be distinguished from MF and pseudo-T-cell lymphomas and also peripheral T-cell lymphoma (NOS) to avoid inappropriately aggressive therapy.

Pathology
There are dense nodular or diffuse infiltrates of small to medium-sized pleomorphic T cells within the dermis, often extending into the subcutis [1]. Occasional larger pleomorphic cells may be present but are a minority. Epidermotropism is variable.

Immunophenotype
The tumour cells are CD4+ and CD3+ but a loss of some T-cell antigens is common [1,5]. CD30 and CD8 are negative and cytotoxic proteins are not expressed. Tumour cells invariably express CXCL13, ICOS and PD1 consistent with a follicular helper T-cell origin [2–4]. Clonal TCR gene rearrangements are present [6].

Clinical features
Patients usually present with solitary or rarely a few small plaques, nodules or tumours, often on the upper trunk or head and neck, without typical polymorphic patches or plaques of MF. Patients are HTLV-1 negative. Systemic involvement has not been reported.

Disease course and prognosis
The estimated 5-year survival is 100%, based on small series [1,5].

Management (Table 139.10)
In view of the excellent prognosis, superficial radiotherapy is appropriate for solitary lesions either as primary treatment or after surgical excision [5,6].

Primary cutaneous acral CD8+ T-cell lymphoma (provisional)

Definition
This is a low-grade indolent CD8+ T-cell lymphoma which is usually solitary and affects acral sites [1].

Pathophysiology
The underlying pathogenesis is unknown but this should always be distinguished on the basis of the clinicopathological features from other CTCL variants such as CD8+ MF and aggressive epidermotropic CD8+ CTCL [1–3]. This entity should not be classified as primary cutaneous peripheral T-cell lymphoma (NOS).

Pathology
There is a dense dermal infiltrate of atypical CD8+ T cells with a cytotoxic phenotype and no epidermotropism.

Immunophenotype
The tumour cells are CD2+, CD3+ and CD8+ with variable loss of other T-cell markers and they express cytotoxic markers including TIA-1, perforin and granzyme B. EBV is negative. CD68 highlights tumour cells with dot-like perinuclear Golgi positivity. Clonal TCR gene rearrangements are detected [1,2].

Clinical features
Patients present with solitary red papules or nodules invariably only affecting the acral sites and in particular the earlobe (Figure 139.34). Rarely patients may present with multifocal skin lesions [3].

Disease course and prognosis
The long-term prognosis is excellent with only very rare cases developing systemic progression. Staging scans are appropriate. Skin recurrences are rare [3].

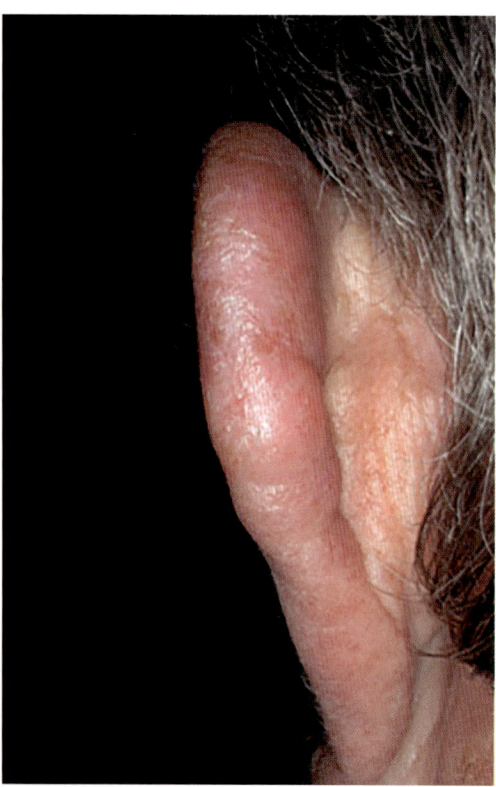

Figure 139.34 Acral CD8+ cutaneous T-cell lymphoma on the earlobe. Reproduced from Beltraminelli *et al.* 2010 [1] with permission of John Wiley & Sons.

Management (Table 139.10)

Patients can be managed conservatively with surgical excision and/or low-dose radiotherapy.

Adult T-cell leukaemia–lymphoma (HTLV-1 associated)

Definition

Adult T-cell leukaemia–lymphoma is a mature T-cell leukaemia–lymphoma caused by the human T-lymphotropic retrovirus type 1 (HTLV-1).

Epidemiology

Infection with HTLV-1 is prevalent in certain parts of the world, including Japan, central Africa, the Caribbean, southeastern states of the USA and in native Australians, and consequently ATLL is endemic in these regions. Sporadic cases are found throughout the world. The disease has a long latency period (15–20 years) and the incidence of ATLL among HTLV-1 carriers has been estimated to be 2.5% [1]. The virus can be transmitted in breast milk and in blood products. There is a slight male predominance and the median age of onset is 55 years [1]. Paediatric cases are rare, but not unknown, and are assumed to follow perinatal infection. In immunosuppressed patients, such as following organ transplantation, progression to ATLL can be rapid.

Pathophysiology

Human T-cell leukaemia virus 1 infects CD4+ T cells and is the underlying cause of ATLL. The virus is randomly integrated into the host genome following expression of viral reverse transcriptase, and the viral tax protein is a potent transactivation factor that induces expression of numerous host genes and specifically the key transcription factor NFκB leading to T-cell activation, differentiation and proliferation [2]. Extensive next generation sequencing studies have shown that additional molecular abnormalities produce the malignant phenotype and these driver gene mutations are similar to those implicated in MF/SS [3], although a specific IRF4 variant has only been identified in ATLL [3]. Unlike MF/SS, there is no characteristic UV mutational signature, which is consistent with the underlying viral transformation [4]. The HTLV-1 proviral DNA is clonally integrated, confirming a pathogenetic role for the virus in individual cases [5,6]. Tumour burden can be assessed by monitoring viral RNA expression levels [5].

Pathology

In the skin, a prominent epidermotropic infiltrate is usually found, consisting of medium to large cells with a pleomorphic nuclear morphology, particularly in the acute and lymphomatous variants (Figure 139.35) [7,8]. Blast-like cells may be present. Pautrier-like microabscesses and a cerebriform nuclear morphology can be seen, simulating MF. However, the degree of cellular atypia may also be mild, causing diagnostic difficulties. Eosinophilia is often present. Granulomatous features have been rarely described. In the peripheral blood, the tumour cells have polylobulated nuclei ('flower cells'). Lymph nodes usually show a leukaemic pattern of infiltration, with preservation and dilatation of lymph node sinuses containing tumour cells. Rarely, Hodgkin-like features are present within an expanded lymph node paracortex containing a diffuse infiltrate of small, mildly atypical lymphocytes and scattered CD30+, CD15+ and Reed–Sternberg-like EBV-positive cells resulting from expansion of EBV-positive cells as a consequence of a relative T-cell immunodeficiency [8].

Immunophenotype

Tumour cells are CD2+, CD3+, CD5+ and CD7–. Most tumour cells are CD4+, although CD8+ and CD4–, and CD8– variants also occur [8]. Leukaemic cells have a similar immunophenotype. CD25 expression is almost universal. Large blast-like cells can be CD30+ but are ALK negative. Cytotoxic proteins are not expressed. Analysis of TCR genes shows clonal TCR gene rearrangements.

Clinical features

Patients with ATLL often have extensive lymph node and peripheral blood involvement but the skin is the most common extranodal site of disease (50% of patients) and primary cutaneous disease can occur [7,9]. Other extranodal sites of disease include bones, lungs, liver, gastrointestinal tract and the CNS. Cutaneous involvement is characterised by widespread or solitary papules, nodules, tumours or erythroderma, often associated with intense pruritus (Figure 139.36). Patients may present with patches and plaques that are clinically indistinguishable from MF.

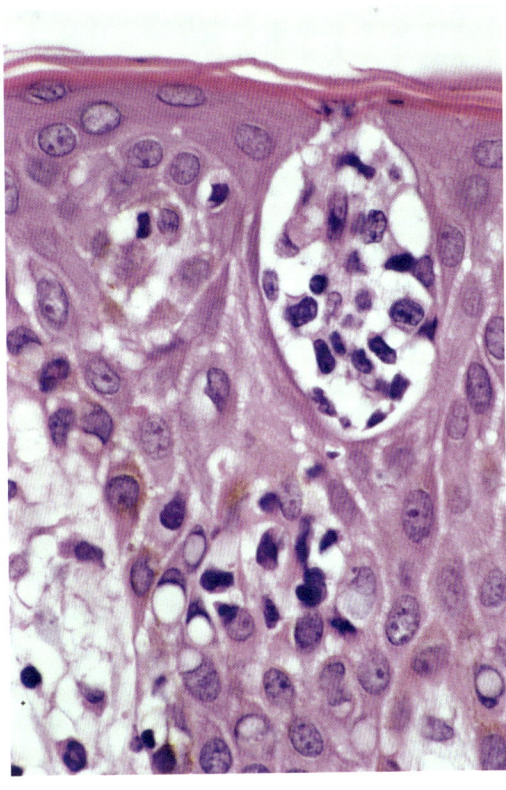
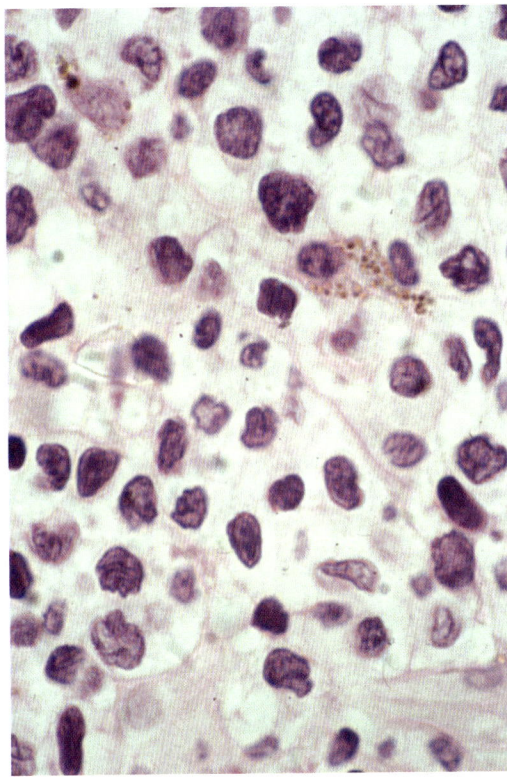

Figure 139.35 Adult T-cell leukaemia–lymphoma: prominent atypical cells forming a Pautrier microabscess and large pleomorphic cells within the dermis.

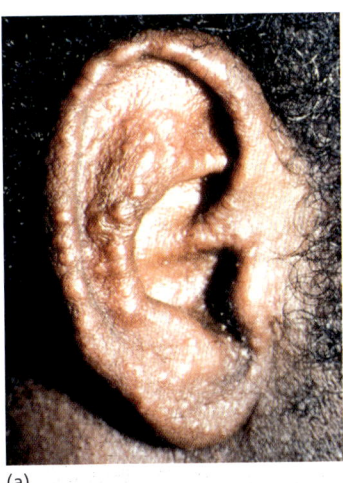
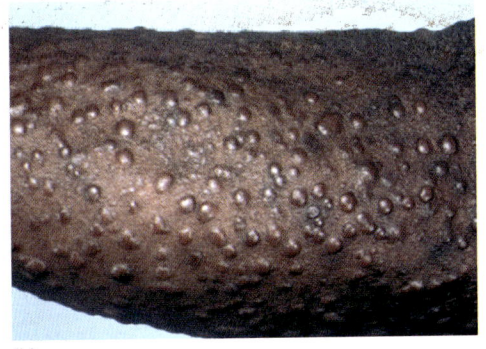
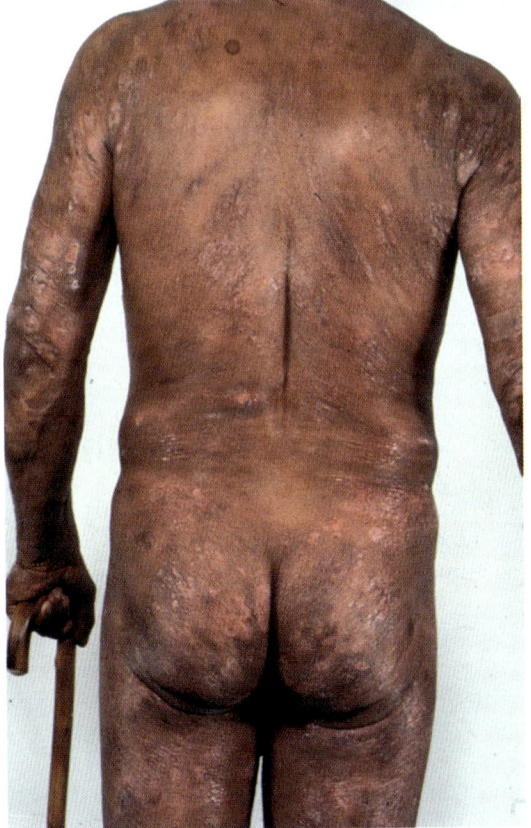

(a)

(b)

(c)

Figure 139.36 Three clinical presentations of cutaneous adult T-cell leukaemia–lymphoma: (a) a pruritic papular eruption confined to the auricle, (b) an extensive nodular eruption on the forearm, and (c) superficial patches and plaques involving the limb–girdle area similar to mycosis fungoides.

Clinical variants

Several clinical variants have been defined [8]. An acute variant is characterised by a leukaemic phase with generalised lymphadenopathy and hepatosplenomegaly often associated with cutaneous involvement and hypercalcaemia with lytic bone lesions. Opportunistic infections are common. A lymphomatous variant is similar but with the absence of peripheral blood involvement. The chronic variant is typically characterised by cutaneous disease and a peripheral blood lymphocytosis without hypercalcaemia. The smouldering variant is also characterised by prominent cutaneous disease without overt peripheral blood involvement. Pulmonary lesions may occur. Progression from the chronic and smouldering variants to acute disease occurs in at least 25% of cases but often only after a long duration. Patients with cutaneous ATLL have shown marked photosensitivity mimicking actinic reticuloid [10].

HTLV-1 infection has also been associated with an inflammatory myopathy, which may show features suggestive of dermatomyositis. However, this inflammatory myopathy responds poorly, if at all, to systemic corticosteroids or other immunosuppressive drugs. Other skin conditions that occur in association with HTLV-1 infection include xerosis and acquired ichthyosis, seborrhoeic dermatitis and non-infectious dermatitis. An infective dermatitis is often seen in children (Chapter 25).

Complications and co-morbidities

Opportunistic infections secondary to reduced immunity are common in ATLL and include scabies, dermatophytosis, onychomycosis, bacterial skin infections including leprosy, warts and strongyloidiasis and tuberculosis.

Disease course and prognosis

Acute and lymphomatous variants have a poor prognosis with less than 10% 5-year survival. In contrast, patients with the chronic (30% 5-year survival) and smouldering (65% 5-year survival) variants can have a prolonged course, although disease transformation eventually occurs for most patients [8].

Investigations

Patients require full staging investigations including PET/CT scans and bone marrow trephine biopsies as well as viral load assays of peripheral blood. HTLV-1 serology is invariably positive [8] and confirmed by detecting antibodies to the virus in a serum sample (enzyme-linked immunosorbent assay first and then immunoblot to distinguish between HTLV-1 and -2). Cultivation and detection of the virus is only available in specialist laboratories but confirmation of infection is possible using PCR methods. Hypercalcaemia is a common and characteristic finding of acute variants.

Management

Cutaneous disease can respond to skin-directed therapy but patients with the acute and lymphomatous variants have a poor prognosis and require combination chemotherapy. Combination azacytidine and IFN therapy is a standard of care for those with chronic and smouldering variants of ATLL [11,12]. Mogamulizumab (anti-CCR4) is an established treatment for ATLL but is only licensed in Japan [13]. Younger patients may be candidates for stem cell transplantation [14].

Extranodal NK/T-cell lymphoma (nasal type)

Definition

This rare type of extranodal EBV-positive angiocentric lymphoma preferentially involves the nasal cavity and naso-pharynx but also shows a predilection for the skin. It used to be referred to as polymorphic reticuloses or angiocentric immunoproliferative lesion [1,2]. Most cases are derived from NK cells but rare cases have a cytotoxic T-cell phenotype. Some cases represent hydroa vacciniforme-like lymphoma (HVLL) or arise in patients with hypersensitivity to mosquito bites [3].

Epidemiology

The disease is more prevalent in Asia and Central and South America.

Pathophysiology

Epstein–Barr virus is present in almost all cases of extranodal NK/T-cell lymphoma, whether CD56+ or CD56– [1]. EBV is present in a clonal episomal form, suggesting that the virus has a critical pathogenetic role. No disease-specific cytogenetic abnormality has been identified but deletions of 6q and isochromosome 6q are common and genomic abnormalities are distinct to those found in NK-cell leukaemias [4,5].

Reports have implicated EBV-infected cytotoxic T cells in the pathogenesis of both the photosensitive disorder hydroa vacciniforme and hypersensitivity to mosquito bites in patients from Asia and South America [3,6]. Furthermore, there is now substantial evidence that such patients are at risk of developing extranodal NK/T-cell lymphomas with a fatal outcome [7–10] such as HVLL [3]. This suggests that in genetically susceptible individuals, an EBV-driven NK/T-cell lymphoproliferative disorder has the potential to transform into an aggressive EBV-associated NK/T-cell lymphoma [6], but the precise relationship between classic hydroa vacciniforme and NK/T-cell lymphoma has yet to be clarified.

Recurrent gene mutations resulting in activation of the JAK-STAT pathway and epigenetic modifiers have been detected in extranodal NK/T-cell lymphomas [11].

Pathology

There is a diffuse infiltrate in the dermis and often the subcutis with prominent angiocentricity and angiodestruction [1,2]. Extensive necrosis is common. Tumour cells can show a variable morphology with small/medium and large pleomorphic/anaplastic cells. An associated heavy mixed inflammatory infiltrate is common and pseudoepitheliomatous hyperplasia may be found, which can lead to diagnostic confusion.

Immunophenotype

Tumour cells are derived from NK cells and are CD56+, CD2+, surface CD3– and cytoplasmic CD3+. Most cases express cytotoxic proteins, namely granzyme B, perforin and TIA-1 [1,2]. Rare cases are CD30+ and this may confer a more favourable prognosis. TCR genes are in a germline configuration consistent with an NK-cell origin. However, rare cases of extranodal NK/T-cell lymphomas have a CD56–, CD3+ cytotoxic phenotype and show a clonal TCR gene rearrangement consistent with derivation from a cytotoxic T cell [2,12,13].

Clinical features
Involvement of the nasal cavity, naso-pharynx, paranasal sinuses, orbit and oro-pharynx is associated with tissue destruction ('lethal midline granuloma'). Secondary involvement of other extranodal sites including the skin and gastrointestinal tract occurs but primary cutaneous disease is rare. Cutaneous plaques, nodules and tumours may ulcerate and become necrotic. Purpura, bullous lesions, a cellulitis-like rash and diffuse maculopapular rashes have been described. A haemophagocytic syndrome can develop rarely and systemic symptoms are common. Bone marrow and peripheral blood involvement is rare but such cases can be indistinguishable from aggressive NK-cell leukaemia.

Disease course and prognosis
The multidrug resistance phenotype is often expressed and the median survival for patients presenting is 12–15 months although the prognosis may be better for those patients with only cutaneous involvement (27 months) [12,13].

Management
The prognosis is poor despite aggressive chemotherapy, particularly for those patients with disease outside the nasal cavity [2].

Table 139.11 American Joint Committee on Cancer staging classification of non-mycosis fungoides/Sézary syndrome primary cutaneous lymphomas.

TNM stage	Description
Tumour	
T1:	Solitary skin involvement
T1a	Solitary lesion <5 cm diameter
T1b	Solitary lesion >5 cm diameter
T2:	Regional skin involvement; multiple lesions limited to one body region or two contiguous body regions
T2a	All-disease-encompassing in a <15 cm diameter circular area
T2b	All-disease-encompassing in a >15 and <30 cm diameter circular area
T2c	All-disease-encompassing in a >30 cm diameter circular area
T3:	Generalised skin involvement
T3a	Multiple lesions involving two non-contiguous body regions
T3b	Multiple lesions involving ≥ three body regions
Node	
N0	No clinical or pathological lymph node involvement
N1	Involvement of one peripheral lymph node region that drains an area of current or prior skin involvement
N2	Involvement of two or more peripheral lymph node regions or involvement of any lymph node region that does not drain an area of current or prior skin involvement
N3	Involvement of central lymph nodes
Metastasis	
M0	No evidence of extracutaneous non-lymph node disease
M1	Extracutaneous non-lymph node disease present

Adapted from Kim *et al.* 2007 [6].

PRIMARY CUTANEOUS B-CELL LYMPHOMAS

Introduction and general description

Primary cutaneous B-cell lymphomas constitute approximately one-quarter of all primary cutaneous lymphomas [1]. The WHO classification defines three specific subtypes of primary cutaneous B-cell lymphoma: marginal zone lymphoma (MZL), follicle centre cell lymphoma (FCL) and diffuse large B-cell lymphoma (LBCL) [1,2]. Full staging investigations are essential for patients with a cutaneous B-cell lymphoma to exclude secondary cutaneous involvement with a nodal lymphoma although bone marrow involvement is very rare in MZL and FCL [3,4]. Most primary cutaneous B-cell lymphomas are indolent with an excellent long-term prognosis, with the exception of primary cutaneous LBCL [1,5].

An ISCL–EORTC TNM classification has been proposed for staging primary cutaneous lymphomas other than MF and SS (Table 139.11) [6]. This staging classification has shown prognostic relevance for primary cutaneous LBCL as multifocal disease appears to be a poor prognostic feature, but the value of staging the skin tumour burden in primary cutaneous MZL (PCMZL) and primary cutaneous FCL (PCFCL) has not yet been shown to have an impact on prognosis [7,8]. Recent ISCL–EORTC consensus recommendations for the management of primary cutaneous B-cell lymphomas have been published and conservative management is appropriate for PCMZL and PCFCL, but more aggressive therapy may be required for primary cutaneous LBCL (Table 139.12). Distinction between cutaneous B-cell pseudolymphomas and MZLs can be particularly difficult. Systemic B-cell non-Hodgkin lymphomas such as small-cell lymphocytic lymphoma and mantle cell lymphomas are only found within skin as secondary cutaneous involvement associated with underlying nodal disease, although very rarely mantle cell lymphomas can be restricted to the skin.

The pathogenetic relationship between these primary cutaneous B-cell lymphomas and their nodal counterparts remains unclear (Table 139.13). Specific translocations characteristic of MALT lymphomas of nodal and extranodal origin have been detected in a minority of PCMZLs. Genomic abnormalities detected in nodal diffuse LBCLs have been identified in primary cutaneous LBCL, suggesting a similar pathogenesis [2]. However, PCFCLs appear to be distinct pathogenetically from nodal follicular lymphomas [2].

In 1982, Burgdorf *et al.* suggested that Lyme disease was caused by the tick *Ixodes ricinus*, and subsequently the spirochete *Borrelia burgdorferi* was recognised as being the vehicle responsible for carrying infection from the tick to humans. Prior to the publication by Burgdorf *et al.*, it had been recognised that patients with acrodermatitis chronica atrophicans, now known to be part of the cutaneous spectrum of Lyme disease, could develop low-grade cutaneous B-cell lymphomas. These patients developed multiple plaques and nodules superimposed on lesions of acrodermatitis chronica atrophicans. In a small number of reported cases, the

Table 139.12 Treatment algorithm for cutaneous B-cell lymphomas.

Prognostic group (stage)	First line	Second line
Primary cutaneous FCL/MZL:		
Localised T1–T2b	Excision	RT
	Expectant	Intralesional rituximab
	RT	
Extensive T2c–T3	Chlorambucil	Rituximab
	RT	CVP-R or CHOP-R
Advanced N1–N3 or M1	CVP-R or CHOP-R	RT
	R-bendamustine	High-dose chemotherapy/auto-SCT
Primary cutaneous diffuse LBCL – leg	CHOP-R for 3–6 cycles ± RT	Second line chemotherapy
		RT
	RT as palliation	High-dose chemotherapy/auto-SCT
Primary cutaneous diffuse LBCL – other (including anaplastic/pleomorphic T-cell/histiocyte-rich and intravascular large B-cell lymphoma)	CHOP-R ± RT RT as palliation	High-dose chemotherapy and auto-SCT

auto-SCT, autologous stem cell transplant; CHOP-R, cyclophosphamide, doxorubicin, vincristine, prednisolone and rituximab; CVP-R, cyclophosphamide, vincristine, prednisolone and rituximab; FCL, follicle centre cell lymphoma; LBCL, large B-cell lymphoma; MZL, marginal zone lymphoma; R, rituximab; RT, local skin radiotherapy.

Table 139.13 Summary of cytogenetic findings in primary cutaneous B-cell lymphomas.

Cytogenetic abnormality	PCMZL	PCFCL	PCLBCL
t(14;18) IgH : MALT1	22% (21/95)	0% (0/6)	0% (0/14)
t(14;18) IgH : BCL2	11% (9/80)	17% (24/143)	7% (4/54)
t(11;18) AP12 : MALT1	4% (4/96)	0% (0/1)	0% (0/6)
t(1;14) BCL10 : IgH	0% (0/63)	ND	ND
t(8;14) MYC : IgH	0% (0/9)	0% (0/6)	36% (5/14)
t(3;14) BCL6 : IgH	0% (0/9)	6% (2/33)	14% (2/14)
Trisomy 3	17% (11/63)	ND	ND
Trisomy 18	6% (4/63)	ND	ND
BCL2/MALT1 amplification	0% (0/11)	8% (2/25)	60% (12/20)
BCL10 mutation	3% (1/33)	50% (2/4)	ND
BCL6 mutation	0% (0/9)	37% (7/19)	47% (15/32)
cMYC amplification	0% (0/9)	0% (0/6)	17% (3/18)
cREL amplification	ND	25% (3/12)	63% (12/19)
9p21.3 (p16/p14ARF) deletion	ND	0% (0/19)	62% (43/64)

ND, not determined; PCFCL, primary cutaneous follicle centre cell lymphoma; PCLBCL, primary cutaneous diffuse large B-cell lymphoma; PCMZL, primary cutaneous marginal zone lymphoma.

lesions of acrodermatitis chronica atrophicans cleared with antibiotic therapy, but the B-cell lymphoma often persisted. Nevertheless, this suggested the possibility that *Borrelia* might have a role in the pathogenesis of PCMZL. For those patients without clinical evidence of acrodermatitis the causal relationship has been more controversial, with some studies detecting positive *Borrelia* serology and the presence of *Borrelia* in tumour DNA using PCR [9,10] and others consistently reporting negative results [11]. Nevertheless, *B. burgdorferi* infection has been established as the cause of a reactive lymphoid hyperplasia (Borrelial lymphocytoma) which tends to preferentially affect the head and neck, breast and genital area and resolves after oral antibiotics [12].

Primary cutaneous marginal zone lymphoma

Definition

This is an indolent cutaneous B-cell lymphoma derived from post-germinal centre cells and characterised by a proliferation of small lymphocytes, marginal zone B cells (small centrocyte-like), lymphoplasmacytoid cells and plasma cells with monotypic cytoplasmic immunoglobulin [1–3]. PCMZL is considered part of the spectrum of extranodal marginal zone B-cell lymphomas that often involve mucosal sites (MALT lymphomas).

This category also includes primary cutaneous immunocytoma [4] and rare primary cutaneous plasmacytoma without overt evidence of underlying myeloma or localised bony or other extramedullary involvement. Extraosseous lesions in multiple myeloma are common, and the skin is infiltrated in approximately 10% of cases, but primary involvement of the skin without evidence of bone involvement is extremely rare.

Epidemiology

There is a slight male predominance and younger adults are more commonly affected.

Pathophysiology

Primary cutaneous MZL is considered to be part of the spectrum of extranodal marginal zone B-cell lymphomas that were first described in the stomach, the so-called MALT lymphoma, and have since been described in the thyroid, salivary gland, orbit and lung as well as the skin.

As would be expected, PCMZL shows a plasma cell signature in a subset of cases [5]. No disease-specific cytogenetic abnormalities have been identified in PCMZL, although CGH techniques have shown amplification of the *BCL2* locus on chromosome 18 [6]. *FAS* mutations have rarely been described [7]. Studies have demonstrated that approximately 50% of PCMZLs have translocations identical to those found in other extranodal MALT lymphomas, including the t(14;18) translocation involving the *IgH* gene locus and *MALT1* gene, which is mostly found in monocytoid variants (Table 139.13) [8–10]. Trisomy 3 and 18 have also been detected in up to 40% of cases [10,11]. The t(11;18) translocation, which produces a fusion protein involving the *AP12* gene and the *MALT1* gene, has also been detected in PCMZL [11,12], although other studies have failed to detect this translocation [7,10]. Other translocations found in extranodal marginal zone B-cell lymphomas, such as the t(1;14) involving the *Bcl-10* gene on 1q, have not yet been identified in PCMZL [7,10,11]. The t(14;18) translocation involving *Bcl-2* has also not been consistently detected in PCMZL [10] except in isolated reports, but this does not have any specific impact on survival [8]. A high frequency of *FAS* gene mutations has been identified which are likely to impair FAS-mediated apoptosis [13].

The development of immunocytomas has been reported in patients with acrodermatitis chronica atrophicans and has led to speculation about the role of *B. burgdorferi* producing chronic antigen stimulation, leading to neoplastic transformation. The detection of *Borrelia* DNA in some cutaneous lesions of PCMZL, using PCR, has provided support for this role. The frequency of positivity varies

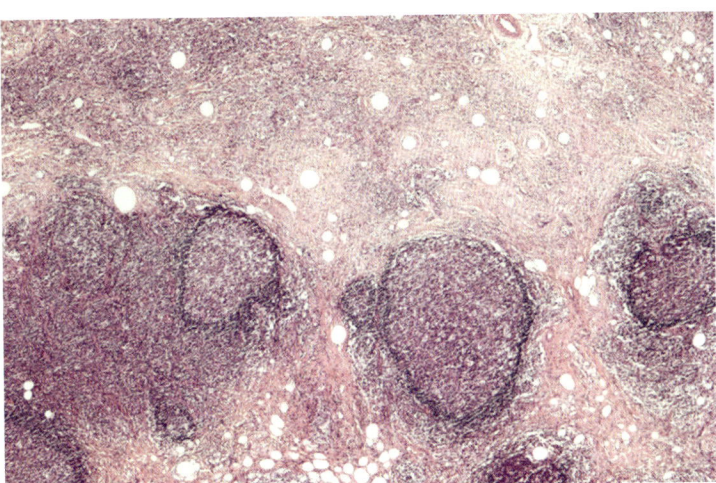

Figure 139.37 Marginal zone primary cutaneous B-cell lymphoma: reactive germinal centres with a non-epidermotropic monomorphic infiltrate of lymphoplasmacytoid cells and mature plasma cells.

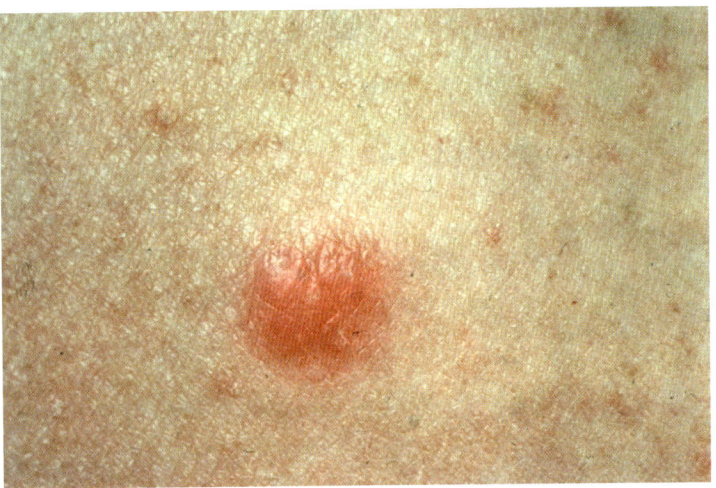

Figure 139.38 Marginal zone primary cutaneous B-cell lymphoma: typical urticated dermal red papules and plaques predominantly situated on the trunk.

considerably in different geographic regions, with positive results in central Europe and Scotland, but no evidence of an association in the USA. To date, most cases of PCMZL associated with *Borrelia* have been κ light chain positive.

Pathology
Histology is characterised by nodular or diffuse dermal infiltrates of small to medium-sized lymphocytes, marginal B cells (centrocyte-like), lymphoplasmacytoid cells and plasma cells, often with a reactive T-cell infiltrate [1–4]. There is no epidermotropism. Reactive follicular structures are often present and tumour cells present within expanded marginal zones and interfollicular areas may colonise these follicular structures (Figure 139.37). This pattern has to be distinguished immunophenotypically from rare follicular patterns of PCFCL. Occasional scattered centrocytes, centroblasts and immunoblasts may be present. Tumour cells, characterised by monotypic κ or λ positive, large, pale lymphoplasmacytoid cells, are concentrated at the periphery of the cellular aggregates or residual follicular structures. Periodic acid–Schiff-positive intranuclear or intracytoplasmic inclusions may be present [1–3]. Cases with a monomorphic infiltrate of plasma cells (immunocytoma-like) are included [4]. Very rare cases of cutaneous plasmacytoma associated with monoclonal gammopathy of uncertain significance have to be distinguished from benign reactive plasma cell infiltrates (plasmacytosis) by identifying monotypic light chain expression.

Immunophenotype
Tumour cells express CD20, CD79a and Bcl-2, but are Bcl-6, CD5 and CD10 negative [3]. PCMZL of the skin should be distinguished from cutaneous infiltrates of chronic B-lymphocytic leukaemia, which are CD5+. Plasma cells are CD138+ and CD79a+ (but CD19– and CD20–) and the infiltrate usually shows either κ or λ light chain restriction (although this can often be difficult to detect in cutaneous sections because of non-specific staining of collagen). Reactive follicles are Bcl-6+ and CD10+ but Bcl-2–.

Clonal immunoglobulin gene rearrangements are detected in most cases. The demonstration of light chain restriction and/or a clonal immunoglobulin gene rearrangement represents a critical technique for distinguishing these low-grade cutaneous lymphomas from reactive cutaneous B-cell infiltrates (pseudolymphomas).

Clinical features
These lymphomas present as asymptomatic solitary or multiple dermal papules, plaques or nodules on any body site, although the trunk is most often involved (Figure 139.38) [1–4]. Spontaneous resolution can occur. Anetoderma associated with individual lesions has been described [14].

Disease course and prognosis
The estimated 5-year survival is 98–100% [3,4,15].

Investigations
Full staging investigations are indicated and a benign monoclonal paraproteinaemia may be present. The differential diagnosis includes plasmacytoma where skeletal surveys are required to exclude underlying myeloma, and Waldenström macroglobulinaemia characterised by an immunoglobulin M (IgM) paraprotein and a clonal proliferation of lymphoplasmacytoid B cells.

Management (see Table 139.12)
Radiotherapy (low dose) is the standard treatment option but some patients may be managed simply by observation in view of the excellent long-term prognosis [16]. Surgical excision may be used for isolated small lesions. The role of IFN-α has not been established but it may be effective either systemically or intralesionally [16]. In cases associated with *B. burgdorferi*, relevant antibiotic therapy can be appropriate but the current evidence for antibiotic usage in *Borrelia*-positive PCMZL is lacking [17]. In patients with multifocal disease chlorambucil may be appropriate [16]. Cutaneous recurrences are common and can be treated in a similar manner.

Primary cutaneous follicle centre cell lymphoma

Definition and nomenclature
This is an indolent primary cutaneous B-cell lymphoma derived from follicle centre cells and consisting of a mixture of centrocytes (small/large cleaved cells) and centroblasts (larger non-cleaved cells).

> **Synoyms and inclusions**
> - Crosti lymphoma

Pathophysiology
The relationship between PCFCL and both nodal systemic follicular and diffuse large B-cell lymphomas remains unclear. While there are morphological similarities, PCFCL follows an indolent clinical course and the immunophenotypic features are distinct (CD10 expression is mostly confined to PCFCL with an exclusively follicular growth pattern and Bcl-2 is usually negative or rarely only weakly positive). Microdissection of tumour cells has also confirmed the germinal centre cell origin of PCFCL Bcl-2-negative tumour cells, with no evidence of the t(14;18) translocation, suggesting a different pathogenesis to nodal follicular lymphoma. Gene expression studies have detected a germinal centre B-cell signature in PCFCL [1] distinct from the activated B-cell signature detected in primary cutaneous diffuse LBCL [2]. While the t(14;18) translocation – characteristic of nodal systemic follicular lymphoma and a significant proportion of diffuse LBCLs – has not been consistently detected in most studies of PCFCL, other studies have detected the t(14;18) in a proportion of CD10+ and Bcl-2-positive PCFCL with a follicular growth pattern. This suggests that there might be an unexplained geographic or histological subset distinction although there are no obvious prognostic differences. A study using a FISH-based technique has detected the t(14;18) translocation involving *Bcl-2* in 41% of 27 cases in which a PCR-based technique failed to identify any *Bcl-2* rearrangement [3]. However, this study restricted the cases of PCFCL to those with a follicular growth pattern only. Other studies have also detected rare t(14;18) translocations in PCFCL using FISH techniques with both Bcl-2 and MALT1 involved as translocation partners [4].

CGH studies have also identified patterns of chromosomal gains and losses associated with specific oncogene abnormalities in PCFCL, including *c-REL* amplification, but a consistent pattern has not yet emerged [5,6]. FISH studies have not identified chromosomal breakpoints involving the IgH, *myc* or *bcl-6* loci although one study did show a t(3;14) in two of 33 cases involving *Bcl-6* and IgH in PCFCL (Table 139.13) [3]. Inactivation of both the cyclin-dependent kinase inhibitors, namely the *p15* and *p16* genes, by promoter hypermethylation has been detected in a proportion of cases but the clinical significance is unclear. A study has identified aberrant somatic hypermutation affecting certain oncogenes in PCFCL including *BCL6*, *PAX5*, *MYC* and *RhoH/TTF* similar to findings in nodal and primary cutaneous LBCL.

At present, a detailed characterisation of the molecular abnormalities in PCFCL is required to clarify the pathogenetic relationship between PCFCL and both nodal follicular and diffuse large B-cell lymphomas.

Pathology
The histology of PCFCL is variable but the infiltrate shows no epidermotropism and there is a clear Grenz zone in the papillary dermis. In the reticular dermis and subcutaneous fat there is a 'bottom heavy' nodular or diffuse infiltrate composed of a mixture of centrocytes (small/large cleaved cells), centroblasts (large, non-cleaved cells with prominent nucleoli) and a prominent infiltrate of reactive T cells with the remnants of poorly formed germinal centres [7–9]. Some tumour cells show a 'strap-like' or 'fibroblast-like' morphology. The growth pattern may be follicular, follicular and diffuse, or diffuse. Individual patients may show different histological patterns in biopsies from the same group of lesions. PCFCL has to be distinguished from MZLs with follicular colonisation of reactive germinal centres. Prominent larger tumours tend to show a more diffuse infiltrate of larger centrocytes, centroblasts and occasional immunoblasts with fewer reactive T cells and no evidence of follicular structures. Such lymphomas should be distinguished from primary cutaneous LBCL, although the presence of a monotonous infiltrate of centroblasts and immunoblasts should be classified as the latter [9]. A subset of PCFCL shows neoplastic follicular structures with an expansile growth pattern, a thin, poorly formed mantle zone and an absence of tingible body (starry sky) macrophages similar to nodal follicular lymphoma although the phenotypic and molecular features are distinct [10].

Immunophenotype
The tumour cells express B-cell-associated markers such as CD19, CD20, CD22 and CD79a but are CD5 negative [9]. CD10 and monotypic cytoplasmic and/or surface immunoglobulin are variably expressed by the neoplastic cells. Follicular structures can be more clearly defined by identifying networks of CD21+ and CD23+ follicular dendritic cells. The tumour cells are mostly Bcl-2 negative, in contrast to systemic nodal follicular lymphoma and diffuse LBCL in which a significant proportion of the tumour cells are CD10+ and Bcl-2 positive [4]. In those cases with a follicular growth pattern, CD10 may be expressed and Bcl-2 may be weakly positive. In contrast, Bcl-6 is usually expressed by PCFCL tumour cells and is indicative of somatic mutation, as also seen in nodal follicular lymphoma and diffuse LBCL [11]. *MUM-1* and *FOXP1* are usually negative but may be rarely expressed [12,13]. Clonal immunoglobulin gene rearrangements are present in most cases. Extensive somatic mutation of variable region genes has been identified, which is also consistent with an origin from germinal centre cells.

Clinical features
Patients present with clinically non-specific solitary or grouped papules, nodules, plaques or tumours, most commonly on the head and neck or trunk [7–9], although any body site may be involved (Figure 139.39). A gradual increase in size of pre-existing lesions and the appearance of new nodules over a period of years is likely without treatment [7–9]. Rarely, multifocal lesions may occur.

Primary cutaneous B-cell lymphomas

Disease course and prognosis
The estimated 5-year survival of PCFCL is 94–97% [9,11].

Investigations
Staging investigations including PET/CT scans of the chest, abdomen and pelvis, and bone marrow aspirate and trephine biopsies are required at the time of diagnosis to exclude a systemic B-cell lymphoma with secondary cutaneous involvement.

Management (Table 139.12)
Superficial radiotherapy is the treatment of choice for solitary, recurrent and multifocal cutaneous disease, except in rare cases with very extensive cutaneous disease or systemic involvement when single-agent treatment with chlorambucil or combination chemotherapy may be indicated [14,**15**]. Single-agent rituximab can be effective and produce durable responses [16,17]. Solitary lesions may be excised, although subsequent radiotherapy is probably advisable to reduce the risk of local recurrence. Recurrences occur in approximately 30% of cases, are usually confined to the skin and do not signify a worse prognosis. Therefore, treatment options remain similar.

Primary cutaneous diffuse large B-cell lymphoma

Definition
Primary cutaneous diffuse LBCL is a rare primary cutaneous lymphoma characterised by a diffuse proliferation of large B cells consisting of centroblasts and immunoblasts, occurring most commonly on the leg [1]. It is closely related to systemic nodal diffuse LBCL, which is the most common form of non-Hodgkin lymphoma.

Epidemiology
Primary cutaneous diffuse LBCL affects an elderly population with a female predominance.

Pathophysiology
Although primary cutaneous diffuse LBCL by definition arises *de novo* in the skin, some tumours might result from high-grade transformation of a low-grade primary cutaneous B-cell lymphoma such as PCFCL. When primary cutaneous LBCL presents at sites other than the leg, it is important to distinguish this from diffuse forms of PCFCL, because PCFCL has an excellent prognosis.

Clonal rearrangements of immunoglobulin genes are present in most cases. No disease-specific cytogenetic abnormalities have been identified. The t(14;18) translocation has not been identified in Bcl-2-positive cutaneous cases, except in rare cases from one series [2]. The t(14;18) translocation is a common feature of nodal diffuse LBCL reflecting a likely transformation from nodal follicular lymphoma and is found in nodal diffuse LBCL with secondary cutaneous involvement. Unlike PCFCL and PCMZL, 6q losses and 2p, 12 and 18q gains are characteristic findings in primary cutaneous LBCL and chromosomal amplification of the *bcl-2* gene may account for Bcl-2 overexpression in primary cutaneous LBCL [2–4]. In addition, inactivation of the *CDKN2A/B* genes by promoter

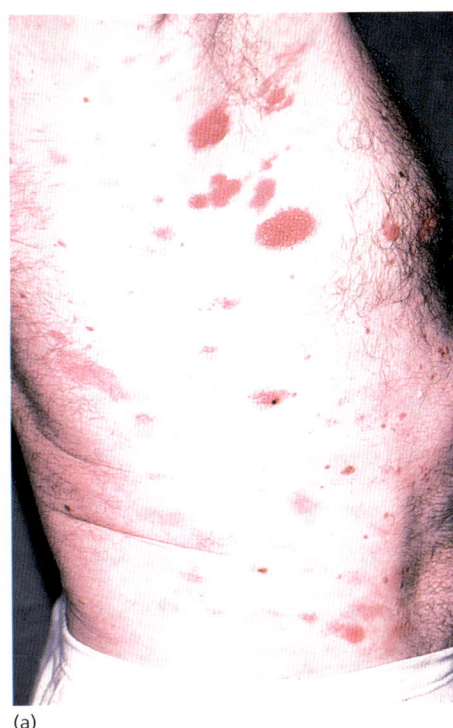
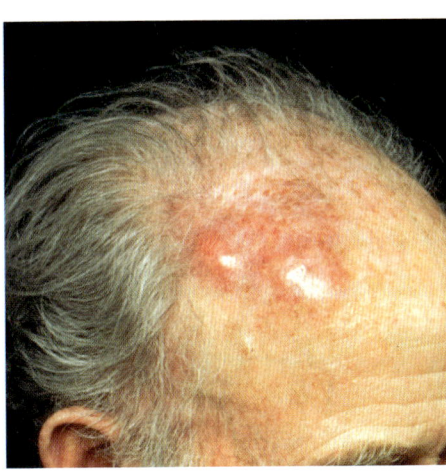
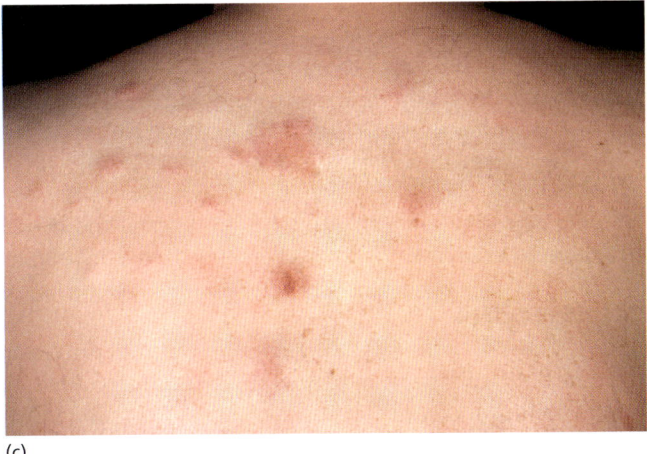

Figure 139.39 Primary cutaneous follicle centre cell lymphoma. (a) Extensive red plaque and nodular lesions on the lower back. (b) Typical clinical presentation on the scalp. (c) Cutaneous presentation of a systemic follicular t(14;18) lymphoma on the trunk with subtle dermal papules and plaques.

hypermethylation and deletion of the 9p21.3 locus containing the *CDKN2A/B* genes has been detected [4,5]. CGH studies have also identified specific oncogene abnormalities including *c-REL* and *MALT1* gene amplification [3,4]. Studies suggest that *p16* loss may have prognostic significance [6]. Studies have also shown rare translocations involving *myc* and IgH in primary cutaneous LBCL in contrast to PCFCL (Table 139.13) [2]. *BCL6* rearrangements have not been detected in primary cutaneous LBCL [8] but mutations of the *BCL6* gene have been detected and this provides an alternative explanation for overexpression of Bcl-6.

Recent studies in nodal diffuse LBCL using microarray technology have confirmed that these tumours are heterogeneous in origin. Three distinct gene expression profiles have been detected that also have prognostic significance: one characteristic of germinal centre cells; one with an expression profile consistent with activated peripheral blood B cells; and one with an indeterminate profile. Studies have shown that primary cutaneous LBCL has an origin from activated B cells, compared with PCFCL which shows a germinal centre B-cell gene expression profile.

Somatic mutations identified include a highly recurrent gene mutation *MYD88* gene variant encoding a Toll-like receptor-associated adapter protein, and other genes affecting B-cell signaling, NFκB activation and chromatin modification [7].

Pathology
There is a diffuse non-epidermotropic infiltrate of large cells with morphological similarity to centroblasts and immunoblasts that may extend to involve the subcutis (Figure 139.40). The infiltrate is monotonous with relatively few associated inflammatory cells or reactive T cells present. Germinal centres are not apparent and mitoses are prominent. Morphological variants recognised in cutaneous disease include cleaved and round cell types but the reproducibility of this distinction is poor [8]. Initially, it was reported that the presence of round cell morphology was an adverse prognostic feature. However, this may be explained by subsequent recognition that the cleaved cell type, showing a predominance of large centrocytes and multilobated cells, represents diffuse PCFCL (Crosti lymphoma) [9].

Immunophenotype
The tumour cells are CD19+, CD20+, CD22+ and CD79a+ with monotypic expression of surface and/or cytoplasmic immunoglobulin in some cases [9]. Tumour cells are usually strongly Bcl-2 positive [9], and Bcl-6 is also expressed in most cases with evidence of *Bcl-6* gene mutations [5,7]. CD10 expression is only rarely detected in primary cutaneous LBCL. MUM-1 and FOX-P1 are invariably expressed by tumour cells in primary cutaneous LBCL in contrast to PCFCL. EBV-positive diffuse LBCL of the elderly can rarely present as a primary cutaneous B-cell lymphoma and is distinguished by expression of EBV (ICD-11: 407807101).

Clinical features
These lymphomas tend to develop on the lower limbs, predominantly as large dermal nodules or tumours, which are either solitary or multifocal and rapidly enlarging (Figure 139.41) [1]. Primary cutaneous LBCL can also rarely occur at other cutaneous sites (non-leg type) [9].

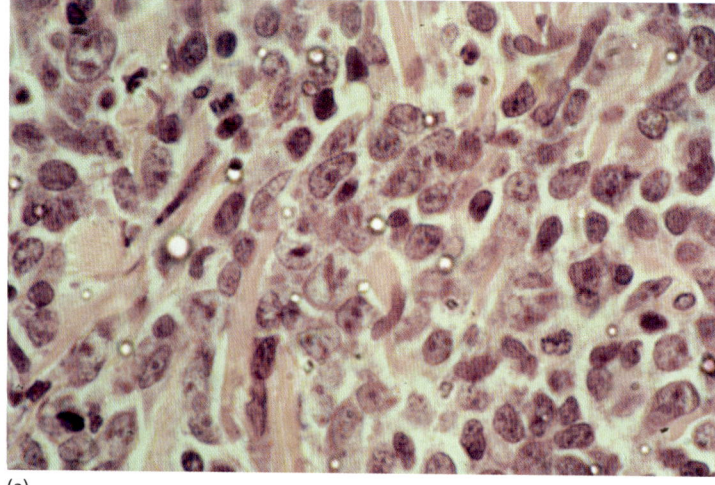

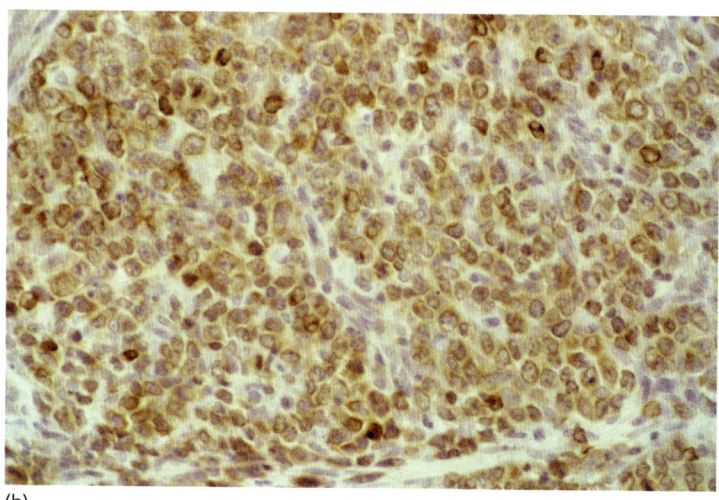

Figure 139.40 Primary cutaneous large B-cell lymphoma (a) showing a diffuse pattern of large mononuclear cells (b) and strong Bcl-2 positivity.

Disease course and prognosis
The prognosis of primary cutaneous LBCL is poor, with a 5-year survival of 41–58% but this is generally better than for nodal diffuse LBCL [1,8,9]. Although studies initially suggested that *Bcl-2* expression was associated with a worse prognosis [8], the prognostic significance of *Bcl-2* expression has since been disputed. Recent studies have shown that multifocal disease and location on the leg are associated with a worse prognosis in multivariate analysis [9].

Investigations
Full staging investigations including PET/CT scans and bone marrow trephine biopsies are critical to exclude systemic involvement.

Management (Table 139.12)
In elderly patients with solitary tumours, radiotherapy may be appropriate but multiagent chemotherapy is usually required, especially for multifocal disease [10]. The role of rituximab (anti-CD20 antibody) as a single agent in cutaneous disease has yet to be determined, but CHOP chemotherapy (CHOP plus rituximab (CHOP-R)) is now the standard of care in nodal diffuse LBCL with subsequent involved field radiotherapy and is an appropriate

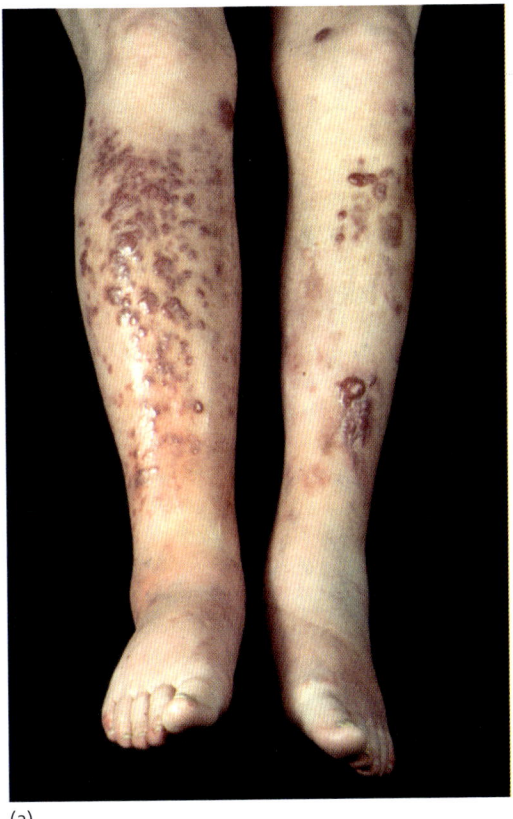
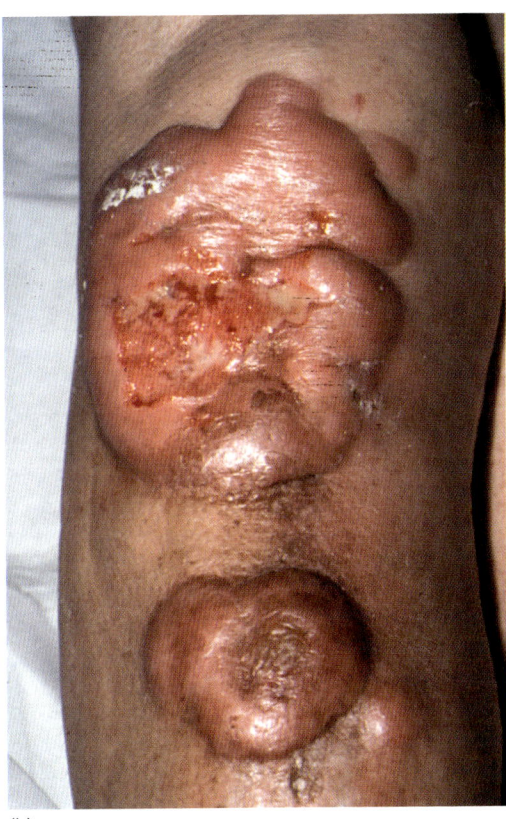

Figure 139.41 (a, b) Clinical presentation of primary cutaneous large B-cell lymphoma on the legs.

consideration for patients with primary cutaneous LBCL. Intralesional rituximab may prove to be effective for selected patients in whom radiotherapy or CHOP-R is not possible.

SECONDARY CUTANEOUS B-CELL LYMPHOMAS

Intravascular large B-cell lymphoma

Definition and nomenclature
This is a very rare extranodal B-cell lymphoma characterised by the accumulation of large B cells within small blood vessels [1]. This tumour usually involves multiple extranodal sites including the CNS, lung and skin, and symptoms and/or signs at these sites may be the presenting feature [2].

Synonyms and inclusions
- Malignant angioendotheliomatosis
- Angiotrophic lymphoma

Pathophysiology
Pathology
The tumour cells are large and show striking atypia with an occasional anaplastic morphology. These cells are situated entirely within dilated vessel lumina in the dermis and subcutis

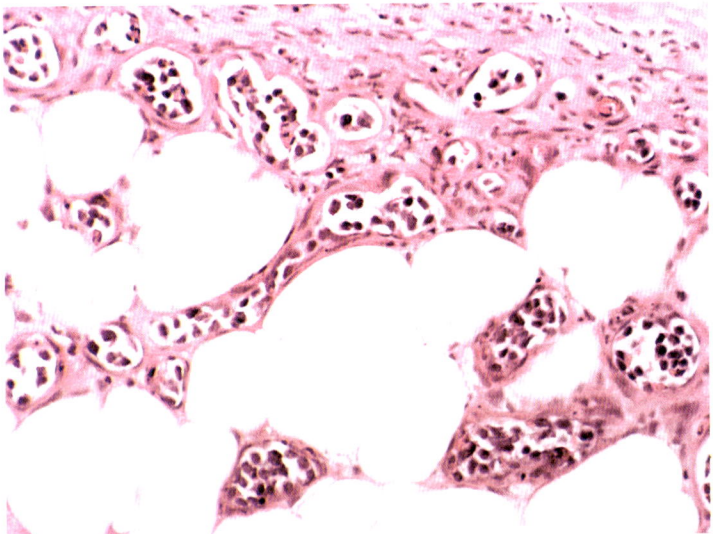

Figure 139.42 Histology of angiocentric B-cell lymphoma showing B cells within small vascular channels in the dermis. These are stained with membrane markers for B cells, not with membrane markers for endothelial cells. Courtesy of Eduardo Calonje.

(Figure 139.42). Vessels may be occluded by tumour cells and fibrin thrombi.

Immunophenotype
The tumour cells are positive for B-cell-associated antigens consistent with an origin from a peripheral post-germinal centre B cell. Clonal immunoglobulin gene rearrangements are present.

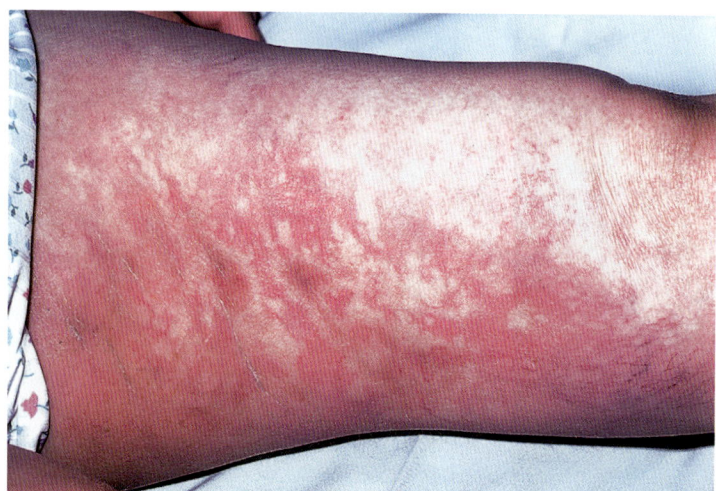

Figure 139.43 Angiocentric B-cell lymphoma. Note the marbled appearance of the inner thigh, which was woody hard on palpation.

Rare cases are derived from T cells and show a clonal TCR gene rearrangement.

Clinical features
Patients present with diffuse, tender, hard, infiltrated plaques, commonly on the thigh (Figure 139.43). The clinical appearance may suggest a sclerotic connective tissue disorder or panniculitis [2]. A variety of clinical features may occur as a consequence of the occlusion of small vessels including telangiectatic skin lesions. Colonisation of benign haemangiomas by tumour cells has been reported.

Disease course and prognosis
The prognosis is poor, although rare cases with disease confined to the skin may have a better outlook with a 3-year survival of 56% versus 22% if spread is beyond the skin [2].

Management
There are some reports of a partial response to combination chemotherapy, but the disease has a poor prognosis and is usually fatal [2].

Lymphomatoid granulomatosis

Definition
This is an angiocentric and angiodestructive extranodal EBV-positive B-cell lymphoma, which invariably involves the lungs and may involve the skin and CNS [1,2].

Pathophysiology
Lymphomatoid granulomatosis is an EBV-driven B-cell lymphoproliferative disorder that can be associated with immunodeficiency states including post-transplantation and with long-term therapies such as methotrexate for rheumatoid arthritis [3,4]. This lymphoma should be distinguished from extranodal NK/T-cell lymphoma (nasal type), which is also EBV positive and characterised by angiodestructive histology.

Pathology
The striking feature is the angiocentricity of the infiltrate and gross vessel destruction sometimes accompanied by fibrinoid necrosis (angiodestruction). The infiltrate is polymorphous and contains both lymphocytes and histiocytes with pleomorphic or large (immunoblast-like) tumour cells and often a prominent reactive T-cell infiltrate. Multinucleated cells may be present although well-formed granulomas are rare. The presence of large transformed cells is associated with a worse prognosis.

Immunophenotype
The tumour cells are EBV positive, express CD20 and are variably CD79a+. CD30 may be expressed but the cells are negative for CD15. Clonal immunoglobulin gene rearrangements can be detected in most cases and the presence of clonal episomal EBV is characteristic.

Clinical features
Patients most frequently present with pulmonary symptoms associated with systemic malaise, arthralgias, weight loss and fever. The skin (50% of cases), CNS and kidneys are also often directly involved. The cutaneous lesions described are diverse but include subcutaneous nodules and plaques, more superficial plaques and a diffuse dusky maculopapular eruption (Figure 139.44) with epidermal atrophy and purpura [3,4]. Necrosis and ulceration may also occur.

Disease course and prognosis
Some patients have a fluctuating course with spontaneous remissions but eventually progressive disease develops. Those cases occurring in patients on long-term methotrexate for conditions such as rheumatoid arthritis may have a better outcome, with resolution of disease on withdrawal of the methotrexate [5].

Management
Although some patients have spontaneous remissions, the development of high-grade disease is associated with a median survival of

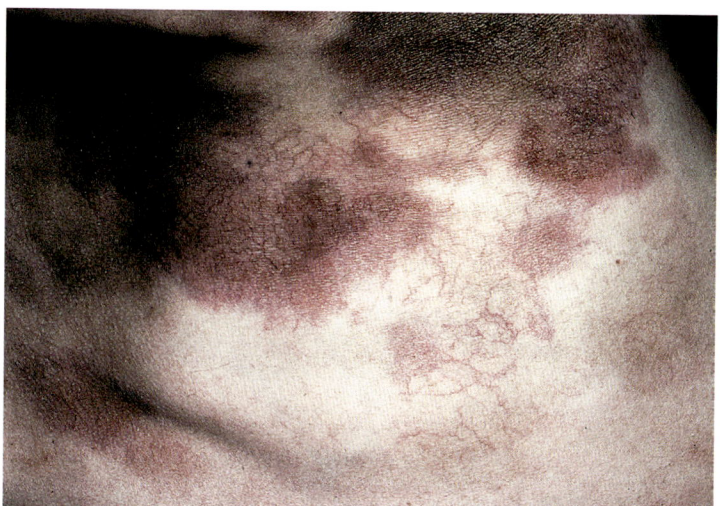

Figure 139.44 Clinical features of lymphomatoid granulomatosis showing extensive purpuric, bruise-like lesions on the trunk.

less than 2 years. Short-lived remissions with high-dose chemotherapy have been described. There are reports of responses to cyclophosphamide and IFN-α.

SECONDARY CUTANEOUS T-CELL LYMPHOMAS

Angioimmunoblastic T-cell lymphoma

Definition and nomenclature
This is a nodal T-cell lymphoma derived from follicular helper T cells and associated with a complex dysregulation of B cells [1]. Extranodal involvement of sites, including the skin, is well recognised [2].

Synonyms and inclusions
- Angioimmunoblastic lymphadenopathy

Pathophysiology
Clonal rearrangements of TCR genes are detected in a majority of cases but additional monoclonal or oligoclonal IgH rearrangements are often found, consistent with the characteristic EBV-positive B-cell proliferation seen in lymph nodes from patients with angioimmunoblastic T-cell lymphoma (AILT) [1]. CXCL13 and ICOS/PD1 expression by tumour cells in AILT confirms a derivation from follicular helper T cells [1].

Pathology
The nodal pathology is characterised by hyperplastic follicles and a prominent arborising vascular proliferation with expanded follicular dendritic cells. There is an associated polymorphous infiltrate with clusters of large clear cells [1]. The infiltrate consists of CD10+ T cells and an expansion of EBV-infected B cells (EBV-encoded small RNA (EBER) positive). Cutaneous involvement is characterised by variable features; a non-specific perivascular lymphocytic infiltrate with minimal atypia and capillary hyperplasia can be found in some biopsies, or more prominent dermal perivascular infiltrates showing cytologically atypical pleomorphic T cells and occasionally more obvious dense infiltrates of atypical T cells are present [3]. Granulomatous infiltrates and vasculitis have been reported [3]. There is no epidermotropism. Necrotising granulomas with abundant histiocytes and eosinophils have been described in some cutaneous infiltrates of AILT. The atypical cells express T-cell antigens and are also CD10+.

Clinical features
Patients may present with systemic and/or peripheral lymphadenopathy, often accompanied by 'B' symptoms [2]. Splenomegaly occurs in over 50% of cases and many patients will have advanced disease and bone marrow involvement at diagnosis [2]. Autoimmune phenomena are common, including neurological abnormalities, arthritis, hypergammaglobulinaemia, haemolytic anaemia and thrombocytopenic purpura [2]. Cutaneous extranodal involvement is common (45% of cases) and rarely can be a presenting feature [2]. Skin changes are highly variable and can be subtle, including maculopapular and papulonodular eruptions. Erythroderma, haemorrhagic and urticarial eruptions have been described as well as dermal plaques. Occasionally, cutaneous involvement in AILD can mimic drug eruptions and infections.

Management
The disease can be indolent but transformation is associated with a poor prognosis and multiagent chemotherapy regimens are invariably required. Immunomodulatory therapies have been used successfully including ciclosporin, steroids, thalidomide and angiogenesis inhibitors such as bevacizumab [1].

OTHER DISORDERS

Blastic plasmacytoid dendritic cell neoplasm (CD4+/CD56+ haematodermic neoplasm)

Definition
This is a rare haematological malignancy that is derived from plasmacytoid dendritic cells and shows a predilection for extranodal sites, particularly the skin, and a tendency to leukaemic dissemination. Previously this tumour was erroneously thought to be derived from NK cells because of CD56 expression.

Epidemiology
Elderly male patients are mostly affected.

Pathophysiology
Epstein–Barr virus has not been detected in tumour cells and no disease-specific cytogenetic abnormality has been detected [1,2]. CGH techniques and gene expression studies have shown a distinct pattern of chromosomal abnormalities and overexpression of the oncogene, *FLT3*, and loss of expression of the *Rb1* gene similar to myeloid malignancies [3–5]. High throughput sequencing and transcriptomic studies have shown mutations characteristic of myeloid and myelodysplasia in a majority of cases and mutations typical of lymphoid malignancies in a minority [6].

Pathology
A dense monomorphic infiltrate of medium-sized tumour cells with a fine chromatin resembling lymphoblasts is seen throughout the dermis with a well-defined Grenz zone (Figure 139.45) [1]. Occasionally, tumour cells show a rosette pattern. Necrosis and angiocentricity are usually absent.

Immunophenotype
Tumour cells are CD56+ with variable expression of CD4, CD45RA and CD43 but do not express surface CD3. CD2, CD7 and cytoplasmic CD3 are usually negative [1]. Cytotoxic proteins may be rarely expressed. Rare cases are CD34+, CD68+ and TdT+. Because

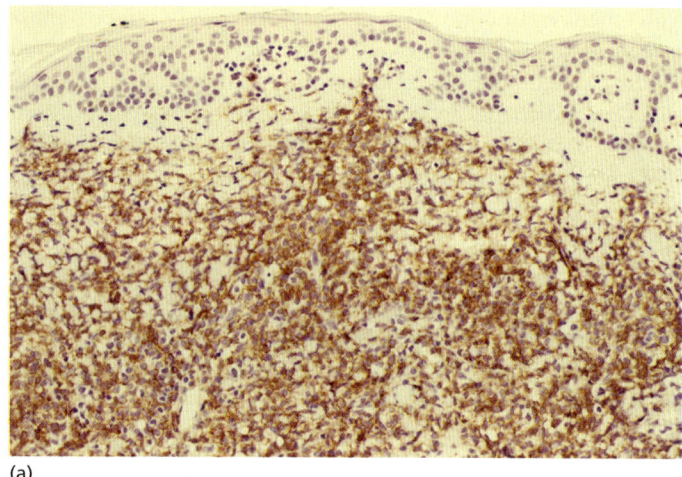
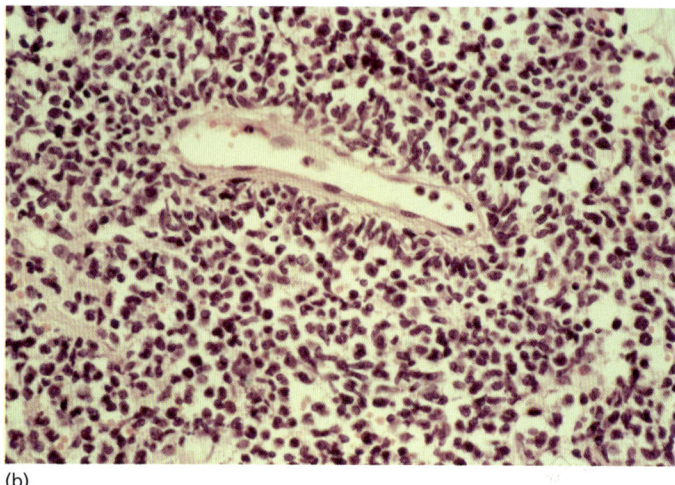
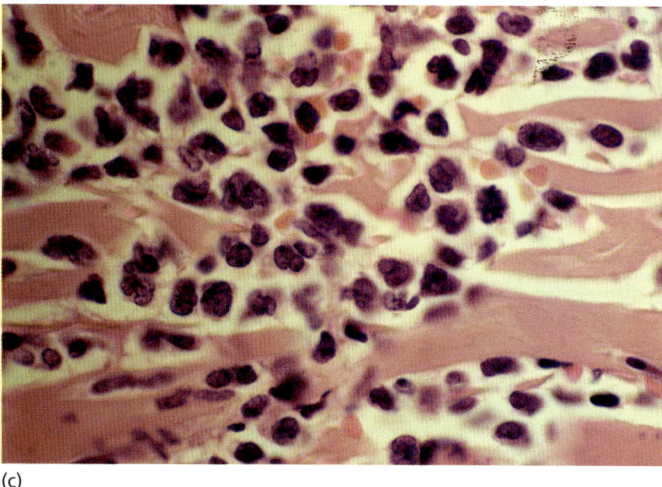

Figure 139.45 Extranodal natural killer/T-cell lymphoma in the skin: (a) CD56 positivity; (b) rosetting of blood vessels; and (c) large atypical mononuclear cells.

of a morphological resemblance to myeloblastic and precursor T-lymphoblastic leukaemia, which also express CD56, it is important to confirm that the tumour cells are negative for surface CD3, CD33 and myeloperoxidase/lysozyme. TCR gene analysis reveals a germline pattern for all TCR genes consistent with a non-lymphoid origin [1,2]. The tumours are CD123+ and TCL1a+, confirming a derivation from rare peripheral blood plasmacytoid dendritic cells [7,8]. Tumour cells may express CXCL12 which might also indicate a potential for leukaemic progression.

Clinical features

Patients usually present with multiple, and rarely solitary, large, dusky mauve, dermal tumours, which can become ulcerated (Figure 139.46). There is no specific site predilection but the upper trunk is often affected. Primary cutaneous disease is common but lymphadenopathy and peripheral blood/bone marrow involvement is likely during the course of the disease [1,9]. This neoplasm must be differentiated from myelomonocytic leukaemia.

Disease course and prognosis

The prognosis is poor with a median survival of 14 months reported. Survival may be better in patients less than 40 years old and with high TdT expression.

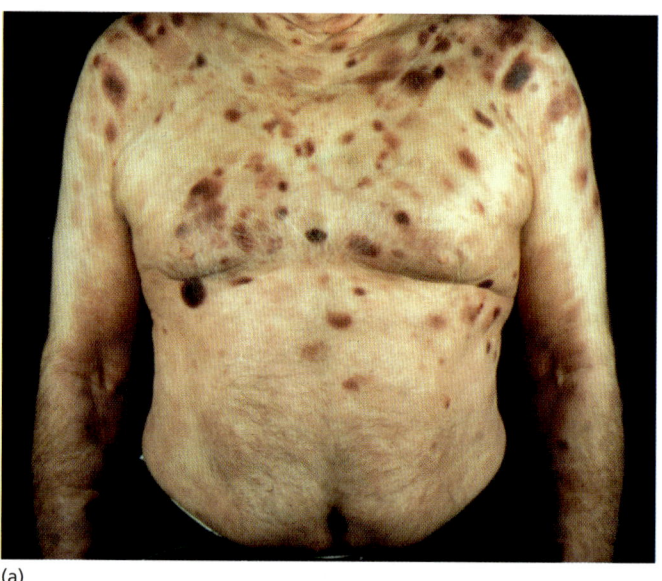
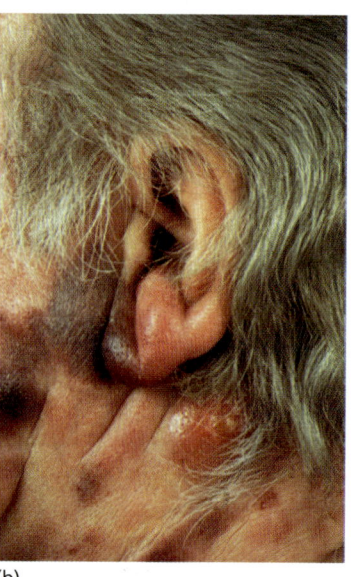

Figure 139.46 Typical clinical presentations of blastic lymphoma in the skin with large mauve and pigmented dermal plaques involving (a) the trunk and (b) the head/neck.

Management
Combination chemotherapy and radiotherapy including TSEBT can produce a partial remission, which is invariably short lived. Myeloid leukaemia protocols are appropriate and transplantation options should be considered [10,11].

Post-transplant lymphoproliferative disorder

Definition
This represents lymphoproliferative disorders occurring in solid organ transplant recipients on immunosuppressive therapy.

Epidemiology
The incidence varies according to the organ transplanted (renal transplant rates of 10%) and although extranodal lymphomas are over-represented in post-transplant lymphoproliferative disorder (PTLD), primary cutaneous involvement is rare [1,2].

Pathophysiology
B-cell PTLD is associated with EBV infection, and progression from an early reactive phase can be identified. Three distinct types of PTLD are recognised: (i) plasmacytic hyperplasia is a polyclonal proliferation associated with multiple copies of EBV and occurs early after transplantation; (ii) polymorphic lymphoproliferative disorder occurring several years after transplantation is a monoclonal EBV proliferation with a single copy of EBV but without secondary genomic abnormalities; and (iii) malignant lymphoma is a monoclonal EBV proliferation with a single copy of EBV and associated secondary genomic abnormalities and widespread disease. Rare cases of primary cutaneous B-cell PTLD have been associated with human herpesvirus 8 (HHV-8) infection [3].

In contrast, viral associations are not consistently described for systemic or cutaneous T-cell PTLD although rare EBV-positive T-cell lymphomas have been reported. Primary cutaneous presentations can also occur in non-organ transplant recipients such as human immunodeficiency virus (HIV) positive patients or those with other forms of profound immunodeficiency. Similarly, EBV-positive lymphoproliferative disorders can develop in patients who have undergone high-dose chemotherapy for primary lymphomas. In rare cases, the transplanted donor organs can be the source of the lymphoma.

Pathology
There are diffuse dermal infiltrates extending to the subcutis and consisting of large pleomorphic lymphocytes or centroblasts. Plasmacytoid differentiation and plasmablasts may be a feature. Necrosis may be present. For primary cutaneous B-cell PTLD the tumour cells express B-cell antigens while primary cutaneous T-cell PTLD may be CD30+, but histological features mimicking all types of CTCL have been described [2,4].

Clinical features
The clinical features described are diverse; solitary or multiple plaques, nodules or tumours, with or without ulceration, have been described affecting any site. Systemic involvement and in particular involvement of the transplanted organ must be excluded in patients with primary cutaneous PTLD. Spontaneous resolution has been reported. For primary cutaneous T-cell PTLD, erythroderma is the most common clinical presentation, but all clinical types of CTCL have been described [4].

Management
While surgery and radiotherapy can be used, reduction in immunosuppression is often effective [5]. Both chemotherapy and rituximab have been reported to be effective. While the prognosis for B-cell PTLD is generally good [6], both primary cutaneous and systemic T-cell PTLD have a poor prognosis.

Leukaemia cutis

Definition
Leukaemia cutis is characterised by solitary or multiple dermal skin lesions due to cutaneous infiltration by leukaemic cells [1].

Introduction and general description
The diagnosis of the specific type of leukaemia depends on a detailed examination of the blood and bone marrow. The cutaneous infiltrate rarely indicates the type of leukaemia involved. Specific cutaneous lesions occur most often in chronic lymphocytic leukaemias, myelomonocytic leukaemias, hairy cell leukaemias and T-cell malignancies such as T-cell prolymphocytic leukaemia and T-cell acute lymphoblastic leukaemia (T-ALL) (Box 139.3). Cutaneous involvement in the other forms of leukaemia is unusual as a presenting feature, and usually appears after the diagnosis has been established. There are a few cases where the diagnosis of leukaemia has been established first by analysis of the skin lesions.

> **Box 139.3 Types of leukaemia causing leukaemia cutis**
>
> - Chronic lymphocytic leukaemia
> - Myelomonocytic leukaemia
> - Hairy cell leukaemia
> - T-cell prolymphocytic leukaemia
> - T-cell acute lymphoblastic leukaemia

Epidemiology
A report of 289 cases of lymphocytic leukaemia with skin lesions described tumours in 50% – the head being the most common site [2]. Erythroderma was present in 25%, herpes zoster in 26%, prurigo-like papules in 21%, bullae in 10% and varicelliform eruptions and urticaria in 3%. Haemorrhagic gangrene of the skin has also been recorded. The usual age at presentation of patients with lymphocytic leukaemia is 45–54 years, but those with cutaneous lesions tend to be older. Skin lesions in myelogenous leukaemia are much less frequent. When the skin is involved the prognosis is poor.

Pathophysiology
Pathology

The diagnosis of leukaemia cutis is based on pathological examination of material from the blood, bone marrow, lymph nodes and skin. Skin infiltration tends to favour the lower dermis and subcutaneous fat, with prominent involvement of the adnexal structures, nerves and vessels of the superficial and deep plexus. Cellular atypia may be prominent and mitotic figures are variable. Immunohistochemical studies may show variable expression of specific leukaemic antigens such as myeloid markers (CD13, CD33, CD117 and myeloperoxidase) and markers of monocytic differentiation (CD11b, CD11c, CD14, CD64, CD68 and lysozyme) in myelomonocytic leukaemic cutaneous infiltrates [3]. In contrast expression of B-cell markers may be detected in chronic lymphatic leukaemia and hairy cell leukaemia, whereas T-cell markers are expressed in T-cell prolymphocytic leukaemia and T-ALL.

Clinical features

Skin lesions are generally asymptomatic and consist of small, reddish or violaceous/grey-blue macules, papules or nodules, which may be fleeting or persistent. Leukaemia cutis occurs in about 20% of patients with acute monocytic leukaemia, and extramedullary involvement is often a poor prognostic feature [4]. Gum involvement occurs in 25–50% of patients. Cutaneous involvement usually occurs after the diagnosis of the underlying haematological malignancy but rarely can occur as the presenting feature.

Non-specific lesions are common. Generalised pruritus may be a presenting symptom and prurigo-like papules develop in some cases. Disseminated or unusually severe herpes zoster is common. In multiple myeloma, both generalised and local amyloidosis is common.

Sweet syndrome and bullous pyoderma can be a non-specific manifestation of an underlying leukaemia (Chapter 49). Thrombocytopenic purpura is a characteristic symptom of acute leukaemias and may occur on the skin or mucous membranes, often as the presenting symptom (Figure 139.47).

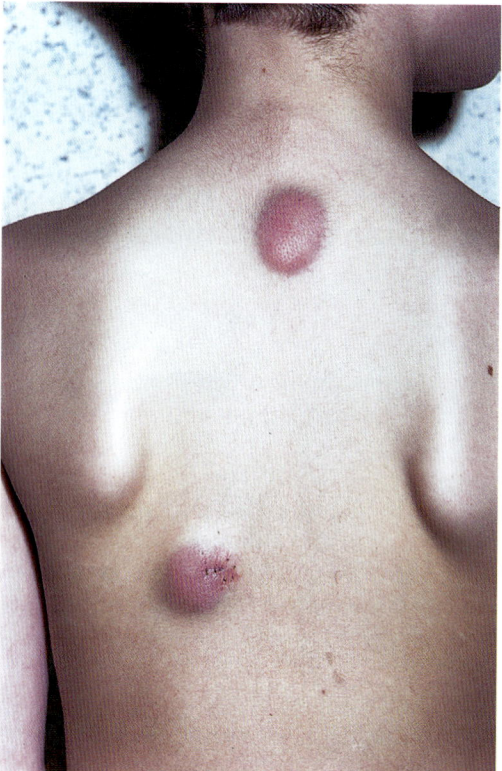

Figure 139.48 Specific deposits in a child with leukaemia. Note the two large nodular lesions on the back.

Differential diagnosis

Clinically, skin lesions may resemble Sweet syndrome, sarcoidosis, panniculitis, other granulomas or cutaneous lymphoma (Figure 139.48). Ulceration, especially around the ankles, simulating gravitational ulceration, has been described in chronic lymphocytic leukaemia and may represent the development of a leukaemic deposit in an area of low vascular resistance. Erythroderma has been recorded in association with an underlying T-cell leukaemia including T-cell prolymphocytic leukaemia and chronic T-cell lymphocytic leukaemia [2], which must be distinguished from Sézary syndrome. There is usually marked exfoliation and the skin may be markedly thickened, especially over the face. Specific leukaemic infiltrations of herpetic scars may occur and bullous lesions have been recorded.

Management

The treatment for leukaemia cutis is management of the underlying disease, with symptomatic measures for the skin lesions when required [5]. Superficial radiotherapy can provide useful palliation for symptomatic skin lesions. Some cutaneous lesions may spontaneously regress.

Cutaneous manifestations of Hodgkin disease

Hodgkin disease does not originate in the skin but rarely can spread to the skin in a contiguous manner as a direct extension

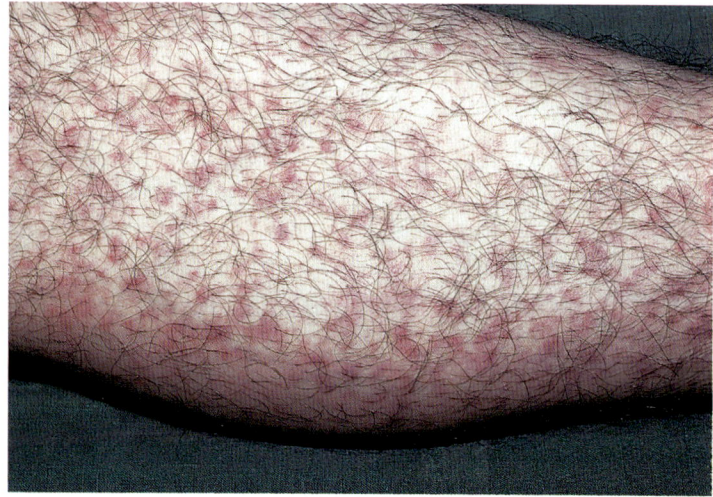

Figure 139.47 Purpuric lesions in an adult patient with myelocytic leukaemia.

from an underlying involved regional lymph node [1]. Cutaneous lesions consist of solitary plaques or tumours that may be ulcerated. Appropriate staging investigations, including CT scans and lymph node biopsies, should be performed. In view of the cytological similarity between primary cutaneous CD30+ lymphoproliferative disorders and Hodgkin disease, this differential diagnosis must be excluded on the basis of clinical and pathological assessment including immunophenotyping of the infiltrate (only Hodgkin cells are CD15+) [2,3].

Non-specific cutaneous signs associated with Hodgkin disease [4] are very common and occur in 3–50% of cases. These include pigmentation, pruritus, prurigo, atrophy, alopecia, exfoliative dermatitis and herpes zoster.

Pigmentation. This is melanin pigmentation and is very common. It resembles the pigmentation of Addison disease, being most marked in areas that normally show some darkening such as the axillae, groins and around the nipples. Less often it is more widespread, and occasionally figurate pigmentation occurs. The mucous membranes are usually spared.

Pruritus. This often occurs together with pigmentation. Pruritus is not infrequently the presenting feature of the disease, and may precede the presence of palpable nodes by months or years. It tends to start on the legs. It is especially severe in patients who show other general symptoms such as fever and weight loss. Both pigmentation and pruritus in association with enlarged mediastinal or retroperitoneal glands should prompt consideration of a diagnosis of Hodgkin disease.

Prurigo. This is a development from pruritus. In addition to the widespread irritation, there are excessively itchy papules which are excoriated until the skin surface is removed and is replaced by a blood crust. The papules and crusts are usually found on the trunk. When present in association with enlarged superficial glands, this forms a very characteristic picture, often called Hodgkin prurigo.

Ichthyosiform atrophy. An acquired ichthyosis occurring in the course of a chronic wasting disease is fairly common. Hodgkin disease is probably the most common condition to be associated with this change. It usually starts on the legs and may remain restricted, but in severe cases progresses until it becomes universal. It resembles ichthyosis vulgaris, with thin, dry and rather firmly attached scales. It is not static and may regress for a time, only to return later. Red streaks are often visible between the scales. The patient is usually wasted and severely ill. Malabsorption from the gut may occur in some cases and contribute to this problem.

Alopecia. Hair loss is common in Hodgkin disease. It can be caused by rubbing or scratching to relieve itching. It may also be part of the ichthyosiform atrophy or be caused by endocrine dysfunction, when specific infiltration occurs in organs such as the pituitary or adrenal.

Exfoliative dermatitis. Erythroderma and exfoliative dermatitis can occur in Hodgkin disease. Most recorded cases would probably be more correctly included under ichthyosiform atrophy.

Herpes zoster. Herpes zoster is common in the course of Hodgkin disease, but disseminated zoster is much less likely to occur in Hodgkin disease than in leukaemias.

Key references

The full list of references can be found in the online version at https://www.wiley.com/rooksdermatology10e

Introduction
2 Willemze R, Cerroni L, Kempf W et al. The 2018 update of the WHO-EORTC classification for primary cutaneous lymphomas. *Blood* 2019;133:1703–14.

Primary cutaneous T-cell lymphomas
Mycosis fungoides
Pathophysiology
Predisposing factors
3 Jones C, Degasperi A, Grandi V et al. Spectrum of mutational signatures in T-cell lymphoma reveals a key role UV radiation in cutaneous T-cell lymphoma. *Scientific Reports* 2021;11:3962–75.

Pathology
5 Agar N, Wedeworth E, Crichton S et al. Survival outcomes and prognostic factors in mycosis fungoides/Sézary syndrome: validation of the revised International Society for Cutaneous Lymphomas/European Organisation for Research and Treatment of Cancer staging proposal. *J Clin Oncol* 2010;28:4730–9.

Molecular features of mycosis fungoides and Sézary syndrome
1 Jones C, Degasperi A, Grandi V et al. Spectrum of mutational signatures in T-cell lymphoma reveals a key role UV radiation in cutaneous T-cell lymphoma. *Scientific Reports* 2021;11:3962–75.
9 Park J, Yang J, Wenzel AT et al. Genomic analysis of 220 CTCLs identifies a novel recurrent gain-of-function alteration in RLTPR (p.Q575E). *Blood* 2017;130:1430–40.

Management of mycosis fungoides and Sézary syndrome
3 Gilson D, Whittaker S, Child F et al. British Association of Dermatologists and UK Cutaneous Lymphoma Group guidelines for the management of primary cutaneous lymphomas 2018. *Br J Dermatol* 2019;180:496–526.

Primary cutaneous CD30+ lymphoproliferative disorders
Introduction and general description
3 Kempf W, Pfaltz K, Vermeer MH et al. EORTC, ISCL, and USCLC consensus recommendations for the treatment of primary cutaneous CD30-positive lymphoproliferative disorders: lymphomatoid papulosis and primary cutaneous anaplastic large-cell lymphoma. *Blood* 2011;118:4024–35.

Primary cutaneous T-cell lymphoma variants
Introduction and general description
1 Willemze R, Cerroni L, Kempf W et al. The 2018 update of the WHO-EORTC classification for primary cutaneous lymphomas. *Blood* 2019;133:1703–14.

Primary cutaneous aggressive epidermotropic CD8+ T-cell lymphoma
1 Willemze R, Cerroni L, Kempf W et al. The 2018 update of the WHO-EORTC classification for primary cutaneous lymphomas. *Blood* 2019;133:1703–14.

Primary cutaneous γδ T-cell lymphoma
1 Willemze R, Cerroni L, Kempf W et al. The 2018 update of the WHO-EORTC classification for primary cutaneous lymphomas. *Blood* 2019;133:1703–14.

Primary cutaneous CD4+ small/medium pleomorphic T-cell lymphoproliferative disorder (provisional)
1 Willemze R, Cerroni L, Kempf W et al. The 2018 update of the WHO-EORTC classification for primary cutaneous lymphomas. *Blood* 2019;133:1703–14.

Adult T-cell leukaemia–lymphoma (HTLV-1 associated)

4 Jones C, Degasperi A, Grandi V et al. Spectrum of mutational signatures in T-cell lymphoma reveals a key role UV radiation in cutaneous T-cell lymphoma. *Sci Rep* 2021;11:3962–75.

Primary cutaneous B-cell lymphomas
Introduction and general description

1 Willemze R, Cerroni L, Kempf W et al. The 2018 update of the WHO-EORTC classification for primary cutaneous lymphomas. *Blood* 2019;133:1703–14.

Primary cutaneous follicle centre cell lymphoma

15 Senff N, Noordijk E, Kim Y et al. European Organization for Research and Treatment of Cancer and International Society for Cutaneous Lymphoma consensus recommendations for the management of cutaneous B-cell lymphomas. *Blood* 2008;112:1600–9.

Primary cutaneous diffuse large B-cell lymphoma

9 Willemze R, Cerroni L, Kempf W et al. The 2018 update of the WHO-EORTC classification for primary cutaneous lymphomas. *Blood* 2019;133:1703–14.

CHAPTER 140

Basal Cell Carcinoma

Carl Vinciullo[1] *and Vishal Madan*[2]

[1]Department of Dermatology, Royal Perth Hospital, Perth, Western Australia, Australia
[2]Dermatology Centre, Salford Royal NHS Foundation Trust, Salford, UK

| Basal cell carcinoma, 140.1 | Bazex–Dupré–Christol syndrome, 140.21 | Key references, 140.21 |
| Naevoid basal cell carcinoma syndrome, 140.18 | | |

Basal cell carcinoma

Definition and nomenclature

Basal cell carcinoma (BCC) is the most common human malignancy. Although there are distinct clinical and pathological differences between BCC and squamous cell carcinomas (SCC) (Chapter 141), they are both carcinomas that share lineage with keratinocytes, thus when considered collectively they are termed most accurately keratinocyte carcinomas (KCs) [1,2]. KCs account for more than 97% of all skin cancers [3]. Traditionally BCC has accounted for approximately 80% of KCs (4:1 ratio) but evidence points to an increasing incidence of SCC with a ratio of BCC to SCC of 2.5:1. One study in the USA using data from the Medicare population aged 65 years and older showed a ratio of 1:1 [3].

Introduction and general description

Basal cell carcinomas are nearly as common as all other human cancers combined [4]. Despite difficulties in capturing and registering data, leading to underreporting of BCC, it is clear that there is at least a 10% per year rise in the incidence of BCC worldwide. KCs exceed the prevalence of all other cancers combined, with the average number of lesions per individual varying between 1.87 and 1.64 in Australia and the USA [3,5]. It is estimated that 40–50% of patients with a primary BCC will develop at least one or more BCCs within 5 years. The estimated incidence of KC in the USA using Medicare data is over 2.4 million affected individuals per year with over 4 million lesions, and at least 50% of these are BCC [3]. Despite their slow-growing and indolent nature, BCC have a major impact on western health economies [6]. In the USA, the annual average cost for the treatment of KC increased by 126% from 2006 to 2011 reaching $8.1 billion, while the cost for all other cancers combined increased by 25% [7]. The Global Burden of Disease Study 2013 found that KCs accounted for 12.9 disability-adjusted life years (DALY) per 100 000 persons; although a reduction of 6.2% from 2005, this still equated to 0.13 years lived with disability (YLD). Overall KCs accounted for only 0.03% of the overall total global burden of skin disease morbidity and mortality of 1.79% [8].

Epidemiology

Incidence and prevalence

Due to the high volume and multiplicity of BCCs, these carcinomas have frequently been excluded from national cancer registries and statistics. In order to validate improved data collection methods in the UK, National Cancer Registration and Analysis Service (NCRAS) data were used in a cohort study from 2013 to 2015 to more accurately document the incidence of BCC [9]. This demonstrated the absolute first BCC count per person per annum increased in the 3-year period from 145 817 to 166 448, an increase of 14%; of these 85% were in England. The European age-adjusted incidence rate was 352 per 100 000 person-years in males and 219 in females [9]. The estimated annual percentage change was 5% in England, but much lower in Northern Ireland (0.3%).

The incidence of BCC has also been noted to be increasing in other European countries. An observational study from the Netherlands noted a quadrupling of incidence of BCC in 37 years from 1973 to 2009 [10]. The increase was more marked from 2002 until 2009 with an estimated annual percentage change of 6.8% for men and 7.9% for women. While ultraviolet (UV) exposure may have a direct role, improved screening measures are also likely to contribute to the increased incidence of BCC [11]. In Germany the most current reporting shows an incidence of 200 per 100 000 person-years, reflecting a steady increase in recent years [12].

Worldwide, the incidence for BCC varies widely. In the USA, incidence has increased an average of 4–8% annually with the most recent data from 2006 showing an age-adjusted incidence rate of 1488 per 100 000 person-years in males and 1019 in females [13,14]. In Australia, the most recent data are from 2002 showing age-standardised incidence rates to have increased by 35–42% from 1985 to 2002, with the rate in males 1041 per 100 000 person-years and in females 745 [15]. There are regional differences in the average incidence rates of BCC within countries. In the UK, the highest BCC rates were observed in southwest England (362 per 100 000 person-years) and the lowest in Dumfries and Galloway in the north (39 per 100 000 person-years) due to geographical differences whereby a higher latitude is associated with lower UV irradiance [9].

Rook's Textbook of Dermatology, Tenth Edition. Edited by Christopher Griffiths, Jonathan Barker, Tanya Bleiker, Walayat Hussain and Rosalind Simpson.
© 2024 John Wiley & Sons Ltd. Published 2024 by John Wiley & Sons Ltd.

The age shift in the population has contributed to an overall increase in the total number of skin cancers as the incidence of BCC increases with advancing age. Indeed, 80% of cases occur in people aged 60 years and over and age is an independent risk factor, with the median age of 71 years at time of diagnosis [9,16].

Compared with women, the incidence of BCC is higher in men. Patients diagnosed with a BCC are at a higher risk of a subsequent one. The 5-year cumulative risk of developing one or more subsequent BCCs is 29.2% [17,18]. This risk is highest in the first 6 months after first BCC diagnosis. Males are at a 30% higher risk of developing multiple BCCs compared with females. Patients aged 65–79 years have a more than 80% higher risk of developing subsequent BCC compared with patients younger than 50 years [17].

An individual's risk for the development of BCC depends upon genotypic, phenotypic and environmental factors. This risk is higher in residents living in areas of high ambient solar irradiance with markers of UV susceptibility such as fair skin colour, red hair and inability to tan [18]. Markers of chronic photodamage are positively associated with BCC [18]. Having more than 10 actinic keratoses confers a fivefold increase in the risk of BCC. Other factors, including solar elastosis, solar lentigines and telangiectasia, have weaker but positive associations with BCC [19].

The geographical variability of KC incidence correlates with the amount of ambient sun irradiance and skin type, the reported incidence of KC in white populations being about five- to sevenfold higher in the USA and Australia than in Europe [9,13–15]. Proximity to the equator is known to be a strong predictor of KC risk and incidence. There is also a strong inverse association between geographical latitude and the risk of BCC [20].

UV radiation is the most important risk factor in the pathogenesis of KC; however, there appears to be a significantly greater effect of increasing sun exposure on the risk of developing SCC than BCC [21]. Unlike SCC, for which cumulative lifetime sun exposure shows a strong dose–response relationship, for BCC intermittent sun exposure and exposure during childhood may be more important [22,23].

Pathophysiology
Predisposing factors
The primary risk factors for BCC development are UV light exposure and genetic predisposition. Other significant risk factors include Fitzpatrick skin types I and II, immunosuppression, advancing age, male sex, previous BCCs and chronic arsenic exposure [24]. Other risk factors are listed in Box 140.1.

Pathology
The tumour cells resemble those of the basal layer of the epidermis and the matrix cells of the appendages, in the relatively small amount of cytoplasm they possess and in their ability to interact with the dermis adjacent to them. Their nuclei are compact, rather darkly staining and closely set. Their cytoplasm is scanty and ill-defined and the cell margins are rather indistinct. Adjacent cells are connected by bridges. The sparsity of keratin fibrils gives these connections a different appearance from the 'prickles' of the Malpighian layer, but the presence of desmosomes and tonofibrils has been shown by electron microscopy. The interaction with the dermis, which is one of the principal functions of the normal epidermal basal cell, produces the characteristic marginal palisade of tumour cells and the well-organised stroma that surrounds it. The dependence of the tumour on its stroma has been shown by transplantation experiments [25]. The cells within the palisade usually show little evidence of organisation or differentiation. Mitotic figures may be frequent, and it is speculated that the combination of large numbers of mitoses and a slow growth rate results from a high rate of apoptosis. Data on cell kinetics indicate that a considerable proportion of cells in the tumour die fairly rapidly [26]. In some tumours, the cells may become acantholytic. Amyloid may be identified [27].

In early lesions, the tumour buds can be seen arising from the epidermis. In very small lesions, multiple buds may be seen. These very soon become confluent, and the three-dimensional examination of superficial BCC shows a coherent margin of tumour with a reticular pattern of growth along the interpapillary ridges and larger, more discrete masses centrally [28]. As the tumour progresses, the masses extend into the dermis, and may separate from each other and from their point of origin. Growth in one area may be accompanied by involution of the tumour in nearby areas leaving an atrophic epidermis. It is difficult to prove a purely adnexal origin for BCC, but some lesions behave as though this were so. In all considerations about the origin of the tumour, one must remember that the tumour can either sever its connection with epithelial structures or establish a secondary connection to structures to which it has grown close.

The variability of the natural history of BCC is reflected in its pattern of growth. Most tumours are composed of rounded expansile islands. These throw out small buds that grow in the same way to produce multilobular masses with thin strands or septa of fibrous tissue penetrating them [28,29]. In some regions, a limited capacity to grow around and enclose adjacent connective tissue may be associated with a reticular or cystic pattern of growth. The capacity to invade in thin strands is often accompanied by an excessive and almost exclusive fibroblastic response, in contrast with the lymphocytic response around the expansile masses. Invasive strands may spread for long distances along nerve sheaths. BCC is truly invasive in only a small proportion of cases. In these, the tumours show no

---

Box 140.1 Risk factors for basal cell carcinoma

Intrinsic factors
- Fitzpatrick skin type I, II
- Iatrogenic immunosuppression
- Human immunodeficiency virus (HIV), acquired immune deficiency syndrome (AIDS)
- Chronic lymphocytic leukaemia, non-Hodgkin lymphoma
- Previous history of basal cell carcinoma
- Photosensitising drugs, azathioprine

Extrinsic factors
- High solar ultraviolet (UV) radiation
- Tanning bed, solarium use
- PUVA, narrow-band UVB phototherapy
- Ionising radiation
- Outdoor occupation
- Chronic arsenic exposure

PUVA, psoralen and UVA.

tendency to grow as rounded masses, have no palisade or organised stroma, and penetrate the dermis and deeper structures, destroying them as they go. Such tumours are almost always ulcerated, usually from an early stage. In the less invasive tumour, ulceration occurs when the epidermis is replaced by the tumour. An eroded vegetating type of growth is rather uncommon.

Most BCCs induce a round-cell inflammatory reaction of some degree. It increases in extent with ulceration and is often conspicuous in the papillary body, with superficial patterns of growth. Mast cells are often present in numbers among the fibroblasts of the stroma, and Langerhans cells have been demonstrated within and near the tumour. This infiltrate has recently been correlated with the aggressive nature of the tumour [30].

The diversity of histological patterns of BCC is caused in part by features that have no direct bearing on the clinical course of the tumour. Not infrequently, melanocytes proliferate within the tumour. The melanin they produce causes the tumour to be pigmented, and numerous melanophages collect in the stroma, and sometimes in cystic cavities. Mucin is commonly found in the stroma, particularly at the margin of the tumour, and may be encysted within it. Cystic cavities also form when the centrally placed cells undergo necrosis. There is no evidence that such cavities represent glandular differentiation. Evidence of true sebaceous or sweat gland differentiation has been reported, but is exceptional. Within some tumours there are strands of fusiform cells with more abundant eosinophilic cytoplasm, which may form whorls or keratinising cysts, and which probably represent rudimentary hair follicle differentiation. Histochemical and electron microscopy investigations show little evidence of differentiation of the tumour cells. However, *in vitro* culture of tumour cells from nodular tumours produces evidence of keratinisation after 30 days, suggesting that the cells possess the biochemical mechanisms for keratinisation but that some factor, possibly dermal in origin, inhibits them.

Clinical and histological differentiation between BCCs and trichoepitheliomas (Chapter 137) can be difficult. The progress of immunohistochemistry to differentiate such tumours has stalled in recent years. Markers which may be useful in differentiating BCCs from trichoepitheliomas include CD-10, Bcl-2, cytokeratin 20 and cytokeratin 15 [31].

Histopathological patterns of BCC include superficial, nodular, infiltrative, micronodular and pigmented types (Figure 140.1) [32].

Superficial basal cell carcinoma. Proliferating atypical basaloid cells form an axis parallel to the epidermal surface. Typical features include palisading basal cells which form slit-like spaces containing Alcian blue-positive stromal mucin. Often, however, only clefting is seen as the mucin is washed away during processing. The atypical basaloid cells rarely show mitoses or apoptotic cells but may extend to the hair follicles and rarely the eccrine adnexal structures.

A band-like lymphoid infiltrate may be present and regression is often seen with areas of papillary dermal fibrosis and mild inflammation. This should prompt a careful search through multiple levels looking for foci of atypical basaloid cells in skin biopsies from suspected superficial BCC.

Nodular basal cell carcinoma. Nodular BCC presents histologically as larger nests/lobules of basaloid cells in the papillary or reticular dermis. The nests are separated from the stroma by a slit-like retraction artefact. The surrounding stroma shows myxoid change, and calcification may be seen focally within nests of tumour cells. As in superficial BCC, which may be coexistent in a third of the cases, mitoses and apoptosis are uncommon. Processing of the specimen may result in drop-out of the tumour nests from the stroma which may lead to 'retraction artefact'.

Micronodular basal cell carcinoma. The tumour nests are much smaller than those in nodular BCC and more widely and asymmetrically dispersed in the dermis and/or subcutis and deeper structures. Subtle stromal proliferation is seen around nests of tumour cells. This type of BCC consists of collagen and rare fibroblasts. Retraction artefact is not usually seen around nests of tumour cells. Perineural invasion may be seen.

Infiltrative basal cell carcinoma. Infiltrative BCC typically shows elongated tumour cell strands, five to eight cells in thickness, which present histologically as irregularly sized and shaped nests which are poorly circumscribed and may show invasion of the subcutis and adjacent muscular and other structures. Like the morpheaform variant, these nests show sharp angulation of their peripheral contours with rare foci of slit-like retraction. Mitotic activity and apoptosis are variable. The stroma is frequently fibrotic with stromal fibroblasts. These tumours are more often associated with perineural invasion.

Morphoeaform basal cell carcinoma. This is also known as sclerosing BCC, and displays columns one to two cells thick of basaloid cells enmeshed in a dense collagenous stroma. Such sharply angulated cords of basaloid cells show marked cell necrosis and mitotic activity. A desmoplastic stroma consisting of dense collagen is present. Invasion of the deep dermis and subcutis is another feature of morphoeaform BCC. Perineural invasion is often seen.

Basosquamous or metatypical basal cell carcinoma. This is a very poorly delineated variant of BCC. In reality, there is a paucity of any meaningful publications on the subject to define the entity and its behaviour in an accurate manner. This variant represents a BCC with true areas of SCC. It is extremely rare, and cases of keratotic BCC are often classified under this rubric. Although it has been suggested that these lesions have a more aggressive behaviour, this has not to date been substantiated with any large series with adequate long-term follow-up.

Genetics

Naevoid BCC syndrome (NBCCS or Gorlin syndrome) is an autosomal dominant disorder with distinct clinical and systemic features with multiple BCCs from an early age. Insight into the molecular pathogenesis of BCC derives from the study of patients with NBCCS, which results from germline mutations in patched-1 (*PTCH1*), a segment polarity gene (9q22.3) with tumour suppressor functions [33]. *PTCH1* was originally identified in the fruitfly *Drosophila melanogaster* and is known to play a critical role in vertebrate development. *PTCH1* encodes a 12-pass putative transmembrane protein, which acts like the receptor of the diffusible morphogen protein sonic hedgehog (SHH) [34].

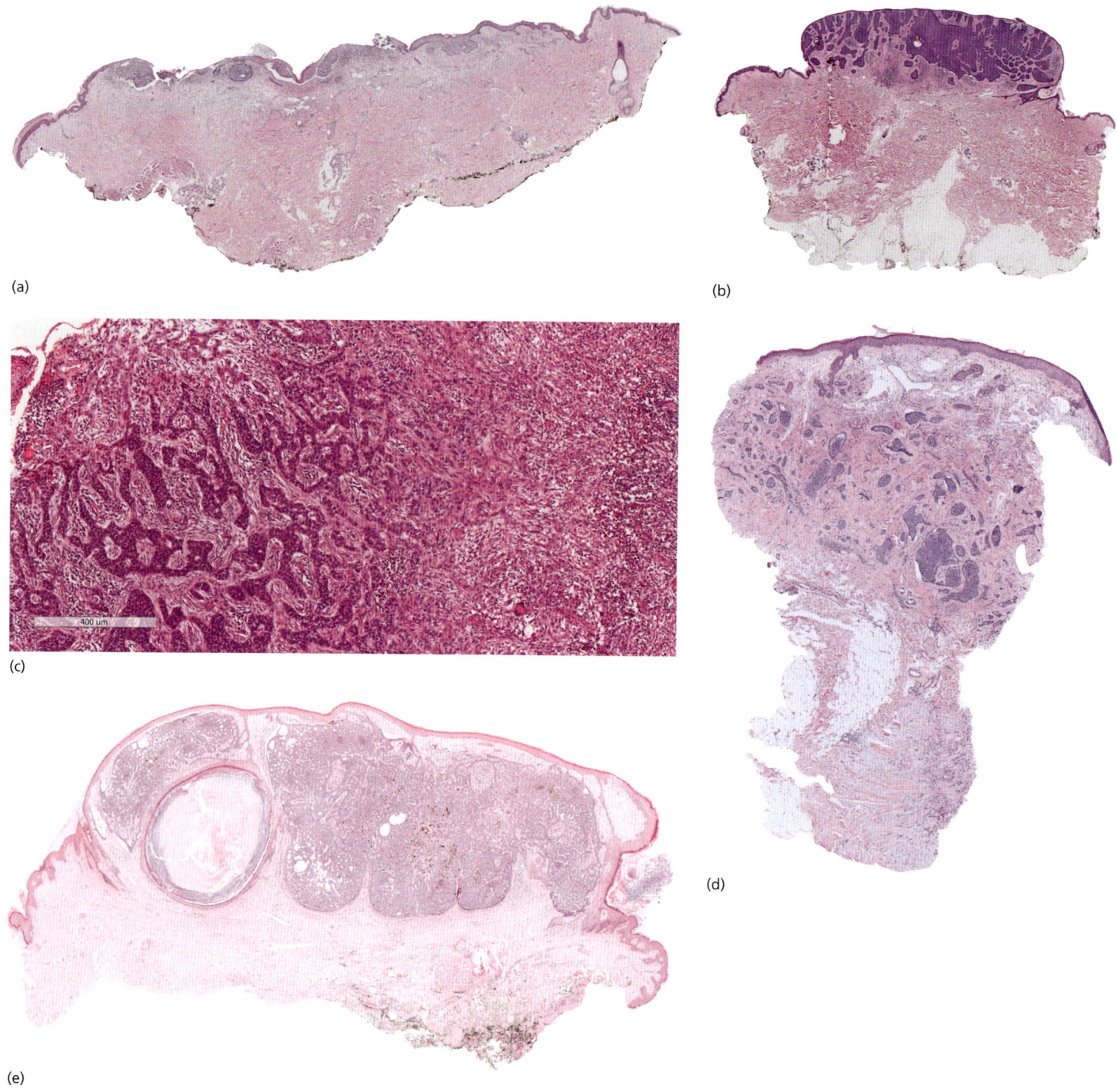

Figure 140.1 Histopathological patterns of basal cell carcinoma (BCC). (a) Superficial. Skin with small islands and downgrowths of basaloid cells arising from multiple points from the epidermis with artefactual clefting. Superficial BCC is usually confined to the papillary dermis. (b) Nodular. Exophytic lesion with large solid islands of basaloid cells, some showing focal central cystic degeneration. Peripheral palisading is present and artefactual clefting focally. (c) Micronodular. Basaloid tumour with numerous small nests in the deep dermis displaying a degree of infiltration at the edge compared with larger nests in the upper dermis which represent a nodular pattern. (d) Infiltrative. Irregular elongated strands and basaloid islands embedded in a variably fibrotic stroma with chronic inflammation. Note extensive involvement of the dermis, subcutis and skeletal muscle. (e) Pigmented. Large solid islands of basaloid cells with central pigmentation. Peripheral palisading is a prominent feature. This lesion may clinically be mistaken for a melanocytic proliferation. (a, b, d, e) Courtesy of Dr Calonje.

PTCH1 acts as a tumour suppressor, repressing the G-protein-coupled receptor smoothened (Smo). Loss-of-function mutations of *PTCH1* result in reduced suppression of Smo which activates the Gli family of transcription factors and promotes their importation into the nucleus, resulting in sustained activation of target genes. Gli proteins are bound by Sufu, loss of which produces constitutive activation of Gli (Figure 140.2).

Atypical protein kinase C iota/lambda (aPKC-ι/λ), a novel Gli regulator, and its polarity signalling partners co-localise at the centrosome and form a complex with missing-in-metastasis (MIM),

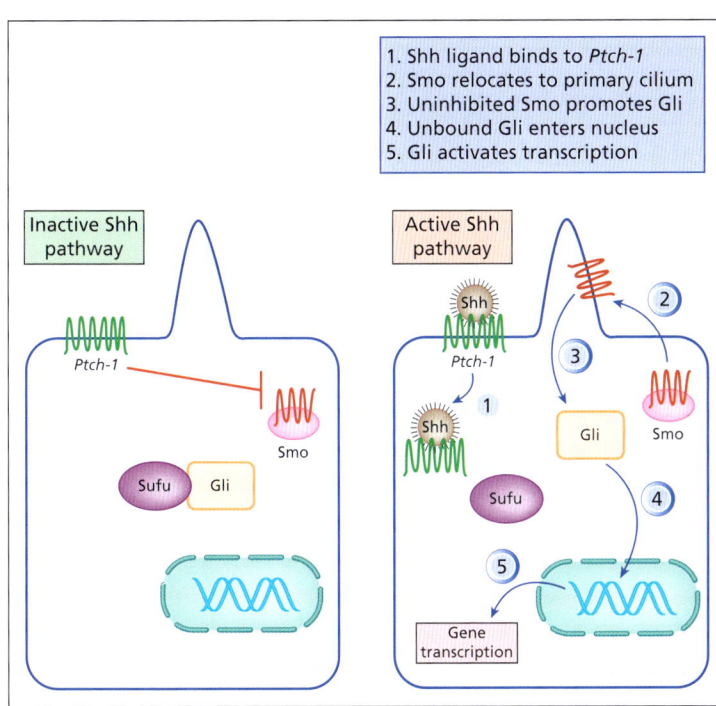

Figure 140.2 The sonic hedgehog (SHH) pathway in the pathogenesis of basal cell carcinoma.

a scaffolding protein that potentiates Hh signalling. Activated aPKC-ɩ/λ is upregulated in Smo-inhibitor-resistant tumours and targeting aPKC-ɩ/λ suppresses signalling and growth of resistant BCC cell lines [35].

Somatic *PTCH1* mutations have a high frequency in familial BCC [36]. Sporadic BCC tumours also demonstrate loss of function of *PTCH1* in 80–90% and Smo in 10–20% of cases [37].

The melanocortin-1 receptor (*MC1R*) gene variants *ASIP* and *TYR* are associated with fair skin, red hair and melanoma risk. Recent evidence suggests that they may also be independent risk factors for BCC [38]. Similarly, the role of the p53 tumour suppressor gene has been examined as 50% of BCCs carry a p53 mutation [11,39].

Both cytochrome P450s (CYP) and glutathione S-transferases (GST) catalyse the detoxification of the products of oxidative stress (e.g. lipid and DNA hydroperoxides). Polymorphism in GST and *CYP2D6* (the gene encoding CYP) have been associated with BCC susceptibility and some allelic variants of *CYP2D6* are associated with a multiple presentation phenotype of BCC [41].

Unlike normal cells, most immortal and tumour cells exhibit significant levels of telomerase activity and show no net loss of telomere length during proliferation, a phenomenon that has also been observed in BCC [42].

The finding that β-catenin and MT1-MMP are increased in high-risk BCC tumour cells may indicate that they play an important role in locally invasive and highly destructive growth behaviour of high-risk BCCs [43].

Immunosuppression
In the general population, BCCs are two to four times more common than SCCs. This ratio reverses in immunosuppressed patients such as solid-organ transplant recipients, where SCCs occur more frequently [44,45]. White-skinned transplant recipients have a 10–16-fold higher risk of developing a BCC compared with the non-transplanted population. Human immunodeficiency virus (HIV)-infected patients and those with chronic lymphocytic leukaemia also have more aggressive KC [46]. Chronic lymphocytic leukaemia patients are 14 times more likely to suffer recurrences of BCC following Mohs surgery [47].

Other risk factors
Chronic exposure to inorganic arsenic through drinking water has been associated with the development of BCC [48]. Other risk factors for the development of BCC include UVB phototherapy [49] and ionising radiation [50]. Besides NBCCS, multiple early-onset BCC may be seen in other syndromes (Tables 140.1 and 140.2) [51].

Environmental factors
The mechanism of UV light-induced mutagenesis has been extensively studied. Daylight UVA or UVB but not UVC induces a characteristic mutation known as solar UV signature mutation occurring preferentially at methyl CpG sites [52].

Daylight UVA and UVB induce indirect DNA damage via the formation of reactive oxygen species (ROS) by a 'photo-oxidative stress' mediated mechanism. The ROS interact with lipids, proteins and DNA to generate intermediates that combine with DNA to form adducts [53]. Several complex DNA repair systems are needed to prevent the deleterious effects of these premutagenic adducts [54]. UV-induced DNA damage normally results in DNA repair or apoptosis; only very rarely does it lead to tumourigenesis. Patients with xeroderma pigmentosum, where DNA repair mechanisms are impaired, can have an up to 2000-fold increased risk of skin cancer [55].

BCCs have been shown to be the most mutated human cancers, with the majority being UV signature mutations. BCCs from anatomical regions with chronic UV exposure are associated with higher mutation rates than those with intermittent exposure. The greater mutational burden facilitates an increased antitumour immunological response which results in a less aggressive phenotype [33].

Clinical features
Unlike SCC, there is no recognised premalignant stage of BCC. A typical BCC runs a slow progressive course of peripheral extension, which produces a thread-like 'pearly' border and a nodule with or without a central depression or expanding ulceration. There may be spontaneous fluctuation in size, and areas of scarring and regression. Traditionally, rapid growth has been thought to be unusual. However, a prospective study looking at periocular BCC showed surprisingly rapid growth in this cohort with a mean increase in size of 1.46 mm in length (area 22 mm^2) every 30 days, with one BCC enlarging by 10 mm in length (area 168 mm^2) in the same time period. The only significant risk factors found for rapid growth were recurrent tumours and greater size at first examination, with surprisingly no additional effect of aggressive pathological features. Whether these findings can be generalised to other facial sites is unknown [56,57].

Approximately 80% of all BCCs occur on the head and neck, and clinical diagnosis is relatively straightforward [58]. Early BCCs are usually small, translucent or pearly nodules, with raised telangiectatic edges. However, the presentation may be varied and small lesions can be lichenoid, keratotic, excoriated or ulcerated.

Table 140.1 Genetic syndromes with basal cell carcinoma (BCC) as a prominent feature.

Condition	Inheritance	Gene(s)	Main additional cutaneous feature(s)	Main additional extracutaneous feature(s)	Main additional neoplasm(s)	Published diagnostic criteria	Available diagnostic test
Naevoid BCC syndrome	AD	PTCH1	Epidermoid cysts, milia, palmoplantar pits	Calcifications of the falx cerebri, coarse face, jaw keratocysts, macrocephaly, spine, limb and oro-facial malformations	Medulloblastomas, rhabdomyosarcomas	Yes	Yes (DNA testing)[a]
Bazex–Dupré–Christol syndrome	XL	Unknown	Flexural hyperpigmentation, follicular atrophoderma, hypohidrosis, hypotrichosis, milia	None	Trichoepitheliomas	No	No
Rombo syndrome	AD	Unknown	Atrophoderma vermiculatum, red lesions, hypotrichosis, milia, telangiectasias	None	Trichoepitheliomas	No	No
Xeroderma pigmentosum (Chapter 76)	AR	XPA-XPG, POLH	Actinic keratosis/cheilitis, lentigines, atrophy, photosensitivity, telangiectasias, mottled hypo-/hyperpigmentation	DD/MR, eye anomalies, movement disorder, peripheral neuropathy, photophobia	Melanomas, squamous cell carcinomas, brain and visceral neoplasms	No	Yes
Generalised follicular basaloid hamartoma syndrome	AD	Unknown	Comedones, hypohidrosis, hypotrichosis, milia	None	None	No	No
Happle–Tinschert syndrome (Chapter 73)	Sporadic	Unknown	Lesions over Blaschko lines, atrophy, hyperpigmentation, teeth abnormalities	Body asymmetry, DD/MR, spine and limb malformations	Brain tumours	No	No

Reproduced from Castori et al. 2012 [51] with permission of John Libbey Eurotext.
[a] In the presence of developmental delay, craniosynostosis, hydrocephalus, overgrowth and seizures, consider the 9q22.3 microdeletion syndrome.
AD, autosomal dominant; AR, autosomal recessive; DD/MR, developmental delay/mental retardation or intellectual disability; XL, X-linked.

More advanced lesions can present as the classic 'rodent ulcer' with an indurated edge and an ulcerated centre. Pigment, when present, is usually unevenly distributed throughout the tumour.

Certain features will classify BCC into high- and low-risk groups for aggressive behaviour, incomplete excision and recurrence which may influence the choice of management (see Tables 140.4 and 140.5 later in this chapter).

Clinical variants

There are a number of BCC variants that are clinically distinctive and can be easily classified. These include nodular, superficial, morphoeic and ulcerative types. Between 10% and 40% of BCCs contain a mixed pattern of two or more of these subtypes, highlighting the need for a clinicopathological diagnosis [59,60]. The status of so-called fibroepithelial BCC (fibroepithelioma of Pinkus/premalignant fibroepithelial tumour) is heavily disputed, with an emerging consensus that this entity is best regarded as a variant of trichoblastoma [61,62].

Other described types such as infiltrative, infundibulocystic, micronodular and basosquamous are histologically distinctive but do not have distinguishing clinical features.

Nodular basal cell carcinoma. Nodular BCC (Figure 140.3) is the commonest subtype of BCC with a predilection for the head and neck. The surface contour of this lesion usually becomes more irregular as the lesion grows. The degree of vascularity varies. There may be surface arborising telangiectasia (a characteristic feature) over a flesh-coloured, shiny nodule with rolled borders or the tumour may be pink or red in colour. Some or all of the component nodules may have cystic centres, which add to the translucent appearance. Nodular BCC may contain pigmentation (Figure 140.4) seen more deeply in the cystic centre rather than the peripheral parts. This may cause diagnostic confusion with melanoma.

Superficial basal cell carcinoma. Superficial BCC (Figure 140.5) is predominantly present on the trunk and limbs. These are thin plaques or patches bounded by a well-circumscribed, slightly raised, thread-like margin which is irregular in outline and may be deficient at part of the circumference. The epidermis covering the central zone is usually scaly and may demonstrate central clearing or atrophy. This, combined with an increased vascularity, gives a resemblance to SCC *in situ*/Bowen disease and Paget disease of the nipple. There may be a series of thickened papular islands of growth within the margin, and these may be crusted or eroded. Patients with truncal BCC of superficial histology demonstrate the highest rate of increasing BCC numbers [63]. Superficial BCCs are often pigmented and can sometimes be difficult to differentiate from psoriasis, discoid eczema or Bowen disease (Chapter 141).

Morphoeic basal cell carcinoma. Morphoeic BCC (Figure 140.6) is also known as morphoeaform, sclerodermiform or desmoplastic, so

Table 140.2 Genetic syndromes with basal cell carcinoma (BCC) as an ancillary feature.

Condition	Inheritance	Gene(s)	Main additional cutaneous features	Main additional extracutaneous features	Main additional neoplasms	Published diagnostic criteria	Genomic testing
Genomic instability syndromes							
Bloom syndrome (Chapter 77)	AR	RECQL3	Café-au-lait spots, photosensitivity, telangiectasias	Diabetes, gastro-oesophageal reflux, growth delay, myelodysplasia, recurrent/chronic infections	Leukaemias, lymphomas, epithelial cancers	No	Yes
Werner syndrome (Chapter 70)	AD (atypical), AR	LMNA (atypical), RECQL2	Atrophy, calcifications, painful callosities, premature greying, scleroderma	Cataract, diabetes, hypogonadism, peripheral neuropathy, premature atherosclerosis and osteoporosis, typical face	Melanomas, (osteo-)sarcomas	No	Yes
Rothmund–Thomson syndrome (Chapter 75)	AR	RECQL4	Hypotrichosis, nail dystrophy, palmoplantar keratoderma, photosensitivity, poikiloderma, teeth anomalies	Cataract, growth delay, myelodysplasia, osteoporosis, patellar hypoplasia, radial ray defects	Bowen disease, osteosarcomas, SCC	Yes	Yes
Muir–Torre syndrome (Chapter 141)	AD	MSH2, MLH1	None	None	Keratoacanthomas, gastrointestinal, urinary and endometrial neoplasms	No	Yes
Disorders of the folliculo-sebaceous unit							
CYLD-associated syndromes (Chapter 137)	AD	CYLD	None	None	Cylindromas, trichoepitheliomas, spiroadenomas, adenomas of salivary glands	No	Yes
Schöpf–Schulz–Passarge syndrome (Chapter 137)	AR	WNT10A	Eyelid cysts, hypohidrosis, hypotrichosis, nail dystrophy, milia, palmoplantar keratoderma, teeth anomalies, telangiectasias	None	Apocrine cystoadenomas, eccrine syringofibroadenomas, eccrine poromas, SCC	No	Yes
Cowden syndrome (Chapter 137)	AD	PTEN	Acral pseudoverrucoid lesions, acrochordons, fibromas, lipomas, oral and lip papillomas, vascular malformations	Breast fibrocystic disease, Lhermitte–Duclos disease, macrocephaly, thyroid dysfunction	Breast cancer, gastrointestinal polyps, ovarian cancer, thyroid cancer, trichilemmomas, uterine cancer	Yes	Yes
Syndromes with immunodeficiency							
Cartilage–hair hypoplasia (Chapters 65, 66, 70)	AR	RMRP	Hypotrichosis/alopecia	Disproportionately short stature, metaphyseal dysplasia, peripheral joint laxity, pudgy extremities	Non-Hodgkin lymphomas	No	Yes
Epidermodysplasia verruciformis (Chapter 25)	AR	EVER1, EVER2	Polymorphic, red lesions, wart-like/flat papules	None	Bowen disease, SCC	No	Yes
Disorders of melanin biosynthesis							
Oculocutaneous albinism (Chapters 63, 68)	AR	MATP TYR, TYRP1 OCA 1/2	Hair, skin and iris hypopigmentation	Photophobia, reduced colour vision, strabismus, visual loss	Melanomas, SCC	No	Yes
Hermansky–Pudlak syndrome (Chapter 68)	AR	HPS1-HPS8	Hair, skin and iris hypopigmentation	Bleeding diathesis, granulomatous colitis, photophobia, pulmonary fibrosis, reduced colour vision, strabismus, visual loss	Melanomas, SCC	No	Yes

Reproduced from Castori *et al.* 2012 [51] with permission of John Libbey Eurotext.
AD, autosomal dominant; AR, autosomal recessive; SCC, squamous cell carcinoma.

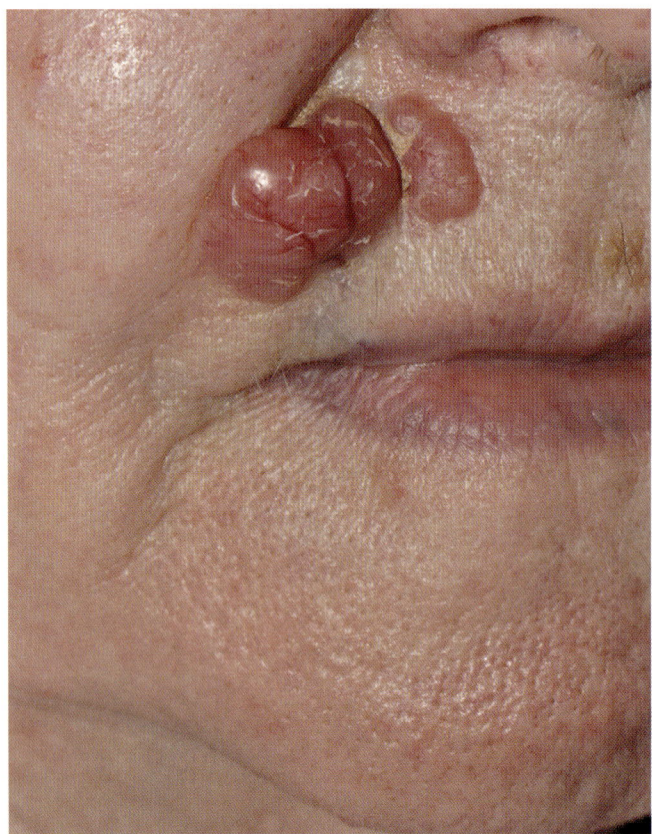

Figure 140.3 Nodular basal cell carcinoma.

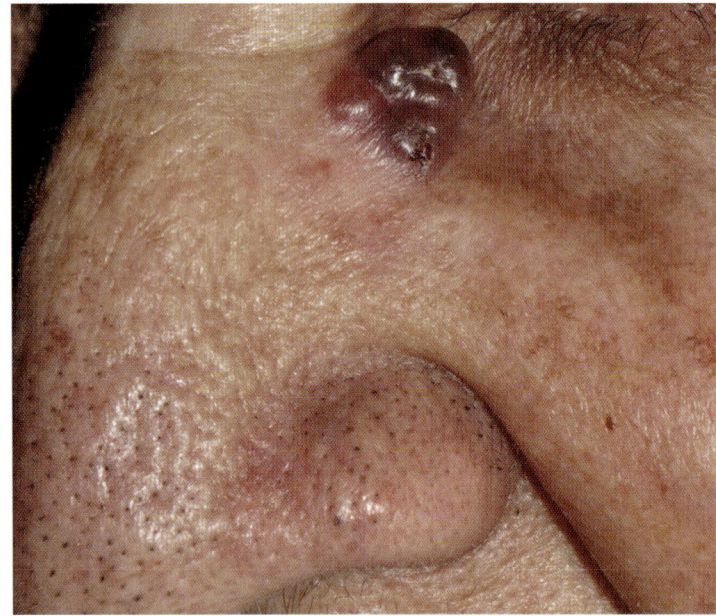

Figure 140.4 Pigmented basal cell carcinoma.

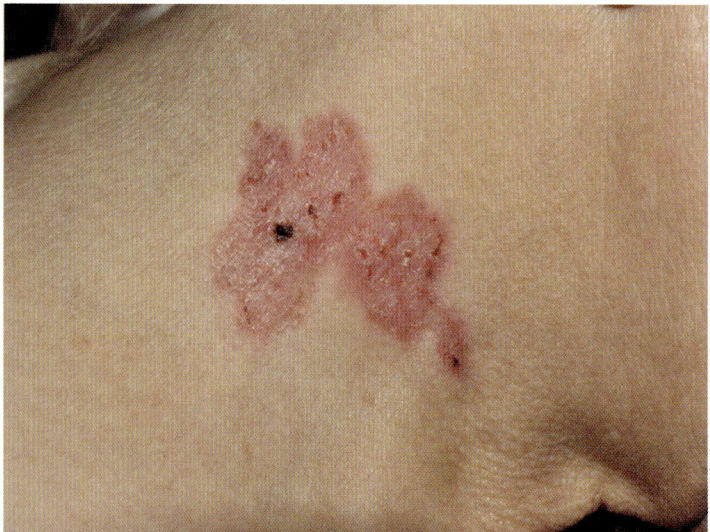

Figure 140.5 Superficial basal cell carcinoma.

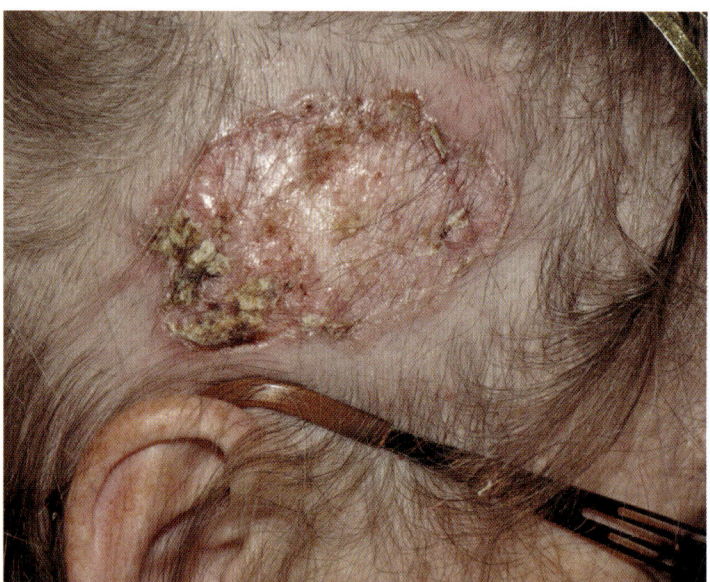

Figure 140.6 Morphoeic basal cell carcinoma.

named because dense fibrosis of the stroma produces a thickened plaque rather than a tumour.

Morphoeic BCCs account for 5% of all BCCs, have ill-defined borders, can be difficult to diagnose clinically and often present late. The exact margin of the lesion is near impossible to define, but palpation reveals a firm skin texture that extends irregularly beyond the visible changes. The surface is smooth and may be slightly raised above, or sometimes slightly depressed below, the normal level. The colour is yellowish. Ulceration is uncommon and only very superficial when it does occur. Many patients and health care providers may take little notice of this type of BCC until its slow extension produces a sizeable lesion with extensive subclinical spread. These lesions can be mistaken for scars.

Ulcerative basal cell carcinoma. Any BCC may ulcerate over time so it is not entirely clear that this is a specific clinical subtype. However some BCCs may start as a small macule or papule but with expansion of the thread-like margins, the attenuated surface ulcerates at an early stage (Figure 140.7). The edge is usually indurated. Such an ulcerated lesion may have begun as a nodule, but more frequently it is crusted or eroded from an early stage of its evolution. If left, the tumour and its following ulcer may spread

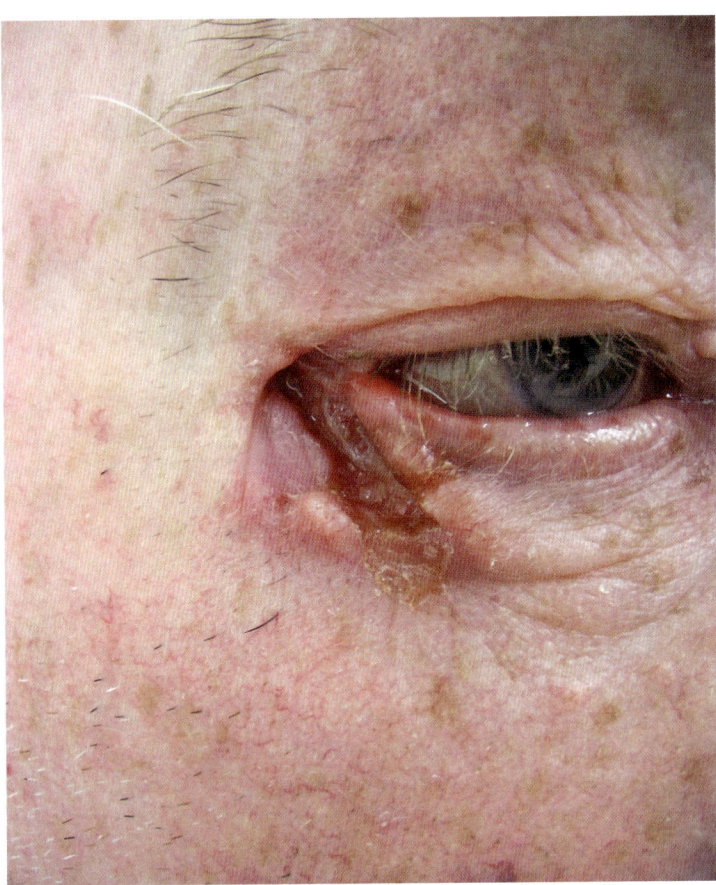

Figure 140.7 Ulcerated basal cell carcinoma.

deeply and cause great destruction, especially around the eye, nose or ear. Advanced cases justify the title 'ulcus terebrans' (penetrating ulcer).

Risk factors for advanced disease

Perineural invasion (PNI) is a sign of increased aggressiveness of BCC. In a large Mohs surgery cohort in Australia 2.7% of patients demonstrated PNI [64], so it can be expected that the incidence of PNI in the general population of patients with BCC is lower. When PNI is asymptomatic it is classified as microscopic PNI and carries a much better prognosis than clinical PNI where neurological symptoms are present or there is imaging evidence of perineural spread.

Risk factors for advanced disease (Figure 140.8) and metastasis include prolonged neglect, which is often associated with fear of medical treatment, psychosocial factors, lack of access to care, multiple recurrences following treatment, clinical perineural invasion (neurological symptoms present and/or imaging evidence of perineural spread is found), large lesion size and aggressive histopathological subtypes. Advanced BCCs are encountered at a rate of 1–2% [65]. Mutilation of the face or scalp, with destruction of the nose or eye and exposure of the paranasal sinuses or the skull, dura or brain may eventually result in death [66]. Progression of advanced BCC to a metastatic form is extremely rare (0.0028–0.55% of BCC) [67]. Authentic cases of bloodstream metastasis are on record in which, for example, deposits in the viscera or spinal column have caused the presenting symptoms of the terminal illness. Other cases have spread via the lymphatics to the regional lymph nodes before disseminating [68]. Basosquamous (metatypical) BCC has an increased risk of metastasis in comparison with other BCC subtypes. Up to 38.1% of primary BCCs that metastasise have this subtype despite basosquamous representing <3% of all BCCs [69].

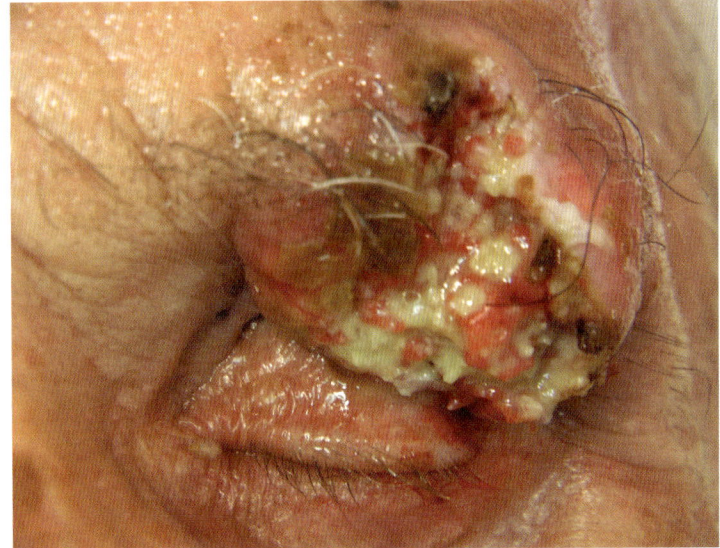

Figure 140.8 Advanced basal cell carcinoma with orbital invasion.

Differential diagnosis

It may be difficult to differentiate nodular BCC from melanocytic naevus (especially when pigmented), or sebaceous hyperplasia on clinical evaluation alone. Naevi can be distinguished if hairs grow from the surface, and in sebaceous hyperplasia there is a central keratin-filled pit (Table 140.3).

Scaling or crusting on the surface of BCC can make differentiation from warts, keratoacanthoma or SCC difficult. In these cases, the debris can usually be easily removed. The friable, relatively avascular tissue beneath is characteristic.

Darkly pigmented tumours with or without ulceration may be occasionally confused with malignant melanoma. The margin of BCC is usually rolled, telangiectatic and multinodular, and there is no pigmented halo. The colour tends to be more definitely brown, in contrast with the dusky greyish brown of malignant melanoma, but this is not a reliable indicator. Dermoscopy can be diagnostic. If diagnostic confusion remains, the lesion is better excised in entirety if possible or a representative partial biopsy or deep shave undertaken.

Superficial BCC can be similar morphologically to patches of eczema, psoriasis or Bowen disease (see Chapter 141). A thread-like margin on stretching the edge will often reveal the true diagnosis. Careful inspection will almost always rule out eczema or psoriasis, which the patient's history will have also made unlikely. There are some cases, however, where distinction from Bowen disease can be made only after biopsy. The consistency of a morphoeic BCC may resemble morphoea or scar; the outline is usually less sharp and the evolution more gradual and relentless.

Chondrodermatitis nodularis helicis (Chapter 106) is usually tender. Some BCCs may not display the typical clinical features. Surface ulceration or excoriation may hinder accurate diagnosis. Clinical diagnostic accuracy in the diagnosis of BCC can be greatly

Table 140.3 Differential diagnosis of basal cell carcinoma.

Diagnosis	Distinguishing clinical features	Image
Naevi	Lack of rolled telangiectatic edge. May be hairy	
Sebaceous hyperplasia	Central depression, usually multiple on a background of sebaceous-quality skin	
Keratoacanthoma	A central keratin plug is typical, with a history of rapid evolution followed by involution	
Squamous cell carcinoma	Shorter history and indurated base (better felt on palpation)	
Bowen disease	Scaly edge and lack of thread-like margin	
Psoriasis	Silvery scales and response to topical antipsoriatic therapy	
Eczema	History of eczema and response to topical eczema therapy	
Melanoma	Grey-black discoloration and pigment spill. Shorter history	
Chondrodermatitis nodularis helicis	Usually tender	
Viral warts	Keratotic 'warty' surface	

enhanced with the application of dermoscopy. Adding dermoscopy to naked eye examination increases the sensitivity of diagnosis in expert hands from 66.9% to 85% ($P = 0.0001$) and specificity from 97.2% to 98.2% ($P = 0.006$) with the greatest benefit seen with pigmented BCC [70].

Investigations

The diagnosis of BCC is primarily clinical. In clinically challenging cases, a biopsy is advisable to guide treatment selection. In nodular BCC, a shave biopsy is easily undertaken. A punch biopsy or incisional biopsy allows for a larger specimen and decreased sampling error which may be more appropriate in identifying aggressive subtypes such as morphoeic lesions. The accuracy of punch biopsy in identifying BCC subtypes in mixed tumours is poor, with concordance between biopsy and subsequent excision only 60.9% [71]. It has been reported that at the time of Mohs surgery upstaging in diagnosis from the preoperative biopsy diagnosis occurs in up to 31% of cases [72].

Dermoscopy using non-polarised or cross-polarised light is an indispensable clinical adjunct in the diagnosis of BCC and differentiation from other tumours and inflammatory conditions (Figure 140.9). Vascular structures consist of arborising vessels and short fine telangiectasia. Pigment structures include maple-leaf-like areas, spoke-wheel areas, multiple blue-grey globules, in-focus dots and concentric structures. Other non-vascular/non-pigmented structures include ulceration, multiple small erosions, shiny white-red structureless areas and white streaks. Arborising vessels are the most noteworthy structures. Dermoscopic criteria for each BCC subtype have been described, however the greatest utility of the technique is to help differentiate BCC from benign naevi, Bowen disease, SCC and melanoma [73].

Other experimental techniques for the non-invasive diagnosis of BCC include high-frequency ultrasound, optical coherence tomography using infrared light and *in vivo* reflectance confocal microscopy [74].

High-definition optical coherence tomography (HD-OCT) is a high-resolution imaging tool, with micrometre resolution in both transverse and axial directions, enabling visualisation of individual cells up to a depth of around 570 μm [75]. Features for four different BCC subtypes were described in both transverse and axial directions. Subepidermal or intradermal aggregations of cells forming islands are surrounded by a less refractile border. This corresponds with palisading and peritumoral mucin production on histology (Figure 140.10). Although still in the experimental stages and not yet widely used in clinical practice, both optical coherence tomography and reflectance confocal microscopy may have a potential role in presurgical margin assessment and non-histological assessment of BCC, respectively, however their use can be limited by optical resolution, steep learning curves and high costs [74,75,**76**].

In confocal microscopy, cellular morphology can be observed in real time, in thin optical sections and high-resolution individual images which are stitched together to create mosaics that display low magnification of large areas of tissue as required for Mohs surgery (Figure 140.11) [76]. Contrast agents such as acridine orange in fluorescence and acetic acid in reflectance confocal microscopy have been used in *ex vivo* imaging to enhance nuclear contrast.

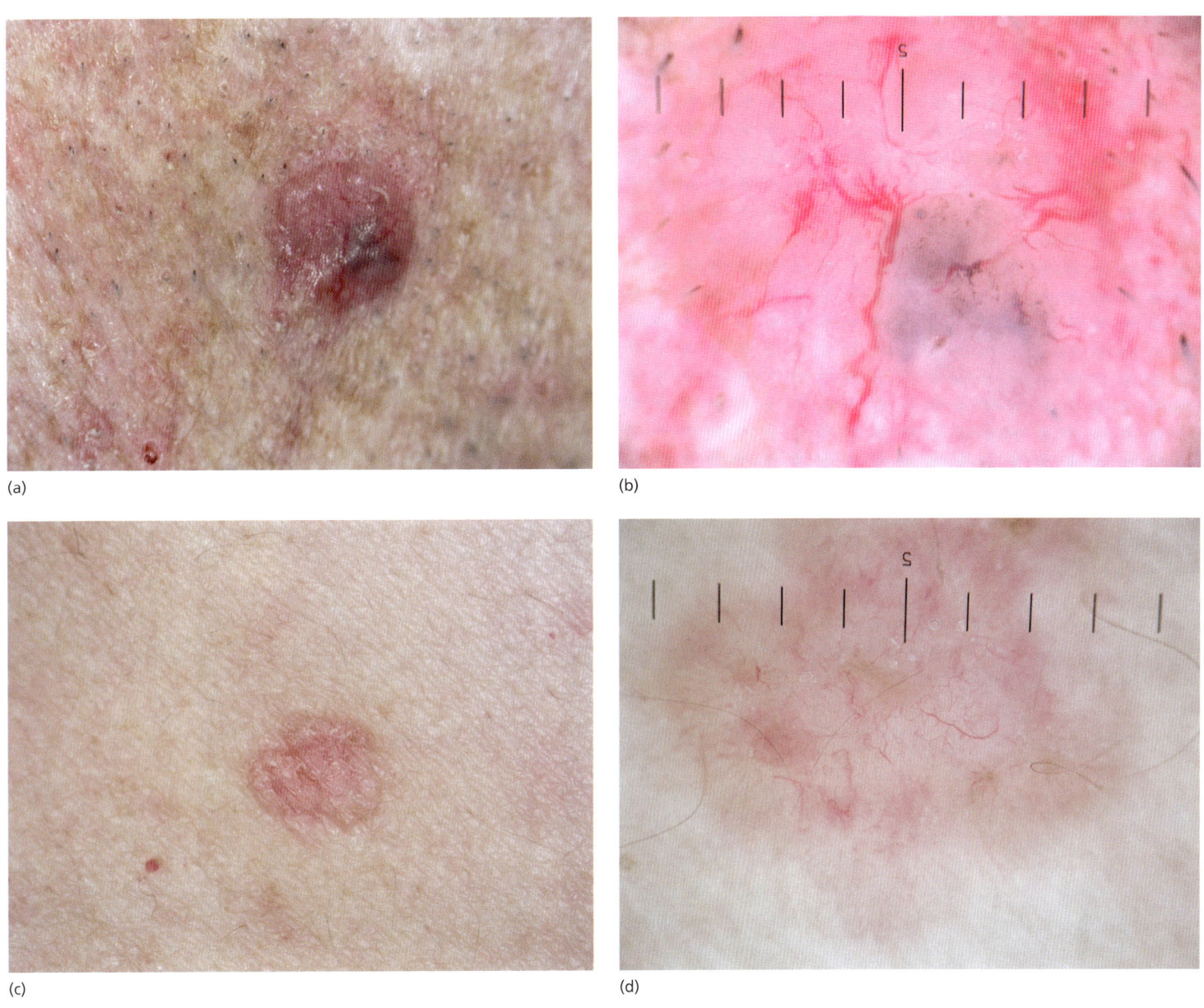

Figure 140.9 Dermoscopic images of basal cell carcinoma (BCC). (a) Nodular BCC. (b) Corresponding dermoscopic image showing white and grey-brown structureless areas, blue-grey globules and telangiectactic vessels. (c) Superficial BCC. (d) Corresponding dermoscopic image showing spoke-wheel areas, concentric structures, arborising, comma and telangiectactic vessels.

Management

Both tumour (including clinical and histological subtype, size and site) and patient (including immunosuppression, previous psoralen and UVA (PUVA) or radiotherapy) factors must be considered. Stratification of BCC into those at low or high risk of tumour recurrence guides the choice of treatment modality (Tables 140.4 and 140.5). Other factors include local experience and availability of treatments, which may indirectly depend upon the cost. Treatment options for BCC have been systematically reviewed and guidelines for the management of BCC have been published by national and international bodies [77–79] with a number of contemporaneous revisions [80–82]. The recommended approach to the treatment of a patient with a BCC is illustrated in Tables 140.6, 140.7 and 140.8.

An evidence-based review of the literature has shown that the best results in the treatment of BCC are obtained with surgery [79] but that radiotherapy is an alternative or adjunct in selected cases. As with any malignancy, the primary aim of treatment is the complete removal or destruction of the BCC. Achieving a functional and acceptable cosmetic outcome is an important secondary goal. For some low-risk BCCs, superficial therapies such as topical treatments and photodynamic therapy (PDT) can be considered, as can cryosurgery. While the cosmetic outcome can be superior with some of these modalities, the cure rate is lower and should not come at the cost of higher risk of recurrence. High-risk BCC should not be treated with curettage and electrodessication, cryosurgery or superficial therapies other than in exceptional circumstances as histological examination of the excision margins is essential.

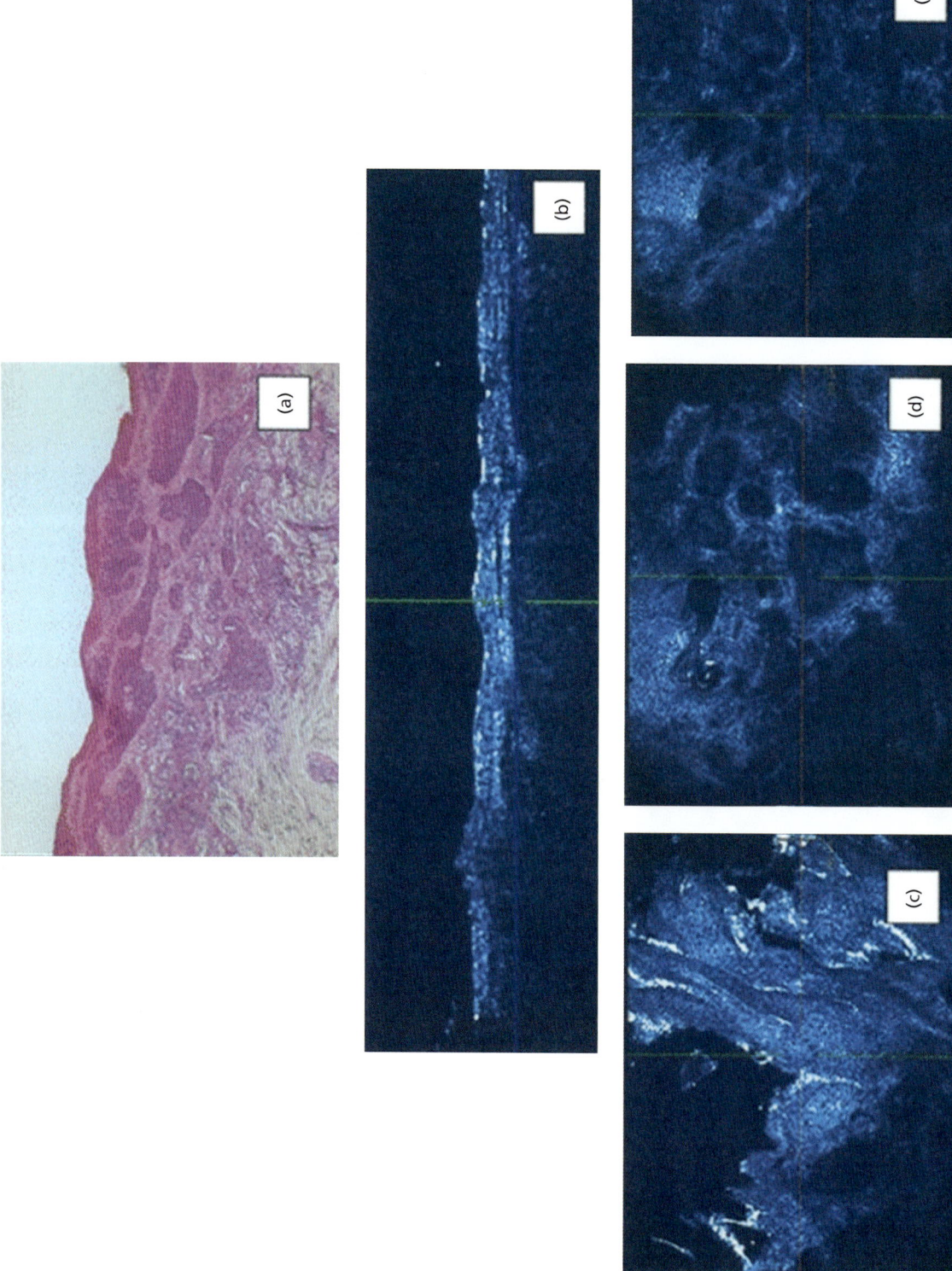

Figure 140.10 Nodular basal cell carcinoma (BCC). (a) H&E stained histological section shows actinic changes in the overlying epidermis and islands of basaloid cells with palisading. These islands are surrounded by an abundant mucinous stroma with separation of the tumour cells from the surrounding stroma (clefting). There is a prominent peritumoural stromal reaction. (b) In high-definition optical coherence tomography (HD-OCT) slice mode, lobular patterns of abnormal architecture are seen with dilated blood vessels and high-reflective margins. (c) In HD-OCT *en face* mode, the overlying epidermis presents an architectural disarray with parakeratosis, pleomorphism and some degree of keratinocyte atypia with variably sized nuclei at the basal cell layer. (d) In *en face* HD-OCT imaging, the nodular BCC islands of tumour cells are noted with intervening areas of low refractility. Inside this low-refractile zone, tumour cells are more refractile. Abundant blood vessels are seen juxtaposed to the islands. (e) *En face* HD-OCT imaging shows a variable refractile stroma with inflammatory cells. Reproduced from Boone *et al.* 2012 [74] with permission of John Wiley & Sons.

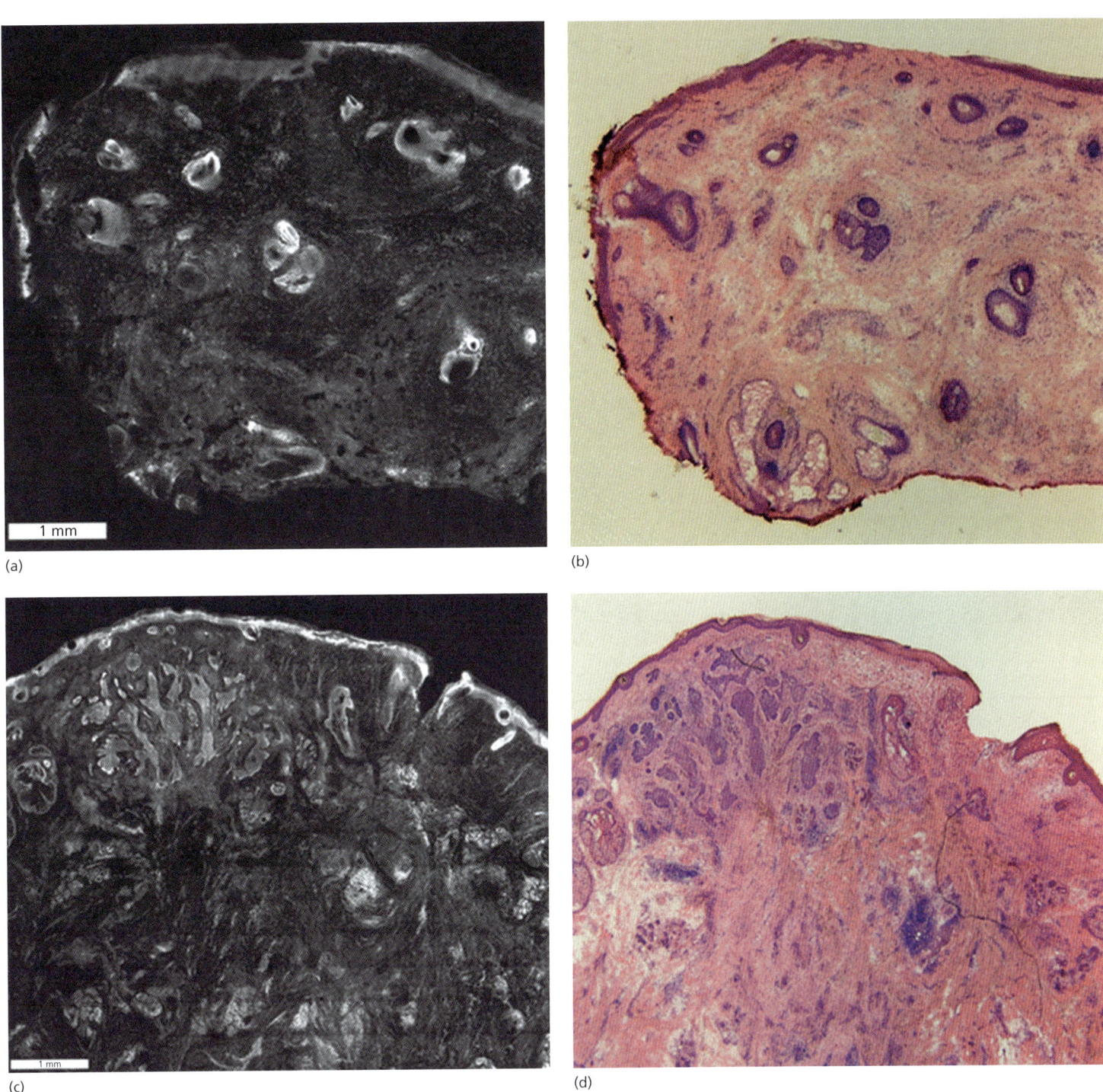

Figure 140.11 Fluorescent confocal submosaics (a, c) and the corresponding H&E-stained Mohs frozen sections (b, d) at 4× magnification. The submosaic and frozen section of a negative Mohs stage shows no residual basal cell carcinoma (BCC) (a, b); positive Mohs stage shows residual BCC within the upper dermis (c, d). There is good correlation between the mosaics and the corresponding frozen sections with respect to the overall size, shape, location and morphology of benign and malignant skin structures. Reproduced from Karen et al. 2009 [76] with permission of John Wiley & Sons.

Superficial treatments

Imiquimod. Imiquimod stimulates Toll-like receptors 7 and 8 expressed on dendritic cells and monocytes, leading to an increased production of cytokines and chemokines. These in turn promote both Th1 innate and adaptive cell-mediated immune responses which are crucial in the recognition and destruction of the tumour cells [83].

Topical 5% imiquimod cream, applied five times per week over 6 weeks, is effective in clearing 69–100% of superficial BCC and 42–76% of nodular BCC on the trunk and limbs [24,84]. There is a lower response rate in nodular BCC and thicker superficial BCC as well as those in high-risk anatomical sites such as the face [85,86]. One study suggests that superficial BCC <0.4 mm in Breslow thickness may be better suited to treatment with imiquimod as

Table 140.4 Investigatons for the diagnosis and risk stratification of basal cell carcinomas (BCCs).

Clinical examination	Investigation	Diagnosis	Risk status for incomplete excision/recurrence	Management
Lesion suspicious for keratinocyte carcinoma Full history Full cutaneous examination	Skin biopsy Imaging (including CT or MRI if there is a suspicion of deep or advanced disease)	BCC	Low risk (Table 140.5)	See Table 140.6
		BCC BCC with involvement of deep soft tissue, perineural invasion, bony erosion or metastasis	High risk (Table 140.5) Advanced disease (Table 140.8)	See Table 140.7 See Table 140.8

Adapted from National Comprehensive Cancer Network Guidelines Version 1.2020 with permission.
CT, computed tomography; MRI, magnetic resonance imaging.

Table 140.5 Stratification of basal cell carcinoma (BCC) into low and high risk.

Feature	Low-risk BCC	High-risk BCC
Location/size	Area L^a <20 mm Area M^b <10 mm	Area L >20 mm Area M >10 mm Area H^c any size
Border	Well defined	Poorly defined
Primary/recurrent	Primary	Recurrent
Immunosuppression	No	Yes
Site of prior radiotherapy	No	Yes
Pathology subtype	No high-risk features Superficial, nodular	Aggressive pattern Infiltrative, micronodular, morphoeic/sclerosing, basosquamous/metatypical
Perineural invasion	No	Yes

Adapted from National Comprehensive Cancer Network Guidelines Version 1.2020 with permission.
^{a} Area L: trunk and extremities excluding the hands, nail units, pretibial, ankles and feet.
^{b} Area M: cheeks, forehead, scalp, neck and pretibial.
^{c} Area H: 'mask' areas of the central face, eyelids, eyebrows, periorbital, nose, lips (cutaneous and vermilion), chin, mandible, pre- and postauricular, temple, ear, genitalia, hands and feet.

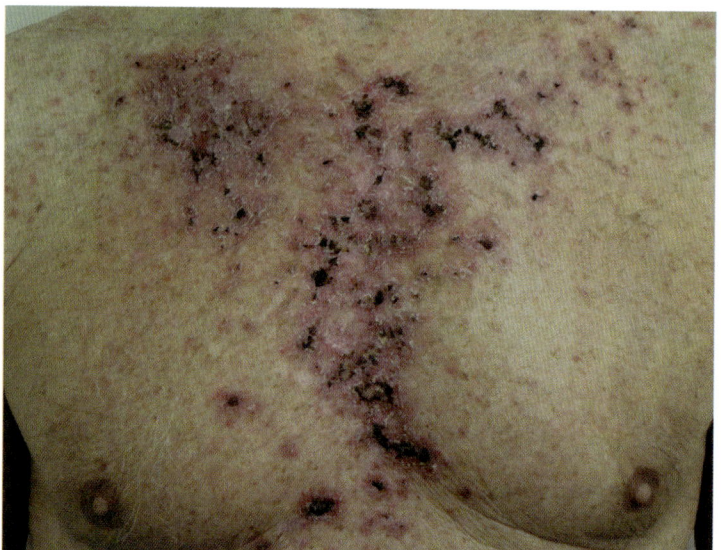

Figure 140.12 Skin reaction to topical imiquimod therapy for superficial basal cell carcinoma.

such lesions are most likely to respond [86]. When compared with PDT, imiquimod may be more effective in treating superficial BCC [87]. Imiquimod is recommended for use in superficial BCC in immunocompetent adults, with a maximum tumour diameter of 2.0 cm.

Patients may experience flu-like symptoms such as fever, chills, body aches and lymphadenopathy. This may be severe enough to warrant discontinuation of treatment. Reddening of the skin, pruritus, erosion, ulceration, dyspigmentation and crusting are commonly observed side effects of topical imiquimod therapy (Figure 140.12).

5-Fluorouracil. Topical 5-fluorouracil (5-FU) disrupts DNA and RNA synthesis by inhibiting the enzyme thymidylate synthetase. This prevents purine and pyrimidine from becoming incorporated into DNA during the S-phase of the cell cycle [88]. When compared with imiquimod in the treatment of superficial BCC, 5-FU cream (5%) has similar efficacy and safety [87]. Like imiquimod, 5-FU is not recommended for the treatment of nodular and high-risk BCC, and local irritation and skin reaction resulting in redness, swelling, desquamation and tenderness are also similar.

Photodynamic therapy. Photodynamic therapy consisting of the application of a photosensitising agent (5-aminolaevulinic acid, methyl aminolaevulinate) to the tumour followed by irradiation with red or blue light relies on the production of ROS, which results in necrosis or apoptosis of tumour cells. A systematic review and meta-analysis of 1583 treated low-risk BCCs has shown an 86.4% complete clearance rate with good to excellent cosmetic outcomes [89]. However, PDT was found to be inferior to both imiquimod and 5-FU other than for superficial BCC below the knee in elderly patients [87]. The complete role of PDT in the treatment of BCC is discussed in Chapter 22.

Intralesional interferon α2b (IFN-α2b). The need for treatment to be delivered in multiple sessions and the high associated costs limit the use of peri- and intralesional IFN-α2b treatment of BCC. This treatment has otherwise high reported cure rates approaching 98% at 12 years and good cosmetic outcomes [90].

Surgical treatments

Cryosurgery. The application of liquid nitrogen to skin lesions to cause destruction of the tissue and a margin of surrounding tissue requires the achievement of lesional temperatures of −50

Table 140.6 Management of low-risk basal cell carcinoma (BCC).

Invasive non-surgical treatment	Superficial treatment	Standard surgical excision	Postoperative pathology margin assessment	Action	Further action	Radiotherapy
Curettage and electrodessication (avoid terminal hair-bearing areas: the scalp, pubic, axillae, beard areas) If adipose tissue is exposed proceed to surgical excision CO_2 laser ablation with curettage Cryosurgery	Imiquimod cream 5-fluorouracil cream Photodynamic therapy (PDT) Intralesional interferon	4 mm clinical margin Postoperative margin assessment Second intention healing or primary linear repair, skin graft or flap	Negative margins	Clinical follow-up by the referring doctor/family physician/general practitioner or dermatologist		Patients where surgery is contraindicated due to medical comorbidities, unacceptable surgical risk, antithrombotic therapy, high risk of bleeding, advanced age, surgical refusal or risk of unacceptable scarring
			Positive margins	Mohs micrographic surgery or Excision with complete circumferential peripheral and deep margin assessment (CCPDMA) or Wide re-excision if feasible or Radiotherapy if surgery is not possible	Positive margins: see Table 140.7	

Adapted from National Comprehensive Cancer Network Guidelines Version 1.2020 with permission.

Table 140.7 Management of high-risk basal cell carcinoma (BCC).

Surgery	Postoperative pathology margin assessment	Action	Further action
Mohs micrographic surgery or Excision with complete circumferential peripheral and deep margin assessment (CCPDMA)	Negative	Clinical follow-up by the referring doctor/family physician/general practitioner or dermatologist If perineural invasion involving nerves >0.1 mm in diameter is seen, consider postoperative radiotherapy and/or multidisciplinary team (MDT) review	
	Positive	Consider MDT meeting to discuss options Re-excision if feasible or Radiotherapy or Systemic therapy (SHHi)	
Wider standard excision with postoperative pathology margin assessment and delayed repair	Negative	Clinical follow-up 6 monthly If perineural invasion is seen consider postoperative radiotherapy	
	Positive	Mohs micrographic surgery or Excision with CCPDMA	Consider MDT meeting to discuss options Radiotherapy or Systemic therapy (SHHi)

Adapted from National Comprehensive Cancer Network Guidelines Version 1.2020 with permission.
SHHi, Sonic hedgehog inhibitor.

to −60°C. Like curettage and electrodessication, liquid nitrogen cryosurgery is considered appropriate for the treatment of some low-risk primary BCCs (see Table 140.6). Published studies are limited by low levels of evidence and anecdote. A double 30 s freeze–thaw cycle for superficial BCC has been reported to have a 95.3% cure rate [91]. A systematic review of recurrence rates found a cumulative risk of 4–17% with an average 5-year follow-up [92]. Compared with standard surgical excision for low-risk primary BCC, cryosurgery may achieve a similar recurrence rate but at the expense of a worse cosmetic outcome as hypopigmentation is a frequent consequence of cryosurgery [93]. While freezing with liquid nitrogen is a quick and relatively tolerable

Table 140.8 Management of advanced basal cell carcinoma (BCC).

Status	Action
No clinical recurrence	Clinical review, for example 6–12 monthly
	Patient education, sun protection, self-examination for new primary BCC
Locally recurrent BCC	See Table 140.7
Nodal or distant metastatic BCC	Consider multidisciplinary team meeting to discuss options, including surgical resection or
	Radiotherapy or
	Systemic therapy (SHHi) or
	Clinical trial recruitment

Adapted from National Comprehensive Cancer Network Guidelines Version 1.2020 with permission.
SHHi, sonic hedgehog inhibitor.

procedure that does not require local anaesthesia, it can be associated with significant morbidity, particularly when tumours selected for treatment require prolonged freeze times to ensure adequate treatment.

Curettage and electrodessication. Curettage and electrodessication (syn. curettage and cautery or C&C) is widely employed for the treatment of BCC as it is fast and can be cost-effective, especially in the treatment of multiple superficial BCCs on the trunk and limbs. However, studies on effectiveness are mostly old and limited by a low evidence base. Reported 5-year cure rates vary from 91–97% for selected primary BCCs through to 73–81% where higher-risk BCCs are selected [92,94–96]. Low-risk superficial non-facial BCCs are best suited for treatment with curettage and electrodessication and should not be employed for the treatment of high-risk BCC. Hair-bearing areas should be avoided due to potential follicular involvement. The results are highly operator dependent and cure rates with the technique likely reflect the experience of the operator [97].

The principal limitation of this technique that must be seriously considered is that histological margins cannot be assessed and the true histological subtype may not be accurately reported. The friable nature of some low-risk BCCs allows removal of abnormal tissue with a dermal curette. The technique involves repeated scraping until firm dermis is reached, followed by electrodessication/cautery to denature any remaining tumour that cannot be identified clinically. Up to three repeated cycles are usual. A modified technique of curettage alone can be an effective way of delineating the extent of some tumours before standard surgical excision or Mohs surgery. However, if performed prior to standard surgical excision, the formal excision pathology specimen is more limited and the interpretation of the pathology potentially affected. The procedure should not breach the dermis. If fat is exposed then the site should be formally excised.

Healing can be unpredictable and is site dependent, with the anterior chest, upper back and shoulders all sites highly prone to hypertrophic scars or keloid following the technique. Mild scarring consisting of some textural change in the skin associated with depigmentation is usual. However, when vigorous diathermy is employed the cosmetic results are less satisfactory.

Standard surgical excision. Standard surgical excision using a 4 mm clinical margin with postoperative margin evaluation is the most effective treatment for low-risk BCC (Table 140.6) [98], with reported 5-year recurrence rates of 0.7–5% [98,99]. A randomised prospective clinical trial with 10-year follow-up showed primary BCCs of the face, excised with 3 mm margins, had 18% of excisions incomplete and a 12.2% recurrence rate. If the BCC was recurrent, standard surgical excision showed 32% incomplete excision with a 13.5% recurrence rate [94].

Primary repair and flap or graft reconstruction following excision can lead to good cosmesis and function, but caution regarding the adequacy of margin clearance is required particularly where tissue rearrangement with flap surgery is undertaken. Aggregated data from an extensive review of all published studies reporting positive histological margins following excision show a mean recurrence rate of 27% if left untreated [100]. So if feasible, wider re-excision should be undertaken or, ideally, Mohs micrographic surgery or resection with complete circumferential peripheral and deep margin assessment (CCPDMA).

Standard surgical excision with wider margins can be considered for high-risk BCC, however the reported surgical margins may need to be up to 15 mm. The current evidence base is insufficient for the margin for high-risk BCC to be accurately specified due to the great range in tumour and patient factors. A meta-analysis of the literature consisting of over 16 000 lesions treated with standard surgical excision showed 4 or 5 mm surgical margins for BCC result in negative margins on pathology in only 85% of cases, with a relative risk of recurrence of 4.2 with a 4 mm margin [100]. One conclusion of this study was that 'Mohs micrographic surgery offers the smallest overall defect size with the lowest recurrence rate for BCC and is the standard against which other treatments are compared'. An alternative when Mohs surgery is unavailable for high-risk BCC is wide resection with CCPDMA.

Mohs micrographic surgery. This is discussed in Chapter 20.

Laser therapy (Chapter 23). The tissue-heating properties of superpulsed CO_2 laser can be used to ablate tumours including BCC. The effects are non-specific and usually need to be combined with curettage to remove the resultant char and any residual friable tumour. Repeated cycles are necessary until all friable tissue is vaporised and firm dermal tissue remains. At this point, any further application of laser results in tissue contraction rather than vaporisation. A single retrospective study showed 100% histological clearance and no recurrences with 3-year follow-up [101]. However, while high clinical cure rates have been reported, with CO_2 laser ablation the lack of histological confirmation of tumour clearance means that its use should be restricted to low-risk non-facial BCC [101,**102**]. Recurrences following CO_2 laser ablation can be more challenging to treat as a dense scar often results, with a longer disease interval to diagnosis and a more aggressive histological pattern compared with primary BCC [**103**].

The pulsed dye laser has also been employed in the treatment of superficial BCC. A randomised placebo-controlled trial showed histological clearance at 6 months in 78.6% of cases [104]. However, the high incomplete clearance rate precludes the use of this technology in the treatment of BCC [105].

A large retrospective study of pulsed neodymium laser therapy for facial BCC showed a low recurrence rate of only 1.8% with follow-up of 3 months to 5 years [106]. However, the lack of histological assessment in these high-risk BCCs and risk of late recurrence and delayed treatment preclude the use of this technology as well.

Radiotherapy (Chapter 24). External beam radiotherapy (EBRT) consisting of superficial X-rays (low-voltage X-ray therapy with energy in the range of 40–200 kV and a 50% depth dose (D50) of 7–10 mm), orthovoltage (deep X-ray therapy with values of 150–400 kV and D50 50–80 mm) and megavoltage X-rays, electrons and protons (with values of >1000 kV and D50 10–200 mm) can be used for the treatment of BCC. Brachytherapy (BT) delivered using radionucleotide iridium-192 moulds or, in more recent times, electronically using a miniature X-ray source (50–100 kV) is another option for smaller, more superficial, low-risk BCCs and some selected high-risk primary BCCs. EBRT is an effective therapeutic strategy in selected cases with primary or surgically recurrent BCC or incompletely excised BCC where further surgical excision would be complex or contraindicated. EBRT also plays an important role as adjuvant postoperative treatment in those with high-risk BCC features such as perineural invasion. Those patients with high- or low-risk BCC who are unwilling or unable to tolerate surgery due to medical co-morbidities or when antithrombotic therapy is a contraindication may also be considered for radiotherapy [107,108]. A meta-analysis of BT versus EBRT in the treatment of keratinocyte carcinoma showed better cosmesis with BT over EBRT when using doses ranging from 50 Gy/15 fractions to 64 Gy/32 fractions, and similar recurrence rates with a median local recurrence of 2% at 1 year and 14% at 5 years [109]. Radiotherapy may be used as a palliative modality in improving the quality of life in patients with advanced and/or inoperable disease [110]. Incomplete clearance of BCC and recurrences after radiotherapy are higher and cosmesis poorer when compared with surgical excision [**111**].

Radiotherapy should not be employed in the treatment of recurrent BCC where the primary treatment was radiotherapy or for treating patients with NBCCS as they have an increased sensitivity to radiation and a tendency to develop multiple BCCs in the irradiated field [112]. Radiotherapy should be used cautiously in patients under the age of 65 years in view of the risk of latent tumours in radiotherapy-treated sites [113]. Radiotherapy should be used with caution or best avoided on the distal upper and lower limbs. The inconvenience and practical difficulties of multiple appointments over many weeks required for a full fractionated course of radiotherapy need to be taken into account when it is considered as an alternative to conventional surgical approaches.

Electrochemotherapy. Electrochemotherapy (ECT) is a local treatment purportedly aimed at enhancing the effects of chemotherapy. The procedure is performed with the patient under general or local anaesthesia with sedation. Chemotherapeutic agents (e.g. bleomycin or cisplatin) are administered either intravenously or directly into the tumour. Shortly after drug administration, brief and intense electric pulses are delivered around or directly into the tumour using either surface plates or needle electrodes. This is meant to make the cell membranes more permeable to the chemotherapy drugs so that the cytotoxic effect is increased.

In the UK, although the National Institute for Health and Care Excellence (NICE) states that ECT may be useful in managing inaccessible or otherwise difficult to treat primary BCCs in carefully selected patients, it is *not* in widespread use, as data from randomised controlled trials are notably lacking. The role of ECT, if any, in dermatological management of BCC remains to be determined and as such remains somewhat controversial given the high cure rates offered by other treatment modalities.

Sonic hedgehog pathway inhibitors. Most spontaneous BCCs have mutations in components of the hedgehog pathway that promote aberrant signalling (see the section on genetics earlier in this chapter). In 85–90% of BCCs inactivating mutations are seen in *PTCH1*, with the remaining 10% having activating mutations in *SMO*. These mutations result in the unchecked activation of the hedgehog pathway, resulting in unregulated proliferation of basal cells leading to BCC development (see Figure 140.1) [**34**]. These findings have been confirmed with genomic profiling using whole exome sequencing. Molecular therapies that downregulate hedgehog pathway signalling impede BCC tumourigenesis and consist of Smo inhibitors and transcription factor-mediated (Gli) inhibitors, a class known as SHHis [114].

Two oral SHHis, vismodegib and sonidegib – both Smo inhibitors – have been developed and used in the treatment of metastatic and locally advanced BCC not considered suitable for surgery or radiotherapy. Other drugs with a mild effect on hedgehog signalling include the azole antifungal itraconazole, but limited data exist on its use [115]. Currently, a new semi-synthetic hedgehog pathway inhibitor, patidegib, also known as saridegib or IPI-926, is undergoing phase II and III clinical trials for the treatment of advanced BCC. Although initial data appear encouraging, longer-term analysis is awaited.

A rigorous meta-analysis [116] has found that the use of vismodegib is favoured over sonidegib in clinical practice. Compared with sonidegib, vismodegib has a higher overall response rate (ORR) of 68.8% versus 56.6%, and complete response rate (CRR) of 30.9% versus 3.0% for locally advanced BCC, and higher ORR of 39.7% versus 14.7% for metastatic BCC with fewer gastrointestinal and muscle side effects. Resistance to both agents involves similar mechanisms. Remarkable responses to SHHis can be seen in cases of both locally advanced disease and metastasis that would otherwise have led to premature death or mutilating surgery, including the avoidance of orbital exenteration (Figure 140.13). Prolongation of therapy leads to better responses but may require breaks of weeks to months in therapy to reduce side effects without compromising response. Localised recurrences at the edges of the regressed tumour are seen but are able to be effectively treated with standard surgical excision in most cases.

The side effects of SHHis can be incapacitating but are mostly reversible. Up to 25% of patients discontinue therapy due to side effects. These include muscle spasms, dysgeusia, decreased appetite, alopecia, weight loss, fatigue, nausea, myalgia, increased creatinine kinase, skin SCC (approximately 4%), diarrhoea and amenorrhoea.

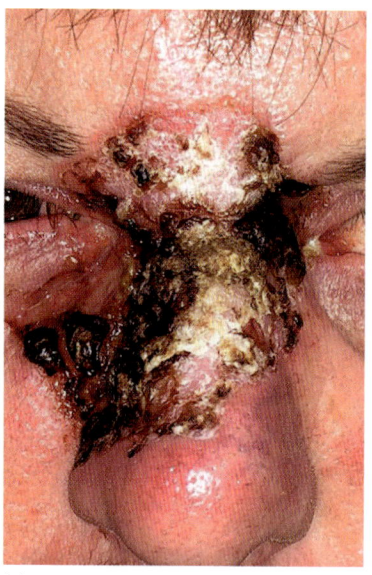

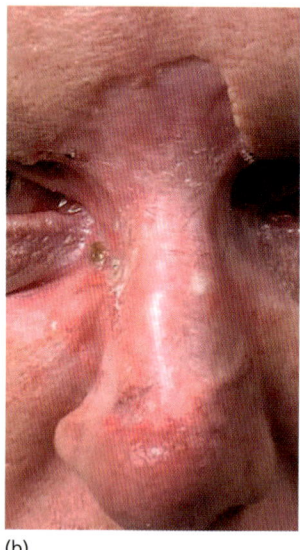

Figure 140.13 (a) Advanced basal cell carcinoma with orbital invasion prior to treatment with vismodegib. (b) Following treatment with vismodegib.

Naevoid basal cell carcinoma syndrome

Definition and nomenclature

This is a rare autosomal dominant familial cancer syndrome in which affected individuals are predisposed to the development of multiple BCCs at an early age, typically around puberty, and a variable combination of other phenotypic abnormalities. These abnormalities include highly characteristic facies (with large forehead/frontal bossing), bifid or otherwise misshapen ribs, vertebral and other skeletal anomalies, keratocystic odontogenic tumours, pits of the skin of the palms and soles, dysgenesis of the corpus callosum, calcification of the falx cerebri (at an earlier age than is seen in non-affected individuals) and macrocephaly. It is also known as Gorlin syndrome or Gorlin–Goltz syndrome.

Epidemiology
Incidence and prevalence

The estimated prevalence of this condition is 1 in 57 000 to 1 in 164 000 without any sex predilection [1]. The high rate of new mutations and the variable expressivity of the condition make full assessment difficult particularly in mildly affected individuals where there is no family history of the condition.

Skin lesions including BCC may develop in infancy but more frequently develop between puberty and 35 years of age, with an average age of onset at 25 years [2].

Pathology

The histopathological appearance of BCCs from patients with NBCCS are indistinguishable from those seen in sporadic forms. The tumours may induce a fibrous stroma as occurs with trichoepithelioma or nodular BCC, and the lesions may become papular or pedunculated. Deeper penetration as a result of greater aggressiveness, ulceration and invasion can occur, with lymphocytic infiltration seen. There may be pigmentation in and around the tumour bulk. The presence of calcification and the general architecture can resemble trichoepithelioma. Palmoplantar pits show focal absence of the stratum corneum with vacuolisation of the spinous layer. At an ultrastructural level, pits show evidence of premature desquamation with a reduction in desmosomes and tonofibrils resulting from delay in maturation of the epidermal basal cells [3,4]. BCCs have developed in palmar pits [3–6].

Genetics

The *NBCCS* gene has been mapped to chromosome 9q22.3-3.1 and, like other tumour suppressor genes, shows frequent deletion in both sporadic and familial BCCs [7]. The *NBCCS* gene was identified in 1996 with the identification of mutations in the *PTCH1* gene in the germline of NBCCS patients and in sporadic BCC tumour samples [8]. *PTCH1* is the human homologue of protein patched homologue, which was first identified as a key regulator of the evolutionarily conserved SHH signalling pathway in elegant genetic studies of embryonic segmentation and imaginal disc specification in *Drosophila*. This finding was the first reported example of a link between genes important in normal development and cancer, and provided a completely new insight into the molecular pathways important in the development of this common skin cancer. The importance of hedgehog signalling during normal development explains many of the other phenotypic abnormalities seen in patients with NBCCS and these features are consistent with findings from studies of heterozygote *PTCH1* knock-out mice [9]. The *PTCH1* mutation rate in NBCCS in published studies appears to range between 40% and 80%. A variety of mutations have been described in these studies including nonsense mutations, in-frame deletion, frame shifts due to deletions and insertions and splice-site mutations [10]. In addition to point mutations, a small number of patients have been described with larger deletions detected by comparative genomic hybridisation methodologies. These patients tend to present with additional clinical features which may be caused by co-deletion of other genes in addition to *PTCH1* [11,12].

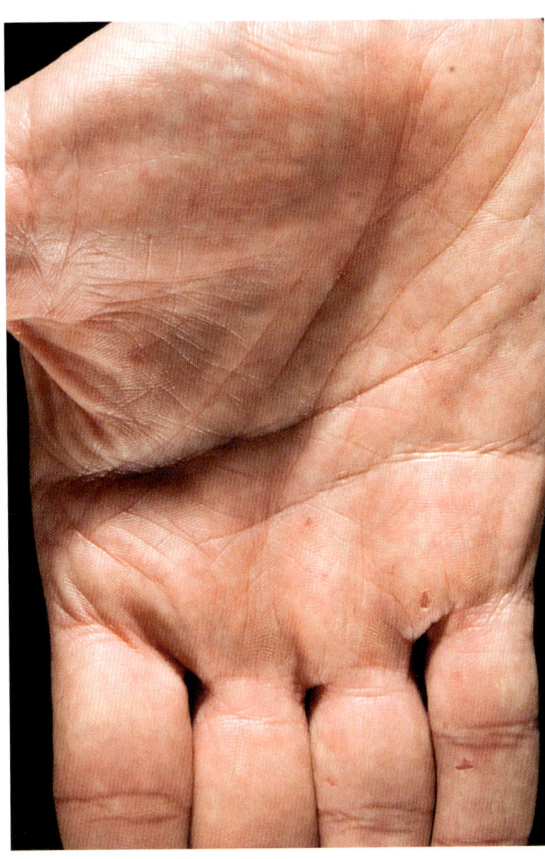

Figure 140.14 Palmar pits in a patient with naevoid basal cell carcinoma syndrome.

Clinical features

The skin manifestations of the syndrome are varied and include BCCs, skin tags, palmoplantar pits (Figure 140.14), milia, epidermoid cysts and lesions that clinically resemble dermal naevi. Affected individuals may develop up to 500 BCCs in their lifetime and these are more common in the fair-skinned population, particularly in areas of high UV irradiation [13]. The BCCs are often smaller and most commonly located on the face and trunk and to a lesser extent on the limbs [14]. The eyelids, nose, cheeks and forehead are the usual sites, but the neck, trunk and axillae are quite frequently involved. The scalp and limbs are usually spared. The individual BCCs are smooth surfaced, rounded, elevated papules, flesh coloured or pigmented, varying in size from 1 to 15 mm in diameter. The lesions tend to increase in size and number up to late adolescence. There may be fine telangiectasia and milium-like bodies just below the surface. Those involving the axillae, neck and eyelids tend to be pedunculated. Most lesions appear to behave in a relatively benign fashion with barely discernible growth or evidence of clinical progression.

As is the case for patients with sporadic BCC, some patients with NBCCS develop more aggressive BCC which can be more difficult to treat and may cause significant morbidity or, rarely, death resulting from extensive invasion or recurrence following treatment. The proportion of NBCCS patients who develop very aggressive tumours and the risk factors for this have not been established. Aggressive tumours appear to occur more frequently on the eyelids or nose, and can cause gross destruction. In one study, four of five cases with aggressive BCCs in a series of 36 NBCCS patients received radiotherapy as the initial therapy, which suggests that radiotherapy may be a contributing factor to tumour aggressiveness in some NBCCS patients [15]. A variety of other skin manifestations have also been described, including multiple epidermoid cysts, milia and palmoplantar pits. The pits are a useful diagnostic feature that occur in about 65% of adults with NBCCS but are relatively rare in children. They are characterised by small, more or less circular pits, which may have a reddish base and are usually 1–2 mm deep. In a recent study, re-examination of the skin phenotype in the context of data implicating hedgehog signalling in hair follicle biology led to the identification of discrete patches of unusually long, pigmented hair on the skin of three patients with NBCCS from two unrelated families with confirmed heterozygous mutations in the PTCH gene [16].

In many cases, the skin lesions resemble melanocytic naevi, von Recklinghausen neurofibromatosis or skin tags rather than BCC, and their true nature may be suspected only because of associated features or family history. The correlation between the clinical and pathological features of the range of skin lesions seen in NBCCS patients is still poorly understood, which makes it difficult to draw firm conclusions about the natural history of the different skin lesions in these patients.

Other diagnostically useful phenotypic abnormalities in NBCCS patients include keratocystic odontogenic tumours (KOT), highly characteristic facies (broad nasal root, hypertelorism, frontal bossing), bifid or otherwise misshapen ribs, vertebral and other skeletal anomalies, dysgenesis of the corpus callosum, calcification of the falx cerebri (Figure 140.15) (at an earlier age than is seen in

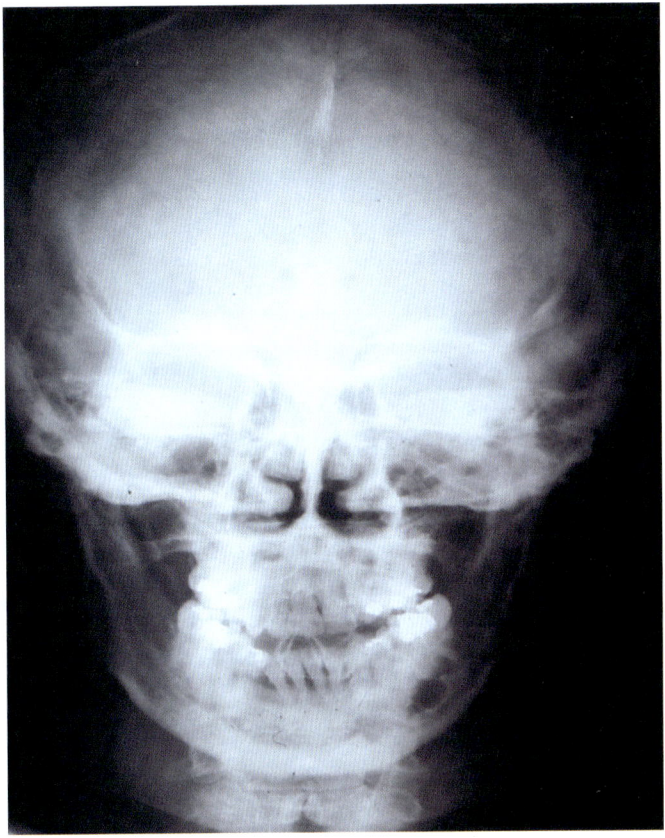

Figure 140.15 Skull X-ray with calcified falx cerebri and a keratocystic odontogenic tumour of the mandible.

non-NBCCS individuals) and macrocephaly [17]. The KOT typically occur in the posterior mandible, are usually unilocular, present with radiological lucency and are associated with the crown of an unerupted tooth. Histologically, they show basal cell palisading and hyperplasia. Skeletal abnormalities include spina bifida occulta, bifid or splayed ribs, scoliosis or kyphosis [18]. Less commonly associated anomalies include syndactyly, shortened metacarpals, cleft lip and palate, bicornuate uterus, hypogonadism in males, lymphatic cysts of the mesentery, ocular abnormalities including dystopia canthorum, cataracts and congenital blindness, and a variety of neurological disorders [18–23]. In addition to BCCs, the syndrome is associated with an increased susceptibility to other neoplasms including rhabdomyosarcoma, ovarian and cardiac fibromas and, in particular, medulloblastoma. Approximately 3% of NBCCS patients develop medulloblastomas, and approximately 3% of patients with medulloblastomas have NBCCS [24]. Atypical clinical features such as brachydactyly, pulmonary valve stenosis and neurodevelopmental disability should prompt consideration of a contiguous gene deletion syndrome.

Diagnostic criteria
A final consensus on diagnostic criteria has been refined to include the need for either two major criteria, one major and two minor criteria, or one major with molecular confirmation (Box 140.2) [25,26].

Investigations
Suspected cases of NBCCS require a full clinical history and examination, imaging including orthopantogram, spinal, chest and skull X-ray, cardiac and pelvic (female) ultrasound and baseline brain magnetic resonance imaging.

Box 140.2 Diagnostic criteria for naevoid basal cell carcinoma syndrome (NBCCS)

Major criteria
- Basal cell carcinoma (BCC) before 20 years of age or excessive numbers of BCCs out of proportion to prior sun exposure and skin type
- Keratocystic odontogenic tumour before 20 years of age
- Palmar or plantar pitting
- Lamellar calcification of the falx cerebri
- Medulloblastoma typically desmoplastic
- First-degree relative with NBCCS

Minor criteria
- Rib abnormalities
- Other specific skeletal malformations and radiological changes (vertebral anomalies, kyphoscoliosis, short fourth metacarpals, postaxial polydactyly)
- Macrocephaly
- Cleft lip or palate
- Ovarian or cardiac fibroma
- Lymphomesenteric cysts
- Ocular abnormalities (strabismus, hypertelorism, congenital cataracts, glaucoma, coloboma)

Adapted from Bresler et al. 2016 [26] with permission.

Molecular genetic testing for heritable pathogenic variants of the *PTCH1* and *SUFU* genes can be undertaken with the probability of detection in up to 60% of cases depending on the clinical diagnostic criteria. Genetic testing does not alter the care of individuals meeting the clinical criteria, but may be helpful in the identification and management of their clinically unaffected relatives. It is also useful in confirming the diagnosis in those not meeting all the clinical criteria [27,28].

Frequent dermatological screening is recommended with radiological screening for medulloblastoma in those under the age of 8 years and with KOT, usually performed annually.

Management
As NBCCS is a complex multisystemic disease, a multidisciplinary approach may be required in the management of these patients. Other than dermatology, multidisciplinary teams might include oral maxillo-facial surgery, oncology, genetics and psychiatry [29].

The large number of BCCs in patients with NBCCS means that standard surgical excision of all lesions is not always practicable. Low-risk BCC can be treated with non-invasive surgical procedures such as curettage and electrodessication and cryosurgery or with superficial therapies in order to keep treatment as simple as possible. Surgery is a mainstay of treatment (see Table 140.6). High-risk BCC requires Mohs surgery or CCPDMA (see Table 140.7), as with sporadic BCC. The psychosocial impact of the relentless development of new BCCs along with frequent surgical procedures from a very young age cannot be underestimated. Fear of pain, needles and surgery often develops and can be extremely problematic, leading to treatment refusal or long delays in definitive management of aggressive lesions in these patients. Radiotherapy is contraindicated as an accelerated rate of development of new BCCs within the irradiated field can occur, and where recurrences do occur, they frequently are more aggressive and difficult to manage than the initial primary tumour.

The value of systemic chemoprevention strategies in the management of patients with NBCCS is still unclear. A few studies suggest that systemic retinoids (isotretinoin >4 mg/kg and etretinate 0.7–1 mg/kg) may reduce the rate of development of new BCCs [30]. The clinical benefits, however, appear small relative to those seen in patients with multiple cutaneous SCCs.

With the advent of therapy targeting aberrant hedgehog signalling, the efficacy of vismodegib in patients with NBCCS has been tested in a randomised double-blind placebo-controlled trial [31,32]. The primary end point was a reduction in the incidence of new BCCs that were eligible for surgical resection with vismodegib versus placebo after 3 months. Secondary end points included a reduction in the size of existing BCCs. After a mean of 8 months' treatment, BCCs eligible for surgical excision were significantly reduced to two per patient in the treatment group versus 29 in the placebo group, as well as a significant reduction in the size of existing BCCs in the treatment group. No tumours progressed while on treatment.

However, patients routinely had grade 1 or 2 adverse events including loss of taste, muscle cramps, hair loss and weight loss. Overall, over half of the patients (54%) receiving vismodegib discontinued drug treatment owing to adverse events. Another issue that might arise is treatment resistance with alterations in the inhibitor pocket of SMO as has been seen with sporadic BCC [33]. Studies are required to assess other treatment regimens to enable more patients to receive the drug for longer. In particular, the use of intermittent dosing schedules, other modes of drug delivery such as topical patidegib, second-generation inhibitors such as sonidegib, different drugs targeting the hedgehog pathway such as itraconazole, and multidrug regimens need to be further investigated.

Bazex–Dupré–Christol syndrome

Definition and nomenclature
Bazex–Dupré–Christol syndrome (BDCS) is a rare genodermatosis that predisposes affected individuals to multiple BCCs, typically with onset in the second decade of life. Approximately 20 cases have been reported in the literature. Additional clinical features include dysgenesis of the hair follicles resulting in follicular atrophoderma and hypotrichosis as well as hypohidrosis. It is also known as follicular atrophoderma and basal cell carcinoma (Bazex) syndrome.

Pathophysiology
Genetics
The BDCS is an X-linked dominantly inherited disorder. In 1995, a linkage of three families to a 23.3 Mb region on chromosome Xq24-27 was reported [1]. These findings were later confirmed with the critical region further elucidated to an 11.4 Mb interval on chromosome Xq25-27.1 [2].

Clinical features
Only females are affected, with no skeletal abnormalities or other organ systems involved. Follicular atrophoderma, hypotrichosis and hypohidrosis are the main presenting features. Follicular atrophoderma is present at birth or in early childhood, and shows as 'ice-pick marks', enlarged follicular ostia on the dorsa of the hands, elbows, feet and face. The follicular changes are not caused by injury or inflammation but there may be facial eczema soon after birth. There may be anhidrosis of the face and head, and hypotrichosis. Milia have been reported as an associated feature [3]. The BCCs appear predominantly on the face typically in the second decade and resemble naevi [4]. Pigmented BCC may be seen as early as age 5 years [1].

The presence of multiple BCCs at an early age raises the likelihood of NBCCS. However the presence of cutaneous abnormalities with a lack of associated skeletal abnormality or tumours involving other organ systems can be seen in a variety of rare inherited disorders including BDCS.

Management
The management of BDCS does not require the intensive follow-up and imaging seen with NBCCS. The management of the BCCs is, however, the same.

Key references

The full list of references can be found in the online version at https://www.wiley.com/rooksdermatology10e

Basal cell carcinoma

6 Cakir BÖ, Adamson P, Cingi C. Epidemiology and economic burden of non-melanoma skin cancer. *Facial Plast Surg Clin North Am* 2012;20:419–22.

22 Kricker A, Armstrong BK, English DR, Heenan PJ. Does intermittent sun exposure cause basal cell carcinoma? A case–control study in Western Australia. *Int J Cancer* 1995;60:489–94.

23 Rosso S, Zanetti R, Martinez C et al. The multicentre south European study 'Helios' II: different sun exposure patterns in the aetiology of basal cell and squamous cell carcinomas of the skin. *Br J Cancer* 1996;73:1447–54.

24 Madan V, Lear JT, Szeimies RM. Non-melanoma skin cancer. *Lancet* 2010; 375:673–85.

33 Jayaraman SS, Rayhan DJ, Hazany S, Kolodney MS. Mutational landscape of basal cell carcinomas by whole-exome sequencing. *J Invest Dermatol* 2014;134:213–20.

34 Stone DM, Hynes M, Armanini M et al. The tumour-suppressor gene patched encodes a candidate receptor for Sonic hedgehog. *Nature* 1996;384:129–34.

70 Reiter O, Mimouni I, Gdalevich M et al. The diagnostic accuracy of dermoscopy for basal cell carcinoma: a systematic review and meta-analysis. *J Am Acad Dermatol* 2019;80:1380–8.

76 Karen JK, Gareau DS, Dusza SW et al. Detection of basal cell carcinomas in Mohs excisions with fluorescence confocal mosaicing microscopy. *Br J Dermatol* 2009;160:1242–50.

77 Telfer NR, Colver GB, Morton CA; British Association of Dermatologists. Guidelines for the management of basal cell carcinoma. *Br J Dermatol* 2008; 159:35–48.

78 Bath-Hextall FJ, Perkins W, Bong J, Williams HC. Interventions for basal cell carcinoma of the skin. *Cochrane Database Syst Rev* 2007;Issue 24:CD003412.

79 Bath-Hextall F, Leonardi-Bee J, Somchand N, Webster A, Delitt J, Perkins W. Interventions for preventing non-melanoma skin cancers in high-risk groups. *Cochrane Database Syst Rev* 2007;Issue 4:CD005414.

102 Humphreys TR, Malhotra R, Scharf MJ et al. Treatment of superficial basal cell carcinoma and squamous cell carcinoma in situ with a high-energy pulsed carbon dioxide laser. *Arch Dermatol* 1998;134:1247–52.

103 Jung DS, Cho HH, Ko HC et al. Recurrent basal cell carcinoma following ablative laser procedures. *J Am Acad Dermatol* 2011;64:723–9.

111 Avril M, Auperin A, Margulis A et al. Basal cell carcinoma of the face: surgery or radiotherapy? Results of a randomized study. *Br J Cancer* 1997;76:100–6.

Naevoid basal cell carcinoma syndrome

2 Gorlin RJ. Nevoid basal cell carcinoma syndrome. *Dermatol Clin* 1995;13:113–25.

7 Evans DG, Howard E, Giblin C et al. Birth incidence and prevalence of tumor-prone syndromes: estimates from a UK family genetic register service. *Am J Med Genet A* 2010;152:327–32.

10 Bale AE, Gailani MR, Leffell DJ. The Gorlin syndrome gene: a tumor suppressor active in basal cell carcinogenesis and embryonic development. *Proc Assoc Am Phys* 1995;107:253–7.

13 Kimonis VE, Goldstein AM, Pastakia B et al. Clinical manifestations in 105 persons with nevoid basal cell carcinoma syndrome. *Am J Med Genet* 1997;69:299–308.

15 Wilson LC, Ajayi-Obe E, Bernhard B et al. Patched mutations and hairy skin patches: a new sign in Gorlin syndrome. *Am J Med Genet A* 2006;140:2625–30.

24 Evans DG, Farndon PA, Burnell LD et al. The incidence of Gorlin syndrome in 173 consecutive cases of medulloblastoma. *Br J Cancer* 1991;64:959–61.

Bazex–Dupré–Christol syndrome

1 Vabres P, Lacombe D, Rabinowitz LG et al. The gene for Bazex–Dupré–Christol syndrome maps to chromosome Xq. *J Invest Dermatol* 1995;105:87–91.

2 Parren LJ, Abuzahra F, Wagenvoort T et al. Linkage refinement of Bazex–Dupré–Christol syndrome to an 11.4-Mb interval on chromosome Xq25-27.1. *Br J Dermatol* 2011;165:201–3.

4 Bazex A, Dupré A, Christol B. Atrophodermie folliculaire proliférations baso-cellulaires et hypotrichose. *Ann Dermatol Syphiligr* 1966;93:241–54.

CHAPTER 141

Squamous Cell Carcinoma and its Precursors

Girish Gupta[1,2] *and Thomas Dirschka*[3,4]

[1]Department of Dermatology, Royal Infirmary of Edinburgh, Edinburgh, UK
[2]University of Edinburgh, Edinburgh, UK
[3]CentroDerm Clinic, Wuppertal, Germany
[4]Faculty of Health, University Witten-Herdecke, Witten, Germany

---

Introduction, 141.1

LESIONS WITH UNCERTAIN OR UNPREDICTABLE MALIGNANT POTENTIAL, 141.1
Actinic keratosis, 141.1
Cutaneous horn, 141.12
Arsenical keratosis, 141.13
Post-ionising radiation keratosis, 141.14
Disseminated superficial actinic porokeratosis, 141.15

***IN SITU* CARCINOMA OF THE SKIN, 141.18**
Bowen disease, 141.18
Anal, vulval, penile and perianal intraepithelial carcinoma, 141.24

SQUAMOUS CELL CARCINOMA OF THE SKIN, 141.26

KERATOACANTHOMAS AND ASSOCIATED SYNDROMES, 141.38

Keratoacanthoma, 141.38
Multiple self-healing squamous epithelioma, 141.41
Generalised eruptive keratoacanthoma, 141.43
Muir–Torre syndrome, 141.44
Acknowledgement, 141.45

Key references, 141.46

Introduction

Keratinocyte cancer (KC) is the most common human cancer. The term encompasses basal cell carcinoma (BCC) (Chapter 140) and squamous cell carcinoma (SCC) of the skin, which are both derived from epidermal keratinocytes. Although these tumours are clinically and pathologically distinctive, they share some characteristics and are frequently classified under the term KC for health care planning, cancer registry reporting and epidemiological purposes. In contrast to other common epithelial cancers, KCs rarely metastasise, which means that the case fatality rate for these cancers is low. This low mortality from KC has contributed to the widespread underreporting of this cancer to disease registries in many countries, which makes it challenging to quantify accurately the morbidity and health care costs associated with this disease. Nevertheless, given the increasing prevalence of KC (especially amongst those on immunosuppressive medication), and the frequent occurrence of multiple primary tumours in affected individuals, there is little disagreement amongst dermatologists that KC is an important and frequently underestimated public health problem.

Patients at risk for development of KC are also predisposed to the development of actinic keratoses (AK) and Bowen disease, which are partial- or full-thickness epidermal dysplastic lesions that show some of the histological characteristics of SCC. The prevalence of AK and the multiplicity of lesions within individual subjects are considerably greater than that for KC. While there is some controversy about the premalignant potential of AK and Bowen disease and their relationship to SCC, these lesions are, in themselves, an important clinical problem for three reasons. First, they need to be distinguished from SCC; second, they cause concern and anxiety in patients, particularly in those with a previous history of KC; and, third, the scaling and inflammation associated with these lesions is an important contributor to the overall morbidity associated with photoageing.

LESIONS WITH UNCERTAIN OR UNPREDICTABLE MALIGNANT POTENTIAL

Actinic keratosis

Definition and nomenclature

Actinic keratoses (AK) are skin lesions or areas that are highly variable in terms of size, extent, keratosis and overall clinical presentation. They emerge from expanding atypical basal keratinocytes. AK occur on chronically UV-exposed adult skin and carry a variable and, so far, unpredictable risk of progression to invasive SCC.

Synonyms and inclusions
- Solar keratosis
- Keratosis senilis

Introduction and general description

AK are common and found chiefly on UV-exposed skin [1]. The spectrum of clinical presentation varies in terms of keratosis (light to severe), area of involvement (a few millimetres to larger areas like the whole scalp), distribution (single lesions, coalescent lesions, small fields, large fields), and colour (white, pink/red, pigmented). Sometimes lesions are more easily palpable than seen because of their sandpaper-like keratotic surface.

Besides chronic UV-exposure, further risk factors comprise fair skin-type (Fitzpatrick I and II), age, male gender, immunosuppression, DNA repair disorders like xeroderma pigmentosum and certain drugs (e.g. thiazide diuretics).

In early AK, atypical keratinocytes are restricted to the basal layer of the epidermis and later either extend to full-thickness atypia of the epidermis and/or protrude into the upper papillary dermis. These atypical keratinocytes resemble the cytomorphological and genetic changes of invasive cutaneous SCC, and the transition into this is characterised by penetration through the basement membrane.

Clinically, the concept of 'field cancerisation' has been described in the context of AK, with evidence of subclinical lesions in an area of photodamaged skin, which strengthens the case to treat the whole field rather than the individual AK [2].

Epidemiology

Incidence and prevalence

In many countries, the prevalence of AK is high and is influenced by the amount of ambient UV radiation, the proportion of susceptible individuals in the population, the age distribution of the population and the time spent in outdoor occupations and recreations. Despite the frequency of AK in clinical practice, there are hardly any reliable population-based data on worldwide epidemiology.

In a white population in northwest England the overall prevalence was 15.4% in men and 5.9% in women. It showed that prevalence was strongly age-related. In men and women aged 70 years and above 34.1% of men and 18.2% of women had AK [3]. In Australia, a country with high ambient UV irradiation and susceptible fair-skinned inhabitants, AK were found in 40–60% of people aged 40 years and older [4,5]. Further data from Australia also show an age-related increase in prevalence of AK from 20% in men aged 60 years and above to 52% in men over the age of 70 years [6]. In contrast, the prevalence of AK in Japan was relatively low ranging from 0.2% in an urban area to 0.8% in a rural area [7]. Beside ambient UV irradiation in the country of origin, travelling and leisure activities are playing an increasingly important role [8].

Age

AK are more common in the elderly. Various studies show an increase in prevalence with increasing age [9].

Sex

AK are common in both sexes but there is a distinct preponderance in men.

Ethnicity

The condition is much more common in the white population, particularly in those who live or have lived in areas of high sunlight exposure. In these areas, such as Australia, there is a prevalence rate of 43% with 18% (of a population of 197) having more than 10 AK [10].

Associated diseases

Patients may present with other UVR-induced skin cancers and full examination of the skin should be undertaken. A large European case–control study showed that patients presenting with AK have coexisting SCCs in 58%, BCCs in 30%, *in situ* melanoma in 12% and invasive melanoma in 6% of cases [11].

Concomitant medication

In addition to immunosuppressive drugs, thiazide diuretics have been reported to be significantly associated with AK due to their photosensitising action [12].

Pathophysiology

Chronic UV exposure is the central driver in the pathogenesis of AK. UVB directly damages DNA, causing the formation of cyclobutene pyrimidine dimers and pyrimidine-pyrimidone 6,4-photoproducts. DNA mutations can lead to a malfunction of tumour suppressor proteins such as TP53 which is located on chromosome 17p13.1. It helps to either repair UV-induced cellular DNA damage or induce apoptosis of irreversibly damaged cells. Mutations of TP53 are frequently seen in AK [13].

p16 is also a tumour suppressor protein encoded by the *CDKN2A* gene in the 9p21 region. It is involved in the arrest of the cell cycle at G1, suppressing the entry into the S-phase. p16 mutations can also be caused by UVR [14]. Inactivation of p16 leads to continuous cell cycling and it is thought that inactivated p16 advances AK to SCC [15].

UVB irradiation can also affect the Erk1/Erk2 signalling pathway leading to increased cellular proliferation. Mutations of the Ras-Oncogene H-RAS in codons 12, 13 and 61 lead to a change in the gene product, a GTP-binding protein, leading to a continuous stimulation of the signalling pathway [16].

UVA irradiation also intervenes in gene regulation. A downregulation of Notch1, Notch2 and HES1, and an upregulation for expression of c-Jun have been demonstrated. The Notch/CSL signalling pathway plays a role in tumour suppression and controls differentiation, apoptosis and proliferation of keratinocytes. Notch1 induces p21 which inhibits the cell cycle leading to uncontrolled proliferation. Hence, downregulation of Notch1 leads to an increase in AK and SCC [17].

Investigation focusing on the epithelial-to-mesenchymal transition (EMT) have demonstrated that this interaction is characterised by atypical basal and suprabasal keratinocytes at the epithelial zone [18].

Human papillomavirus (HPV) infection plays an important role in the development of AK and SCC. Similar to mucosal high-risk HPV carcinogenesis, β-HPV types are involved and in particular the viral E6 and E7 oncoproteins from some cutaneous β-HPV types exert transforming activities. It has been demonstrated that these β-HPV types can alter the networks regulated by the tumour suppressor gene products retinoblastoma (pRb) and p53, leading to loss of cell cycle control, apoptosis and DNA repair. Moreover, β-HPV E6 oncoprotein has been shown to deregulate the Notch signalling pathway. In association with UV radiation, these oncoproteins block UV-induced apoptosis and promote cellular proliferation. This highlights the role of cutaneous β-HPV types in the initiation of carcinogenesis but not in its maintenance (the 'hit-and-run' theory) [19,20]. Besides this oncogenic effect of HPV, the loss of T cell immunity against cutaneous β-HPV in the immunocompromised has been demonstrated to contribute to an increased risk of AK and SCC [21].

Predisposing factors

The vast majority of AK occur on light-exposed sites in fair-skinned people who have had excessive exposure to UVR. These AK are commoner in people who have worked outdoors, which carries a fourfold increase in risk compared with outdoor hobbies, which carries a 1.3 times higher risk [11]. AK are commoner in people with red hair and those with blue eyes [11]. People with brown eyes and/or black hair carry the lowest risk for AK development.

Men and people over the age of 70 years carry a higher risk in developing AK. The geographical location of the place of residence is of major relevance: the closer to the equator, the higher the risk [3,22–24].

Chronic immunosuppression is a major factor for the development of AK and cutaneous SCC. Pharmacological immunosuppression has been studied most comprehensively in solid organ transplant recipients (OTRs) exhibiting an estimated 250-fold increased incidence for cutaneous SCC. Calcineurin inhibitors such as ciclosporin and tacrolimus are amongst the drugs most strongly promoting carcinogenesis. Azathioprine is also associated with increased skin cancer risk. In contrast, the mammalian target of rapamycin (mTOR) inhibitors have demonstrated direct antitumour properties qualifying them as an alternative for OTRs. Oral glucocorticosteroids are associated with an up to threefold increase in KC [25]. Beside pharmacological immunosuppression, chronic lymphatic leukaemia has been identified to have an eightfold increased risk for non-melanoma skin cancer [26].

Pathology

AK are mainly diagnosed clinically. Diagnostic biopsies are only undertaken in a small percentage of cases, typically to rule out SCCs. Generally, there is a variable loss of the normal orderly arrangement of the epidermis characterised by different degrees of cellular atypia. Lesional keratinocytes reveal loss of polarity, nuclear crowding, nuclear hyperchromatism, pleomorphism and nucleolar prominence. Epidermal mitotic activity is increased and there are occasional dyskeratotic cells. Focal parakeratosis with loss of the underlying granular layer is a characteristic feature of AK. Acrosyringia are uninvolved creating funnel-shaped columns of orthokeratosis.

Early changes are characterised by a crowding of atypical keratinocytes along the basement membrane (Figure 141.1). Atypical keratinocytes can later extend throughout the upper epidermis and/or protrude into the papillary dermis without breaching the basement membrane. Intraepidermal expansion and budding or papillary sprouting into the papillary dermis can be combined. Acantholysis can sometimes be observed. Solar elastosis is a regular finding but not always present. The papillary vessels are irregularly increased and there is a variably dense lymphoid infiltrate

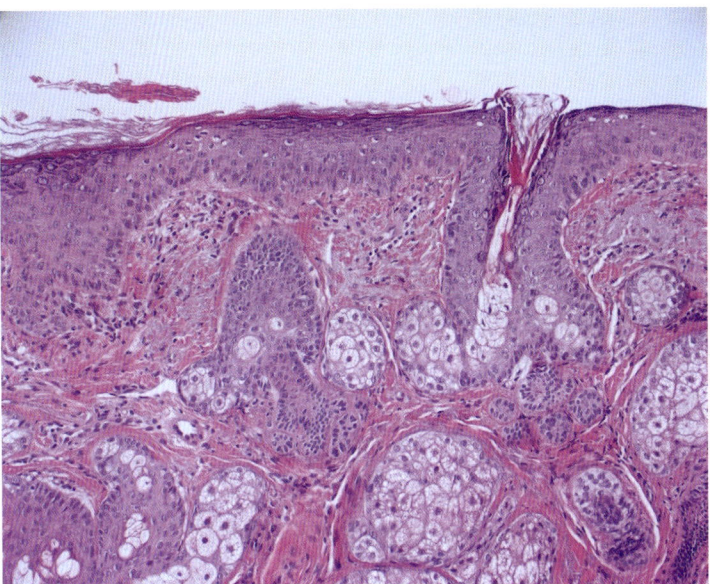

Figure 141.1 Pathological features of early, non-proliferating actinic keratosis showing crowding of atypical keratinocytes in the basal epidermis. H&E, ×20.

beneath the lesion. Numerous plasma cells may form part of the inflammatory cell infiltrate, particularly in lesions from the scalp and lips (actinic cheilitis) and in ulcerated lesions. Histological variants of AK include atrophic, hypertrophic, lichenoid, acantholytic, pigmented and bowenoid [27].

Röwert-Huber graded the extent of atypical keratinocytes throughout the epidermis. In grade AK I, atypical keratinocytes are restricted to the lower third of the epidermis. In grade AK II, atypical keratocytes extend to the lower two-thirds of the epidermis and in grade AK III full thickness atypia of the epidermis is present [28]. Recently, the basal proliferative growth pattern of AK has been used to establish a different grading system. In this, crowding of atypical keratinocytes in the basal epidermis has been termed Pro I, budding of small round nests of atypical keratinocytes Pro II and spiky or filiform papillary elongation of atypical keratinocytes into the papillary dermis without penetrating the basement membrane has been described as Pro III (papillary sprouting) (Figure 141.2) [29]. Basal proliferative AK as well as AK I lesions are most commonly found adjacent to invasive SCC [30,31].

Bowenoid AK differs histologically from Bowen disease by a poor lateral demarcation and gradual transition into actinic field disease. Bowenoid AK shows an alternating pattern of parakeratosis and orthokeratosis. Sparing of the basal keratinocytes in Bowen disease (the so-called 'eyeliner sign') is a characteristic phenomenon in early lesions. It suggests that atypical keratinocytes may have a suprabasal origin. In contrast, the basal keratinocytes are always atypical in AK. Solar elastosis is not always observed in Bowen disease. AK may demonstrate architectural complexity and assessment of early dermal invasion may be difficult. Careful examination of several sections is required to confirm the presence of intraepidermal dysplasia only.

Environmental factors

There is a direct relationship between AK and chronic sun exposure [11]. AK are also more common following iatrogenic phototherapy,

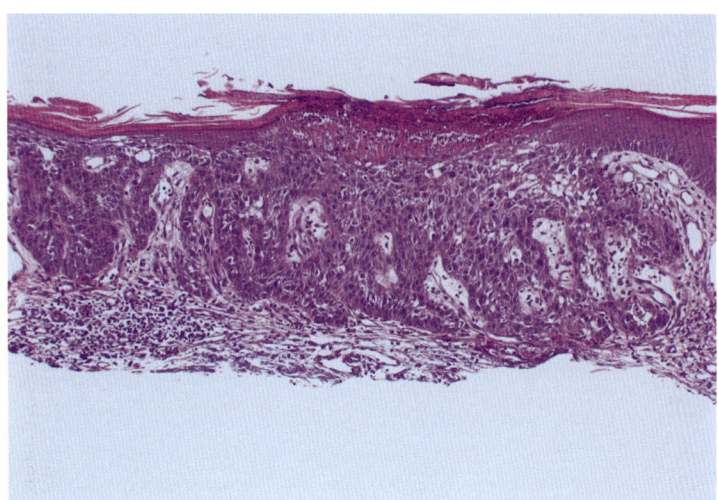

Figure 141.2 Pathological features of proliferating actinic keratosis showing papillary sprouting of atypical keratinocytes. H&E, ×20.

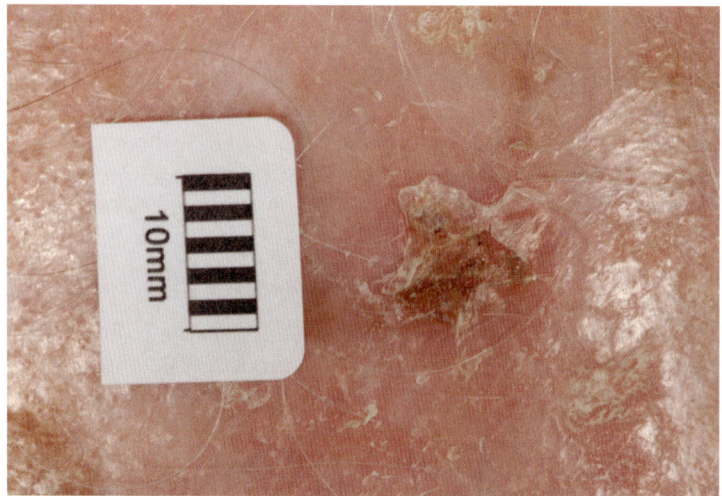

Figure 141.3 Actinic keratosis.

ionising radiation and sunbed usage. Historically, arsenic and chemicals from coal distillation increased the risk of AK development.

Clinical features
History
Patients are usually middle-aged or elderly and develop rough scaly areas on sun-exposed sites, which are either asymptomatic or painful on palpation. Many patients give a history of relapsing and/or remitting lesions, which often disappear either spontaneously or after sun avoidance and regular use of sunscreens.

Presentation
AK are commonly present on sun-exposed areas such as the face, scalp and dorsa of the hands. The sides of the neck are involved in both sexes, but the ears predominate in men. The vermilion of the lower lip and in few cases the upper lip may also be involved and with a much higher incidence in men than in women. Lesions are usually multiple and comprise either macules or papules with a rough scaly surface resulting from disorganised keratinisation and a variable degree of inflammation. Lesions vary in size from less than 1 mm to over 2 cm and are usually asymptomatic. In many individuals, the number of lesions can be better appreciated by skin palpation, which is a sensitive way of detecting the characteristic roughness associated with smaller lesions. Many of these small lesions may pass unnoticed by most patients and the diagnostic changes often only appear later as a dry rough adherent and often yellow- or brown-coloured scale (Figure 141.3).

The adherent scale can only be picked off with difficulty, revealing a hyperaemic base with punctate bleeding points. In some cases, scaling may be prominent and in time may become thick and horny. If individual lesions exist, the edge of the AK is usually sharply demarcated, and the reddening is usually closely confined to the area immediately below the area of abnormal scaling.

In many cases AK do not exist as discrete entities but often coalesce across the affected field, making it difficult to assess AK numbers accurately. This represents a clear limitation in clinical trials as many are based on lesion counts [32]. The area surrounding visible AK is often associated with 'field change', characterised by areas of photodamage, skin atrophy, telangiectasia and pigmentary change. This has been designated 'field cancerisation' but a better term would be 'actinic dysplastic field', which is often prone to develop clinically visible or further recurrent AK [33]. Histology of this 'field change' has shown evidence of epithelial dysplasia with *TP53* mutations consistent with 'subclinical disease' [2].

Clinical variants
Several clinical variants of AK have been described. The hyperplastic (hypertrophic) form, found predominantly on the dorsum of the hands and the forearms, is characterised by thick AK lesions. Hyperkeratosis can limit penetration of topical treatments for AK and many drugs are confined to be used in thin to moderately hyperkeratotic AK. Acantholytic variants can mimic superficial BCC. The flat, atrophic, or lichenoid variety are most commonly seen on the face. Pigmented AK can be found on any sun-exposed skin. Pigmented lesions can show collision with solar lentigo or melanoma *in situ*. Recently it has been shown that AK which are painful on palpation are more treatment resistant and often show a basal proliferative pattern on histopathology [34].

Differential diagnosis (Table 141.1)
The diagnosis is usually based on clinical findings which consider the morphology of individual lesions and the clinical setting. For lesions less than 3 mm, clinical discrimination from an early SCC may be difficult. This diagnostic uncertainty, particularly for small lesions, is one of the reasons why it is difficult to establish accurate rates of progression for AK to SCC. Clinical pointers favouring the diagnosis of an early invasive SCC include the presence of tenderness, induration or a raised shoulder that extends beyond the area of disorganised scaling. Other diagnoses that need to be considered, particularly in patients with large confluent areas of pink/red skin and scaling, include discoid lupus erythematosus. The pink/brown colour of lichenoid AK can easily be mistaken for focal areas of lichen planus or lichen planus-like keratosis, particularly when these lesions have only minimal scaling (Figure 141.4). When an AK is pigmented, it may resemble a superficial seborrhoeic

Lesions with uncertain or unpredictable malignant potential

Table 141.1 Common clinical differential diagnoses of actinic keratosis (AK).

Diagnosis	Differentiating features	Image
Seborrhoeic keratosis	May mimic pigmented AK Usually larger, darker and multiple Raised 'greasy' warty surface 'Stuck on' appearance Dermoscopy: horn cysts	Figures 141.5 and 141.6
Squamous cell carcinoma	Enlarging lesion Induration Raised shoulder or nodule Tenderness	Figure 141.7
Bowen disease	Usually larger and solitary Irregular erythematous base Mainly occur on lower legs in females	Figure 141.8
Keratoacanthoma	Enlarging lesion Rapid growth Central hyperkeratotic crater Generally larger and solitary Usually more hyperkeratotic than AK	Figure 141.9
Basal cell carcinoma	Often solitary with pearly, rolled border Usually less hyperkeratotic than AK Irregular erythematous base	Figure 141.10

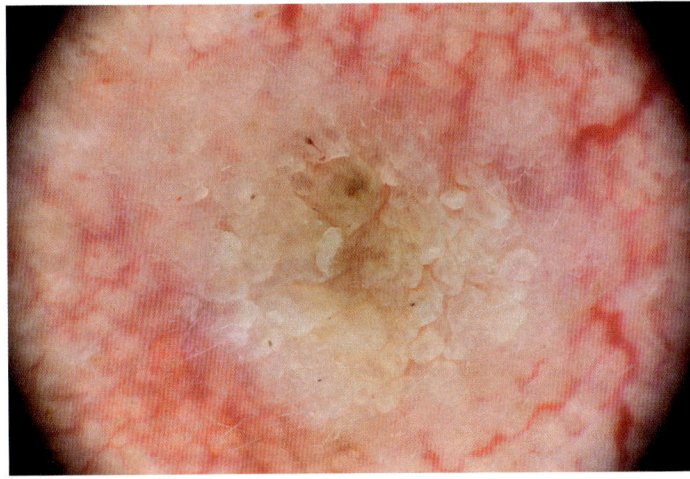

Figure 141.6 Dermoscopy showing thickened warty appearance of seborrhoeic keratosis.

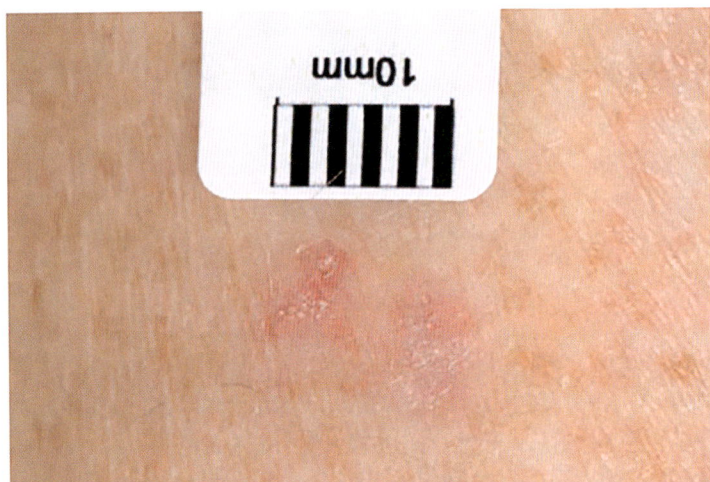

Figure 141.4 Lichenoid actinic keratoses.

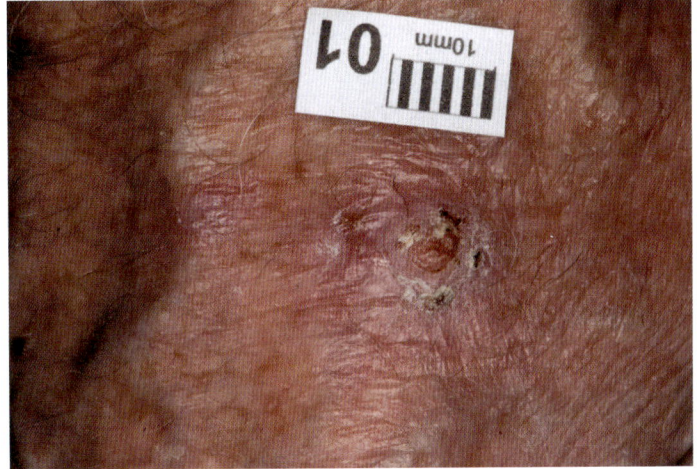

Figure 141.7 Squamous cell carcinoma showing hyperkeratosis with a raised nodule.

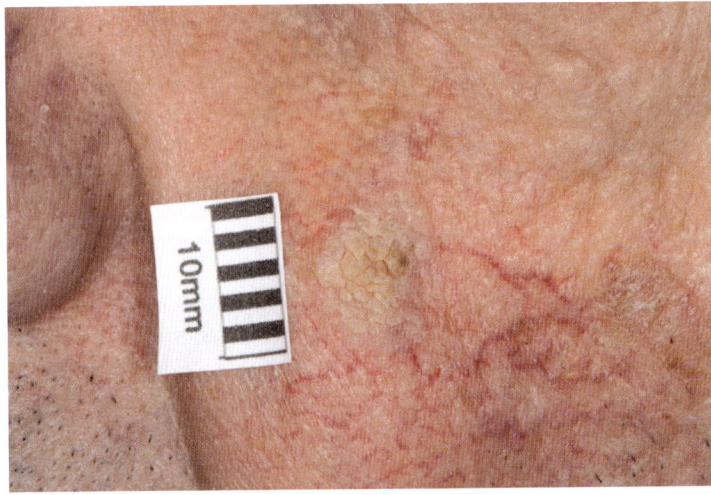

Figure 141.5 Seborrhoeic keratosis.

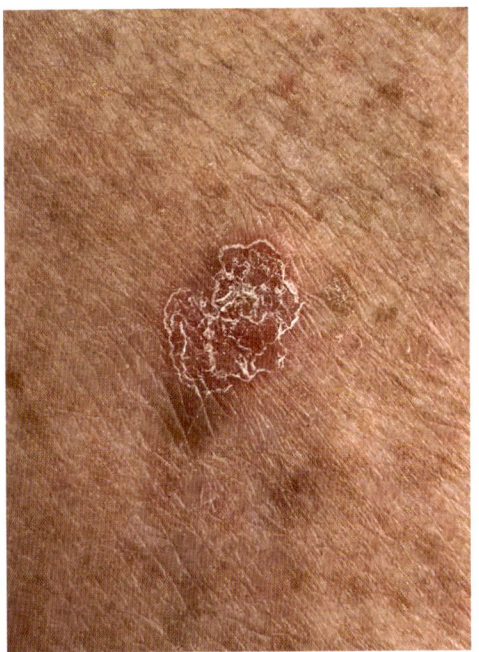

Figure 141.8 Bowen disease, which is usually larger than actinic keratoses with an irregular erythematous base.

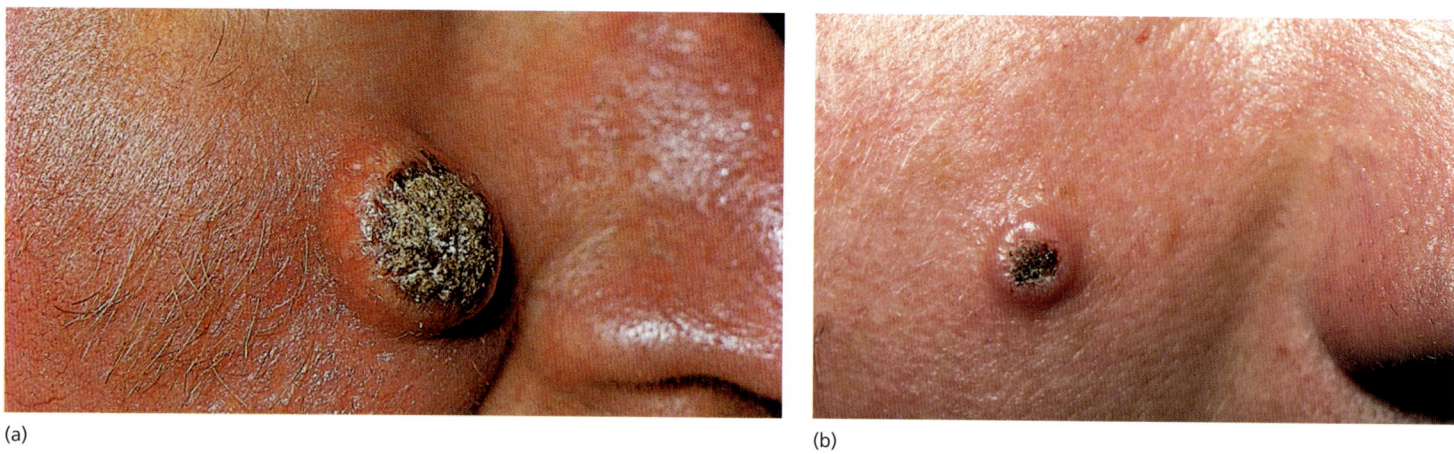

Figure 141.9 (a,b) Keratoacanthoma, which is often larger and more hyperkeratotic than actinic keratosis.

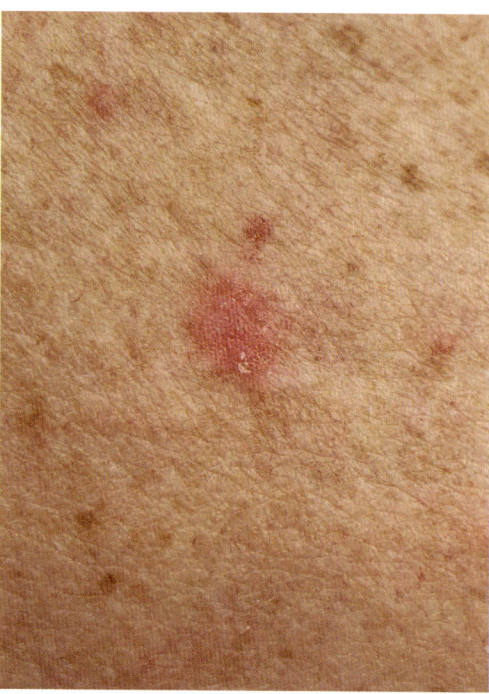

Figure 141.10 Solitary basal cell carcinoma with pearly edge and minimal hyperkeratosis.

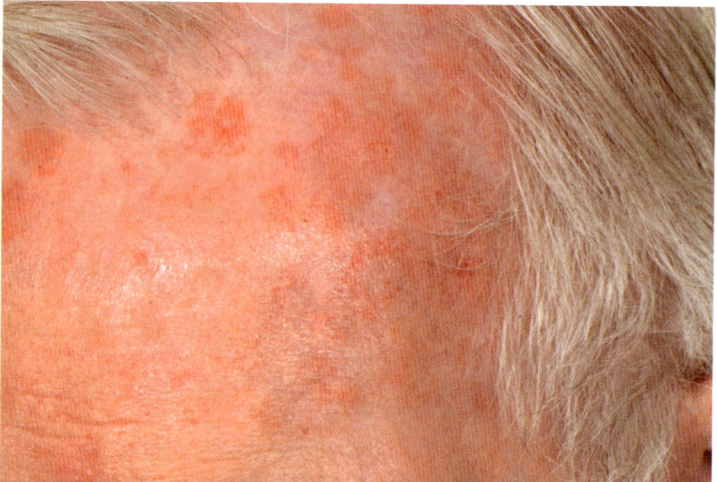

Figure 141.11 'Low-risk' disease characterised by several thin actinic keratoses.

keratosis, but can usually be distinguished from such lesions by the lack of organisation of the hyperkeratosis and on dermoscopy (Figures 141.5 and 141.6). Bowen disease and superficial BCC usually have a more irregular contour and pink/red base.

Classification of severity

A number of clinical and histopathological classifications have been proposed but none has shown accurate clinicopathological correlation. The AK I–III histopathological classification is based on the extension of atypical keratinocytes throughout the epidermis. However, there is poor clinical correlation with this pathological staging [28]. Some dermatologists describe the clinical thickness of disease by using the term 'mild' with thin slightly palpable disease to 'moderate' where AK are easily seen and felt, to 'thick', but this does not correlate with pathological changes [35].

Many studies measure AK counts, but because of the varied clinical presentation of AK, counts have shown to be imprecise [36], the Actinic Keratosis Area and Severity Index (AKASI) was developed with the intent of characterising the severity of AK across a field. It stratifies AK on the face and scalp in a similar manner to the Psoriasis Area Severity Index (PASI) score in psoriasis. Three parameters are the basis to calculate AKASI: area (scalp, forehead, right/left face), percentage of actinically damaged skin in each area and the extent of clinical AK severity, including redness, thickness and distribution. Higher scores indicate more severe disease [32] and correlate with the incidence of cutaneous SCC [37].

The risk of SCC has been reported to increase with the number of thick AK, previous KC and immunosuppression. It would be reasonable to divide AK into 'low risk': immunocompetent individuals with few thin AK and no history of KC (Figure 141.11); and 'high risk' individuals with numerous thick AK with or without a history of immunosuppression and previous KC (Figures 141.12 and 141.13) (Box 141.1).

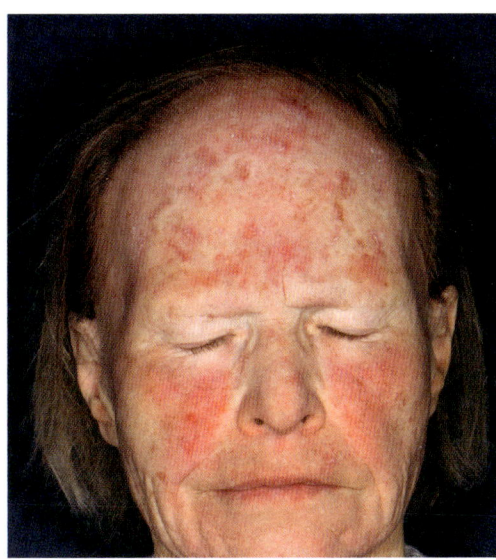

Figure 141.12 'High-risk' disease characterised by field cancerization with multiple thick actinic keratoses.

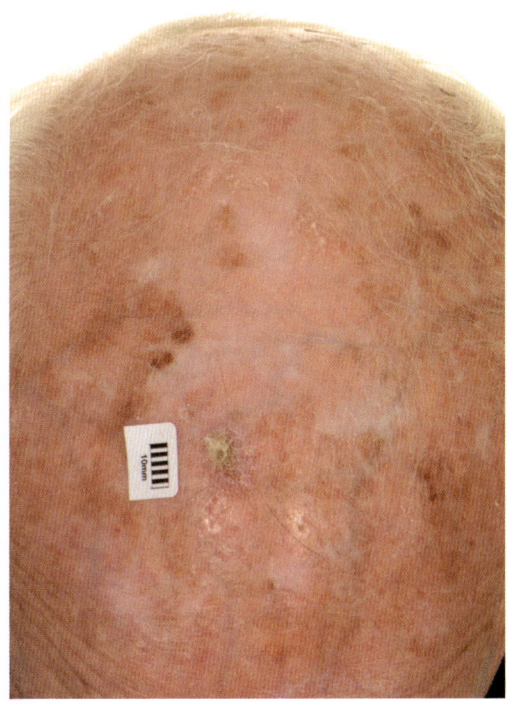

Figure 141.13 'High-risk' disease characterised by multiple thick actinic keratoses in an immunosuppressed patient on ciclosporin.

Complications and co-morbidity

AK are usually asymptomatic but patients may complain of local pruritus and discomfort. AK can be painful on palpation, in particular if they histologically demonstrate basal proliferation (34). Most patients find them a cosmetic nuisance. Patients with AK are at a higher risk of concurrent SCC, BCC, *in situ* and invasive melanoma [7]. Quality of life (QoL) may be affected and can be determined using the AKQoL questionnaire [38].

Disease course and prognosis

Longitudinal studies with patients of AK have established firstly, that there is a high probability of developing new lesions and secondly, lesions may undergo spontaneous resolution [39]. Rates of regression of single lesions have been reported to range from 15% to 63% after one year. Data available on recurrence rates of single lesions one year after regression indicate a recurrence rate of 15–53% [40]. Although the rate of progression of an individual AK to invasive SCC has been estimated to be low (less than 1 in 1000/year), an individual with an average of 7.7 AK has a probability of around 10% of one AK transforming to a SCC over a 10-year period [41]. The presence of AK is therefore an important biomarker of excessive UV exposure and increased skin cancer risk.

Treatment resistance in AK is histologically linked to basal proliferation which can be observed adjacent to cutaneous SCCs. Therefore, lesions that do not respond to treatment may have an increased risk to transform into SCC [34].

Box 141.1 High-risk clinical features of actinic keratosis (AK)

The presence of one or more of these features may increase the risk of progression to squamous cell carcinoma but evidence for some individual factors such as extensive actinic damage, although reasonable, is lacking.
- Multiple thick AK
- High AKASI score
- Basal proliferation on histology
- Past history of KC
- Extensive actinic damage
- Immunosuppression
- Tender enlarging lesion(s)
- Lesions resistant to treatment

Investigations

Diagnosis of AK is made on clinical grounds, but a skin biopsy may be necessary to differentiate from a SCC, BCC or Bowen disease in case of clinical suspicion. Dermoscopy can be a useful tool to increase diagnostic precision. Facial non-pigmented AK are characterised by a pink-to-red pseudo network and white-to-yellow surface scales. In the case of facial pigmented AK, slate-grey-to-dark brown dots and globules, annular granular structures and a brown-to-grey pseudo-network can be observed [42]. More recently, non-invasive techniques such as reflectance confocal microscopy and high-definition optical coherence tomography have been used to determine the optical features of AK and differentiate these from SCC [43]. Dynamic optical coherence tomography, a novel angiographic variant of optical coherence tomography, may aid in distinguishing AK from Bowen disease and cutaneous SCC [44].

Management

Management of patients with AK needs to begin with a thorough explanation of the nature, natural history and risks associated with the presence of these lesions (Figure 141.14, Tables 141.2 and 141.3),

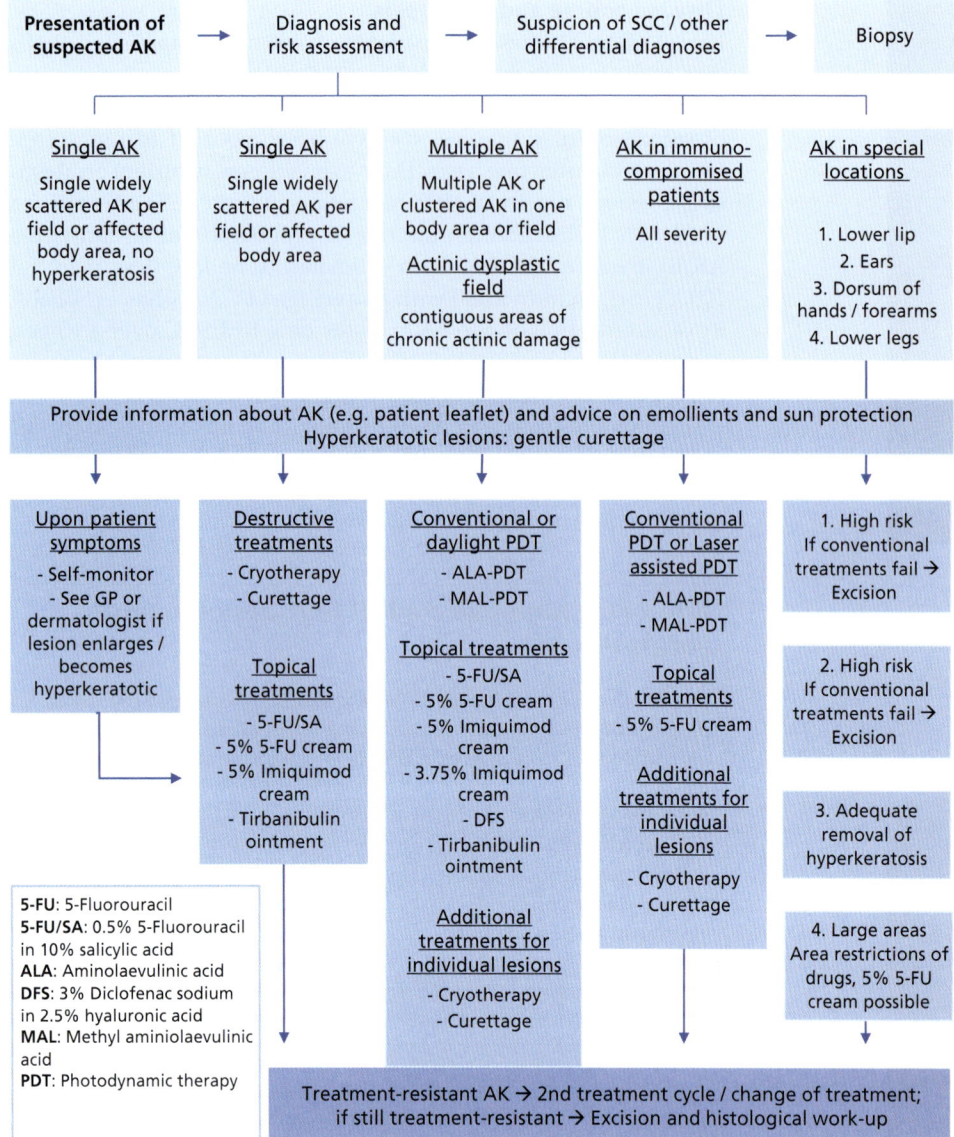

Figure 141.14 Actinic keratoses management algorithm.

as AK are a highly sensitive marker of levels of UV exposure capable of producing malignant change. Many treatments of AK can achieve effective lesion clearance for a short term. However, it remains uncertain if the efficacy can be sustained over a longer period of time without further intervention. AK represent chronic disease and therefore sequential therapy and follow-up is likely to be required.

The main goal of treatment is to reduce the number of AK and to prevent the progression of AK to invasive SCC. Other concerns such as the negative impact on QoL or aesthetic aspects can be secondary drivers of treatment considerations. For this, the spectrum of approach ranges from advice on sun protection to more aggressive topical treatments or surgical interventions. It remains, however, a basic problem with AK that it cannot be foreseen precisely which lesions will progress to SCC. Individual AK remain enigmatic and the spectrum includes spontaneous resolution to malignant transition into SCC.

First line

All patients with AK need to be instructed on avoidance of direct sun exposure and personal sun protective equipment like a hat, clothing and use of sunblocks. Regular sunscreen use has shown to reduce the rate of development of new AK [45]. Asymptomatic patients with 'low-risk' disease and few thin AK may decide that self-monitoring is a reasonable option. Other patients may wish to simply use emollients and sunblocks.

The armamentarium to treat AK comprises numerous topical agents, destructive treatments such as cryotherapy or surgical techniques (e.g. curettage, cautery) and selective treatments such as photodynamic therapy (PDT). The selection of a suitable therapy depends on various factors such as patient preference, local expertise, availability of the particular therapy and cost.

Some topical treatments for AK are limited to a maximum application area of 25 cm² by license. These are 5% imiquimod cream, 0.5% fluorouracil with 10% salicylic acid and tirbanibulin ointment.

Table 141.2 Treatment options for actinic keratoses (AK).

Lesion characteristics/ distribution	Treatment
Single AK lesions	• Cryotherapy[a] • Curettage • Ablative laser (CO$_2$ / Er:YAG)[a,c] • 5% 5-fluorouracil (Efudix®) • Imiquimod 5% (Aldara®)[b] • 0.5% 5-fluorouracil/10% salicylic acid (Actikerall®)[b] • Tirbanibulin 1% ointment (Klisyri®)
Multiple AK lesions	• 0.5% 5-fluorouracil/10% salicylic acid (Actikerall®)[b] • 5% 5-fluorouracil (Efudix®) • Diclofenac 3% (Solaraze®) • Imiquimod 5% (Aldara®)[b] • Imiquimod 3.75% (Zyclara®)[b] • Tirbanibulin 1% ointment (Klisyri®) • PDT (conventional /daylight) (Ameluz® / Metvix®)[c]
Field cancerisation	• Diclofenac 3% (Solaraze®) • 5% 5-fluorouracil (Efudix®) • Imiquimod 3.75% (Zyclara®)[b] • Tirbanibulin 1% ointment (Klisyri®) • PDT (conventional / daylight) (Ameluz® / Metvix®)[c]
AK in immunocompromised patients	• 5% 5-fluorouracil (Efudix®) • PDT (conventional) (Ameluz® / Metvix®)[c]

[a] By experienced practitioner.
[b] Topical therapy without specific licence for trunk/limb AK.
[c] Usually initiated in specialist dermatology department.
PDT, photodynamic therapy.

Treatment recommendations have therefore been divided into three treatment arms: single lesions, small field (maximum 25 cm^2), and large field (>25 cm^2) [8]. From a clinical point of view, AK are rarely limited to 25 cm^2 so that this division appears artificial.

Cryotherapy. Treatment with liquid nitrogen is effective for patients with a small number of lesions. Patients must be informed about blistering, oedema, crusting and soreness as short-term side effects. Long-term side effects mainly comprise hypopigmentation or scarring as a consequence of excessive treatment. Generally, cryotherapy gives good cosmetic results. This treatment does require a visit to a clinic and only targets specific treated lesions. Cryotherapy is difficult to standardise because of the many variables involved such as duration of freeze, duration of thaw and number of freeze–thaw cycles.

Curettage and cautery. This is a destructive therapy which can be useful for larger hyperkeratotic lesions. It has the advantage of providing a specimen for histological assessment. Gentle superficial curettage of scale and crust represents an important pretreatment for other therapies, e.g. PDT. In this context, care should be taken to avoid bleeding.

3% diclofenac in 2.5% hyaluronic gel. This non-steroidal anti-inflammatory drug's mechanism of action in AK is not known but may be related to the inhibition of the cyclo-oxygenase pathway leading to reduced prostaglandin E2 (PGE2) synthesis. It is licensed for application twice daily for 60–90 days.

In randomised placebo-controlled double-blind studies, complete clearance rates of 47% compared with 19% for placebo were observed at 30 days follow-up after 90 days of treatment [46]. Allergic contact dermatitis to diclofenac has been reported in few cases.

5% 5-fluorouracil cream. The mechanism of action is not clear, but it is believed to act through inhibition of DNA synthesis and possibly RNA function, leading to cell apoptosis.

5% 5-fluorouracil cream has shown good efficacy. It has the advantage that it can be applied to large areas up to 500 cm^2 and often causes an inflammatory response with crusting. In a comparative trial on treatment of AK on the head, 5% 5-fluorouracil cream demonstrated superiority over 5% imiquimod cream, MAL-PDT and the now withdrawn 0.015% ingenol mebutate gel [47].

0.5% 5-fluorouracil combined with 10% salicylic acid. The addition of salicylic acid in the 0.5% formulation leads to a keratolytic effect and reduces the hyperkeratosis associated with AK. The treatment area is limited to 25 cm^2 by license. In a randomised double-blind study comparing 0.5% 5-fluorouracil combined with 10% salicylic acid with 3% diclofenac in 2.5% hyaluronic acid and placebo, complete clearance rates were 55.4%, 32% and 15.1%, respectively, at 8 weeks follow-up after 12 weeks of treatment [48].

3.75% and 5% imiquimod cream. Imiquimod is a toll-like receptor 7 (TLR7) and TLR8 agonist that upregulates the expression of pro-inflammatory genes. Specifically, it induces translocation of several transcription factors, most importantly nuclear factor (NF)-κB, to the nucleus that activates expression of a multitude of pro-inflammatory genes. Ultimately, there is generation of tumour necrosis factor (TNF) α, interferon (IFN) α, interleukins and chemokines. It also upregulates the pro-apoptotic CD95 receptor that is known to be downregulated in AK and SCCs.

In randomised double-blind studies, 3.75% imiquimod cream was compared with placebo in large treatment areas with clearance rates of 35.6% and 6.3%, respectively, at 8 weeks follow-up after two cycles of 2-week treatment with a 2-week rest period between each cycle [49].

5% imiquimod cream has been compared with placebo in a randomised double-blind study, which showed complete clearance rates of 55% and 2.3%, respectively, at 8-week follow-up after one or two cycles of three times per week over 4 weeks of treatment [50]. While 3.75% imiquimod cream can be applied to either whole scalp or whole face, 5% imiquimod cream is limited to a treatment area of 25 cm^2 by license. Both treatments can cause marked inflammatory reactions which settle within a few weeks (Figure 141.15a–c).

Tirbanibulin ointment. This is a synthetic inhibitor of tubulin polymerisation leading to microtubular disruption and along with Src kinase signalling inhibition, results in cellular apoptosis.

In two phase 3, randomised, double-blind, vehicle-controlled trials, pooled rates of complete clearance and partial (≥75%) clearance

Table 141.3 Topical therapy for actinic keratosis (AK).

Therapy	Protocol	Limitations	Specific features
Diclofenac 3% gel (Solaraze®, Almirall)	Twice daily for 60–90 days	Maximum area 200 cm^2, only Olsen grade I/II lesions	Isolated cases of allergic contact dermatitis and renal affection
5% 5-fluorouracil (Efudix®, Mylan)	Once or twice daily for 3–4 weeks	Maximum area 500 cm^2	Inflammatory reaction in the second week of application followed by short necrotic phase and healing
0.5% 5-fluorouracil combined with 10% salicylic acid (Actikerall®, Almirall)	Once daily for maximum of 12 weeks, optimal effect may not be evident for up to 8 weeks after cessation	Maximum area: 25 cm^2, only Olsen grade I/II lesions	Painted on each lesion and film peeled off following day
Imiquimod 5% (Aldara®, Mylan)	Apply three times a week to AK on face or scalp for 4 weeks. Assess after a 4-week interval, repeat cycle if required	Maximum area: 25 cm^2, only Olsen grade I/II lesions, only in immunocompetent adults	Local inflammatory reactions are common. There is an association between clearance and intensity of reaction. Advise rest period of several days if inflammation is severe. Flu-like symptoms possible
Imiquimod 3.75% (Zyclara®, Mylan)	Once daily for 2 treatment cycles of 2 weeks, each separated by a 2-week interval	Up to two sachets per application, full face or balding scalp, only Olsen grade I/II lesions, only in immunocompetent adults	Rest period if required. Flu-like symptoms possible
Tirbanibulin 1% (Klisyri®, Almirall)	Once daily for 5 consecutive days to AK on face and scalp	Maximum area: 25 cm^2, only Olsen grade I/II lesions, only in immunocompetent adults	Mostly mild to moderate reaction with slight redness and swelling, which generally peaks at day 8
Conventional PDT (Ameluz®, Biofrontera or Metvix®, Galderma)	Ameluz® (nanoemulsion of 5-ALA), Metvix® (methylester of 5-ALA)	Only non-pigmented Olsen grade I/II lesions on the face and scalp; Ameluz®: also, in the body regions trunk, neck or extremities	Applied under occlusion for 3 hours before illumination with red light. Only to be administered by healthcare professionals trained in PDT. Pain/burning sensation is common during PDT. Some redness common after treatment and scab formation
Daylight PDT (Ameluz®, Biofrontera or Metvix®, Galderma)	Ameluz® (nanoemulsion of 5-ALA), Metvix® (methylester of 5-ALA)	Only non-pigmented Olsen grade I/II lesions on the face and scalp; clear weather, ambient temperature should exceed 10°C	Apply to scalp/face; patients should be outdoors within 30 minutes. Patients should stay outside for two continuous hours in full natural daylight. Single treatment, repeat at 3 months if required

5-ALA, 5-aminolaevulinic acid.
PDT, photodynamic therapy.

were reported at day 57 of treatment to be 49% and 72%, respectively. Treatment was applied to the face or scalp and local skin reactions were reported to be mostly mild to moderate peaking at day 8 and mostly resolved by day 29 [51].

Conventional photodynamic therapy. This is a treatment modality involving the administration of photosensitising compound, which selectively accumulates in the hyperproliferative target cells, followed by local irradiation with visible light, causing selective damage to target tissue by necrosis and apoptosis. The procedure is quite time consuming and requires approved illumination devices. In most cases, irradiation of the treatment area is felt to be very painful which is a relevant disadvantage of conventional PDT.

5-aminolaevulinic acid (ALA)-PDT and its methyl ester, MAL-PDT, have been licensed and approved for the treatment of AK. In a large randomised double-blind study comparing ALA-PDT to placebo-PDT, complete clearance rates were 64% and 11%, respectively [52]. When ALA-PDT was compared with MAL-PDT and placebo-PDT in a large randomised double-blind study, complete response rates were 78.2%, 64.2% and 17.1%, respectively [53]. An open-label non-sponsored randomised controlled trial comparing MAL-PDT to 3% diclofenac in 2.5% hyaluronic gel for the treatment of multiple face and scalp AK, showed that patient complete response was 68% with MAL-PDT and 27% with 3% diclofenac in 2.5% hyaluronic gel at 3 months. At 12 months, of the patients who had a complete response 37/67 (55%) and 7/25 (28%) remained clear, respectively. MAL-PDT was superior in efficacy, cosmetic outcome and overall patient satisfaction. The authors concluded that while MAL-PDT was more expensive, it was also more cost-effective than 3% diclofenac in 2.5% hyaluronic gel [54].

Daylight photodynamic therapy. ALA-PDT and MAL-PDT are both approved for daylight PDT in the EU and UK. The advantages of using daylight PDT are that no specific illumination device is required and there is no pain during irradiation.

Daylight PDT is confined to non-hyperkeratotic AK. After application of an organic sunscreen on all sun-exposed areas, crusts and scales are gently removed. MAL or ALA is then applied on the treatment area and the 2-hour exposure to daylight has to start within 30 minutes after application. ALA-daylight PDT with an approved ALA nanoemulsion was non-inferior to MAL-daylight PDT reaching clearance rate of 79.8% and 76.5% respectively [55].

Lesions with uncertain or unpredictable malignant potential

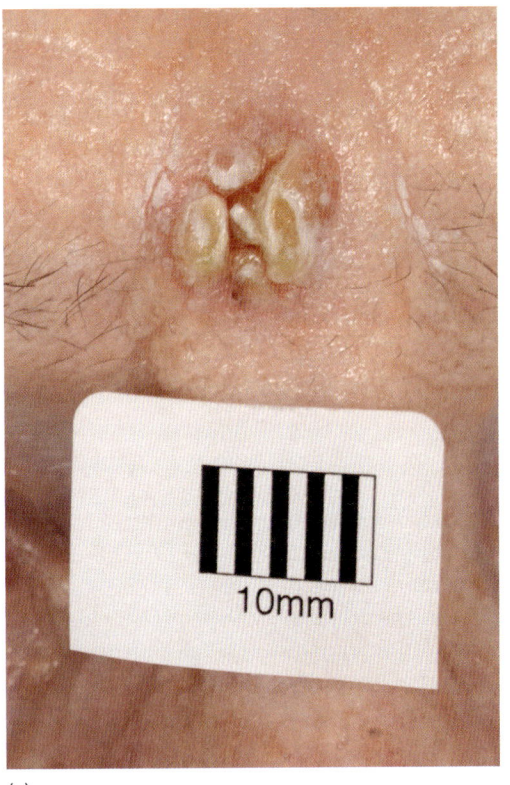
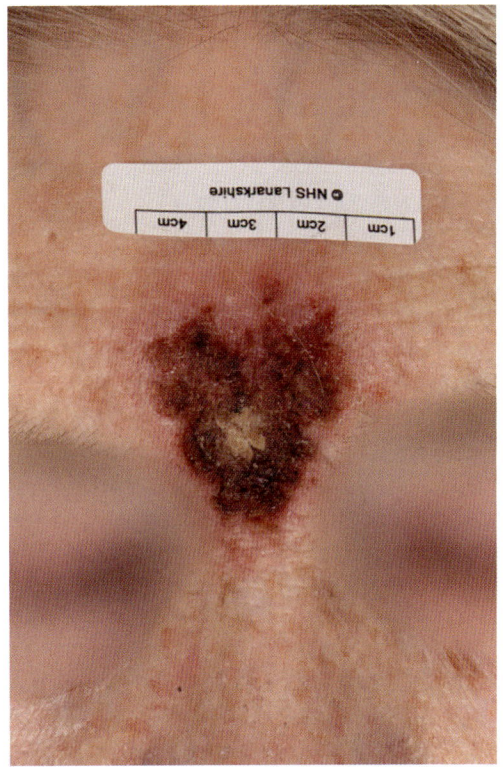
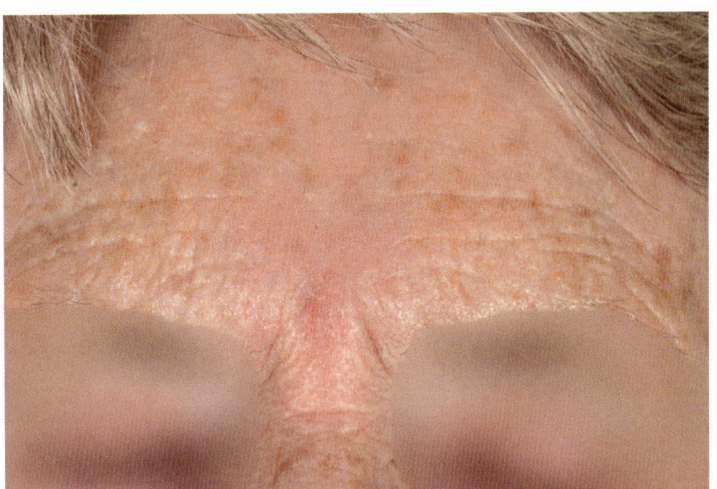

Figure 141.15 (a) Hyperkeratotic actinic keratosis before treatment with 5% imiquimod cream. (b) Four weeks into treatment with 5% imiquimod cream. (c) Post-treatment.

Daylight PDT requires strict adherence to the protocol and adequate illumination conditions (>10°C, clear conditions, two hours of illumination under sufficient ambient light).

Second line
Topical retinoids have been used to treat AK with limited benefit in small case series. Oral retinoids (acitretin) and oral nicotinamide have shown some benefit in reducing number of AK in OTRs but evidence remains poor.

Third line
Laser treatments, preferably with CO_2- or Er:YAG-lasers, dermabrasion and chemical peels can be used for field-directed treatment of AK. Clinical trials comparing these treatments with placebo or no treatment are required. These treatments may be used in combination with other treatments especially in extensive field cancerisation [56].

Resources

Further information
Dirschka T, Gupta G, Micali G *et al*. Real-world approach to actinic keratosis management: practical treatment algorithm for office-based dermatology. *J Dermatolog Treat* 2017;28;431–42.
Werner RN, Sammain A, Erdmann R *et al*. The natural history of actinic keratosis: a systematic review. *Br J Dermatol* 2013;169:502–18.

Berker D, McGregor JM, Mohd Mustapa MF et al. British Association of Dermatologists' guidelines for the care of patients with actinic keratosis 2017. Br J Dermatol 2017;176:20–43.

Cutaneous horn [1]

Definition
Cutaneous horns are hard conical projections from the skin, made of compact keratin. They arise from benign, premalignant or malignant skin lesions.

Introduction and general description
This is a clinical and not a pathological diagnosis. Horny plugs or outgrowths may be caused by various epidermal changes, such as an epidermal naevus, a viral wart, molluscum contagiosum, a keratoacanthoma (KA), a seborrhoeic keratosis, or a marsupialised trichilemmal or epidermoid cyst. In most of these cases, the primary diagnosis is suggested by the appearance and clinical course and, in most, the horn has a friable quality. Cutaneous horns are generally small and are usually localised to the face or hands but can occur on any body part (Figure 141.16).

Epidemiology
Incidence and prevalence
There are no published epidemiology studies but a large retrospective series of 643 cutaneous horns over a 19-year period suggested an incidence of 32 new cases per year [2].

Age
Cutaneous horns are more common in the older population with a peak incidence in those between 60 and 70 years. There is an increased chance of finding premalignant or malignant change in the base with increasing age [2].

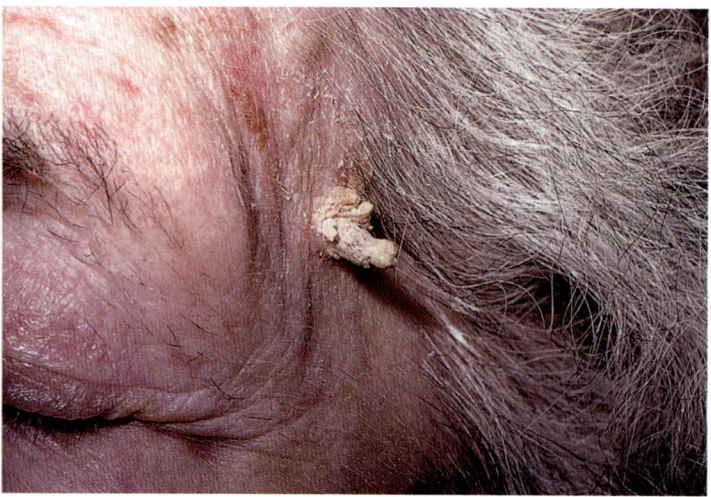

Figure 141.16 Typical cutaneous horn. Underlying this lesion, a carcinoma *in situ* was identified after biopsy.

Sex
In one large series, cutaneous horns were commoner in females [2], although other reports have not confirmed this finding [3,4]. However, cutaneous horns with premalignant or malignant pathology at the base were more common in males [2].

Ethnicity
They are more common in Fitzpatrick skin types I and II.

Pathophysiology
Pathology
The gradual continuing development from relatively normal-looking skin to a hard keratotic protrusion resembling an animal horn in miniature is the result of dysplastic epidermal changes similar to those seen in AK. Histologically, there is usually no atypicality or loss of polarity of the epidermal cells, but the granular layer may be deficient or absent. Histological examination of the base should confirm the cause of the horn. In long-established lesions there may be budding from the basal layer, indicating early development of a SCC.

Causative organisms
There is a possible association with the HPV family, particularly HPV-2 subtype [5].

Environmental factors
Exposure to UVR may trigger the onset, as evidenced by a higher rate of lesions occurring on light-exposed sites.

Clinical features
A cutaneous horn has been defined as a keratotic lesion with its height at least half the widest diameter of its base [3]. Most cutaneous horns have a benign pathology at their base, such as a seborrhoeic keratosis, viral wart or a trichilemmal cyst. However, just under 40% have premalignant or malignant change, usually a SCC, at their base [2]. In horns with premalignant or malignant aetiology, the lesions are commoner on light-exposed sites and in older men [2].

History
They are often solitary and asymptomatic.

Presentation
Cutaneous horns generally present as curved hard, yellow to brown keratotic outgrowths with circumferential ridges, which are surrounded either by normal-looking epidermis or by an acanthotic collarette. Recurrent injury may cause the base to be inflamed; a combination of inflammation and induration beneath the horn is suggestive of malignant transformation. The lesions are most common on the exposed areas, particularly the upper part of the face and the ears. They are commonly single, but may be multiple; it is usual to find some more typical AK or other evidence of UVR damage. Cutaneous horns with a wide base or a low height-to-base ratio have been reported to show either premalignant or malignant base

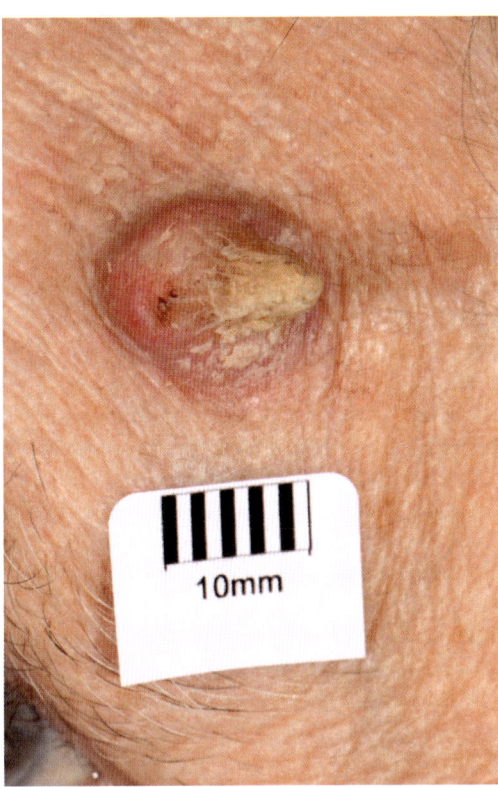

Figure 141.17 Cutaneous horn with low height-to-base ratio. Pathology showed squamous cell carcinoma at the base.

pathology (Figure 141.17). The coexistence of other premalignant or malignant skin lesions increases the likelihood of finding a horn with similar base pathology [2].

The size of the horn may vary from a few millimetres to several centimetres. They are often asymptomatic but malignant change is suggested by pain and redness, induration at the base, increase in size and a wide base or low height-to-base ratio.

Differential diagnosis
The common differential diagnoses to consider are viral warts and AK but others such as seborrhoeic keratosis, KA and invasive SCC may resemble cutaneous horns.

Disease course and prognosis
Most horns have benign base pathology but in a large series approximately 9% showed SCC pathological features at the base [2]. Other cancers reported in the literature include sebaceous gland carcinoma [4], malignant melanoma [6], BCC [7], Merkel cell carcinoma [8], Kaposi sarcoma [9] and cutaneous metastasis from renal cell carcinoma [10].

Management
A cutaneous horn is diagnosed by its clinical appearance. Histological examination of the horn base is crucial to rule out malignancy, as there are no diagnostic clinical features that can definitively distinguish benign lesions from skin cancer.

Surgical excision is usually advised to obtain pathology and rule out malignancy.

Arsenical keratosis [1]

Definition
A corn-like, punctate keratosis caused by arsenic, characteristically affecting the palms and soles, which may progress to SCC.

Introduction and general description
Inorganic arsenic has been classified as a class 1 human carcinogen by the International Agency for Research on Cancer (IARC). Arsenic, which is absorbed into the bloodstream predominantly via contaminated drinking water, has been linked to a variety of adverse health outcomes, including cancers of the skin, lung, bladder, liver and kidney [2,3,4].

Epidemiology
Incidence and prevalence
Groundwater contamination with arsenic and its resultant severe health effects have been reported in populations from different parts of the world, including Taiwan, Mexico, Chile, Argentina, Thailand, USA, Canada, Hungary, Japan, Bangladesh and India. The problem is greatest in parts of Bangladesh, West Bengal and Taiwan resulting from well water contamination [5]. A considerable proportion of any population exposed to chronic arsenic intoxication develops keratoses, the frequency increasing with the degree of intoxication and its duration [6]. A dose-dependent increase in skin lesions, including pigmentary change and keratoses, has been reported with increasing arsenic exposure [7] and between skin cancer prevalence and chronic arsenic exposure [8].

Age
Changes in the skin due to arsenic exposure can occur at any age. However, the incidence of skin lesions, including keratoses, has been reported to be higher in older individuals [7].

Sex
Males have been shown to have an increased incidence of developing skin lesions, including keratoses, following chronic arsenic exposure [7,9] but the dose-dependent association between arsenic exposure and lesion status is more pronounced in females [7].

Ethnicity
The prevalence is greatest in Bangladesh, parts of India and Taiwan.

Pathophysiology
Several *in vitro* and *in vivo* studies have shown that the DNA repair system is compromised by arsenic exposure. Individuals with the tumour protein 53 (*TP53*) arginine homozygous genotype (Arg/Arg) exhibit more DNA damage and this is not repaired as quickly as in those with other genotypes [10]. Recent studies have revealed the role of arsenic-induced epithelial alterations [11] with antihistone proteins (*H3K79me1*) being possible novel epigenetic signatures of arsenic-induced skin lesions [12].

Predisposing factors
Nutritional deficiencies such as retinol, calcium, fibre, folate, iron, riboflavin, thiamin and vitamins A, C and E, have been reported in

patients with keratotic skin lesions but not with non-keratotic skin lesions, and this observation is greater in females [9]. The strongest evidence is for low intakes of retinol equivalents, calcium, vitamin A and riboflavin in females with severe keratoses [9]. These deficiencies may have an adverse effect on arsenic metabolism.

Chronic liver disease [8] and smoking [13] have also been reported to increase the risk of developing keratoses and skin cancer. UVR and sodium arsenite can interact synergistically to enhance mutagenesis [14] but arsenical keratoses differ from UVR-induced keratoses as they tend to occur on light-protected areas, such as the palms and soles.

Chinese herbal medicine and Ayurvedic medicine may rarely contain arsenic resulting in similar clinical features [15,16].

Pathology
A range of changes may be seen from a benign-looking hyperplasia or dysplasia, through mild or moderate atypia, to frank Bowen disease [17,18]. There is no microscopic feature that allows a positive diagnosis of arsenic as the cause. In most lesions, there is no elastotic degeneration of the upper dermis.

Clinical features
History
Skin lesions appear a few years after exposure and usually progress through stages. Typically, the progression begins with hyperpigmentation of the skin (melanosis) in a 'raindrop' pattern. This is often accompanied with multiple hypopigmented areas (leukomelanosis). Palmar and plantar keratoses develop and can progress to generalised thickening of the palms and soles. Mees lines (transverse white bands) may be seen in the fingernails.

Presentation
The keratoses usually begin on the palms or soles as small areas of hyperkeratosis resembling corns. These enlarge, thicken and increase in number. The fingers, backs of the hands and more proximal parts of the extremities may be involved. Induration, inflammation and ulceration occur when the lesion becomes malignant. There may be areas of Bowen disease in other sites and multiple BCC, mainly of the trunk, may occur in association.

Differential diagnosis
Punctate keratosis, such as disseminated punctate keratoderma, usually appears in early life. Darier disease and lichen planus usually have characteristic lesions elsewhere. Plantar warts differ in being papillomatous.

Complications and co-morbidity
Arsenic exposure predisposes individuals to cancer in a number of organs, including the skin, lung and bladder. Individuals without palmar hyperkeratosis have a low excess risk of subsequent internal malignancy [19]. However, in individuals with keratoses, a significant associated risk of bladder cancer and lung cancer exists, particularly in those who are smokers [13]. Besides tumours, prolonged arsenic exposure can lead to its accumulation in the liver, kidneys, heart, lungs, muscles, nervous system and gastrointestinal tract.

Disease course and prognosis
The keratotic lesions usually progress over time with increasing numbers, which may coalesce. Individual lesions may develop malignant change and there is a higher risk of developing Bowen disease, BCC and SCC. A study from Taiwan reported the overall prevalence of skin cancer to be 6.1% and this was associated with liver dysfunction and undernourishment [8].

Investigations
In endemic areas, sampling of the drinking water is useful to ascertain levels of contamination. Level of arsenic exposure may be quantified by blood and spot urine tests. Hair and nail samples may be useful as deposits are found with chronic exposure. A skin biopsy usually shows non-specific change but may show keratinocyte dysplasia.

Management
There are a number of public health campaigns helping to reduce arsenic exposure in endemic areas. As there is an association with smoking and malnutrition, individuals should be advised to stop smoking and to eat a well-balanced diet, which may be difficult in poor economic areas.

The multiplicity of the keratoses makes treatment difficult. All affected patients should be examined periodically for evidence of malignant change and for signs of visceral malignancy.

First line
Individuals with solitary or few keratoses often respond to cryotherapy or curettage and cautery. Where individuals have multiple keratoses, oral retinoids, such as acitretin have been reported to improve the keratoses and associated Bowen disease [20]. Oral retinoids can also be used in combination with keratolytic agents [21].

Second line
Imiquimod cream (5%) once daily for 6 weeks or once daily three to five times per week for 8 weeks has been reported to improve arsenical keratoses and associated Bowen disease and BCC [22,23].

Post-ionising radiation keratosis

Definition
These may occur following accidental exposure to ionising radiation or after therapeutic radiotherapy.

Introduction and general description
These may occur in an area of scarring following radiotherapy or excessive fluoroscopy where there is obvious dermal damage. They may also be seen in radiologists, surgeons, dentists and others who have exposed their skin to frequent small doses of X-rays, although such cases are now rare.

Epidemiology

Incidence and prevalence
Radiation effects on the skin are a common consequence of accidental ionising radiation exposure or following routine clinical radiotherapy, but radiation keratoses are uncommon [1,2].

Age
All ages can be affected.

Sex
Both sexes can be affected.

Associated diseases
There is an increased incidence of bone marrow suppression and internal malignancy in those who have been accidently exposed to large doses of ionising radiation.

Pathophysiology
In vitro studies have demonstrated that exposure of skin cells to ionising radiation causes an acute inflammatory response which is mediated by an upregulation of inflammatory markers such as β1 integrin (CD29) and intercellular adhesion molecule 1 (ICAM-1) [3–6].

Pathology
The epidermal changes are similar to AK. Histologically, the dermis shows a much more extensive replacement of collagen by scar and elastotic material, obliterative changes in the vessels and, at times, the presence of abnormally large and irregular fibroblasts (Figure 141.18).

Environmental factors
Accidental exposure to ionising radiation or following therapeutic radiotherapy.

Clinical features

History
Keratoses are the late effects of ionising radiation. They usually occur months to years following exposure. They are commoner on the limbs but may also occur on covered body sites following accidental ionising radiation exposure [1].

Presentation
Cutaneous signs of ionising radiation include keratoses, telangiectasia, vasculitis, radiation ulcers, haemangiomas, destruction of the lymphatic network, regional lymphostasis and subcutaneous sclerosis of the connective tissue. Pigmentary changes and pain are often present.

Differential diagnosis
Post-ionising radiation keratoses may resemble AK but other signs of radiation damage will be present.

Disease course and prognosis
Keratotic lesions may increase in number and skin cancer is possible in subsequent years.

Investigations
A skin biopsy may be necessary to confirm the diagnosis and to exclude malignant change.

Management
Immediate reduction in exposure to ionising radiation is necessary. *In vitro* studies have demonstrated that 1α,25-dihydroxyvitamin D_3 modulates the human keratinocyte response to ionising radiation exposure and may be useful in reducing the reaction following therapeutic radiotherapy [7]. Individual lesions may be treated with cryotherapy.

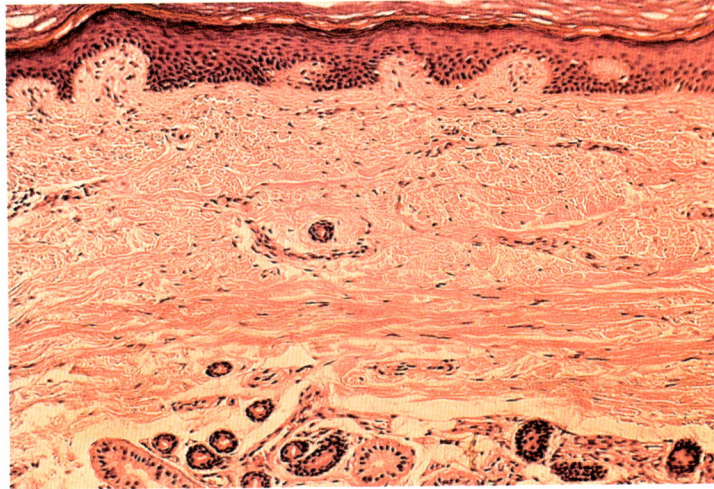

Figure 141.18 Pathology of post-ionising radiation keratosis.

Disseminated superficial actinic porokeratosis

Definition
Disseminated superficial actinic porokeratosis (DSAP) is the most common clinical type of porokeratosis (Chapter 85), characterised by hyperkeratotic papules surrounded by a thread-like elevated border. It appears on sun-exposed areas becoming more prominent in summer and may improve in winter.

Introduction and general description
DSAP was first recognised in Texas [1,2], and is common in Australia [3]. DSAP is an autosomal dominant disorder with incomplete penetrance early in life [4–6]. Mutations in the mevalonate pathway which involves mevalonate kinase (*MVK*), mevalonate diphosphate decarboxylase (*MVD*), farnesyl diphosphate synthase (*FDPS*) amongst others have been reported in Chinese patients with familial and sporadic DSAP [6–8]. DSAP demonstrates the

Knudson 'two-hit' hypothesis, where in the presence of monoallelic germline mutations of causative genes, a second hit results in genetic change in the wild-type allele of those genes [9]. On a background of germline mutations in *MVK* and *MVD*, it has been demonstrated that a second hit causes somatic homologous recombinations that render the monoallelic mutation biallelic or causes C to T transition mutations (C>T) in the wild-type allele [10].

Epidemiology
Incidence and prevalence
This is an uncommon epidermal keratinisation disorder.

Age
DSAP is rare in childhood with the earliest reported age of onset being 10 years [11]. The average age at which patients first notice DSAP is about 40 years, and its frequency in members of affected families increases with age.

Sex
Both sexes are affected with a female preponderance. In a study with 248 Chinese family members, 41 had DSAP and of these 26 were males and 15 females, suggesting geographical gender variations [4].

Ethnicity
This condition is commoner in those who have lived or live in areas of high sunlight exposure such as the USA and Australia. More recently, Chinese patients with familial and sporadic DSAP have been reported.

Associated diseases
It has been reported to coexist with other types of porokeratosis, such as linear hyperkeratotic and verrucous variants [12–14]. It has been reported that this coexistence forms a type II segmental manifestation of an autosomal dominant disorder [15].

Pathophysiology
Predisposing factors
Risk factors for developing DSAP include genetic factors, UVR exposure and immunosuppression [16,17]. DSAP commonly occurs on light-exposed skin and has also been reported to occur after narrow-band UVB therapy and after psoralen and UVA (PUVA) therapy [16,18–20].

Pathology
There is no microscopic feature that separates this disorder from porokeratosis of Mibelli, and both have been explained as the result of localised clones of abnormal epidermal cells [21], an idea supported by the successful autotransplantation of the disseminated superficial variety [22].

The distinctive pathological feature of porokeratosis is the cornoid lamella at the margin (Figure 141.19). This is a narrow column of altered or parakeratotic keratin, seated in a slight depression in the

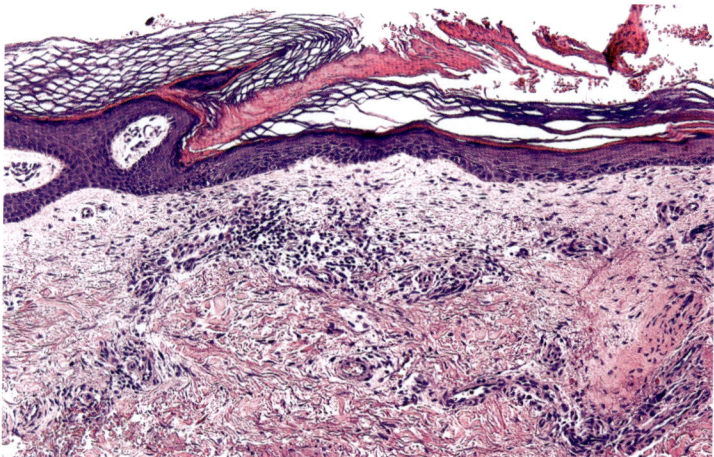

Figure 141.19 Cornoid lamella with parakeratotic column overlying epidermal dyskeratotic and vacuolated cells, representing the clinically visible raised margin seen in disseminated superficial actinic porokeratosis.

epidermis and directed obliquely inwards in some cases. It may involve the ostia of follicles and sweat ducts. The granular layer of the indented epidermis is usually missing and there may be dyskeratotic cells. The epidermis enclosed by the ridge is usually thinned, the interpapillary ridges and dermal papillae may be flattened, and the basal cells may show liquefaction degeneration. In addition to solar elastosis, decrease in collagen and telangiectasia, the upper dermis may have a non-specific inflammatory infiltrate with vascular proliferation, oedema and fibrosis.

Genetics
Several genetic loci for DSAP have been reported in large Chinese families with familial and sporadic DSAP. These include 12q23.2-24.1 [4], 12q24.-24.2 [23], 15q25.1-26.1 [5], 1p31.3-31.1 [24] and 16q24.1-24.3 [25]. The *MVK* gene maps to chromosome 12q24.11 and DNA sequencing has identified *MVK* mutations in 33% of familial and 16% of sporadic cases [7]. All of these mutations were heterozygous and did not affect ethnically matched normal controls, five patients with porokeratosis of Mibelli, two with linear porokeratosis and four with DSAP [7]. Mutations have also been found in the *MVD* gene which maps to chromosome 16q24.2 and the *FDPS* gene on chromosome 1q22 [8]. On a background of heterozygous germline mutations in *MVK* and *MVD*, it has been demonstrated that a second hit causes somatic homologous recombinations that render the monoallelic mutation biallelic or causes C>T transition mutations in the wild-type allele [10]. As most lesions occur on light-exposed skin, it is likely that this second hit is caused by ultraviolet radiation (UVR).

The mevalonate pathway is regulated by *MVK*, *MVD* and *FDPS* genes amongst others and these are expressed in many tissues, including skin epidermal cells. The *MVK* gene catalyses the phosphorylation of mevalonic acid to 5-phosphomevalonate and functions downstream of 3-hydroxy-3-methyl-glutaryl-coenzyme A reductase (HMG-CoA) [26]. *MVK* mutations are reported to alter the gene expression of keratin 1 and apoptosis of cells [26]. The mevalonate pathway is vital for multiple cellular processes, providing cells with essential bioactive molecules and involved in the biosynthesis of cholesterol and isoprenoid. Loss of function mutations lead to reduction in its end products including cholesterol and accumulation of toxic metabolites. Cholesterol deficiency leads to increased keratinocyte sensitivity to apoptosis, and premature apoptosis along with dysregulated keratinocyte differentiation has been found in porokeratosis [27].

Environmental factors
It commonly occurs on light-exposed skin.

Clinical features
History
DSAP usually affects light-exposed sites appearing mainly on the distal extremities. The malar regions and the cheeks may be affected but it is not seen on areas habitually covered by clothes, or on the palms or soles. Patients often notice multiple enlarging rough lesions. These tend to be asymptomatic but may be mildly pruritic, particularly after sun exposure and patients often complain of the lesions being unsightly.

Presentation
The lesion begins as a 1–3 mm conical papule, brownish red or brown in colour, and usually around a follicle containing a keratotic plug. It expands and a sharp slightly raised keratotic ring, a fraction of a millimetre thick, develops and spreads out to a diameter of 10 mm or more. The skin within the ring is somewhat atrophic and mildly reddened or hyperpigmented, but a hypopigmented ring may be seen just inside the ridge. The ridge itself is sometimes darkly pigmented. The central thickening usually disappears, but it may persist with an attached scale, follicular plug or central depression. Sweating is absent within the lesions. In sunny areas, lesions may be present in very large numbers and may change from a circular to a polycyclic outline. In less sunny climates, such as the UK, patients have fewer lesions, which tend to remain circular (Figure 141.20). In a few cases, the centre of the area becomes considerably inflamed and covered by thick hyperkeratosis or may ulcerate and become crusted.

Clinical variants
Porokeratosis variants (Chapter 85) include porokeratosis of Mibelli, linear porokeratosis, disseminated superficial porokeratosis, porokeratosis palmaris and plantaris diffusa and punctate porokeratosis.

The rim of DSAP is very much smaller than in Mibelli porokeratosis and never contains a cleft. The onset of Mibelli porokeratosis is often in childhood, and the lesions are usually solitary or few in number and do not necessarily affect exposed parts.

Differential diagnosis
DSAP may need to be differentiated from AK particularly if they are present on the face but AK may be present on other light-exposed sites such as the dorsal surface of the hands and do not possess the marginal ridge seen in DSAP. DSAP on the legs may resemble Bowen disease but this too lacks the marginal ridge and bowenoid lesions tend to be larger with surface change throughout the lesion. Superficial BCC (sBCC) may resemble DSAP but sBCC lack the marginal ridge and tend to be fewer in number.

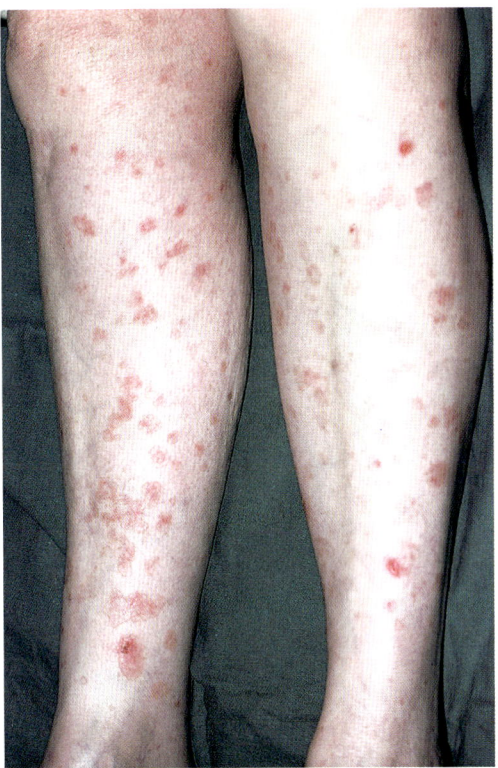

Figure 141.20 Disseminated superficial actinic porokeratosis on the lower legs.

Disease course and prognosis
The number of lesions tends to increase over time but the risk of malignant change remains very low. In a review of 281 cases with all forms of porokeratosis, the incidence of Bowen disease and SCC was 3.4% in the DSAP group [12] but others have found no increase in invasive malignancy [28].

Investigations
The diagnosis of DSAP is generally a clinical one and further investigations are not required but a skin biopsy may be necessary to confirm diagnosis.

Management
Patients should be reassured and given advice on the use of emollients and high factor broad spectrum sunscreen. There are no published controlled trials to date and evidence is taken from case reports and case series [29].

Lesions may respond to cryotherapy with liquid nitrogen, but new lesions tend to develop [2,3]. For numerous lesions, treatment with topical diclofenac gel [30,31], vitamin D_3 analogues [32,33], 5% 5-fluorouracil cream [34], 5% imiquimod cream [35] and PDT [36,37] has been reported with varying degrees of success.

Case reports with the use of lasers such as erbium [38], carbon dioxide [39], Q-switched ruby laser (QSRL) [40] and neodymium: yttrium-aluminium-garnet (Nd:YAG) [41] have been published showing some degree of success. More recently, individual cases with DSAP have been reported to have been successfully treated with topical 2% cholesterol/2% lovastatin cream but not with cholesterol cream alone [42] and 2% cholesterol/2% simvastatin cream [43]. Future pathogenic-directed treatment may therefore include cholesterol replacement along with HMG-CoA inhibitors and further trials are required.

IN SITU CARCINOMA OF THE SKIN

Bowen disease

Definition and nomenclature
Bowen disease (BD) is a form of intraepidermal (*in situ*) SCC. Most cases are characterised by a persistent, non-elevated, non-infiltrated, red, scaly or crusted and sharply defined patch. These patches range from a few millimetres to many centimetres in diameter and have a small potential for invasive malignancy [1]. Progressive growth is usual but spontaneous partial regression occurs occasionally.

> **Synonyms and inclusions**
> - Intraepithelial carcinoma
> - SCC *in situ*

Introduction and general description
BD can be found in any part of the skin. It is mostly asymptomatic and expands slowly and centrifugally. The risk of malignant transformation is low (3–5%). Beside the typical clinical patch-like presentation, verrucous, nodular, eroded, and pigmented variants occur.

Epidemiology
Incidence and prevalence
The incidence in the UK is estimated to be approximately 15/100 000 population per year but this is based on USA data and so may reflect a higher incidence due to increased sun exposure [2,3]. In the white North American population, it is reported to range from 14.9/100 000 to 27.8/100 000 [3,4]. More recent data from the Netherlands have shown a statistically significant increase in the annual age-standardised incidence rates per 100 000 people from 8.1 in 2003 to 68.9 in 2013 [5].

Age
BD can occur at any age in adults, but it is rare in those under the age of 30 years and much more common in patients over the age of 60 years. In the UK, the peak age of onset has been reported to be the seventh decade [6,7].

Sex
The division of BD between the sexes is judged controversially in the literature [5,8–10].

Ethnicity
This condition is much more common in the white population, particularly in those who have lived or live in areas of high sunlight exposure [3,4].

Associated diseases
Patients may present other UVR-induced skin cancers and full examination of the skin should be undertaken. In studies, 30–50% of BD cases had other previous or subsequent skin cancers, mainly BCC [10,11]. The standardised incidence ratio for subsequent KC and lip cancer was 4.3 and 8.2, respectively [12].

Pathophysiology
Predisposing factors
Several large studies have identified a link between BD and ingestion of arsenic, which can pre-date the onset of the disease by several decades [13,14]. Historically, arsenic was found in Fowler solution used for psoriasis and Gay solution to treat asthma. Agricultural workers may be exposed to arsenic salts used in fungicide, weedkiller, sheep dip or pesticide. Drinking of water contaminated with arsenic is regarded as the major route of human exposure. In some countries, notably parts of Argentina, Bangladesh, Chile, China, India, Mexico, Taiwan and the USA, the water supply was contaminated in the past [15]. Long-term arsenic exposure results in impaired immunity characterised by oxidative DNA damage of peripheral polymorphonuclear leukocytes and impaired macrophage function in adults with skin lesions [16].

Immunosuppression following solid-organ transplant, haematological malignancies, in particular chronic lymphocytic leukaemia or HIV, increases the risk of developing SCC and premalignant skin conditions but the exact risk for BD has not yet been determined. There are reports, however, of multiple areas of BD occurring in a younger age group in those under immunosuppressive treatment following solid-organ transplantation [17,18].

There are also reports of BD following therapeutic and other ionising radiation and following skin injury or chronic inflammation, such as lupus vulgaris and chronic lupus erythematosus [19].

Pathology
BD is characterised by sharply demarcated, puzzle-like arranged polymorphous atypical keratinocytes within the epidermis and sometimes the pilosebaceous epithelium. Since the basal layer of the epidermis is often spared (so called 'eyeliner sign'), the frequently used designation 'full thickness atypia' cannot be generalised. Mitoses and multinucleated keratinocytes can be observed at different levels. Most cases show a loss of the granular layer and overlying parakeratosis and hyperkeratosis (Figure 141.21). Clear cell change may be observed due to increased intracytoplasmic glycogen, which can be highlighted by a PAS stain. HPV-associated viral cytopathic changes are not uncommon.

Several histological subtypes have been described and sometimes these subtypes appear side by side within the same lesion. The psoriasiform subtype shows regular acanthosis and parakeratosis. Moreover, atrophic, verrucous-hyperkeratotic, papillated type, pigmented and a pagetoid type have been described, according to the overall morphology.

In contrast to AK, BD usually involves the acrosyringium and often spares the basal layer of the epidermis. The latter phenomenon has been called 'eyeliner sign' which never occurs in AK.

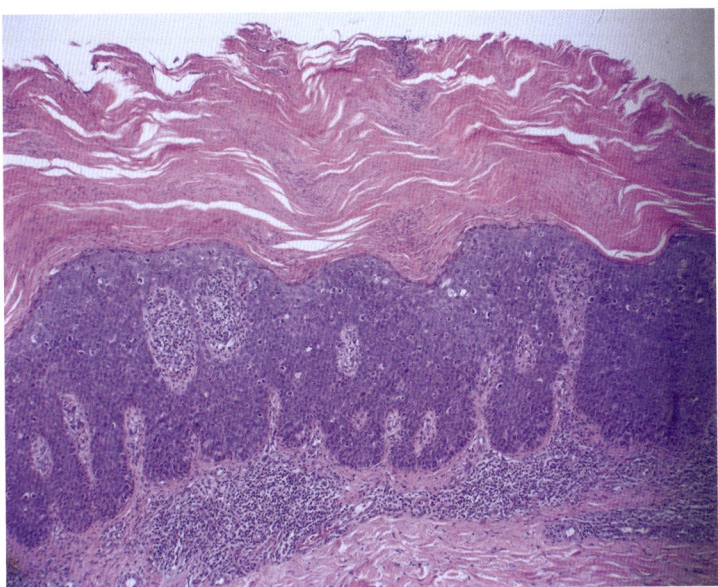

Figure 141.21 Pathology of Bowen disease showing full thickness atypia of the epidermis and the presence of atypical mitoses, giant cells and inflammatory cell infiltrate. H&E, ×10.

The superficial dermis can show an inflammatory cell infiltrate that is frequently quite dense and sometimes mimics lichenoid dermatoses. Actinic elastosis can be present in chronically light exposed areas.

The histopathology of bowenoid papulosis may be indistinguishable from BD. Sometimes numerous mitoses in metaphase and koilocytes can be observed. HPV-related cytopathic changes are seen, although they may be subtle. These changes include hypergranulosis and coarse keratohyaline granules with surrounding haloes.

Causative organisms

Viral agents have been implicated in the aetiology of BD. Interest has centred around HPV with reports of a number of HPV types being present. HPV DNA has been demonstrated in extragenital BD in varying amounts from 4.8% to 60% [20–23]. Larger studies have failed to confirm these findings, except for HPV16 and HPV18, which are both commoner in anogenital BD and HPV16 has also been implicated in 60% of palmoplantar and periungual lesions [24–26].

Environmental factors

BD is more common on light-exposed sites such as the lower legs, suggesting a relationship with chronic UV damage from solar or iatrogenic sources [8,9].

Clinical features

History

Patients usually present a solitary plaque but in 10–20% of cases there may be multiple lesions. In typical cases in white populations, lesions of BD are found on the lower legs of elderly women. However, BD can be found on any site and recent reports suggest an increased incidence on the head and neck [7,27]. It can occur on

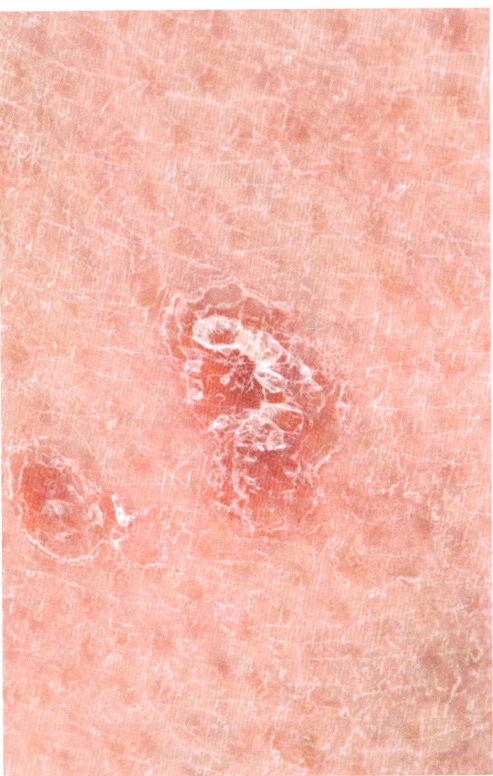

Figure 141.22 Bowen disease.

the perianal skin, subungual region, palms and soles uncommonly, and rarely it is found on mucosal surfaces such as the oral mucosa. BD arising in mucosal genital skin is described separately (Chapters 109, 110 and 111).

Presentation

The initial change is a small, pink/red, non-infiltrated and slightly scaly area, which is symptomless and gradually enlarges in irregular fashion. The white or yellowish scale is detached without much difficulty to expose a moist, reddened and at times granular surface. In contrast to psoriasis plaques, the BD uncommonly produces bleeding when detaching the scale. The margin is well demarcated and the lesion slightly raised; the surface is usually flat but may become hyperkeratotic or crusted (Figure 141.22). There may be several lesions, either widely spread or sometimes close together and becoming confluent with extension (Figure 141.23). Ulceration is usually a sign of the development of invasive carcinoma and may be delayed for many years after the appearance of the intraepidermal change.

Clinical variants

BD on perianal skin carries a higher risk of invasion, recurrence, and an association with cervical and vulval dysplasia. BD of the nail unit (subungual, periungual) affects younger women and is associated with high-risk HPV types such as HPV16 [25]. There is a higher risk of invasion and recurrence (Figure 141.24). Pigmented BD is uncommon (1.7% of cases in one study) and usually found in the flexures, perianal or subungual sites. Verrucous BD is rare and may raise the suspicion of SCC.

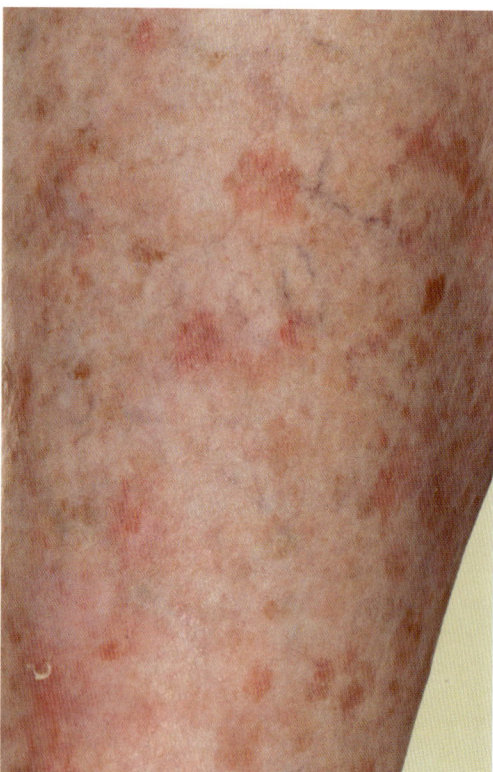

Figure 141.23 Multiple areas of Bowen disease on the lower leg.

Table 141.4 Common clinical differential diagnoses of Bowen disease.

Diagnosis	Differentiating features	Image
Seborrheic keratosis	Usually larger, darker, and multiple Appear 'stuck on' the skin Raised 'greasy' warty surface Common presence of horn cysts	Figures 141.5 and 141.6
Basal cell carcinoma	Superficial variant may mimic Bowen disease Usually less hyperkeratotic Often bigger lesions	Figure 141.25
Squamous cell carcinoma	Enlarging lesion Induration Raised shoulder or nodule Tenderness	Figure 141.26
Discoid dermatitis	Often large multiple plaques Pruritus is main symptom	Figure 141.27
Psoriasis	Thickened plaque with marked scale Bleeding upon removal of scale typical Often multiple, large and on other body sites	Figure 141.28

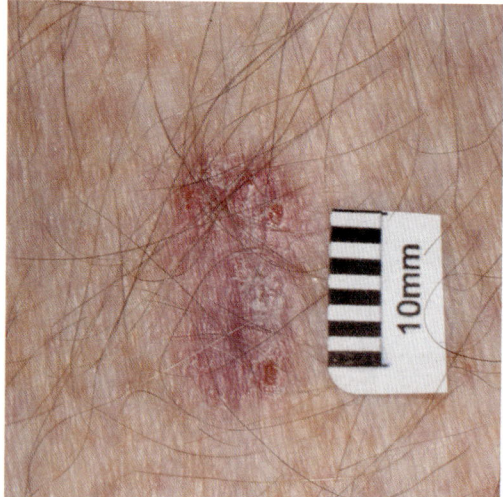

Figure 141.25 Superficial basal cell carcinoma mimicking Bowen disease.

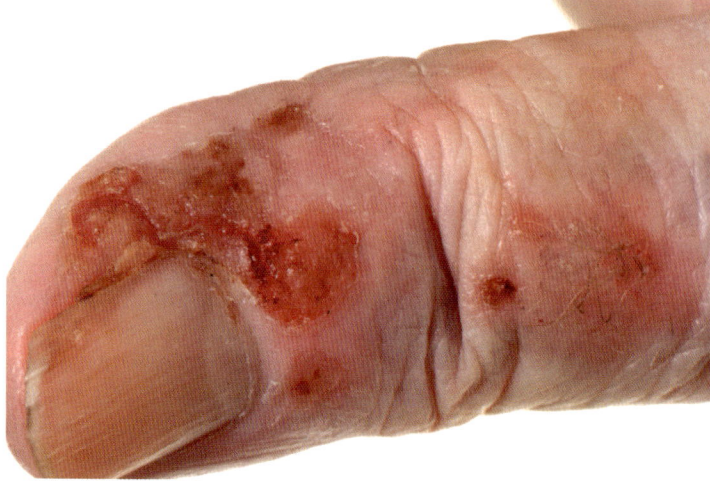

Figure 141.24 Periungual Bowen disease.

Differential diagnosis (Table 141.4)

BD has to be differentiated from KC, particularly sBCC (Figure 141.25) and early SCC. sBCC may present a solitary plaque or multiple scaly plaques but usually they have a pearly whipcord edge. Early invasive SCC may suggest a diagnostic challenge but generally patients give a history of change and the plaque may have evolved to form a small nodule or develop ulceration. Firm infiltration is a characteristic of SCC (Figure 141.26). Small bowenoid papules/plaques may mimic AK but AK tend to be scaly, hyperkeratotic, multiple and often painful while scratching. BD may also need to be differentiated from inflammatory dermatoses, such as psoriasis, lichen simplex and discoid dermatitis, particularly if it is pruritic (Figures 141.27 and 141.28). Tinea corporis, nummular eczema and seborrheic keratosis may also resemble BD. Paget disease, in particular the extramammary type, can be confused with BD, both clinically and histologically. BD of the nail unit may appear similar to viral warts, but viral warts tend to be multiple.

Bowenoid papulosis may resemble BD, but this is usually found on genital skin in younger sexually active people. Bowenoid papulosis tends to run a benign course with spontaneous regression occurring within several months, although recurrences are not uncommon [28]. A more protracted course may occur in older patients lasting as long as 5 years or more. The lesions tend to be asymptomatic but can be inflamed, pruritic or painful. Bowenoid papulosis presents as solitary or multiple, small, pigmented (red, brown or flesh coloured) papules with a flat to verrucous surface. The bowenoid papulosis lesions can coalesce into larger plaques (Figure 141.29). Lesions occur most commonly on the shaft of the penis or the external genitalia of females, although they can occur anywhere on the genitalia and in the perianal region, with

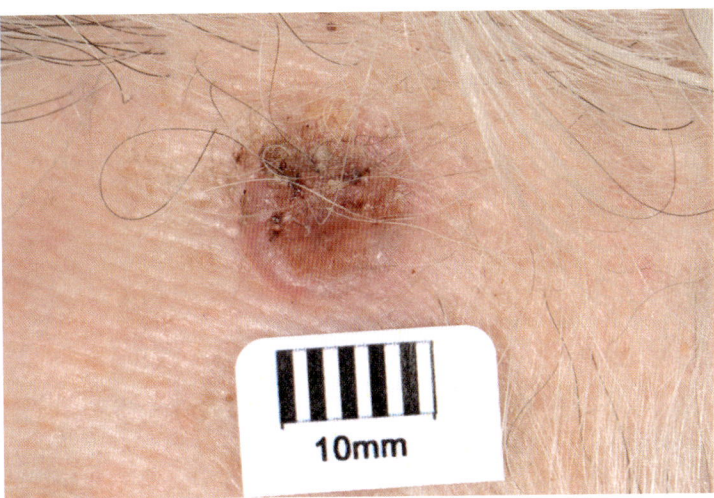

Figure 141.26 Squamous cell carcinoma with hyperkeratosis and raised thickened edge.

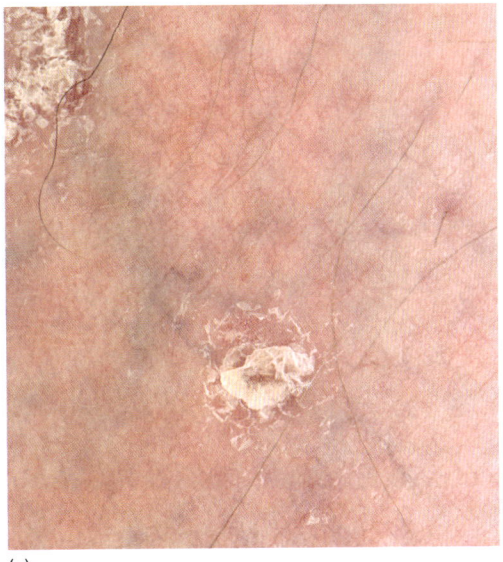

(a)

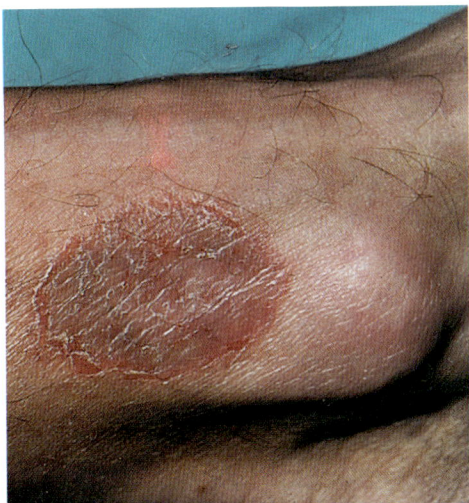

Figure 141.27 Discoid dermatitis of the lower leg. Courtesy of Dr W.A.D. Griffiths, Epsom Hospital, Surrey, UK.

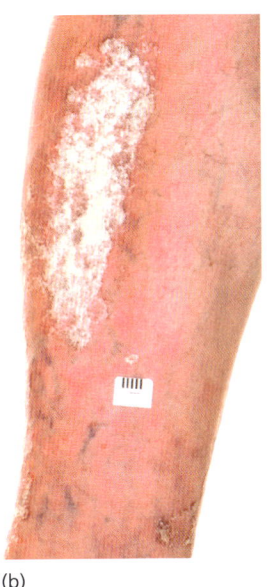

(b)

Figure 141.28 (a,b) Plaque with thick scale. Examination elsewhere shows typical scaly plaques seen in psoriasis.

occasional reports of them found on non-genital skin [29,30]. A number of HPV types, particularly HPV16 and HPV18, have been linked closely to bowenoid papulosis. Consequently, the risk of acquiring bowenoid papulosis is identical to that for other genital HPV-associated conditions via sexual contact or, possibly, via vertical transmission from mother to newborn [31,32].

Complications and co-morbidities

BD tends to be persistent with a low lifetime risk of malignant transformation of about 3–5%, although studies are generally retrospective and the evidence relatively poor [3,4]. Where there is malignant transformation, it results in an invasive SCC, which may metastasise if left untreated. Clinical signs of invasiveness are firm infiltration, ulceration and lesion tenderness. SCC arising from BD tend to be more aggressive than those evolving from AK.

Due to the recurrent nature of perianal and subungual BD, surgery with wide excision for perianal disease and digital amputation or Mohs micrographic surgery (MMS) for nail unit disease may be necessary [33].

Disease course and prognosis

Most patients with BD run a chronic course with the development of single or multiple lesions over time. Complications are few and the prognosis excellent, except in cases of SCC transformation. BD is a marker of UV-induced skin damage and so patients are at a higher risk of developing other UV-induced premalignant and malignant lesions. Evidence for follow-up duration is poor but in uncomplicated cases patients could be discharged following treatment.

Investigations

The condition must be distinguished from chronic inflammatory dermatoses and if the diagnosis is uncertain on first examination, the lack of improvement when steroids are applied is suggestive of BD. Where diagnosis remains in doubt, a skin biopsy is necessary to confirm the diagnosis. Dermoscopy features have been described

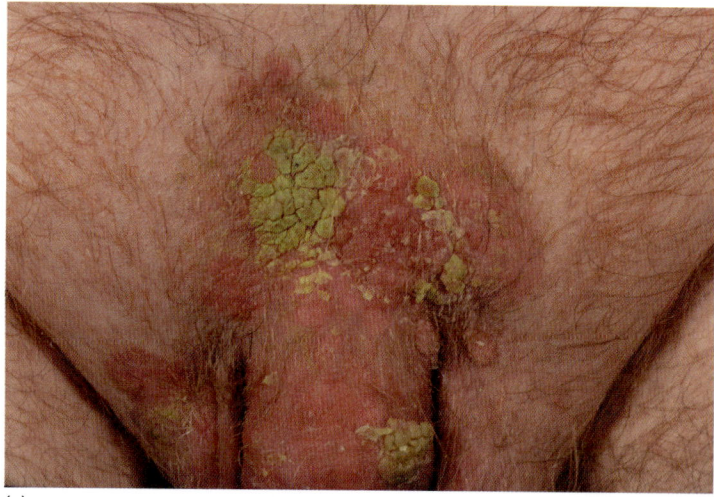

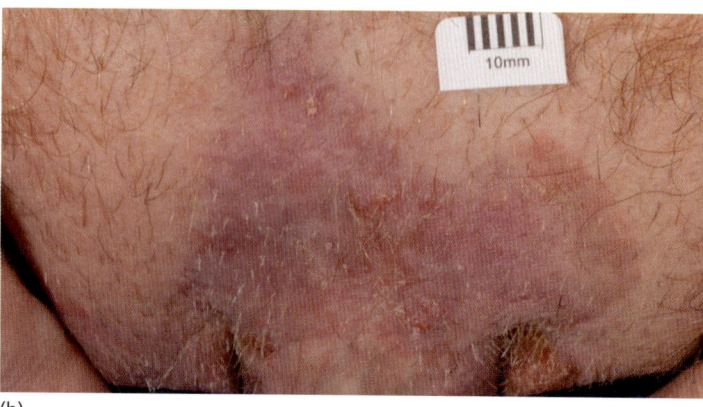

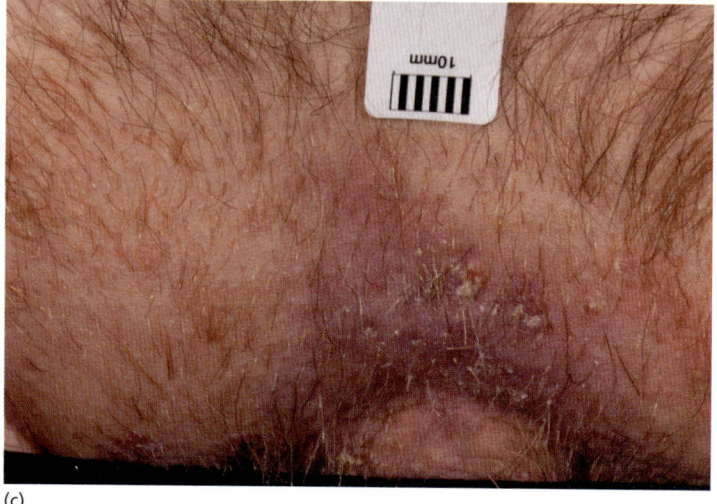

Figure 141.29 (a) Large confluent areas of bowenoid papulosis. (b) Following treatment for 6 weeks with 5% imiquimod cream. (c) Marked improvement seen at follow-up.

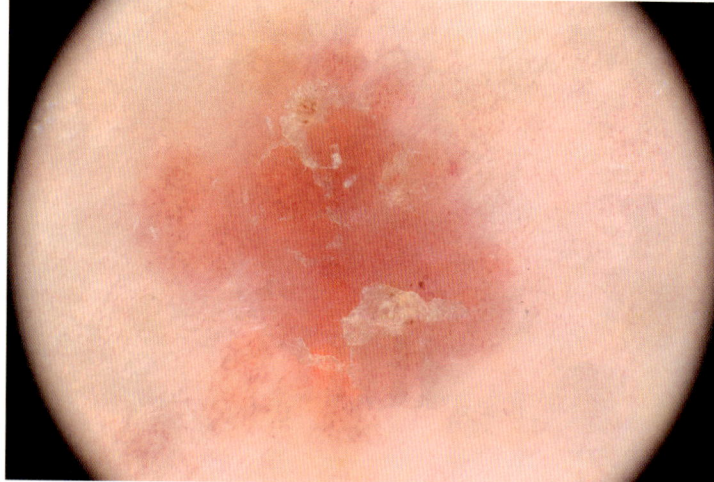

Figure 141.30 Dermoscopy of Bowen disease showing irregular erythematous base, mild hyperkeratosis with vascular structures throughout the lesion.

in BD, particularly the presence of vascular structures, which if persistent following topical treatment, suggests residual disease. Clearance of these structures correlates with clinical clearance and reappearance suggests recurrent disease [34] (Figure 141.30). Recently, dynamic optical coherence tomography has become a useful tool in the diagnosis of BD, especially when it comes to differentiating it from AK and SCC. Vascular shapes (so-called 'blobs') have been determined to be characteristic features of dynamic optical coherence tomography of BD [35].

Management

In most patients the diagnosis is made on clinical grounds aided by pathology where diagnosis has been in doubt. Advice on high factor broad spectrum sunscreen should be provided. There is a wide range of therapeutic options available for the treatment of BD (Table 141.5) [36]. The preferred treatment option is based on a number of factors including the size of the lesion, site, previous treatment, experience of the various treatments and number of lesions. Destructive therapies such as curettage and cautery or cryotherapy are widely used in clinical practice. Comparison of the relative effectiveness of different therapies and regimens is difficult as published studies do not fully control factors such as site and size and there are inconsistencies between treatment regimens used at different centres. A Cochrane review on treatment of BD concluded that specific recommendations for therapy could not be made on the current evidence [37]. In some cases, particularly with thin plaques and multiple co-morbidities, active surveillance may be a reasonable option [36].

First line

For solitary or for a small number of lesions on good healing sites, cryotherapy, curettage, topical 5% 5-fluorouracil, 5% imiquimod cream or PDT would be the treatments of choice (Table 141.5) [36]. Small lesions on poor healing sites could also be treated with these modalities or, if solitary, could be excised. PDT, topical 5% 5-fluorouracil or 5% imiquimod cream would be reasonable options for large lesions on poor healing sites (Table 141.5) (Figure 141.31) [36].

Cryotherapy. Cryotherapy using liquid nitrogen is a simple, inexpensive and quick method of treating BD (Figure 141.32). Clearance rates have varied widely probably reflecting differences in the techniques and regimens used, with failure rates in the order of 5–10% in the larger series. Cryotherapy using a single freeze–thaw

Table 141.5 Summary of the main treatment options for Bowen disease. The suggested scoring of the treatments listed takes into account the evidence for benefit, ease of application or time required for the procedure, wound healing, cosmetic result and current availability/costs of the method or facilities required. Evidence for interventions based on single studies or anecdotal cases is not included. Adapted from [36].

Lesion characteristics (small <2 cm)	Topical 5–fluorouracil	Topical imiquimod[b]	Cryotherapy	Curettage	Excision	PDT	Radiotherapy	Laser
Small, single/few, good healing[a]	3	3	2	1	3	3	5	4
Large, single, good healing[a]	3	3	3	4	5	2	4	–
Multiple, good healing[a]	2	3	2	3	5	3	4	4
Small, single/few, poor healing site[a]	2	2	3	2	2	2	5	–
Large, single, poor healing site[a]	3	2	5	4	5	1	6	–
Facial	3	3	4	2	4	3	4	–
Digital	3	3	4	5	2	3	3	3
Nail bed	–	4	–	–	2[c]	3	4	4
Penile	3	3	4	5	4[c]	3	3	3
Lesion in immunocompromised patients	5	4	3	3	4	3	–	–

[a] Clinician's perceived potential for good or poor healing at the affected site.
[b] Does not have a product licence for squamous cell carcinoma in situ.
[c] Consider micrographic surgery for tissue sparing or if poorly defined or recurrent.
Key:
1: Probably treatment of choice.
2: Generally good choice.
3: Generally fair choice.
4: Reasonable but not usually required.
5: Generally poor choice.
6: Probably should not be used.
–: Insufficient evidence available.

cycle (FTC) of 30 seconds, two FTCs of 20 seconds with a thaw period, or up to three single treatments of 20 seconds at intervals of several weeks have been reported [37–41]. However, such doses can cause significant discomfort and may cause ulceration.

In the largest, prospective open study, a single 30 second FTC on one to eight lesions, more than half of which were on the calf, achieved a clearance rate of 100% and recurrence rate of 0.8%, with follow-up periods ranging from 6 months to 5 years [39]. However, in a retrospective comparison study the use of a 20 second FTC on 91 lesions resulted in lower clearance rates of 68% after one treatment and 86% after retreatment of lesions [40]. It would appear from the existing literature that the more aggressive approach consisting of a freeze of 30 seconds at least once, or 20 seconds at least twice, yields better results, but the optimum freeze time, the number of freezes in one treatment cycle and the role of retreatment visits are not clear. Other complications include poor healing, the risk of ulceration particularly on the lower legs and hypopigmented scarring.

Curettage. Curettage and cautery is a simple, inexpensive method of treating BD, especially in patients who have large hyperkeratotic lesions, who are unable to tolerate cryotherapy and, due to oedematous legs, are at higher risk of ulceration, or those who are unable to apply topical therapy over a prolonged period. In a prospective but non-randomised trial of curettage and cautery (44 lesions) compared with cryotherapy (36 lesions) involving 67 patients with 74% of lesions on the lower leg, curettage was preferable in terms of pain, healing and recurrence rate [42]. Median time to healing with cryotherapy was 46 days (90 days on the lower leg), compared with 35 days (39 days on the lower leg) for curetted lesions, and reported pain was significantly greater with cryotherapy. Recurrences were more likely following cryotherapy (36%, 13/36) compared with curettage (9%, 4/44) during a median follow-up period of 2 years, although the cryotherapy regimen was less aggressive than in most other studies.

No treatment. As the lifetime risk of malignant transformation is low, in some patients with slowly progressive thin lesions, especially on the lower leg of elderly patients where healing is poor, there is an argument for observation rather than intervention. Patients should be trained to recognise changes in good time. They should also be advised to use regular emollients, which can help reduce scaling. Routine follow-up is generally not required but could be scheduled if there are any changes to the lesion.

5% 5-fluorouracil cream. This is a widely used treatment for multiple BD, but the number of treatment applications and the time durations vary. The typical regimen in current clinical use is once- or twice-daily application for 3–4 weeks, repeated if required. Topical 5% 5-fluorouracil cream, applied once daily for 1 week, then twice daily for 3 weeks, was compared with both MAL-PDT and cryotherapy in a large European multicentre randomised controlled trial [43]. At 3 months following the last treatment, 83% of lesions treated by 5% 5-fluorouracil cream showed complete response, compared with 93% with PDT and 86% with cryotherapy. Treatment may be difficult if patients are unable to apply the cream regularly and treatment may cause significant inflammation with the risk of ulceration.

5% imiquimod cream. There are a number of small case series of 5% imiquimod cream in the treatment of BD but the best evidence comes from a small randomised controlled trial demonstrating 73% histologically proven clearance with once-daily application for 16 weeks, compared with no response in the placebo group [44]. Imiquimod cream can cause marked inflammation but may be useful to treat multiple lesions on the lower legs.

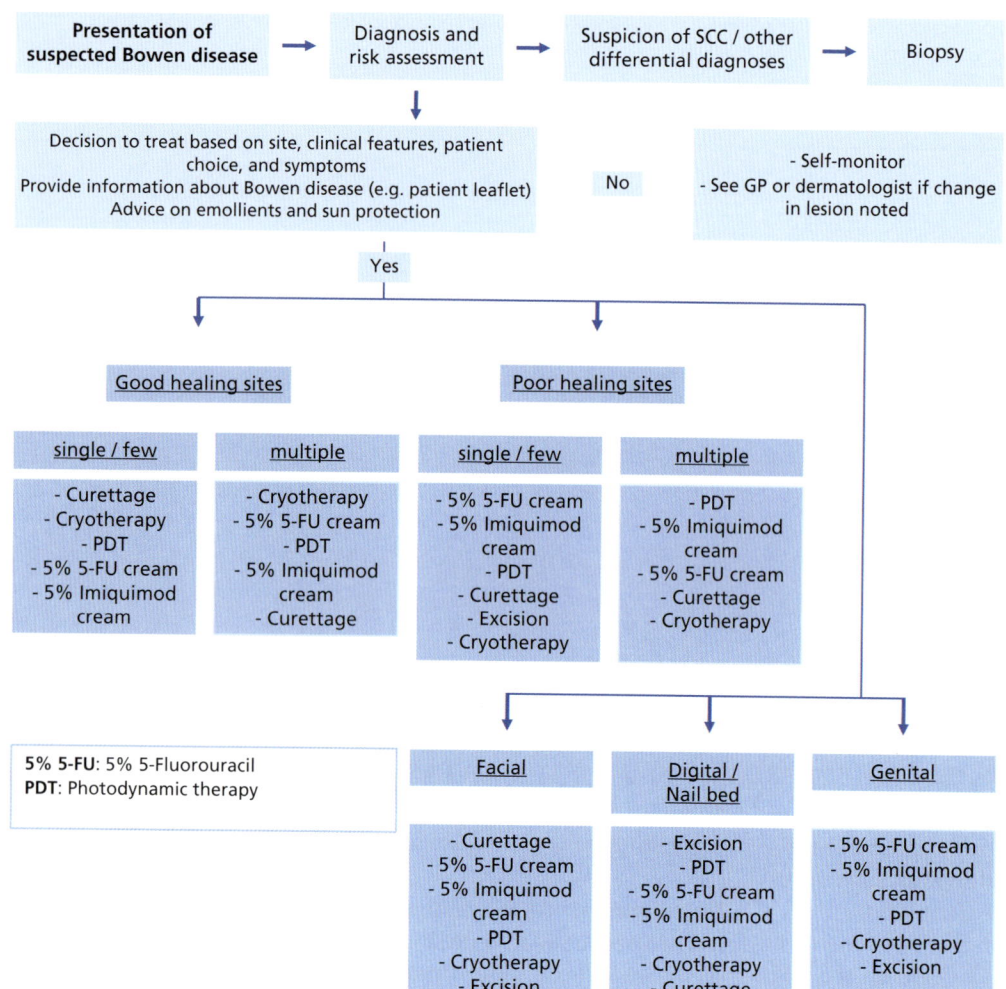

Figure 141.31 Bowen disease treatment algorithm.

Photodynamic therapy. PDT can be used to treat large multiple lesions on poor healing sites with less risk of side effects except pain. A multicentre randomised study comparing MAL-PDT with cryotherapy or 5% 5-fluorouracil cream in 225 patients with 275 BD lesions showed complete response rates of 93% for MAL-PDT, 86% for cryotherapy and 83% for 5% 5-fluorouracil cream. PDT gave superior cosmetic results compared with cryotherapy or 5% 5-fluorouracil [43]. However, PDT is an out-patient delivered treatment requiring hospital visits, time for lesion preparation and treatment, which may be difficult for some patients.

Second line
Radiotherapy using both high- and low-dose regimens has been reported with equal efficacy [45] but the evidence in trials remains poor. Impaired healing on the lower leg was observed in a large retrospective study [40]. The use of combination therapy has been reported but the studies included a small number of patients and were generally underpowered [36]. The evidence for treating BD of the nail unit and perianal region is poor but surgical techniques including margin-controlled excision are recommended due to the higher risk of malignant change.

Third line
There are case reports or case series of topical 3% diclofenac in 2.5% hyaluronic acid gel, phenol peels, 0.1% tazarotene gel and oral retinoids (acitretin) in the treatment of BD with varying degrees of success [36].

Resources

Further information

Bath-Hextall FJ, Matin RN, Wilkinson D, Leonardi-Bee J. Interventions for cutaneous Bowen's disease. *Cochrane Database Syst Rev* 2013;6:CD007281.

Morton CA, Birnie AJ, Eedy DJ. British Association of Dermatologists' guidelines for the management of squamous cell carcinoma in situ (Bowen's disease) 2014. *Br J Dermatol* 2014;170:245–60.

Riddel C, Rashid R, Thomas V. Ungual and periungual human papillomavirus associated squamous cell carcinoma: a review. *J Am Acad Dermatol* 2011;64:1147–53.

Anal, vulval, penile and perianal intraepithelial carcinoma (see Chapters 109, 110 and 111)

Definition and nomenclature
These conditions result from dysplasia of the intraepithelial portion of skin or mucosal surface. Classification depends on the amount and severity of dysplasia with a higher risk of malignant

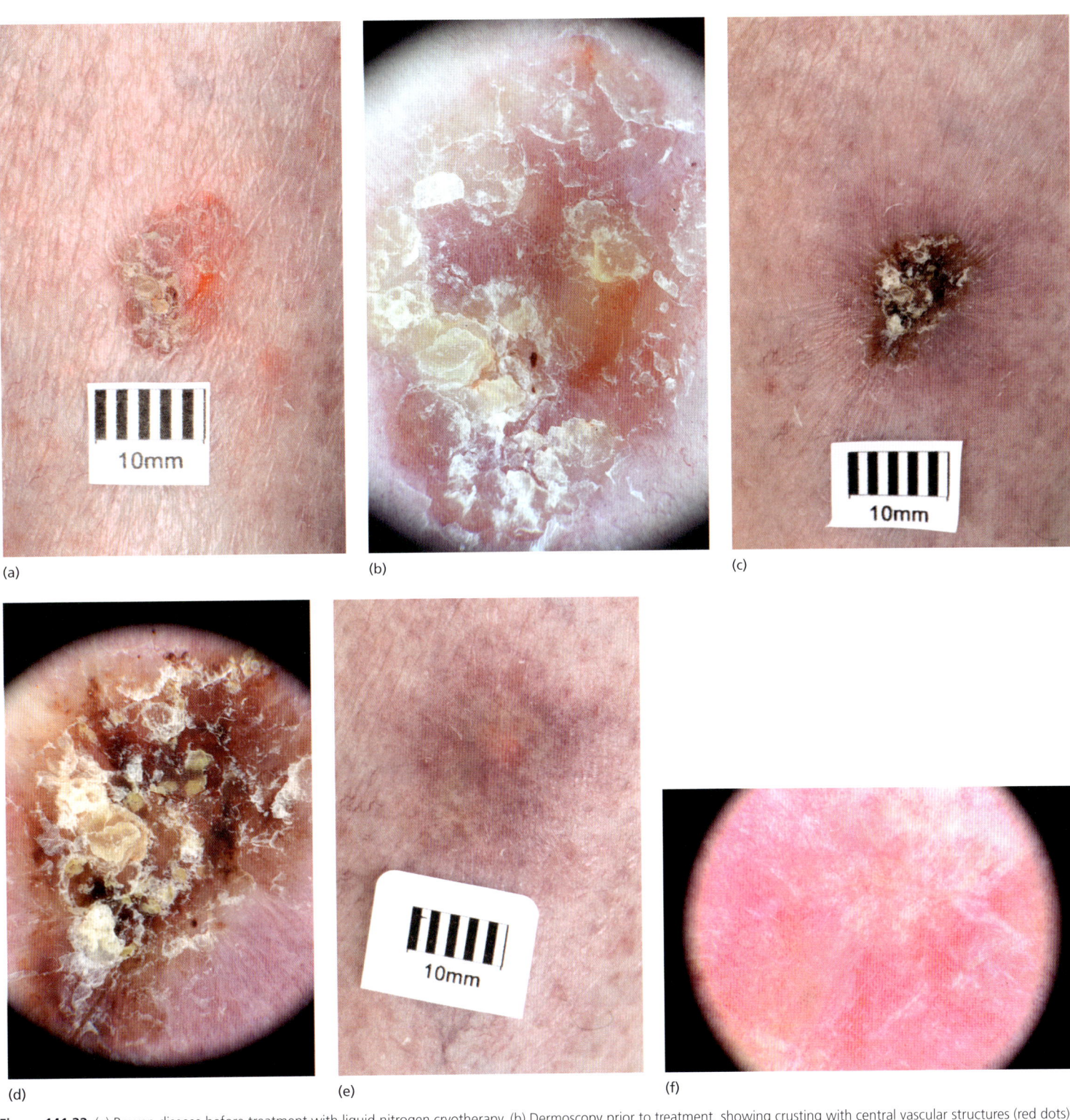

Figure 141.32 (a) Bowen disease before treatment with liquid nitrogen cryotherapy. (b) Dermoscopy prior to treatment, showing crusting with central vascular structures (red dots). (c) Inflammation following cryotherapy. (d) Dermoscopy showing marked crusting following cryotherapy. (e) Post-treatment showing clearance. (f) Dermoscopy showing clearance of lesion and central vascular structures (red dots).

transformation in severely dysplastic disease. These have recently been reclassified as non-HPV or HPV-associated squamous intraepithelial lesions (SIL) which are site specific [1].

> **Synonyms and inclusions**
> - Squamous intraepithelial lesions
> - Anal intraepithelial neoplasia
> - Vulval intraepithelial neoplasia
> - Penile intraepithelial neoplasia
> - Bowen disease
> - Bowenoid papulosis
> - Erythroplasia of Queyrat
> - In situ SCC

Introduction and general description

Anal intraepithelial dysplasia (anal SIL) can affect the perianal skin and anal canal. Anal SIL has been subdivided into low-grade SILs (anal LSIL; AIN-1) and high-grade SILs (anal HSIL; AIN-2, AIN-3) [2,3]. There is continuing discussion on AIN-2 grade and it is suggested that those positive with p16 should be upstaged to AIN-3 and those negative to AIN-1 [4]. Anal LSIL is now not considered to be a precursor of anal carcinoma but may progress to anal HSIL. Patients with anal LSIL may require multiple biopsies to confirm diagnosis and then observed if asymptomatic [5]. Patients with anal HSIL have an estimated long-term risk of malignant transformation in the range of 8.5–13% [6,7].

Vulval intraepithelial neoplasia (VIN) has also been subdivided into low risk (vulval LSIL; VIN-1), high risk (vulval HSIL; VIN-2, VIN-3) and differentiated-type VIN (dVIN) [8]. VIN-1 has been dropped from the classification as this rarely leads to invasive change. Most cases of vulval HSIL are of the 'usual' type (uVIN) with a rate of progression to SCC of 9–16% for untreated cases and 3% for treated cases. dVIN is non-HPV-related and occurs in older women, often associated with lichen sclerosus or lichen planus. It has a higher risk of progression to malignant transformation than HSIL [9,10].

Penile intraepithelial dysplasia (PeIN) is similar to VIN and has been subdivided into 'differentiated' and 'undifferentiated'. Differentiated PeIN is non-HPV-related, often associated with lichen sclerosus and tends to affect the mucosal surface of the foreskin. Undifferentiated PeIN is HPV-related and previously termed PeIN-3 [11]. Malignant transformation is estimated at 10–30% in untreated cases with SCCs being more common in differentiated disease [11,12].

Overall, genital intraepithelial neoplasia is strongly associated with HPV infection, mainly HPV-16 and HPV-18 types. Other risk factors include iatrogenic or acquired immunosuppression, chronic skin disease, i.e. genital lichen sclerosus or lichen planus, smoking and increased number of sexual partners, particularly in the HPV-associated group [13].

Treatment in low-risk disease may be simple observation but in cases where the risk is higher, there are a number of options depending on the extent, severity and co-morbidities. Surgery is generally performed to excise the tissue and so prevent local invasion. Other options include topical 5% 5-fluorouracil cream, 5% imiquimod cream, cryotherapy, PDT and laser ablation or diathermy [8,11,13].

Immunisation with the HPV vaccine has resulted in a decrease in the risk of developing genital warts and VIN [14]. In men who have sex with men, the use of the quadrivalent vaccine against HPV types 6, 11, 16 and 18 has led to a decrease in high-grade anal intraepithelial neoplasia and HPV infection 2 years after vaccination [15]. Administration of vaccines prior to sexual activity appears to provide the greatest benefit for prevention of AIN and anal carcinoma [16].

SQUAMOUS CELL CARCINOMA OF THE SKIN

Definition and nomenclature

SCC is a malignant tumour arising from epidermal keratinocytes or its appendages.

This section includes primary cutaneous SCC only. In general SCCs have a low rate of local, regional and distant spread. However, risk stratification is important as 'high-risk' SCCs carry greater risks of metastasis. This section aims to delineate the high-risk features of SCC and its management and prognosis. SCCs arising in genital areas from intraepidermal dysplasia are described separately.

> **Synonyms and inclusions**
> - Squamous cell epithelioma

Introduction and general description

Cutaneous SCC is a heterogeneous disease both in its aetiology and clinically, with different risk factors implicated in its development in different populations. The epidemiology of the disease has changed over the last 50 years, with a decrease in the importance of occupational exposure to chemical carcinogens and an increase in the proportion of cases caused by recreational sun exposure and an ageing population. In addition, diseases such as HIV infection, chronic lymphocytic leukaemia, PUVA therapy and therapeutic advances with the introduction of effective immunosuppressive therapies to prevent rejection of transplanted organs and targeted treatments for other cancers such as *BRAF* inhibitors for melanoma, have resulted in the emergence of new populations that are highly susceptible to SCC development.

Epidemiology

Incidence and prevalence

SCC is the second commonest skin cancer after BCC and worldwide its incidence has been increasing since 1960 [1]. National cancer registries generally exclude the registration of KC or record only the first tumour, so accurate figures for SCC are not available. Pooled data from England suggest an average annual incidence of SCC to be 22.65/100 000 person-years, with the lowest incidence in London (14.98/100 000 person-years) and the highest in south-west England (33.02/100 000 person-years), possibly reflecting variations in ethnicity [1]. The incidence in Wales has been reported to be between 15.1 and 19/100 000 person-year [2,3] and in Scotland the incidence rate has increased from 16.1 in 1979 to 36.9/100 000 person-years in 2003 [4]. The incidence is much higher in the USA and Australia with rates of 290 and 387/100 000 person-years, respectively [5,6]. The Netherlands Cancer Registry cohort study assessing the incidence of first SCC between 1989 and 2017 and multiple SCCs per patient diagnosed in 2017 showed that the incidence continues to increase, particularly in females. The European Standardised Rate (ESR) for first SCC increased from 40/100 000 person-years in 1989 to 107.6/100 000 person-years in 2017 in males and from 13.9/100 000 person-years to 68.7/100 000 person-years in 2017 in females. For those with multiple SCCs, the ESR increased by 58.4% in males and 34.8% in females with estimated further increases of 23% for males and 29.4% for females to the year 2027 [7]. With an increasingly ageing population, the workload of managing KC in the UK has been predicted to increase by 50% by 2030 [8]. In addition, OTRs, who are at an increased risk due to immunosuppression, are at a 153-fold excess risk for developing SCC and dying from it compared with the general population [9].

Age
The incidence of SCC increases with age. Data from the Swedish National Cancer Registry has shown that the age-adjusted incidence is highest in males and females aged ≥85 years (26.9/100 000 person-years) as compared with an incidence of 4.02/100 000 person-years in those who are ≤64 years and 9.0/100 000 person-years in those aged 65–84 years, with SCC occurring on both, light-exposed and covered sites [10].

Sex
Males are more at risk of developing SCC, possibly due to outdoor employment and differences in sun avoidance behaviour than females [10,11]. SCC incidence has increased in males and females on both covered and light-exposed sites but the overall increase has generally been greater in females [7,10,11]. Males develop more SCCs on the head and neck than females [12].

Ethnicity
SCC is predominantly a disease of white populations and is especially prevalent in this group in areas of high ambient sun exposure [12,13]. Although the incidence is low in non-white populations, SCC is still the most common skin cancer in these populations but shows differences in the anatomical location of the tumours, recognised aetiological factors and prognosis [14]. Factors implicated in the pathogenesis of cutaneous malignancy in Africans and African Americans include trauma, albinism, burn scars, ionising radiation, chronic inflammation and chronic discoid lupus erythematosus [14]. There is a high incidence of SCC in Nigerian people with albinism, but no evidence of an increased incidence in vitiliginous skin of black people [15].

Associated diseases
Patients may present with other UVR-induced skin cancers and full examination of the skin should be undertaken. Precursor lesions such as AK or BD may often be present and patients are more susceptible to developing other UVR-induced skin cancers. A population-based Dutch cohort study assessing the incidence of SCC *in situ* and subsequent risk of developing SCC compared with the general population, from 1989 to 2017, showed an increasing incidence of SCC *in situ*, highest in 2017 (71.7 cases per 100 000 person-years for females and 540.9 cases per 100 000 person-years for males aged 80 years and older), with the most common site affected being the face in females (15.9 cases per 100 000 person-years) and scalp and/or neck in males (12.3 cases per 100 000 person-years). After 5-year follow-up, there was a significant difference in those with SCC *in situ* compared with the general population developing SCC, with a cumulative risk of 11.7% (95% CI 11.6–11.9%) in males and 6.9% (95% CI 6.8–7.0%) in females [16].

Pathophysiology
A complex network of genetic and epigenomic alterations along with dysregulated molecular pathways have been implicated in SCC development. SCC carries a high mutational burden and classical tumour suppressor genes (tumour protein 53 (*TP53*), NOTCH1, NOTCH2, CDKN2A and FAT1) are consistently mutated in SCC (Figure 141.33) [17]. *TP53* located on chromosome 17p13.1 is a tumour suppressor gene, which helps to repair cells when DNA is damaged by UVR and causes cell apoptosis when the damage cannot be repaired. Mutations of *TP53* caused by UVR leading to pyrimidine dimers are frequently seen in AK and approximately 90% of SCCs [18,19]. The vast majority of *TP53* mutations are C>T and CC>TT tandem double transition mutations, considered the 'mutational signature' of UV exposure [20]. These mutations have a strong tendency to occur at methylated cytosines and studies have shown that this methylation process increases the frequency of UVB-induced cyclobutane pyrimidine dimer formation by 1.7-fold, confirming that methylation per se influences the probability of cell damage [21]. These altered DNA methylation patterns are considered to be a classic hallmark of cancer [22] and studies using high-resolution methylation profiles analysing methylomes of SCC have shown two distinct subgroups, defined by stem cell-like and keratinocyte-like methylation patterns with similar results seen in AK, suggesting that AK and SCC arise from two different cell types of origin, likely to be from two (or more) differentiation stages of epidermal stem cells [23].

Somatic mutations of NOTCH receptors (NOTCH1 and NOTCH2) have been implicated in about 75% of SCCs. Most NOTCH mutations in SCCs result from a G>A transition induced by UVR after homozygous *TP53* loss, consistent with evidence of its role in tumour progression [24,25].

p16 is also a tumour suppressor protein encoded by the *CDKN2A* gene in the 9p21 region. It is involved in the arrest of the cell cycle at G1, suppressing the entry into the S phase. p16 mutations can also be caused by UVR [26]. Inactivation of p16 leads to continuous cell cycling and it is thought that inactivated p16 advances AK to SCC [27].

Whole exome sequencing studies have shown several chromosomal abnormalities that are shared between AK and SCC, including losses at chromosome 3p, 5q, 8q, 9p, 11p, 13q, 17p and 18p. However, there are molecular differences between them with SCC having more complex karyotypes with higher intra-sample heterogeneity [28,29]. When compared with AK, there were more mutations found in immune-related and TGFβ signalling pathways [29].

Signalling pathways implicated in SCC include RAS-RAF-MEK-ERK and P13K/AKT/mTOR cascades (Figure 141.34) [30].

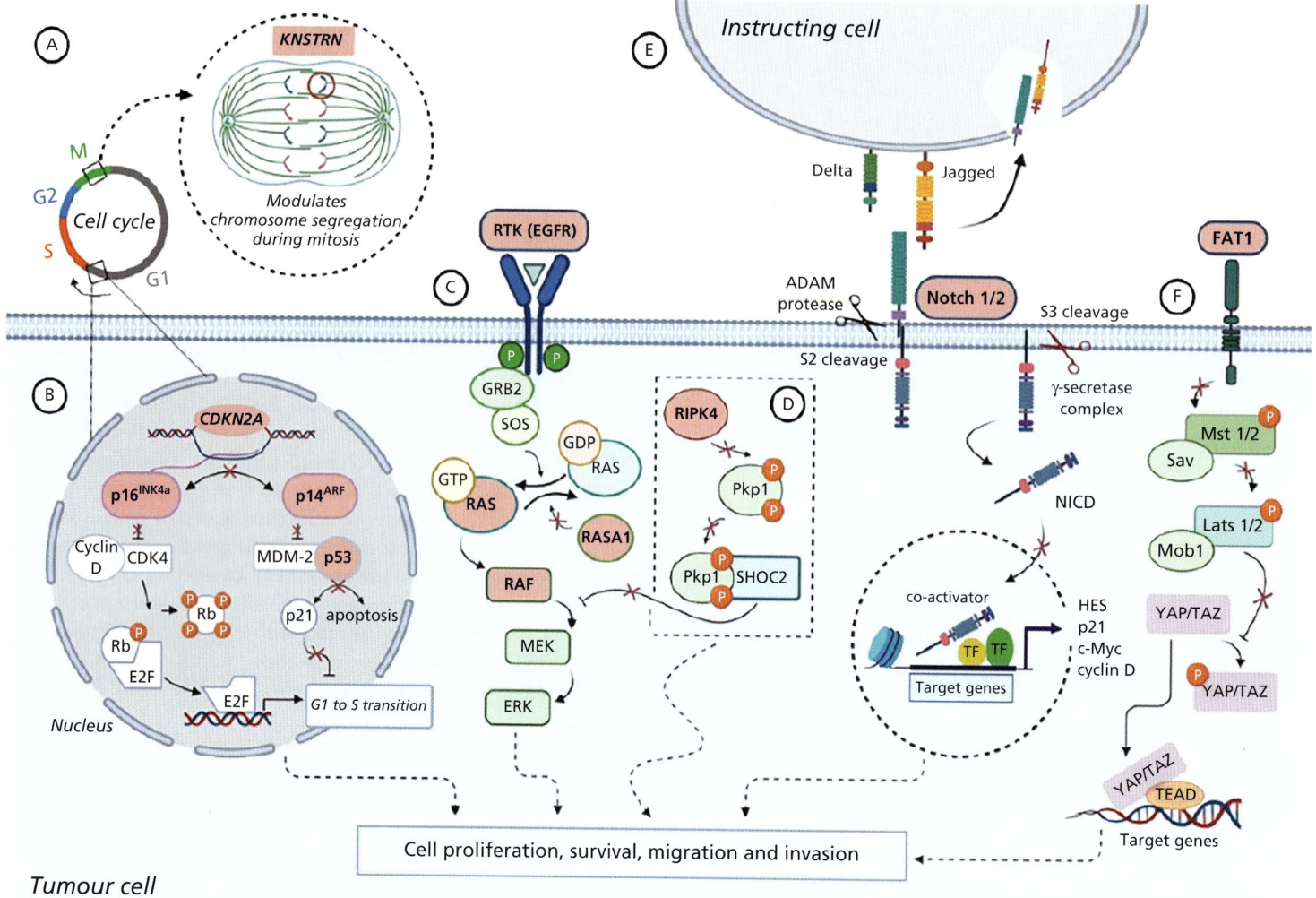

Figure 141.33 Molecular alterations that drive cutaneous squamous cell carcinoma (cSCC) proliferation, survival and metastasis through aberrant signalling (highlighted in pink). (A) Alterations in KNSTRN expression promote abnormal chromosome segregation during mitosis. (B) CDKN2A encodes for cell-cycle regulatory proteins p16^{INK4A} and p14^{ARF}, involved in retinoblastoma (RB) and p53 pathways. Loss of heterozygosity (LOH), mutations or deletions of CDKN2A leads to functional loss of: (i) p16^{INK4A}, which allows phosphorylation of RB by CDK4-Cyclin D complex and release of E2F transcription factors, that can then transcribe S phase promoting genes; (ii) p14^{ARF}, which allows MDM-2 to bind p53 and inhibit apoptosis. (C) Activating mutations in EGFR, RAS and RAF or inactivation of negative regulator RASA1 promotes cell proliferation and survival through constitutive activation of MAPK pathway. (D) Proposed model for RIPK4 action in skin carcinogenesis that depicts the phosphorylation of PKP1 by RIPK4, which promotes binding to scaffold protein SHOC2 and blocking of RAS/MAPK signalling. In the absence of functional RIPK4, the complex cannot assemble and the signalling pathway remains active, thus facilitating SCC development. (E) Inactive precursor is cleaved in the Golgi by a furin-like convertase (S1 cleavage) and translocated into the cell membrane, where binding of a NOTCH ligand (Delta, Jagged) to the receptor induces the second cleavage (S2) by a member of the disintegrin and metalloproteinases (ADAM) family. This results in a formation of a membrane-tethered NOTCH truncated fragment, which is further cleaved (S3) by a presenilin-dependent γ-secretase complex, generating the NOTCH intracellular domain (NICD). The active form of the NOTCH receptor (NICD) can now enter into the nucleus, where it exerts its transcriptional activity. Inactivation of NOTCH 1/2 favours SCC progression. However, the specific functional significance of this mutation has yet to be described. (F) The molecular mechanisms that contribute to tumour development in the context of FAT1 functional loss are poorly understood in SCC. However, a model proposed for HNSCC suggests FAT1 acts as a scaffold for Hippo kinases, favouring the activation of the complex and the phosphorylation of YAP, which is sequestered in the cytoplasm or degraded. Absence of FAT1 dismantles the Hippo core complex leading to YAP dephosphorylation and its translocation to the nucleus, where it interacts with TEAD to induce the expression of genes promoting tumour progression. Reproduced from [17]/Public Domain/MDPI.

RAS-RAF-MEK-ERK signalling cascade represents the mitogen-activated protein kinase (MAPK) pathway and animal models have shown that MAPK [31] along with a number of other pathways, including *HRAS* [32], Wnt/β-catenin/TCF [33] and STAT3 [34] are either mutated or activated resulting in SCC formation. *HRAS* mutations are uncommon in human SCC at a frequency of 3–30% but *HRAS* mutated stem cells are found in human skin, demonstrated by the fact that patients with melanoma treated with *BRAF* (V-raf murine sarcoma viral oncogene homologue B1) inhibitor, vemurafenib, develop *Ras*-mutated (mostly *HRAS* codon 61) KA and SCC within several weeks after starting treatment [32]. Another mechanism of controlling *TP53* function in human SCC is through the aberrant activation of epidermal growth factor receptor (EGFR) and *Fyn*, a Src-family tyrosinase kinase (*SFK*). These kinases downregulate *TP53* mRNA and protein levels through a c-Jun-dependent mechanism [35,36]. The oncogene *PIK3CA* was found to be mutated in nearly 50% of SCCs and activating mutations in this gene result in the activation of the P13K/AKT/mTOR pathway [29] which is commonly found in other organ SCCs [37].

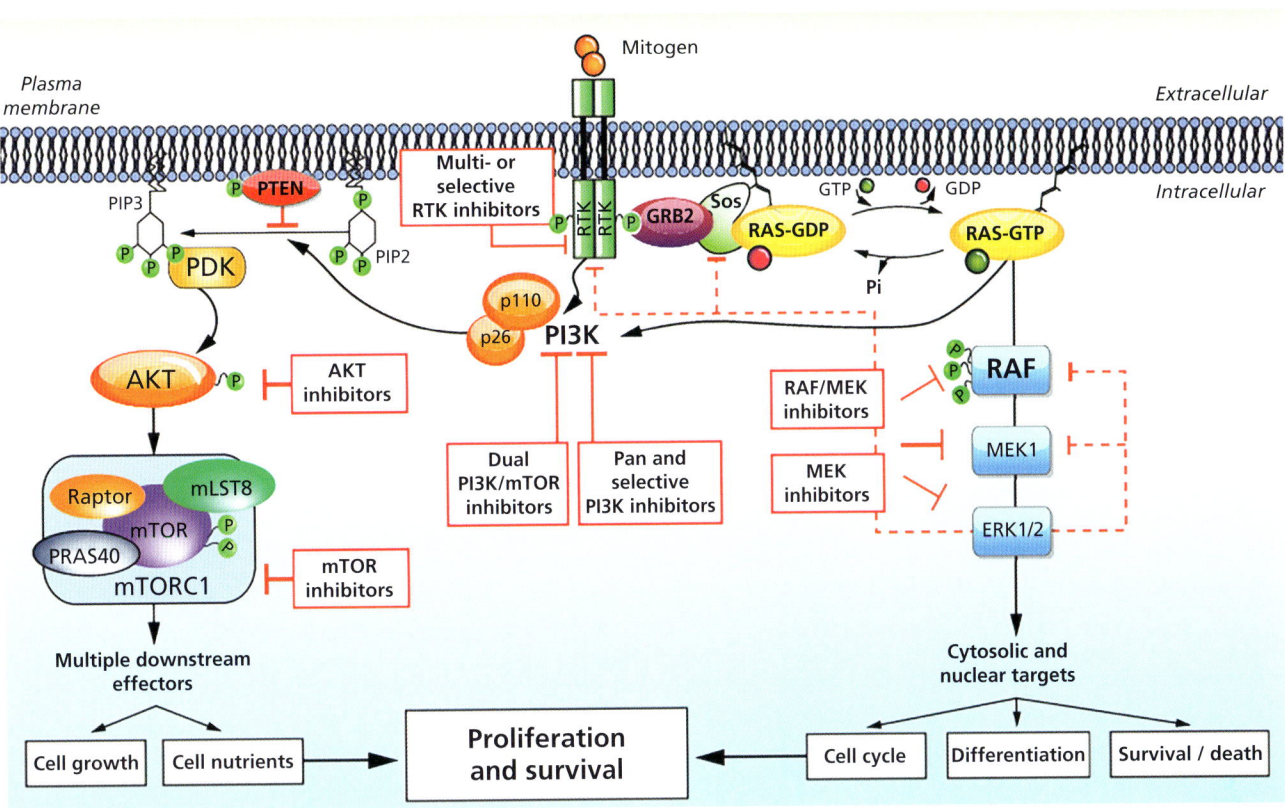

Figure 141.34 The interconnected signalling network between MAPK and PI3K/AKT pathways via sharing inputs like tyrosinase kinase receptors (RTK) and RAS. The PI3K catalytic subunit exhibits a Ras-binding motif that stimulates optimal kinase activity following Ras-activated protein linkage. Thus, either MAPK/ERK or PI3K pathways can be activated by mutant RAS as part of a compensatory mechanism that could drive resistance to therapeutic targeting strategies Reproduced from [30] with permission from John Wiley & Sons.

Predisposing factors

Immunosuppression in OTRs or patients on azathioprine or ciclosporin have an increased risk of developing SCC [9,38] (see Chapter 147). The SCC risk in OTRs is determined by the age at transplantation, duration of transplant, level of immunosuppression and previous solar damage. The normal ratio of BCC:SCC is reversed and SCC is more common. The lesions are most numerous on light-exposed sites and are frequently multiple. They may clinically be deceptively banal and resemble either a KA or AK. All such lesions should be regarded with suspicion in OTRs and biopsied to establish their true nature. Patients with compromised immunity such as haematological malignancy, chronic lymphocytic leukaemia or HIV are also at an increased risk of developing multiple tumours which may display a more aggressive behaviour [39].

SCC is an uncommon complication of longstanding chronic ulceration and post-radiation [40]. SCC may also be associated with other diseases such as hidradenitis suppurativa [41], morphoea [42], lymphoedema [43], Hailey–Hailey disease [44] and recessive dystrophic epidermolysis bullosa [45].

Pathology

Invasive SCC begins when atypical keratinocytes breach the epidermal basement membrane and invade the dermis (Figure 141.35). Differentiation from precursor lesions is thus architectural rather than cytological and is based on the presence of either descending strands of morphologically malignant keratinocytes or single atypical keratinocytes, which can no longer be regarded as distorted interpapillary ridges. The distinction may be further complicated by the phenomenon of pseudoepitheliomatous hyperplasia, which may occur at an ulcer margin or over certain inflammatory or neoplastic states in the dermis.

Histological variants of SCC have been described: classic/no special type, acantholytic, spindle cell, desmoplastic, basaloid, verrucous, pseudovascular and follicular.

The classic/no special type is the most common variant. The cells of SCC vary from large, polygonal cells with vesicular nuclei, prominent nucleoli and an abundant cytoplasm, overt evidence of keratinisation and well-developed intercellular bridges (well-differentiated lesions) to pleomorphic cells which provide no clear cytological evidence of their origin (poorly differentiated lesions). Histological grading of the differentiation of the tumour is required, as it guides the pathological staging, prognosis and treatment options. The Royal College of Pathologists (RCPath UK) recommends that the degree of differentiation of an individual tumour is recorded according to the worst component identified within the lesion regardless of the proportion of the tumour that displays those characteristics [46].

The possibility of metastatic SCCs (not necessarily cutaneous) should be considered when an *in situ* component is not identified.

The histological diagnosis of some poorly differentiated SCCs and these variants (particularly the spindle cell variant) relies on the identification of *in situ* tumour and expression of cytokeratin markers by the tumour cells on immunohistochemistry.

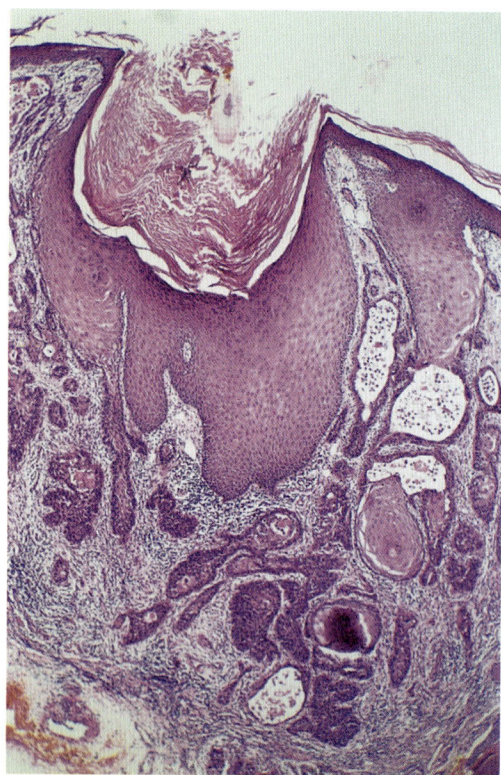

Figure 141.35 Pathological features of well-differentiated, early invasive squamous cell carcinoma, showing differentiated keratinocytes invading the underlying dermis.

KA is a matter of controversy in dermatopathology. For some it is a subtype of SCC. There are no reliable histological features to distinguish between KA and early invasive well-differentiated SCC with a crater-like architecture. The current recommendation from the RCPath UK is to record lesions with a KA-like morphology as KA-like SCC and lesions should be managed as well-differentiated SCC [46].

The histopathological report of excision specimens for SCC should include macroscopic diameter, tumour type, grade of differentiation, tumour thickness, level of invasion, perineural invasion (PNI), lymphovascular invasion, excision margins and pathological stage.

Causative organisms

HPV infection plays an important role in the development of SCC and β-HPV types are present in significant numbers, although the precise mechanism by which HPV infection contributes to SCC development is not fully understood. There is an excess risk of SCC associated with all β-HPV types and this risk increases with increasing number of β types that are present. In particular, the viral E6 and E7 oncoproteins from some cutaneous β-HPV types exert transforming activities. It has been demonstrated that these β-HPV types can alter the networks regulated by the tumour suppressor gene products retinoblastoma (pRb) and p53, leading to loss of cell cycle control, apoptosis and DNA repair. Moreover, β-HPV E6 oncoprotein has been shown to deregulate the Notch signalling pathway. In association with UV radiation, these oncoproteins block UV-induced apoptosis and promote cellular proliferation. This highlights the role of cutaneous β-HPV types in the initiation of carcinogenesis but not in its maintenance (the 'hit-and-run' theory)

[47,48]. Besides this oncogenic effect of HPV, the loss of T cell immunity against cutaneous β-HPV in the immunocompromised has been demonstrated to contribute to an increased risk of AK and SCC [49].

Genetics

Patients with Fitzpatrick skin types I and II, particularly those with freckling, high UVR exposure and on immunosuppression are most at risk [50].

Environmental factors

Most SCCs develop on the light-exposed areas of the head and neck, and the cumulative lifetime exposure to UVR from sunlight and artificial tanning lamps strongly correlates with the development of SCC [51,52].

Clinical features
History

The most common sites for SCC are those most exposed to the sun. They occur on the backs of the hands and forearms, the upper part of the face and, especially in males, on the lower lip and pinna.

The evolution of SCC is usually faster than that of BCC but is generally slower than that of KA, which may attain the same size in as many weeks as SCC does in months. Often these are solitary nodules which may be tender on palpation.

Presentation

SCCs often arise in photodamaged skin (Figures 141.36 and 141.37). The first clinical evidence of malignancy is induration. The area may

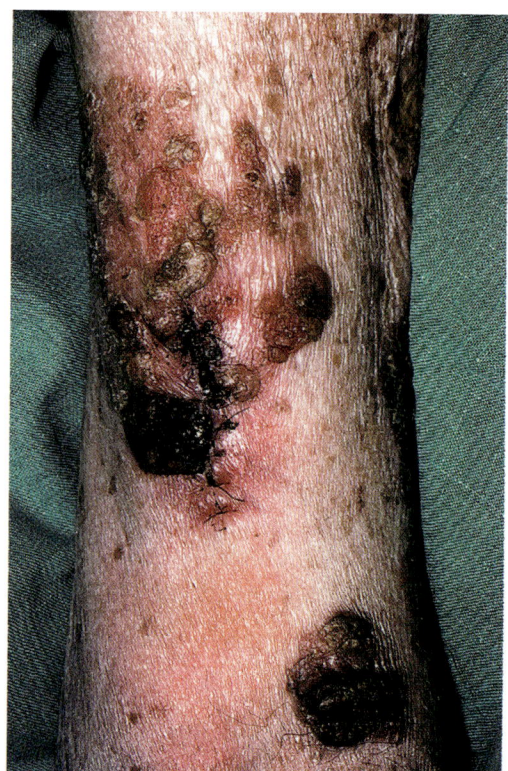

Figure 141.36 Multiple invasive squamous cell carcinomas in a patient with a history of exposure to arsenic.

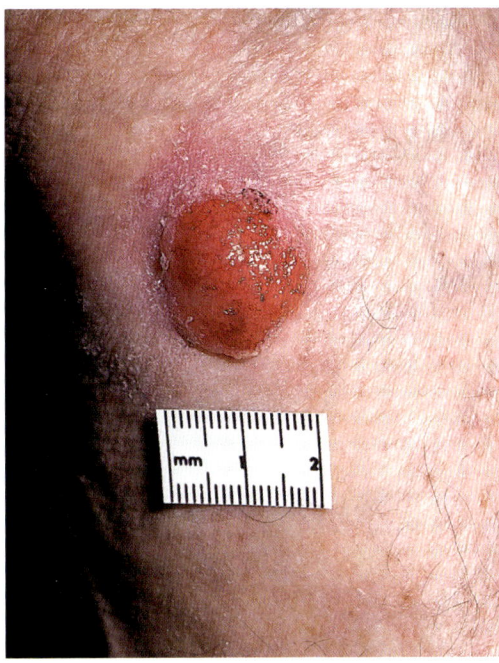

Figure 141.37 Raised erythematous invasive squamous cell carcinoma in an elderly patient on a light-exposed site.

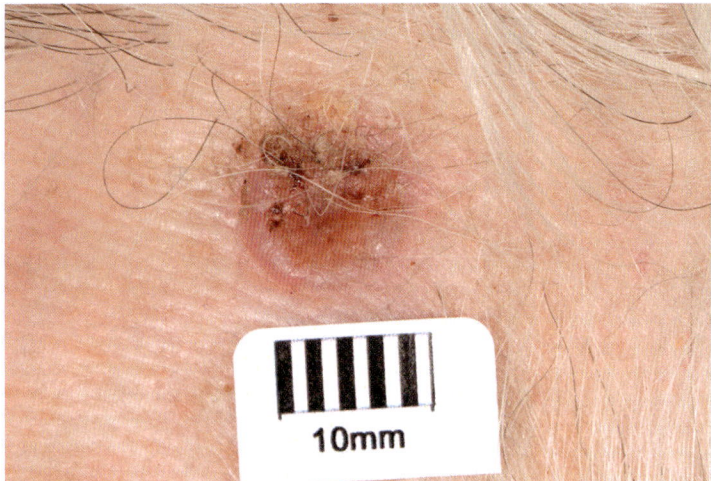

Figure 141.38 Well-differentiated squamous cell carcinoma with even circumscribed edge and central crusting.

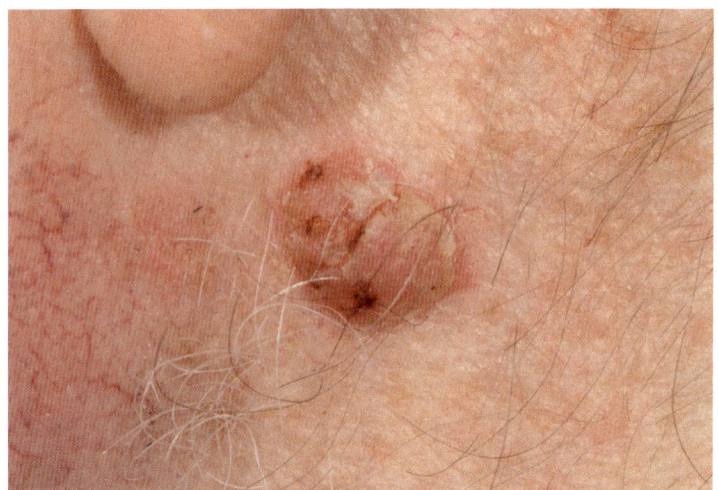

Figure 141.39 Seborrhoeic keratosis mimicking squamous cell carcinoma.

be plaque-like, verrucous, tumid or ulcerated, but in all cases the lesion feels firm when pressed between the finger and thumb. The limits of the induration are not sharp and usually extend beyond the visible margin of the lesion. The resistance to pressure is much greater than that given by an inflammatory lesion or benign epithelial hyperplasia.

The tissue around the tumour is inflamed and the edge is an opaque yellowish red colour. The better-differentiated tumours are usually papillomatous and are capped by a keratotic crust in the earlier stages. This may be shed later to reveal an ulcer or eroded tumour with an indurated margin and a purulent exuding surface that bleeds rather easily. The outline may be rounded, but is often irregular, and in premalignant lesions the induration and elevation is often asymmetrical at first. On mobile structures such as the lip or genitalia the presenting sign may be a fissure or small erosion or ulcer which fails to heal and bleeds recurrently.

Clinical variants
Verrucous carcinoma of the foot has been called epithelioma cuniculatum. This is a slow-growing well-differentiated SCC which rarely metastasises [53]. The tumour is characterised by an exophytic verruciform appearance; however, it may exhibit hyperkeratosis, ulceration or a malodorous discharge [53]. The aetiology of verrucous carcinoma is unknown but it can develop in areas of chronic inflammation. HPV has been associated with this tumour and specifically HPV types 11 and 16 have been described in plantar lesions [54,55].

Differential diagnosis
The indurated well-differentiated SCC arising in photodamaged skin is usually easily diagnosed (Figure 141.38). Typical KA have a faster rate of growth and involute to leave a scar. AK tend to be multiple and lack a dermal component on palpation. BCC, amelanotic melanoma and skin metastases from internal malignancy may resemble a SCC. Warty lesions such as viral warts or seborrhoeic keratoses (Figure 141.39) are not indurated and are frequently multiple. SCC on the lip may be mistaken for oral HSV and unsuccessfully treated with antivirals.

Classification of severity
SCC has a low rate of metastasis of about 5% [56]. Low-grade tumours carry an excellent prognosis but the risk of developing metastasis increases significantly in a SCC displaying 'high-risk' features [57]. SCCs are classified as low-risk, high-risk and very high-risk based on their clinical, pathological, tumour-nodes-metastasis (TNM) staging and margin criteria [58]. Figure 141.40 shows factors associated with poor disease outcome and guidance on referral to multidisciplinary teams (MDT) as well as follow-up [58].

Staging systems should reliably stratify patients according to their risk of developing local and/or disseminated disease. There are three main staging systems currently used: The American Joint Committee on Cancer 8 (AJCC8) [59], the Union for International Cancer Control 8 (UICC8) [60] and the Brigham and Women's Hospital (BWH) criteria [61], with the UICC8 staging system

	Low risk	High risk	Very high risk
Tumour factors	Tumour diameter ≤20 mm (= pT1) Tumour thickness ≤4 mm Invasion into dermis No perineural invasion Well differentiated or moderately differentiated histology No lymphovascular invasion (ALL ABOVE FACTORS SHOULD APPLY to denote a low-risk tumour)	Diameter >20–40 mm (= pT2) Thickness >4–6 mm Invasion into subcutaneous fat Perineural invasion present – dermal only; nerve diameter <0.1 mm Poorly differentiated histology Lymphovascular invasion Tumour site ear or lip Tumour arising within scar or area of chronic inflammation (ANY SINGLE FACTOR denotes a high-risk tumour)	Diameter >40 mm (= pT3) Thickness >6 mm Invasion beyond subcutaneous fat Any bone invasion Perineural invasion present in named nerve; nerve ≥0.1 mm; or nerve beyond dermis High-grade histological subtype – adenosquamous, desmoplastic, spindle/sarcomatoid/metaplastic In-transit metastasis (ANY SINGLE FACTOR denotes a very high-risk tumour)
Margin status	Clear pathology margins in all dimensions (≥1 mm)	One of more involved or close (<1 mm) pathology margin in a pT1 tumour. Close pathology margins (<1 mm) in a pT2 tumour.	One or more involved or close (<1 mm) pathology margin in a high-risk tumour
Patient factors	Immune-competent	Iatrogenic immunosuppression or biological therapies; frailty and/or comorbidities likely to cause some degree of immune compromise; HIV infection stabilised on HAART	AS FOR HIGH-RISK especially solid organ transplant recipients; haematological malignancies such as chronic lymphocytic leukaemia or myelofibrosis; other significant immunosuppression.
Referral to MDT (Scotland has no LSMDT / SSMDT division)	LSMDT discussion not needed	LSMDT discussion of patients with close or involved pathology margins; if margins are not involved other factors alone may not require LSMDT discussion unless more than one factor pertains. Patient factors increase risk, but do not mandate LSMDT discussion in absence of tumour risk factors.	SSMDT discussion should be considered for all patients with very high-risk tumours except those which require straightforward standard surgical excision. A referral to or opinion from an appropriate site-specific MDT may be required to ensure the best management.
Follow-up	Follow-up in secondary care not needed after single post-treatment appointment, where appropriate. Full skin check, examination of regional lymph node basin, discussion of diagnosis and patient education. This may take place before the histological diagnosis. Patient education about sun protection and skin surveillance is advised. Patients and their GPs should be informed of the risk of further cSCCs. There is a 40% risk of a further keratinocyte cancer within 5 years. If this is suspected, refer via the 2-week wait pathway.	4-monthly for 12 months (+ 6-monthly for the second year) especially if several risk factors apply. Full skin check examination of regional lymph node basin.* discussion of diagnosis and patient education. Advise patient education about sun protection and skin surveillance. Patients with more than one prior keratinocyte carcinomas have an 80% risk of a further keratinocyte cancer within 5 years.	4-monthly for 2 years and 6-monthly for a third year. Full skin check, examination of regional lymph node basin,* discussion of diagnosis and patient education. Advise patient education about sun protection and skin surveillance. Patients with more than one prior keratinocyte carcinomas have an 80% risk of a further keratinocyte cancer within 5 years.

Figure 141.40 Guidance for referral to local skin cancer multidisciplinary teams (LSMDTs) and specialist skin cancer multidisciplinary teams (SSMDTs). This referral guidance relates to primary cutaneous squamous cell carcinoma (cSCC), where treatment has been excisional surgery with curative intent. Factors associated with risk of poor disease-related outcomes (local recurrence, nodal metastasis, disease-specific death) in multiple studies using univariate or multivariate analysis. Reproduced from [58] with permission from John Wiley & Sons. GP, general practitioner; HAART, highly active antiretroviral therapy; HIV, human immunodeficiency virus; MDT, multidisciplinary team.

(Tables 141.6 and 141.7) being adopted by UK dermatologists and pathologists as AJCC8 covers head and neck SCC only. The BWH staging system showed that of all the high-risk features reported, four were more accurate in predicting tumour spread, when compared with AJCC7 and UICC7 staging systems (Table 141.8) [61]. Further comparative work performed by the same group has confirmed these findings, with the addition of PNI with a calibre size of ≥0.1 mm [62]. Population-based studies are now required to validate these findings against UICC8 criteria.

These staging systems, although widely used, have limited positive predictive value in identifying those at greatest risk of developing metastases. The gene expression profile (GEP) of primary cutaneous SCC with known outcomes has been used to develop and validate the 40-GEP test for predicting risk of metastasis from localised high-risk SCC, based on BWH metastasis risk: class 1 (low risk), class 2A (high risk), and class 2B (highest risk). The 3-year metastasis-free survival rates were 91.4%, 80.6% and 44.0%, respectively. A positive predictive value of 60% was achieved for the highest-risk group (class 2B), which is an improvement over current staging systems. A negative predictive value, sensitivity and specificity were shown to be comparable to current AJCC8 and BWH staging systems [63].

Complications and co-morbidities

SCC will generally progress by local invasion if left untreated, leading to metastasis. If diagnosis or treatment are delayed, the resultant surgery to excise the tumour may result in large scars or skin grafts on cosmetically visual sites. In some patients, multiple or large tumours may develop, requiring extensive surgery.

Disease course and prognosis

SCCs, in the absence of high-risk features, carry an excellent prognosis and following definitive treatment patients may be discharged from regular hospital follow-up after one visit [38,57,58]. SCCs with high-risk features (Figures 141.41 and 141.42) have a greater potential for local invasion and to develop metastases. In a

Table 141.6 TNM8 (tumour-nodes-metastasis) classification for cutaneous squamous cell carcinoma (SCC). Reproduced from [60] with permission from John Wiley & Sons.

T categories

T1	≤2 cm in greatest dimension
T2	>2–4 cm in greatest dimension
T3	>4 cm in greatest dimension or minor bone erosion or specified perineural invasion (≥0.1 mm in diameter and/or deeper than the dermis and/or a named nerve) or deep invasion (thickness >6 mm and/or beyond the subcutaneous fat)
T4a	Tumour with gross cortical bone/marrow invasion
T4b	Tumour with skull base or axial skeleton invasion including foraminal involvement and/or vertebral foramen involvement to the epidural space

N categories for non-head and neck

N1	Metastasis in a single node ≤3 cm in greatest dimension
N2	Metastasis in a single ipsilateral lymph node >3 cm but ≤6 cm or in multiple ipsilateral nodes with none >6 cm in greatest dimension
N3	Metastasis in a lymph node >6 cm in greatest dimension

N categories for head and neck region

N1	Metastasis in a single ipsilateral lymph node ≤3 cm in greatest dimension without ENE*
N2a	Metastasis in a single ipsilateral lymph node >3 cm but <6 cm in greatest dimension without ENE
N2b	Metastasis in multiple ipsilateral lymph nodes, where none are >6 cm in greatest dimension without ENE
N2c	Metastasis in bilateral or contralateral lymph nodes, where none are >6 cm in greatest dimension without ENE
N3a	Metastasis in a single or multiple lymph nodes >6 cm in greatest dimension without ENE
N3b	Metastasis in a single or multiple lymph nodes with ENE

M categories

M0	No distant metastasis
M1	Distant metastasis (including contralateral nodes in non-head and neck cSCC)

[a] Extranodal extension (ENE) can be clinical or pathological.

Table 141.7 TNM8 (tumour-nodes-metastasis) stage groups for cutaneous squamous cell carcinoma (SCC). Reproduced from [60] with permission from John Wiley & Sons.

Stage	T	N	M
I	T1	N0	M0
II	T2	N0	M0
III	T3	N0	M0
	T1, T2, T3	N1	M0
IVA	T1, T2, T3	N2, N3	M0
	T4	Any N	M0
IVB	Any T	Any N	M1

Table 141.8 Discriminating prognostic indicators and risk of local recurrence, nodal metastases or disease-specific death based on the number of high-risk factors present.

High–risk features[a]

Diameter >2 cm
Perineural involvement
Poorly differentiated or undifferentiated tumour
Involvement beyond fat

Stage	Risk of local recurrence, nodal metastases or disease-specific death based on the number of high-risk features (%)[a]	
T1	No high-risk features	4/134 (3%)
T2A	1 high-risk feature	9/67 (13%)
T2B	2–3 high-risk features	37/49 (76%)
T3	4 of 4 high-risk features	8/8 (100%)

[a] Based on a cohort of 256 cutaneous squamous cell carcinomas.

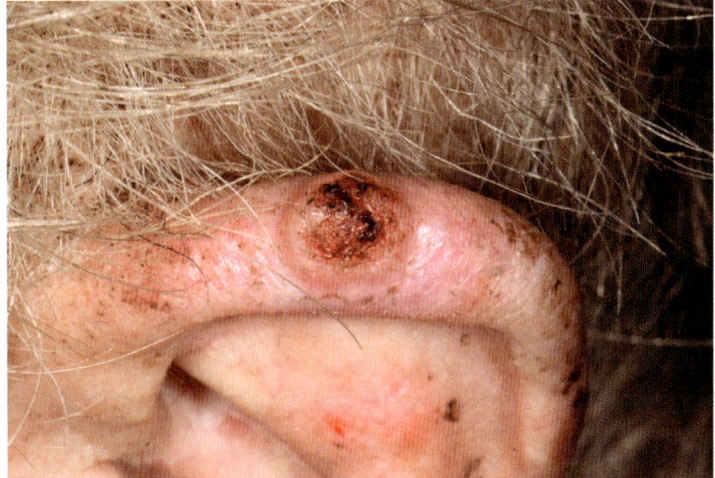

Figure 141.41 Well-differentiated squamous cell carcinoma on the helix of the ear (high-risk site).

prospective study of 615 primary SCCs with a median follow-up of 43 months (1–165 months), 3% of high-risk SCCs were locally invasive and of these 65% developed recurrence in the first year [57]. In a retrospective Mohs micrographic surgery (MMS) case review of 200 patients, 25 (12.5%) developed metastases, which occurred by year 1 in 14/25 (56%) patients, by year 2 in 18/25 (72%) patients and by year 3 in 20/25 (80%) patients [64]. A review of the literature from 1940 to 1990 identified 10 studies and showed that 75% of local recurrence and 84% of metastases occur within 2 years with 83% of local recurrence and 91% of metastases occurring within 3 years [56]. The risk is higher with an increasing number of high-risk factors (see Table 141.8) [61]. SCC behaves more aggressively in immunosuppressed OTRs and in a retrospective study, lymph node metastases (9% vs 3%) were more common than in immunocompetent patients and distant metastases (3%) occurred in the OTR group only. Two-year disease-specific survival of the OTR group was lower (93% vs 100%) [65]. Recommendations for follow-up of high-risk SCC, based on existing evidence, suggest at least a 2-year period with longer follow-up for those on immunosuppression, those with very high-risk disease (Figure 141.40) or multiple tumours [38,58].

Patients who develop progressive disease, defined as locally advanced, recurrent or metastatic disease, should be discussed at an appropriate MDT (Figure 141.43) [58]. Those who develop regional lymph node disease should be offered regional lymphadenectomy, with adjuvant radiotherapy reserved for the high-risk pathology group (Table 141.6: UICC8 >N1) [58]. Immune checkpoint inhibitors (ICI) should be considered in those with locally advanced SCC where surgery or radiotherapy is not a reasonable option, or

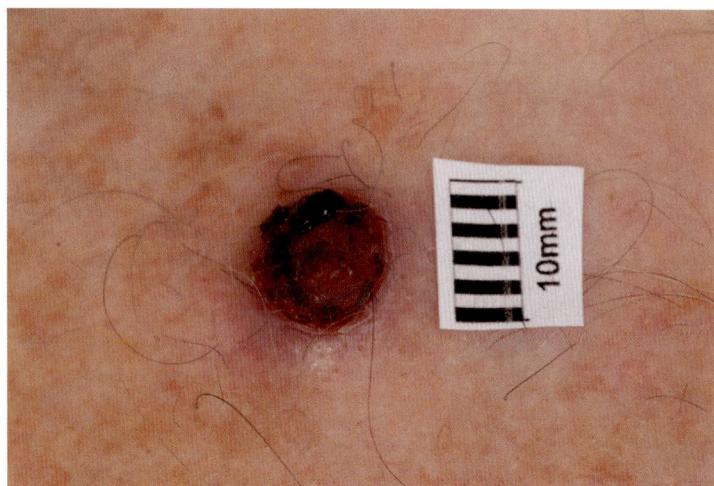

Figure 141.42 Poorly differentiated squamous cell carcinoma presenting as a nodule and lacking typical keratin centre.

those with metastatic SCC [58]. A systematic review showed that the evidence for their use remains poor but results with cemiplimab and pembrolizumab look encouraging [66]. Other therapeutic options, if ICIs are contraindicated, include systemic chemotherapy, EGFR inhibitors or best supportive care [58].

Investigations

Where there is diagnostic doubt, a skin biopsy is the standard technique to establish the diagnosis of SCC. A number of new techniques such as reflectance confocal microscopy and high-resolution optical coherence tomography are currently being evaluated but image quality is variable due to hyperkeratosis seen in SCC, thickness of the tumour and illumination not adequately reaching deeper structures resulting in unreliable images [67] (see also Chapter 40 in this volume). There is no evidence for performing sentinel lymph node biopsy (SNLB) in patients with primary SCC and SNLB should be conducted as part of a clinical trial [38,58].

An editorial review of the role of imaging in the management of high-risk SCC extrapolated evidence from the use of cross-sectional imaging in the management of head and neck cancers. Magnetic resonance imaging (MRI) is widely accepted as the imaging of choice in detecting PNI as it has been shown to have a sensitivity of 95% for detecting PNI in head and neck cancers. This decreases to 63% when used to detect the entire extent of PNI. MRI may be supplemented by computed tomography (CT) when there is a concern around potential nerve involvement at the skull base as CT scans are superior to MRI in outlining bony anatomy [68]. Traditionally, CT, MRI and ultrasound scans have been the main imaging modalities used in the evaluation of skin cancer. Other imaging techniques such as high-resolution micro-coil MRI [69], single-photon emission CT and positron emission tomography/computed tomography (PET/CT) may have an increasing role in the future [70].

There are no clear indications for when radiological imaging is warranted to search for nodal metastases. Conventional CT and MRI scans add little to the clinical examination of a node-negative region. However, in cases where an SCC is deemed very high risk, particularly when drainage is to the parotid nodes or there is evidence of in-transit metastasis, MRI is useful to stage disease and high-resolution ultrasound has also been shown to be a sensitive and accessible method of evaluating lymph nodes especially when combined with a guided fine-needle aspiration (FNA) or core biopsy [58,68]. When there is clinical evidence of locally advanced, recurrent or metastatic disease, imaging with CT or MRI should be performed prior to treatment initiation [58].

Management

Patients should be given a thorough explanation of the diagnosis and signs to observe should any future tumours arise. They should be provided with sun-avoidance information, detailed information about their tumour and self-examination of the skin and lymph nodes. The aims of any therapy selected for the treatment of SCC is to ensure complete removal and destruction of the primary tumour and to prevent metastasis (Figure 141.44). A Cochrane review found the evidence to base decisions on the best therapeutic option to achieve this to be poor, with only one randomised controlled trial comparing recurrence between groups receiving either adjuvant 13-cis retinoic acid and interferon-α after initial surgery or no adjuvant therapy [71]. UK guidelines for the treatment of SCC recommends surgical excision, including MMS, if appropriate, as the main form of therapy (Figure 141.43) [58]. However, the authors emphasise that clinicians need to be aware of other factors that could influence success when choosing a treatment modality [58]. In the absence of high-quality randomised controlled trials, a systematic review and pooled analysis of observational studies reported 118 publications covering seven different treatment modalities; standard surgical excision, MMS, external radiotherapy, brachytherapy, adjuvant radiotherapy, curettage and electrodesiccation, cryotherapy and PDT [72]. Meta-analysis of data showed that pooled estimates of recurrence of SCCs were lowest after cryotherapy (0.8% (95% confidence interval 0.1–2%)) and curettage and electrodesiccation (1.7% (0.5–3.4%)) but most treated SCCs were small low-risk tumours and these data should be treated with caution. After MMS, the pooled estimate of local recurrence was 3% (2.2–3.9%), which was non-significantly lower than the pooled estimate of local recurrence for standard surgical excision (5.4% (2.5–9.1%)) and external radiotherapy (6.4% (3–11%)). The pooled estimate of local recurrence for PDT was significantly higher (26.4% (12.3–43.7%)). There was very limited evidence for topical and laser therapy [72].

While surgical techniques may be the best therapeutic option, based on current literature and evidence it is important to risk-stratify SCC, depending on the presence or absence of high-risk features, and manage the lesion appropriately (Figure 141.43) [58]. In summary, for high-risk tumours surgical excision should be the first therapeutic choice, while curettage and cautery is a treatment option for low-risk tumours (Figure 141.43) [58].

First line

Low-risk squamous cell carcinoma. Most studies of curettage and cautery in the literature are small and retrospective and report on the use of a blunt curette. There were no studies identified which reported on the use of a single-use sharp ring curette [38]. Most studies also did not state the number of treatment cycles performed [72]. However, on the basis of limited evidence, curettage

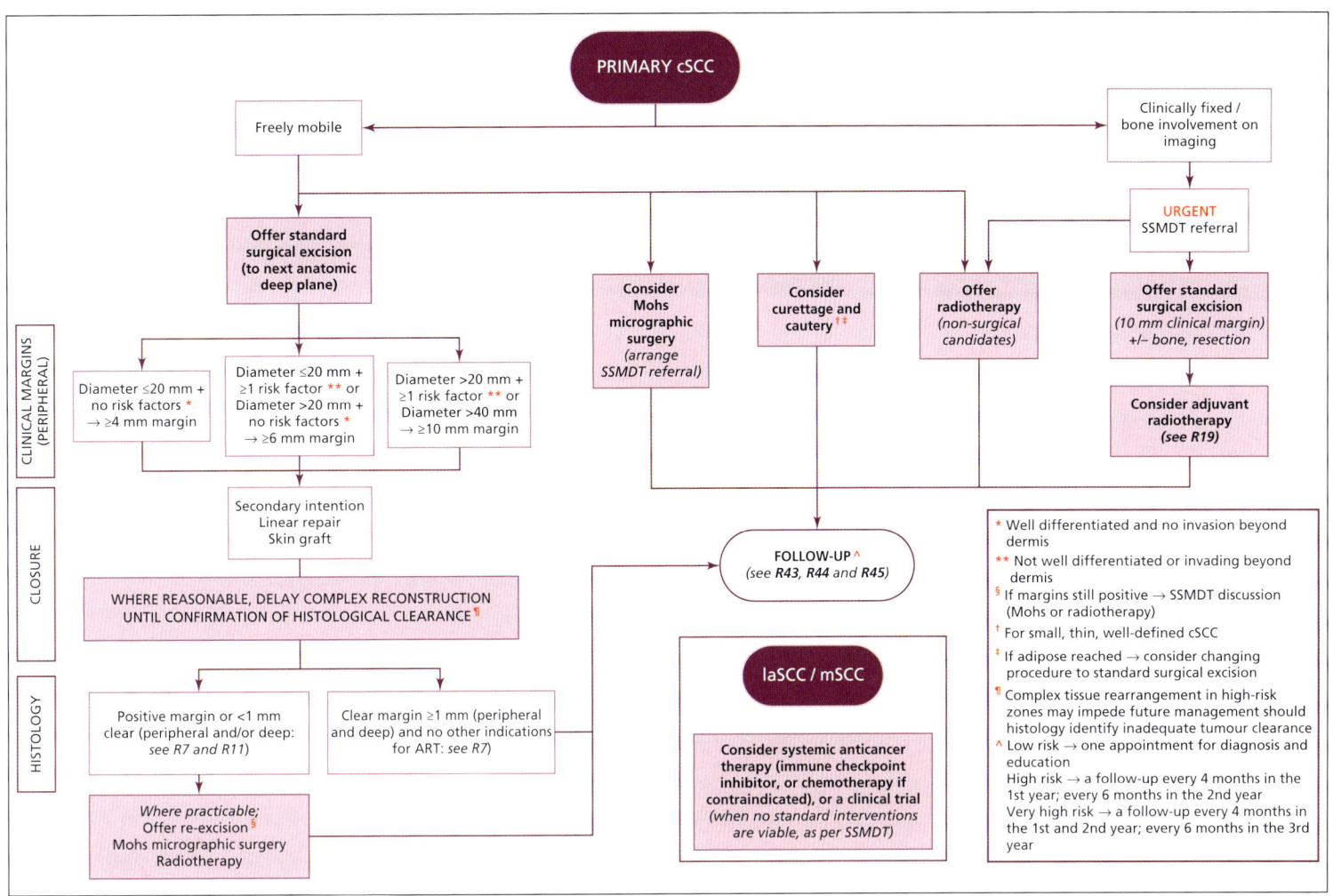

Figure 141.43 Treatment pathway for primary cutaneous squamous cell carcinoma (cSCC) in adults. Reproduced from [58] with permission from John Wiley & Sons. ART, adjuvant radiotherapy; laSCC, locally advanced squamous cell carcinoma; mSCC, metastatic squamous cell carcinoma; SSMDT, specialist skin cancer multidisciplinary team.

and cautery may be an acceptable and appropriate treatment for low-risk tumours [38,58,72].

Cryotherapy has been reported particularly in the treatment of low-risk tumours [72]. Of the eight case series identified, one used nitrogen peroxide and four used curettage followed by cryotherapy. Only three used liquid nitrogen spray methodology; treatment duration and number of cycles were poorly reported [38,72]. There is insufficient evidence to recommend cryotherapy as a treatment option for SCC [58].

PDT, using topical or systemic photosensitisers, has been reported in 14 studies but the evidence remains poor. A pooled estimate of recurrence at 6–38 months was 26.4% (95% CI 12.3–43.7%) based on 119 tumours [72]. Until further research is performed, PDT is not an appropriate treatment option for SCC [38,58].

There is also currently insufficient evidence to base any recommendations for laser treatment, intralesional 5-fluorouracil or interferon-α, and topical treatment with 5% imiquimod cream or 5-fluorouracil cream in concentrations of 5%, 10% or 20% [38,58].

High and very high-risk squamous cell carcinoma. Surgical excision or MMS are recommended due to the higher risk of tumour spread [38,58]. In the absence of prospective randomised controlled trials, the choice between the two treatments should be based on the number, size and site of tumours, local expertise, patient preference and access to MMS, which may be limited in some geographical regions. Patients should be offered wide local excision and complete margin assessment by pathology. The aim should be to completely excise the tumour taking a peripheral and deep margin of normal skin. Table 141.9 shows the overall pooled recurrence rates following excision surgery and MMS [72]. While data for MMS appear to show lower rates of local recurrence and death, this should be interpreted with caution as most studies assessed in this pooled analysis were retrospective and of variable quality or follow-up; prospective randomised controlled trials comparing MMS with excision surgery, based on SCC risk stratification, with long-term follow-up, are required [72]. MMS has the advantage of real-time margin assessment potentially allowing narrower surgical margins and confirmation of complete tumour excision, along with tissue preservation, particularly on functionally sensitive sites such as the eyelid or lip.

In a prospective study of MMS in 111 patients with 141 SCCs, initial margins of 2 mm were taken and then increased by 2 mm increments to 6 mm. Clearance rates for margins of 2 mm, 4 mm and 6 mm were 78%, 96% and 99%, respectively. When high-risk

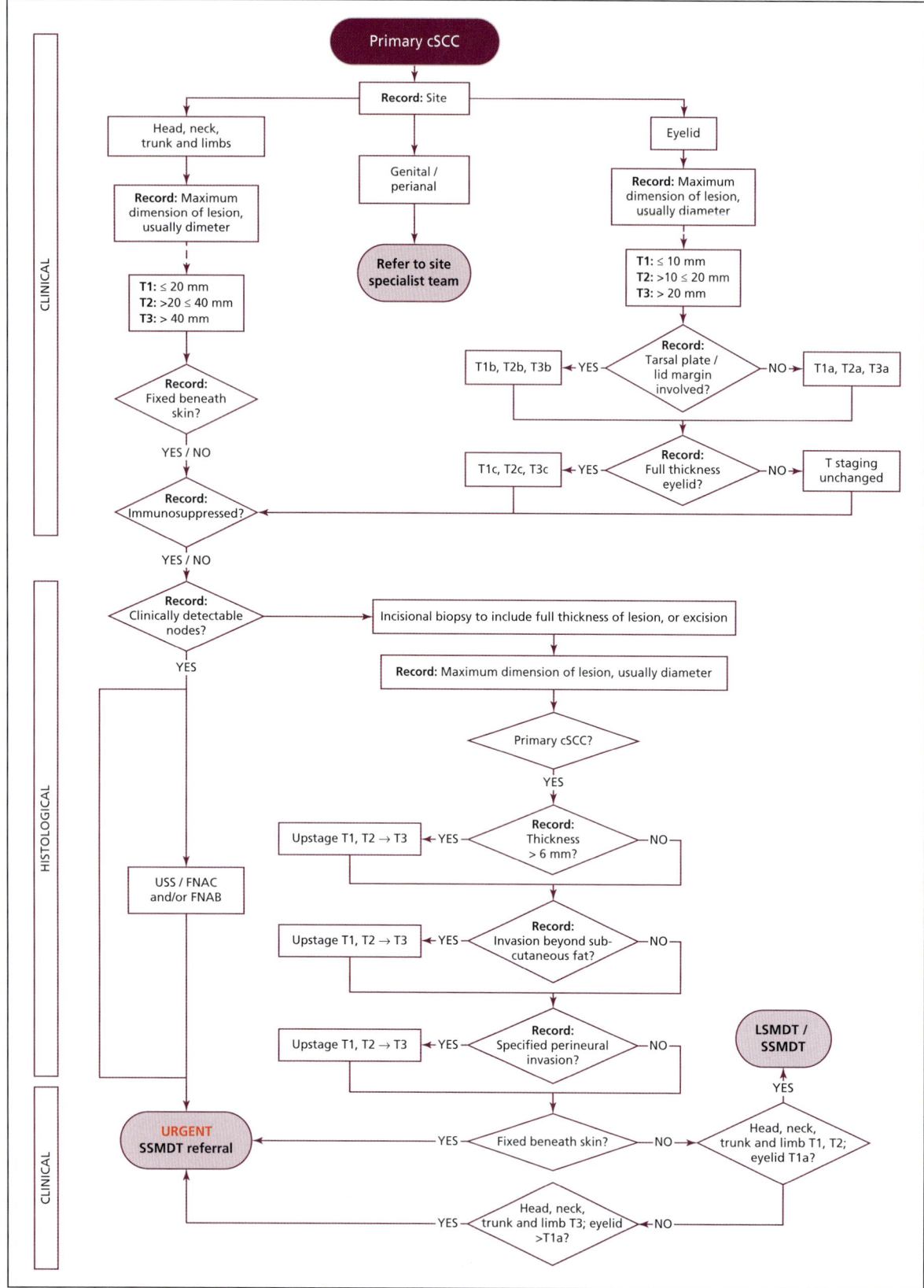

Figure 141.44 Staging and management pathway of primary cutaneous squamous cell carcinoma (cSCC). Reproduced from [58] with permission from John Wiley & Sons. FNAB, fine-needle aspiration biopsy; FNAC, fine-needle aspiration cytology; LSMDT, local skin cancer multidisciplinary team; SSMDT, specialist skin cancer multidisciplinary team; USS, ultrasound scan.

Table 141.9 Overall pooled recurrence rates for squamous cell carcinoma (SCC) following excision surgery and Mohs micrographic surgery (MMS). Adapted from [58,71].

	Pooled estimate of recurrence			
	Local (95% CI)	Regional (95% CI)	Distant/unspecified[a] (95% CI)	Death (95% CI)
Excision surgery	5.4% (2.5–9.1%)	4.4% (2.4–6.9%)	5.4% (0.7–27.6%)	4.1% (1.7–7.6%)
Number of studies (total number of patients)	12 studies (1144 patients)	8 studies (786 patients)	4 studies (146 patients)	8 studies (485 patients)
MMS	3.0% (2.2–3.9%)	4.2% (2.3–6.6%)	4.7% (0.7–11.7%)	1.1% (0.2–2.6%)
Number of studies (total number of patients)	10 studies (1572 patients)	6 studies (1162 patients)	5 studies (766 patients)	4 studies (941 patients)

[a] Data represents recurrence at unspecified location.
CI, confidence interval.

features and clearance rates were analysed separately, the results showed that a 2 mm margin was associated with a poor clearance rate of high-risk tumours. A 4 mm margin gave better peripheral clearance but only 90% deep clearance if there was subcutaneous involvement [73]. Based on current evidence, a clinical peripheral margin of 4 mm is recommended when excising low-risk SCC, 6 mm for high-risk SCC and 10 mm for very high-risk SCC, where it is surgically achievable and clinically appropriate [58]. Evidence for deep margins remains inconclusive but the tumour should be excised at the anatomical plane deep to the clinically apparent level of tumour invasion [38,58].

Second line

Primary radiotherapy has been reported in one prospective and 13 retrospective studies but the radiation source, dosage, number of fractions, field size and follow-up period were not uniform. A meta-analysis of these studies showed a pooled estimate of local recurrence to be 6.4% (95% CI 3–11%) [72]. Radiotherapy is relatively contraindicated in previously irradiated sites and for genodermatoses predisposing to skin cancer but should be considered in patients where surgery is contraindicated or in elderly patients with multiple co-morbidities [38,58].

Adjuvant radiotherapy may be an effective therapeutic option in decreasing the risk of tumour progression when a SCC has been excised with close or involved margins, or where completely excised T3 tumours have multiple high-risk features including PNI, depth of >6 mm and/or invasion beyond fat [58]. Adjuvant radiotherapy has been reported in nine studies; five with PNI and four without. The pooled recurrence rate in the five studies with PNI was 18.2% (95% CI 3.9–39.8%). In the four studies without PNI but with other high-risk features, the pooled recurrence rate was 11.1% (95% CI 2.4–25%) [72]. Comparative studies assessing the presence of perineural involvement, size, extent and site of nerves affected are required. A retrospective study of 167 patients with cutaneous SCC with metastases to head and neck lymph nodes treated with either surgery or surgery and adjuvant radiotherapy, showed that patients in the combined group had a lower rate of locoregional recurrence (20% vs 43%) and a significantly better 5-year disease-free survival rate (73% versus 54%, $P = 0.004$) [74].

Secondary prevention

In OTRs with high-risk SCCs, a reduction or substitution of immunosuppression has shown to be beneficial in two large studies [75,76]. A study of 155 renal transplant recipients with a history of SCC had a significant risk reduction of developing new SCCs at 1 year (HR 0.50, 95% CI 0.28–0.9, $P = 0.021$) but this was not significant at 2 years (HR 0.76, 95% CI 0.48–1.2, $P = 0.255$) [75]. In a multicentre randomised controlled trial of 120 OTRs with a history of SCC maintained on ciclosporin or converted to sirolimus, a significantly longer tumour-free survival was demonstrated in the sirolimus group (15 versus 7 months, $P = 0.02$), with a relative risk of new SCCs in the sirolimus group of 0.56 (95% CI 0.32–0.98) [76].

A systematic review of studies, examining the role of oral retinoids (acitretin) in the secondary prevention of skin cancers in OTRs identified three studies, with inconsistencies in dose and effect. Acitretin at 25 mg/day reduced the development of SCCs compared with placebo. In all studies, acitretin was poorly tolerated with adverse effects of oral retinoids [77–79]. Oral nicotinamide should also be considered if oral retinoids cannot be used [80] and in the very high risk OTR group with multiple SCCs, combination therapy may be considered but there are no published studies. Other treatments with limited evidence include topical 5% 5-fluorouracil [81], topical 5% imiquimod cream [82], and PDT [83].

Resources

Further information

Keohane SG, Botting J, Budny PG *et al*. British Association of Dermatologists guidelines for the management of people with cutaneous squamous cell carcinoma 2020. *Br J Dermatol* 2021;184:401–14.

Lansbury L, Bath-Hextall F, Perkins W, Stanton W, Leonardi-Bee J. Interventions for non-metastatic squamous cell carcinoma of the skin: systematic review and pooled analysis of observational studies. *BMJ* 2013;347:f6153.

Lansbury L, Leonardi-Bee J, Perkins W, Goodacre T, Tweed JA, Bath-Hextall FJ. Interventions for non-metastatic squamous cell carcinoma of the skin. *Cochrane Database Syst Rev* 2010;4:CD007869.

Scottish Intercollegiate Guidelines Network (SIGN). *Management of primary cutaneous squamous cell carcinoma*. Edinburgh: SIGN, 2014, SIGN publication no. 140. Cited 16 June 2014.

KERATOACANTHOMAS AND ASSOCIATED SYNDROMES

Keratoacanthoma

Definition and nomenclature
Keratoacanthoma (KA) is a rapidly evolving tumour of the skin, composed of keratinising squamous cells originating in pilosebaceous follicles and resolving spontaneously if untreated. KA has been reclassified as a well-differentiated SCC (keratoacanthomatous type) in the World Health Organization (WHO) classification [1] but more recently, in the RCPath UK classification, remains as a separate diagnostic clinicopathological entity, if classical features are present [2], although management of KA is similar to well-differentiated SCC.

> **Synonyms and inclusions**
> - Well-differentiated SCC (keratoacanthomatous type) [1]
> - Molluscum sebaceum

Introduction and general description
KA has historically been classified as a benign tumour which resolves spontaneously. In most cases, the diagnosis is made on clinical features but in some cases it may be indistinguishable from invasive SCC and there has been considerable debate as to whether KA is a benign tumour or a variant of SCC, particularly as metastases have been described in the literature [3]. However, a systematic review of 455 cases showed that there were no reports of metastasis or deaths [4].

Epidemiology
Incidence and prevalence
This is a relatively common tumour found in the white population. The incidence is higher in immunosuppressed patients and increases in places with higher levels of UVR such as North America and Australia. The incidence rate of 104 per 100 000 person-years has been previously reported from Hawaii [5] and more recently a rate of 409 per 100,00 person-years from Queensland, Australia [6].

Age
The adjusted age distribution shows that it is most frequent in older age groups and in a large Australian population-based study was more common in those aged 60 or over [6].

Sex
KA is more common in males with reported male to female ratios ranging from 1.2:1 to 2:1 [6].

Ethnicity
It is uncommon in dark-skinned races and is relatively common in the white population, occurring with about one-third of the frequency of SCC [6].

Associated diseases
Patients may present with other UVR-induced skin cancers and full examination of the skin should be undertaken.

Pathophysiology
Predisposing factors
Epidemiological data suggest that the incidence of KA is related to sun exposure, and the localisation of the tumours mainly on the head and upper limb supports this. Contact with tar and mineral oil has also been shown to cause an increased incidence [7] and very similar lesions have been produced in animals by painting with carcinogenic hydrocarbons. In some cases, the lesion follows injury to the skin, which suggests that wound healing may play a part in its origin, a view supported by the occurrence of multiple KAs in skin grafts of patients with the tumour in the recipient site [8], the donor site [9] or both [10]. KAs have also reported following tattoos, laser treatment, chemical peels, hyaluronic acid and collagen fillers [11]. KAs are more commonly found in immunosuppressed patients and there are reports of KA associated with carcinoma of the larynx [12], multiple internal malignancy [13], leukaemia [14], deficient cell-mediated immunity [15] and in transplant recipients [16]. The solid tumour multikinase inhibitor, sorafenib, has also been reported to lead to the development of KA, which resolved or stopped developing when therapy was discontinued. More recently, there have been reports of KA following treatment of metastatic melanoma with *BRAF* inhibitors, vemurafenib [17] and dabrafenib. A meta-analysis of 20 trials of dabrafenib-treated melanoma cases showed that the incidence of KA and SCC was 20% and 16%, respectively [18]. KA has also been reported with programmed cell death 1 (PD-1) inhibitor therapy [19] and in the treatment of locally invasive BCC with the Hedgehog signalling pathway inhibitor, vismodegib [20].

Pathology
The diagnosis of KA is one that requires close clinicopathological correlation. Examination of the whole/intact lesion is ideal in order to assess its architecture reliably [21]. The histological features vary with the stage of evolution. Early-stage KA is characterised by an exo-endophytic growth pattern that evolves into a symmetrical central structure that contains keratin. Peripheral epidermal lipping is a feature. The endophytic component is usually composed of curving or blunt epithelial down growths. Frank dermal invasion or solid growths of atypical cells are not KA features (Figure 141.45a). The proliferating keratinocytes show relatively mild cytonuclear atypia and they are present in the lower layers of the epidermis with evolution into more mature keratinocytes towards the centre of the lesion (Figure 141.45b). These maturing cells have abundant eosinophilic glassy cytoplasm and no significant nuclear abnormalities (Figure 141.45c). Transition between maturing and proliferating cells may be abrupt. Keratinisation is present. The lesion does not extend beyond the level of the sweat glands or into the subcutis. Although mitotic activity may be brisk, the presence of atypical mitotic figures should be viewed with caution.

Intraepithelial microabscesses and intraepidermal elastic fibres may be observed, but it is important to highlight that these features

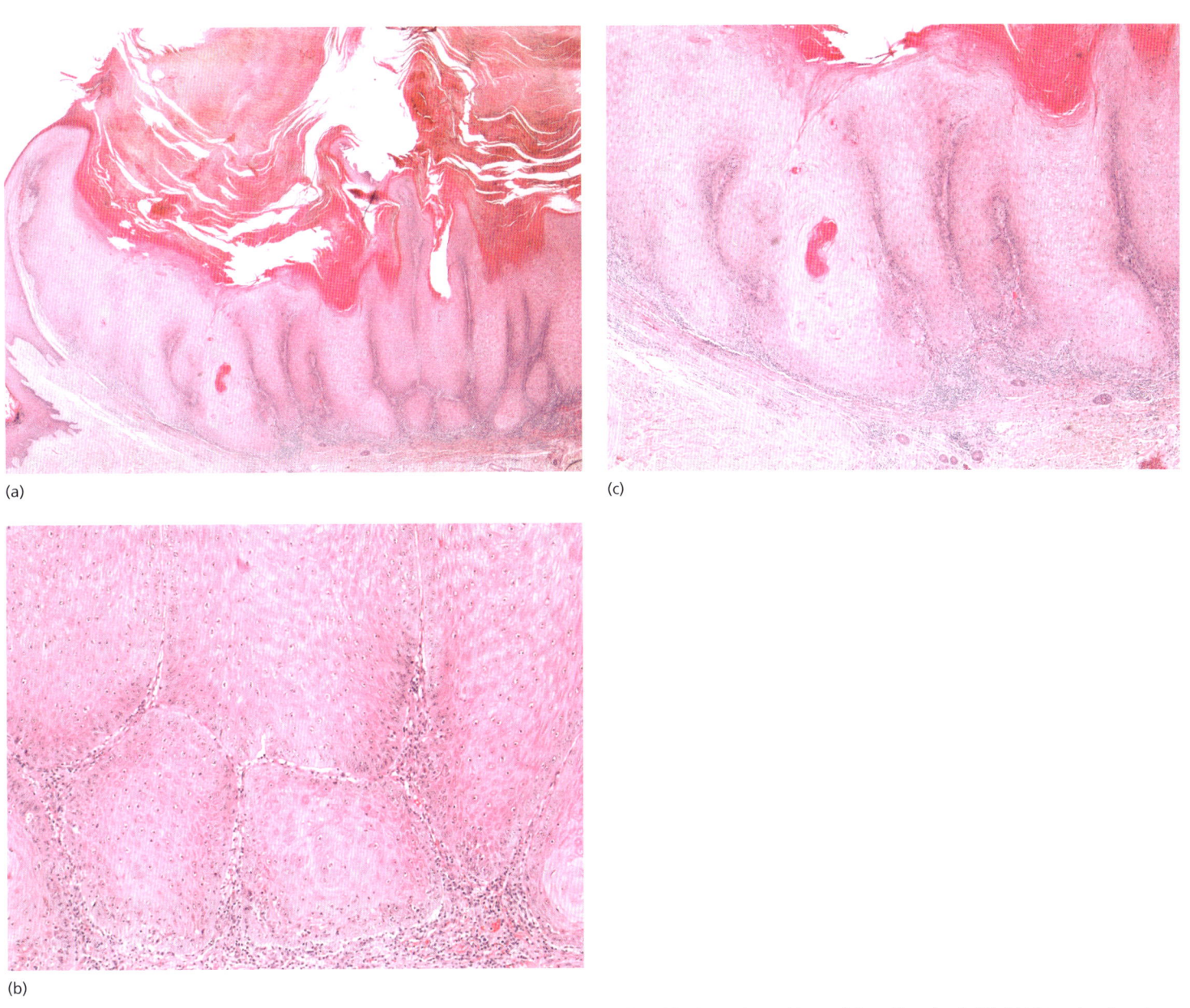

Figure 141.45 (a) Pathology of keratoacanthoma showing endophytic growth pattern with epidermal lipping and no evidence of dermal invasion (×20). (b) Mature keratinocytes seen towards the centre with mild cytonuclear atypia (×100). (c) Cells containing abundant eosinophilic glassy cytoplasm and no significant nuclear abnormalities (×40). All images courtesy of Dr M. Agarwal, Monklands Hospital, Lanarkshire, UK.

are not pathognomonic of KA. The underlying dermal tissue frequently shows inflammation with lichenoid features. Stromal desmoplasia should not be present.

In regressing lesions, the crater-like low-grade morphology of the lesion is preserved; however, the epidermis is attenuated and the underlying tissue shows fibrosis, lichenoid inflammatory changes and foci of foreign-body type granulomatous inflammation to free keratin.

Perineural invasion has been reported in KA, particularly in lesions from the face. This feature does not appear to be linked to metastatic disease [22].

Multiple and eruptive KA have a more readily identifiable follicular origin and the interfollicular epidermis is unremarkable.

Causative organisms

Virus-like particles have been seen under electron microscopy. However, there is no evidence of human polyomaviruses present [23], except for one small case series showing 42.3% of KA reported to have human polyomavirus 6 on polymerase chain reaction [24]. HPV has also been demonstrated [25] but no predominant HPV type has been found [26].

Genetics

KA behaves differently from invasive SCC clinically and there is considerable debate whether KA is a separate entity or a variant of SCC. Molecular markers to discriminate between the two have proved to be either inconclusive or not sensitive. However, more recently, using array comparative genomic hybridisation techniques to analyse the differences between KA and SCC, some degree of genetic aberrations have been found with significant differences in the aberrant clone and recurrent aberrations between KA and SCC. Tumour size, fibrosis and inflammation related to the development stages of KA showed significant association with aberrations of selected genomic regions suggesting chromosomal instability during the life cycle of KA [25]. It is now postulated that UV-mutated or activated committed infundibular stem cells are driven by a combination of two molecular pathways: oncogenic RAS pathway and the Wnt/beta-catenin pathway responsible for skin stem cell maintenance, hair follicle development and wound healing [26,27].

Environmental factors
KA are more common on light-exposed sites such as the head and extensor surface of the arms and the dorsal aspects of the hands. UV exposure increases risks particularly in those who are immunosuppressed. Patients exposed to tars and mineral oil are also at an increased risk.

Clinical features
History
KA evolves in three clinical phases: proliferative, maturing and resolving. The first evidence of KA is a firm, rounded, flesh-coloured or reddish papule, which may resemble molluscum contagiosum or, if keratotic, a viral wart. The patient rarely seeks advice at this stage. There is then a rapid growth phase and in a few weeks it may become 10–20 mm across. There is no infiltration at the base. The epidermis over the nodule is smooth and shiny; the lesion is skin coloured to red with telangiectasia just beneath the surface. The centre contains a horny plug or is covered by a crust which conceals a keratin-filled crater (Figure 141.9). As the lesion matures, the accumulating keratin expands the outermost part making the edge overhang the base, but the radial symmetry is usually well preserved. The keratin may project like a horn or it may soften and break down. Spontaneous resolution is achieved by the epidermal covering receding towards the base and the horny core being shed. The base is revealed as irregular and puckered and the edge may remain as soft but thickened epidermis, either as a continuous rim or a series of papillomatous tags. The process of spontaneous healing usually takes about 3 months.

Presentation
The most frequently affected area is the central part of the face: the nose, cheeks, eyelids and lips. The dorsum of the hand, wrist and forearm are commonly affected; the thigh, chest, shoulder and scalp less so; and the ano-genital area uncommonly except in those exposed to occupational hazards. Lesions have occurred subungually [28], on the vermilion of the lips and on the buccal mucosa.

In most cases, the tumour presents as a solitary lesion. Multiple or recurrent tumours are more likely to be present in patients who are immunosuppressed, those treated with phototherapy or with targeted therapies for melanoma metastasis. There may be recurrences after curettage or excision, more frequently in lesions on the lips and fingers and when treatment is carried out in the early stages. Recurrence may happen after spontaneous resolution [29].

Clinical variants
A small proportion of KA grow to much larger dimensions with 5 cm or more in diameter being not exceptional on the forearm. Giant KA, keratoma centrifugum marginatum, measuring 15–20 cm, have been rarely described in the literature [30]. In some cases, the maximum size may be reached in a month or two; others may enlarge over many months. After growth ceases, involution may not occur for some months or may occur at part of the periphery while growth continues elsewhere.

Differential diagnosis
Molluscum contagiosum and viral warts may mimic KA in the very early stage. Cutaneous horn and hypertrophic AK may appear similar in the proliferative stage. Invasive SCC is the commonest differential diagnosis in the maturation phase but KA generally starts to involute spontaneously in the resolution stage.

In patients with multiple KA, a family history should be sought to exclude multiple self-healing squamous epithelioma (MSSE). The lack of symptoms such as pruritus and multiple KA only on exposed sites should help exclude generalised eruptive KA (Grzybowski syndrome).

Xeroderma pigmentosum and Muir–Torre syndrome (MTS) are also associated with KA but other features of MTS include a family history, sebaceous neoplasms and internal malignancy, most commonly carcinoma of the colon. Secondary deposits from non-cutaneous malignancies can also occasionally mimic KA.

Complications and co-morbidities
KA will resolve to leave a pitted or unsightly scar. KAs have been rarely reported to metastasise.

Disease course and prognosis
KA typically resolves spontaneously but can recur within the scar infrequently. Often patients may develop further KA, particularly those who are immunosuppressed.

Investigations
Investigations are generally not necessary but a skin biopsy may be taken or the lesion excised when diagnosis is in doubt or the lesion persists without typical spontaneous resolution. Dermoscopy of KA has been reported to show hairpin vessels, linear-irregular vessels, targetoid hair follicles, white structureless areas, a central mass of keratin and ulceration, but these features were also found in invasive SCC and therefore not diagnostic of KA [31].

Management
Most tumours regress spontaneously leaving a scar. Patients should be advised on the signs of new tumour development and what to look out for: red or flesh-coloured crusted lesions usually on light-exposed sites. Advice on high factor broad spectrum sunscreen should be provided.

First line
Most lesions are solitary and surgical excision or curettage and cautery are the best treatment options for those that have not resolved completely. Small lesions possess a low risk of invasion

and so could be treated with curettage and cautery particularly if they are less than 2 cm in diameter. For larger lesions over 2 cm in diameter, subungual lesions and where diagnosis is not clear then surgical excision would be recommended [2].

Second line
Radiotherapy shortens the course and improves the scar, and can be used in patients who refuse surgery.

The application of 5% 5-fluorouracil cream twice daily may reduce the time taken for natural resolution and diminish scarring [32]. Topical 5% imiquimod cream has also been reported to clear KA. A systematic review of non-surgical treatments reported that topical 5% 5-fluorouracil cream led to faster time to heal than 5% imiquimod cream [33].

Third line
In a patient with multiple KA due to vemurafenib, systemic retinoids (acitretin) at a dose of 25 mg on alternate days along with intralesional fluorouracil have been reported to clear and reduce the development of new KA [17]. Intralesional methotrexate has also shown improvement but in a systematic review, intralesional 5-fluorouracil led to faster healing times than intralesional methotrexate [33]. PDT has also been reported in a similar case with significant clinical regression of KAs [34].

Resources

Further information

Elder DE, Massi D, Scolyer RA, Willemze R, eds. *WHO Classification of Skin Tumours*, 4th edn. Lyon, France: IARC Press, 2018.

Slater DN, Barrett P. Dataset for the histological reporting of primary cutaneous squamous cell carcinoma and regional lymph nodes. Available at: https://www.rcpath.org/uploads/assets/9c1d8f71-5d3b-4508-8e6200f11e1f4a39/Dataset-for-histopathological-reporting-of-primary-invasive-cutaneous-squamous-cell-carcinoma-and-regional-lymph-nodes.pdf (last accessed 21 July 2022).

Multiple self-healing squamous epithelioma

Definition and nomenclature
Multiple self-healing squamous epithelioma (MSSE) is an autosomal dominant condition characterised by the intermittent development of spontaneously regressing skin tumours which are histologically identical to well-differentiated SCCs. Susceptibility to MSSE is conferred by heterozygous loss-of-function mutations in the *TGFBR1* gene and variants at a second linked locus on the long arm of chromosome 9.

Synonyms and inclusions
- Familial multiple KAs
- Ferguson-Smith disease

Introduction and general description
This autosomal dominant condition was first described by Ferguson-Smith in 1934 in a single case. Patients develop multiple tumours mainly on sun-exposed sites which spontaneously regress a few weeks later.

Epidemiology

Incidence and prevalence
The incidence is unknown but the condition is extremely rare. Two large Scottish kindreds are well described in the literature [1–3], and accurate genetic pedigree analysis has suggested that the condition may have arisen in these two families from a single mutation around 1790. Haplotype analysis for polymorphic markers segregating with MSSE in non-Scottish and Scottish families has shown differences which suggest that MSSE may not be caused by a founder mutation and that the syndrome may be more common than originally thought [4].

Age
Age of onset is highly variable ranging from childhood to the ninth decade (median 28 years) but the first tumours usually appear in the second decade of life. The mean age of onset in women is 25.5 and in men 26.9 years [3].

Sex
Males and females are equally affected.

Ethnicity
MSSE was first described in the Scottish population, although there are reports of MSSE in non-Scottish families. MSSE mainly affects white patients with Scottish cases outnumbering cases from the rest of the world [3].

Pathophysiology

Pathology
See pathology section of KA.

Genetics
Initial linkage studies had initially mapped MSSE to chromosome 9q22.3 in a region of less than 4 Mb between the markers D9S197 and D9S1809 [5–7]. Further molecular analysis of tissue has shown loss of heterozygosity of the MSSE region with loss of the normal allele, indicating that the *MSSE* gene is likely to be a tumour suppressor gene [5]. Linkage analysis has confirmed a highly significant association between MSSE and the *TGFBR1* gene mutations with a LOD (maximum $\log_{10}$ odds) score of 16.9. Eighteen different families with 67 affected individuals were studied and found to have *TGFBR1* mutations in all cases [8]. Eleven different heterozygous mutations were found, which occurred in either the extracellular ligand-binding domain or in the serine/threonine kinase (STK) domain of the protein and all were predicted or demonstrated to result in loss of receptor function.

More recently, variants in an adjacent region of chromosome 9q22.3 to known *TGFBR1* mutations have been demonstrated suggesting a digenic or multilocus aetiology [9]. Haplotype comparisons suggest the second locus lies proximal to the XPAC gene on chromosome 9q22.3 over 1.5 Mb from *TGFBR1* but this locus is as yet unidentified [9,**10**].

MSSE therefore results from loss of function mutations in the extracellular ligand-binding domain or truncating mutations in the STK domain, with evidence of a second locus near *TGFBR1*. Missense mutations in the STK domain have been reported in Loeys-Dietz syndrome (LDS). LDS is an autosomal dominant disorder and has characteristics similar to Marfan syndrome with aortic aneurysm and dissection. Patients with LDS also exhibit hypertelorism, bifid uvula, cleft palate, arterial tortuosity and aneurysms, although there is a spectrum of features found [11]. Although MSSE and LDS have different disease pathogenesis and are considered separate conditions, there are two reports of patients having both with splice junctional mutations in the STK domain [10,12].

In MSSE, the wild-type *TGFBR1* allele acts as a tumour suppressor and it is postulated that its somatic deletion by a classic 'second hit' could then lead to carcinogenesis. As most lesions occur on light-exposed sites, it is likely that this 'second hit' is caused by UVR. *TGFBR1* affects the TGFß signalling pathway and loss of *TGFBR1* expression through loss of wild-type allele could lead to increased cell proliferation as seen in MSSE [8]. TGFß is a known tumour suppressor and in a phase 1 study using a human anti-TGFß monoclonal antibody for advanced melanoma or renal cell carcinoma, 4 of 29 patients developed multiple KA or SCC-like tumours which, when not removed, spontaneously resolved when treatment was discontinued [13]. The spontaneous regression of tumours in MSSE has, however, still not been adequately explained using molecular genetics.

Environmental factors
The lesions develop most frequently on light-exposed skin and it is postulated that UVR is an important co-factor in the development of these tumours.

Clinical features
History
The first lesions usually appear in the second decade of life, and each patient tends to have a fairly specific pattern of development, duration and evolution. Knowledge of the 'normal' pattern for the patient is of great value in the management of individual lesions.

Presentation
The lesions develop predominantly on exposed skin and may cluster around the nose or ears. In the majority of reported cases, one or more lesions have been present on the scalp, a site rarely affected by KA. A small raised red nodule is the first sign of a new lesion. This may grow over 2–4 weeks to a diameter of 2–3 cm and may become crusted or ulcerated. The lesion may then remain unchanged for 1–2 months, and then gradually shrinks, leaving behind a very characteristic and unsightly crenellated scar (Figure 141.46). Lesions develop singly or in crops.

Clinical variants
In one case, lesions were strikingly confined to half of the body [14].

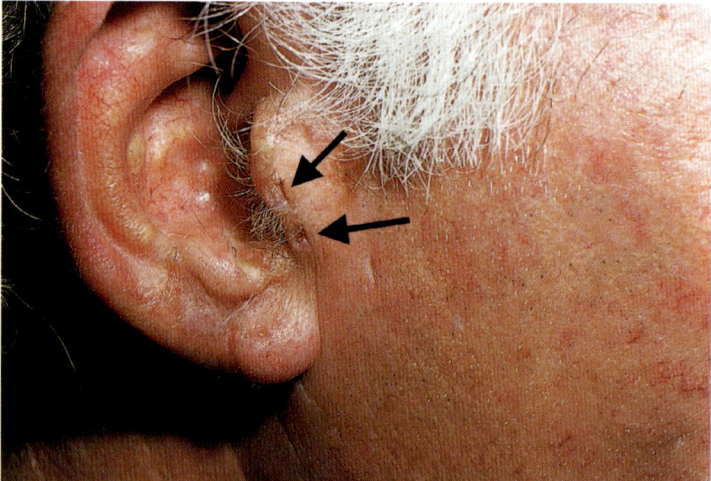

Figure 141.46 Scarring seen in a patient with multiple self-healing squamous epitheliomas.

Differential diagnosis
The differential diagnosis of MSSE includes generalised eruptive KA (Grzybowski syndrome) but in cases of MSSE there is generally a family history and an earlier age of onset. Witten and Zac also described a single case who developed multiple eruptive KA on exposed and covered sites along with severe pruritus, buccal mucosal change with white streaks and hoarseness. The case had many features similar to those described in Grzybowski syndrome [15]. Multiple KAs have also been described in Muir–Torre syndrome but this is associated with internal malignancy, most commonly carcinoma of the colon.

Complications and co-morbidities
Marked unsightly scars are left when the tumours regress.

Disease course and prognosis
This is a chronic condition with patients developing multiple tumours in their lifetime. There are occasional reports in the literature suggesting that radiotherapy may exacerbate the development of further new tumours and so should be avoided [16,17].

Investigations
Generally, investigations are not required to reach a diagnosis, particularly when there is a family history of MSSE.

Management
Most tumours regress spontaneously leaving a scar. Patients should be advised about signs of new tumour development and what to look out for: red or flesh-coloured nodules usually on light-exposed sites. Advice on high factor broad spectrum sunscreen should be provided. Radiotherapy should be avoided.

If the tumour is solitary, surgical excision or curettage would be appropriate allowing for the best cosmetic result.

Oral retinoids (acitretin) have been used successfully in a few reports to prevent and control the development of new tumours. Dosage has varied but 10–20 mg has been used to control disease [16].

Generalised eruptive keratoacanthoma

Definition and nomenclature
Generalised eruptive KA of Grzybowski is a rare condition with approximately 40 cases being reported in the literature since its first description in 1950 [1]. Numerous small, 1–3 mm in diameter, flesh-coloured umbilicated papules resembling KAs develop abruptly and may persist for several months. Spontaneous regression may occur, which leads to atrophic scars. The mucosal surfaces may be affected as well. Other associated findings include severe pruritus, a Koebner reaction, mask-like facial appearance, ectropion and hoarseness due to nodules on the larynx.

Synonyms and inclusions
- Grzybowski syndrome

Introduction and general description
This rare condition was first described in 1950. Patients develop hundreds of small KAs often with mucosal involvement, associated with pruritus. The cause is not known.

Epidemiology
Incidence and prevalence
The incidence is unknown but the condition is extremely rare, with about 40 cases reported in the literature.

Age
It mainly affects adults in the fifth to seventh decades of life.

Sex
Males and females are equally affected.

Ethnicity
Mainly described in the white population.

Pathophysiology
Pathology
See pathology section of KA.

Causative organisms
As some of the lesions appear warty and behave like viral warts, they have been analysed for HPV infection but evidence for a viral association has not been found [2] with only rare reports on HPV-16 and HPV-39 DNA isolated from lesional skin [3,4], thought to be coincidental.

Environmental factors
UVR may be a co-factor in the development of these tumours.

Clinical features
History
The first lesions usually appear in the fifth to seventh decade of life, with patients developing hundreds of KAs on light-exposed skin but also on covered body sites.

Presentation
The KAs develop abruptly often with mucosal involvement and may koebnerise. Patients often complain of severe pruritus. They may develop a mask-like face, present with an ectropion and have hoarseness due to nodules in the larynx. The lesions grow rapidly, last a few weeks and then regress spontaneously leaving atrophic scarring.

Clinical variants
There are several published case reports of KAs with limited skin involvement, mainly of the lower extremities. In these cases, there was evidence of infundibulocystic hyperplasia which developed in the context of hypertrophic lichen planus [5,6].

Differential diagnosis
The differential diagnosis of generalised eruptive KA (Grzybowski syndrome) includes MSSE but in cases of MSSE there is generally a family history and an earlier age of onset. Although Witten and Zac reported a single case of multiple eruptive KA with features similar to Grzybowski syndrome [7], there is a report of familial eruptive KA with overlapping features described by Witten and Zac and those found in MSSE [8]. Muir–Torre syndrome is also associated with multiple KAs but other features include sebaceous neoplasms and internal malignancy, most commonly carcinoma of the colon.

Complications and co-morbidities
Patients develop multiple tumours over their lifetime resulting in marked unsightly scars.

Disease course and prognosis
This is a chronic condition with patients developing multiple lesions over time. It generally runs a benign course without spread to the lymph nodes.

Investigations
Investigations are generally not required but biopsy of a nodule may be necessary to help with the diagnosis.

Management
Most tumours regress spontaneously leaving a scar. Patients should be advised about signs of new tumour development and what to look out for: red or flesh-coloured nodules usually on light-exposed sites. Advice on high factor broad spectrum sunscreen should be provided. The resulting ectropion may need surgical correction.

If there are a small number of tumours, surgical excision or curettage would be appropriate allowing for the best cosmetic result.

Oral retinoids (acitretin) in doses of 10–25 mg have been used to control the development of multiple new tumours either alone [3,4] or in combination with methyl aminoleavulinate PDT (MAL-PDT) [9]. Other options include isotretinoin, methotrexate, intralesional corticosteroid [10] and cyclophosphamide at doses of 100–200 mg daily [11].

Resources

Further information

Nofal A, Assaf M, Nofal E, Alradi M. Generalized eruptive keratoacanthoma: proposed diagnostic criteria and therapeutic options. *J Eur Acad Dermatol Venereol* 2014;28:397–404.

Muir–Torre syndrome

Definition and nomenclature

Muir–Torre syndrome (MTS) is an autosomal dominant inherited condition which is best regarded as a phenotypic variant of the Lynch II cancer family syndrome [1]. It is characterised by the development of one or more sebaceous neoplasms (sebaceous adenoma, sebaceous epithelioma or sebaceous carcinoma) and/or KA along with one or more visceral malignancies [2,3].

Synonyms and inclusions
- Hereditary non-polyposis colorectal cancer
- Lynch II syndrome

Introduction and general description

This autosomal dominant syndrome was originally described by Muir *et al.* in 1967 in a single case with KA on the face and primary carcinomas of the colon, duodenum and larynx [4]. Family history of visceral malignancy was not observed. Torre in 1968 described a patient with multiple sebaceous adenomas and multiple primary visceral tumours [5].

Epidemiology

Incidence and prevalence
MTS is rare with only several hundred cases being described in the literature. The majority of cases are familial but sporadic cases have been described.

Age
Although described from the second decade, most cases present with cutaneous and/or internal tumours after the fifth decade [6].

Sex
There is no reported sex bias, although there are infrequent reports of male preponderance [7].

Ethnicity
There are more reports in white patients.

Pathophysiology

Pathology
See pathology section of sebaceous tumours in Chapter 137.

Genetics
MTS is caused by germline mutations on one of four DNA mismatch repair (*MMR*) genes. In about 90% of cases, the mutation occurs in the Mutator S homologue 2 (*MSH2*) gene which maps to chromosome 2p; similar to findings in Lynch syndrome [8]. In fewer than 10% of cases, the mutation is found in the Mutator L homolog 1 (*MLH1*) gene which maps to chromosome 3p [9]. Rarely mutations are found in the Mutator S homolog 6 (*MSH6*) gene [9] and in post-meiotic segregation increased 2 (*PMS2*) gene [6]. There is close interplay between these proteins and several different mutations have been described for each *MMR* gene but the outcome is similar with loss of expression of the protein. This results in micro-satellite instability (MSI) in tumour tissue following a somatic inactivation of the corresponding second mismatch repair allele 'second hit', which is not due to loss of heterozygosity. There is one report of a large deletion involving exons 1–6 of the *MSH2* gene [10]. MSI has been reported in 46–100% of tumours associated with MTS [6].

In patients with MTS, there was a 95% concordance between *MMR* protein immunohistochemical staining profile in sebaceous neoplasms and underlying germline mutations, particularly if the sebaceous neoplasms were on extra-facial sites where the concordance was 100% [11].

In a small study of six lesions, whole exon sequencing from *MMR*-deficient sebaceous lesions in patients known to have *MSH2* gene mutations were compared to a similar number of *MMR*-proficient sebaceous lesions in those individuals without Lynch syndrome, showing that tumour mutational signatures 6 and 15 were effective in differentiating Lynch-related from non-Lynch sebaceous lesions [12].

MSH6 germline mutations are usually associated with a lower incidence of colon cancer and its later onset but with a higher incidence of extracolonic malignancies, mainly endometrial carcinoma which has an earlier age of onset than colonic carcinoma [13].

BRAF gene mutations can be associated with somatic mutations in the *MMR* gene and have been found in sebaceous hyperplasia of patients with mutator Y homologue (*MYH*)-associated polyposis [14]. Further studies are required in tumours from Muir–Torre patients.

Clinical features

History
The majority of patients have a family history of cutaneous tumours and/or internal malignancy. Patients often develop multiple sebaceous tumours and multiple primary internal carcinomas, mainly colorectal carcinoma, in more than 50% of cases [15]. Immunosuppression following renal transplantation has been reported to exacerbate tumour development [16] and switching from tacrolimus to a sirolimus-based regimen resulted in arrest of new sebaceous tumour development [17].

Presentation
Cutaneous tumours. Most patients are disease free until their second/third decade when cutaneous tumours may start to arise before internal malignancy (22–32% of cases), concomitantly (6–12%) or after internal malignancy has been diagnosed (56–59%). Sebaceous adenomas are found in 25–68% of patients, sebaceous epitheliomas

in 31–86% and sebaceous carcinomas in 66–100% of cases with MTS [6]. In a single report, all 13 patients with MTS, with mutations in *MLH1* and *MSH2* genes, had Fordyce granules in the oral mucosa, mainly on the vestibular aspect, which may constitute an additional parameter in diagnosing MTS [18].

KA may occur in about 20% of patients with MTS and may be multiple, on light-protected sites and may occur in younger age groups [6,9]. Solitary KA has been described in this condition. A number of other skin tumours, including SCC, BCC and AK, have also been described in patients with MTS.

Internal malignancy. Most patients develop colorectal carcinoma and nearly 50% have two or more visceral carcinomas. Ten per cent have more than four primary tumours and patients with up to nine tumours have been reported in the literature. Other internal malignancies include carcinoma of the endometrium, stomach, small bowel, genitourinary tract, breast, ovary, pancreas, liver and kidney [6]. There are single reports of an association with non-small cell carcinoma of the lung.

Visceral tumours in MTS are usually low-grade malignancies, which tend to permit prolonged survival. The sebaceous carcinomas in this syndrome, like the visceral malignancies, are less aggressive than their counterparts that occur independently.

Differential diagnosis
In patients presenting with solitary or few sebaceous tumours or KAs, it may be difficult to diagnose MTS without a family history or a history of internal malignancy.

A few cases of MTS with Turcot syndrome, where the patient developed colon carcinoma, sebaceous carcinoma and malignant astrocytoma, have been reported. There is an overlap between the two syndromes with both exhibiting mutations in the *MLH1* and *PMS2* gene but in Turcot syndrome there is a higher risk of developing tumours of the brain [19].

In familial adenomatous polyposis, patients develop colon carcinoma, colon polyps and other features not usually seen in MTS, including hepatoblastoma, thyroid, pancreatic, adrenal and bile duct tumours, along with osteomas, unerupted or extra teeth, congenital hypertrophy of the retinal pigment epithelium, desmoid tumours and benign skin lesions, epidermoid cyst and fibromas.

Gardner syndrome is a subtype of familial adenomatous polyposis with a higher risk of colon carcinoma and multiple colon polyps. However, patients may also develop sebaceous cysts, epidermoid cysts, fibromas, desmoid tumours and osteomas, not features of MTS.

Complications and co-morbidities
Main complications are due to internal malignancies, particularly in those who have multiple primary tumours.

Disease course and prognosis
The frequency of cutaneous change and internal malignancy increases with age with most patients presenting in the fifth decade and upwards [6]. The cumulative risk of developing sebaceous carcinoma and SCC significantly increased at age 70 years compared with the general Dutch population. Univariate analysis of this group showed that only mutation status with mainly mutations in *MLH1* and *MSH2* genes was associated with this risk [20]. Although patients may develop multiple tumours, prognosis is generally better than in those who do not have MTS [21].

Patients and their family members should receive genetic screening and counselling.

Investigations
The diagnosis is generally made on clinical grounds but genetic screening to look for germline mutations in the four DNA *MMR* genes is required, particularly in those who develop multiple sebaceous adenomas or sebaceous carcinomas.

Management
Patients and their family members should be managed using a multidisciplinary approach, mainly between gastroenterologists and dermatologists, with other specialists becoming involved should tumours arise at other body sites. Although evidence for screening is relatively poor, the general recommendations are for patients to have an annual clinical examination, chest radiography and urine cytology. The frequency of performing colonoscopy varies from once every 3 years to every 1–2 years, particularly in higher risk patients [22]. Female patients require an annual cervical smear and carcinoembryonic antigen testing, along with mammography every 1–2 years up to age 50 and then annually thereafter. Endometrial biopsy has also been recommended every 3–5 years [3]. In one report, two patients presenting with cutaneous signs only were found to have colonic malignancy with positron emission tomography/computed tomography (PET/CT) and further studies are required to assess the reliability of this in detecting occult malignancy [23].

Surgical clearance of internal tumours and sebaceous carcinoma should be performed where possible. For patients with solitary or few cutaneous lesions, surgery in the form of excision or curettage and cautery would be appropriate.

For patients with multiple benign cutaneous lesions, isotretinoin has been reported to prevent new tumour development [24].

Resources

Further information
Fernandez-Flores A. Considerations on the performance of immunohistochemistry for mismatch repair gene proteins in cases of sebaceous neoplasms and keratoacanthomas with reference to Muir–Torre syndrome. *Am J Dermatopathol* 2012;34:416–22.

Lynch HT, Lynch PM, Pester J, Fusaro RM. The cancer family syndrome. Rare cutaneous phenotypic linkage of Torre's syndrome. *Arch Intern Med* 1981;141:607–11.

Vasen HF, Blanco I, Aktan-Collan K *et al*. Revised guidelines for the clinical management of Lynch syndrome (HNPCC): recommendations by a group of European experts. *Gut* 2013;62:812–23.

Acknowledgement

The authors are grateful to Dr Luisa Motta, Consultant Dermatopathologist, Salford Royal NHS Trust, for her help in critically appraising the pathology section.

Key references

The full list of references can be found in the online version at https://www.wiley.com/rooksdermatology10e

Lesions with uncertain or unpredictable malignant potential
Actinic keratosis

11 Traianou A, Ulrich M, Apalla Z et al. Risk factors for actinic keratosis in eight European centres: a case–control study. Br J Dermatol 2012;167:36–42.
29 Schmitz L, Gambichler T, Gupta G et al. Actinic keratoses show variable histological basal growth patterns – a proposed classification adjustment. J Eur Acad Dermatol Venereol 2018;32:745–51.
32 Dirschka T, Pellacani G, Micali G et al. A proposed scoring system for assessing the severity of actinic keratosis on the head: actinic keratosis area and severity index. J Eur Acad Dermatol Venereol 2017;31:1295–302.
45 de Berker D, McGregor JM, Mohd Mustapa MF et al. British Association of Dermatologists' guidelines for the care of patients with actinic keratosis 2017. Br J Dermatol 2017;176:20–43.

Cutaneous horn

2 Yu RC, Pryce DW, MacFarlane AW, Stewart TW. A histopathological study of 643 cutaneous horns. Br J Dermatol 1991;124:449–52.

Arsenical keratosis

4 Chen CJ, Chen CW, Wu MM, Kuo TL. Cancer potential in liver, lung, bladder and kidney due to ingested inorganic arsenic in drinking water. Br J Cancer 1992;66:888–92.

Post-ionising radiation keratosis

1 Peter RU, Braun-Falco O, Birioukov A et al. Chronic cutaneous damage after accidental exposure to ionizing radiation: the Chernobyl experience. J Am Acad Dermatol 1994;30:719–23.

Disseminated superficial actinic porokeratosis

10 Kubo A, Sasaki T, Suzuki H et al. Clonal expansion of second-hit cells with somatic recombinations or C>T transitions form porokeratosis in MVD or MVK mutant heterozygotes. J Invest Dermatol 2019;139:2458–66.
26 Li M, Min W, Wang J et al. Effects of mevalonate kinase interference on cell differentiation, apoptosis, prenylation and geranylgeranylation of human keratinocytes are attenuated by farnesyl pyrophosphate or geranylgeranyl pyrophosphate. Exp Ther Med 2020;19:2861–70.
42 Atzmony L, Lim YH, Hamilton C et al. Topical cholesterol/lovastatin for the treatment of porokeratosis: a pathogenesis-directed therapy. J Am Acad Dermatol 2020;82:123–31.

In situ carcinoma of the skin
Bowen disease

30 Fleury FJ. Bowenoid papulosis of the genitalia. Arch Dermatol 1980;116:274.
36 Morton CA, Birnie AJ, Eedy DJ. British Association of Dermatologists' guidelines for the management of squamous cell carcinoma in situ (Bowen's disease) 2014. Br J Dermatol 2014;170:245–60.

Anal, vulval, penile and perianal intraepithelial carcinoma

1 Darragh TM, Colgan TJ, Thomas C et al. The lower anogenital squamous terminology standardization project for HPV-associated lesions: background and consensus recommendations from the College of American Pathologists and the American Society for Colposcopy and Cervical Pathology. Int J Gynecol Pathol 2013;32:76–115.
14 FUTURE I/II Study Group. Dillner J, Kjaer SK, Wheeler CM et al. Four year efficacy of prophylactic human papillomavirus quadrivalent vaccine against low grade cervical, vulvar, and vaginal intraepithelial neoplasia and anogenital warts: randomised controlled trial. BMJ 2010;341:c3493.

Squamous cell carcinoma of the skin

29 Thomson J, Bewicke-Copley F, Anene CA et al. The genomic landscape of actinic keratosis. J Invest Dermatol 2021;141:1664–74.
30 Di Nardo L, Pellegrini C, Di Stefani A et al. Molecular genetics of cutaneous squamous cell carcinoma: perspective for treatment strategies. J Eur Acad Dermatol Venereol 2020;34:932–41.
38 Scottish Intercollegiate Guidelines Network (SIGN). Management of primary cutaneous squamous cell carcinoma. Edinburgh: SIGN, 2014, SIGN publication no. 140. Cited 16 June 2014.
46 Slater DN, Barrett P. Dataset for the histological reporting of primary cutaneous squamous cell carcinoma and regional lymph nodes. Available at: https://www.rcpath.org/uploads/assets/9c1d8f71-5d3b-4508-8e6200f11e1f4a39/Dataset-for-histopathological-reporting-of-primary-invasive-cutaneous-squamous-cell-carcinoma-and-regional-lymph-nodes.pdf (last accessed 21 July 2022).
58 Keohane SG, Botting J, Budny PG et al. British Association of Dermatologists guidelines for the management of people with cutaneous squamous cell carcinoma 2020. Br J Dermatol 2021;184:401–14.
59 Califano JA, Lydiatt WM, Nehal KS et al. Cutaneous squamous cell carcinoma of the head and neck. In: Amin MB, Edge SB, Greene FL, Byrd DR, Brookland RK et al., eds. AJCC Cancer Staging Manual, 8th edn. New York: Springer, 2017:171–81.
60 Brierley JD, Gospodarowicz MK, Wittekind C. Skin tumours. In: Brierley JD, Gospodarowicz MK, Wittekind C, eds. TNM Classification of Malignant Tumours, 8th edn. Chichester: John Wiley and Sons, 2017:131–49.
61 Jambusaria-Pahlajani A, Kanetsky PA, Karia PS et al. Evaluation of AJCC tumor staging for cutaneous squamous cell carcinoma and a proposed alternative tumor staging system. JAMA Dermatol 2013;149:402–10.
72 Lansbury L, Bath-Hextall F, Perkins W, Stanton W, Leonardi-Bee J. Interventions for non-metastatic squamous cell carcinoma of the skin: systematic review and pooled analysis of observational studies. BMJ 2013;347:f6153.

Keratoacanthomas and associated syndromes
Keratoacanthoma

1 Elder DE, Massi D, Scolyer RA, Willemze R, eds. WHO Classification of Skin Tumours, 4th edn. Lyon, France: IARC Press, 2018.
2 Slater DN, Barrett P. Dataset for the histological reporting of primary cutaneous squamous cell carcinoma and regional lymph nodes. Available at: https://www.rcpath.org/uploads/assets/9c1d8f71-5d3b-4508-8e6200f11e1f4a39/Dataset-for-histopathological-reporting-of-primary-invasive-cutaneous-squamous-cell-carcinoma-and-regional-lymph-nodes.pdf (last accessed 21 July 2022).
27 Kossard S. Keratoacanthoma, committed stem cells and neoplastic aberrant infundibulogenesis integral to formulating a conceptual model for an infundibulocystic pathway to squamous cell carcinoma. J Cutan Pathol 2021;48:184–91.

Multiple self-healing squamous epithelioma

10 Goudie D. Multiple self-healing squamous epithelioma (MSSE): a digenic trait associated with loss of function mutations in TGFBR1 and variants at a second linked locus on the long arm of chromosome 9. Genes (Basel) 2020;11:1410.
12 Sirisomboonwong KE, Martindale J, Keefe M, Goudie D, Poke G. Features of multiple self-healing squamous epithelioma and Loeys-Dietz syndrome in a patient with a novel TGFBR1 variant. Am J Med Genet A 2018;176:2892–5.

Generalized eruptive keratoacanthoma

1 Schwartz RA, Blaszczyk M, Jablonska S. Generalized eruptive keratoacanthoma of Grzybowski: follow-up of the original description and 50-year retrospect. Dermatology 2002;205:348–52.

Muir–Torre syndrome

11 Nguyen CV, Gaddis KJ, Stephens MR, Seykora JT, Chu EY. An intrapatient concordance study of mismatch repair protein immunohistochemical staining patterns in patients with Muir–Torre syndrome. JAMA Dermatol 2020;156:676–80.
22 Vasen HF, Blanco I, Aktan-Collan K et al. Revised guidelines for the clinical management of Lynch syndrome (HNPCC): recommendations by a group of European experts. Gut 2013;62:812–23.

CHAPTER 142

Melanoma Clinicopathology

Jean Jacques Grob and Caroline Gaudy-Marqueste

Service de Dermatologie et Cancérologie Cutanée, Hôpital de la Timone, Aix-Marseille Université, Marseille, France

Key references, 142.25

Definition
A malignant tumour arising from melanocytes.

Epidemiology

Descriptive epidemiology
Melanoma (MM), which only represents 4% of skin cancers, accounts for 80% of skin cancer deaths. White fair-skinned populations are mainly affected whereas incidence rates are low in dark-skinned populations. The global incidence of invasive MM is about 287 000 new cases per year with 60 000 deaths [1]. The highest incidence rates are currently recorded in Australia and New Zealand with up to 70 cases per 100 000 inhabitants per year [2] whereas the lowest rates are found in Asia and Africa [3]. These different figures are easily explained by sun gradients and phenotypic differences, with the highest rate in the most sunny areas and in those with fair skin. An opposite gradient is observed in European countries with the highest incidence rates in the North (23 cases per 100 000) rather than in the South (around 12 cases per 100 000) [4,5], probably related to the high economic level of northern populations who have more access to recreational travel and have a lighter skin type than southern Mediterranean populations.

Large disparities also exist in neighbouring countries (Poland/Germany or Hungary/Romania) despite apparently common environmental risk factors and phenotypic characteristics. This may be accounted for by differences in the collection and reporting of data as well as economic factors [1,4,6].

The diagnosis of MM can be made at any age except very early in life (0.6% of MM diagnosed under the age of 20) with a median age at diagnosis around 65 in the USA [7] and 9.0% of patients >85 years. Men seem to be more affected in high-incidence countries and in central, eastern and southern European countries, whereas females are predominantly affected in western and northern European countries [8–11]. The incidence is generally higher in women than men up to the age of approximately 50 years, after which higher rates prevail in men [9]. Differences in anatomical distribution by sex are also observed, with more lesions in the lower limb in females before mid-life and more lesions of the head and neck in males following mid-life [8]. Behavioural differences in relation to sun exposure might account for these differences as well as different susceptibility of melanocytes on different body sites as suggested by the divergent pathway hypothesis [8,12].

Epidemiological trends in incidence and mortality
The incidence of MM has been rising worldwide in developed countries over the past five decades, usually attributed to an increase in recreational sun exposure [1,3–6,13,14]. Annual incidence rates have increased among all populations, ranging from 3% to 7%, which results in a doubling every 10–20 years [3,9]. After a peak in 2005, data have shown a decrease of MM incidence in younger birth cohorts in several countries, contrasting with an increase of MM incidence in older adults, especially in males aged >60 years [2,5,8,13–17]. However, women in the 20–39 years age group appeared to have twice the risk of MM of young adult men [17] suggesting gender-related factors, either environmental or endogenous, are implicated in early-onset MM [16]. The trend of median tumour thickness towards thinner MM has been reported in Central Europe, the USA and Australia during recent decades [5,6,18]. However, a stable or increased incidence of thick MM (>4 mm) is also observed in most countries [5,19–23].

An overall increase in MM mortality has been observed over the past 30 years with notable variation between countries, males and females, and different age groups. The highest mortality rates are observed in Australia and Norway and among males and older age groups [14,24]. In contrast, a stabilisation or decrease in MM mortality was reported in Australia in the period 1994–2015, except in men aged 60 or over [2]. MM is currently the fifth leading cancer in males and the sixth in females [7,25]. In the USA, the numbers of deaths in the white population from 2014 to 2018 were 3.4/100 000 per year in males and 1.4/100 000 per year in females with a median age at death of 71 [7]. In Australia, mortality rates were around 5.72/100 000 and 2.53/100 000 per year in males and females, respectively, during the 2013–2015 period [26], whereas in Europe, estimated age standardised mortality rates for 2020 were 4.6/100 000 and 2.6/100 000 per year, respectively, with large disparities ranging from 1.6 to 5.3 in women, and from 2.8 to 9.6 in men [27].

Rook's Textbook of Dermatology, Tenth Edition. Edited by Christopher Griffiths, Jonathan Barker, Tanya Bleiker, Walayat Hussain and Rosalind Simpson.
© 2024 John Wiley & Sons Ltd. Published 2024 by John Wiley & Sons Ltd.

Current situation and public health consequences

Although the situation is much more favourable in countries where prevention campaigns and early detection interventions have been conducted, the situation is far from satisfactory. MM is one of the only cancers for which neither the incidence nor mortality is decreasing overall, except in very limited geographical, sex and age subgroups. Although there appears to be a more favourable trend in young generations, uncertainty remains. The decreasing trend in median tumour thickness [5,6,19,23] contrasting with the stability of thick MM and the relative stability of mortality rates [6] suggests that there might be a subtype of aggressive MM which causes mortality even when detected early with a thin Breslow thickness. This suggests that we cannot rely on early detection alone and that we need to develop new approaches to impact directly on the natural history of these aggressive tumours (see later).

Pathophysiology
Predisposing factors

The role of melanoma precursors. The proportion of cutaneous melanomas (CMs) which originate from normal skin or from a pre-existing naevus is uncertain [28]. A recent prospective study found that naevus remnants (of any type) were associated with more than half of MM cases, while other estimations consider that 80% of melanomas arise from normal skin [29]. In lentigo maligna melanoma and acral lentiginous melanoma no benign precursor lesion may be identified. A certain number of naevi have been suspected as having a higher risk than others of transforming into MM (dysplastic, congenital and a few others).

Searching for the 'missing link' between a naevus and MM. Genomic analysis of melanocytic lesions displaying intermediate morphological characteristics between benign naevi and MM has further confirmed the clonal origin of MM from adjacent naevi [30]. Distinct evolutionary trajectories have been established, with pathways incrementally perturbed by multiple independent genetic alterations. Common naevi typically showed a single activating mutation in the MAPK pathway, most commonly the BRAF V600E mutation, while MM, particularly in the advanced stages, typically harbours multiple alterations [30,31,**32**], suggesting that progression from benign lesions to advanced MM may depend on sequential acquisition of abnormalities involving oncogenes and tumour suppressors, as well as other classes of genes. *TERT* promoter mutations are the earliest secondary alterations, already emerging in intermediate lesions and MM *in situ* [30]. Such mutations were initially thought to be absent in benign naevi but they have been identified in benign melanocytic lesions and are thus considered as 'intermediate' [30–33]. However, whole genome sequencing data revealed that *TERT* promoter mutations were also present in morphologically benign naevi in subclonal populations and could not therefore serve as a molecular surrogate of malignancy [34]. Thus, the acquisition of step-by-step abnormalities leading to malignancy seems stochastic and therefore no naevus can be individualised as a privileged precursor of melanoma. In this regard, the so-called 'dysplastic' naevus should no longer be considered dysplastic, but only a common morphological variant of growing naevi.

The term 'melanocytoma' was recently introduced to define melanocytic neoplasms displaying an increased cellularity and/or atypia, i.e. additional molecular events compared with a common naevus [35]. Although melanocytomas are said to have an increased (although generally still low) probability of turning into an MM, this neologism is perhaps more a way to cover potential diagnostic uncertainty, rather than an identification of a real MM precursor. Similarly, several rare morphological entities like deep penetrating naevus (DPN), pigmented epithelioid melanocytoma (PEM) and BAP1-inactivated melanocytic neoplasms (BIM) showing distinctive histology owing to *CTNNB1/APC*, *PRKAR1A* and *BAP1* mutational hits, respectively [35,36], cannot be considered as frequent precursors, despite a seemingly high risk of local recurrence.

Congenital naevi. There is little doubt that congenital melanocytic naevi (CMN) may be precursors of MM, but the magnitude of risk of malignant transformation in MM (Chapter 73) remains controversial [37] and seems to be linked to the size of the lesion [38]. Therefore, CMN are arbitrarily classified as large, medium and small. For large CMN (defined by a largest diameter >20 cm), the lifetime risk of MM transformation has been estimated to be between 5 and 15% [39–42] but is probably lower (around 2.5–2.8%) [43,44]. Melanoma-associated large CMN are more often located on the trunk and present with satellites and a largest diameter of >40 cm [45] (Figure 142.1). Such lesions, sometimes also affecting the central nervous system, are more closely aligned to complex congenital malformations than to common naevi. Molecular investigations suggest that CMN are driven by mutations which are different from those of common naevi of adulthood [46]. NRAS mutation is the most common genetic hit underlying CMN pathogenesis but other molecular events can occur [46–48]. Whole genome sequencing data also show that while the UV radiation (UVR) mutational signature 7 is predominant in acquired naevi, mutational signatures 1 and 5 are predominant in CMN [34]. Malignant transformation of large CMN most often occurs during childhood [37–39,42,45] and more rarely later, from the skin but also within the central nervous system (CNS) [49]. Primary MM growing on the CNS accounts for approximately one-third of melanoma occurring in patients with CMN [50]. However, the real risk is difficult to quantify, given the difficulties in differentiating congenital neurological abnormalities from true CNS MM. The risk of MM appears to be higher in those with congenital abnormalities of the CNS [51].

The risk of transformation of small- or medium-sized CMN is even more controversial. The lifetime risk of transformation has been estimated to be between 2.6 and 4.9% in CMN <4.5 cm in diameter [52] but more likely similar to that of common naevi.

Common naevi. The annual risk of transformation of a naevus into a MM is very low and has been estimated to be around 1/200 000 before the age of 40 in both sexes and 1/30 000 for men older than 60 [53]. For a 20-year-old individual, the estimated lifetime risks of transformation of any given mole are about 1/3000 for males and 1/10 000 for females.

Atypical/dysplastic naevi. Atypical/dysplastic naevi (AN/DN) (Chapter 131) are acquired pigmented lesions which have been

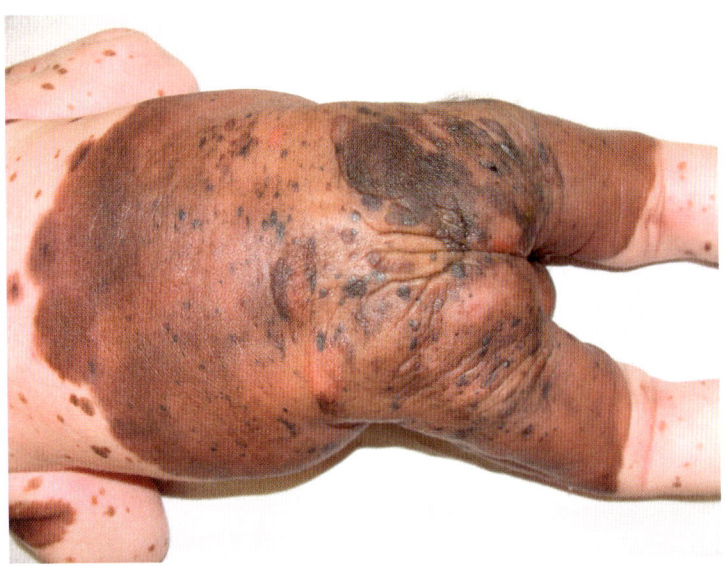

Figure 142.1 Large congenital naevus.

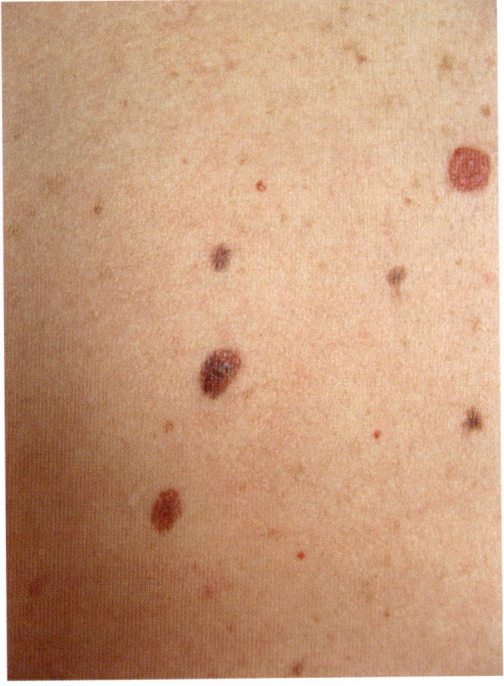

Figure 142.2 Atypical/dysplastic naevi.

isolated among common acquired naevi by either pathological (the concept of 'dysplastic naevi') or clinical features (the concept of 'atypical naevi'), although not all DN are AN and vice versa [54]. Such naevi are common in clinical practice, with DN representing approximately 5% of cutaneous pathological reports [55]. AN are characterised by a usually large size (>5 mm) with irregularly distributed colours (Figure 142.2) and a tendency to emerge even after a young age. These features may be considered clinically suspicious and often lead to excision for fear of an MM. From a pathological viewpoint, DN have some distinct patterns which may be interpreted either as a pattern of naevus growth or as a premalignant status (thus giving rise to the name dysplastic) [56,57].

Diagnostic criteria for DN have been developed and validated by the International Melanoma Pathology Study Group (IMPSG) [58]. They include a subset of lesions supposedly intermediate between a naevus and melanoma that are characterised by cytological and architectural atypia, and additional molecular events (in contrast to common acquired naevi which only have a single mutated gene) [30]. Mutation of the *TERT* promoter seems to be an early event in any progression towards melanoma *in situ*, but the correlation between this genetic alteration and the degree of morphological dysplasia is still unknown [30].

Although the number of AN/DN is a phenotypic risk factor for MM (risk increases with the number of DN in the same patient) [59,60], the risk of MM transformation of any single AN/DN is very low [61], and probably not higher than most other common naevi. Annual AN/DN transformation rates have been estimated to be around 1 in 30 000 moles and 1 in 40 000 moles for males and females, respectively [53]. In conclusion, although 'dysplastic naevi' have been the subject of scrutiny in the literature, they are, in essence, common large and flat naevi that should perhaps no longer be referred to as 'dysplastic' because they are neither frequent melanoma precursors nor an intermediate step to melanoma.

Practical consequences. Currently, the prophylactic surgical excision of naevi to prevent MM cannot be recommended, since none of the subtypes of naevi that we can identify fulfils the rate of transformation which would make it a cost-efficient or desirable exercise. Only the preventative removal of selected large congenital naevi may be desirable for risk reduction and cosmesis, although often surgery is impossible in practice due to the size and neurological extension of these lesions.

Genetics

Familial melanoma. Data on the prevalence of a reported family history of MM range from 1.3% in northern European studies to 15.8% in Australian studies. In a large meta-analysis [62], a family history of MM was associated with a twofold increased risk of MM development.

Phenotypic traits

Skin pigmentation and tanning abilities. Skin pigmentation and the ability to tan, reflecting the skin's sensitivity to sunlight exposure, are well-known risk factors for MM. In a meta-analysis, the pooled estimates of relative risk are around twofold for skin type I compared with skin type IV (Fitzpatrick's classification) [63]; approximately twofold for fair versus dark skin colour; around 1.5 for blue eyes versus dark eyes; 3.5 for red versus dark hair colour; and around twofold for a high density of freckles [64].

Naevus phenotype. Naevus phenotype may be defined by the number and features of naevi, which is dependent on the genetic background of the individual, but also on the amount of sun exposure since birth [65,66]. There is a spectrum of phenotypic expressions from virtually no naevi, to 10–30 small naevi, up to the so-called atypical or dysplastic naevus syndrome (DNS) characterised by a large number of atypical/dysplastic naevi

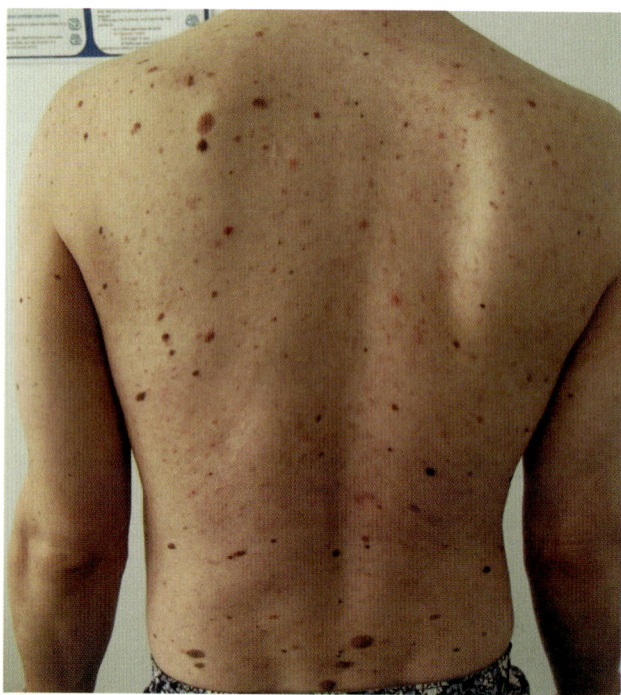

Figure 142.3 Atypical/dysplastic naevus syndrome.

(Figure 142.3). DNS was first described in 1978 [67] and subsequently described under various denominations such as atypical naevus syndrome [54,68,69], with or without a familial history of MM [70].

Among white people, a fairly large body of evidence suggested that the naevus phenotype (number, size and features of melanocytic naevi) represents a very good predictor for CM. The risk of MM rises with an increasing number of clinically atypical naevi. For example, a high naevus count (100–120 common naevi) is associated with an approximate sevenfold increased risk of MM compared to having fewer than 15 naevi. The presence of any clinically atypical naevi gives a relative risk of 4, increasing to more than 6 for patients carrying more than five atypical naevi as compared to non-carriers [71]. The cumulative risk of melanoma in members of families affected by a familial form of AN/DN syndrome is estimated to be 49% in individuals 10–50 years old and 82% in individuals 72 years old [72].

Genes associated with melanoma risk [73]

General understanding of genetically driven risk factors. A few major high penetrance genes confer a very high risk of MM and lead to familial aggregation of MM by a simple transmission of the gene. However, they account only for a minority of MM. Most sporadic cases of MM may be genetically driven to a certain extent by the convergence in a given individual of different alleles of low penetrance genes, which contribute to facilitate MM development via different mechanisms (pigmentation, molecular repair, control of melanocytes, etc.). This genetic background interacts with environmental factors, and as with all cancers, the stronger the genetics, the fewer the environmental factors there needs to be for a naevus to progress to MM.

Major melanoma susceptibility genes (high penetrance genes). High penetrance germline mutations in susceptibility genes are rare, but when present, confer on the carrier a high probability of developing at least one MM.

The cyclin-dependent kinase (CDK) inhibitor 2A gene (*CDKN2A*), located on chromosome 9p21, is the best known high-risk locus for MM susceptibility. *CDKN2A* encodes, via alternative splicing, two proteins involved in cell cycle regulation: p16/Ink4a and p14/Arf. These both act as tumour suppressors through the Rb and p53 cancer pathways, respectively [74]. *CDKN2A* mutations are found in approximately 40% of individuals with familial MM [75]. The probability of finding a mutation increases with the number of MM cases within the family [76], with a young age at diagnosis (<50 years) [77], and in the presence of individuals with multiple MM.

Germline mutations in *CDKN2A* increase the risk of MM development 65-fold [76]. MM occurs approximately 15 years earlier in *CDKN2A* mutation carriers compared with the general population [78]. An excess of pancreatic [77], upper digestive cancers and cancer involving the respiratory tract, and even more rarely breast cancers, has also been reported [79–82]. Patients with *CDKN2A* mutations affecting the p14ARF transcript (exon 1) may also develop tumours of the CNS [83,84].

Excluding multiple-case MM families, *CDKN2A* mutations have also been identified in patients presenting with multiple MM but with no family history, at a frequency of around 10% [85,86]. The penetrance of *CDKN2A* mutations is 30% by the age of 50 and 67% by the age of 80 and can be influenced by the naevus phenotype (number and type) and the geographical location. The highest penetrance is observed in regions with the highest MM incidence [87]. This variation as a result of geographical location suggests that other factors, such as the degree of sun exposure or other co-inherited gene modifiers, also contribute to the overall risk [88]. The impact of *CDKN2A* germline mutations on MM survival remains controversial with some reports suggesting worse survival in carriers versus wild-type patients [89,90], while no difference in overall survival or MM-specific survival was reported in an Italian population [91].

The *CDK4* gene located on chromosome 12q13 encodes the kinase targeted by p16/Ink4a. Any mutation of this gene abolishes the binding domain of p16/Ink4a. Only a single activating mutation in *CDK4* is necessary for tumourigenesis [92]. *CDK4* germline mutations are rare [93–95]. Only 2% of the families exhibited these mutations in the most extensive study of familial MM conducted by the Melanoma Genetics Consortium (GenoMel) [92], with fewer than 20 families reported in the literature. Similarly to *CDKN2A* mutations, *CDK4* germline mutations predispose to early-onset multiple primary MM and an increased number of atypical naevi [96]. An increased risk of other cancers has also been reported [80,96].

BAP1 is a tumour suppressor gene belonging to a subfamily of deubiquitinating enzymes involved in the removal of ubiquitin from proteins, in addition to the regulation of transcription, cell cycle and growth, response to DNA damage and chromatin dynamics. Germline mutations in the *BAP1* gene have been identified in families with hereditary cancers [97,98]. The clinical phenotype of *BAP1* hereditary cancer predisposition syndrome includes uveal MM (UM), mesothelioma, CM, renal cell carcinoma and atypical melanocytic tumours/naevi [99,**100**]. Several other tumours were also reported in these families including cholangiocarcinomas, meningiomas and basal cell carcinomas [73,99]. The high frequency of germline *BAP1* mutations in patients presenting with metastatic disease suggests that UM is more aggressive in these patients [101]. Recent data suggest that penetrance of *BAP1* mutation is fairly high and more than 80% of gene carriers are ultimately affected by at least one type of cancer [102]. The occurrence of the main *BAP1*-tumour types in carriers of null and missense variants respectively are, in decreasing order, UM (24.7% and 24%), mesothelioma (20.4% and 14.0%), CM (17.0% and 36%) and renal (10.2% and 12.0%) [103]. *BAP1*-inactivated naevi are present in up to 90% of mutation carriers. Their clinical presentation is distinctive with multiple, skin-coloured to reddish-brown, dome-shaped to pedunculated papules [99] appearing early in life and increasing in number with age [104]. Typical histological presentation is a dome-shaped, exclusively or predominantly intradermal melanocytic proliferation with spitzoid epithelioid cells frequently associated with a common naevus component [73,103,105].

TERT is one of the main components of telomerase and plays an important role in appropriate telomere length maintenance [106]. Telomeres are highly implicated in tumourigenesis and germline and somatic mutations of *TERT* are common in human cancer [73,107]. Somatic mutations in *TERT* are one of the earliest secondary mutations following *BRAF* or *NRAS* driver mutations and are found in 30–70% of somatic MM [30,73,108]. Germline mutations in the *TERT* promoter are rare but predispose to early-onset MM and other tumour types including ovarian, renal cell, bladder, breast and bronchial cancers [73,108,109]. Germline mutations in *ACD*, *TERF2IP* and *POT1*, encoding other member of the shelterin family involved in the regulation of telomere processing and stability, have also been reported to cause hereditary MM as well as several other human cancers [73,80,110–112]. Overall, germline mutations in *POT1*, *ACD* and *TERF2IP* are detected in approximately 9% of high-density families without mutations in known high penetrance genes [113].

Other susceptibility genes (intermediate penetrance genes). The melanocortin-1 receptor (*MC1R*) gene, a key regulator of skin pigmentation located on chromosome 16q24, is considered as a moderate-risk gene for MM. *MC1R* encodes the receptor protein for melanocyte-stimulating hormone (MSH). Losses in function are thus associated with a switch in melanin production from eumelanin to phaeomelanin. The *MC1R* gene locus is highly polymorphic. In one meta-analysis, variant *MC1R* alleles have been shown to double the risk of developing MM [114]. Recent data suggest a 1.5–4-fold increased risk of MM and a three- to fourfold risk of thick MM in *MC1R* variant carriers [115,116]. MM risk is increased in individuals carrying multiple-variant alleles compared with those with single variants [116]. Within 20 allelic variants [117], some are associated with the 'red hair, pale complexion, burn easily' phenotype [118], but some carry the risk of MM independent of skin type [115,119]. Several *MC1R* variants also serve as modifier alleles on the *CDKN2A* gene [120,121]. The penetrance of *CDKN2A* mutations increases from 50% to more than 80% among patients with *MC1R* variants and the age of onset of MM is significantly reduced (by 20 years) [122].

Missense variants of *ASIP*, encoding the agouti-signalling protein, have been identified in both European [122,123] and Australian populations [124] with an odds ratio ranging from 1.45 [125] to 1.7 [126]. Variants in *TYR*, encoding tyrosinase protein, have also been reported to slightly increase MM risk [114]. Among the several other low penetrance genes involved in pigmentation and naevus count [92], some appear to confer protection from MM: *SLC45A2B* (*MATP*) [114,122,126] and *TYRP1* [114,122]. Others increase the risk: *OCA2* [127,128] and *MYO7A* [128].

The combination of single nucleotide polymorphisms (SNPs) in five loci (*MC1R*, *SLC45A2*, *OCA2*, *TYR* and *ASIP*) has been shown to explain roughly one-third to one-half of the variation in the risk due to observed pigmentation phenotype [129]. Several other genes related to the production or transport of melanin, hair colour, tanning ability, naevus count or melanocyte proliferation, differentiation and survival are currently being studied [126] but more studies are needed to assess their definitive effects on MM susceptibility.

MITF (microphthalmia-associated transcription factor) is a master regulator gene of melanocyte development and differentiation. Several *MITF* target genes are known to regulate cell cycle and survival [130]. *MITF* appears to protect against oxidative stress [131]. Carriers of the *E318K* variant have a three- to fivefold increased risk of MM [132,133]. The mutation has also been detected in patients affected by multiple primary MM or presenting with both MM and renal cell carcinoma [133,134]. Carriers with a personal or familial history of pancreatic cancer have a 31-fold increased risk for developing a CM, while this increase is eightfold for those with a personal or familial history of renal cancer [134].

Variants in the DNA repair genes *XPF* and *ERCC1* have been shown to increase MM risk [135,136], whereas *XRCC3* variants appear to be protective [137]. An association of *XRCC1* and *ERCC1* variants with an increased rate of survival has also been demonstrated [137,138].

Genes involved in the metabolism and detoxification of oxygen radicals (*CYP2D6* and glutathione-S-transferases (GSTs)) as well as immune response genes (*IL10*, *IL1α*, *TNFβ*, *IL6R*, HLA class II alleles and *ICAM1*) have been investigated as possible MM susceptibility genes with conflicting results [92]. Vitamin D receptor polymorphisms data remain contradictory [139–141].

Environmental factors

Role of UV and sun exposure in melanoma. Sun exposure has been identified as an environmental risk factor for MM development, on the basis of epidemiological data. To date, although this remains the only definitive environmental factor associated with MM, the attributable risk is not at all at the level of smoking and lung cancer for instance [142]. The association of sun (UV) exposure with MM appears complex and uncertainties remain regarding the timing of vulnerable periods of sun exposure, the respective aetiological role of continuous versus intermittent UV exposure, and the interactions of sun exposure with phenotypic factors (e.g. skin, hair and eye colour, etc.) [125,143,144]. In addition, there are probably different types of MM which may develop depending on an individual's sun exposure [145–149].

Biological data. MM has been shown to contain significantly elevated numbers of UVR signature mutations compared with internal cancers [150]. A series of studies has confirmed that sun-exposed

MM had markedly more UVR-like C>T somatic mutations compared with sun-shielded acral lentiginous, mucosal and UM. UVR signatures have been identified in driver mutations [151–153]. Due to their low basal DNA repair capacity leading to the retention of 'damaged' cells [154], genomic damage from intermittent sun exposure during childhood and adolescence seems to have more consequences in melanocytes than keratinocytes [143,154]. Animal models tend to confirm this hypothesis [155].

Epidemiological data. Demographic data have indicated that, within countries, MM incidence and mortality among white people correlate inversely with the latitude of residence and the dose of UV radiation, the highest rates being nearest the equator [156]. Multiple case–control studies have shown that patients with fair complexions (light skin types) are at a greater risk of developing an MM [64]. Ambient exposure studies have reported that fair-skinned people born and raised in environments of low solar irradiation exhibited significantly lower risks of CM than people of similar complexion born and raised in sunny environments [157]. Many case–control studies converge to demonstrate that sun exposure as a whole confers a risk of MM, although this risk is relatively low [**142**], ranging between 1.2 and 2.

Type of sun exposure. Meta-analysis from multiple case–control studies suggests that MM risk is mainly related to intermittent sun exposure and a history of sunburn [**142**]. The pattern of sun exposure varies according to the anatomical location of the MM. Trunk MM are preferentially associated with intermittent patterns of sun exposure while head and neck MM, like lentigo maligna, are preferentially associated with chronic patterns of sun exposure [151]. The impact of chronic and/or cumulative exposure to sunlight is also documented.

The presence or history of pre-malignant and cancerous lesions (actinic keratosis, squamous cell carcinoma and basal cell carcinoma) confers a risk of 4.28 and the presence of actinic damage indicators such as solar lentigines and elastosis, a risk of 2.02 [64,**142**]. However, separating intermittent from chronic and cumulative exposure to sunlight is somewhat of an artificial oversimplification. For example, lentigo maligna on the face of elderly people may also be influenced by an accumulation of intermittent sun exposure [158].

Sun exposure in childhood. Repeated intermittent sun exposure during childhood is considered an important risk factor for MM [143,157]. Migrant studies have provided evidence that childhood and adolescence are critical periods for future MM development. Young Australian migrants arriving before the age of 10 years to sunny climates had an increased risk of MM compared with later migrants (>15 years or older) [159,160]. There were similar findings for European patients [161] and Israeli males [162]. Studies of location of residence provided further evidence: an increased risk of MM was found in women whose residence between 15 and 20 years of age was more equatorial in latitude [163] or in those who lived near the coast before the age of 15 [164]. In a meta-analysis pooling results from 51 independent study populations for those who had experienced even a single sunburn episode and risk of CM, the risk was highest in childhood (1.9 times), followed by adolescence (1.6 times) and adulthood (1.4 times) [165]. Despite all the evidence, separating the role of childhood from adult exposure is artificial as people tend to keep their sun habits in childhood throughout their life, and earlier exposure also implies an increase of cumulative exposure at any age.

Artificial sources of UV: sunbeds and therapeutic UV. Indoor tanning is a widespread practice in most developed countries, particularly in northern Europe and the USA. Although initial studies [166–168] did not initially establish evidence of a risk associated with sunbed use, sunlamp usage or attendance at a tanning salon, the use of artificial UV sources was later shown to be significantly associated with melanoma after adjusting for potential confounding variables, with a higher risk in younger populations [169–171].

A meta-analysis extended to studies published up to May 2012 demonstrated a relative risk of MM of around 1.2 if artificial UV sources were used [172]. This risk increased by 1.8% for each additional session of sunbed use per year and reached 42% in cases of intensive use. The first use of sunbeds before the age of 35 years is also associated with a higher risk [172,173]. Indoor tanning has been banned in Australia and some other states, and regulation has been reinforced in many countries with restricted teenage access. In the USA, the Food and Drug Administration (FDA) established a requirement for sunlamp products to carry a visible black-box warning on all devices stating that the sunlamp product should not be used on persons under the age of 18 years.

Therapeutic UV can also be involved in MM risk. Patients receiving psoralen and ultraviolet A (PUVA) therapy often develop lentigines [174]. As PUVA has been shown to induce CM in mice [175] and as it stimulates the growth of MM cells *in vivo* [176], there is reason to believe that PUVA treatment may cause MM [177].

Stern *et al.* were the first to report that there might be an increased risk for MM in a 16-centre prospective study of 1380 patients treated with high cumulative dosages of PUVA [178]. The increased risk began 15 years after first exposure to PUVA and was significantly higher in the study patients than in an age- and gender-matched US population. There was also a significant link between a high level of exposure to PUVA (at least 250 sessions). In the most recent assessment from the same PUVA follow-up cohort, after adjustment for age and gender, the incidence of both invasive and *in situ* MM more than doubled among patients exposed to at least 200 PUVA treatments compared with cohort patients exposed to lower doses. When the time since first treatment was >15 years compared with <15 years, the risk for MM increased approximately five times in patients treated with high doses of PUVA [179]. These results were not confirmed in European cohorts [177,180,181]. However, the power to detect an increased risk may have been affected by a shorter follow-up period [182]. Despite the limitations of the available studies in terms of sample size, duration of follow-up and exposure classification, no increased risk of MM has been suggested following narrow-band UVB therapy [183–186].

Prevention

Primary prevention of melanoma

This involves the identification of individuals particularly at risk of melanoma using genetic and/or phenotypic tools, and utilising information about the general population with the aim of reducing the risk linked to the sun exposure.

Phenotypic tools to identify population at risk.
Many algorithms have been proposed to distinguish those with a high risk of MM based on hair and skin colour, sun sensitivity and number of naevi [187–191]. However, it is impossible to clearly define a population from which most MM will develop, and even more challenging discerning those from which the most aggressive ones may occur.

People with fair skin colour and high density of naevi have a higher risk of MM, but most aggressive MM do not develop in these patients. Genetic testing and treatment of large data by artificial intelligence may help in the future to characterise people at risk not identifiable on the basis of these current phenotypic criteria.

Genetic tools to identify population at risk.
The assessment of MM predisposing mutations is not currently part of routine clinical practice. Mutations of *CDKN2A* are rare and thus have a low probability of detection in unselected populations. A guide by which to select patients for genetic testing according to the incidence of MM and prevalence of mutations in each region has been proposed by Leachman *et al.* [192].

For moderate to high MM incident areas (such as the USA and northern Europe), individuals currently considered appropriate candidates for genetic testing are those with three or more primary MM and/or families with at least one invasive MM and two or more other diagnoses of MM and/or pancreatic cancer among first- or second-degree relatives on the same side of the family.

For low MM incidence areas (such as southern Europe), appropriate candidates are individuals with two primary MM and/or families with at least one invasive MM and one or more other diagnoses of MM and/or pancreatic cancer among first- or second-degree relatives on the same side of the family.

CDKN2A genetic testing in patients with DNS without a positive family history of MM is not justified based on current data. At present, genetic testing in cases of familial MM can neither provide certainty to non-carriers, nor give additional information to individuals already recognised as at risk by their phenotype or allow a more discriminative detection of patients at risk in the general population.

Indeed, in large cohorts of families carrying mutations in *CDKN2A*, the incidence of MM may be increased in some individuals not carrying mutations in *CDKN2A* (probably due to the co-inheritance of other less penetrant susceptibility genes and the existence of environmental risk factors), while some individuals carrying mutations may never develop MM [193].

Genetic testing including low or intermediate penetrance genes is mostly a field of research, with so far little impact on daily practice. Patients with a strong family history but negative for *CDKN2A* and *CDK4* mutations can be tested for *BAP1* in the presence of typical cutaneous melanocytic nevi, uveal MM or other associated cancers or *MITF* in the presence of renal cell carcinoma [113]. A surveillance plan for germline *BAP1* mutation carriers has been proposed by Star and colleagues but remains controversial [194].

Campaigns for sun avoidance.
Reducing UV exposure is the basis of primary prevention of MM. Phenotypic risk factors help to tailor the sun protection message to the individual. The challenge of influencing the incidence of MM by sun protection is a difficult one. It is important to note that sun protection campaigns have reduced the dramatic increase in MM incidence, but so far failed to actually decrease the incidence of MM [195]. This is probably linked to the difficulty in changing societal trends, which have promoted sun-related UV exposure in the last 60 years as a source of pleasure, associated with fashion, sport, health and other positive values. The awareness of the risk of sun-related UV exposure has considerably improved but changing the behaviour of a population is difficult and slow, especially in the context of a society which places value on the sun, tanning and the ability to travel. The role of sunscreens is difficult to define. The protection spectrum of current sunscreens is likely to cover the radiation at risk in MM, and cohort studies have suggested that sunscreen use could protect against MM [**196**]. However, most people do not use sunscreens in a way which could be protective [197,198]. If they were using them correctly for the whole body, the large quantities may also be a risk via penetration of filters or nanoparticles – although this remains highly controversial. They can thus be promoted as a complement to clothing. So far, no drug has shown efficacy in chemoprevention of MM [199].

Pathology
Histological assessment remains the gold standard for MM diagnosis. Features captured on histology such as depth of invasion and ulceration can also guide appropriate treatment.

Histoclinical subtypes.
The first classification system was proposed by McGovern *et al.* in 1973 [200] into four main types: nodular melanoma (NM), superficial spreading melanoma (SSM), lentigo maligna melanoma (LMM) and acral lentiginous melanoma (ALM). This classification is based on the hypothesis that these patterns reflect the way the tumour grows. All MM first expand along the basal membrane (radial growth phase) [201] before penetrating into the dermis (vertical growth phase), which gives rise to the potential metastatic process. NM, SSM, LMM and ALM can now be understood as four points within a continuous spectrum of tumours. At one end of the spectrum there are MM with a long horizontal phase (LMM and ALM), and thus plenty of time to detect them before they turn into an aggressive vertical phase. At the other end of the spectrum, NM have virtually no horizontal phase and turn rapidly into vertical progression. In this regard, many studies have confirmed that NM have a poorer prognosis than the other histoclinical subtypes. Between the two ends of the spectrum, SSM represent the most frequent intermediate situation with a horizontal phase followed more or less rapidly by a vertical growth. Although used in everyday practice, this classification is not very informative about the biological aggressiveness of the tumour and has little practical input to the assessment of prognosis. It will hopefully be replaced by a classification with more reliable prognostic value and perhaps therapeutic indications.

New approaches for primary melanoma classification
Several classifications have emerged over the past few years.

Epidemiological classification. In an attempt to explain the complex epidemiological data, a 'dual pathway' hypothesis and classification were proposed by Whiteman et al. [202]. In people with a high naevus count (presumed to have melanocytes with genetically high proliferative potential), sun-related UV exposure is required only to initiate MM development, after which other host factors drive progression to cancer. In contrast, in people with low propensity to develop naevi, a lot of sun-related UV exposure is necessary to drive melanocytes into MM [12,203].

Classification based on tumour kinetics and aggressiveness. It is clear that all primary MM do not have the same biological behaviour, with some behaving very aggressively and others as slow indolent tumours. The suggestion that this 'aggressiveness' could be estimated by the kinetics of the tumour has been proposed and confirmed to be valid. The growth rate calculation, based on the Breslow thickness and self-reported information from the patient about the time taken for the MM to develop [204], has been shown to be a prognostic marker predictive of aggressiveness independent of tumour thickness [204]. An aggressive, fast-growing subtype of MM can thus be individualised. These MM are associated with clinical features that are not those usually described by algorithms like ABCD (asymmetry, border, colour, diameter), and they are more often nodular, developing on the trunk, with specific risk factors (elderly males presenting with few melanocytic naevi and freckles, no clear excessive sun exposure in childhood and higher rate of past history of non-melanoma skin cancers) [205–209]. Biological features of aggressiveness are also found in these fast-growing melanomas such as high mitotic rate, high expression of proliferation markers [210] and a higher frequency of *NRAS* and *TERT* promoter mutations [211,212]. The challenge is now to find molecular markers for these aggressive MM, which may be dangerous even when detected early and warrant early drug intervention.

Molecular classification. Over the past 15 years, molecular studies have provided strong genetic support for the existence of distinct molecular pathways to MM [151,213,214].

Mutations in proteins along the RAS-RAF-MEK-ERK pathway resulting in the aberrant activation of the mitogen-activated protein kinase (MAPK) pathway are present in the most common MM histoclinical subtypes, covering over 80% of primary MM [213,214]. The three most frequently activated oncogenes in CM are *BRAF* (40–50%), *NRAS* (15–28%) and *NF1* (14%) [215–217]. A genomic classification into four subtypes, mutant *BRAF*, mutant *RAS*, mutant *NF1* and Triple-WT (wild-type), was proposed in 2015 [218], and further expanded in 2018 by the World Health Organization (WHO) classification of cutaneous tumours [35] (see later).

Desmoplastic MM usually lacks activating mutations in the MAPK pathway and instead harbours *NF1* mutations in combination with amplifications of kinases such as *EGFR*, *MET*, *ERBB2* and inactivation of *RB1*, *CDKN2A* [219].

Malignant Spitz tumours (Spitzoid MM) also usually lack mutations in the MAPK pathway and instead display mutually exclusive kinase fusions of *ROS1*, *ALK*, *BRAF*, *NTRK1*, *NTRK3*, *MET*, *RET* [220].

The mutational landscape of mucosal MM is significantly different [221,222]. Approximately 28% of mucosal MM harbour *BRAF*-V600 mutations (6% *BRAF*, 8% *NRAS* and 14% *NF1*) versus 94% of CMs. *KIT* and *SF3B1* mutations are also frequent (up to 20% of *KIT* mutations and 15% of *S3BF1* mutations in mucosal MM vs 7% and 8% respectively for CM) [215,217,218,221,222].

Uveal MM shows a different pattern of driver mutations. Alterations in the heterotrimeric G proteins (GNAQ) or GNA11 which couple seven-transmembrane domain receptors to intracellular signalling machinery are found in up to 50% of the tumours [223,224]. The activating *GNAQ/11* mutations are also present in benign choroidan naevi and are therefore thought to be precursor events requiring a 'second hit' in order to lead to malignant transformation [225]. A second layer of mutations consists of mutations in *BAP1*, *SF3B1* and *EIFIAX* (present respectively in 33%, 23% and 13% of the 80 uveal MM samples analysed in the TCGA uveal MM project) [225]. These mutations were usually mutually exclusive and were associated with distinct prognoses [225].

WHO classification of cutaneous tumours. This classification proposed in 2018 distinguishes nine subsets of MM based on their epidemiology, clinical and histological morphology, and genomic characteristics. MM are divided into those considered aetiologically related to sun exposure and those that are not, as determined by their mutational signatures, anatomical site and epidemiology. MM on sun-exposed skin are further divided according to the histopathological degree of associated solar elastosis of the surrounding skin into low-CSD (chronically sun-damaged), including SSM, and high-CSD, including lentigo maligna and desmoplastic MM. The 'non-solar' category includes acral MM, MM arising in congenital naevi, MM in blue naevi, Spitzoid MM, mucosal MM and uveal MM [35].

Any classification that integrates epidemiological, clinical, histological and genomic characteristics should ideally inform us of the intrinsic aggressiveness of the primary MM. To date, the genetic profiling of tumours does not yet permit a real operational classification.

However, some correlations have been found between some mutation profiles and histoclinical subtypes: more *BRAF* mutation in SSM, *NRAS* in NM, *KIT* mutations in ALM, LMM and mucosal MM and *NF1* mutations in desmoplastic MM; age (more *BRAF* mutations in young people and *NRAS* in older); location (higher *BRAF* mutation rates for primary tumours developed on the trunk and limb and *KIT* in acral or mucosal sites); sun damage (more *BRAF* and *NRAS* mutations in tumours developed on intermittent sun-exposed sites and *KIT* on chronically sun-exposed areas) [215–218,226,227]. Molecular profiling by new sequencing techniques may thus help to characterise MM subtypes with prognostic and therapeutic applications in the future.

Clinical features

General principles of early clinical diagnosis

Early diagnosis of MM is considered the best way to save a patient's life. However, early MM are usually discrete and may be difficult to distinguish from benign pigmented lesions. The challenge is to have a high sensitivity for MM but also a reasonable specificity to avoid the inappropriate excisions of benign lesions. Clinicians determine the likelihood that a given pigmented lesion may or may not be an MM, by making an analysis of colour distribution and shapes, based on the fact that an MM is more likely to display a disordered and changing pattern of colour compared with a benign naevus. Consciously or subconsciously the following four general principles are applied: analytical examination, pattern recognition, comparative analysis and dynamic analysis.

Analytical examination and algorithms. This is the most commonly described diagnostic clue, known as the ABCD algorithm [228] (Box 142.1), which assumes that if a naevus is *A*symmetrical, with irregular *B*orders and inhomogeneous *C*olour, with a *D*iameter over 6 mm, it may be considered as a potential MM. More recently, the addition of 'E' to denote lesion 'Evolution' has been added to the algorithm. More complex algorithms such as the seven-point checklist [229] have been developed in order to help clinicians, but also the public for MM detection. However, a large number of seborrhoeic keratoses and atypical naevi fulfil the ABCD criteria whereas many MM (in particular NMs) do not.

> **Box 142.1 ABCDE algorithm**
>
> - Asymmetry
> - Border irregularity
> - Colour variegation
> - Diameter >6 mm
> - Evolution

Pattern recognition. The human brain recognises any object by a cognitive strategy based on a holistic recognition of the image. When an individual sees a new object, a cognitive pattern, or a representation for this object, is built subconsciously, which will then be used to recognise it when faced with the object again. Thus, those who see more MM will more easily recognise a new one. Indeed, the diagnostic accuracy of dermatologists in pigmented lesions has been shown to rely much more on overall pattern recognition than on the application of a combination of criteria such as ABCDE [230–233].

Intra-individual comparative analysis ('ugly duckling' sign). This cognitive process is based on the human brain's ability to recognise any object that does not fit in its environment. Naevi in a given individual tend to share morphological characteristics [233] that the human brain has the ability to perceive [230], and which differ from the naevi in another individual. A naevus which does not fit into any of the few dominant patterns of naevi of a given individual deserves attention even though it may not appear highly suspicious in a separate analytical analysis. This 'ugly duckling' (UD) sign [232], which has been subconsciously used by dermatologists for decades, is now widely recognised as a major sign for MM suspicion [**234**]. Conversely, a naevus that fits into one of the dominant clusters of naevi in a given individual is unlikely to be an MM, even though it may be considered as such in an isolated analysis.

Dynamic analysis. Naevi grow and change, but slowly (over years) and mainly in the first two decades, while contrastingly most MM tend to grow and change faster or appear *de novo*. Therefore, dynamic assessment either of the changes, in the size, colour or shape of pre-existing pigmented lesions, or of any new growing skin lesion is an important criterion for suspecting an MM.

This led to the implementation of the *E* (*Evolution*) in the ABCDE rule. Although patients and their families can perceive a change in naevi, dynamic assessment is highly facilitated when there is a document like a 'whole body photograph' to refer to, in order to ascertain the reality and the rapidity of a change in any skin lesion, as well as the appearance of a new lesion. This is particularly important in people with a lot of atypical naevi, in which analysis and even pattern recognition may fail.

Diagnostic tools

Several tools have been developed to increase the accuracy of visual examination.

Dermoscopy (Chapter 145). This is a simple non-invasive method allowing magnified *in vivo* observation of the skin. Dermoscopy, which increases the granularity of observation, has been shown to improve the diagnostic accuracy for MM in comparison with inspection by the unaided eye with a 10–27% increase in sensitivity [235].

One of the major impacts is to reduce unnecessary excisions of benign lesions, by increasing specificity. Despite these advantages, one has to keep in mind that dermoscopy has the same limits as visual examination because it is mainly based on an analysis of colour distribution, which is not a perfect reflection of malignancy. The four principles of diagnosis are exactly the same as in clinical diagnosis. Dermoscopy experts have developed several analytical examination criteria, describing as many encountered patterns as possible. However, this becomes increasingly complex for the non-expert and reduces reproducibility among non-specialists. Ultimately, the intuitive interpretation of dermoscopy relies on pattern recognition, comparative analysis (UD) and dynamic analysis, which ultimately contribute to the final dermatoscopic diagnosis. As in clinical examination, success depends on the training and ultimate experience of the clinician.

Computerised dermoscopy devices. With the storage of high-resolution images, such devices permit sequential digital dermatoscopic monitoring of lesions, and thus improve dynamic analysis, which is particularly useful in patients with multiple (atypical) naevi.

Other source of images

Reflectance confocal microscopy. This uses a near infrared laser to obtain *in vivo* imaging of the top layers of the skin. The device produces horizontal sections at nearly histopathological resolution. Specific morphological patterns are observed, allowing for differentiating between benign and malignant lesions, but also melanocytic from non-melanocytic lesions such as pigmented basal cell carcinoma. Specific algorithms have been proposed for MM detection [236–238].

The main application of this is in the targeting of the optimal region to biopsy in the case of a large equivocal lesion when located on a cosmetically sensitive area [239,240]. The main limitations are the time spent for assessment of one lesion and the low penetration within the skin.

Optical coherence tomography (OCT). OCT uses a low-coherence source of light to image non-transparent tissues. It allows examination of skin lesions at a structural resolution (approximately 10 µm) and generates serial axial images reaching deep down to the reticular dermis (at a depth of approximately 2 mm) [241]. This technique has been used to analyse non-melanocytic tumours, with a large number of studies on basal cell carcinoma [242]. The technology is still under development for the analysis of melanocytic lesions [243].

Other non-invasive techniques based on a wide range of concepts are currently under investigation [244]. For example, multispectral analysis uses a specific software to process images obtained from different wavelengths; electrical impedance spectroscopy assumes that cancer cells have electrochemical properties that are distinct from those of healthy cells.

Other sources of diagnostic information. Genomic analysis of the squames uses an adhesive tape to sample cells from the stratum corneum (tape stripping) and analyses the expression of targeted genes. Mass spectrometry analysis is based on protein expression profile.

Computer-aided diagnostic systems (CAD). CAD systems utilise dermatoscopic images for monitoring pigmented skin lesions. Some systems have demonstrated good performance in an experimental setting. The practical benefit of such devices in a real-world clinical setting is still under investigation. Early studies relied on hand-crafted feature engineering and segmentation masks, but recent advances in computer science and the introduction of convolutional neural networks and deep-learning-based approaches have revolutionised the classification of medical image analysis [245].

Despite numerous breakthrough studies that demonstrate expert-level accuracy of CAD for MM [245,246–248], many limitations exist including quality, diversity and lack of generalisability of the training data sets. As a consequence, existing devices or applications are not widely used in current practice [249]. Approaches relying on human–computer collaboration [250,251], utilising artificial intelligence algorithms, are likely to be the way forward in the future. Artificial intelligence could also permit the integration of other sources of information about the tumour other than visible light and dermoscopy (for example, ultrasound and OCT, etc.) and factors other than morphology such as an individual's phenotypic trait, to make the best use of such systems.

Presentation

The most common clinicopathological situations in early diagnosis of melanoma are described.

Situation 1: 'an atypical naevus' (superficial spreading MM). In most cases (60–70% of MM), which usually correspond to the SSM histoclinical subtype, MM presents like an atypical naevus, i.e. a flat pigmented macule (Figure 142.4a–c) which progressively becomes more and more irregular in shape and colour (Figure 142.5a) with shades of brown, black, grey and red as well as depigmented areas (regression) over several months or more rarely years. This situation represents one of the best uses of dermoscopy, since the main differential diagnosis is the AN/DN, which is very common and shares most of the morphological characteristics (ABCD) to some degree. It is a real challenge in people with multiple atypical naevi, who are at risk of developing such an MM. In these situations, monitoring by digital dermoscopy is the most effective technique although it can be labour intensive.

At the earliest stage, the 'atypical naevus-like lesion' may in fact correspond to an MM *in situ* (MM cells migrating only in the epidermis), or to a focal malignant transformation in the middle or the border of a pre-existing naevus. As growth continues, the diagnosis will become obvious; the lesion will become palpable with the development of a nodule, reflecting the vertical growth phase, that may bleed (Figure 142.5b), and is no longer an early diagnosis.

Situation 2: 'a pigmented or red nodule' (nodular melanoma). Between 10 and 20% of MM may present as a regular, symmetrical, elevated, dome-shaped papulo-nodule. Infrequently it appears polypoid or sometimes pedunculated in nature (Figure 142.6a–c). Its colour ranges from black, dark brown to red. NM belong to the fast-growing subgroup of MM and are therefore usually thick tumours at diagnosis. Ulceration and bleeding are commonly seen. Lesions to consider in the differential diagnosis especially when the lesion is not pigmented are basal cell carcinoma, angioma and dermatofibroma. The rule should be to biopsy any fast-growing nodule. Dermoscopy is less helpful in these nodular lesions, especially in those with little or no pigmentation.

Situation 3: 'a lentigo of the face in the elderly' (lentigo maligna melanoma). This type of MM presents as a flat, brown or black, irregularly shaped lesion which grows slowly over months and years on chronically sun-exposed areas of the skin (e.g. the face, neck, forearms) in the elderly (Figure 142.7a–e). It corresponds in most cases to the LMM histoclinical subtype and is part of the slowly growing MM subgroup with a prolonged radial growth phase. This situation is challenging since MM, especially in the early intraepidermal phase known as a lentigo maligna (Hutchinson's melanotic freckle; melanosis circumscripta precancerosa of Dubreuilh), can be mistaken for a solar lentigo, a pigmented actinic keratosis or a flat seborrhoeic keratosis. In time, a nodule may develop, making the diagnosis of MM obvious.

Situation 4: 'a pigmented stain on the sole' (acral lentiginous melanoma). The initial presentation is of a discrete light brown or black macule, often described as a 'dirt-like stain', with indistinct borders on the soles of patients usually aged over 60 years. The frequency differs by race ranging from 2% to 10% of MM in white to 60% to 72% in dark-skinned populations. This situation corresponds in most cases to the ALM subtype (Figure 142.8a–d), and in a substantial proportion to the *KIT* mutated group. Because of the discrete position, the diagnosis is often delayed by years. In darker-skinned populations, benign pigmentation on the soles is frequent and may be confusing. At later stages, a nodule or ulceration can develop (Figure 142.9), which should make the diagnosis more apparent, but may still be confused with warts or trophic ulceration.

Situation 5: 'pigmentation in the nail' (subungual melanoma). This form represents approximately 2–3% of MM in white-skinned individuals but a higher proportion in darker-skinned populations. The first sign is a brown to black linear discoloration in the nail bed,

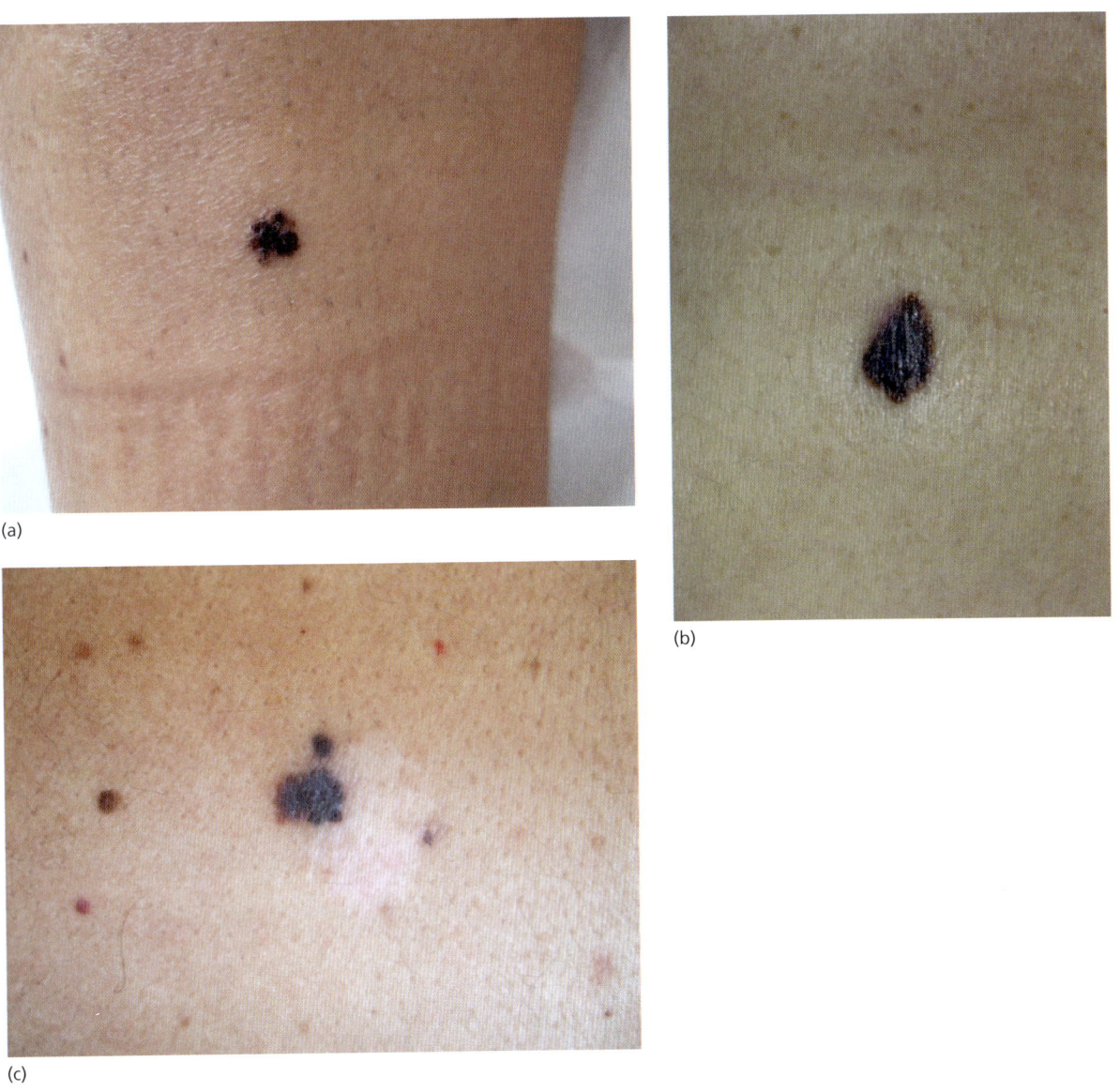

Figure 142.4 (a–c) Superficial spreading melanoma (early presentation).

which is hard to differentiate from benign melanonychia, which is quite common, especially in darker skin (Figure 142.10). ALM will often present as an irregular band, but it remains a diagnostic challenge not to miss an MM and to avoid over-biopsying the nail bed with consequent permanent nail disfigurement. Dermoscopy may be of some use, but changes in the width and colour of the nail band should raise suspicion of an MM. Later, symptoms become prominent with Hutchinson's sign (pigmentation in the adjacent skin) and inflammatory or pigmented paronychia being seen (Figure 142.11a–c). However, distinguishing ALM from other benign nail pathology such as onychomycosis, paronychia, subungual haemorrhage, benign naevus and pyogenic granuloma is not always straightforward.

Other clinical situations

Pigmented lesion of the vulva or the mouth. Primary MM arising from the mucosal epithelia lining the respiratory, alimentary and genito-urinary tracts are quite rare (<5%). MM of the mouth and vulva are the most frequent. They present as irregular macular pigmentation (Figure 142.12a,b). The diagnosis may be readily apparent but requires a chance gynaecological or stomatological examination, unless the patient themselves specifically notices such changes. Ulceration and bleeding are common at later stages. The prognosis is often poor due to a late diagnosis and should therefore prompt clinicians to undertake routine mucosal examination when screening for melanoma.

Melanoma arising within congenital naevi. Detection of MM within giant congenital naevi is often difficult because of the frequent verrucous and lobulated surface of these naevi, and because benign nodular flare-ups are sometimes observed. The development of MM in the deep portions of the naevus (within the dermis and subcutaneous fat) makes the diagnosis very challenging.

Ocular melanoma. Ocular MM, arising from melanocytes situated in the conjunctival membrane and uveal tract of the eye, is the

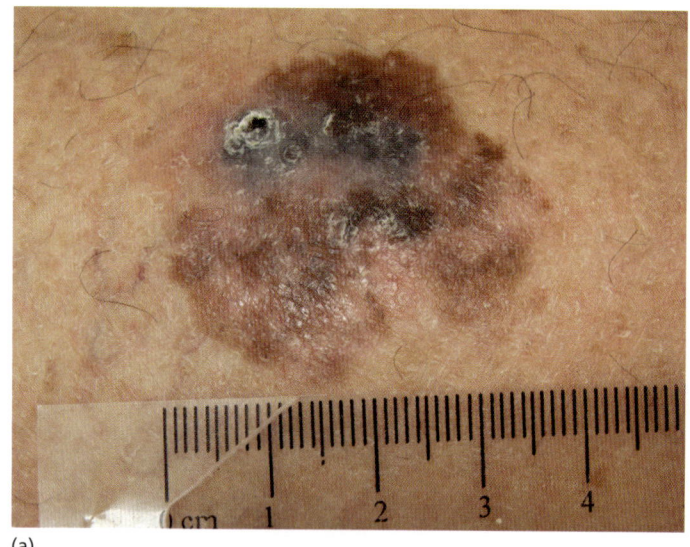

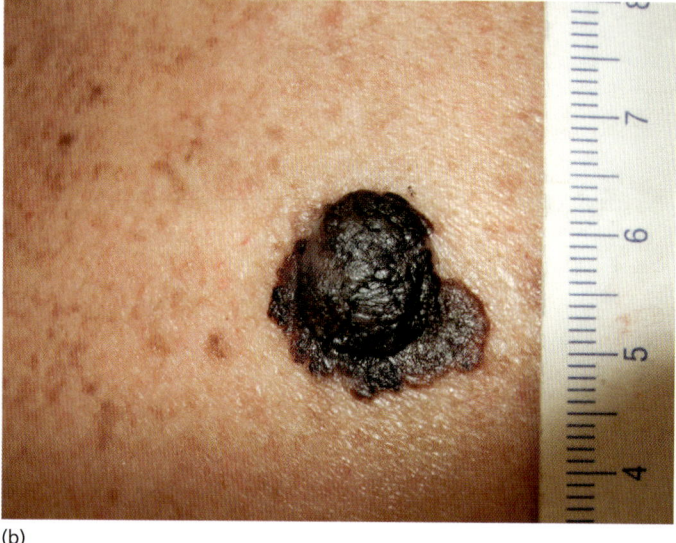

Figure 142.5 (a, b) Superficial spreading melanoma (late presentation).

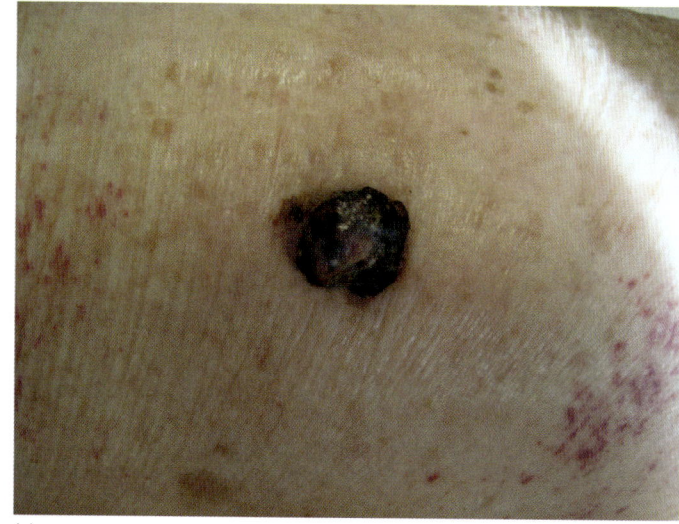

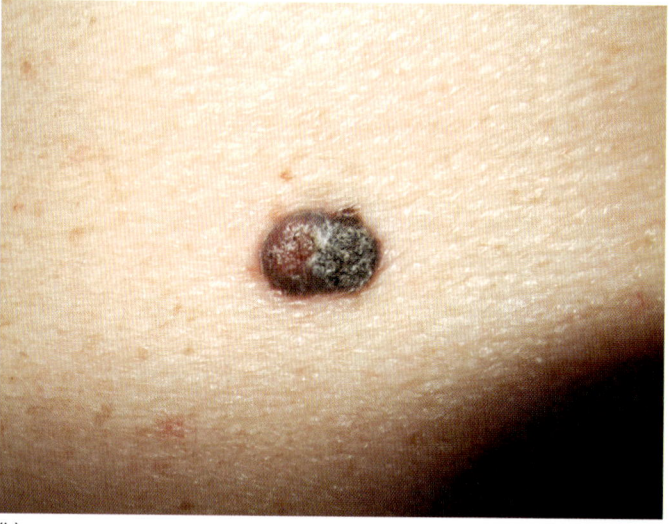

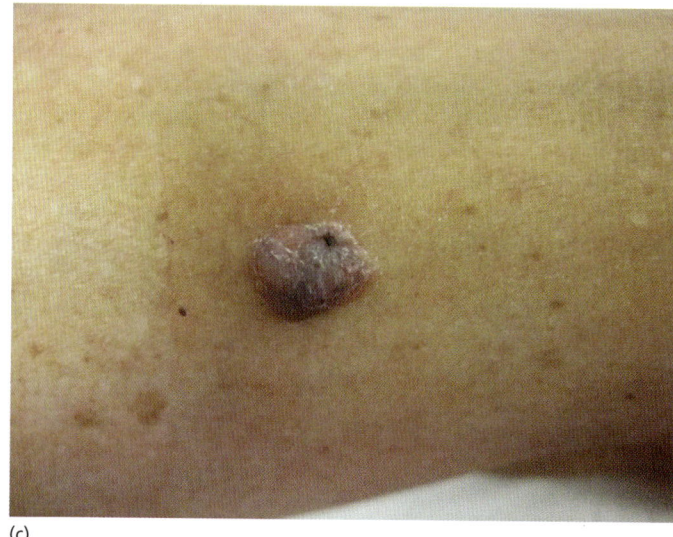

Figure 142.6 (a–c) Nodular melanomas.

second most common type of MM after cutaneous. Uveal MM can affect any part of the uveal tract, but choroidal MM is predominant (86.3%), while iris and ciliary body MM are far less frequent [252]. The presentation of uveal MM mainly depends on the size and location of the tumour and can vary from asymptomatic (detected incidentally on eye examination), to the development of various visual disturbances including visual loss in the affected eye. Conjunctival MM is very rare [253]. It usually presents as a raised pigmented lesion often surrounded by prominent feeder blood vessels. Multifocal lesions are present in almost one-third of patients [254]. Amelanotic lesions are very challenging.

Challenging clinical situations. This category of MM are either in hidden areas (not assessed during a routine clinical examination), have a non-suspicious clinical appearance or mimic another (benign) lesion. Subsequently, either they are not suspicious for MM and an unexpected histopathological diagnosis is made, or more

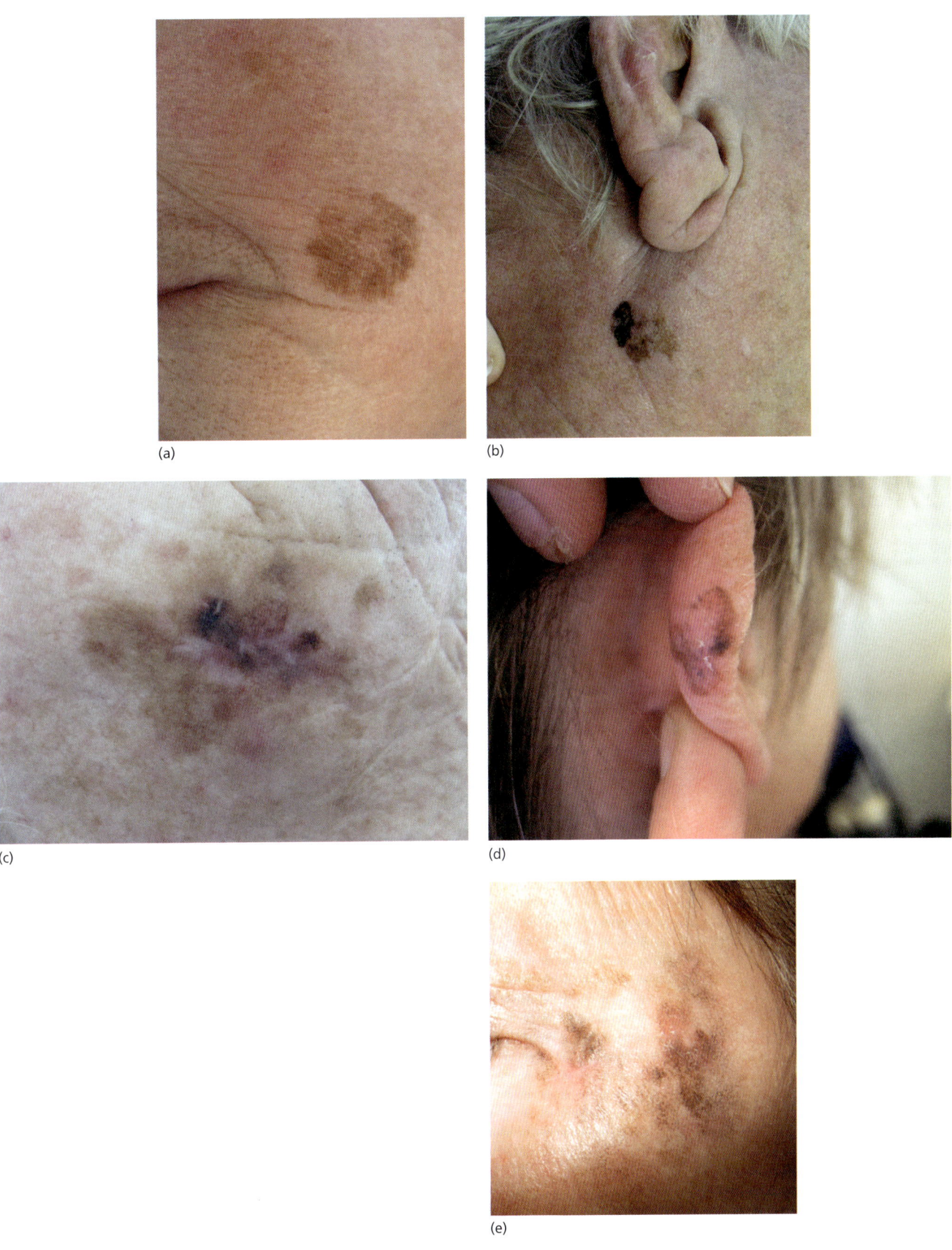

Figure 142.7 (a–e) Lentigo maligna melanomas.

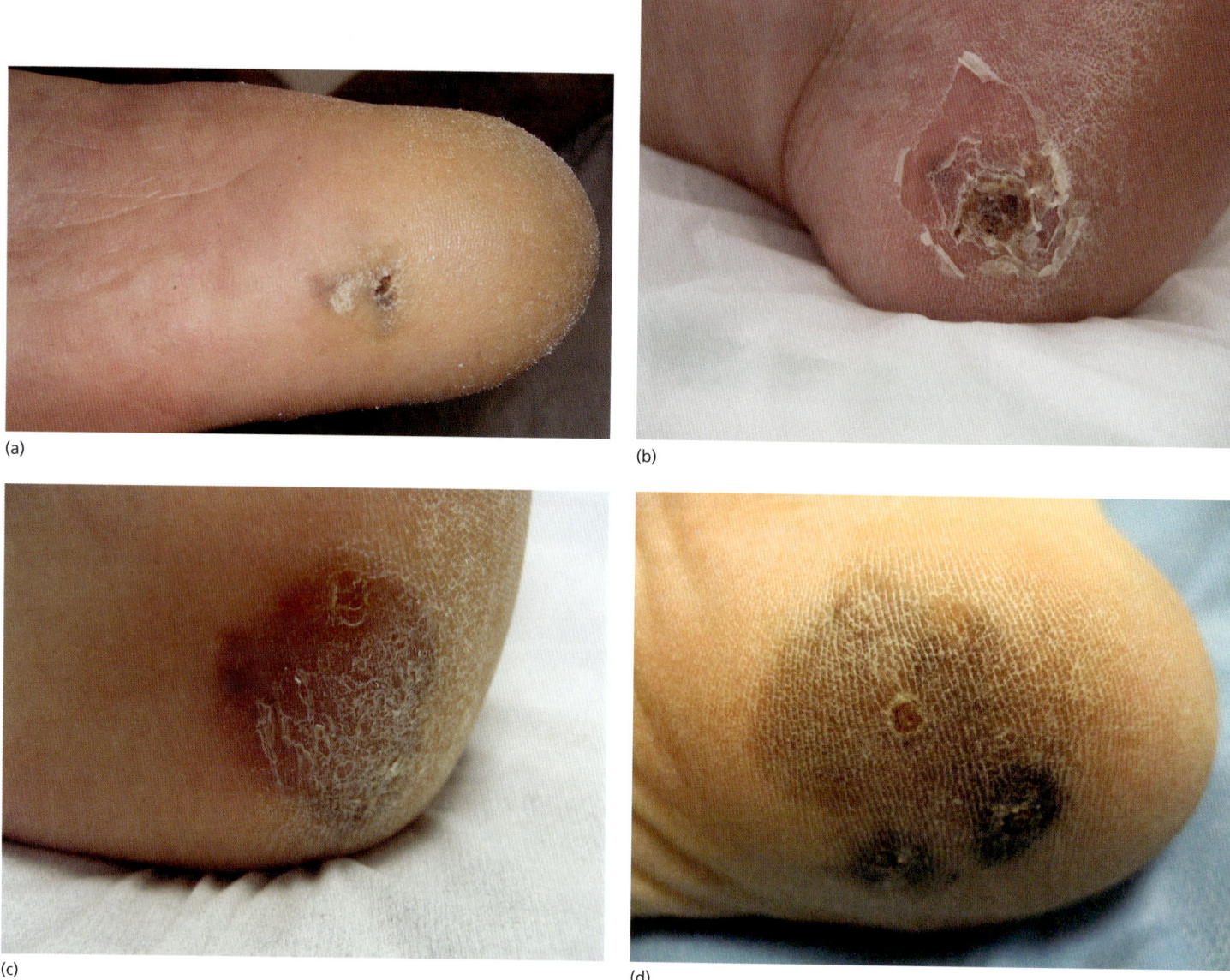

Figure 142.8 (a–d) Acral lentiginous melanomas.

commonly they are not even biopsied since they are considered as benign.

Amelanotic melanoma (Figures 142.13a,b and 142.14a,b). As the diagnosis of MM is often suggested by abnormal pigmentation, amelanotic MM can be easily missed even by the most experienced of clinicians. Such lesions may mimic inflammatory lesions, poromas, angiomas, sarcomas, squamous cell carcinomas, basal cell carcinomas or others. They may be hardly visible, especially on the soles, until a warty or nodular lesion reveals them, but by then it is often late and associated with a poor prognosis.

Regressive melanoma. Inflammation can lead to a focal regression of an MM, which is usually visible as an irregular focus of hypopigmentation (Figure 142.15a,b). However, when the regression is more severe, the MM may no longer be visible. Up to 8% of MM present as metastatic disease from an unknown primary [255,256]. In some patients, a previous history of a pigmented lesion which cleared spontaneously is elicited. In others, no primary MM can be found. As naevus cells may be seen in the subcapsular area of lymph nodes it is postulated that MM may arise *de novo* in a lymph node [257].

Malignant blue naevus (Chapter 131). Excessive dermal pigment makes the clinical and dermoscopic analysis of such lesions problematic. The suspicion of a neoplastic process arises primarily from dynamic criteria, i.e. a rapid development or a rapid change in an otherwise common blue naevus.

Sinonasal melanoma. Epistaxis and nasal obstruction are the most common presenting symptoms leading to the initial suspicion of inflammatory sino-nasal disease. The diagnosis of MM is usually delayed when the patient presents with bleeding or extension of the lesion to the adjacent structures such as the orbit, brain or

Melanoma clinicopathology 142.15

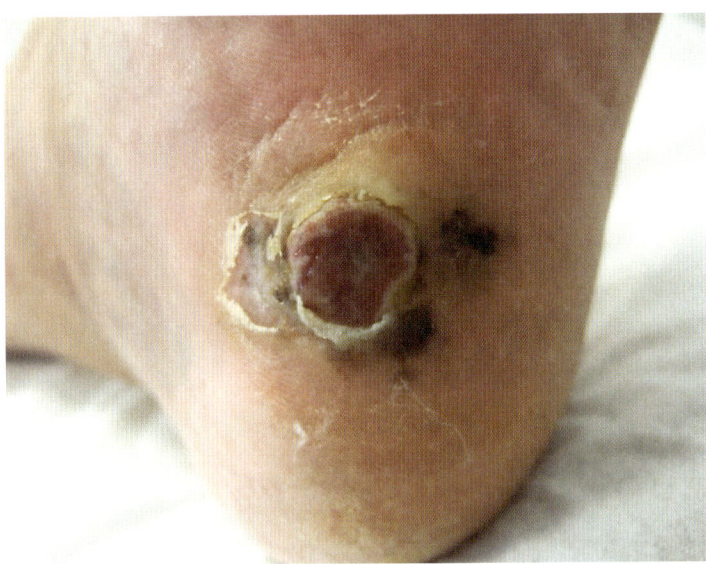

Figure 142.9 Acral lentiginous melanoma of the sole (late presentation).

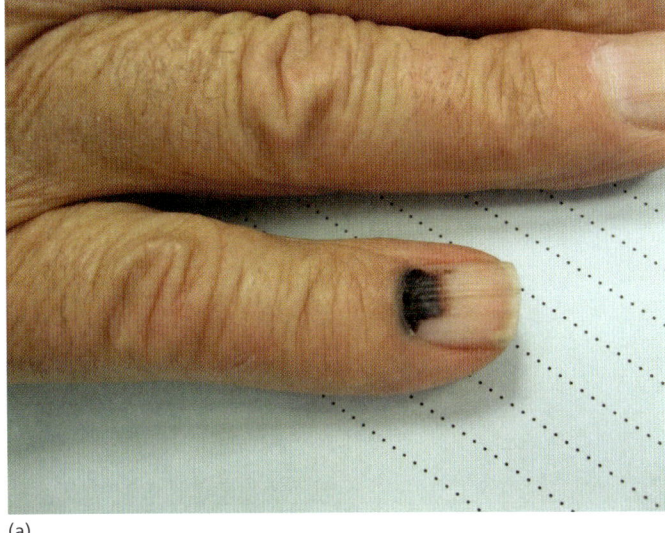

(a)

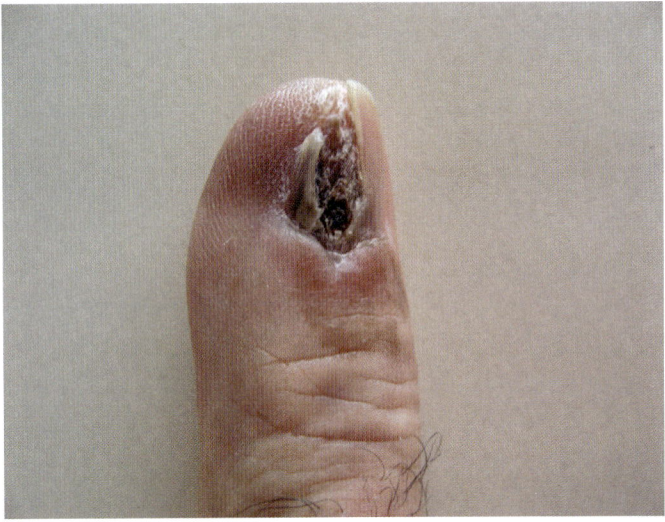

(b)

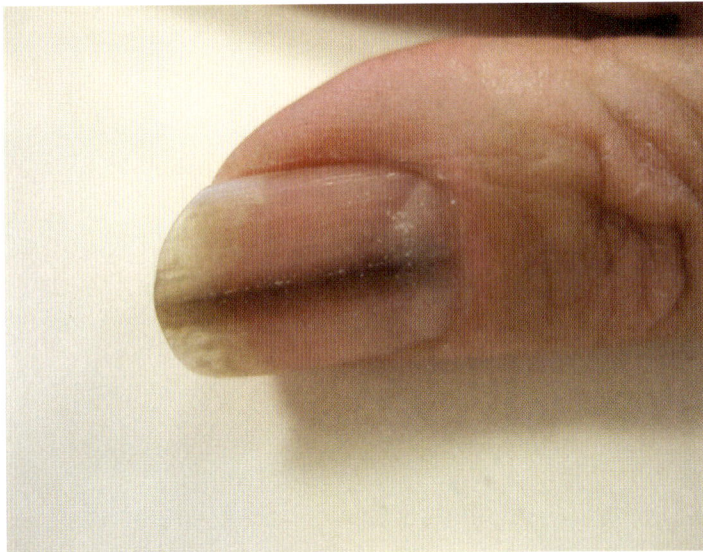

Figure 142.10 Acral lentiginous melanoma in the nail area. Early presentation as a longitudinal melanonychia.

cranial nerves. Therefore, the prognosis at the time of diagnosis is usually poor.

Strategies for early detection

General principles. The early detection of MM is crucial, as it clearly improves prognosis. Skin cancer is externally visible, and this has led to the conviction that mortality may be reduced by regular clinical surveillance of high-risk populations. However, mortality has not decreased due to two important factors, which are often underestimated: the different biological aggressiveness of different MM, and the limited proportion of overall MM that arise within the high-risk groups.

Limits of early detection. Contrary to intuitive perceptions, Breslow thickness does not always correlate directly with delay in

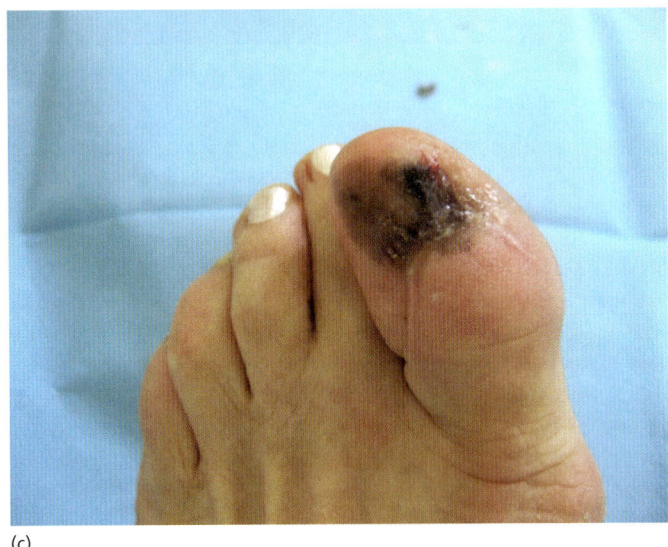

(c)

Figure 142.11 (a–c) Acral lentiginous melanomas in the nail area. Late presentation.

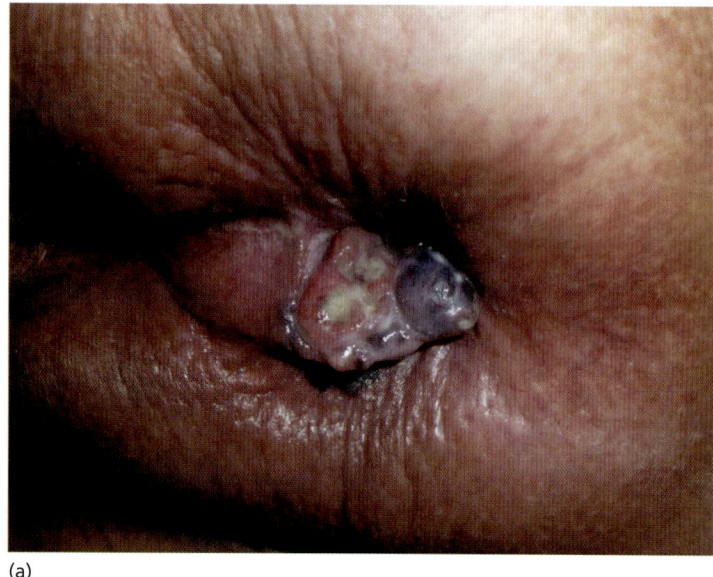
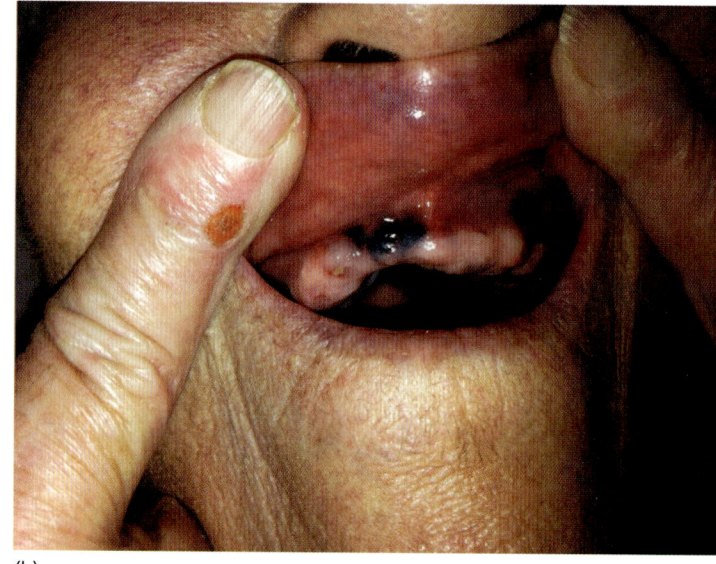

(a) (b)

Figure 142.12 Mucosal melanomas. (a) Anal; (b) oral.

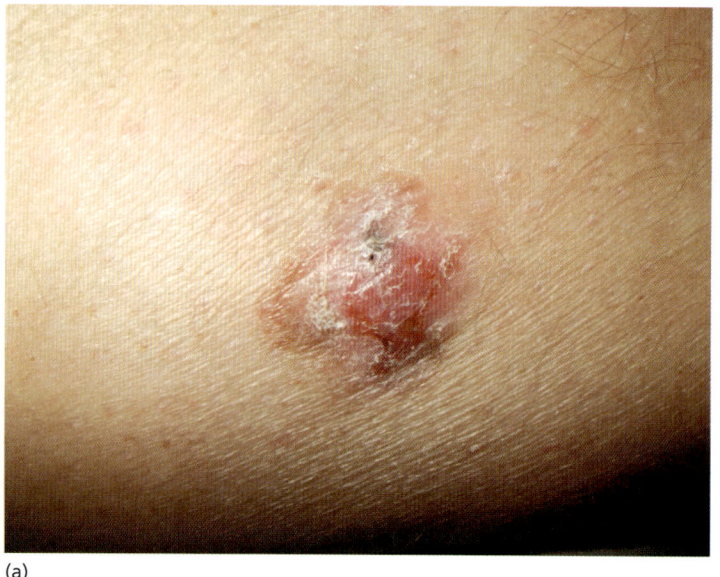
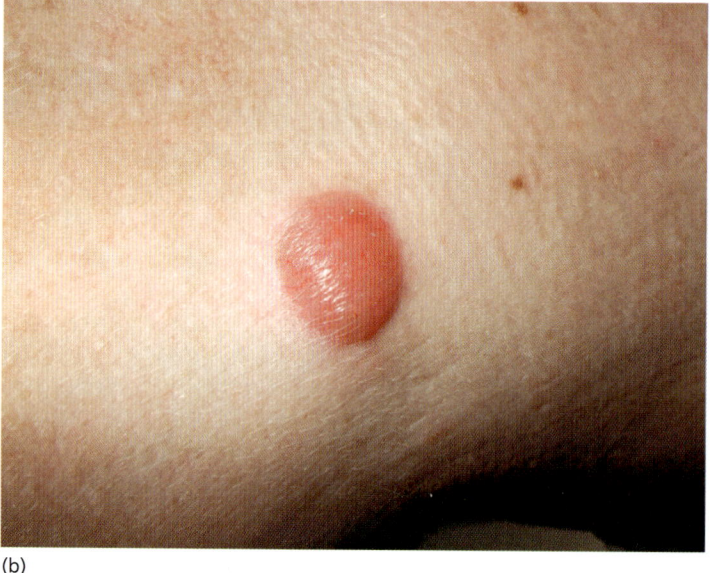

(a) (b)

Figure 142.13 Amelanotic melanoma. (a) Amelanotic superficial spreading melanoma. (b) Amelanotic nodular melanoma.

diagnosis [258–261]. This is understandable, once it is acknowledged that there are different kinetics of growths in primary MM. The most aggressive tumours tend to be fast growing and thus are more likely to have a high Breslow thickness, even when they are detected very early. In contrast, less aggressive, slowly growing primary MM are likely to have a low tumour thickness, even with a late detection. Furthermore, the inverse relationship between tumour thickness and prognosis is not that simple for the same reasons. Even with an opportunistic early detection and a low tumour thickness, there is no certainty that the prognosis of an aggressive fast-growing melanoma is altered by early surgery [204]. Conversely, even with relatively late detection and a high Breslow thickness, a slowly growing melanoma may not have a poor prognostic outcome. Thus, despite an overall benefit of early detection attested by the improvement of prognosis in countries which have promoted early detection, the proportion of primary MM, in which the prognosis is significantly influenced by early detection, is actually unknown.

What place for artificial intelligence? Machine learning (ML) has recently matched the diagnostic performance of dermatologists for melanoma detection, albeit in somewhat artificial situations. Algorithms are currently under investigation utilising clinical and dermoscopic images. The place of these new tools to augment the performance of primary care clinicians and trained specialists, and/or to automatise repeated tasks in order to save medical time in screening, is the challenge of the next decade. Ensuring sensitivity and specificity across all skin types is the biggest challenge in ML, as most preliminary data to date have utilised algorithms trained on white-skinned populations.

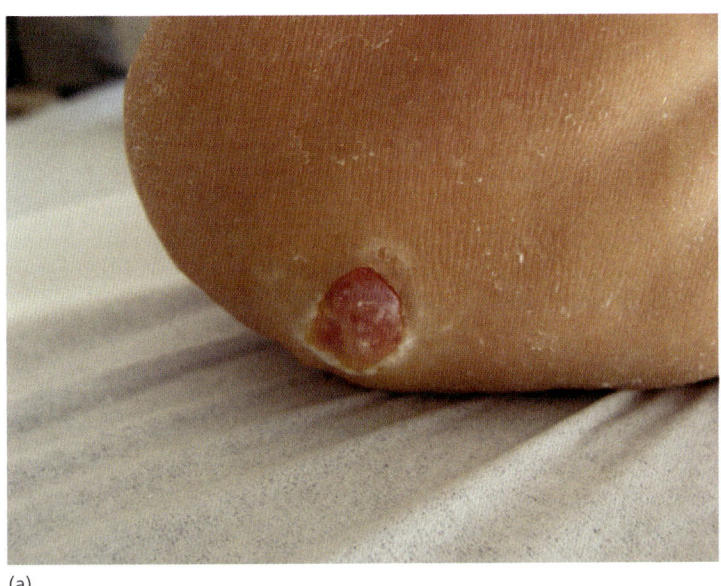

Figure 142.14 (a, b) Amelanotic acral lentiginous melanomas.

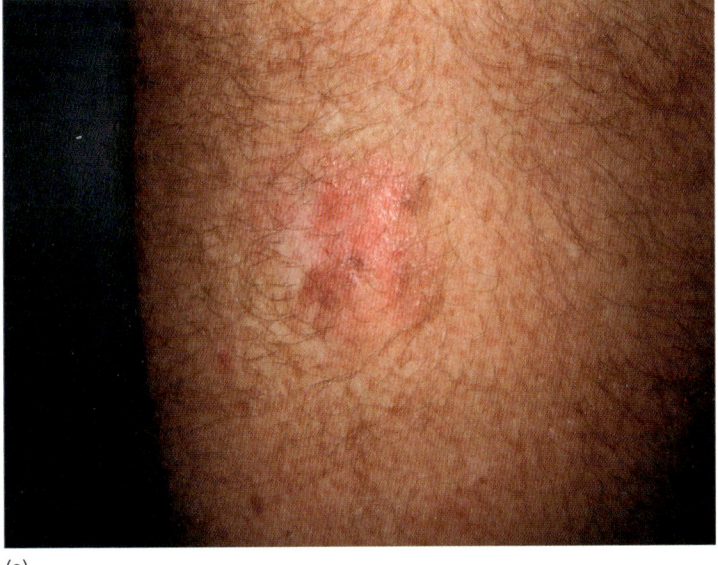
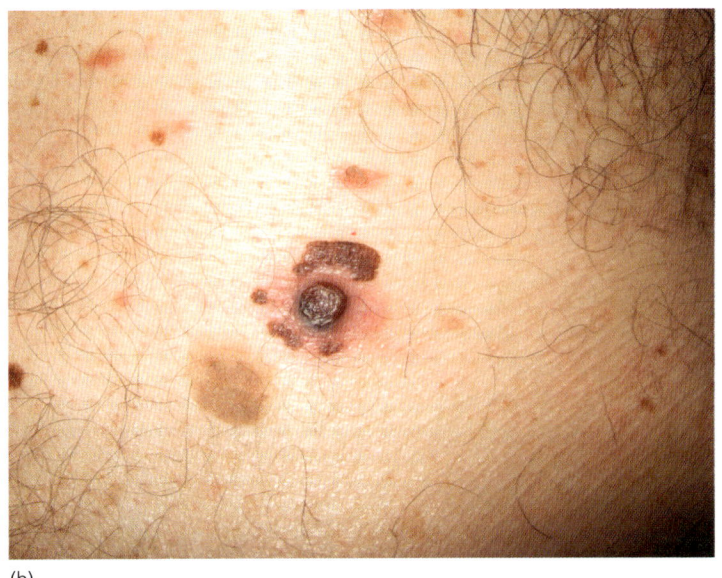

Figure 142.15 Regressive melanomas. (a) Quasi-total regression. (b) Partial regression.

Difficulty in targeting the right population. Any successful screening strategy must address the high-risk population defined by phenotypic criteria such as fair skin type, high number of naevi, etc. It cannot, however, be restricted solely to that group as the majority of MM will not arise in this high-risk group, especially the most aggressive type of MM.

Medical system organisation in different countries, plus societal and psychological factors, explains why some populations (e.g. elderly white men) have a poorer prognosis by virtue of their late presentation [262,263]. Such groups would likely benefit from specific targeting [264].

Screening in the high-risk population. Screening for MM in a high-risk population is a cost-effective intervention. However, it probably fails to pick up the majority of the most aggressive tumours, which develop in patients who are not identified as high risk by virtue of their phenotype. This is demonstrated for instance by the fact that NMs are more common in patients without multiple naevi [265], and by an inverse association of fast-growing MM with this skin phenotype [205].

Dermatological periodic monitoring. Such monitoring may be performed either by full body clinical examination, by comparison with reference total body photographs or by computerised dermoscopy, which permits individual naevus follow-up. Such monitoring is highly efficacious, but very time-consuming. There is no agreement as to the frequency of this monitoring and to which population this should be applied to. Very high-risk patients, i.e. those with a past personal or familial history of MM, a high naevus count or atypical mole syndrome, should undergo systematic examination of the entire skin more than once a year. The risk of 'over-excising' benign lesions remains high, especially if such monitoring practices are performed by less experienced clinicians.

Education on self-detection and skin self-examination. This remains essential in the prevention and early detection of MM. It is neither possible nor cost-effective for dermatologists to monitor all of the high-risk population frequently. The interval between two successive examinations can be covered by self-examination, which has been proven to be effective [266,267]. Self-surveillance can now be assisted by smartphone apps, although their accuracy remains highly controversial.

Periodic screening in the general population. MM is not confined just to high-risk groups, thus screening of the general population makes rational sense. However, there is no evidence that a yearly skin examination of the whole population would be efficient, or even feasible. Periodic screening in the whole population is a high-cost intervention with a high demand in terms of medical interventions. An experiment in Schleswig-Holstein [268] has shown encouraging data including reduction in mortality. However, there was no difference in other close areas where there was no intervention, and a return to pre-screening mortality rates was noted [269]. It is thus unlikely that any transient reduction in mortality was linked to systematic screening. Thus routine screening is not currently recommended by most health authorities. The US Preventive Services Task Force and most national authorities have not made any formal recommendations for widespread skin cancer screening given the lack of prospective evidentiary trials.

Occasional screening sessions. 'MM days' or similar services have been conducted in most developed countries in the last few decades. They have virtually no direct impact and only detect a few MM. Their major interest is to increase the awareness of the population and doctors about sun protection and MM and non-MM skin cancers.

Opportunistic screening. The random detection by a primary care physician or medical professional (e.g. nurse, physiotherapist) is important, but is dependent on their general skill and on the frequency they see people with skin exposed. These two conditions are not necessarily met in everyday practice.

Public health education. Improving the ability of patients to recognise MM and to seek medical advice for suspicious lesions is crucial for early detection and improvement of MM prognosis in the general population [270,271]. First, patients are responsible for most of the delay in MM diagnosis (due to late presentation) [272]. Second, two-thirds of MM are self-detected and only a third detected by doctors [273]. Third, the most dangerous MM [204,207] probably grow so fast that only patients can detect them early enough. Therefore, this strategy of education of the community is most reasonable in terms of cost-efficiency and gives the best chance to impact on mortality. Most campaigns worldwide have used analytical algorithms such as the ABCDE rule [229,274]. However, presenting pictures of MM to the population has been shown to be better than education with ABCDE criteria [231] and can be used in a real-world campaign [275]. The Internet offers an easy opportunity to promote such cognitive training in the general population.

Basis for melanoma diagnosis
Histopathological diagnosis [276–280]

Pathological examination remains the gold standard for MM diagnosis, despite many attempts to use molecular approaches to replace it. Any lesion suspicious for MM must be completely removed and sent for pathological examination. The pathological analysis aims at confirming the malignancy and the melanocytic origin of the proliferation, but also to collect major prognostic information.

There is a great variability in the morphology and pattern of benign naevi as well as MM, which has resulted in the description of a great number of naevi, as well as many MM pathological subtypes. There remain ambiguous situations where there is doubt between a benign and malignant melanocytic tumour, some covered by a panel of terms which do not always clarify the position. In this complex situation, a few criteria should be highlighted which are the basis of the differential diagnosis between naevus and MM, none of them being specific.

Pathological criteria of malignancy

Architectural. The most important is probably architectural. In naevus and MM, melanocytes organise along the dermo–epidermal junction and within the dermis and usually tend to form aggregates or nests. MM does not have the overall symmetrical (well-organised) structure of naevi and is characterised by a general asymmetry, loss of architecture, and heterogeneity in the size, shape and placement of nests, along with confluence or fusion of the nests. At the dermal level, the architecture of MM is distinct from a naevus by the lack of so-called maturation gradient, which is a top-down morphological gradient from epithelioid to neuroid.

Pagetoid spread. Another criterion for malignancy is the upward individual migration of atypical melanocytes (pagetoid spread) within the epidermis, which is unusual in most benign naevi. Malignant melanocytes are not confined to the basal layer like normal melanocytes, but spread upwards, in a disordered manner, into the epidermis.

Cytology. This is variable but the usual malignancy criteria such as nuclear pleomorphism, enlargement and hyperchromatism, prominent nucleoli and mitotic activity are important diagnostic features. The abrupt change in cell types observed in MM contrasts with the gradual linear cytological changes observed in melanocytic naevi and is also an important clue to the diagnosis.

Brisk and asymmetrical host inflammatory response. This is often present in MM. Regression figures, i.e. focal disappearance of melanocytes replaced by pigment, dermal fibrosis, verticalisation of the blood vessels and lymphocytic inflammation, are frequently observed and interpreted as an immune reaction against MM.

Difficulties in diagnosis. The aforementioned 'malignancy criteria' are not always present and in some cases can be observed in truly benign naevi, and an MM can also arise from a naevus. This creates diagnostic ambiguities.

A number of neologisms have been proposed to denominate lesions in this grey zone, such as 'naevoid MM' [281], 'MELTUMP' (melanocytic tumours of uncertain malignant potential) [282] and 'MANIAC' (melanocytic acral naevus with intraepidermal ascent of cells) [283]. They do not simplify the practical management of the ambiguous lesions, which need to be managed according to the worst hypothesis, i.e. that they are in fact MM.

Main situations for the pathologist. There is a vast spectrum of morphologies: at one end there are MM which develop upfront as a tumoural dermal proliferation raising the epidermis (nodular pattern), while at the other end there are tumours showing a long-lasting horizontal intraepidermal growth (lentiginous pattern) before they invade the dermis. In between sits the majority of tumours with a junctional pattern made up of nests and pagetoid migration, usually combined with dermal invasion (superficial spreading pattern). These features are the radial and vertical growth phase of MM.

Melanomas presenting as a predominantly dermal proliferation.
These share some characteristics. They tend to constitute a nodular mass raising the epidermis with little or even no junctional/pagetoid spread (which is probably the geometric result of a fast centrifuge growth of the invasive dermal component), which is pushing the epidermis upwards. This is the typical appearance of 'nodular MM' (Figure 142.16). In non-pigmented lesions the differential diagnosis includes non-melanoma anaplastic tumours such as lymphoma and Merkel cell carcinoma. In these situations, histochemical markers are useful. Cutaneous metastases from an MM can also be nodular. Typically, skin metastases are less likely to push towards the epidermis and instead form a nodule just below the epidermis or within the deep dermis, but pathological examination cannot always exclude a metastasis, especially with a history of a prior MM. Radiological examination is required to search for other signs of metastases.

Melanoma presenting as flat proliferation of melanocytes with a typical lentiginous pattern.
These are characterised by malignant melanocytes spreading out along the dermo–epidermal junction, which then appears crowded, with a propensity to follow appendageal structures, and with some tendency to form nests of dendritic or spindle-shaped cells. Dermal invasion is only seen in tumours removed late and is usually also characterised most commonly by dendritic or spindle-shaped cells. This pattern is mainly seen in two very different situations, MM of the soles, and MM of chronically sun-exposed areas in the elderly. These two situations modulate the overall lentiginous pattern. The location in the soles and subungual areas, described as ALM (Figure 142.17), shows some tendency to intraepidermal isolated migration, epidermal acanthosis and elongation of the rete ridges. The location on the skin of always sun-exposed areas (face) in elderly people, described as lentigo maligna (LM) when it is strictly intraepidermal and lentigo maligna melanoma (Figure 142.18) when there is dermal invasion, is logically associated with elastosis and epidermal atrophy. The early stages of LM may be difficult to distinguish from some solar lentigos.

Melanomas presenting as an atypical junctional and intraepithelial pattern.
A strictly intraepithelial melanocytic proliferation made of nests and intraepithelial pagetoid spread confined to the epidermis is usually called *in situ* MM when isolated. It is often later

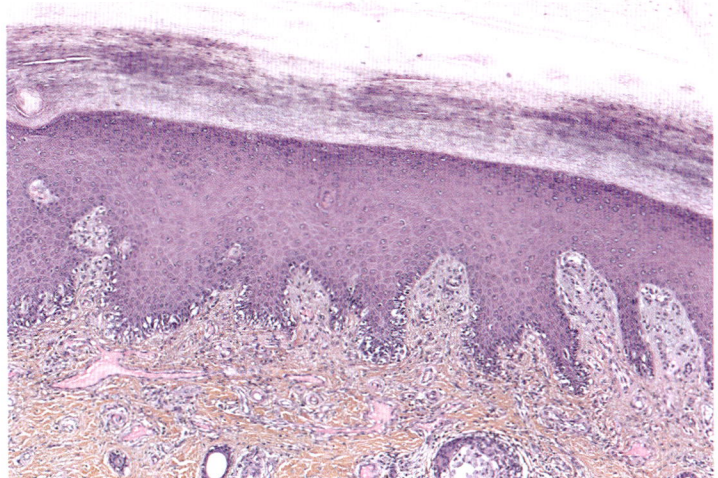
Figure 142.17 Acral lentiginous melanoma with typical lentiginous pattern.

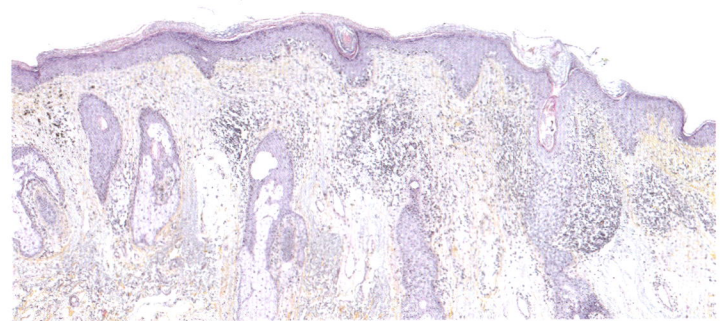
Figure 142.18 Lentigo maligna melanoma.

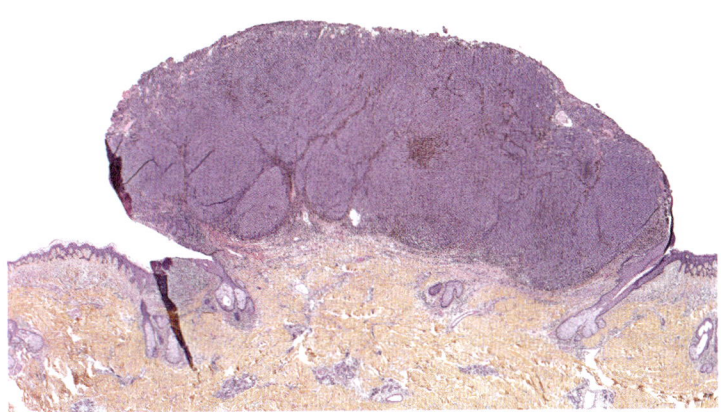
Figure 142.16 Nodular melanoma.

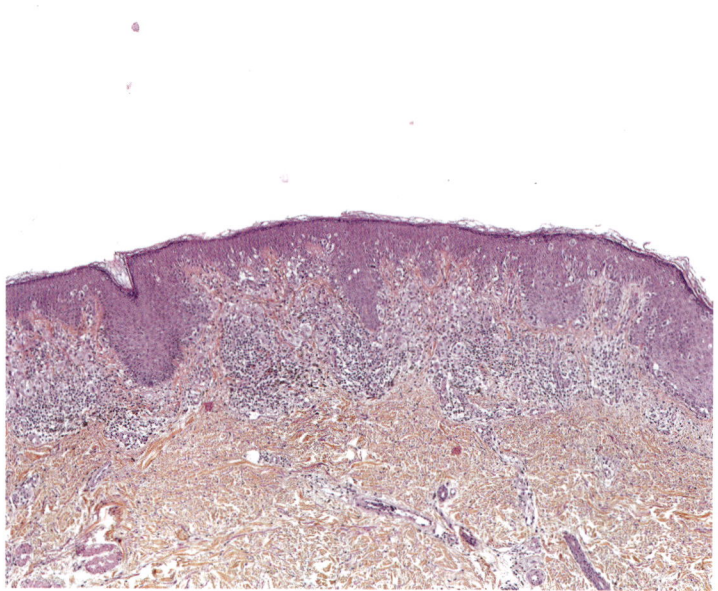

Figure 142.19 Superficial spreading melanoma.

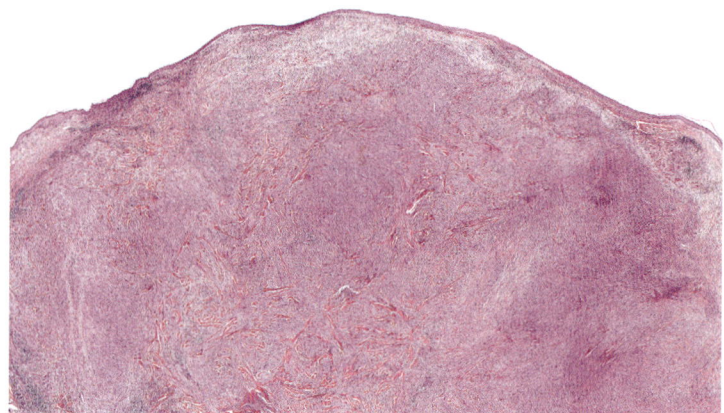

Figure 142.20 Desmoplastic melanoma.

associated with a dermal component usually with an epithelioid cytology corresponding to the SSM clinicopathological subtype of MM (Figure 142.19), with the horizontal and vertical two-step growth phases as described. Initially, the overall appearance is similar to an atypical/dysplastic junctional naevus, both showing some degree of cellular atypia resulting in a frequent diagnostic challenge. Symmetry, lamellar fibrosis and bridging of nests are more likely in an atypical naevus, whereas intraepithelial pagetoid migration of melanocytes, asymmetry, ulceration, mitotic figures and poor maturation of the dermal component are more likely seen in an MM.

Rare challenging melanoma patterns.

1 *Desmoplastic melanoma*. This is a proliferation of spindle-shaped melanocytes with no or little pigmentation, with scar-like fibrosis in the dermis associated with a conspicuous inflammatory infiltrate (Figure 142.20). It can display at the same time attributes of melanocytic, fibroblastic and schwannian differentiation, often variably intermingled [284]. The differential diagnosis includes cutaneous sarcomas or spindle-cell squamous cell carcinoma. Staining with SOX10 and/or S100 protein usually marks the spindle-shaped cells whereas Melan-A and HMB-45 antigen staining are always negative.
2 *Spitzoid neoplasms*. In a malignant Spitz tumour, the tumour cells harbour a Spitzoid cytology, resembling a neoplasm within a Spitz spectrum. This is characterised by large epithelioid or spindle-shaped melanocytic cells, often amelanotic, associated with epidermal hyperplasia, and even mitoses [285,286].

  In the context of this Spitz spectrum, the diagnosis between a Spitz naevus and a Spitzoid MM is particularly difficult and uncertain on morphological grounds. It is often determined on genomics. The Spitz spectrum is characterised by gene fusion involving *ALK*, *ROS1*, *MET*, *RET*, *NTRK1*, *NTRK3*, *MAP3K8* and always lacks mutations in the MAPK pathway, such as canonical *BRAF*, *NRAS*, *KIT*, *GNAQ* or *GNA11* mutations. Searching for the latter can help classify a lesion as non-Spitz MM, despite its Spitzoid morphology. The prognosis of a lesion within the Spitz spectrum is better assessed using cytogenetics, involving FISH fluorescence *in situ* hybridisation (FISH) techniques or array comparative genomic hybridisation (aCGH) [287–289].
3 *Regressive melanoma*. This can be challenging, when the residual tumour associated with the lymphocytic infiltrate no longer has characteristics of MM. It may be mistaken for a regressive Sutton naevus, or be labelled non-diagnostic in cases of total or subtotal regression. SOX10 can be expressed in scars and constitutes a diagnosis pitfall.
4 *Melanoma arising in a blue naevus (malignant blue naevus)*. This is difficult to diagnose, because it is very rare as compared with a blue naevus, with which it shares most of the organisational characteristics, and because pigment deposits obscure the cytology (Figure 142.21). Blue naevus-like MM (malignant blue naevus) is molecularly related to uveal MM and shares many molecular and cytogenetic similarities. An integrated histomolecular diagnosis is based on canonical alteration of *GNAQ*, *GNA11*, *PLCB4* or *CYSLTR2* mutations [290,291], with additional alterations on SF3B1 or BAP1 [292]. Redundant cytogenetic alterations with gains in 6p and/or 8q, monosomy 3, and loss in 1p are similar to those detected in uveal MM [293].
5 *Pigmented epithelioid melanocytoma/pigment synthesising melanoma (animal-type melanoma)*. These are rare melanocytic tumours (melanocytoma), considered as intermediate in nature, with metastatic potential limited to the regional lymph nodes, although this is not clear at all. Histologically, they show heavily pigmented spindle-shaped or epithelioid melanocytes which mimic MM, composed of heavily pigmented epithelioid or dendritic cells. These lesions usually harbour both BRAF V600E mutations and loss-of-function alterations affecting *PRKAR1A* or *PRKCA* gene fusion [294,295]. Such lesions can occur in a sporadic setting or in patients affected with Carney complex.

Immunohistochemistry in the diagnosis of melanoma. Immunohistochemistry is not necessary for the diagnosis of a melanocytic neoplasm. However, it can be used to assess prognosis or specific molecular subtype, or in the setting of amelanotic or poorly

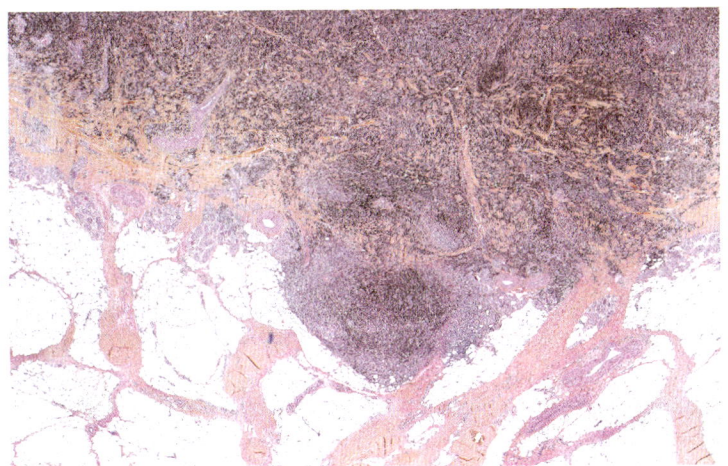

Figure 142.21 Malignant blue naevus.

differentiated MM. S100 protein is expressed by 99% of all MM and melanocytic naevi [296] but also by several other tumours that harbour cartilaginous, nervous or myoepithelial differentiation. A more recent marker is SOX10, which displays the same or a slightly higher sensibility compared with S100, with a different pattern of specificity, staining the nuclei of neoplastic cells, which can aid in asserting ascents of cells and nuclear pleomorphism. Mart-1 (Melan-A) and HMB-45 are more specific, but lack some sensitivity [297], and in particular do not stain desmoplastic MM. Many other markers are useful in the diagnosis of MM, including MITF [298]. Next-generation antibodies, directed against canonical molecular alterations, such as NTRK, ALK, ROS1, MET, RET, BRAF V600E, NRAS Q61R, HRAS and PRKAR1A, are particularly used by referral centres as a substitute for genetic testing [299].

PRAME expression might be useful in distinguishing >90% of benign versus malignant melanocytic neoplasms. PRAME is particularly useful in assessing the margins of lentiginous MM such as LM and ALM. Clonal loss of expression of p16, associated or not with copy number aberrations of the CDKN2A locus by FISH or aCGH, has been reported as highly specific for borderline and malignant Spitzoid neoplasms [300].

Introducing novel techniques in the diagnosis of primary melanoma

Techniques that may assist in the pathological diagnosis in difficult cases have been extensively researched over recent years. Their real impact on the classification of ambiguous cases remains to be proven.

Fluorescence *in situ* hybridisation. Fluorescence *in situ* hybridisation (FISH) detects copy number changes as well as chromosomal translocations [301] and allows the direct visualisation of tissue histology [302,303]. When performed with a panel of four probes, FISH seems to represent a sensitive and molecular tool for the diagnosis of non-ambiguous melanocytic lesions [304], whereas in the context of ambiguous melanocytic tumours, results are still controversial [305]. FISH is also a useful tool to detect gene fusions for Spitz neoplasms, some of which have an important prognostic and theragnostic value [306].

RNA sequencing. Chromosomal rearrangements leading to the formation of fusion transcripts are a frequent driver in the Spitz group of neoplasms (*ALK, BRAF, NTRK1, NTRK3, ROS1, MET, MAP3K8* and *RET*) and some PEM (*PRKCA*). Transcriptome sequencing (RNA-seq) has emerged as an effective method to detect fusion transcripts and is now considered the most reliable method to detect fusions, while immunohistochemistry and FISH are cost-effective alternatives in some cases [307,308].

Comparative genomic hybridisation (CGH). This technique detects copy number changes, including chromosomal gains or losses of the whole genome on the tissue target [302]. A significant limitation is the close dependence on the purity of the analysed specimen and on the number of cells showing the chromosomal aberration. aCGH is very helpful in challenging situations and is currently part of routine diagnosis for referral centres.

Machine learning as a way to augment human performance in diagnosis. There are attempts to utilise machine learning (ML) for diagnostic purposes in MM. ML is able to recognise and extract information from digital slides that human experts do not take into account. These classifiers may improve and standardise expert accuracy in the near future or help a non-expert to reach a good level of accuracy.

Prognostic markers

Primary MM have different abilities to metastasise to any organ or tissue [309]. The initial site of metastasis is most commonly the skin or subcutaneous tissue, but 18–27% of the initial recurrences involve a distant organ [309–311]. Lung, brain, liver and bones are the most common metastasis sites. Predicting the risk of a patient is crucial to indicate adjuvant treatment and monitor the patient. Pathological characteristics have been the only prognostic marker for years, but new biomarkers such as interferon gamma signature, tumour mutation load and others are entering the field.

Classic pathological markers (Box 142.2). There are a number of pathological characteristics in primary MM which are statistically correlated to the risk of recurrence and overall survival. The detection of clinically undetectable nodes in the first draining nodes, which can be detected by the sentinel node technique, is

---

Box 142.2 Main prognostic factors for primary melanoma

- Thickness (Breslow index)***
- Sentinel node status***
- Ulceration**
- Mitotic rate** (pejorative value especially in thin tumours)
- Regression* (underestimation of Breslow)
- Age* (more pejorative for older age)
- Sex* (more pejorative for males)
- Location* (more pejorative for head and neck)

Prognostic value from *** high to * low.

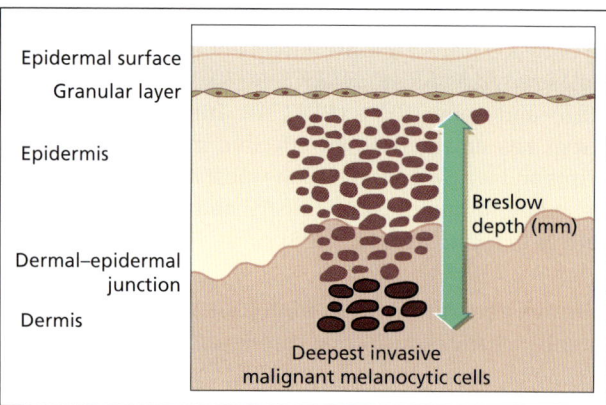

Figure 142.22 Breslow depth.

also linked to prognosis. The most important prognostic factor in primary MM is provided by the tumour (Breslow) thickness (Figure 142.22), corresponding to the measurement (in millimetres) of the distance between the overlying epidermal granular layer and the deepest level of invasion of the primary lesion [312–315]. Thicker tumours have a higher metastatic potential, peaking early after the diagnosis of the primary MM, while thinner tumours are less prone to metastasise, but late recurrences can occur after a disease-free interval of 10 or 20 years [316].

Other important markers include mitotic rate, which becomes a particularly relevant indicator in thin tumours [315,317–322] and the presence of ulceration, which is not only a negative marker whatever the tumour thickness, but also indicates the biological subtype of the primary MM. Indeed, adjuvant therapy with interferon has been proven to be more efficacious in MM with ulceration [323,324]. Other attributes that have relevance to prognosis include lymphovascular invasion, perineural invasion, presence of regression and Clark's level of invasion [325,326]. However this latter is less reproducible among pathologists and has a lower accuracy in providing prognostic information compared with tumour thickness [327,328]. Sex, age and anatomical location [326,329–333] are other prognostic factors (worst prognosis is for head and neck MM in elderly males) but these correlate with the thickness and are thus of less interest.

Positivity of sentinel node status (Chapter 143) is an indicator of prognosis correlating with recurrence rates, disease-free survival and overall survival [334–336]. The status of the sentinel node is currently required to indicate adjuvant therapy because the benefit of modern adjuvant therapies has been so far only studied in patients with a positive sentinel node biopsy [337–340].

However, the utility of the sentinel node is being increasingly debated and may disappear when other non-invasive biomarkers substitute for it as a prognostic marker.

The delay of the scintigraphic appearance time could be a relevant factor for the prediction of sentinel node involvement (low probability of sentinel node involvement for long scintigraphic appearance time) [341,342].

Towards new individual prognostic and predictive biomarkers.
None of the usual pathological markers is an absolute predictor of individual risk of relapse (prognostic marker) or of the likelihood of responding to adjuvant strategies (predictive marker). A tumour with good prognostic pathological markers may still metastasise, while another with poor prognostic markers may never relapse. New biomarkers are thus needed to assess the objective risk of patients, guide the use of adjuvant therapy and tailor the surveillance in each individual. There are several approaches. Firstly, simple clinical biomarkers so far not used in practice, such as the assessment of the kinetics of the primary MM according to the patient description, have been shown to be good prognostic indicators [204]. ML could help extract best prognostic multiparameter models from electronic patient records including a huge amount of potentially underutilised information.

Secondly, gene expression profiling in primary MM has been extensively investigated and several panels are already proposed for commercialisation (e.g. Decision DX, Melagenix, Skyline Dx) but their prospective validation is awaited to enter everyday clinical practice) [343,344]. They all have to be validated to predict not surrogate steps like the status of the sentinel node, but the relapse itself [345]. Gene expression profiling can be combined with other pathological biomarkers such as T stage or sentinel node status within multiparameter prognostic nomograms. Thirdly, liquid biopsies such as circulating tumour cells, circulating free DNA and cytokine levels have the major advantage of assessing the tumour and the host reaction, and of being non-invasive, thus easy to repeat. They are, however, probably biomarkers more adapted to advanced stages than to primary MM.

Management

Management of melanoma after excision of the primary
See Chapter 143 on melanoma surgery.

Staging primary melanoma
The 8th American Joint Committee on Cancer (AJCC) melanoma staging system was published in 2018, on the basis of an analysis of more than 46 000 patients with stages I, II and III melanoma and 7972 patients with stage IV melanoma (the latter were kept from the 7th edition) [346] (Tables 142.1 and 142.2). Modifications from the 7th edition include:
- Tumour thickness measurement to be recorded to the nearest 0.1 mm (not 0.01).
- Revision of the T1a and T1b stages with mitotic rate no longer a T category criterion.
- Revision of pathological stage IA.
- Redefinition of the N category descriptors 'microscopic' and 'macroscopic' in 'clinically occult' and 'clinically apparent'.
- Increase of the number of the stage III category from three into four subgroups (IIIA–IIID).
- Revision of the N subcategories.
- Descriptors for LDH in each M1 subcategory (0 or 1).
- New M1d subcategory in case of CNS metastases.

In patients with localised MM (stage I and II), tumour thickness and ulceration are retained as the most dominant prognostic factors with 5-year and 10-year survival rate estimates ranging from 99% and 98% for patients with stage IA MM (Breslow <0.8 mm without ulceration) to 82% and 75%, respectively, for patients with stage IIC MM (Breslow >4 mm with ulceration). All patients

Table 142.1 TNM staging categories for cutaneous melanoma.

Classification	Thickness (mm)	Ulceration status/mitoses
T		
Tis	N/A	N/A
T1	<0.8	a: Without ulceration
		b: With ulceration
T2	1.01–2.00	a: Without ulceration
		b: With ulceration
T3	2.01–4.00	a: Without ulceration
		b: With ulceration
T4	>4.00	a: Without ulceration
		b: With ulceration
N	**No. of regional lymph nodes**	**Nodal metastatic burden**
N0	0	N/A
N1	1	a: Clinically occult detected by SLN biopsy
		b: Clinically detected
		c: No regional lymph node but presence of in-transit, satellites and/or microsatellite metastasis
N2	2–3	a: Clinically occult detected by SLN biopsy
		b: At least one clinically detected
		c: One clinically occult or clinically detected and presence of in-transit, satellites and/or microsatellite metastasis
N3	≥4	a: Clinically occult detected by SLN biopsy
		b: At least one clinically detected or presence of any number of matted nodes
		c: Two or more clinically occult or clinically detected and/or presence of any number of matted nodes
M	**Site**	**Serum LDH**
M0	No distant metastases	N/A
M1a	Distant skin, subcutaneous or nodal metastases	Normal M1a(0)/elevated M1a(1)
M1b	Lung metastases	Normal M1b(0)/elevated M1b(1)
M1c	Other visceral metastases excluding CNS	Normal M1c(0)/Elevated M1c(1)
M1d	CNS metastases	Normal M1d(0)/Elevated M1d(1)

From Gershenwald et al. 2017 [346].
CNS, central nervous system; LDH, lactate dehydrogenase; N/A, not applicable; SLN, sentinel lymph node.

Table 142.2 Anatomical stage groupings for cutaneous melanoma.

	Clinical staging				Pathological staging		
	T	N	M		T	N	M
0	Tis	N0	M0	0	Tis	N0	M0
IA	T1a	N0	M0	IA	T1a	N0	M0
IB	T1b	N0	M0	IB	T1b	N0	M0
	T2a	N0	M0		T2a	N0	M0
IIA	T2b	N0	M0	IIA	T2b	N0	M0
	T3a	N0	M0		T3a	N0	M0
IIB	T3b	N0	M0	IIB	T3b	N0	M0
	T4a	N0	M0		T4a	N0	M0
IIC	T4b	N0	M0	IIC	T4b	N0	M0
III	Any T	N > N0	M0	IIIA	T1a/b–T2a	N1a/N2a	M0
				IIIB	T0	N1b/N1c	M0
					T1a/b–T2a	N1b/c–N2b	M0
					T2b/T3a	N1a–N2b	M0
				IIIC	T0	N2b, N2c, N3b, N3c	M0
					T3b–T4a	Any N ≥ N1	M0
					T4b	N3 a/b/c	M0
				IIID	T4b	N3a/b/c	M0
IV	Any T	Any N	M1	IV	Any T	Any N	M1

From Gershenwald, et al. 2017 [346].

with nodal metastases including micrometastases detected by immunohistochemistry (i.e. sentinel node involvement) are classified as stage III. The number of tumour-bearing nodes, tumour burden at the time of staging (i.e. clinically occult versus clinically detected), the presence or absence of primary tumour ulceration and thickness of the primary MM, are the most accurate predictive factors for survival in these patients. The 5-year survival rates are 93%, 83%, 69% and 32% for patients with stage IIIA, IIIB, IIIC and IIID MM, respectively (Table 142.3). CT scanning is mainly useful as a reference for subsequent follow-up.

Table 142.3 Estimated 5- and 10-year survival rates according to the American Joint Committee on Cancer (AJCC) staging.

	5-year survival (%)	10-year survival (%)
Stage IA	99	98
Stage IB	97	94
Stage IIA	94	88
Stage IIB	87	82
Stage IIC	82	75
Stage IIIA	93	88
Stage IIIB	83	77
Stage IIIC	69	60
Stage IIID	32	24
Stage IV	15–20	10–15

From Gershenwald, et al. 2017 [346].

The role of sentinel lymph node biopsy in staging is covered in Chapter 143.

Compared with AJCC 7th edition guidance, the main difference is the improvement of prognosis of the IIIA group, due to its new definition. Secondly, other series [347] have suggested that AJCC database prognosis may be a little optimistic as to prognosis for most of the groups.

Follow-up

The main purpose of any follow-up is to detect any local recurrence around the scar of the excised MM, to palpate the draining lymph nodes for any clinically detectable evidence of nodal spread and to examine the rest of the skin for second primary MM. Such second primary MM have been reported to develop in 1.0–4.4% of patients diagnosed with a first MM [348]. All patients should be taught self-examination in order to detect early recurrence, how to palpate for lymph nodes and how to detect a second primary MM. Patients should have a point of contact to enable early review in case recurrence is suspected. Guidance on follow-up after surgery varies between countries, because there is no clear evidence that routine follow-up examinations or periodic CT scans have an impact on mortality. The majority of patients detect recurrence between medical visits, so intervals and duration of follow-up are usually adapted to the estimated risk of metastases based on prognostic markers (Breslow thickness and sentinel node status), but also on the actual risk at a given period after primary MM resection [349]. Medical surveillance is usually proposed every 3–6 months for the first 3–5 years after diagnosis. Comparison of follow-up guidelines in Table 142.4 [350] shows that, in the absence of comparative trials, there are divergent points of view.

Table 142.4 Comparison of recommended follow-up guidelines for patients with melanoma based on the American Joint Committee on Cancer (AJCC) stage of the primary lesion.

Melanoma AJCC stage	Follow-up interval			
	NCCN	ACN	ESMO	CCO/CMA
Stage 0	Annual skin examination	Annual skin examination	Generally does not have strong recommendations for follow-up, but suggests every 3 months during first 3 years, and every 6–12 months thereafter mainly for psychological support. Patients recommended to perform lifelong self-examinations of skin and peripheral lymph nodes	Annual skin examination
Stage IA	Comprehensive H&P every 3–12 months for 5 years, annually thereafter	Comprehensive H&P every 6 months for 5 years, annually thereafter		Every 6–12 months for 1 year, then annually thereafter
Stage IB				Every 6 months for 3 years, annually for the following 2 years, then as clinically indicated
Stage IIA		Comprehensive H&P every 3–4 months for 5 years, annually thereafter		
Stage IIB	Comprehensive H&P every 3–6 months for 2 years, every 3–12 months for the following 3 years, annually thereafter			
Stage IIC				
Stage III				Every 3–6 months for 3 years, every 4–12 months for the following 2 years, annually thereafter
Stage IV				

Reproduced from Fong and Tanabe 2014 [350].
ACN, Australian Cancer Network; CCO, Cancer Care Ontario; CMA, Canadian Medical Association; ESMO, European Society for Medical Oncology; NCCN, National Comprehensive Cancer Network; H&P, history and physical examination.
Radiographic imaging is not recommended at baseline but is appropriate at the discretion of the physician or when clinically indicated. Blood tests (S100B, lactate dehydrogenase) are generally not indicated routinely for follow-up.

Periodic radiological examinations in asymptomatic patients are not considered useful, although they are performed in many countries. At the time of chemotherapy, early diagnosis of metastases was not considered a benefit, due to the lack of efficacy of treatments. With the development of recent very active molecules (targeted therapy and immune therapies) there is no clear demonstration that early diagnosis of metastasis may confer an advantage to patients compared with those who will be treated some time later. Other factors are part of the debate: toxicity of repeated irradiations for imaging, medicolegal issues, impact on patient quality of life and patient anxiety, etc.

The follow-up for patients with MM *in situ* (stage 0) is less stringent and most individuals can be discharged after appropriate surgery and education on self-examination and sun protection. However, there are different situations with MM *in situ* which deserve particular attention. Many patients with MM *in situ* for example may harbour a large number of clinically atypical moles and may thus warrant remaining under surveillance for detection of an additional secondary MM.

Management of patients with advanced disease is discussed in Chapter 144.

Key references

The full list of references can be found in the online version at https://www.wiley.com/rooksdermatology10e

32 Shain AH, Joseph NM, Yu R *et al*. Genomic and transcriptomic analysis reveals incremental disruption of key signaling pathways during melanoma evolution. *Cancer Cell* 2018;34:45–55.e4.

73 Toussi A, Mans N, Welborn J, Kiuru M. Germline mutations predisposing to melanoma. *J Cutan Pathol* 2020;47:606–16.

100 Wiesner T, Obenauf AC, Murali R *et al*. Germline mutations in BAP1 predispose to melanocytic tumors. *Nat Genet* 2011;43:1018–21.

108 Horn S, Figl A, Rachakonda PS *et al*. TERT promoter mutations in familial and sporadic melanoma. *Science* 2013;339(6122):959–61.

142 Gandini S, Sera F, Cattaruzza MS *et al*. Meta-analysis of risk factors for cutaneous melanoma: II. Sun exposure. *Eur J Cancer* 2005;41:45–60.

196 Green AC, Williams GM, Logan V, Strutton GM. Reduced melanoma risk after regular sunscreen use: randomized trial follow-up. *J Clin Oncol* 2011;29:257–63.

204 Grob JJ, Richard MA, Gouvernet J *et al*. The kinetics of the visible growth of a primary melanoma reflects the tumor aggressiveness and is an independent prognostic marker: a prospective study. *Int J Cancer* 2002;102:34–8.

234 Gaudy-Marqueste C, Wazaefi Y, Bruneu Y *et al*. Ugly duckling sign as a major factor of efficiency in melanoma detection. *JAMA Dermatol* 2017;153:279–84.

245 Esteva A, Kuprel B, Novoa RA *et al*. Dermatologist-level classification of skin cancer with deep neural networks. *Nature* 2017;542(7639):115–18.

346 Gershenwald JE, Scolyer RA, Hess KR *et al*. Melanoma staging: evidence-based changes in the American Joint Committee on Cancer eighth edition cancer staging manual. *CA Cancer J Clin* 2017;67:472–92.

CHAPTER 143

Melanoma Surgery

Noah R. Smith, Kelly B. Cha, Timothy M. Johnson and Alison B. Durham

Michigan Medicine Department of Dermatology, Ann Arbor, MI, USA

Biopsy, 143.1	Lentigo maligna melanoma and lentigo maligna melanoma *in situ*, 143.3	**Patient selection for sentinel lymph node biopsy, 143.5**
Wide local excision, 143.1	**Sentinel lymph node biopsy, 143.4**	**Future work, 143.6**
Melanoma *in situ*, 143.3	**Completion lymph node dissection, 143.5**	**Key references, 143.6**

Biopsy

Early detection of melanoma is associated with thinner tumours with better prognosis and outcomes. While melanoma is most commonly detected by the patient or a significant other, physician detection is more frequently associated with thinner lesions [1]. Historical features that raise suspicion in a lesion include a change in size, shape or colour, or lesion pruritus [1,2]. Ulceration, tenderness and bleeding are later signs. On physical examination, criteria such as the ABCD checklist can help identify suspicious lesions (Chapter 142) [3,4]. An E for evolving may be added as a reminder of the importance of a history of a changing lesion [5]. Additionally, an overall assessment of the skin in which a lesion appears unique or different compared with the patient's other lesions (the ugly duckling sign) raises concern for melanoma [6].

Any lesion suspicious for melanoma on the basis of the history or clinical examination requires a biopsy to provide a diagnosis and direct appropriate treatment. The ideal biopsy is a prompt, narrow 1–3 mm margin excision of the entire clinically apparent lesion. This may be performed as a sutured ellipse or punch biopsy or deep saucerisation at least 2 mm in depth. This allows determination of diagnosis, key melanoma parameters and accurate staging, while preserving the accuracy of sentinel lymph node biopsy (SLNB), should this be indicated. The biopsy should be orientated with definitive wide excision in mind and, for the arms and legs, more parallel to the extremity to facilitate SLNB if indicated. A wide local excision (WLE) or flap closure as the initial biopsy may prevent the option of subsequent SLNB or grossly overtreat a benign melanoma mimic. Palpation of the regional lymph nodes on the day of biopsy is indicated.

For many lesions, size, location or other practical considerations such as time, surgical experience or low suspicion may preclude complete excisional biopsy. In these cases, an incisional biopsy usually via punch, ellipse or deep saucerisation through the thickest, darkest portion is performed. Identification of the most suspicious area to biopsy may also be facilitated by dermoscopy or confocal microscopy. Incisional biopsies are not associated with an increased risk of metastasis [7]. However, a partial incisional biopsy is subject to sampling error in diagnosis, Breslow depth and other staging factors. The ability to accurately predict the deepest portion by clinical inspection or incisional biopsy is not always reliable. In one study involving 1783 consecutive patients, 250 of whom presented with ≥50% residual clinical lesion after incisional biopsy, removal of the remainder of the lesion altered staging and prognosis in 21%, and 10% became candidates for SLNB based upon a new Breslow depth of ≥1 mm revealed in the residual lesion [8]. Therefore, if treatment recommendations might change upon further information gained on complete sampling, a narrow-margin excision to remove the remainder of the lesion for accurate microstaging is recommended prior to proceeding with definitive treatment.

Review of biopsy material by a dermatopathologist experienced in melanoma and pigmented lesions is crucial for optimal patient management [9–11]. Once melanoma is diagnosed, a number of histopathological features are necessary for staging and treatment recommendations [12]. These include pathological primary tumour (T) stage, Breslow thickness rounded to the nearest 0.1 mm, ulceration status, status of peripheral and deep margins, microsatellitosis status, pure desmoplasia if present, lymphovascular/angiolymphatic invasion, and Clark level (for lesions ≤1 mm where mitotic rate is not determined). Additional characteristics include anatomical body site location, regression, dermal mitotic rate (number per mm^2), tumour infiltrating lymphocytes, growth phase, neurotropism, histological subtype classification and coexisting naevus status [12]. Molecular testing may be indicated for equivocal lesions.

Wide local excision

Any patient with a new diagnosis of melanoma requires a history and physical examination prior to WLE. The history should include

Table 143.1 Prospective, randomised trials investigating appropriate clinical margins for excision of melanoma.

Trial	Number of participants	Tumour thickness (mm)	Surgical margins (cm)		Median follow-up (years)
			Narrow	Wide	
WHO Melanoma Group Trial [13–15]	612	≤2	1	≥3	12
Swedish Melanoma Trial Group [16]	989	>0.8 to ≤2	2	5	11 (survival), 8 (recurrence)
Intergroup Melanoma Surgical Trial [17]	468	1–4	2	4	10
French Group of Research on Malignant Melanoma Trial [18]	337	<2.1	2	5	16
UK Melanoma Study Group Trial [19]	900	≥2	1	3	9
Multicentre European Trial [20,21]	936	>2	2	4	20

preoperative co-morbidity factors which impact surgical approach and a melanoma-focused review of systems for metastatic disease. A total body skin inspection is indicated since the patient is at risk for additional primary melanoma that may occur anywhere on the skin surface. The regional draining lymph node basins require palpation to detect metastatic disease, with biopsy most commonly via fine-needle aspirate prior to WLE if enlarged nodes are noted.

Most newly diagnosed melanomas are clinically localised to the primary site. Surgical resection of the primary tumour or the diagnostic biopsy site with a clinical margin of normal skin is indicated for biopsy-proven melanoma. The intention of resection is to prevent local recurrence from persistent microscopic disease. Excessively wide margins result in significant morbidity and costs. In contrast, excessively narrow margins may be associated with unacceptable rates of local recurrence with potential for lethal consequence. The appropriate margin of resection has been investigated in six prospective randomised trials (Table 143.1).

The World Health Organization conducted a prospective randomised study to assess the efficacy of narrow (1 cm) excision for thin melanoma [13–15]. In this trial, 612 patients with melanoma ≤2 mm in thickness on the trunk, arms or legs were randomised to receive narrow (1 cm) or wide (≥3 cm) excision. Of note in this trial, excision margins in the subcutaneous fat and muscular fascia were 1–2 cm greater than at the skin surface. The patients were followed for a median of 12 years. Local recurrence, defined as within 1 cm of the scar, was analysed. Eleven patients recurred locally. Eight were in the narrow excision group; five of these had melanoma 1.1–2 mm in depth. The difference in local recurrence between the narrow and wide excision groups was not statistically significant.

The Swedish Melanoma Study Group performed a prospective randomised study of 989 patients with melanoma of the trunk and extremities, tumour thickness >0.8 mm and ≤2 mm, to evaluate the efficacy of a 2 cm versus 5 cm margin excision [16]. With a median follow-up of 8 years for recurrence, patients who received excision with 2 cm margins fared as well as those with wide 5 cm margins. Local recurrence in this trial was defined as recurrence within the scar or graft. Of five patients who experienced local recurrence as a first event, four were in the wide excision group and one in the narrow excision group. Of the total of eight patients who experienced local recurrence at any time, five were in the wide excision group and three in the narrow excision group.

The Intergroup Melanoma Surgical Trial conducted a prospective randomised trial to examine differences in outcomes in patients with intermediate-thickness melanoma treated with 2 cm versus 4 cm excision margins [17]. In this trial, 468 patients with melanoma located on the trunk or proximal extremities with tumour depth of 1–4 mm were randomised to receive excision with 2 cm or 4 cm margins. Local recurrence in this trial was defined as any melanoma recurrence within 2 cm of the surgical scar. After a median of 10 years of follow-up, 11 patients experienced local recurrence, which did not correlate with excision margin (local recurrence of 2.1% ($n = 5$) with 2 cm margin and 2.6% ($n = 6$) with 4 cm margin).

The French Group of Research on Malignant Melanoma prospectively randomised 337 patients with melanoma ≤2 mm in depth to receive excision with 2 cm or 5 cm margins [18]. Patients with lentigo maligna melanoma, acral lentiginous melanoma, aged >70 or with melanoma on the toe, nail or finger were excluded. Sixteen-year follow-up data were published. Local recurrence was defined as tumour occurring within 2 cm of the excision, which affected five patients (one in the narrow excision arm, four in the wide excision arm).

The multicentre trial performed by the UK Melanoma Study Group prospectively randomised 900 patients with melanoma ≥2 mm on the trunk and extremities, excluding the palms and soles, to treatment with excision with 1 cm or 3 cm margins [19]. Local recurrence was defined as recurrence within 2 cm of the primary excision site, and in-transit recurrence defined as beyond 2 cm. 'Locoregional' recurrence was defined by combining the rates of local, in-transit and regional nodal recurrence into a single category. When these three different types of recurrence were pooled into a single end point, a significant increase in 'locoregional' recurrence was noted for the 1 cm margin group compared with the 3 cm margin group ($P = 0.05$), possibly influenced by a larger number of nodal recurrences in the 1 cm margin group. No statistically significant difference was found for the rates of local, in-transit or nodal recurrence when each was considered alone (15 local recurrences for 1 cm margin versus 13 for 3 cm margin).

Finally, a sixth multicentre European trial prospectively randomised 936 patients with trunk or extremity melanoma >2 mm depth to receive WLE with 2 cm versus 4 cm margins. No significant difference was noted in local recurrence, melanoma-specific nor overall survival at 6.7 and 19.6 year follow-up [20,21].

A meta-analysis of five of these six randomised prospective trial data performed by the Cochrane Collaboration found no significant difference in local recurrence, overall survival or recurrence-free survival [22]. Although none of these trials individually had enough statistical power to detect a small benefit, these trials represent the best available evidence regarding WLE margins for melanoma.

Table 143.2 Recommended clinical margin for wide local excision of melanoma.

Melanoma tumour thickness	Recommended clinical margin[a]
Melanoma in situ	0.5–1 cm
Breslow depth ≤ 1.0 mm	1 cm
Breslow depth 1.0–2.0 mm	1–2 cm
Breslow depth > 2.0 mm	2 cm

Adapted from National Comprehensive Cancer Network Guidelines – Melanoma: Cutaneous (Version 1.2021). Margins may be modified to accommodate individual anatomical or functional consideration.
[a] For lentigo maligna pattern melanoma, especially on the head and neck, wider margins with more comprehensive histological margin analysis may be required for tumour clearance.

Based on current best available evidence, surgical recommendation for melanoma *in situ* is a 0.5–1 cm margin; for invasive melanoma <1.0 mm thick, 1 cm margin; for melanoma 1.0–2.0 mm thick, 1–2 cm margin; and for melanoma >2.0 mm, 2 cm margin (Table 143.2) [12,23]. A feasibility pilot international study involving 400 patients from 17 centres in five countries comparing a 1 cm versus 2 cm surgical margin with sentinel node biopsy for patients with primary melanoma >1 mm was reported in 2018 [24]. Based on this trial, a definitive multicentre randomised control trial investigating 1 cm versus 2 cm wide excision margins for pT2b-pT4b (American Joint Committee on Cancer, 8th edition) primary cutaneous melanoma is accruing patients (ClinicalTrials.gov Identifier: NCT03860883) [25]. The appropriate depth for any melanoma resection is also debated but typically recommended to extend to the deep adipose tissue for melanoma *in situ* and thin melanoma, and through the subcutaneous fat to the plane of the muscular fascia for deeper melanomas. Surgical resection of melanoma on special sites such as the face, hands and feet may require amendment of the recommended margin due to anatomical considerations. However, tumour clearance is the highest priority, followed by cosmesis. When considering the morbidity of treatment, one should not ignore the morbidity of recurrence. Coordination with multiple specialties may be optimal.

It is important to note that, to date, all studies of margins for melanoma that inform current practice guidelines used clinically measured margins, not histologically measured margins. Therefore, margin size recommendations are based on clinical margin. Histopathological evaluation of the excision specimen is required to demonstrate negative margins. If the margin is deemed positive, re-excision is warranted.

Melanoma *in situ*

For melanoma *in situ*, current practice guidelines recommend a clinical margin of 0.5–1 cm [12,23]. The pathological finding of regression in melanoma *in situ* may represent invasive melanoma that has been obscured or obliterated by the host immune response, suggesting the potential, albeit small, for locoregional or metastatic disease. Therefore, consideration may be given to a margin of 1 cm when regression is noted in melanoma *in situ* [26]. Although extremely infrequent, melanoma *in situ* without regression may also metastasise, presumably due to occult microinvasion noted with immunohistochemistry and more serial sectioning in up to one-third of specimens in an investigative setting [27,28].

Lentigo maligna melanoma and lentigo maligna melanoma *in situ*

Lentigo maligna pattern invasive (LMM) and *in situ* melanoma (LM) warrant special consideration, especially on the head and neck. This pattern is seen most commonly in chronically sun-damaged skin on the head and neck and may be associated with clinically ill-defined borders with potentially wide occult extension beyond the visible clinical margin [29]. Several techniques for treatment of LM/LMM have been reported to mitigate between the subclinical extension on the one hand and the cosmetic sensitivity on the other. Options include standard excision with side-to-side closure versus delayed reconstruction to allow for permanent section margin analysis; Mohs surgery with immunostaining; and permanent sectioning mapped (i.e. 'slow Mohs') or staged mapped (i.e. 'square') techniques. Distinguishing between the trailing edge of the melanoma and background sun damage requires high dermatopathology expertise and clinical pathological correlation. To date, permanent section analysis with dermatopathologist expertise represents the gold standard for margin analysis for melanoma [30], but Mohs with immunohistochemistry shows promise [31].

Staged excision using permanent section tissue processing with complete peripheral margin assessment or Mohs surgery with immunohistochemistry should be considered for high local control rates with tissue preservation for LMM/LM on the head and neck [12,29]. Several staged excision methods with slight variability using complete permanent section margin assessment without immunohistochemistry, such as the 'square' procedure, have been described [29]. The largest study with prospectively collected single institution data reported 834 consecutive LMM/LM lesions on the head and neck in 806 patients, with a median follow-up of 9.3 years. The local recurrence rate was 1.4% at 5 years, 1.8% at 7.5 years and 2.2% at 10 years. The mean margin for clearance was 9.3 mm for melanoma *in situ* and 13.7 mm for invasive melanoma. Forty-one percent of melanoma *in situ* was histological margin tumour-free after ≤5 mm surgical margins and 75% after ≤10 mm surgical margin. For invasive melanoma, histological margins were tumour-free after surgical margins of ≤5 mm in 3%, 52% after ≤10 mm margins. Factors associated with greater surgical margins required to achieve tumour-free histology included invasive versus *in situ* disease, increasing clinical lesion size and previous incomplete excision [29]. Importantly, 36% of local recurrences in this cohort occurred after 5 years, highlighting the importance of longer follow-up periods for accurate evidence assessment, which is lacking in the majority of staged excision and Mohs surgery publications.

Consistent with staged permanent section margin methods, studies of Mohs surgery with immunohistochemistry report 0.9–1.5 cm surgical margins were histological margin tumour-free in 95–97% of melanoma *in situ* lesions on the head and neck, with a 0.5 cm margin clearing 65% of these lesions [32]. Mohs surgery with immunohistochemistry used to treat melanoma in all body locations continues to rise, from 2.6% in 2001 to 7.9% in 2016 [31]. Various publications report local recurrence rates of 1–2% but must be interpreted with caution. Evidence assessment is restricted due to considerable variability of Mohs technique from paper to paper, relatively small patient numbers with many trunk and extremity melanomas included, and follow-up time ranging from 1 month to 5 years. Equivocal histology with Mohs frozen sections requires permanent section confirmation. Inaccurate staging may occur due to failure to detect occult invasive disease after the Mohs procedure has started and may result in a suboptimal treatment approach if unsuspected deeper invasion is noted. High local recurrence rates of 33% are reported with Mohs surgery without immunohistochemistry [33]. Still, Mohs surgery continues to evolve and improve with technique modification and optimisation, resulting in high local control rates achieved by those with the highest levels of specialty training and expertise.

Sentinel lymph node biopsy

Optimal treatment of melanoma involves WLE with appropriate margins, and also consideration and completion of SLNB for nodal staging in appropriate patients, because the most frequent site of first metastasis for melanoma is the regional nodal basin. SLNB was first introduced in 1992 by Morton *et al.* as a minimally invasive procedure to identify patients with occult nodal disease [34].

When metastatic cells enter the lymphatic system, they typically first involve only one node (or possibly a small number of nodes) within the regional nodal basin. Clinicians can identify the first node of potential involvement, the sentinel node, by utilising tracers, typically radiocolloid and vital blue dye, injected intradermally at the site of the primary lesion (Figure 143.1). These tracers travel to and collect in the sentinel node(s) allowing for identification of the most likely site of microscopic metastasis. This node (or nodes) is removed and evaluated thoroughly with serial sectioning and both haematoxylin and eosin and immunohistochemical stains [35]. Since the introduction of the technique, multiple studies worldwide have confirmed the high accuracy of the procedure. Even within the head and neck region, where complex lymphatic drainage may make SLNB more difficult, SLNB has high accuracy when performed by an experienced surgeon and centre [36,37]. Particularly within the head and neck, use of single photon emission computed tomography/computed tomography (SPECT/CT), a three-dimensional, precise imaging modality, improves sentinel node identification rates compared with standard SLNB without SPECT/CT [38]. Accuracy may be decreased if SLNB is performed after WLE or a flap closure at any site but particularly in ambiguous drainage areas like the head, neck or central trunk. Thus, SLNB is ideally performed at the time of WLE to allow tracers to be injected near the true site of the initial lesion [39].

While numerous publications detail known and potential benefits of SLNB, there is currently one prospective randomised controlled trial comparing WLE plus SLNB with immediate completion lymph node dissection (CLND) for a positive sentinel node versus WLE plus observation with CLND upon the development of regional disease. This trial, the Multicenter Selective Lymphadenectomy Trial-I (MSLT-I), began in 1994 across 18 centres worldwide, funded by the National Cancer Institute, National Institutes of Health and the Australia and New Zealand Melanoma Trials Group (ClinicalTrials.gov number, NCT00275496; last update posted 2 September, 2015). The main aims were to determine if SLNB could be used to identify patients with subclinical regional nodal disease and whether immediate CLND in those with occult disease could result in improved outcomes compared with observation and subsequent CLND upon the development of clinically apparent regional disease. Interim outcomes data were published in 2006 [40]. In 2014, the final analysis of outcomes data from MSLT-I was published [41].

In the final analysis, the 10-year melanoma-specific survival rate for intermediate-thickness melanoma, defined as Breslow depth 1.2–3.5 mm, was 85% for patients with a negative sentinel node versus 62% for patients with a positive sentinel node (hazard ratio, 3.09; P <0.001), confirming the prognostic value of sentinel node

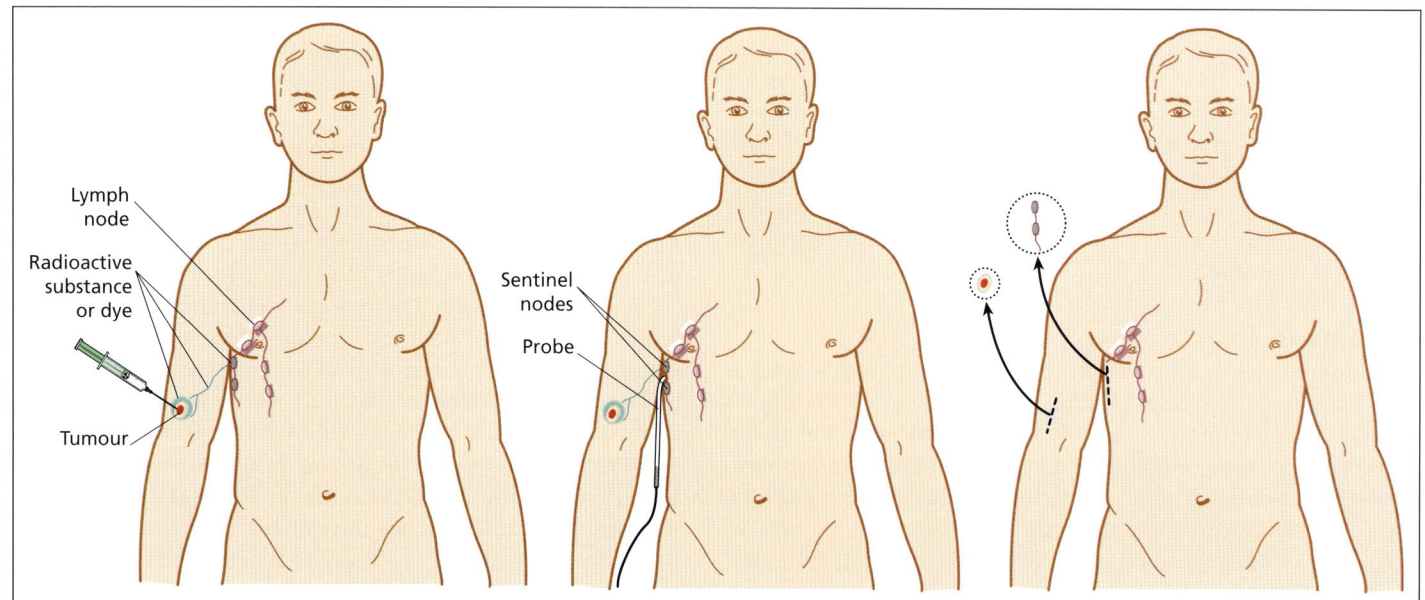

Figure 143.1 (a–c) Sentinel lymph node biopsy allows detection of melanoma micrometastases in regional lymph nodes. Radioactive tracer and dye are injected intradermally at the primary melanoma tumour site and follow the lymphatic drainage pathway to the first, or sentinel, regional lymph node. Intraoperatively, a probe is used to detect the target node, which is then surgically excised for pathological evaluation. Courtesy of Hensin Tsao, Skin Cancer Genetics Laboratory/Wellman Center for Photomedicine, Boston, MA, USA.

status. Among patients with thick melanoma, this rate was 65% for patients with a negative sentinel node versus 48% for patients with a positive sentinel node (hazard ratio, 1.75; $P = 0.03$). Sentinel node status was the most powerful prognostic factor in multivariate analysis [41].

For those patients with nodal disease, identification through SLNB was associated with a reduction in the total number of tumour-positive nodes identified following completion lymphadenectomy (1.4 versus 3.3, $P < 0.001$) [40]. These findings support disease progression and greater tumour burden with observation. At 10 years, a comparison of the estimated cumulative incidence of nodal metastasis melanoma was similar between the two arms: 19.5% in the observation arm compared with 21.9% in the SLNB arm for intermediate-depth melanoma and 41.4% in the observation arm compared with 42.0% in the SLNB arm for thick melanoma, indicating that concerns about false positive results with SLNB are unfounded and melanoma identified by SLNB is clinically meaningful [41].

The overall rate of nodal disease within the study was 20.8%, meaning that the majority of randomised participants could not benefit from SLNB. Therefore, it was neither surprising nor unexpected that the 10-year melanoma-specific survival rate was not different between the two arms overall. Ten-year disease-free survival improved in the SLNB arm: 71% versus 65% for patients with intermediate-thickness melanoma (1.2–3.5 mm Breslow depth) ($P = 0.01$); and 51% versus 41% for patients with thick melanoma (≥ 3.5 mm Breslow depth) ($P = 0.03$) [41].

A secondary latent subgroup analysis was used to determine if there was a survival benefit associated with early, SLNB-directed CLND for patients with nodal metastasis. This analysis compared outcomes between patients treated with CLND following identification of occult nodal disease with SLNB to patients treated with CLND upon development of clinically apparent disease. Acknowledging controversy regarding subgroup analysis validity, within the subset of patients with intermediate-thickness melanoma and nodal disease, early identification and intervention with CLND for a positive sentinel node were associated with improved 10-year melanoma-specific survival. Among patients with intermediate-thickness melanoma, the survival rate was 56% for patients with CLND in the SLNB arm (including those patients with a false negative SLNB) versus 42% for patients in the observation arm (hazard ratio for death from melanoma, 0.56; $P = 0.04$). Among patients with thick melanoma and nodal disease, a treatment-related difference was not demonstrated: 10-year melanoma-specific survival rates were 48% for patients in the SLNB arm versus 46% for patients in the observation arm ($P = 0.78$) [41].

Completion lymph node dissection

The majority of patients who undergo completion lymph node dissection (CLND) after positive SLNB have no positive non-sentinel nodes, raising the question of whether patients with a positive SLNB could be monitored closely and CLND performed only upon identification of nodal disease recurrence. Two randomised controlled trials, the Multicenter Selective Lymphadenectomy Trial-II (MSLT-II) and the German Dermatologic Cooperative Oncology Group Trial (DeCOG-SLT), were designed to answer this question. In MSLT-II, after primary treatment with WLE and positive SLNB, patients in the observation arm had clinical examination with nodal ultrasound of the positive nodal basin every 4 months for 2 years, then every 6 months during years 3–5. Subsequently, patients had clinical examination annually. In DeCOG-SLT, patients in the observation arm underwent clinical examination and ultrasound evaluation from the site of the primary site scar to and including the regional lymph node basin every 3 months for 3 years and additionally had blood tests and imaging (CT, MRI, PET-CT or chest X-ray and abdominal ultrasound) every 6 months for 3 years. Of note, patients with melanoma on the head and neck were excluded from DeCOG-SLT and accounted for only approximately 14% of those patients enrolled in MSLT-II.

The interim data from MSLT-II were published in 2017. The 3-year rate of melanoma-specific survival was 86% in both the treatment and observation arms, at a median follow-up time of 43 months ($P = 0.42$). The risk of lymphoedema was higher in the immediate CLND group, compared with the observation arm (24.1% vs 6.3%). The rate of disease-free survival was better with immediate CLND at 3 years (68% vs 63%, $P = 0.05$), which was felt to be due to improved rate of disease control in the regional nodal basin (92% vs 77%, $P < 0.001$ by the log-rank test) [42].

In the final analysis of DeCOG-SLT, 5-year distant metastasis-free survival (67.6% vs 64.9%, hazard ratio (HR) 1.08; $P = 0.87$), recurrence-free survival (HR 1.01) and overall survival (HR 0.99) were similar between the treatment and observation arms. Adverse events were only recorded for the immediate CLND arm, with lymphoedema (grade 3 and 4 toxicity) reported in 8.3% [43].

Although limitations exist with both MSLT-II and DeCOG-SLT, including a high proportion of enrolled patients with minimal disease burden in the sentinel lymph node and few patients studied with head and neck melanoma, the data from these trials show that patients with a positive SLNB may defer immediate CLND in exchange for close clinical follow-up without negative impact on melanoma-related outcomes. These trial results have led to significant changes in surgical management of the affected nodal basin after discovery of a positive SLNB, with observation being preferred over CLND in the majority of cases [44,45].

Patient selection for sentinel lymph node biopsy

Thankfully, the majority of melanomas worldwide are diagnosed at early stages and do not require treatment beyond WLE. However, given the available evidence, health care providers managing patients with melanoma should identify patients who may benefit from staging with SLNB and discuss with them the benefits, risks and limitations of the procedure. In general, SLNB should be recommended in relatively healthy patients with primary localised lesions ≥ 1.0 mm Breslow depth. For patients with American Joint Committee on Cancer, 8th edition T1b melanoma (Breslow depth 0.8–1.0 mm without ulceration or < 1.0 mm with ulceration), SLNB may be considered on a case-by-case basis. Currently, many clinicians will consider performing SLNB for T1b lesions if other adverse parameters are present, such as young age as a continuous variable centred around 40–45; the presence of angiolymphatic invasion, ulceration or increased mitotic rate as a continuous variable starting at $1/mm^2$; a positive deep margin usually on shave biopsy such that the true Breslow depth is unknown; and dermal regression to 1 mm thickness [44,46–48].

In summary, SLNB is a valid staging test to identify occult melanoma in the lymph nodes in appropriate candidates. Patients who undergo SLNB staging benefit from prognostic information gained, which forms the basis for follow-up strategies which now include use of nodal ultrasound for monitoring of the regional nodal basin, often in conjunction with other staging imaging to monitor for distant disease development. Importantly, use of SLNB to detect occult nodal disease also identifies those patients eligible for treatment with adjuvant systemic therapy.

Future work

The field of melanoma care, including surgical management, is continuously evolving. Future research will expand our understanding of the biology of melanoma and allow us to determine additional characteristics of the patient and primary lesion that can guide optimal patient selection for biopsy, local excision and SLNB. This chapter presents the most relevant current treatment guidelines. In the coming era of personalised medicine and the global research pipeline, sweeping changes in treatment options and evolution of guidelines will undoubtedly occur to improve clinical practice.

Key references

The full list of references can be found in the online version at https://www.wiley.com/rooksdermatology10e

2 Liu W, Hill D, Gibbs AF *et al*. What features do patients notice that help to distinguish between benign pigmented lesions and melanomas? The ABCD(E) rule versus the seven-point checklist. *Melanoma Res* 2005;15:549–54.
23 Swetter SM, Tsao H, Bichakjian CK *et al*. Guidelines of care for the management of primary cutaneous melanoma. *J Am Acad Dermatol* 2019;80:208–50.
29 Moyer JS, Rudy S, Boonstra PS *et al*. Efficacy of staged excision with permanent section margin control for cutaneous head and neck melanoma. *JAMA Dermatol* 2017;153:282–8.
31 Miller CJ, Giordano CN, Higgins HW, 2nd. Mohs micrographic surgery for melanoma: as use increases, so does the need for best practices. *JAMA Dermatol* 2019;155:1225–6.
40 Morton DL, Thompson JF, Cochran AJ *et al*. Sentinel-node biopsy or nodal observation in melanoma. *N Engl J Med* 2006;355:1307–17.
41 Morton DL, Thompson JF, Cochran AJ *et al*. Final trial report of sentinel-node biopsy versus nodal observation in melanoma. *N Engl J Med* 2014;370:599–609.
42 Faries MB, Thompson JF, Cochran AJ *et al*. Completion dissection or observation for sentinel-node metastasis in melanoma. *N Engl J Med* 2017;376:2211–22.
43 Leiter U, Stadler R, Mauch C *et al*. Final analysis of DeCOG-SLT Trial: no survival benefit for complete lymph node dissection in patients with melanoma with positive sentinel node. *J Clin Oncol* 2019;37:3000–8.
44 Coit DG. *NCCN Clinical Practice Guidelines in Oncology* (NCCN Guidelines). Cutaneous melanoma. Version 1.2020, 2020.
45 Garbe C, Amaral T, Peris K *et al*. European consensus-based interdisciplinary guideline for melanoma. Part 2: Treatment – update 2019. *Eur J Cancer* 2020;126:159–77.

CHAPTER 144

Systemic Treatment of Melanoma

Reinhard Dummer and Simone M. Goldinger

Department of Dermatology, University Hospital Zurich, Zurich, Switzerland

---

Introduction, 144.1
Treatment options in local and systemic therapy of melanoma, 144.1
Local therapies, 144.1
Immunotherapy, 144.2
Targeted therapy, 144.4

Chemotherapy, 144.5
Other therapies, 144.5
Therapeutic approach for systemic management of melanoma, 144.5
Neoadjuvant systemic treatment, 144.6

Adjuvant systemic treatment, 144.6
Systemic therapy for metastatic disease, 144.6
Systemic therapy in special circumstances, 144.7
Cutaneous side effects of systemic therapies, 144.9

Key references, 144.12

Introduction

The systemic treatment paradigm for melanoma has rapidly evolved over the past decade. Therapy options include oncolytic, immune-directed and targeted therapies. Multiple well-designed international clinical trials have demonstrated improved progression-free and overall survival of melanoma patients. Although chemotherapy is still available, it has mainly been replaced by these new regimens. In addition, most treatment options are now used not only for advanced melanoma but also in the adjuvant or even neoadjuvant setting. Overall, these therapeutic shifts have had a positive impact on both patients' prognosis and quality of life. At the same time, new emerging ranges of adverse effects require specific knowledge and appropriate management. Improved patients' survival and prolonged treatment periods can also lead to new financial burdens that need to be taken into account when managing the disease. Additional novel approaches for the management of advanced melanoma are under continuous development. Patients should be referred to tertiary skin cancer centres that can offer clinical trial participation. They should be encouraged to enrol in clinical trials whenever possible.

This subchapter is divided into three parts:
1 Treatment options in local and systemic therapy of melanoma.
2 Therapeutic approach for the systemic management of melanoma:
 - Neoadjuvant systemic therapy: treatment for localised disease before surgical resection in stage III.
 - Adjuvant systemic therapy: specific treatment approaches in stage III/N2–3 disease.
 - Systemic therapy for metastatic disease: treatment for advanced stage IIIB/IIIC and stage IV disease.
 - Systemic therapy in special circumstances: treatment for brain metastasis and mucosal or uveal melanoma.
3 Cutaneous side effects of systemic melanoma therapies

Treatment options in local and systemic therapy of melanoma

Over the past decade, melanoma therapies have undergone an impressive boost. From interferon and standard chemotherapy, the treatment options have now expanded and improved.

Local therapies
Surgery
Surgical resection is often the first treatment option when isolated melanoma recurrences are detected. This topic is discussed extensively elsewhere. It is critical to emphasise the importance of tissue sampling any recurrences as this is a key step for molecular genetic profiling and for the assessment of specific markers (such as programmed cell death protein 1 (PD-L1)). The results of these investigations are usually required for choosing appropriate further systemic treatment in advanced melanoma patients.

Oncolytic virus therapy
Talimogene laherparepvec (T-vec) is a genetically engineered herpes simplex virus. It is injected directly into tumour lesions. By producing granulocyte–macrophage colony-stimulating factor gene (GM-CSF), the attenuated oncolytic virus is believed to initiate local tumour cell destruction as well as enhancing local and systemic cellular antitumour responses [1].

In a pivotal phase III trial, 436 melanoma patients were randomised and treated either with T-vec or with GM-CSF [2]. All the patients had unresectable, injectable stage III or IV melanoma with a limited visceral disease burden. T-vec was injected intralesionally every 2 weeks and GM-CSF was administered subcutaneously daily for 2 weeks every month. Patients treated with T-vec had significant longer response rates compared with GM-CSF, defined as 6 months or longer (16.3% versus 2.1%). Antitumour effect was observed in the uninjected lesions and at visceral sites. The response

---

Rook's Textbook of Dermatology, Tenth Edition. Edited by Christopher Griffiths, Jonathan Barker, Tanya Bleiker, Walayat Hussain and Rosalind Simpson.
© 2024 John Wiley & Sons Ltd. Published 2024 by John Wiley & Sons Ltd.

rate was significantly higher (26.4% versus 5.7%). Overall survival was only improved in a subset of patients (stage III or IVa) [2]. The most common adverse effects of this treatment included fatigue, chills, pyrexia, nausea, influenza-like illness and pain at the injection site. While T-vec monotherapy is mainly indicated for a subset of patients with locally advanced melanoma with injectable lesions, promising data suggest that oncolytic virotherapy may improve the efficacy of immunotherapy by changing the tumour microenvironment [3,4].

Radiotherapy

Radiotherapy can be considered in melanoma patients in certain circumstances. Despite not having an impact on overall survival (OS) and progression-free survival (PFS), radiotherapy has been used in certain settings such as inoperable desmoplastic melanoma or after lymph node dissection to prevent local recurrences. With the advent of new therapeutic options influencing survival, radiotherapy is now primarily evaluated in symptomatic metastatic lesions and brain metastasis. Overall, stereotactic radiotherapy is favoured over whole brain radiotherapy. Patients considered for radiotherapy should be discussed in a multidisciplinary team and will include melanoma patients with multiple or large lymph node metastasis, extranodal involvement, symptomatic metastasis or brain metastasis. Of note, in the era of immunotherapy, stereotactic radiotherapy has been postulated to have both synergistic properties when used during checkpoint inhibitor therapy as well as the potential to consolidate the effect of immune-directed treatment.

Electrochemotherapy

Electrochemotherapy (ECT) is an anticancer treatment that uses a small electric current (electroporation) to increase chemotherapeutic drug uptake into the tumour. Bleomycin is commonly used. It is primarily used for tumour control in ulcerating skin metastasis aiming to improve the patient's quality of life [5].

Isolated limb perfusion

Isolated limb perfusion (ILP) is a technique used to perfuse anticancer agents into an extremity. The flow of blood to and from the limb is temporarily stopped with a tourniquet, and melphalan and/or tumour necrosis factor α (TNF-α) are injected directly into the blood of the limb. It is mainly used to palliate disease. It may be considered a treatment option if the tumour is limited to an extremity or in an adjuvant setting after surgical tumour resection. Although ILP does decrease the incidence of both in transit and local recurrences and has resulted in long-term survival in a small number of patients, clinical trials have not demonstrated significant improvement in survival [6]. Of note, there is significant associated morbidity with approximately 1% risk for limb loss [7] and its use should therefore be restricted to centres of excellence. ILP is not used in common practice any more. The role of ILP in the context of immunotherapy is currently being investigated (NCT01323517, NCT02115243).

Immunotherapy
Interferons

Interferon α (IFN-α) and pegylated IFN-α (peg-IFN-α) were the first recombinant cytokines used to treat metastatic melanoma [8]. They are pleiotropic proteins produced by white blood cells other than lymphocytes. The term pegylation describes the conjugation of a molecule with polyethylene-glycol (peg), which is used to alter the physical and chemical profile of a molecule. Pegylation increases the stability and solubility of a drug. Interferons were used in the era before the introduction of checkpoint inhibitors. There has never been general agreement on the optimal dosage, nor about the treatment duration in melanoma. Of note, particularly high-dose regimens were associated with numerous severe side effects, including acute constitutional symptoms, chronic fatigue, myelosuppression, hepatotoxicity and neurological and psychological side effects. With the development of new treatment options, immunotherapy with IFN-α and peg-IFN-α is generally no longer used for the treatment of melanoma.

Checkpoint inhibitors

Immune checkpoints are a normal part of the immune system. They are a group of co-stimulatory and inhibitory pathways that regulate T-cell immune responses. Their role is to prevent an immune response overreacting and destroying healthy cells of the body (autoimmune reaction). Thus, they are considered as either positive or negative regulators of the immune system (Figure 144.1).

Some cancer cells, including melanoma cells, are able to stimulate immune checkpoints by expressing certain surface proteins that bind to partner proteins on T cells. This results in a downregulation of the immune system and prevention of tumour cell destruction.

Checkpoint inhibitors shift the immune system response, aiming to increase its alertness against tumour cells. Ipilimumab is a monoclonal antibody-blocking cytotoxic T-lymphocyte-associated antigen 4 (CTLA-4) promoting T-cell priming against tumour cells. Nivolumab and pembrolizumab, in turn, target PD-1 on T cells and play a key role during the effector phase of antigen recognition. By blocking the interaction between PD-1 and its ligand (PD-L1), these checkpoint inhibitors can restore or even increase the antitumour immune response. They are used either as monotherapy or in combination with other molecules. Currently, they are considered the gold standard treatment for advanced melanoma.

Checkpoint inhibitors typically induce immune-related adverse effects [9], probably as a direct result of limiting immune tolerance against antigens that belong to the affected person. Upon early detection and when following specific treatment guidelines, these side effects are manageable and reversible most of the time [10,11]. The side effects follow a fairly specific timeline pattern and include dermatitis, colitis/diarrhoea, autoimmune endocrinopathies such as hypophysitis and hepatitis; uveitis, nephritis, pneumonitis and inflammatory myopathy also have been reported occasionally [12,13]. Their cutaneous side effects are further elucidated later in this chapter.

Combination therapies

Combination therapies of immunotherapy with local options such as radiotherapy and virotherapy as well as with systemic treatments including kinase inhibitors and chemotherapy have been investigated aiming to improve the outcome of the use of monoclonal antibodies alone.

Radiotherapy has often been used for local tumour control, particularly in draining lymph node basins as well as for

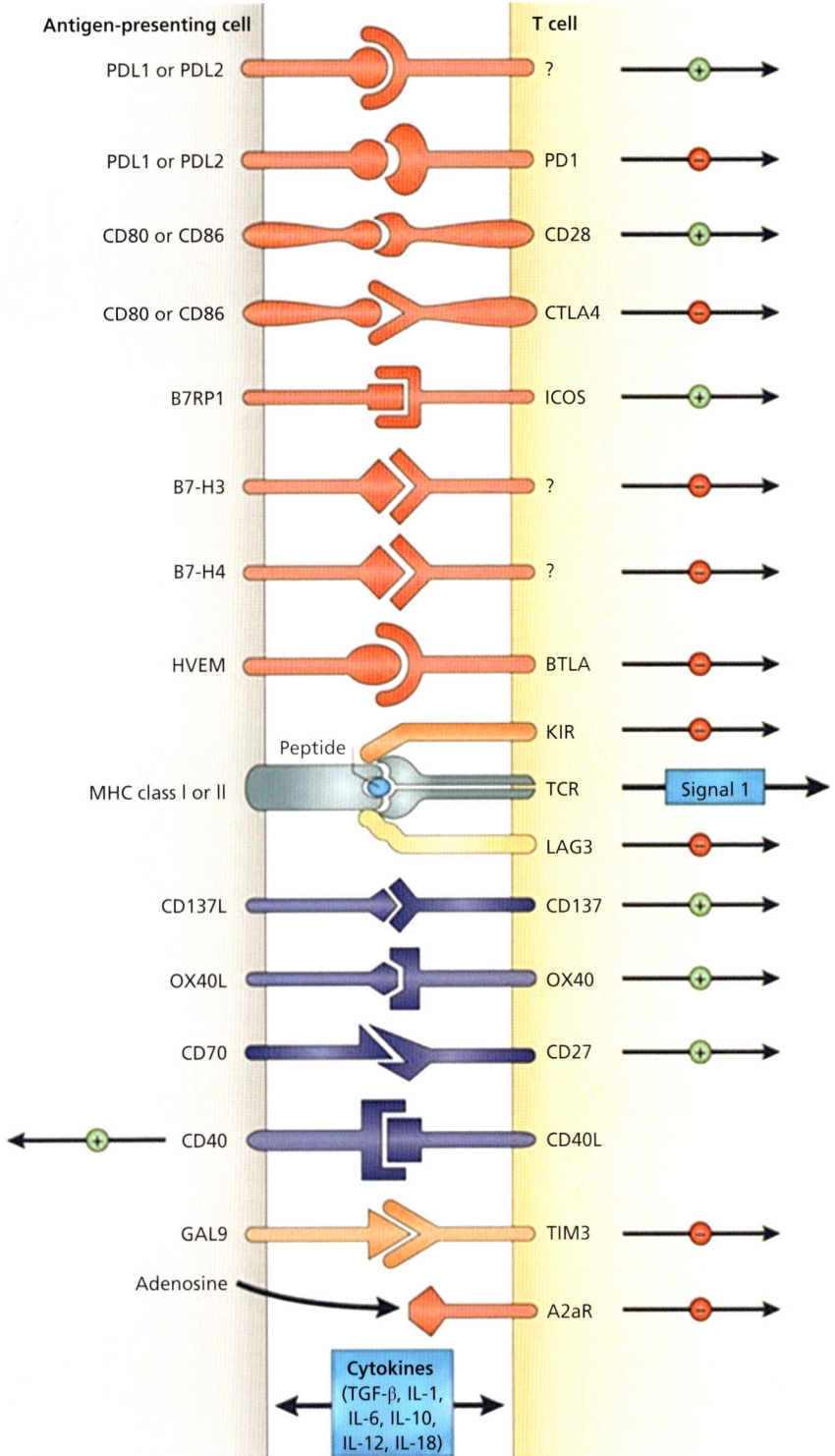

Figure 144.1 Checkpoints with relevant antibodies showing ligand–receptor interactions between T cells and antigen-presenting cells. These interactions regulate the T-cell response to antigen exposure and can be targeted by checkpoint inhibitors. The responses are bidirectional and can occur during the initiation phase in lymph nodes (priming of T cells) or in peripheral tissues or tumours (effector phase). A2aR, adenosine A2a receptor; B7RP1, B7-related protein 1; BTLA, B and T lymphocyte attenuator; CTLA4, cytotoxic T-lymphocyte-associated protein 4; GAL9, galectin 9; HVEM, herpesvirus entry mediator; ICOS, inducible T-cell co-stimulator; IL, interleukin; KIR, killer cell immunoglobulin-like receptor; LAG3, lymphocyte activation gene 3; MHC, major histocompatibility complex; PD1, programmed cell death protein 1; PDL, PD1 ligand; TCR, T-cell receptor; TGF-β, transforming growth factor β; TIM3, T-cell membrane protein 3. Reproduced from Pardoll 2012 [72].

symptomatic metastases, such as brain or bone metastases [14]. Radiotherapy causes local inflammation of the treated area that in turn leads to an increased influx of lymphocytic cells. There are preclinical and clinical data supporting the synergistic effect of immunotherapy with radiotherapy [15–17]. The abscopal effect, defined as enhanced antitumoural response rates both within as well as outside of the irradiated sites, has been controversially discussed in cancer therapy. Overall, the combined use of immunotherapy with fractionated radiotherapy is a potential treatment enhancement in melanoma therapy [18,19]. This can be a useful combination in situations where tumour response shows a mixed response or when metastases in critical locations need to be addressed [20]. Patients need to be monitored for potential serious side effects such as radionecrosis [21]. There are several trials currently investigating the combination of checkpoint inhibitors and radiotherapy.

Oncolytic virotherapy may improve the efficacy of anti-PD-1 therapy by changing the tumour microenvironment [3]. T-vec is considered to be a promoter of local tumour cell destruction, which is concomitant with increased tumoural antigen release and therefore an indirect cause of enhanced immune cell influx. The tumour-specific immune activation is further boosted by the presence of checkpoint-inhibitor antibodies that redirect the immune system towards an improved antigen presentation and T-cell priming. Similar to radiotherapy, antitumoural response in non-T-vec-injected tumour lesions has been described. The prerequisite for this treatment combination is the presence of at least one injectable tumour lesion. T-vec has been studied both in combination with anti-CTLA-4 [4] and anti-PD-1 antibodies [3]. This combination appears to increase objective response rates by approximately 50% in phase I studies. The results of the phase III trial component of the study comparing pembrolizumab with either T-vec or placebo (Keynote-034, NCT02263508) do not, however, support these observations.

Combinations of other checkpoint inhibitors such as the combination of anti-PD-1 antibodies with relatlimab, targeting lymphocyte activated gene 3 (LAG-3) protein, are more efficient than monotherapy with anti-PD-1 antibodies. This combination also shows less toxicity than the well-established anti-CTLA-4 and anti-PD-1 combination [22–24].

The combination of immunotherapy and targeted therapy is reserved for patients with a *BRAF* mutation and is discussed in the section on *BRAF* and *NRAS* mutations later in this chapter.

Finally, combinations with chemotherapy have been assessed. The alkylating agents dacarbazine and temozolomide were investigated in combination with ipilimumab, investigating possible enhancement of antitumor activity [25–27]. However, in the context of emerging treatment options in both targeted and immune-directed therapy, this type of combination has not been further prioritised in melanoma patients.

Targeted therapy

The mitogen-activated protein kinase (MAPK) pathway is a key regulator for gene expression that drives melanocytic gene differentiation such as *MITF*, proliferation and cell survival by suppressing apoptotic pathways. It plays a main role in oncogenic signalling in the majority of melanoma patients. The MAPK pathway consists of serine/threonine-specific kinases including RAS (rat sarcoma), RAF (rapidly accelerated fibrosarcoma), MEK (mitogen-activated protein kinase kinase) and ERK (extracellular signal-related kinase) (Figure 144.2).

BRAF and NRAS mutations

The presence of activating mutations in *BRAF* in about 50% and in *NRAS* in about 20% of all melanomas offers additional therapeutic opportunities. Selective kinase inhibitors targeting RAF and MEK are available for *BRAF* V600 mutation-positive melanoma patients. In a majority of these patients, BRAF inhibition produces rapid tumour regression [28,29,30]. This is especially important for patients with extensive tumour burden and disease-related symptoms [31].

Selective MEK inhibitors have shown efficacy in patients with *BRAF* mutant melanoma as well. In particular trametinib has

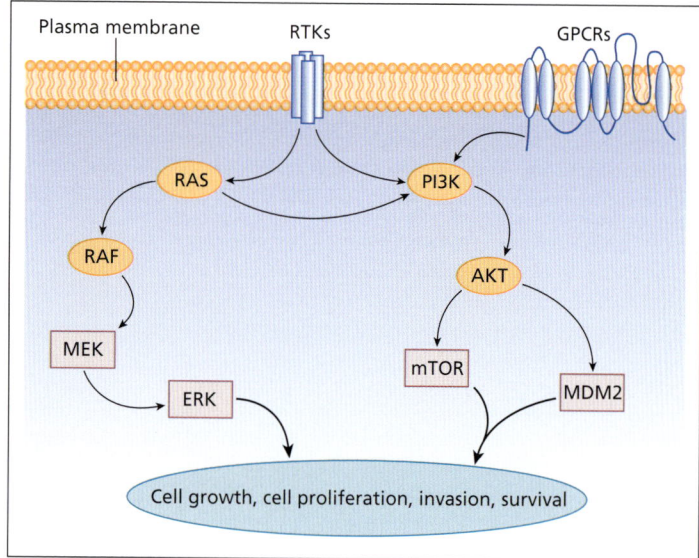

Figure 144.2 The mitogen-activated protein kinase (MAPK) pathway with targetable drugs. The MAPK pathway is one of the most important signalling pathways in melanoma. It consists of serine/threonine-specific kinases including RAS (rat sarcoma), RAF (rapidly accelerated fibrosarcoma), MEK (mitogen-activated protein kinase kinase) and ERK (extracellular signal-related kinase). In addition, the PI3K/AKT/mTOR pathway is important for cell apoptosis and longevity. It includes PI3K (phosphoinositide 3 kinase), AKT (protein kinase B) and mTOR (mammalian target of rapamycin). Both signalling pathways are a very important platform for the development of new drugs leading to an interaction with this signalling cascade. GPCR, G-protein-coupled receptor; RTK, receptor tyrosine kinase.

shown reasonable objective response rates (25%) and an improved survival (median OS of 14.2 months for trametinib in patients who were not previously treated with a BRAF inhibitor) compared with chemotherapy in *BRAF* mutant melanoma [32]. Binimetinib, another highly selective MEK inhibitor, was investigated in *NRAS* mutant melanoma [33–35]. Despite demonstrating some disease control in highly advanced melanoma patients, particularly with intermittent dosing, MEK inhibitors as monotherapy are not used outside of clinical trials.

Simultaneous inhibition of BRAF and MEK improves response rates and survival compared with BRAF inhibition alone. The addition of MEK inhibition not only improves survival, it also reduces resistance development and decreases the cutaneous toxicity seen with single-agent BRAF inhibition [36,37]. In particular, the incidence of squamous cell carcinomas and keratoacanthomas, classically emerging with single-agent BRAF inhibitors, are significantly reduced with the combination [38,39]. Available oral combinations include dabrafenib plus trametinib, vemurafenib plus cobimetinib and encorafenib plus binimetinib. The three combinations show similar efficacy data [40,41,42]. The side effects on the other hand vary, with pyrexia and fatigue being most common with dabrafenib and trametinib, photosensitivity being observed with vemurafenib and cobimetinib, and gastrointestinal adverse effects being slightly more common with encorafenib and binimetinib. The decision on which combination regimen to use should be based on each individual patient's lifestyle as well as the local regimen availability.

A subset of patients with *BRAF* mutation have long-term benefits from targeted therapy. Retrospective survival data analysis from two large pivotal trials confirmed that 34% of *BRAF* mutated melanoma patients treated with dabrafenib and trametinib were alive at 5 years, and approximately 20% of these patients did not progress at this landmark. Similar durable responses were demonstrated with the other combinations as well [43,44–47]. Relevant prognostic factors include lactate dehydrogenase, higher performance status and less than three organ sites with metastases [31].

In contrast to immunotherapy, targeted therapy is generally administered indefinitely. Discontinuation of targeted therapy might lead to tumour regrowth. Interestingly, however, data also suggest that resistance to targeted therapy may be partially reversed by intermittent dosing or by drug holiday [35,48–51].

KIT and GNA11/GNAQ mutations

A small subset accounting for approximately 10% of acral and mucosal melanomas expresses mutations in KIT (v-kit Hardy–Zuckerman 4 feline sarcoma viral oncogene homologue) and a minor portion of uveal melanomas exhibit mutations in GNA11/GNAQ (guanine nucleotide binding protein (G protein), q polypeptide) (approximately 1%) [52,53].

Only approximately one-third of melanomas with KIT mutations are responsive to targeted therapy. Patients with activating mutations in KIT have had clinically meaningful responses in small trials with agents such as imatinib and nilotinib [54–58]. Mutations in exon 11 and 13 of c-KIT (particularly L576P mutation in exon 11) seem to be associated with higher response rates, whereas amplifications of KIT typically do not respond to KIT inhibition.

Overall, targeted KIT inhibition is not used as a first line therapy option in advanced melanoma. Combination with immunotherapies can be considered, ideally in the context of clinical trials.

Combination therapies

Targeted therapies can be combined with other local or systemic agents. Several groups have evaluated the combination of radiotherapy and targeted therapy in BRAF mutant melanoma patients, mainly in the context of present brain metastases. Despite concerns due to radiation sensitisation previously reported with BRAF monotherapy [59–61], radiotherapy-associated toxicity does not seem to increase when radiotherapy is combined with BRAF and MEK inhibitors [17,62–65]. The results of further prospective clinical trials (NCT02392871, NCT02974803) are pending while writing this chapter.

Given immunotherapy and targeted therapy have both positively influenced survival, the combination of these agents have captured increasing interest in BRAF mutant melanoma patients [66,67]. Atezolizumab is a PD-L1 inhibitor that was investigated in combination with vemurafenib and cobimetinib and has recently shown a modest improved PFS compared with targeted therapy alone [68]. Other trials assessing for example the PD-1 inhibitor spartalizumab as well as pembrolizumab in combination with dabrafenib and trametinib appear similarly effective (NCT02967692, NCT02130466).

Combination with chemotherapy on the other hand is not recommended in daily practice.

Chemotherapy

Chemotherapy has been used for many years in melanoma with little efficacy [14]. In particular, dacarbazine was considered as the reference drug to compare new agents for the treatment of melanoma. However, it has shown little benefit, with a median OS in the first line setting of only a few months [15,16] and historical 5-year survival of less than 10% [17]. Other chemotherapeutic agents include temozolomide and fotemustine, which given their properties to cross the blood–brain barrier were often prescribed in patients with brain metastasis [14]. The combination carboplatin and paclitaxel was another regimen commonly prescribed. In a phase III trial including 823 stage IV melanoma patients, the median OS for first line treatment with carboplatin and paclitaxel was 11.3 (95% confidence interval (CI) 9.8–12.2 months) [15]. Taxanes disrupt the microtubule function and thus inhibit cell division. They have been used in several cancer types including melanoma. More recently, in a pivotal phase III trial including 529 melanoma patients, the protein-bound paclitaxel, nab-paclitaxel, showed improvement in PFS and disease control rate compared with dacarbazine: 4.8 versus 2.5 months (95%CI 0.631–0.992; $P = 0.044$) and 39% versus 27% ($P = 0.004$) for nab-paclitaxel and dacarbazine, respectively [69]. Given the advent of checkpoint inhibitors and targeted agents, this treatment never became a standard therapy for melanoma.

In contrast to immunotherapy and targeted therapy, cytotoxic chemotherapy has not been shown to increase survival or to induce durable remissions. Even after checkpoint inhibitor failure, chemotherapy has a low response rate in metastatic melanoma [70]. Therefore, chemotherapy is generally limited to patients who are not candidates for further treatment with either immunotherapy or targeted therapy and for whom there is no appropriate clinical trial. In exceptional cases, chemotherapy can be contemplated as bridging treatment option.

Other therapies

Adjuvant chemotherapy, mistletoe extracts and hormone therapies are not beneficial and should therefore not be recommended [71].

Therapeutic approach for systemic management of melanoma

The choice for the appropriate treatment stage, regimen and sequence has become more challenging over the past few years given emerging data and effective drugs influencing patients' survival. Personalised medicine and the introduction of targeted and immune-directed therapies has led to several new options and strategies compared with the previous chemotherapy era. Whereas former focus was mainly on achieving disease stabilisation, the research community currently is focusing on limiting primary and secondary resistance development, identifying biomarkers and improving quality of life of affected patients. Overall, the aim to achieve long-term remission and eventually to cure melanoma has become more tangible over the last decade.

Tumour tissue should be tested for the presence or absence of a driver mutation and PD-L1 expression wherever possible. The presence of such mutations determines whether a patient is likely to respond to certain treatments and, hence, can be a relevant factor in choosing and sequencing therapies for patients with advanced melanoma.

Neoadjuvant systemic treatment

Patients with advanced stage III melanoma with macrometastases are good candidates for neoadjuvant therapy, preferentially in a clinical trial. They are considered a high-risk patient population for developing metastatic disease. Neoadjuvant therapy is currently an active area of research for melanoma with many completed and ongoing trials [1]. This will have further practical and therapeutical implications in the near future.

Adjuvant systemic treatment

For patients who have undergone a complete resection of a cutaneous melanoma, the decision of whether or not to recommend adjuvant therapy depends on the risk of disease recurrence. The stage at diagnosis, age, co-morbidities and personal preferences should all be considered and discussed in a multidisciplinary team.

In the adjuvant setting, ipilimumab significantly improved relapse-free survival (RFS) in comparison with placebo (26.1 versus 17.1 months, hazard ratio (HR) 0.75) [2]. The OS rate at 5 years was significantly higher as well (65.4% versus 54.4%, HR for death 0.72; 95%CI 0.58–0.88; $P = 0.001$). Contrary to interferon, this benefit was also confirmed for N1b and higher stages. Notably, the treatment regimen in this pivotal trial differed from the previously studied and approved one, with higher doses (10 mg/kg) and more than four infusions. It is therefore not surprising that severe and partially long-lasting adverse reactions, including colitis and endocrinopathies, were reported. Due to better safety profiles, anti-PD-1 therapy or dabrafenib and trametinib are the preferred adjuvant treatment options.

Both pembrolizumab and nivolumab have demonstrated RFS benefit in stage III melanoma. Nivolumab was compared with high-dose ipilimumab and showed a 4-year rate RFS of 51.7% (95%CI 46.8–56.3) versus 41.2% (95%CI 36.4–45.9), respectively (HR 0.71; 95%CI 0.60–0.86; $P = 0.0003$). The 4-year OS for nivolumab was 77.9% (95%CI 73.7–81.5) [3,4]. Pembrolizumab was compared with placebo in a slightly different adjuvant melanoma population [5]. At a median follow-up of 15 months, pembrolizumab was associated with significantly longer RFS than placebo (1-year RFS of 75.4% (95%CI 71.3–78.9) versus 61.0% (95%CI 56.5–65.1), respectively (HR 0.57; 98.4%CI 0.43–0.74; $P <0.001$) [5].

Given the successful use of immunotherapy in stage III disease, both pembrolizumab and nivolumab have been studied in stage II disease as well (NCT03553836 [6], NCT04309409). Notably, first results demonstrate significant risk reduction for recurrence (RFS and distant metastasis-free survival (DMFS)) in patients with primary melanoma stage IIB and IIC treated with pembrolizumab or nivolumab [7]. These results that adjuvant immunotherapy should be expanded to this patient population.

Dabrafenib with trametinib is another treatment option in the adjuvant setting for *BRAF* mutant melanoma patients. Compared with placebo, this combination showed an improved estimated RFS of 58% versus 39% at 3 years (HR 0.47; 95%CI 0.39–0.58; $P <0.001$) in high-risk melanoma patients with stage IIIA (with lymph node metastasis diameter >1 mm), IIIB or IIIC [8]. OS was 86% with dabrafenib and trametinib versus 77% with placebo (HR 0.57; 95%CI 0.42–0.79; $P = 0.0006$) [9,10–12].

There is no direct efficacy comparison between targeted versus immune-directed therapy. Therefore, treatment decisions for *BRAF* mutated melanoma patients should be individually discussed.

Systemic therapy for metastatic disease

Both immunotherapy and targeted therapy have markedly improved survival compared with the use of chemotherapy regimens. Despite striking therapeutic progress for melanoma patients in addressing and treating melanomas that are resistant to these therapy options, inclusion in clinical trials should remain the number one priority in all settings.

First line treatment options for unresectable stage III and IV are anti-PD-1-based therapies (nivolumab, pembrolizumab alone or in combination with ipilimumab) [13,14,16]. For melanoma patients harbouring a *BRAF* mutation, targeted therapy with BRAF and MEK inhibitors (dabrafenib plus trametinib, vemurafenib plus cobimetinib or encorafenib plus binimetinib) is an additional valuable treatment option that is recommended as a second line option except in symptomatic patients (Table 144.1) [17–19]. Lastly for early advanced stages with cutaneous metastases (stages IIIB and C, and stage IV), T-vec injections can be considered [20,21].

Pembrolizumab and nivolumab can be administered either as monotherapy (200 mg IV every 3 weeks and 240 mg IV every 2 weeks) or in combination with ipilimumab (1 mg/kg IV every 3 weeks followed by ipilimumab 3 mg/kg for the first four infusions; 3 weeks after the last combined treatment session continue with 240 mg IV every 2 weeks). Response rates ranged from 35% to 60% of treated patients. The combination treatment demonstrated higher response rates, higher duration of response and greater rates of PFS and OS up to a 4-year follow-up [13,14]. In the comparative pivotal trial, median PFS for the combination arm was 11.5 months (95%CI 8.7–19.3) and 6.9 months (95%CI 5.1–10.2) for nivolumab. Median OS was not reached for nivolumab plus ipilimumab (95%CI 38.2 to NR (not reached)) and was 36.9 months (28.3 to NR) with nivolumab; both significantly higher than ipilimumab (19.9 months, 95%CI 16.9–24.6) [14]. OS rates at 5 years were 52% in the nivolumab plus ipilimumab group and 44% in the

Table 144.1 Common checkpoint inhibitor and targeted therapy regimens for BRAF mutated (BRAFmut) and BRAF wild-type (BRAFwt), NRAS wild-type (NRASwt) or NRAS mutated (NRASmut) melanoma patients.

Mutation	Treatment/regimen options	Standard dose
BRAFmut	Vemurafenib + cobimetinib	960 mg (4 × 240 mg tbl) BD + 60 mg (3 × 20 mg tbl) QD 21/28
	Dabrafenib + trametinib	150 mg (2 × 75 mg tbl) BD + 2 mg QD
	Encorafenib + binimetinib	450 mg (6 × 75 mg tbl) QD + 45 mg (3 × 15 mg tbl) BD
	Vemurafenib + cobimetinib + atezolizumab	720 mg (3 × 240 mg tbl) BD + 60 mg (3 × 20 mg tbl) QD 21/28 + 840 mg IV every 2 weeks
BRAFmut and BRAFwt NRASmut and NRASwt	Nivolumab	3 mg/kg every 2 weeks IV
	Pembrolizumab	2 mg/kg every 3 weeks IV or 200 mg every 3 weeks IV
	Nivolumab + ipilimumab	1 mg/kg + 3 mg/kg every 3 weeks IV (total four doses), followed by nivolumab 3 mg/kg IV every 2 weeks
	Pembrolizumab + ipilimumab	2mg/kg + 1 mg/kg every 3 weeks IV (total four doses), followed by pembrolizumab 2 mg/kg IV every 3 weeks

BD, twice daily; QD, once daily; tbl, tablet.

nivolumab group, as compared with 26% in the ipilimumab group [22]. Despite being numerically superior, patients undergoing the treatment combination need to be selected carefully given the significant increase in amount and severity of adverse effects. Overall, individual treatment decisions for each patient should be discussed in a multidisciplinary team meeting.

Targeted therapy options include oral dabrafenib (150 mg BD) plus trametinib (2 mg QD), oral vemurafenib (960 mg BD) plus cobimetinib (60 mg QD for 21 days in a 28-day cycle) and oral encorafenib (450 mg QD) plus binimetinib (45 mg BD). Given this is a selective treatment option, response rates for targeted therapy were higher ranging from 59% to 76%. Exemplary for kinase inhibitors, the combination of dabrafenib and trametinib demonstrated PFS rates of 21% (95%CI 17–24) at 4 years and 19% (95%CI 15–22) at 5 years. OS rates were 37% (95%CI 33–42) and 34% (95%CI 30–38) at 4 and 5 years, respectively. Complete response occurred in 19% of the investigated patients and was associated with OS rates of 71% (95%CI 62–79) at 5 years [19]. Single-agent BRAF inhibitors should be used only in case of an absolute contraindication for MEK inhibitors. Currently there is no direct comparison between targeted and immune-directed therapy. Based on prospective trial results, current data suggest that long-term survival may be more beneficial in patients treated with immunotherapy up front [23,24]. Interesting preliminary data suggest that a sandwich treatment with targeted and immune-directed therapy might be a good strategy option for *BRAF* mutant patients [25].

Recently, the combination of both immunotherapy and targeted therapy has captured increasing attention [26]. Atezolizumab is a PD-L1 inhibitor that was investigated in combination with vemurafenib and cobimetinib in a double-blinded, placebo-controlled, multicentre study with over 500 untreated, advanced *BRAF V600* mutant melanoma patients [27]. With the triplet regimen, the complete response rate was 15.7%, the partial response rate was 50.6% and the stable disease rate was 22.7% compared with 17.1%, 48.0% and 22.8% in the placebo arm, respectively. PFS was 15.1 months with the triplet regimen (95%CI 11.4–18.4) compared with 10.6 months (95%CI 9.3–12.7) in the placebo arm [27]. Based on these results, the triple-combined therapy was recently US Food and Drug Administration (FDA) and Swissmedic approved and may be beneficial for a minority of patients with *BRAF* mutated melanoma. Many clinical trials are currently in progress exploring open questions about optimal timing, immune biomarkers and eligible patients for these combination regimens.

Systemic therapy in special circumstances

There are certain situations that need to be addressed specifically and are therefore discussed separately. These special circumstances include patients with brain metastases, patients with mucosal and ocular melanomas as well as patients who have achieved complete response after undergoing systemic therapy.

Systemic treatment of brain metastases

Brain metastases are a frequent complication in patients with advanced melanoma and are an important cause of both morbidity and mortality. The approach to these patients is particularly challenging and is rapidly evolving. Due to concerns of drug penetration through the blood–brain barrier and symptoms such as intracranial bleeding resulting in life-threatening consequences, most clinical trials have historically excluded patients with brain metastasis. Recent studies have confirmed that both targeted therapies and immunotherapies can be safely and efficiently used in patients with brain metastases [28,29]. With an overall response rate of 46% in patients with asymptomatic brain metastases as well as a PFS of >50% at 18 months, a combination of anti-PD-1 and anti-CTLA-4 antibodies should be favoured whenever possible [28,30]. In addition, systemic treatment can be combined with neurosurgical techniques as well as radiotherapy, particularly stereotactic radiosurgery [31–33]. With the advent of successful systemic therapies, whole brain radiotherapy should generally not be further recommended given its lack of efficacy and long-term toxicities [34,35].

Systemic treatment of mucosal melanoma

Mucosal melanomas are rare and distinct from cutaneous melanomas [36]. The common drivers such as BRAF and NRAS found in cutaneous melanoma have lower mutation rates in mucosal melanoma. In contrast, KIT is more common in mucosal melanoma, in particular in genital mucosa [37]. Treatment options for advanced mucosal melanoma historically have been very limited. Studies of standard chemotherapy regimens such as dacarbazine and paclitaxel and carboplatin showed limited response rates.

For patients harbouring a mutation in *KIT*, durable responses with imatinib (400 mg BD) were observed in 16% of a 51 patient cohort [38]. In another phase II trial with 43 patients with *KIT* mutations or amplification, 23% of patients had objective responses [39]. Nilotinib (400 mg BD) also demonstrated some responses, including in patients who were previously treated with imatinib [40–42]. In contrast, the response rate to dasatinib (70 mg BD) was low among *KIT* mutated melanoma patients [43].

Immunotherapy in mucosal melanoma patients has generally lower response rates compared with cutaneous melanoma. In a pooled analysis of mucosal melanoma patients treated with anti-PD-1 monotherapy, PFS was 3.0 months (95%CI 2.2–5.4) with objective response rates of 23.3% (95%CI 14.8–33.6) [44]. In patients treated with nivolumab and ipilimumab, PFS was 5.9 months (95%CI 2.8 to NR), with objective response rates of 37.1% (95%CI, 21.5–55.1) [44]. Although lower, complete response to immunotherapy has been described [45]. Overall, and whenever possible, combined immunotherapy should be considered for these patients.

Systemic treatment of uveal melanoma

Most primary uveal melanomas are treated with radiotherapy. Enucleation is often necessary for large tumours. Approximately half of the patients develop distant – typically hepatic – metastasis despite local tumour control. MEK inhibitors have shown discrete responses in patients with uveal melanoma [46,47]. Attempts to utilise other targeted therapies and chemotherapies as well as combinations of targeted and immune-directed therapies are ongoing [48,49].

Recently, the combination of nivolumab and ipilimumab demonstrated activity in metastatic uveal melanoma [50]. In a prospective study, 35 patients had a response rate of 18% with PFS of 5.5 months (95%CI 3.4–9.5), and OS of 19.1 months (95%CI 9.6

to NR) [51]. Similar benefits were observed in other retrospective analyses [52,53]. The response rates were lower than the ones observed in cutaneous melanoma. Unless a patient is included in a clinical trial, nivolumab and ipilimumab should be considered for metastatic uveal melanoma patients.

Practice-changing data influencing the survival of metastatic uveal melanoma patients have been recently released for patients treated with tebentafusp (IMCgp100) (NCT03070392). At a median follow-up of 14.1 months, the OS with tebentafusp was 21.7 months (95%CI 18.6–23.6) versus 16.0 months (95%CI 9.7–19.4) with the investigator's choice of pembrolizumab, ipilimumab or dacarbazine. OS rates at 1 year were 73.2% versus 58.5%, respectively [54].

Patients achieving complete response after systemic therapy

A subset of patients will achieve complete response upon following systemic therapy. Quality of life and inclination to cease therapy

Table 144.2 Incidence, timing and systemic immunosuppression use within 7 days following cutaneous diagnosis in patients treated with immune-checkpoint inhibitors (ICIs).

Cutaneous diagnosis	Number of patients who developed disease (%)	Median time of onset (IQR) (days)	Number of patients who received systemic immunosuppression (%)
Any of the following diseases*	2171 (25.1%)	113.0 (42.0–254.0)	109 (5.0%)
Rash and other non-specific eruption†	779 (9.0%)	121.0 (42.0–259.0)	44 (5.6%)
Pruritus†	416 (4.8%)	139.0 (56.0–328.8)	16 (3.8%)
Drug eruption or other non-specific drug reaction†	359 (4.2%)	133.0 (45.5–277.5)	20 (5.6%)
Actinic keratosis	335 (3.9%)	215.0 (82.0–442.0)	4 (1.2%)
Squamous cell carcinoma of the skin	207 (2.4%)	197.0 (80.5–406.5)	9 (4.3%)
Xerosis	180 (2.1%)	215.5 (85.0–481.0)	3 (1.7%)
Spongiotic dermatitis	145 (1.7%)	175.0 (90.0–388.0)	8 (5.5%)
Mucositis†	128 (1.5%)	144.0 (64.0–346.3)	4 (3.1%)
Erythroderma†	98 (1.1%)	212.0 (64.3–393.3)	2 (2.0%)
Acral erythema	83 (1.0%)	273.0 (123.5–473.0)	1 (1.2%)
Maculopapular eruption†	76 (0.9%)	187.0 (98.0–310.5)	4 (5.3%)
Hyperhidrosis	68 (0.8%)	260.0 (97.0–449.3)	2 (2.9%)
Xerostomia	63 (0.7%)	170.0 (59.5–290.5)	4 (6.3%)
Dermatomyositis	59 (0.7%)	113.0 (52.5–215.5)	2 (3.4%)
Urticaria	59 (0.7%)	225.0 (73.5–429.0)	4 (6.8%)
Vitiligo†	57 (0.7%)	294.0 (196.0–489.0)	1 (1.8%)
Eczema or atopic dermatitis	48 (0.6%)	206.5 (77.3–377.8)	0 (0.0%)
Psoriasis and related conditions	47 (0.5%)	220.0 (91.0–399.0)	2 (4.3%)
Lichen planus†	45 (0.5%)	213.0 (124.0–354.0)	1 (2.2%)
Rosacea	42 (0.5%)	320.0 (116.5–575.3)	1 (2.4%)
Paronychia	40 (0.5%)	219.5 (92.5–345.8)	0 (0.0%)
Dyspigmentation	33 (0.4%)	321.0 (199.0–545.0)	0 (0.0%)
Keratoacanthoma	27 (0.3%)	244.0 (165.0–442.5)	1 (3.7%)
Sarcoidosis or granulomatous disease of the skin	27 (0.3%)	341.0 (102.5–467.5)	2 (7.4%)
Pemphigoid†	26 (0.3%)	294.0 (231.0–530.0)	2 (7.7%)
Photosensitivity	24 (0.3%)	374.5 (107.5–453.0)	0 (0.0%)
Pemphigus	23 (0.3%)	191.0 (123.0–387.5)	1 (4.3%)
Onycholysis	22 (0.3%)	275.5 (134.8–450.5)	1 (4.5%)
Hyperkeratosis	20 (0.2%)	249.0 (194.0–659.3)	0 (0.0%)
Grover disease†	18 (0.2%)	266.5 (112.0–384.3)	0 (0.0%)
Vasculitides	13 (0.2%)	118.0 (87.0–226.0)	1 (7.7%)
Erythema multiforme	10 (0.1%)	106.0 (53.0–130.0)	0 (0.0%)
Granuloma annulare	10 (0.1%)	223.5 (178.8–273.8)	1 (10.0%)
Panniculitis	7 (0.1%)	413.0 (205.5–699.0)	0 (0.0%)
Erythema nodosum	4 (0.0%)	382.5 (299.3–647.0)	1 (25.0%)
Neutrophilic dermatosis, Sweet disease or pyoderma gangrenosum	4 (0.0%)	257.0 (134.5–500.8)	0 (0.0%)
SJS/TEN	4 (0.0%)	84.0 (29.8–219.0)	0 (0.0%)
Subacute cutaneous lupus erythematosus	4 (0.0%)	81.0 (48.0–148.3)	0 (0.0%)
Alopecia areata	2 (0.0%)	242.5 (233.8–251.2)	0 (0.0%)
Scleroderma or CREST syndrome	2 (0.0%)	266.0 (188.0–344.0)	0 (0.0%)
Linear IgA dermatosis	1 (0.0%)	183.0 (183.0–183.0)	0 (0.0%)
Parapsoriasis	1 (0.0%)	55.0 (55.0–55.0)	0 (0.0%)

Reproduced from Wongvibulsin et al. 2022 [17].
*Patients with more than one cutaneous immune-related adverse event were counted only once.
†Cutaneous diagnoses of interest were defined as dermatological diagnoses with an IRR >1 for the ICI cohort compared with the control group and an adjusted P value of <0.05 after multiple comparison correction.
CREST, calcinosis, Raynaud phenomenon, oesophageal dysmotility, sclerodactyly and telangiectasia; IgA, immunoglobulin A; IQR, interquartile range; IRR, incidence rate ratio; SJS/TEN, Stevens–Johnson syndrome/toxic epidermal necrolysis.

are increasingly important topics while managing metastatic melanoma patients [55,56]. In 67 patients who stopped pembrolizumab after achieving complete response, over 90% did not relapse after 2 years [57]. Moreover, extended follow-up confirmed durable response [58]. Based on these results and based on a consensus of 32 melanoma experts, stopping treatment in patients achieving complete response who have received at least 6 months of anti-PD-1-based therapy can be considered [59,60].

There are limited data regarding stopping targeted therapy in patients with a complete response. Relapse rates in over half of the patients were reported in small cohort studies after stopping BRAF or a combination of BRAF and MEK inhibitors [61,62]. Therefore, discontinuation of targeted therapy is not recommended outside of clinical trial settings.

Cutaneous side effects of systemic therapies

Both immunotherapies and targeted therapy have cutaneous side effects that dermatologists should recognise and manage. They can range from mild pruritus to the development of secondary skin cancers or severe cytotoxic drug reactions. Regular dermatological follow-up should be compulsory in melanoma patients treated with systemic antitumour therapies.

The most common dermatological side effects of treatment with immune-checkpoint inhibitors include lichenoid dermatitis, pruritus and vitiligo (Table 144.2; Figures 144.3 and 144.4) [1]. A spectrum of bullous disorders from autoimmune to toxic have been reported [2,3]. Rarer dermatological conditions such as alopecia, keratoacathomas and eosinophilic fasciitis have been described as

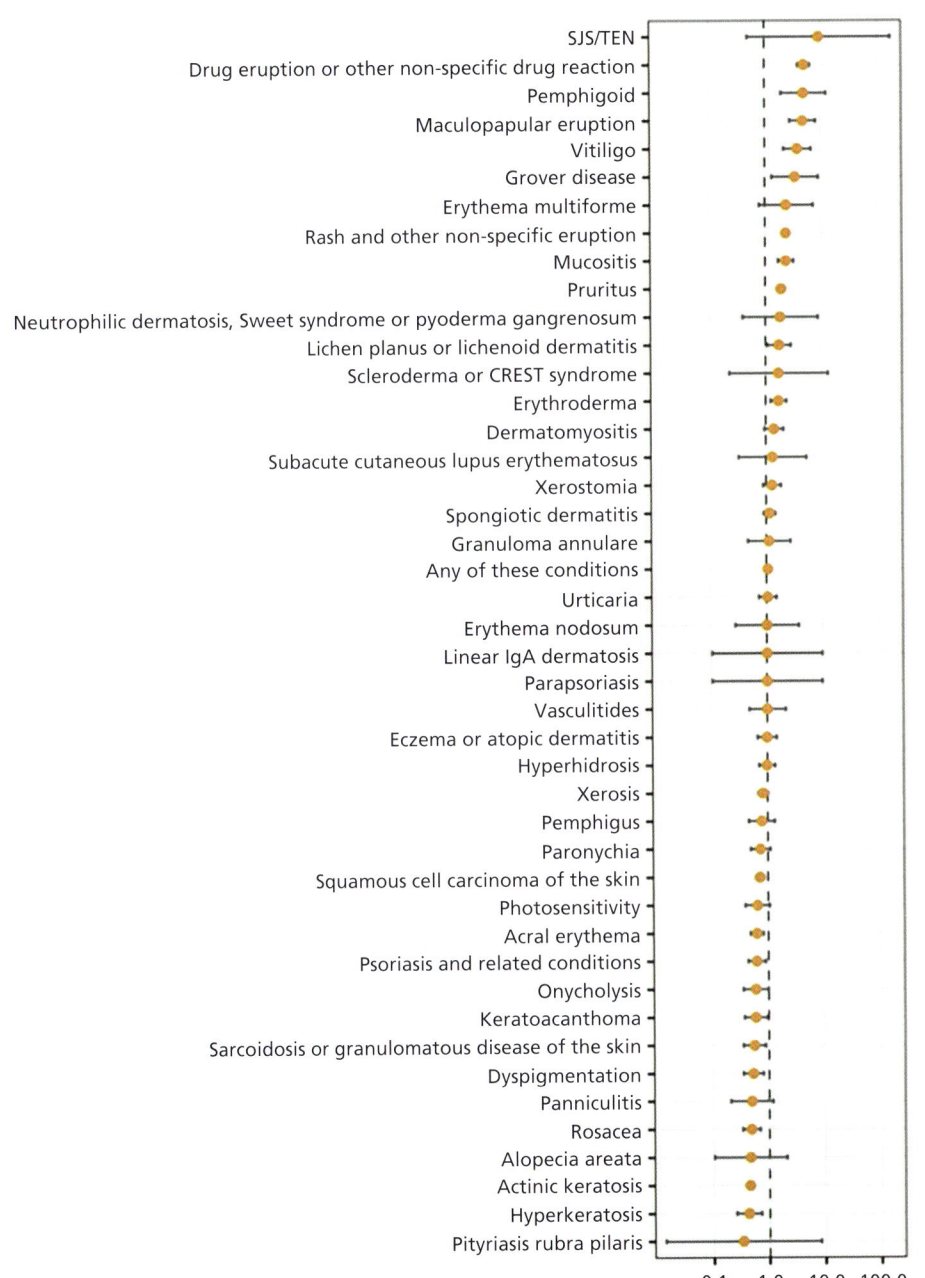

Figure 144.3 Cutaneous adverse events with checkpoint inhibitor therapy Incidence rate ratios for cutaneous diagnoses previously reported as immune-related adverse events for immune-checkpoint inhibitor group compared with the control group. CREST, calcinosis, Raynaud phenomenon, oesophageal dysmotility, sclerodactyly and telangiectasia; IgA, immunoglobulin A; SJS/TEN, Stevens–Johnson syndrome/toxic epidermal necrolysis. Reproduced from Wongvibulsin et al. 2022 [17].

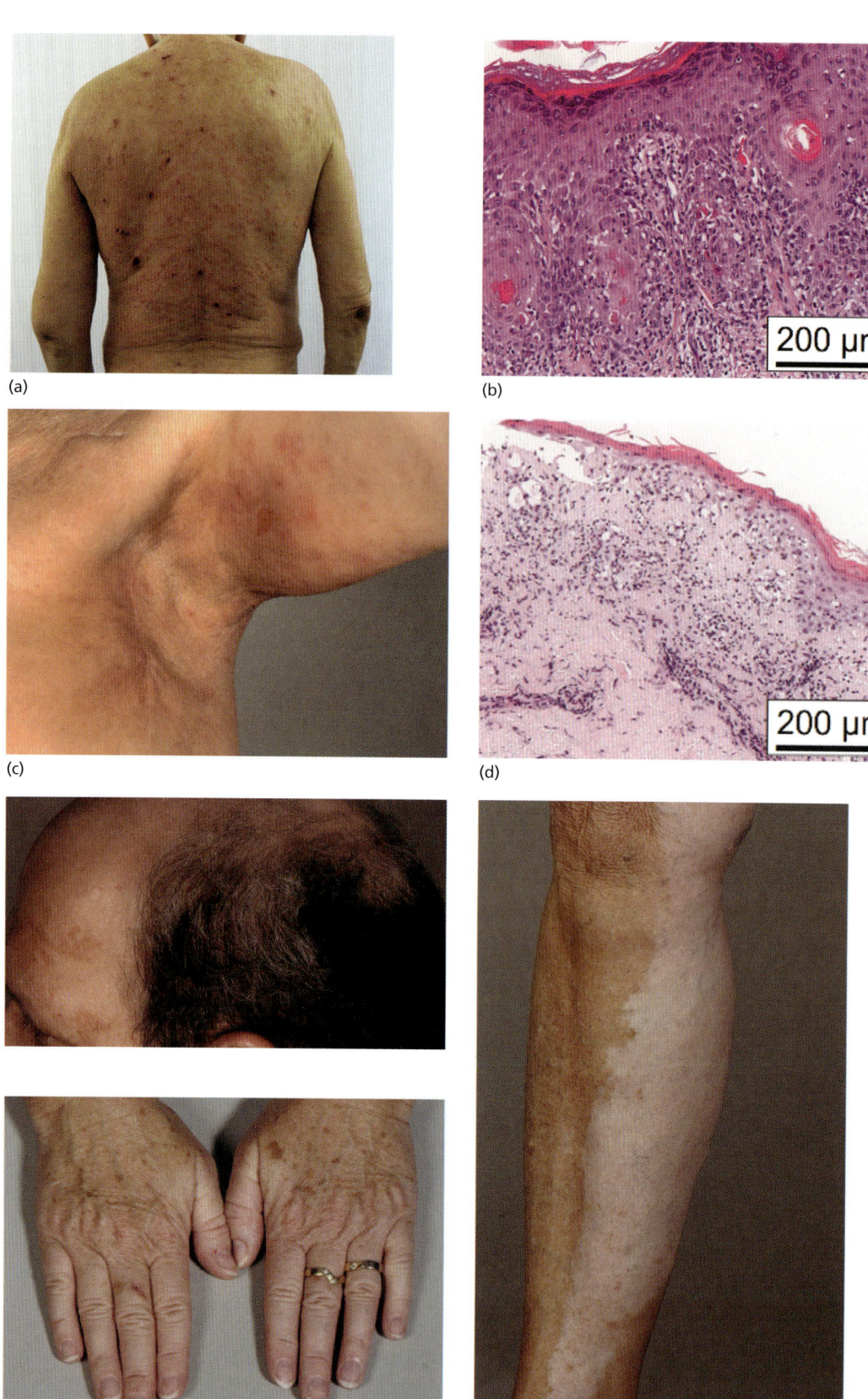

Figure 144.4 Cutaneous adverse events with checkpoint inhibitor therapy. (a, b) Lichenoid reaction during treatment with anti-PD-1 antibodies: (a) clinical presentation and (b) histopathology demonstrating lichenoid changes (H&E). (c, d) Maculopapular skin reaction including focal epidermal detachment during checkpoint inhibitor treatment: (c) clinical presentation and (d) histopathology demonstrating epidermal damage with apoptotic keratinocytes, subepidermal lymphocytic infiltrates and dermal–epidermal cleavage (H&E). (e, f) Vitiligo-like depigmentation during checkpoint inhibitor therapy.

Table 144.3 Cutaneous adverse events (cuAEs) with targeted therapy: comparison of different cutaneous adverse event profiles with different kinase inhibitors.

	Number of patients with cuAE (%)*					
	MEKi		BRAFi		Combination BRAFi and MEKi	
	Binimetinib (n = 25)	Trametinib (n = 8)	Encorafenib (n = 24)	Vemurafenib (n = 6)	Dabrafenib plus trametinib (n = 11)	Encorafenib plus binimetinib (n = 49)
Keratinocytic proliferations						
Acanthopapilloma	0	0	2 (8.3%)	5 (83%)	0	2 (4.1%)
Actinic keratosis	0	1 (12.5%)	0	0	0	0
Squamous cell carcinoma	0	0	1 (4.1%)	2 (33.3%)	0	1 (2.0%)
Xerosis cutis	8 (32%)	2 (25%)	4 (16.7%)	0	0	1 (2.0%)
Keratosis pilaris	0	0	5 (20.8%)	2 (33.3%)	0	1 (2.0%)
Inflammatory disorders						
Palmoplantar erythrodysaesthesia	0	0	14 (58.3%)	3 (50%)	0	0
Palmoplantar hyperkeratosis	1 (4%)	0	13 (54.2%)	3 (50%)	0	5 (10.2%)
Drug-induced papulopustular eruptions	16 (64%)	6 (75%)	0	0	1 (9.1%)	0
Macular and maculopapular exanthemas	5 (20%)	1 (12.5%)	8 (33.3%)	4 (66.7%)	2 (18.2%)	3 (6.1%)
Granuloma pyogenicum	0	0	1 (4.1%)	0	0	0
Panniculitis	1 (4%)	0	0	1 (16.7%)	1 (9.1%)	1 (2.0%)
Photoallergic and phototoxic reactions	0	0	0	1 (16.7%)	0	1 (2.0%)
Eczematous eruptions	5 (20%)	0	2 (8.3%)	0	0	2 (4.1%)
Erythema multiforme	2 (8%)	0	0	0	0	0
Erythema anulare-like eruptions	0	0	0	0	2 (18.2%)	1 (2.0%)
Hair changes						
Alopecia	2 (8%)	2 (25%)	11 (45.8%)	2 (33.3%)	0	4 (8.2%)

Reproduced from Graf et al. 2019 [10].
a Total n = 123.
BRAFi, BRAF inhibitors; MEKi, MEK inhibitors.

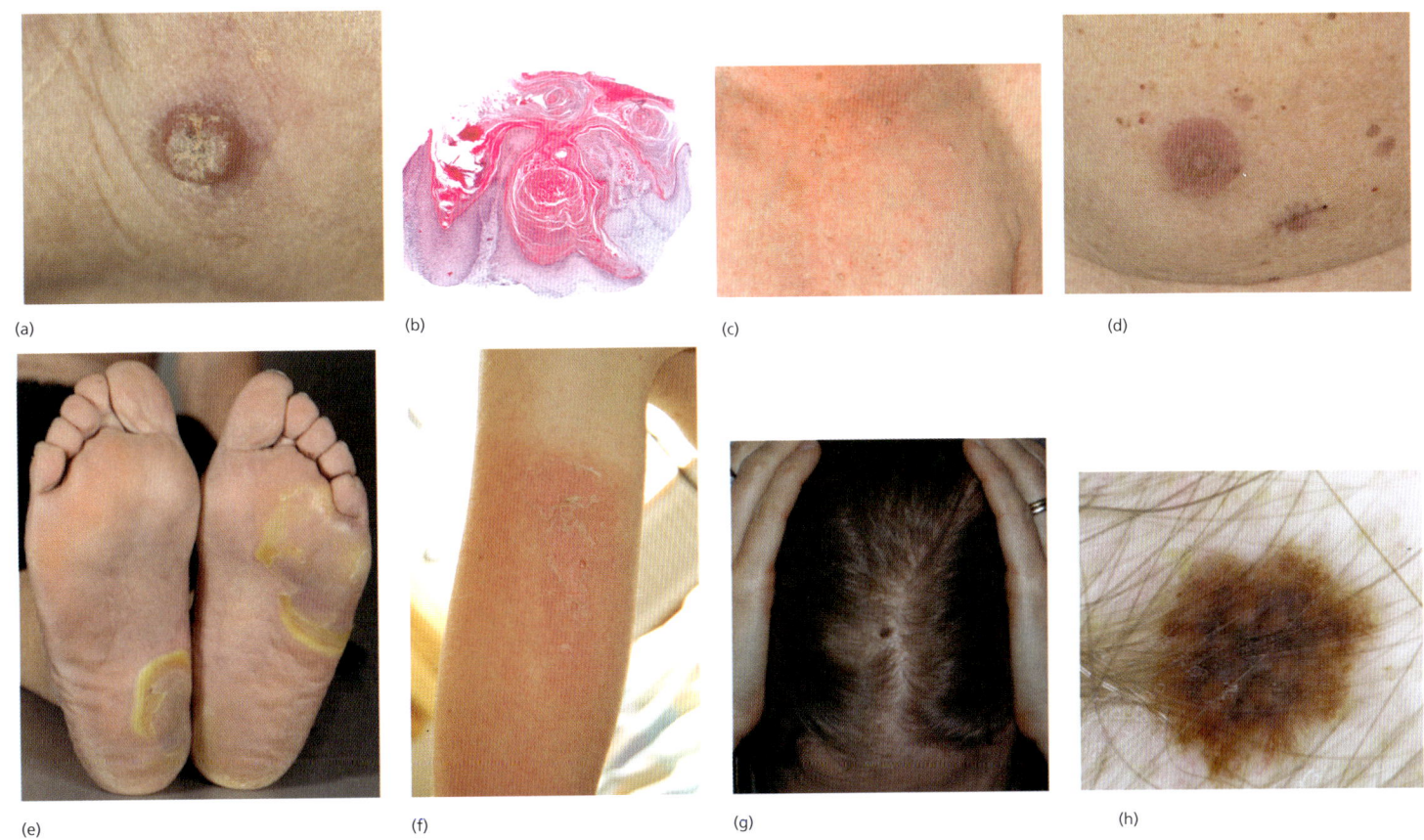

Figure 144.5 Cutaneous adverse events with targeted therapy. (a, b) Keratoacanthoma developing during targeted therapy treatment: (a) clinical presentation and (b) histopathology demonstrating a well-differentiated squamous cell carcinoma of the keratoacanthoma type. (c) Multiple small acanthopapillomas on the chest. (d) Mammillary hyperkeratotic eczema. (e) Plantar hyperkeratosis. (f) Photosensitivity reaction induced by ultraviolet exposure during targeted therapy. (g, h) Melanocytic proliferation during targeted therapy: (g) clinical presentation and (h) dermoscopy of a newly developed superficial spreading melanoma with Breslow thickness 0.45 mm on a patient treated with a BRAF inhibitor.

well [4–6]. Management primarily involves the use of topical corticosteroids for mild to moderate cutaneous side effects. Systemic corticosteroids should be considered for severe immune-related cutaneous side effects. For patients developing severe cytotoxic reactions to immunotherapy, treatment discontinuation has to be evaluated [3].

Both BRAF and MEK inhibitors have a very particular side effect profile (Table 144.3; Figure 144.5). BRAF inhibitors are characterised by similar cutaneous findings found in patients with germ line mutations of RAS as well and can be termed as RASopathic [7]. Melanocytic disorders and proliferations have been described [8]. Cutaneous reactions predominantly start to appear during the first weeks of treatment and persist during BRAF inhibition. Vemurafenib causes clinically relevant ultraviolet A (UVA) dependent phototoxicity that requires adequate UV protection [9], whereas phototoxic reactions have not been described with dabrafenib and encorafenib [10,11]. MEK inhibitors, on the other hand, partly overlap with cutaneous adverse effects observed with epidermal growth factor receptor inhibition. In addition, pigmentation of the skin and hair is affected. The interruption of the MEK signalling pathway results in an acute keratinocytic stress response with disturbed epidermal homeostasis, inflammation and tissue damage [12]. MEK inhibitors typically cause xerosis cutis and papulopustular rashes in the first 2–6 weeks of treatment. In this situation, local steroids and systemic administration of doxycycline should be evaluated. The topical administration of acne treatment (i.e. benzoyl peroxide) may worsen the clinical picture and should not be prescribed. Moreover, self-limiting, retinopathy-like, dose-dependent retinal disorders with early onset have been described [13,14]. Overall, the combination of BRAF and MEK inhibitors reduces both severity and frequency of cutaneous adverse events [10,15,16].

Key references

The full list of references can be found in the online version at https://www.wiley.com/rooksdermatology10e

Treatment options in local and systemic therapy of melanoma

12 Geisler AN, Phillips GS, Barrios DM et al. Immune checkpoint inhibitor-related dermatologic adverse events. *J Am Acad Dermatol* 2020;83:1255–68.

30 Long GV, Trefzer U, Davies MA et al. Dabrafenib in patients with Val600Glu or Val600Lys BRAF-mutant melanoma metastatic to the brain (BREAK-MB): a multicentre, open-label, phase 2 trial. *Lancet Oncol* 2012;13:1087–95.

40 Dummer R, Ascierto PA, Gogas HJ et al. Overall survival in patients with BRAF-mutant melanoma receiving encorafenib plus binimetinib versus vemurafenib or encorafenib (COLUMBUS): a multicentre, open-label, randomised, phase 3 trial. *Lancet Oncol* 2018;19:1315–27.

43 Dummer R, Hauschild A, Santinami M et al. Five-year analysis of adjuvant dabrafenib plus trametinib in stage III melanoma. *N Engl J Med* 2020;383:1139–48.

Therapeutic approach for systemic management of melanoma

3 Ascierto PA, Del Vecchio M, Mandala M et al. Adjuvant nivolumab versus ipilimumab in resected stage IIIB-C and stage IV melanoma (CheckMate 238): 4-year results from a multicentre, double-blind, randomised, controlled, phase 3 trial. *Lancet Oncol* 2020;21:1465–77.

5 Eggermont AMM, Blank CU, Mandala M et al. Adjuvant pembrolizumab versus placebo in resected stage III melanoma. *N Engl J Med* 2018;378:1789–801.

9 Dummer R, Hauschild A, Santinami M et al. Five-year analysis of adjuvant dabrafenib plus trametinib in stage III melanoma. *N Engl J Med* 2020;383:1139–48.

13 Wolchok JD, Chiarion-Sileni V, Gonzalez R et al. Overall survival with combined nivolumab and ipilimumab in advanced melanoma. *N Engl J Med* 2017;377:1345–56.

22 Larkin J, Chiarion-Sileni V, Gonzalez R et al. Five-year survival with combined nivolumab and ipilimumab in advanced melanoma. *N Engl J Med* 2019;381:1535–46.

27 Gutzmer R, Stroyakovskiy D, Gogas H et al. Atezolizumab, vemurafenib, and cobimetinib as first-line treatment for unresectable advanced BRAF(V600) mutation-positive melanoma (IMspire150): primary analysis of the randomised, double-blind, placebo-controlled, phase 3 trial. *Lancet* 2020;395:1835–44.

30 Tawbi HA, Forsyth PA, Algazi A et al. Combined nivolumab and ipilimumab in melanoma metastatic to the brain. *N Engl J Med* 2018;379:722–30.

CHAPTER 145

Dermoscopy of Melanoma and Naevi

Natalia Jaimes[1] and Ashfaq A. Marghoob[2]

[1] Dr Phillip Frost Department of Dermatology & Cutaneous Surgery and Sylvester Comprehensive Cancer Center, University of Miami Miller School of Medicine, Miami, FL, USA
[2] Dermatology Service, Memorial Sloan-Kettering Cancer Center, New York, NY, USA

Introduction, 145.1	Dermoscopic patterns seen in intradermal naevi, 145.6	Melanomas on special locations, 145.9
Dermoscopic patterns associated with naevi, 145.1	Dermoscopic patterns encountered in Spitz naevi, 145.6	Melanomas displaying an organised pattern, 145.13
Dermoscopic patterns frequently observed in acquired and small congenital naevi (excluding intradermal naevi), 145.4	Dermoscopy of melanoma, 145.7	Conclusion, 145.15
	Melanomas on non-glabrous and non-facial skin, 145.7	Key references, 145.16

Introduction

The well-known ABCD (asymmetry, border irregularity, colour variegation and diameter >6 mm) morphology-related mnemonic, created to help detect melanoma and differentiate it from naevi has limitations in both sensitivity and specificity for early melanoma detection. Some melanoma variants, such as nodular, amelanotic, naevoid, spitzoid, desmoplastic, among others, often lack the ABCD features and escape detection if one were to rely only on the ABCD rule. In contrast, naevi including so-called dysplastic naevi (large acquired naevi, Clark naevi) can reveal some or all of the ABCD features, potentially resulting in many of these naevi being subjected to unnecessary biopsies if the ABCD rule was used to differentiate naevi from melanoma.

Fortunately, use of the dermoscope can improve diagnostic accuracy by up to 30% compared with naked eye examination. In the hands of experienced users this improved diagnostic accuracy translates into a significant reduction in their benign to malignant biopsy ratio [1–11]. This enhanced ability to identify melanoma and differentiate them from naevi is dependent on the assessment of global dermoscopic patterns and specific dermoscopic structures. A set of dermoscopic structures have been identified that are more commonly associated with melanoma and are called the melanoma-specific structures. In addition, a group of organised patterns have been identified and shown to be associated with naevi. These benign patterns do require context for their interpretation but in the correct context they have proven to be strongly associated with benignity.

This chapter is structured to provide the reader with an overview of the structures and organised patterns associated with naevi, including the relevant contextual features required to confidently assign them to a benign category. Unlike naevi, most established melanomas are easy to identify since they usually display a disorganised pattern and reveal at least one melanoma-specific structure. This chapter will discuss the melanoma-specific structures that have consistently been found to be associated with a higher odds ratio for melanoma. Lastly, although there exist subsets of melanomas that will display an organised pattern on dermoscopy these melanomas will usually not mimic one of the benign naevus patterns and instead will display at least one of two patterns, one of two structures or one of four colours. This chapter will discuss the patterns, structures and colours encountered in these melanomas.

Dermoscopic patterns associated with naevi

Numerous subsets of naevi have been identified, differing from each other by morphology, driver mutation signature and other patient-related factors. These subtypes of naevi range from small to large congenital naevi to acquired naevi including the so-called atypical/dysplastic naevi (Clark naevus, large acquired naevus), blue naevus, combined naevus, intradermal naevus of the Unna or Miescher type, epithelioid and spindle cell naevus (Spitz and Reed naevi), balloon cell naevi, BAP1-deficient naevi, among numerous others [12,13–16]. This chapter outlines the patterns seen in the most common naevi encountered in clinical practice that frequently manifest morphological features overlapping with those of melanoma [17]. In addition, dermoscopic features commonly seen in other naevus subtypes are described in Table 145.1.

The first goal when evaluating a melanocytic lesion is to determine whether the lesion manifests one of the *benign patterns* commonly seen in naevi (Figures 145.1–145.3 and 145.4). Overall, patterns are determined by the distribution of colours and structures within the lesion. In general, naevi tend to exhibit dermoscopic symmetry in the distribution of colours and structures, while melanomas tend to manifest an asymmetrical, disorganised and chaotic pattern with at least one of the melanoma-specific structures. Benign patterns seen in naevi are formed by the combination of three main structures, including network, globules and homogeneous areas (Figure 145.1).

Rook's Textbook of Dermatology, Tenth Edition. Edited by Christopher Griffiths, Jonathan Barker, Tanya Bleiker, Walayat Hussain and Rosalind Simpson.
© 2024 John Wiley & Sons Ltd. Published 2024 by John Wiley & Sons Ltd.

Table 145.1 Dermoscopic characteristics of different naevi subtypes.

Naevus subtype	Dermoscopic characteristics
Halo naevus [70]	The naevi that involute via a halo phenomenon usually have a globular or homogeneous pattern The halo of depigmentation surrounds the globular naevus and over time the globular naevus becomes smaller and eventually disappears. The area of depigmentation can eventually repigment and resemble normal skin It takes approximately 8 years for a halo naevus to completely involute [71]
Meyerson (or eczematous) naevus	Usually, the eczematous reaction does not significantly distort the dermoscopic pattern of the naevus
Cockade naevus	Targetoid appearance: darker, central globular or homogeneous pattern, surrounded by a hypopigmented homogeneous structureless inner rim and a peripheral darker reticular outer rim [72]
Recurrent naevus [14]	Pigmentation usually confined to the scar, displaying a centrifugal growth pattern (i.e. symmetric radial lines) that does not traverse from the scar into the surrounding normal skin Pigmented structures are usually arranged contiguously and centrifugally
Naevus arising in lichen sclerosus [73]	Naevus: parallel, globular or homogeneous pattern (a multicomponent pattern is not uncommon) Lichen sclerosus: porcelain-white structureless areas, with or without comedo-like openings, and with or without vessels or shiny white lines
Balloon cell naevus [13]	Three or more aggregated white-to-yellow globules (visualised with polarised and non-polarised light)
Epidermolysis bullosa naevus [74]	Not infrequently EB naevi can demonstrate dermoscopic features that overlap with those seen in melanoma, including a multicomponent pattern, with atypical pigment network, irregular dots and globules, and milky-red areas.
BRCA1-associated protein 1 (BAP1)-inactivated melanocytic tumours [75]	Dome-shaped pink papules with pink-to-tan structureless areas and atypical dots/globules or network

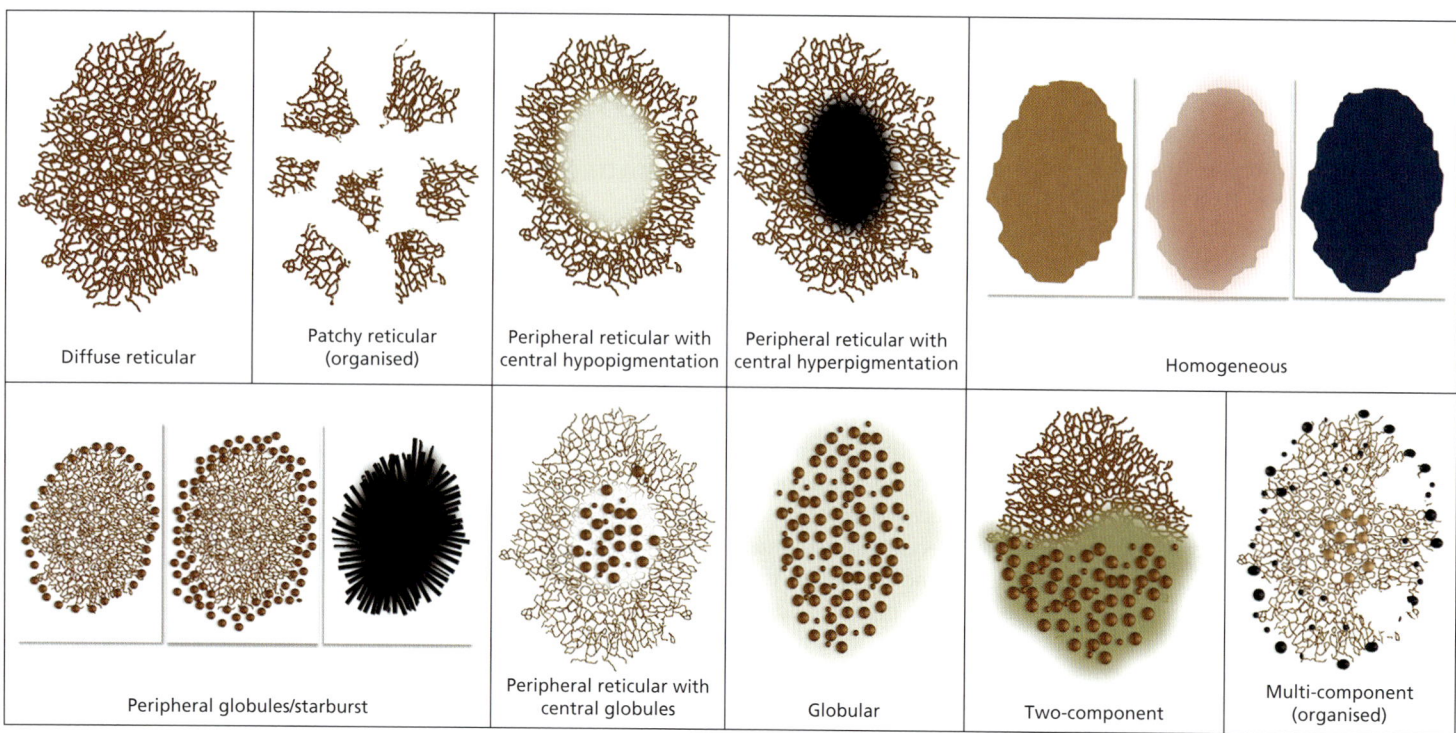

Figure 145.1 Dermoscopy naevi patterns.

Once the dermoscopic pattern of the lesion is determined, it is valuable to evaluate other naevi in the patient (comparative approach) [18]. Most individuals demonstrate a predominant or signature naevus pattern with one or two of the abovementioned patterns being displayed in most of their naevi [18,19,20]. If the lesion of concern does not adhere to the signature naevus pattern displayed by the other naevi in the patient, then the lesion is considered an *outlier lesion*, which may be one that deserves closer scrutiny and perhaps a biopsy. On the other hand, lesions manifesting the same pattern as the predominant naevus pattern may be safely monitored [18]. Yet, a final clinical dermoscopy interpretation of any skin lesion should only be established after appropriate integration of the dermoscopy findings, in addition to other contextual factors, including age of the patient, skin phenotype, past medical

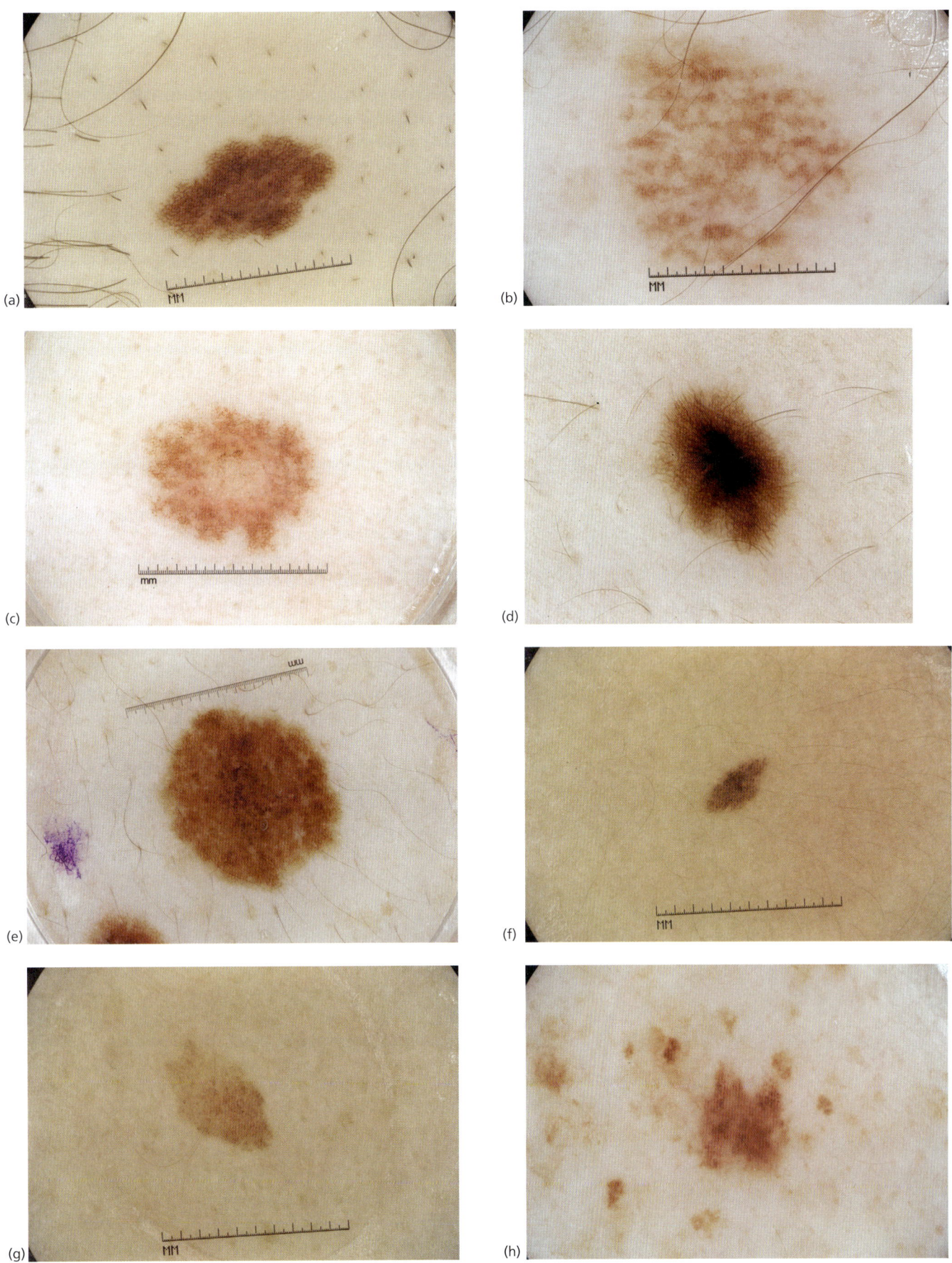

Figure 145.2 (a) Reticular diffuse naevus. (b) Reticular patchy naevus. (c) Peripheral reticular with central hypopigmentation naevus. (d) Peripheral reticular with central hyperpigmentation naevus. (e) Peripheral reticular naevus with central globules. (f) Naevus with globular pattern. (g) Two-component pattern naevus. (h) Multicomponent pattern naevus.

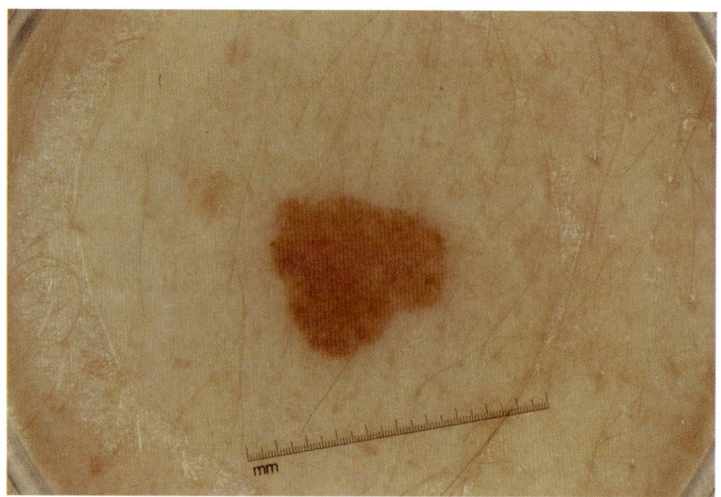

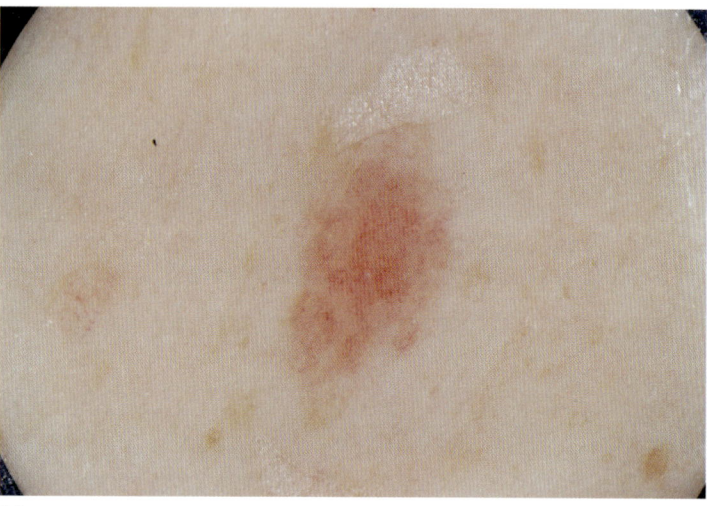

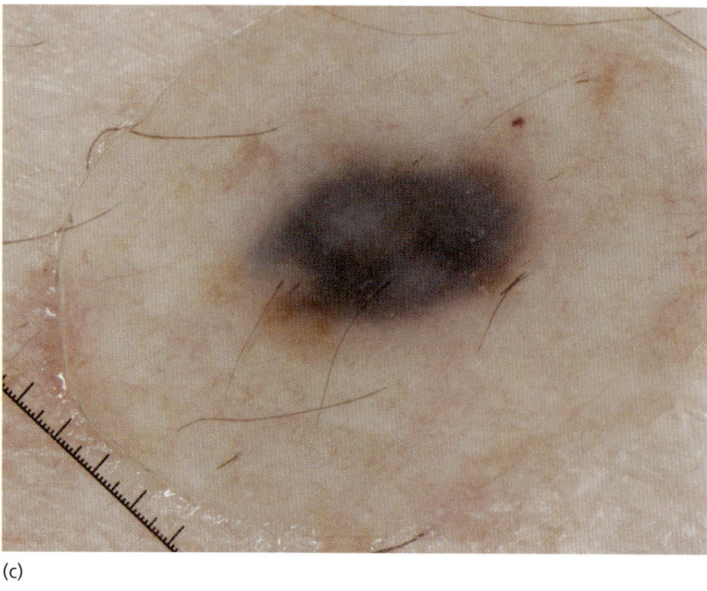

Figure 145.3 Homogeneous pattern naevi: (a) homogeneous brown; (b) homogeneous pink; and (c) homogeneous grey-blue.

history, any complaint and other clinical characteristics (e.g. size, location, outlier lesion) [21].

Dermoscopic patterns frequently observed in acquired and small congenital naevi (excluding intradermal naevi)

Network/reticular pattern, including diffuse and patchy

The *diffuse reticular pattern* consists of an organised network with minimal variation in its thickness and colour and the holes of the network are relatively uniform in their appearance (regular/typical network). The *patchy network pattern* consists of islands of typical network distributed in an organised manner. The network patches all have the same type of network with minimal variability in the thickness and colour of the lines (Figures 145.1 and 145.2).

Key contextual feature: melanoma on sun-damaged skin can sometimes appear as isolated large lentiginous lesions with a network or patchy network pattern. The *clues* to the diagnosis of melanoma include older age, the relative large size of these lesions, their presence as isolated lesions on sun-damaged skin and that the network is usually not distributed in an organised fashion [22].

Peripheral network with central hypo- or hyperpigmentation

The peripheral network is typical/regular in both of these naevi. In one the central portion is hypopigmented (i.e. the area is lighter in colour compared with the network but darker than the surrounding skin); in the other the central portion is hyperpigmented (i.e. blotch). The blotch in naevi with peripheral network and central hyperpigmentation is often due to the accumulation of melanin-laden corneocytes in the stratum corneum (black lamella), which can usually be tape stripped off revealing an underlying typical network (Figures 145.1 and 145.2).

Key contextual feature: naevi with central hypopigmentation are usually seen in patients with lighter skin colour and naevi with central hyperpigmentation are seen in patients with darker skin phenotypes. Thus, lesions displaying central hypopigmentation in dark skin phenotypes and lesions with central hyperpigmentation in light skin phenotypes should raise the possibility of melanoma [21,23,24].

Reticular pattern with peripheral globules (Figures 145.1 and 145.3)

This pattern consists of a typical network with one peripheral rim of regular brown globules. This pattern is associated with the radial growth phase of Clark/dysplastic naevi and is commonly encountered in younger patients with the atypical mole syndrome. On histopathology, these naevi correspond to dysplastic naevi with mild to moderate atypia. Naevi with peripheral globules can also display a multi-tiered peripheral globular pattern at the periphery. This multi-tiered peripheral globular pattern corresponds on histopathology with dysplastic naevi that display at least some degree of spitzoid morphology.

The *key contextual features* in naevi with peripheral globules are age and location. Since these naevi are most common on the torso of younger to middle-aged patients, newly acquired lesions displaying peripheral globules should be viewed with caution if seen in older individuals, especially if the lesion is located on an extremity, or reveals a melanoma-specific structure [21,25–27].

Naevi with globules including central brown globules with peripheral network and globular pattern including cobblestone globular naevi

Central brown globules with peripheral network pattern consists of naevi displaying a typical network at the periphery of the lesion and central brown globules that are regular with minimal variation in their size and colour. Naevi with a *globular pattern* display only round to oval globules throughout the lesion with minimal variability in globule size and colour (i.e. regular/typical) and are distributed in an organised manner within the lesion. Occasionally, the globules can be white, as seen in balloon cell naevi. While black and blue globules can on occasion be seen in congenital naevi, their presence should raise suspicion for melanoma. When globules are very large they take on the appearance of cobblestones creating the *cobblestone globular pattern*. This is a specific type of globular pattern that consists of large brown angulated globules that create a pattern reminiscent of cobblestones and is associated with congenital naevi (Figures 145.1 and 145.2).

Key contextual feature: naevi with globules in their centre or throughout are usually congenital and are usually found on the head/neck or torso. Thus, newly acquired lesions with a globular morphology occurring in an older individual and especially if the lesion is located on an extremity should raise concern for melanoma [21,28,29].

Starburst pattern

The starburst pattern is an easy to recognise pattern, consisting of a darkly pigmented naevus with a symmetric distribution of streaks around its perimeter. This pattern is associated with Reed naevi that are in their radial growth phase (Figures 145.1 and 145.3).

The *key contextual feature* with starburst naevi is age. Although streaks can also be encountered in superficial spreading melanoma, such melanomas are extremely rare in pre-adolescent individuals. Thus, lesions with a starburst pattern seen in children have an extremely high pre-test probability for being Reed naevi, whereas lesions with a starburst pattern seen in older individuals have a heightened pre-test probability for melanoma [12].

Homogeneous blue

A homogeneous blue colour with a whitish veil that encompasses the entire lesion's surface is the hallmark of a blue naevus. The blue colour and white veil in blue naevi will display minimal variation in blue hue, especially if visualised with non-polarised light. If there are multiple hues (i.e. heterogeneous blue colour or non-homogeneous veil) then one should consider the diagnosis of melanoma (Figures 145.1 and 145.4).

The *key contextual feature* in a lesion with a presumed blue naevus pattern is a previous history of an invasive melanoma because epidermotropic metastasis can mimic blue naevi [30].

Homogeneous brown

A homogeneous brown pattern consists of a lesion displaying a brown colour with minimal to no variation in its hues. While it is usually devoid of any other structures, on rare occasions one can see

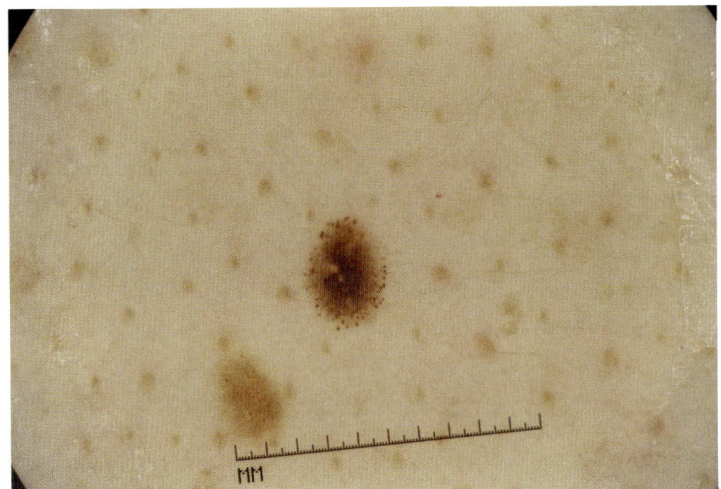

(a)

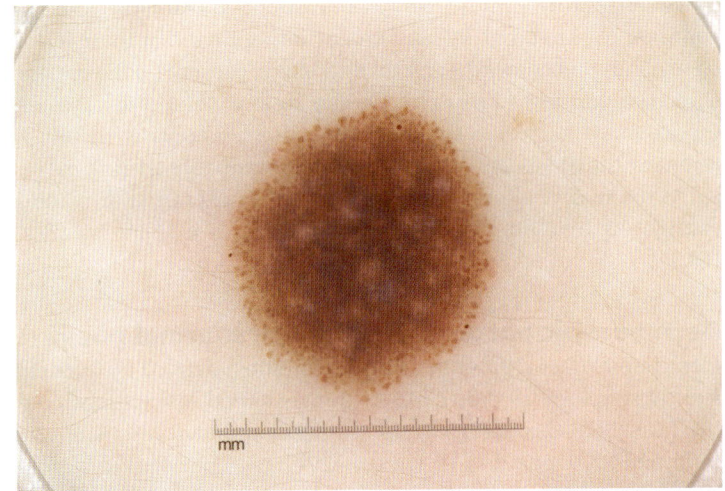

(b)

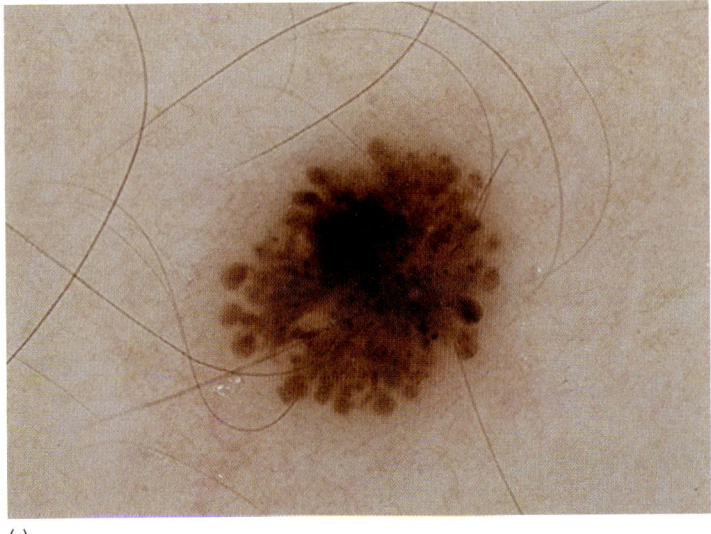

(c)

Figure 145.4 Naevi with peripheral globules: (a) growing naevus with a single row of globules; (b) Spitz naevus with multiple rows of globules; and (c) Spitz naevus with streaks giving the appearance of an exploding star.

few regular dots/globules and fragments of network (Figures 145.1 and 145.4).

Key contextual feature: a homogeneous brown pattern is associated with small to medium congenital naevi. These naevi are usually present at birth or develop within the first few years of life and are stable lesions. Thus, newly acquired homogeneous brown lesions in adults should be viewed with caution. Such lesions, if not palpable, can be digitally monitored and biopsied if they display change [31].

Homogeneous tan/pink

These naevi display a featureless tan-to-pink colour but some can also display vessels (Figures 145.1 and 145.4).

The *key contextual feature* in naevi with a homogeneous tan/pink pattern is skin phenotype. These naevi are seen predominantly in individuals with skin types I–II. Thus, newly acquired naevi with a homogeneous tan-to-pink colour occurring in darker skinned individuals should raise concern for amelanotic or hypomelanotic melanoma. Furthermore, since amelanotic melanomas are also common in skin types I–II, it remains imperative that these lesions be evaluated in context with the other naevi present on the patient's skin (comparative approach). Outlier lesions should always raise the index of suspicion for melanoma. If melanoma is in the differential diagnosis and the lesion is non-palpable then it may be subjected to digital monitoring. Lesions that are raised or manifest change on follow-up should be viewed with extreme suspicion [18,31].

Dermoscopic patterns seen in intradermal naevi

Intradermal naevi (IDN) are first and foremost defined by their clinical morphology as either raised dome-shaped lesions located on the face (Miescher naevi) or as sessile mamillated lesions located on the torso (Unna naevi). These naevi have preserved skin markings and may have hair emanating from their surface. IDN usually reveal one or more of the following features on dermoscopy [15,32,33]:

- Predominantly comma-shaped vessels or a polymorphous vascular pattern with at least some comma-shaped vessels.
- Brown halo.
- Globules, including cobblestone-type globules.
- Small foci of tan to brown structureless pigment and/or hypopigmented areas.

IDN, especially of the Miescher type, can sometimes be challenging to differentiate from basal cell carcinoma (BCC) [34]. One of the main reasons for this is that IDN can at times reveal arborising vessels, which raises the concern for BCC. There are, however, clinical and dermoscopic *clues* that can assist in differentiating an IDN from a BCC [35].

Clinical clues
- IDN tend to have been present on the skin for many years, without any history of change and they do not spontaneously bleed.
- The skin markings in an IDN tend to be preserved whereas in BCC they are lost, thus resulting in BCCs having a shiny surface.
- If hair is present within the lesion then it is highly suggestive of an IDN.

Dermoscopic clues
- IDN wobble on dermoscopy and BCC tend not to wobble [36]. Placing the dermoscope over the lesion (i.e. contact mode) and then applying horizontal pressure in a back-and-forth motion will show that an IDN wobbles, whereas lesions without a dermal component will slide and not wobble.
- A closer look at the arborising vessels will reveal that the extent of arborisation in IDN tends to be much less than in BCC. In fact, in IDN there may only be one arborising point created a 'Y'-shaped vessel [15].
- The vessels in BCC tend to be much sharper in focus and have a much brighter red colour.
- Unlike BCC, IDN do not reveal any shiny white blotches and strands on polarised dermoscopy.

Dermoscopic patterns encountered in Spitz naevi

Spitz naevi are benign neoplasms that clinically and dermoscopically display features most commonly associated with melanoma. This makes it difficult to differentiate Spitz naevi from melanoma confidently based on morphology alone. Heavily pigmented Spitz naevi (also known as Reed naevi) display morphological structures resembling superficial spreading melanoma. These structures include atypical network, streaks, shiny white lines, and/or atypical globules. The archetypal iconic dermoscopic pattern of a Reed naevus is the starburst pattern, which represents the radial growth phase of this naevus. In contrast, amelanotic or hypomelanotic Spitz naevi display dermoscopic features associated with nodular melanoma including shiny white lines, reticular depigmentation and/or atypical vessels. Given the morphological overlap between Spitz naevi and melanoma, decisions regarding management rely heavily upon context including age of patient, pattern of growth and anatomical location, among others [12,37].

Dermoscopic patterns

Most Spitz naevi display an organised dermoscopic pattern, but the colours and structures of atypical Spitz naevi can be distributed in an extremely disorganised manner, making it impossible to exclude melanoma from the differential diagnosis.

1. *Starburst pattern*. Dark homogeneous pigmentation with peripheral streaks (i.e. pseudopods or radial streaming) or multiple rows of peripheral globules (i.e. tiered globules) surrounding the entire perimeter of the lesion, usually in a symmetric fashion. The central portion of the lesion will often have a blue-white veil and shiny white lines.
2. *Globular pattern*. Globules of different size, shape and/or colour throughout the lesion.
3. *Homogeneous pattern*. Diffuse homogeneous colour (i.e. pigmented vs non-pigmented/pink) throughout the lesions, with or without vascular structures (i.e. dotted vessels). These lesions can also display shiny white lines or reticular depigmentation. The pigmented variant often has a central blue-whitish veil.
4. *Negative network pattern*. Negative network that is symmetrically distributed throughout the lesion. A variant of the negative network, known as reticular depigmentation, can also be seen in these lesions.
5. *Reticular pattern*. Thickened dark network throughout the lesion. The background colour of the naevus often has a blue-whitish hue.

6 *Atypical or multicomponent pattern.* The colours and structures tend to be asymmetrically distributed. These lesions are difficult, if not impossible, to differentiate from melanomas based on morphology alone.

Dermoscopy of melanoma

Melanomas on non-glabrous and non-facial skin

Melanomas usually present themselves as lesions with a disorganised dermoscopy pattern. In addition, most melanomas will display at least one of the melanoma-specific structures listed in Table 145.2. The pattern, colours and structures manifest by melanoma can vary depending on factors such as anatomical location, histopathological subtype, growth phase, tumour thickness, sun-exposure and genetic mutation profile. While naevi tend to manifest one of the aforementioned benign patterns, melanomas almost always manifest a disorganised, asymmetric and chaotic pattern that deviates from those seen in naevi [38–40] and reveal at least one of the following melanoma-specific structures (Table 145.2; Figure 145.5):

1 *Atypical network.* An atypical network consists of a web of lines of varying colours and thicknesses, with holes of varying diameters. The colour of the atypical network ranges from brown to black or grey and it can appear smudged or seemingly out of focus. An atypical network correlates with the expansion of malignant melanocytes at the rete ridges and can often be found focally at or near the edge of a superficial spreading melanoma (SSM) [41,42]. The atypical network is often associated with the *in situ* component and may be the only specific feature of an early thin SSM [41,42] (Figure 145.5a,b).

2 *Negative network.* A negative network (reverse network) consists of hypopigmented serpiginous interconnecting lines that surround irregularly shaped pigmented structures resembling elongated curvilinear globules [42,43]. Histology reveals bridging or elongation of rete ridges in association with large melanocytic nests in the papillary dermis [43]. It can be seen in melanoma, Spitz naevi, dysplastic naevi or melanomas arising in association with naevi [44] (Figure 145.5c).

3 *Angulated lines.* Angulated lines are usually associated with melanomas on sun-damaged skin [22]. They appear as brown to grey linear structures that intersect at acute angles creating geometric structures or a zig-zag pattern. Angulated lines can coalesce together forming polygonal structures, including rhomboidal structures that may or may not obliterate the adnexal openings. Histologically, angulated lines correspond to confluent proliferation of junctional atypical melanocytes in the basal layer, pagetoid spread of melanocytes and underlying papillary dermal melanin either in melanophages or free in the dermis (Figure 145.6).

4 *Atypical streaks, including pseudopods and radial streaming.* Streaks consist of linear/radial projections at the periphery of the lesion, arising from the tumour and radiating towards the normal skin. Their presence represents the radial growth phase of either a pigmented Spitz naevus or a SSM. On histology, streaks correlate with confluent radial nests of melanoma at the dermo-epidermal junction. In general, typical streaks, as seen in Spitz naevi, tend to be evenly distributed around the entire perimeter of the lesion in a relatively symmetric manner (Figure 145.3c). In contrast, atypical streaks, as seen in melanomas, are irregularly and focally distributed at the periphery of the lesion (Figure 145.5d). However, since spitzoid lesions can be difficult to differentiate from melanoma, an excision biopsy is recommended in patients older than 12 years presenting with symmetric spitzoid lesions.

5 *Shiny white lines.* Shiny white lines (formerly known as crystalline structures) consist of short, bright, white lines that are usually orientated parallel or orthogonal to each other and can only be seen with polarised light. Histologically, they correspond to stromal alteration and dermal fibrosis. When seen in a melanocytic neoplasm, the differential diagnosis lies between a Spitz/Reed naevus and a melanoma [45] (Figure 145.5b).

6 *Atypical dots and/or globules. Dots* are black or brown round structures measuring less than 0.1 mm in diameter. Atypical dots tend to be distributed randomly, are often found towards the periphery of the melanoma, and they may or may not be associated with a network, but if a network is present it is often atypical. On histology, black dots represent malignant melanocytes found at or near the stratum corneum and represent the pagetoid spread as seen in SSM. *Globules* are round to oval pigmented structures larger than 0.1 mm in diameter. Atypical globules present with varying size, shape and/or colours, and may be distributed in a disorganised fashion within the lesion. On histology, globules correspond to nests of melanocytes at the dermo-epidermal junction or dermis (Figure 145.5e).

7 *Regression structures (i.e. scar-like areas and peppering or granularity. Scar-like areas* appear as white or porcelain-white structureless areas that are lighter than the surrounding normal skin. The scar-like areas tend not to reveal any blood vessels on dermoscopy. *Peppering or granularity* appears as blue-grey fine dots (Figure 145.5a,b). Histologically, the scar-like depigmentation corresponds to dermal fibrosis peppering and the peppering corresponds to melanophages or free melanin in the papillary dermis. Regression areas displaying peppering in association with scar-like depigmentation can manifest a blue-whitish colour; however, in contrast to the blue-white veil, this blue-white colour is usually seen in macular lesions, as opposed to the blue-white veil, which is seen in raised or palpable lesions.

8 *Blue-white veil.* Blue-white veil consists of a blue colour in association with an overlying white ground glass haze. In contrast to the homogeneous steel-blue colour seen in blue naevi, which occupy the entire lesion, blue-white veil in melanomas does not encompass the entire surface of the lesion and it often displays multiple hues of blue (Figure 145.5f). Histologically, the blue-white veil correlates with melanocytes in the deeper dermis with an overlying compact orthokeratosis.

9 *Peripheral light brown structureless areas.* Peripheral light brown structureless areas are seen as homogeneous light brown areas of variable size and shape located at the periphery of the lesion and occupying more than 10% of its surface (Figure 145.5) [46]. Histologically the areas are due to relative flattening of the rete ridges in combination with pagetoid melanoma cells.

10 *Atypical blotch.* A blotch consists of a dark-brown to black, usually homogeneous area with varying hues of pigment that

Table 145.2 Melanoma-specific structures.

Dermoscopic structure	Definition
Atypical network	Increased variability in the width of the network lines, their colour and distribution. The hole sizes also have increased variability. The network can appear broken up (non-contiguous), appearing as branched streaks, and the network may end abruptly at the periphery
Angulated lines	Brown to bluish grey dots and/or lines arranged in an angulated linear pattern
Negative network	Serpiginous interconnecting hypopigmented lines, which surround irregularly shaped pigmented structures that resemble elongated curvilinear globules. It can be seen diffusely throughout the lesion or focally and asymmetrically located within the lesion
Streaks, including pseudopods and radial streaming	Radial projections located at the periphery of the lesion, extending from the tumour toward the surrounding normal skin. The presence of irregular, asymmetrical and focally distributed streaks are highly suggestive of melanoma. *Pseudopods* are finger-like projections with small knobs at their tips, whereas *radial streaming* are the same structures without the knobs. Because both structures represent confluent junctional nests of melanocytes, they are now both categorised under the term streaks
Shiny white lines	Shiny white linear streaks that are often orientated parallel or orthogonal to each other
Atypical dots or globules	*Dots* are small, round structures, which may be black, brown and/or blue-grey in colour. In melanoma, dots vary in size, colour and distribution, tending to be located towards the periphery of the lesion, and are not associated with the pigmented network lines. *Globules* consist of 3–5 or more clustered, well-demarcated, round to oval structures that may be brown, black, blue and/or white in colour and that are larger than dots. In melanoma they are usually multiple and of differing sizes, shapes and colours. They are often asymmetrically and/or focally distributed within the lesion
Atypical blotch, including off-centre blotch or multiple asymmetrically located blotches	Dark-brown to black, usually homogeneous areas with varying hues of pigment that obscure visualisation of any other structures. In melanoma, blotches are asymmetrically and/or focally located towards the periphery of the lesion or can present as multiple blotches. Eccentric peripheral hyperpigmentation is often found in melanoma
Regression structures (white scar-like depigmentation and/or blue-grey granularity or peppering)	Consist of granularity (also known as peppering) and scar-like areas. When both are present together, it gives the appearance of a blue-white veil over a macular area. In melanoma, regression structures tend to be asymmetrically located and often involve more than 50% of the lesion's surface area
Blue-white veil	Confluent blue pigmentation of varying hues with an overlying white 'ground glass' haze, which tend to be asymmetrically located and seen over a raised area of the lesion.

(continued)

Table 145.2 (continued)

Dermoscopic structure	Definition
Atypical vascular structures	*Dotted vessels* over milky-red background suggests melanoma or Spitz naevus *Serpentine vessels*: linear and irregular *Polymorphous vessels*: two or more vessel morphologies within the same lesion *Corkscrew vessels*: usually seen in nodular or desmoplastic melanoma, and melanoma metastases
Peripheral tan structureless areas	Structureless light brown area/s located at the periphery of the lesion and encompassing more than 10% of a lesion's surface area

obscure visualisation of any other structures. An atypical blotch includes an off-centre blotch or multiple asymmetrically located blotches (Figure 145.5a,b,d,f).

11 *Atypical vessels*. Assessment of vascular structures/vessels include the evaluation of the (i) morphology; (ii) arrangement; and (iii) other features (e.g. halo, background colour). To enhance the ability to visualise the blood vessels one should use non-contact polarised dermoscopy. If non-polarised dermoscopy is used then efforts need to be taken to prevent the blanching of vessels, which can easily occur when too much pressure is applied to the skin when the scope is placed in direct contact with the lesion. An easy way to avoid blanching the vasculature is to use a gel interface between the scope and the lesion; the scope can then be placed in contact with the lesion with minimal pressure being applied to the lesion [45,47]. With the exception of intradermal naevi displaying comma-shaped vessels, blood vessels seen in melanocytic tumors should raise concern for melanoma. Vessels considered atypical include comma-shaped vessels in lesions that do not appear as intradermal naevi on clinical inspection, dotted, linear irregular or corkscrew vessels, also milky-red globules and milky-red areas. The most common vessel pattern seen in melanoma is the polymorphous pattern, which includes two or more vessel morphology within the same lesion [48,49,50,51].

Melanomas on special locations

Melanomas developing on special sites, including volar skin, face, mucosae, nails, or those on chronically sun-damaged skin can reveal any of the abovementioned melanoma-specific structures (Table 145.2; Figure 145.5), but usually display a different set of dermoscopic structures (Tables 145.3, 145.4 and 145.5; Figures 145.6 and 145.7).

Melanomas on facial skin or chronically sun-damaged skin
[22,52–55] (Table 145.3; Figure 145.6)
- Annular–granular pattern, formed by slate-grey dots/granules surrounding adnexal openings.
- Asymmetric follicular openings, consisting of an asymmetric distribution of colour (tan-brown to grey) surrounding follicular openings.
- Angulated lines, defined as multiple, confluent greyish to brown lines meeting at acute angles and coalescing to form polygonal shapes such as rhomboids. The lines can be formed by confluent granules or dots and this may at times be the only criterion present to indicate malignancy [15–17].
- Rhomboidal structures consist of homogeneous darkly pigmented areas (brown, grey, or black) around the adnexal or follicular openings.
- Blotches form when the melanoma starts to obliterate the adnexal openings creating areas of dark pigment where the pigment is so dark that it precludes the ability to see any other structures in the area.
- Concentric isobar pattern or circle within a circle, defined as concentric pigmented rings encircling each other around hair follicles.

Early signs of melanomas on facial or chronically sun-damaged skin (i.e. lentigo maligna) include an annular granular pattern, asymmetric follicular openings, granularity, angulated lines or dots aggregated around adnexal openings. As lesions progress, these dermoscopic features are replaced by homogeneous dark areas or blotches with obliteration of adnexal openings [15]. Most melanomas on chronic sun-damaged skin will reveal a disorganised pattern with at least one of the features mentioned above. However, some can be featureless tan macules and others can just reveal network structures. Any acquired, isolated, large lentiginous lesion on chronic sun-damaged skin should raise concern for melanoma, even if it only reveals network structures. The network in these melanomas tends to be quite normal in appearance but close scrutiny will usually reveal that the network is distributed as small islands with intervening structureless areas and these islands of network tend to be distributed in a patchy and disorganised manner. In structureless melanomas on sun-damaged skin, digital dermoscopy follow-up may assist in correctly identifying the melanoma based on change.

Melanoma on volar skin of palms and soles

During the dermoscopic evaluation of lesions on palms and soles it is imperative to identify the furrows and ridges of the dermatoglyphics. Pigment predominantly localised to the ridges

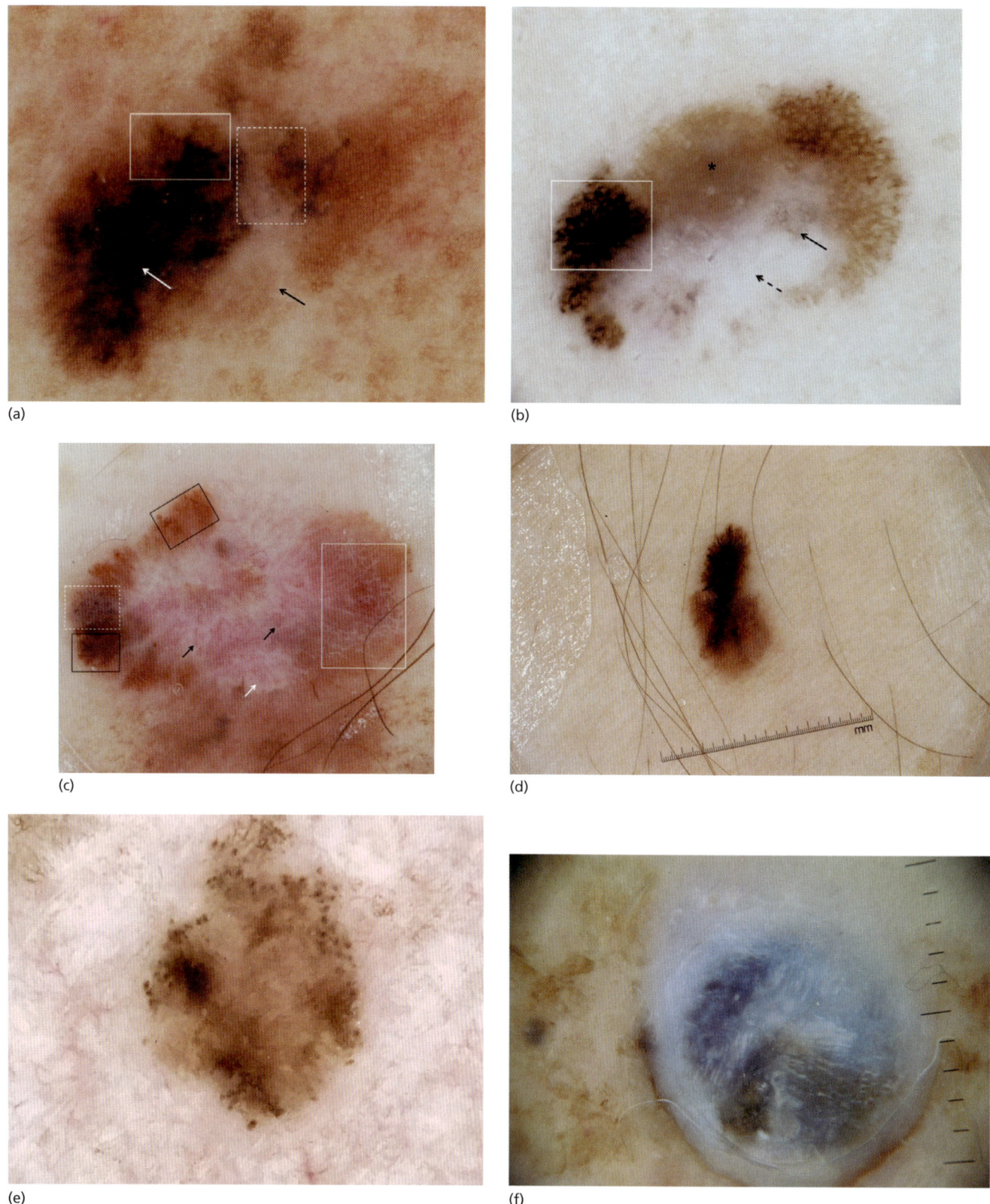

Figure 145.5 (a) Dermoscopic image of a melanoma on the lower back revealing an atypical network (solid box), regression structures including granularity and scar-like depigmentation (dashed box), peripheral tan structureless area (black arrow) and atypical blotch (white arrow). (b) Dermoscopic image of a melanoma located on the leg with an atypical network (solid box), regression structures (arrows) with the solid arrow pointing to granularity/peppering and the dashed arrow pointing to scar-like depigmentation. The lesion also has a peripheral tan structureless area (asterix). (c) Dermoscopic image of a melanoma located on the abdomen, with an atypical network (black solid boxes), atypical globules (white dashed box), negative network (white solid box), scar-like areas (white arrow) and atypical vessels including serpentine, dotted and irregular hairpin vessels (black arrows). (d) Dermoscopic image of a melanoma located on the thigh with atypical peripheral streaks (i.e. radial streaming). (e) Dermoscopic image of a melanoma *in situ* displaying atypical globules and peripheral tan structureless areas. (f) Dermoscopic image of a melanoma displaying a blue-white veil. (f) Courtesy of The International Skin Imaging Collaboration.

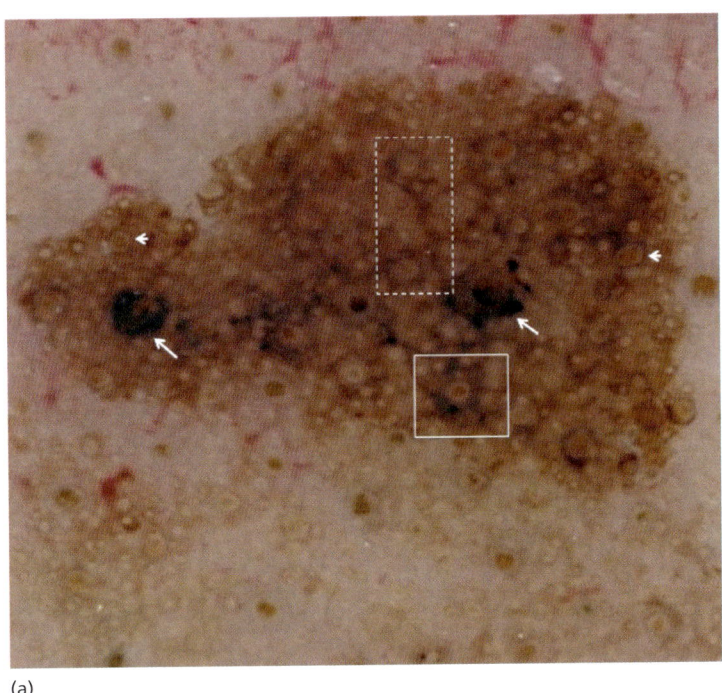
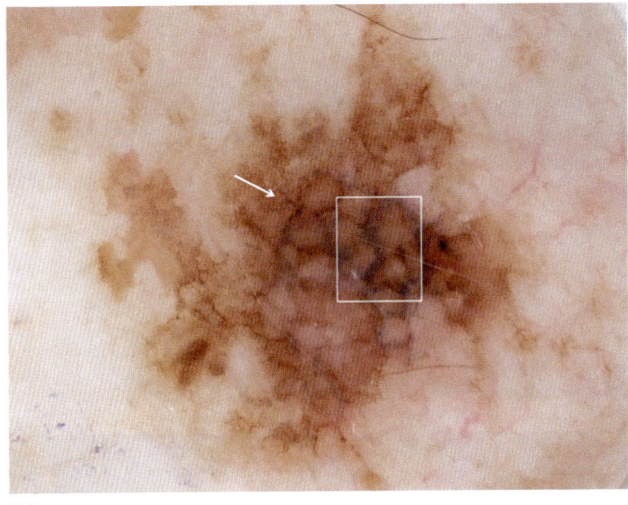

(a) (b)

Figure 145.6 (a) Dermoscopic image of a lentigo maligna located on the nose with perifollciular granularity and asymmetrical grey perifollicular openings (solid box), polygonal structures (dashed box), rhomboidal structures (solid arrows) and circle within a circle (arrowheads). (b) Dermoscopic image of a melanoma located on chronic sun-damaged skin on the shoulder, revealing perifollciular granularity and asymmetrical grey perifollicular openings (solid box) and polygonal structures (white arrow).

Table 145.3 Melanoma structures seen on facial or on sun-damaged skin.

Dermoscopic structure	Definition	Schematic illustration
Asymmetrical perifollicular openings	Dots or grey granularity aggregated around hair follicles in an asymmetrical fashion. This asymmetrical distribution often creates a crescent shape around the hair follicles	
Angulated lines (i.e. polygonal lines, zig-zag lines)	Brown to bluish grey dots and/or lines arranged in an angulated linear pattern	
Rhomboidal structures	Hyperpigmented brown and grey lines surrounding hair follicles and creating shapes like rhomboids	
Follicle obliteration	Rhomboidal structures become broader, obliterating hair follicles	
Circle within a circle (isobar pattern)	Concentric pigmented rings encircling each other	

Table 145.4 Melanoma structures in acral melanoma (melanomas on volar skin).

Dermoscopic structure	Definition	Schematic illustration
Parallel ridge pattern	Pigmentation located on the ridges of palms and soles	
Irregular diffuse pigmentation	Irregular, diffuse pigmentation with different shades of tan, brown, black and/or grey	
Irregular/atypical fibrillar pattern	Any fibrillar pattern on the palms or fibrillar pattern on the soles that reveals an increased variability in the thickness or colours of the lines. Line colour other than brown is also considered atypical	
Large-diameter lesion	Newly acquired lesion greater than 7–10 mm in diameter, especially in individuals over the age of 50 years	

(i.e. parallel ridge pattern) is highly suggestive of melanoma (Table 145.4; Figure 145.7a,b); however, in darker skin the ridges can be normally pigmented and thus this feature cannot be relied upon to differentiate melanoma from benign pigmented macules. Clues to assist in recognising the ridges include:

- The ducts of the eccrine glands open on the surface of the skin overlying the ridges and are seen as tiny white dots aligned in rows.
- Ridges are wider than the furrows.
- The ink test, described by Braun *et al.* [56] and Uhara *et al.* [57], in which ink applied to the skin highlights the furrows and ridges and even the eccrine openings.

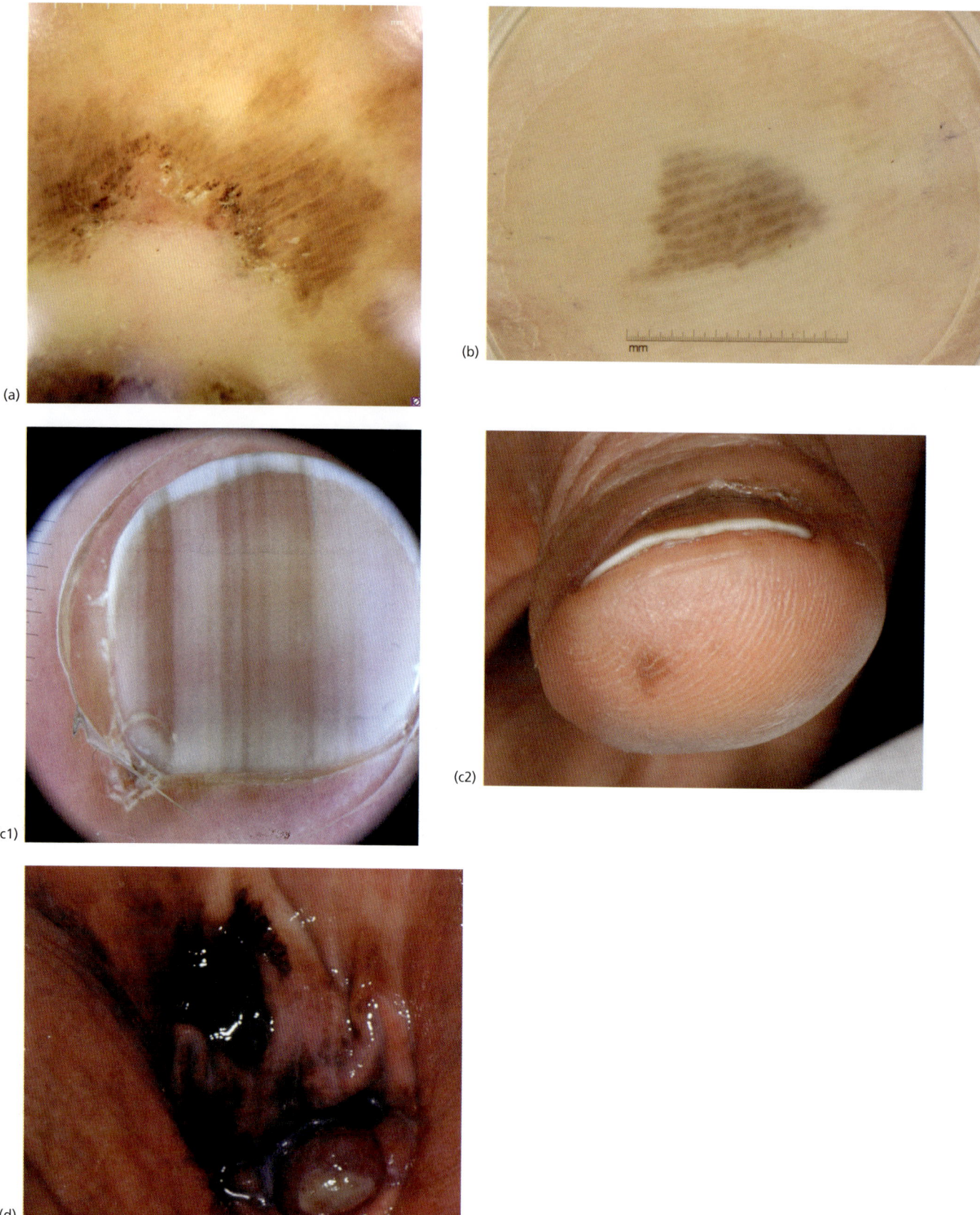

Figure 145.7 (a, b) Dermoscopic images of melanomas located on the soles with a parallel ridge pattern. (c) Dermoscopic image (c1) of a melanoma, 0.6 mm in thickness, involving the nail unit with multiple, longitudinal, irregular, brown bands with irregular spacing and thickness and the micro-Hutchinson sign Also present is irregular pigmentation on the hyponychium (clinical image, c2). (d) Dermoscopic image of a vaginal (mucosal) melanoma, demonstrating the presence of blue, grey and white colours within the lesion, and a multicomponent pattern composed by irregular brown-black globules and blue-white veil.

Dermoscopy structures suggestive of acral/volar melanoma, include (Table 145.4; Figure 145.7a,b):
- *Parallel ridge pattern*. The presence of a parallel ridge pattern has a diagnostic accuracy of 82% for melanoma, with a sensitivity of 86%, specificity of 99%, a positive predictive value of 94% and a negative predictive value of 98% [58,59]. Exceptions to the ridge pattern exist with some benign lesions manifesting a parallel ridge pattern, for example some congenital naevi and lesions seen in Peutz–Jegher syndrome, Luzier Hunziger syndrome, subcorneal haemorrhage and race-related pigmentation. In contrast to melanoma, most naevi reveal patterns with pigment predominantly located in the dermatoglyphic furrows (i.e. parallel furrow and lattice-like patterns).
- *Homogeneous pattern* displaying multiple shades of brown and/or other colours such as black, red, white, grey and blue [58,60].
- *Atypical/irregular fibrillar pattern*. An atypical fibrillar pattern consists of lines with increased variability in thickness, spacing and colour [61]. In addition, a lesion displaying a fibrillar pattern on the palms should be viewed with suspicion.

If the volar lesion does not reveal any of the aforementioned diagnostic features, management relies on the maximal diameter of the lesion. Lesions greater than 7–10 mm in diameter should be considered for biopsy, especially in patients older than 50 years, whereas lesions smaller than 7–10 mm in diameter can either be biopsied or digitally monitored [62].

Melanoma involving the nail unit

Evaluation of melanonychia striata requires inspection of the nail plate, cuticle, paronychium and hyponychium. Pigment on any of the three latter sites, in association with an acquired melanonychia striata, is highly suggestive of melanoma (Table 145.5; Figure 145.7c).

Clinical findings are (Table 145.5):
- Hutchinson sign: pigmentation on the proximal nail fold visualised with the naked eye.
- Triangular shape: the width of the melanonychia is wider at the proximal end of the nail plate compared with the distal end. A wider diameter at the proximal end, resulting in a triangular shape can be seen in rapidly growing tumours, including melanomas [60].
- Nail dystrophy with complete or partial destruction of the nail plate.

Dermoscopy structures suggestive of nail melanoma (Table 145.5; Figure 145.7c):
- Micro-Hutchinson sign: pigmentation on the proximal nail fold or cuticle, only visualised with dermoscopy. The micro-Hutchinson sign needs to be differentiated from the pseudo-Hutchinson sign, which occurs when the pigment located in the nail matrix/nail plate is visible through a relatively translucent and normal cuticular skin and which has no diagnostic significance.
- Hyponychial pigmentation with any melanoma-specific structure (Tables 145.2 and 145.4): pigmentation on the hyponychium should be evaluated in the same manner as described for acral/volar melanomas. For example, pigmentation on the hyponychium with a parallel ridge pattern would be highly suggestive for melanoma.
- Irregular band pattern: an irregular pattern consists of multiple longitudinal bands of different colours and thicknesses. Lines are spaced at irregular intervals and demonstrate disruption of the parallelism [60].

Although some authors have suggested that applying dermoscopy directly to the nail matrix and nail bed after nail avulsion can help in identifying nail matrix melanoma [63], this is not a practical method for the routine evaluation of melanonychia striata. Instead, dermoscopic examination of the nail plate can provide valuable, albeit indirect, clues regarding the nature of the nail matrix lesion.

Melanomas displaying an organised pattern

There exists a subset of melanomas that will display an organised pattern. Some of these melanomas include the nodular, naevoid, desmoplastic, spitzoid, featureless/structureless and amelanotic subtypes (Figure 145.8); also epidermotropic metastases can demonstrate an organised pattern. These 'organised' melanomas will usually not mimic one of the benign naevi patterns and instead will display at least one of two patterns, one of two structures or one of four colours [64,65].

Two patterns

1 *Streaks or globules forming a starburst pattern*: a starburst pattern can be seen in Spitz/Reed naevi, but also in melanoma. Thus, this pattern should be considered suspicious, especially if found in individuals over the age of 12 years (Figure 145.9).
2 *Negative network pattern*: both Spitz naevi and melanomas can display a negative network throughout the lesion. Thus, this

Table 145.5 Melanoma-specific structures of the nail unit.

Dermoscopic structure	Definition	Schematic illustration
Hyponychial pigment with any features described in Table 145.2 and 145.4	Irregular pigmentation on the distal periungual skin, with any of the features associated with melanomas on acral skin	
Hutchinson or micro-Hutchinson sign	Pigmentation of the proximal nail fold that can be seen with the naked eye (Hutchinson) or only with dermoscopy (micro-Hutchinson)	
Triangular shape	Width of the melanonychia striata is wider at the proximal end of the nail plate	
Irregular band pattern	Multiple, longitudinal, irregular bands of different colours (i.e. black, brown, grey) with irregular spacing, thickness and disruption of parallelism	
Nail dystrophy	Complete or partial nail destruction and/or absence of the nail plate	

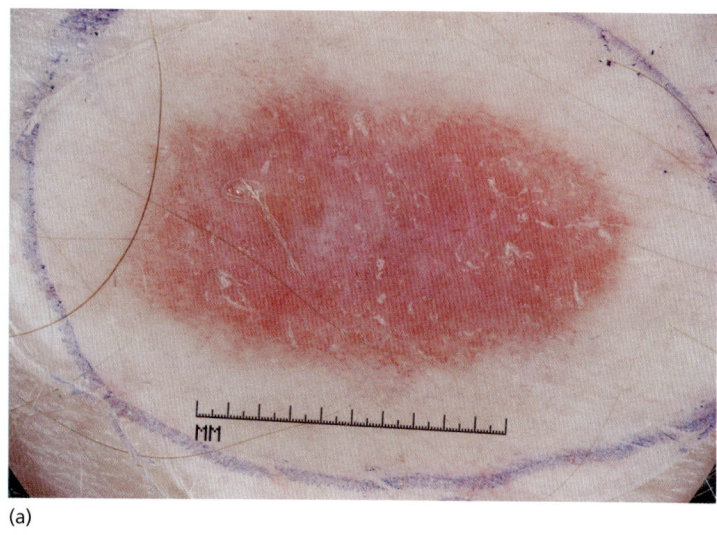
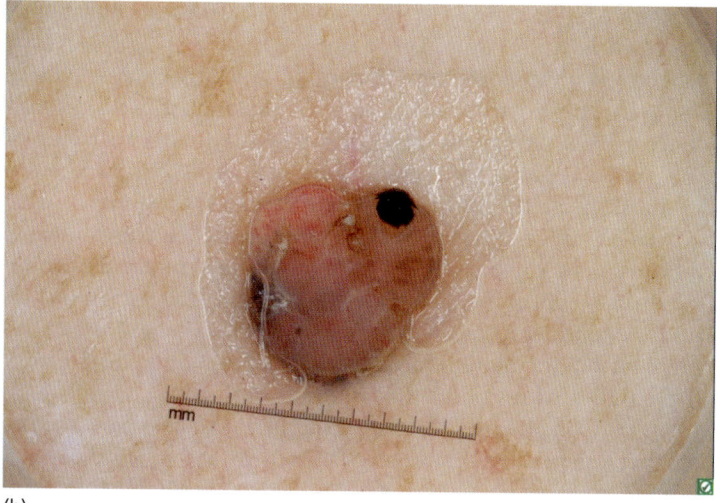
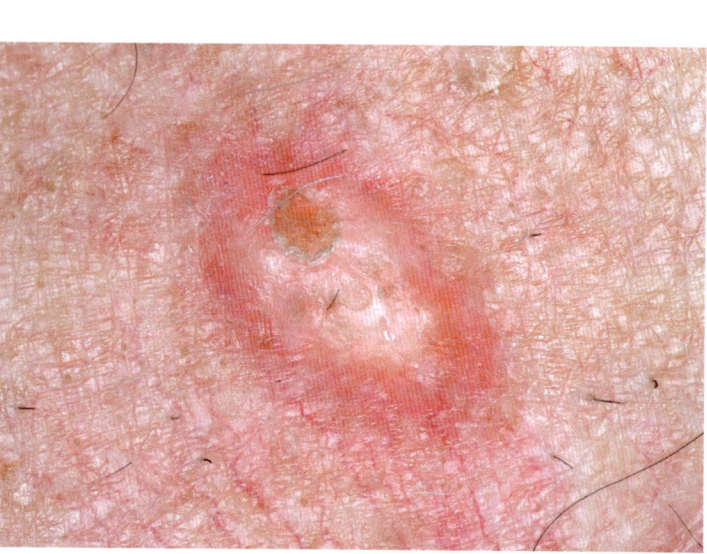
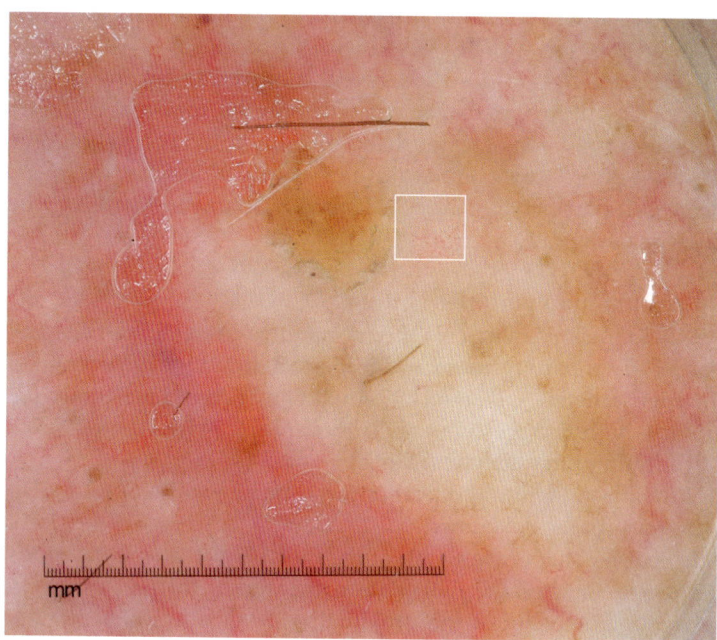

Figure 145.8 (a) Dermoscopic image of an amelanotic melanoma that is not of the nodular subtype, showing serpentine vessels, dotted vessels and vascular blush throughout the lesion. (b) Dermoscopic image of a nodular, amelanotic melanoma displaying atypical vessels (i.e. serpentine and hairpin vessels) within pseudo-lagoons characterised by pink lacuna-like structures that are not separated from each other by septae. (c) Clinical image of a 6.1 mm pure desmoplastic melanoma. (d) Dermoscopic image of the same melanoma showing subtle dotted vessels (box). A biopsy was performed revealing a 6.1 mm pure desmoplastic melanoma with no associated epidermal component.

pattern should be considered suspicious in post-adolescence and a biopsy should be considered (Figure 145.10).

Two structures

1 *Vessels:* lesions revealing any vascular structure, including vessels of any morphology, should be considered concerning.
2 *Ulceration:* a lesion with ulceration or erosions should always be considered suspect.

Four colours

1 *Blue-black colour (1,2):* the presence of blue-black colour has been shown to have high sensitivity for nodular melanoma [4] (Figure 145.5).
2 *Grey (3):* grey colour is an important clue for skin cancer, in particular for melanomas on sun-damaged skin [5]. Therefore, any organised lesion revealing blue-black or grey colour should be considered suspicious [10,11].
3 *White (4):* white structures include shiny white lines, which can only be seen with polarised light. Although all white structures including shiny white structures have a strong association with malignancy [12,13,14], there are benign lesions, such as dermatofibromas, lichen planus-like keratoses and Spitz naevi that may also reveal these structures. However, for the purpose of lesion triage it is advisable that any lesion displaying white colour be viewed with suspicion [64] (Figures 145.5 and 145.10).

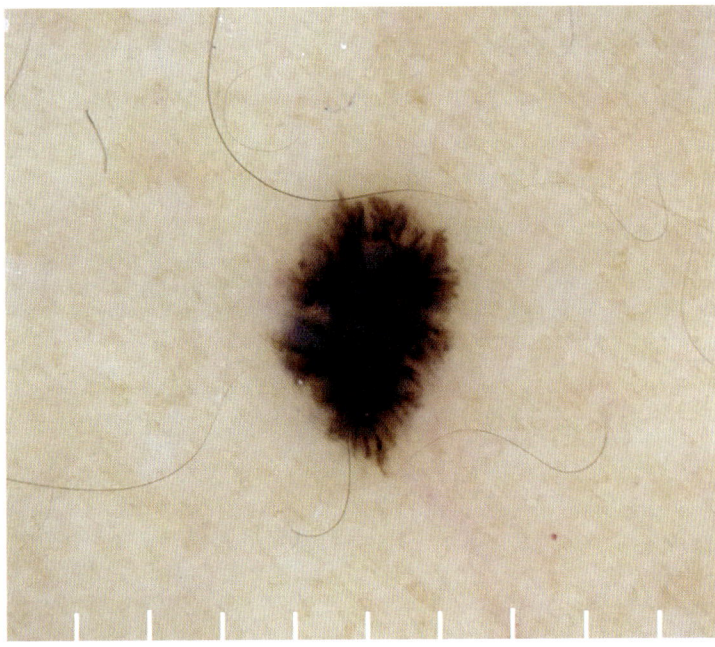

Figure 145.9 Melanoma *in situ* presenting with a starburst pattern.

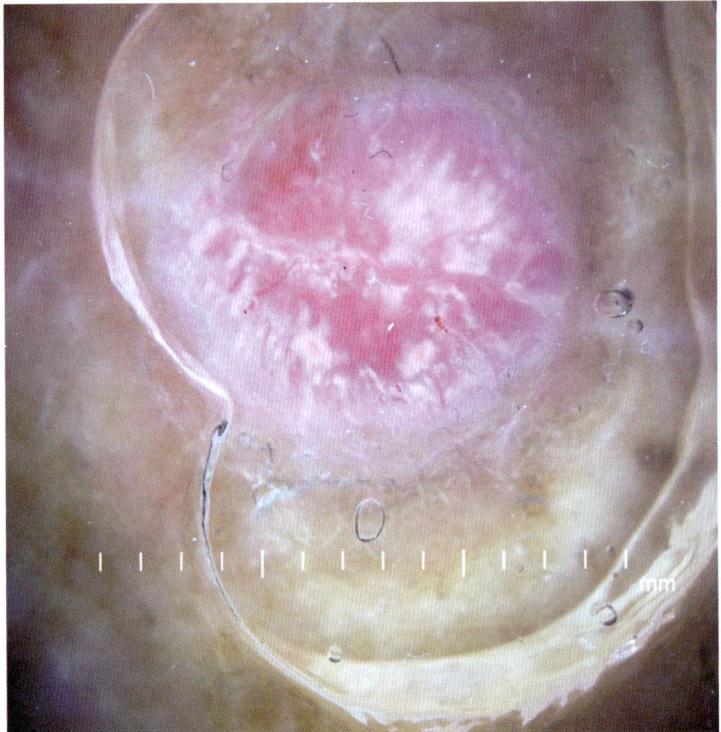

Figure 145.10 Nodular amelanotic melanoma presenting with an 'organised pattern'; dermoscopy reveals shiny white structures and atypical vessels.

Conclusion

While the clinical morphology of naevi and melanoma may overlap, the visualisation of colours and structures under dermoscopy has shown to improve our ability to discriminate between these two entities. Overall, naevi tend to display symmetrical and organised dermoscopic patterns while melanomas tend to manifest asymmetrical and disorganised patterns that display at least one melanoma-specific structure. The most common naevi patterns encountered in clinical practice have been discussed in this chapter. There are, however, other less common types of naevi with their own signature dermoscopic features that have not been discussed, including balloon cell naevi, BAP deficient naevi, epidermolysis bullosa naevi, naevi arising in lichen sclerosus, recurrent naevi, Meyerson naevi and halo naevi among others (Table 145.1). In addition, there is a group of naevi that manifest a disorganised and multicomponent dermoscopy pattern, which can be impossible to differentiate from melanoma based on the clinical and dermoscopy morphology alone.

In this chapter we have also provided an overview of the melanoma-specific structures including an atypical network, a negative network, angulated lines, streaks, shiny-white lines, atypical dots/globules, off-centre blotches, blue-white veils, regression structures, atypical vessels and peripheral tan structureless areas. Some studies have suggested that the constellation of dermoscopic structures within a melanoma can be used to predict its thickness [66]. In addition, the clinical morphology of the melanoma, its location and the dermoscopic structures it manifests can help predict the melanoma subtype, from lentigo maligna to superficial spreading melanoma, nodular melanoma, verrucous melanoma, desmoplastic melanoma, naevoid melanoma, spitzoid melanoma and recurrent melanoma amongst others. However, for the purpose of this chapter we have chosen to highlight the features seen in any melanoma subtype, irrespective of whether *in situ*, micro-invasive or deeply invasive.

The established use of dermoscopy has improved our benign-to-malignant biopsy ratio due to fewer naevi being removed and more melanomas being found. The melanomas discovered because of dermoscopy are primarily those that lack the clinical ABCDs, have smaller diameters and are *in situ* or microinvasive. In addition, with sequential digital monitoring, the featureless melanomas can also be discovered based on changes noted during serial digital dermoscopy monitoring [67]. All this effort has likely saved countless lives but probably has also contributed to the overdiagnosis of this cancer [68]. Future research will need to focus on deciphering which of the melanomas found with dermoscopy will behave in an aggressive manner and which will behave in an indolent manner during the course of the patient's life. Much effort is currently being directed towards training artificial intelligence (AI) neural networks in differentiating naevi from melanoma. Although multiple studies utilising selected melanocytic tumour images have shown that AI's diagnostic accuracy approaches and even surpasses expert dermoscopy readers [69], their performance in real-world settings and their impact on patient management are lacking. Besides investigating AI's role in the diagnostic process, researchers are actively looking at ways for AI to direct human vision to focal areas or structures within a lesion that may have diagnostic significance, ensuring that the human observer has in fact seen the area of interest before rendering a final diagnosis. Over the next decade we are likely to see diagnostic AI programs or AI programs designed to augment human intelligence penetrate the clinical care environment.

Key references

The full list of references can be found in the online version at https://www.wiley.com/rooksdermatology10e

12 Lallas A, Apalla Z, Ioannides D *et al*. Update on dermoscopy of Spitz/Reed naevi and management guidelines by the International Dermoscopy Society. *Br J Dermatol* 2017;177:645–55.

18 Argenziano G, Catricala C, Ardigo M *et al*. Dermoscopy of patients with multiple nevi: improved management recommendations using a comparative diagnostic approach. *Arch Dermatol* 2011;147:46–9.

31 Kittler H, Guitera P, Riedl E *et al*. Identification of clinically featureless incipient melanoma using sequential dermoscopy imaging. *Arch Dermatol* 2006;142:1113–19.

45 Balagula Y, Braun RP, Rabinovitz HS *et al*. The significance of crystalline/chrysalis structures in the diagnosis of melanocytic and nonmelanocytic lesions. *J Am Acad Dermatol* 2012;67:194.e1–8.

46 Annessi G, Bono R, Sampogna F, Faraggiana T, Abeni D. Sensitivity, specificity, and diagnostic accuracy of three dermoscopic algorithmic methods in the diagnosis of doubtful melanocytic lesions: the importance of light brown structureless areas in differentiating atypical melanocytic nevi from thin melanomas. *J Am Acad Dermatol* 2007;56:759–67.

49 Menzies SW, Moloney FJ, Byth K *et al*. Dermoscopic evaluation of nodular melanoma. *JAMA Dermatol* 2013;149:699–709.

50 Menzies SW, Kreusch J, Byth K *et al*. Dermoscopic evaluation of amelanotic and hypomelanotic melanoma. *Arch Dermatol* 2008;144:1120–7.

62 Koga H, Saida T. Revised 3-step dermoscopic algorithm for the management of acral melanocytic lesions. *Arch Dermatol* 2011;147:741–3.

64 Jaimes N, Marghoob AA. Triage amalgamated dermoscopic algorithm. *J Am Acad Dermatol* 2020;82:1551–2.

66 Sgouros D, Lallas A, Kittler H *et al*. Dermatoscopic features of thin (≤2 mm Breslow thickness) vs. thick (>2 mm Breslow thickness) nodular melanoma and predictors of nodular melanoma versus nodular non-melanoma tumours: a multicentric collaborative study by the International Dermoscopy Society. *J Eur Acad Dermatol Venereol* 2020;34:2541–7.

CHAPTER 146

Merkel Cell Carcinoma

Jürgen C. Becker[1], Isaac Brownell[2] and Thibault Kervarrec[3]

[1] Translational Skin Cancer Research (TSCR), German Cancer Consortium (DKTK) Site Essen/Düsseldorf, Essen; Deutsches Krebsforschungsinstitut (DKFZ), Heidelberg, Germany
[2] Dermatology Branch, National Institute of Arthritis and Musculoskeletal and Skin Diseases, National Institutes of Health, Bethesda, MD, USA
[3] Department of Pathology, University Hospital Center of Tours, Tours, France

Merkel cell carcinoma, 146.1	Epidemiology, 146.1	Investigations, 146.7
Definition, nomenclature and classification, 146.1	Pathophysiology, 146.2	Management, 146.8
Introduction and general description, 146.1	Clinical features, 146.5	**Key references, 146.10**

Merkel cell carcinoma

Definition, nomenclature and classification

Synonyms and inclusions
- Cutaneous neuroendocrine carcinoma
- Primary neuroendocrine carcinoma of the skin
- Trabecular carcinoma of the skin

Classification
- ICD-10-CM: C4A.0–C4A.39
- ICD-10: C44 (ILDS C44.L44)
- ICD-9: 209.31–209.36
- ICD-O: M8247/3
- Snomed CT: 5052009
- Orphanet: ORPHA79140

Introduction and general description

Merkel cell carcinoma (MCC) is a highly aggressive carcinoma of the skin with neuroendocrine differentiation demonstrating high rates of recurrence and metastasis. Indeed, the 5-year rate for MCC-specific survival in the USA is only about 76% for localised, 53% for regional and 19% for distant disease. The clinical appearance of MCC is usually that of a rapidly growing, reddish, spherical tumour with a smooth, shiny surface and a firm consistency, but there are exceptions such as plaque-like or ulcerated tumours. Spontaneous, often complete, regression of MCC is observed sporadically. Complete regression of the primary tumour may explain cases in which only lymph node or distant metastases are found at the time of initial diagnosis.

Although the incidence of MCC has been rapidly increasing since its first description, it is still a very rare tumour. In 1972 Toker reported five patients with unusual skin tumours characterised by histologically anastomosing trabeculae and cell nests; he therefore named these tumours 'trabecular carcinoma of the skin' [1]. This histological feature already suggested a neuroendocrine origin, and this notion was substantiated by the discovery of electron-dense neurosecretory granules in the tumour cells. In 1982 Rywlin suggested naming this tumour Merkel cell carcinoma due to the morphological similarities of the tumour cells to Merkel cells [2]. In addition, Merkel cells and MCC tumour cells share similar immunophenotypical features.

Merkel cells are thought to function as slowly adapting mechanoreceptors in the basal layer of the epidermis and appendage structures [1], and belong to the amine precursor uptake and decarboxylation system. Although they were suspected for a long time to have a neural crest origin, it has now been demonstrated that mammalian Merkel cells derive from epidermal stem cells in the skin [2,3]. Immunophenotypical similarities between Merkel cells and MCCs generated speculation that Merkel cells may be the cells of origin for MCC. However, several reports have identified non-neuroendocrine epithelial cells and sarcomatous elements in some MCCs [4]. This suggests that MCC may arise from primitive, pluripotent/stem epidermal stem cells, which are able to differentiate into different cell lineages.

Epidemiology

Only a small fraction of all cutaneous malignancies are MCCs. In a study comprising 3720 MCC patients from the Surveillance, Epidemiology and End Results (SEER) database diagnosed between 2012 and 2016, the age-adjusted annual incidence rate was 0.66 per 100 000, representing a 3.5-fold increase over the period between 1987 to 1991. MCC is a tumour of advanced age with the highest incidence rate observed in those 85 years or older, with an age-adjusted rate of 14.6 per 100 000 for males and 5.5 for females. The increasing MCC incidence over time can be attributed to changing environmental risk factors, an ageing population and improving diagnostic tools. Although the birth cohort effect (risk factors) and

Rook's Textbook of Dermatology, Tenth Edition. Edited by Christopher Griffiths, Jonathan Barker, Tanya Bleiker, Walayat Hussain and Rosalind Simpson.
© 2024 John Wiley & Sons Ltd. Published 2024 by John Wiley & Sons Ltd.

age effects have continued to increase over time, the era of diagnosis effect has begun to plateau [5]. Notably, earlier studies also reported an increase in MCC incidence during the 1990s, but also suggest a more recent stabilisation of rate [6–8]. Thus, increased detection of MCC by improved diagnostics and disease awareness is having a waning influence on disease incidence, whereas changes in the ageing population continue to drive the growing incidence.

MCCs are most often found on the sun-exposed skin areas of the white population who are older than 50 years. Indeed, MCC is much more common in white than in black patients, i.e. 0.31 and 0.01 per 100 000 persons, respectively [6]. Albeit not specifically reported, it may be hypothesised based on other ultraviolet (UV)-induced tumours that the rates in Asian or Hispanic patients will be somewhere between these two.

The mean age of patients at the time of initial diagnosis is about 76 years for women and 73 years for men. In fact, 71.6% of patients are older than 70. MCC predominates in men (61.5%).

MCC occurs much more frequently in severely immunosuppressed populations, such as organ transplant patients, patients with haematolymphoid disorders or acquired immune deficiency syndrome (AIDS) [9–11]. Indeed, the mean age at diagnosis in organ transplant recipients is almost 20 years lower compared with immunocompetent patients. In organ transplant recipients, MCCs tend to develop 7–8 years post-transplantation and affect the head and neck areas, often in the presence of other UV-induced skin cancers.

Patients diagnosed with MCC bear an increased risk for being diagnosed with a second primary cancer when compared with the general population [12]. The increase in the risk of developing a second primary cancer may, in part, be due to shared aetiological factors between the cancers. Nonetheless, clinicians treating MCC patients should be aware of these associations.

Pathophysiology
Pathogenesis
The carcinogenesis of MCC is associated either with the clonal integration of Merkel cell polyomavirus (MCPyV) DNA into the host genome or UV-induced DNA mutations, both resulting in similar cellular aberrations.

Intially, Merkel cells were thought to be the cells of origin for MCC due to similarities in morphology and protein expression. Merkel cells are located at the epidermal–dermal junction, mostly in association with appendage structures, and act as light touch receptors [1]. However, the deep dermal location of most MCC tumours, the lack of MCPyV detection in Merkel cells and their post-mitotic state have raised serious doubts about this theory [13]. An alternative hypothesis is that Merkel cell-like features are acquired by tumour cells during oncogenesis, comparable to the neuroendocrine transformation of other tumour entities [14]. Indeed, inactivation of pRB either by MCPyV T-antigen expression or somatic mutations is expected to induce the expression of several transcription factors involved in Merkel cell differentiation such as SOX2 (SRY-box 2) and ATOH1 (Atonal homolog 1) [**15**,16,17]. An oncogenic transdifferentiation hypothesis has been proposed for a number of potential MCC cells of origin including pluripotent/stem cells of the epidermis and appendages and dermal fibroblasts, as well as pre-/pro-B cells [18–21]. Moreover, significant variation in morphology and genetic variants has suggested that MCPyV-positive and -negative cases might derive from distinct cellular ancestries [22]. Although several lineage tracking experiences in mouse models failed to identify the MCC cell of origin [23,24], recent investigation by massive parallel sequencing of a rare combined MCC associated with a benign adnexal neoplasm strongly suggests that MCPyV integration in an epithelial progenitor can give rise to MCC. These observations argue in favour of an epithelial origin of MCPyV-positive tumours which might derive either from the epidermis or from appendages [25]. In addition, detection of high tumour mutation burden, prominent UV signature and frequent association with squamous cell carcinoma and precursors support an epidermal origin for MCPyV-negative MCC [26–28].

Predisposing factors, causative organisms and environmental factors
The mean age of patients at the time of initial diagnosis is above 70 years [5]. Notably, there is a 5–10-fold increase in incidence after the age of 65. It has been proposed that an age-related impairment of immune functions, that is, immunosenescence, may explain this age predisposition. Immune control of MCC is supported by a number of observations. For example, MCC occurs more frequently and at younger ages in severely immunocompromised populations, such as organ transplant patients, patients with haematolymphoid disorders or human immunodeficiency virus (HIV) infected individuals [9–11]. Moreover, the prognosis of MCC in immunocompromised patients is much worse; an association that is independent of the stage at diagnosis [9]. Finally, there are numerous case reports of spontaneous regressions of MCCs, even in metastatic stages, particularly when any form of immune-suppressive therapy is ceased [29].

Given the increased risk of MCC in immunocompromised patients a causative infectious agent was hypothesised, leading to the discovery in 2008 of a novel human polyomavirus, MCPyV, by whole transcriptome sequencing [30]. The presence of MCPyV in a large fraction of MCC cases – particularly in patients living in regions with a higher latitude – has been confirmed in several studies [31]. MCPyV is the first polyomavirus directly linked to human cancer. The assumed viral carcinogenesis of MCC explains several of the features of MCC including its outstanding immunogenicity. MCPyV DNA is clonally integrated into the host genome of the MCC tumour cells; moreover, virus-positive MCC tumour cells require continued MCPyV oncoprotein expression to survive (Figure 146.1) [32]. The integrated viral genomes of each tumour contain unique mutations in the large T-antigen gene viral oncogene that incapacitates viral DNA replication [33,34]. Both humoral and cellular immune responses have been demonstrated against virally encoded proteins. Notably, while immune responses against MCPyV capsid proteins can be readily detected in the general population, responses against viral oncogens are mostly restricted to MCC patients [35,36]. Indeed, increased antibody titres against the viral oncogenes have been proposed as a biomarker for tumour burden in MCC patients [37].

The observation that the incidence rates for MCCs increase for persons living in areas of lower latitudes, and that MCC is most often found on the sun-exposed skin of white people, suggest UV exposure as one of the major environmental risk factors [6]. Additional lines of evidence are the increased MCC incidence

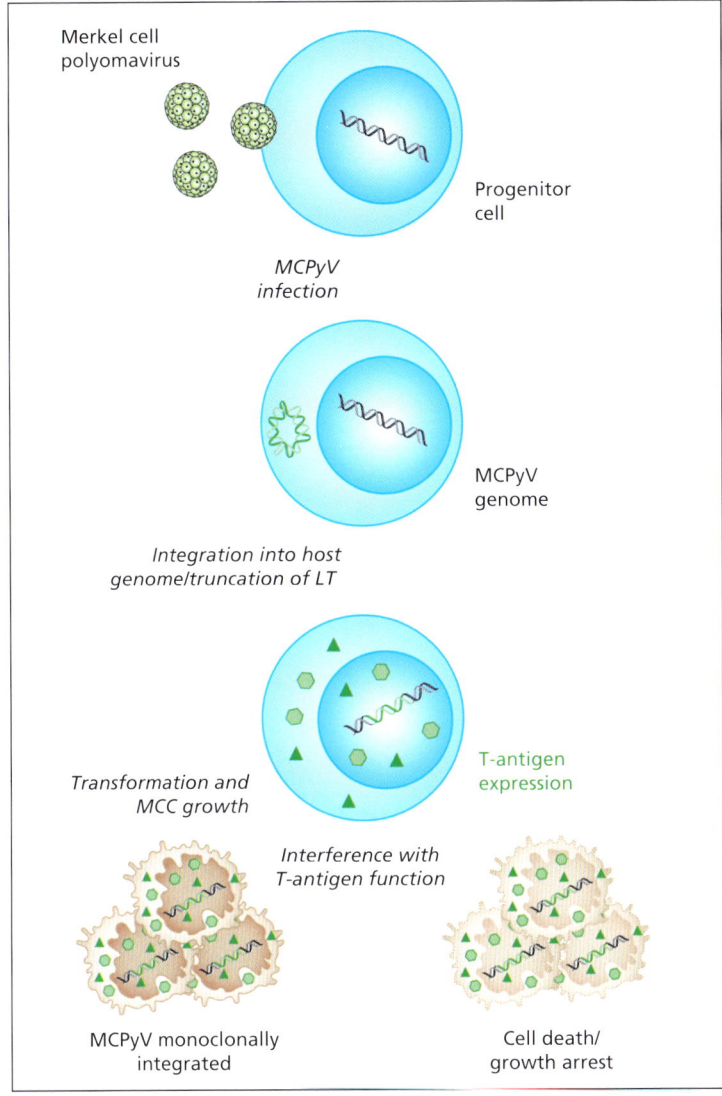

Figure 146.1 Proposed viral carcinogenesis of Merkel cell carcinoma (MCC). Merkel cell polyomavirus (MCPyV) must enter host cells by endocytosis and navigate through various intracellular compartments, where they undergo sequential conformational changes, which enable them to uncoat and deliver the DNA genome into the nucleus. Since the MCPyV genome is found clonally integrated in all MCC lesions of one patient, it is assumed that integration occurs prior to transformation. The interference with the function of the virally encoded early genes, that is, the small and large T antigen (LT) in MCPyV-positive MCC cell lines, caused growth arrest and cell death; thus, such interference may represent a therapeutic approach to tackle MCC.

in individuals treated with UVA photochemotherapy and the observation that many patients with MCC have a history of other skin cancers associated with sun exposure [38,39]. Whether UV light contributes to MCC development directly or indirectly by immunosuppression is probably different for MCPyV-positive and -negative MCCs [40]. It is generally accepted that UV exposure can suppress immune responses and permit progression of immunogenic tumours, whereas MCPyV-negative MCCs carry a molecular UV signature (DNA mutations that are typically caused by UV damage, such as C to T transitions that occur in the context of dipyrimidines: C[C>T]N and N[C>T]C), suggesting a direct role for UV in tumour carcinogenesis.

Pathology

From a histological point of view, MCC is defined as a primary malignant tumour of the skin harbouring both epithelial and neuroendocrine differentiation. Under microscopic examination, MCC almost always infiltrates the dermis and/or subcutaneous tissues without connection with the overlying epidermis, although connections with appendages might be observed (Figure 146.2) [41]. Classic MCC tumour cell features include a high nucleocytoplasmic ratio, scant cytoplasm, round nucleus with frequent nuclear moulding and fine, vesicular chromatin (so-called 'salt and pepper'). Mitotic figures and large areas of necrosis are frequent and reflect tumour aggressiveness. Most MCCs already demonstrate lymphatic and vascular invasion at the first histopathological diagnosis. Trabecular, diffuse or solid architectures have been described without prognostic impact and are frequently intermixed in tumour specimens [41]. Histological features of the tumours associated with poor outcome include tumour size (≥5 mm), extension into the subcutaneous tissue, vascular invasion and a blurred boundary. Notably, quantification of the CD8(+) tumour infiltrating lymphocytes was identified as an additional relevant marker to predict patient outcome, particularly if combined with T-cell receptor repertoire analysis [42,43]. Indeed, T-cell lymphocytes targeting MCPyV T antigens are often present in the tumour microenvironment of MCC patients [44], and therefore CD8 density is likely to reflect the antitumour immune response [42]. In contrast, the prognostic impact of MCPyV in MCC is currently controversial, with virus-negative tumours tending to present at more advanced stages and thus having worse outcomes.

Since MCC belongs to the spectrum of 'basophilic, round tumour cell' proliferations, the differential diagnosis includes haematological malignancies, naevoid/small cell variants of melanoma and rare superficial forms of sarcomas, notably Ewing sarcoma. In this context immunohistochemistry is mandatory for MCC diagnosis confirmation (Table 146.1), demonstrating dual epithelial and neuroendocrine differentiation [41]. Indeed, MCC tumours coexpress epithelial markers, notably cytokeratins and epithelial cell adhesion molecule (EPCAM), and neuroendocrine markers, including chromogranin A, synaptophysin, CD56 and INSM1 [45]. Of note, frequent positivity of MCC tumour cells for markers observed in haematological (PAX5 (a B-cell-specific activating protein) and TdT (terminal desoxynucleotidyl transferase)) [19] and soft tissue malignancies (CD99) [46] should not lead to misdiagnoses.

Morphological similarities and shared dual epithelial and neuroendocrine differentiation make metastasis of an extracutaneous neuroendocrine carcinoma, mostly from the lung, the most challenging differential diagnosis for MCC. Immunohistochemistry is a crucial tool in resolving these entities. Cytokeratin 20 expression with a paranuclear dot-like pattern as well as neurofilament and SATB2 are hallmarks of MCC [41,47], whereas these markers are almost lacking in extracutaneous neuroendocrine tumours. By contrast, expressions of thyroid transcription factor 1 (TTF-1) and cytokeratin 7 are frequently observed in extracutaneous cases, and are restricted to only a small subset of MCC (<10%) [47]. The detection of MCPyV either by immunohistochemistry or polymerase chain reaction (PCR) is an additional performant tool to confirm the primary skin origin of MCC [48]. Importantly, a combination of immunohistochemical panel and virus detection is crucial in cases of MCC of the lymph nodes without a detectable skin primary, which should

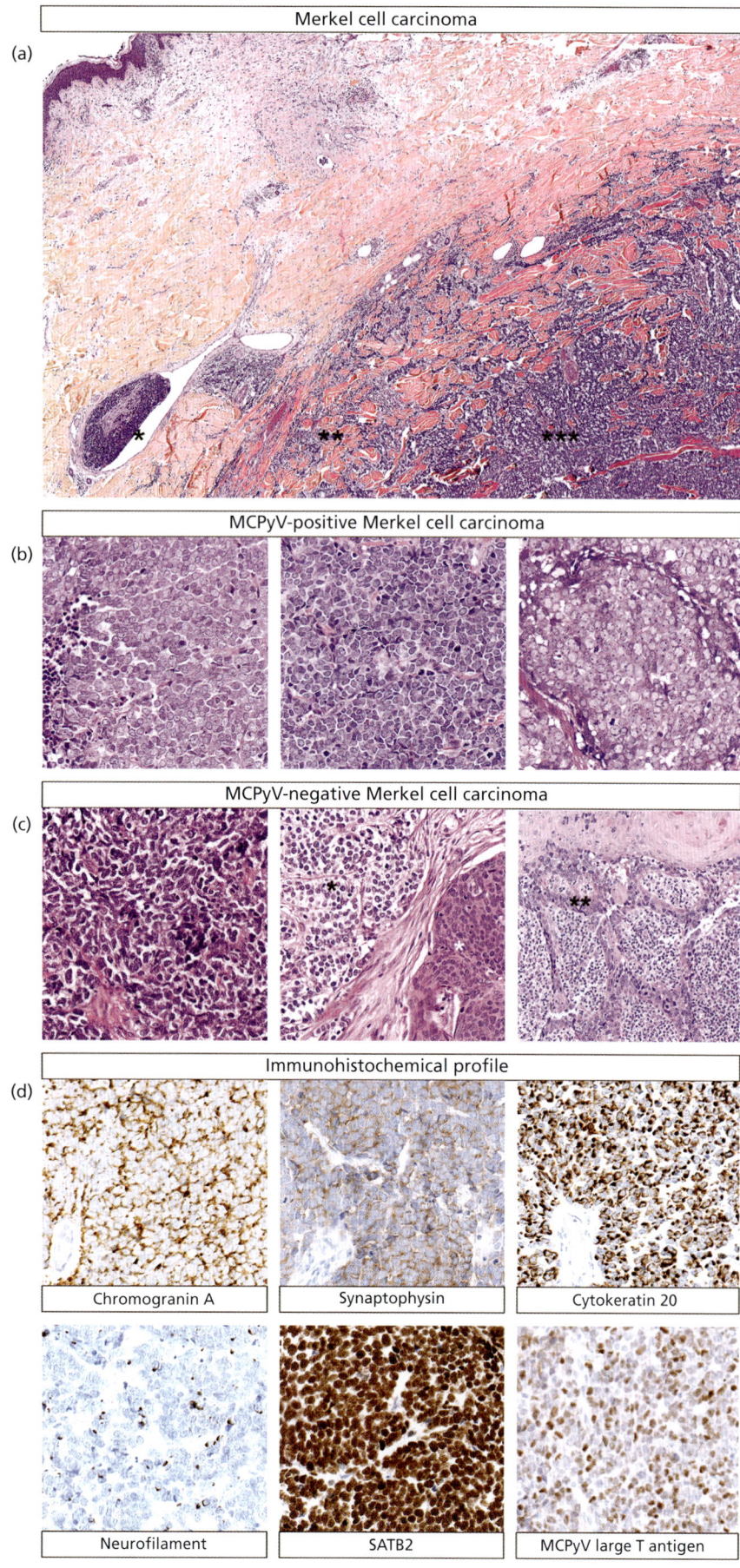

Figure 146.2 Histomorphological and immunophenotypical features of Merkel cell carcinoma (MCC). (a) General morphological features of MCC. At low magnification MCC appears a malignant proliferation of tumour cells invading the dermis and subcutaneous tissues without connection with the overlining epidermis. Vascular invasion is present (*). The tumour cells harbour both trabecular (**) and solid (***) patterns. Magnification 1.25× (haematein–phloxin–saffron). (b) Morphological features of Merkel cell polyomavirus (MCPyV)-positive MCC. MCPyV-positive tumour cells have a high nucleocytoplasmic ratio, round to oval nuclei and clear and dusty so-called 'salt and pepper' chromatin. (c) Morphological features of MCPyV-negative MCC. MCPyV-negative cases harbour irregular spindle nuclei and more abundant clear cytoplasm. Combined tumours consisting of MCPyV-negative MCC (black *) and squamous cell carcinoma (white *) may be seen. In addition, MCPyV-negative MCC might harbour an epidermotropic component (**). Magnification 20× (H&E). (d) Immunophenotypical features of MCC. MCC sections were stained with the indicated antibodies, which were visualised by 3,3′-diaminobenzidine (DAB) stain. Magnification 20×.

Table 146.1 Immunohistochemical markers of Merkel cell carcinoma (MCC).

Antigen	MCPyV(+) MCC	MCPyV(–) MCC	Lymphoma	Melanoma	eNEC	BCC
Cytokeratins	+	+	–	–	+	+
Synaptophysin	+	+	–	–	+/–	+/–
Chromogranin A	+/–	+/–	–	–	+/–	+/–
Melan-A/MART-1	–	–	–	+	–	–
CD45	–	–	+	–	–	–
Cytokeratin 20	+	+/–	–	–	–	–
SATB2	+	+/–	+/–	–	–	–
Neurofilament	+	+/–	–	–	–	–
LTA	+	–	–	–	–	–
Cytokeratin 7	–	+/– (weak)	–	–	+	+/–
TTF-1	–	+/– (weak)	–	–	+	–
BerEP4	+	+	–	–	–	+

BCC, basal cell carcinoma; eNEC, extracutaneous neuroendocrine carcinoma; LTA, large T antigen; MCC, Merkel cell carcinoma; MCPyV, Merkel cell polyomavirus.

be distinguished from other metastatic neuroendocrine carcinomas due to the significant variations in prognosis and management [49]. On a small-sized biopsy, an additional potential pitfall is to misdiagnose MCC as basal cell carcinoma due to a partial overlap in morphology and immunohistochemical profile [50]. Indeed, the expression of BerEP4, a well-known basal cell carcinoma marker, is observed in the majority of MCC cases, and neuroendocrine marker positivity is frequent in basal cell carcinoma. In addition, neuroendocrine differentiation might be observed in rare endocrine mucin-producing sweat gland carcinoma and in the closely related low-grade neuroendocrine tumours of the skin [51]. No expression of cytokeratin 20, special AT-rich sequence-binding protein 2 (SATB2) or neurofilament, however, has been detected in these entities.

Depending on MCC aetiology, several phenotypic variations can be detected. Features mostly observed in MCPyV-negative tumours are irregular/spindle nuclei, abundant clear cytoplasm, the presence of ulceration [52], intraepidermal involvement [53] and association with epidermal tumours or the presence of a divergent differentiation [22,54]. Although the ability of cytological analysis to predict virus status remains to be tested, association of MCC with *in situ* or invasive squamous cell carcinoma is highly suggestive of a MCPyV-negative tumour. In addition, an 'aberrant' immunophenotype, with frequent negativity for cytokeratin 20 (9%) and/or neurofilament (25%) and weak positivity for cytokeratin 7 (8%) and TTF-1 (11%), are more frequently observed in MCPyV-negative MCC cases than in others [41,47]. Importantly, in this setting the use of a large immunohistochemical panel as well as the detection of an *in situ* component, and negativity of the extended work-up, allow the confirmation of a primary cutaneous origin of the tumour in most cases.

Clinical features
History and presentation
MCC is a fast-growing, asymptomatic solitary, firm, non-sensitive, flesh to red to violaceous nodule with a smooth, shiny surface (Figure 146.3) [55]. MCC usually develops and grows rapidly over weeks to months on chronically sun-damaged skin. Thus, the predominant sites are the head and neck (more than half of cases) and extremities (one-third of cases), whereas the trunk as well as the oral and genital mucosa are involved in less than 10% of cases. The clinical appearance of MCC results from the fact that the tumour usually grows hemispherically in depth, so that the intact epidermis is stretched. In addition to the most common nodular type of MCC, rarely plaque-like variants occur, especially on the trunk. Ulceration of primary MCC tumours is rarely observed and mostly occurs in advanced disease. In contrast, satellite metastases are frequently observed (Figure 146.4). They often exhibit overlying telangiectasia, making MCC lesions easily confused with basal cell carcinoma. Altogether, the clinical presentation of MCC may be ambiguous and can be confused with a number of either benign (cysts, lipomas, dermatofibromas, vascular lesions) or malignant (basal cell carcinoma, lymphoma, sarcoma, cutaneous metastases) conditions. Thus, clinical diagnosis of MCC can be challenging. To aid the clinical diagnosis, the acronym AEIOU has been proposed to describe the most common clinical characteristics of MCC: *a*symptomatic, *e*xpanding rapidly, *i*mmune suppression, *o*lder than 50 years, *u*ltraviolet-exposed site on fair skin. Almost 90% of MCCs exhibit at least three of these five features (Table 146.2) [56].

Disease course and prognosis
In addition to the prognostic histopathological markers discussed earlier, several favourable prognostic factors have been identified, including primary tumour size ≤2 cm, local disease, female gender and primary tumour localised on the upper limb [57]. In addition, several studies confirmed the prognostic significance of unimpaired immune function [58]. However, lymph node status is the most important independent predictor including occult microscopic nodal involvement, which is present in one-third of patients [59–61].

Staging
The first consensus staging system for MCC was published in 2010 by the American Joint Committee on Cancer (AJCC), which replaced a number of older systems that are no longer generally accepted [57]. The AJCC staging system is based on 4700 MCC cases from the National Cancer Database (NCDB) and defines four stages (I to IV) based on clinical and pathological characteristics; stages I to III are further subdivided. Stage is determined from information about the primary tumour (T), regional lymph nodes (N) and metastases (M) at the time of initial diagnosis by grouping cases with similar prognoses (Table 146.3).

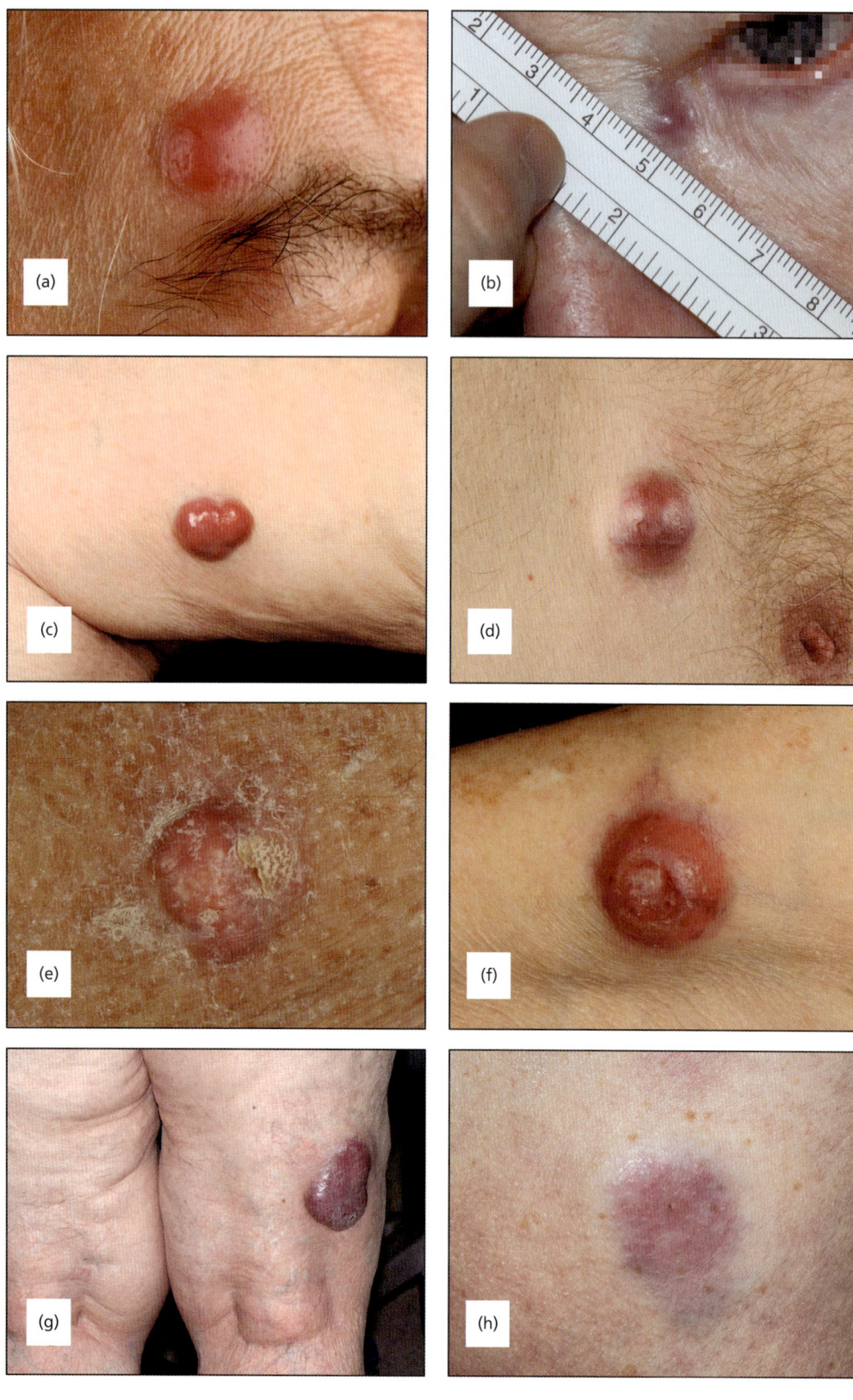

Figure 146.3 Primary tumour. (a–d) Primary Merkel cell carcinoma (MCC) appears as a fast-growing, asymptomatic, solitary, firm, non-sensitive, flesh to red to violaceous nodule with a smooth, shiny surface. (e, f) Ulcerations of MCC primaries are rarely observed and mostly occur in advanced tumours. (g, h) Besides the more frequent nodular type of MCC, plaque-like variants occur, especially on the trunk and the lower extremities.

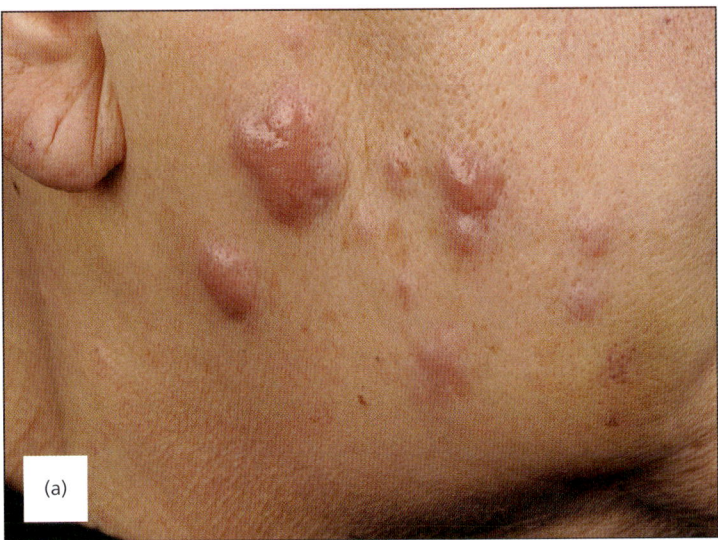

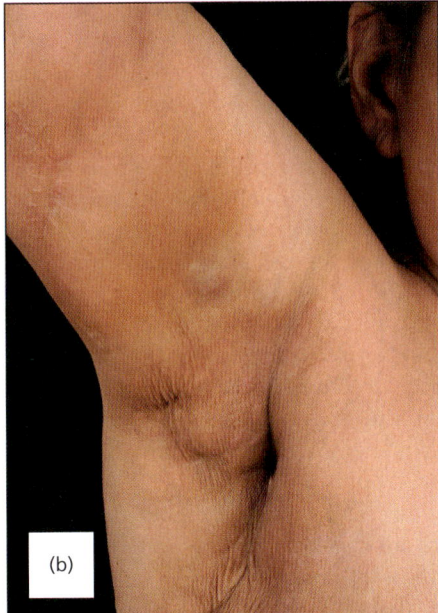

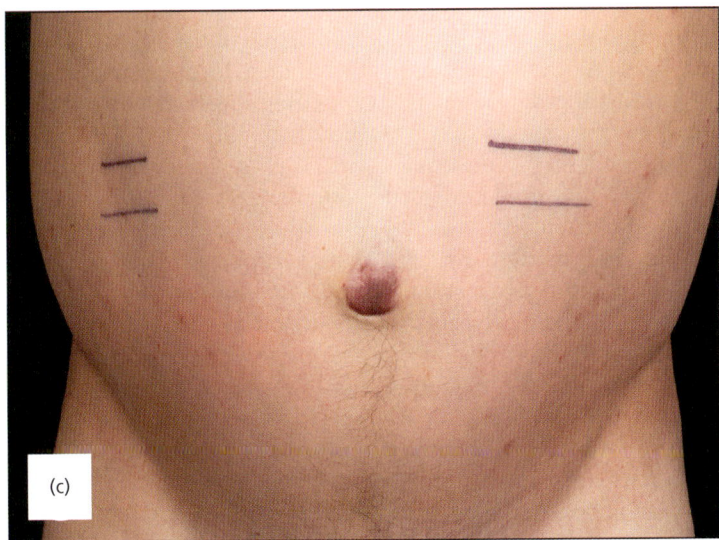

Figure 146.4 Metastatic Merkel cell carcinoma (MCC): (a) satellite, (b) lymph node and (c) distant cutaneous metastases. The latter appeared as a 'Sister Mary Joseph nodule' in a patient suffering from peritoneal carcinogenesis causing severe ascites.

Table 146.2 Summary of the most common clinical characteristics of Merkel cell carcinoma (MCC).

AEIOU parameter	Percentage
Asymptomatic	88%
Expanding rapidly	63%
Immune suppressed	7.8%
Older than age 50	90%
UV exposed	81%
No. of criteria met by primary MCC:[a]	
≥3 criteria	89%
≥4 criteria	32%
5 criteria	7%

Adapted from Heath et al. 2008 [56].
[a] For those where all five criteria are known.

The T category is classified by measuring the maximum dimension of the primary tumour: 2 cm or less (T1), more than 2 but less than 5 cm (T2) and more than 5 cm (T3); extracutaneous invasion into bone, muscle, fascia or cartilage is classified as T4. Increasing tumour size is associated with a modestly poorer prognosis.

The N category is related to the nodal tumour burden. Due to the high propensity for clinically inapparent lymph node metastases, true lymph node negativity by pathological evaluation (pN0) alludes to a better prognosis compared with patients whose lymph nodes are only evaluated by clinical or ultrasound examination (cN0). N1a represents microscopic and N1b macroscopic (i.e. clinically apparent) lymph node metastases. N2 refers to the presence of in-transit metastases.

The M category for distant metastatic disease comprises three groups: M1a includes distant skin, subcutaneous tissues or lymph nodes; M1b is lung; and M1c all other visceral organ sites or brain metastases.

The prognostic groups defined by these categories are summarised in Table 146.3 with corresponding 3-year and 5-year survival rates [62]. However, it should be kept in mind that these rates are based on the NCDB and unfortunately do not allow the calculation of disease-specific survival. This is a significant limitation for a disease such as MCC that affects predominantly older individuals who frequently suffer from significant co-morbidities. In a recent study from two high-volume centres, overall and disease-specific survivals (OS and DSS, respectively) for 409 patients were analysed, revealing a 5-year OS of 70% whereas the 5-year DSS was 84% [63].

Investigations

After a confirmed diagnosis of a primary MCC, clinically indicated imaging may be useful in identifying distant metastases considering the metastatic potential of this tumour. In general, it is currently recommended to perform at least an ultrasound of the draining lymph nodes and the abdomen as well as a chest X-ray [64]. It should be noted, however, that the main value of chest X-ray at the time of diagnosis is to provide a basis of comparison for future diagnostics. Positron emission tomography/computed tomography (PET/CT) scanning is gaining importance in diagnostic imaging of MCC and may be preferred even at initial diagnosis [61]. Due to the high frequency of lymphatic metastases, sentinel lymph node biopsy (SLNB) is generally advised to allow pathological evaluation

Table 146.3 Staging of Merkel cell carcinoma (MCC) and predicted 3- and 5-year survival rates.

Stage		Primary tumour	Nodes	Distant metastases	3-year survival	5-year survival
I	A	≤2 cm (T1)	Pathological negative (pN0)	None (M0)	86%	79%
	B	≤2 cm (T1)	Clinical negative (cN0)	None (M0)	70%	60%
II	A	≥2 cm (T2/T3)	Pathological negative (pN0)	None (M0)	64%	58%
	B	≥2 cm (T2/T3)	Clinical negative (cN0)	None (M0)	58%	49%
	C	Extracutaneous invasion (T4)	Negative (N0)	None (M0)	55%	47%
III	A	Any T	Micrometastasis (N1a)	None (M0)	50%	42%
	B	Any T	Macrometastasis (N1b) or in transit metastasis (N2)	None (M0)	34%	26%
IV		Any T	Any N	Beyond regional nodes (M1)	20%	18%
	A	Any T	Any N	Skin, soft tissue, distant nodes (M1a)		
	B	Any T	Any N	Lung (M1b)		
	C	Any T	Any N	All other visceral sites (M1c)		

Adapted from Lemos et al. 2010 [62].

of the sentinel lymph nodes, especially since micrometastases seem to denote poorer prognosis (see earlier) [62]. When distant metastases are suspected, the appropriate organ imaging should be performed. The most frequently involved organ systems are the skin, lymphatics and liver; however, all organ systems may be potentially affected including the central nervous system. Somatostatin-receptor scintigraphy is not well suited for determining disease spread; the usefulness of DOTATOC (DOTA^0-Phe^1-Tyr^3 octreotid) and fluorodeoxyglucose (FDG) PET/CT scans has not yet been conclusively shown, although recent studies suggest their high sensitivity in detecting organ metastases [65,66].

Management
General principles of management
There is a consensus that the mainstay of therapy for patients with newly diagnosed primary MCC is surgery [67]. Apart from this, the optimal therapy management strategy for MCC is controversially discussed, and there is no broad consensus on for example margins of excision, adjuvant radiotherapy, and palliative systemic therapy in stage IV. Owing to the rarity of MCC, there remains a lack of randomised trials to determine the most appropriate therapy in any stage. Thus, a multidisciplinary approach to the treatment of MCC is essential to optimise outcomes.

Primary tumour and locoregional metastases
For primary tumours without signs of organ metastases, complete surgical excision is considered basic therapy. Given the high rate of local recurrences, which generally are due to subclinical satellite metastases, the National Comprehensive Cancer Network recommends excision with 1–2 cm margins around the clinically apparent primary tumour if this does not result in functional impairment. A recent study analysing more than 6000 patients confirmed that clinical margins larger than 1.0 cm were associated with an improved OS, which was independent of tumour subsite or adverse pathological features for stage I to stage II MCC [68]. However, patients with excision margins of less than 1.0 cm who received adjuvant radiotherapy experienced OS rates that were similar to those of patients with larger margins who did not receive radiotherapy [68].

At certain locations, in which only a small safety margin is possible, complete histological inspection of the margins of the excised material (e.g. with 3D histology), including immunohistochemistry, should be performed [69]. Unfortunately, prospective studies of such situations are still lacking. Furthermore, it should be noted that most of the recurrences are due to satellite or in transit metastasis than to incomplete excision of the primary tumour and that the correct histological diagnosis of MCC on frozen section is challenging. For local recurrences, surgical resection is also the treatment of choice; here, the treatment intention is still curative.

Due to the high frequency of lymphogenous metastasis, an SLNB should be performed for risk stratification [60,61,70]. Whether the indication for an SLNB should be based on tumour size or on other characteristics is still under discussion. The majority of publications report lymph node involvement even with small tumours, so that an SLNB is generally recommended for all patients [71]. Given the very high rate of lymphogenous metastasis of MCC in the head and neck region, an SLNB should not be performed, but rather a functional neck dissection should be considered [72]. If the SLNB is positive, a therapeutic lymphadenectomy of the affected region is warranted, although there are currently no prospective studies demonstrating a benefit from this procedure [73,74].

MCCs are usually highly sensitive to ionising radiation therapy (RT) (Figure 146.5). Retrospective analyses have shown that high local rates of recurrence after a R0 resection of the primary tumour can be significantly reduced by combined locoregional adjuvant RT (irradiating the skin area surrounding the excision scar with a 3 cm safety margin as well as the next regional lymph node station) [75]. Indeed, literature reviews on 1254 patients demonstrated that adjuvant RT reduced local recurrence from 39% to 12% and regional recurrence from 56% to 23%, respectively [56]. Similarly, multivariate analysis demonstrated that postoperative RT is the only significant predictive factor for relapse-free survival. Hence, for primary MCCs and local recurrences adjuvant RT of the tumour region and regional lymphatic drainage area are recommended (depending on the anatomical proximity, either together or separately). In the only randomised study on additive RT of the lymphatic drainage area, RT achieved a significant reduction in regional recurrences [76]. It is still uncertain whether, given histologically negative sentinel nodes, one can forgo treatment of the regional lymphatic drainage region [73,77,78]. Thus, in many hospitals and clinics, an expectant approach is taken for involvement of the axilla and groin, while an active approach is taken for the head and neck region.

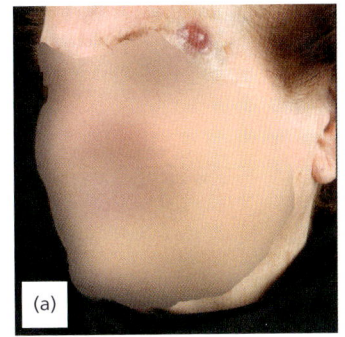
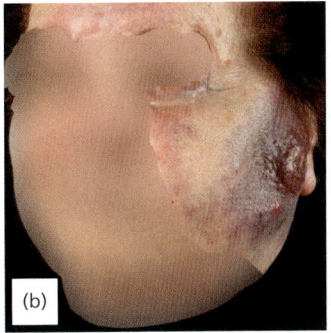
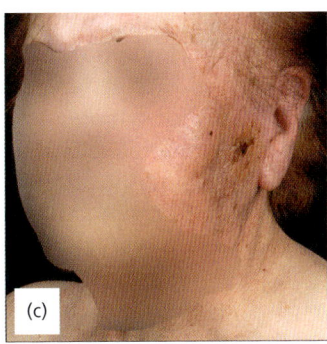

Figure 146.5 Response to radiotherapy. Primary tumour (a) and subsequent locoregional metastases prior (b) and after (c) radiation therapy.

If an R0 resection is not possible in locoregional tumour manifestations, RT may be considered [79,80]. The total dose for adjuvant treatment is ≥50 Gy with a single dose of 2 Gy five times a week [81]. The literature currently tends to report on the higher dosage level, without demonstrating a significant additional improvement in local tumour control. For prevention of lymph node metastasis, there are still not sufficient data showing the advantage of adjuvant RT of the lymphatic drainage area. However, if there are clinically detectable metastases present and a complete lymph node dissection is not possible, a total dose of ≥55 Gy can achieve good local control [81].

Some studies also advocate the use of RT for primary tumours instead of surgery [82–84]. Indeed, when RT was used as the exclusive treatment for unresectable disease, the control rate was found to be similar to that observed for conventional treatment combining wide excision and RT. Only a few reports on the effect of RT dose and volume in the treatment of MCC either in the adjuvant (both primary and nodal) or palliative setting (for gross primary and/or nodal disease) have been published. In a retrospective analysis of 112 patients, a different dose–response correlation was observed for subclinical and gross MCC: doses of 50 Gy or more for subclinical disease and 55 Gy or more for gross disease provided the best disease control rates [81].

The therapeutic usefulness of adjuvant chemotherapy has not yet been demonstrated. Hence, outside of controlled studies, a recommendation in this regard cannot be made.

Distant metastases – stage IV

Until the first reports on the high efficacy of immunotherapy [85,86,87,88], MCC was treated like other high-grade small cell neuroendocrine cancers with chemotherapy agents such as cisplatin and etoposide. MCC has a high rate of initial response to chemotherapy (c.65%), but the responses are seldom durable and average OS was less than 1 year for metastatic disease.

While most of the attention with respect to tumour immunology and immunotherapy of skin cancer was focused on melanoma, the notion that immunosuppressed patients have a dramatically higher risk of developing MCC than melanoma already suggested a possible success of immunotherapeutic strategies in MCC [10,11]. Moreover, the disease in immunosuppressed patients displays an increased aggressiveness, with higher recurrence rates, increased rate of regional metastasis, impaired response to therapy and higher mortality [89]. Conversely, even metastatic MCC lesions may regress upon cessation of immunosuppression [90]. Viral carcinogenesis of MCC and the oncogenic addiction to continuous expression of viral oncogenes explain the exquisite immunogenicity of the majority of MCCs. The remaining virus-negative MCCs are characterised by a high mutational burden with a UV signature, resulting in numerous neoantigens. Adaptive immune responses may induce PD-L1 expression on tumour and stroma cells causing exhaustion of tumour-specific T cells, which is particularly relevant in patients with a constricted T-cell receptor repertoire such as elderly patients. Thus, reversal of this immune evasion mechanism through PD-1/PD-L1 blocking antibodies was predicted to be highly efficacious in MCC patients.

Indeed, several clinical trials confirmed the efficacy of immune checkpoint blocking antibodies in the treatment of patients with advanced MCC, resulting in the registration of avelumab and pembrolizumab for this indication. A clinical trial using the PD-L1 inhibitor avelumab in patients who had previously progressed after chemotherapy reported response rates of 33% and a 1-year OS of 52% [85,86]. Avelumab was subsequently tested in treatment-naïve patients, inducing response rates of 62% [91]. The fact that PD-L1 inhibition was less effective when used after chemotherapy suggests that the cytotoxic agents may harm immune effector cells and attenuate the response to subsequent immunotherapy. An impressive therapeutic effect of inhibiting the PD-1/PDL-1 checkpoint axis in MCC was further confirmed with the PD-1 inhibitor pembrolizumab [87,88]. The response rate in treatment-naïve patients was 56%, including 24% complete responders. Importantly, the responses to immunotherapy are not only frequent, but have a rapid onset (days to weeks) and are durable. Due to these characteristics, pembrolizumab and avelumab are now considered the current standard of care for first line treatment of metastatic MCC; up to now these drugs have not been directly compared against each other. While the efficacy of immune checkpoint inhibitors in advanced MCC is impressive, a significant proportion of patients still do not respond at all (primary resistance) or progress after initial clinical benefit (secondary resistance) [92]. Whereas possible biomarkers predicting resistance are emerging, they still have not been validated in prospective cohorts [93]. Thus, there still is a significant unmet need for these patients. Multiple clinical trials are investigating RT, other checkpoint inhibitors, oncolytic viruses, Toll-like receptor agonists, cytokine therapy, vaccines, adoptive T-cell therapy, inhibition of the MDM2 protein or epigenetic modifiers as ways to augment immunotherapy responses in MCC.

Actively recruiting trials can be searched at http://clinicaltrials.gov and https://eudract.ema.europa.eu (both last accessed February 2022).

For MCC patients refractory to immunotherapy, irradiation as part of a multimodal treatment approach along with surgical excisions and/or systemic chemotherapy may be considered [94]. Particularly for symptomatic patients refractory to immunotherapy and not eligible for clinical trials, chemotherapy may provide symptom control and thus improve the quality of life even if only for a limited time. This procedure should be considered on an individual case-by-case basis, however, and is generally performed with a palliative intent.

MCC, similar to other neuroendocrine tumours, is a primarily chemosensitive tumour [95]. However, regarding the toxicity of most chemotherapy agents, doses and regimens should be adjusted for elderly patients (limited liver and renal function as well as haematopoiesis), that is, it is essential to take into account the principles of geriatric oncology [62]. A standard chemotherapy treatment for MCC has not yet been established. In the past, various schemes were often selected that were primarily established for the treatment of small cell lung cancer. Anthracyclines, antimetabolites, taxanes, bleomycin, cyclophosphamide, etoposide and platinum derivatives can be used either as monotherapy or as combined effective systemic treatments [95]. Although combination treatments can achieve relatively high response rates, given the generally short period of remission there is no significant improvement in survival (median survival of 8 months) [95]. To date, there is no apparent correlation known between the treatment intensity and response; however data from various prospective studies are not available. An alternative to combination therapy is sequential monochemotherapy. Well-tolerated monotherapy options are taxanes, etoposide and anthracyclines [95].

Follow-up

At present there are no scientifically validated studies on the follow-up care of MCC patients [96–98]. In general, clinical follow-ups at 3-month intervals are performed given the high risk of local recurrences or regional lymph node metastases in the first 2 years after removal of the primary tumour. However, in high-risk patients 6-weekly clinical follow-ups may be considered. After 2 years, follow-up is recommended at 6-month intervals and may later be prolonged into semiannual visits. At every second visit, besides the clinical examination including lymph node palpation, imaging of the regional lymph node stations should be performed. Once a year, an upper abdominal ultrasound and a chest radiograph or CT scans may be considered. The usefulness of FDG- or DOTATOC-PET studies as a part of follow-up has not yet been established [99]. The follow-up period is generally restricted to 5 years given that the majority of recurrences occur during this time.

Resources

Guidelines
AWMF (Working Group of Scientific Medical Societies): www.awmf.org.
National Cancer Institute: https://www.cancer.gov/types/skin/patient/merkel-cell-treatment-pdq.
National Comprehensive Cancer Network: www.nccn.org.

Clinical trials
ClinicalTrials.gov: http://clinicaltrials.gov.
EudraCT (European Union Drug Regulating Authorities Clinical Trials Database): https://eudract.ema.europa.eu.

Patient resources
merkelcell.org: www.merkelcell.org.
National Cancer Institute, Merket cell carcinoma treatment (PDF®) – patient version: http://www.cancer.gov/cancertopics/pdq/treatment/merkelcell/patient.
(All last accessed February 2022.)

Key references

The full list of references can be found in the online version at https://www.wiley.com/rooksdermatology10e

5 Jacobs D, Huang H, Olino K et al. Assessment of age, period, and birth cohort effects and trends in Merkel cell carcinoma incidence in the United States. *JAMA Dermatol* 2021;157:59–65.

15 Starrett GJ, Thakuria M, Chen T et al. Clinical and molecular characterization of virus-positive and virus-negative Merkel cell carcinoma. *Genome Med* 2020; 12:30.

30 Feng H, Shuda M, Chang Y, Moore PS. Clonal integration of a polyomavirus in human Merkel cell carcinoma. *Science* 2008;319:1096–100.

32 Houben R, Shuda M, Weinkam R et al. Merkel cell polyomavirus-infected Merkel cell carcinoma cells require expression of viral T antigens. *J Virol* 2010;84: 7064–72.

49 Kervarrec T, Zaragoza J, Gaboriaud P et al. Differentiating Merkel cell carcinoma of lymph nodes without a detectable primary skin tumor from other metastatic neuroendocrine carcinomas: the ELECTHIP criteria. *J Am Acad Dermatol* 2018;78:964–72.e3.

58 Yusuf MB, Gaskins J, Rattani A et al. Immune status in Merkel cell carcinoma: relationships with clinical factors and independent prognostic value. *Ann Surg Oncol* 2021;28:6154–65.

68 Andruska N, Fischer-Valuck BW, Mahapatra L et al. Association between surgical margins larger than 1 cm and overall survival in patients with Merkel cell carcinoma. *JAMA Dermatol* 2021;157:540–8.

74 Hruby G, Guminski A, Thompson JF. Management of regional lymph nodes in patients with Merkel cell carcinoma following a positive sentinel node biopsy: less may be more, but is either enough? *Ann Surg Oncol* 2019;26:315–17.

87 Nghiem PT, Bhatia S, Lipson EJ et al. PD-1 blockade with pembrolizumab in advanced Merkel-cell carcinoma. *N Engl J Med* 2016;374:2542–52.

93 Spassova I, Ugurel S, Terheyden P et al. Predominance of central memory T cells with high T-cell receptor repertoire diversity is associated with response to PD-1/PD-L1 inhibition in Merkel cell carcinoma. *Clin Cancer Res* 2020;26: 2257–67.

95 Nghiem P, Kaufman HL, Bharmal M, Mahnke L, Phatak H, Becker JC. Systematic literature review of efficacy, safety and tolerability outcomes of chemotherapy regimens in patients with metastatic Merkel cell carcinoma. *Future Oncol* 2017;13:1263–79.

CHAPTER 147

Skin Cancer in the Immunocompromised Patient

Catherine A. Harwood[1], Rubeta N. Matin[2] and Charlotte M. Proby[3]

[1]Department of Dermatology, The Royal London Hospital, London; Centre for Cell Biology and Cutaneous Research, Blizard Institute, Barts and London School of Medicine and Dentistry, Queen Mary University of London, London, UK
[2]Department of Dermatology, Churchill Hospital, Oxford University Hospitals NHS Foundation Trust, Oxford, UK
[3]Division of Molecular and Cellular Medicine, School of Medicine, University of Dundee, Ninewells Hospital, Dundee, UK

Introduction, 147.1
Skin cancer in primary and acquired immunodeficiency: an overview, 147.1
Primary immunodeficiency diseases, 147.1
Acquired immunodeficiency diseases, 147.2
Pathogenesis, 147.5
Ultraviolet radiation and genetic changes, 147.5
Reduced tumour immune surveillance, 147.5
Host genetic predisposition, 147.6
Drugs, 147.6
Oncogenic viruses, 147.8
Ionising radiation, 147.9
Graft-versus-host disease, 147.9
Donor-derived skin malignancy, 147.10
Clinicopathological features of specific skin cancers, 147.10

Keratinocyte cancers, 147.10
Squamous cell carcinoma, 147.10
Actinic keratoses, Bowen disease, field cancerisation and porokeratosis, 147.11
Basal cell carcinoma, 147.12
Melanoma, 147.13
Kaposi sarcoma, 147.14
Merkel cell carcinoma, 147.14
Primary cutaneous lymphoma, 147.15
Skin appendage tumours, 147.16
Sarcomas, 147.16
Sarcomas, 147.16
Management, 147.16
Keratinocyte cancers, 147.16
Melanoma, 147.21
Kaposi sarcoma, 147.23

Merkel cell carcinoma, 147.23
Skin cancer screening and surveillance, 147.24
Initial post-transplant assessment, 147.24
Risk stratification and post-transplant surveillance protocols before first skin cancer, 147.24
Skin cancer follow-up protocols, 147.25
Pre-transplantation screening, 147.25
Surveillance in other immunocompromised patient cohorts, 147.25
Organisations for patients and health care professionals, 147.25
Conclusions, 147.25

Key references, 147.26

Introduction

The immune system plays a critical role in skin cancer initation, progression, recognition and elimination. Compelling epidemiological evidence for this is provided by the significantly increased risk of skin cancers among immunocompromised individuals. Skin cancers in these patient cohorts represent a growing challenge in terms of their frequency and diversity as well as their atypical and often aggressive nature. Associated morbidity and mortality are often considerable, pathogenesis is multifactorial and an evidence base to guide their management is lacking in many key areas.

Skin cancer in primary and acquired immunodeficiency: an overview

Certain primary immunodeficiencies predispose to skin cancer but the greatest burden of disease is associated with acquired immunodeficiency, including immunosuppressive drug therapy (including that required after solid-organ and haematopoietic cell transplantation and for immune-mediated inflammatory disorders) or disease-associated immunosuppression (including non-Hodgkin lymphoma/chronic lymphocytic leukaemia (NHL/CLL) and human immunodeficiency virus (HIV) infection).

Primary immunodeficiency diseases

Primary immunodeficiency diseases (or primary inborn errors of immunity) may predispose to skin cancer. The spectrum of such primary immunodeficiencies associated with skin cancer underscores the complexity of the immunological basis of skin cancer development [1,2]. This is illustrated by the following selected examples.

Epidermodysplasia verruciformis

Epidermodysplasia verruciformis (EV) is a rare genodermatosis characterised by predisposition to persistent infection with beta human papillomavirus (β-HPV) infection [3]. Disseminated plane warts, multiple common warts and pityriasis versicolor-like lesions appear from early childhood. Cutaneous squamous cell carcinomas (cSCCs) develop on ultraviolet (UV) exposed sites in up to 60% of patients from the third decade onwards, with no other abnormalities in most patients. Invasive cSCCs are mainly located on UV-exposed sites, particularly the forehead; they develop slowly and may be locally destructive, but rarely metastasise. Primary EV is considered to be typical genetic EV when β-HPV cutaneous infection results from mutations in genes important in keratinocyte intrinsic immunity (*EVER1/TMC6*, *EVER2/TMC8* and *CIB1*) with no other evidence of compromised T-cell-mediated immunity. Atypical genetic EV is seen with some inborn errors of T-cell immunity, for example due to deficiency in RHOH and MST1, and patients are vulnerable to other infections. Acquired T-cell-deficiency disorders such as HIV and haematological malignancy may also confer an EV-like phenotype [5]. EV is discussed in more detail in Chapter 25.

Severe combined immunodeficiency

Severe combined immunodeficiency (SCID) is caused by deficiency and impaired function of T cells and, in some forms, additional reduction or dysfunction of natural killer (NK) cells and/or B cells. It results from diverse molecular defects in genes including *IL-7R*, *CD45*, *IL-2Rγ*, *JAK3*, *RAG1*, *RAG2*, *ARTEMIS* and *ADA* [1]. An EV-like phenotype may occur in JAK3- and IL-2Rγ-deficient patients after bone marrow transplantation [6]. A similar HPV association is reported in other SCID-like immunodeficiencies such as WHIM syndrome (warts, hypogammaglobulinaemia, infections and myelokathexis) caused by autosomal gain-of-function mutations in CXC chemokine receptor 4 (CXCR4) in which vulvar SCC, basal cell carcinoma (BCC) and cutaneous T-cell lymphoma (CTCL) are reported [7,8]. Autosomal recessive mutations in *DOCK8* cause a combined immunodeficiency syndrome characterised by low T, B and NK cells, elevated serum immunoglobulin E (IgE) levels, depressed IgM levels, eosinophilia, sinopulmonary infections, cutaneous viral infections (HPV, herpes simplex virus and molluscum contagiosum [9]) and malignancy [10]. Mucocutaneous SCCs occur in 19% and are often associated with viral warts. Aggressive CTCL, diffuse large B-cell lymphoma and cutaneous microcystic adnexal carcinoma have also been reported [10].

Common variable immunodeficiency

Common variable immunodeficiency (CVID) encompasses a group of genetic disorders characterised by a failure of B-cell maturation, and are the most common primary immunodeficiencies in adults. The principal defect is in antibody formation and is characterised by hypogammaglobulinaemia, recurrent bacterial infections, autoimmune diseases and malignancy – particularly lymphoma and gastric cancer – with rare reports of cSCC, CTCL and melanoma [2,11,12].

Wiskott–Aldrich syndrome

This is a severe X-linked immunodeficiency caused by mutations in the gene encoding WASP, a key regulator of signalling and cytoskeletal reorganisation in haematopoietic cells. Clinical manifestations include congenital thrombocytopaenia, eczema, recurrent infections and an increased incidence of autoimmunity and malignancy, including head and neck SCC and Kaposi sarcoma (KS) [13].

Dyskeratosis congenita

Dyskeratosis congenita is an inherited bone marrow failure syndrome caused by abnormal telomere maintenance which, in 60% of patients, results from germline mutations in one of at least 11 telomere biology genes. Nail dystrophy, reticulate skin pigmentation and oral leukoplakia are characteristic and patients are at high risk of bone marrow failure, pulmonary fibrosis, liver disease and mucocutaneous SCC [14,15].

Netherton syndrome

This is due to mutations in *SPINK5* and is an autosomal recessive disorder characterised by congenital ichthyosiform erythroderma, trichorrhexis invaginata, atopy, food allergies and asthma [16]. Cutaneous SCCs are reported, with some cases associated with β-HPV infections [17,18].

Acquired immunodeficiency diseases

The total burden of skin cancer resulting from acquired immunodeficiency is far greater than that associated with primary immunodeficiency disorders [**19**]. The exact magnitude is difficult to quantify because accurate population-based data on incidence rates of many skin cancers, particularly keratinocyte carcinomas (KCs), are incomplete [20]. The spectrum of acquired immune-related conditions associated with increased skin cancer risk is broad [21] and includes people living with HIV infection (PLWH), haematological malignancy (particularly non-Hodgkin lymphoma/chronic lymphocytic leukaemia), immunosuppressive drug therapy (e.g. following solid-organ or haematopoietic cell transplantation) and immune-mediated inflammatory disorders (e.g. inflammatory bowel disease and rheumatoid arthritis) (Table 147.1).

HIV infection (Chapter 31)

Worldwide there are an estimated 37.9 million people living with HIV (https://www.hiv.gov/hiv-basics/overview/data-and-trends/global-statistics; last accessed March 2023). They have a 1.5–2-fold elevated risk of malignancy [22] and the proportion of adult PLWH aged 65 years or older is projected to triple between 2010 and 2030, with a consequent further increase in this burden [23]. Antiretroviral therapy (ART) has reduced the incidence of acquired immune deficiency syndrome (AIDS) defining cancers (ADC) include KS, NHL and cervical cancer, with a shift to predominantly non-AIDS-defining cancers (NADC) [22–24].

KCs are among the most common cutaneous NADCs with standardised incidence ratios (SIRs) of 2.1–5.4, which are lower in patients on ART [25,26,**27**]. In contrast to solid-organ transplant recipients (SOTRs), in whom there is a reversal of the usual BCC : cSCC ratio of 3–4 : 1 seen in the general population, this ratio is maintained in PLWH who have CD4 counts >500 cells/μL. The duration of HIV infection is the main risk factor for skin cancer [27]. In a Danish cohort there was evidence that the increased risk of BCC in PLWH is restricted to men who have sex with men (MSM), possibly related to increased recreational UV exposure [26]. cSCCs may arise in the context of an EV-like phenotype [28] and appear to predominate when nadir CD4 falls below 200 cells/μL [29,30] and with higher viral load [30], suggesting that immune dysfunction contributes to risk. The incidence of HPV-related anal, penile and vulvar SCC is also increased with SIRs of 19.1, 5.3 and 9.4, respectively [31].

Although the incidence of KS has decreased significantly with ART in PLWH, SIRs approach 500 in the USA, with a prevalence of 6% which is highest in MSM [31]. Merkel cell carcinoma (MCC) incidence is increased 11–13-fold in PLWH [32], but there are conflicting data regarding the increased risk of melanoma, with reported SIRs of between 0.5 and 4 [33]. Recent cohort studies suggest there is no clear association of melanoma with immune dysfunction but rather as association with age and UV exposure in PLWH [21,26].

Table 147.1 Risk estimates for skin cancers in the immunosuppressed.[a]

Cancer SIR	OTR	NHL/CLL	HSCT	HIV/PLWH	IBD	RA
cSCC	65–480	5–8	18	2.6–4	1.2–5	1.5–1.7
BCC	4.5–10	4–8	3	2.1	1.2	
Melanoma	1.35–5	2–8	5	0.8–12.6	1.09	1.2–2.3
Kaposi sarcoma	40–200	3–5	3–5	450–3640	2–3	2.5
Merkel cell carcinoma	24–142	3–10		12–13.4	2–4	1.4–2.4
Appendageal malignancies	20–100			3.3–7.5		
Vulva/vagina cSCC	7–24			4.4–6.8		
Penis	4.5–25			4–8		

[a] The numbers given summarise risk ranges from references cited in the text.
BCC, basal cell carcinoma; CLL, chronic lymphocytic leukaemia; cSCC, cutaneous squamous cell carcinoma; HIV, human immunodeficiency virus; HSCT, haematopoietic stem cell transplantation; IBD, inflammatory bowel disease; MCC, Merkel cell carcinoma; NHL, non-Hodgkin lymphoma; OTR, organ transplant recipient; PLWH, person living with HIV; RA, rheumatoid arthritis; SIR, standardised incidence ratio.

HIV may have direct cellular and molecular effects that contribute to the development of skin cancer, including activation of proto-oncogenes, alterations in cell cycle regulation, inhibition of tumour suppressor genes, induction of microsatellite instability and promotion of pro-angiogenesis signalling [27]. In addition, there is an increased risk of infection with other skin cancer-associated viruses, including human herpesvirus 8 (HHV-8), Epstein–Barr virus (EBV) and β-HPV [27].

Non-Hodgkin lymphoma/chronic lymphocytic leukaemia

Non-Hodgkin lymphoma is a lymphoproliferative malignancy and includes CLL, which is a clonal B-cell disorder accounting for 25% of all leukaemias [34]. These malignancies are associated with innate defects in both cell and humoral-mediated immune responses, which may be exacerbated by therapy; the overall risk for second malignancies is more than double that of the general population [35,36]. KC risk is increased 4–8-fold and increases with time after diagnosis [37–39], with higher risk in CLL compared with non-CLL NHL and cumulative incidence by 20 years in a US cohort of 43.2% for cSCC and 30.6% for BCC [37]. The risk association between skin cancer and NHL is reciprocal: there is a 2–4-fold increase in melanoma in patients with CLL compared with the general population [40–42] and a similar increased risk for CLL occurs in patients with previous cSCC [43]. More aggressive CLL at the time of diagnosis is predictive of worse cSCC prognosis [39,44] and a previous history of skin cancer increases risk as does male sex, age and previous T-cell immunosuppressive treatments [39,45]. The melanoma standardised mortality ratio (SMR) for patients with CLL is 2.8 in the USA rising to almost 5 in Australia [46], where the overall SMR for KC is 17 [47]. Risk of MCC is increased eightfold and patients are almost four times more likely to develop metastases [46,48]. Risk of KS is increased 2–3-fold and patients with non-CLL NHL have a greater risk of overall and cause-specific death than expected [49]. The incidence of other rare skin malignancies such as sebaceous carcinoma, malignant fibrous histiocytoma and dermatofibrosarcoma protuberans is also increased [40].

Solid-organ transplantation

Skin cancer is a well-recognised complication of immunosuppressive drug treatment. SOTRs, in whom long-term immunosuppressive therapy is required to prevent allograft rejection, represent the largest and most comprehensively studied group. Organ transplantation is a highly successful treatment for end-stage organ failure, with 160 000 organ transplants perfomed worldwide in 2019 (www.transplant-observatory.org; last accessed March 2023). Survival continues to steadily increase, as does the risk of malignancy which is 2–6-fold greater than that of the general population, with a disproportionate increase in four tumour types: KC, post-transplant lymphoproliferative disorders (PTLDs), ano-genital malignancy and KS, with smaller but significant increases in hepatocellular and renal cancers and some sarcomas [50,51].

Spectrum of skin cancers post-transplant

Keratinocyte carcinoma accounts for more than 95% of all post-transplant skin cancer [52,53]. cSCCs predominate with SIRs ranging from 45 to 480, a risk which is significantly greater for those under 50 years and increases with time post-transplant, reaching more than 200 and 300 in renal and cardiac organ transplant recipients (OTRs), respectively, at 10–20 years post-transplant (Table 147.1) [52,53–55,56,57,58]. BCCs are the second most common skin cancer: incidence is increased 5–10-fold, with reversal in the usual 3 or 4 : 1 ratio of BCC : cSCC seen in the general population. This ratio is influenced by time from transplantation since BCC shows a more linear increase compared with an exponential rise in SCC [54]. OTRs with KC also have a threefold increased risk of developing internal malignancies [59]. However, there is recent evidence that KC risk may be declining. A cohort study from Norway showed a significant decline in OTRs transplanted between 1983 and 1992 compared with 2003–2012, and a similar trend was seen in a recent cohort study from Ireland. The reasons for this decline are uncertain, but may include changes in immunosuppressive drug regimens and increased awareness and surveillance [60,61]. Melanoma incidence is increased 2.1–8-fold [55,62–64], with evidence that the risk has increased over the past two decades, in contrast to KC [65]. KS risk is increased approximately 40–200-fold [55], appendageal tumours 20–100-fold [52,66] and MCC up to 60-fold [66,67]. Primary cutaneous lymphoma (PCL) and sarcomas such as dermatofibrosarcoma protuberans (DFSP) and atypical fibroxanthoma (AFX) are also overrepresented, although population-based studies quantifying this risk are few [68,69].

Tumour burden and accrual

The high incidence of skin cancers in OTRs is compounded by their multiplicity, which increases with duration post-transplantation. In a UK OTR cohort, almost 30% of all OTRs who had been transplanted for a median of 10 years had developed skin cancer, rising from 10% at 5 years to almost 75% at 30 years. Two-thirds of affected individuals had more than one skin cancer, with an average of six tumours per patient; a minority of OTRs contributed disproportionately to the total cohort tumour burden, with more than 50% of the total number of cSCCs arising in just 3.4% of individuals [52]. Once the first KC has developed, more than 30% will develop a further KC by 1 year and almost 75% by 5 years [43,70–72] compared with 14.5% and 40.7%, respectively, in the general population [73]. OTRs in one Australian cohort developed an average of 3.35 ± 4.29 tumours per year at 20 years' post-transplant [74]. In a UK cohort, the time interval between subsequent KCs shortened progressively from 24 months to a second cancer, 14.7 and 8.4 months to a third and fourth, respectively; patients with 10 or more tumours developed a new cancer every 3 months and were at increased risk for metastastic disease [52]. Lung OTRs generally require the most intense immunosuppression and consequently develop the highest skin cancer burden [75–77]. A prospective study from Queensland, Australia calculated age-standardised incidence rates of 447 (cSCC) and 281 (BCC) per 1000 person-years: this is 77 times higher than the estimated cSCC incidence rate in the Queensland general population, which is already the highest in the world [77]. Use of voriconazole as prophylaxis for fungal lung infections compounds this risk [77,78].

Population diversity and geographical and environmental influences

Comparisons between studies of post-transplant skin cancer may be complicated by differences in population diversity including skin phototype and ethnicity, in addition to environmental factors – particularly UV and viral exposure – due to geographical location [79]. White people living in Australia have the highest incidence of post-transplant KC, affecting more than 80% of those transplanted for 20 years and the SMR for malignancy is highest for cSCC [80]. Japan and Taiwan report a low incidence of KC and KS, and although also low in Korea, the incidence of KC is still significantly greater than in the general population [81–83]. Two London- and Philadephia-based OTR cohorts that included a significant proportion of OTRs with skin of colour and from diverse countries of origin [52,58,84] reported skin cancer across all groups, although this varied with skin type and country of birth. OTRs with darker skin types were disproportionately affected by malignant genital tumours [84] and KS was more common in those from HHV-8 endemic areas [52,58]. Similarly, post-transplant KS is most common in OTRs from the Mediterranean and from sub-Saharan Africa and is the most common post-transplant malignancy in Saudi Arabia [58,85,86].

Paediatric organ transplant recipients

The spectum of malignancies developing after paediatric organ transplantation differs from that seen in adult OTR populations and skin cancer is rare [87–89]. KC is the most frequent malignancy following renal transplantation, with an average time of onset of 12–18 years post-transplant, and in other organ transplants is the second most common after PTLD [89]. Benign melanocytic naevi are increased [88], and melanoma at an average of 14–16 years post-transplant is proportionately more common in paediatric OTRs, accounting for 15% of all skin cancers [62].

Type of solid-organ transplant

In a population-based study of more than 10 000 OTRs over 20 years, cSCC risk appears to be greatest after cardiac and/or lung transplantation, followed by renal transplantation with risk lowest in liver transplant recipients, possibly related to intensity of immunosuppression [55]. Incidence is particularly high after simultaneous pancreas and kidney transplants, with cSCC reported to be 6.2-fold higher than age- and sex-matched renal transplant recipients [90]. The number of renal transplantations does not appear to increase risk [91], although risk remains elevated during periods on dialysis between transplants [92]; and for patients with a history of cSCC who are then retransplantated, prognosis appears to be worse [93].

Cause of end-stage organ disease

End-stage organ failure itself is associated with a small increased risk of cancer: in one study, the SIR for malignancy was 1.16 before renal replacement therapy, 1.35 during dialysis and 3.27 after renal transplant [50]. A Danish registry study also reported a SIR of 4.8 for cSCC among patients with renal failure, but not for cardiac, lung or liver failure [94]. There is some evidence that the cause of end-stage renal disease may also impact on skin cancer risk. For example, polycystic kidney disease confers a higher risk than diabetic renal disease [95], but no association was identified with causes for end-stage liver disease in a French series [96]. HIV-related organ failure may be predicted to significantly increase risk, but early evidence indicates that rates of skin cancer are relatively low, although HPV-related anal neoplasia may be at an increased risk of progression [97] and KS risk is increased compared with the non-HIV OTR population in a French study [98]. Prerenal transplant immunosuppression in an Australian study increased the risk of ano-genital cancer, NHL and breast and urinary tract cancer but not melanoma or KS, although KC was not included [99].

Vascularised composite tissue allografts

Since the 1990s vascularised composite allotransplantation has aimed to replace non-vital tissues lost usually following severe trauma and has included the hands, forearms and face. Vascularised composite tissue allografts (VCAs) are highly immunogenic and require lifelong immunosuppression, with the accompanying risks of infection and malignancy, and there have been several case reports of BCC and cSCC occurring post-VCA [100].

Haematopoetic stem cell transplantation

Survival after haematopoietic stem cell transplantation (HSCT) for haematological malignancy has increased steadily over the past two decades and secondary solid cancers are an increasingly important late complication. Skin cancers are among the most common neoplasms, accounting for 0–58.5% of secondary neoplasms, and occur in both adult and paediatric populations [101–103]. Chronic graft-versus-host disease (cGVHD), ionising radiation and treatment-related immunosuppression are all recognised as risk

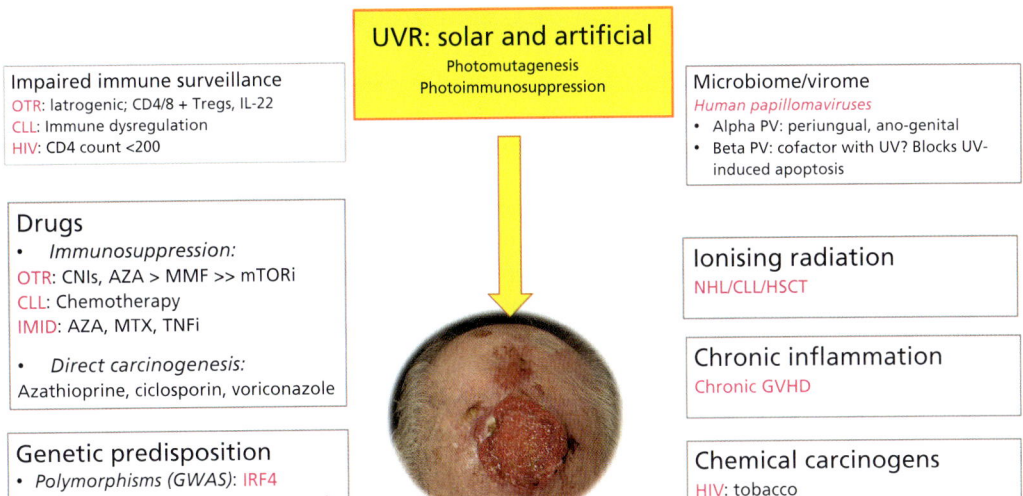

Figure 147.1 Mechanisms contributing to increased skin carcinogenesis in the immunosuppressed. AZA, azathioprine; CLL, chronic lymphocytic leukaemia; CNI, calcineurin inhibitor; GVHD, graft-versus-host disease; GWAS, genome-wide association study; HIV, human immunodeficiency virus; HLA, human leukocyte antigen; HLA-DR, HLA donor–recipient; HSCT, haematopoetic stem cell transplantation; IL-22, interleukin 22; IMID, immune-mediated inflammatory diseases; IRF4, interferon regulatory factor 4; MMF, mycophenylate mofetil; mTORi, mammalian target of rapamycin inhibitor; MTX, methotrexate; NHL, non-Hodgkin lymphoma; OTR, organ transplant recipient; PV, papillomavirus; TNFi, tumour necrosis factor inhibitor; Tregs, regulatory T-lymphocytes; UVR, ultraviolet radiation.

factors. Cumulative incidence estimates for BCC and SCC in one large study at 20 years were 6.5% and 3.4%, respectively [104]. Median time from HSCT to diagnosis is 7.3–9.4 years for BCC and 2.1–7.0 years for cSCC and patients often develop multiple tumours [105]. In one large single centre study, 40 of 209 (19%) patients with secondary malignancy developed a further tumour, including 13 patients with local skin cancer recurrences and 12 patients who presented with cSCC or BCC before other solid malignancies; 22% of long-term survivors' deaths were attributable to secondary neoplasms and four out of five metastatic cSCCs were reported to be the cause of death [106]. Melanoma incidence is also increased with SIRs between 3.5 and 8.3 and half occurring after 1–4 years [107–109].

Immune-mediated inflammatory diseases

Immune-mediated inflammatory diseases (IMIDs) are a clinically diverse group of conditions which include inflammatory bowel disease (IBD, Crohn disease and ulcerative colitis), rheumatoid arthritis (RA), cutaneous inflammatory conditions (e.g. psoriasis), connective tissue disorders (e.g. systemic lupus erythematosus) and autoimmune conditions (e.g. multiple sclerosis) [110] and many are associated with an increased risk of skin cancer [111]. This may be partly due to intrinsic immune dysregulation and other disease-specific pathomechanisms including chronic inflammation. However, most studies have focused on the role of non-biological immunomodulatory and antiproliferative drugs (e.g. azathioprine, ciclosporin, methotrexate), biological immune-targeted therapies particularly the antitumour necrosis factor (anti-TNF) agents (infliximab, adalimumab, etanercept, certolizumab, golimumab) and small-molecular-based immune-targeted therapeutics including Janus kinase (JAK) inhibitors (e.g. tofacitinib, baricitinib, ruxolitinib). This is discussed further in the section on drugs later in this chapter.

Pathogenesis

The pathogenesis of skin cancer arising in the context of immunosuppression is likely to be multifactorial and current evidence suggests a complex interplay primarily between UV radiation (both solar and artificial/therapeutic), altered immune surveillance, drugs, oncogenic viruses, host genetic susceptibility, chronic inflammation and additional environmental carcinogens such as tobacco and ionising radiation (Figure 147.1) [112,113].

Ultraviolet radiation and genetic changes

As in the general population, UV radiation (UVR) is a significant carcinogen and the most important environmental risk factor for skin cancer (Chapter 10). Consistent with this, immunosuppression-associated KC is more prevalent in regions of high ambient UVR, 75% occur on photoexposed body sites, and they are more common in those with fair skin phenotype and a history of both chronic UVR exposure and acute sunburn [52,112–114]. As in the immune-competent population, cSCC and BCC from immunosuppressed individuals have a high prevalence of UV-induced mutations and although there are no clear differences in the spectrum of genetic changes present in tumours from immunocompromised individuals, some of the drugs used in these patients (e.g. ciclosporin, azathioprine, voriconazole) may interact with UVR and directly or indirectly enhance its carcinogenic effects, as may HPV [112,115–117] (see the section on drugs later in this chapter).

Reduced tumour immune surveillance

Ultraviolet exposure has long been known to have profound effects on immune function [118,119] and a deregulated immune system underpins carcinogenesis. However, the additional immune dysregulatory mechanisms in patients immunosuppressed by drugs or disease are not well understood [120]. In general, the incidence of KC in OTRs is proportional to the level of immunosuppression and is associated with lower peripheral CD4 counts [121,122]. Reduction of immunosuppression in OTRs reduces the rate of subsequent accrual of skin cancers [123] (particularly virus-related cancers) and synergy between viral oncogenesis and immune dysregulation (e.g. by enhanced viral replication or integration) may provide additional mechanisms in immunosuppression [124]. The immunophenotype differs in cSCC in OTRs, with higher numbers of circulating T-regulatory cells (Tregs) predictive for new cSCC development [125]. In HIV, the risk of cSCC but not BCC may increase with lower CD4 counts [29]. NHL/CLL is associated with innate immune dysregulation involving complex defects of both humoral and cell-mediated immunity which, independent of treatment-related risk factors, may be sufficient to account for the increased skin cancer risk [37].

In addition to systemic immune dysregulation, the immune tumour microenvironment is also altered in OTR cSCC. The tumour-associated inflammatory infiltrate appears to be reduced with reduced CD4+ T-cell infiltration, decreased cytotoxic CD8+ T cells and increased regulatory T cells in some but not all studies [125–129] and is predicted to lead to a 'cancer permissive' tumour microenvironment with decreased immune surveillance. In addition, impaired antigen presentation through reduced CD123+ plasmacytoid dendritic cells [127] and increased exposure to interleukin 22 (IL-22) may accelerate tumour growth [129] and potentially contribute to the aggressive nature of some OTR cSCC. Elevated CD57 expression on circulating T cells reflecting immunological senescence is also linked to increased OTR skin cancer development and may represent a predictive biomarker for cSCC risk [130].

Host genetic predisposition

Germline single nucleotide polymorphisms (SNPs) associated with an increased risk of skin cancer have been evaluated at the individual SNP level and in genome-wide association studies (GWAS) both in the general population [131–134] and in OTRs [112].

SNPs in pigmentation genes have been extensively studied in the general population. In Norwegian OTRs, variation in the key signalling regulator *MC1R*, but not other pigmentation-associated genes, was associated with a twofold increased cSCC risk, independent of hair colour and skin phototype [135]. Eight pigmentation genes were investigated in relation to time to first cSCC post-transplant: an increased risk was associated with a polymorphism in *IRF4* and a decreased risk with polymorphism of *SLC45A2* [568]. A significant association was also identified between p53 codon 72 arginine homozygosity in cSCC in OTRs but not immunocompetent individuals [136]. Associations have been identified in OTRs with polymorphisms in detoxifying enzymes glutathione-*S*-transferase [137,138] and IL-10 [139], human leukocyte antigen (HLA) alleles and polymorphisms [140,141], *COX2* gene regulatory region variants [142], methylenetetrahydrofolate reductase polymorphisms [143,144], *PTCH1* gene haplotypes [145] and cytochrome P450 enzymes involved in drug metabolism including CYP1A1 [146] and CYP2C19 [147]. Polymorphisms in vitamin D receptor, epidermal growth factor receptor (EGFR), Toll-like receptor 4, 7 and 8 [143] and DNA mismatch repair genes *MSH2* and *MLH1* [148] are not associated with OTR skin cancer.

Until recently none of these genetic alterations were sufficiently robust to use in skin cancer prediction algorithms in OTRs [52,149,150]. However, studies in the general population have demonstrated that polygenic risk scores (PRSs) incorporating SNPs derived from GWAS analyses for BCC and cSCC confer significant predictive value for KC risk beyond clinical variables [151–154]. PRSs derived from the general population have also been evaluated in OTR populations both in low UV and high UV settings. A study from Ireland found that PRS was the most significant predictor of time to post-transplant KC [155,156] and a PRS derived from UK Biobank and 23andMe datasets also improved predictive accuracy for KC in OTRs in an Australian population [157]. The possibility that shared genetic risk factors between CLL and KC contribute to their observed association was explored in a meta-analysis of PRS generated for CLL, BCC and cSCC susceptibility loci. A higher CLL PRS increased BCC risk (but not the reverse) and increased CLL risk was increased with higher cSCC PRS and this was driven by shared genetic susceptibility at the 6p25.3 (IRF4/EXOC2) risk locus [158]. PRS-based approaches may therefore have future clinical utility in improving KC risk stratification in OTRs and in other immunocompromised individuals in combination with clinical risk factor evaluation.

Drugs

Immunosuppressive drugs and transplantation

Current immunosuppressive drug regimens used in transplantation usually use a combination of agents with differing actions at specific sites of the T-cell activation cascade. Immunosuppressive protocols generally consist of two phases: a perioperative induction phase (e.g. OKT3, antithymocyte globulin, basiliximab, daclizumab) followed by a long-term maintenance phase with regimens including calcineurin inhibitors (CNIs) (e.g. ciclosporin, tacrolimus), purine antagonists (e.g. azathioprine, mycophenolate mofetil (MMF)), mammalian target of rapamycin (mTOR) inhibitors (e.g. sirolimus, everolimus) and cytotoxic T-lymphocyte associated protein 4 (CTLA4) inhibitors (e.g. belatacept) [159]. Characteristics of immunosuppressive regimens including duration, use of induction therapy and type of maintenance therapy may all be important risk factors for skin cancer, but establishing the degree of risk conferred by individual drugs is challenging [112].

The overall level of immune suppression may be more important than the effects of specific drugs. Both duration and dose intensity of immunosuppressive drug therapy are relevant: triple versus dual versus monotherapy and higher versus lower dose ciclosporin regimens are associated with increased risk [121], whereas less intensive immunosuppression in liver transplant recipients may account for their lower rates of skin cancer compared with other OTRs [160]. Similarly, the lower skin cancer risk in HSCT recipients reflects the generally shorter duration of immunosuppressive drug use post-transplant compared with OTRs [161]. However, even prolonged use of single-agent oral corticosteroids and azathioprine is associated with a 2–4-fold increased risk of KC [162,163]. In addition to reduced tumour immunosurveillance, certain immunosuppressants have direct effects on carcinogenesis and tumour progression [112]. Azathioprine and ciclosporin have synergistic pro-carcinogenic interactions with UVB and UVA, whereas mTOR inhibitors have direct anticarcinogenic properties [112,164]. Examples of direct pro- and anticarcinogenic mechanisms are discussed in more detail here.

Specific immunosuppressive drugs and skin cancer risk
Purine antagonists
Azathioprine and MMF inhibit the purine pathway and are antiproliferative [164]. A systematic review of skin cancer risk in OTRs confirmed a significantly increased risk of cSCC (but not BCC) (odds

ratio (OR) 1.56, 95% confidence interval (95%CI) 1.11–2.18) when treated with azathioprine compared with other immunosuppressive agents [165]. Observational and clinical trial data in IBD also document an increased risk of KC particularly associated with thiopurine use, although the relative risk is smaller than for OTRs. In a retrospective registry study the adjusted OR was 3.56, rising to 4.27 where thiopurines are used for more than 12 months [163]. A similar effect of thiopurines was confirmed in a separate retrospective cohort study [166], a prospective observational cohort study [167] and a meta-analysis [168]. The risk is higher for cSCC compared with BCC [169,170], and this increased cSCC risk is also seen in patients on biological therapy with previous or concurrent thiopurine use [171,172]. Increased cSCC risk in patients with RA has similarly been shown for azathioprine [173]. MMF replaced azathioprine from the mid-1990s and there is a signal that the risk of cSCC is reduced compared with azathioprine use [174], although this may be confounded by era effects with, for example, patients receiving MMF also benefitting from greater screening and photoprotection advice than earlier cohorts on azathioprine.

In addition to its immunosuppressive properties, azathioprine is also associated with UVA photosensitivity and the generation of mutagenic oxidative DNA damage [175]. The azathioprine metabolite, 6-thioguanine, replaces a proportion of DNA guanine in replicating cells and becomes a strong UVA chromophore, interacting with UVA to generate reactive oxygen species, in turn causing direct DNA damage and widespread protein oxidation, the latter increasing UVB mutagenicity by damage to proteins involved in DNA repair [176]. Azathioprine-induced UVA photosensitivity has been confirmed in clinical studies and is reversed by switching from azathioprine to MMF [177,178]. Mutational signature analysis of cSCC in azathioprine-exposed patients has identified the novel signature-32 which is predominantly C>T (75%), in combination with C>A, T>A and T>C mutations [117].

Calcineurin inhibitors
Calcineurin inhibitors (ciclosporin and tacrolimus) also have synergistic pro-carcinogenic interactions with UVB and UVA [164]. The diverse mechanisms involved include UVA induction of oncogenic activating transcription factor 3 [179,180], inhibition of UVB-induced DNA repair and apoptosis [181–183] in addition to UV-independent mechanisms including upregulated tumour growth factor-β signalling [184–186] and suppression of p53-dependent senescence, mitochondrial permeability transition pore (MPTP) and phosphatase and tensin homologue (PTEN) inhibition [187,188]. There is no clear evidence that tacrolimus, which was introduced in 1994 to replace ciclosporin, is associated with a reduced skin cancer risk [174].

Mammalian target of rapamycin inhibitors
The mTOR inhibitors (e.g. rapamycin/sirolimus, everolimus) were introduced in 1999 and have potentially anticarcinogenic properties that include suppression of angiogenesis, autophagy-mediated DNA repair and promotion of memory T-cell function [189–193]. There is clear evidence from prospective randomised controlled trials (RCTs) that mTOR inhibitors confer reduced skin cancer risk, especially if the conversion from CNI to mTOR inhibitor occurs after the development of a first cSCC [**194**,195–198]. Their antiproliferative, anti-angiogenic activities are especially helpful in virally driven skin malignancies such as KS [199,200]. The role of conversion to mTOR inhibitors in skin cancer treatment and prevention is discussed in more detail in the section on the management of KC later in this chapter.

Belatacept
The skin cancer risk of many newer immunosuppressive drugs remains uncertain. For example, belatacept, which causes selective T-cell co-stimulation blockade by its anti-CTLA4 properties, has been used as an alternative to ciclosporin since 2011. There is some evidence that it may be associated with a reduced risk of cSCC but not BCC in kidney OTRs [201].

Biologic immune-targeted drugs
Data relating to use of biologics in IMIDs and skin cancer are conflicting. Overall, the evidence suggests an increased risk for KCs, predominantly cSCC, for patients with IMIDs receiving the anti-TNF therapies etanercept and adalimumab. However, this increase has not been demonstrated with the non-TNF-targeted biologics in psoriasis, RA and IBD [202–206] and some systematic reviews and meta-analyses indicate no increased risk with the newer anti-TNF agents certolizumab and golimumab [207], although longer term studies are required. It is likely that discrepancies between studies may be due to methodological differences including inappropriate comparator arms and failure to account for important confounding factors, such as prior phototherapy for psoriasis [203]. In hidradenitis suppurativa, the increased skin cancer risk noted in the PIONEER randomised control trial was similar in the intervention and placebo arms and could be disease-specific rather than therapy-driven [208]. Increased cSCC risk in patients with RA has similarly been shown for both azathioprine [173] and anti-TNF agents [201,209].

Melanoma risk may also be increased in IMIDs. In an observational study, biological therapy was associated with an excess risk of melanoma particularly in Crohn disease, with an OR of 1.88 [210]. Increased melanoma risk was reported to be increased for RA with an OR of 2.3 [211]. However, this has not been confirmed in a more recent large European collaborative project evaluating anti-TNF, rituximab, tocalizumab and abatacept therapy in RA [212]. Similarly, melanoma risk was not increased for patients with spondyloarthritis treated with anti-TNF drugs [213].

Small-molecule-based immune-targeted drugs
Inhibition of the JAK/STAT pathway causes immunosuppression due to impaired T-cell signalling and JAK inhibitors are approved in specific IMIDs (including RA, psoriasis and ulcerative colitis), acute GVHD, haematological conditions (including myelofibrosis and polycythaemia rubra vera), and are in trials for a range of additional IMIDs and malignancies [214]. Although skin cancer is predicted to be associated with the use of JAK inhibitors, data from clinical trials do not yet consistently support an increased risk [215–217]. However, there are multiple case reports of aggressive cSCC associated with their use [218,219] and larger studies with longer term outcomes are required [214].

Methotrexate
Data reporting an association between KC risk and methotrexate are inconsistent [202–204]. Some but not all data suggest a small increased risk of melanoma with methotrexate [220–222].

Disease-modifying drugs in multiple sclerosis
Fingolimod is an oral sphingosine-1-phosphate receptor inhibitor that sequesters lymphocytes in lymph nodes, leading to systemic lymphopenia. Natalizumab is a monoclonal antibody blocking VLA4 and inhibits transmigration of lymphocytes across the blood–brain barrier. Although there are reports of melanoma [223–225], MCC [226–228] and cutaneous lymphoma [229–232], this has not been confirmed in all studies [569].

Other drugs
Other drugs commonly used in transplantation and in other immunocompromised individuals may also affect skin cancer risk.

Chemotherapeutic drugs
Data are conflicting on whether chemotherapy for CLL/NHL affects the incidence of skin cancers. Although it has been suggested in CLL that cytotoxic chemotherapy contributes to skin cancer risk [233], most studies indicate a relationship with skin cancer that is unlikely to be primarily iatrogenic [35,234,235].

Antifungal drugs
Voriconazole is a triazole antifungal often used in the treatment and prophylaxis of invasive fungal infections such as aspergillosis in OTRs – particularly lung transplant recipients – and in HCT recipients [78]. Like azathioprine, voriconazole is a photosensitiser for UVA: it was first reported to induce cSCC in 2007 [237] and there have been multiple subsequent reports documenting an association with cSCC which may be multiple and aggressive [78,238–242]. The mechanisms underlying carcinogenesis are likely to involve initiation by reactive oxygen species generated by voriconazole metabolites and UVA which results in epidermal DNA damage, in addition to tumour promotion by voriconazole itself which stimulates aryl hydrocarbon receptors with upregulation of COX-2 [243,244]. Retrospective studies have identifed it as an independent risk factor for cSCC in lung transplant recipients which is both dose- and drug-duration dependent [77,244,245]. In a French series of 19 cases, a multistep process was common, with acute phototoxicity in the first year, actinic keratosis (AK) in the second/third year and cSCC by the third year onwards [239], underscoring the importance of photoprotection and vigilant skin cancer surveillance in patients receiving voriconazole prophylaxis. In a population-based cohort study of almost 10 000 lung OTRs, cSCC risk was estimated to be increased threefold after 15 months of voriconazole exposure compared with OTRs not receiving the drug, and a small increased risk was observed with the related antifungal itraconazole [246]. In the same study, there was a signal that both itraconazole and posaconazole but not voriconazole were associated with an increased risk of BCC, although the authors speculate that this finding may be in part confounded by prescribing practices [246].

Statins
Statins are hydroxymethylglutaryl-coenzyme A reductase inhibitors that lower blood cholesterol. Although they have antiproliferative, pro-apoptotic, antimetastatic and anti-inflammatory properties in preclinical studies, they may also be photosensitising and immune-modulating, which has led to concerns that skin cancer risk may be increased [247,248]. The evidence for this is currently inconsistent. No effect on KC risk was identified in a one meta-analysis [249], whereas another meta-analysis of observational studies, but not RCTs, showed a possible increased risk [250]. The risk therefore remains uncertain, but is unlikely to be large [251,252].

Hydrochlorthiazide diuretics
These are among the most frequently prescribed antihypertensive drugs and have photosensitising properties. Multiple studies have confirmed an increased risk of cutaneous cSCC which is dose- and duration-dependent [253–256]. BCC risk is increased in some studies [255,257,258], but not all [256,259], and there is evidence for an association with melanoma, MCC and adnexal skin tumours with high doses [255,258,260]. The association with cSCC is not increased for other thiazides such as bendroflumethiazide and thiazide-like drugs such as indapamide, although indapamide may be associated with an moderately increased risk of melanoma [259].

Non-steroidal anti-inflammatory drugs
Non-steroidal anti-inflammatory drugs have been proposed to have a possible protective effect against skin cancer [261], but this was not confirmed in a large meta-analysis [262].

Oncogenic viruses
The most common immunosuppression-associated malignancies are those due to known or suspected oncogenic viruses and in the skin these include KS (HHV-8), post-transplant lymphoproliferative disorders (EBV) and MCC (Merkel cell polyomavirus, MCPyV). HHV-8, EBV and MCPyV viral oncogenesis are discussed in more detail elsewhere (Chapters 25, 138, 139 and 146). Given its significantly increased frequency in immunosuppression, a cofactor role for a viral carcinogen has been sought in cSCC. There has been a particular focus on HPV for many years, and although there are supportive epidemiological and molecular data, its role in cSCC remains controversial but has potentially important preventative and therapeutic implications [263–266].

Human papillomaviruses and cSCC
Human papillomaviruses are double-stranded DNA viruses that infect the skin and mucosal epithelium of vertebrates. Human papillomaviridae are organised into five genera (alpha, beta, gamma, mu and nu) and further classified into species and types: more than 450 individual human HPV types are currently recognised [267]. All genera infect skin and alphapapillomaviruses (alphaPV) also contain types that preferentially infect oral and genital mucosa. Specific oncogenic or 'high-risk' mucosal papillomaviruses (including HPV types 16 and 18) are important carcinogens in ano-genital SCC, in a proportion of head and neck SCC and in periungual SCC [267]. AlphaPV vaccination programmes have had a substantial impact on ano-genital HPV infections, ano-genital warts and grade 2+ cervical

intraepithelial neoplasia [268]. Beta- and gammaPVs are ubiquitous in the skin of healthy individuals, with a likely reservoir in hair follicle stem cells; they are usually acquired in infancy, increase with age and are considered to be part of the normal skin microbial flora [267,269,270]. Immunosuppression is associated with an increased prevalence in the skin of beta- and gammaPVs and coinfection with multiple HPV types and higher HPV seropositivity are also observed [271].

In the genodermatosis EV, betaPV (particularly HPV-5 and -8) are detected in more than 90% of cSCC and are co-carcinogenic with UVR [3,272]. Independent epidemiological and molecular studies have also provided evidence of a role for betaPV in promoting non-EV cSCC, particularly in immunosuppressed individuals in whom cutaneous HPV infection is often widespread and HPV-associated histological features may be evident in cSCCs [112,264,266]. Epidemiological studies of HPV serological responses in OTRs and HPV DNA in eyebrow hair follicles of OTRs have shown that the presence of betaPV is associated with an approximately twofold increased risk of cSCC – of the same order as that conferred by skin phototype [273]. HPV serology and DNA are not always concordant, but when they are there appears to be a dose effect in that OTRs with five or more different betaPV types have 1.7 times the risk of cSCC compared with those with 0–4 different types [274]. A positive seroresponse to betaPV at the time of transplantation is also predictive for subsequent skin cancer risk, with a hazard ratio of 2.9 [275]. BetaPV DNA is detected in more than 80% of OTR cSCC versus 30–50% of immunocompetent cSCC, although HPV detection methodologies vary in sensitivity and ability to detect diverse HPV types [276]. HPV viral gene expression has been observed in cSCC with *in situ* hybridisation [277], but viral load is usually <1 copy per cell and higher in AK compared with cSCC [278]. This, together with the apparent lack of viral transcriptional activity reported in other studies [279,280], has been taken as evidence that HPV may only be required in early stages of cSCC development, the so-called 'hit and run' hypothesis [264,266,272]. In this respect, it differs significantly from alphaPV-induced ano-genital cancers. Furthermore, in contrast with HPV in ano-genital cancer, no clear hierarchy of cancer-associated HPV types has been defined in cSCC [271].

High-risk alphaPVs are oncogenic through integration of the virus into the host genome with consequent upregulated expression of the early viral proteins E6 and E7, which act as oncoproteins through a myriad of host cellular pro-carcinogenic interactions. For example, E7 proteins bind and degrade retinoblastoma protein (pRb), and E6 proteins degrade p53 and PDZ polarity proteins and upregulate telomerase [267]. Conversely, betaPVs rarely integrate and their early proteins E6 and E7 do not directly target p53 and pRb. However, there is a significant evidence base that some betaPVs are pro-carcinogenic in cooperation with UVR by, for example, abrogating UVR-induced apoptosis, delaying repair of UV-induced DNA damage and cell cycle arrest and interfering with NOTCH tumour suppression pathways. It is postulated that alterations in these cellular pathways cause genetic instability in keratinocytes and facilitate enhanced accumulation of UV-induced mutations in oncogenic driver genes leading to malignant transformation. From this stage, the virus is dispensable for maintaining the malignant phenotype, explaining the apparently low viral load and lack of viral transcriptional activity in cSCC [112,264,266,272]. Further support for the role of betaPV in cSCC is provided by transgenic mouse models in which the viral E2, E6 and E7 proteins from betaPV types 8 and 38 are oncogenic, and also the mouse *Mastomys coucha* model. The latter provides mechanistic evidence for cooperation between UVB and betaPV infection with loss of viral DNA during squamous carcinogenesis progression [281]. An alternative role for HPV in cSCC has more recently been proposed [265]. These authors argue that T-cell immunity against commensal betaPV may actually prevent cSCC. However, their study was conducted in mouse models and the conclusions of this study remain controversial [266].

Ultimately, clarification of the part played by HPV in cSCC development may be revealed if vaccination strategies for betaPV can be developed. This is a potential new direction for cSCC treatment and prevention and could become important for the immunosuppressed patient. Vaccination is not yet possible as current HPV vaccines only confer type-restricted protection against the high-risk alphaPV types [282]. Although these vaccines are thought to have the potential to eliminate 90% of cervical cancer and 50% of other alphaPV-associated cancers, they have limited cross-protection against non-alphaPV types [267]. Despite the occasional case report of possible activity of current HPV vaccines in AK/cSCC [283,284], it is likely that future HPV vaccine development for cSCC will need to focus on formulations that confer protection against a broad range of betaPV types. In mouse models at least, there is evidence that such an approach may prevent cSCC [285,286]. Currently, licensed highly effective alphaPV vaccines are all based on L1 virus-like particles and confer almost no cross-reactivity to other HPV types including cutaneous HPVs. Second generation vaccines based on L2 are likely to provide much broader based protection, but L2 peptides are less successful at inducing neutralising antibodies and augmenting broad-based anti-HPV immunity is an area of active current research [287].

Ionising radiation
Radiotherapy may contribute to skin carcinogenesis in immunocompromised individuals. Increased melanoma risk persists for more than 20 years after radiotherapy for Hodgkin lymphoma and, as not all tumours arise within the irradiated field, radiation may have an additional systemic effect [288]. In HSCT, total-body irradiation conditioning regimens increase BCC risk; those exposed to radiation at an age of less than 10 years show significantly greater risk than older individuals [103,104]. Studies in non-immunosuppressed populations suggest that exposure to therapeutic radiation [289] or occupational exposure [290] is associated with BCC but not with cSCC.

Graft-versus-host disease
The pathogenesis of skin cancers after HSCT is multifactorial, but both therapy (radiation or chemotherapy) and GVHD contribute [103]. A meta-analysis of 50 951 HSCT recipients showed that chronic GVHD was associated with an increased incidence of BCC (relative risk (RR) 1.95) and cSCC (RR 5.31) but not melanoma, and acute GVHD alone was not associated with an increased risk of skin cancer [291]. A case–control study of 24 011 HSCT recipients reported that the risk of cSCC was almost threefold higher in those

Table 147.2 Risk factors for skin cancer development in solid organ transplant recipients.

Risk factors for time to first skin cancer	Risk factors for total numbers of skin cancers	Other patient-related risk factors	Transplant-related risk factors
Duration of immunosuppression	Duration of immunosuppression	Smoking – inconsistent	Allograft type (lung/cardiac > renal > liver)
Age at transplant	Age at transplant	Alcohol – inconsistent	Cause of end-stage organ disease
History of five or more sunburns pre-transplant	Sunburn pre-transplant	Genetic polymorphisms	
Ethnicity (white versus non-white)	Chronic UV exposure	CD4 count	
Skin cancer pre-transplant	Skin phototype	β-HPV DNA/serology concordance	
	Male sex		
	Number of keratotic lesions (AKs and verrucokeratotic lesions)		
	Voriconazole		

Based on the following studies: [**52**,77,78,95,114,149,**150**,273,274,299,320].
AK, actinic keratosis; HPV, human papillomavirus; UV, ultraviolet light.

with chronic GVHD and even higher with previous acute GVHD. Treatment of GVHD with azathioprine, ciclosporin, corticosteroids and psoralen and ultraviolet A (PUVA) increased the risk for SCC 18–50-fold [161].

Donor-derived skin malignancy

The presence of donor-derived cells has been reported as potentially pathogenic in HSCT-related oral malignancies [292] and has also been reported for donor-derived mycosis fungoides [293]. In OTR it has been reported to induce KCs [294,295] and KS [296], although the mechanisms involved remain unclear. Donor transmitted melanoma is discussed in the section on melanoma later in this chapter.

Clinicopathological features of specific skin cancers

The clinical presentation and histological features of skin tumours arising in immunosuppression may be atypical and their clinical course may be altered compared with the immunocompetent population. This section provides an overview of clinicopathological features and clinical course for specific skin cancers that differ in the setting of immunosuppression.

Keratinocyte cancers

Cutaneous SCCs are usually reported to be up to 150-fold more common in OTRs compared with immunocompetent populations, with a lower but significantly increased risk in other immunocompromised groups (Table 147.1). Fewer data are available for immunosuppression-associated cSCC premalignancies including AK, Bowen disease (squamous carcinoma *in situ*, CIS) and possibly porokeratosis. BCCs are up to 10-fold more common in OTRs and the cSCC : BCC ratio seen in the immunocompetent population is generally reversed, although this is not necessarily the case in all immunocompromised patient groups.

The impact of skin cancers on health-related quality of life in OTRs is unclear. In one US study, the number of skin cancers correlated with higher levels of anxiety although this did not quite reach significance [297], while in a cohort from Ireland, skin cancer impacted less on quality of life than certain benign dermatoses associated with transplantation [298].

Clinical risk factors (Table 147.2)

Cohort studies have identified clinical features associated with an increased risk of developing KCs [149] and the most significant form the basis for two risk stratification classifications reported for OTRs in the UK [**52**] and USA [**150**].

- *Age at transplant*. This is a significant predictor of both time to first skin cancer and cumulative skin cancer burden. In a UK cohort, risk was increased 12-fold in OTRs transplanted at 55 years or above compared with those younger than 34 years, with median time to diagnosis of 8, 12 and 19 years for those transplanted at age >55 years, 45–54 years and 35–44 years, respectively [**52**].
- *UV exposure and skin phototype*. Skin phototype and a history of five or more pre-transplant sunburns, particularly sunburn in childhood, were associated with time to first KC; chronic UV exposure was associated with cumulative KC burden [**52**].
- *Male sex*. cSCC risk is higher in males, even when adjusted for other risk factors [**150**].
- *Organ type*. The risk is higher in thoracic versus abdominal transplants [**150**].
- *History of pre-transplant skin cancer*. Time to first cancer is reduced from 105 to 71 months if there is a history of a pre-transplant KC [**52**].
- *Actinic keratoses*. These are a significant biomarker of cSCC risk in OTRs [114,300–302].
- *Duration of immunosuppression*. Approximately 30–50% of OTRs have developed skin cancer by 20 years post-transplant in Europe [**52**,58,90], with even higher rates in Australia [76,77,80]. Similarly, in CLL the cumulative incidence by 20 years in the USA is more than 40% for cSCC and 30% for BCC [40].

Squamous cell carcinoma

As in the general population, cSCCs are mainly located on UV-exposed sites, but are more common on non-head and neck sites in immunocompromised compared with immunocompetent individuals [126]. Although diagnosis is usually made clinically, appearances may be atypical and a high index of suspicion is required (Figure 147.2) [303]. Pain is a useful symptom of invasive malignancy in this context [304,**305**]. Differential diagnoses include AK, Bowen disease, appendageal malignancies and infections, in particular viral warts which may be clinically and

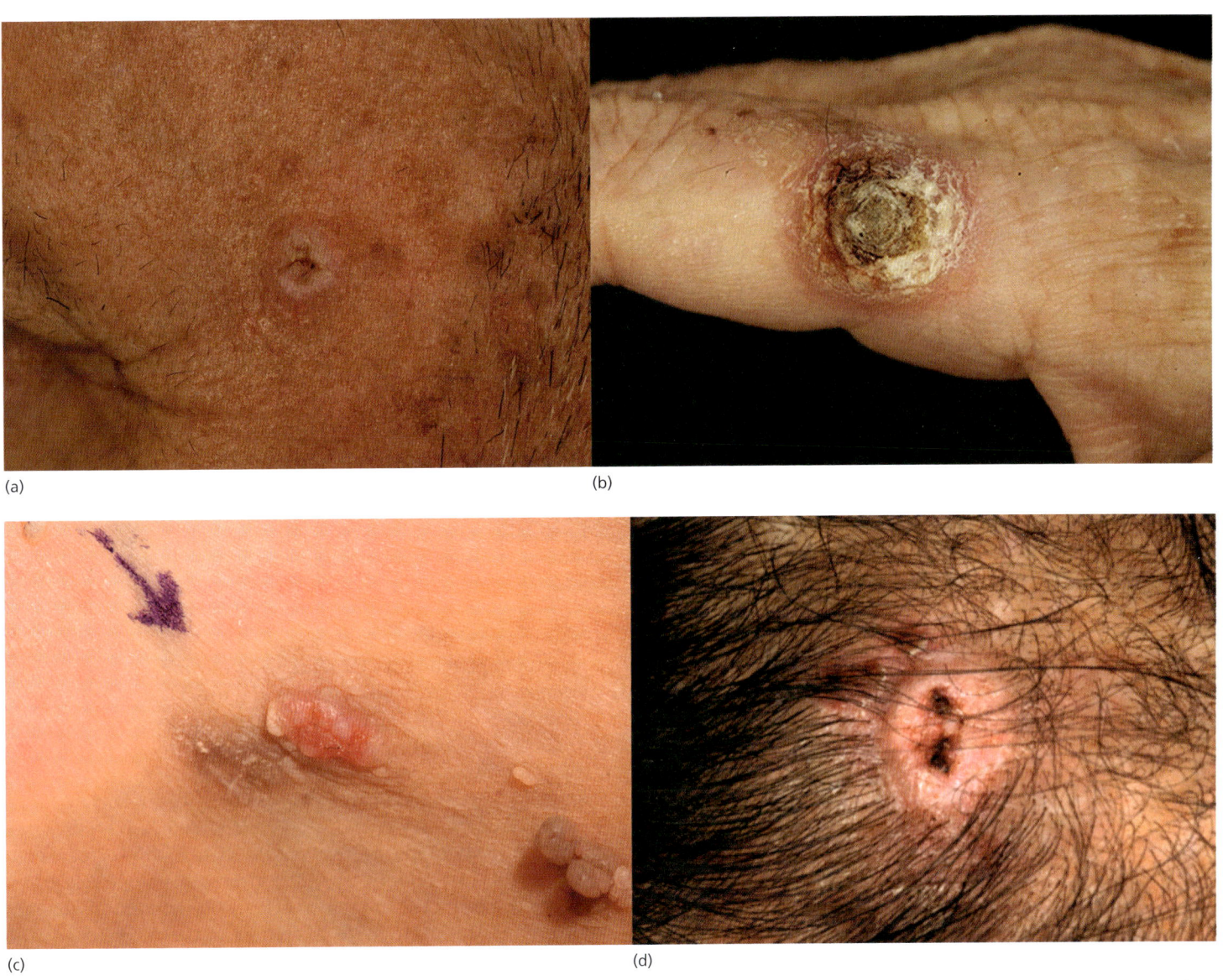

Figure 147.2 Examples of cutaneous squamous cell carcinomas (cSCCs) in organ transplant recipients (OTRs). (a) Clinically typical cSCC on the left temple and (b) right index finger in OTRs with Fitzpatrick skin types 1 and 2. (c) Clinically atypical cSCC on the upper medial arm and (d) scalp in OTRs with Fitzpatrick skin types 1 and 5.

histologically atypical (Figure 147.3), chronic herpes simplex and atypical mycobacterial infections.

There is an estimated metastatic risk of up to 7% for cSCC in immunosuppressed individuals, which is more than twice that in the general population [20,306]. Metastatic disease has a worse prognosis in immunosuppressed individuals [307] with, for example, a median 3-year survival of 56% in OTRs [308] which is even worse in OTRs from countries with a high incidence of KC, such as Australia [80], and in cardiac and lung transplant recipients [77,309–311]. In transit metastases are also more common in OTRs, particularly on the scalp [303,312]. cSCCs have worse outcomes in patients with CLL and HIV: locoregional recurrences are sevenfold more common than in the general population and metastases occur in 18% [27,37,313].

Although for individual immunosuppressed patients a potentially worse prognosis for cSCC is evident, it is less clear whether the increased rate of metastasis is a result of increased tumour burden rather than the increased aggression of individual tumours: metastatic risk increases in patients with 10 or more cSCCs, many of whom are immunosuppressed [314]. In terms of histological risk factors, differentiation status is not usually significantly different, but there is a reported increased depth of invasion, reduced inflammatory infiltrate and increased rates of spindle cell morphology, perineural invasion, lymphatic invasion and acantholysis [126,315–317]. There is also evidence that aggressive subclinical extension is more common in OTRs and CLL [318].

Actinic keratoses, Bowen disease, field cancerisation and porokeratosis

The true SIR of AK and CIS in immunocompromised individual OTRs is not known, with reported prevalence ranging from 28% to 50% [300,319]. The presence of AK increased cSCC risk by more than 30-fold in one UK study [300] and in Australia the OR for cSCC over a 12-month period was almost 4 in OTRs with 10 or more AKs [301].

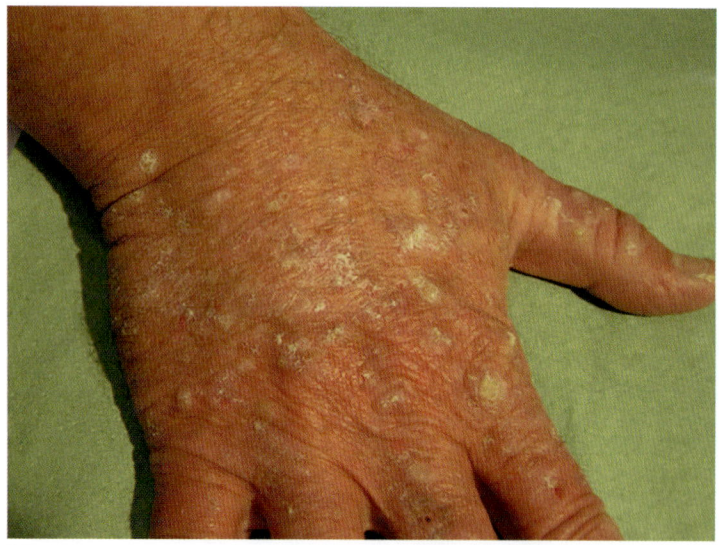

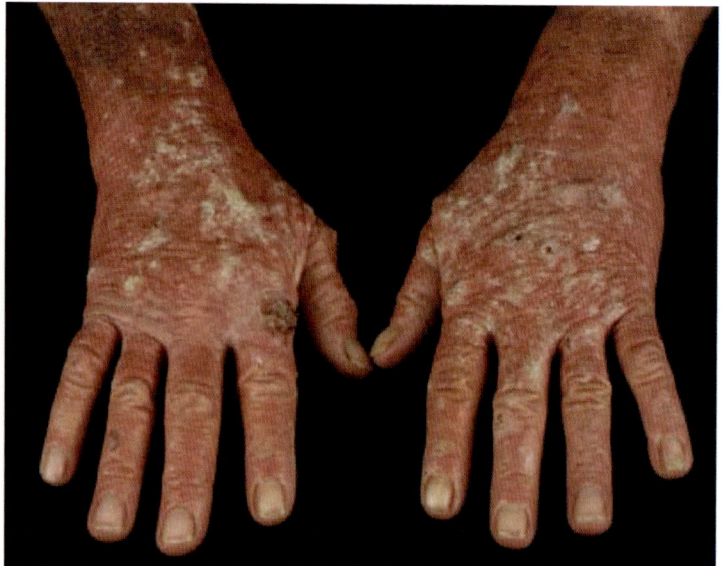

Figure 147.4 Field cancerisation in a patient with Crohn disease who was taking azathioprine for many years. Confluent actinic keratoses and Bowen disease (field cancerisation/field change) are present and a squamous cell carcinoma has developed on the dorsum of the right hand.

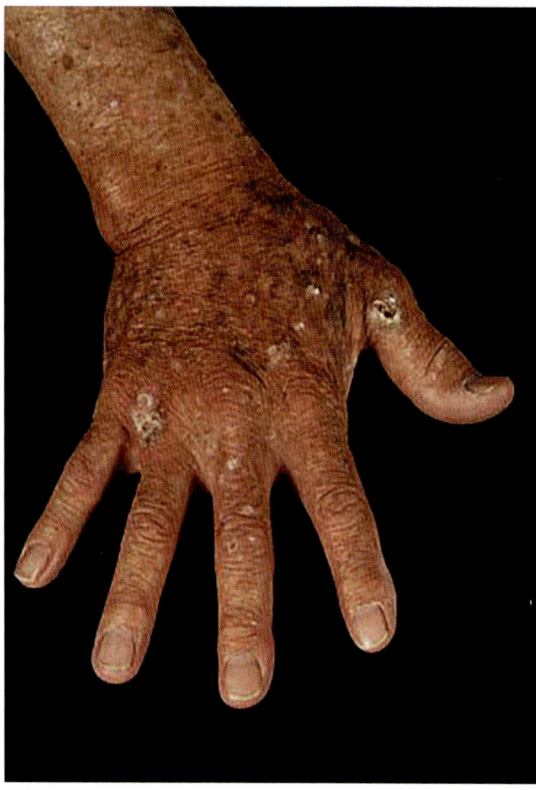

Figure 147.3 Dorsal aspect of hands in organ transplant recipients (OTR) with (a) Fitzpatrick type 1 skin and (b) with Fitzpatrick type 5 skin. In both, typical and atypical viral warts and verrucokeratotic lesions coexist with actinic keratoses and Bowen disease (squamous carcinoma *in situ*) and early cutaneous squamous cell carcinoma.

Field cancerisation – areas of confluent AK/CIS – is a common problem in immunosuppression (Figure 147.4) and is associated with an even higher risk of cSCC. About 70% of cSCC developed within areas of field cancerisation in one UK study of renal OTRs, with an OR for cSCC of 20 for discrete AK versus 93 for field cancerisation [300]. In an Australian case–control study, the presence of AK patches was associated with an OR for cSCC of greater than 6 [302].

AK may be difficult to distinguish clinically from viral warts at non-palmoplantar sites in immunosuppression and they are often termed 'verrucokeratotic' lesions (Figure 147.3). They are often contiguous on the dorsum of the hands and forehead. In a large multicentre European study there was a 12-fold increased risk of cSCC for 50 or more verrucokeratotic lesions, a fourfold increase for BCC, and common palmoplantar warts were associated with an cSCC OR of 1.6 but were not associated with BCC [114]. In contrast, a French study found cSCCs were associated with verrucokeratotic lesions but not common warts [320]. Certain histological features are reported to be more common in OTR versus immunocompetent AK, including mitotic activity, parakeratosis and verrucous change [321].

Porokeratosis is considered to have premalignant potential and is well documented in association with immunosuppression [322,323]. Up to 10% of OTRs are affected and it is also described in post-stem cell transplant and in association with GVHD, HIV [324,325] and with several other immunosuppressive drugs [326]. Progression to cSCC is rare, but metastatic disease has been reported [327–329].

Basal cell carcinoma (Chapter 140)

The anatomical location of BCC differs from that of cSCC in OTRs [330]: in a UK cohort BCCs were twice as common as cSCCs on the trunk (22.2% versus 8.5%) and less common on the hands and forearms (5.2% versus 36.3%) [52,126]. Truncal superficial BCCs are also more frequent in PLWH [27] and although this may indicate pathogenetic differences, it may also be in part due to increased indoor tanning or as a consequence of more intense surveillance of these patient groups [331]. High-risk BCC subtypes (infiltrative/morphoeic, micronodular and basosquamous) appear not to be overrepresented in OTRs, but are more frequent in PLWH [27,126,332]. Immunosuppression-associated BCCs have reduced inflammatory infiltrate and increased squamous differentiation, but tumour depth, perineural and vascular invasion are similar to immunocompetent BCCs [126,330]. Aggressive subclinical extension (defined as 3 Mohs micrographic surgery stages with final surgical margins of at least 10 mm) is almost twofold more common in immunosuppression and is highest in OTRs (particularly lung and cardiac OTRs) and haematological malignancy compared with PLWH [318]. Differential diagnoses include sebaceous gland hyperplasia, which is more common in OTRs, often in association with CNI use [333], molluscum contagiosum in PLWH, and rare infections such as cryptococcus which are more common in immunosuppression [334]. Recurrence rates for BCCs are significantly increased after conventional and Mohs surgery in both HIV and CLL, and this may result from dense lymphocytic infiltrate obscuring the tumour margins and perineural invasion; worse outcomes are not reported in OTRs [27,335–337].

Melanoma (Chapters 142–145)

The immune system has an important role in melanoma pathogenesis and progression and this is reflected in the higher incidence and generally worse outcomes for melanoma in immunocompromised individuals [21,33,40–42,62–65,166,338,339].

Melanoma in organ transplant recipients

Melanoma is recognised to occur in one of three main clinical scenarios in OTRs: most commonly *de novo* post-transplant melanoma, occasionally a history of pre-transplant melanoma and, in rare but often devastating cases, as melanoma transmitted from an organ donor [339,340].

De novo post-transplant melanoma

Most studies report SIRs of 2–8 for post-transplant melanoma and melanoma *in situ*, which is higher in cardiac and lung OTRs but significantly lower than for cSCC [56,62–65,338,339,341,342]. SIRs of more than 17 are reported in African American OTRs compared with the general population [343]. In paediatric OTRs, a relative risk of 4.5 was reported in one cohort study with diagnosis at a median of 19 years post-transplant [344]. There is evidence that unlike cSCC, post-transplant melanoma risk may be increasing [60,61,65]. Also in contrast to KCs, this risk does not appear to correlate as closely with duration of transplantation [64,345]. In a US registry study the risk of presentation with primary cutaneous melanoma at diagnosis was stable over time but presentation with stage III/IV disease was approximately fourfold more common in OTRs and was increased significantly within the first 4 years after transplantation and thereafter declined [64]. These findings were similar to those reported in a Swedish registry study [346]. In an Australian registry study, primary melanoma risk was highest in the second year of transplantation and subsequently declined linearly, consistent with the authors' hypothesis that immunosuppression acts as a tumour promoter in high-risk individuals with pre-neoplastic lesions [345].

Risk factors for post-transplant melanoma include indicators of high personal UV exposure and UV sensitivity [345]. Current immunosuppression is also a strong risk factor and, unlike KCs, this risk reverts to baseline within 2 years of returning to dialysis [345]. The use of T-cell lymphocyte depleting antibodies may increase risk [345] as may voriconazole [240], and mTOR inhibitors may be protective [347]. Data are limited on the role of other immunosuppressive drugs [339].

Clinicopathological characteristics of post-transplant melanoma are broadly similar to those of melanoma in immunocompetent patients [348,349]. However, there are suggestions of a possible increased incidence of mucosal melanoma [339]. Reduced tumour infiltrating lymphocytes has been reported in one study and was associated with worse outcomes [346]. Some reports indicate an increased association with pre-existing melanocytic naevi, possibly suggesting that melanocytic precursors present before the transplant progress rapidly with intense immunosuppression post-transplant [341,342,346,348]. A lower BRAF mutation rate was found in 10 post-transplant melanomas compared with non-OTR tumours [350], but this was not observed in a larger study [351]. Reports of reduced CD8, FoxP3, PD1 and PD-L1 and enhanced expression of the potent immunosuppressive enzyme indoleamine 2,3-dioxygenase (IDO) may be indicative of an immunosuppressed tumour microenvironment possibly induced by IDO [351].

Outcomes for post-transplant melanomas are generally worse compared with those for immunocompetent individuals. In a multicentre European study of 100 OTRs, melanomas with a Breslow depth of less than 2 mm had a similar prognosis to matched controls from the American Joint Committee on Cancer (AJCC) melanoma database, but melanomas of 2 mm or thicker were associated with higher mortality [348]. A subsequent US registry study of 724 tumours reported worse prognosis for melanomas with a Breslow depth of 1.5–3 mm [352], and a smaller Australian study in 75 post-transplant melanomas adjusted for stage also found an increased melanoma-specific mortality (hazard ratio (HR) 1.74) [353]. A similar HR of 1.93 was reported in a Canadian study of 50 OTRs [349], and in larger Swedish and US studies adjusted HRs were even higher at approximately 3.0 [64,346].

Pre-transplant melanoma

Historic data have suggested recurrence rates of 20% in patients with pre-transplant melanoma [354]. Several subsequent studies did not confirm worse outcomes, although these studies were relatively small, tumour stage was often not reported and possible selection bias was likely [348,352,355]. In a more recent, larger, US registry study, outcomes in 336 OTRs with pre-transplant melanoma were evaluated [356]. The risk of melanoma-specific mortality post-transplant was significantly increased (HR 27, 95%CI 11–64, $P < 0.0001$) compared with OTRs without pre-transplant melanoma. Although this is a seemingly large increased risk, the difference in 5-year mortality was just 1.2% as, in absolute terms, melanoma-specific death is rare in OTRs [356].

Donor-transmitted melanoma

Cancers related to organ transplantation may be donor-derived (arising in the allograft itself) or donor-transmitted (a donor malignancy that is transmitted by the allograft) [357]. The risk of occult donor malignancy is estimated at 1.3% and transmission to a recipient occurs in 0.2%. Together with renal cancer and lymphoma, melanoma is one of the most common donor-transmitted malignancies; however, the prognosis is much worse, with a 5-year overall survival of 43% [357,358]. The development of metastatic disease occurs within 12 months of transplantation in the vast majority of cases [357,359] and the donor origin of metastatic melanoma may be established by polymerase chain reaction-based DNA analysis for microsatellite markers, HLA typing, immunohistochemistry or fluorescent *in situ* hybridisation [360]. In most cases, the donor was not known to have had melanoma and the cause of the donor's death in such occult cases is often cerebral haemorrhage, which in retrospect was secondary to brain metastases [357]. However, transmission of known melanoma resected in a donor decades previously has also been reported [341,361]. Any past history of melanoma is therefore considered to be an absolute contraindication to organ donation in many guidelines such as those in the USA, but this remains controversial and, given the shortage of donors, very early-stage melanoma and melanoma *in situ* are permitted by other guidelines, such as those in the UK [362].

Melanoma in other immunosuppressed individuals

In PLWH, the SIR for melanoma is approximately 1.15–2.6 in most studies and this does not appear to have changed in the pre-ART versus post-ART eras [26,33,51,363], although some more recent studies have suggested the incidence is not increased compared with the general population [21,26]. It has been suggested that HIV-induced immune dysfunction has less effect on melanoma development compared with KC and and older age. Higher UVB exposure, rather than CD4 and HIV RNA, were associated with increased melanoma incidence [21]. However, as in OTRs, stage at presentation is reported to be more advanced and melanoma-specific mortality is increased independent of stage [26,363]. Melanoma risk is increased approximately 2–7 times in CLL/NHL and overall survival is worse, with a SMR of more than 7 in Australia: the risk is bidirectional, with worse prognosis if the melanoma is diagnosed before CLL/NHL [38,41,42,62]. Allogeneic HSCT recipients in one Danish study had a threefold higher risk of melanoma compared with OTR [26], and in an Australian study the risk was highest in the first 4 years post-transplant, as in solid OTRs [364].

Eruptive melanocytic naevi

Increased numbers of melanocytic naevi have been observed in paediatric OTRs [365,366] and in individuals with HIV [367]. The entity of eruptive melanocytic naevi (EMN) describes the rapid simultaneous appearance of multiple melanocytic naevi on previously uninvolved sun-exposed skin. Although reported in otherwise healthy individuals and bullous dermatoses, it may also be associated with drugs (including immunosuppressants), chemotherapy, targeted cancer therapy such as BRAF inhibitors and melanocyte stimulators such as α-melanocyte-stimulating hormone analogues [368,369]. EMN are particularly associated with immunosuppression in OTRs [370,371], HIV [372,373], IBD, psoriasis and myasthenia gravis [374,375] and post-chemotherapy [376]. Regression on the withdrawal of immunosuppression is reported [377]. BRAF *V600E* gene mutations have been detected in EMN in the setting of immunosuppression, but association of EMN with melanoma remains uncertain [369,378,379].

Kaposi sarcoma (Chapter 138)

Kaposi sarcoma is a multifocal neoplasm of lymphatic endothelium-derived cells infected with HHV-8 [380]. Of the five recognised subtypes – classic, endemic, iatrogenic (post-transplant), epidemic (HIV-related) and KS in HIV-negative MSM – the types more clearly related to immunosuppression (iatrogenic and epidemic) are generally the most aggressive forms [380]. KS is an AIDS-defining disease and was the most common skin malignancy in PLWH in the pre-ART era, with a SIR in excess of 400–500 [380,381]. The KS risk is increased sevenfold in haematological malignancy and the risk is reciprocal [38]. The incidence of KS in OTRs mirrors geographical HHV-8 seroprevalence and is therefore most common in patients from sub-Saharan Africa, the Mediterranean and Middle East [380].

In OTRs, the SIR for KS is more than 200: it is usually due to reactivation of latent virus, with prevalence in OTRs from highly endemic areas reported as 3.2–5.3%, representing 35–88% of all post-transplant malignancy in these locations [380,382]. Post-transplant acquisition, for example through blood transfusion or donor transmission (particularly after liver transplantation), is much less common but also recognised [380,382,383]. Recent evidence suggests that the epidemiology of post-transplant KS is changing. Cohort studies from the USA [384], Italy [200] and Egypt [385] have reported a decreasing incidence in recent years. The reasons for this are unclear: a more frequent use of steroid-free or mTOR inhibitor regimens and cytomegalovirus prophylaxis are plausible explanations but remain to be validated [200,384,385]. Conversely, there is evidence that the risk of donor-transmitted KS may be increasing even if KS due to latent HHV-8 reactivation is decreasing. This is possibly driven by a rise in 'increased risk donors', for example those with a history of high-risk sexual behaviour. Outcomes in donor-transmitted KS appear to be worse [386].

Cutaneous KS typically presents with purplish, reddish blue or dark/brown macules, plaques and/or nodules that may ulcerate, bleed, become hyperkeratotic or verrucous. Lymphoedema may precede the appearance of typical skin lesions, and in high-risk OTRs from sub-Saharan Africa presentation is often with a preceding leg lymphoedema (often unilateral) (Figure 147.5) [52,387]. A multicentre, European retrospective analysis of 145 OTRs reported that the median onset of KS was 17 months post-transplant; this is consistent with the majority being the result of HHV-8 reactivation, as is the observation that more than half were of sub-Saharan African or Caribbean origin [387]. Although the majority of OTRs had cutaneous KS, one-third had nodal KS, 36% gastrointestinal KS and 20% pulmonary involvement. KS-specific mortality was low in this series with a 5-year overall survival of 82%, but graft loss was reported in 23% and KS-specific death in 3% [387]. Outcomes for donor-transmitted KS appear to be worse [386], but KS outcomes in OTRs who are HIV positive – an increasingly common clinical scenario – were similar to non-HIV-positive OTRs in a French study [98]. In contrast, patients with KS associated with non-CLL/NHL had a worse prognosis than expected [49].

Merkel cell carcinoma (Chapter 146)

At least 10% of all MCCs arise in immunocompromised individuals [388], most often in OTRs and patients with CLL/NHL [48]. In OTRs, SIRs of more than 20 and, in a study from Ireland, as high as 97, are reported: incidence increases with duration of transplantation, the majority of tumours are on UV-exposed sites and patients frequently have multiple other skin cancers [48,66,389–391]. SIRs are approximately 11–13 in PLWH [32,392] and risk is also increased in autoimmune disease [32,48]. In NHL/CLL, SIRs are 18 with reciprocal increases in CLL for patients diagnosed with MCC [38]. MCC should be considered in the differential diagnosis of rapidly enlarging nodules and plaques in immunosuppressed patients and, as in the general population, diagnosis is based on histology, although

Clinicopathological features of specific skin cancers

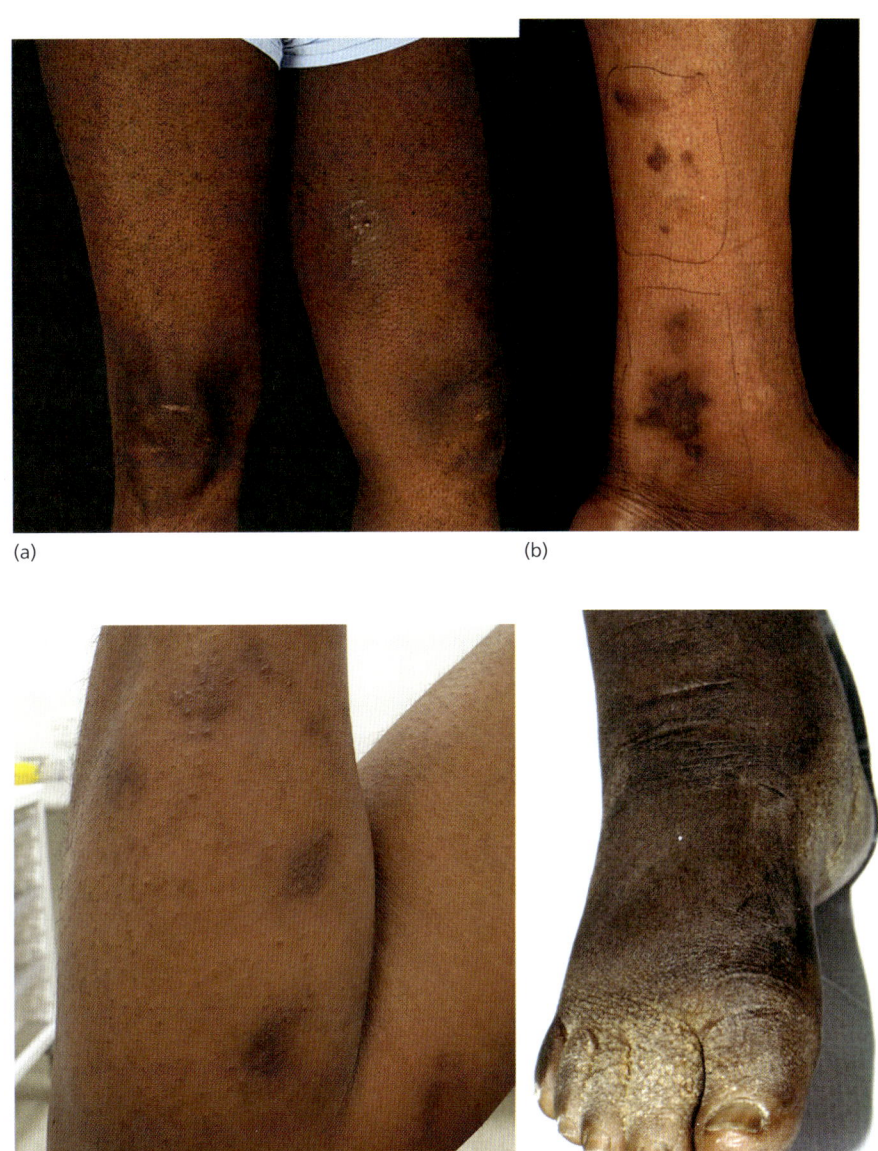

Figure 147.5 Kaposi sarcoma (KS) in organ transplant recipients: (a) unilateral left leg oedema with a plaque of KS on the left thigh, (b, c) KS plaques on the lower legs and arms, and (d) chronic lymphoedema secondary to KS.

overlapping marker expression between MCC and haematological neoplasms may cause diagnostic challenges [393].

Immunosuppression appears to facilitate both UV- and MCPyV-associated MCC carcinogenesis [388]. Although virally driven cancers are more common in immunosuppression and despite data indicating higher MCPyV viral loads in normal skin of immunosuppressed individuals, there is increasing evidence that MCPyV-negative MCC may be significantly more common than in the general population. Eighty per cent of immunosuppressed MCCs were MCPyV negative in one series [394] and immunosuppressed patients with MCC were more often seronegative [395]. The reasons for these apparently counterintuitive observations are unclear and require confirmation, but there is some evidence that MCPyV-negative MCC may behave more aggressively and this may therefore be relevant to outcomes in immunosuppression [396].

In a US registry study of 969 patients with MCC, the median age of MCC diagnosis was significantly younger in OTRs and PLWH than in other immunosuppressed groups and stage at presentation was also more advanced [48]. MCC-specific survival (MSS) and overall survival are worse in the context of immunosuppression, particularly in OTRs and PLWH, and this is independent of stage [32,48,66,389–392,397,398]. MCC independent of stage at diagnosis was the most common cause of death in immunosuppressed patients with MCC, despite competing co-morbidities [48]. MCC patients with HIV/AIDS had the worst MSS and overall survival, corresponding to the observation that the majority of first recurrences were distant and not curable [48].

Primary cutaneous lymphoma (Chapter 139)

Immunosuppression is associated with an increased risk of systemic lymphoma. However, PCLs are uncommon. In OTRs, PTLD presenting in the skin without systemic involvement is rare [399]. In a multicentre European study, the spectrum of disease in 35 OTRs with PCL was similar to that seen in the general population: 69% were T-cell and 31% B-cell lymphomas, the majority of which were EBV positive [69]. The prognosis of CD30-positive CTCL was worse than post-transplant mycosis fungoides and its counterpart in the immunocompetent population [69]. Most lymphomas are B cell in PLWH, but PCLs include CD30-positive anaplastic T-cell lymphoma, which may have a worse prognosis than in the general population [400,401]. PCLs in NHL/CLL are also overrepresented and overall survival is worse for those who develop CLL prior or concurrent to CTCL [402,403].

Skin appendage tumours (Chapter 137)

An increased incidence of tumours of eccrine, apocrine, follicular and sebaceous origin in OTRs was first reported in 2003 [404] and is now well established [66,329,405]. Appendageal tumours are also overrepresented in HIV [406] and in CLL/NHL [49].

Sebaceous carcinomas were the most common appendageal tumours in a US registry study: risk is significantly increased with duration of transplantation and overall SIRs of 25–30 were reported, increasing to almost 50 in lung OTRs and more than 100 in OTRs with a previous history of cSCC [66,407]. Sebaceous carcinoma has been linked to both UV exposure and dysregulated DNA mismatch repair with microsatellite instability similar to that observed in Muir–Torre syndrome (MTS) [408]. However, MTS was confirmed in fewer than 5% of OTRs in one series [407]. Mismatch repair deficiency resulting from chronic azathioprine exposure was proposed as a cofactor in OTRs [409], but remains unconfirmed [410]. HIV infection may exacerbate skin tumour development in known MTS [411] and a possible role for HPV or other novel viruses has also been proposed [412]. Decreased overall survival and mortality of 4.3% was observed in one OTR series [407], and in non-CLL/NHL is associated with worse outcomes [49]. Porocarcinomas are also more common (Figure 147.6) [404] as are other eccrine tumours [66], and there is some evidence that potentially aggressive squamoid eccrine ductal carcinomas may be associated with immunosuppression [413].

Establishing the diagnosis of appendageal malignancies prospectively may be challenging. These tumours often arise in individuals who have many other skin cancers and may simulate more common skin cancers. Diagnosis is usually only on the basis of histology but should be considered in the differential diagnosis of any suspected but atypical skin cancers in immunosuppressed individuals [405].

Sarcomas

Sarcomas other than KS are more common in immunocompromised individuals [66,67]. The size of this increased incidence is difficult to assess given the rarity of these tumours in the general population, but SIRs of almost 7 have been estimated in OTRs [66]. Atypical fibroxanthoma and pleomorphic dermal sarcoma (undifferentiated pleomorphic sarcoma (previously malignant fibrous histiocytoma)) are reported in OTRs, HIV and NHL/CLL, with some evidence for increased rates of recurrence and metastasis compared with the general population [40,49,68,414–416], and with evidence for atypical clinical presentations [416]. Dermatofibrosarcoma protuberans is reported [40,417,418] and cutaneous leiomyosarcomas and angiosarcomas occur disproportionately in HIV and OTRs [419]. Leiomyosarcomas are frequently EBV positive and angiosarcomas appear to have a particular predilection for arteriovenous fistula sites [419].

Management

There are relatively few RCTs and limited non-randomised prospective and retrospective studies to guide decision making in the management of skin cancers arising in immunocompromised individuals. A multidisciplinary approach plays a key part in delivering comprehensive and patient-centred care for OTRs, with close dialogue and shared decision making between patients, their carers, dermatologists, oncologists, surgeons, transplant clinicians and other relevant health care professionals. The same principles apply to the management of skin cancer in other immunocompromised patient groups including those with haematological malignancies and PLWH [19,420].

Keratinocyte cancers
Primary cSCC and BCC

Important gaps exist in our understanding of optimal management of primary KC in immunosuppression. There is little prospective, randomised evidence to suggest that primary BCC and cSCC/cSCC *in situ* require significantly different management approaches to the general population [112,421]. However, the index of suspicion for possible malignancy should be high and the threshold for biopsy correspondingly low, particularly in areas of field cancerisation [19,422,423]. Most guidelines recommend that cSCC in immunocompromised individuals should be considered potentially 'high risk' for the purposes of management decision making [424].

Staging

The Brigham and Women's Hospital cSCC staging criteria better risk stratify cSCC for risk of nodal metastasis and risk of local recurrence in immunosuppressed patients compared with AJCC7, with the majority of poor outcomes occurring in low T stages [425] while the AJCC8 risk stratification appears to be similar for immunosuppressed and non-immunosuppressed patients [426]. There is limited

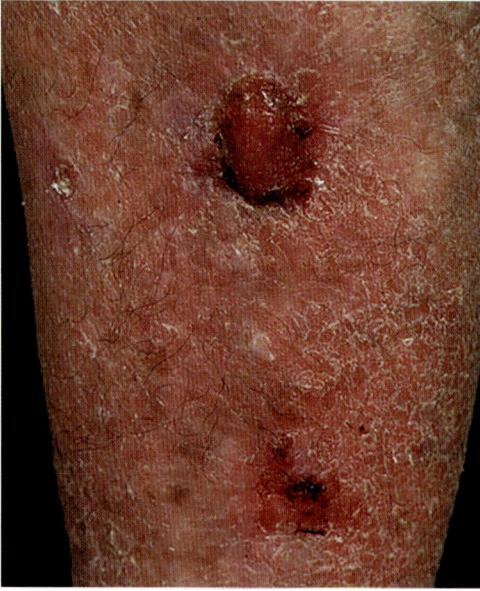

Figure 147.6 Eccrine porocarcinoma on the leg of an organ transplant recipient.

evidence on the role of staging investigations such as sentinel lymph node biopsy in cSCC, and prospective studies are required, but this may be considered for selected cSCC on a case-by-case basis [421,427]. There are some data to suggest that positron emission tomography/computed tomography (PET/CT) may be promising in nodal staging of cSCC in patients with CLL [428].

Surgery
Excision is the most appropriate option for the majority of tumours. It is usually recommended that high-risk OTR tumours require more 'aggressive' surgery, but optimal excision margins and the role of MMS/intraoperative margin assessment in immunosuppression have not been clearly defined [19,421,429,430]. Some immunosuppressed patients have a higher rate of subclinical margin extension, particularly OTRs and patients with haematological malignancy, suggesting that MMS may be preferable but prospective, randomised trials are required to confirm this [318,431]. Rates of recurrence may also be higher after MMS for certain KCs, for example BCC arising in patients with CLL [335,432]. Curettage and electrocautery may provide satisfactory clearance rates for selected low-risk tumours, including well-differentiated SCC, and may be considered in certain clinical situations for reasons of cosmesis and convenience [433]. Few data exist on postoperative complications in immunosuppressed patients, including rates of infection and the need for prophylactic antibiotics [434]. Sirolimus is associated with an increase risk of surgical dehiscence, but the associated morbidity does not usually justify stopping sirolimus before primary skin cancer excision [430,435].

Radiotherapy
Radiotherapy is not the first option for most primary tumours in immunosuppressed individuals, who tend to be younger and more likely to develop multiple primary tumours at specific anatomical sites, precluding its use subsequently at those sites. The uncertain risk of carcinogenesis is also a consideration. However, as in non-immunosuppressed patients, it is an important option when surgery is not possible [430]. There are no RCTs evaluating the use of adjuvant radiotherapy for high-risk cSCC, and its role remains uncertain [436]. The potential for poorer outcomes in immunosuppressed patients provides a rationale for its use, although this should be considered on a case-by-case basis [430].

Other non-surgical modalities
Non-surgical approaches including cryotherapy, photodynamic therapy (PDT), imiquimod (IMIQ) cream and 5-fluorouracil (5-FU) cream may have a therapeutic role in selected cases, particularly for BCC and cSCC *in situ* and in patients with multiple low-risk malignancies in whom repeated surgery is otherwise required. Although response rates may be lower, there is no evidence that these agents carry additional significant risk (see later in this chapter).

Locally advanced and metastatic KC
There are currently no standards of care for the management of regionally advanced and metastatic cSCCs in OTRs and current practice is based largely on consensus recommendations. The use of both surgery and radiotherapy is broadly similar to their use in the general population. However, there are important considerations relating to the use of chemotherapy, targeted therapy and immunotherapy and sequencing of these strategies in some immunosuppressed groups compared with the general population [430]. Additional strategies of immunosuppression reduction, conversion to mTOR inhibitors and, in some cases, complete withdrawal of immunosuppression in locally advanced and metastatic KC are further detailed later in this chapter [19,430,437].

Conventional chemotherapy
There are few data relating to responses in immunosuppression for conventional cSCC chemotherapeutic agents including systemic 5-FU, platinum-based compounds (e.g. cisplatin, carboplatin) and taxanes (e.g. paclitaxel) [430,438,439]. Consideration should be given to transplant-directed dosage adjustment, close monitoring of allograft function and potential interactions with drugs such as CNIs and antiretroviral medications [437].

Targeted therapy: EGFR and hedgehog inhibitors
Data on the use of anti-EGFR inhibitors such as cetuximab are limited to case reports in OTRs and CLL [440,441]. Complications relevant to immunosuppressed individuals include neutropenia, infection and liver dysfunction [437]; fatal pulmonary toxicity reported in lung transplant recipients with cetuximab suggest that particular caution should be taken with this drug [442]. In advanced BCC, responses to hedgehog inhibitors have been described in OTRs and PLWH; a potential interaction of vismodegib with ciclosporin requires monitoring of drug levels [443–446].

Immune checkpoint inhibitor therapy
Anti-PD1 immunotherapy (cemiplimab approved in Europe, cemiplimab and pembrolizumab in the USA) has revolutionised treatment of metastatic cSCC in immunocompetent patients [447,448]. Pivotal clinical trials excluded immunosuppressed individuals and information on their safety and efficacy is restricted to case reports and retrospective series; most experience derives from the use of immune checkpoint inhibitor (ICI) in immunosuppressed patients with melanoma, but increasing data are now available for cSCC [449–456]. Currently, no consensus guidelines exist for the use of anti-PD1 immunotherapy in immunosuppressed patients with advanced cSCC and use should be considered on a case-by-case basis in multidisciplinary consultation with the patient and their health care team. Key considerations include the high risk of allograft rejection in OTRs, the type of allograft and the options for replacement therapy should the allograft fail and the possibility that treatment efficacy may be reduced by immune compromise.

In OTRs, PD1 blockade threatens allograft rejection as the PD1 pathway is critical in maintaining allograft tolerance [449]. The effects of immune-related adverse events on graft function and possible reduced antitumour activity of ICI in the presence of immunosuppressive drugs are also relevant [430]. Data from at least 35 OTRs with metastatic cSCC have been reported to date: disease control rates (complete response, partial response and stable disease) are promising and range from 30% to 50%, but graft rejection was observed in up to 40% [449–459]. The role of reducing/stopping CNIs and/or converting to mTOR inhibitors in preventing rejection is unclear in metastatic cSCC, but recent reports using this approach and also using peri-infusional steroids provide a signal that this may mitigate rejection [456,458,460]. However, in advanced melanoma where experience is more extensive, the benefit of significant reduction in immunosuppression has been questioned [461]. Encouragingly, successful transplantation after ICI therapy for metastatic cSCC has been reported in one case [462]. PD1 blockade for metastatic cSCC has also been reported in PLWH and in patients with haematological malignancies in whom disease control rates appear to be lower than for PLWH and OTRs [463].

Further studies are now a priority and a clinical trial examining cemiplimab in kidney and stem cell transplant patients which includes peri-infusional prednisone and conversion to mTOR inhibitor (NCT04339062) is ongoing, as is another trial evaluating tacrolimus, nivolumab and ipilimumab in OTRs with unresectable/metastatic cancers including cSCC (NCT03816332). Major challenges for the future include a better understanding of how to uncouple alloreactive immunity from antitumour immunity in OTRs, biomarkers for identifying OTRs likely to benefit from immunotherapy and early detection of allograft rejection [430].

Pre-transplant KC and transplantation
Patients with a history of KC being considered as candidates for transplantation (or other iatrogenic immunosuppression) is an increasingly common clinical scenario. Organ stewardship requires a reasonable 5-year post-transplant survival to prevent futile use of scarce organs [464]. However, multidisciplinary decision making in consultation and on a case-by-case basis is crucial [464,567]. Based on considerations of the risk and kinetics of cSCC metastasis, consensus recommendations from the International Transplant Skin Cancer Collaborative (ITSCC) are that no waiting time is required for low-risk cSCC, 2 years is required for high-risk cSCC without perineural invasion, 2–4 years for high-risk cSCC with perineural invasion and two or more other risk factors and 5 years for cSCC with nodal metastasis; and that for distant metastasis, transplantation is almost always contraindicated [19,464]. However, with the introduction of more effective treatments for advanced cSCC, this is a rapidly changing landscape [462]. Time to first KC is much shorter in OTRs with pre-transplant KC and similar to the interval between first and second cancers in those without pre-transplant KC [52]. The role of mTOR immunosuppressives and systemic retinoids in delaying this onset is not established, but close surveillance is warranted [52]. For OTRs with a history of post-transplant KC being considered for retransplantation, the observed increased risk of developing aggressive cSCC associated with higher mortality also needs to be taken into consideration [93].

Keratinocyte cancer prevention
Primary prevention for immunosuppression-associated KC has focused mainly on photoprotection. Secondary prevention strategies include treatment of premalignant skin lesions, modification of immunosuppression and use of systemic chemoprevention. However, the current evidence base for guiding decision making and clinical practice is limited, particularly in terms of selecting the most effective treatments and the thresholds at which to initiate and sequence each strategy [420,466].

Photoprotection
Most expert consensus guidelines for OTRs recommend strict photoprotection, with behavioural, clothing and sunscreen advice [429,466,467,468]. In the general population there is convincing evidence that sunscreens reduce AK, cSCC and melanoma risk, but there is no equivalent evidence that their use post-transplant has the same effect [469–471]. The only significant study is a non-randomised, prospective, open-label trial of a liposomal sunscreen which showed a significant reduction at 24 months in AK and cSCC, but not BCC [472]. Vitamin D levels were lower in the sunscreen group in this study and monitoring of levels in OTRs is advisable [473]. For patients on azathioprine, there is a good rationale for using sunscreen with significant UVA protection all year round in view of the UVA-sensitising properties of azathioprine [117,175]. The same applies for lung transplant recipients on prophylactic voriconazole. A systematic review of behavioural interventions (written material, text messages, mobile apps and videos) in OTRs showed benefit in improving sun protection behaviour, knowledge, attitudes and biological measures of UV exposure, but which method was most effective in delivering photoprotection education and whether this translates into CSCC prevention has not been confirmed [420].

Treatment of pre-malignant lesions
Actinic keratosis and field cancerisation are significant risk factors for immunosuppression-associated cSCC, providing a rationale for treatment as a secondary prevention approach. Multiple lesion-directed and field-directed treatments are available [474], but there are few RCT data for their use in immunosuppressed individuals [466,475–477]. Although it may be valid to extrapolate data from the general population, AKs arising in the context of immunocompromise may progress to cSCC more rapidly, new AKs may arise more frequently and immunosuppression may reduce treatment efficacy, particularly those dependent on an immune response [474,477]. A systematic review of topical AK interventions in OTRs identified only eight RCTs: participant numbers were usually low with significant heterogeneity in treatment regimens, variable AK quantification and short durations of follow-up [476]. PDT and IMIQ were the most frequent treatments studied, with only a handful of studies assessing 5-FU, diclofenac and ingenol mebutate [477]. Although not directly compared, there is some suggestion that responses are lower than in the general population and also that spontaneous regression of AKs is less common [476]. Patient preferences are important in ensuring acceptability and adherence to self-delivered topical AK/field interventions. This was highlighted in a discrete choice experiment that included OTRs and which demonstrated significant variation in perceived utility of treatment and willingness to trade some reduction in efficacy to reduce the burden of the treatment regimen and adverse effects [478].

Surgery and cryosurgery. Excision and grafting of areas of severe field carcinogenesis within which cSCCs are developing is reported in OTRs [479]. Cryosurgery is also widely used although there are few reports of its efficacy compared with the immunocompetent population [466].

5-Fluorouracil (5% and 0.5%). In the general population there is RCT evidence that 5-FU is more effective than IMIQ, PDT and ingenol mebutate in AK clearance [480] and that 5-FU prevents cSCC in high-risk immunocompetent populations [481]. Until recently, there have been fewer data for immunosuppressed populations; however, an RCT comparing treatment in 40 OTRs with 5% 5-FU, IMIQ and sunscreen for AKs (SPOT study) found that 5-FU (1–2 times a day for 4 weeks, repeated after 4 weeks if required) was more effective than IMIQ (3–5 times a week for 4 weeks, repeated after 4 weeks if required) or SPF30+ sunscreen in clearing AKs and preventing new AKs after 12 months of follow-up [477]. Local skin toxicity was higher for 5-FU but there were otherwise no safety concerns with either 5-FU or IMIQ. A 4-day course of 5-FU combined with calcipotriol ointment has proved to be effective in clearing AKs and preventing head and neck cSCC in immunocompetent individuals, but its effects in immunosuppression have not been evaluated [482,483].

Imiquimod (5% and 3.75%). Although there is a theoretical risk of immunostimulation and allograft rejection with topical IMIQ, its use appears to be safe in OTRs at least when limited to 25–50 mg/day [477,484,485]. In a placebo-controlled RCT in 21 OTRs, IMIQ significantly reduced dysplasia [485] and in a multicentre RCT of 43 OTRs, IMIQ used three times a week for 16 weeks gave an overall clearance at 8 weeks post-treatment of 74% [484]. Despite the longer duration of treatment, this was a similar rate to that found in the SPOT study, but lower than the clearance achieved with 5-FU [477].

Diclofenac 3% in 2.5% hyaluronic acid gel. The only study in OTRs was an RCT of 32 patients treated twice daily for 16 weeks: complete response was achieved in 41% but recurrent AKs were noted at 24 months in 55% [486].

Ingenol mebutate. In a prospective, non-randomised study in 20 OTRs, complete and partial responses were achieved in 40% and 60% at 8 weeks post treatment [487]. Although there were no short-term safety issues in OTRs, ingenol mebutate use was suspended in January 2020 in Europe and the USA by the European Medicines Agency (EMA) pending a review of safety and skin cancer risk.

Photodynamic therapy. PDT is the best-studied AK intervention in OTRs and most RCTs have been within-patient [475,476]. In a comparative RCT of 5-aminolevulinic acid PDT (ALA-PDT) with violet light in 40 OTRs, new keratotic lesions were reduced over 2 years although there was no reduction in cSCC [433]. New keratotic lesions were also reduced using methyl aminolaevulinate PDT (MAL-PDT) with red light [488]. Clearance rates of 77% [489] and 90% [490] were reported with MAL-PDT at 3–4 months compared with 95% and 54% with 5-FU and IMIQ, respectively, in the SPOT study [477]. Complete responses in 35 OTRs were also higher with MAL-PDT in an RCT comparing it with IMIQ [491]. The efficacy of daylight PDT was equivalent to MAL-PDT in another study and ablative fractional laser increased the efficacy of both [492,493].

Tirbanibulin. This microtubule inhibitor is the most recent topical treatment for AK, although cSCC prevention has not been evaluated [494]. There are no particular theoretical concerns relating to its use in immunosuppression, although this has not yet been reported.

Modification of immunosuppression

The incidence of KC is usually reduced when immunosuppression is minimised or discontinued. Modification of immunosuppression is therefore a potential approach to secondary skin cancer prevention, but there is limited evidence regarding when this should be initiated or how exactly it should be undertaken. These decisions should be adjusted for factors such as the type of allograft, the risk status of individual tumours and the rate of accrual of tumours [123,421,**466**]. The main approaches usually considered are: (i) minimisation of drug doses for some/all drugs; (ii) discontinuation of specific drugs; (iii) conversion to alternative immunosuppressive drugs (usually mTOR inhibitors); or (iv) combinations of all three strategies [**19**,420,**466**].

Revision of immunosuppression. The overall intensity of immunosuppression may be as important as the role of individual drugs, but a major barrier to decision making is the lack of a robust measure for immunosuppressive intensity to guide appropriate reductions in some/all immunosuppressive drugs [**466**]. There is also relatively limited evidence to guide which specific drugs should be reduced or discontinued. As discussed in the section on drugs earlier in this chapter, there is growing evidence that azathioprine confers a particularly high skin cancer risk, and that this is higher than the alternative purine antagonist, MMF [**174**].

Conversions to alternative immunosuppressive drugs. Lung OTRs who were moved from azathioprine to MMF appeared to have a lower risk of cSCC in a retrospective cohort analysis [495]. However, there is less evidence for significant differences between the CNIs, and lung OTRs who were switched from ciclosporin to tacrolimus did not have a reduced risk [**174**,495]. Conversion from CNIs to the selective T-cell co-stimulatory blockade agent, belatacept, is associated with a lower risk of cSCC [201].

Conversion to mTOR inhibitors. Most evidence exists for conversion to mTOR inhibitors (sirolimus/rapamycin, everolimus). Retrospective registry data, observational series and *post hoc* analyses of immunosuppressive drug RCTs demonstrate reduced levels of malignancy overall, but particularly cSCCs, in OTRs receiving mTOR inhibitors [437,496]. Discontinuation of CNIs and conversion to mTOR inhibitors was first described as an approach to treatment in OTRs with KS [**497**]. There is now considerable RCT evidence for KC prevention: RCTs have demonstrated that conversion from CNIs to mTOR inhibitors after a first cSCC reduces the risk of subsequent tumours [**194**,195–197,498] with reduction in the thickness and peritumoural vascularisation of the cSCC [499]. However, in patients with multiple cSCCs, a non-significant reduction of subsequent cSCCs was seen with mTOR inhibitor conversion [**194**,195]. The effect on BCC reduction is less significant, possibly because of differential expression of phospho-mTOR in BCC and cSCC [500]. There is no evidence that mTOR inhibitors have a primary protective effect against post-transplant KC [496,501].

Although they have advantages in terms of malignancy reduction, mTOR inhibitors are not standard first line immunosuppressive drugs as their adverse effect profile (including delayed wound healing, diarrhoea, mucositis and peripheral oedema), often leads to them being poorly tolerated with high rates of discontinuation

[437]. A 56% reduction in KCs and 40% reduction in malignancies overall with mTOR inhibitor use was confirmed in a meta-analysis of 5876 OTRs from 21 RCTs, but an overall increase in mortality (HR 1.4) was also reported [502]. However, it is possible that mortality was associated with high-dose mTOR inhibitors used in early trials as it was not evident in low-dose mTOR inhibitor studies [502], nor was there an increased mortality in subsequent studies of mTOR inhibitors [503].

Systemic chemoprevention

Nicotinamide, retinoids and capecitabine are the main systemic agents that have been evaluated in immunosuppression for their KC chemoprevention potential [420,474,504].

Retinoids. The chemopreventive mechanisms of action for oral vitamin A analogues are thought to be through induction of differentiation, antiproliferative and antiapoptotic effects, immunomodulation and possibly arrest of HPV replication [505]. Their use in chemoprevention for OTRs with KC were first described in 1988 with etretinate [506] and subsequently in multiple case series, usually with acitretin [507–510]. Three RCTs have confirmed significant reduction in AK and/or cSCC in OTRs [511–513]. A systematic review of retinoid use in kidney transplant recipients calculated a 56% overall reduction in KC (mean of 0.68 per patient per year), with a 54% reduction in cSCC (mean of 0.57 per patient per year) and a 73% reduction in BCC (mean of 0.10 per patient per year) [514].

In most studies, the reported adverse effects which may be dose limiting are cheilitis, xerosis, alopecia, headache, musculoskeletal complaints and hyperlipidaemia [514–517]. In a systematic review, almost all OTRs experienced mucocutaneous side effects and overall 14% discontinued therapy [514]. A rebound increased incidence of cSCCs was also consistently observed 3–4 months after discontinuation of retinoids [510,516]. There is a theoretical risk of allograft rejection given their immunomodulatory properties, but this has not been reported [518]. Whether isotretinoin has similar chemopreventive properties in OTRs in whom a retinoid with a shorter half-life is more appropriate (e.g. women of child-bearing age) is unclear. There are also few data relating to their use in other immunosuppressed patient groups such as patients with haematological malignancy or IBD or PLWH.

Despite their widespread use, there is currently no US Food and Drug Administration (FDA) or EMA approval for the use of retinoids in KC chemoprevention, and no formal prescribing guidelines exist. Further research is needed to clarify indications for their initiation, as well as the tolerability and efficacy of optimal dosing regimens [466]. However, consensus opinion recommends starting at low dose (e.g. 10 mg/day acitretin) and escalating as tolerated to an effective maintenance dose (e.g. up to 30 mg/day acitretin) [517]. Because of potential rebound cSCC development, when discussing initiation with patients, retinoid chemoprevention should be viewed as long-term strategy requiring laboratory monitoring (liver function tests, lipids) [510]. Whether nicotinamide or retinoids should be considered as first line systemic chemoprevention in OTRs is currently not clear [515,519].

Nicotinamide. Nicotinamide is an amide form of vitamin B_3 and the precursor of nicotinamide adenine dinucleotide, which is an essential cofactor for adenosine triphosphate (ATP) production. Laboratory and preclinical studies confirm that it boosts cellular energy and enhances repair of UV-induced DNA damage by preventing UV-associated ATP depletion and glycolytic blockade; it also reduces UV-induced DNA damage-associated immunosuppression [520,521]. In phase II RCTs in immuncompetent, sun-damaged Australians, nicotinamide 500 mg twice daily reduced AKs by 35% at 4 months [522]. ONTRAC (Oral Nicotinamide to Reduce Actinic Cancer), a multicentre, phase III RCT, compared the efficacy of oral nicotinamide 500 mg twice daily with placebo over 12 months in high-risk Australian immunocompetent patients: cSCC rates were reduced by 30% ($P = 0.05$), AK by 13% ($P = 0.001$) and BCC by 20% ($P = 0.12$) with few side effects although – as for systemic retinoids – there was a rebound in KC when nicotinamide was discontinued [523].

In OTRs, two small studies have provided a signal of efficacy but were underpowered to show a significant KC chemoprevention effect [524,525]. In a study in 38 Italian OTRs, a significant reduction in AK size ($P > 0.05$) and non-significant trend to reduction in cSCC was observed with nicotinamide 500 mg once daily over 6 months [525]. In 22 Australian OTRs, nicotinamide 500 mg twice daily over 6 months resulted in a 35% reduction in KCs and a 16% reduction in AKs, results similar to those seen in the ONTRAC study but insufficiently powered to reach significance [524]. In 2022, there were phase III RCTs in OTRs ongoing in Australia and Canada.

In comparison to systemic retinoids, nicotinamide had few adverse effects in clinical trials and does not require laboratory monitoring [515]. It is also available over the counter and is cheap in countries such as the USA where retinoids require prescription and are relatively costly by comparison [514]. In a systematic review of the limited clinical trial data available, there is a suggestion that retinoids and nicotinamide are equally effective in KC chemoprevention [519]. Given the adverse effect profile and requirements for monitoring with retinoids, it has been argued that nicotinamide should be the first line systemic chemopreventive agent [515]. However, for OTRs and other immunosuppressed groups, this remains to be established in prospective RCTs [466].

Capecitabine. Capecitabine is an oral prodrug that is converted into the antimetabolite 5-FU in a three-step enzymatic process requiring thymidine phosphorylase, which is selectively overexpressed in human cancer cells. Patients treated with capecitabine for cancer were observed to develop inflammation of pre-existing AK and there are limited data from uncontrolled case reports/series that it reduces the incidence of AK, cSCC and BCC in OTRs [526–528]. However, it has significant dose-limiting side effects including fatigue, hand–foot syndrome, diarrhoea, nausea/vomiting, mucositis, anaemia and hyperuricaemia/gout resulting in discontinuation in 43% of patients. It is also associated with possible rebound cSCC development on discontinuation, but no evidence of allograft rejection [526]. As with both retinoids and nicotinamide, it is not FDA/EMA approved as a KC chemopreventive agent and optimal dosing regimens are not established [526], but intermittent regimens such as 500 mg twice daily every other week for 1–3 months or 1000 mg twice daily for days 1–14 of a 21-day cycle have been proposed [474]. It may have a role when other chemopreventive agents are not appropriate or are insufficient, but further clinical trials are required to establish optimal patient selection, dosing, safety and long-term efficacy [474,526].

Sequencing of KC prevention approaches

The thresholds at which to initiate each of these potential KC chemopreventive approaches and which approaches are superior in immunosuppressed individuals are an important area of clinical decision making for which there are currently considerable gaps in our evidence base [421]. These gaps have been highlighted in recent consensus-based recommendations on the prevention of cSCC in OTRs [466]. In this e-Delphi process, 48 international experts aimed to reach consensus over three rounds on management at each of six stages in the evolution of cSCC in OTRs [466]. As summarised in Table 147.3, consensus was reached on photodamage, discrete AK and diffuse AK/cSCC *in situ*, although 5-FU was not universally adopted despite existing evidence because of concerns around patient adherence. It was notable that no consensus was reached for prevention strategies after the first invasive cSCC, despite RCT evidence for mTOR inhibitor conversion; this was largely because of concerns regarding mTOR inhibitor adverse effects. For OTRs with low accrual rates of multiple cSCC, modification of immunosuppression was recommended along with systemic chemoprevention, although there was no agreement as to which chemoprevention to use; perceived lack of evidence in OTRs around nicotinamide was cited as a barrier for its routine use. With higher rates of cSCC accrual (>10/year), acitretin was recommended and was similarly the first choice for high-risk cSCC [466].

Melanoma

Primary melanoma

Initial surgical approaches in immunocompromised individuals, including the use of sentinel lymph node biopsy, follow the same principles as in the general population, although data are limited [339,340]. In OTRs, the reduction of immunosuppression and consideration of mTOR inhibitor conversion while maintaining good graft function is recommended, although evidence is limited. The level of reduction will depend on the type of graft as well as the stage and perceived risk from the melanoma [340].

Advanced melanoma

In advanced melanoma, multidisciplinary management is particularly essential. The safety and efficacy of targeted therapies and immunotherapy were not evaluated in immunocompromised individuals in pivotal RCTs. However, experience with their use for metastatic disease is emerging through case reports and case series and several clinical trials are now underway. Few data are available regarding use in the adjuvant setting.

Targeted therapy

Responses to BRAF and MEK inhibitors in metastatic melanoma in OTRs, PLWH and those with CLL appear to be acceptable with few signals beyond those reported in pivotal trials [529,570]. Targeted therapy has also been successfully used in donor-transmitted melanoma [530]. Consideration should be given to potential effects on allografts and drug interactions [437]. Given the risk of rejection with ICIs in OTRs, targeted treatments are theoretically a safer approach to adjuvant therapy, although data are currently lacking.

Immune checkpoint inhibitors

Immune checkpoint inhibitors present potentially significant problems in both metastatic and adjuvant settings [531]. In PLWH, activity appears to be comparable to that reported in pivotal clinical trials with no treatment-related increases in viral load, although hepatitis B prophylaxis should be considered in patients also positive for hepatitis B surface antigen because of the potential for reactivation [529,531,546]. In pre-existing autoimmune diseases, responses may be lower in those on immunosuppressive drugs, autoimmune side effects are more common and anti-PD1 therapy-associated flares in pre-existing autoimmune disease is most common in rheumatological conditions and with ipilimumab most common in IBD [531]. In haematological malignancy, retrospective multicentre data suggest similar responses to those in the general population [463,532].

OTRs are the immunosuppressed group in whom use of ICIs poses the greatest challenge [531]. Multiple systematic reviews and case series of retrospective, non-RCT data are now available [450–453,463]. Very broadly, these data indicate disease control rates (complete response, partial response and stable disease) in the order of 30–40%, which are generally lower than those from pivotal trials in the non-immunosuppressed population. Graft rejection rates are approximately 40% and usually occur within 3–4 weeks of treatment. Although early data suggested lower rejection rates with anticytotoxic T-lymphocyte-associated protein 4 treatment [449,461], newer data have not shown significant differences in rejection rates; deaths from disease progression are, however, greater than those for rejection [450–455,463]. Identifying OTRs at risk of rejection is an area of major clinical need and monitoring of donor-derived cell-free DNA has been proposed as a possible approach [533]. Whether immunosuppression should be modified when starting ICIs is also uncertain: in many cases, CNIs are stopped and mTOR inhibitors started, but there is increasing evidence that aggressive reduction of immunosuppression is associated with higher levels of rejection and whether this is appropriate is an important area of uncertainty [461].

Talimogene laherparepvec

Several cases of the successful use of talimogene laherparepvec intralesional immunotherapy in metastatic melanoma have been reported in heart and kidney transplant recipients with no apparent graft rejection, although data are limited [534–536].

Pre-transplant melanoma

Although less common than pre-transplant KC, a previous history of melanoma is likely to become an increasingly common clinical scenario for transplant candidates and the benefits of transplantation need to be carefully balanced against the risk of recurrence [356]. Consensus expert opinion produced by the American Society for Transplantation was modelled on post-transplant survival thresholds, AJCC8 survival curves and the kinetics of cancer recurrence. If a melanoma-specific survival threshold of 80% at 5 years is accepted, then the recommendations are that melanoma *in situ* is not a contraindication to transplantation and waiting times should be 12 months for stage IA–IIA melanoma, 1–2 years for IIIA, and 2–4 years for IIB, IIC and IIIB (acknowledging that data are limited for patients treated with adjuvant immunotherapy). No consensus

Table 147.3 Suggested management protocol for primary skin cancers in organ transplant recipients based on published literature summarised in the text and an expert consensus Delphi exercise.

Stage	Therapeutic considerations	Surveillance
Pre-transplant	Risk assessment Education Photoprotection Treatment of precancerous lesions	
Post-transplant	Baseline risk assessment (risk stratified by age at transplantation, skin phototype, number of sunburns) Education Photoprotection	Within 6–12 months of transplantation
No lesions	Education, photoprotection	Surveillance according to risk levels 1–5 (Figure 147.7)

AK/Bowen disease	Photoprotection
	Lesion-directed therapy:
	  Cryotherapy for isolated or hyperkeratotic AK
	  Surgery if clinically suspicious (e.g. pain, bleeding, nodule)
	Field-directed therapy (for grouped thin AK), e.g. topical 5-FU 5% cream, imiquimod 5% cream, diclofenac 3% gel, PDT/daylight PDT
		12 months
		
		Evidence (limited) supports 5-FU-based regimens first line

Field cancerisation	For thick grouped AK and field cancerisation use cryotherapy first (or 10% salicylic acid ointment) plus field-directed therapy with 5-FU-based treatment (5-FU 5% cream)	6 months

Invasive keratinocyte skin cancers:
BCC
	Infiltrative, nodular: surgery (excision, Mohs micrographic surgery)
	Superficial:
	  Surgery (excision, curettage/cautery)
	  Non-surgical (cryotherapy, 5-FU, imiquimod, PDT)
		6 months (Table 147.4)

First invasive cSCC	Surgery (excision, curettage/cautery) Treatment of AK/Bowen disease/field cancerisation No consensus on oral chemoprevention or modification of immunosuppression	4 months (Table 147.4)
Multiple low-risk cSCC (>3–5)	Rigorous treatment of AK/Bowen disease/field cancerisation Low rate (1 cSCC per year): consider oral chemoprevention (acitretin) High rate (10 cSCCs per year): acitretin and discussion with transplant team regarding modification of immunosuppression	 3 months 2–3 months
High-risk or very high-risk cSCC	Surgery (excision, Mohs micrographic surgery); may need to consider sentinel node biopsy, adjuvant radiotherapy; discussion with transplant team regarding modification of immunosuppression	2–3 months (some evidence that mTOR inhibitors are more effective if introduced after first cSCC)
Multiple high-risk cSCC, >10 cSCCs	Aggressive treatment of individual lesions (as above) Strong indication for modification of immunosuppression Strong indication for oral chemoprevention with systemic retinoids	2 months
Other moderate-risk skin cancers: Melanoma Early KS	Treatment of individual lesions as per standard guidelines Consider revision of immunosuppression (minimisation or switch to mTOR inhibitor) – discuss with transplant clinicians	3 months
Very high-risk skin cancer	Aggressive treatment of individual lesions as indicated above	2 months (Table 147.4)
AJCC stage IIA and above melanoma; extensive KS; MCC; appendageal tumours	Strong indication to revise immunosuppression (minimisation or switch to mTOR inhibitor) – discuss with transplant clinicians	2 months

Adapted from Harwood *et al.* 2013 [52] and Massey *et al.* 2021 [466].
AJCC, American Joint Committee on Cancer; AK, actinic keratosis; BCC, basal cell carcinoma; cSCC, cutaneous squamous cell carcinoma; FC, field cancerisation; 5-FU, 5-fluorouracil 5% cream; KC, keratinocyte cancer; KS, Kaposi sarcoma; MCC, Merkel cell carcinoma; mTOR, mammalian target of rapamycin; PDT, photodynamic therapy.

Table 147.4 Suggested surveillance protocol in organ transplant recipients with skin cancer.

Risk level	Surveillance intervals
First SCC	4, 8 and 12 months; then annually if no further cancers
First BCC	6 and 12 months; then annually if no further cancers
Second/third cancer	3, 6, 9 and 12 months; then annually if no further cancers
>10 cancers or very high-risk skin cancer	2 monthly

Adapted from Harwood et al. 2013 [52].

was reached for melanoma stage IIIC and above, but waiting times of at least 5 years should be considered on a case-by-case basis [537].

Donor transmitted melanoma

Once molecular confirmation of the donor origin of metastatic melanoma in a transplant recipient is confirmed both the recipient and coordinating transplant organisation should be rapidly informed as other recipients from the same donor will also be at high risk [360,538]. There are no consensus recommendations for optimal management and this will particularly depend on the type of allograft and the patient's wishes. For kidney OTRs in whom there is the option of returning to dialysis, immunosuppression is usually withdrawn and the allograft resected. This is not possible for most non-kidney allografts, although successful treatment with targeted therapy and checkpoint inhibitors has been described [530,539,540].

Kaposi sarcoma (Chapter 138)

Diagnosis and staging

The diagnosis of suspected KS is primarily based upon clinical features, but confirmation by histology and immunohistochemistry is particularly important in the context of immunosuppressed patients in whom the differential diagnosis may include atypical infections and other skin tumours [541]. The significant nodal and visceral disease observed in immunosuppression [387] underscores the importance of screening for non-cutaneous involvement. Cross-sectional imaging is usually recommended at baseline together with upper gastrointestinal endoscopy and lung imaging/bronchoscopy in selected cases [387,541].

Treatment

This depends on whether disease is localised and non-aggressive, locally aggressive or disseminated and is aimed at achieving disease control and preserving graft function [541]. Although there are no prospective RCTs in post-transplant KS, European guidelines provide consensus management recommendations for OTRs [541]. In addition to local modalities used in the general population such as surgery, radiotherapy and IMIQ, current recommendations are based on three main axes: immunosuppression reduction, conversion to mTOR inhibitor and chemotherapy [541]. Reduction of immunosuppression usually involves minimising or discontinuing CNIs and this alone can lead to approximately 50% complete or partial regression although it may take months to stabilise [387].

Switching to a mTOR inhibitor, such as sirolimus, was described in 2005 to induce 100% remission in 15 patients [497], although subsequent reports have highlighted relapse and resistance in some cases [542,543]. Chemotherapy including anthracyclines (e.g. pegylated liposomal doxorubicin) and taxanes (e.g. paclitaxel) are used in extensive disease, although preservation of graft function may be an important consideration with some agents [541]. Interferon is not recommended in OTRs as it may be associated with rejection risk, as may PD1 blockade immunotherapy which has shown promise in endemic and classic subtypes [387,541]. Most HIV-related KS responds to ART as first line treatment, but systemic therapy is recommended for more extensive disease [541]. Antiangiogenic agents (e.g. pomalidomide, lenalidomide/bevacizumab) have shown activity in HIV-related KS [544,545] and objective response rates of approximately 63% have been obtained with ICIs in case reports [546].

HHV-8 screening

In HHV-8 seropositive OTRs, viral reactivation with the development of KS occurs in up to 13% after transplant, and transplantation from a seropositive donor to an HHV-8-negative recipient results in seroconversion in up to 30%, although fewer than 4% will develop KS [383,541,547,548]. However, current serological assays have significant limitations and HHV-8 serological screening of donors and recipients pre-transplant is not routine, although it may be indicated in donors and recipients from endemic areas or as targeted screening for high-risk groups in low prevalence regions [541]. Similarly, in recipients who are HHV-8 positive or have a positive donor, viral load monitoring appears to be of limited value in predicting or managing post-transplant KS: 50% or more patients with post-transplant KS may test negative for HHV-8 DNA. There is also no proven role for antivirals, or for tailoring immunosuppression, but it is important to advise patients on potential risk [382,387,541].

Pre-transplant KS and retransplantation

Few data are available regarding transplantation in a patient with a history of KS and this should be considered on a case-by-case basis with possible early introduction of mTOR inhibitor. Post-transplant KS does not automatically preclude retransplantation. Encouragingly, a retrospective review from France found a 25% (2/8) KS recurrence rate after a second kidney transplant in those patients who had post-transplant KS after their first transplant, and recurrent KS usually resolved with modification of immunosuppression [549].

Merkel cell carcinoma
Primary MCC
Surgery and staging

Data on the management of MCC and rare cancers occurring in immunosuppression are limited. There are few data to guide decision making other than the consideration of the higher risk of poorer outcomes. Initial management approaches in terms of surgery, adjuvant radiotherapy and imaging are therefore generally similar to those in the general population (Chapter 146). Although sentinel lymph node biopsy positivity is higher in immunocompromised than immunocompetent patients (31% versus 21%, $P = 0.042$) [550], the implications of this on overall survival are not clear

[550,551]. Nonetheless, accurate nodal staging may inform treatment decisions around optimising regional disease in this high-risk population [550].

Radiotherapy
Responses to radiotherapy are significantly worse in immunosuppression: in patients treated with curative intent for stages I–III MCC, radiotherapy improved recurrence-free survival in immuncompetent but not in immunocompromised patients [552].

Advanced MCC
As for cSCC and melanoma, immunosuppression was an exclusion criterion in pivotal RCTs of anti-PD-L1 therapy in MCC. However, real world data from the expanded access programme for anti-PD-L1 avelumab included patients with CLL, PLWH and OTRs. Although responses were possibly reduced compared with immunocompetent patients, they provide a signal of activity [553], as do data from multicentre retrospective studies in CLL [463] and case series in HIV [546]. Prospective RCTs are required.

Pre-transplant MCC
Although there are currently no reported studies of transplant candidates with MCC, consensus recommendations based on 5-year survival and kinetics of recurrences are for a 2-year minimum waiting time for stage IIb or less (tumour size >2 cm, negative nodal status). For stage III and higher (regional nodal disease), transplantation is not currently recommended [464].

Skin cancer screening and surveillance

Skin cancers in immunocompromised patients pose a significant and growing burden of disease on affected individuals and resource-limited health care systems. Health education, skin cancer screening and risk-stratified surveillance, skin cancer risk prediction, targeted implementation of preventative strategies and rapid access to diagnosis and treatment may all contribute to reducing the impact of skin cancers. In the UK, the National Institute for Health and Care Excellence (NICE) has recommended that immunosuppressed individuals with pre-cancerous lesions or invasive skin cancer should be seen in dedicated clinics, and skin surveillance in these patient groups is increasingly being delivered by such specialist clinics [554–556,573,574].

Most national and international post-transplant clinical practice guidelines (CPGs) advise that all OTRs should be offered skin cancer surveillance at least annually, with full skin examination performed by a dermatologist or trained specialist [557]. There is limited evidence to validate the effectiveness of these expert opinion-based CPG recommendations on reducing skin cancer incidence and improving outcomes. Adherence to surveillance is often low and the health care resource implications of providing universal annual monitoring are considerable [558,573]. Consequently, more risk-stratified approaches to surveillance have been proposed based on observed skin cancer risk in cohort analyses [52,150]. The Covid-19 pandemic and high vulnerability of many of these patient groups has highlighted further the need for rationalising the timing and nature of such routine surveillance.

Initial post-transplant assessment
Following transplantation, baseline assessment of skin cancer risk and health educational advice focusing on photoprotection, self-skin examination and early detection of suspicious lesions is recommended for all patients. Potentially, an initial risk assessment can be done at the time of transplantation using simple clinical information based on age, sex, race and organ type [558]. Recommendations on the optimal timing of subsequent dermatology/specialist skin cancer screening varies and will depend on this initial risk assessment and may be within 12 months post-transplant [52] extended to 2–5 years if the initial risk assessment and educational advice are provided by the transplant team [558].

Evidence from several studies indicates that skin cancer awareness is improved and photoprotective advice better recalled and implemented if health educational advice is provided in a specialist clinical setting [554,555]. The advice provided should be individualised and take into account patient preferences and priorities in order to improve adherence [420,571]. Photoprotection advice, in particular, should be tailored to skin type [58]. Advice may be further optimised by strategies such as the use of written and audiovisual material [420]. Reinforcement of educational messages both improves recall and adherence to advice [420,559–561,572]. Optimal timing for delivering this information is uncertain: in one study patients expressed a preference for receiving information pre-transplant which was then regularly repeated post-transplant [562], while in another, post-transplant intervention was preferred [563].

Risk stratification and post-transplant surveillance protocols before first skin cancer
Understanding the predictors of post-transplant skin cancer enables health care providers to direct targeted surveillance, prevention and management strategies towards higher risk individuals [149]. Several clinical risk prediction models have been described and used to inform the development of risk-stratified surveillance programmes [52,149,150]. Clinical risk factors are also being combined with polygenic risk scores to further improve identification of patients at the highest skin cancer risk.

Clinical risk stratification
The established clinical risk factors for post-transplant skin cancer have been used in a number of risk stratification models from which surveillance protocols have been derived [52,74,149,**150**,564]. For example:
- A risk stratification tool based on a UK OTR cohort assessed the cumulative incidence of skin cancer over time post-transplant to construct five risk groups based upon three risk factors: skin phototype (Fitzpatrick 1–4 versus 5–6), age at transplant (<35, 35–45, 45–55 and >55 years) and sunburn history (<5 versus ≥5 incidents). Clinical surveillance intervals were derived for each group, aiming to keep the estimated cumulative incidence of KC below 5% after baseline assessment; surveillance intervals were also assessed for patients after the first and subsequent skin cancers (Figure 147.7) [52].
- SUNTRAC (Skin and UV Neoplasia Transplant Risk Assessment Calculator) was based on a larger US cohort and defined four risk groups based upon five weighted risk factors: white race, age at

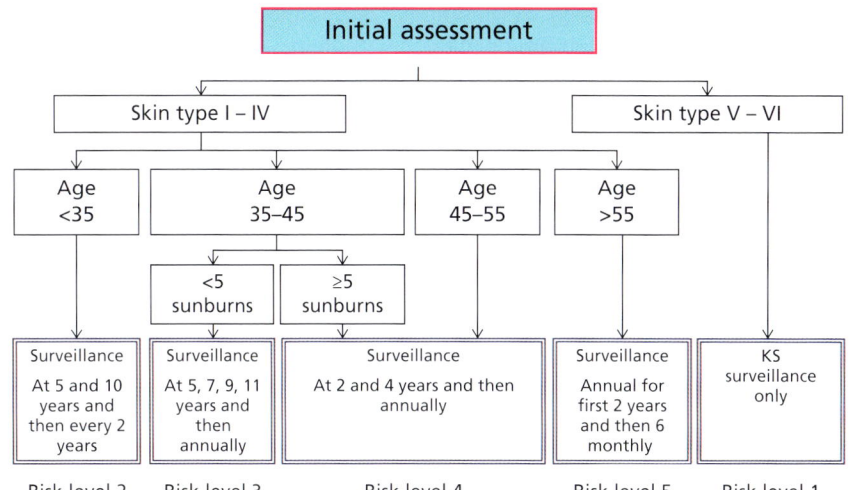

Figure 147.7 Screening and surveillance post-transplant until first skin cancer. KS, Kaposi sarcoma. Adapted from Harwood et al. 2013 [52].

transplant >50 years, history of pre-transplant skin cancer, male versus female and heart/lung versus renal/liver transplant. The 5-year cumulative incidence for skin cancer for low, medium, high and very high SUNTRAC categories was 1.01%, 6.15%, 15.14% and 44.75%, respectively, and surveillance intervals were derived for each risk category based on a minimum 2% skin cancer incidence threshold screening [150].

- In cardiac OTRs, a risk prediction model for cSCC was generated in a multivariate model (age, male sex, white race, recipient and donor HLA mismatch level, malignancy at listing, diagnosis with restrictive myopathy or hypertrophic myopathy, heart retransplant, and induction therapy with OKT3 or daclizumab) with good concordance between the predicted and actual risk at 5, 8 and 10 years post-transplant [564].

Polygenic risk scores

As discussed in more detail earlier in this chapter, polygenic risk scores have been developed that can identify OTRs at a high absolute risk of developing KC in both low and high UV environments [155–157] and may improve KC risk stratification approaches to surveillance in OTRs. However, their cost-effectiveness needs to be validated.

Skin cancer follow-up protocols

Once premalignancy lesions (AK, SCC *in situ*) have developed, annual review is usually recommended and appropriate follow-up after a first invasive skin cancer should be guided by known accrual rates after an initial BCC or cSCC [52,70,72]. For example, a surveillance protocol ensuring cumulative KC risk remains below 15% recommends initial intervals of 4–6 months depending on skin cancer type, reducing to 3–4 monthly or more frequently in those with multiple or very high-risk tumours (Table 147.4) [52].

Pre-transplantation screening

Potential risk reduction strategies such as educational advice on photoprotection and treatment of AK may be most effective if initiated in the pre-transplant period [420]. KC risk stratification pre-transplant, identification of patients with pre-transplant skin cancer and determination of HHV-8 status in patients at risk of KS, may also provide an opportunity for decision making relating to post-transplant immunosuppressive drug regimens and intensity of skin surveillance [464,465]. However, the cost-effectiveness of such pre-transplantation screening strategies has yet to be validated.

Surveillance in other immunocompromised patient cohorts

Most research on risk stratification, screening and surveillance in immunocompromised patient cohorts has focused on OTRs. However, there is increasing recognition that other immunocompromised groups may also potentially benefit, and this has been particularly promoted in patients with CLL and IBD [45,565,566].

Organisations for patients and health care professionals

Several special interest organisations with a focus on skin cancer in immunocompromised individuals exist internationally for patients, carers and health care providers. In Europe, SCOP*E* (Skin Care in Organ Transplant Patients *Europe*, www.scopenetwork.org) coordinates clinical research initiatives and, with ITSCC (International Immunosuppression and Transplant Skin Cancer Collaborative, http://www.itscc.org/), has produced expert consensus guideline documents for the management of post-transplant skin cancer. The AT-RISC Alliance (After Transplantation – Reduce Incidence of Skin Cancer, www.at-risc.org) is linked to ITSCC and has developed educational resources for both patients and health care providers. In the UK, BSSCII (British Society for Skin Care in Immunosuppressed Individuals, www.bsscii.org.uk), aims to fulfil a similar role with a broad remit across all immunocompromised patient groups (all websites last accessed March 2023).

Conclusions

Skin cancers in immunocompromised patients represent a significant burden of disease for affected individuals and a major and escalating clinical challenge for health care providers. Management requires a multidisciplinary approach with integrated decision making between dermatology, dermatological surgery, medical oncology, radiation oncology, pathology and specialist clinical teams (e.g. transplant, HIV, haematology), as well as shared decision making with patients and their carers. Risk stratification together with appropriate counselling, surveillance, access to rapid diagnosis and treatment and preventative strategies may reduce the incidence and impact of these skin cancers in the future. Although there have been advances in the diagnosis and treatment of skin cancer in these patient groups, the evidence base in many key areas is limited. Further clinical and translational research efforts are urgently required to address these gaps. These high-risk patients arguably present a model of accelerated skin carcinogenesis and are an important population in whom to further investigate pathogenesis, therapeutic and preventative approaches in skin cancer. Indeed, it is likely that many future advances in improving patient outcomes for skin cancer, particularly cSCC, will come from research in immunocompromised patient populations.

Key references

The full list of references can be found in the online version at https://www.wiley.com/rooksdermatology10e

19 Collins L, Quinn A, Stasko T. Skin cancer and immunosuppression. *Dermatol Clin* 2019;37:83–94.

27 Venanzi Rullo E *et al*. Non-melanoma skin cancer in people living with HIV: from epidemiology to clinical management. *Front Oncol* 2021;11:689789.

44 Velez NF *et al*. Association of advanced leukemic stage and skin cancer tumor stage with poor skin cancer outcomes in patients with chronic lymphocytic leukemia. *JAMA Dermatol* 2014;150:280–7.

48 Cook M *et al*. Differential outcomes among immunosuppressed patients with Merkel cell carcinoma: impact of immunosuppression type on cancer-specific and overall survival. *Am J Clin Oncol* 2019;42:82–8.

52 Harwood CA *et al*. A surveillance model for skin cancer in organ transplant recipients: a 22-year prospective study in an ethnically diverse population. *Am J Transplant* 2013;13:119–29.

56 Garrett GL *et al*. Incidence of and risk factors for skin cancer in organ transplant recipients in the United States. *JAMA Dermatol* 2017;153:296–303.

58 Kentley J *et al*. The burden of cutaneous disease in solid organ transplant recipients of color. *Am J Transplant* 2021;21:1215–26.

60 Rizvi SMH *et al*. Long-term change in the risk of skin cancer after organ transplantation: a population-based nationwide cohort study. *JAMA Dermatol* 2017;153:1270–7.

150 Jambusaria-Pahlajani A *et al*. Predicting skin cancer in organ transplant recipients: development of the SUNTRAC screening tool using data from a multicenter cohort study. *Transpl Int* 2019;32:1259–67.

174 Coghill AE *et al*. Immunosuppressive medications and squamous cell skin carcinoma: nested case–control study within the skin cancer after organ transplant (SCOT) cohort. *Am J Transplant* 2016;16:565–73.

175 O'Donovan P *et al*. Azathioprine and UVA light generate mutagenic oxidative DNA damage. *Science* 2005;309:1871–4.

194 Euvrard S *et al*. Sirolimus and secondary skin-cancer prevention in kidney transplantation. *N Engl J Med* 2012;367:329–39.

305 Bouwes Bavinck JN *et al*. Pain identifies squamous cell carcinoma in organ transplant recipients: the SCOPE-ITSCC PAIN study. *Am J Transplant* 2014;14:668–76.

387 Delyon J *et al*. Management of Kaposi sarcoma after solid organ transplantation: a European retrospective study. *J Am Acad Dermatol* 2019;81:448–55.

466 Massey PR *et al*. Consensus-based recommendations on the prevention of squamous cell carcinoma in solid organ transplant recipients: a Delphi consensus statement. *JAMA Dermatol* 2021;157:1219–26.

497 Stallone G *et al*. Sirolimus for Kaposi's sarcoma in renal-transplant recipients. *N Engl J Med* 2005;352:1317–23.

PART 13
Systemic Disease and the Skin

CHAPTER 148

Cutaneous Markers of Internal Malignancy

Lennart Emtestam[1] *and Karin Sartorius*[2]

[1] Department of Medicine Huddinge, Karolinska Institutet, Stockholm, Sweden
[2] Department of Clinical Sciences and Education, Karolinska Institutet, Stockholm; and Department of Dermatology, Södersjukhuset, Stockholm, Sweden

Introduction, 148.2

MULTISYSTEM AND HAEMATOPOIETIC TUMOURS THAT INVOLVE THE SKIN, 148.2

TUMOUR SPREAD FROM ADJACENT AND DISTANT TISSUES, 148.2
DIRECT TUMOUR SPREAD AND INVASION, 148.2
CUTANEOUS METASTASIS, 148.4
Paget disease, 148.6
Paget disease of the breast, 148.6
Extramammary Paget disease, 148.7

GENODERMATOSES ASSOCIATED WITH INTERNAL MALIGNANCIES, 148.7
Howel–Evans syndrome, 148.7
Naevoid basal cell carcinoma syndrome, 148.7
Familial melanoma syndrome, 148.8
Melanoma–astrocytoma syndrome, 148.9
Xeroderma pigmentosum, 148.9
Von Hippel–Lindau disease, 148.9
Neurofibromatosis types 1 and 2, 148.9
Tuberous sclerosis complex, 148.10
Multiple endocrine neoplasia syndromes, 148.10
Multiple endocrine neoplasia type 1, 148.10
Multiple endocrine neoplasia type 2A, 148.10
Multiple endocrine neoplasia type 2B, 148.10
Carney complex, 148.11
PTEN hamartoma tumour syndrome, 148.11
Sebaceous tumours, keratoacanthomas and visceral malignancy, 148.12
Hereditary leiomyomatosis and renal cell carcinoma syndrome, 148.12
Bloom, Rothmund–Thomson and Werner syndromes, 148.12
Bloom syndrome, 148.13
Rothmund–Thomson syndrome, 148.13
Werner syndrome, 148.13

IMMUNODEFICIENCY AND NEOPLASIA SYNDROMES, 148.13
Wiskott–Aldrich syndrome, 148.13
Chediak–Higashi syndrome, 148.13
Ataxia-telangiectasia, 148.13
Dyskeratosis congenita, 148.14
Fanconi anaemia, 148.14

PARANEOPLASTIC PHENOMENA INVOLVING THE SKIN, 148.14
ACANTHOTIC AND ICHTHYOTIC EPIDERMAL DISORDERS, 148.14
Acanthosis nigricans, 148.14
Acanthosis palmaris, 148.15
Sign of Leser–Trélat, 148.16
Florid cutaneous papillomatosis, 148.16
Acquired ichthyosis, 148.17
OTHER EPIDERMAL DISORDERS, 148.17
PARANEOPLASTIC PIGMENTATION, 148.17
HAIR, NAILS AND SKIN APPENDAGES, 148.17
Paraneoplastic hypertrichosis lanuginosa acquisita, 148.17
Clubbing of nails, 148.18
Hyperhidrosis, 148.18

DERMATOSES ASSOCIATED WITH INTERNAL MALIGNANCIES, 148.19
Acrokeratosis paraneoplastica, 148.19
Migratory erythemas, 148.19
CONNECTIVE TISSUE AND RHEUMATOLOGICAL DISORDERS, 148.20
Dermatomyositis, 148.20
Lupus erythematosus, 148.21
Systemic sclerosis and other inflammatory fibrosing conditions of the dermis and subcutis, 148.21
BULLOUS DISORDERS ASSOCIATED WITH INTERNAL MALIGNANCY, 148.21
Paraneoplastic pemphigus, 148.21
Bullous pemphigoid, 148.22
Pemphigus, 148.22
OTHER BLISTERING DISORDERS, 148.22
Dermatitis herpetiformis, 148.22
Linear IgA disease, 148.22
Epidermolysis bullosa acquisita, 148.22
Porphyria cutanea tarda and variegate porphyrias, 148.22
DEPOSITION DISORDERS, 148.22
OTHER DERMATOLOGICAL DISORDERS, 148.23
Lichen planus, 148.23
Urticaria, 148.23
Erythroderma and exfoliative dermatitis, 148.23
Granuloma annulare, 148.23
Insect bite-like reactions, 148.23
Cutis verticis gyrata, 148.23
Mental neuropathy, 148.23
Pyoderma gangrenosum and neutrophilic dermatoses, 148.23
Multicentric reticulohistiocytosis, 148.24

VASCULAR DISORDERS ASSOCIATED WITH INTERNAL MALIGNANCY, 148.24
Raynaud phenomenon and digital ischaemia, 148.24
Erythromelalgia, 148.25
Palmar erythema, 148.25
Vasculitis, 148.25
Chilblain-like lesions, 148.25
Flushing, 148.25
Carcinoid syndrome, 148.25
Mastocytosis, 148.26
Phaeochromocytomas, 148.26
Medullary carcinoma of thyroid, 148.26
CANCER-ASSOCIATED THROMBOSIS, 148.26
Migratory thrombophlebitis, 148.26
Deep-vein thrombosis, 148.26
Mondor disease, 148.26
Venous or lymphatic obstruction, 148.27

PARANEOPLASTIC PRURITUS, 148.27
Generalised pruritus, 148.27
Localised pruritus, 148.27

Key references, 148.27

Introduction

There is a great variation of skin change associated with internal malignancy, and the connection between systemic neoplasia and associated skin conditions are so numerous that to report all documented associations here is impracticable. However, the following categories entail most associations and interactions between skin and internal malignancy:

1. Multisystem and haematopoietic tumours that involve the skin.
2. Tumour spread.
3. Genetically determined syndromes with cutaneous manifestations where there is a recognised predisposition to internal malignancy (also termed 'genodermatoses with malignant potential'). This category also includes the hamartoneoplastic syndromes.
4. Paraneoplastic disorders: cutaneous reaction patterns that have an association with neoplasia involving various internal organ systems.
5. Indirect cutaneous markers of internal malignancy (for example dermatological features of exposure to carcinogens).

Potential cutaneous markers of internal malignancy vary in their reliability for predicting underlying neoplasia. The extent and intensity of the investigations for malignancy should therefore be tempered by a general assessment of the patient. Cutaneous adverse reactions to drugs used to treat malignancy are covered in Chapter 119.

MULTISYSTEM AND HAEMATOPOIETIC TUMOURS THAT INVOLVE THE SKIN

This group includes several tumours in which the skin is involved as part of a multisystem neoplasm. The contributions from dermatologists are important since the diagnosis may present with skin lesions, or the skin may be the easiest accessible site for biopsies. The types of skin involvement that may occur in such disorders range from non-specific signs, such as purpura reflecting thrombocytopenia, to specific features such as cutaneous deposits of the malignancy. This type of involvement of the skin as part of a multisystem tumour is somewhat different from that of metastases from solid tumours, both in mechanism and in lesion distribution. For example, skin involvement is an important component of haematopoietic malignancies, including lymphoma and Langerhans cell histiocytosis [1,2]; specific cutaneous infiltrations of the skin may occur with myeloproliferative disorders, such as lymphoma and leukaemia (Figure 148.1) [3].

TUMOUR SPREAD FROM ADJACENT AND DISTANT TISSUES

DIRECT TUMOUR SPREAD AND INVASION

Other than primary skin neoplasms, the skin may be involved by tumour either through direct invasion, or through local metastasis, or from cutaneous metastases from an internal tumour.

Direct invasion of the skin from a deeper tumour usually causes nodular infiltration, ulceration or inflammation, but may present in less obvious ways: dermal infiltration causing sclerosis (carcinoma en cuirasse), vascular changes (carcinoma telangiectodes), a *peau d'orange* (orange peel) appearance and, more rarely, a carcinoma erysipeloides (inflammatory metastatic carcinoma) pattern (Figures 148.2 and 148.3). Although these patterns may occur as distant metastases, they most commonly occur in the skin in the vicinity of the primary tumour (most commonly associated with breast cancer) and are therefore usefully considered as a rather different pattern from those tumours that metastasise to distant sites. All of these patterns may be difficult to diagnose unless there is clinical suspicion.

Carcinoma en cuirasse. This may have an early inflammatory stage, and may include some nodularity (Figure 148.2b), but at a later stage is sclerodermoid in appearance (Figure 148.2c). A particular diagnostic problem arises when a breast cancer has been treated with radiotherapy as this may cause postirradiation morphoea. The latter is relatively well documented but the early inflammatory phase of postirradiation morphoea that occurs in some patients is much less well recognised and may be alarming clinically. Carcinoma en cuirasse may also occur with lung, gastrointestinal, renal and other malignancies [1].

Carcinoma erysipeloides. This resembles erysipelas, presenting as an extensive, warm, oedematous, tender plaque but without pyrexia or toxaemia (Figure 147.2d). This pattern accounts for nearly a third of cases of cutaneous metastases from breast cancer [2], the malignancy with which it is most commonly associated [3]. Similar presentations have been reported in melanoma, mesothelioma and carcinomas of the lung, prostate, oesophagus, bladder, colon, larynx, rectum, stomach, cutaneous squamous and pancreas [3–23]. In the majority of cases, the clinical picture is due to the plugging of dermal lymphatics by tumour cell emboli rather than

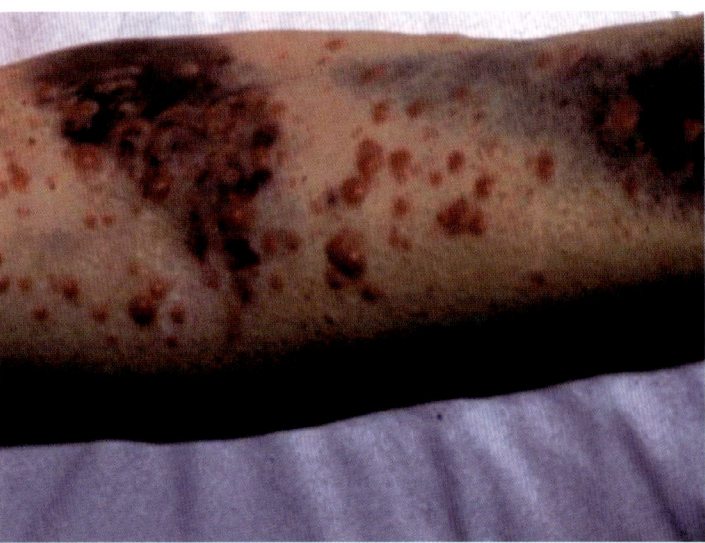

Figure 148.1 Leukaemia cutis (acute myeloid leukaemia) and purpura.

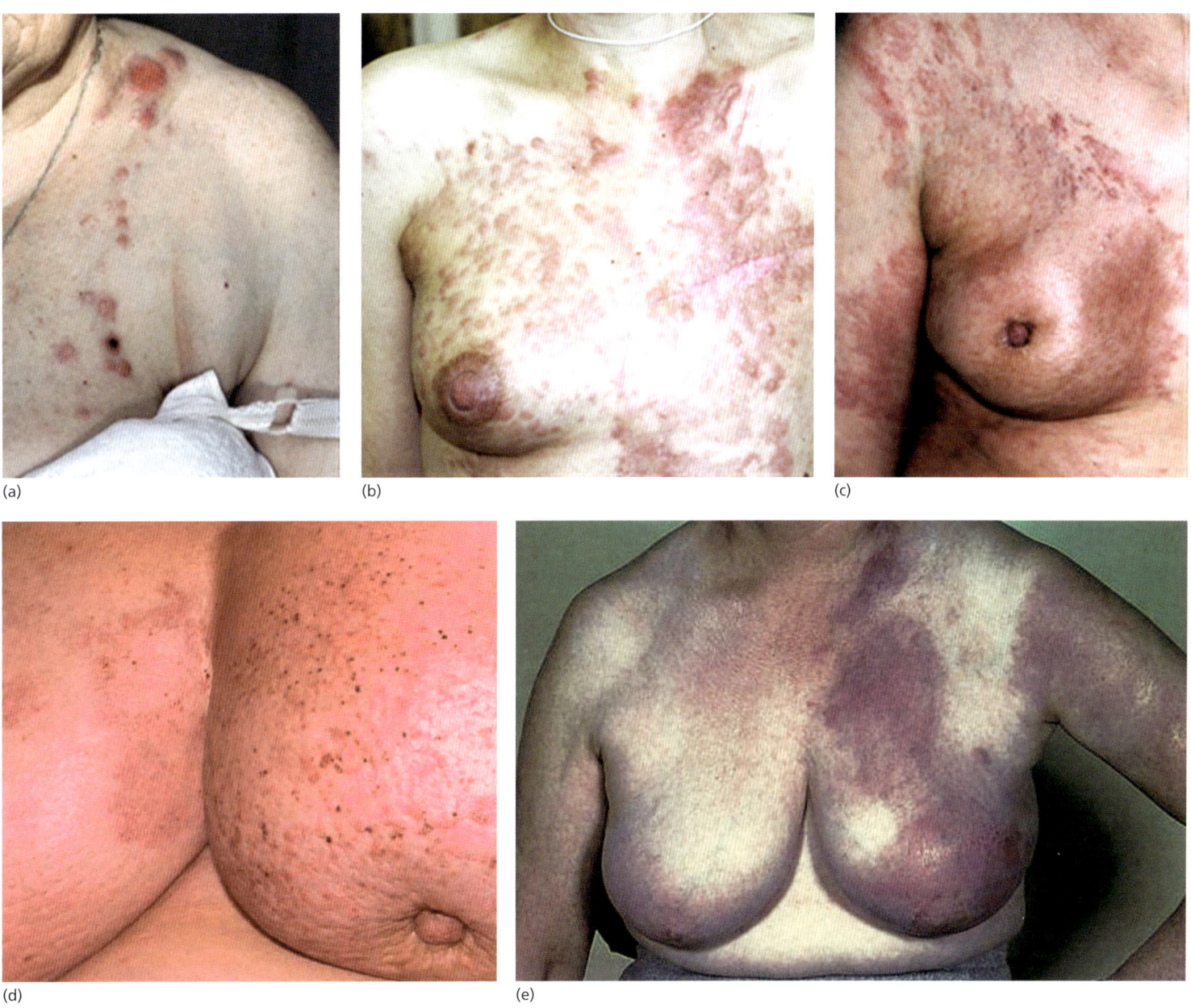

Figure 148.2 Patterns of skin infiltration by carcinoma of the breast. (a, b) Limited (a) and extensive (b) nodular infiltration. (c) Sclerotic infiltration (carcinoma en cuirasse) of breast skin and telangiectatic infiltration (carcinoma telangiectodes) extending beyond the breast. (d) *Peau d'orange* appearance due to infiltrative carcinoma skin of left breast. (d, e) Erysipelas-like changes (carcinoma erysipeloides) involving the right breast at an early stage (d) and at an advanced stage involving the left upper extremity as well as the breast (e). Note also nipple retraction in parts (c) and (d). (a–c) Courtesy of Dr Olga Mikheeva, Moscow Region Oncological Dispensary, Russia. (d) Courtesy of Dr Ken Tsai; (e) Courtesy of Dr R. Emmerson, Royal Berkshire Hospital, Reading, UK.

to intratumoural lymphatic invasion [2,24]. Histologically, there is plugging of the dermal lymphatics at all levels by aggregates of carcinoma cells (Figure 148.4).

Telangiectatic metastatic carcinoma. Telangiectatic metastatic carcinoma is typically associated with breast cancer and may be difficult to diagnose as tumour cells may be quite scanty and the telangiectasia quite subtle. The vascular changes may be more florid and lesional skin can resemble angiosarcoma.

Less common patterns of direct tumour invasion include breast carcinoma presenting as an inframammary intertrigo-like pattern, and lymphatic obstruction by pelvic tumours or lymphadenopathy, which may be accompanied by extensive tumour cells within the lymphatics presenting as skin nodules. Oral tumours, usually squamous cell carcinomas, may extend to directly involve the skin of the face.

Local and in-transit metastases from primary epidermal tumours are discussed in the relevant chapters in this book; melanoma is the most important tumour in this context. It is a particular feature of malignant lymph node metastases (e.g. breast carcinoma, melanoma), and occasionally arises after diagnostic or therapeutic interventions such as needle aspiration of a tumour, pleural biopsy, drainage of malignant ascites or placement of other drains in the

148.4 Chapter 148: Cutaneous Markers of Internal Malignancy

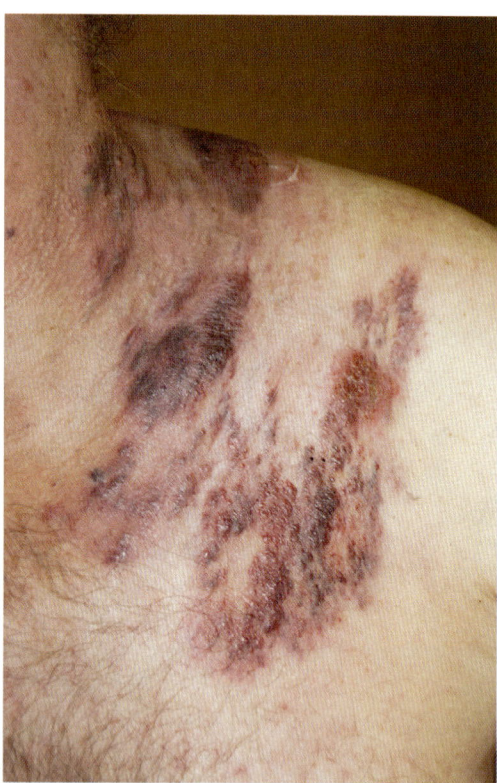

Figure 148.3 Metastatic bronchial carcinoma resembling cutaneous angiosarcoma. Courtesy of Dr Olga Mikheeva, Moscow Region Oncological Dispensary, Russia.

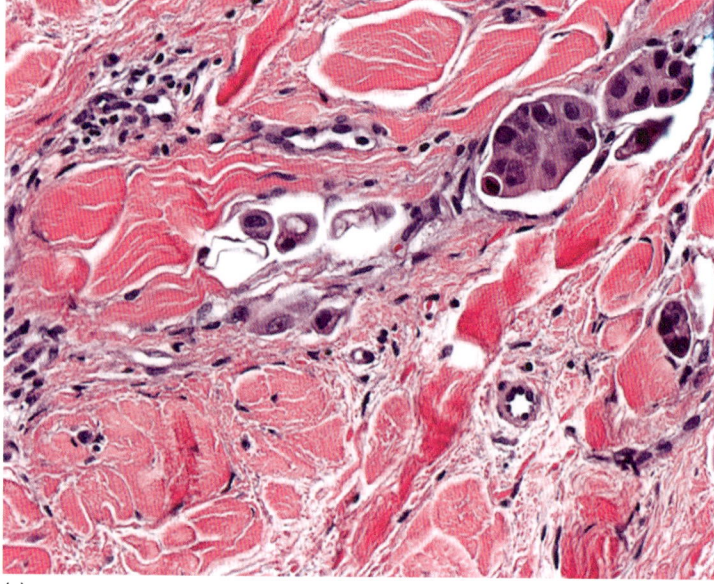

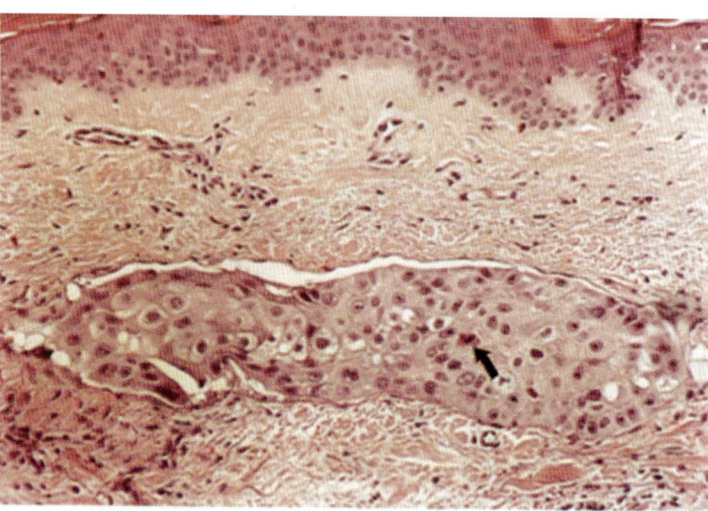

Figure 148.4 Carcinoma erysipeloides. (a) Small aggregates of large epithelioid carcinoma cells within the dilated lymphatics. (b) Dermal lymphatic completely occluded by poorly differentiated epithelioid cells. Note tumour cell necrosis (arrow). (a) Courtesy of Dr K. Tsai. (b) Reproduced from Finkel and Griffiths 1993 [22] with permission of John Wiley & Sons.

vicinity of a tumour. 'Tumour spillage' is the direct contamination of wounds with tumour cells during a laparoscopy or surgical procedure. This was common previously but the rates of laparoscopic port site metastasis and laparotomy wound metastasis from tumour inoculation are now both approximately 0.8% [25].

CUTANEOUS METASTASIS

Frequency of skin metastases

Metastasis to the skin is not as common as metastasis to the liver, lung or bone. Autopsy studies suggest that up to 9% of patients with internal cancer have had skin metastases; a large analysis indicated that 5% is usual [1], and in about 0.5–1% a metastasis is the presenting feature of internal cancer [2,3]. Of patients with metastatic cancer, 10% have cutaneous metastases [4]. Studies vary in cited frequency of skin metastases in part because some include metastasis from cutaneous melanoma whilst others exclude this and only refer to internally originating tumours. Additionally, it can sometimes be difficult to know whether skin involvement is from close proximity with a primary tumour of a different organ, that is, direct invasion not metastasis [5]. The most common sources of cutaneous metastases are, in generally accepted order of frequency: breast, melanoma, lung, colon, stomach, upper aerodigestive tract, uterus and kidney. The most common skin metastases from a previously unknown primary tumour originate from the kidney, lung, thyroid or ovary [3,6,7].

Appearance of skin metastases

Cutaneous metastases generally present as painless, firm to hard nodules, which may be skin coloured, blue-brown or reddish purple. The commonest pattern presents with a solitary nodule (Figure 148.5), which is twice as frequent as multiple nodules (Figure 148.6). Dermal or subcutaneous nodules may be more readily detected by palpation as they may not initially be apparent or symptomatic (Figure 148.7) [6]. The ulceration of nodules may occur but is not usually a feature at initial presentation. Other patterns include morphoea-like sclerotic plaques, scar infiltration, erysipelas-like diffuse skin infiltration, infiltrated areas of alopecia (alopecia neoplastica) and embolic metastasis to digits (Figure 148.8).

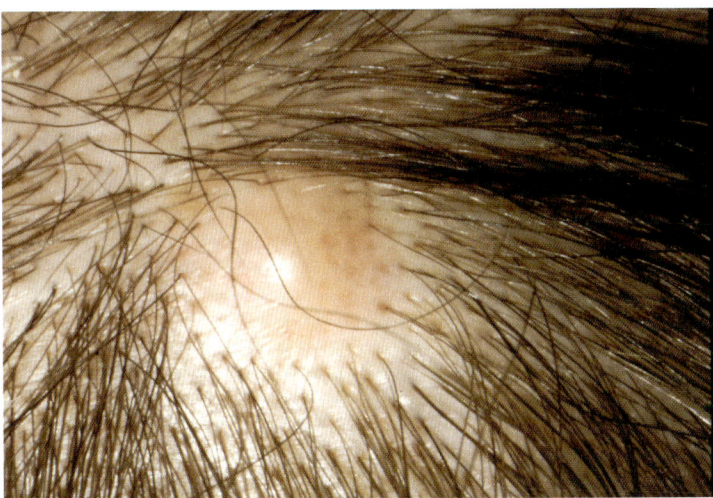

Figure 148.5 Solitary metastasis of squamous carcinoma to the scalp from an unknown primary.

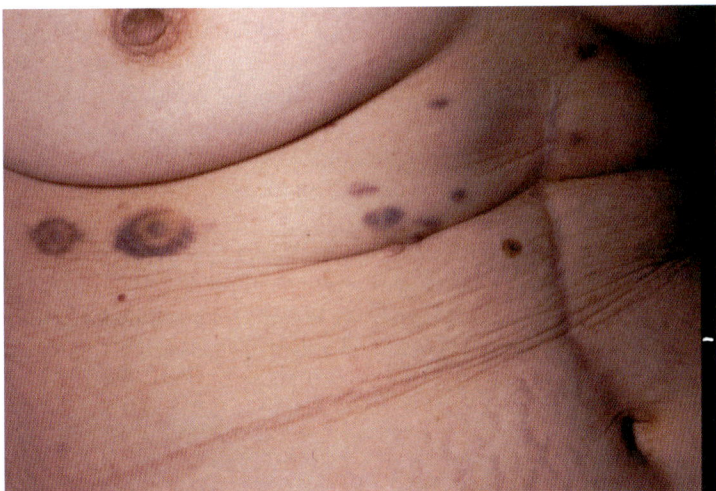

Figure 148.6 Metastatic pancreatic carcinoma manifesting as haemorrhagic nodules in the skin.

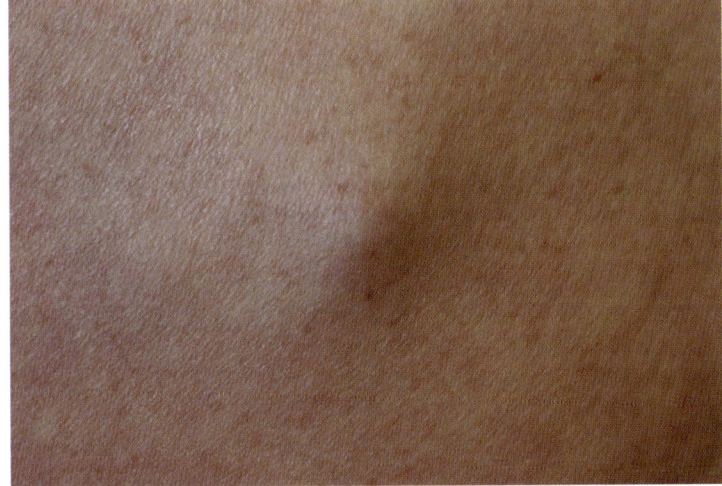

Figure 148.7 Subcutaneous metastasis from lung carcinoma. These metastases are typically multiple and multiple firm nodules can usually be palpated if the patient is carefully examined.

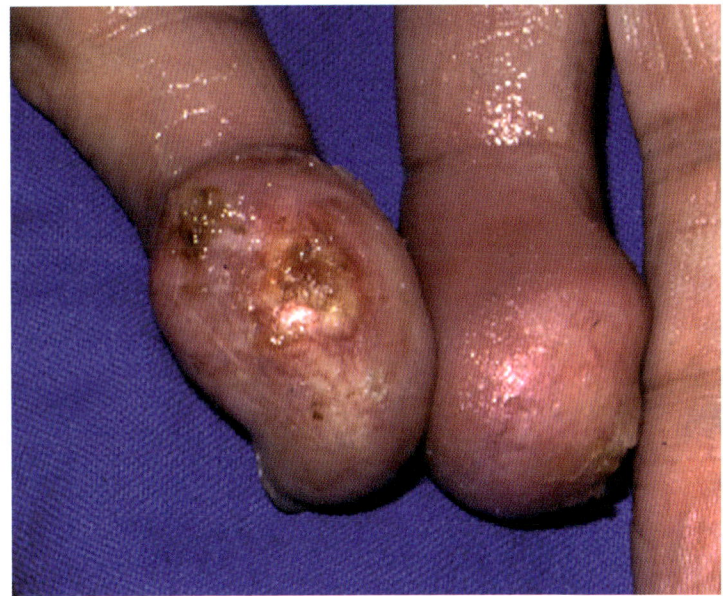

Figure 148.8 Embolic metastasis to the fifth digit of each hand from carcinoma of the oesophagus.

Mechanisms and distribution

Metastasis to the skin occurs as a result of lymphatic or haematogenous dissemination of tumour. The distribution pattern on the skin is not random [3,5]. Indeed, 75% of metastases are found on the head, neck and upper trunk, which together constitute only 25% of the body surface area [3]. The clinical pattern of metastases may provide clues to the route of metastasis. For example, metastases to extremities suggest intra-arterial embolic spread, widespread skin metastases suggest that tumour cells are present in the general circulation, whilst metastases to the skin in the vicinity of the affected organ is more suggestive of dissemination by lymphatic vessels or by veins (Figure 148.9). Retrograde lymphatic spread may occur from pelvic tumours causing metastases in the perineal area or on the legs. In general, the head, neck and upper trunk are disproportionately affected by tumours that metastasise to the skin [3,6–8], possibly because of the high vascularity of this area. The tumour and host factors involved in metastasis, both generally and organ-specific, are not fully understood but recent studies indicate that non-coding RNAs in tumour-derived exosomes influence the metastatic spread [9,10].

Other than the scalp, notable sites for skin metastasis include the umbilicus (Sister Mary Joseph nodule related most commonly to bowel tumours) [7,11,12] and recent operative scars. Scar metastasis is most often related to surgery for the primary tumour, and with the low frequency of 'tumour spillage' presumably represents spread by local lymphatic or venous drainage. However, recent but distant scars (e.g. skin graft donor sites [13,14]) may be a site of metastases. Metastases have also been reported that are localised to a site of irradiation of the skin [15]. An additional, unusual phenomenon is 'tumour-to-tumour metastasis', in which metastases localise to another (usually benign) tumour [16]. Most such metastases occur within quite vascular neoplasms, such as thyroid or adrenal adenomas, but metastasis to lipoma and to basal cell carcinoma have both been reported rarely and are relevant to dermatologists [17].

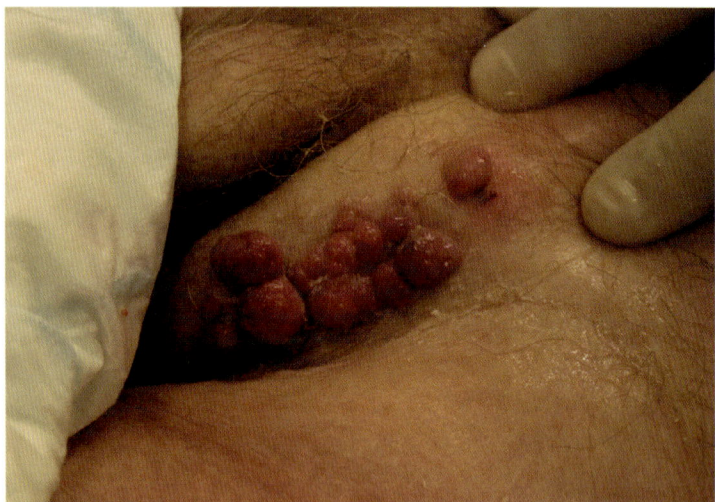

Figure 148.9 Metastasis to the groin in a patient with extensive pelvic prostatic carcinoma.

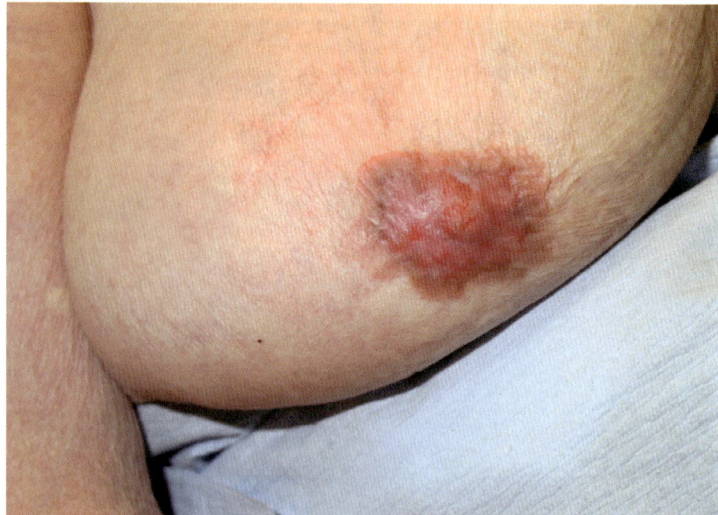

Figure 148.10 Paget disease of the breast causing destruction of the right nipple.

Metastases to the scalp may give rise to focal alopecia, usually from carcinomas of the breast, lung or kidney. Renal and thyroid cancer metastases may be quite vascular in appearance, both clinically and pathologically [18], and are occasionally misdiagnosed as benign haemangiomas or pyogenic granulomas. Metastases from renal cell carcinoma may even be pulsatile. Cutaneous metastases may be mistaken for cysts or inflammatory lesions, and alopecia over a scalp 'cyst' should alert the physician to the possibility of malignancy.

Histopathology

Biopsy of a suspected skin metastasis will usually successfully confirm or exclude malignancy. It is not, however, always useful in determining the organ of origin if the tumour cells are poorly differentiated. Recent work has uncovered the unique biology of metastasis-initiating cells that results in tumour growth in distant organs, the evasion of host immune surveillance and co-option of metastatic microenvironments [19]. Occasionally it may be difficult, even with the use of various types of molecular tumour markers, to distinguish reliably between primary skin tumours and metastatic disease. Although the cells of a metastasis usually resemble the cells of the primary tumour, some patterns may prove diagnostically difficult. Spindle cell tumours and tumours comprising 'small blue cells' cause particular difficulty and may need a panel of molecular markers to aid in diagnosis, both between primary skin lesions and metastases or between different origins of an internal tumour.

In some instances there may be marked oedema or dilated lymphatic vessels that makes diagnosis difficult. In some specific tumours such as renal cell carcinoma or in some clinical patterns such as carcinoma telangiectodes, the tumour cells may either be scanty or the vascular proliferation may dominate the histopathological appearance. Lymphatic spread of tumour cells may lead to an 'Indian filing' appearance in some cases, sometimes with fibrosis.

Prognosis

Cutaneous metastases usually occur in subjects with a known cancer but may be the first indication of an internal neoplasm, especially in the case of lung cancers. They are usually suggestive of disseminated disease and hence indicate a poor prognosis: survival with disseminated skin metastases is typically only about 3 months [4]. Patients with solitary metastases without other evidence of dissemination may have a better survival rate [20]. Infrequent cases of tumour regression after primary tumour removal have been documented [21]. It is noteworthy that cutaneous metastases do not necessarily relate to a prior, documented tumour. The histological pattern, localisation and temporal relationship may occasionally point to a second primary [22].

Treatment options, depending on the primary tumour, may include excision or other destructive therapy (e.g. laser destruction, radiotherapy, photodynamic therapy) for limited numbers of lesions, and chemotherapy or other systemic treatment for disseminated lesions.

Paget disease

Paget disease occurs in mammary and extramammary forms. Paget disease of the breast occurs due to an underlying ductal tumour [1]. Extramammary Paget disease may occur without an underlying tumour, or distant to a tumour, and so does not have the close link with direct tumour spread of the mammary pattern [2].

Paget disease of the breast

This condition presents with scaling and redness, sometimes with oozing and crusting, on or around the nipple (Figure 148.10). It is generally viewed as a direct epidermal extension of an underlying ductal adenocarcinoma, and is important as the underlying tumour is usually small and superficial so early recognition may allow curative intervention. However, of the 30–50% of patients with a palpable underlying lesion, half will have axillary lymph node involvement. The reason for the epidermotropic spread of tumour cells is uncertain but a keratinocyte-derived chemoattractant for Paget cells, termed heregulin-α, was proposed [2]. The main pathogenetic hypothesis for those cases that do not have an underlying carcinoma is derivation from Toker cells within the epidermis of the nipple and areola [2].

Eczema, psoriasis, hyperkeratosis and erosive adenomatosis of the nipple are in the clinical differential diagnosis of mammary

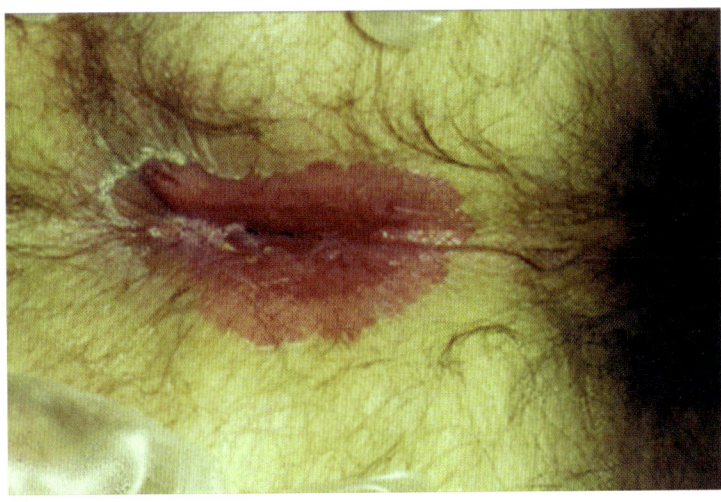

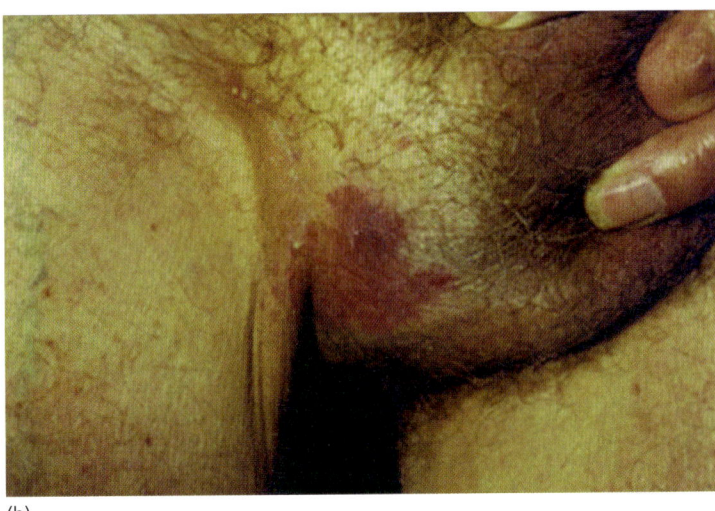

Figure 148.11 Extramammary Paget disease. (a, b) Well-defined red plaques involving the perianal skin (a) and the scrotum (b). Reproduced from Wagner and Sachse 2011 [8] with permission of John Wiley & Sons.

Paget disease. Histologically, there may be diagnostic problems from other disorders with Pagetoid spread, such as some melanomas or Bowen disease, and also from a benign proliferation of Toker cells (clear cell papulosis). Useful histopathological markers for mammary Paget disease include epithelial membrane antigen (EMA), carcinoembryonic antigen (CEA) and cytokeratins (CK8/18) as well as mucins such as MUC1 [3,4].

Extramammary Paget disease

Extramammary Paget disease (EMPD) occurs in apocrine gland-bearing areas such as ano-genital and axillary sites (Chapters 109 and 110). About 60% of cases are vulval, 20% perianal and 15% penile or scrotal. There is thus a female preponderance, although some populations, such as the Japanese [3], have a male preponderance. The histogenesis is less certain and only about 25% of patients appear to have an associated invasive malignancy. Of the malignancies associated with vulval Paget disease, less than 50% arise locally from apocrine sweat glands or Bartholin glands; the remainder arise from the vagina, cervix, bladder, ovary, colon or rectum, or occasionally from more distant sites such as the breast or gallbladder [4,5]. Perianal Paget disease (Figure 148.11a) is associated with an adnexal tumour in about 10% and a distant tumour in about 25% (rectum, stomach, ureter, breast) [4,5]. Male genital Paget disease (Figure 147.11b) is associated with carcinoma of the prostate, bladder, ureter, kidney or testes in about 10% of cases [4,5]. In other cases, EMPD arises locally in the epidermis.

Most patients are over 60 years of age. Clinical features include itch, a burning sensation, oedema, bleeding and reddish brown (or sometimes hypopigmented) plaques, often with a prominent margin. The margin may, however, be obscured by secondary infection and may be difficult to define in vaginal mucosa. Genital EMPD is often mistaken for an eczematous process, psoriasis or tinea. Histological and immunohistochemical features are similar to those of mammary Paget disease; the antigen RCAS1 seems particularly sensitive [6]. The prognosis is determined by the underlying tumour, if present, and whether or not this is amenable to curative treatment. For associated malignancies of a local epidermal origin, the depth of invasion and lymphatic spread dictate the prognosis, and serum CEA is a useful indicator of survival [3]. CK19 fragment 21-1 is a promising new marker for the same purpose [7].

GENODERMATOSES ASSOCIATED WITH INTERNAL MALIGNANCIES

There are many genodermatoses that are associated with an increased risk of internal malignancy (Table 148.1) [1–5,**6**,7,8,**9**,10]. A number of mechanisms are involved and these include chromosomal instability, faulty DNA repair mechanisms, abnormal lymphocyte function and immunosurveillance, and in some cases a combination of these processes.

Howel–Evans syndrome

This syndrome is the association of autosomal dominantly inherited focal palmoplantar keratoderma (tylosis) with the eventual development of oesophageal carcinoma (Chapter 63). Oral leukoplakia also frequently occurs in Howel–Evans syndrome [1–9].

Naevoid basal cell carcinoma syndrome

Synonyms and inclusions
- Gorlin syndrome

Naevoid basal cell carcinoma syndrome is the association between basal cell carcinomas, mandibular odontogenic keratocysts, skeletal anomalies, abnormal calcification and dyskeratotic pits of palms and soles (Chapter 140). Patients with this syndrome are at risk of developing medulloblastoma and ovarian tumours. Other rare

Table 148.1 Examples of genodermatoses associated with internal malignancies.

Main organ affected or usual mode of presentation (many are multisystem disorders)	Genodermatosis	Main neoplasms (may be limited to few families in some of the disorders listed)
Gastrointestinal tract	Gardner syndrome Bannayan–Riley–Ruvalcaba syndrome Turcot syndrome (mismatch repair cancer syndrome)	Gastrointestinal polyposis and carcinomas, central nervous system tumours
	Peutz–Jeghers syndrome	Gastrointestinal polyposis and carcinomas, pancreatic carcinoma, genital tumours (especially Sertoli cell, sex cord and cervix), breast cancers, lung cancers
Neurological	Ataxia–telangiectasia	Lymphomas, leukaemias
	Neurofibromatosis	Neurological tumours, sarcomas, phaeochromocytoma
Skin	Xeroderma pigmentosum	Skin cancers, sarcomas, central nervous system tumours, leukaemia, various solid organ tumours
	Naevoid basal cell carcinoma syndrome (Gorlin)	Basal cell carcinomas of skin, medulloblastoma
	Bazex–Dupré–Christol syndrome	Basal cell carcinomas of skin, possible leukaemia
	Porphyria cutanea tarda	Hepatocellular carcinoma
	Tylosis	Oesophageal carcinoma
	Sclerotylosis (Huriez syndrome)	Squamous cell carcinoma of skin; oral and bowel cancers also reported
	Muir–Torre syndrome	Colo-rectal tumours, sebaceous carcinoma
	Birt–Hogg–Dubé syndrome and Hornstein–Knickenberg syndrome	Medullary carcinoma of thyroid, renal cell carcinoma
	Familial leiomyomas (also uterine)	Renal cell carcinoma, others (see text)
	Incontinentia pigmenti	Wilms tumour, rhabdomyosarcomas (renal, paratesticular), retinoblastoma, leukaemias
	Familial atypical naevi and melanoma	Pancreatic carcinoma, cutaneous and ocular melanoma
	Melanoma–astrocytoma syndrome	Melanomas, astrocytomas and other central nervous system tumours
	Supernumerary nipples	Genito-urinary tumours: renal cell carcinoma, Wilms tumour, bladder, testicular, prostate
	Ichthyoses (autosomal dominant and X-linked)	Testicular carcinoma
Endocrine	Multiple endocrine neoplasia syndromes	Medullary carcinoma of thyroid, phaeochromocytoma
Growth/skeletal	Werner syndrome	Many tumours especially sarcomas
	Rothmund–Thomson syndrome	Skin cancers, osteosarcoma
	Bloom syndrome	As for general population but early onset
	Maffucci syndrome	Chondrosarcomas, gliomas, ovarian cancers
	Goltz syndrome	Chondrosarcomas, giant cell tumour of bone
	Fanconi anaemia (usually presents due to congenital malformations)	Myelodysplastic syndrome, acute myelogenous leukaemia, hepatic carcinoma
Haematopoietic	Dyskeratosis congenita	Mucosal squamous cell carcinoma, haematopoietic malignancy and others
Immunological	Wiskott–Aldrich syndrome	Lymphoreticular malignancies
	Chediak–Higashi syndrome	Lymphoreticular malignancies
Multisystem	Cowden (multiple hamartoma and neoplasia) syndrome	Breast, thyroid, gastrointestinal, cerebellum, endometrial and renal carcinomas
	Carney complex	Myxomas, schwannomas, testicular Sertoli cell tumour, pituitary adenomas, thyroid cancer
	Von Hippel–Lindau disease	Phaeochromocytoma, renal carcinoma, haemangioblastoma, pancreatic carcinoma
	Beckwith–Wiedemann syndrome (exomphalos–macroglossia–gigantism syndrome)	Wilms tumour, adrenal carcinoma, hepatoblastoma, pancreatoblastoma and others (especially in patients with hemihypertrophy)

central nervous system (CNS) tumours have been reported in naevoid basal cell carcinoma syndrome [1–5,**6**,7–10].

Familial melanoma syndrome

Typically, there is one or more of the following: a family history of melanoma, a personal history of multiple atypical melanocytic naevi or a family history of multiple atypical melanocytic naevi (Chapter 142). Large, multiple and irregular naevi are the norm, with an early onset of melanoma. Multiple primary melanomas may occur and, in some pedigrees, there is an increase in non-cutaneous malignancies.

The mode of inheritance is probably polygenic. Higher risk susceptibility genes have been identified, a *CDKN2A* germline mutation in the 9p21 gene region is the most common [1–3]. Mutations that impair p16 function are linked with an increased risk in pancreatic cancer, and specific mutations have been linked with breast cancer in some populations [2,3]. Cases with pancreatic, gastrointestinal, lung, breast and laryngeal cancers are published.

Melanoma–astrocytoma syndrome

This syndrome comprises an association of melanomas with astrocytomas or other CNS tumours, meningiomas, ependymomas and peripheral nerve tumours such as malignant schwannoma [1–4] (Chapter 142). Deletions of chromosome 9p21, which includes tumour suppressor and cell cycle regulating genes, are implicated. Several genetic loci have been implicated in different families including all or parts of the p16, p19 and p15 gene cluster (*INK4* locus), which includes *CDKN2A* and *CDKN2B* [1–3], and a specific deletion of p14(ARF) [4].

Xeroderma pigmentosum

Xeroderma pigmentosum (XP) characteristically presents at an early age with severe photosensitivity (Chapter 76). Patients display a marked congenital reduction in threshold for sunburn and present with myriads of lentigines, principally in a sun-exposed distribution. Early onset of photoageing is found in infants, followed by sun-induced dysplasias, basal and squamous cell carcinomas and malignant melanomas, commencing in the first decade of life [1].

The mode of inheritance is autosomal recessive. The mutations causing XP cause abnormal fibroblast sensitivity to ultraviolet radiation, in most cases (complementation groups A–G) resulting from a defective DNA nucleotide excision repair process. Inactivation of tumour suppressors and activation of oncogenes due to these mutations results in the development of multiple tumours [2].

Ocular neoplasms, both melanoma and non-melanoma, occur in 10–20% of individuals with XP. However, there is also a 10–20-fold increased incidence of internal malignancy in XP including CNS sarcomas, leukaemia and carcinomas of the lung, breast, pancreas, stomach and testes [3].

Von Hippel–Lindau disease

Von Hippel–Lindau disease is an autosomal dominantly inherited condition that carries a high risk of internal malignancy and is associated with non-specific cutaneous manifestations such as haemangiomas and café-au-lait spots [1,2]. It is characterised by benign and malignant tumours of various systems, particularly haemangioblastomas of the CNS, angiomatosis of the retinae, phaeochromocytoma (which may be bilateral) [1], renal carcinoma [3], pancreatic adenoma, carcinoma and cysts [4] and epididymal cystadenomas.

The VHL gene has been located on the short arm of chromosome 3, although different mutations have been found to be causative. The gene is a tumour suppressor gene following the Knudson two-hit hypothesis. Families may be characterised by the absence of phaeochromocytoma (type 1, deletions/protein-truncating mutations) or the presence of phaeochromocytoma (type 2, missense mutations) [5,6].

Neurofibromatosis types 1 and 2

Synonyms and inclusions
Neurofibromatosis type 1
• Von Recklinghausen disease

There are two main forms of neurofibromatosis: type 1 (NF1) and type 2 (NF2) and both have an autosomal dominant inheritance. In a proportion of affected individuals the condition is due to a *de novo* mutation.

The abnormal function of neural crest cells in NF1 leads to the development of multiple peripheral neurofibromas as well as CNS tumours, notably optic glioma (which is one of the diagnostic criteria for NF1) and café-au-lait macules [1,2–4]. Clinical overlap between NF1 and NF2 occurs particularly in children, who may have café-au-lait macules and peripheral nerve tumours; flexural freckling is indicative of NF1. Café-au-lait macules occur in NF2 but only in half of affected subjects, and there are usually fewer than six in number (six or more being one of the diagnostic criteria for NF1). Lisch nodules (pigmented iris hamartomas) are found with slit lamp analysis in 90% of adult patients with NF1 and are fairly specific for NF1. Around 80% of patients with NF2 have posterior subcapsular cataracts, including about a third of affected children. It was recently shown in mice that the NF1 mutation drives neuronal activity-dependent intiation of optic gliomas [5].

The associations with benign tumours, malignant tumours and systemic manifestations are varied but patients with NF1 have a 2.5-fold increase in risk of developing a malignancy [4]. NF2 patients develop vestibular and peripheral nerve schwannomas (the vestibular schwannomas characteristically being bilateral), together with CNS tumours such as meningiomas [3,4]. Spinal schwannomas, astrocytomas or ependymomas eventually occur in about three-quarters of patients with NF2. If meningiomas occur in children, NF2 should be suspected. Perhaps the commonest neoplasm associated with neurofibromatosis is a malignant neurofibrosarcoma [6]. Most superficial neurofibromas have a low malignant potential, change occurring more often in the deep plexiform neurofibromas and those in continuity with peripheral nerves, designated schwannomas. Benign tumours such as acoustic neuromas, dumb-bell tumours and optic gliomas can result in disastrous sequelae when occurring in confined, pressure-sensitive sites. The commonest CNS malignancy is an astrocytoma. Other malignancies include nephroblastoma (Wilms tumour), fibrosarcoma, rhabdomyosarcoma and leukaemia, especially in children [3,4,6–8]. There is an association between NF1 and juvenile myelomonocytic leukaemia and juvenile xanthogranulomas [9]. Monosomy 7 myelodysplastic syndrome may also occur [10]. There is an increased frequency of phaeochromocytomas and carcinoid tumours [4] and ocular melanoma has been reported [11].

Tuberous sclerosis complex

Synonyms and inclusions
- Bourneville disease

Tuberous sclerosis complex (TSC) consists of angiokeratomas, epilepsy and learning difficulties. It may be associated with multisystem tumour involvement, mostly hamartomatous [1]. TSC is an autosomal dominant condition but there is a high spontaneous mutation rate which accounts for over 50% of cases. There are two known causative genes: *TSC1* on chromosome 9q34 (encoding hamartin) and *TSC2* on chromosome 16p13.3 (encoding tuberin) and both genes function as tumour suppressor genes. There are large numbers of different mutations, with *TSC2* mutations being more common and causing more severe disease compared with *TSC1* mutations.

Other than skin lesions, the CNS, renal and cardiopulmonary systems are most significantly affected [2–4]. Angiomyolipomas (of vessels, fat and smooth muscle) all show the same loss of heterozygosity at the *TSC1* or *TSC2* loci. Malignant sarcomatous change can occur particularly with angiomyolipomas and rhabdomyomas, but is uncommon and metastases are unusual [5]. Renal cell carcinoma is a recognised, infrequent complication [4–7].

Multiple endocrine neoplasia syndromes

Multiple endocrine neoplasia type 1

Synonyms and inclusions
- Wermer syndrome

This is a familial cancer syndrome with parathyroid, pancreas and pituitary gland tumours as well as cutaneous findings. Dermatological features in multiple endocrine neoplasia type 1 (MEN1) are typically multiple facial angiofibromas (22–88%) and collagenomas (0–72%). Lipomas may occur in more than 33% of patients with MEN1. Café-au-lait macules are also encountered [1–3].

It is caused by mutations in the *MEN1* gene, located on chromosome 11q13, which codes for the production of the menin protein.

MEN1 is characterised by tumours of the parathyroid, anterior pituitary, pancreatic islet cells, cells of neuroendocrine origin, foregut carcinoid and adrenal cortex. It is associated with 20–25% of cases of Zollinger–Ellison syndrome (ZES). In MEN1, 60–100% of cases have gastroenteropancreatic lesions, especially pancreatic islet tumours, also referred to as pancreatic neuroendocrine tumours (NETs). The incidence of tumours is as follows: ZES 54%, insulinoma 21%, glucagonoma 3% and VIPoma (vasoactive intestinal peptide) 1%. In MEN1, associated endocrine disease consists of parathyroid hyperplasia in over 95%, anterior pituitary adenomas in 15–50%, adrenal adenomas in 30% and carcinoid tumours in more than 3% (carcinoid tumours are located in the bronchi, gastrointestinal tract, pancreas or thymus). The pituitary adenomas secrete prolactin in 60%, growth hormone in less than 25% and adrenocorticotrophic hormone (ACTH) in 5%. The commonest tumours in MEN1 secrete parathyroid hormone or gastrin.

Metastases from malignant neuroendocrine tumours, in particular malignant pancreatic NETs and thymic carcinoid tumours, are one of the commonest causes of mortality in patients with MEN1 [1–4,**5**,6].

Multiple endocrine neoplasia type 2A

Synonyms and inclusions
- Sipple syndrome

Both MEN2A and MEN2B principally involve the thyroid and parathyroid glands, and the adrenal medulla, and are linked with familial medullary thyroid carcinoma [7,8]. MEN2A lacks the mucosal neuromas and skin lipomas of MEN1 and MEN2B. Café-au-lait macules are only present in those with a combined phenotype of MEN2A with NF1. In MEN2A there may be symmetrical, bilateral, pruritic skin lesions found overlying the scapular area, with hyperpigmentation and hyperkeratosis clinically suggestive of amyloidosis; deposits of keratin-derived amyloid are typically found histologically [4,6,9].

MEN2A and MEN2B are caused by mutations of the *RET* proto-oncogene locus (10q11.2) [10–12]. Both are autosomal dominant but 50% of cases with MEN2B are due to spontaneous mutations. RET testing has replaced calcitonin screening to diagnose MEN2 carrier status. The specific RET codon mutation will delineate the course of the disease and degree of aggression [4,**5**,1–13]. Screening of all first-degree relatives should be performed in order to identify RET-mutated gene carriers.

The main internal disorders in MEN2A, described as the triad of cardinal manifestations, are medullary thyroid carcinoma (MTC), phaeochromocytoma and hyperparathyroidism (due to either hyperplasia or adenomas). Other hamartomas and tumours include cerebellar haemangioblastomas, cervical neuroblastoma, pituitary adenomas and pinealomas [9].

Multiple endocrine neoplasia type 2B

This is characterised by mucosal neuromas that are apparent at birth or in the first years of life [14]. Neuromas manifest as asymptomatic, soft, flesh-coloured papules or nodules. They cause a characteristic facial appearance with soft, lumpy ('blubbery'), protuberant lips; everted, thickened, bumpy eyelids; and prominent eyebrows. Neuromas typically affect the mucosal surfaces, especially the anterior border of the tongue and the buccal mucosa inside the commissures of the lips; gingival, palatal and pharyngeal surfaces may occasionally be affected. Cutaneous nodules or plaques, often linear in shape and hyperpigmented, are occasionally reported, with the histopathological picture of dermal nerve hypertrophy and clinical hyperpigmentation due to chronic scratching and trauma [14]. About 75% of patients have a Marfanoid appearance; muscle weakness and musculoskeletal anomalies (especially kyphoscoliosis, pes cavus and bilateral slipped upper femoral epiphysis) may also be present [10].

Hyperparathyroidism due to parathyroid hyperplasia or adenomatosis is much less common than in MEN1 and MEN2A. Intestinal ganglioneuromatosis is more common in type 2B than 2A, occurring in 30% and often presenting early in life due to constipation or abdominal pain.

MEN2B is associated with MTC in 75% of cases, and phaeochromocytoma in almost 50%. MTC in type 2B presents earlier and more aggressively than in type 2A. The MTC is often multicentric and bilateral occurring in a background of calcitonin-producing cell hyperplasia. Early lymphatic spread may occur and 75% have metastases at presentation [10]. Phaeochromocytomas are often bilateral but the mortality is greater from MTC than from phaeochromocytoma.

Carney complex

Synonyms and inclusions
- Myxoma syndrome
- Carney complex/myxoma syndrome

This is a group of disorders in which there are cutaneous pigmented lesions associated with cutaneous, subcutaneous and internal myxomas and associated endocrinopathy (mainly tumours), including involvement of one or more of the adrenal cortex, thyroid, pituitary and gonads [1]. The NAME syndrome consists of *n*aevi (congenital melanocytic), *a*trial myxomas, *m*yxoid neurofibromas and *e*phelides. The LAMB syndrome consists of *l*entigines, *a*trial myxomas, *m*ucocutaneous myxomas and *b*lue naevi. The association with myxomas has led to many other names; some prefer to use myxoma syndrome, or the combined term Carney complex/myxoma syndrome [2].

Three of the major diagnostic criteria involve the skin: spotty cutaneous pigmentation (lips, conjunctiva, eyelids, genital mucosa), mucocutaneous myxomas and multiple blue naevi [3]. Cardiac myxomas occur in 61% [4]. The adrenal tumours in Carney complex are typically of the primary pigmented nodular type, an otherwise rare condition. Various other gonadal and endocrine hormone-secreting tumours, including pituitary tumours producing growth hormone, prolactin or ACTH, are found. Ovarian tumours are associated and both benign and malignant thyroid tumours (usually of follicular type) also occur [5,6]. Testicular tumours (often large-cell calcifying Sertoli cell tumours) occur in about 30% of males and are often bilateral and multicentric. Psammomatous melanotic schwannoma, usually of the upper gastrointestinal tract or of the paravertebral sympathetic nerves, is very suggestive of this syndrome. Myxoid fibroadenomas of the breast and mammary ductal adenomas may be found [2], and myxoid leiomyomas and uterine tumours are described. Lentiginosis occurs in 70–75% and blue naevi in about 50% of patients with Carney complex [2,3]. Skin myxomas occur in over a third of cases [4]. Multiple mucocutaneous myxomas are the most specific cutaneous marker for Carney complex, however these lesions are difficult to recognise clinically [3].

PTEN hamartoma tumour syndrome

Synonyms and inclusions
- Cowden disease

This rare, cancer-associated genodermatosis was first described by Lloyd and Dennis and was named after their patient Rachel Cowden [1,2].

Pathognomonic criteria for the PTEN (phosphatase and tensin homologue) hamartoma tumour syndrome are mucocutaneous lesions, facial trichilemmomas (at least three), acral keratosis (at least six palmar lesions), papillomatous lesions and mucosal lesions. These are found in over 90% of patients. The mucosal lesions comprise a warty, 'cobblestone' hyperplasia of the mucosal surfaces, particularly affecting the tongue and buccal mucosa (Figure 148.12). Periorificial facial papules, acral warty keratoses and palmoplantar, semitranslucent, punctate keratosis are characteristic. The lesions are grouped especially around the mouth, nose and ears and have a hyperkeratotic, flat-topped, wart-like appearance similar to many lesions elsewhere. Histologically, these are mostly trichilemmomas or related benign tumours of the follicular infundibulum [3–7]. Multiple hamartomatous lesions of ectodermal, endodermal and mesodermal origin occur. The other cutaneous lesions include ganglioneuromas, lipomas, fibromas, angiomas, angiolipomas, epidermoid cysts and a variety of pigmentary changes. Craniomegaly is common; there may be an adenoid facies, kyphoscoliosis and a high-arched palate.

Seizures and learning difficulties occur (the latter is a minor diagnostic criterion) and there may be an association with meningioma.

Only about one-third of patients meeting the clinical diagnostic criteria for the syndrome actually have a detectable *PTEN* mutation.

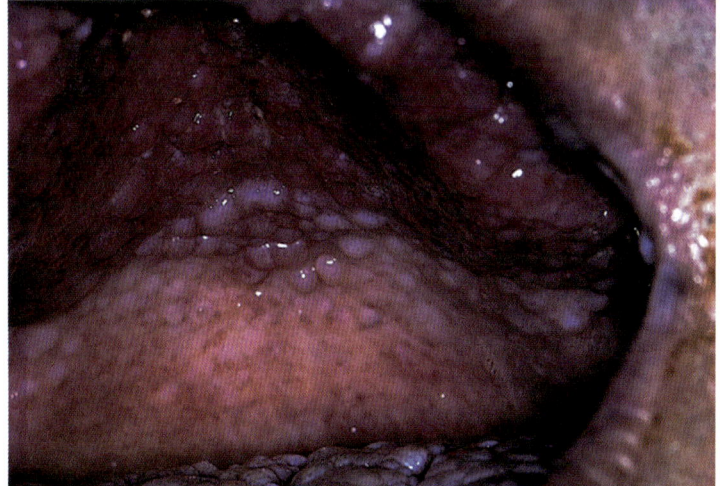

Figure 148.12 Warty papillomatosis of the hard palate in PTEN hamartoma tumour syndrome. Courtesy of Dr R. Emmerson, Royal Berkshire Hospital, Reading, UK.

Benign internal anomalies are numerous and most commonly affect the breast (severe fibrocystic disease occurs in the majority of women) and the thyroid (mainly multinodular goitres and adenomas). Gastrointestinal polyposis and cysts or polyps of the female genito-urinary system are also frequent.

The cumulative risk of developing cancer in patients with PTEN hamartoma tumour syndrome is elevated, especially in women [8]. The most frequently reported cancers are female breast cancer (bilateral in almost 50% of cases) and thyroid cancer [8]. Fibrocystic breast disease and cancers may have an early onset and screening of at-risk family members is therefore recommended. Breast, endometrial and thyroid cancers all contribute to a higher mortality in females. Renal carcinomas have also been linked with this syndrome and an increased likelihood of melanoma has been suggested.

Sebaceous tumours, keratoacanthomas and visceral malignancy

Synonyms and inclusions
- Lynch syndrome
- Muir–Torre syndrome

This is a cancer-associated genodermatosis in which there is an association between sebaceous lesions, and to a lesser extent keratoacanthomas, and internal malignancy (Chapter 137). Inheritance of this syndrome is autosomal dominant with variable expression, males being affected more commonly than females [1–3].

Sebaceous tumours are usually multiple but occasionally solitary. Although sebaceous adenoma is the commonest, sebaceous carcinoma and epithelioma frequently occur, and within the same patient a variety of different pilosebaceous-derived skin lesions including keratoacanthomas may arise. Most skin tumours occur in middle age and keratoacanthomas occur in a quarter of affected subjects. Multiple or early onset of keratoacanthomas are suggestive of this diagnosis, as are multiple (especially eyelid) sebaceous tumours.

Up to 60% of affected individuals develop sebaceous neoplasms preceding visceral malignancies [4]. It has been suggested that when a sebaceous neoplasm is identified individuals should be screened for internal malignancies [4]. Criteria for diagnosis (Amsterdam and Bethesda criteria) and recommendations for screening of patients and relatives have been reviewed [5].

The most important internal malignancy is colonic adenocarcinoma, which occurs in almost 50%, often at a relatively young age (around 10 years earlier than in the normal population) and most commonly in the region of the splenic flexure. Rectal adenocarcinomas also occur but only in about 5% [6,7]. Uro-genital malignancies are also common, occurring in 25% [6]; bladder, renal, pelvis and endometrial cancers each account for about 5% of cancers in this syndrome. Nearly 50% of affected patients have two or more internal malignancies [8,9]. Other notable malignancies are breast cancers, haematological malignancies [6], small intestine adenocarcinoma, head and neck squamous cell carcinoma and lung carcinoma [7]. Despite the high risk of malignancy, both the malignant cutaneous sebaceous tumours and the colonic tumours tend to have relatively indolent behaviour (50% survival time for colonic cancers is 12 years [2]) and the incidence of metastases is relatively low.

A clinical scoring system to identify patients with sebaceous neoplasms at risk for the Muir–Torre variant of Lynch syndrome has been published by Roberts *et al*. [10].

Hereditary leiomyomatosis and renal cell carcinoma syndrome

Synonyms and inclusions
- Multiple cutaneous and uterine leiomyomas syndrome
- Reed syndrome

Hereditary leiomyomatosis and renal cell cancer (HLRCC) forms an autosomal dominant tumour syndrome caused by heterozygous germline mutations in the fumarate hydratase (FH) gene [1,2].

The syndrome comprises multiple cutaneous leiomyomas with uterine leiomyomas. In some cases there is also an association with aggressive renal cell carcinoma, mainly of the papillary cell type. For cutaneous leiomyomas, the indication for treatment is the alleviation of cosmetic and pain-related complications. For solitary tumours, surgical excision is commonly applied. Multiple painful lesions require management by medical measures [3].

Lifetime risk for renal cancer in FH mutation carriers is estimated to be 15% [4]. Most women with HLRCC syndrome develop uterine leiomyomas (fibroids) with early onset. One study of 35 FH mutation carriers found that cutaneous leiomyomas were present in all subjects older than 40 years. Eleven out of 21 female mutation carriers underwent surgical treatment for symptomatic uterine leiomyomas, at an average of 35 years. Two of the FH mutation carriers had renal cancer [1].

Several other tumours have been reported in FH mutation carriers, including benign ovarian mucinous cystadenomas, renal cysts, adrenal gland adenomas, thyroid lesions, uterine leiomyosarcomas, breast, bladder and brain tumours, lymphoid malignancies and basal cell carcinomas.

The main focus of management in HLRCC is prevention of disease and death due to renal cancer. A surveillance protocol has been proposed [4,5].

Bloom, Rothmund–Thomson and Werner syndromes

The Bloom, Rothmund–Thomson and Werner syndromes are rare (≤1/50 000 live births), autosomal recessive diseases. These conditions are considered together as they are all caused by RecQ helicase gene mutations and they all predispose to abnormal growth, premature ageing and increased incidence of site-specific malignancies [1,2] (Chapters 75, 76 and 77).

Bloom syndrome

Affected subjects have small stature and slight build, a sun-sensitive telangiectatic facial rash and café-au-lait macules. Minor congenital anatomical abnormalities commonly occur. Deficient cellular and humoral immunity is common.

Mutations of the gene designated *BLM* on chromosome 15q26.1 lead to inhibition of the function of the protein product, a DNA helicase enzyme. This loss of function allows genomic instability with the occurrence of significantly increased exchanges between DNA strands during mitosis, including an increase in sister chromatid exchanges, such that mutations occur throughout the genome.

The occurrence of lymphoproliferative neoplasia (approximately equally divided between leukaemias and lymphomas) and epithelial tissue cancers, particularly of the aerodigestive tract and lower gastrointestinal tumours, is very high; they typically occur at an early age and the mean age of death is 23 years [3]. Cervical cancer and Wilms tumour are additional risks. There is a predisposition to malignancy through mutations in other target genes [4].

Rothmund–Thomson syndrome

This autosomal recessive disease is characterised by developmental abnormalities in the skin and skeletal systems, with photosensitivity, poikiloderma, small stature, premature ageing and juvenile cataracts. There is a predisposition to certain malignancies including a 30% incidence of osteosarcoma. Fibrosarcoma, myelodysplasia and non-melanoma skin cancer may also occur [5–8].

Werner syndrome

> **Synonyms and inclusions**
> - Adult progeria

This is a condition of premature ageing with onset in the second to third decade of life. The key clinical findings include short stature, early greying and loss of hair, bilateral cataracts and scleroderma-like skin changes. Werner syndrome is a chromosome instability syndrome and, as with XP, ataxia-telangiectasia, Bloom syndrome and Fanconi anaemia, is associated with a high incidence of neoplasia [9,10]. Neoplasms develop in about 10% of cases although the commonest cause of death is arteriosclerosis. Sarcomas, melanomas, leukaemia, meningiomas and a variety of epithelial-derived carcinomas have been reported [9–15].

IMMUNODEFICIENCY AND NEOPLASIA SYNDROMES

See also Chapter 80.

Wiskott–Aldrich syndrome

Wiskott–Aldrich syndrome is an X-linked recessive immunodeficiency syndrome. The Wiskott–Aldrich syndrome protein (WASp) is expressed in all haematopoietic cells and mutations cause defective T-cell function and thrombocytopenia. In addition to bleeding and susceptibility to infections, severe eczema may occur. Older patients also reveal an increased risk of autoimmune disorders and lymphoid malignancies [1]. Non-Hodgkin lymphoma occurs in almost all subjects who survive infections or bleeding due to thrombocytopenia, usually by the age of 30 years. Lymphoma (especially large cell or immunoblastic) and leukaemia also occur; the small intestine is a particular site for lymphomatous involvement. Cerebral tumours such as astrocytoma and various sarcomas have also been reported [2,3,4]. Recently, haematopoietic stem cell transplantation treatment with good outcome has been reported [1,5] and attempts of therapy by gene correction are ongoing [6].

Chediak–Higashi syndrome

This is a fatal, autosomal recessive disorder with features of oculocutaneous albinism, silvery hair, photophobia, neurological abnormalities and severe, recurrent bacterial infections. There is extensive organ infiltration with lymphoid and histiocytic cells. Patients develop fever, jaundice, hepatosplenomegaly, lymphadenopathy, leukaemia-like gingival lesions and sloughing of the oral mucosa, pancytopaenia and neurological deterioration. Although strongly suggestive of lymphoma, the infiltrate of affected organs is reported to be of a reactive, diffuse, mononuclear cell type, rather than neoplastic [1]. About 85% of patients develop an accelerated 'lymphomatous' phase which may be triggered by viral infections, especially Epstein–Barr virus [2].

Ataxia-telangiectasia

This is an autosomal recessive condition characterised by progressive cerebellar ataxia and oculocutaneous telangiectasia. Premature ageing of the skin and hair is noted in almost 90% of individuals. Non-infectious cutaneous granulomas, with a tendency to ulcerate, are frequent [1]. The skin findings do not usually occur until 3–6 years of age and are preceded by ataxia [2]. Peripheral blood lymphocytes are abnormal and there is a variable but progressive immune deficiency of both the cell-mediated and humoral types [1,3]. Chronic and recurrent sinopulmonary infections occur in a majority of patients with ataxia-telangiectasia and represent the most common cause of death [1].

Most families have one of many different germ-line mutations in the large *ATM* gene at chromosome 11q22.3. The product, ATM protein, is involved in the handling of chromosome strand breaks and activation of multiple targets, among them the p53 oncogene [1,2], and has been considered to be a 'caretaker' of the genome and tumour suppressor. Mutations are mainly inactivating in type but may be missense [4] and allow unregulated DNA synthesis, with DNA predisposed to instability and hypersensitivity to ionising radiation [2].

There is a high incidence of neoplasia (approximately 30% lifetime risk) usually in or before the teenage years and causing death in 15% of affected individuals [2,3,5–8]. The majority (80%) of tumours are lymphoproliferative or leukaemic, although carcinomas of various sites also occur mainly in older subjects [6–8]. Most haematological malignancies are B-cell lymphomas but 25% are leukaemias, notably chronic T-cell leukaemia with chromosome 14 translocations in older patients. However, T-cell leukaemias do occur in younger patients and both T-cell lymphomas and B-cell leukaemias are also encountered. Most tumours have early onset and may precede diagnosis of ataxia-telangiectasia from the cutaneous features. This is of considerable importance as standard radiotherapy doses are contraindicated. Heterozygotes (carriers) have a 5–10-fold increased risk of tumours, usually not lymphoid, and a 5-fold increase in risk of breast malignancy in females [2,5].

Dyskeratosis congenita

Dyskeratosis congenita (DC) is a multisystem inherited syndrome, with clinical and genetic heterogeneity, characterised by mucocutaneous abnormalities, bone marrow failure and a predisposition to cancer. Most cases have X-linked recessive inheritance but autosomal recessive and autosomal dominant forms also occur [1].

A triad of abnormalities are the most consistent and diagnostic mucocutaneous features, comprising reticulate hyperpigmentation of the skin, nail dystrophy and leukoplakia of the mucous membranes. Dental, skeletal, ocular and gastrointestinal abnormalities are common; learning difficulties, short stature and premature ageing also occur. Aplastic anaemia occurs in 50%, typically in the early teens, and is the main cause of mortality.

The DC genes have been characterised and the majority are important in telomere maintenance, which is defective in DC patients who usually have very short telomeres. The genetic advances in the last decades have led to the unification with several other severe multisystem disorders, including the Hoyeraal–Hreidarsson and Revesz syndromes, as well as a subset of patients with aplastic anaemia, myelodysplasia, leukaemia and idiopathic pulmonary fibrosis [2].

Oro-pharyngeal carcinomas secondary to the mucous membrane lesions are the commonest form of malignancy. There is also increased incidence of internal malignancy, particularly gastrointestinal, including pancreatic adenocarcinoma and other haematological disorders, similar to those found in Fanconi anaemia [3,4].

Fanconi anaemia

This is a genetically and phenotypically heterogeneous recessive disorder, characterised by diverse congenital malformations, progressive pancytopenia and predisposition to haematological malignancies and solid tumours [1]. The underlying defect in Fanconi anaemia is one of increased DNA cross-linkage (especially radiation induced) and defective DNA repair. The main role of Fanconi anaemia proteins is the repair of DNA interstrand cross-links and the maintenance of genomic stability. More than a dozen genes have been identified as mutated in these patients and many more interacting genes have been discovered [2,3].

Dermatologically, Fanconi anaemia is characterised by pigmentary abnormalities that may be diffuse (with accentuation around the neck and over joints), mottled, often with scattered darker macules and sometimes just exhibiting localised café-au-lait macules. Scattered areas of hypopigmentation are also a common finding.

The main abnormality is progressive pancytopenia, which may lead eventually to the development of leukaemia. Multiple skeletal abnormalities occur including digital hypoplasias, scoliosis and short stature. The relative risk of cancer in Fanconi anaemia is exceedingly high in comparison with the incidences expected in the general population [3]. Acute myeloid leukaemia and solid tumours are common, especially head and neck or gynaecological squamous cell carcinomas.

PARANEOPLASTIC PHENOMENA INVOLVING THE SKIN

Paraneoplastic dermatoses are skin conditions that have an association with internal malignancy but are not themselves malignant. At least one of the following defining characteristics should be present in order to consider a dermatosis as being related to an underlying malignancy:

1. The malignancy and the cutaneous disorder should occur concurrently.
2. The two disorders should follow a parallel course.
3. There should be a specific tumour site or cell type associated with the cutaneous disease.
4. There should be a statistical association between the two processes.
5. There should be a genetic association between the two processes.

Paraneoplastic dermatoses may be classified in a variety of ways. Some authors include genodermatoses within the spectrum of paraneoplastic disorders [1] whilst others view these as a separate group [2,3], or distinguish between paraneoplastic dermatoses [4], hereditary paraneoplastic syndromes [5] and hormonally mediated paraneoplastic syndromes [6]. They may be classified according to strength of association with malignancy, association with certain types of malignancy [7], by the type of eruption that occurs (e.g. papulosquamous, vascular) or by the apparent mechanism (e.g. hormone secretion, autoimmune, cytokine/growth factor).

The likelihood of finding a neoplasm in some of the better known paraneoplastic disorders may be graded as high, intermediate or low (Table 148.2). Nonetheless the evidence supporting paraneoplastic phenomena is highly variable. The majority of the literature is based on case reports or case series: most of the data are hypothesis-generating in nature and only rarely supported by studies of epidemiology or pathogenetic pathways [7–13,**14**].

ACANTHOTIC AND ICHTHYOTIC EPIDERMAL DISORDERS

Acanthosis nigricans

Acanthosis nigricans may be divided into two important categories, benign and malignant, although Schwartz [1] described eight types

Table 148.2 Strength of correlation of some potentially paraneoplastic dermatoses with internal malignancy.

Strength of correlation	Type of reaction pattern	Examples
Strong	Papulosquamous and figurate eruptions	Bazex syndrome
		Erythema gyratum repens
		Necrolytic migratory erythema
	Epidermal conditions	Acanthosis palmaris (tripe palms)
		Florid cutaneous papillomatosis
	Deposition disorders	Primary amyloidosis
		Scleromyxoedema
		Necrobiotic xanthogranuloma
		POEMS syndrome
	Others	Acquired hypertrichosis lanuginosa
		Paraneoplastic pemphigus
		Carcinoid syndrome
		Trousseau syndrome
Moderate	Papulosquamous and neutrophilic eruptions	Sweet syndrome
		Pyoderma gangrenosum
		Dermatomyositis
	Others	Multicentric reticulohistiocytosis
		Pityriasis rotunda
Weak	Epidermal conditions	Acanthosis nigricans in isolation
		Acquired ichthyosis (unless widespread, deeply fissured, truncal pattern)
		Eruptive seborrhoeic keratoses (sign of Leser–Trélat)
	Deposition disorders	Scleroedema
		Calcinosis cutis
	Others	Vasculitis, Raynaud phenomenon, digital ischaemia
		Erythromelalgia
		Relapsing polychondritis
		Erythroderma/exfoliative dermatitis
		Digital clubbing (unless with hypertrophic osteoarthropathy)
		Pruritus
		Erythema annulare centrifugum
		Cushing syndrome

POEMS, polyneuropathy, organomegaly, endocrinopathy, M-protein and skin changes.

including benign, obesity associated, syndromic, malignant, acral, unilateral, medication induced (especially nicotinic acid) and mixed types.

Benign acanthosis nigricans is often associated with obesity or insulin resistance and is common and usually mild (Chapter 85). It has been documented in up to 7% of children, mainly in the teenage years. Virtually all childhood cases are of the benign type although malignant acanthosis nigricans (functional adrenocortical tumour) has been reported in a paediatric patient [2].

Malignancy-associated acanthosis nigricans is much less common. It may have a rapid onset and progression to produce symmetrical, hyperpigmented, rugose, velvety plaques (Figure 148.13) [1–6]. The axillae and other flexures are particularly affected, along with the areolar area and nape of the neck and, less commonly, mucosal surfaces. The hands and feet may also be affected [7]. There may be prominent acrochordon-like papillomatosis arising from the plaques; the sign of Leser–Trélat and acanthosis palmaris (tripe palms) may coexist [6]. *De novo* development of acanthosis nigricans in adults, especially if progressive and associated with weight loss, should raise suspicions that there is an underlying neoplasm, although cases have been described in which acanthosis nigricans has preceded a malignancy by 10 years or more [3]. If there is also generalised pruritus or the skin changes of tripe palms, then a malignancy is even more likely. Production by tumour cells of either transforming growth factor α or cytokines that activate insulin-like growth factors or their cutaneous receptors have been proposed as the pathogenetic mechanism.

By far the commonest site of underlying neoplasm is the gastrointestinal tract (70–90%), most frequently gastric adenocarcinoma [1–7]. A number of different malignancies have been reported, nearly all being adenocarcinomas, in other parts of the intestine, liver or bile duct. Other tumours include lung, breast, endometrium, kidney, bladder, prostate, testis, cervix, thyroid and adrenal. Most are solid organ tumours but lymphoma has been recorded. Sarcomas occur rarely. The prognosis with malignant acanthosis nigricans is related to the survival rate from the neoplasia concerned. However, the skin changes may improve or resolve with eradication of the cancer [8,9]. Acanthosis nigricans may precede the diagnosis of the malignancy (20%), appear simultaneously (60%) or after tumour detection (20%) [9].

Acanthosis palmaris

Synonyms and inclusions
- Tripe palms
- Pachydermatoglyphy

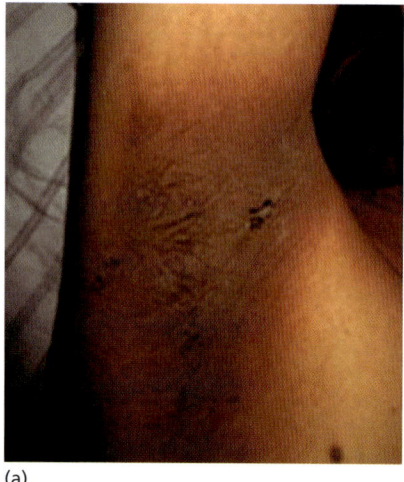
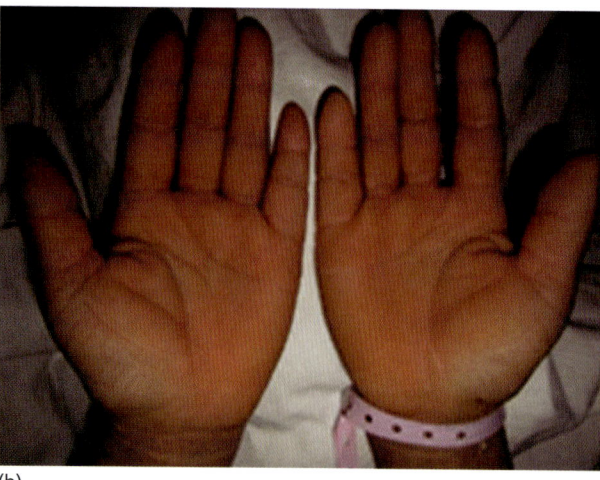

Figure 148.13 (a, b) Paraneoplastic acanthosis nigricans. Gastric adenocarcinoma was found after investigation of this woman with a 1-year history of velvety thickening of the skin of the palms, soles and flexures.

Acanthosis palmaris describes thickened skin of the palms and occasionally the soles with an enhanced dermatoglyphic change, causing a velvety (Figure 148.13b) or less commonly a pitted, honeycombed pattern of the hand. It is associated with neoplasia in about 90% of cases and may be the only paraneoplastic manifestation in 30–40%. It may also occur with one or both of malignant acanthosis nigricans or the sign of Leser–Trélat [1–3], or with florid cutaneous papillomatosis [4]. It occurs particularly in men, especially when the underlying tumour is a lung cancer [2]. However, it can occur in isolation without neoplasia, or as a pattern of exfoliative psoriasis or eczema [1,2], and has been reported with bullous pemphigoid.

As the condition frequently is associated with an internal neoplasm, usually of solid organ type, it requires appropriate evaluation and investigation. In the majority of cases, the onset of tripe palms precedes or occurs concurrently with the detection of a previously unsuspected malignancy [3]. Most commonly, the underlying tumour is bronchial or gastric, together accounting for over 50% of the associated malignancies. Many other sites are reported including tumours of the genito-urinary tract, as well as carcinomas in the breast and other organs [2,3]. Acanthosis palmaris occurring alone is more often associated with bronchial carcinoma compared with combined acanthosis nigricans and acanthosis palmaris, in which gastric carcinoma is more common [3]. If nail clubbing is also present (especially in a male patient), then bronchial carcinoma is very likely [2]. Interestingly, the appearance or exacerbation of tripe palms in a known cancer patient may be a sign of recurrence of the malignancy [3].

Sign of Leser–Trélat

This is the sudden development of numerous seborrhoeic keratoses in an eruptive fashion, with or without pruritus, as an indicator of internal malignancy. However, the significance of eruptive seborrhoeic keratoses remains unclear, with strong proponents and opponents of its importance [1–4]. Multiple seborrhoeic keratoses are extremely common, especially in elderly people, and may be pruritic or rapidly erupting without any apparent cause. They may also occur in other situations [4,5] such as human immunodeficiency virus (HIV) infection, acromegaly and in the resolving phase of erythrodermic dermatoses [6].

Of the cases reported with a neoplasm, 50% of the tumours are adenocarcinomas and one-third of all the associated tumours arise in the gastrointestinal tract; this is similar to the distribution of tumours in acanthosis nigricans, which may coexist. Carcinomas of the breast are also frequent, although this may just reflect the incidence of these tumours in an age group who are also likely to have seborrhoeic keratoses. Rare associations have been documented with a variety of other neoplasms including malignant haemangiopericytoma [7], malignant melanoma [8], renal carcinoma [5] and transitional cell carcinoma of the bladder [9]. Lymphoproliferative disorders, which are rarely associated with acanthosis nigricans, have been more commonly reported with the sign of Leser–Trélat, accounting for about 20% of associated tumours [5]. Eruption of seborrheic keratoses over the upper body occurred in a young patient with relapse of a previously treated pre-B-cell acute lymphocytic leukaemia [10]. Six multiple metachronous cancers in a patient with the sign of Leser–Trélat has been reported [11].

Genuine sudden development of multiple seborrhoeic keratosis, especially in younger patients and if associated with pruritus or with acanthosis nigricans, warrants investigation. However, the mere presence of many seborrhoeic keratoses is unlikely to be linked with malignancy and the strength of this sign as a marker of internal malignancy must be viewed as uncertain.

Florid cutaneous papillomatosis

This rare paraneoplastic phenomenon is characterised by a widespread, often pruritic, eruption of warty papules associated with an underlying malignancy, particularly gastric adenocarcinoma [1,2]. The eruption closely resembles disseminated human papillomavirus infection (Figure 148.14) but no evidence of this is found on histological or ultrastructural examination. It may appear concomitantly with other paraneoplastic phenomena, particularly paraneoplastic acanthosis nigricans (see earlier), and the underlying mechanisms are presumed to be similar.

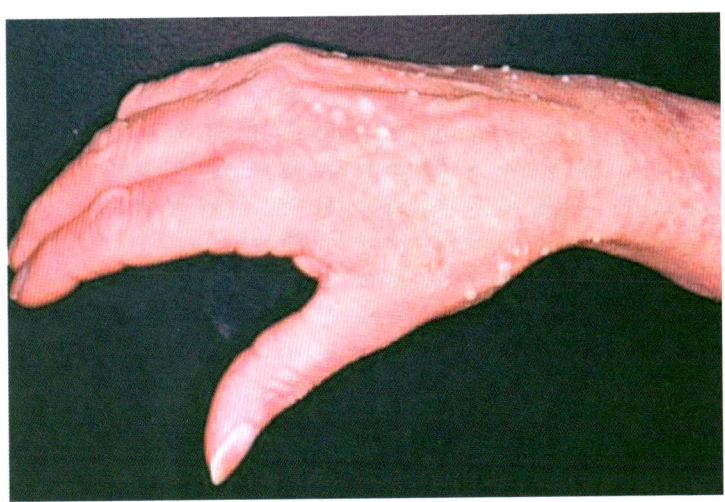

Figure 148.14 Florid cutaneous papillomatosis. Reproduced from Janniger and Schwartz 2010 [1] with permission of John Wiley & Sons.

Acquired ichthyosis

Many systemic diseases may be associated with acquired ichthyosis including nutritional deficiencies, sarcoidosis, leprosy, HIV infection, hypothyroidism, lupus erythematosus, graft-versus-host disease and drug reactions (Chapter 85) [1].

However, more sudden onset of ichthyosis similar to the pattern of ichthyosis vulgaris in adult life or with a generalised eczema craquelé appearance suggests the possibility of internal malignancy, particularly if it occurs in a younger age group. Paraneoplastic ichthyosis is typically very extensive, affecting the trunk and having quite prominent fissuring. Other paraneoplastic signs have been reported to be present in conjunction with acquired ichthyosis, including erythema gyratum repens, Bazex syndrome and dermatomyositis [2,3]. The strongest association is with Hodgkin disease (accounting for over 70% of cases) and other lymphoreticular tumours, including T-cell lymphomas, leukaemias, myelodysplastic syndrome, multiple myeloma and polycythaemia vera [1,2,3]. Cases linked with solid tumours are also well documented, including cancers of the ovary, kidney, liver and breast, as well as leiomyosarcoma [1,2,3]. A course paralleling that of an underlying lymphoma (including resolution related to treatment) is usual [4,5].

OTHER EPIDERMAL DISORDERS

Pityriasis rotunda is a fixed, annular, scaly dermatosis that has been associated with neoplasia, particularly hepatocellular carcinoma. However, it may also be seen in other systemic diseases and in leprosy [1] (Chapter 85).

Transient acantholytic dermatosis (Grover disease; Chapter 85) has been linked with internal malignancy, particularly with myelogenous leukaemia [2,3] and carcinoma of the genito-urinary tract. However, this may be linked in part with therapy [4], or simply because it may go unrecognised unless it is specifically considered [2].

Acquired seed-like keratoses of the palms and soles are a common normal finding in healthy subjects (36%) over 50 years old but are apparently more common in individuals with carcinoma of the bladder or bronchus [5]. Punctate keratoderma occurring in Cowden syndrome and seed-like keratoses with arsenic ingestion may also be associated with internal malignancy.

PARANEOPLASTIC PIGMENTATION

The ectopic ACTH syndrome (extracutaneous neuroendocrine melanoderma) occurs due to production of an ACTH-like hormone from tumours; small cell bronchial carcinoma is the cause in over 50% (Table 148.3). Other reports have described the same condition resulting from gastric, pancreatic, oesophageal and ovarian cancers, as well as in thymoma, phaeochromocytoma, carcinoid syndrome and in various APUD (amine precursor uptake and decarboxylation) tumours. The pigmentation in ectopic ACTH syndrome is Addisonian in distribution, diffuse (but with photoaccentuation) and greater prominence over pressure points and in flexures, genital skin, scars and the oral mucosa [1].

In Carney complex, lentiginosis is typically centrofacial but may be widespread at almost any body site; the buccal mucosa is affected in only 5% of cases. Rarer sites include the conjunctivae and labia minora; the palms, soles and penis are rarely affected. Blue naevi, usually few in number, occur on the face, trunk or limbs but rarely on the extremities [2].

HAIR, NAILS AND SKIN APPENDAGES

Paraneoplastic hypertrichosis lanuginosa acquisita

The development of paraneoplastic hypertrichosis lanuginosa acquisita tends to affect the face initially, extending down the body with time. The hair is of fine, downy lanugo type. The mechanism is unclear but prolongation of the anagen growth phase has been proposed. Resolution of hypertrichosis lanuginosa occurs after treatment of the underlying tumour and regrowth can be related to recurrence of the neoplasm. There may be associated acanthosis nigricans, hypertrophy of the papillae of the tongue and glossitis [1] and disturbances of taste or smell also occur [2]. However, the glossitis in at least some patients may be a manifestation of vitamin deficiency rather than a specifically malignancy-related condition [3].

About 70% of cases occur in women, usually aged 40–70 years and most patients have metastatic tumours at presentation, with correspondingly poor prognosis. The commonest tumour sites in men are lung followed by colo-rectal, and in women are colo-rectal followed by lung and breast. Other reported sites or tumour types include endometrium (7–8% of cases), ovary, cervix, renal, prostate, bladder,

Table 148.3 Pigmentary abnormalities associated with internal malignancy.

Pigmentary change	Pattern	Examples
Hyperpigmentation	Diffuse, or diffuse with localised accentuation (Addisonian pattern of pigmentation)	Melanoma (rarely causes diffuse slate grey pigmentation)
		Phaeochromocytoma (Addisonian pattern)
		Ectopic ACTH syndrome (Addisonian pattern)
		POEMS syndrome (diffuse or semiconfluent speckled pattern)
		Hyperpigmentation with scleromyxoedema and gammopathy
		Diffuse mastocytosis
		Lymphomas (uncommon)
		Ependymoma (mild increase in pigmentation)
		Werner syndrome (localised or diffuse pigmentation)
		Cachexia due to neoplasia
	Patchy or reticulated	Fanconi anaemia (various pigmentary changes)
		Dyskeratosis congenita (reticulate pigmentation)
	Other distributions	Carcinoid syndrome (photodistributed)
		Pancreatic, gastric and renal tumours (erythema ab igne due to local application of heat)
	Lentigines and freckles	Peutz–Jeghers syndrome (lentigines)
		Carney complex (lentiginosis is characteristic, freckles also occur)
		Xeroderma pigmentosum (freckles)
		Neurofibromatosis (flexural freckle-like macules) (Chapter 78)
		Cowden disease and Bannayan–Riley–Ruvalcaba syndrome (genital lentigines)
		Gardner syndrome (freckles)
		Paraneoplastic acral lentiginosis
	Café-au-lait macules	Neurofibromatosis
		Bloom syndrome
		Multiple endocrine neoplasia types 1 and 2B
		Fanconi anaemia
		Von Hippel–Lindau disease
	With epidermal hyperplasia	Acanthosis nigricans
	Melanocytic naevi and melanoma	Associated with pancreatic neoplasia, astrocytomas and other cerebral neoplasms in some families
		Blue naevi and ordinary naevi occur in Carney complex
Mixed hyper- and hypopigmentation	Poikiloderma	Dermatomyositis (speckled pigmentation on hypopigmented background)
		Rothmund–Thomson syndrome (photodistributed poikiloderma)
Hypopigmentation	Generalised	Chediak–Higashi syndrome
	Localised, multiple	Tuberous sclerosis complex (ash leaf macules)
		Mycosis fungoides (hypopigmented variant)
		Halo depigmentation around primary tumour or metastases
	Melanoma-associated (other than regression within the primary lesion)	Distant leukoderma, usually with centrifugal spread starting on the trunk

ACTH, adrenocorticotrophic hormone; POEMS, polyneuropathy, organomegaly, endocrinopathy, M-protein and skin changes.

adrenal gland, stomach, gallbladder, skin (including melanoma), parotid gland, sarcoma, lymphoma and leukaemia [2,4–6].

Clubbing of nails

In clubbing, there is increased transverse and longitudinal nail curvature with hypertrophy of the soft-tissue components of the digit pulp (Chapter 93). Both clubbing and associated hypertrophic osteoarthropathy have been documented with many neoplasms, and the commonest is carcinoma of the bronchus. In patients with lung cancer, clubbing has been reported in 29%, especially in females, and most lung tumours are squamous cell carcinoma or adenocarcinoma [1]. Resolution of the clubbing after tumour resection has been reported [2]. Clubbing has also been associated with gastrointestinal tumours and tumours metastatic to the lung [3].

A high incidence of hypertrophic osteoarthropathy occurs particularly with mesothelioma but it may also occur with malignancies of the pulmonary, cardiovascular, gastrointestinal and hepato-biliary systems [4]; overall it is much less common than clubbing.

Hyperhidrosis

Generalised hyperhidrosis may rarely be associated with malignant disease (Chapter 92). It is an almost consistent finding in phaeochromocytoma, in which it may be limited to night-time or may occur at any time. Nocturnal hyperhidrosis ('night sweats') may also occur in lymphoma and carcinoid syndrome as well as in non-neoplastic conditions such as thyrotoxicosis, chronic infections and others [1]. Localised hyperhidrosis may occur in the POEMS syndrome (polyneuropathy, organomegaly, endocrinopathy, M-protein and skin changes).

Specific distributions of localised hyperhidrosis may also be important. Hyperhidrosis with autonomic dysreflexia is associated with spinal cord lesions above T6. It is characterised by episodic sweating of the face, neck and upper trunk with vasodilatation in the same distribution, and is accompanied by headache, hypertension and piloerection. Most cases are due to injury or cord compression but intracranial posterior fossa neoplasms can produce similar symptoms [1]. A case of intramedullary thoracic spinal cord ganglioglioma in a 16-year-old patient presented with abnormal sweating on the right side of the neck, chest and right arm for 6 years [2].

Paroxysmal unilateral hyperhidrosis of the face and neck, usually severe and unrelated to stimuli such as eating, may be due to an ipsilateral thoracic tumour (adenocarcinoma, squamous cell carcinoma or mesothelioma) compressing or infiltrating the sympathetic trunk. Associated features may include Horner syndrome, facial weakness, sensory disturbance and other features of the primary tumour [1].

DERMATOSES ASSOCIATED WITH INTERNAL MALIGNANCIES

Acrokeratosis paraneoplastica

Synonyms and inclusions
- Bazex syndrome

Acrokeratosis paraneoplastica is a rare paraneoplastic condition which is more common in males. It is particularly associated with squamous cell carcinoma of the upper respiratory or gastrointestinal tracts, especially when there are metastases in the cervical lymph nodes.

The cutaneous changes develop gradually, often in several phases, initially with violaceous coloration, redness and scaling on the peripheries, especially the helices of the ears, tip of the nose, hands and feet (particularly the distal area of the digits). The eruption then becomes more hyperkeratotic with a keratoderma on the hands and feet and subsequently the eruption may become generalised. Nail dystrophy and paronychia are often present. Changes on the face may appear eczematous or lupus erythematosus-like, whereas acral changes are often psoriasiform. The differential diagnosis can include dermatitis, especially seborrhoeic or contact allergic types, acral psoriasis or reactive arthritis (Reiter syndrome). The histological changes are non-diagnostic but essentially reflect the clinical appearance with hyperkeratosis, parakeratosis, focal spongiosis and a mixed inflammatory cell infiltrate [1–3,4,5].

More than 60% of tumours arise in the oro-pharynx or larynx or are cervical squamous cell carcinoma metastases with an unknown primary site; lung, oesophageal and other primary or metastatic lesions above the diaphragm make up most of the remainder [5]. Rare associations such as metastatic adenocarcinoma of the prostate and transitional cell carcinoma of the bladder have been reported [6,7]. The lesions often appear before the cancer is diagnosed [8]. The course mostly parallels the underlying neoplasm. Resolution may occur with successful tumour resection and recurrence may develop on relapse of malignancy. Various skin-directed therapies can be helpful to control symptoms such as itching and pain but usually show a weak improvement of the lesions. Systemic retinoids may improve the hyperkeratosis [9,10].

Migratory erythemas (Chapter 47)

This descriptive term is applied to a variety of annular and figurate eruptions. Two variants are erythema gyratum repens and necrolytic migratory erythema, which have a clear association with internal neoplasia. Other migratory erythemas are less clearly associated with neoplasia and erythema annulare centrifugum is usually *not* associated with neoplasia [1,2]. If an underlying malignancy is found, a myeloproliferative disorder, specifically lymphoma or leukaemia, is most often reported [2]. There are also reports of subacute cutaneous lupus erythematosus-like annular and figurate rashes, linked with myeloproliferative disorders and carcinoma of the lung, liver, breast, larynx and oesophagus in individual cases.

Erythema gyratum repens is a rare, bizarre, cutaneous eruption consisting of mobile, concentric, often palpable, erythematous, wave-like bands, which give a 'wood-grain' appearance to the skin (Figure 148.15). A peripheral scale or collarette may be present. The complete torso is frequently affected. There is often associated severe pruritus, sometimes ichthyosis, and occasionally bullae within the redness. The lesions migrate from day to day, usually changing position by about 1 cm daily. It has a strong association with internal malignancy (over 80% of cases), particularly lung cancer [3,4] which is present in about a third of cases. Other cancer sites include oesophagus, breast, bowel, uterus, cervix, kidney, pancreas and haematological neoplasia [4]. Occasional cases without associated malignancy have been reported [5,6] but it is important to be aware that 6% are found to have a tumour of unknown primary origin [4]. Identification and resection of the tumour often results in resolution of the eruption.

Necrolytic migratory erythema (NME) is strongly associated with a glucagon-secreting α-cell tumour of the pancreas [7]. It presents as a widespread, painful, migratory rash with repeated eruptions of irregular polycyclic, intensely inflammatory red patches with

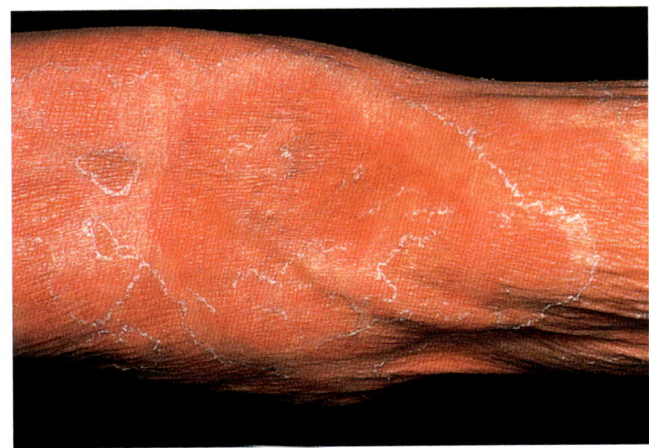

Figure 148.15 Erythema gyratum repens of the arm secondary to carcinoma of the bronchus.

expanding scaling margins; these blister and break down with superficial epidermal necrosis and crusting. It may affect any skin site but has a predilection for the ano-genital region and trunk. NME is strongly associated with the presence of an underlying glucagon-secreting pancreatic islet cell adenoma, although cases have been described where this was not found. NME is one of the components of the glucagonoma syndrome along with weight loss, diabetes, stomatitis and diarrhoea [7]. If glucagon levels can be restored to normal either by surgery or by the long-acting somatostatin analogue octreotide the rash will usually resolve.

CONNECTIVE TISSUE AND RHEUMATOLOGICAL DISORDERS

Malignancies have been reported in association with many disorders that overlap between dermatology and rheumatology. Those that fall into the connective tissue disease group are discussed here.

Dermatomyositis

Dermatomyositis (Figure 148.16) and polymyositis may be associated with internal malignancy in adults (Chapter 52). The reported likelihood of finding a neoplasm varies widely, but around 25–30% has been reported in various studies of dermatomyositis, hence indicating a significant association with underlying malignancy [1–3,4,5]. The association with neoplasia is much stronger for dermatomyositis than for polymyositis or dermatomyositis/autoimmune disease overlap conditions [6]. Malignancy is an uncommon cause of dermatomyositis in subjects less than 40 years of age; however, paediatric cases with neoplasia have been reported [7]. As there is a lower incidence of malignancy in the younger age group, and there are no age-matched comparative studies against a control population in children, it is difficult to judge the strength of the association in this age group [3].

The temporal association of dermatomyositis with neoplasia varies. In one report approximately equal proportions had: (i) a known malignancy at the time that dermatomyositis presented; (ii) a malignancy found due to investigation when dermatomyositis was diagnosed; or (iii) a malignancy found during follow-up (usually in the first 6 months after diagnosis of dermatomyositis) [4]. The risk of malignancy is higher in the first year after the dermatomyositis diagnosis, then decreases through 5 years, but remains slightly elevated in comparison with the general population even after 5 years [8,9].

Accounts of specific malignant associations may be subject to bias by rare case reporting, and in larger series the malignancies identified generally reflect tumour prevalence in the general population: lung cancer in men, breast and gynaecological tumours in women, and colorectal cancers in both sexes. In South-East Asia there is a higher frequency of naso-pharyngeal carcinoma, which probably also reflects the background risk of this type of neoplasm. The one exception to this generalisation is ovarian carcinoma, which appears to be significantly overrepresented and potentially overlooked [2,4,5]. Despite the increase in the relative risk of ovarian

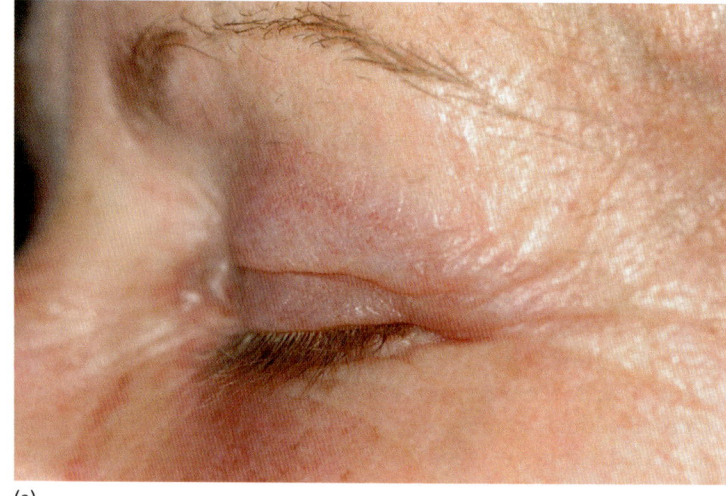

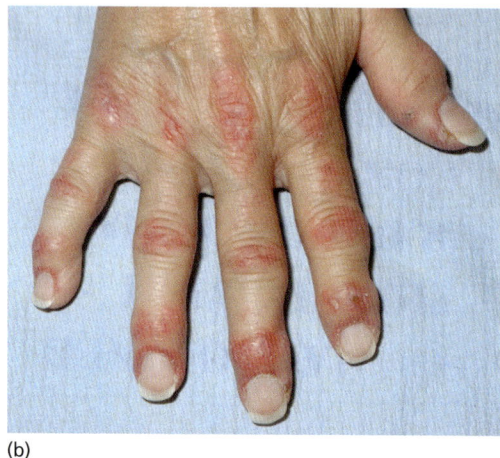

Figure 148.16 Dermatomyositis with typical changes: (a) heliotrope rash affecting the eyelids and (b) Gottron papules on the hands.

cancer, patients with dermatomyositis are still more likely to have the more common cancers, such as lung and breast cancer [9].

The value of extensive screening for neoplasia in dermatomyositis is questionable. Several authors have stressed that the emphasis should be attached to thorough clinical evaluation, simple investigations and then specific investigations if indicated [1,4]. There should certainly be a low threshold for further or repeated investigations, as indicated at the time of diagnosis or during follow-up, if previous neoplasia has been present, when the therapeutic response is poor or if new symptoms develop. There is also an argument for ongoing screening for ovarian cancers throughout follow-up of female patients [2].

In general, subjects with amyopathic dermatomyositis (dermatomyositis sine myositis) or who have a connective tissue overlap syndrome appear less likely to have an underlying malignancy. However, some patients with amyopathic disease at the outset do eventually develop myositis and tumours have been reported in all such variants, so screening investigations should still be performed [10]. In one study, patients with malignancy were found to have a more rapid onset of dermatomyositis, higher mean creatine kinase and erythrocyte sedimentation rates, and a lower frequency of Raynaud phenomenon compared with patients without an underlying malignancy [11]. Vasculitis or necrosis manifesting clinically or in histopathology specimens has also been associated with an increased risk of an associated neoplasm [12,13]. Several characteristics may influence cancer development among patients with dermatomyositis and polymyositis: old age at diagnosis, male sex, cutaneous necrosis and dysphagia all increased the risk; arthritis and interstitial lung disease decreased the risk of malignancy [14].

It has been demonstrated that anti-NXP-2 (nuclear matrix protein 2) and anti-TIF-1γ (transcription intermediary factor 1γ) antibodies are frequent in dermatomyositis (found in 55% of patients with dermatomyositis) and that either of them is present in most patients (83%) with cancer-associated dermatomyositis, especially in males [15]. Anti-MDA-5 (melanoma differentiation-associated protein 5) antibodies are found in approximately 10–20% of dermatomyositis patients and are associated with interstitial lung disease [15,16]. Progress in serotype–phenotype associations may help to determine which patients require more extensive investigation for malignancy [17].

Lupus erythematosus (Chapter 51)

The possibility of an increased risk of internal malignancy in systemic lupus erythematosus (SLE) [1–3] and subacute cutaneous lupus erythematosus (SCLE) [4,5] has been debated for many years and still remains controversial. There are individual cases in which a close temporal relationship has been documented [4], and large cohort and population studies have mainly produced results in favour of an increased risk. Studies that have supported an association with malignancy have suggested increases in lymphomas, monoclonal gammopathy and in cervical, lung, hepato-biliary and breast cancer [3,6–8], although the latter has been shown to be decreased [6,9]. The majority of large studies suggest an increase in non-Hodgkin lymphoma [3,6], particularly diffuse large B-cell lymphoma (DLBCL) [7]. The evidence for an association between autoimmune conditions and lymphoma is supported by a large study of 3055 patients with non-Hodgkin lymphoma and matched controls; significant associations were found with rheumatoid arthritis, primary Sjögren syndrome and SLE, again documenting the specific association with DLBCL [10]. Treatment with antimalarials has been suggested to have a protective effect against the development of cancers in SLE [11] and in a recent large multicentre cohort study antimalarial drugs were associated with a lower risk of breast and non-melanoma skin cancer [12].

Rare patterns of lupus erythematosus, such as lupus erythematosus gyratum repens, may carry a higher risk of internal malignancy [13], although this condition is generally reported as isolated cases so this conclusion is uncertain. Individual reports suggest an association of an SCLE-like eruption with tumours of various organs including myeloproliferative disorders causing a neutrophilic lupus-like figurate erythema and an SCLE-like rash associated with tumours of the lung, liver, larynx, breast and oesophagus [14,15]. Potential clues to this association are an SCLE-like rash in males, SCLE in an older age group than usual and therapy-resistant SCLE.

Systemic sclerosis and other inflammatory fibrosing conditions of the dermis and subcutis

Like SLE, systemic sclerosis (SSc) has been linked with the occurrence of internal malignancy [1,2] (Chapter 54). A meta-analysis of population-based studies revealed increased risks for lung, liver, haematological and bladder cancers, although absolute risks were relatively low [3]. Recent studies have confirmed the increased risk of cancer in SSc compared with the general population, in particular the risk of breast, lung and skin cancer [4].

Likewise, eosinophilic fasciitis has occasionally been linked with contemporaneous diagnosis of a neoplasm [5]. Many of the cases described are not entirely classic or 'usual' SSc, some cases having a more aggressive course of fibrosis than anticipated, an unusual distribution, extensive fibrotic changes in the subcutaneous fat or progressive arthritis. To reflect these features, more recent cases have been described under the terms palmar fibrosis/arthritis [6,7] or cancer-associated fasciitis/arthritis [6,7] or cancer-associated fasciitis–panniculitis syndrome [8,9]. The commonest tumour types documented are ovarian and lung; breast, prostate and pancreatic tumours have also been reported.

Panniculitis may occur in patients with acinar cell carcinoma of the pancreas, in whom a syndrome of panniculitis, polyarthritis and eosinophilia can occur. Eosinophilic panniculitis has also been reported in association with other solid tumours or pre-leukaemia [10,11].

Scleroderma-like skin changes may also be a cutaneous manifestation of carcinoid syndrome, the differential diagnosis from SSc being suggested by the presence of flushing and the absence of Raynaud phenomenon.

BULLOUS DISORDERS ASSOCIATED WITH INTERNAL MALIGNANCY

See also Chapter 50.

Paraneoplastic pemphigus

Paraneoplastic pemphigus is a heterogeneous, multiorgan, autoimmune syndrome in which patients display a spectrum of mucocutaneous manifestations including pemphigus-like, pemphigoid-like, erythema multiforme-like, graft-versus-host disease-like or lichen planus-like patterns, characteristically with oral involvement [1] (Chapter 50). In addition, there is an association with small-airways occlusion [2] and the deposition of autoantibody complexes in different organs. The mucosal disease is often severe and progressive.

Associated neoplasms in one large review series were mainly B-cell proliferations and thymoma or thymoma-like neoplasms; specific neoplasms included non-Hodgkin lymphoma (42%), chronic lymphocytic leukaemia (29%), Castleman tumour (10%), thymoma (6%), spindle cell neoplasms (6%) and Waldenström macroglobulinaemia (6%) [3].

Paraneoplastic pemphigus is distinguished from pemphigus by its clinical features and by the presence of serum autoantibodies to a range of antigens (bullous pemphigoid antigen and a range of desmosomal and hemidesmosomal proteins). Direct immunofluorescence of skin biopsies is usually positive for immunoglobulin G (IgG) and C3 but may be negative in some cases. High sensitivity and specificity for this differential diagnosis has been reported by taking account of the association with a lymphoproliferative disorder, by finding antibodies to desmoplakin on indirect immunofluorescence using rat bladder urothelium, or envoplakin and/or periplakin bands on immunoblotting [4–6].

Bullous pemphigoid

Data about the association of bullous pemphigoid with overall cancer risk is conflicting. Isolated reports have suggested an association between bullous pemphigoid and underlying neoplasia [1,2,3]. However, larger series do not support a significant association with malignant disease [4,5]. Despite this, the issue remains controversial and more selective studies have shown there may be a correlation when immunofluorescent findings are negative and mucosal involvement is present [4]. Historical reports are difficult to evaluate with certainty, as some cases may have been epidermolysis bullosa acquisita or even bullous pemphigoid-like paraneoplastic pemphigus, which can now be separated from bullous pemphigoid by current immunological techniques. Malignancies have been reported from the breast, lung, thyroid, larynx, skin, soft tissue, stomach, colon, lymphoreticular system, prostate, cervix, bladder, kidney and uterus. Recently, registry-based studies showed that patients with bullous pemphigoid are at increased risk of developing cutaneous squamous cell cancer and lymphoma [6,7]. Another study revealed that patients with BP do not experience an overall increased risk of developing solid malignancies, however they are more likely to have uterine cancer [8].

Pemphigus

Historically, pemphigus has been linked with various tumours. Some cases, such as those associated with thymoma and Castleman tumour, would probably now be found to have the features of paraneoplastic pemphigus. Pemphigus foliaceus has been associated with acanthosis nigricans-like lesions and hepatocellular carcinoma [1], and pemphigus in Japanese subjects has been associated with lung cancer. The concurrence of internal malignancy and pemphigus may, as with bullous pemphigoid, be a true association [2], although some suggest this to be coincidence [3].

In more recent studies pemphigus has been found to be significantly associated with chronic leukaemia, multiple myeloma and non-Hodgkin lymphoma, as well as solid malignancies of the larynx, oesophagus and colon [4–6].

OTHER BLISTERING DISORDERS

Dermatitis herpetiformis

Dermatitis herpetiformis (DH) has been documented in some studies to have a link with internal malignancy of various types, especially lymphoma [1–5]. There is logic for an indirect link with lymphoma; DH is always associated with some degree of gluten-sensitive enteropathy and the latter has a well-documented association with small bowel lymphoma. One group of authors who initially found an increased risk of lymphoma in DH [4] later, in a larger study, documented that the overall risk of mortality in DH was lower than in the general population [6] but that the risk of non-Hodgkin lymphoma was increased, with a standardised incidence ratio of 6.0. In this study, one in seven lymphomas in DH was an enteropathy-associated T-cell lymphoma associated with inadequate dietary compliance [6], supporting the earlier documentation that a gluten-free diet reduces the risk of small bowel lymphoma in patients with DH [7]. There may be a difference between DH and coeliac disease; in coeliac disease, the lymphoma risk is limited to enteropathy-associated T-cell lymphoma in the small bowel, whereas B-cell lymphomas predominate in DH [8].

Linear IgA disease

This also appears to have a higher than predicted association with lymphoproliferative malignancy, although this is much less well documented [9]. The most frequent tumours associated with linear IgA dermatosis are lymphoproliferative malignancies, especially non-Hodgkin lymphoma and Hodgkin lymphoma. Other associated malignancies include oesophageal, renal, thyroid and bladder cancer [10].

Epidermolysis bullosa acquisita

Epidermolysis bullosa acquisita is commonly linked with autoimmune diseases but has also been reported to occur in association with neoplasia, particularly myeloma and lymphoma [11–14].

Porphyria cutanea tarda and variegate porphyrias

These disorders have mainly been associated with hepatocellular carcinoma [12,15,16] (Chapter 58).

DEPOSITION DISORDERS

Dermal deposition disorders, such as mucinoses, xanthomas, amyloidosis and calcification, may be linked with internal malignancy

[1–3]. Some of the most important deposition disorders, and their potentially associated internal malignancy, are listed in Table 148.4.

Calcinosis cutis is a rare complication of internal carcinoma. However, it should be noted that many cancers cause hypercalcaemia, and that metastatic calcification may occur in other organs, such as the lung or kidney, even if not in the skin. The commonest underlying malignancies are carcinoma of the oesophagus, myeloma, breast cancer, lymphoma or any other tumour responsible for osteolytic metastases [2].

OTHER DERMATOLOGICAL DISORDERS

Lichen planus

Lichen planus may rarely be associated with neoplasia (Chapter 37) [1]. There is also an increased risk, particularly in males, of oral squamous cell carcinoma; this may be due to a combined direct effect and co-factors such as smoking [2]. In a recent meta-analysis evaluating the cancer development in oral lichen planus, malignant transformation was reported to be 1.14%. The risk of malignant transformation was increased by localisation on the tongue, the presence of erosive and/or atrophic areas, the consumption of tobacco and/or alcohol and hepatitis C infection [3].

Urticaria

Except for cold urticaria and peripheral gangrene as a result of circulating cryoglobulins, where there is a possible but uncommon link with myeloma and lymphoma [4], associations of urticaria and neoplasia are difficult to evaluate (Chapter 42). Certainly, it cannot be regarded as an established paraneoplastic phenomenon other than in Schnitzler syndrome (Chapter 45), a distinct autoinflammatory disorder characterised by chronic urticarial whealing, bone pain, hyperostosis, high erythrocyte sedimentation rate, monoclonal IgM gammopathy (usually IgM-κ) and a significant risk of AA amyloidosis. Although the overall prognosis is reasonable, around 10–15% of patients develop a B-cell lymphoproliferative disorder [5].

Erythroderma and exfoliative dermatitis

Exfoliative dermatitis has been linked with malignancy [6,7]. In most such cases (around 10% in most reported series), the neoplasm is mycosis fungoides or its leukaemic variant, Sézary syndrome (Chapter 139). These cases are really a representation of a systemic neoplasm rather than a truly paraneoplastic disorder. However, there are a small number of patients who have neither condition, but present with erythroderma and eventually develop lymphoma or leukaemia [8]. Immunophenotypic studies do not appear to help distinguish benign from malignant cases [9]. There are additional reported cases of erythroderma with cancers of the liver, lung, colon, stomach, pancreas, thyroid, prostate and cervix [6,7,10]. Ofuji papuloerythroderma is a rare condition that has been associated with solid malignancies and haematological neoplasms [11].

Granuloma annulare

Granuloma annulare has been reported in association with lymphomas, other haematological malignancies and uncommonly with solid tumours [12] (Chapter 95). However, a causal relationship in such cases is uncertain. Among recent studies one case–control study on the prevalence of malignancy in generalised granuloma annulare (GGA) showed that the prevalence was identical in patients with and without GGA [13], and one retrospective cross-sectional study did not show that granuloma annulare was associated with solid organ malignancy [14].

Insect bite-like reactions

Florid insect bite reactions are reported in haematological malignancy, usually chronic lymphocytic leukaemia [15].

Cutis verticis gyrata

This may occasionally occur as a paraneoplastic phenomenon [16].

Mental neuropathy

Mental neuropathy or 'numb chin syndrome' has several benign causes, but may occur as a feature of metastatic disease and is considered an indicator of poor prognosis [17]. Relevant tumours include breast, thyroid, renal, lung, prostate, lymphomas and melanoma. Also, a case of numb chin syndrome as the presenting sign of acute myeloid leukaemia was recently reported [18].

Pyoderma gangrenosum and neutrophilic dermatoses

Pyoderma gangrenosum, particularly the superficial and bullous forms, has been associated with myeloproliferative diseases, including acute and chronic myeloid leukaemia, acute lymphocytic leukaemia, myeloid metaplasia, polycythaemia rubra vera, multiple myeloma, lymphoma and myelofibrosis (Figure 148.17) [19] (Chapter 49). The association of pyoderma gangrenosum with monoclonal gammopathy is uncertain, but it does occur at a frequency higher than expected in the general population and is usually of IgA type, whereas IgG gammopathy is the commonest type overall.

Solid tumours reported include pharynx, gastric, ileum, colorectal, renal, breast and lung cancer [20].

Sweet syndrome has likewise been associated with several malignancies, especially haematopoietic (Chapter 149). Cutaneous

Table 148.4 Some deposition disorders that are linked with internal malignancy.

Material deposited	Disorder	Associated internal malignancies	Comments
Amyloid proteins (Chapter 56) [1]	Primary and myeloma-associated systemic amyloidosis (AL protein deposition)	Paraproteinaemia, myeloma	Amyloidosis occurs in about 15% of patients with myelomatosis
	Secondary amyloidosis (AA protein deposition)	Lymphomas, especially Hodgkin lymphoma, hypernephroma, other solid tumours	
Mucin/proteoglycans and fibromucinoses (Chapter 57)	Scleromyxoedema/lichen myxoedematosus	Paraproteinaemia, typically a 'slow gamma region'	Paraprotein is present in most cases
	Papular mucinosis	Paraproteinaemia	Uncommon
	Scleroedema	Paraproteinaemia	More commonly associated with diabetes or streptococcal infection
	POEMS syndrome	Paraproteinaemia	Features are polyneuropathy, organomegaly, endocrinopathy, M-protein and skin changes (POEMS)
Lipids (as foamy macrophages)	Necrobiotic xanthogranuloma	Paraproteinaemia, usually monoclonal IgG-κ, present in about 70% of cases	Also associated with cryoglobulinaemia, myeloma, marrow dyscrasias and rarely leukaemia; some cases apparently occur in isolation
	Normolipaemic plane xanthomatosis	Myeloma	Usually IgG paraprotein
	Xanthoma disseminatum	Gammopathy, bone marrow dyscrasias	Usually IgG paraprotein
Calcium	Metastatic calcification	Lung and other squamous carcinomas	Due to ectopic parathyroid-like hormone secretion
		Due to primary hyperparathyroidism; may be associated with multiple endocrine neoplasia syndromes	
	Dystrophic calcification	Pancreatic carcinoma	Calcification of fat

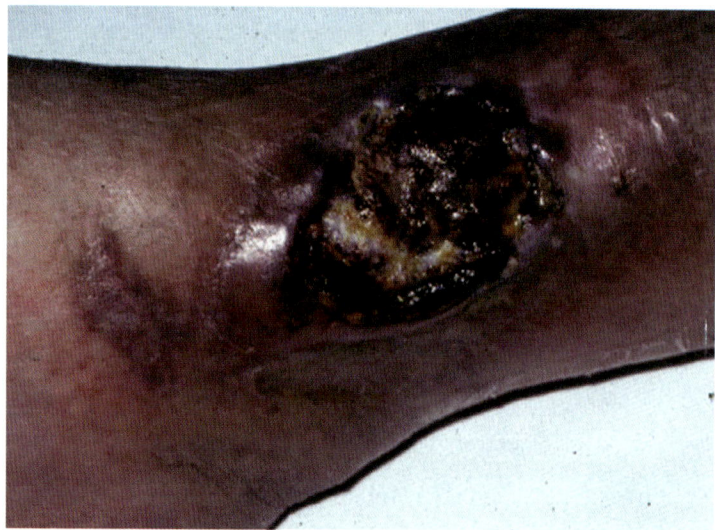

Figure 148.17 Pyoderma gangrenosum of the lower leg in a patient with myelodysplastic syndrome.

manifestations usually occur months to years before the diagnosis of the haematological malignancy, but may also be concomitant with the onset, and may recur during relapses after clinical remission [21]. Chronic recurrent Sweet syndrome appears to have a particularly strong link with myelodysplastic disorders [22].

Multicentric reticulohistiocytosis

This is a rare condition usually occurring in adult life and characterised by papulonodular lesions of the fingers or other extremities, the face and sometimes mucous membranes. Its synonyms include lipoid dermatoarthritis and reticulocytoma cutis. Papules around the nail fold have been termed the 'coral bead sign' (Chapter 135). A severe, symmetrical polyarthritis especially affecting the hands is frequently associated. Approximately 25% of cases are associated with internal neoplasia with both solid tumours, and haematological malignancies [23–26].

VASCULAR DISORDERS ASSOCIATED WITH INTERNAL MALIGNANCY

Raynaud phenomenon and digital ischaemia

Synonyms and inclusions
- Paraneoplastic acral vascular syndrome

Persistent, painful digital ischaemia, with an unusual Raynaud syndrome-type appearance but often progressing to gangrene, has been linked to a variety of solid tumours and reticuloendothelial neoplasms [1–3]. The process may have a vasculitic element [4].

Hyperviscosity syndromes such as polycythaemia vera, leukaemias or myeloma-linked cryoglobulinaemia may give rise to cutaneous ischaemia and phlebitis by microvascular occlusion. Cancer-associated coagulopathy may also cause vascular occlusion [5].

Hypereosinophilic syndrome, for which there is increasing evidence of a malignant clonal proliferation, has also been associated with acrocyanosis, cutaneous microthrombi, digital infarction and gangrene [6–8].

Erythromelalgia

This condition is linked with myeloproliferative disorders, most commonly polycythaemia vera or essential thrombocythaemia in over a third of adult cases (Chapter 101). In a large series of patients with erythromelalgia linked with haematological malignancy, the feet were most affected, with severe burning pain and redness; symptoms may occur 2 years or more before the haematological disorder is documented [9,10]. The mechanism involves microvascular occlusion (typically with platelet aggregates, termed 'white thrombi'); Raynaud phenomenon may occur.

Palmar erythema

This is rarely linked with malignancy, but an interesting association was observed in a series of patients with cerebral malignancies, in whom nearly 20% had palmar and (to a lesser extent) plantar redness, either diffuse or mottled. This occurrence seemed to be linked with the vascularity of the tumour, and was particularly seen with high-grade astrocytomas and glioblastomas; a role for vascular endothelial growth factor was proposed [11].

Vasculitis

There appears to be an association of cutaneous vasculitis with neoplasia, particularly in myeloproliferative disorders [12,13] and myeloma [14,15], although solid tumours have also been reported [4,16,17] (Chapter 100). About 5% of cutaneous vasculitis occurs in patients with underlying malignancies. The majority (90%) of these patients have an underlying haematological malignancy including chronic myelomonocytic leukaemia, non-Hodgkin lymphoma, Hodgkin disease, B-cell chronic lymphatic leukaemia and multiple myeloma. It rarely occurs in patients with solid tumours. The most common of these are renal, breast and lung carcinomas [18].

In a study of 200 patients with antineutrophil cytoplasmic antibody-positive vasculitis (granulomatosis with polyangiitis or microscopic polyangiitis) published in 2004, the relative risk of malignancy preceding or concurrent with vasculitis was sixfold greater than that for the local population. Patients with Henoch–Schönlein purpura ($n = 129$) had a fivefold relative risk, but only five of 333 patients with SLE had a malignancy [17]. A much lower relative risk of approximately 1.5 was found in a study of 535 patients. The authors speculated whether this may be due to a reduced reliance on cyclophosphamide in current treatment protocols [19].

The dermatological manifestations include palpable purpura and maculopapular, urticarial and petechial lesions; these presumably reflect a small-vessel vasculitis or even, when ulceration occurs, a necrotising vasculitis [4,11]. When linked with a haematological malignancy, vasculitis often antedates bone marrow involvement,

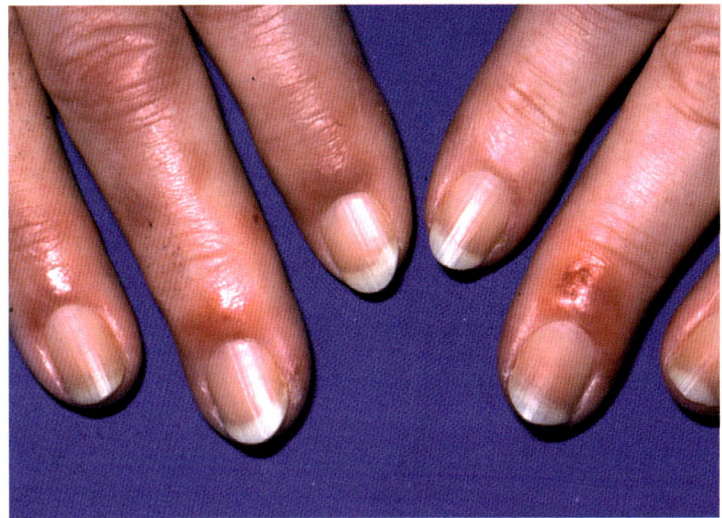

Figure 148.18 Chilblain-like lesions in acute myeloid leukaemia.

as opposed to the more predictable purpura due to thrombocytopenia, which reflects bone marrow infiltration by myeloproliferative disease or carcinoma. It is difficult in some reports to distinguish between microvascular occlusion (for example, by a monoclonal type I cryoglobulin) versus primary vasculitis or therapy-related vessel injury.

Chilblain-like lesions

Lesions resembling perniosis may be a manifestation of leukaemias and myeloproliferative disorders (Figure 148.18) [20,21]. They are persistent rather than episodic, tend to be refractory to treatment with drugs (such as calcium channel blockers) and on biopsy may show blast cells as well as vascular changes. Metastasis from breast carcinoma has also been documented as resembling chilblains [22].

Flushing

This is a normal physiological response and may be a problematic menopausal symptom (Chapter 104). However, it may be a feature of carcinoid syndrome, mastocytosis, phaeochromocytoma, medullary carcinoma of the thyroid, hypogonadism in males, pancreatic tumours producing vasoactive intestinal peptide (VIPomas), basophilic leukaemia, horseshoe kidney (Rovsing syndrome) and renal cell carcinoma [23–25]. It is also a feature of POEMS syndrome, which is associated with myeloma. Plethora, but not flushing, may be apparent in polycythaemia vera.

Carcinoid syndrome

This may be difficult to diagnose at an early stage, as flushing is typically provoked by common triggers of physiological flushing such as emotional stress or alcohol ingestion (Chapter 150). Only about 10% of patients with a carcinoid tumour have a malignant carcinoid syndrome and paroxysmal flushing is present in virtually all cases;

episodes typically last a few minutes and may be more widespread than emotional flushing, sometimes involving the whole body. Nearly 75% of carcinoid tumours are gastrointestinal (especially involving the appendix and ileum), 25% are bronchial, and a small number arise at other sites including the larynx, pancreas, gallbladder and ovary [25,26]. Flushing is described as varying according to the site of the neoplasm. The most common midgut tumours (appendix and ileum) are associated with a gradual development of fixed cyanotic erythema in the flushing distribution, whereas foregut tumours (stomach, pancreas, lung) are associated with a brighter pink flush. This may reflect the production of different mediators; gastric carcinoids typically cause flushing by the production of histamine, whereas midgut carcinoids produce serotonin, bradykinin and prostaglandins. Other symptoms such as diarrhoea, abdominal pain, dyspnoea, wheezing and occasionally syncope may occur with progression of the tumour, usually not occurring until liver metastases have developed. Persistent erythema with or without telangiectasia, scleroderma-like change, pigmentary anomalies and a pellagra-like dermatitis eventually develop.

Mastocytosis

This is most commonly limited to the skin but may be systemic, in which case it may be classified into four groups: (i) indolent; (ii) associated with a clonal, haematological, non-mast cell lineage disease (myeloproliferative or myelodysplastic disorders); (iii) aggressive (lymphadenopathic with eosinophilia); and (iv) mast cell leukaemia (Chapter 45) [26]. A majority of patients with mastocytosis have mutations in the gene for *c-kit* [25]. The more aggressive forms tend not to be associated with cutaneous mast cell lesions, but flushing, dyspnoea, chest pain, abdominal cramps, palpitations, syncope and other systemic reactions due to mast cell degranulation may occur. Serum tryptase is a useful screening test that may suggest systemic disease. However, the proportion of bone marrow mast cells, eosinophilia (especially in bone marrow) and alkaline phosphatase level are of greater prognostic importance than levels of mast cell mediators [27,28].

Phaeochromocytomas

Phaeochromocytomas may cause pallor with rebound flushing [23–25] but the more typical dermatological feature is hyperhidrosis.

Medullary carcinoma of thyroid

Medullary carcinoma of thyroid, like phaeochromocytomas, may occur as part of a MEN syndrome but can also occur in isolation. The flushing involves the face and upper extremities, and can occur with perspiration, discoloration and telangiectasias [25].

CANCER-ASSOCIATED THROMBOSIS

Three main patterns need to be considered: migratory thrombophlebitis, deep venous thrombosis and Mondor disease (a specific and distinct pattern of thrombophlebitis). Arterial thrombosis may also occur as a paraneoplastic entity, but is much less common. The aetiology of cancer-associated thrombosis is multifactorial [1]. The interaction of macrophages with cancer cells causes the release of tumour necrosis factor and interleukin 6 (IL-6), which damage endothelium creating a prothrombotic situation. The same interaction causes activation of platelets and clotting factors X and XII [2]. Some tumour proteases are also procoagulant, especially 'tissue factor' which activates factor VII, and sialic acid moieties of mucin (released from adenocarcinomas) which activate factor X [2].

Migratory thrombophlebitis

Unlike superficial thrombophlebitis confined to the lower limbs, thrombophlebitis associated with neoplasia is often recurrent and migratory (Trousseau sign). A variety of sites, especially the upper extremities and trunk, can be involved and lesions are usually multiple. Migratory thrombophlebitis is associated with malignancy in 50% of cases. The mechanism in most cases is an intravascular, low-grade hypercoagulation, which responds poorly to anticoagulant therapy; heparin is usually more effective than warfarin [3]. As well as an altered level or function of prothrombotic and anticoagulant proteins, the coagulation and thrombotic process may involve cytokines, angiogenic factors or mucin secretion by tumours. Altered blood viscosity, vascular endothelial changes and production of small tumour emboli may also be contributory. Migratory thrombophlebitis can be associated with any cancer, but particularly occurs with carcinomas of the pancreas, stomach, colon and lung. Pancreatic carcinoma accounts for about 50% of all cases. Leukaemias and lymphomas are less commonly associated with migratory thrombophlebitis. Causative tumours are often highly malignant and metastatic with a poor prognosis.

Deep-vein thrombosis

This is not commonly the presenting feature of malignancy [4,5], although cancers have a significant risk of causing thrombosis. The likelihood of finding a malignancy is increased by about fourfold in patients with a deep-vein thrombosis (DVT) of the leg compared with expected population rates; the overall risk of such an association is about 10%. By contrast, DVT of the upper limb is more commonly linked with neoplasia (in some cases the reason is obstruction by an apical lung tumour), and DVT is identified postmortem in half of patients who died due to cancer. Tumours associated with DVT are usually adenocarcinomas in the gastrointestinal tract, uro-genital tract, breast or lung. Mucin secretion, as noted, causes non-enzymatic activation of factor X to factor Xa, initiating the thrombotic cascade. An older age of patients with DVT has been proposed as a factor that should be associated with a lower threshold for malignancy screening.

Mondor disease

This is a rare condition in which a cord-like lesion is palpable in the subcutaneous tissue of the anterior or lateral thorax, or sometimes abdomen. The underlying lesion is a thrombophlebitis of thoracic or epigastric veins, usually unilateral but occasionally bilateral, which may occur as a result of trauma, inflammation or postsurgery. However, 10–15% of patients may have an associated breast carcinoma [4–7] so careful examination and mammography are indicated unless an alternative cause is obvious.

Venous or lymphatic obstruction

In addition to vasculitis and the thrombotic intravascular occlusion described earlier, vessels of different types may become occluded by intravascular tumour cells or may be compressed by an adjacent tumour. The facial and upper limb suffusion of superior vena caval obstruction is well known. Obstruction of venous flow from the head and neck may also occur due to benign retrosternal thyroid gland enlargement and is typically seen when the arms are elevated (Pemberton sign). Lymphatic obstruction typically occurs at the main lymph node sites such as in the axilla due to a breast carcinoma, lymphoma or limb melanoma. Arterial obstruction by tumours is much less common, although tumour emboli may occur.

PARANEOPLASTIC PRURITUS

Internal carcinoma is a non-specific, rare but important cause of pruritus (Chapter 81) [1]. Many mechanisms may be involved including secondary metabolic effects such as uraemia or cholestasis, or itch related to iron deficiency anaemia, acquired ichthyosis or xerosis. Other mechanisms such as those that link brain tumours with pruritus are less well understood. Unfortunately, senile pruritus and asteatosis are not uncommonly encountered in elderly patients, a group who are more at risk from malignancy. It is therefore difficult to dissociate chance from true association which can lead to difficulties in deciding whether screening is justified [2].

Generalised pruritus

In a 6-year study of 125 patients with generalised pruritus, Paul et al. [2] found no significant increase in malignancy, although of the eight patients with malignancy detected, two had lymphoma which is a higher than expected incidence. Other studies support the likelihood of a genuine association of haematological disorders and lymphoma with generalised pruritus. Generalised itching may occur in more than 25% of patients with Hodgkin disease and around 15% in non-Hodgkin lymphoma [3,4]. Other haematological disorders including Sézary syndrome, mycosis fungoides, myelomatosis and leukaemia may also cause generalised pruritus [1,3–5]. Aquagenic pruritus may be encountered in polycythaemia vera as well as in lymphoproliferative diseases (T-cell lymphoma, myelodysplasia) [1]. Many visceral carcinomas can cause pruritus including breast and gastrointestinal cancers and carcinoid syndrome [4] and again the mechanisms are poorly understood. Generalised itching can also sometimes occur with intracranial neoplasia [6].

Treatment of pruritus in malignancy is often difficult. In addition to standard topical agents such as moisturisers, current systemic treatment strategies to reduce the itch include blocking of afferent transmission via peripheral and central neural mechanisms [1,4]. Opioid antagonists, antidepressants and neuroleptics are some of the therapeutic options [1,4].

Localised pruritus

Nerve damage by a tumour at any site can cause neuropathic pain or pruritus. The patterns that are most likely to present to a dermatologist are brachioradial pruritus and localised facial or nasal pruritus [6,7]. Cases with localised pruritus in the neck–shoulder–arm region due to a spinal tumour have been reported with rapid resolution of symptoms after treatment [8]; in one child it was the sole manifestation of an intramedullary tumour [9].

Brain tumours are an uncommon cause of pruritus localised to the face [6]. Variations that have been recorded include unilateral pruritus and pruritus limited to the nostril as well as trigeminal neuralgia [7].

Key references

The full list of references can be found in the online version at https://www.wiley.com/rooksdermatology10e

Multisystem and haematopoietic tumours that involve the skin

1 English JC III, Huen AC, Patton TJ, Grandinetti LM, eds. *Skin and Systemic Disease: a Clinicians Guide*. New York, CRC Press, 2015.
2 Callen J, Jorizzo J, Zone J, Piette W, Rosenbach M, Vleugels RA. *Dermatological Signs of Systemic Disease*, 5th edn. Edinburgh: Elsevier, 2017.

Genodermatoses associated with internal malignancies

6 Ladd R, Davis M, Dyer JA. Genodermatosis with malignant potential. *Clin Dermatol* 2020;38:432–54.
9 Hamid RN, Akkurt ZM. Hereditary tumor syndromes with skin involvement. *Dermatol Clin* 2019;37:607–13.

Naevoid basal cell carcinoma syndrome
6 John AM, Schwartz RA. Basal cell naevus syndrome: an update on genetics and treatment. *Br J Dermatol* 2016;174:68–76.

Neurofibromatosis types 1 and 2
1 Riccardi VM. *Neurofibromatosis: Phenotype, Natural History, and Pathogenesis*, 2nd edn. Baltimore: Johns Hopkins University Press, 1992:213–23.

Multiple endocrine neoplasia syndromes
5 Brandi ML, Agarwal SK, Perrier ND et al. Multiple endocrine neoplasia type 1: latest insights. *Endocrinol Rev* 2021;42:133–170.

Immunodeficiency and neoplasia syndromes

Wiskott–Aldrich syndrome
2 Schaffer JV, Makhija M, Paller AS. Immunodeficiency syndromes. In: Hoeger PH, Kinsler V, Yan AC, eds. *Harper's Textbook of Pediatric Dermatology*, 4th edn. Oxford: Wiley-Blackwell, 2019.

Paraneoplastic phenomena involving the skin

14 Wick MR, Patterson JW. Cutaneous paraneoplastic syndromes. *Semin Diagn Pathol* 2019;36:211–28.

Acanthotic and ichthyotic epidermal disorders
Acquired ichthyosis

1 Patel N, Spencer LA, English JC, III, Zirwas MJ. Acquired ichthyosis. *J Am Acad Dermatol* 2006;55:647–56.

Dermatoses associated with internal malignancies
Acrokeratosis paraneoplastica

4 Moore RL, Devere TS. Epidermal manifestations of internal malignancy. *Dermatol Clin* 2008;26:17–29.

Connective tissue and rheumatological disorders
Dermatomyositis

4 Cox NH, Lawrence CM, Langtry JA *et al*. Dermatomyositis: disease associations and evaluation of screening investigations for malignancy. *Arch Dermatol* 1990;126:61–5.

Bullous disorders associated with internal malignancy
Bullous pemphigoid

1 Hodge L, Marsden RA, Black MM *et al*. Bullous pemphigoid: the frequency of mucosal involvement and concurrent malignancy related to indirect immunofluorescence findings. *Br J Dermatol* 1981;105:65–9.

CHAPTER 149

The Skin and Disorders of the Haematopoietic and Immune Systems

Tanya N. Basu[1] and Austin Kulasekararaj[2]

[1] Department of Dermatology, King's College Hospital, London, UK
[2] Department of Haematology, King's College Hospital, London, UK

Introduction, 149.1

SKIN MANIFESTATIONS OF HAEMATOLOGICAL DISORDERS, 149.2

SKIN DISORDERS CAUSED BY INFILTRATION OF THE SKIN WITH NEOPLASTIC CELLS, 149.2

Leukaemia cutis, 149.2
Lymphomatous skin infiltrates, 149.4
Malignant infiltration of the skin in plasma cell disorders, 149.4
Extramedullary haematopoiesis, 149.5

PARANEOPLASTIC MANIFESTATIONS OF MYELOID MALIGNANCIES, 149.5

Sweet syndrome, 149.6
VEXAS syndrome associated with cutaneous Sweet syndrome and myelodysplasia, 149.7
Pyoderma gangrenosum, 149.7
Neutrophilic eccrine hidradenitis, 149.7
Behçet-like syndrome associated with trisomy 8 myelodysplasia, 149.8

PARANEOPLASTIC MANIFESTATIONS OF LYMPHOID MALIGNANCIES, 149.8

Insect bite-like reaction or exaggerated insect bite reaction, 149.8
Lymphomatoid papulosis, 149.9
Paraneoplastic pemphigus, 149.9
Paraneoplastic pruritus, 149.9

SKIN MANIFESTATIONS ASSOCIATED WITH PLASMA CELL DISORDERS, 149.9

SKIN MANIFESTATIONS AND SYNDROMES DUE TO THE BIOLOGICAL ACTIVITY OF PARAPROTEINS, 149.10

Scleromyxoedema, 149.10
Scleroedema of Buschke, 149.10
Necrobiotic xanthogranuloma and normolipaemic xanthoma, 149.11
AESOP syndrome, 149.11
POEMS syndrome, 149.11
TEMPI syndrome, 149.12
Schnitzler syndrome, 149.12

DISORDERS OF PARAPROTEIN DEPOSITION, 149.13

Extravascular paraprotein deposition, 149.13
Cutaneous macroglobulinosis, 149.13
Primary systemic or amyloid light-chain amyloidosis (extravascular), 149.13
Linear IgA disease, 149.13
Intravascular paraprotein deposition, 149.13
Type I cryoglobulinaemia (intravascular) and perniosis, 149.13
Paraprotein-associated vasculitis, 149.14

GENODERMATOSES AND RARE SYNDROMES INVOLVING SKIN ASSOCIATED WITH HAEMATOLOGICAL CANCERS, 149.14

Neurofibromatosis type 1, juvenile xanthogranuloma and juvenile chronic myeloid leukaemia, 149.14
Other rare syndromes involving skin associated with haematological cancers, 149.14
GATA2 deficiency, 149.14

Clericuzio-type poikiloderma with neutropenia, 149.14
Dyskeratosis congenita, 149.14
Ataxia-pancytopenia syndrome, 149.15

ANAEMIAS AND HAEMOGLOBINOPATHIES, 149.15

Nutritional anaemias, 149.15
Haemoglobinopathies, 149.15

TRANSFUSION REACTIONS, 149.16

Allergic transfusion reactions, 149.16
Transfusion-associated graft-versus-host disease, 149.16
Post-transfusion purpura, 149.16

SKIN AND DISORDERS OF THE IMMUNE SYSTEM, 149.16

SKIN MANIFESTATIONS IN IDIOPATHIC LYMPHADENOPATHIES, 149.16

Kikuchi–Fujimoto disease, 149.16
Kimura disease, 149.17
Rosai–Dorfman disease, 149.17
Immunoglobulin G4-related disease, 149.17

SKIN MANIFESTATIONS IN PRIMARY IMMUNODEFICIENCIES, 149.18

Mucocutaneous candidosis, 149.18
Bacterial infections, 149.19
Persistent human papillomavirus infections, 149.19
Other skin conditions associated with immunodeficiencies, 149.19

SKIN MANIFESTATIONS IN ACQUIRED IMMUNODEFICIENCIES, 149.20

Acknowledgement, 149.20

Key references, 149.22

Introduction

In this chapter the cutaneous manifestations of malignant and benign haematological disease are reviewed, as well as skin disorders associated with primary and acquired immunodeficiency. Patients with malignant haematological disease often present with concomitant dermatological conditions. These can occur before, during or after diagnosis of the haematological disorder. Hence, cutaneous findings can point to a new haematological diagnosis or be a harbinger of transformation of existing haematological malignancy. Prompt recognition that there may be an underlying haematological condition can improve patient outcomes. Thus, it is paramount that a dermatologist can recognise cardinal cutaneous manifestations of haematological disease. Skin changes can be due to direct neoplastic infiltration of the skin, a paraneoplastic phenomenon, or indeed iatrogenic. This chapter also highlights the skin signs associated with benign haematological disorders including haemoglobinopathies and acquired anaemias. Finally,

---

Rook's Textbook of Dermatology, Tenth Edition. Edited by Christopher Griffiths, Jonathan Barker, Tanya Bleiker, Walayat Hussain and Rosalind Simpson.
© 2024 John Wiley & Sons Ltd. Published 2024 by John Wiley & Sons Ltd.

the constellations of skin signs that can point to an inherited or acquired immunodeficiency are outlined. The vast array of skin manifestations associated with disorders of the haematopoietic and immune systems emphasise the importance of close collaboration between dermatology, haematology and immunology teams to deliver optimal multidisciplinary patient care.

Other related diseases are described in separate chapters: primary cutaneous lymphomas (Chapter 139), mastocytosis (Chapter 46), histiocytic neoplasms (Chapter 135), purpura and disorders of coagulation (Chapter 99), antiphospholipid syndrome (Chapter 51), skin manifestations of graft-versus-host disease (Chapter 38) and skin reactions to the drugs used for the treatment of haematological diseases (Chapters 117, 118 and 119).

Table 149.1 Infiltration of the skin with neoplastic cells

Condition	Associated haematological disease
Leukaemia cutis	Acute myeloid leukaemia
	Myeloproliferative neoplasms
	Myelodysplastic syndrome
	Chronic lymphocytic leukaemia
	Adult T-cell leukaemia/lymphoma
Lymphomatous skin infiltrates	T-cell prolymphocytic leukaemia
	Mantle cell lymphoma
	Follicular lymphoma
	Intravascular lymphoma
	Lymphomatoid granulomatosis
	Hodgkin lymphoma
Plasma cell infiltrates (plasmacytomas)	Multiple myeloma
	Waldenström macroglobulinaemia
Malignant extramedullary haematopoiesis	Myelodysplastic syndrome

SKIN MANIFESTATIONS OF HAEMATOLOGICAL DISORDERS

There are three broad categories of cutaneous manifestations of haematological neoplasms. In the first, skin lesions are caused directly by the infiltration of the skin with malignant cells. The second category comprises cutaneous manifestations that are indirectly caused by the underlying malignancy or by-products of malignant cells (e.g. paraproteins), such as in the paraneoplastic conditions, infiltration of the skin or dermatological syndromes. The third category includes skin manifestations caused by treatment of haematological cancers (e.g. graft-versus-host disease after allogeneic bone marrow transplantation (Chapter 38), infections due to immunosuppression or adverse effects of anticancer therapies (Chapters 117, 118 and 119)).

Benign haematological disorders such as nutritional anaemias and haemoglobinopathies also lead to cutaneous signs. Disorders of haem biosynthesis, the porphyrias, are described in Chapter 58.

SKIN DISORDERS CAUSED BY INFILTRATION OF THE SKIN WITH NEOPLASTIC CELLS

Haematological malignancies are neoplasms that originate from cells in the haematopoietic tissue of the bone marrow, lymph nodes or thymus. The myeloid malignancies are a heterogeneous group of diseases including myelodysplastic syndromes, myeloid leukaemias, the myeloproliferative disorders and the rare blastic plasmacytoid dendritic cell neoplasm that often presents in the skin [1]. Lymphoproliferative malignancies originate from the lymphocytes or their precursors and include mature B-cell lymphomas (such as chronic lymphocytic leukaemia), mature T-cell lymphomas, Hodgkin lymphoma and post-transplant lymphoproliferative disorders (often driven by Epstein–Barr virus (EBV)). Mature B-cell neoplasms also encompass plasma cell neoplasms such as multiple myelomas, Waldenström macroglobulinaemia and pre-cancerous monoclonal gammopathy of uncertain significance (MGUS) [2].

Four different classes of haematological malignant deposits can present in the skin: leukaemia cutis, lymphomatous skin infiltrates, malignant plasma cell infiltrates and malignant extramedullary haematopoiesis (Table 149.1).

Leukaemia cutis

Definition and nomenclature
Leukaemia cutis is an infiltration of the skin by myeloid or lymphoid neoplastic leukocytes resulting in clinically identifiable cutaneous lesions [3]. When made up of malignant granulocytic precursor cells, leukaemia cutis lesions are also called myeloid sarcoma, and formally granulocytic sarcoma or chloroma (named due to the greenish hue of the skin lesions, derived from myeloperoxidase granules in the neoplastic cells).

Epidemiology
Skin lesions mostly develop after or concurrently with the diagnosis of a myeloid disorder (60% and 25%, respectively) and only in approximately 5% of cases do they develop before any detectable bone marrow or blood involvement as an aleukaemic leukaemia cutis [4,5]. In chronic lymphocytic leukaemia (CLL), leukaemia cutis may be the first sign of the disease in 16% of cases [6]. In patients with chronic disease, such as chronic myelomonocytic leukaemia (CMML), skin involvement may be a sign of disease progression and blastic transformation [7]. The likelihood of developing leukaemia cutis depends on the type of underlying haematological neoplasm (Table 149.2). Leukaemia cutis is most common in patients with myeloid neoplasms (10–15%) [7], especially in acute myeloid leukaemia (AML) (2.5–9.1% patients) [8,9] and in leukaemias with monocytic differentiation, such as CMML [4,10]. Leukaemia cutis associated with AML accounts for 60–70% of all cases [4]. The risk of leukaemia cutis is higher in AML with neoplastic cells displaying the chromosomal translocation t(8,21) [11]. In patients with a particular subtype of AML (acute myelomonocytic or M4/M5 by the French–American–British (FAB) classification) gingival infiltration of leukaemic deposits can be seen in the mouth; hence it is important to consider a diagnostic biopsy with unexplained gingival enlargement [12]. Within the lymphocytic neoplasms, the risk of leukaemia cutis is relatively high for mature T-cell neoplasms such as adult T-cell leukaemia/lymphoma and T-cell prolymphocytic leukaemia (20–70%) [13,14,**15**] and CLL (4–20%) [5,**15**]. In other

Table 149.2 Leukaemia cutis and lymphomatous skin infiltrates in the setting of a haematological neoplasm.

Condition	Probability of clinically apparent skin involvement[a]
Myeloid neoplasms	
All types	++ (10–15%)
	Higher risk in congenital leukaemia and paediatric leukaemia
AML (acute myeloid leukaemia)	++ (2.5–9.1%)
	Higher incidence in AML with t(8;21) translocations
Other myeloid neoplasms[b]	+
Lymphoid leukaemias	
CLL (chronic lymphocytic leukaemia)	+++ (4–20%)
Adult T-cell leukaemia/lymphoma	+++ (20–70%)
T-cell prolymphocytic leukaemia	+++
Other lymphocytic leukaemias	+
Lymphomas	
Hodgkin lymphoma	+ (0.5–3.4%)
Lymphoblastic lymphoma	+
Mantle cell lymphoma	+++
Follicular lymphoma	++
Diffuse large B-cell lymphoma – intravascular type	+++
Lymphomatoid granulomatosis	+++ (40–50%)

[a] Strength of association: +, occasional <4%; ++, frequent 5–14%; +++, very frequent >15%.
[b] Myeloid neoplasms comprise over 30 well-defined clinicopathological entities in five major groups: myeloproliferative neoplasms (chronic myeloid leukaemia, polycythaemia vera, primary myelofibrosis, essential thrombocythaemia, mastocytosis), myeloid neoplasms with eosinophilia, myelodysplastic neoplasms (e.g. juvenile myelomonocytic leukaemia) and myelodysplastic syndrome [16].

lymphocytic leukaemias, such as acute B- and T-cell lymphoblastic leukaemias (ALLs), the incidence of leukaemia cutis is much lower (below 3%) [5,15].

The incidence of leukaemia cutis is higher in children with leukaemia, and in congenital leukaemias it may be as high as 30% [17]. Isolated leukaemia cutis seems to be more frequent in patients who relapse after allogeneic bone marrow transplant, where frequencies of 8–20% have been reported [18].

Pathophysiology

The molecular basis underlying the migration of leukaemic cells to the skin in leukaemia cutis is not fully understood. Homing of malignant cells to the skin may depend on specific chemokine receptors, such as chemokine receptor 4 (CCR4) interacting with specific intercellular adhesion molecules such as intercellular adhesion molecule 1 (ICAM-1) [19]. Cutaneous leukocyte antigen expressed on acute myelomonocytic cells in 14 patients out of 18 in one study may have accounted for skin homing [15,16].

Pathology

In leukaemia cutis associated with myeloid neoplasms, skin infiltration is typically both superficial and deep, and consists of proliferating immature myeloid cells (myeloblasts, monoblasts, promonocytes or promyelocytes) [20]. The infiltrate may also be quite subtle and resemble non-specific dermatitis [21], granuloma annulare, histiocytoid Sweet syndrome [4], vasculitis [22] or multicentric reticulohistiocytosis [23]. Immunohistological profiling is therefore an essential part of the diagnostic work-up. The most sensitive markers are CD43, CD68 and lysozyme. Other useful markers are myeloperoxidase, CD33, CD34, CD117 and CD68 [4,20,21] but CD117 and myeloperoxidase immunostaining are usually negative in monoblastic skin infiltrates. It is also noteworthy that the immune profile of the circulating leukaemic cells may vary from those in the skin infiltrates, which probably reflects different clonal evolution of the malignant cells in different anatomical compartments [16]. Myeloid leukaemia cutis should be differentiated from blastic plasmacytoid dendritic cell neoplasm that may present in the skin and which is characterised by plasmacytoid CD4+ CD56+ cells thought to derive from dendritic cell precursors (Chapter 139). Other differential diagnoses comprise some poorly differentiated solid tumours such as metastatic malignant melanoma, Ewing sarcoma or medulloblastoma and histiocytic sarcomas, which may be positive for CD68 and lysozyme but are negative for CD33 and CD13.

The skin infiltrate of CLL comprises small monomorphic lymphocytes with an aberrant marker pattern (CD20+5+43+) in a lichenoid, perivascular or nodular pattern [6]. Analysis of monoclonal immunoglobulin heavy chain (IgH) gene arrangement may be a useful aid to the diagnosis [24].

Clinical features

Leukaemia cutis typically presents as single or multiple monomorphic violaceous, dark red or haemorrhagic skin nodules, especially on the legs, arms and face (Figures 149.1 and 149.2) [15]. In skin of colour, there may be varied colours at presentation. The lesions have a predilection for sites of trauma (e.g. central line insertion sites) or previous inflammation (e.g. herpes zoster) (Figure 149.3) but may present anywhere on the skin. Other presentations range from small asymptomatic papules or a maculopapular rash to diffuse skin infiltration, ulceration or even erythroderma. It may mimic a variety of benign conditions such as venous leg ulcer, dyshidrotic eczema, cutaneous vasculitis, Jessner lymphocytic infiltration, granuloma annulare or rosacea [4,15,21,25]. The appearance of the skin lesions is not specific for the particular subtype of leukaemia.

Prognosis

The prognostic significance of leukaemia cutis has not been firmly established. In some studies, the presence of leukaemia cutis did not appear to affect the 5-year survival of patients with AML [7,18] but in others it was associated with a significantly poorer survival both in AML (75% 1-year mortality) [18] and in CMML [23]. The presence of leukaemia cutis does not affect the prognosis of CLL; indeed CLL cells will often seed to the skin alongside an inflammatory skin eruption or squamoproliferative lesion, so the presence of CLL cells in a skin biopsy of a patient with known CLL does not indicate a worse prognosis [24]. The exception is when there is large-cell transformation of CLL (Richter syndrome) where prognosis is grave in the presence of large blastic cells in the infiltrate [6,26].

Management

Leukaemia cutis is a cutaneous manifestation of an underlying systemic disease. Hence, treatment should be guided by the underlying leukaemia with supportive care for the skin lesions. However, the skin lesions may be less responsive to chemotherapy than the

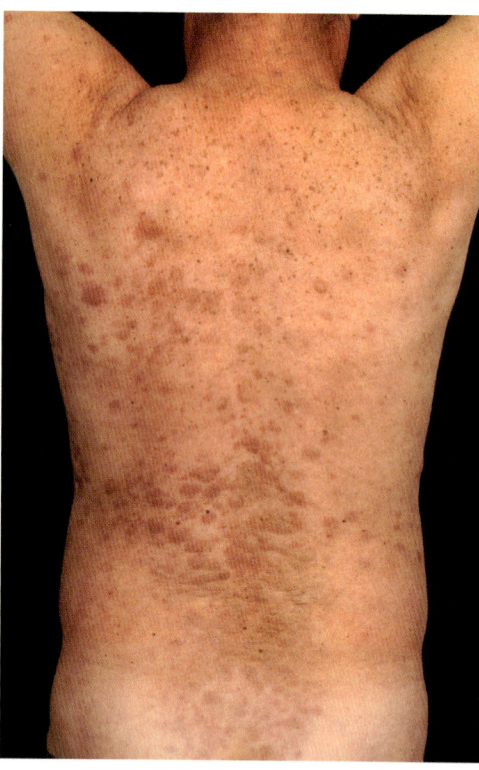

Figure 149.1 Leukaemia cutis in acute myeloid leukaemia: extensive infiltrative, papulonodular lesions over the back. Courtesy of Professor Lorenzo Cerroni, University of Graz, Austria.

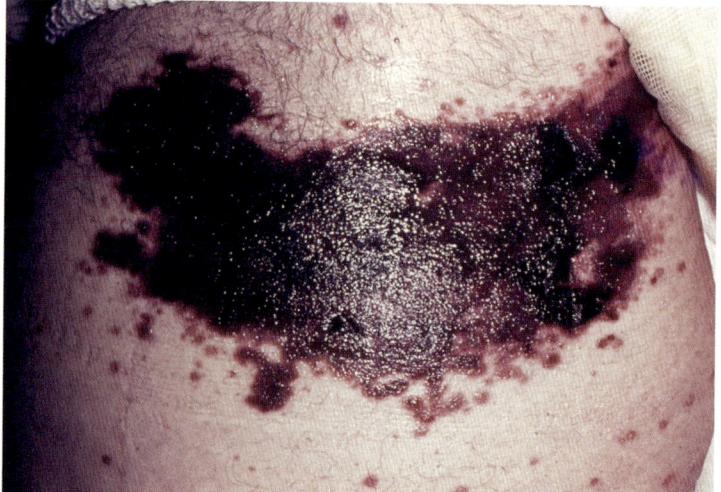

Figure 149.3 Haemorrhagic leukaemic infiltration at the site of thoracic herpes zoster in an elderly man with chronic lymphatic leukaemia.

involvement in non-Hodgkin lymphomas is more frequent, especially for mantle cell lymphoma and lymphomatoid granulomatosis (lymphoid dyscrasia caused by EBV) [28–30].

In Hodgkin lymphoma, the skin infiltrate does not always faithfully replicate the nodal disease. Reed–Sternberg cells in the skin are CD30+ CD45–. In a minority of cases, the neoplastic cells in the skin may be negative for CD15 even in patients with nodal CD15 positivity [27]. The major differential diagnoses are primary cutaneous CD30+ lymphomas and CD30+ transformation of mycosis fungoides.

In Hodgkin lymphoma, the majority of patients die within a few months following the development of skin lesions [27]. Therefore, skin involvement is considered to be an indication of stage IV disease.

Malignant infiltration of the skin in plasma cell disorders

The most common plasma cell malignancies are multiple myeloma and Waldenström macroglobulinaemia. Both conditions are characterised by the presence of >10% malignant plasmacytic cells in the bone marrow and an associated monoclonal gammopathy. It is thought that these malignancies are preceded by a premalignant stage in which bone marrow infiltration with abnormal plasma cells is below the threshold of detection (<10%) and the identifiable feature is a monoclonal gammopathy, known as MGUS. MGUS is detected in approximately 3% of the general population aged 50 years or older and is associated with a 1% per year risk of progression to multiple myeloma or Waldenström macroglobulinaemia [31,32]. According to the type of gammopathy, there are three major classes of MGUS: the immunoglobulin M (IgM) type (progressing to Waldenström macroglobulinaemia), the non-IgM type (IgG or IgA) and light-chain MGUS which may progress to multiple myeloma [31].

Apart from the bone marrow, neoplastic plasma cells may also develop in extramedullary locations as solitary plasmacytomas,

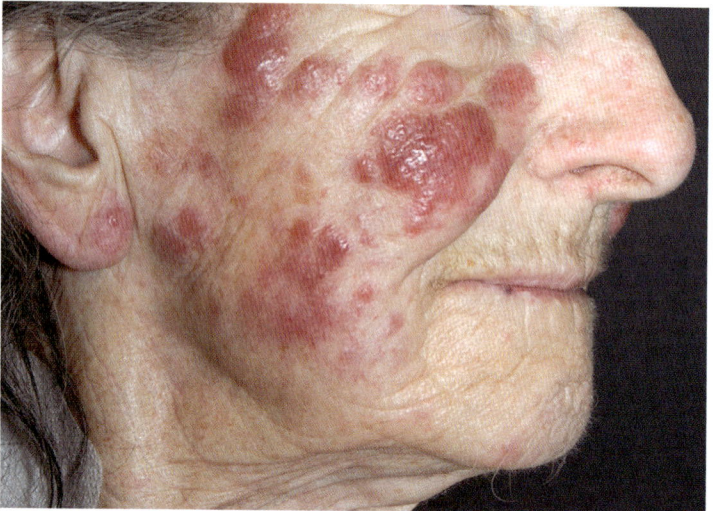

Figure 149.2 Leukaemia cutis in chronic lymphocytic leukaemia: infiltrated nodules and plaques on the cheek. Courtesy of Professor Lorenzo Cerroni, University of Graz, Austria.

disease in the bone marrow or the blood [25]. Radiotherapy with photons or electron beam can be beneficial to treat focal leukaemic skin infiltrates.

Lymphomatous skin infiltrates

In Hodgkin disease, specific skin involvement is uncommon, with an estimated prevalence of 0.5–3.4% [27]. Lymphomatous skin

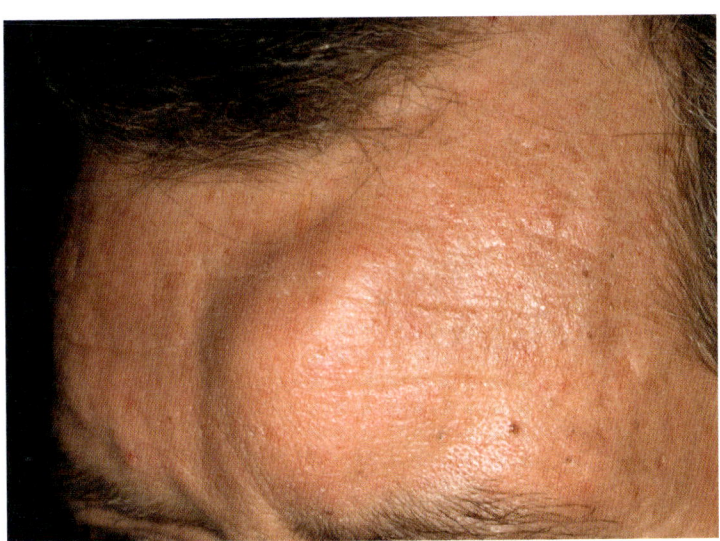

Figure 149.4 Plasmacytoma cutis. Courtesy of Professor Lorenzo Cerroni, University of Graz, Austria.

most commonly in the bone or upper respiratory tract. In exceptional situations, a plasmacytoma may be confined to the skin (Figure 149.4). Plasmacytomas may result in MGUS and may progress to multiple myeloma if untreated. Cutaneous plasma cell infiltration in pre-existing multiple myeloma and Waldenström macroglobulinaemia is a very rare phenomenon, with approximately 100 cases described in the literature [33,34]. The risk of cutaneous involvement does not depend on the immunoglobulin isotype produced by the neoplastic plasma cells [34]. The lesions are described as firm, smooth, violaceous papules and nodules, sometimes with secondary ulceration. The most frequent sites affected are the trunk, followed by the scalp and face. Rarely there can be a hyperpigmented cutaneous patch overlying the plasmacytoma (see AESOP syndrome later in this chapter).

Histopathologically, the infiltrates are diffuse or nodular aggregations of lymphoplasmacytic cells showing a strong immunoreactivity for CD79a and CD138 and an aberrant expression of CD43 and CD56. In multiple myeloma, the cells are usually negative for pan-B-cell markers such as CD19 and CD20. This is in contrast to Waldenström macroglobulinaemia where the neoplastic cells are often CD19+ CD20+. Differential diagnosis includes primary plasmacytoma cutis and EBV-related plasmacytoid hyperplasia which develops in immunosuppressed transplant patients [35]. In only exceptional cases do these conditions present in the skin [36]. In most cases, skin lesions appear relatively late in the course of multiple myeloma or Waldenström macroglobulinaemia and indicate an unfavourable outcome.

Extramedullary haematopoiesis

Extramedullary haematopoiesis is the formation of cellular blood components outside the bone marrow. It can be a pathological feature of chronic myeloproliferative syndromes such as primary myelofibrosis [37]; foci commonly occur in the spleen and may in rare instances occur in the skin [38]. The process is probably caused by seeding of abnormal haematopoietic stem cells outside the bone marrow and subsequent aberrant proliferation. Skin manifestations include pink to red or violaceous (angioma-like) papules, nodules, tumours and ulcers, often on the torso, that may appear soon after diagnosis with myelofibrosis (and sometimes following splenectomy). Skin lesions may resemble leukaemia cutis [38] from which they should be differentiated. Histologically, skin lesions are characterised by a polymorphous dermal infiltrate of myeloid and erythroid cell precursors, often with the presence of dysplastic megakaryocytes and occasionally few myeloblasts [39,40].

Prolonged dermal extramedullary haematopoiesis can also occur in neonates without a haematological neoplasm but as a reactive phenomenon to an infection commencing *in utero*, such as one of the TORCH group of infections (toxoplasmosis, other (e.g. syphilis, varicella-zoster, parvovirus B19), rubella, cytomegalovirus and herpes infections). The generalised haemorrhagic, purpuric eruption that ensues has led to the term 'blueberry muffin baby'. In children and adults, reactive extramedullary haematopoiesis may also accompany thalassaemias, sickle cell anaemia or thrombocytopenic purpura but skin involvement in adults is exceptionally rare [39].

PARANEOPLASTIC MANIFESTATIONS OF MYELOID MALIGNANCIES

Paraneoplastic syndromes (described in detail in Chapter 148) may be associated with myeloid or lymphoid malignancies. Diagnosis of any of these paraneoplastic conditions warrants an active search for a possible underlying haematological malignancy. Paraneoplastic conditions may precede the haematological neoplasm by months or years [41] and the history is therefore an important first step in linking the skin symptoms to an underlying malignancy. Drug intake at the time of disease onset should be determined, as some drug reactions may mimic the paraneoplastic conditions.

Diagnostic screening may include clinical examination of the peripheral lymph nodes, analysis of the peripheral full blood count, blood film and lactose dehydrogenase, protein electrophoresis to detect monoclonal paraproteins, a bone marrow biopsy (if a myeloid disorder is suspected), and combined ^{18}F fluorodeoxyglucose positron emission and X-ray computed tomography (FDG-PET/CT) scanning. The latter has been found to be a good screening tool, especially for lymphoma and leukaemia [42,43]. However, not all haematological neoplasms (in particular low-grade lymphomas) will be detected by this technique [44]. Many of these paraneoplastic skin conditions remain refractory to treatment until management of the underlying haematological malignancy is addressed [45].

Myelodysplasias are the skin manifestations of myeloid disorders. They are a heterogeneous collection of clonal stem cell abnormalities characterised by ineffective haematopoiesis, with cytopenias with fatigue (due to anaemia), bruising (thrombocytopenia) and infections (leukopenias), but a hypercellular bone marrow. There is a tendency for leukaemic transformation to AML [46]. Patients are often elderly with a median age of 72 years; young patients do present with myelodysplasia but usually with an underlying genetic disorder such as GATA-2 deficiency [47,48]. In low-risk myelodysplasia, a proinflammatory cytokine milieu and a tendency towards autoimmune disorders, including systemic lupus erythematosus, as well as inflammatory neutrophilic dermatoses, is now well recognised [49].

Sweet syndrome

Sweet syndrome is an acute, febrile, neutrophilic dermatosis (Chapter 49). It may be drug induced or paraneoplastic (in 20% of cases [50]), or no cause is found in other cases which are labelled idiopathic. The paraneoplastic form is predominantly associated with haematological neoplasms, particularly myeloid leukaemias and myelodysplasias. Sweet syndrome may precede the development of a haematological malignancy by over a decade [51]. The pathogenesis of paraneoplastic Sweet syndrome has not been elucidated, but a hypersensitivity reaction to tumour antigens or an autoinflammatory interleukin 1 (IL-1) mediated process have been suggested as putative mechanisms [52–55]. Moreover, heterozygous mutations in the gene *MEFV* known to cause familial Mediterranean fever have been reported in two patients with concurrent Sweet and myelodysplastic syndrome, suggesting there may be an underlying genetic tendency to develop Sweet syndrome in a subset of patients with evolving myeloid malignancies (see the next section on the VEXAS syndrome) [56]. An important variant of Sweet syndrome is histiocytoid Sweet syndrome, where the dermal infiltrate is composed of immature myeloid precursors that resemble histiocytes; some studies suggest the dermal infiltrates are clonal [57], exhibiting the same mutations as the associated myelodysplasia clone. Hence, whilst these lesions are not leukaemia cutis [58], they may well be clonal myeloid precursor lesions.

The clinical features of paraneoplastic Sweet syndrome are variable. The classic presentation with myelodysplasia is a relapsing and remitting condition with episodes of fever, arthralgia and an eruption of tender, red or violaceous papules and nodules surmounted by pseudovesicles. In skin of colour, varied colours may be observed. However, paraneoplastic Sweet syndrome has a tendency to involve extracutaneous sites more often than the idiopathic type. Mucosal lesions (see section on the Behçet-like syndrome later in this chapter), neurological complications (parkinsonism) and ophthalmological complications (optic neuritis, chorioretinitis) are more common in patients with myeloproliferative diseases than in idiopathic Sweet syndrome [51]. Other clinical variants include acute necrotising, isomorphic and subcutaneous varieties and the neutrophilic dermatosis of dorsal hands. In the acute necrotising variant, there is a fulminant onset of oedematous, pink to red plaques accompanied by necrosis of the skin and soft tissues [59]. Isomorphic Sweet syndrome develops at the site of the trauma such as radiation fields or surgery scars. Subcutaneous Sweet syndrome is a variant overlapping with pyoderma gangrenosum and seems to be particularly associated with myeloproliferative diseases: it presents with tender nodules with a predilection for the buttocks and lower extremities without tissue necrosis and has a tendency to resolve spontaneously [60]. Neutrophilic dermatosis of the dorsal hands is a localised variant of Sweet syndrome that has been described to occur in the context of a variety of malignancies including the haematological neoplasms (Figure 149.5) [61,62].

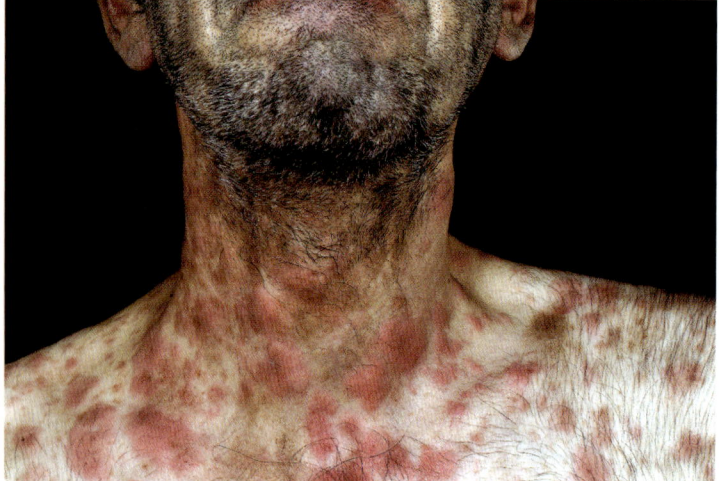

Figure 149.5 Extensive odematous plaques of histiocytoid Sweet syndrome in a patient with VEXAS syndrome.

Table 149.3 Drugs used in the management of patients with haematological malignancies with known association with Sweet syndrome.

Drug group	Examples
Cytotoxic anticancer agents	Proteasome inhibitors (bortezomib)
	Mitoxantrone
	Cytarabine
Other anticancer drugs and biological response modifiers	Tyrosine kinase inhibitors (imatinib mesylate)
	Lenalinomide
	Granulocyte colony-stimulating factor
	All-*trans*-retinoic acid
	Interferon-α
Antibiotics	Clindamycin
	Tetracyclines
	Quinolones
	Trimethoprim with sulfamethoxazole
Antivirals	Abacavir
	Aciclovir

Paraneoplastic Sweet syndrome should be differentiated from other neutrophilic paraneoplastic conditions (neutrophilic eccrine hidradenitis, pyoderma gangrenosum), as well as vasculitis, erythema elevatum diutinum, infectious neutrophilic panniculitis, panniculitic id reaction, early erythema nodosum and leukaemia cutis. The differential diagnosis may be challenging since paraneoplastic Sweet syndrome has a tendency to coexist with other neutrophilic paraneoplastic conditions in the same patient [51]. Moreover, drug-induced Sweet syndrome should be borne in mind since a number of drugs used in the treatment of haematological malignancies have the potential to precipitate Sweet syndrome (Table 149.3).

A skin biopsy of a lesion in Sweet syndrome often shows a dense dermal neutrophilic infiltrate. However, the histiocytoid variant of Sweet syndrome can easily be missed if the histopathologist is not alerted to this possible diagnosis. In histiocytoid Sweet syndrome, the histiocytoid cells are actually myeloid precursors, and can be identified with myeloperoxidase (MPO) staining.

In myelodysplasia, the skin lesions of Sweet syndrome are often extremely refractory to treatments including dapsone and colchicine; oral corticosteroids are often the only treatment to help initially. In corticosteroid-refractory disease, 5-azacytadine therapy (a cytadine analogue used to treat myelodysplasia) often resolves the lesions, supporting the idea of a myeloid clonal dermal infiltrate driven by the underlying myelodysplasia [63]. However, this therapy can itself cause a flare of Sweet syndrome [64] (hence corticosteroid cover can be required during the 5-azacytadine therapy).

VEXAS syndrome associated with cutaneous Sweet syndrome and myelodysplasia

In 2020, a new X-linked autoinflammatory syndrome called VEXAS (vacuoles E1 enzymes, X-linked, autoinflammatory, somatic) was described. In this, Sweet syndrome lesions develop (Figure 149.5) with myelodysplasia with severe systemic symptoms of pyrexias and arthritis, and a poor prognosis [65]. As well as Sweet syndrome, patients can have concurrent cutaneous vasculitis, polychondritis and thrombocytopenia [66] (Chapter 45). In VEXAS sydrome, it seems that the Sweet syndrome lesions are clonal and derived from the myeloid clone proliferating in the bone marrow [67]. Of note, VEXAS patients often show a flare of systemic and skin symptoms with IL-1 inhibitor anakinra [65]. Treatment with 5-azacytadine therapy to target the underlying myeloid clone shows promise in case reports [68]. Many patients with Sweet syndrome and myelodysplasia have a good prognosis [41], so it is unlikely that VEXAS accounts for all cases of myelodysplasia-associated Sweet syndrome; it is likely that other myeloid-restricted genes that predispose to Sweet syndrome will be identified.

Pyoderma gangrenosum

Pyoderma gangrenosum (Chapter 49) is another neutrophilic dermatosis and is classified into four clinical types: classic ulcerative, bullous, pustular and vegetative types. It has been estimated that between 20% and 60% of cases of pyoderma gangrenosum are associated with a haematological malignancy [69,70]. The non-classic presentations are overrepresented in paraneoplastic pyoderma [69]. The bullous variant is associated with haematological neoplasms in more than 70% of cases (Figure 149.6) [71,72].

MGUS, myelodysplastic syndromes and myeloid leukaemias are the most common underlying diseases. Pyoderma gangrenosum and Sweet syndrome may coexist in the same patient with a myeloproliferative disorder. It has been proposed that these entities and neutrophilic eccrine hidradenitis constitute a pathogenic continuum (see earlier in this chapter) [73].

The development of pyoderma gangrenosum in a patient with a myeloproliferative disease may have a negative prognostic significance. For example, the 1-year mortality for patients with AML and pyoderma gangrenosum is 75% after the appearance of the skin lesions [74]. Pyoderma gangrenosum has been reported in the context of myelodysplasia transforming the AML [75] so the patient's haematologist should be alerted to the possibility of associated disease progression.

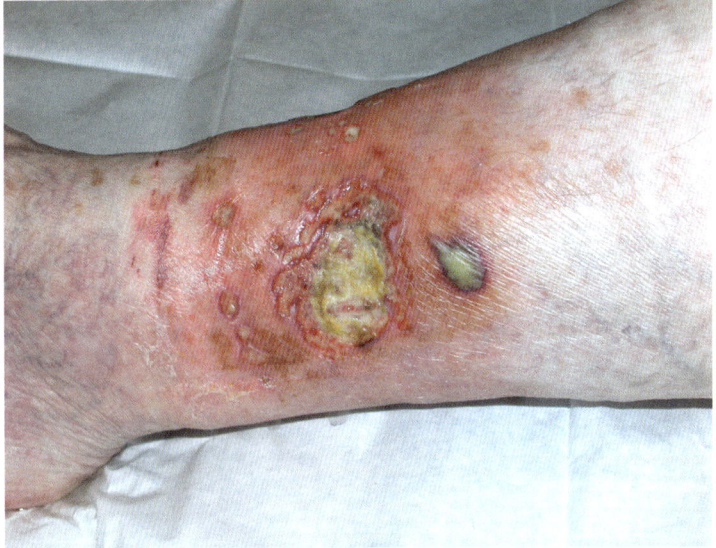

Figure 149.6 Bullous pyoderma gangrenosum in patient with IgA paraproteinaemia. Courtesy of Dr Ian Coulson, Burnley General Hospital, UK.

Neutrophilic eccrine hidradenitis

This condition is one of the rarest of the family of paraneoplastic neutrophilic dermatoses that also includes Sweet syndrome and pyoderma gangrenosum. It is characterised by neutrophilic infiltrates around the eccrine glands and coils [76]. The condition has a very strong association with an underlying cancer since 90% of patients with neutrophilic eccrine hidradenitis have an underlying haematological malignancy, especially AML. Neutrophilic eccrine hidradenitis has also been reported in association with CLL, Hodgkin lymphoma and a variety of nodal non-Hodgkin lymphomas and multiple myeloma. It has been debated whether neutrophilic eccrine hidradenitis is a drug-induced condition rather than a paraneoplastic one. However, in 20% of cases, neutrophilic eccrine hidradenitis develops before the onset of therapy and may even precede the presentation of the haematological malignancy, which would indicate that certainly in some cases the condition is paraneoplastic.

In approximately 80% of patients, the occurrence of neutrophilic eccrine hidradenitis can be linked to drug exposure. The offending drugs are similar to those implicated in Sweet syndrome (Table 149.3). The most common agent is cytarabine followed by decitabine [77], vincristine, imatinib mesylate, topotecan [78], granulocyte colony-stimulating factor (G-CSF) and antibiotics and antiviral agents [68]. The median time from drug exposure to the onset of symptoms is 9 days [76].

Neutrophilic eccrine hidradenitis can be caused by other factors, especially infections (*Staphylococcus aureus*, *Serratia marcescens*, *Enterobacter* spp.), and has been reported in association with human immunodeficiency virus (HIV) infection (Chapter 31).

The classic clinical features are infiltrated pink to red papules and plaques with a predilection for the periorbital area and face,

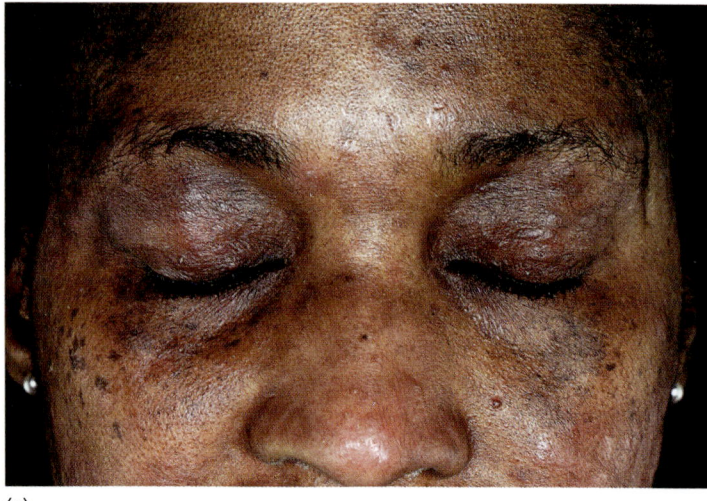

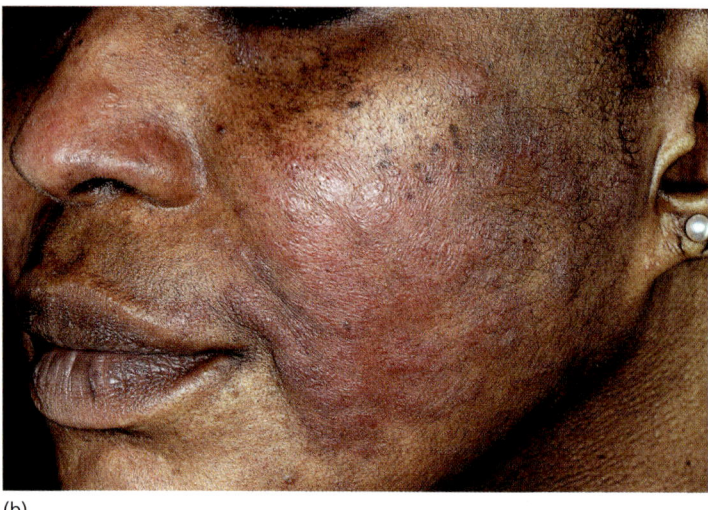

Figure 149.7 Neutrophilic eccrine hidradenitis (NEH) in a patient with an immunoglobulin κ light chain paraprotein. (a) Characteristic dusky periorbital infiltration and (b) red polycyclic plaques of NEH on the cheek.

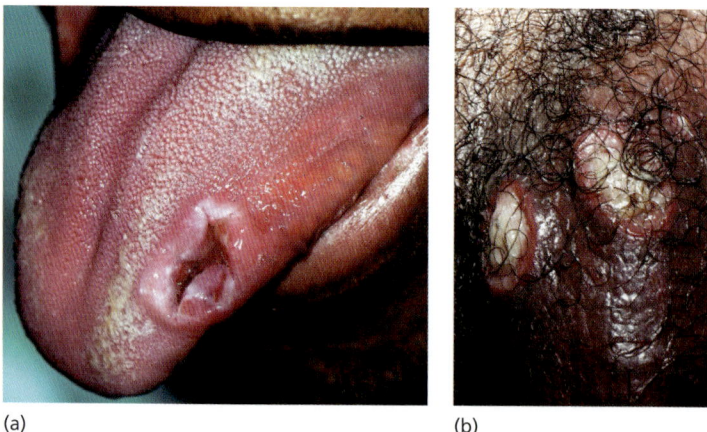

Figure 149.8 Behçet-like syndrome in a patient with trisomy 8 myelodysplasia. (a) A tender oral ulcer and (b) well-demarcated scrotal ulcers.

but there is substantial heterogeneity in its clinical manifestations (Figure 149.7). The lesions may also involve the upper trunk, arms, thighs and palmoplantar skin. They may be annular or linear and may resemble erythema multiforme or Sweet syndrome, from which they should be differentiated. An infectious aetiology should be excluded during differential diagnosis.

The optimal treatment depends on the underlying cause. In some cases, the disease resolves spontaneously, especially after the discontinuation of the offending drug. Therapeutic effects of non-steroidal anti-inflammatory drugs (NSAIDs), systemic steroids or dapsone have been reported in single cases.

Behçet-like syndrome associated with trisomy 8 myelodysplasia

In the trisomy 8 variant of myelodysplasia (where the myeloid clone exhibits trisomy of chromosome 8), a Behçet-like syndrome is recognised [79]. Patients develop oral ulceration (sometimes with pyostomatitis vegetans), gastrointestinal tract ulceration and neutrophilic genital ulceration but no pathergy or arthritis (Figure 149.8). This variant of Sweet syndrome carries a poorer prognosis compared with Sweet syndrome on non-mucosal sites [80].

PARANEOPLASTIC MANIFESTATIONS OF LYMPHOID MALIGNANCIES

Insect bite-like reaction or exaggerated insect bite reaction

An insect bite-like reaction has been described as a paraneoplastic phenomenon associated with lymphoproliferative neoplasms. This condition is also reported as an exaggerated insect bite reaction but is not usually precipitated by an actual arthropod bite, but rather occurs spontaneously, mimicking an insect bite reaction both clinically and histologically. Eosinophilic dermatosis of haematological malignancy is another reported name [81]. The pathogenesis is not well understood but the skin reaction may be related to immune dysregulation associated with conditions such as CLL; external factors such as cancer-related immunosuppression and pyogenic infection exacerbate the reaction. In a minority of patients, this reaction precedes the malignancy, but in most cases insect bite-like reactions occur within 2 years after the diagnosis of the underlying malignant disease. Insect bite-like reactions may also occur in immunosuppressed patients (e.g. in the course of HIV infection, congenital agammaglobulinaemia, natural killer lymphocytosis or EBV infection).

The patient develops red infiltrated plaques and, as the condition progresses, vesicles, bullae and skin ulceration (Figure 149.9). CLL is the most commonly associated disease, followed by mantle cell lymphoma, ALL, acute monocytic leukaemia, Burkitt lymphoma and myelodysplastic syndrome [27,82]. The therapeutic response is often unsatisfactory; oral corticosteroids may produce partial response whereas topical corticosteroids and phototherapy provide only marginal benefit [77]. Oral ciclosporin therapy can be helpful [83]. The prognostic significance is unknown; in CLL patients,

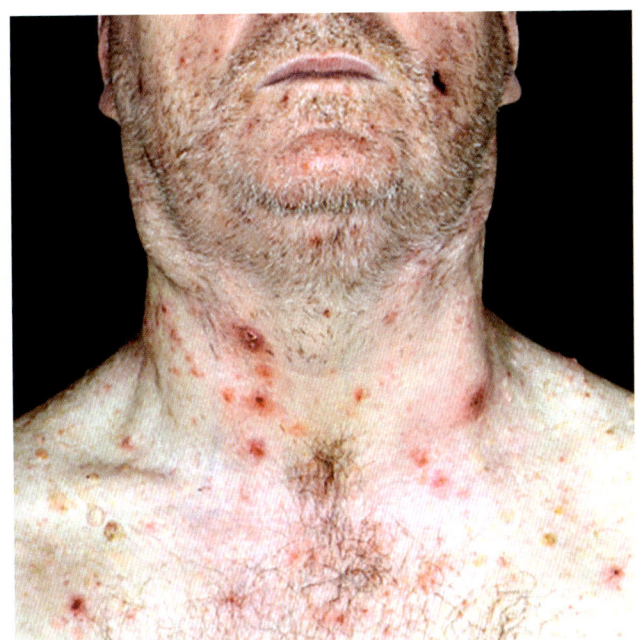

Figure 149.9 Exaggerated insect bite-like reaction in chronic lymphocytic leukaemia.

the course of the skin eruption is not related to CLL activity or the course of the haematological disease [84,85]. The treatment of CLL with the Bruton tyrosine kinase inhibitor ibrutinib has been reported to induce remission of the insect-bite like reaction [86].

Lymphomatoid papulosis

Lymphomatoid papulosis, a CD 30+ lymphoproliferative condition where crops of papulonecrotic skin lesions come and go, can be associated with primary cutaneous or nodal CD30+ large-cell anaplastic T-cell lymphoma and Hodgkin disease in 10–20% of cases (or run a benign course) [87]. Furthermore, in some patients, lymphomatoid papulosis-like lesions follow known Hodgkin disease [88,89]. Patients with lymphomatoid papulosis may also have coexisting or pre-existing cutaneous T-cell lymphoma [90] (Chapter 140).

Paraneoplastic pemphigus

This disorder entity is reviewed in Chapter 50. Paraneoplastic pemphigus is almost exclusively associated with haematological malignancies, particularly of lymphocytic origin. The strongest association is with non-Hodgkin lymphoma (approximately 40%), followed by CLL (20%), Castleman disease and thymoma (20%) [91]. The pathogenesis is unknown, but postulated mechanisms include epitope spreading, antigen mimicry or IL-6 dysregulation by tumour cells [92]. Early histopathology can be lichenoid, making direct and indirect immunofluorescence studies paramount to confirm diagnosis [93]. Untreated paraneoplastic pemphigus has a mortality approaching 90% at 2 years following diagnosis. Treatment of the underlying disease may lead to remission; rituximab, the anti-CD20 monoclonal antibody therapy, has produced both partial and complete remissions in a number of cases.

Paraneoplastic pruritus

Chronic pruritus, defined as a skin itch of longer duration than 6 weeks, is well known to be associated with haematological neoplasms, in particular lymphomas (Chapters 83 and 139) [94]. Paraneoplastic pruritus may precede the clinical signs of lymphoma by weeks or months. Its intensity varies from mild to severe and nocturnal exacerbation is typical. The itch may be accompanied by ichthyosiform skin changes on the extremities. The most commonly associated haematological malignancies are Hodgkin lymphoma (30% incidence of paraneoplastic pruritus), non-Hodgkin lymphomas (10–20%), multiple myelomas and lymphatic leukaemia. Aquagenic pruritus is strongly associated with myelodysplastic syndromes (most notably polycythaemia vera and myelofibrosis) and T-cell lymphomas. Suspicion of underlying lymphoma or myelodysplasia should be high in those over 60 years old with less than 1 year of itch [95].

The mechanism of paraneoplastic pruritus is largely unknown. Antihistamines and local steroids are largely ineffective. There is recent evidence that paraneoplastic pruritus can be ameliorated by aprepitant [96], nalfurafine [97] and butorphanol [98]. Short courses of oral steroids, ultraviolet B (UVB) phototherapy, thalidomide, gabapentin and serotonin–norepinephrine reuptake inhibitors (SNRIs) have been effective in single cases [94,99].

SKIN MANIFESTATIONS ASSOCIATED WITH PLASMA CELL DISORDERS

A myriad of rare but noteworthy skin manifestations are driven by plasma cell disorders that should alert the dermatologist to check for a paraprotein and refer to a haematologist to consider continued joint management. Whilst the reasons for these intriguing disorders are often poorly understood, it is still helpful to group these cutaneous manifestations by pathogenetic mechanism (Table 149.4). Clonal plasma cell deposits causing extramedullary tumours in the skin have already been discussed. Other cutaneous manifestations are due to the biological activity of the excess paraproteins, or due to deposits of paraproteins within blood vessels or outside of blood vessels.

Management should be aimed at treating the underlying paraprotein. Some patients with paraprotein-driven skin manifestations may have haematological disease that fits the criteria for intervention. For example, in multiple myeloma, where an individual has a paraprotein of more than 3 g/dL and organ (often renal) impairment, lytic bone lesions or hypercalcaemia, or in smouldering myeloma (no organ impairment), treatment would be offered [100]. However, often patients have MGUS with only a small clone of paraprotein (less than 3 g/dL) that does not warrant active treatment [101]. Whereas the 5-year life expectancy with multiple myeloma is 53%, only a small percentage of MGUS patients progress to multiple myeloma so often no treatment is required. In the last

Table 149.4 An approach to cutaneous manifestations of plasma cell disorders by pathogenesis.

Pathogenetic mechanism	Disorder
Biological activity of the paraprotein	Scleromyxoedema
	Scleroedema of Bushke
	Necrobiotic xanthogranuloma
	AESOPS syndrome
	POEMS syndrome
	Neutrophilic dermatoses
	Autoinflammatory disorders
Extravascular paraprotein deposits	Cutaneous macroglobulinosis
	Amyloidosis
	Linear IgA disease
Intravascular paraprotein deposits	Cryoglobulinaemia
	Perniosis
	Vasculitis
Plasma cell deposits	Plasmacytomas

AESOP, adenopathy and extensive skin patch overlying a plasmacytoma; IgA, immunoglobulin A; POEMS, polyneuropathy, organomegaly, endocrinopathy, monoclonal protein and skin changes

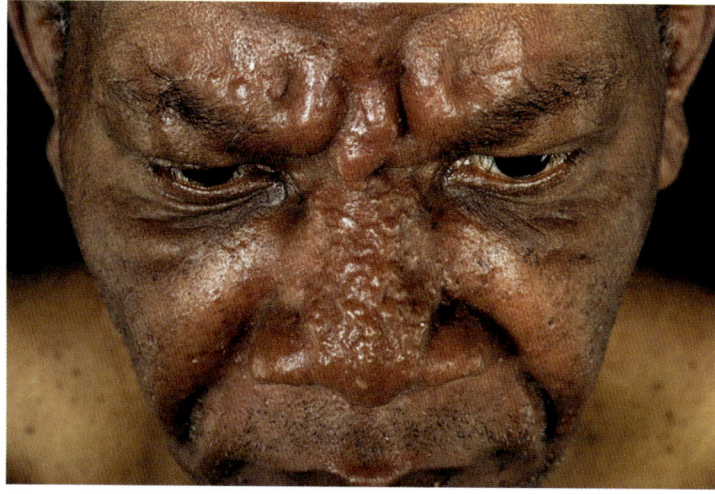

(a)

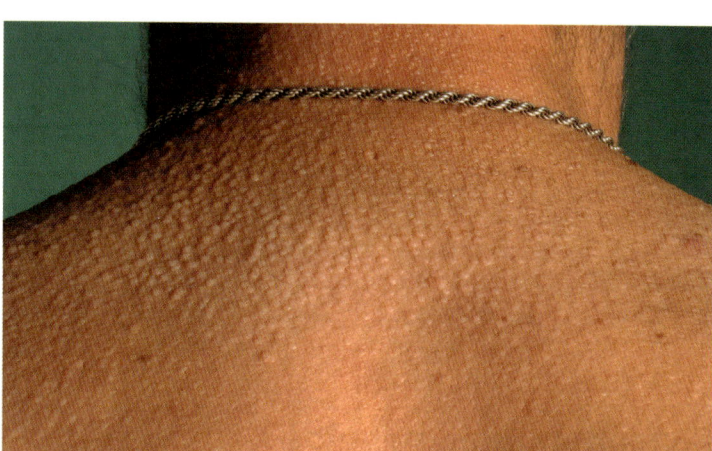

(b)

Figure 149.10 (a) Scleromyxoedema with waxy coalescing papules and leonine facies in a patient with an IgG-κ paraprotein. Sourced by Dr Tanya Basu. (b) Scleromyxoedema in patient with MGUS (monoclonal gammopathy of undetermined significance).

few years, a term in the literature has emerged, 'a monoclonal gammopathy of clinical or cutaneous significance' [102,103]. This is an extremely helpful term because haematologists recognise this entity and are more willing to consider active treatment for a debilitating paraprotein-driven skin condition, even if haematological criteria for paraprotein treatment are not fulfilled [104,105].

SKIN MANIFESTATIONS AND SYNDROMES DUE TO THE BIOLOGICAL ACTIVITY OF PARAPROTEINS

Scleromyxoedema

Scleromyxoedema is a rare generalised cutaneous mucinosis resulting from increased mucin (heavily glycosylated proteins made by fibroblasts) synthesis and deposition following fibroblast proliferation (Chapter 57). In the absence of thyroid disease, scleromyxoedema develops almost invariably in patients with monoclonal gammopathies, either associated with MGUS, multiple myeloma or plasmacytomas [76,77]. Over 80% of patients have an IgG-λ paraproteinaemia [39,78]. The paraneoplastic mechanism of fibroblast activation and mucin synthesis by paraproteins remains unknown. Overexpression of mucin genes, such as *MUC1*, is associated with many cancers [79].

Clinically, there is a widespread papular and sclerodermatous eruption with a particular predilection for the face, ears and dorsal hands. The papules are firm, slightly translucent and waxy in appearance (Figure 149.10). There are no epidermal changes and inflammation is minimal or absent. Histologically, collagen fibres in the dermis are separated widely by mucin deposits; increased fibroblast numbers and fibrosis are observed.

Extracutaneous manifestations are multiple and significantly contribute to the morbidity of scleromyxoedema. The most common are dysphagia, hoarseness and aspiration due to laryngeal involvement, proximal or generalised myopathy, polyarthritis, central nervous system involvement (encephalopathy, seizures, vertigo, psychosis), arrhythmia or myocardial infarction due to myocardial involvement and dyspnoea due to lung involvement.

The course is progressive and mortality is substantial, varying between 15% and 50% [106,107]. The main causes of death are the progression of the haematological disease or central nervous system involvement [107]. Intravenous immunoglobulin provides a rapid response in at least 50% of patients and may be considered first line treatment. Other options are melphalan, systemic corticosteroids, thalidomide and plasmapheresis [107,108]. Treatment of the underlying paraproteinaemia with agents such as bortezomib [109] and autologous haematopoietic stem cell transplant can be beneficial [110].

Scleroedema of Buschke

Scleroedema is a rare skin-thickening disorder, characterised by woody induration and non-pitting oedema, typically localised to the face and neck with subsequent spread to the scalp and upper trunk (Figure 149.11). The hands and feet are usually spared

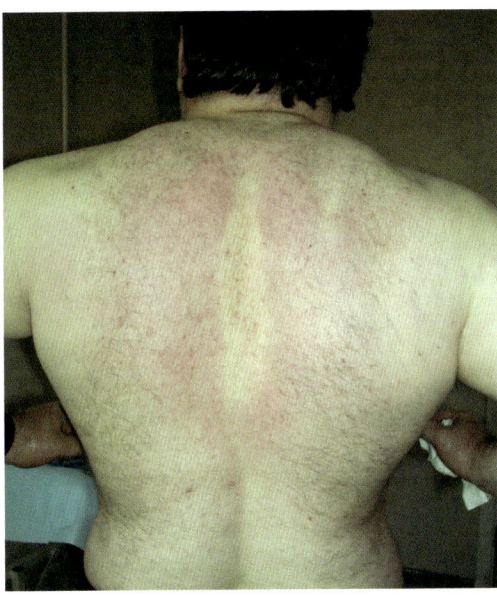

Figure 149.11 Scleroedema in a patient with MGUS (monoclonal gammopathy of undetermined significance). Courtesy of Dr Ian Coulson, Burnley General Hospital, UK.

(Chapter 57). Three clinical variants of scleroedema are recognised: the classic type (55% of cases) precipitated by a febrile illness, diabetes-associated scleroedema and paraneoplastic scleroedema (25% of cases). The latter develops in a setting of monoclonal gammopathy or a B-cell lymphoma [111,112]. In contrast to scleromyxoedema, scleroedema may arise in the context of IgG2-κ, IgG3-κ or IgA-κ paraproteins (rather than IgG1-λ) [111,112]. The paraneoplastic pathogenesis is not clear but there is dermal and subcutaneous thickening due to an increase in glycosaminoglycans separating collagen fibres. No mucin protein deposition is observed in scleroedema. Paraneoplastic scleroedema does not resolve spontaneously like the classic variant of the disease. Internal organs may be involved, in particular the heart, joints and eye [113,114]. An association with the POEMS syndrome (polyneuropathy, organomegaly, endocrinopathy, monoclonal protein and skin changes) has been reported [115]. Treatment is challenging, but psoralen and vitamin A (PUVA) [116], electron beam radiation [111], intravenous immunoglobulins [117], broadband UVA (UVA1) phototherapy [118] and extracorporeal photopheresis [119] have been used with benefit in single patients. Successful treatment of scleroedema with bortezomib-based regimens for the underlying paraprotein is reported [120,121].

Necrobiotic xanthogranuloma and normolipaemic xanthoma

Diffuse normolipaemic xanthoma and necrobiotic xanthogranuloma (NXG) are non-Langerhans histiocytic paraneoplastic conditions without coexisting hyperlipidaemia (Chapter 135) [122]. NXG accounts for two-thirds of paraneoplastic xanthomas. NXG may result from a foreign-body giant cell reaction to cutaneous (and extracutaneous) deposition of serum paraprotein complexed with lipids. Normolipaemic xanthomas resemble classic hyperlipaemic xanthomas clinically, whereas NXGs are firm nodules, papules or plaques in the periorbital area or at any site, often with ulceration, crusting or telangiectasia [123]. The upper extremities and the upper trunk are affected in less than half of cases. Exceptionally, extracutaneous sites such as the oral mucosa, eyes, bones, liver or lungs can be affected [122]. The histopathological features of normolipaemic xanthogranuloma are similar to the hyperlipaemic variant whereas NXG shows a granulomatous inflammation with lymphocytes, foreign body-like giant cells, Touton giant cells and foci of collagen necrobiosis [123].

NXG and normolipaemic xanthoma are associated with monoclonal gammopathy in 80–90% cases. The majority (80%) of these are IgG paraproteinaemias, in particular MGUS (approximately 50%) and multiple myeloma (approximately 40%). The remainder are associated with Waldenström macroglobulinaemia, CMML, CLL or non-Hodgkin lymphoma [122]. In almost all cases, xanthomas are the first sign of the haematological disease.

The differentiation between paraneoplastic NXG and other types of xanthoma can be achieved on the basis of clinical manifestations and histology. However, the separation between normolipaemic xanthoma and hyperlipaemic xanthoma may be difficult due to overlapping clinicopathological features and the frequent presence of hyperlipidaemias in patients with monoclonal gammopathies. It has been proposed that low levels of complement C4 and C1 inhibitor are indicative of a paraneoplastic basis [122].

Therapeutic options beyond the treatment of the underlying disease are limited. Surgical excision may provide symptomatic relief in some patients. A multicentre cross-sectional study shows intravenous immunoglobulin, antimalarials, intralesional triamcinolone and lenalidomide regimens [124] have been effective in single patients [123,125,126].

AESOP syndrome

The AESOP syndrome is an acronym of adenopathy and extensive skin patch overlying a plasmacytoma [127]. Very few cases have been described. The cardinal features are slowly enlarging violaceous skin patches or plaques, and enlarged regional lymph nodes (Figure 149.12). A biopsy from the cutaneous patch overlying the plasmacytoma shows increased dermal mucin and vascular hyperplasia. In all described cases, the skin lesion was overlying a solitary plasmacytoma of bone. The patient may share features with the POEMS syndrome, in particular the polyneuropathy. AESOP syndrome, when recognised at an early stage, may lead to the detection of a curable solitary plasmacytoma of bone.

POEMS syndrome

The POEMS syndrome develops in the context of a monoclonal plasma cell disorder (virtually always of the λ light-chain type). The acronym stands for polyneuropathy, organomegaly, endocrinopathy, monoclonal protein and skin changes. In addition there may be oedema, ascites, pleural effusion, osteosclerotic bone lesions,

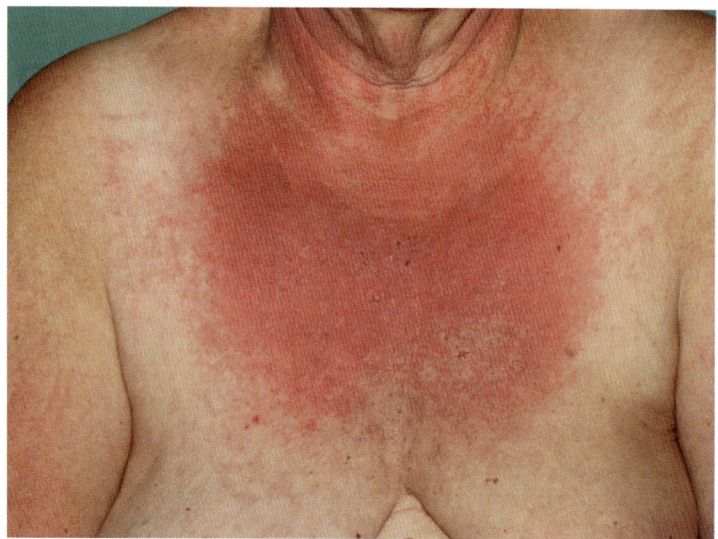

Figure 149.12 AESOP syndrome: a presternal red-brown patch overlying a sternal plasmacytoma.

Table 149.5 Diagnostic criteria for POEMS syndrome[a].

Major criteria	Minor criteria
Mandatory	Organomegaly
Polyneuropathy	Extravascular volume overload (oedema, ascites, pleural effusion)
Monoclonal gammopathy (λ chain restricted)	Endocrinopathy
	Skin changes
Other	Papilloedema
Castleman disease	Thrombocytosis or polycythaemia
Osteosclerotic lesions	
Elevated serum or plasma vascular endothelial growth factor levels	

Adapted from Dispenzieri 2011 [131].
[a] For a diagnosis of POEMS syndrome, the two major mandatory criteria and one additional major criterion and one minor criterion must be recognised.

Table 149.6 Frequency of signs in POEMS syndrome.

Feature	Frequency (%)
Polyneuropathy	100
Monoclonal plasma cell dyscrasia	100
Organomegaly (hepatomegaly, splenomegaly or other)	45–85
Lymphadenopathy	26–74
Castleman disease	11–25
Endocrinopathy	67–84
Papilloedema	29–64
Extravascular volume overload	29–87
Bone lesions	27–97
Thrombocytosis	54–88
Skin changes:	68–89
Hyperpigmentation	46–93
Acrocyanosis	19
Hypertrichosis	26–74
Skin thickening	5–43

Adapted from Dispenzieri 2011 [131].

Castleman disease and thrombocytosis [128]. Skin changes comprise hyperpigmentation, eruptive haemangiomas, hypertrichosis, acrocyanosis, leukonychia, sclerodermoid changes, finger clubbing and facial flushing. The cause of POEMS syndrome is not known but the overproduction of vascular endocrine growth factor (VEGF) by plasma cells, and pro-inflammatory cytokines are major features [129]. An association with a monoclonal IgG4 has been noted in one patient [130]. The known symptoms of POEMS syndrome and the diagnostic criteria are summarised in Table 149.5 [131]. The diagnosis of POEMS syndrome is a multidisciplinary task (Table 149.6).

The course of the disease is chronic with a reported median survival of nearly 14 years. The total number of POEMS features does not affect survival, but fingernail clubbing, effusions, oedema, ascites and respiratory symptoms have been associated with a significantly shorter overall survival [131]. The treatment of the underlying paraproteinaemia and plasma cell disorder is essential. Isolated lesions of plasmacytoma may be treated by radiation. Bortezomib with dexamethasone is considered an effective therapy regimen [132]. Some success has been reported with lenalinomide and autologous haematopoietic stem cell transplantation. The latter modality has become the first line treatment for younger patients with normal organ function [128,131].

TEMPI syndrome

The TEMPI syndrome is another rare multisystem syndrome associated with monoclonal gammopathy. The acronym describes the following constellation of symptoms: telangiectasia, elevated erythropoietin and erythrocytosis, monoclonal gammopathy, perinephric fluid collections and intrapulmonary shunting [133]. Recent genome-wide sequencing suggests a role of duplication defects of the gene encoding the MIF protein (macrophage migratory inhibitory factor) in TEMPI; levels of MIF protein, produced by monoclonal plasma cells, are upregulated, as seen in three patients [134]. The MIF protein is pro-inflammatory, and promotes angiogenesis. Males and females aged 35–56 years are affected. Skin manifestations are telangiectasiae on the face, neck and upper trunk. Patients with TEMPI syndrome are at risk of cerebral thrombosis and venous thrombosis. Untreated, TEMPI syndrome has a progressive course, but responses to plasma cell-directed therapy with bortezomib have been described [133,135,136].

Schnitzler syndrome

Schnitzler syndrome is an autoinflammatory skin disease occurring in the context of a monoclonal paraproteinaemia, typically IgM and rarely IgG [137] (Chapter 45). The patients are usually adults aged 40–60 years who develop a recurrent urticarial rash accompanied by systemic symptoms (fever, arthralgia, myalgia, lymph node enlargement and hepatosplenomegaly) (Figure 149.13). Laboratory tests usually show leukocytosis and an elevated erythrocyte sedimentation rate (ESR) and level of C-reactive protein (CRP).

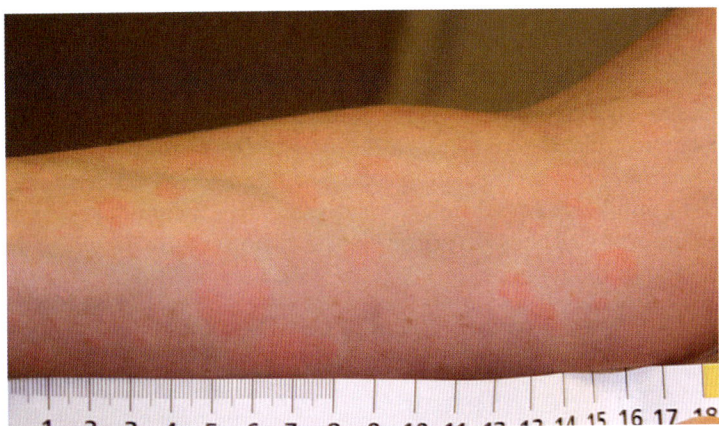

Figure 149.13 Urticaria in Schnitzler syndrome in a patient with MGUS (monoclonal gammopathy of undetermined significance).

The differential diagnoses include urticaria and urticarial vasculitis, systemic adult-onset Still disease and a number of rare autoinflammatory skin diseases, especially adult-onset cryopyrin-associated periodic syndrome (CAPS) [138] and mevalonate kinase deficiency (hyper-IgD syndrome). Diagnosis is often delayed, but timely treatment with IL-1 receptor antagonists such as anakinra or canakinumab can alleviate symptoms and halt end-organ damage [139]. The anti-IL-6 antibody, tocilizumab, may also be partially effective in selected cases [140]. Untreated disease may result in AA amyloidosis, a deposition disease of serum amyloid A (SAA) protein. The patients should be monitored with periodic checks of SAA protein levels and quantification of the monoclonal paraprotein.

DISORDERS OF PARAPROTEIN DEPOSITION

Circulating abnormal immunoglobulins produced by neoplastic plasma cells in MGUS, multiple myeloma or Waldenström macroglobulinaemia may accumulate in the skin. If the immunoglobulin deposition is extravascular, the major manifestations of this phenomenon are macroglobulinaemia cutis, amyloid light-chain amyloidosis and linear IgA disease. If the immunoglobulins collect in intravascular spaces, the main manifestations are type I cryoglobulinaemia, perniosis and leukocytoclastic vasculitis [141,142].

Extravascular paraprotein deposition

Cutaneous macroglobulinosis

This disorder (also termed macroglobulinaemia cutis) is defined by deposition of IgM paraproteins in the skin associated with IgM paraproteinaemia or Waldenström macroglobulinaemia. This may produce two distinct patterns of disease: IgM storage papules and immunobullous cutaneous macroglobulinosis [143]. Both presentations are very rare. IgM storage papules are translucent flesh-coloured papules, usually localised on the extensor surfaces of the extremities. The deposits are periodic acid–Schiff (PAS) positive and stain positively for IgM on direct immunofluorescence but are negative for amyloid [107,144,145]. In rare instances, the IgM paraproteins show affinity for the plasma membrane and result in blistering (immunobullous cutaneous macroglobulinosis) [146–148]. Pathological paraprotein deposition at the dermal–epidermal junction is readily detectable by direct immunofluorescence. Immunobullous cutaneous macroglobulinosis has been treated successfully by rituximab, bendamustine [149] or multiagent chemotherapy [146].

Primary systemic or amyloid light-chain amyloidosis (extravascular)

Amyloid light-chain amyloidosis is a devastating, life-threatening disease that develops as a result of abnormal processing and degradation of the variable portion of monoclonal light chains (Chapter 56). Over 90% of patients have a monoclonal gammopathy, most commonly MGUS or multiple myeloma, and occasionally Waldenström macroglobulinaemia or solitary plasmacytoma. Amyloid light-chain amyloidosis may involve multiple organs and result in nephrotic syndrome, renal failure, congestive heart failure and peripheral neuropathy. Skin symptoms are common (40% of patients) and are very characteristic with purpura and ecchymoses, typically in the perioral and periorbital areas, waxy papules and plaques with sclerodermatous or bullous change. Macroglossia is another typical manifestation [107,145], along with patchy alopecia and generalised oedema. The differential diagnosis for bullous purpura in the context of a paraprotein includes type I cryoglobulinaemia, bullous vasculitis and linear IgA disease. Optimal treatment remains unclear [150]; treatment regimens include high-dose melphalan followed by autologous haematopoietic stem cell transplantation or oral melphalan with dexamethasone [151]. Median survival without treatment is 12–18 months, and poorer if congestive heart failure is present at diagnosis; a multidisciplinary team approach to treatment is warranted [152,153].

Linear IgA disease

The immunobullous disorder linear IgA disease can rarely be a presenting feature of IgA plasma cell disorders, such as IgA multiple myeloma [154,155] (Chapter 50).

Intravascular paraprotein deposition

Type I cryoglobulinaemia (intravascular) and perniosis

Type I cryoglobulinaemia may develop in the context of any plasma cell disorder with paraproteinaemia. It results from the microvascular deposition of abnormal monoclonal immunoglobulins (usually IgM and less often IgG and IgA) that can precipitate out at low temperatures. This in turn leads to microvascular occlusion in the skin and other tissues. The incidence ranges from 5% for patients with multiple myeloma to 37% for Waldenström macroglobulinaemia [107,145]. Typical clinical manifestations comprise purpura, cutaneous ulceration, infarction (often on the lower legs or the face), cold urticaria, Raynaud phenomenon, livedo reticularis, perniosis and inflammatory macules and papules. Horn-like filiform spicules in the follicular ostia of the face, particularly the nose (termed follicular spicules of the nose), have been reported to be a sign of myeloma-associated cryoglobulinaemia [34]. Systemic manifestations include neuropathy, nephropathy and, more rarely, gastrointestinal disturbances [156]. Some patients develop the hyperviscosity syndrome with neurological (headache, confusion), ocular (blurred vision, visual loss), rhino-otological (epistaxis, hearing loss) and renal involvement [156]. An association with reactive angiomatosis has been reported in single cases [157]. It may result in multiorgan failure and thus requires urgent therapy.

The diagnosis of type I cryoglobulinaemia is typically made by direct measurement of cryoglobulins in the serum and is supported by typical clinical features and skin biopsy showing intravascular PAS-positive hyaline material [107,145]. A paraprotein check should be considered in patients with refractory Covid-19-induced perniosis [158]. Type I cryoglobulinaemia should be differentiated from other cryoglobulinaemias (Chapter 124). Plasma exchange, rituximab and bortezomib-based therapy regimens were successful treatments in a single-centre study [159].

Paraprotein-associated vasculitis

Whilst plasma cell disorders can certainly cause a non-immune-mediated occlusive vasculopathy, it is becoming clear that refractory leukocytoclastic vasculitis associated with a paraprotein is also a phenomenon, thought to be intravascular due to immune complex deposition [160,161]. If other causes of vasculitis have been excluded, this should be considered a MGUS. The vasculitis is often refractory to immunosuppressive therapy; treatment should be aimed at the underlying paraprotein [142].

GENODERMATOSES AND RARE SYNDROMES INVOLVING SKIN ASSOCIATED WITH HAEMATOLOGICAL CANCERS

Neurofibromatosis type 1, juvenile xanthogranuloma and juvenile chronic myeloid leukaemia

Over 10% of children with juvenile myelomonocytic leukaemia have a clinical diagnosis of neurofibromatosis type 1 (NF1) and the risk of leukaemia in a child with NF1 is 200–500 times above normal [162,163]. The association with chronic myeloid leukaemia (CML) is even more pronounced (additional 20–30-fold) for those children with concurrent findings of NF1 and juvenile xanthogranulomas [164]. The child presents with multiple (>6) café-au-lait patches and at least one juvenile xanthogranuloma. This neurocutaneous syndrome is caused by activation of Ras proteins due to defective neurofibromin (the product of the *NF1* tumour suppressor gene) causing an increased risk of malignant transformation of haematological and neural crest-derived cells [163,165].

Other rare syndromes involving skin associated with haematological cancers

A number of rare inherited syndromes with a predisposition to haematological neoplasms have been described. A significant proportion of affected patients may present with skin changes. The genetic defect has been defined in many of these syndromes [166,167]. The main mechanisms involved are the DNA double-stranded break repair defects (Fanconi anaemia, ataxia telangiectasia, Bloom syndrome, Nijmegen breakage syndrome) or defects in proteins regulating cell signalling and cell differentiation (NF1 and Legius syndrome). It is notable that café-au-lait spots are common to all these syndromes, the main features of which are shown in Table 149.7.

GATA2 deficiency

GATA2 deficiency or MonoMac syndrome is a rare disorder associated with a familial tendency to myeloid malignancy, immunodeficiency and problems of the lymphatic system [168] (Chapter 73). Loss-of-function mutations in the gene that encodes a zinc-finger transcription factor essential for haematopoiesis and lymphatic angiogenesis, cause the syndrome [169]. Cutaneous signs include lymphoedema (Emberger syndrome) and viral warts in an adolescent, and susceptibility to other viral and non-tuberculous mycobacterial infections. A low monocyte count may point to this disorder. Patients may develop myelodysplasia or AML, and may have a strong family history of myeloid cancers [170]. Allogeneic stem cell transplant can be curative [171,172].

Clericuzio-type poikiloderma with neutropenia

This autosomal recessive congenital poikiloderma is due to loss-of-function mutations in the *USB1* gene, which encodes a phosphodiesterase enzyme essential in spliceosome RNA modification [173] (Chapter 75). Patients present as infants with an acute-phase papular, red rash that then settles leaving widespread poikiloderma. Unlike in Rothmund–Thomson syndrome, the main differential diagnosis, there is no alopecia or photodistribution of the poikiloderma in Clericuzio-type poikiloderma [174]. Patients have non-cyclical neutropenia [175] so are prone to sino-pulmonary infections. Prompt recognition is important as the neutropenia may progress to myelodysplasia or AML as patients become young adults [173].

Dyskeratosis congenita

This rare, collection of inherited bone marrow failure disorders are due to various mutations (e.g. TERC and TERT mutations) that allow telomere shortening (Chapter 77). Skin features may be subtle but include poikiloderma and reticulate dyspigmentation with nail dystrophy in adolescence. Up to 93% of patients develop cytopenias. Patients have an increased risk of hypoplastic myelodysplasia [176] and acute myeloid leukaemia [177].

Table 149.7 Rare syndromes associated with haematological malignancies and skin signs [166,167].

Condition	Skin signs	Other clinical features	Associated haematological neoplasias	Genetic inheritance and defect
Bloom syndrome (Chapter 77)	Ultraviolet hypersensitivity, skin redness and maculopapular rash in sun-exposed areas, café-au-lait macules, pigmentary abnormalities	Cranio-facial dysmorphism, low birth weight, retarded growth, 50% risk for cancer	15% risk for leukaemia (myelodysplastic syndrome, AML, ALL); 15% risk for lymphoma	Autosomal recessive. BLM gene encoding helicase
Nijmegen breakage syndrome (Chapter 80)	Café-au-lait macules	Microcephaly, prominent midface, recurrent infections, marrow failure	30% risk for lymphoma; 5% risk for leukaemia	Autosomal recessive NBS1 gene
Ataxia telangiectasia (Chapter 76)	Café-au-lait macules, mucocutaneous telangiectasia, poikiloderma, premature canities (hair greying) and skin ageing	Cerebellar degeneration, immunodeficiency, hypogonadism, insulin resistance, predisposition to cancer (35% incidence by the age of 20 years)	High risks of leukaemia and non-Hodgkin lymphoma	Autosomal recessive ATM gene
Fanconi anaemia (Chapter 76)	Pigmentary changes and café-au-lait macules	Short stature, eye malformations, deafness, malformations of the heart, uro-genital system and central nervous system, haematopoietic abnormalities	25% cumulative risk of haematological malignancy by age 45 years (A<L, myelodysplastic syndrome)	Autosomal recessive (FANC genes: A, D1, D2, E, F, G, I, J, L, M, N, RAD51C) or X-linked (FANCB)
Neurofibromatosis type 1 (Chapter 78)	Neurofibromas, café-au-lait macules, axillary freckling	Scoliosis, epilepsy, glial tumours, learning disabilities, ocular hamartomas	Juvenile myelomonocytic leukaemia	Autosomal dominant (acquired mutation in 50% of cases) NF-1 gene
Legius syndrome (Chapter 78)	Axillary and inguinal freckling, café-au-lait macules, neurofibromas, schwannomas	Brain tumours	Juvenile myelomonocytic leukaemia	Autosomal dominant SPRED1 gene
Clericuzio-type poikiloderma with neutropenia (Chapter 75)	Widespread poikiloderma, acral hyperkeratosis, nail dystrophy, skin ulceration	Short stature, mid-facial hypoplasia, osteopenia, hypergonadotropic hypgonadism	Myelodysplasia and AML	Autosomal recessive USB1 loss-of-function mutations
GATA2 deficiency syndrome	Lymphoedema, recalcitrant viral warts	Autoimmune diatheses, pulmonary alveolar proteinosis	Monocytopenias precede myelodysplasia, AML (familial) or CMML	Autosomal dominant GATA2 gene mutation with haploinsufficiency
Dyskeratosis congenita	Reticulate dyspigmentation, skin atrophy, subtle poikiloderma, leukoplakia, nail dystrophy	Pulmonary fibrosis	Hypocellular myelodysplasia and AML	Autosomal dominant (TERC, TERT mutations), autosomal recessive (NOP10, NHP2) or X-linked (DKC1) inheritance, or sporadic mutations that cause telomere instability

AML, acute myeloid leukaemia; ALL, acute lymphoblastic leukaemia; CMML, chronic myelomonocytic leukaemia

Ataxia-pancytopenia syndrome

This novel syndrome is caused by germline mutations in *SAMD9* and *SAMD9L* genes located in tandem on chromosome 7. Partial loss of chromosome 7 also leads to a tendency to myelodysplasia [178]. Intractable pruritus is noted in some patients [179].

ANAEMIAS AND HAEMOGLOBINOPATHIES

Nutritional anaemias

Anaemia (decreased haemoglobin compared with an age-matched control) can be the result of a deficiency of iron (microcytic), vitamin B_{12} or folate (macrocytic). Vigilance for nutritional anaemia is warranted in patients who follow a vegan or vegetarian diet [180]. It causes pallor of the skin and mucosae. It is caused by peripheral vasoconstriction in response to reduced oxygen supply to the skin. Palmar pallor is particularly useful for recognising anaemia in children <5 years of age at a primary care level [181,182]. Pallor of the palmar creases is visible at haemoglobin levels below 70 g/L. Pruritus is reported in 15% of females and 5% of males with iron deficiency anaemia [183]. Glossitis and ulcerative stomatitis are associated with megaloblastic anaemia and vitamin B_{12} deficiency [181,184]. The prevalence of oral mucosal symptoms in megaloblastic anaemia is as high as 65% [181]. Glossitis and ulcerative stomatitis are not linked to other types of anaemia, but oral candidosis is more prevalent in iron deficiency anaemia [185].

Fingernail abnormalities such as trachyonychia and koilonychia have been traditionally linked to iron deficiency anaemia [181].

Haemoglobinopathies

Sickle cell anaemia and thalassaemias are associated with skin ulceration in approximately 5–10% of patients [186]. Skin ulcers resemble venous ulcers and are characteristically localised in the

Table 149.8 Transfusion reactions with skin involvement

Reaction	Skin lesions
Acute allergic reaction	Rare. Urticaria, angio-oedema and redness which occur during or immediately after transfusion
Transfusion-associated graft-versus-host disease	Redness, maculopapular rash 2–30 days after transfusion
Post-transfusion purpura	Thrombocytopenic purpura within 2 weeks after transfusion

gaiter area of the lower extremities [187]. The pathogenesis of ulceration is probably microvascular obstruction and hypoxia by abnormal erythrocytes, which are dehydrated, dense and inelastic. Treatment with compression therapy and biomaterial dressings containing the arginine–glycine–aspartate (RGD) peptide seem to be effective [187,188].

TRANSFUSION REACTIONS

Transfusion reactions with skin manifestations are very rare and fall into one of the following classes: acute allergic reactions, transfusion-associated graft-versus-host disease (GVHD) and post-transfusion purpura (Table 149.8) [189].

Allergic transfusion reactions

The incidence of allergic reactions to transfused platelets and red blood cells is 3.7% and 0.15%, respectively, and only a minority of those have skin manifestations such as acute urticaria or redness (or variations in skin of colour). Plasma proteins (especially IgA and haptoglobin) are the most frequent allergens and these reactions are more common in patients with IgA deficiency (IgA levels <0.5 mg/L). Haptoglobin deficiency is more prevalent in South-East Asia and may contribute to transfusion reactions in populations from this region. Chemical and food allergens have been reported as causes of allergic transfusion reactions [189]. Examples include methylene blue, used for viral inactivation of fresh plasma, and passive transfer of peanut allergens.

Transfusion-associated graft-versus-host disease

Transfusion-associated GVHD is caused by alloreactive donor leukocytes present in the transfusion product. It presents within 2–30 days after transfusion with a pink to red maculopapular rash, often associated with systemic symptoms such as liver enzyme elevation, jaundice, diarrhoea or vomiting [190,191]. The diagnosis is supported by skin biopsy and human leukocyte antigen (HLA) typing. Prognosis is poor and the condition is often fatal, especially if gastrointestinal GVHD develops. Immunosuppressed patients and the individuals receiving blood products from related donors are at a higher risk. Various methods for eliminating transfusion-associated GVHD have been adopted in different countries including γ-irradiation, X-ray irradiation and leukoreduction of blood products. GVHD is discussed in greater detail in Chapter 38.

Post-transfusion purpura

Post-transfusion purpura is a rare adverse reaction to a transfusion of any platelet-containing product such as packed red blood cells, platelets or granulocyte infusions. It is caused by the production of antibodies to introduced platelet alloantigens, often in a woman previously sensitised by pregnancy [192]. The patient develops antiplatelet antibodies that destroy both the introduced platelets and, surprisingly, their own platelets (the mechanism is unclear) causing sudden-onset thrombocytopenia and thrombocytopenic purpura within 4–11 days after transfusion [193]. Treatment with intravenous immunoglobulin infusions and systemic steroids produces satisfactory responses within 2 months after onset [193,194].

SKIN AND DISORDERS OF THE IMMUNE SYSTEM

SKIN MANIFESTATIONS IN IDIOPATHIC LYMPHADENOPATHIES

This group of diseases comprises four distinct entities: Kikuchi–Fujimoto disease, Kimura disease, the histiocytic disorder Rosai–Dorfman disease (also known as sinus histiocytosis with massive lymphadenopathy) [1] (Chapter 135) and immunoglobulin G4-related disease (IgG4-RD). Castleman disease [2] is not included here as it does not involve the skin directly. The underlying aetiologies of these conditions remain an area of active research. They present with lymphadenopathy clinically mimicking lymphoma or histiocytosis, and are associated with pathologies in other tissues and organs including the skin.

Kikuchi–Fujimoto disease

Also known as Kikuchi disease or Kikuchi histiocytic necrotising lymphadenitis, this is a rare benign condition of unknown cause that is seen predominantly in East Asia. Whilst originally described in young women, the disorder does occur in male and female adults and young children. The clinical course and histological changes suggest a histiocytic and T-cell response to an infectious agent, such as EBV, HIV, mycoplasma [3] and parvovirus [4]. Clinical presentation is often with painful cervical lymphadenopathy, fever and leukocytosis in a previously well patient. Skin involvement

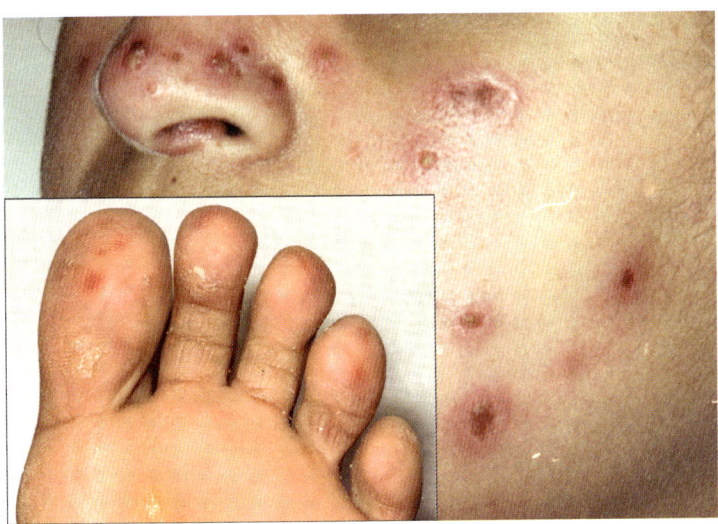

Figure 149.14 Kikuchi–Fujimoto syndrome in a 37-year-old South Asian female patient who presented with a 6-day history of malaise, sweating, pyrexia and painful left-sided cervical lymphadenopathy associated with an eruption of ulcerated papules on the face and macules resembling the Janeway lesions of bacterial endocarditis on the toes (inset).

is present in 25% of patients. The cutaneous manifestations are heterogeneous and include papules, plaques, acneiform lesions or pseudo-targetoid lesions, often localised on the face and upper trunk (Figure 149.14) [5]. The diagnosis is based on an excisional biopsy of an affected lymph node which, depending on the stage of the disease, may reveal proliferative, necrotic or xanthogranulomatous changes [6]. Kikuchi–Fujimoto disease resolves spontaneously within 3–4 months [7]. No effective treatment is established but in patients with severe or refractory symptoms, high-dose corticosteroids with intravenous immunoglobulin have been used [8].

Kimura disease

This is a rare, benign, chronic inflammatory condition seen predominantly in younger males of East Asian descent. There is a 3–6-fold male preponderance with a median age at onset of 32 years [9]. The classic clinical presentation is with bilateral, cervical lymphadenopathy, occasionally with fever, accompanied by peripheral blood eosinophilia and elevated IgE. Skin involvement is common and ranges from specific infiltration with characteristic histology and presenting as subcutaneous masses, particularly around the head and neck, to a variety of non-specific manifestations including itch, urticaria and chronic eczema. Other sites of involvement are the orbit, oral cavity and nasal sinuses. Kidney involvement has prognostic significance since 12–16% of patients with Kimura disease develop nephrotic syndrome [10].

Histologically, Kimura disease usually displays an inflammatory infiltrate with eosinophils and follicular hyperplasia, fibrosis and arborising vascular proliferation of the postcapillary venules. The most important differential diagnoses are other diseases with eosinophilic infiltrates including parasitic infections, drug reactions, angiolymphoid hyperplasia with eosinophilia, Castleman disease and eosinophilic granulomatosis with polyangiitis (Churg–Strauss syndrome).

Kimura disease has a chronic and relapsing course. There is no effective treatment but the available options are localised radiotherapy (20–45 Gy), local excision of affected tissues, corticosteroid therapy, ciclosporin and low-dose imatinib mesylate [11].

Rosai–Dorfman disease

This rare non-Langerhans histiocytic disorder is also known as Rosai–Dorfman–Destombes disease or sinus histiocytosis with massive lymphadenopathy. It affects adults and children and is more frequently seen in males (Chapter 135). Rosai–Dorfman disease can be associated with lymphomas including follicular and diffuse large B-cell splenic lymphoma [12,13]. Increasing evidence suggests the disorder is driven by pathogenic mutations in the extracellular signal-regulated kinase (ERK) pathway activating histiocyte proliferation [14–16]. The characteristic clinical presentation is with significant but painless lymphadenopathy (mainly cervical, mediastinal and axillary), fever, anaemia, neutrophilia and polyclonal hypergammaglobulinaemia [11,17]. The skin is a common extranodal site of involvement and skin lesions are observed in approximately 10% of cases [11]. Lesions are brownish plaques, papules and nodules, and may resemble xanthomas; subcutaneous plaques can be studded with cutaneous papules. In some patients, the lesions are deeper and may mimic morphoea or panniculitis. The key to the diagnosis is the histopathological examination of an affected lymph node that shows dilated sinuses containing neutrophils, lymphocytes, plasma cells and large S100+ CD11c+ CD68+ histiocytes [18]. The main differential diagnoses are lymphoma, Kikuchi–Fujimoto disease and the IgG4-RD.

The course is indolent but protracted. The disease may disappear spontaneously. Therapies such as systemic corticosteroids, radiotherapy and thalidomide have each been advocated [18–20] and consensus guidelines for treatment have been established [21].

Immunoglobulin G4-related disease

Immunoglubulin G4-RD is an increasingly recognised fibroinflammatory multiorgan disease affecting predominantly middle-aged and elderly males [22–24]. The pathogenesis is uncertain but an autoimmune basis seems likely and various putative autoantigens have been identified including galectin-3, laminin-111 and annexin-A11 [25]. Further confirmatory studies are, however, required [26]. IgG4 itself does not seem to play a pathogenic role but is likely an epiphenomenon, perhaps involved in the anti-inflammatory disease response [22,27,28]. The disorder has been associated with both Hodgkin and non-Hodgkin lymphoma, as well as other B-cell neoplasms and multiple myeloma [29]. The hallmark is sclerosing, autoimmune pancreatitis, retroperitoneal fibrosis, pituitary inflammation (hypophysitis) [30], lymphadenopathy and elevated IgG4 levels. The skin is involved in less than 50% of cases. Patients present with nodules or plaques in the head and neck region. Histologically, the lesions may resemble pseudolymphoma; however, there is stromal fibrosis with dermal and subcutaneous infiltration by lymphocytes, IgG4-positive plasma cells and eosinophils. Other common sites of involvement are the hepato-biliary tract, the orbit and the lacrimal and salivary glands. Virtually any organ including the central nervous system may be affected.

The major differential diagnosis is multicentric Castleman disease, which has an abrupt onset and systemic symptoms with a high mortality rate. IgG4 serum and tissue levels may also be elevated in multicentric Castleman disease (which does not itself affect the skin) [31]. The other differential diagnosis is cutaneous Rosai–Dorfman disease where there may also be an increased proportion of IgG4-positive cells in the dermal infiltrate. IgG4-RD can mimic systemic lupus erythematosus and Sjögren disease. The mainstay of treatment for IgG4-RD is corticosteroid therapy with rituximab to induce remission [32].

SKIN MANIFESTATIONS IN PRIMARY IMMUNODEFICIENCIES

Primary immunodeficiencies are a heterogeneous group of disorders caused by mutations in the genes encoding functional proteins of the immune cells. They are discussed in detail in Chapter 80. The skin is very often involved with, most commonly, recalcitrant, relapsing bacterial or fungal infections. These infections respond poorly to antibiotics and antifungals and have a tendency to recur. Skin infections are accompanied by infections in other organs. Multiple episodes of otitis media, pneumonia, deep abscesses or other recurring serious infections are considered warning signs that may portend a primary immunodeficiency (Box 149.1).

> **Box 149.1 Warning signs heralding primary immunodeficiency**
>
> **Infectious signs**
> - Infections with atypical or opportunistic organisms, recurrent or persistent infection
> - >6 episodes of otitis media per year
> - Resistance to antibiotics (no effect after >2 months of antibiotic treatment)
> - >2 episodes of pneumonia over a year
> - Deep infections and abscesses
>
> **Other signs**
> - Family history of primary immunodeficiency
> - Diarrhoea
> - Failure to thrive
>
> Reproduced from Sillevis Smitt *et al.* 2005 [33].

The most common cutaneous infections in immunodeficient patients are caused by *Candida, Staphylococcus aureus, Molluscum contagiosum* and human papillomavirus (HPV) (Table 149.9).

Table 149.9 Skin diseases and symptoms accompanying primary immunodeficiencies.

Infection/disorder	Symptoms
Fungal infections	*Candida*: oral candidosis, mucocutaneous candidosis, *Candida* paronychia, granulomatous candidosis
	Other: disseminated dermatophytosis, aspergillosis, blastomycosis, coccidioidomycosis, cryptococcosis, histoplasmosis, paracoccidioidomycosis, mucormycosis, sporotrichosis
Bacterial infections	*Staphylococcus aureus*: impetigo, persistent folliculitis, furunculosis, cellulitis
	Ecthyma gangrenosum (*Pseudomonas*), streptococcal cellulitis and deep cutaneous infections, atypical cellulitis (*Helicobacter* spp., *Campylobacter* spp., *Haemophilus influenzae*)
	Atypical mycobacterial infections, disseminated *Mycobacterium marinum*, extensive Bacillus Calmette–Guérin (BCG) reaction
Viral infections	Molluscum contagiosum, severe infections with varicella-zoster virus (and other herpes viruses), human papillomavirus (extensive warts)
Eczema	Dermatitis resembling atopic eczema
	Erythrodermic dermatitis
Vasculitis	Small-vessel vasculitis resembling IgA (Henoch–Schönlein) vasculitis
Autoimmune conditions	Systemic lupus erythematosus-like disease
	Vitiligo

Mucocutaneous candidosis

Chronic mucocutaneous candidosis is the most typical and common phenotype but recalcitrant candidosis may also provide an important clue to the presence of other forms of immunodeficiency (Figure 149.15). Cutaneous *Candida* species infections are a very sensitive sign of T-cell deficiencies, in particular those affecting Th17 and Th22 cells. Thus, any global T-cell deficiency disorder, such as Di George syndrome, Omenn syndrome or severe combined immunodeficiency is associated with chronic or recurrent candidosis.

In the autosomal dominant form of hyper-IgE syndrome, in which 80% of patients have mucocutaneous candidosis, Th17 cells are suppressed. The cause of hyper-IgE syndrome is a mutation of the transcription factor STAT3. In a physiological situation, STAT3 mediates the expression of RORγt, which in turn causes Th17 cell differentiation. In hyper-IgE syndrome, this differentiation pathway is impaired. These patients have low numbers of circulating Th17 cells (CD4+ CCR6+) and have reduced levels of antimicrobial proteins, such as β-defensin 2 and histatins, the expression of which is stimulated by IL-17 [34].

Deficiency of mannan-binding lectin (MBL) has been linked to recurrent vaginal candidosis but whether it is also connected to skin candidosis has not been shown conclusively [35].

Non-syndromic mucocutaneous candidosis may be caused by mutations in the genes coding for IL-17 receptor or in the genes coding the pattern recognition receptors capturing *Candida* antigens, such as dectin-1 and CARD9 (Table 149.10). Another interesting mechanism is the gain-of-function STAT1 mutations that cause

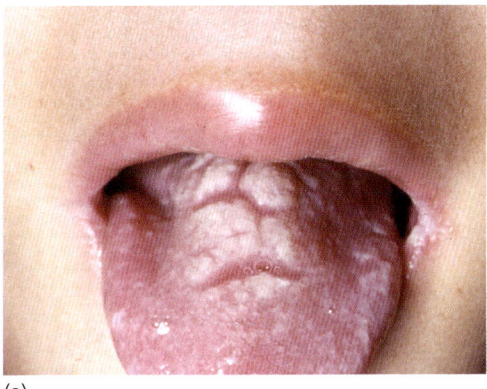
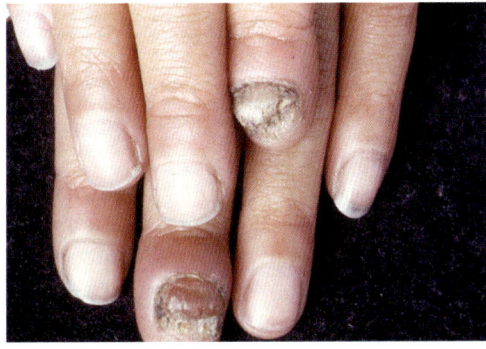
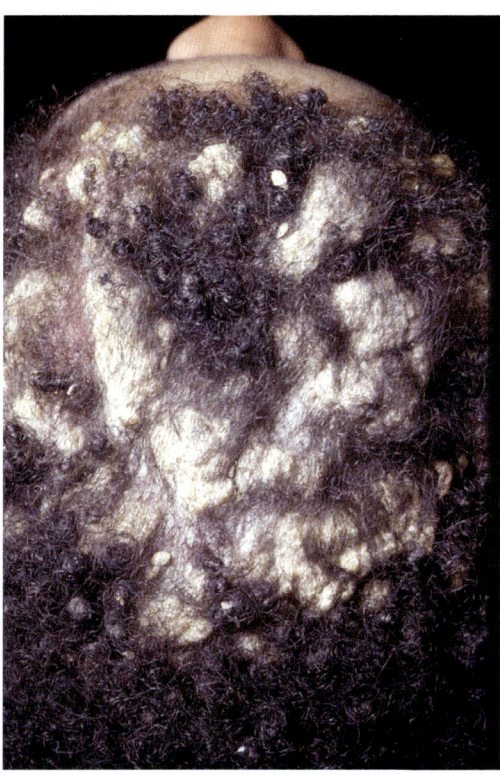

Figure 149.15 Chronic mucocutaneous candidosis in a 6-year-old boy with involvement of (a) the tongue and (b) the fingernails, and (c) severe hyperkeratosis of the scalp.

enhanced responses to Th17 suppressors (interferon γ (IFN-γ), IL-27 and IFN-α) with a consequent decrease in Th17 [36,37].

Bacterial infections

Pyogenic skin infections are common in immunodeficiencies. Recalcitrant *Staphylococcal* impetigo, folliculitis and abscesses are the most common manifestations. Bacterial infections are a sensitive marker of immunodeficiencies of the innate immune system targeting granulocytes and cytotoxic T cells (Chediak–Higashi syndrome, Hermansky–Pudlak syndrome, Griscelli syndrome, Wiskott–Aldrich syndrome, chronic granulomatous disease or cyclic haematopoiesis).

Mycobacterial infections are associated with impaired cellular immunity, in particular that mediated by IL-12 and interferons. IL-12 receptor mutations and IFN-γγ receptor are strongly associated with atypical mycobacterial skin infections, including *Mycobacterium ulcerans*, *M. avium* and *M. marinum* [38].

Persistent human papillomavirus infections

Persistent viral warts are associated with suppressed T-cell responses. Examples are congenital CD4 deficiency and the WHIM syndrome (warts, hypogammaglobulinaemia, infections and myelokathexis (congenital deficiency of white blood cells leading to chronic leukopenia and neutropenia)) where persistent viral

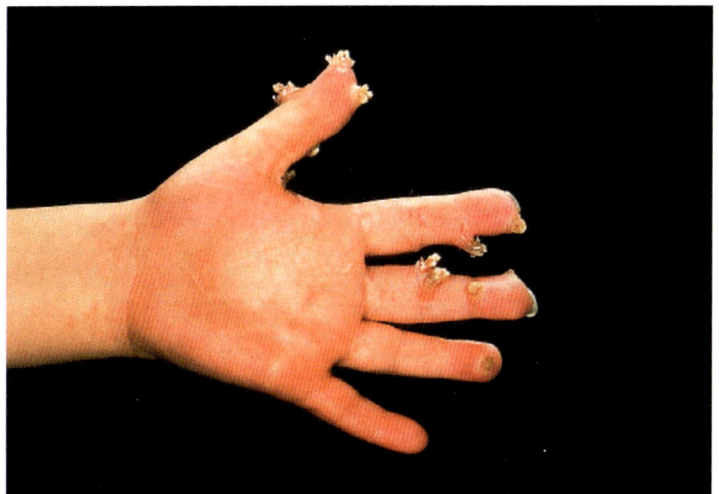

Figure 149.16 Unusually large and rapidly proliferating viral warts in a child with CD4 deficiency.

warts are the dominating symptom (Figure 149.16). Haematopoietic stem cell transplantation can be an effective treatment for this syndrome [39].

Other skin conditions associated with immunodeficiencies

Eczematous skin conditions accompany some immunodeficiencies, in particular hyper-IgE syndrome, Omenn syndrome,

Table 149.10 Immunodeficiencies caused by mutations in cytokines and signalling proteins.

Target protein (and reference)	Symptoms	Remarks
IL-17 receptor deficiency [37,55]	Mucocutaneous candidosis Staphylococcal folliculitis and abscesses	Mutation of IL-17R and abolition of the responses to IL-17A and IL-17F
Dectin-1 deficiency [56]	Mucocutaneous candidosis	Stop codon mutation in the pattern recognition receptor dectin-1, which recognises *Candida* antigens. Reduced production of IL-17, TNF-α and IL-6 in response to *Candida*
CARD9 [57,58]	Mucocutaneous candidosis	CARD9 mediates dectin-1 signalling and the disease is a phenocopy of dectin-1 deficiency
IFN-γ receptor 1 deficiency [59]	Mycobacterial skin granulomas (*M. bovis*, *M. avium intracellulare*, *M. fortuitum*, *M. ulcerans*) Lymphoedema	Mutations in IFN-γR1
IL-12p40 and IL-12 receptor β1 deficiencies [47]	Mycobacterial infections including the skin Mucocutaneous candidosis (25% patients) Salmonellosis	
STAT1 gain of function [36,60,61]	Mucocutaneous candidosis, staphylococcal infections, susceptibility to viral infections	Inhibition of Th17 cells due to enhanced STAT1-dependent cellular responses to Th17 repressors (IFN-γ, IL-27 and IFN-α)

IL, interleukin; IFN, interferon; TNF, tumour necrosis factor.

Wiskott–Aldrich syndrome, common variable immunodeficiency, selective IgA deficiency and X-linked agammaglobulinaemia (Table 149.11). Erythrodermic eczema in a child may be caused by a primary immunodeficiency in up to 30% of cases [40] and is a constant feature of Omenn syndrome.

Vasculitis associated with primary immunodeficiencies is often of small-vessel type and presents as purpura resembling Henoch–Schönlein disease (IgA vasculitis). It is most typically a feature of Wiskott–Aldrich syndrome.

Paradoxically, autoimmune diseases are overrepresented in people with immunodeficiency disorders. Systemic lupus erythematosus is associated with hyper-IgE syndrome and chronic granulomatous disease.

SKIN MANIFESTATIONS IN ACQUIRED IMMUNODEFICIENCIES

Human immunodeficiency virus infection, diabetes, cancer and iatrogenic immunosuppression are the leading causes of acquired immunodeficiency in adults, and their dermatological manifestations have been described in detail (Chapters 31, 62 and 147). Immunodeficiency may also develop in an adult due to the antibodies against cytokines and their receptors (Table 149.12). The clinical symptoms are similar to those seen in children with genetic errors in cytokine receptor genes (Table 149.11). Patients with thymoma may occasionally develop antibodies against the IL-12 p35 and p40 subunits, type I interferons and, more rarely, against IL-1α, IL-17A and IL-22 [41]. In 5–10% of patients with thymoma, the immunodeficiency is syndromic (Good syndrome) comprising hypogammaglobulinaemia and variable lymphopenia [42]. The clinical picture is more severe than in those with anticytokine antibodies alone and resembles X-linked agammaglobulinaemia and common variable immune deficiency. Mucocutaneous candidosis is a prominent feature of this condition [42].

Anti-IL-17A, anti-IL-17F or anti-IL-22 autoantibodies in patients with mucocutaneous candidosis may also develop in the setting of the APECED (autoimmune polyendocrinopathy, candidosis and ectodermal dystrophy) syndrome [43–45].

Finally, different anticytokine antibodies have been observed in immunodeficient patients [43]. Reported cases include antigranulocyte–macrophage CSF (anti-GM-CSF), IFN-γ [46], anti-IL-17 [45], IL-22 [43] and anti-IL-6 [47]. Naturally occurring anti-IFN-γ autoantibodies are associated with cutaneous mycobacterial infections and coccidioidomycosis [48,49], as could be predicted from the paediatric phenotypes of genetic immunodeficiencies. Anti-IL-6 autoantibodies have been linked to *Staphylococcal* cellulitis and subcutaneous abscesses. Emerging pathogens such as the multidrug resistant Gram-negative bacterium *Stenotrophomonas maltophilia* should be considered in atypical or subcutaneous soft tissue infection [50]. An incisional skin biopsy for bacterial and mycology cultures may be helpful. Serum procalcitonin can be a useful serum maker to delineate bacterial infection from other causes of febrile neutropenia in the immunocompromised [51].

Fungal infections such as *Mucor* mycosis, causing a necrotic sinusitis or paranasal cellulitis, and *Fusarium* causing ecthyma gangrenosum lesions [52] that can be mistaken for pseudomonal ecthyma, or periorbital cellulitis should be borne in mind in the immunocompromised patient. Serum fungal markers such as beta-D glucan can be helpful in diagnosis [53].

Refractory or multi-dermatomal varicella-zoster infection can be seen with iatrogenic immunosuppression. Aciclovir-resistant herpes simplex virus (HSV), which may be haemorrhagic or vegetative, can be seen in up to 17% of stem cell transplant patients; therapy with foscarnet is often required (Figure 149.17) [54].

Acknowledgement

We thank Professor Robert Gniadecki, who wrote this chapter for the 9th edition of this volume.

Table 149.11 Skin manifestations of primary immunodeficiency syndromes.

Syndrome	Skin manifestations	Other symptoms	Pathogenesis
Chediak–Higashi syndrome	Hypopigmented skin, silvery hair (partial albinism) Pyogenic and fungal infections	Neuropathy Neutropenia	Mutations in the CHS1 gene (also called LYST) causing defective vesicular transport, melanosome and phagolysosome formation and secretion of cytotoxic granules
Hermansky–Pudlak syndrome	Oculo-cutaneous albinism	Platelet coagulopathy, bleeding Pulmonary fibrosis Granulomatous colitis	Autosomal recessive Mutations in genes HPS1-7 play a role in lysosome and melanosome biosynthesis
Griscelli syndrome	Albinism Pyogenic skin infections	Hepatosplenomegaly Neutropenia Thrombocytopenia	Autosomal recessive Mutations in MYO5 (type 1), RAB27A (type 2) and MLPH (type 3) Defective secretion of T-cell cytotoxic granules
Wiskott–Aldrich syndrome	Eczema Recurrent staphylococcal skin infections	Coagulopathy due to thrombocytopenia Leukaemia, lymphoma Reduced IgM levels	X-linked, recessive WAS gene Disorder of actin polymerisation, cytoskeletal rearrangement and immunological synapse disruption
Omenn syndrome	Graft-versus-host-like symptoms Eczematous lesions Hyperkeratosis and desquamation Erythroderma Persistent bacterial skin infections	Diarrhoea Hepatosplenomegaly Leukocytosis Lymphadenopathy Elevated IgE	Autosomal recessive Recombination activated genes RAG1 and RAG2 Dysfunction of B and T cells
DiGeorge syndrome	Mucocutaneous candidosis Cutaneous calcification	Thymic hypoplasia Absence of T cells Congenital heart disease Seizures and hypocalcaemic tetany Facial features (short philtrum, low-set ears, hypertelorism)	22q11.2 deletion syndrome Haploinsufficiency of Tbx1
Hyper-IgE syndrome	Eczematous skin changes Staphylococcal folliculitis and abscesses Mucocutaneous candidosis	Retained primary teeth Characteristic facial features (prominent forehead, deep-set eyes, broad nasal bridge) Scoliosis Increased IgE and eosinophilia	Autosomal dominant (STST3 mutation) Autosomal recessive (DOCK8) Defective cytokine signalling
Chronic granulomatous disease	Pyogenic and fungal skin infections Perioral dermatitis Granulomatous cheilitis	Lymphadenopathy	Variable mutations (X-linked recessive gp91phax, autosomal recessive p47phax) resulting in a defect in neutrophil respiratory burst
Congenital CD4 deficiency	Persistent viral warts	Increased risk of lymphoma (primary effusion lymphoma (PEL), MALT lymphoma, Burkitt lymphoma, diffuse large-cell lymphoma) Low numbers of CD4+ cells (<300 cells/μL) on two or more measurements over at least 6 weeks Less than 20% of T lymphocytes are CD4+	Unknown
WHIM syndrome (warts, hypoimmunoglobulinaemia, infections, myelokathexis)	Multiple, large viral warts Recurrent skin bacterial infections	B-cell dysfunction Neutropenia	CXCR4 gene
Cyclic haematopoiesis	Recurrent aphthous stomatitis Staphylococcal skin infections Periodontitis	Periodic failure of haematopoietic progenitor cells resulting in dramatic oscillations in neutrophil, monocyte, eosinophil, platelet and reticulocyte counts, often in periods of 20 days Fever	Autosomal dominant neutrophil elastase gene ELA2
Common variable immunodeficiency	Recurrent pyogenic skin infections Eczema	Recurring infections in different organs Bronchiectasis and asthma Viral infections, enlarged lymph nodes and spleen Hypogammaglobulinaemia: low levels of IgG, IgA, IgM	Variable aetiology: different mutations in six different types of the disease
X-linked agammaglobulinaemia	Recurrent pyogenic skin infections	Various infections, as in common variable immunodeficiency	X-linked Mutation in Btk kinase Lack of mature B cells and low levels of immunoglobulins

Ig, immunoglobulin; MALT, mucosa-associated lymphoid tissue.

Table 149.12 Acquired immunodeficiencies due to immunosuppressive antibodies.

Condition (and reference)	Antibodies against	Clinical findings
Thymoma [41]	IL-12 (p35 and p40) subunits, type I interferons, IL-1α, IL-17A, IL-22	Mucocutaneous candidosis Mycobacterial infections
Good syndrome [42]	IL-12, IL-22, IL-17A	Cutaneous candidosis Recurrent bacterial and fungal infections Hypogammaglobulinaemia Lymphopenia
APECED syndrome [43–45]	IL-17A, IL-17F or anti-IL-22	Autoimmune polyendocrinopathy Cutaneous candidosis Ectodermal dystrophy (APECED)
Spontaneous appearance of immunosuppressive antibodies [37,43,47,62]	IFN-γ	Mycobacterial infections Coccidioidomycosis
	IL-6	Staphylococcal cellulitis Abscesses
	IL-17, IL-22	Mucocutaneous candidosis Dermatophytosis

APECED, autoimmune polyendocrinopathy, candidosis and ectodermal dystrophy; IFN, interferon; IL, interleukin.

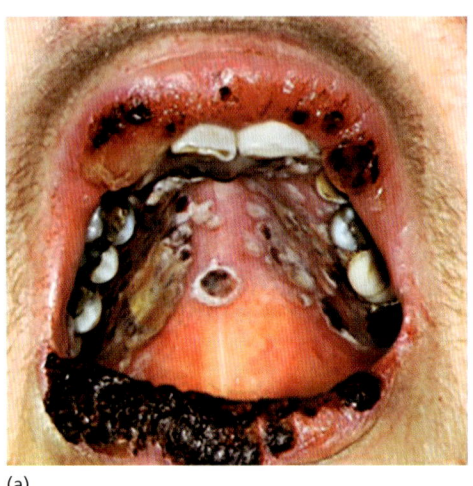 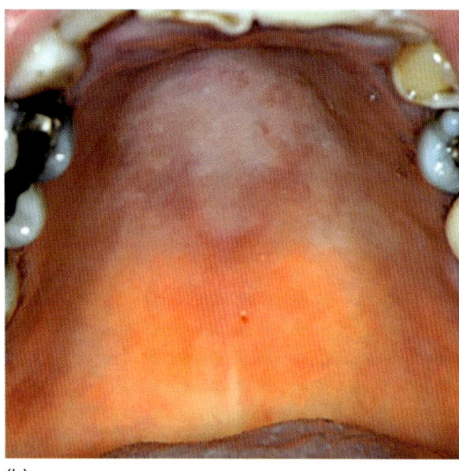

Figure 149.17 (a) Haemorrhagic aciclovir-resistant mucosal herpes simplex virus 1 (HSV1) infection, sparing the soft palate, in the mouth of a patient with myelodysplasia on prophylactic aciclovir. (b) The same patient following intravenous foscarnet therapy.

Key references

The full list of references can be found in the online version at https://www.wiley.com/rooksdermatology10e

Skin disorders caused by infiltration of the skin with neoplastic cells

3 Wagner G, Fenchel K, Back W et al. Leukemia cutis – epidemiology, clinical presentation, and differential diagnoses. *J Dtsch Dermatol Ges* 2012;10:27–36.
15 Cho-Vega JH, Medeiros LJ, Prieto VG, Vega F. Leukemia cutis. *Am J Clin Pathol* 2008;129:130–42.
41 Kulasekararaj AG, Kordasti S, Basu T et al. Chronic relapsing remitting Sweet syndrome – a harbinger of myelodysplastic syndrome. *Br J Haematol* 2015;170:649–56.
45 Fogo A, du Vivier A. The cutaneous manifestations of haematological malignancy. *Clin Med (Lond)* 2009;9:366–70.

58 Alegría-Landa V, Rodríguez-Pinilla SM, Santos-Briz A et al. Clinicopathologic, immunohistochemical, and molecular features of histiocytoid Sweet syndrome. *JAMA Dermatolo* 2017;153:651–9.
65 Beck DB, Ferrada MA, Sikora KA et al. Somatic mutations in UBA1 and severe adult-onset autoinflammatory disease. *N Engl J Med* 2020;383:2628–38.
79 Wesner N, Fenaux P, Jachiet V et al. [Behçet's-like syndrome and other dysimmunitary manifestations related to myelodysplastic syndromes with trisomy 8.] *Rev Med Interne* 2021;42:170–6.
103 Lipsker D. Monoclonal gammopathy of cutaneous significance: review of a relevant concept. *J Eur Acad Dermatol Venereol* 2017;31:45–52.

Skin and disorders of the immune system

11 O'Malley DP, Grimm KE. Reactive lymphadenopathies that mimic lymphoma: entities of unknown etiology. *Semin Diagn Pathol* 2013;30:137–45.
33 Sillevis Smitt JH, Wulffraat NM, Kuijpers TW. The skin in primary immunodeficiency disorders. *Eur J Dermatol* 2005;15:425–32.

CHAPTER 150

The Skin and Endocrine Disorders

Ralf Paus[1,2,3] and Yuval Ramot[4]

[1] Dr Phillip Frost Department of Dermatology & Cutaneous Surgery, University of Miami Miller School of Medicine, Miami, FL, USA
[2] Centre for Dermatology Research, Institute of Inflammation and Repair, University of Manchester, Manchester, UK
[3] Department of Dermatology, University of Münster, Münster, Germany
[4] Department of Dermatology, Hadassah Medical Center and the Faculty of Medicine, Hebrew University of Jerusalem, Jerusalem, Israel

---

Introduction and overview, 150.1
Biological basis of dermatoendocrinology, 150.2
Principles of endocrinology, 150.2
Skin as a (neuro-)endocrine organ, 150.5
Skin as a hormone target, 150.5
Neuroendocrine stress response systems in human skin and the brain–skin axis, 150.8
Human skin and hair research models as discovery tools for general neuroendocrinology, 150.9
(Neuro-)endocrine contributions to cutaneous pathogenesis, 150.9
Basics of clinical dermatoendocrinology, 150.10

How to evaluate a patient for a suspected (neuro-)endocrine disorder, 150.10
Endocrinological considerations in skin therapy, 150.12
Systematic review of clinical dermatoendocrinology, 150.15
Hypopituitarism, 150.15
Hyperpituitarism, 150.16
Adrenal hyperfunction, 150.17
Adrenal insufficiency (Addison disease), 150.18
Hyperandrogenism, 150.18
Hypoandrogenism, 150.18
Hyperoestrogenism, 150.18

Hypo-oestrogenism, 150.18
Phaeochromocytoma, 150.19
Carcinoid, 150.19
Glucagon and glucagonoma, 150.19
Polyendocrine disease, 150.19
Diabetes, 150.19
Hyper- and hypothyroidism, 150.19
Hyperparathyroidism, 150.20
Hypoparathyroidism, 150.20
Future perspectives, 150.21

Key references, 150.21

Introduction and overview

When classic endocrine glands and their systemically secreted products (hormones) were originally recognised, it was quickly realised that excessive or insufficient circulating levels of these hormones could affect the skin. It was much later that the specific receptors for these steroid and peptide hormones were identified and the molecular basis of interactions between hormonal ligands and their receptors was better understood. This is when it was realised that cutaneous responses to endocrine abnormalities reflect the fact that all constituent cell populations of human skin express multiple cognate receptors, not just for these hormones, but also for many other neuromediators. Though the mechanisms involved are still insufficiently understood, the visible effects of abnormal ligand–receptor interactions on the skin provide important diagnostic clues to underlying endocrine disease. However, the importance of hormones in dermatology extends well beyond this.

The field of dermatoendocrinology has undergone a major revolution over the past two decades: human skin and its appendages are recognised not only as prominent hormone target tissues, but also as major endocrine organs themselves. Human scalp hair follicles (HFs) have provided a model for exploring this relatively recent research frontier in investigative dermatology and for identifying 'novel' functions of classic neurohormones, particularly as they represent exquisitely hormone-sensitive mini-organs [1,**2**,**3**,4–6,**7**]. Therefore, where appropriate, HFs will be used as models for illustrating and exploring general principles.

This chapter reviews the key elements of the biological basis of dermatoendocrinology to help clinicians understand how general skin signs and symptoms such as pruritus, skin dryness, hair loss, hypertrichosis, hirsutism, hyperhidrosis and/or hyperpigmentation result from defined endocrine disorders. Also discussed are the characteristic skin manifestations of underlying endocrine disease and a practical approach to skin patients with suspected underlying hormonal problems, with special emphasis on thyroid and pituitary disorders and mention of dermatologically relevant drugs which may cause endocrine abnormalities that affect the skin. Diabetes (Chapter 62) and hormonally active vitamins (hyper- or hypovitaminosis A or D) (Chapter 61) are discussed elsewhere.

This chapter concludes by examining why the skin operating as a complex (neuro-)endocrine organ has important practical implications for future dermatological therapy: the clinical significance and biomedical fascination of dermatoendocrinology extends beyond providing diagnostic clues to the identification of underlying endocrine disease.

Rook's Textbook of Dermatology, Tenth Edition. Edited by Christopher Griffiths, Jonathan Barker, Tanya Bleiker, Walayat Hussain and Rosalind Simpson.
© 2024 John Wiley & Sons Ltd. Published 2024 by John Wiley & Sons Ltd.

Biological basis of dermatoendocrinology

Principles of endocrinology

Enshrined as a concept by Bayliss and Starling's famous Croonian Lecture [8], 'hormones' have generally come to be understood as relatively stable secreted molecules that are released into the bloodstream to reach and modulate the function of distant tissue targets. This 'endocrine' secretory activity is distinguished from 'paracrine' hormone secretion that targets adjacent cells, 'autocrine' signalling which describes the autostimulation of a cell with a hormone released by that cell itself and 'intracrine' signalling whereby the hormone in question does not leave the cell that has produced it and therefore acts intracellularly [9].

Classic endocrine signalling operates along several central axes through which the brain controls key functions of 'professional' endocrine glands. The most familiar of these are the hypothalamopituitary–adrenal (HPA) and the hypothalamopituitary–thyroid (HPT) axes; central nervous system (CNS) controlled signalling axes dominated by prolactin, growth hormone (GH), catecholamines or acetylcholine are also well known (Figure 150.1). If hormone imbalances within these central axes lead to excessive or insufficient serum levels of key hormones, peripheral tissues such as the skin will be affected if they express cognate hormone receptors. Such imbalances can result from a wide range of disorders including hormone-secreting tumours, autoimmune attack, biochemical abnormalities, environmental or nutritional signals, drugs, psychological and emotional stress, or the physiological consequences of puberty, menopause or ageing on systemic hormone levels.

The term endocrine was originally coined to distinguish the control of organ function by secreted hormones from those exerted more directly by the nervous system. With increased knowledge, however, the borders between endocrinology, neuroendocrinology, neuropharmacology and other neuroscience disciplines have become indistinct. Hormones can act both locally and at distant body sites as well as on the nervous system, and the distribution of high-affinity hormone receptors is far more widespread than previously thought. Unsurprisingly, all hormones and neuromediators exert many more biological activities than had been apparent during the early years following their discovery. For example, classic steroid hormones generated outside the CNS or administered therapeutically exert profound neurochemical effects in the brain, while classic neurohormones, neuropeptides and neurotransmitters have an impact not only on the growth, regeneration and other

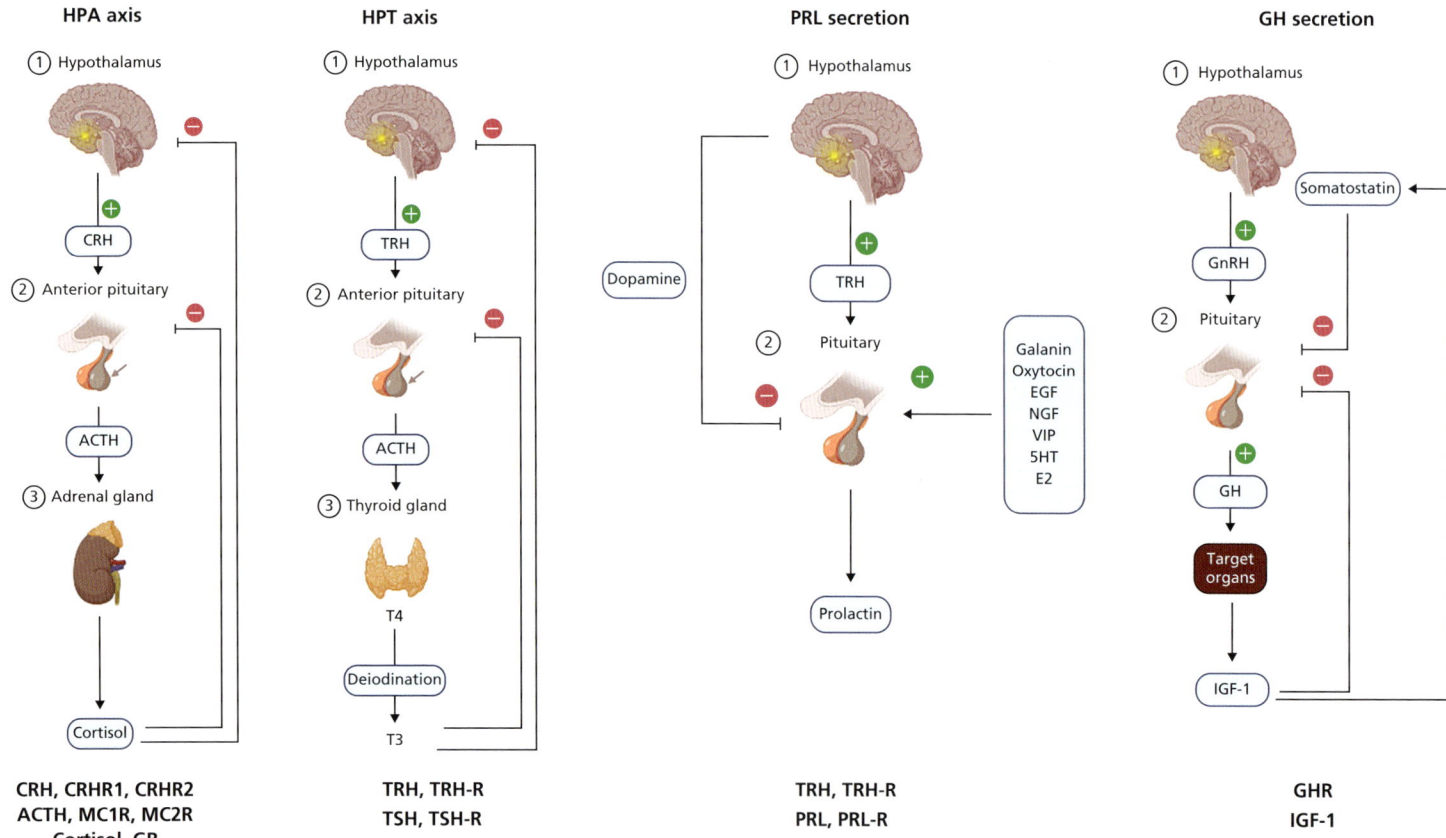

Figure 150.1 Schematic representation of four hypothalamopituitary axes that have a role in the skin: the hypothalamic–pituitary–adrenal, hypothalamic–pituitary–thyroid, prolactin, and growth hormone axes. ACTH, adrenocorticotropic hormone; CRH, corticotropin-releasing hormone; CRHR, corticotropin-releasing hormone receptor; E2, oestrogen; EGF, epidermal growth factor; FGF, fibroblast growth factor; GH, growth hormone; GR, glucocorticoid receptor; 5-HT, 5-hydroxytryptamine; HPA, hypothalamic–pituitary–adrenal; HPT, hypothalamic–pituitary–thyroid; IGF-1, insulin-like growth factor 1; MCR, melanocortin receptor; NGF, nerve growth factor; PRL, prolactin; PRLR, prolactin receptor; TRH, thyrotropin-releasing hormone; TRH-R, thyrotropin-releasing hormone receptor; TSH, thyroid-stimulating hormone; TSH-R, thyroid-stimulating hormone receptor; VIP, vasoactive intestinal polypeptide. Reproduced from [3] with permission from Elsevier.

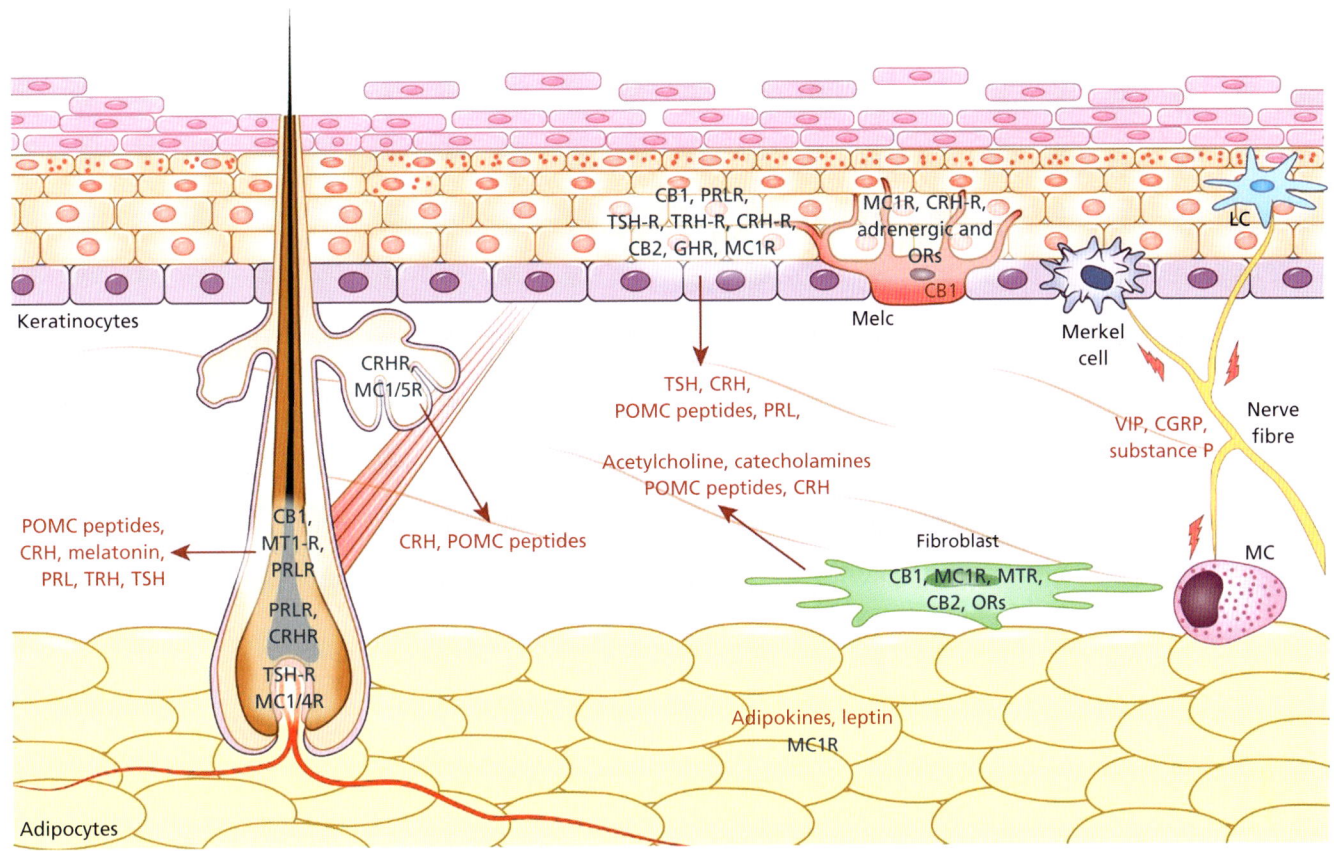

Figure 150.2 Human skin and the hair follicle (HF) as a (neuro-)endocrine microcosm. The HF, sebaceous gland and each layer of the skin (epidermis, dermis and hypodermis) secrete and react to many neuroendocrine mediators. This forms a complex neuroendocrine activity, complete with positive and negative feedback loops. All this activity occurs alongside and often within the same tissue compartments, as does the metabolism and/or synthesis of steroid hormones such as retinoids, androgens, oestrogens, progesterones and vitamin D derivatives. These hormones modulate the synthesis of numerous other signalling molecules such as cytokines, growth factors, leukotrienes and antimicrobial peptides, and in turn are modulated by additional signals received from the HF's vasculature and innervation. Specifically, the HF is a prominent source and target of neurohormones (2). All of them are secreted from the HF epithelium, namely the outer root sheath (ORS), where also their receptors are located. Just as is seen in the interactions between the hypothalamus, the pituitary and the adrenal glands, the ORS produces and secretes CRH, which stimulates ACTH production and thereby local cortisol synthesis; cortisol in turn down-regulates intrafollicular CRH production. Thus it remains one of the great enigmas of skin biology how all this signalling activity is coordinated and controlled within a tiny mini-organ. α-MSH, α-Melanocyte-stimulating hormone; ACTH, adrenocorticotropic hormone; CB1 and CB2, cannabinoid receptors 1 and 2; CGRP, calcitonin gene-related peptide; CRH, corticotropin-releasing hormone; CRHR, corticotropin-releasing hormone receptor; GHR, growth hormone receptor; LC, Langerhans cell; MC, mast cell; MelC, melanocyte; MT-1, melatonin 1 receptor; OR, opioid receptor; PRL, prolactin; PRLR, prolactin receptor; TSH, thyroid-stimulating hormone; TSH-R, thyroid-stimulating hormone receptor; TRH, thyrotropin-releasing hormone; TRH-R, thyrotropin-releasing hormone receptor; VIP, vasoactive intestinal polypeptide. Reproduced from [3] with permission from Elsevier.

specific functions of epithelial and mesenchymal tissues but are also produced by them. Essentially, all tissues and organs, including human skin and its appendages, can generate a wide range of hormones and neuromediators.

Human epidermal and HF keratinocytes, sebocytes and subcutaneous adipocytes are recognised as potent sources of steroid and peptide hormones as well as of a steadily growing list of neuromediators (Figure 150.2, Table 150.1 and see later) [3,7]. *In situ*, many of these were first discovered in human scalp HFs [2].

Current evidence suggests that inflammation, oxidative and psycho-emotional stress, UV irradiation, microbiomal signals, certain nutritional and sensory stimuli and some drugs can influence intracutaneous hormone and neuromediator production, often in a similar though not necessarily identical manner to the regulation of central hormone production [3,4,7,10–23,24,25–27]. Thus, endocrine organs, the CNS, the peripheral nervous system and peripheral tissues such as the skin share and generate a comparable spectrum of hormonal and neuromediator ligands and express a very similar repertoire of cognate receptors which together facilitate intersystem communication, even though the subtype and preferred intracellular signal transduction pathways may differ (e.g. between the brain and the skin). Hormones such as prolactin and leptin also exert potent cytokine-like effects in addition to their classic endocrine activities [28–34], while steroid hormones, which regulate the function of multiple non-neuronal cells outside the nervous system, double as profound neuromodulators and neurotransmitters [35].

Key elements of the three major central endocrine signalling axes, i.e. the HPA axis, the HPT axis and the regulatory system of pituitary prolactin release, have been identified in other peripheral tissues together with negative and positive feedback regulatory loops. In conclusion, the traditional distinctions between hormones, neuropeptides, neurotransmitters and cytokines have ceased to be meaningful.

Table 150.1 Key components in the human cutaneous (neuro-)endocrine signalling mechanism. For a comprehensive review and additional relevant ligands and receptors see references [2,3,14,22,23].

Ligand	Intracutaneous receptor	Selected activities	References
Generated within human skin and/or its appendages			
CRH	CRHR1, CRHR2	Stress response coordinator, controls skin HPA axis equivalent and both mast cell activation and local maturation, HF cycling and melanogenesis, inhibits sebocyte proliferation and induces lipid synthesis in sebaceous glands	**7**,22,23,36–38
ACTH	MC2R (MC1R)	Stimulates intracutaneous cortisol synthesis, activates mast cells, controls HF melanogenesis	23,36–38
α-MSH	MC1R	Stimulates pigmentation, maintains HF immune privilege, multiple immune-inhibitory, anti-allergic, tolerogenic and oxidative damage-protective functions, regulates collagen synthesis; possibly also has antimicrobial activities	**7**,37,39–43
β-endorphin	μ-opioid receptor	Key role in itch modulation, mast cell secretagogue, stimulates pigmentation	20,22,37,44–46
Cortisol	GR	Regulates cell metabolism, epidermal barrier function, skin and pilosebaceous immune homeostasis (maintenance of relative immunoinhibition)	**2**,22,23,36,47
Androgens (DHT)	AR	DHT synthesis controlled by 5-α-reductase, AR stimulation of HFs results in either TGF-β or IGF-1 secretion (location dependent); stimulate sebaceous gland	**7**,48–52,**53**,54,55
Oestrogens (17-β-oestradiol)	ER	17-β ER synthesis controlled by aromatase, large sex-dependent differences in response to ER stimulation, promote wound healing; inhibit sebaceous gland	52,56,**57**,58,59
Vitamin D3 and its metabolites	VDR	Pleiotropic effects (e.g. inhibit keratinocyte proliferation, stimulate keratin expression, anti-inflammatory)	46,47,60,61
Retinoids	RAR, RXR	Pleiotropic effects	
PPARγ ligands (small lipids)	PPARγ	Inhibit keratinocyte proliferation and hair growth, but maintain epithelial stem cells; anti-inflammatory; control of mitochondrial energy metabolism in the HF; promote melanogenesis; regulation of sebaceous gland function	62–67,**68**,69
Endocannabinoids (e.g. anandamide, 2-AG)	CB1, CB2	CB1 stimulation inhibits hair growth and excessive mast cell degranulation/maturation, but stimulates sebogenesis; controls barrier integrity, possesses anti-inflammatory effects, and controls keratin expression and mitochondrial function; CB1 signalling is required for stem cell survival	70–77
Catecholamines (also derived from intracutaneous nerve fibres)	α-/β-adrenergic receptors	Regulate skin perfusion and sweating; inhibit mast cell degranulation, retard keratinocyte migration and wound healing; regulate melanocyte functions	78–87
Acetylcholine receptor ligands (also derived from intracutaneous nerve fibres)	Nicotinic and muscarinic acetylcholine receptors	Regulate keratinocyte proliferation, differentiation, migration, adhesion and apoptosis; activate/attract neutrophils; stimulate sweating; regulate sebocyte lipid production	79,88–92
Melatonin	MT-1, MT-2	Oxidative damage control, DNA damage repair, immunoregulatory effects, collagen production regulation, protection of HF immune privilege and melanogenesis	**1**,**24**,93–100
TRH	TRH-R	Promotes hair growth and keratinocyte mitochondrial function, stimulates HF pigmentation; regulates keratin expression; stimulates epidermal TSH expression; regulates intracutaneous prolactin expression	4,101–106
TSH	TSH-R	Stimulates keratinocyte mitochondrial activity and biogenesis; regulates keratin expression; induces fibroblast proliferation	**2**,105,107–109
Prolactin	PRL-R	Inhibits or promotes hair growth (species- and sex-dependent), stimulates sebum production; immunomodulatory; regulates keratin expression; regulation of cutaneous wound healing; modulation of sebaceous gland function	1,**2**,4,33,34,104,110–112
PTH/PTHrp	PTH/PTHrp receptor	Regulates keratinocyte proliferation and differentiation; modulates hair growth (mice); regulates skin angiogenesis	113–117
Generated (mainly) outside the skin (transported via nerve fibres or blood vessels)			
Substance P	NK1	Activates mast cells; pro-inflammatory; induces collapse of HF immune privilege	16,38,118–121
CGRP	CGRP-R	Anti-inflammatory and tolerogenic; guardian of HF immune privilege	122–124
Dopamine	DR 1	Hair growth inhibitory	125,126
Thyroid hormones (T3, T4)	TRα, TRβ	Regulate keratin expression; prolong anagen; promote wound healing; stimulate keratinocyte mitochondrial activity and heat production; regulate epithelial stem cell functions; promote hair growth and peripheral clock	105,127–130,**131**,132–134

For additional relevant (neuro-)endocrine ligands and their receptors in human skin, see the following references: proenkephalin [135], dynorphin [136], galanin [137], somatostatin [138–140], oxytocin [141], neuropeptide Y [142–144], serotonin [97,145,146], leptin [30,147,148], endovanilloids [148–154], erythropoietin [155–158] and growth hormone (GH) [159,160].

ACTH, adrenocorticotropic hormone; AR, androgen receptor; CB1/2, cannabinoid receptors 1/2; CGRP/CGRP-R, calcitonin gene related protein/CGRP receptor; CRH, corticotropin-releasing hormone (synonym: CRF); CRHR1/R2, CRH receptors 1/2; DR1, dopamine receptor type 1; ER, oestrogen receptor; GR, glucocorticoid receptor; MC1R/2R, melanocortin receptors 1/2; α-MSH, α-melanocyte-stimulating hormone (synonym: melanotropin); MT1/2, melatonin receptors 1/2; NK1, neurokinin receptor 1; PPARγ, peroxisome proliferator activator receptor γ; PRLR, prolactin receptor; PTH, parathyroid hormone; RAR/RORα/RXR, retinoid receptors; TRs, thyroid hormone receptors; TRPV1/3/4, transient receptor potential ion channels of vanilloid type 1/3/4; VDR, vitamin D receptor.

Skin as a (neuro-)endocrine organ

Human skin contains integral functional equivalents of the HPA axis (CRH → ACTH → cortisol) [2,3,22,23,36] and key elements of the HPT axis (TRH→TSH) [2,3,107,109]. In addition, human skin displays complete cholinergic and adrenergic signalling systems [79,83,88–90] with potentially important functions in the control of wound healing [80,81,87,161,162], epidermal immunity [163] and skin cancer [38,164]. Human skin also metabolises numerous hormones and neuromediators, including glucocorticoids, androgens, oestrogens, neuropeptides such as substance P, and lipid neuromediators such as endocannabinoids [2,3,21–23,47,75,76,120,121].

Human skin and its pilosebaceous units and sweat glands also produce a bewildering range of steroid and peptide hormones, ranging from vitamin D, androgens, oestrogens and retinoids to erythropoietin, and classic neurohormones such as corticotrophin-releasing hormone (CRH), thyrotropin-releasing hormone (TRH), thyroid-stimulating hormone (TSH), adrenocorticotrophic hormone (ACTH), α-MSH, β-endorphin and other opioids, melatonin and prolactin, along with multiple other neuromediators. This is complemented by lipid mediators such as endocannabinoids and endovanilloids, which exert neuromediator and many other functions (Tables 150.1 and 150.2) [2,3,7,17,21,22,49,60,77,**165**,166,167]. Intriguingly, human scalp HFs have been shown to be an important component of the neuroendocrine biology of human skin and show prominent expression/production of and/or sensitivity to a surprisingly wide range of neuromediators (Table 150.3), some of which are shown in Figure 150.2.

Human keratinocytes not only express functional adrenergic and cholinergic receptors but also synthesise and metabolise corresponding ligands (catecholamines, acetylcholine). Additionally, the skin displays a complex endocannabinoid and endovanilloid neuroendocrine signalling system, complete with intracutaneously expressed cannabinoid and vanilloid receptors, locally produced (typically lipid-based) ligands and a refined enzymatic machinery for synthesising and degrading the latter. This machinery controls the intracutaneous level of these versatile neuromediators. The list of human skin functions known to be modulated by these systems is growing steadily: to name a few, it currently includes the regulation of keratinocyte and sebocyte proliferation, migration, apoptosis, differentiation, cytokine secretion and lipid production; mast cell differentiation from resident precursors and mast cell degranulation; control of epidermal and/or hair pigmentation; and the modulation of immune responses (Tables 150.1 and 150.2). This list is bound to grow.

These multipurpose neuromediators are complemented by an array of intraepithelially generated classic (neuro-)hormones such as melatonin [1,**24**,93–100,256], the pro-opiomelanocortin (POMC) products, α-MSH, ACTH and β-endorphin [7,23,36–43,46], as well as CRH [7,22,23,36–38], erythropoietin [155–158], neuropeptides released by sensory nerve fibres (mainly substance P, calcitonin gene related peptide (CGRP) and vasoactive intestinal peptide (VIP) [16,38,118–124,257]) and cytokine-like hormones released by skin adipocytes (adipokines, e.g. leptin) [30,147,148], with important differences in the secretory profile of what is now called 'dermal adipose tissue' and adipocytes of the deeper subcutis [258,259]. These neuromediators both exert long-distance effects (e.g. regulation of the hypothalamic controls of feeding behaviour) and regulate skin physiology and repair in a para- and autocrine manner via the stimulation of locally expressed specific receptors.

In addition, human skin and its appendages synthesise opioids and enkephalins, and express corresponding receptors. Apart from the long-recognised role of these neuromediators in the modulation of itch and pain they are now recognised as regulating numerous other aspects of skin biology. Examples of these are listed in Table 150.1, along with corresponding references.

Since Merkel cells engage in substantial neuroendocrine secretory activities [40,143,260,261], their local functions within skin epithelium are likely to extend well beyond their role as mechanosensory cells [260–264].

This complex hormone and neuromediator-based dermatoendocrinological signalling mechanism intimately links specialised (neuro-)endocrine glands, the nervous system and peripheral tissue physiology, and is further complicated by the fact that the same hormones and neuromediators also regulate immune responses. Many of these substances are generated and secreted by immunocytes such as mast cells, T cells and macrophages [265–267]. These immunocytes alter peripheral tissue function in the skin and elsewhere, not only under conditions of infection, inflammation or tumour growth but also 'around the clock', thereby contributing to skin homeostasis [15,16,22,268].

To illustrate this, skin mast cells are highly sensitive to neuroendocrine stimuli (e.g. by CRH, ACTH, endocannabinoids, substance P and catecholamines) and are often in intimate physical contact with sensory nerve fibres that release neuropeptides [12,16,72,118,269–273]. Mast cells regulate T-cell function [274–276], angiogenesis [277–280], connective tissue turnover [281], wound healing [282,283] and hair growth; they also detoxify venoms [284–286]. Thus, the neuroendocrine controls that these key protagonists of innate immunity are subjected to have a profound impact on skin immune responses and other aspects of skin function in health and disease. We can assume that every resident and transient cell found in human skin can respond to different hormones and neuromediators, can generate, secrete and/or metabolise many of these, and can engage in complex endocrinologically and neuroimmunologically relevant signalling interactions with its neighbours. Some of these signals can reach distant organs via the bloodstream or even the CNS by manipulating the firing sequence of action potentials generated by sensory skin nerve fibres.

Skin as a hormone target

Insight into the complexities of the skin's endocrine and neuroendocrine pathways provides the practising dermatologist not only with a better understanding of how hormones exert their therapeutic action but also with assistance in recognising classic endocrine and neuroendocrine diseases that can affect the skin.

The classic signalling scenarios consist in either stimulation of specific cell surface receptors (e.g. by peptide hormones, neuropeptides, neurotransmitters or lipid neuromediators), resulting in rapid cell responses or binding to nuclear hormone receptors, which produce slightly less immediate responses (as seen with all steroid

Table 150.2 Examples of (neuro-)endocrine contributions to cutaneous pathogenesis.

Mediator	Condition	Action	References
Androgens +, Insulin −	Wound healing	Impairment	58,128,168–177
T3/T4 −	Wound healing	Impairment	128,**131**
T3/T4 +	Telogen effluvium	Promotion	50,130,133,134,178,179
Oestrogens +	Melasma	Promotion	180–182
	Chemotherapy-induced alopecia	Promotion of hair regrowth?	183
DHT +	Androgenetic alopecia	Essential for pathogenesis	172,184
	Seborrhoea	Promotion	48,50
	Acne vulgaris	Promotion	185,186
Prolactin +	Psoriasis	Aggravation (see text)	4,187–189
	Psoriatic arthritis		29,187,190–192
	Seborrhoea	Promotion	**7**
	Systemic lupus erythematosus	Aggravation (see text)	193–195
	Female pattern androgenetic alopecia	Aggravation	196,197
Substance P +	Atopic eczema	Triggering/aggravation via induction of neurogenic inflammation	12,198
	Psoriasis		**2**,118,199,200
	Urticaria		201,202
	'Stress'-induced telogen effluvium		154
	Alopecia areata		201,203
	Prurigo nodularis		204,205
	Chronic pruritus		119,206,207
	Rosacea		206,208
Cortisol +	Cushing syndrome	Induction	180
	Acne	Induction, aggravation	180
ACTH +	Hyperpigmentation	Induction	180
	Hypertrichosis		180
α-MSH +	Hyperpigmentation	Induction	180
	Melanoma	Potential suppression of anti-tumour immunity	41
		Autocrine secretion as survival factor for MM cells?	209
		Increased risk after Melanotan® therapy?	210–213,225–227
	Psoriasis	Potential induction of tolerogenic dendritic cells and T-regs	214
	Chemotherapy-induced alopecia	Protective effect?	40
	Melanocytic/dysplastic naevi	Increased growth after Melanotan® or α-MSH therapy	215–217
α-MSH −	Alopecia areata	Insufficient maintenance of hair bulb immune privilege	42,218
	Lichen planopilaris	Insufficient maintenance of bulge immune privilege	219
	Acne vulgaris	α-MSH analogue may be therapeutically beneficial	**7**,220
	Scleroderma	Insufficient α-MSH-mediated signalling and therapeutic effect of α-MSH postulated	221
MC1R variants	Melanoma	Increased risk	222–227
		Antagonising MC1 signalling as antimelanoma strategy?	222
	Vitiligo	Association discussed in text	228–230
CRH +	Atopic eczema	Stress-related triggering/aggravation via induction of neurogenic inflammation (see text)	23,231
	Alopecia areata	Abnormalities in the intrafollicular equivalent of the central HPA stress response-axis	232
	Acne vulgaris	Promotion (see text)	233,234
CGRP +	Atopic eczema	Increased IL-13 secretion (see text)	122
	AIDS	Inhibits HIV transmission from Langerhans to T cells	235
	UV-associated immunosuppression	Mediated by CGRP (mice)	236
	Allergic contact dermatitis	Induction of hapten-specific tolerance (mice)	236,237
GH +	Acromegaly	Induction	238
	Seborrhoea	Promotion	**7**,239
	Melanocytic naevi	Increased growth	240,241
Somatostatin	Merkel cell carcinoma	Growth inhibition by therapy with somatostatin analogue	242,243
	Alopecia areata	Important for HF immune privilege?	138
β-endorphin	Atopic eczema	Increased serum level	244–246
	Psoriasis		247
Bradykinin	Hereditary angio-oedema	Receptor antagonist may be therapeutically beneficial	248,249
β2-adrenergic receptor (BAR)	Atopic eczema	Reduced signalling due to BAR point mutation	85
		Reduced catecholamine synthesis and increased catecholamine degradation in atopic epidermis	84
	Vitiligo, psoriasis	Insufficient BAR signalling (see text)	250
TRPVs	Rosacea	TRPVs overexpressed	251,252
		Can be stimulated by recognised rosacea trigger factors	206
	Pruritus	Stimulation can promote itch	150,153,154,253–255

+, Increased; −, reduced. Abbreviations: see Table 150.1.

Table 150.3 When to suspect a hormonal basis for a skin disease: general signs and symptoms.

Sign/symptom	Underlying (neuro-)endocrine causes
Anaemia	Anaemia caused by insufficient renal production of erythropoietin (tumour anaemia, diabetic nephropathy and other renal diseases)
Body odour (unpleasant)	Acromegaly (due to enlarged apocrine glands)
Dryness	Thyroid dysfunction (mainly hypothyroidism)
Exophthalmus	Hyperthyroidism (Graves disease)
Extremities enlarged (notably fingers and toes, 'spade-like' hands)	Acromegaly
Facial features (overall change)	*Coarse features*: acromegaly (look also for other signs of acromegaly (Tables 150.4 and 150.5) and bone and cartilage abnormalities (e.g. prognathism, frontal bossing, enlarged hands/feet))
	'Moon facies': hypercortisolism (Cushing syndrome)
Hyperhidrosis (Chapter 92)	Hyperthyroidism; acromegaly (enlarged eccrine glands)
Hair, dry/brittle (Chapter 87)	Hypothyroidism
Hair, loss or gain of (effluvium, alopecia, hirsutism, hypertrichosis) (Chapter 87)	Virilising tumour, adrenogenital syndrome, polycystic ovary syndrome
	Insufficient oestrogen serum level
	Hypo- or hyperthyroidism, hyperprolactinaemia
	ACTH-secreting tumour (e.g. pituitary tumour or small cell bronchial carcinoma)
Joints, swollen	Sometimes associated with acromegaly (note thickening of phalangeal joints), hyper- or hypoparathyroidism, hypothyroidism
Libido (loss of) and impotence	Hypopituitarism
Menorrhoea	Hyperprolactinaemia, hypogonadism
Pigmentary abnormalities (Chapter 86)	*Hypo-/hyperpigmentation*: Addison disease, ACTH-secreting tumour, hypopituitarism
	Yellow tint of skin: hypercarotenaemia in association with hypothyroidism or diabetes
	Pallor with yellow tint: hypopituitarism
Pruritus (Chapter 81)	Diabetes, thyroid dysfunction, anaemia due to insufficient erythropoietin production (see later)
Psychological and neuropsychiatric disturbances (Chapter 84)	Hypo- and hyperthyroidism, hypercortisolism
Skin texture thickened	Acromegaly
Skin thinning/atrophy (increased skin vulnerability to minor trauma)	Cushing disease
Weight loss or gain	Thyroid dysfunction, Cushing syndrome
Wound healing impaired	Androgen excess or relative lack of oestrogens
	Diabetes, hypothyroidism, hypercortisolism

hormones) [9,287,288]. While the effects of hormones and other mediators are commonly ascribed to their interaction (or lack of interaction) with cognate intracutaneously expressed receptors, it is unclear how exactly a given hormone or neuromediator induces any of the defined skin phenomena discussed later. Tables 150.1 and 150.2 list examples of important receptors for which there is persuasive either clinical or preclinical evidence of a significant impact on human or mutant mice skin physiology or pathology.

When examining the skin as a hormone target, one needs to consider the many different means by which a given hormone or neuromediator can signal. Some steroid hormones (e.g. glucocorticoids, calcitriols and oestradiol) can exert very rapid and transient signalling effects via cell surface receptors as well as slower responses via classic interaction with hormone response elements in nuclear DNA. In addition, steroid hormones typically show dose-dependent 'promiscuous' effects, because they can also bind to receptors other than their chief signalling partner and can then influence the binding properties of these receptors to their main ligands [9,35]. Such receptor promiscuity and cross-regulation have also been shown to occur with some peptide hormones and lipid-based neuromediators [9,35,287,289].

Many of the biological effects of hormones depend on the extent to which a cell stimulated by a given hormone generates secondary mediators, such as the production of insulin-like growth factor 1 (IGF-1) by insulin and GH (synonym: somatotropin (STH)), or whether the stimulation of an HF with the potent androgen dihydrotestosterone (DHT) results predominantly in the production of hair growth inhibitory growth factors (e.g. TGFβ1, TGFβ2) or the hair growth promoting factor IGF-1 [50]. Thus, to understand the role of GH in human epidermal physiology [290] or of androgens in scalp HF biology [50,291] it will be necessary to separate the direct from the indirect and perhaps clinically even more important growth factor-mediated effects of these hormones.

Another important factor is the extent to which a given target tissue in the skin is capable of transforming a prohormone into active metabolites [292]. This can make a significant difference to the biological outcome of hormone stimulation of a defined skin cell population or structure and has been extensively studied for intracutaneous steroid hormone metabolism. Examples include the conversion of testosterone into the highly active androgen DHT by 5-α-reductase and of androgens into oestrogens as well as vitamin D metabolism [21,60,293–296]. Key examples for intracutaneous neurohormone metabolism are the conversion of POMC by prohormone convertases to either ACTH, α-MSH or β-endorphin [21,22,46]. In addition, ligands produced in the skin (e.g. sex steroids, glucocorticoids, retinoids and β-endorphin) can pass through the blood–brain barrier to the CNS, where they may be further metabolised, producing complex neuropsychological and neuroendocrine responses with potential effects directed back at the skin.

Other ligands can exert additional, receptor-independent effects, such as the direct, intra- and extracellular scavenging of reactive oxygen species by melatonin [1,**24**,98,100], or the modulation of tyrosinase activity by α-MSH [37,292]. Finally, the specific biological activities exerted by most hormones or neuromediators in a given skin territory depend on how quickly they are degraded by local enzymes (e.g. degradation of substance P by neutral endopeptidase and angiotensin-converting enzyme), the activity of which may vary from one specific skin territory to another. All these signalling variations are again influenced by the simultaneous presence of other ligands, co-factors, decoy receptors, binding proteins and the overall cytokine signalling milieu (e.g. whether or not there is inflammation).

There are also sex and/or regional differences in the response of human skin and its appendages to a given hormone or neuromediator. While this has been appreciated for androgens, as for example reflected in the 'paradoxical' response to DHT of beard versus temporofrontal scalp HFs [50,291], it also applies to hormones such as 17-β-oestradiol [**57**,297,298] and prolactin [29,111]. Another example is cutaneous wound healing, which is promoted by oestrogens but inhibited by androgens [106,168,169,171].

This level of (neuro-)endocrine signalling complexity explains why it is often extremely difficult to pinpoint exactly how a given hormone or neuromediator has induced the human skin phenomena we observe. Conversely, it also explains why the same dose of the same agent used in hormonal dermatotherapy (e.g. in the management of acne or psoriasis) can produce such distinct clinical results in different individuals, despite belonging to the same sex and age group and having a comparable medical background. Dermatologists need to be aware of these hidden (neuro-)endocrine dimensions in their daily work.

Additional reasons why dermatoendocrinological considerations are inescapable in routine dermatological practice are as follows:
- Key dermatological symptoms and signs such as pruritus, flushing, redness, eczema and whealing, and complex skin parameters such as skin barrier function, wound healing, hair growth, pigmentation and skin immune status, are influenced by the characteristics of this intracutaneous (neuro-)endocrine signalling mechanism.
- The intraepithelial endocrine and neuroendocrine signalling milieu that is created under physiological circumstances in human epidermis and HFs is probably predominantly immunoinhibitory [**2**,**3**,22,23,47], and this may be a prerequisite for skin homeostasis: evidence suggests that maintenance of this signalling milieu plays a key role in preventing excessive skin inflammation and itch that would otherwise result from the continuous onslaught of environmental stressors. Imbalances in this neuroendocrine signalling system may influence dermatoses where neurogenic skin inflammation plays a significant role and which are known to be triggered or aggravated by environmental stressors (e.g. psoriasis, atopic eczema, alopecia areata (AA), urticaria, pruritus).
- The skin's response to excessive or deficient systemic hormone levels is influenced by underlying systemic and local factors, ranging from UV exposure, humidity, barrier function via inflammation and microbiological colonisation of the skin to a patient's psychoemotional status, medication and concomitant chemical or physical skin trauma. All these factors impact on the endocrine and neuroendocrine signalling concert of human skin.
- Stress-associated neuropeptides such as substance P and CGRP may modulate the composition of the skin microbiome [299,300].
- Ageing is associated with significant changes in systemic hormone levels, particularly in circulating androgens and oestrogens. These changes affect human skin on many more levels than were previously recognised, ranging from changes in overall skin architecture, skin immune responses and cutaneous microbiology via altered skin barrier function, cutaneous drug absorption and metabolism to hormone-dependent effects on hair growth, sebum production and wound healing [37,63,**68**,75,100, 301–306].

Neuroendocrine stress response systems in human skin and the brain–skin axis

The importance of hormones in dermatology is underscored when considering the role of psychoemotional stress as a triggering or aggravating factor in common dermatoses such as psoriasis, atopic eczema, urticaria, nodular prurigo, lichen planopilaris or AA. Solid experimental and clinical data can explain how major neuroendocrine stress mediators such as CRH, ACTH, prolactin and substance P may trigger or aggravate skin disease [1,11,15,16,23,120,154,203,289,307,308]. Stress-induced neurogenic skin inflammation represents the best-defined neuroendocrine explanation for how psychoemotional stress influences dermatoses such as psoriasis, atopic eczema or urticaria [12,15,16, 201,204,309–312].

Pro-inflammatory activities of skin mast cells assume a 'central switchboard' role in neurogenic skin inflammation. Mast cells undergo enhanced degranulation after direct stimulation by increased levels of stress-associated mediators such as CRH, ACTH, nerve growth factor (NGF) and substance P, all of which act as secretagogues for human skin mast cells. The latter are often found in close proximity to sensory nerve fibres and neuropeptide-releasing sensory neurons are stimulated by NGF to synthesise substance P for transport via sensory nerve fibres to the skin, where it can provoke or exacerbate inflammation [15,119,121,154]. Simultaneously, psychoemotional stress can upregulate the intracutaneous generation of stress-response hormones, such as CRH and ACTH [12,16,154,199,203,309,313,314].

Certain stress-associated hormones are an important element of 'foetal programming', a process during which maternal stress impacts on the offspring's stress responses in later life [315–317]. For example, an inverse association between the maternal serum progesterone level and the risk of girls subsequently developing atopic eczema has been described. Since progesterone is thought to operate as an endocrine foeto-maternal 'stress sentinel' and to promote foetal tolerance it is, thus, conceivable that a lowered maternal progesterone level may predispose the foetus to the development of atopic eczema [318].

These interactions along the brain–skin axis [3,**7**,11,15,119,269,313, 319–321] can recruit a cascade of secondary inflammatory events, thus conspiring to trigger or aggravate inflammatory, pruritic and/or hyperproliferative dermatoses. Conversely, most recent neuro-imaging evidence suggests that chronic skin inflammation can exert profound retrograde pro-inflammatory effects on the human brain, for example in patients with psoriasis [322]. This may even negatively affect their cognitive performance [323], although being still controversial [324,325].

Human skin and hair research models as discovery tools for general neuroendocrinology

A (neuro-)endocrinological approach to the investigation of skin disease has already contributed to major translationally relevant progress in general endocrine and neuroendocrinological research, e.g. by organ-culturing intact human skin and scalp HFs and by studying human keratinocyte and sebocyte cell cultures.

Apart from the discovery that the skin and its pilosebaceous units rank among the most endocrinologically active organs of the human body and display regulatory neuroendocrine signalling loops that parallel in complexity those found in the central HPA and HPT axes [2,3,7,19,20,22,23,47,61], this line of research has identified novel neuroendocrine controls of pigmentation [14], e.g. the discovery of β-endorphin as melanotropin [44], and of TRH as a promoter not only of human hair pigmentation [102] but also of human epidermal re-epithelialisation following a wound [106], suggesting that TRH is involved in the control of wound healing.

Human skin and hair research has helped to show that α-MSH exerts multiple anti-inflammatory activities [326] and acts as a powerful immune privilege guardian in human skin [40,43,218,219, 327–329]. Mouse research suggests that α-MSH may also act as a potential antifibrotic neurohormone. This may be of relevance to the pathogenesis of systemic sclerosis [221,330] and studies on human skin *in situ* are awaited to see whether α-MSH might promote the development of tolerogenic dendritic cells and/or regulatory T cells [214]. Preclinical evidence suggests both that α-MSH may exert local antiallergic activity by inhibiting human basophils *in vitro* [39] and that it may promote systems that limit UV-induced oxidative damage [330,331].

Prolactin and thyroid hormones have also been shown to act as stimulators of human HF epithelial stem cells *in situ* [112,127,129]. TRH, TSH, prolactin and the cannabinoid system have all recently surfaced as novel neuroendocrine regulators of keratin gene and protein expression [4,76,332–334].

The systematic dissection of vitamin D metabolism in human skin [60,335,**336**] has also identified a new line of secosteroids with intriguing therapeutic potential [46,47,61,337,338]. The analysis of PPARγ-mediated signalling in human skin has shown that these nuclear hormone receptors and their agonists operate as important 'guardians' of human epithelial (HF) stem cells [63–66,**68**,69,339] and enhance mitochondrial energy metabolism in the HF [67], and as molecular curbs on excessive skin inflammation [63,**68**,340]. PPARγ stimulation may also help to reduce skin ageing induced by photo-oxidative damage [341].

Finally, recent research in healthy organ-cultured human epidermis and HFs has revealed that TRH and TSH act as potent neuroendocrine stimulators of human mitochondrial activity and even mitochondrial biogenesis [103,105,342]. This insight into the neuroendocrine control of mitochondria had been missed by mainstream mitochondrial and neuroendocrinology research, which has traditionally focused on tissues other than skin. Given the central role of mitochondrial dysfunction in ageing and in many degenerative diseases [343–348], this discovery opens up interesting new avenues for clinical research (see later).

These examples demonstrate that the study of skin from a (neuro-)endocrinological perspective promises benefits well beyond the integument. They also show that human skin and pilosebaceous research models provide excellent discovery tools for exploring the full range of physiological activities in which neurohormones and other neuromediators play a part in human biology [2,3,4,7,22]. In this respect, important clues may be drawn from the study of evolutionarily much older vertebrate skin, namely that of frogs, which generates a striking variety and quantity of neurohormones and neuropeptides. An understanding of these may help to reveal evolutionarily conserved but unappreciated functions common to both frog and human skin [106,349,350].

(Neuro-)endocrine contributions to cutaneous pathogenesis

The example of stress-induced neurogenic skin inflammation has already illustrated how neuroendocrine and neuro-immunological mechanisms can contribute to the pathogenesis and course of stress-triggered or aggravated human skin diseases. Table 150.2 lists selected dermatoses for which a neuroendocrine contribution to disease pathogenesis has been postulated. For example, modulation of immune responses by neurohormones, neuropeptides and neurotransmitters may contribute to the development and/or clinical course of psoriasis, atopic eczema, urticaria, pruritus, AA, systemic lupus erythematosus, systemic sclerosis, impaired wound healing and melanoma (Table 150.3).

However, conclusive proof that neuroendocrine mechanisms contribute fundamentally, rather than peripherally, to the primary pathogenesis of the most common human skin diseases such as atopic eczema and psoriasis, as opposed to playing a role in triggering or aggravating them, is still missing. Regrettably, a stringent neuroendocrine approach is rarely adopted when investigating human skin diseases. Mainstream neuroendocrinology research has been slow to recognise and adopt human skin and its appendages as instructive research objects and experimental models.

One notable exception is the long line of research that has shed light on a significant β-adrenergic signalling defect in atopic eczema. Starting from Szentivanyi's β-adrenergic theory of atopy [351], this has arguably come very close to demonstrating primary relevance for the pathogenesis and neuropharmacological management of atopic diseases, including atopic eczema [84,85,352–354]. While the role of β-adrenergic receptors in haemangioma pathogenesis remains ill understood, the therapeutic response seen with β-blocker administration in haemangioma [355,356] serves as an additional encouragement to undertake a systematic re-exploration of the role of catecholamines and their receptors in human skin physiology and pathology [78,82–87,90,161,357–365]. It opens the possibility that adrenergic receptor agonists and antagonists, which have already been used for decades in clinical medicine, may yet find new roles in the management of skin disease.

A second important exception is the melanocortin receptor type 1 (MC1R), the chief receptor for α-MSH, whose loss-of-function polymorphisms (found in red-haired individuals) are associated with a significantly increased risk of developing melanoma [222–225,366–368] (Chapter 142). α-MSH also operates as a powerful immune privilege guardian in human skin [43,218,329]. A relative insufficiency of α-MSH/MC1R-mediated signalling may contribute to the collapse of immune privilege in the anagen hair bulb, a key element in the pathogenesis of AA [43,218,369,370]. Likewise, it has been speculated that insufficient α-MSH/MC1R-mediated signalling at the HF bulge, the repository of follicle stem cells, contributes to the pathogenesis of lichen planopilaris, facilitating the collapse of immune privilege at that site [219].

A third area where endocrine research has contributed to an understanding of skin disease pathogenesis is the study of endogenous or exogenously administered vitamin D and vitamin A derivatives in a wide range of dermatoses. It would not be surprising to find that abnormalities in intracutaneous calcitriol and retinoid synthesis and metabolism have an impact on an individual's susceptibility to skin diseases such as skin cancer, alopecia, impaired wound healing and acne, or on that individual's response to therapy with steroid hormones. The first examples of this new endocrine dimension in dermatology have already emerged [10,60,371–377].

It is in this context of widely underappreciated progress in cutaneous (neuro-)endocrinology that traditional clinical dermatoendocrinology is still unfolding.

Basics of clinical dermatoendocrinology

How to evaluate a patient for a suspected (neuro-)endocrine disorder

Hormones may control general body characteristics such as height, weight, body contour and posture, mood, agility, nervousness, hair phenotype, and food and fluid intake. Being alerted to changes in such general characteristics will help to identify a potential endocrinological dimension in patients presenting with a skin complaint. At the very least, when a patient presents with any of the lead signs or symptoms in Table 150.3, a hormonal basis for the dermatological problem should be considered and systematically confirmed or excluded.

Some characteristic skin signs provide invaluable indicators of specific endocrine diseases (Table 150.4). Additional 'diagnostic pearls' that will greatly help in identifying a potential underlying endocrine pathology are summarised in Table 150.5.

Comparing a patient's current facial appearance with an older photograph can offer rapidly collectable information about changes in overall facial features, as may occur from acromegaly or Cushing disease.

Given the increasing incidence and prevalence of diabetes, it is important to consider this as a factor. The cutaneous features of diabetes (Box 150.1) are discussed elsewhere (Chapter 62).

Table 150.4 Characteristic skin signs indicating specific endocrine diseases.

Sign	Figure	Associated endocrine disease/condition
Acanthosis nigricans (Chapter 85)	Figure 150.3	Puberty, diabetes, other causes of insulin resistance including HAIR-AN syndrome of young black females (hyperandrogenism, insulin resistance, acanthosis nigricans; often associated with polycystic ovary syndrome, hirsutism and others signs of androgen excess), acromegaly
Acne (Chapter 88)	Figure 150.4	Cushing syndrome, glucocorticoid therapy, ACTH-secreting tumours (e.g. small cell bronchial carcinoma, acromegaly)
Cutis verticis gyrata (Chapter 105)	Figure 150.5	Acromegaly
Flushing (Chapter 104)	Figure 150.6	Menopause-associated hot flushes Phaeochromocytoma, carcinoid
Galactorrhoea		Hyperprolactinaemia (e.g. due to prolactinoma, tumour-associated ectopic prolactin production or medication with neuroleptic drugs, oral contraceptives, tricyclic antidepressants)
Granuloma annulare (Chapter 95)		Diabetes (Chapter 62)
Gynaecomastia (usually, but not always, symmetrical)	Figures 150.7 and 150.8	Puberty, hypogonadism (e.g. Klinefelter syndrome), pituitary and gonadal tumours (e.g. prolactinoma, testis carcinoma), excessive endogenous oestrogen production (e.g. oestrogen-secreting tumours), insufficient oestrogen metabolism (e.g. liver cirrhosis), drugs (e.g. oestrogens, spironolactone, isoniazid, resumption of normal hypophyseal gonadotropin secretion after a long period of hunger, extreme diet, or major consumptive disease), hypopituitarism
Hyperpigmentation	Figure 150.9	Addison disease
Hypertrichosis (Chapter 87)		Excess ACTH production (tumour, Cushing disease), hyperthyroidism (often in association with myxoedema in Graves disease)
Melasma (Chapter 86)	Figure 150.10	Pregnancy, oral contraceptives, oestrogen-secreting tumour
'Moon facies'		Cushing syndrome
Myxoedema, pretibial (Chapter 57)	Figure 150.11	Hypo- or hyperthyroidism (notably in Graves disease)
Necrobiosis lipoidica (Chapter 95)		Diabetes (search for additional cutaneous complications of diabetes in Box 150.1 and in Chapter 62)
Necrolytic migratory erythema (Chapter 148)	Figure 150.12	Glucagonoma
Palmar erythema		Hyperthyroidism
Scleredema adultorum (Buschke) (Chapter 57)		Diabetes
Stretch marks (striae distensae) (Chapter 94)	Figure 150.13	Cushing disease, glucocorticoid therapy, ACTH-secreting tumours (e.g. small cell bronchial carcinoma); pregnancy, contraceptive therapy, puberty (growth spurt, namely in adipose individuals)

Adapted from Braverman 1998 [180], Du Vivier 2002 [378] and Luger and Böhm 2012 [379] © John Wiley.

Table 150.5 Additional 'diagnostic pearls' in clinical dermatoendocrinology.

Sign/symptom	Figure	Consider presence/role of ...
Alopecia areata (Chapter 87)		Thyroid autoimmune disease
Alopecia, rapidly progressing pattern balding (especially in female patients)		Virilising tumour, adrenogenital syndrome; pregnancy or discontinuation of oral contraceptive; thyroid dysfunction, hyperprolactinaemia
Axillary hair, diminished growth		Panhypopituitarism
'Buffalo hump'		Cushing syndrome
Digital clubbing (Chapter 93)		Hyperthyroidism (thyroid acropachy), hyper- or hypoparathyroidism (periosteal formation of new bone)
Epidermoid cysts		Acromegaly
Eyelids, thickened/oedematous		Acromegaly
Gingival or oral hyperpigmentation	Figure 150.14	Addison disease (gingival hyperpigmentation: consider also hyperthyroidism and Cushing disease; distinguish from ephelide-like hyperpigmentation of Peutz–Jeghers syndrome)
Hair, repigmentation of grey hair		ACTH-producing tumour (e.g. pituitary, or ectopic ACTH production by small cell bronchial carcinoma)
Macroglossia (tongue often also fissured)	Figure 150.15	Acromegaly; hypothyroidism (usually less pronounced than in acromegaly)
Mastitis, neonatal		Temporary stimulation of mammary gland by maternal hormones
Nails, thickened and hardened		Acromegaly
Sebaceous gland hypertrophy (Chapter 91)		Acromegaly
Seborrhoea		Virilising tumour, hyperprolactinaemia
		Parkinson disease (→ insufficient dopamine production, associated with hyperprolactinaemia)
Skin tags (acrochordons)		Acromegaly
Telogen effluvium (Chapter 87)		Thyroid dysfunction, hyperprolactinaemia, virilising tumour, adrenogenital syndrome; polycystic ovary syndrome; pregnancy or discontinuation of oral contraceptive
Ulcer, gangrene		Diabetes
Urticaria (Chapter 42)		Chronic urticaria associated with thyroid hormone abnormalities (due to Hashimoto thyroiditis or Graves disease)
Vitiligo (Chapter 86)	Figure 150.16	Can be associated with thyroid autoimmune disease and Addison disease

Adapted from Braverman 1998 [180], Du Vivier 2002 [378], Luger and Böhm 2012 [379], Jabbour 2003 [388] and Jabbour 2010 [386] © John Wiley.

> **Box 150.1 Cutaneous complications of diabetes** (Chapter 62)
>
> - Infections (notably, oral and genital candidiasis, *Candida* intertrigo, recurrent folliculitis, abscess and erysipelas)
> - Ulcers and gangrene (as secondary skin changes due to diabetic microangiopathy and neuropathy)
> - Necrobiosis lipoidica
> - Diabetic rubeosis
> - Lipoatrophy/lipohypertrophy (including postinsulin injection)
> - Diabetic dermopathy (Binkley spots)
> - Diabetic sclerodactyly (diabetic stiff skin, diabetic cheiroarthropathy)
> - Diabetic scleredema
> - Diabetic bullae (bullosis diabeticorum)
> - Acanthosis nigricans (including its possible minor/disseminated variant, finger pebbles) [278]
> - Carotenaemia ('aurantiasis cutis', xanthochromia due to β-carotene accumulation in stratum corneum associated with diabetic hypercarotenaemia, especially over the knuckles, elbows, knees and in palmoplantar skin)
> - Acquired perforating dermatosis
> - Eruptive xanthomas
> - Generalised granuloma annulare
> - Vitiligo
> - Cutaneous adverse effects of antidiabetic agents (including phototoxic and photoallergic reactions)
>
> Adapted from Du Vivier 2002 [378] and Luger and Böhm 2012 [379] © John Wiley.

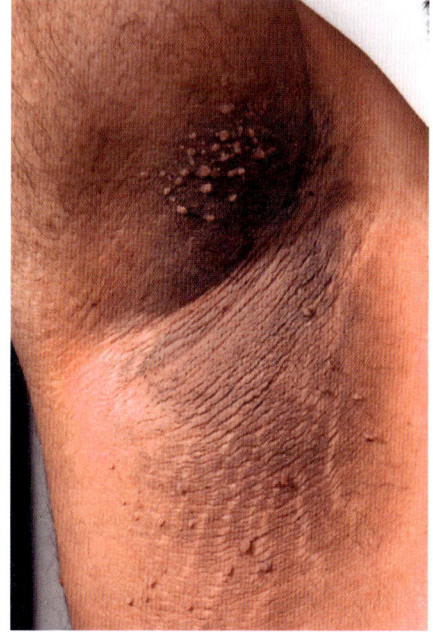

Figure 150.3 Acanthosis nigricans, skin tags and striae in a 41-year-old obese male with type 2 diabetes.

There are also the cutaneous consequences of hypo- or hyperthyroidism to be considered. Finally, it is possible that the observed skin phenomena are caused by a hormone-secreting tumour, such as skin hyperpigmentation, acneiform lesions and/or cushingoid features in ACTH-secreting small cell bronchial carcinoma [380,381], sudden

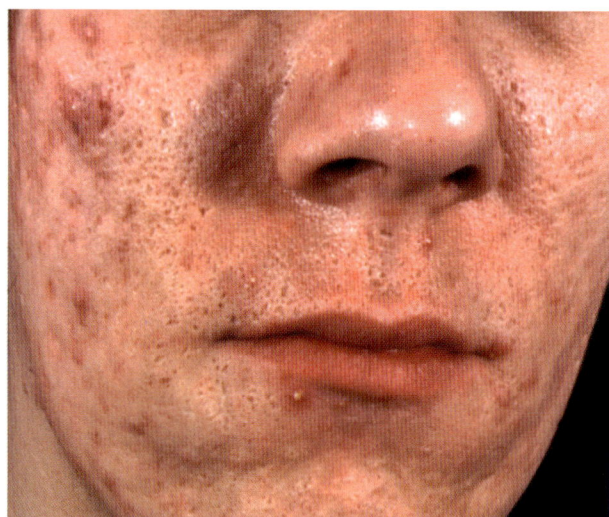

Figure 150.4 Acromegaly: note the coarse features, severe acne and seborrhoea.

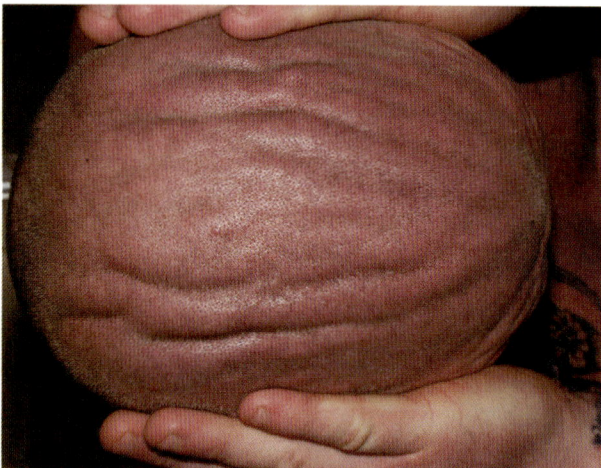

Figure 150.5 Cutis verticis gyrata.

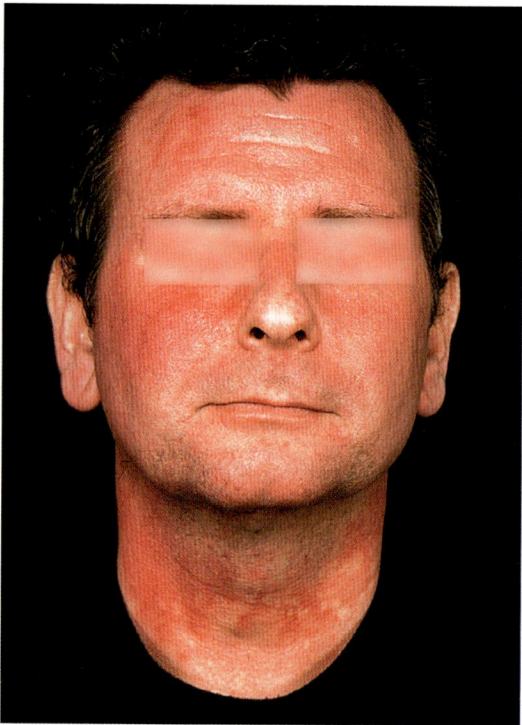

Figure 150.6 Histamine-evoked 'geographic' pattern of flushing due to foregut carcinoid tumour. Courtesy of Professor M. Greaves, London, UK.

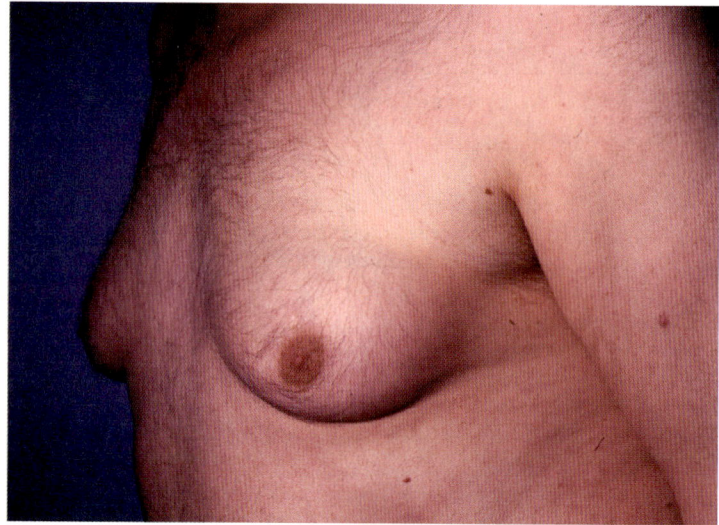

Figure 150.7 Gynaecomastia due to long-term spironolactone therapy given for hypertension.

attacks of hyperhidrosis (typically along with headache, tachycardia and hypertension) in catecholamine-secreting phaeochromocytoma, or necrolytic migratory erythema in glucagonoma syndrome [382–384] (Tables 150.4 and 150.5). (For details on paraneoplastic skin disease, see [385–387] and Chapter 148.)

Endocrinological considerations in skin therapy

Once an endocrinological diagnosis has been made or is suspected, patients should be referred to an appropriate specialist, such as an endocrinologist or neurosurgeon, to undergo further diagnostic procedures and appropriate management. However, even replacement or suppressive therapy may not always result in a rapid return of the skin to its premorbid state. The skin's response to therapeutic interventions can be slow or impossible to achieve, and some endocrine conditions can result in irreversible skin damage.

If a patient is known to have an endocrine disorder, it may also aggravate, increase susceptibility to or alter response to therapy of other skin disorders (Table 150.3), and may also result in accelerated skin ageing. The possibility that neuroendocrine abnormalities associated with psychoemotional stress may have triggered or aggravated a dermatosis via the induction of neurogenic skin inflammation should be considered and discussed with the patient.

Application of exogenous glucocorticosteroid hormone to human skin is likely to impact not only the metabolism and synthesis of *endogenous* steroid hormones in human skin but also intracutaneous neuroendocrine signalling axes, which affect the secretion of potent growth factors/cytokines or the signalling of receptors that are not classic targets of the administered hormone. Glucocorticoids may also affect peripheral clock gene activity in human skin. Given the increasing insight into its regulation of such diverse aspects of

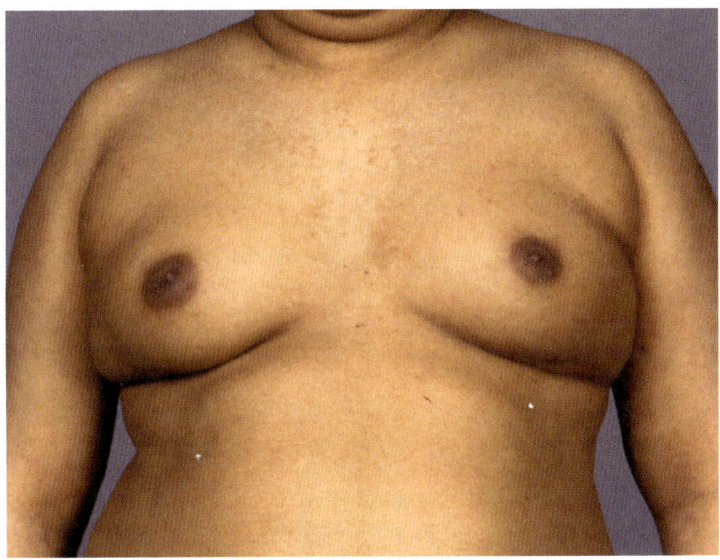
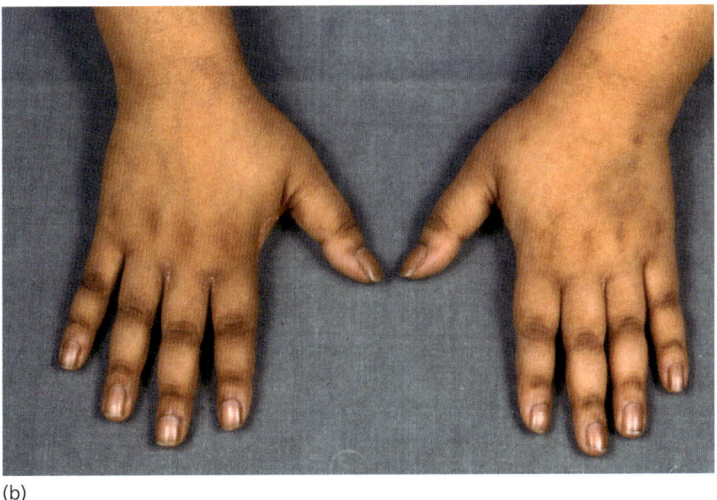

Figure 150.8 An 18-year-old male with pituitary Cushing disease followed by hypopituitarism. (a) Obesity and gynaecomastia. (b) Insulin resistance with acanthosis nigricans of the knuckles, an unusual site in common causes of acanthosis nigricans.

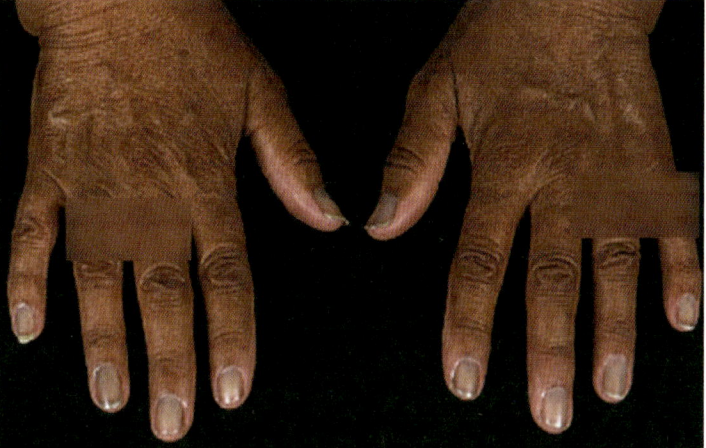
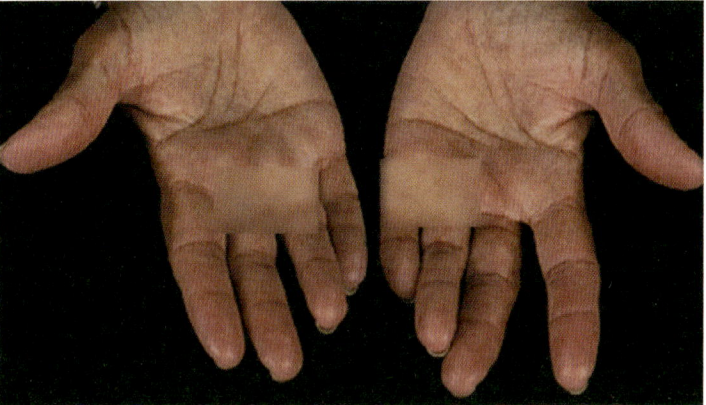

Figure 150.9 Addisonian pigmentation of the palmar creases 37 years after bilateral adrenalectomy for Cushing disease from ACTH-producing pituitary adenoma (Nelson syndrome).

skin physiology as hair growth and pigmentation [37,134,389–394], this chronobiological dimension of glucocorticoid therapy could be more important than previously appreciated.

The dermatologist should be aware of the complex interplay between hormones and the skin. For example, cortisol administration reduces the intrafollicular expression of CRH in human scalp HFs *ex vivo* [36]. Therefore, it is conceivable that chronic glucocorticoid administration reduces the skin and the adrenal gland's CRH-dependent constitutive cortisol synthesis [23,36]. This iatrogenic disruption of the brain–skin axis may contribute to the classic rebound phenomena typically seen after withdrawal of glucocorticoid therapy [2,19,23]. Moreover, all-*trans*-retinoic acid modulates the intrafollicular expression of key growth factors; that is, it upregulates TGFβ1 and TGFβ2, thereby switching scalp HFs from anagen to catagen; this may explain why patients under retinoid therapy can experience a telogen effluvium [395]. Instead, the frequently observed retinoid-associated skin irritation results partly from sensory hypersensitivity induced by retinoid activation of a vanilloid receptor (TRPV1) [396].

Abuse or misuse of hormonally active substances (e.g. anabolic hormones or glucocorticosteroids) may manifest in the skin. A patient's medication may also result in hormonally mediated adverse cutaneous effects. These may be obvious when they result from systemic or high-potency topical glucocorticosteroids or systemic retinoids but less so when due to anabolic agents or hormonal contraceptives. Adverse cutaneous effects may also manifest when a patient has taken novel neuroendocrine agents, such as the synthetic α-MSH analogue, Melanotan, which is used (or abused) for tanning purposes. This agent may also stimulate the appearance of multiple melanocytic naevi and/or dysplastic changes in existing naevi (Table 150.3).

Other medications have less obvious (neuro-)endocrinological effects on the skin. For example, dopamine exerts direct hair growth-inhibitory properties on human scalp HFs [125]. This may explain why bromocriptine, the dopaminergic inhibitor of pituitary prolactin secretion used for treating prolactinoma patients, can cause effluvium in female patients [397]. Neuroleptics and other antipsychotic agents frequently cause hyperprolactinaemia [398]. Therefore, it is reasonable to consider whether skin abnormalities in which excessive prolactin signalling may play a part (Table 150.3) might have been aggravated by such a medication, or whether standard therapy may have been less effective than

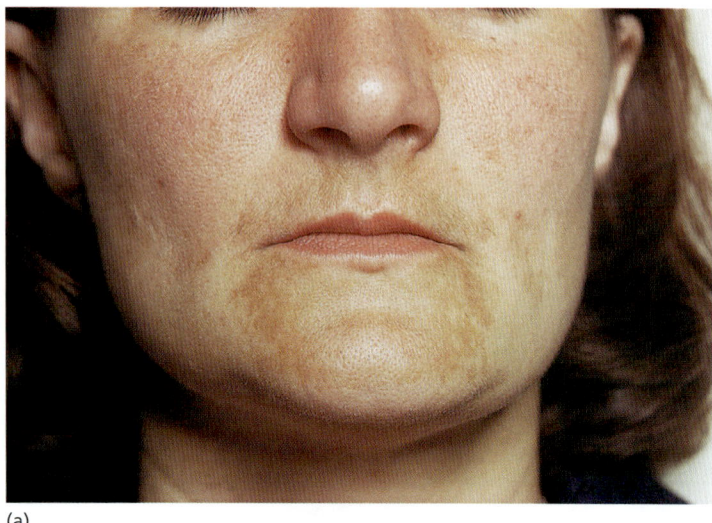

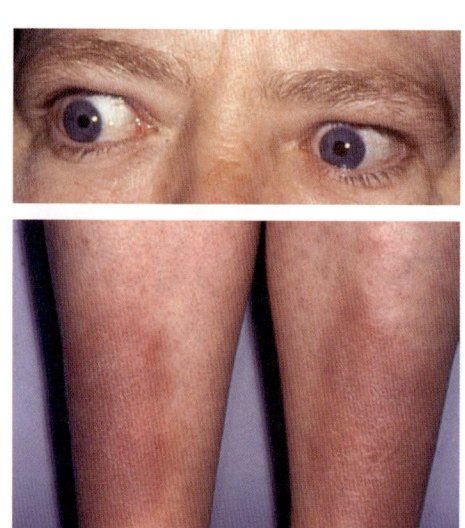

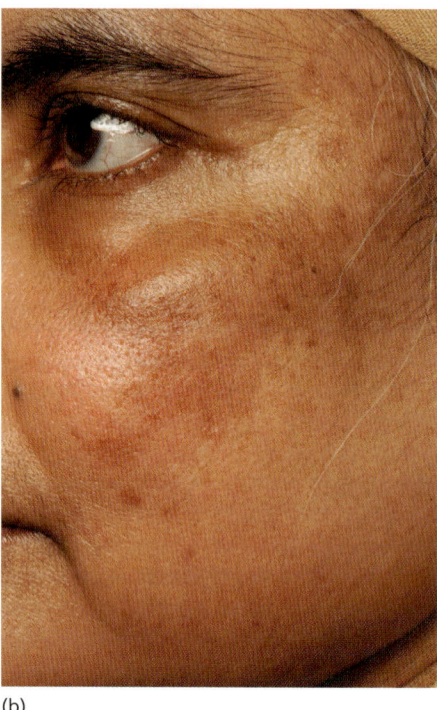

Figure 150.10 Melasma on the face in (a) white skin and (b) skin of colour.

Figure 150.11 A patient with Graves disease with pretibial myxoedema and exophthalmos.

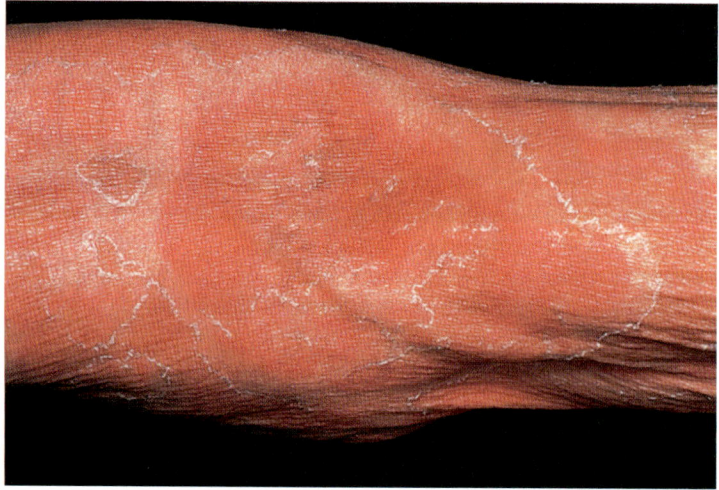

Figure 150.12 Necrolytic migratory erythema. Courtesy of Dr Kristian Thomsen, Finsen Institute, Copenhagen, Denmark.

expected in patients treated with these drugs. Where medically justifiable, it may be worth temporarily discontinuing or reducing such medication.

Long-term ciclosporin therapy can result in hypertrichosis, and rarely in reversible gynaecomastia associated with hyperprolactinaemia [399]. In murine skin, ciclosporin controls HF stem cell activation and thus hair growth in a prolactin receptor-dependent manner [400], while it prolongs the duration of anagen in human scalp HFs [401,402]. It has been suggested, somewhat controversially, that the efficacy of ciclosporin therapy might be enhanced by co-administering bromocriptine, which lowers the serum prolactin level [403], while neuroleptics which cause hyperprolactinaemia may reduce the effectiveness of immunosuppression by ciclosporin [404].

Angiotensin-converting enzyme inhibitors are the leading cause of drug-induced angio-oedema [405–408]. These agents inhibit the intracutaneous degradation of substance P, bradykinin and other pro-inflammatory, vasoactive and mast cell activating neuropeptides that can aggravate neurogenic skin inflammation, vasodilatation and extravasation [12,35,154,409,410].

These considerations illustrate the value of a (neuro-)endocrinological perspective when approaching and managing patients with skin disease. Traditionally, however, it is the diagnostic benefits of such a perspective that secure the place of hormones in the dermatologist's mind.

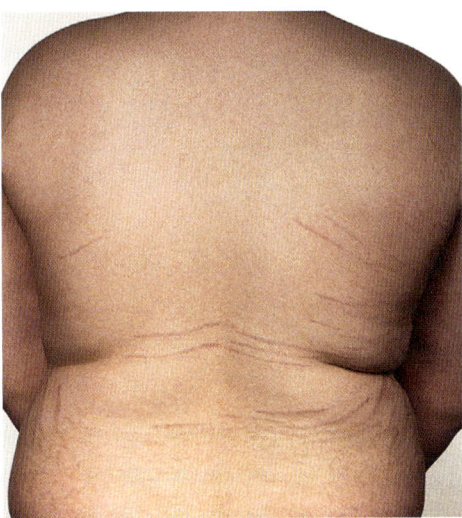

Figure 150.13 Striae due to obesity in a young man.

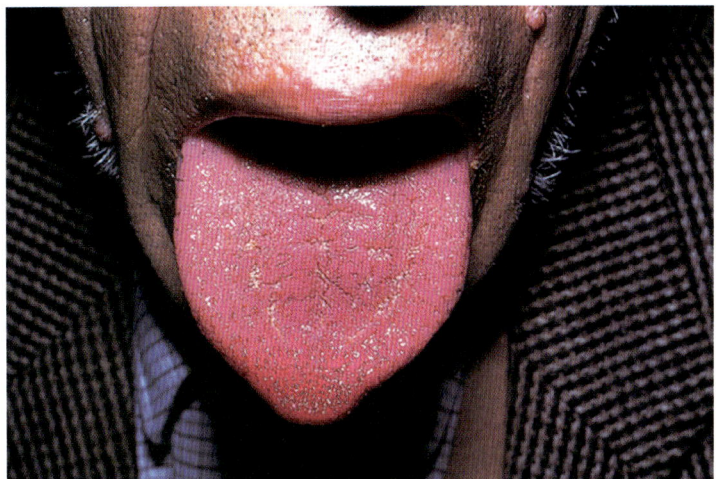

Figure 150.15 Acromegalic macroglossia.

Systematic review of clinical dermatoendocrinology

All the central endocrine signalling axes (Figure 150.1) and (neuro-)endocrine systems described earlier can show abnormalities that result in either excessive or insufficient hormone levels. In the following sections, the skin signs or symptoms summarised in Tables 150.4 and 150.5 are briefly discussed. Further clinical information can be obtained from relevant review articles [119,172,385,386,388,411,412] and Braverman's classic monograph [180]. For clinical illustrations, follow the indicators listed in Tables 150.4 and 150.5.

As the diagnostic confirmation and therapeutic management of the endocrinological disease states listed later typically lie in the hands of endocrinologists, paediatricians, gynaecologists or neurosurgeons, investigation and management are not discussed here: see [9,287,289,413] for details on diagnostic procedures and disease management.

Hypopituitarism

Inherited or acquired insufficiency of pituitary hormone production can result from many different causes. These range from congenital defects in pro-opiomelanocortin (POMC) synthesis [414] or processing, via traumatic brain injury, ionising irradiation, tumours and infection to sarcoidosis and postpartum pituitary necrosis (Sheehan syndrome) [180,388,411,415,416]. The associated skin phenotype is dominated by the main neurohormones that are produced in insufficient amounts.

Given the usually non-hormone-selective nature of hypopituitarism, the levels of several pituitary neurohormones are reduced simultaneously, and the serum levels of other key hormones (e.g. thyroxine, cortisol) and growth factors (e.g. IGF-1) regulated by the former are typically reduced as well. Thus, it is often impossible to discern which hormonal imbalance has caused the observed skin phenotype. It is diagnostically important to identify which pituitary hormone(s) is/are deficient [388,416]. Classically, the absence of melanotropic neurohormones (e.g. ACTH, α-MSH) results in

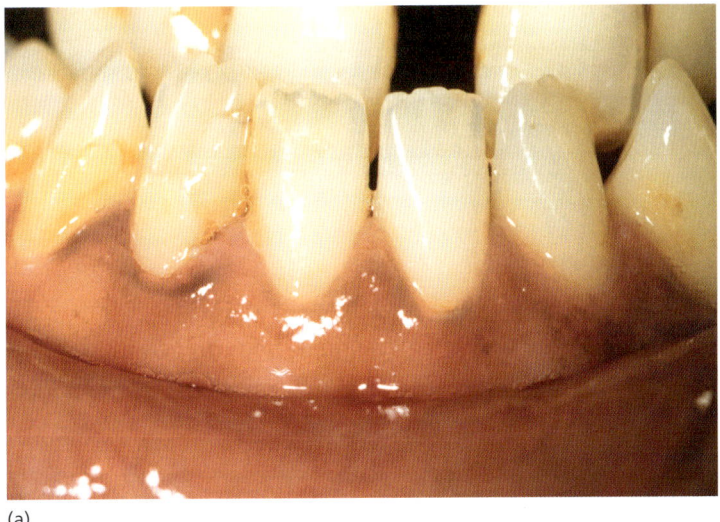

(a)

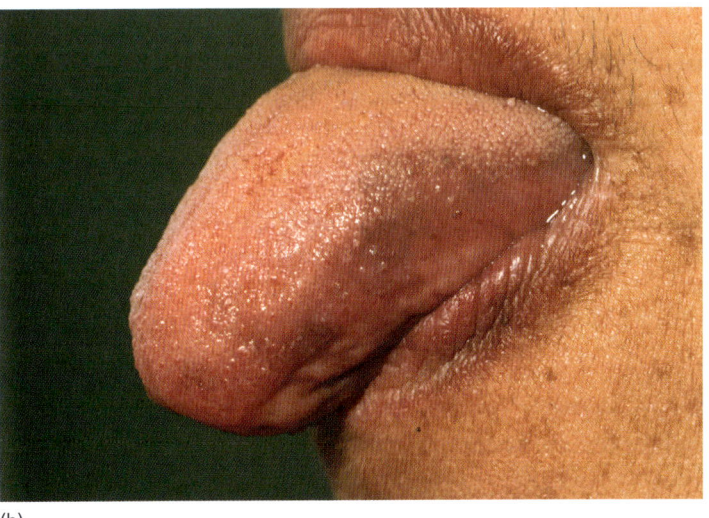

(b)

Figure 150.14 Pigmentation of (a) the gingivae and (b) the tongue in a woman who presented with darkening skin due to Addison disease.

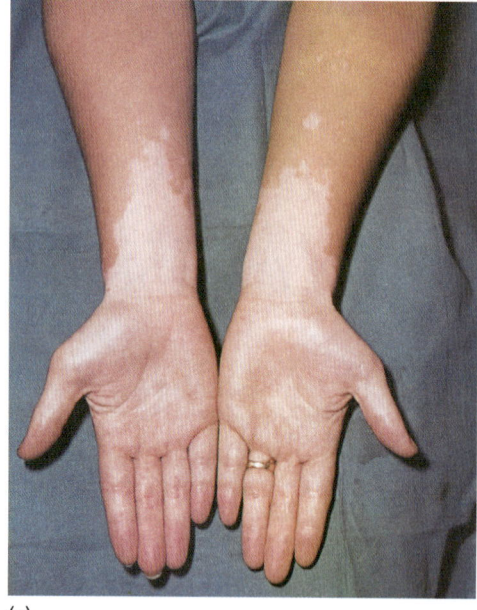

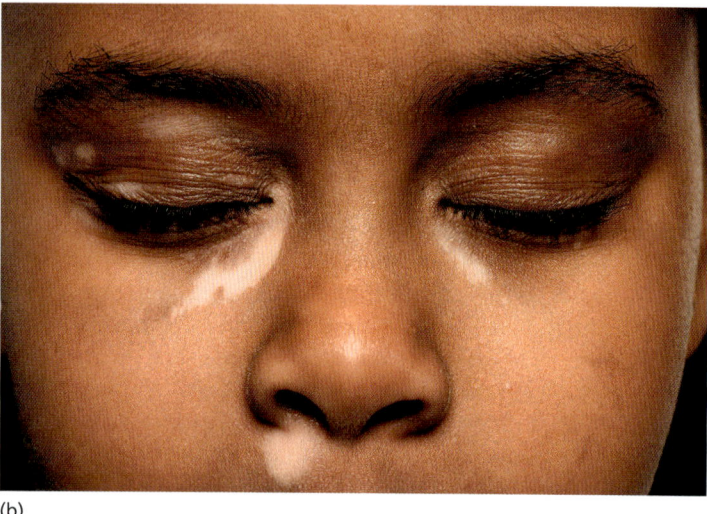

Figure 150.16 Vitiligo on (a) arms and (b) face in skin of colour.

pale hypopigmented skin, not uncommonly with a yellowish tint. Instead, GH (STH) and/or prolactin deficiency gives rise to structural skin changes, e.g. overall skin thinning and reduced sebum and sweat secretion. Rarely, gynaecomastia can be a result of secondary hypopituitarism [417], as in the sarcoidosis patient shown in Figure 150.17.

Isolated GH deficiency or multiple pituitary hormone deficiencies can lead to abnormal elastin fibres, suggesting that GH and other pituitary hormones regulate elastogenesis in human skin [418]. Reduced collagen synthesis has also been seen in patients with hypopituitarism [419]. In GH-deficient patients with Sheehan syndrome, skin capacitance and sebum content were found to be decreased [415]. Patients affected by congenital POMC deficiency [414] are often red-haired and show a pale skin and early onset of obesity.

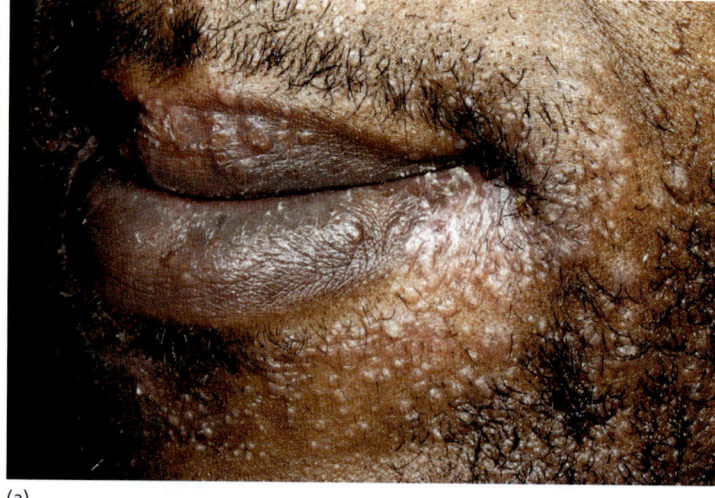

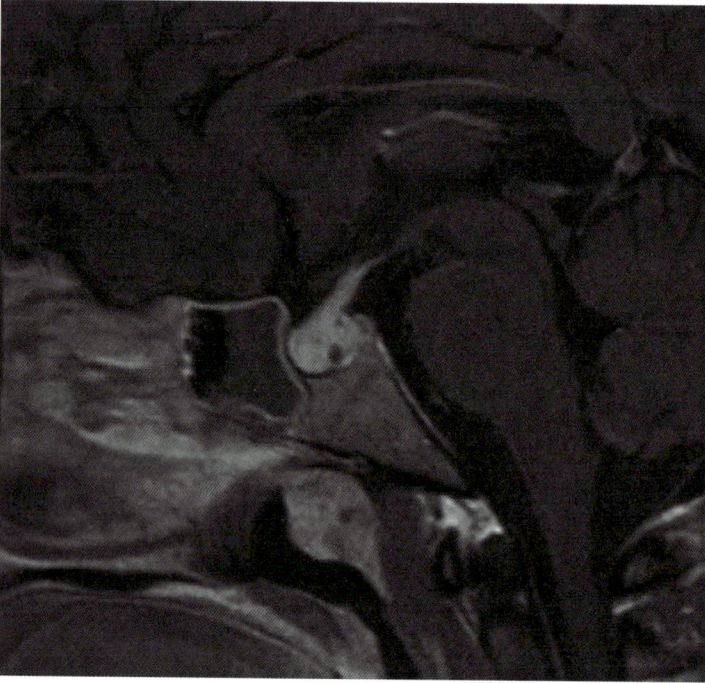

Figure 150.17 Neurosarcoidosis with hypopituitarism presenting as a rash. A diagnosis of cutaneous and pulmonary sarcoidosis was readily established in a 35-year-old man who presented with a widespread undiagnosed papular rash (a) associated with fatigue and shortness of breath. He was, however, incidentally noted to have gynaecomastia and, on further questioning, reduced libido. Endocrinological assessment and pituitary magnetic resonance imaging demonstrated, respectively, hypogonadotrophic hypogonadism and pituitary enlargement (b) in keeping with sarcoid infiltration. Courtesy of Dr S. Walsh, King's College Hospital, London, UK.

Hyperpituitarism

The major disease states resulting from hyperpituitarism (i.e. acromegaly, hyperprolactinaemia and Cushing disease) have very characteristic skin signs.

In *acromegaly*, an excessive GH secretion leads to a secondary rise in IGF-1 serum and tissue levels. It is characterised by excessive growth of acral cartilage and skin with prominent epidermal hyperplasia and dermal glycosaminoglycan accumulation. External manifestations include progressive enlargement of earlobes and fingers ('my gloves don't fit any more'), increasingly coarse facial features with a prominent chin (Figure 150.4) and large frontal skin folds ('thinker's folds'), which may be associated with cutis verticis gyrata (Figure 150.5). Other changes include hypermelanosis, hypertrichosis, seborrhoea, thickened finger- and toenails, acanthosis nigricans, hyperhidrosis and macroglossia (Figure 150.15; Tables 150.4 and 150.5) [9,420–422]. Decreased transepidermal water loss, reduced skin surface temperature and an increase in skin pH and elasticity have also been reported [423,424].

Treatment of acromegaly may partially reverse the cutaneous phenomena. Unfortunately, how these therapies affect human skin have been largely overlooked. It has, however, recently been shown that, surprisingly, GH reduces the growth of female HFs *ex vivo*, presumably by stimulating the expression of TGF-β [160]. Some of the effects of GH on the skin can also be indirect, for example, by upregulating insulin-like growth factor-1 expression [425].

Conversely, GH therapy can enhance the growth of melanocytic naevi [240,241]. Indeed, in murine wound healing studies, treatment with GH-releasing hormone (GHRH) or a GH agonist increased the density of fibroblasts during the early stages of wound healing and accelerated re-epithelialisation. Therefore, the undesired dermatological phenomena seen in acromegaly may well indicate novel strategies for promoting cutaneous wound healing [290]. It has also been proposed that replacement therapy with GH or the key growth factor stimulated by it (IGF-1) represents a potential anti-skin ageing strategy that is worth systematically exploring [306].

Prolonged *hyperprolactinaemia* most frequently results either from a prolactin-secreting micro- or macroadenoma or from drugs (e.g. phenothiazine, dopamine antagonists, oestrogens, morphine derivatives, H_2-antagonists and neuroleptic agents) [2,3,413].

As with GH, a sustained elevation of prolactin serum levels results in increased serum and tissue IGF-1 levels [29]. Thus, there is some limited overlap in the cutaneous phenomena seen in acromegaly and hyperprolactinaemia, namely seborrhoea, though less than expected if increased IGF-1 secretion were the primary mode of prolactin action on human skin. Instead, hyperprolactinaemia in women is typically associated with *s*eborrhoea, *a*cne, *h*irsutism, and *a*ndrogenetic *a*lopecia, termed the SAHA syndrome. SAHA can also be associated with ovarian and adrenal dysfunction (Chapter 88). Hyperprolactinaemia can induce galactorrhoea in both men and women, usually along with gynaecomastia in men.

However, recent research suggests that the prominent effects on the pilosebaceous unit and the mammary gland represent only a small part of prolactin's full range of actions on human skin. These range from the modulation of keratinocyte and sebocyte proliferation, differentiation and apoptosis to the regulation of cytokine secretion and keratin expression, including keratin 15 expression, a key epithelial stem cell marker, indicating a wider role for prolactin in epithelial stem cell biology; moreover, prolactin actions may differ between the sexes [2,3,34,104,111,112,126]. Prolactin can also negatively regulate skin re-epithelialisation during wound healing [33]. If it is confirmed that prolactin also modulates peripheral androgen metabolism [426] and plays a significant role in cutaneous autoimmunity [427], this serves as additional motivation to explore fully the impact of prolactin [104,110,126] on skin physiology.

Most patients affected by Cushing disease suffer from an ACTH-producing tumour, either in the anterior pituitary or in an extrapituitary location. The associated skin phenomena are dominated by the pigmentary effects of ACTH and the hypercortisolism induced by the chronically elevated serum cortisol level [379]. Proximal repigmentation of previously grey/white hair and/or hyperpigmented palmar lines (in pale skin) should indicate screening for an ACTH-secreting tumour or Addison disease.

Adrenal hyperfunction

There are three forms of adrenal hyperfunction.

Hypercortisolism (Cushing syndrome). This is most frequently iatrogenic and results from systemic or occasionally extensive topical glucocorticoid therapy. Less common are ACTH-producing tumours (Cushing disease) and, very rarely, CRH-producing hypothalamic tumours [386,428] or autoimmune stimulation of adrenal ACTH receptors (MC2R) by autoantibodies (Carney syndrome) [429]; the latter is to be distinguished from the Carney complex, an exceptionally rare, dominantly inherited syndrome (Chapter 151) [430–433].

The non-pigmentary skin manifestations of both Cushing disease and Cushing syndrome are thought to result primarily from excessive adrenal cortisol production (hypercortisolism), even though ACTH also stimulates steroidogenesis in human skin and its appendages [36,47]. Therefore, it remains to be explored whether some of the steroid hormone-dependent cutaneous phenomena are due to excessive compensatory intracutaneous steroidogenesis.

The dermatological manifestations of hypercortisolism include facial and neck changes due to altered subcutaneous fat distribution ('moon face', 'buffalo hump') (see Tables 150.4 and 150.5), generalised hypertrichosis, acne and the consequences of increased collagen breakdown, namely skin fragility, stretch marks, vascular fragility with resulting purpura and impaired wound healing. Hypercortisolism can also induce diabetes, thus adding to the spectrum of diabetes-associated skin phenomena (see Box 150.1).

Hyperaldosteronism. Several indications from the experimental literature suggest that hyperaldosteronism (Conn syndrome) can affect human skin and the HF [434–436]. However, prominent skin signs or symptoms have not yet been described in individuals with hyperaldosteronism.

Congenital adrenal hyperplasia. Congenital adrenal hyperplasia (CAH, MIM: 201910) is in most cases due to deficiency of 21-hydroxylase due to mutations in the *CYP21* gene. The cortisol precursor 17-hydroxyprogesterone cannot be metabolised to cortisol but is shunted towards enhanced androgen production instead. This results in virilisation with associated skin signs including acne and hirsutism. ACTH levels are increased as compensation for insufficient cortisol production resulting in hypermelanosis. In women, the clinical features may be difficult to distinguish from those of polycystic ovary syndrome, idiopathic hirsutism or hyperinsulinaemia and the possibility of underlying CAH should not be overlooked: short stature may be a helpful clue [437,438].

Adrenal insufficiency (Addison disease)
Insufficient adrenal cortisol production is most commonly the consequence of autoimmune disease (autoimmune adrenalitis) or of suppression of ACTH secretion following long-term glucocorticoid therapy. Recovery of endogenous ACTH production may be delayed and give rise to the same clinical picture. Infectious diseases (tuberculosis, systemic fungal infection) are also important causes. For a full list of the many rarer causes, endocrinology textbooks should be consulted [9].

Vitamin B_{12} deficiency may rarely result in epidermal hyperpigmentation like Addison disease but is distinguishable by its haematological abnormalities [439–441]. Adrenal insufficiency should be considered in early-onset obesity that is not otherwise explained [442,443], due to a rare loss-of-function mutation in POMC, the precursor hormone of ACTH [414].

Hypermelanosis due to compensatory pituitary (and possibly intracutaneous) oversecretion of ACTH or α-MSH is a prominent component of Addison disease. This is often first and best visible as hyperpigmented palmar skin creases but also affects intertriginous skin, external genitalia, nail beds, oral mucosa and lips (maybe due to higher levels of MC1R or MC2R expression in the melanocytes in these regions) [444].

If Addisonian pigmentation presents in association with vitiligo (Chapter 86) or, rarely, AA (Chapter 87) it may be due to autoimmune adrenalitis; this possibility should then be explored by a specialist. It has been argued that patients presenting with generalised hyperpigmentation of unclear origin should have serum ACTH and mineralocorticoid function checked without delay for undiagnosed primary adrenal insufficiency [445].

Hyperandrogenism
The main adrenal androgens are dehydroepiandrosterone (DHEA) and androstenedione, which are metabolised in their target tissues. The most important enzymatic processes are the conversion of testosterone to DHT by 5-α-reductase and the conversion of androgens to 17-β-oestradiol [48,50]. All relevant enzyme activities and androgen receptors are present in human skin, most prominently in its pilosebaceous units. It is thought that the higher androgen content of male skin partly explains why it is thicker, more hairy and slightly more pigmented than female skin [179,379]. This is in accordance with the skin phenotype seen in hyperandrogenism.

Apart from exogenous androgen use or abuse (e.g. anabolic steroids) and CAH, polycystic ovary syndrome with the production of androgens by ovarian theca cells is the most frequent cause of hyperandrogenism in women [446–449]. Acromegaly, Cushing disease, androgen-secreting (virilising) tumours of the ovary or adrenal gland, and hyperprolactinaemia represent other less common causes.

The cutaneous hallmarks of hyperandrogenism are seborrhoea, severe acne, hirsutism, telogen effluvium and female or male pattern balding [185,450–453]. Hyperandrogenism should be considered as a potential underlying cause of late-onset acne in women. Other signs of virilisation may make the clinical diagnosis of hyperandrogenism straightforward, and a full endocrinological assessment should be undertaken. Polycystic ovary syndrome is often coupled with hyperprolactinaemia and/or increased luteinising hormone levels [446,447,449]. Treatment requires careful consideration [452,454].

Hypoandrogenism
Whether it is caused by castration, tumours, antiandrogen therapy, genetically deficient androgen production (e.g. Klinefelter syndrome) or defective androgen receptor-mediated signalling, the dermatological picture of hypoandrogenism is mainly determined by the timing of androgen deficiency. If hypoandrogenism occurs before puberty, it will manifest as *eunuchoid* habitus, with undeveloped male body habitus, minimal or absent male secondary hair and no acne during puberty. If hypoandrogenism occurs after puberty, there is a progressive loss of male sexual characteristics and androgenetic alopecia does not progress [9,48,287,379].

If androgen deficiency is corrected too aggressively in male patients, features of hyperandrogenism such as seborrhoea, acne and rapidly progressive male pattern balding can develop.

One cause of infertility in hypoandrogenised males, typically with reduced beard and body hair growth, is polymorphism of the androgen receptor [455].

Hyperoestrogenism
Besides oral contraceptives and excessive consumption of phyto-oestrogens, oestrogen-producing tumours are the most common and most serious causes of hyperoestrogenism. The classic skin signs are melasma, spider naevi and increased susceptibility to *Candida* vulvovaginitis. While girls can undergo precocious puberty, boys develop gynaecomastia. Erythema nodosum, porphyria cutanea tarda, pemphigoid gestationis and systemic lupus erythematosus can be seen [180,379,388].

Hypo-oestrogenism
Hypo-oestrogenism due to menopause or ovariectomy may result in female pattern balding. Sometimes this female variant of androgenetic alopecia may follow the male pattern or can also show a mixed phenotype (male and female pattern balding) (Chapter 87). The latter phenotype is associated with postmenopausal hypo-oestrogenism [59] and supports the hypothesis that, in contrast to androgenetic alopecia in males, a relative deficiency in the stimulation of scalp HFs by 17-β-oestradiol is a major factor in female pattern balding [57,196,298,456–462].

This is further supported by observations in iatrogenic hypo-oestrogenism: aromatase inhibitors frequently cause telogen effluvium [463,464] and sometimes may induce male pattern hair loss [459]. Reportedly, skin with high aromatase expression (expected to be associated with elevated local oestrogen levels) also shows thicker elastic fibres [40].

Because 17-oestradiol is a promoter of wound healing [59,106,168,169,301,465], impaired wound healing can be associated with hypo-oestrogenism [171] and 17-β-oestradiol can slow or reverse skin ageing [58,59,239,301,302], hypo-oestrogenism justifies consideration of hormone replacement. The benefits of this must be balanced against the potential adverse effects of oestrogen therapy [466–468].

In contrast to androgens, 17-β-oestradiol restricts sebocyte proliferation and sebum production [56]. Therefore, in addition to genital pruritus and burning mouth syndrome, seborrhoea is another dermatological manifestation of hypo-oestrogenism. If these occur with osteoporosis, menopausal mood swings, paroxysmal hyperhidrosis and flushing, a diagnosis of hypo-oestrogenism is easily reached and can be confirmed by measuring serum hormone levels.

Phaeochromocytoma

Phaeochromocytoma is a life-threating catecholamine-secreting endocrine neoplasm of the adrenal medulla. It can occur bilaterally or may be ectopic; in 10–15% of cases it is malignant. In comparison with its dominant clinical presentations (hypertension, paroxysmal hypertensive crises, headaches, tremor, palpitations, anxiety), its skin manifestations may not be obvious including hyperhidrosis, paroxysmal facial pallor and sometimes aggravation of pre-existing Raynaud phenomenon [180,386,388,469]. Dermatologists should be alert to such systemic signs in patients with these cutaneous features, particularly if they have neurofibromatosis type I [388,469–471].

Carcinoid

Carcinoid is a malignant neoplasm of specialised serotonin-producing epithelial cells of the small intestine and classically presents as paroxysmal flushing of the face and upper torso. These flushes generate a sensation of rapidly ascending heat, which may be accompanied by wheezing and/or diarrhoea [386,412,469,472,473]. It is assumed also that neuropeptides such as substance P and bradykinin are involved in inducing these signs and symptoms.

Flushing occurs in fewer than 25% of patients with carcinoid [379]; therefore, its absence does not rule out the diagnosis. This must be kept in mind, as over the past 30 years the incidence of gastrointestinal carcinoid has been rising faster than that of any other cancer and the 5-year survival rate is only 28% [474,475].

As an extreme rarity, human skin can also produce primary carcinoid tumours [476,477], while visceral neuroendocrine tumours may metastasise to the skin [478].

Glucagon and glucagonoma

Necrolytic migratory erythema (Chapter 148) is the pathognomonic dermatological presentation of glucagonoma [382–384,479,480], a neoplasm which typically arises from α-cells of the pancreas and secretes excessive amounts of glucagon. The associated cutaneous histopathological findings (intercellular epidermal oedema together with hydropic degeneration of epidermal keratinocytes) are shared with pellagra, zinc deficiency and acro-dermatitis enteropathica, even though patients with glucagonoma syndrome have normal zinc serum levels [180].

Besides surgery, somatostatin analogues usually improve the skin eruption [481,482]. Little is known about how somatostatin or glucagon itself affects normal skin physiology or how excessive glucagon levels induce the clinical phenotype in the skin. Interestingly, some frog species generate glucagon and many other neuropeptides in the skin [349]. Somatostatin may play a role in maintaining the physiological immune privilege of the HF [138]. It has been postulated that it may not be glucagon itself but another tumour-secreted peptide that is responsible for necrolytic migratory erythema [180]. Yet, it has been reported that necrolytic migratory erythema can be induced by glucagon therapy alone [483,484].

Glucagon-like peptide-1 (GLP-1) is a gut hormone derived from proglucagon which has affinity for specific GLP-1 receptors in the pancreas and the brain. GLP-1 also inhibits secretion of glucagon, enhances glucose-dependent insulin secretion, and induces a feeling of satiety. Synthetic GLP-1 receptor agonists are employed for treating type 2 diabetes. These drugs appear to be beneficial for psoriasis in diabetic patients with insulin resistance before metabolic improvement can be detected [485–487], highlighting the possible role of GLP-1 in human skin, especially since psoriatic lesions show increased expression of GLP-1 receptors [486,488].

Polyendocrine disease

Multiple endocrine neoplasia (MEN-1 and MEN-2) and the autoimmune polyglandular syndromes (e.g. APS-1, due to a defective *AIRE* gene) can generate several of the skin lesions and symptoms described in this chapter [180,489–495]. They are discussed in more detail in Chapter 148.

Diabetes

The dermatological dimensions of diabetes are described in Chapter 62 and summarised in Box 150.1.

Hyper- and hypothyroidism

Along with diabetes, hyper- and hypothyroidism are the endocrine disorders that most frequently cause skin abnormalities [178, 496,497]. If they occur together, pretibial myxoedema, weight loss, hyperhidrosis and an increased state of nervousness quickly indicate hyperthyroidism. By contrast, the combination of dry skin, telogen effluvium, brittle hair, pallor, weight gain, increased tiredness and decreased alertness is suggestive of hypothyroidism [180,379,497]. Textbooks and reviews therefore traditionally deal with the dermatological aspects of hyper- and hypothyroidism in separate chapters. However, it may be more helpful to consider these conditions jointly, as we do here.

The dermatologist will identify the skin signs and symptoms (Tables 150.3, 150.4 and 150.5) which point to the possibility of thyroid dysfunction; the dermatologist will then request routine thyroid function tests (TSH, free triiodothyronine (T3) and thyroxine (T4)), leaving the establishment of the finer details to the thyroid specialist.

Thyroid hormone receptors are abundantly expressed in human skin and HFs. Organ-cultured human skin and HFs respond directly to thyroid hormone stimulation in multiple ways with effects on keratinocyte proliferation and keratin expression, intracutaneous regulation of neurohormone production and HF epithelial stem cell functions, stimulation of HF pigmentation, keratinocyte energy metabolism and wound healing [37,105,107,128–133,498–500]. Thyroxine also strongly up-regulates expression of core clock genes (genes regulating circadian rhythm) in human skin [134].

Given the importance of peripheral clock activity for many aspects of skin physiology ranging from cell cycle control and cell metabolism via pigmentation to hair growth control [37,389–393, 501], this link between skin endocrinology and chronobiology underscores the importance of hyper- or hypothyroidism from a dermatological perspective. Both excessive and insufficient serum levels of T3 or thyroxine T4 can generate a plethora of dermatological signs and symptoms. However, none of these mechanisms is yet fully understood.

A hyperthyroid state most frequently results from Graves disease, the most prevalent endocrinopathy after diabetes. It primarily affects women or occurs during the initial phase of autoimmune thyroiditis (Hashimoto type) [9,287]. While the latter eventually results in hypothyroidism, its first dermatological presentation can be due to hyperthyroidism. Postpartum thyroiditis also manifests initially as hyperthyroidism, which is then followed by hypothyroidism. Excessive T4 medication or exposure to iodine, hormone-secreting thyroid adenomas, multinodular goitre and, very rarely, a TSH-secreting pituitary adenoma are other important causes of hyperthyroidism. All these can induce the dermatological findings summarised earlier. An additional skin sign is chronic urticaria, which has been postulated to be inducible by IgE autoantibodies against thyroid peroxidase [502,503].

Intradermal TSH receptors may provide the main inciting autoantigen for the generation of stimulatory anti-TSH receptor autoantibodies [13,108]. The stimulation of TSH receptors expressed by skin fibroblasts may induce the characteristic increased production and deposition of glycosaminoglycans responsible for pretibial and eyelid myxoedema as well as exophthalmos. Excessive cutaneous glycosaminoglycans can induce both hypertrichosis and alopecia, possibly depending on whether the deposition of these extracellular matrix components acts on relatively 'quiescent' telogen or maximally proliferating anagen HFs [504]. Both excessive and insufficient thyroid hormone serum levels can be associated with effluvium and alterations in hair shaft structure, elasticity or sheen [13,37,130,133,178]. The cutaneous microcirculation can also be affected in patients with Graves disease [505].

Hashimoto thyroiditis, the main cause of hypothyroidism apart from dietary iodine deficiency, can be associated with a few additional characteristic signs, namely lateral sparseness of the eyebrows (the sign of Hertoghe) and a yellowish hue of the skin due to β-carotene accumulation (aurantiasis cutis) [506]. If these are accompanied by carpal tunnel syndrome, ptosis and brittle, slow-growing nails, this further indicates the presence of hypothyroidism [180,388]. Apart from pretibial myxoedema (Table 150.4) a more generalised myxoedema may also be present, often most prominently on the face, giving it a waxen appearance.

Iatrogenic hypothyroidism can be seen following thyroid surgery, thyroid radiation or thyrostatic drug therapy. Bexarotene, a second line therapy for cutaneous T-cell lymphoma, can also induce significant hypothyroidism [507–510] (Chapter 19).

Hyperparathyroidism

The typical hypercalcaemia associated with hyperparathyroidism causes only mild pruritus and/or skin dryness or no dermatological signs and symptoms. It is therefore easily overlooked by dermatologists.

Primary hyperparathyroidism most commonly results from an autonomous parathormone-secreting adenoma; secondary hyperparathyroidism may arise from vitamin D deficiency or from disturbances of the calcium-phosphate balance. This predisposes to calciphylaxis (calcific uraemic arteriolopathy), though not all patients with this condition have either abnormal parathormone levels or high calcium-phosphate products [9,180] (in such cases, other disorders should be considered, such as hyperoxaluria) [511]. Calciphylaxis is characterised by widespread vascular calcification and thrombotic occlusion of cutaneous blood vessels with resultant extensive tissue necrosis. Calciphylaxis is a frequent complication of end-stage renal insufficiency [512–515]. Given the extremely high mortality of calciphylaxis, its development requires rapid diagnostic action [514–516].

Rarely, hyperparathyroidism may result in metastatic calcification in the dermis and subcutis, which presents as firm papules, nodules or plaques, particularly around large joints or flexural sites. Unlike calciphylaxis it does not lead to tissue necrosis [517–519]. See Chapter 59 for more details.

Primary hyperparathyroidism can also occur as a component of the MEN-1 syndrome [520,521].

Autosomal recessive congenital ichthyosis and epidermolytic ichthyosis in children were found to be associated with increased PTH serum and a higher radiological rickets score compared with common ichthyosis [522,523]. This raises the question of whether some chronic dermatoses, characterised by abnormalities of keratinisation, are associated with increased intracutaneous production of PTH/PTH-related peptide (PTHrp). This possibility deserves systematic investigation.

Hypoparathyroidism

Hypoparathyroidism predominantly arises following thyroidectomy. It is clinically most obvious from the characteristic resultant tetanic muscle cramps. Hypoparathyroidism can also be seen in polyglandular autoimmune endocrinopathies or rare genetic defects, where its onset and progression can be more insidious. In patients with pseudohypoparathyroidism the target tissues show greatly decreased sensitivity to stimulation with PTH.

Hair and nail growth disorders and skin dryness are the most frequently associated dermatological phenomena. Dry, rough skin; coarse, brittle hair; and lustreless, distally split nails [524–527] are common signs in patients with idiopathic hypoparathyroidism.

This hair phenotype corresponds well with the knowledge that both PTH/PTHrp agonists and antagonists modulate rodent HF cycling *in vivo* as well as the HF response to chemotherapy-induced damage [115–117,528]. This may be related to the effects of PTH/PTHrp-mediated signalling on angiogenesis in murine skin [114].

Three concepts are important from a clinical dermatoendocrinological perspective:
1 The interactions between PTH/PTHrp with its receptor constitute a functionally important, intracutaneous hormonal signalling system, the epithelial–mesenchymal interactions of which have an impact on rodent HF growth and skin vasculature.
2 That patients with hypoparathyroidism also show hair growth abnormalities suggests that this signalling system also operates in human skin, is clinically important and might be targeted therapeutically [116,402,529–532].
3 Any hormonal signalling system that modulates both the activities of an entire mini-organ (here, the HF) and angiogenesis is almost guaranteed to have effects on multiple other aspects of skin physiology and pathology. The finding that PTHrp regulates proliferation and differentiation in a human keratinocyte cell line *in vitro* [533] supports this notion.

Thus, hypoparathyroidism illustrates the principle that the skin phenotype seen in patients with a defined hormone deficiency, if interpreted in conjunction with the experimental literature, can highlight clinically relevant novel research frontiers in investigative dermatoendocrinology.

Future perspectives

Recognising the skin signs and symptoms that indicate underlying endocrine abnormalities or conditions remains the core endocrinological challenge for the practising dermatologist. However, owing to the discovery that human skin is a major endocrine organ, the future scope and practice of dermatoendocrinology will change. With increasing insight into previously unsuspected (neuro-)endocrine dimensions of common skin diseases (Table 150.2) and of standard therapeutic agents used to treat them, clinical dermatology cannot escape these important developments.

A few examples for future perspectives of dermatoendocrinology underscore this point:

- All routinely administered hormone-based agents used for treating skin disease (glucocorticoids, retinoids, vitamin D derivatives) can have an impact on the physiological (neuro-)endocrine signalling milieu of the skin. A better understanding of these interactions can help reduce adverse effects and enhance therapeutic efficacy.
- In all endocrine disorders that affect the skin, there are alterations in the ways that relevant (neuro-)hormones and neuromediators are expressed or metabolised in the skin; and receptor-mediated signalling must be altered as a secondary consequence of systemic endocrine abnormalities.
- It remains a matter of speculation how secondary intracutaneous (neuro-)endocrine abnormalities contribute to discernible skin phenotypes associated with classic endocrine disease (Tables 150.4 and 150.5 and Box 150.1).
- Better understanding of how the complex signalling interactions between the individual (neuro-)hormones and neuromediators present in the skin affect its functioning in health and disease should help to develop new strategies for improving skin function, and potentially retarding or even reversing skin ageing [**2**,3,37,59,**68**,132,306].
- Understanding which specific (neuro-)endocrine abnormalities associated with inflamed, hyperproliferating and/or fibrosing skin diseases contribute to the pathogenesis of common dermatoses will identify novel therapeutic targets and management strategies.
- The 'epidemic' of allergic diseases throughout western civilisation [534,535] calls for the development of effective antiallergic strategies. Neuroendocrine strategies are particularly promising in this context. Examples include studies in human skin and HF organ culture which have shown that (i) endogenous and exogenous agonists of cannabinoid receptor 1 have a suppressive effect on mast cell degranulation and the maturation of functional mast cells from resident progenitor cells in human skin and airway mucosa [72,271], while CRH promotes both [**2**,203,270,276]; (ii) SP stimulates human skin mast cell degranulation and neurogenic inflammation [15,16,118,121]; (iii) activation of the kappa-opioid receptor decreases the number of mast cells in human skin *ex vivo* [272]; and (iv) the α-MSH-derived peptide, K(D)PT, inhibits human mast cell degranulation *in situ* [327]. Thus, in addition to neuropeptides, CB1 agonists and CRH and SP receptor (NK1) antagonists are promising candidates for antiallergy therapeutics.
- Antagonising CRH [231,270] or substance P [119–121,203,278,536], or stimulating CGRP receptors [118], holds promise for the future management of inflammatory skin diseases such as atopic eczema by counteracting SP- and/or CRH-driven neurogenic skin inflammation. Although pharmacological antagonists of substance P or CRH have been shown to significantly mitigate neurogenic skin inflammation and its sequelae (e.g. hair growth inhibition, itch, eczema) in animal experiments, this remains to be fully explored in human skin.

Finally, it has long been suspected that the modern penchant for sun exposure, despite its much publicised effects on skin ageing and skin cancer risk, has a habit-forming neuroendocrine component. A recent animal study supports this notion: UV-seeking addictive behaviour in mice was influenced by the UV-induced intracutaneous synthesis of β-endorphin, leading to elevated plasma levels even after low-dose UV irradiation [537]. Narrow-band UV increased β-endorphin synthesis also in human skin *in vivo* [538]. This shows that endorphins synthesised peripherally in mammalian skin can, in principle, reach both the circulation *and* the brain, and can cause behavioural changes [46]. Interestingly, an increase of enkephalin plasma levels has already been reported in patients undergoing UVA phototherapy [539]. Therefore, it has become conceivable that future dermatological therapy will be capable of modulating this brain–skin axis in ways that may help dermatological patients whose skin disease has a major psychological component [46,40].

In addition to its paramount importance for the identification of underlying endocrine disorders, it is for all these reasons that dermatoendocrinology lies at the very heart of modern dermatological practice.

Key references

The full list of references can be found in the online version at https://www.wiley.com/rooksdermatology10e

2 Paus R, Langan EA, Vidali S, Ramot Y, Andersen B. Neuroendocrinology of the hair follicle: principles and clinical perspectives. *Trends Mol Med* 2014;20:559–70.

3 Ramot Y, Bohm M, Paus R. Translational neuroendocrinology of human skin: concepts and perspectives. *Trends Mol Med* 2020;27:60–74.

7 Clayton RW, Langan EA, Ansell DM *et al*. Neuroendocrinology and neurobiology of sebaceous glands. *Biol Rev Camb Philos Soc* 2020;95:592–624.

24 Slominski AT, Hardeland R, Zmijewski MA, Slominski RM, Reiter RJ, Paus R. Melatonin: a cutaneous perspective on its production, metabolism, and functions. *J Invest Dermatol* 2018;138:490–9.

53 Heilmann-Heimbach S, Herold C, Hochfeld LM *et al*. Meta-analysis identifies novel risk loci and yields systematic insights into the biology of male-pattern baldness. *Nat Commun* 2017;8:14694.

57 Ohnemus U, Uenalan M, Inzunza J, Gustafsson JA, Paus R. The hair follicle as an estrogen target and source. *Endocr Rev* 2006;27:677–706.

68 Ramot Y, Bertolini M, Boboljova M, Uchida Y, Paus R. PPAR-gamma signalling as a key mediator of human hair follicle physiology and pathology. *Exp Dermatol* 2020;29:312–21.

131 Paus R, Ramot Y, Kirsner RS, Tomic-Canic M. Topical L-thyroxine: the Cinderella among hormones waiting to dance on the floor of dermatological therapy? *Exp Dermatol* 2020;29:910–23.

165 Bohm M, Paus R. Towards a renaissance of dermatoendocrinology: selected current frontiers. *Exp Dermatol* 2020;29:786–9.

336 Slominski AT, Manna PR, Tuckey RC. On the role of skin in the regulation of local and systemic steroidogenic activities. *Steroids* 2015;103:72–88.

CHAPTER 151

The Skin and Disorders of the Heart

Sonja Molin[1] and Thomas Ruzicka[2]

[1] Division of Dermatology, Queen's University, Kingston, Canada
[2] Department of Dermatology and Allergology, Ludwig Maximilian University, Munich, Germany

Introduction, 151.1
Skin signs of cardiac disease, 151.1

HEREDITARY SYNDROMES, 151.1
Lymphoedema–distichiasis syndrome, 151.2
Fabry disease, 151.2

RASopathies, 151.3
Carney complex, 151.3

CARDIAC INVOLVEMENT IN DERMATOSES OR SYSTEMIC DISEASES WITH SKIN FEATURES, 151.4
INFLAMMATORY DISORDERS, 151.4

INFECTIONS, 151.5
MISCELLANEOUS, 151.5

Key references, 151.6

Introduction

There are several diseases in which both cardiac and skin involvement may be found (Table 151.1). Most of these are part of a syndrome or are systemic disorders affecting other organs as well [1,2]. Disorders of blood vessels are not included here. The effects of skin disease on the heart (e.g. cardiac failure due to erythroderma) and indirect effects, such as anaemia due to immunosuppressive agents used to treat the skin, are not discussed here either. Numerous infections may occasionally cause myocardial disease and may also present with an exanthem (e.g. parvovirus B19), but these are not discussed individually. Drug reactions due to cardiac medications are described in Chapters 117 and 118.

Skin signs of cardiac disease

Dermatological consequences of cardiac disease include skin colour changes such as cyanosis, redness due to secondary polycythaemia, and a combination of the two that may occur in congenital heart disease (and which has been termed erythraemia). Finger clubbing is a consequence of congenital cyanotic heart disease (Figure 151.1) but occurs in other situations as well. A visible pulsation of the nail bed in time with the pulse is a sign of aortic regurgitation due to the wide pulse pressure in this disorder (Quincke pulsation) [1,2].

HEREDITARY SYNDROMES

Cardiac involvement occurs in several congenital and inherited conditions, such as the RASopathies, Carney complex, Fabry disease and Alagille syndrome [1,3], as well as in chromosomal abnormalities such as Turner syndrome and trisomy 13 or 18 [1].

Table 151.1 Conditions that affect the heart and skin.

Disease	Main cardiac features
Congenital/inherited	
Ehlers–Danlos syndrome	Dilated main vessels, mitral or tricuspid insufficiency, cardiac/vascular rupture (type IV)
Cutis laxa	Early CAD, aortic aneurysm, mitral valve prolapse
Marfan syndrome	Aortic aneurysm, aortic regurgitation, mitral valve prolapse or regurgitation
Pseudoxanthoma elasticum	Arterial calcification, CAD, mitral valve prolapse
Werner disease	Early CAD
Progeria	Early CAD
Cockayne syndrome	Early CAD
Cornelia de Lange syndrome	Septal defects, persistent ductus arteriosus, pulmonary stenosis
Fabry disease	Conduction defects, arrhythmias, hypertension, left ventricular hypertrophy, mitral valve prolapse; see main text for further information
RASopathies:	See text for further information
Noonan syndrome	Pulmonary stenosis, septal defects, hypertrophic cardiomyopathy, aortic abnormalities, other features
Noonan syndrome with multiple lentigines (LEOPARD syndrome)	ECG abnormalities (various forms of heart block), pulmonary stenosis, also subaortic stenosis and hypertrophic cardiomyopathy
Neurofibromatosis	Hypertension (renovascular or phaeochromocytoma)
Rubinstein–Taybi syndrome	Aortic coarctation, persistent ductus arteriosus, pulmonary stenosis, septal defects
Tuberous sclerosis	Cardiac rhabdomyomas
Incontinentia pigmenti	Patent ductus arteriosus, tricuspid insufficiency
Alagille syndrome	Pulmonary artery hypoplasia/stenosis
Di George syndrome	Tetralogy of Fallot, aortic arch defects
Lymphoedema–distichiasis syndrome	Tetralogy of Fallot, patent ductus arteriosus
Naxos disease	Arrhythmogenic right ventricular cardiomyopathy
Chromosomal syndromes	Various, includes Down syndrome, Turner syndrome, trisomy 13, trisomy 18
Carney complex	See text for further information

(continued)

Table 151.1 (continued)

Disease	Main cardiac features
Inflammatory diseases, connective tissue disease, vasculitis	
Systemic lupus erythematosus	Vegetations (especially mitral, Libman–Sacks endocarditis), pericarditis, myocarditis, aortic/mitral regurgitation
Neonatal lupus erythematosus	Neonatal heart block (various patterns), septal defects, persistent ductus arteriosus, tricuspid/mitral insufficiency
Systemic sclerosis	Pericarditis and effusion, conduction defects, myocardial fibrosis, cardiomyopathy, cor pulmonale
Limited systemic sclerosis (CREST)	Pulmonary hypertension
Polyarteritis nodosa	Coronary artery vasculitis, ECG abnormalities, hypertension
Behçet disease	Pericarditis, pulmonary and coronary artery aneurysm
Antiphospholipid syndrome	Vegetations, valvular heart disease, coronary artery thrombosis, pericardial effusion, CCF
Degos disease	Pericarditis, pericardial effusion
Eosinophilic granulomatosis with polyangiitis (EGPA; former Churg–Strauss syndrome)	Pericarditis, cardiac fibrosis, pericardial effusion
Granulomatosis with polyangiitis (GPA)	Cardiomyopathy
Cholesterol emboli	Coronary artery occlusion
Other vasculitides	Coronary artery vasculitis
Dermatomyositis	Conduction defects, arrhythmias, cardiomyopathy, CCF, (rarely) pulmonary hypertension
Relapsing polychondritis	Mitral or aortic insufficiency, dissecting aortic aneurysm, pericarditis, myocardial ischaemia, heart block, aortitis
Rheumatic fever	Mitral and aortic valve disease
Kawasaki disease	Conduction defects, coronary artery aneurysms, pericardial effusion, cardiomegaly
Multicentric reticulohistiocytosis	Pericarditis, cardiomegaly, CAD, CCF
Hypereosinophilic syndrome	Eosinophilic endomyocarditis, valvular scarring, CCF, restrictive cardiomyopathy
Sarcoidosis	Conduction defects, arrhythmias, CCF
Reactive arthritis	Conduction defects, aortic regurgitation
Deposition, metabolic and endocrine disorders	
Amyloidosis	Conduction defects, cardiomegaly, CCF
Haemochromatosis	Arrhythmias, cardiomyopathy, CCF
Wilson disease	Arrhythmias, cardiomyopathy
Mucinoses: scleromyxoedema	Cardiomyopathy, CCF
Hyperlipidaemias	CAD
Diabetes	CAD, cardiomyopathy
Hyperthyroidism	Tachycardia, atrial fibrillation, mitral regurgitation
Hypothyroidism	Bradycardia, CAD, pericardial effusion
Acromegaly	Left ventricular hypertrophy, CCF
Carcinoid syndrome	Tricuspid or pulmonary stenosis, right heart failure
Phaeochromocytoma	Variable heart rate, hypertension/hypotension
Mastocytosis	Tachycardia, hypotension, arrhythmia, angina
Homocystinuria	Atherosclerosis
Embolic diseases:	
Infective endocarditis	Vegetations, valvular incompetence
Cholesterol emboli	Usually from proximal arteries rather than cardiac
Atrial myxomas	See text for further information
Infections	
Lyme disease	Myocarditis, heart block
Syphilis	Aortitis, aortic aneurysm, aortic and mitral regurgitation, obstructed coronary arteries
Varicella	Myocarditis
SARS-CoV-2	Tachycardia, haemodynamic shock, myocarditis, decreased left ventricular ejection fraction (LVEF), coronary aneurysm and dilatation
Septicaemia	Pustules, infarcts, disseminated intravascular coagulopathy
Congenital rubella	Pulmonary artery and valve stenosis, patent ductus arteriosus
Whipple disease	Pericarditis, myocarditis, valve deformity (especially mitral valve endocarditis)
Drugs	
Used in cardiology, causing rash	Amiodarone (photosensitivity, pigmentation), amlodipine (ankle oedema)
Cardiotoxic and cause skin eruptions	Doxorubicin (cardiotoxic, anagen effluvium, pigmentation)
Used for skin disease, cardiovascular side effects	Ciclosporin (hypertension), hydroxychloroquine (QT interval prolongation)
Teratogenic, causing both skin and cardiac defects	Alcohol, phenytoin, retinoids
Miscellaneous	
Earlobe crease	CAD
POEMS syndrome	Cardiac failure
Mycosis fungoides, Sézary syndrome	Heart is infiltrated in advanced disease
Kaposi sarcoma	Heart is commonly involved
Diffuse neonatal haemangiomatosis	High-output cardiac failure
Erythroderma, any cause	High-output cardiac failure
Pacemaker reactions	Infection, contact dermatitis, mechanical issues
Clubbing of nails	Cyanotic congenital heart defects
Red lunulae	Occur in CCF

CAD, coronary artery disease; CCF, congestive cardiac failure; CREST, *c*alcinosis, *R*aynaud's phenomenon, *e*sophageal disease, *s*clerodactyly, *t*elangiectasia (syndrome); ECG, electrocardiogram; LEOPARD, *l*entigines, *E*CG abnormalities, *o*cular hypertelorism, *p*ulmonary stenosis, *a*bnormalities of genitalia, *r*etardation of growth, *d*eafness (syndrome); POEMS, *p*olyneuropathy, *o*rganomegaly, *e*ndocrinopathy, *M* protein, *s*kin changes (syndrome); SARS-CoV-2, severe acute respiratory syndrome coronavirus 2.

Lymphoedema–distichiasis syndrome

The lymphoedema–distichiasis syndrome is an autosomal dominant genetic disorder due to mutations in the *FOXC2* gene. Beyond lower-extremity lymphoedema and distichiasis, a condition where eyelashes grow from abnormal locations on the eyelid, it has been linked to cardiac anomalies [4].

Cardiac rhabdomyomas, cardiomyopathy and supraventricular tachycardia are reported in patients with tuberous sclerosis (Chapter 78) [1].

Fabry disease

Synonyms and inclusions
- Angiokeratoma corporis diffusum
- Anderson–Fabry disease

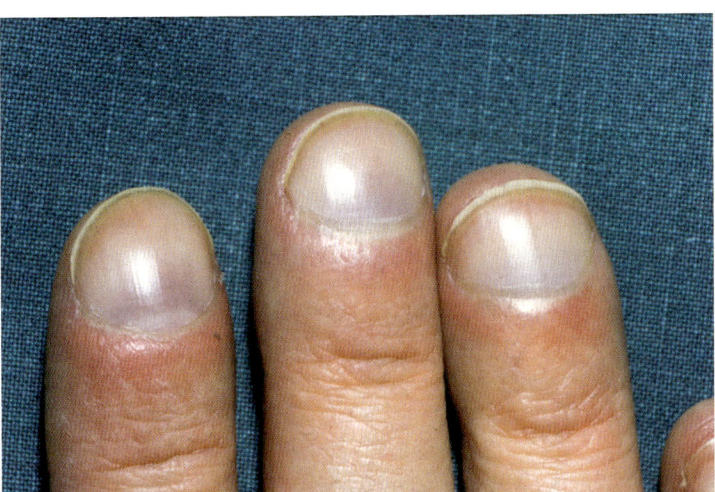

Figure 151.1 Finger clubbing in association with congenital cyanotic heart disease and Eisenmenger syndrome.

In this rare inherited sphingolipidosis, cardiac involvement may be manifest as arrhythmias, hypertrophic cardiomyopathy, valvular abnormalities and coronary artery disease (Chapter 79) [1,2]. The cutaneous features include angiokeratoma corporis diffusum and hypohidrosis or anhidrosis (Figure 151.2) [3].

RASopathies

A number of genetic syndromes have been summarised under the term RASopathies [3]. Amongst them are the Noonan syndrome, Noonan with multiple lentigines syndrome (also known as the LEOPARD syndrome or multiple lentigines syndrome), Costello syndrome, cardiofaciocutaneous syndrome and neurofibromatosis 1. They share the common feature that mutations in the rat sarcoma–mitogen-activated protein kinase (Ras-MAPK) signal transduction pathway are pathogenic and lead to the development of cardiac and cutaneous malformations. The former include hypertrophic cardiomyopathy, pulmonary stenosis and atrial septal defects.

Characteristic for Noonan with multiple lentigines syndrome are widespread lentigines, electrocardiographic abnormalities, ocular hypertelorism, pulmonary stenosis, abnormal genitals, retardation of growth and deafness (hence LEOPARD syndrome). The cardiac involvement includes left axis deviation on an electrocardiogram (ECG), ventricular hypertrophy and arrhythmia.

Carney complex

The Carney complex was previously known as the LAMB (lentigines, atrial myxoma, mucocutaneous myxoma, blue naevi) syndrome or the NAME (blue naevi, atrial myxoma, myxoid neurofibromas, ephelides) syndrome. It is a result of mutations in the *PRKAR1A* gene (protein kinase, cAMP-dependent, regulatory, type I, alpha) [3,5]. The inheritance is autosomal dominant with incomplete penetrance. It is characterised by recurrent myxomas,

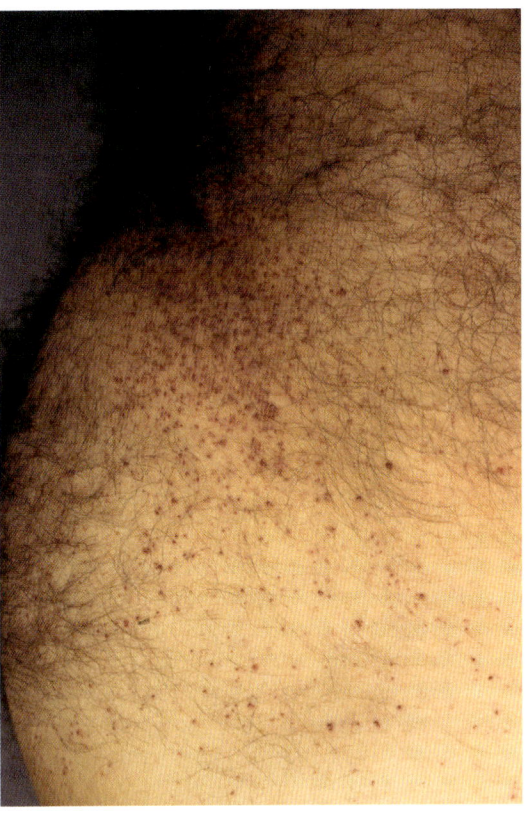

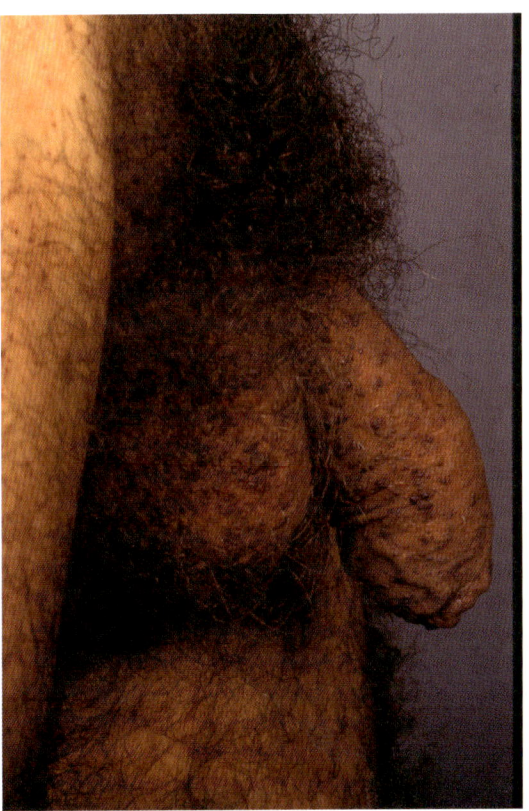

Figure 151.2 Fabry disease in a 46-year-old man with extensive involvement of (a) the buttocks and (b) the genitalia.

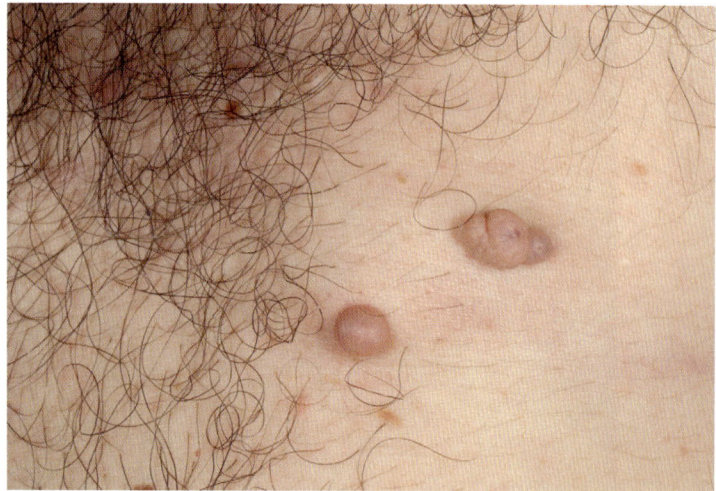

Figure 151.3 Cutaneous myxoma in a patient with Carney complex.

pigmented skin lesions, endocrine overactivity and neoplasms (e.g. growth hormone-producing adenoma often with acromegaly, Sertoli cell tumours and Cushing syndrome) [5]. Nearly 70% of patients have myxomatous cardiac tumours. Mucocutaneous myxomas (eyelids, external ear, breast and oro-pharynx) are present in one-third of patients (Figure 151.3). Pigmentary abnormalities such as blue naevi, café-au-lait macules and lentigines are commonly seen (in 75% of cases) [5].

CARDIAC INVOLVEMENT IN DERMATOSES OR SYSTEMIC DISEASES WITH SKIN FEATURES

INFLAMMATORY DISORDERS

Cardiac involvement is common in systemic disorders such as sarcoidosis (Chapter 96) [6], mixed connective tissue disease (Chapter 53) [7], dermatomyositis (Chapter 52) [7], lupus erythematosus (Chapter 51) [8,9], systemic sclerosis (see Chapter 54) [10] and vasculitis (Chapter 100) [11,12], although it may be underestimated if symptoms are absent.

Sarcoidosis. Up to 25% of patients with sarcoidosis have heart involvement. Sudden death due to conduction defects and ventricular arrhythmias is the most important complication and is particularly well recognised in sarcoidosis. Cardiomyopathy may also occur [6].

Mixed connective tissue disease. Clinically significant pericarditis, myocarditis and pulmonary hypertension may occur in mixed connective tissue disease, but this is rare [7].

Dermatomyositis. The heart may be involved in dermatomyositis or polymyositis with the occurrence of congestive heart failure, coronary artery disease or conduction abnormalities [7].

Systemic lupus erythematosus. Cardiovascular disease is very frequent in systemic lupus erythematosus [8]. A number of cardiac complications occur, especially pericarditis, a high prevalence of atherosclerosis and an increased risk of myocardial infarction.

Neonatal lupus erythematosus. A congenital atrioventricular block (AVB) is the most common cardiovascular symptom of neonatal lupus erythematosus (LE). Mothers of affected children generally express the 52 and 60 kDa anti-SS-A (Ro) antibodies, even if they have no other features of LE [9]. Beyond AVB, the spectrum of heart involvement in neonatal LE varies widely and includes not only valve defects, but also cardiomyopathy or myocarditis.

Systemic sclerosis. Cardiac involvement in systemic sclerosis is not always clinically apparent but is believed to be a poor prognostic factor. Pericarditis, pericardial effusion, arrhythmias, myocardial fibrosis, conduction system defects, endothelial damage to coronary arteries and heart failure due to pulmonary arterial hypertension all occur [10]. Symptoms include heart failure, palpitations and myocardial infarction.

Antiphospholipid syndrome. In the antiphospholipid syndrome [13], about 50% of patients have valvular heart disease, either vegetations or thickening (Chapter 51). The mitral valve is most frequently affected. There is also an increased incidence of atherosclerosis, coronary artery disease and myocardial infarction.

Vasculitides. The major vasculitides that affect the heart belong to one of the following groups: (i) small-vessel vasculitis (granulomatosis with polyangiitis (GPA), eosinophilic GPA (EGPA)); (ii) medium-vessel vasculitis (polyarteritis nodosa, Kawasaki disease); or (iii) large-vessel vasculitis (temporal arteritis, Takayasu arteritis) [11]. Cardiac involvement is commoner in EGPA than in GPA [12].

Amyloidosis. Cardiac involvement is frequent in primary amyloidosis [2,14], causing features of cardiomyopathy such as congestive heart failure, low voltage on an ECG and conduction disturbances. Cutaneous signs, macroglossia and demonstration of amyloid deposition on skin histology support the diagnosis (Chapter 56).

Kawasaki disease. Kawasaki disease (mucocutaneous lymph node syndrome) is an acute febrile disease principally of infants and children (Figure 151.4) and is due to an immune-mediated medium vessel vasculitis that affects the coronary arteries (Chapter 26). Clinical manifestations are prolonged fever and signs of acute inflammation [2]. Coronary artery aneurysms may develop in up to 25% of patients; other cardiac sequelae include myocardial infarction, conduction defects, pericardial effusion and cardiomegaly.

Coronavirus disease in 2019 (Covid-19) led to a global pandemic starting in 2020. Shortly after the onset of the pandemic, first reports of children affected by a Kawasaki-like disease in the context of SARS-CoV-2 (severe acute respiratory syndrome coronavirus 2) infection were published from Europe and North America. This syndrome is referred to as paediatric inflammatory multisystem syndrome temporally associated with SARS-CoV-2

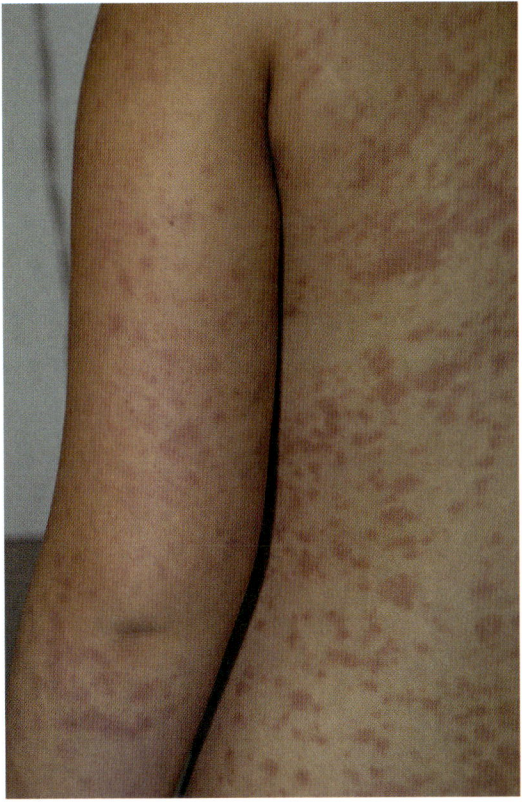
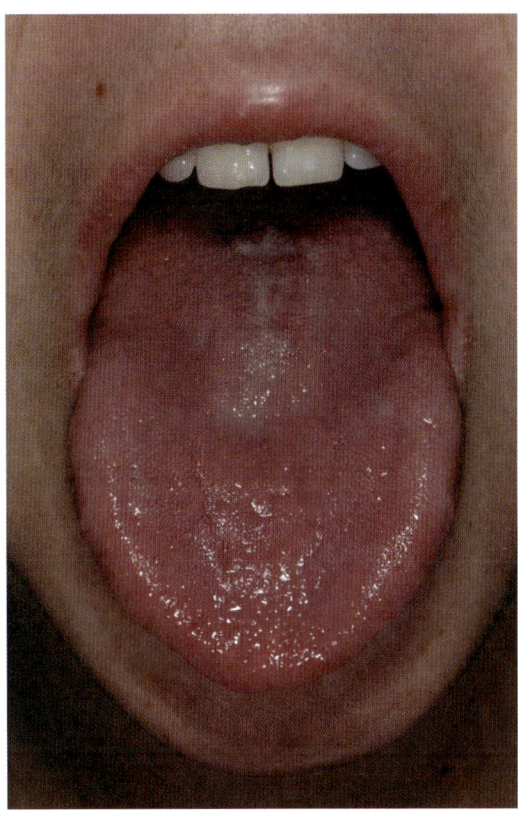

Figure 151.4 Kawasaki syndrome in a 16-year-old girl showing (a) a rash on her body and (b) the characteristic 'strawberry tongue'.

infection (PIMS-TS) or multisystem inflammatory syndrome in children (MIS(-C)) [15]. It predominantly affects the cardiovascular system, gastrointestinal tract or neurological organ systems. A rate of 79% of cardiovascular involvement is described with tachycardia, haemodynamic shock, myocarditis, decreased left ventricular ejection fraction (LVEF) and coronary aneurysm and dilatation [15].

INFECTIONS

Infective endocarditis. Infective endocarditis [2] typically occurs in patients with a past history of heart disease (rheumatic fever, congenital heart disease, degenerative valve disease, heart valve operation), intravenous drug use or recent dental surgery. Around 50% of cases of infective endocarditis develop in patients without a history of valve disease [16]. Up to 80% of cases are caused by staphylococcal or streptococcal infection. Cutaneous lesions may represent either septic emboli or immune complex disease due to circulating bacterial antigens [2]. The skin lesions may be purpuric, pustular or red (note variations in skin of colour) and other patterns are described. Splinter haemorrhages of the nail fold or nail bed occur as well as conjunctival and palatal petechiae. Osler nodes are small, tender, red papules situated mainly on the distal finger and toe pads; Janeway lesions are faint, red, macular lesions on the thenar and hypothenar eminences.

Rheumatic fever. Rheumatic fever is a complication of streptococcal infection [2]. It causes arthritis, carditis, neuromuscular disease (e.g. Sydenham chorea, muscle weakness) and cutaneous lesions. The latter include erythema marginatum and subcutaneous nodules on the extensor surface of the extremities, particularly near the joints. Erythema marginatum is a transitory gyrate redness located mainly on the trunk and proximal extremities (Figure 151.5). Cardiac features include valvular disease, pericarditis, myocarditis and congestive heart failure.

SARS-CoV-2. See Kawasaki disease section under Inflammatory disorders.

MISCELLANEOUS

Coronary artery disease. Coronary artery disease and ischaemic heart disease may occur in premature ageing syndromes such as progeria and Werner syndrome. Premature atherosclerotic vascular disease has also been reported in pseudoxanthoma elasticum [3]. Coronary artery disease may be associated with xanthelasma or xanthomas due to hyperlipidaemia [2]. The presence of a diagonal earlobe skin crease (Frank sign) has been linked with coronary artery disease. This issue has been a matter of controversy over the years but current studies show a high positive correlation [17]. The coronary arteries are also involved in Kawasaki disease.

Skin problems related to cardiac pacemakers and implantable defibrillators. Cutaneous reactions over the site of implanted cardiac pacemakers have been reported. Most of these are either infections or mechanical problems (erosions, extrusions, capsular contracture, exposed generator or electrodes, bronchopleural cutaneous fistulae) and may respond to antibiotics or altered positioning of the pacemaker [18,19]. Contact dermatitis from implanted cardiac

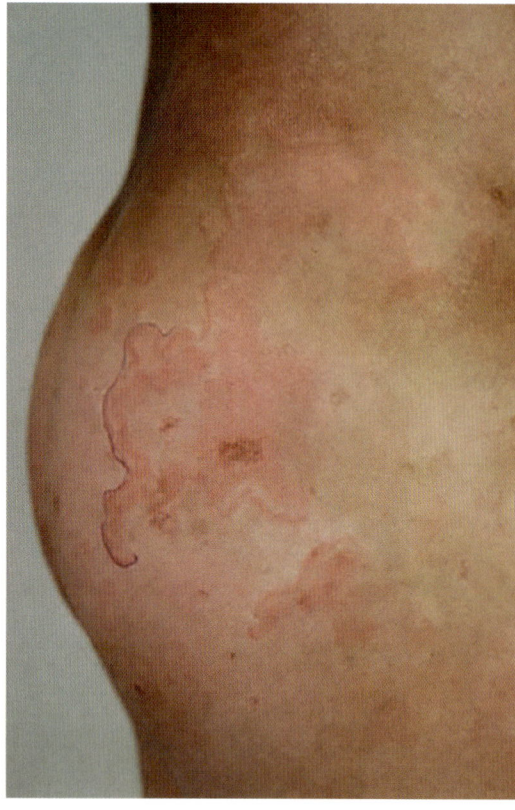

Figure 151.5 Erythema marginatum (rheumatic fever). Reproduced with permission of DermNet New Zealand Trust. https://dermnetnz.org/topics/rheumatic-fever.

rhythm devices is rare; allergies to cobalt, epoxy resin, mercury, nickel, titanium and gold stents have all been described [20].

Key references

The full list of references can be found in the online version at https://www.wiley.com/rooksdermatology10e

1 Abdelmalek NF, Gerber TL, Menter A. Cardiocutaneous syndromes and associations. *J Am Acad Dermatol* 2002;46:161–83.
2 Uliasz A, Lebwohl M. Cutaneous manifestations of cardiovascular diseases. *Clin Dermatol* 2008;26:243–54.
3 O'Neill JL, Narahari S, Sane DC *et al*. Cardiac manifestations of cutaneous disorders. *J Am Acad Dermatol* 2013;68:156–66.
5 Shetty Roy AN, Radin M, Sarabi D *et al*. Familial recurrent atrial myxoma: Carney's complex. *Clin Cardiol* 2011;34:83–6.
8 Frostegård J. Systemic lupus erythematosus and cardiovascular disease. *Lupus* 2008;17:364–7.
11 Jennette JC. Overview of the 2012 revised International Chapel Hill Consensus Conference nomenclature of vasculitides. *Clin Exp Nephrol* 2013;17:603–6.
12 Millet A, Pederzoli-Ribeil M, Guillevin L *et al*. Antineutrophil cytoplasmic antibody-associated vasculitides: is it time to split up the group? *Ann Rheum Dis* 2013;72:1273–9.
15 Hoste L, Van Paemel R, Haerynck F. Multisystem inflammatory syndrome in children related to COVID-19: a systematic review. *Eur J Pediatr* 2021;180:2019–34.
16 Hoen B, Duval X. Clinical practice. Infective endocarditis. *N Engl J Med* 2013;368:1425–33.
17 Shmilovich H, Cheng VY, Rajani R *et al*. Relation of diagonal ear lobe crease to the presence, extent, and severity of coronary artery disease determined by coronary computed tomography angiography. *Am J Cardiol* 2012;109:1283–7.
20 Kang J, Simpson CS, Campbell D *et al*. Cardiac rhythm device contact dermatitis. *Ann Noninvasive Electrocardiol* 2013;18:79–83.

CHAPTER 152

The Skin and Disorders of the Respiratory System

Sonja Molin[1] and Thomas Ruzicka[2]

[1] Division of Dermatology, Queen's University, Kingston, Canada
[2] Department of Dermatology and Allergology, Ludwig Maximilian University, Munich, Germany

Introduction, 152.1	Small-vessel vasculitis, 152.3	NEUTROPHILIC DERMATOSES, 152.5
ALLERGIC DISORDERS, 152.1	Variable-vessel vasculitis, 152.4	OTHER SYSTEMIC DISEASES, 152.5
AUTOIMMUNE DISORDERS, 152.2	INFECTIONS, 152.4	MISCELLANEOUS DISORDERS, 152.6
VASCULITIS, 152.3	CONGENITAL AND INHERITED DISORDERS/GENETIC SYNDROMES, 152.5	Key references, 152.7

Introduction

There are many disorders that affect both the skin and the respiratory system, ranging from common infections and allergies to complex multisystem diseases. This chapter examines the relationship between these two organ systems and discusses selected disorders from amongst the diverse groups of diseases that may affect both (Table 152.1). After a brief discussion of allergic disorders affecting the upper respiratory tract, the chapter focuses on pulmonary involvement in autoimmune disorders, vasculitides, infections and hereditary syndromes.

The mucosa of the upper respiratory tract may be affected by the same processes as the skin in a range of infective and allergic disorders.

Pulmonary disease rarely occurs as a direct consequence of a primary skin disease, except for instances such as metastasis from a primary skin tumour (e.g. melanoma). Similarly, there are relatively few instances in which skin abnormalities occur as a direct consequence of respiratory pathology. Examples include cyanosis due to severe pulmonary disease or intrapulmonary right-to-left shunts, and finger clubbing due to chronic cyanotic lung disease or neoplasm.

Some drugs used for the treatment of pulmonary disease may cause side effects on the skin and vice versa. A very few drugs may cause skin symptoms and respiratory tract disease at the same time (e.g. cisplatin).

ALLERGIC DISORDERS

The respiratory system is frequently involved in allergic reactions, particularly those due to type I allergic sensitisation. Amongst the atopic disorders, *allergic rhinoconjunctivitis* and *allergic asthma*

Table 152.1 Conditions that affect the skin and respiratory system.

Disease	Respiratory system features
Inflammatory	
Sarcoidosis	Pulmonary fibrosis, hilar lymphadenopathy, laryngeal involvement, necrotising sarcoid granulomatosis
Pulmonary vasculitides	See text for further information (in this section)
Systemic sclerosis	Interstitial fibrosis, pneumothorax, pulmonary hypertension
Sjögren syndrome	Decreased secretions, sinusitis, bronchoalveolitis, interstitial lung disease
Lupus erythematosus	Pleuritis, pleural effusion, shrinking lungs syndrome
Mixed connective tissue disease	Fibrosing alveolitis (especially U_1 ribonucleoprotein antibody positive)
Antiphospholipid syndrome	Pulmonary embolism, infarction, thrombosis, haemorrhage
Dermatomyositis	Muscular weakness, pharyngeal dysfunction (aspiration pneumonia), interstitial lung disease, bronchiolitis obliterans
Relapsing polychondritis	Tracheal collapse
Multicentric reticulohistiocytosis	May be associated with bronchial neoplasia, lung infiltration, pleural effusion
Bullous diseases (epidermolysis bullosa, pemphigus, Stevens–Johnson syndrome, toxic epidermal necrolysis)	Upper respiratory tract involvement; paraneoplastic pemphigus is associated with intrathoracic disease, especially Castleman disease, thymoma
Graft-versus-host disease	Restrictive defect, fibrosis
Pyoderma gangrenosum	Neutrophilic nodules in lung, tracheal involvement
Familial Mediterranean fever	Pleurisy
Infections and infestations	
Tuberculosis	Specific skin lesions, erythema nodosum
Mycobacterium avium–intracellulare infection	May disseminate to skin (usually in HIV infection)
Leprosy	Laryngeal involvement
Mycoplasma infection	Causes erythema multiforme (often mucosal)
Dissemination of pulmonary fungal infections	Blastomycosis, coccidioidomycosis, cryptococcosis, aspergillosis, histoplasmosis, melioidosis
Scrub typhus	Pneumonia (common)

(continued)

Rook's Textbook of Dermatology, Tenth Edition. Edited by Christopher Griffiths, Jonathan Barker, Tanya Bleiker, Walayat Hussain and Rosalind Simpson.
© 2024 John Wiley & Sons Ltd. Published 2024 by John Wiley & Sons Ltd.

Table 152.1 (continued)

Disease	Respiratory system features
SARS-CoV-2	Symptoms vary depending on severity of disease course: cold-like symptoms, pneumonia, hypoxaemic respiratory failure/respiratory distress syndrome
	Variety of cutaneous manifestations: pseudo-chilblain lesions, maculo-papular exanthema, urticarial or vesicular lesions
Varicella	Pneumonia
Measles	Pneumonia
Larva migrans	Asthma/bronchitis with eosinophilia
Chronic mucocutaneous candidiasis	Bronchiectasis
Whipple disease	Cough, pleural effusion, pulmonary infiltrate, hilar lymphadenopathy
Congenital/inherited	
Atopic disease	Asthma, hay fever
Cutis laxa	Emphysema, cor pulmonale
Tuberous sclerosis	Rhabdomyomas
Neurofibromatosis	Kyphoscoliosis, intrathoracic neuromas, lung fibrosis, bullae
Ataxia-telangiectasia	Pneumonia, bronchiectasis, pulmonary fibrosis
Hereditary haemorrhagic telangiectasia	Haemoptysis, dyspnoea, cyanosis due to arteriovenous shunting
α_1-antitrypsin deficiency	Emphysema
Darier disease	Lower lobe fibrosis, laryngeal involvement
Dyskeratosis congenita	Interstitial pneumonia, fibrosis
Lipoid proteinosis	Laryngeal involvement
Riley–Day syndrome	Lung infiltrate, pneumonia
Birt–Hogg–Dubé syndrome	Lung cysts, pneumothorax
Hyper-IgE syndrome	Abscesses, pneumonia
Infiltrations and metabolic	
Histiocytoses (Langerhans cell histiocytosis, Rosai–Dorfman disease, haematophagocytic syndrome, necrobiotic xanthogranuloma, sea-blue histiocytosis, others)	Pulmonary nodules and fibrosis, upper respiratory tract infiltration disease, xanthoma disseminatum
Amyloidosis	Cutaneous amyloid deposition secondary to chronic lung disease, lung infiltration in primary amyloidosis
POEMS syndrome	Pleural effusion, bronchospasm
Carcinoid syndrome	Bronchospasm
Hypothyroidism	Laryngeal involvement
Myxoma	Pleurisy
Drugs	
Used in respiratory disease, causing rash, phototoxicity	Co-trimoxazole (drug eruptions), pirfenidone
May cause skin eruptions and respiratory tract disease	Antibiotic-induced toxic epidermal necrolysis, cisplatin (bronchospasm, pigmentation)
Used for skin disease, respiratory side effects	Isotretinoin (bronchospasm), methotrexate (lung fibrosis, pneumonitis), mycophenolate mofetil (lung fibrosis)
Miscellaneous	
Angio-oedema	Upper airway obstruction
Anaphylaxis	Bronchospasm
Pancreatitis	Basal pleural reaction, cutaneous fat necrosis
Yellow nail syndrome	Pleural effusion, bronchiectasis
Mastocytosis	Rhinorrhoea, laryngeal oedema, bronchospasm
Tumours	Metastatic disease, Kaposi sarcoma, lymphomatoid granulomatosis, extensive mycosis fungoides/Sézary syndrome

HIV, human immunodeficiency virus; POEMS, polyneuropathy, organomegaly, endocrinopathy, *M* protein, *skin* changes; SARS-CoV-2, severe acute respiratory syndrome coronavirus 2.

affect the respiratory tract and contribute significantly to the burden of disease in many individuals who also have atopic eczema. Angio-oedema is a component part of urticaria (Figure 152.1) and can cause life-threatening pharyngeal and laryngeal oedema, most commonly in the context of *IgE-mediated anaphylaxis*. These conditions are addressed in Chapters 41, 42 and 43.

AUTOIMMUNE DISORDERS

Amongst autoimmune disorders, it is the connective tissue diseases in particular that may affect both organs.

Respiratory disease is the second most common clinical manifestation of *systemic sclerosis* (Chapter 54), with a prevalence of between 25% and 90% [1]. Systemic sclerosis is associated with interstitial lung disease and pulmonary vascular disease leading to pulmonary hypertension. In addition, bronchiectases are found in up to 68% of patients on high-resolution computer tomography. Pneumothorax, pleural effusion, respiratory muscle involvement and 'splinting' of the chest by sclerotic skin may all occur.

The proportion of patients with *systemic lupus erythematosus* (SLE) (Chapter 51) who develop pulmonary disease is variable in reported series [2]. The clinical manifestations involve all compartments of the respiratory tract (pleura, parenchyma, vessels and airways) and can follow an acute or chronic course. Pleuritis, pulmonary hypertension or interstitial lung disease may be present in *mixed connective tissue disease* [3]. Involvement of the respiratory muscles may lead to diaphragmatic elevation and the '*shrinking lungs*' syndrome [4]. Pulmonary embolism, haemorrhage, infarction and hypertension as well as thrombosis of the lung vessels may occur in patients with the *antiphospholipid syndrome* (Chapter 51) [5].

Relapsing polychondritis (Chapter 155) [6] is due to autoantibodies against type II collagen and is a potentially fatal disease. Dyspnoea and inspiratory stridor occur in over 50% of patients as a result of oedema of the respiratory tract mucosa and collapse of the cartilaginous support of the larynx and trachea. Inflamed nasal and auricular cartilages are present in most patients, with nasal obstruction, arthropathy and a high erythrocyte sedimentation rate. Costal cartilage is involved in one-third of cases. The non-cartilaginous lobe of the ear is classically spared in relapsing polychondritis.

In *dermatomyositis* (Chapter 52), there are three main mechanisms that provide a link with respiratory disease [7]. Firstly, dermatomyositis may occur as a consequence of bronchial carcinoma. Secondly, muscular weakness due to myositis may affect either the intercostal and thoracic musculature, or the larynx and pharynx – involvement of the latter may lead to aspiration pneumonia as a complication. Finally, interstitial lung disease or bronchiolitis obliterans may occur in dermatomyositis. The lung disease is typically associated with the presence of antiaminoacyl transfer RNA (tRNA) synthetase antibodies, such as the histidyl tRNA synthetase (Jo-1) antibody. The *antisynthetase syndrome* consists of dermatomyositis (or polymyositis) with interstitial lung disease, arthritis and Raynaud phenomenon [8]. The presence of antisynthetase antibodies is also associated with the clinical entity of 'mechanics' hands' in dermatomyositis, characterised by hyperkeratotic skin on the lateral aspects of the fingers. Dermatomyositis may also indirectly be associated with lung disease as a

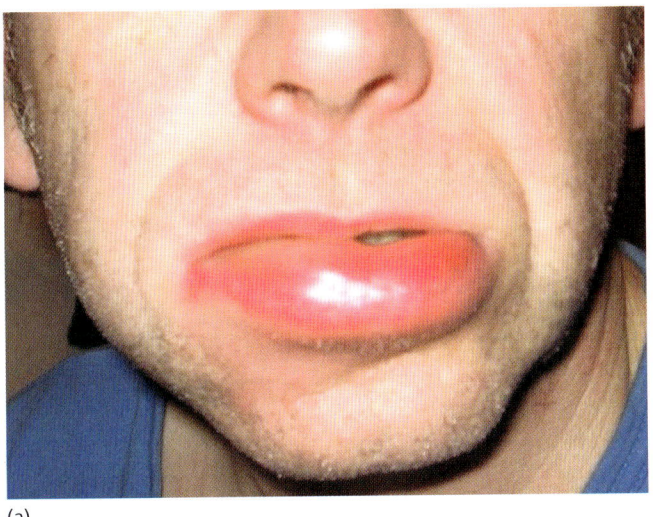
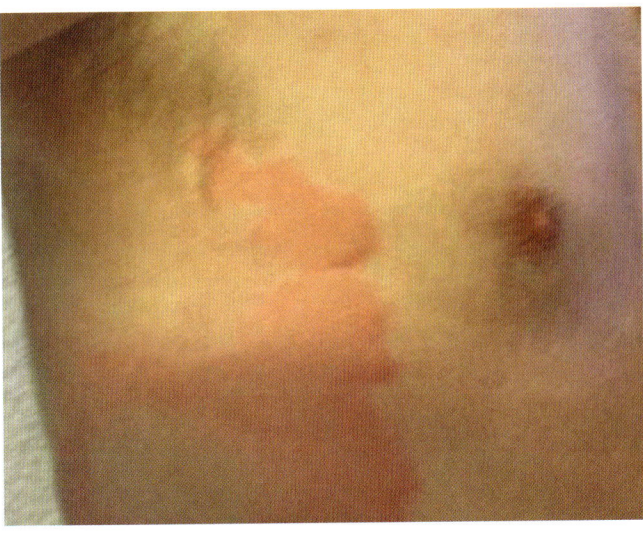
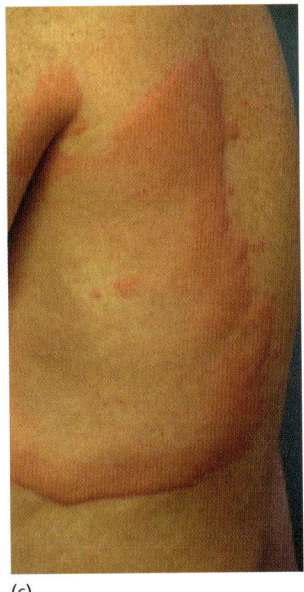

Figure 152.1 Acute angio-oedema and giant urticaria.

consequence of treatment – either infection due to immunosuppression or, rarely, drug-induced pneumonitis (methotrexate), which may cause diagnostic confusion with pulmonary involvement by the disease itself.

In *Sjögren syndrome* (Chapter 53), the frequency of lung involvement varies between 9% and 75%. It can affect the small airways but may also present with interstitial lung disease [9]. Alveolitis can be demonstrated in about 50% of patients but is often asymptomatic.

VASCULITIS

Vasculitis of many types may affect the lung (Chapter 100). The major pulmonary vasculitides belong either to the group of small-vessel vasculitis or variable-vessel vasculitis [10].

Small-vessel vasculitis

Any form of systemic small-vessel vasculitis (SVV) can affect the lung. According to current classifications [10], SVV can be divided into antineutrophil cytoplasmic antibody (ANCA) associated vasculitis and immune complex SVV. The ANCA-associated forms are: granulomatosis with polyangiitis (GPA), eosinophilic GPA (EGPA, formerly the Churg–Strauss syndrome) and microscopic polyangiitis (MPA).

Granulomatosis with polyangiitis [11–13]. This rare disease is characterised by necrotising granulomatous vasculitis of the upper and lower respiratory tracts, necrotising glomerulonephritis, and disseminated vasculitis of various organs. ANCAs directed against proteinase 3 are found in 40–95% of cases. Skin lesions are present in 30–60% of patients, including vasculitis with purpura, subcutaneous nodules and ulcers (Chapter 100). Upper airway disease causes nasal discharge, ulceration and bleeding, and may be associated with oral ulceration. Pulmonary changes are typical with bilateral infiltrates, nodules or cavities. Subglottic or tracheobronchostenosis may also occur. Prognosis is poor in patients with lung or renal disease. Chronic nasal staphylococcal carriage is more frequent in GPA than in healthy controls and is associated with a poorer prognosis and a higher relapse rate [11]. Diffuse alveolar haemorrhage, due to extensive pulmonary capillaritis, is a life-threatening complication of GPA; it also occurs in MPA, and more rarely in SLE, antiphospholipid syndrome, Behçet disease and secondary to drugs such as D-penicillamine [14].

Eosinophilic granulomatosis with polyangiitis (Churg–Strauss syndrome) [12,13]. This rare condition comprises rhinitis, asthma, pneumonitis, fever, malaise, eosinophilia (usually over 10%) and widespread vasculitis, which may cause skin lesions, neuropathy and cardiac or, less commonly, renal disease. Cutaneous lesions include palpable purpura and nodular lesions and are present in up to 70% of patients (Figure 152.2). ANCAs are not present in all cases of EGPA. They may be helpful in differentiating the disease into two subgroups: one with more vasculitic and one with more eosinophilic manifestations. The latter ANCA-negative subgroup is

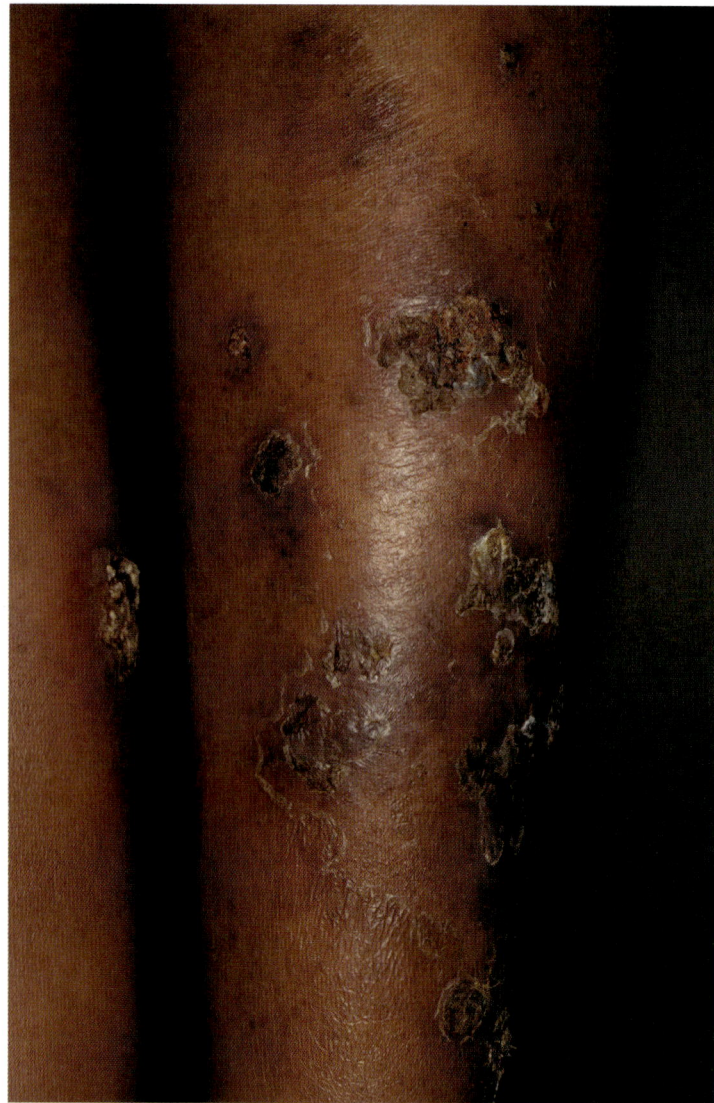

Figure 152.2 Eosinophilic granulomatosis with polyangiitis.

reported to have endomyocardial involvement and lung infiltrates more often [15]. The ANCAs detected in EGPA are directed against myeloperoxidase in 32–92% of cases [11].

Microscopic polyangiitis. ANCAs against myeloperoxidase (MPO-ANCA) can be found in up to 80% of patients with MPA [11]. It is a necrotising form of vasculitis that predominantly affects small vessels: arterioles, venules and capillaries may all be affected. Lung involvement is reported in 20–60% and skin involvement in 40–70% of cases [11]. Common pulmonary clinical symptoms are dyspnoea, cough and haemoptysis. Alveolar haemorrhage can occur in up to a third of MPA patients [16].

Immune complex small-vessel vasculitis. Pathognomonic are vessel wall deposits of immunoglobulin and complement factors that predominantly affect the small vessels. Urticarial vasculitis, cryoglobulinaemic vasculitis and IgA vasculitis (Henoch–Schönlein purpura) belong to this subgroup [10]. In urticarial vasculitis, pulmonary involvement is common and comprises pleuritis and obstructive lung disease [17]. In one large series, over 20% of patients with urticarial vasculitis had lung involvement, either chronic obstructive pulmonary disease or asthma. Although it is not clear that these were always causally related to the vasculitis, obstructive pulmonary disease was more frequent in the group of patients with hypocomplementaemia [18], and pulmonary vasculitis was demonstrated in over 50% of patients with lung disease.

Variable-vessel vasculitis

Behçet disease. Behçet disease has been classified amongst the variable-vessel vasculitis group [10], although it also has many features of an autoinflammatory disease (Figure 152.3) [19]. The frequency of lung involvement in Behçet disease shows a wide variation, from <1% to 18%. Pulmonary involvement can be classified into three groups: pulmonary artery aneurysm, parenchymal changes and a subgroup of diverse pulmonary disorders including pleural effusion. Thrombophlebitis may be a marker for an increased risk of pulmonary artery aneurysm as about 80% of patients with this complication also have thrombophlebitis [20].

INFECTIONS

Numerous infections may involve both the respiratory tract and the skin: a selection of these have been listed in Table 152.1. Many viral infections, for example, may cause upper and sometimes lower respiratory tract symptoms in association with either a non-specific exanthem or with erythema multiforme. *Mycoplasma* infection is particularly associated with Stevens–Johnson syndrome. *Psittacosis* (ornithosis) may be accompanied by erythema nodosum and erythema multiforme.

SARS-CoV-2 (severe acute respiratory syndrome coronavirus 2) led to a global pandemic starting in 2020. Coronavirus disease 2019 (Covid-19) ranges from mild cases with cold-like symptoms to severe cases with pneumonia and hypoxaemic respiratory failure. Shortly after the onset of the pandemic, reports emerged describing various cutaneous manifestations associated with Covid-19. They are discussed in Chapter 25 in more detail. Their morphology and prevalence seem to vary geographically. Pseudo-chilblains, maculo-papular exanthema, vesicular or urticarial lesions, vaso-occlusive lesions like livedo racemosa or retiform purpura have been described [21].

Associations between *tuberculosis* and the skin include non-specific reactions such as erythema nodosum or erythema multiforme, as well as several patterns of specific skin lesions such as lichen scrofulosorum, Bazin disease and papulonecrotic tuberculide (Chapter 27). Several *systemic mycoses* (Chapter 32) are caused by inhalation but may subsequently cause skin lesions, either non-specific reactions including erythema multiforme and erythema nodosum, or specific lesions caused by haematogenous dissemination. Other mycoses may have primary cutaneous lesions with occasional spread to internal organs, including the lung (e.g. sporotrichosis).

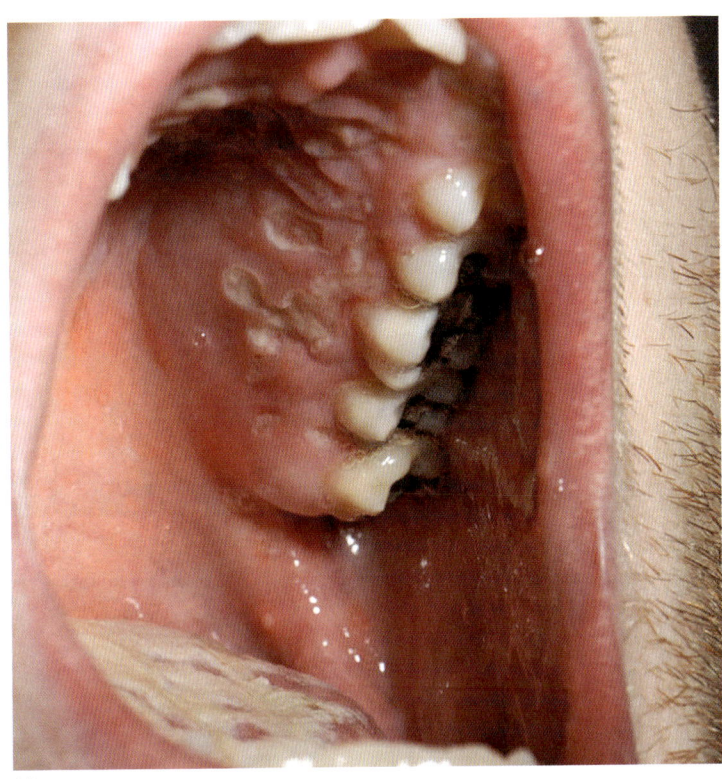

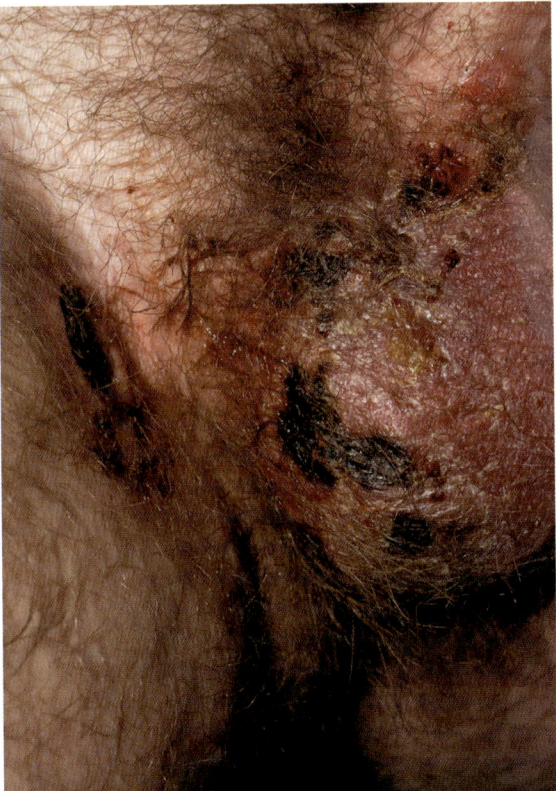

Figure 152.3 Behçet disease with ulceration of (a) the hard palate and (b) the scrotum and perigenital skin.

CONGENITAL AND INHERITED DISORDERS/GENETIC SYNDROMES

Examples are listed in Table 152.1.

Neurofibromatosis 1 (Chapter 78). This is not uncommonly associated with the development of lung disease as a result of kyphoscoliosis. Intrathoracic, intra-abdominal or retroperitoneal diffuse plexiform neurofibromas can also compromise pulmonary function. Fibrosis affects mainly the lower lobes whereas bullous changes may occur in the upper lobes [22].

Tuberous sclerosis. Pleural effusions have been reported in tuberous sclerosis [23] (Chapter 78). Pulmonary involvement is uncommon but, especially in adult female patients, there may be numerous small cysts that represent lymphangioleiomyomatosis [24]. These may be mistaken for tuberculosis or sarcoidosis radiologically.

α_1-antitrypsin deficiency. α_1-antitrypsin deficiency, particularly the ZZ genotype, links cutaneous panniculitis with emphysema and hepatic cirrhosis [25].

Familial dysautonomia. In familial dysautonomia (Riley–Day syndrome), there are acute episodes of bronchopneumonia with profuse mucus secretion causing dyspnoea. Skin changes include multiple excoriations, and pink to red mottling associated with fever and sweating [26]. Radiological features of lung disease [27] may be accompanied by abdominal distension as the 'chest–abdomen' sign [28].

Ataxia-telangiectasia. Ataxia-telangiectasia (Louis-Bar syndrome) may be associated with pulmonary problems, including recurrent pneumonia, bronchiectasis and pulmonary fibrosis [29].

Birt–Hogg–Dubé syndrome. Lung cysts and pneumothorax can occur in Birt–Hogg–Dubé syndrome (Chapters 78 and 154).

NEUTROPHILIC DERMATOSES

Pulmonary and major airway involvement has been described with *pyoderma gangrenosum* and with *neutrophilic dermatoses* [30,31], usually comprising focal, dense neutrophilic infiltrates with scattered radiological opacities. In *Sweet syndrome*, the principal clinical symptoms of lung involvement are dyspnoea, cough and general malaise. Endobronchial involvement may also occur in eosinophilic states such as the *hypereosinophilic syndrome*, although cardiac disease is more important in this condition. See also Chapter 49.

OTHER SYSTEMIC DISEASES

Sarcoidosis (Chapter 96). Hilar lymphadenopathy occurs with erythema nodosum in acute sarcoidosis (Löfgren syndrome). Pulmonary involvement is the major feature in chronic sarcoidosis [32].

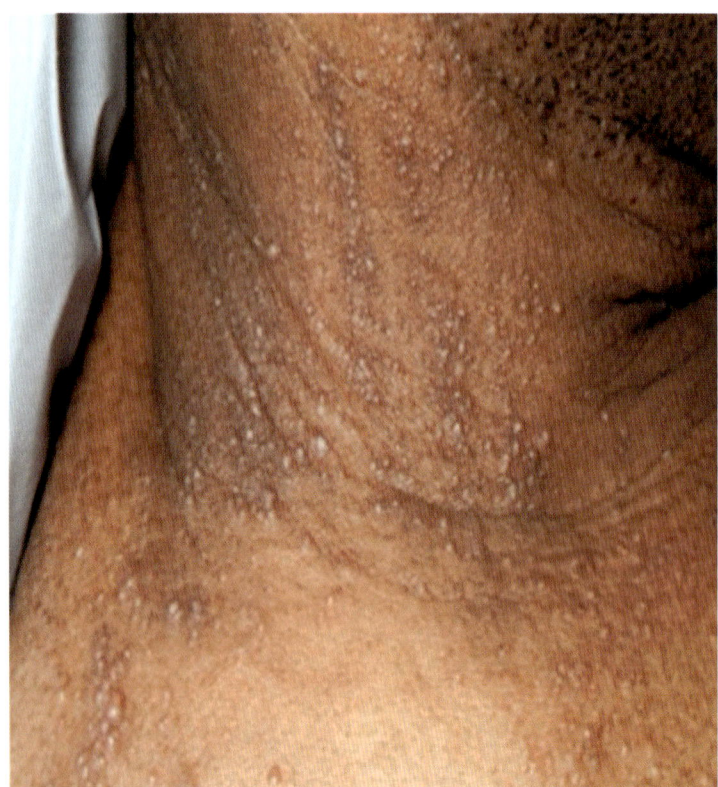

Figure 152.4 Scleromyxoedema with typical linear arrays of dermal papules on the neck.

Necrotising sarcoid granulomatosis. This is a very rare disorder of unknown aetiology [33]. In the respiratory system, a nodular pulmonary infiltrate is typical as well as local pleural thickening or effusion. Extrapulmonary involvement may be ophthalmological (uveitis) but other organs including the skin [34] may be involved, and erythema nodosum or necrosis due to arteritic vascular occlusion may be a feature.

Multicentric reticulohistiocytosis (Chapter 135). Multicentric reticulohistiocytosis is associated with pleural effusion [35]; it may also occur as a paraneoplastic phenomenon.

Scleromyxoedema (Chapter 57). Scleromyxoedema has been associated with lung disease, mainly causing dyspnoea (Figure 152.4) [36].

Amyloidosis (Chapter 56). Involvement of the respiratory tract is common in primary amyloidosis. It may cause dyspnoea but is often asymptomatic.

Lymphomatoid granulomatosis (Chapter 139). This is a rare Epstein–Barr virus infection-driven lymphoproliferative disease in which the lung is involved in more than 90% of patients [37]. Radiology shows multiple small nodules that affect predominantly the periphery of the lower lung fields. Cutaneous lesions are present in 25–50% of cases, typically on the extremities, and consist of infiltrated flat or nodular lesions that may become necrotic and ulcerated.

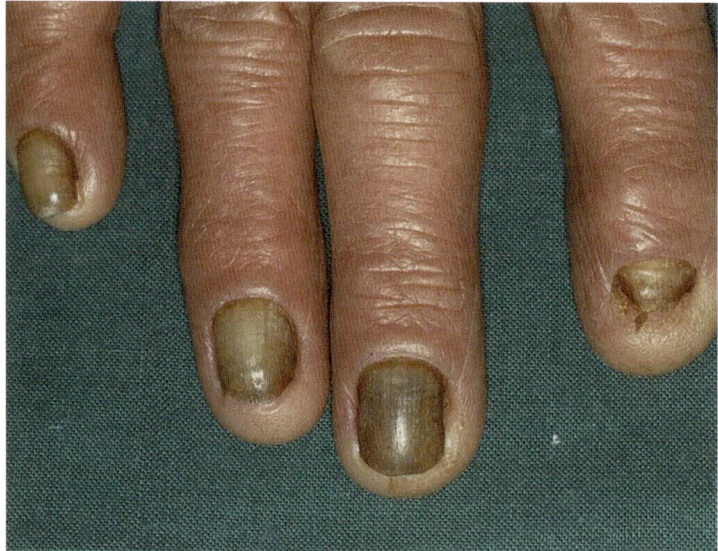

(a)

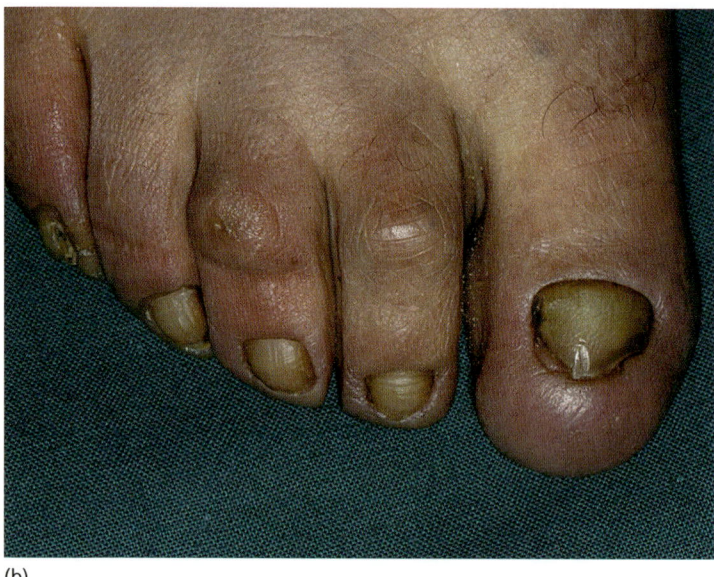

(b)

Figure 152.5 Yellow nail syndrome affecting the nails of (a) the fingers and (b) the toes.

Yellow nail syndrome (Chapter 93). Yellow nail syndrome (Figure 152.5) is associated with a diverse array of respiratory abnormalities including dyspnoea or cough, pleural effusion, bronchiectasis and chronic sinus and lung infections [38].

MISCELLANEOUS DISORDERS

Paraneoplastic pemphigus (Chapter 148). Respiratory failure in paraneoplastic pemphigus (PNP) is particularly important as it might be the cause of death in patients with this disorder. Pathologically, there is a diffuse, segmental, constrictive bronchiolitis of the small bronchioles causing a bronchiolitis obliterans clinical picture. The mechanism may be due to autoantibody-mediated damage, as direct immunofluorescence of bronchial mucosal biopsies may demonstrate linear deposition of IgG and complement in the lamina propria [39]. CD8+ T-lymphocytes may also play a key role in this process [40]. An ectopic expression of desmoglein 3 and other epidermal antigens might explain the pulmonary involvement in PNP [41]. The underlying neoplasm, toxic effects of immunosuppressive therapy and secondary infection may all contribute to the pulmonary morbidity.

> **Box 152.1 Examples of disorders with skin and systemic manifestations that may cause hoarseness of the voice**
>
> - Pachyonychia congenita
> - Cornelia de Lange syndrome
> - Farber disease (disseminated lipogranulomatosis)
> - Lipoid proteinosis
> - Sarcoidosis
> - Secondary syphilis
> - Epidemic typhus
> - Hypothyroidism
> - Relapsing polychondritis
> - Systemic lupus erythematosus
> - Dermatomyositis
> - Mucous membrane pemphigoid
> - Epidermolysis bullosa

Hoarseness as a sign of systemic disease. Hoarseness from laryngeal or tracheal involvement is an important audible sign of certain systemic diseases with skin involvement (Box 152.1) [42]. In particular, a range of inherited or acquired bullous diseases may affect the pharyngeal or laryngeal mucosa, for example mucous membrane pemphigoid, in which chronic inflammation may predispose to carcinoma of the larynx.

Key references

The full list of references can be found in the online version at https://www.wiley.com/rooksdermatology10e

1 Gómez Carrera L, Bonilla Hernan G. Pulmonary manifestations of collagen diseases. *Arch Bronconeumol* 2013;49:249–60.
2 Depascale R, Del Frate G, Gasparotto M *et al*. Diagnosis and management of lung involvement in systemic lupus erythematosus and Sjögren's syndrome: a literature review. *Ther Adv Musculoskelet Dis* 2021;13:1759720X211040696.
3 Gunnarsson R, Aaløkken TM, Molberg Ø *et al*. Prevalence and severity of interstitial lung disease in mixed connective tissue disease: a nationwide, cross-sectional study. *Ann Rheum Dis* 2012;71:1966–72.
8 Vij R, Strek ME. Diagnosis and treatment of connective tissue disease-associated interstitial lung disease. *Chest* 2013;143:814–24.
10 Jennette JC. Overview of the 2012 revised International Chapel Hill Consensus Conference nomenclature of vasculitides. *Clin Exp Nephrol* 2013;17:603–6.
11 Millet A, Pederzoli-Ribeil M, Guillevin L *et al*. Antineutrophil cytoplasmic antibody-associated vasculitides: is it time to split up the group? *Ann Rheum Dis* 2013;72:1273–9.
15 Vaglio A, Buzio C, Zwerina J. Eosinophilic granulomatosis with polyangiitis (Churg–Strauss): state of the art. *Allergy* 2013;68:261–73.
20 Uzun O, Akpolat T, Erkan L. Pulmonary vasculitis in Behcet disease: a cumulative analysis. *Chest* 2005;12:2243–53.
21 Tan SW, Tam YC, Oh CC. Skin manifestations of COVID-19: a worldwide review. *JAAD Int* 2021;2:119–33.

CHAPTER 153

The Skin and Disorders of the Digestive System

Sonja Molin[1] and Thomas Ruzicka[2]

[1]Division of Dermatology, Queen's University, Kingston, Canada
[2]Department of Dermatology and Allergology, Ludwig Maximilian University, Munich, Germany

Introduction, 153.1	PANCREATIC DISEASE, 153.5	Skin complications of stomas, 153.7
	Acute pancreatitis, 153.5	Liver disease and the skin, 153.7
OESOPHAGUS, STOMACH AND INTESTINE, 153.1	Panniculitis/subcutaneous fat necrosis, 153.6	Systemic diseases and the liver, 153.7
Inflammatory bowel disease, 153.1	Migratory thrombophlebitis, 153.6	Pruritus, 153.8
Collagenous colitis, 153.3	Necrolytic migratory erythema, 153.6	Skin pigment changes in liver disease, 153.8
Coeliac disease, 153.3	Other dermatological features	Vascular changes, 153.8
Bowel-associated dermatosis–arthritis syndrome, 153.3	of pancreatitis, 153.6	Hair and nail changes, 153.9
Whipple disease, 153.4	DERMATOLOGICAL MANIFESTATIONS OF OTHER DISORDERS INVOLVING THE DIGESTIVE SYSTEM, 153.6	Porphyria cutanea tarda, 153.9
Intestinal polyposis, 153.4		Other cutaneous lesions associated with liver disease, 153.9
LIVER AND GALL BLADDER, 153.4	Skin disorders associated with gastrointestinal bleeding, 153.6	Drugs and the liver, 153.9
Hepatitis and acute liver disease, 153.4	Gastrointestinal malabsorption and the skin, 153.7	Key references, 153.9
Liver cirrhosis, 153.5		

Introduction

This chapter concentrates on gastrointestinal, hepatic and pancreatic diseases in which cutaneous signs or symptoms are prominent, but also discusses situations either where the skin and the digestive system are affected by the same disease process or where a skin disease itself has an effect on the latter [1,2,3]. Skin changes related to more general effects of gastrointestinal diseases, such as nutritional defects, are discussed elsewhere in this book (Chapter 61).

OESOPHAGUS, STOMACH AND INTESTINE

Bleeding from the gastrointestinal tract may be associated with skin and nail signs of iron deficiency, such as koilonychia, smooth tongue and angular cheilitis (Chapter 61). The association of longstanding iron deficiency anaemia with dysphagia and an oesophageal web is known as Plummer–Vinson or Paterson–Brown-Kelly syndrome [1]; it may predispose to squamous cell carcinoma of the oesophagus.

Cutaneous metastases may occur from tumours of the oesophagus or stomach. Rarely they arise in the umbilicus and look like a firm but mobile nodule(s). This phenomenon has been called Sister Mary Joseph nodules. The most common cancers that metastasise to the umbilicus are those of the stomach, pancreas, colon and ovary [4].

Paraneoplastic eruptions linked to malignant neoplasms of the upper gastrointestinal tract, including palmoplantar keratoderma–oral leukokeratosis–oesophageal carcinoma (Howel–Evans syndrome), acrokeratosis paraneoplastica (Bazex syndrome) and paraneoplastic acanthosis nigricans, are discussed in Chapter 148.

Deficiencies of essential minerals and vitamins may manifest in the skin in a variety of ways. A major cause is impaired absorption from the gastrointestinal tract as the result of specific transport defects (e.g. vitamin B_{12}, zinc), surgery (e.g. gastrectomy, gastrointestinal bypass) or disease (e.g. Crohn disease) [1]. These are discussed in more detail in Chapter 61.

Helicobacter pylori infection has been reported to be associated with a wide variety of skin disorders including chronic urticaria, rosacea, IgA vasculitis, Sweet syndrome, erythema multiforme, alopecia areata, pruritus, nodular prurigo and atopic eczema [5].

Inflammatory bowel disease

Crohn disease (CD) (see Chapter 95) and ulcerative colitis (UC) are the major causes of what is termed inflammatory bowel disease (IBD). Despite several similarities, including their age distribution and incidence rate, these two diseases are distinct in several ways [2]:
1 Inflammatory profile: CD is mediated by TH1 cells, whereas UC is mediated by TH2 cells.

Rook's Textbook of Dermatology, Tenth Edition. Edited by Christopher Griffiths, Jonathan Barker, Tanya Bleiker, Walayat Hussain and Rosalind Simpson.
© 2024 John Wiley & Sons Ltd. Published 2024 by John Wiley & Sons Ltd.

2 Clinical picture: CD can affect the whole gastrointestinal tract, while UC is confined to the colon.
3 Genetic predisposition: HLA-B27 is associated with UC, whereas other genes such as the caspase recruitment domain 15 gene, *CARD15*, predispose to CD.
4 Risk factors: CD is associated with smoking, unlike UC.

According to current classifications, skin involvement in IBD can be grouped into four categories [2,6]: (i) specific conditions; (ii) reactive conditions; (iii) associated conditions; or (iv) complications of treatment of IBD. *Specific lesions* reflect direct skin involvement by IBD and are found only in CD. *Reactive lesions* are induced indirectly by the IBD (in both UC and CD). Immune cross-reactivity between the skin and gut seems to play an important role in their development. Certain skin conditions are *associated* with the HLA predisposition or the chronic inflammatory milieu in IBD. Finally, IBD *complications* or side effects of IBD *treatments* may manifest in the skin. In addition, newer treatments for skin diseases like anti-IL-17 therapy for psoriasis were found to be associated with induction and exacerbation of IBD in some cases [7].

Specific lesions
Direct skin and mucosal involvement
Crohn disease may occur at sites adjacent to the digestive tract, such as the oral cavity or ano-genital region. Anal tags are common. Perineal abscesses, fissures and fistulae occur in about 20–60% of patients with CD and only rarely in UC. They are more commonly seen in patients with CD colitis and may cause severe morbidity ('watering-can perineum'). Oral CD occurs in about 9% of patients with CD and manifests as swelling of the lips (Figure 153.1) or as a nodular 'cobblestone' oedema of the gingivae and oral mucosa; painful ulceration may develop [2,6].

Cutaneous Crohn disease at other sites
Cutaneous CD may also occur at sites distant from the bowel [2]. The lesions have the same histopathology as the gastrointestinal lesions [6]. Lesions of cutaneous CD may be solitary or multiple, and may have varied morphology, including intact or eroded plaques and nodules. The lower extremities are commonly involved, but cutaneous CD may affect the flexures, genitalia, face and other sites.

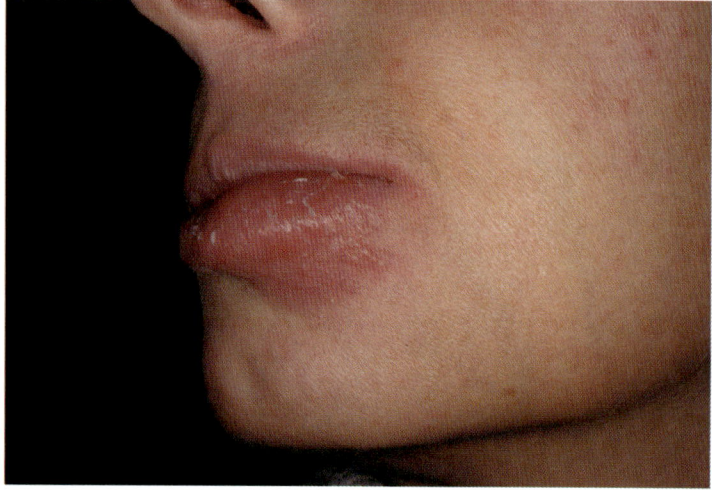

Figure 153.1 Oral Crohn disease.

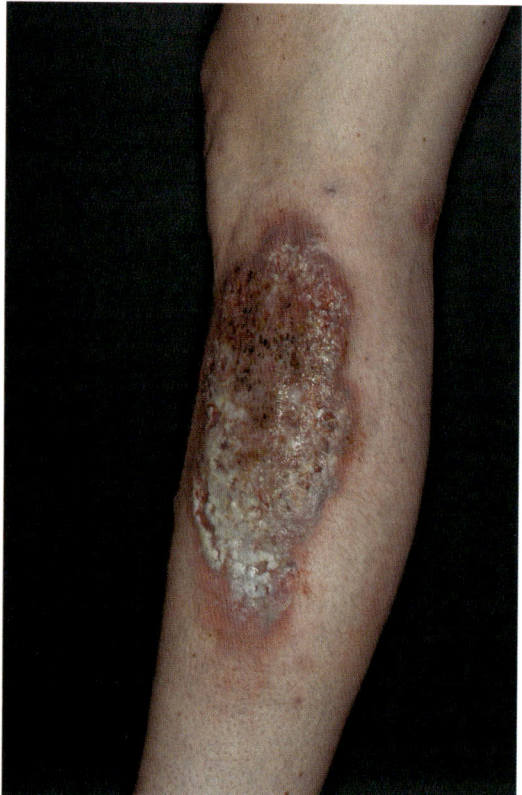

Figure 153.2 Pyoderma gangrenosum in a patient with Crohn disease.

Reactive lesions
A variety of reactive lesions may occur with either UC or CD, usually paralleling the activity of the IBD. All of these are discussed in detail in other chapters of this book. The most common are erythema nodosum and pyoderma gangrenosum [6].

Erythema nodosum (Chapter 97). Three to 10% of patients with UC and 4–15% of patients with CD develop erythema nodosum. It shows a female predilection [6].

Pyoderma gangrenosum (Chapter 47). Pyoderma gangrenosum occurs as a complication of IBD (Figure 153.2), haematological disorders, inflammatory arthritis and other medical conditions. It is estimated to occur in about 5–12% of patients with UC, clearly more often than in those with CD (1–2%). Like erythema nodosum it is more common in females [6].

Acute febrile neutrophilic dermatosis (Chapter 49). Acute febrile neutrophilic dermatosis or Sweet syndrome has been reported to be associated with IBD, especially UC [6].

Pyodermatitis–pyostomatitis vegetans. Pyodermatitis–pyostomatitis vegetans or pyodermite végétante Hallopeau [2,6] is a rare disorder of the oral mucosa and a rare cutaneous manifestation of IBD. Most cases of pyodermatitis–pyostomatitis vegetans are associated with IBD, usually UC. The oral lesions consist of multiple pustules, plaques and erosions, which may have a 'snail-track' appearance. The skin lesions are crusted papules and vegetating plaques with surrounding pustules, mainly affecting the major flexures and the scalp (Chapter 148).

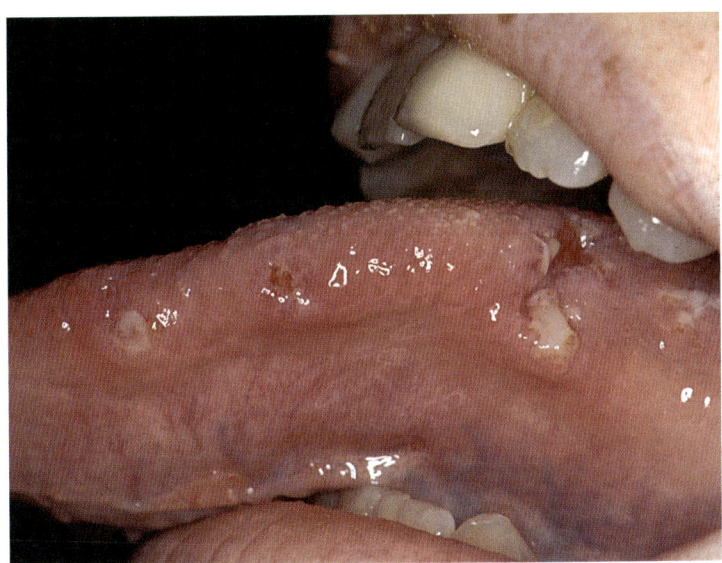

Figure 153.3 Recurrent major aphthae in a 26-year-old man with longstanding severe Crohn disease.

Cutaneous polyarteritis nodosa. This is a vasculitis of small and medium-sized vessels localised in the dermis and subcutis; 10% of cases are associated with IBD [2].

Leukocytoclastic vasculitis. Leukocytoclastic vasculitis may occur in either UC or CD but is more common in the former. The clinical picture is one of a leukocytoclastic vasculitis with palpable purpura, typically affecting the lower legs and sometimes causing nodules or ulceration. It can occur in CD during remission or exacerbation, whereas in UC it normally precedes the onset of bowel disease [6]. Involvement of the gastrointestinal tract is the third most common organ manifestation of IgA vasculitis (Henoch–Schönlein purpura), occurring in 50–75% of patients [2].

Thrombosis. The risk of thrombosis is elevated in patients with IBD and directly correlates with bowel disease activity. It may affect atypical locations, such as the heart or brain and the axillary or subclavian venous systems [2].

Oral aphthous ulcers. Oral aphthous ulcers are typically located on the buccal mucosa and the lips. They are more common in CD (10%) than in UC (4%) (Figure 153.3). In CD they are thought to represent specific rather than reactive lesions, but their pathogenesis in UC remains unclear. It has been postulated that they may sometimes be attributable to malnutrition secondary to IBD rather than to the IBD itself [6].

Associated lesions

Several skin diseases have been reported in the context of IBD, amongst them epidermolysis bullosa acquisita, psoriasis, vitiligo, hidradenitis suppurativa, phlebitis, erythema multiforme, urticaria, lichen planus, secondary amyloidosis, bullous pemphigoid and linear IgA bullous dermatosis. There also appears to be an increased risk of skin cancers such as squamous cell carcinoma [6].

Epidermolysis bullosa acquisita. This has been associated with both CD and UC, but like vitiligo it is very rare in CD and more often found in UC.

Psoriasis. This is more commonly associated with CD (11.2%) than with UC (5.7%) [6].

Collagenous colitis

This is a type of microscopic colitis characterised clinically by diarrhoea and histologically by a band-like collagen deposit [8]. Cases have been described that have evolved into other forms of IBD such as CD and UC. Concomitant coeliac disease has also been reported. It has been linked to the use of a variety of drugs including non-steroidal anti-inflammatory drugs or proton pump inhibitors. It has been associated with pyoderma gangrenosum.

Coeliac disease

Coeliac disease is an immune-mediated gluten-dependent enteropathy [9]. It is the result of a genetically based inappropriate T-cell-mediated immune response against gluten. It causes malabsorption and diarrhoea but diagnosis is often delayed and may first be discovered after a patient presents with dermatitis herpetiformis. The disease shows a strong HLA association: more than 90% of patients express the HLA-DQ ($\alpha 1^*501, \beta 1^*02$) heterodimer (HLA-DQ2) and almost all the remainder have HLA-DQ8. The diagnosis of coeliac disease can be made by serological tests for antigliadin, antiendomysial and tissue transglutaminase antibodies. A strict gluten-free diet is mandatory.

The most common skin manifestation of coeliac disease is dermatitis herpetiformis; the association is described in detail in Chapter 50. Cutaneous signs of malabsorption may be present in patients with severe coeliac disease. There is an increased incidence of autoimmune disorders that manifest in the skin, including psoriasis, alopecia areata, linear IgA bullous dermatosis and vitiligo. Other skin diseases that have been described in the context of coeliac disease include aphthous stomatitis, urticaria, hereditary angio-oedema, cutaneous vasculitis, erythema nodosum and erythema elevatum diutinum [3].

Bowel-associated dermatosis–arthritis syndrome

Bowel-associated dermatosis–arthritis syndrome (BADAS) comprises flu-like symptoms, polyarthralgia and eruptions of papules and pustules [2]. It shows a chronic and recurring course of disease with flares every 4–6 weeks. Its development had initially been linked to bowel bypass surgery for obesity (jejuno-ileal bypass), but now is also reported after modern bariatric procedures as well as in patients with IBD and cases of diverticulitis with sigmoid stenosis or acute appendicitis. The papules and pustules evolve from pink to red macules mainly on the extremities and the upper trunk.

The pathomechanisms leading to the development of the disease have not yet been fully understood. It seems that bacterial overgrowth in the altered parts of the gut and a production of antibodies against peptidoglycans in the bacterial cell wall play an important role. Deposition of immune complexes against peptidoglycan has been observed in patients with BADAS. Treatment mainly aims at reducing the bacterial load with long-term antibiotics or at correction of the blind loop in a jejuno-ileal bypass. Similar clinical features have been reported in association with severe achalasia of the cardia, in which food remnants are retained in the oesophagus for prolonged periods: a similar mechanism has been postulated [10,11].

Whipple disease

Whipple disease is a disorder of the small intestine due to infection with *Tropheryma whippelii*. The disorder usually presents with arthralgia and general malaise. Abdominal pain, diarrhoea and weight loss due to malabsorption occur in most individuals with more advanced disease. Cardiac, pleural, ophthalmic or neurological symptoms also occur [12]. The most common sign of skin involvement is diffuse hyperpigmentation in sun-exposed areas, which is seen in 45–54% of patients. Other cutaneous manifestations are rare and non-specific including subcutaneous nodules, erythroderma, purpura, vasculitis, panniculitis, hyperkeratosis, urticaria, dermatomyositis and eczema [3].

The diagnosis can be confirmed by demonstration of periodic acid–Schiff-positive particles in small bowel biopsies, by polymerase chain reaction examination of synovial fluid or tissue or by immunohistochemistry [12].

Intestinal polyposis

A number of usually inherited gastrointestinal polyposis disorders also have cutaneous features. They are discussed in detail elsewhere. The most important are:
- Peutz–Jeghers syndrome
- Gardner syndrome
- Cowden disease (multiple hamartoma and neoplasia syndrome)
- Bannayan–Riley–Ruvalcaba syndrome
- Cronkhite–Canada syndrome (non-inherited)
- Birt–Hogg–Dubé syndrome
- Naevoid basal cell carcinoma syndrome
- Neurofibromatosis.

LIVER AND GALL BLADDER

Hepatobiliary diseases are frequently associated with abnormalities of the skin, nails and hair [13,14]. However, these are mostly non-specific as they may be present in other diseases and absent even in patients with advanced liver dysfunction. Additionally, many diseases may share the same cutaneous features (e.g. most causes of cirrhosis have common clinical signs), and there is no clear correlation between the degree of the skin changes and the severity of liver dysfunction. However, there may be clinical features that suggest specific diagnoses (e.g. pigmentation, jaundice and xanthomas in primary biliary cirrhosis). The overall clinical presentation of the patient may therefore be as useful as the presence of specific cutaneous signs. Cutaneous features of chronic liver disease are listed in Box 153.1. This section will discuss some of the main groups of hepatobiliary disease, followed by some of the more important symptoms and signs in the following section.

> **Box 153.1 Skin lesions associated with chronic liver disease**
>
> - Spider angiomas and telangiectasia
> - Palmar erythema
> - Dilated abdominal/chest veins (including periumbilical caput medusae)
> - Jaundice
> - Increased melanin pigmentation
> - Thin 'paper-money' skin, striae
> - Excoriations
> - Loss of secondary sexual hair in males
> - Bruising, purpura
> - Nail changes: clubbing, pallor, Muehrcke's bands, Terry's nails
> - Features of malnutrition (Chapter 61)
> - Associated lesions:
>   - Xanthomas
>   - Porphyria cutanea tarda
>   - Vasculitis/capillaritis/pyoderma gangrenosum
>   - Lichen planus

Hepatitis and acute liver disease

Acute hepatic damage is most often due to viral hepatitis, alcohol or drugs. Cutaneous features may be absent or there may be jaundice. This section considers the dermatological associations of infective hepatitis.

Hepatitis A virus infection. This is usually asymptomatic and transient. Dermatological features, if present, are jaundice, urticaria (less than 2%) and exanthema [15]. Chronic liver disease does not occur but a relapsing variant has been described in which itch, purpura and urticarial lesions are present [16]. Histology in such cases demonstrates a small-vessel vasculitis. More severe vasculitis or panniculitis is rare.

Hepatitis B virus (HBV) infection. HBV infection is of major relevance to health care workers as it may be transmitted parenterally. It is also transmitted sexually and HBV infection may be associated with other sexually transmitted diseases. HBV screening and vaccination are recommended for all health care workers. Vaccination can cause dermatological side effects such as provocation of granuloma annulare, lichen planus, Gianotti–Crosti syndrome

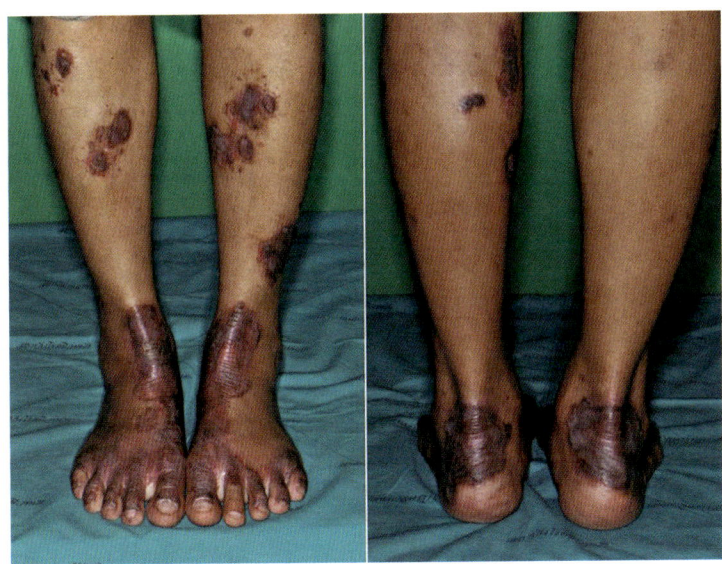

Figure 153.4 Necrolytic acral erythema in patient with longstanding hepatitis C. Courtesy of Dr Vesarat Wessagowit, Institute of Dermatology, Bangkok.

and urticaria, and contact allergy to preservatives [17–19]. Twenty to 30% of patients with acute HBV infection develop a serum sickness-like disease, which occurs weeks before the clinical onset of liver disease. Up to 8% of patients with acute HBV infection develop polyarteritis nodosa. Other dermatoses that have been associated with acute HBV infection include urticaria, erythema multiforme, Gianotti–Crosti syndrome, mixed cryoglobulinaemia, lichen planus and dermatomyositis [13].

Hepatitis C virus (HCV) infection. This is usually transmitted parenterally. Necrolytic acral erythema is a specific feature of acute HCV infection [13]. Well-demarcated, acral (mainly dorsa of the feet), dusky discoloration with peripheral blister formation progresses to form keratotic erythrokeratoderma-like chronic inflammation (Figure 153.4). Histology and the clinical picture are similar to those of other necrolytic erythemas.

Up to 75% of patients with HCV fail to eradicate the virus after the initial infection [13]. Many of these may present with skin disorders. Mixed cryoglobulins can be detected in up to 50% of patients with HCV infection but only a small proportion of patients develop manifest cryoglobulinaemic vasculitis (Chapter 100) [20]. Other dermatological conditions that have been associated with persistent infection include polyarteritis nodosa, porphyria cutanea tarda, lichen planus, sicca syndrome, manifestations of chronic liver disease such as pruritus and prurigo and reactions to antiviral drugs. Less well-corroborated associations with HCV infection include pyoderma gangrenosum, antiphospholipid syndrome, Behçet disease, vitiligo, amyloidosis, sarcoidosis and Sjögren syndrome.

Liver cirrhosis

Skin signs of liver cirrhosis are similar to those seen generally in chronic liver disease. They reflect the various components of functional hepatic impairment and are discussed in the section 'Liver diseases and the skin'.

Haemochromatosis [15]. Haemochromatosis ('bronze diabetes') is a disorder in which iron overload leads to iron deposition in various organs, including the liver and the skin (Chapter 86). Classic idiopathic haemochromatosis usually presents in males over the age of 40 years. An acquired form also occurs, secondary to haemosiderosis or alcohol abuse. Skin pigmentation occurs in up to 90% of patients with haemochromatosis. It typically has a bronze-coloured or grey hue and is most prominent on sun-exposed skin. This pigmentation seems to be a result of elevated melanin production. Stigmata of chronic hepatic failure may also be present. Ichthyosiform dryness of the skin, koilonychia and loss of body hair also occur.

Primary biliary cirrhosis and biliary tract disease. From the dermatological point of view, primary biliary cirrhosis (PBC) is the most important biliary tract disease. Nearly 40% of PBC patients first present with skin signs or symptoms [13]. The cutaneous features of significance are marked itch (discussed in more detail later in this chapter), excoriation, hyperpigmentation and various xanthomatous lesions due to secondary hyperlipidaemia [13]. Xanthelasmas, palmar xanthomas and tuberous xanthomas may all occur. PBC occurs mainly in middle-aged women as an autoimmune disease and is strongly associated with the presence of antimitochondrial antibodies. It can be associated with numerous other autoimmune conditions, among them Raynaud disease, keratoconjunctivis sicca and systemic sclerosis [21]. The constellation of systemic sclerosis and its variants with PBC is also known as Reynolds syndrome [22].

Cholestasis and bile stones may cause acute or chronic jaundice and other features of liver disease. Pigment bile stones may occur due to erythropoietic protoporphyria, a disease which may also rarely cause fulminant hepatic failure [23].

Congenital biliary tract hypoplasia with consecutive cholestasis is a feature of Alagille syndrome (arteriohepatic dysplasia) [13], a dominantly inherited disorder. Affected individuals have a characteristic facies, jaundice, severe pruritus, widespread xanthomas and retardation of growth and mental development. Various skeletal, ocular and vascular defects are associated.

PANCREATIC DISEASE

Apart from jaundice and panniculitis, skin changes associated with pancreatic disease are uncommon. The glucagonoma syndrome is a rare but highly characteristic skin disorder, which is discussed in the section on necrolytic migratory erythema. Skin disorders associated with diabetes are discussed in Chapter 62.

Acute pancreatitis

Jaundice and fat necrosis may both be prominent. Purpura or bruising may occur in patients with acute pancreatitis. Note, however, that none of these is specific for pancreatitis [24]. They may also occur due to retroperitoneal haemorrhage or bleeding from sources such as splenic rupture, ectopic pregnancy, metastatic tumour or

aortic aneurysm. Four eponymous signs occur with retroperitoneal bleeding or the tracking of haemorrhagic fluid:
1 Grey Turner sign: tracks from the pararenal space to the edge of the quadratus lumborum muscle, then through a defect in the fascia to the subcutaneous tissues of the flank (left-sided in pancreatitis).
2 Cullen sign: tracks into the falciparum ligament, then through the connective tissues of the round ligament to the periumbilical area.
3 Fox sign: tracks along the fascia of the psoas and iliac muscles to the subcutaneous tissues of the upper thigh.
4 Bryant sign: tracks to the scrotum to produce the 'blue scrotum' sign [25].

Features related to the aetiology of the pancreatitis may also be present, such as signs of alcohol abuse or hepatic cirrhosis, or xanthomas due to hypertriglyceridaemia.

Panniculitis/subcutaneous fat necrosis

Patients with pancreatic disease develop lobular panniculitis in 2–3% of cases (Chapter 97) [26,27]. It may be associated with acute or chronic pancreatitis, pancreatic carcinoma or other pancreatic diseases [24]. Histopathologically, subcutaneous fat necrosis is pathognomonic together with ghost-like anucleated cells [24]. Arthritis with intraosseous fat necrosis may accompany the pancreatitis and the panniculitis, which together (with polyarthritis) is called PPP syndrome [23]. Nodular lesions are usually 1–3 cm in diameter and are tender or symptomless. The areas of predilection are the lower extremities, but lesions may occur anywhere. Lesions persist for 2–3 weeks and then heal. They may leave atrophic, hyperpigmented scars.

Migratory thrombophlebitis

The highest risk of developing migratory superficial thrombophlebitis seems to be associated with adenocarcinoma of the pancreas [28].

Necrolytic migratory erythema

Necrolytic migratory erythema is the cutaneous manifestation of the glucagonoma syndrome, which results from a glucagon-secreting α-cell tumour of the pancreas (Chapter 148). Necrolytic migratory erythema may also occur without glucagonoma: what has been termed pseudoglucagonoma syndrome has been described in association with zinc and protein deficiency, liver cirrhosis, IBD, pancreatitis and non-pancreatic malignancies [1].

Lesions are annular and pink to red with erosions, crusting, desquamation and hyperpigmentation fluctuating in extent and severity. The rash is itchy or painful and particularly affects sites exposed to friction and pressure including flexural sites on the lower abdomen, groin, buttocks and thighs. In skin of colour, variations of red and even grey to black may be seen.

Apart from elevated serum glucagon levels, the clinical spectrum also includes diarrhoea, weight loss, weakness, thrombosis and psychiatric disturbances.

Other dermatological features of pancreatitis

The main dermatological features of acute and chronic pancreatitis have been described in this chapter or are the result of malabsorption attributable to pancreatic failure (see Gastrointestinal malabsorption and the skin in this chapter). Livedo reticularis has also been described in pancreatitis as the Walzel sign [24].

DERMATOLOGICAL MANIFESTATIONS OF OTHER DISORDERS INVOLVING THE DIGESTIVE SYSTEM

Bullous diseases may affect the pharynx, oesophagus or stomach. Epidermolysis bullosa is of particular relevance as some forms may affect all parts of the digestive system [29].

Immunobullous diseases, particularly those with an IgA basement membrane zone immunoreactant, may cause mucosal blistering and erosions. Examples include mucous membrane pemphigoid, linear IgA disease and the IgA variant of epidermolysis bullosa acquisita. Mucous membrane pemphigoid may also cause oesophageal scarring and stenosis.

Sclerodermatous processes also affect the oesophagus, in particular limited systemic sclerosis, formerly known as CREST (calcinosis, Raynaud phenomenon, oesophageal dysmotility, sclerodactyly, telangiectasia). This disorder is discussed more fully in Chapter 54. Gastrointestinal involvement occurs in up to 90% of patients with diffuse systemic sclerosis [30]. It can affect all parts of the gastrointestinal tract and is associated with decreased peristalsis throughout the bowel, leading to malabsorption, constipation and diverticula. Sjögren syndrome may also cause dysphagia, as may dermatomyositis in cases in which there is involvement of the pharyngeal musculature. Several patterns of cutaneous vasculitis may be associated with mesenteric vasculitis and/or thrombosis, leading to bleeding or ulceration. Various gastrointestinal symptoms have been reported in relation to systemic lupus erythematosus, and include gastro-oesophageal reflux, dysphagia, abdominal pain, impaired digestion, perforation and bleeding [31].

Several other inflammatory disorders such as lichen planus may affect the mouth, pharynx or oesophagus [32].

Skin disorders associated with gastrointestinal bleeding

These are listed in Table 153.1.

Table 153.1 Skin lesions associated with gastrointestinal disorders that may present with bleeding.

Disease	Gastrointestinal lesion	Skin manifestation
Vascular defects and inherited		
Osler–Weber–Rendu disease	Telangiectasia	Telangiectasia
Blue rubber bleb naevus syndrome	Haemangiomas	Haemangiomas
Pseudoxanthoma elasticum	Involvement of visceral arteries	Yellowish papules and plaques
Ehlers–Danlos syndrome (type IV)	Fragility of visceral arteries	Hyperelasticity of skin and joints
Polyposis		
Neurofibromatosis (von Recklinghausen)	Neurofibromas	Café-au-lait spots, neurofibromas
Cronkhite–Canada syndrome	Gastrointestinal polyposis	Diffuse hyperpigmentation, alopecia, nail defects
Gardner syndrome	Polyposis of colon (cancer)	Lipomas, epidermoid cysts
Peutz–Jeghers syndrome	Polyposis, especially small intestine	Hyperpigmentation on lips, circumoral area and fingertips
Cowden's disease	Polyposis	Papules, lipomas, angiomas
Inflammatory bowel disease		
Crohn disease, ulcerative colitis	Inflammatory changes of the intestinal wall	Erythema nodosum
		Aphthous stomatitis
		Pyoderma gangrenosum, other neutrophilic dermatoses
		Necrotising vasculitis
		Epidermolysis bullosa acquisita
		Erythema multiforme
Vasculitis and systemic disease		
IgA vasculitis (Henoch–Schönlein purpura) and other vasculitides	Mesenteric vasculitis, gastric ulcers (polyarteritis nodosa)	Purpura, livedo, nodules, necrosis
Cholesterol emboli	Intestinal arterial occlusion	Vasculitis, necrosis, livedo
Degos disease	Intestinal perforation	White atrophic papules
Amyloidosis	Vascular fragility	Purpuric lesions
Neoplasia		
Primary gastrointestinal cancers	Neoplasm	Metastases, paraneoplastic eruptions, features of polyposis syndromes
Kaposi sarcoma	Kaposi sarcoma of bowel	Kaposi sarcoma of skin

Gastrointestinal malabsorption and the skin

Malabsorption may be associated with skin changes in a number of different ways: (1) malabsorption can cause a skin disorder; (2) a skin disorder can cause malabsorption; (3) skin abnormalities and malabsorption may have a common cause; and (4) skin disease and malabsorption can be related indirectly [33]. The skin changes from the first category may be due to deficiencies of macronutrients, including proteins, fat and carbohydrates, or of micronutrients, including minerals, trace elements and fat-soluble vitamins [34]. Some causes of malabsorption are listed in Box 153.2. Non-specific cutaneous manifestations of malabsorption are listed in Box 153.3. The cutaneous manifestations of specific vitamin and mineral deficiencies are discussed in Chapter 61. Patients presenting with skin changes suggestive of malabsorption should be thoroughly investigated to identify the cause.

Skin complications of stomas

Stomas are most frequently required for the management of gastrointestinal disorders including IBD, bowel cancer, diverticulosis or bowel obstruction (e.g. volvulus or intussusception). There is an increased prevalence of psoriasis in patients with IBD and peristomal psoriasis may cause problems with stoma management in affected patients [35]. Parastomal pyoderma gangrenosum is particularly associated with Crohn disease. Skin problems of stomas are fully discussed in Chapter 112.

Liver disease and the skin

Systemic diseases and the liver

A large number of systemic diseases may affect the liver, many with cutaneous features. Most are discussed in other chapters. For example, sarcoidosis is associated with subclinical hepatic involvement in over 50% of patients but may cause overt hepatomegaly or abnormalities of liver function in conjunction with skin lesions.

Porphyrias (Chapter 58), especially porphyria cutanea tarda, may occur as a consequence of liver disease but severe liver disease is also a feature in some patients with erythropoietic protoporphyria.

Hereditary haemorrhagic telangiectasia, mentioned earlier as a cause of gastrointestinal bleeding, is associated with portal hypertension due mainly to portosystemic shunting, so bleeding in such patients may be from varices [36].

> **Box 153.2 Some causes of intestinal malabsorption**
>
> **Chelating substances in the gut** (phytates)
> **Insufficient digestive enzyme activity** (pancreatitis, mucoviscidosis)
> **Defective micelle formation** (obstructive jaundice, hepatic cirrhosis)
> **Stagnant loop syndrome and bacterial overgrowth** (strictures, surgical blind loops, systemic sclerosis)
> **Gastric resection** (lack of hydrochloric acid production)
> **Bariatric surgery**
> **Defective enzyme activity or carrier function in the intestinal mucosa**
> - Disaccharidase deficiency
> - Coeliac disease
> - Acrodermatitis enteropathica (zinc deficiency)
> - Hartnup disease (pellagra)
>
> **Loss of absorption capacity**
> - Intestinal fistulas, intestinal resection and bypass operations
> - Crohn disease
> - Intestinal lymphoma
>
> **Interference with intestinal lymphatics**
> - Intestinal lymphangiectasia
> - Tuberculous mesenteric adenitis
>
> **Chronic mesenteric ischaemia** (atherosclerosis)
> **Miscellaneous**
> - Cronkhite–Canada syndrome
> - Whipple disease
> - Environmental enteropathy (tropical sprue)
> - Amyloidosis
> - Mastocytosis
> - Protein-losing enteropathy
> - Thyroid disease (hyperthyroidism, hypothyroidism)

> **Box 153.3 Non-specific cutaneous manifestations of gastrointestinal malabsorption**
> - Xerosis and acquired ichthyosis
> - Atrophy of skin and subcutaneous fat
> - Pruritus and prurigo
> - Melanosis (symmetrical hyperpigmentation of the skin)
> - Brittle nails
> - Hair loss

Pruritus

Pruritus is the most common skin symptom associated with liver disease. It may precede the diagnosis of liver disease. Liver diseases in which itch is most prominent are PBC, sclerosing cholangitis and any other biliary tract obstruction, and disorders causing cholestasis. Itch is less prominent in haemochromatosis, alcoholic cirrhosis and autoimmune chronic active hepatitis [37]. The symptoms are generally most severe at acral sites and at areas of tight clothing, and are more prominent nocturnally.

The precise mechanism of itch in cholestatic liver disease remains unclear. There is controversy over whether bile salts contribute to itch. The release of undefined putative pruritogens from the liver in the presence of cholestasis has been proposed as an alternative mechanism. Endogenous opioids and steroid metabolites also seem to be part of the complex process that leads to the development of cholestatic pruritus [38].

Treatment, where possible, is for the underlying cause – for example, drug withdrawal in drug-induced cholestasis, surgery for mechanical biliary obstruction and treatment for chronic HCV infection. Diverse treatment regimens for cholestatic pruritus have been proposed: among them is a stepwise escalation scheme, starting with bile salt-chelating resins, followed in turn by rifampicin then opioid antagonists (e.g. naltrexone), then sertraline and, finally, consideration of other more experimental approaches [36]. UVB phototherapy can be effective [13], but ongoing treatment is generally required. Other treatments that have been used with success include albumin dialysis and plasmapheresis. The problem will normally respond to liver transplantation where this is indicated.

Skin pigment changes in liver disease [12]

A yellowish hue of the sclerae, mucous membranes and skin due to hyperbilirubinaemia is called icterus (jaundice). Green-coloured sweat [39] and green discoloration of the gingivae may accompany jaundice. Melanosis cutis due to excess epidermal melanin is found. A muddy grey pigmentation occurs in chronic liver disease of any cause. It may be blotchy or diffuse, and may be exaggerated in the areolar as well as in the perioral and periorbital areas (resembling melasma); in other cases, it may resemble freckling and it can also localise to the palmar creases. Spotty hypomelanosis may occur on the back, buttocks and extremities, often in relation to spider angiomas. In skin of colour, these typical presentations may be modified with variations in the colours observed.

Vascular changes [13,14]

Spider telangiectases. These are a characteristic feature in patients with severe chronic liver disease (Figure 153.5) and are found in one-third of patients with liver cirrhosis. Hyperoestrogenaemia (which also accounts for the loss of secondary male-pattern hair, gynaecomastia and testicular atrophy) seems to be an important factor for the development of theses vascular changes.

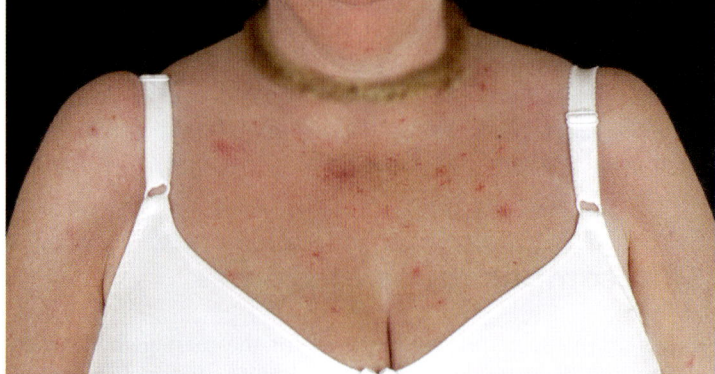

Figure 153.5 Multiple spider telangiectases in 53-year-old woman with alcoholic liver disease.

Palmar erythema. Palmar erythema refers to a bright red discoloration of the palms, which is most pronounced on the hypothenar eminences and may also affect the soles of the feet. None of these vascular features are specific for liver disease. Diffusely scattered tiny telangiectatic vessels are referred to as 'paper-money' skin. Increased peripheral blood flow with dilatation of digital pulp arteriovenous anastomoses is thought to be the cause of finger clubbing.

Bleeding. Purpura, petechiae, ecchymoses and mucosal bleeding (epistaxis, gingival bleeding) may occur due to coagulation defects in patients with liver disease. In progressive liver disease with portal hypertension, collateral blood flow creates visible coiled varicose veins on the abdominal wall. When these are in a pattern radiating from the umbilicus, the appearance is termed 'caput Medusae'.

Hair and nail changes [13,14]

The body hair is often thinned or partially lost, and males tend to develop a female pubic hair pattern, which may be associated with gynecomastia and testicular atrophy.

Various nail changes have been reported in association with chronic liver disease (Chapter 93). They include a diffuse white colour with an invisible lunula, a proximal white colour with distal pink or brownish colour (Terry nails) or paired white bands (Muehrke bands). Altered digital blood flow, soft-tissue overgrowth and hypoalbuminaemia may all contribute. Nail plate changes include clubbing and its milder variant, the 'watch-glass' deformity; flattened nails or koilonychia as well as brittle nails may also occur. These are all non-specific findings that are also found in association with internal diseases of other organ systems.

Porphyria cutanea tarda

Chronic liver disease is involved in the skin changes of porphyria cutanea tarda (Figure 153.6). Lesions consist of bullae, scarring and hyperpigmentation of sun-exposed skin areas and hypertrichosis of the face. This is discussed in more detail in Chapter 58.

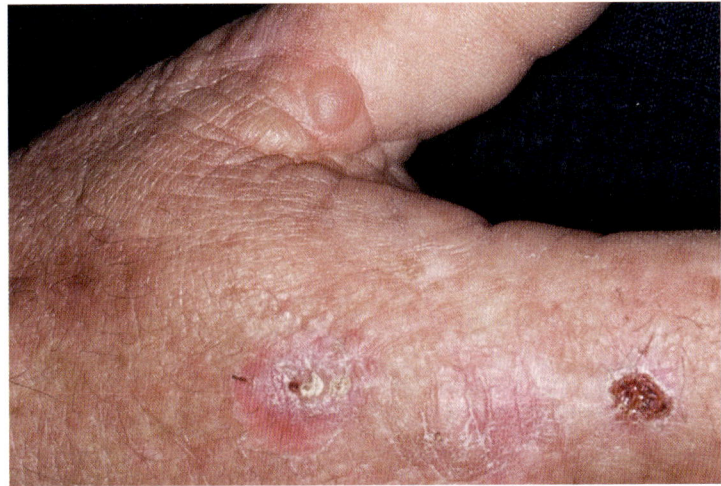

Figure 153.6 Porphyria cutanea tarda of the hand.

Table 153.2 Drug-related links between the skin and the liver.

Mechanism	Examples
Drugs whose hepatic metabolism is altered by liver disease or by other drugs that are also metabolised in the liver	Ciclosporin
Drugs that may cause hepatitis or other liver damage	Azathioprine, methotrexate
Drugs for the treatment or prevention of liver disease causing cutaneous side effects	Penicillamine (elastosis perforans serpiginosa), thimerosal or other preservatives in hepatitis vaccines (local reactions)
Drugs that cause liver changes with secondary cutaneous signs	Oestrogens (porphyria cutanea tarda)
Drugs that may cause concurrent hepatitis and rash	Phenytoin and other anticonvulsants

Other cutaneous lesions associated with liver disease

Lichen planus has been reported in a number of diseases with abnormal immune function. The association of erosive oral lesions in PBC and chronic active hepatitis may be related to a common immunological pathogenesis. There is uncertainty as to whether there is an association between HCV infection and lichen planus [40].

Pyoderma gangrenosum has also been reported in chronic active hepatitis [41]. The Gianotti–Crosti syndrome has been linked to hepatitis. Skin changes simulating classic glucagonoma syndrome have been reported in cirrhosis and termed the pseudoglucagonoma syndrome [1].

Acquired zinc deficiency may occur in chronic liver disease, especially alcoholic liver disease, and is thought to be due to a combination of increased urinary excretion and decreased dietary intake [42].

Drugs and the liver

Examples of drug-related links between the skin and the liver are given in Table 153.2.

Key references

The full list of references can be found in the online version at https://www.wiley.com/rooksdermatology10e

1 Shah KR, Boland CR, Patel M *et al*. Cutaneous manifestations of gastrointestinal disease: part I. *J Am Acad Dermatol* 2013;68:189.e1–21; quiz 210.
2 Thrash B, Patel M, Shah KR *et al*. Cutaneous manifestations of gastrointestinal disease: part II. *J Am Acad Dermatol* 2013;68:211.e1–33; quiz 244–6.
9 Rodrigo L, Beteta-Gorriti V, Alvarez N *et al*. Cutaneous and mucosal manifestations associated with celiac disease. *Nutrients* 2018;10:800.
13 Ghosn SH, Kibbi AG. Cutaneous manifestations of liver diseases. *Clin Dermatol* 2008;26:274–82.
14 Hazin R, Abu-Rajab Tamimi TI *et al*. Recognizing and treating cutaneous signs of liver disease. *Cleve Clin J Med* 2009;76:599–606.
21 Rashtak S, Pittelkow MR. Skin involvement in systemic autoimmune diseases. *Curr Dir Autoimmun* 2008;10:344–58.
32 Fox LP, Lightdale CJ, Grossman ME. Lichen planus of the esophagus: what dermatologists need to know. *J Am Acad Dermatol* 2011;65:175–83.
33 Marks J, Shuster S. Intestinal malabsorption and the skin. *Gut* 1971;12:938–47.
34 Jen M, Yan AC. Syndromes associated with nutritional deficiency and excess. *Clin Dermatol* 2010;28:669–85.
42 Mohammad MK, Zhou Z, Cave M *et al*. Zinc and liver disease. *Nutr Clin Pract* 2012;27:8–20.

CHAPTER 154

The Skin and Disorders of the Kidney and Urinary Tract

Sonja Molin[1] and Thomas Ruzicka[2]

[1] Division of Dermatology, Queen's University, Kingston, Canada
[2] Department of Dermatology and Allergology, Ludwig Maximilian University, Munich, Germany

Introduction, 154.1	Metabolic and systemic disorders, 154.2	SKIN DISORDERS THAT MAY AFFECT THE KIDNEY AND URINARY TRACT, 154.6
HEREDITARY SYNDROMES WITH SKIN AND RENAL INVOLVEMENT, 154.1	Renal failure and dialysis, 154.3	
	Renal transplantation, 154.5	Key references, 154.7
SKIN SYMPTOMS AND SIGNS ASSOCIATED WITH RENAL DISORDERS, 154.2	ACQUIRED DISORDERS WITH SKIN AND RENAL INVOLVEMENT, 154.6	

Introduction

Skin disorders may be associated with disorders of the kidney and, occasionally, of other parts of the urinary tract. This chapter examines these associations, which may be due to hereditary syndromes or acquired disorders affecting both the skin and kidney, the effects of renal failure on the skin, or the effects of skin disease on the kidneys and urinary tract [1–5,**6**]. A selection of renocutaneous syndromes is listed in Box 154.1.

HEREDITARY SYNDROMES WITH SKIN AND RENAL INVOLVEMENT

Fabry disease (Chapter 79). Fabry nephropathy (angiokeratoma corporis diffusum) can develop in early childhood in both sexes, although it may be clinically silent at onset [7]. Symptoms show a wide variation. Affected individuals often may have proteinuria, microalbuminuria, microscopic haematuria and lipiduria. Premature mortality in the condition is often the result of renal failure. Enzyme replacement therapy with α-galactosidase A may not be fully effective if started in the presence of manifest proteinuria or renal impairment. Early diagnosis of Fabry nephropathy is therefore very important.

Neurofibromatosis (Chapter 78). In neurofibromatosis (von Recklinghausen disease) urinary outflow obstruction may develop secondary to an impinging neurofibroma [8,9]. Vascular lesions can result in renal artery thrombosis and subsequent hypertension, which may also develop as a result of an associated phaeochromocytoma or renal artery stenosis.

Box 154.1 Renocutaneous diseases

Hereditary syndromes
- Angiokeratoma corporis diffusum
- Neurofibromatosis
- Tuberous sclerosis
- Nail–patella syndrome
- Birt–Hogg–Dubé syndrome
- Sickle cell disease
- Pseudoxanthoma elasticum
- Oro-facial–digital syndrome
- Von Hippel–Lindau disease
- Hereditary haemorrhagic telangiectasia

Metabolic disorders
- Primary systemic amyloidosis
- Calcinosis

Inflammatory and miscellaneous
- Systemic vasculitis
- Systemic lupus erythematosus
- Polyarteritis nodosa
- Systemic sclerosis
- Nephrogenic systemic fibrosis
- Granulomatosis with polyangiitis
- Erythema multiforme
- IgA vasculitis (Henoch–Schönlein purpura)
- Drug-induced toxic epidermal necrolysis

Nail–patella syndrome (Chapter 67). Renal involvement is present in up to 40% of patients with nail–patella syndrome (Fong syndrome or hereditary osteo-onychodysplasia) [10]. Many affected individuals only present with premature loss of renal function but rarely develop symptomatic kidney failure. Only 5–10% of

Rook's Textbook of Dermatology, Tenth Edition. Edited by Christopher Griffiths, Jonathan Barker, Tanya Bleiker, Walayat Hussain and Rosalind Simpson.
© 2024 John Wiley & Sons Ltd. Published 2024 by John Wiley & Sons Ltd.

nail–patella syndrome patients develop severe renal impairment progressing to end-stage kidney failure [10].

Tuberous sclerosis (Chapter 79). Renal involvement in tuberous sclerosis (Bourneville disease) includes angiomyolipomas, renal cysts and malignant tumours such as clear cell carcinoma [11].

Birt–Hogg–Dubé syndrome (Chapter 78). A seven-fold increase in the incidence of renal tumours is associated with Birt–Hogg–Dubé (BHD) syndrome (Hornstein–Knickenberg syndrome), predominantly various types of renal cell carcinoma. The cutaneous features of BHD include trichofolliculomas, trichodiscomas and skin tags.

Hereditary leiomyomatosis and renal cell carcinoma syndrome (Chapter 78). Multiple cutaneous leiomyomas, which have an inherited predisposition, are linked to uterine leiomyoma (Reed syndrome) and also appear to be associated with an increased incidence of renal cell carcinoma, usually of the papillary cell type [11].

Von Hippel–Lindau syndrome. Renal lesions in von Hippel–Lindau syndrome (familial cerebelloretinal angiomatosis) are either simple cysts or renal cell carcinoma; usually they are a late manifestation [11].

Multiple hamartoma and neoplasia syndrome (Chapter 78). Multiple hamartoma and neoplasia syndrome (Cowden's disease) is associated with an increased incidence of renal cell carcinoma or transitional cell carcinoma of the bladder [12].

Familial Mediterranean fever with urticaria, Muckle–Wells syndrome and tumour necrosis receptor associated periodic syndrome (Chapter 45). These hereditary autoinflammatory syndromes may all be complicated by systemic amyloid A amyloidosis with a significant risk of renal failure [13].

Oro-facial–digital syndrome type 1 [14] (Chapter 65). Oro-facial–digital syndrome type 1 (OFD1) is characterised by the following abnormalities:
- Oral: lobed tongue, hamartomas or lipomas of the tongue, cleft of the hard or soft palate, accessory gingival frenula, hypodontia and other dental abnormalities.
- Facial: ocular hypertelorism or telecanthus, hypoplasia of the alae nasi, median cleft or pseudocleft upper lip and micrognathia.
- Digital: brachydactyly, syndactyly of varying degrees and clinodactyly of the fifth finger; duplicated hallux (great toe); and preaxial or postaxial polydactyly of the hands.
- Brain: intracerebral cysts, corpus callosum agenesis and cerebellar agenesis with or without the Dandy–Walker malformation.

Polycystic disease of the kidneys and liver occurs commonly in this condition. As many as 50% of individuals with OFD1 have some degree of mental impairment, which is usually mild. Almost all affected individuals are female. However, males with OFD1 have been described, mostly as malformed fetuses born to women with OFD1.

SKIN SYMPTOMS AND SIGNS ASSOCIATED WITH RENAL DISORDERS

Metabolic and systemic disorders

Acquired partial lipodystrophy (Chapter 98). In acquired partial lipodystrophy (Barraquer–Simons syndrome), lipoatrophy of the upper part of the body is associated with lipohypertrophy of the thighs and, in about a quarter of cases, with renal disease, usually a membranoproliferative glomerulonephritis. There is a circulating C3 nephritic factor and reduced levels of complement (C3) [15]. Renal failure at an early age is common.

Amyloid A (AA) amyloidosis [16,17]. Proteinuria leading to the nephrotic syndrome or renal insufficiency is often the first clinical manifestation of AA amyloidosis in patients with chronic inflammatory diseases. Secondary AA amyloidosis is associated with various underlying conditions such as chronic infection, rheumatic diseases (rheumatoid arthritis, ankylosing spondylitis, chronic juvenile arthritis), inflammatory bowel disease and many autoinflammatory syndromes including cryopyrin-associated periodic syndromes (e.g. Muckle–Wells syndrome) and familial Mediterranean fever (Chapter 45). These conditions frequently have skin manifestations and may present with specific skin signs. AA amyloidosis is also reported to be a frequent cause of kidney disease in intravenous drug abusers.

Metastatic cutaneous calcification (metastatic calcinosis cutis, calcific panniculitis, benign nodular calcification) (Chapter 59). Metastatic calcification is a rare phenomenon affecting the dermis and subcutis and affecting predominantly uraemic patients with combined hyperphosphataemia and hypercalcaemia, often in the context of hyperparathyroidism. It typically presents as firm papules, nodules or plaques in the dermis or subcutis, particularly around the large joints or flexural sites. Unlike calciphylaxis it does not lead to tissue necrosis [5].

Calciphylaxis (Chapter 59). Calcification of small-vessel walls in calciphylaxis (calcific uraemic arteriolopathy) leads to extremely painful cutaneous necrosis and ulceration (Figure 154.1) [18]. It occurs in up to 4% of patients on long-term haemodialysis, but may also be associated with hyperparathyroidism, liver disease, systemic steroid use, malignancy or connective tissue disease in the absence of renal impairment. Prognosis is poor with a mortality rate of up to 80%, mainly due to the risk of sepsis. Careful wound management is particularly important to prevent wound infection; it may include surgical debridement of necrotic tissue, hydrocolloid dressings and systemic antibiotics. Treatment options aiming at a reduction of calciphylaxis risk include a low phosphate diet, low calcium dialysate fluids, non-calcium phosphate binders, parathyroidectomy and, more recently, drugs such as sodium thiosulphate or cinacalcet, which alter calcium metabolism.

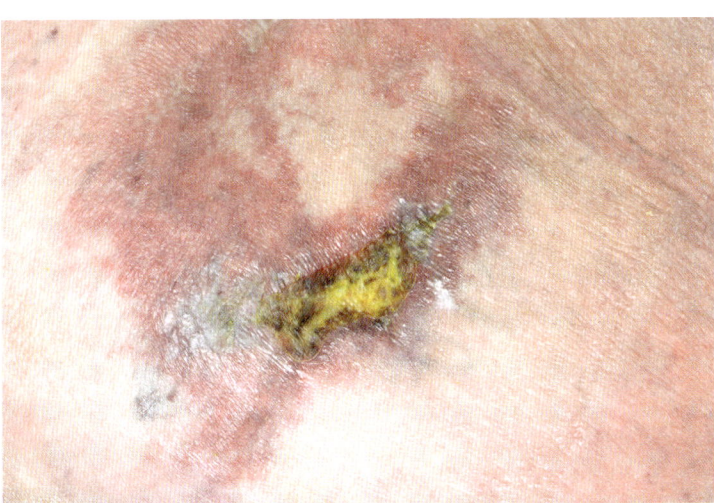

Figure 154.1 Early signs of calciphylaxis with superficial skin necrosis and ulceration.

Renal failure and dialysis

Cutaneous signs of renal failure are mainly related to chronicity of disease. Uraemic frosting [5], in which crystalline urea is deposited on the skin, is now very rare due to the widespread use of haemodialysis, but dry, pigmented skin with excoriations is typical.

Xerosis. Uraemic patients tend to have a dry skin, sometimes with fine scaling. A reduction in the size of the eccrine sweat glands in uraemia may contribute to this effect [5].

Pigmentation [5]. Anaemia presenting as pallor is an early and common sign in renal failure, resulting from reduced erythropoiesis and increased haemolysis (Figure 154.2). Hyperpigmentation is a common clinical sign in patients with end-stage renal disease. The pathomechanisms leading to the development of 'half-and-half'

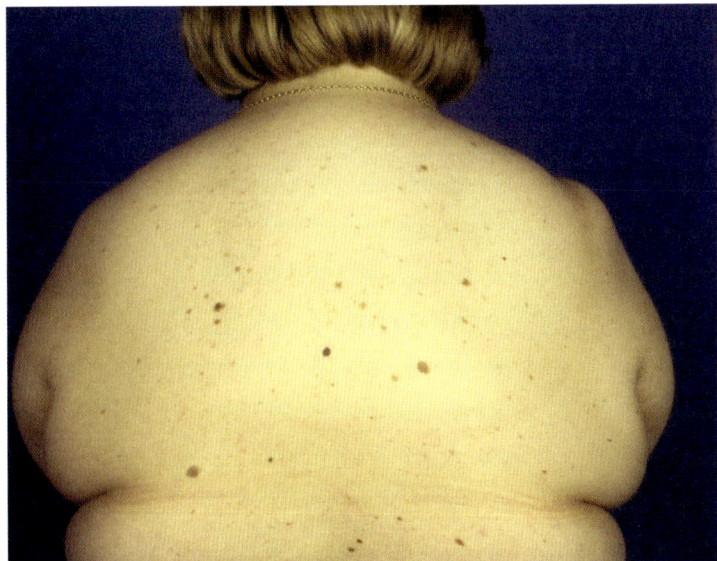

Figure 154.2 Lemon yellow pallor in a 27-year-old woman with end-stage renal failure (creatinine 497 µM/L, Hb 77 g/L) resulting from diabetic nephropathy.

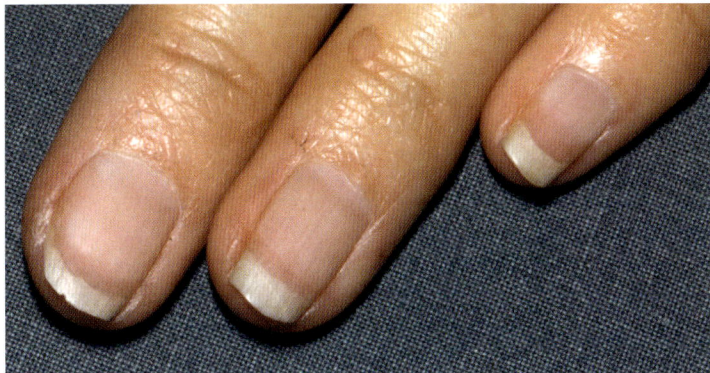

(a)

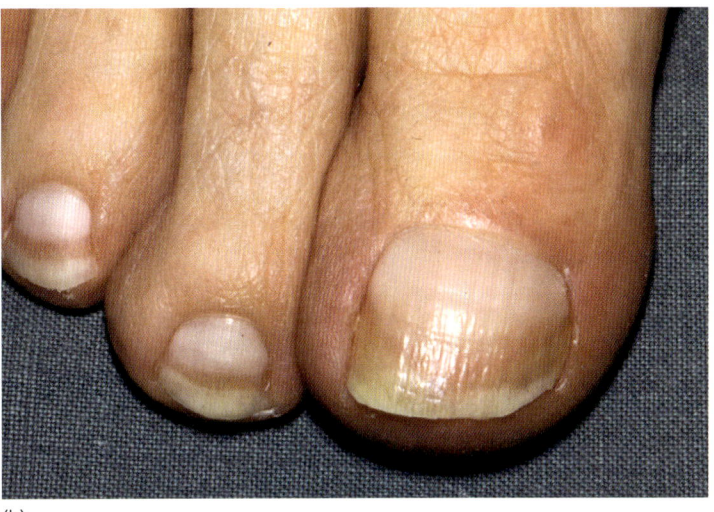

(b)

Figure 154.3 'Half-and-half' nails readily apparent on (a) the fingers and (b) the toes of a patient with uraemia.

nails, a distinctive pattern seen in up to 21% of patients with haemodialysis, are not fully understood. They are characterised by a distal brown or reddish colour, combined with a proximal white appearance (Figure 154.3).

Pruritus [5,6]. Localised (trunk, head) or generalised pruritus occurs in a large proportion of patients with end-stage kidney disease (Figure 154.4). It leads to secondary skin lesions including excoriations, chronic prurigo or acquired perforating dermatosis. The pathogenesis of pruritus in renal failure still remains unclear. Up to 90% of patients on haemodialysis suffer from itching. Other causes of itch should be excluded in every patient. Various treatment modalities have been reported in uraemic pruritus. Among them, topical capsaicin cream has been shown to be effective, as has UVB phototherapy. Parathyroidectomy may be helpful in patients with hyperparathyroidism.

Perforating disorders [5]. The acquired perforating dermatoses have been variously labelled reactive perforating collagenosis, perforating folliculitis, Kyrle disease and elastosis perforans serpiginosa depending on the precise clinicopathological presentation

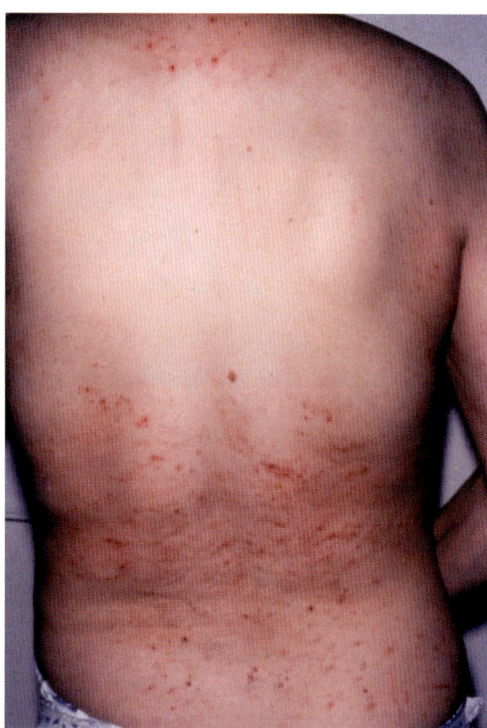

Figure 154.4 Severe uraemic prurigo in a 57-year-old woman with kidney damage following major surgery 1 year earlier. Note the normal skin in areas that cannot be reached to scratch.

(Chapter 94). The first three of these closely related entities occur principally in patients with end-stage renal disease, particularly in the context of longstanding diabetes (Chapter 94). They are characterised by the elimination of altered dermal collagen and elastin admixed with degenerate keratin through the follicular wall and/or the epidermis. Pruritus is nearly always present and up to 11% of dialysis patients may be affected. The cutaneous lesions consist of hyperpigmented papules, plaques and nodules up to 1 cm in diameter with a central keratinous plug. The extensor surfaces of the limbs are more commonly affected but the trunk and face may be involved as well (Figure 154.5).

Bullous diseases [5,6]. Pseudoporphyria is a bullous eruption mimicking porphyria cutanea tarda (PCT) that has been reported in patients with end-stage renal disease (chronic renal failure, haemodialysis), with an incidence rate of between 1% and 18% (Figure 154.6). True PCT due to deficiency of uroporphyrinogen decarboxylase is also reported but is uncommon. Distinguishing these two conditions can be difficult as many patients on haemodialysis have elevated blood porphyrin levels slightly above what is regarded as the normal range. However, patients with pseudoporphyria do not present the same porphyrin profile as patients with PCT. Several drugs such as furosemide, oestrogens and non-steroidal anti-inflammatory drugs have been reported as possible triggers of pseudoporphyria and also UV phototherapy. In all cases, UV protection is important. *N*-acetylcysteine, which acts as an antioxidant, may be of benefit in patients with pseudoporphyria on haemodialysis. These conditions are discussed in greater detail in Chapter 58.

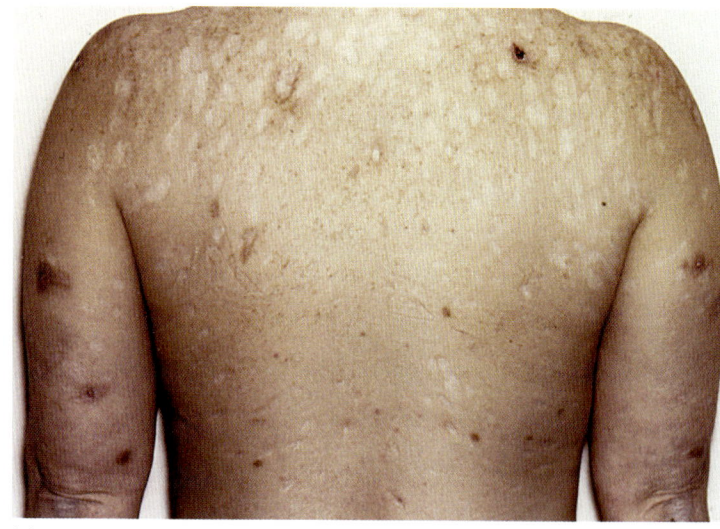

(a)

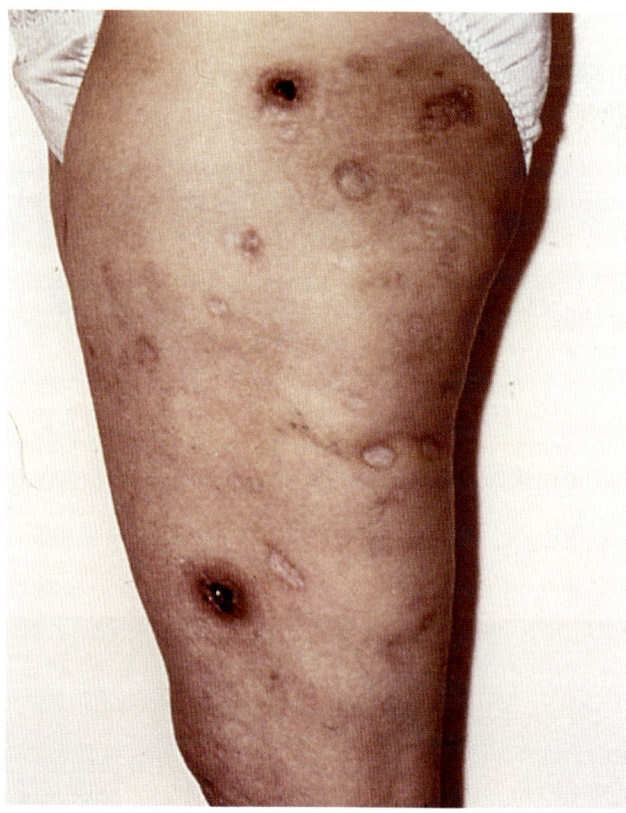

(b)

Figure 154.5 Extensive acquired perforating dermatosis with views of (a) the back and (b) the thigh of a 48-year-old woman with longstanding diabetes complicated by diabetic nephropathy requiring renal transplantation. She had a 12-year history of tender sore areas that broke down before healing with atrophic scars.

Features related to treatment. Premature ageing of the skin and actinic keratoses have been described; this is a reason for avoiding excessive UV therapy for pruritus. This should be distinguished from the numerous viral, dysplastic and (pre-) malignant skin lesions that may develop in immunosuppressed renal allograft recipients. Cutaneous complications affecting the limb of patients

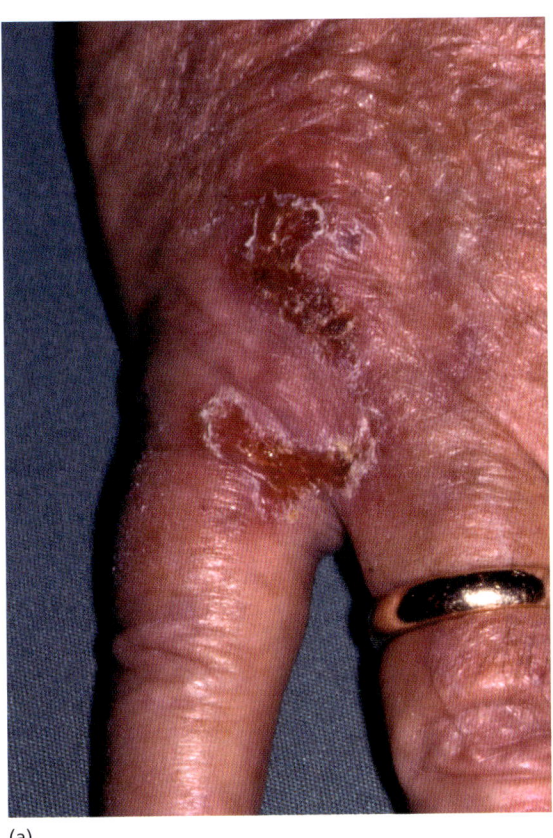
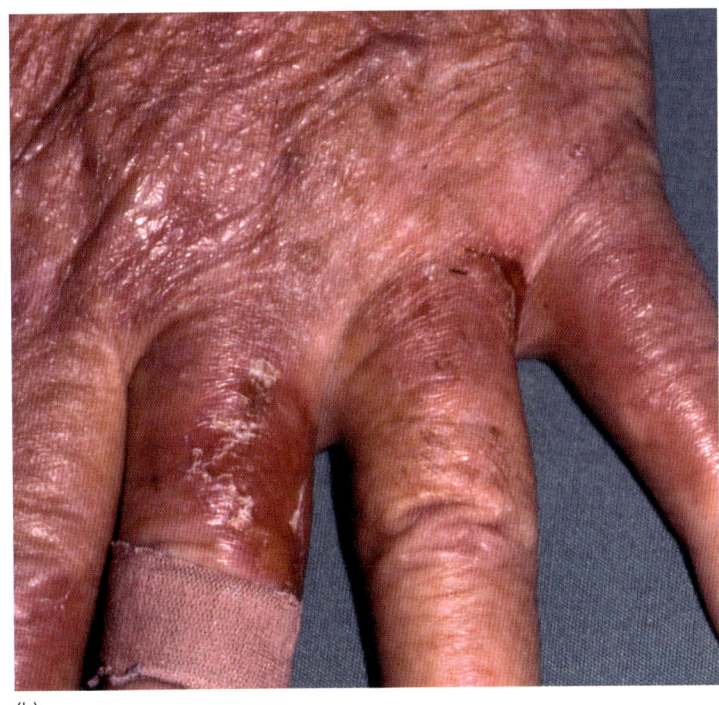

Figure 154.6 Pseudoporphyria on the backs of the hands of a 64-year-old man receiving renal dialysis for end-stage chronic kidney disease. There was no evidence of elevated porphyrins.

in which their haemodialysis arteriovenous shunt is sited include infection, phlebitis and haematoma. Both irritant and allergic contact eczema may also occur [19], as may pseudo-Kaposi sarcoma. A shunt-associated steal phenomenon can lead to distal ulceration and necrosis.

Nephrogenic systemic fibrosis. Nephrogenic systemic fibrosis is linked to renal dysfunction. It was initially described in 2000 as 'nephrogenic fibrosing dermopathy' in patients receiving, or with a history of, haemodialysis [5,20]. It is associated in over 90% of cases with the use of radiocontrast agents containing gadolinium, which are used to enhance magnetic resonance imaging of the blood vessels. Several other risk factors have, however, been suspected to play a role in its development, especially pro-inflammatory conditions including major surgery.

Clinical features include systemic fibrosis, including skin fibrosis with indurated plaques, sometimes with finger-like projections, that may be pink to red, yellowish or skin-coloured. Nodules and contractures occur in more advanced disease. Internal organs that may be involved include the heart, kidney and lungs. A deep skin biopsy down to deep fascia is required for histopathological evaluation. Histological criteria for the diagnosis have been published and include increased spindle cells and compact collagen bundles [20]. As no specific treatment exists, the use of gadolinium should be avoided in patients with significantly impaired renal function.

Renal transplantation

To prevent graft rejection after renal transplantation, immunosuppressive therapy is required. Documentation of the short- and long-term consequences of immunosuppression have been obtained principally from renal transplant recipients. Infections and the development of skin tumours are the most important dermatological consequences.

Infections [21,22]. Fungi, bacteria and viruses all play an important role as causes of cutaneous infections after kidney transplantation. Infections in general are very common in renal transplant patients. They follow a predictable time course after transplantation: within the first month these are mainly donor-derived infections, infections due to surgery-related issues (e.g. wound infection) or nosocomial infections. During the following months, opportunistic infections start to predominate and viral or bacterial infections become more important. By 6 months after transplantation, many patients start to suffer from chronic and progressive infections by, for instance, human papillomaviruses (Figure 154.7).

Other common viral infections include herpes simplex, herpes zoster and molluscum contagiosum. The predominant bacterial infections in renal transplant recipients are impetigo, folliculitis and erysipelas. Cutaneous fungal infections mainly comprise candidosis, dermatophytosis, including onychomycosis and pityriasis

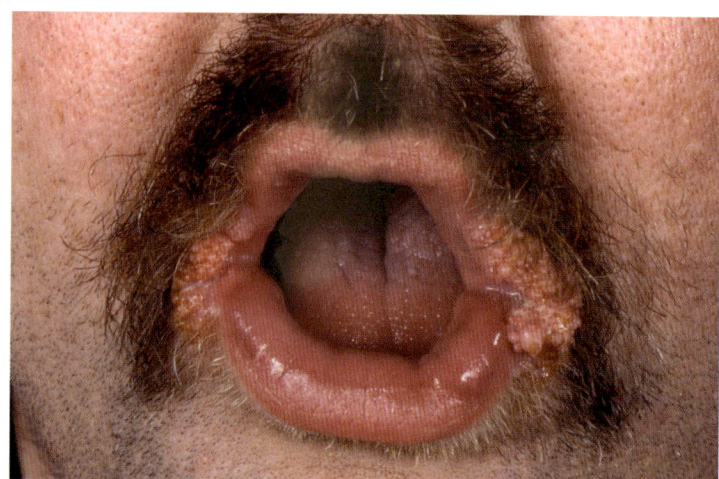

Figure 154.7 Exuberant viral warts at the oral commissures in a 37-year-old man immunosuppressed following renal transplant.

versicolor [22]. Exotic infections attributable to immunosuppression may occur following kidney transplantation, but these are relatively uncommon.

Skin tumours [23,24,25,26]. The incidence of malignancy in renal transplant recipients is particularly high, with skin cancer being the most frequently encountered. This topic is discussed in detail in Chapter 147.

ACQUIRED DISORDERS WITH SKIN AND RENAL INVOLVEMENT

Systemic autoimmune (connective tissue) diseases. Renal involvement is an important feature of many such diseases (Chapters 53 and 54). Although a majority of patients with systemic lupus erythematosus have renal involvement, this can be clinically inapparent. Levels of complement factors C3 and C4 can help to distinguish between active and inactive lupus nephritis: they are lower in active lupus nephritis [27]. Five percent of patients with systemic sclerosis develop scleroderma renal crisis [27]. It is characterised by severe hypertension, progressive decline of renal function and thrombotic microangiopathy.

Sarcoidosis [28]. Nephrolithiasis and nephrocalcinosis can occur in patients with sarcoidosis. Hypercalcaemia may also cause renal impairment and may even precipitate acute renal failure. Renal sarcoidosis can give rise to granulomatous interstitial nephritis due to immune complex deposition. The renal involvement in many cases may, however, remain clinically silent. Rarely, cases of ureteric obstruction, voiding impairment, bladder involvement and sarcoid of the urethra have been reported.

Vasculitis (see Chapter 100). The vasculitides have recently been reclassified due to a better understanding of the different disease entities [29]. The new nomenclature comprises small-, medium-, large- and variable-vessel vasculitis, single-organ vasculitis and vasculitis associated with systemic disease or probable aetiology. Small-vessel vasculitis (SVV) can be further subclassified into antineutrophil cytoplasmic antibody (ANCA) associated vasculitis or immune complex SVV. Granulomatosis with polyangiitis (GPA), microscopic polyangiitis (MPA) and eosinophilic GPA (formerly Churg–Strauss syndrome) belong to the ANCA-associated SVVs, whereas antiglomerular basement membrane (anti-GBM) disease and IgA vasculitis (formerly Henoch–Schönlein purpura) belong to the group of immune complex SVVs. Behçet disease is considered to be a variable-vessel vasculitis [29].

Renal involvement is common in a variety of vasculitides that present with cutaneous lesions and is the main cause of mortality in many of them. IgA vasculitis is a small-vessel leukocytoclastic vasculitis predominantly affecting the skin, joints, gastrointestinal tract and kidneys, especially in children between 3 and 12 years of age [30]. The renal symptoms include haematuria, proteinuria, nephrotic syndrome, renal impairment and hypertension [31]. Renal involvement (mainly rapidly progressive glomerulonephritis) is common in ANCA-associated SVV, mainly in GPA (50–80%) and MPA (90–100%). In eosinophilic GPA it is less frequent (4–51%) [32]. Renal involvement in Behçet disease may include glomerulonephritis, vascular disease, interstitial nephritis or renal failure [33].

SKIN DISORDERS THAT MAY AFFECT THE KIDNEY AND URINARY TRACT

Bullous pemphigoid. Renal disease, including membranous glomerulopathy, diffuse proliferative and mesangioproliferative glomerulonephritis, has been infrequently reported in patients with pemphigoid [34].

Toxic epidermal necrolysis [35]. Deteriorating renal function is a poor prognostic factor in this disorder and is one of the parameters used in the SCORTEN prognostic score.

Epidermolysis bullosa. Renal failure was the second most common cause of death (with a mean age of 35 years) in 12% of adults with generalised severe recessive dystrophic epidermolysis bullosa (Hallopeau–Siemens syndrome) [36]. In epidermolysis bullosa, mucous membrane involvement can be associated with ulceration of the genito-urinary epithelium. Genito-urinary involvement is rare and often asymptomatic, but may clinically present as haematuria, meatal stenosis, sepsis, dysuria and hydronephrosis [37].

Skin infections. *Streptococcal impetigo*: post-streptococcal glomerulonephritis may occur 1–4 weeks after superficial streptococcal skin infections such as impetigo [38]. *Secondary syphilis*: this is a rare cause of the nephrotic syndrome [39]. *Herpes zoster*: if affecting the relevant dermatomes, herpes zoster may cause neurogenic bladder dysfunction leading to acute urinary retention [40].

Key references

The full list of references can be found in the online version at https://www.wiley.com/rooksdermatology10e

6 Kurban MS, Boueiz A, Kibbi AG. Cutaneous manifestations of chronic kidney disease. *Clin Dermatol* 2008;26:255–64.

11 Ferzli PG, Millett CR, Newman MD *et al*. The dermatologist's guide to hereditary syndromes with renal tumors. *Cutis* 2008;81:41–8.

20 Weller A, Barber JL, Olsen OE. Gadolinium and nephrogenic systemic fibrosis: an update. *Pediatr Nephrol* 2014;29:1927–37.

21 Karuthu S, Blumberg EA. Common infections in kidney transplant recipients. *Clin J Am Soc Nephrol* 2012;7:2058–70.

23 Stenz NA, Stampf S, Arnold AW *et al*. Skin cancer development in solid organ transplant recipients in Switzerland (Swiss Transplant Cohort Study). *Dermatology* 2021;237:970–80.

24 Zwald FO, Brown M. Skin cancer in solid organ transplant recipients: advances in therapy and management: part I. Epidemiology of skin cancer in solid organ transplant recipients. *J Am Acad Dermatol* 2011;65:253–61; quiz 262.

27 Kronbichler A, Mayer G. Renal involvement in autoimmune connective tissue diseases. *BMC Med* 2013;11:95.

28 La Rochelle JC, Coogan CL. Urological manifestations of sarcoidosis. *J Urol* 2012;187:18–24.

31 Tizard EJ, Hamilton-Ayres MJ. Henoch Schonlein purpura. *Arch Dis Child Educ Pract Ed* 2008;93:1–8.

33 Akpolat T, Dilek M, Aksu K *et al*. Renal Behçet's disease: an update. *Semin Arthritis Rheum* 2008;38:241–8.

CHAPTER 155

The Skin and Disorders of the Musculoskeletal System

Christopher R. Lovell

Department of Dermatology, Royal United Hospital and Royal National Hospital for Rheumatic Diseases, Bath, UK

Introduction, 155.1
History and examination, 155.1

INFECTIVE ARTHROPATHIES, 155.2
Reactive arthritis, 155.2
Viral arthropathies, 155.2
Bacterial arthropathies, 155.4
Other infective arthropathies, 155.5

INFLAMMATORY ARTHROPATHIES, 155.5
Seronegative arthritis and spondylitis, 155.5
Rheumatoid arthritis, 155.5
Atrophic skin with rheumatoid arthritis, 155.5
Rheumatoid nodules, 155.5
Rheumatoid vasculitis and cutaneous ulceration, 155.6
Rheumatoid neutrophilic dermatosis, 155.6

Other, 155.6
Fibroblastic rheumatism, 155.7
Sarcoidosis, 155.7

OSTEOARTHRITIS, 155.8
Heberden and Bouchard nodes, 155.8

METABOLIC DISORDERS WITH MUSCULOSKELETAL AND CUTANEOUS INVOLVEMENT, 155.9
Haemochromatosis, 155.9
Alkaptonuria, 155.9
Gout, 155.9

AUTOINFLAMMATORY DISORDERS, 155.10
Hereditary autoinflammatory disorders, 155.10
Acquired autoinflammatory disorders, 155.10
Acne, 155.10
Hidradenitis suppurativa, 155.11

INFLAMMATORY CHONDROPATHIES, 155.11
Relapsing polychondritis, 155.11
MAGIC syndrome, 155.13

MISCELLANEOUS DISORDERS INVOLVING THE SKIN AND MUSCULOSKELETAL SYSTEM, 155.13
Mastocytosis, 155.13
Multicentric reticulohistiocytosis, 155.14
Pachydermoperiostosis, 155.14
Interstitial granulomatous dermatosis, 155.14
Intralymphatic histiocytosis, 155.14

CUTANEOUS ADVERSE REACTIONS TO ANTIRHEUMATIC THERAPIES, 155.15

Acknowledgement, 155.16

Key references, 155.16

Introduction

Combined clinics with rheumatology provide a valuable tertiary referral service for patients with complex disease. A combined therapeutic approach can improve the quality of life of patients with psoriatic arthritis for example. Both dermatologists and rheumatologists can learn from each other when discussing the management of autoimmune connective tissue diseases such as lupus erythematosus, dermatomyositis, systemic sclerosis and the vasculitides. A patient with an inborn error of matrix protein synthesis such as Ehlers–Danlos syndrome may present to either specialty. This chapter examines some other specific conditions where skin eruptions and arthropathy play a major part. These include infections, metabolic disorders such as gout, inflammasome disorders and infiltrative conditions such as multicentric reticulohistiocytosis. In addition, this chapter explores cutaneous manifestations of rheumatoid disease, relapsing polychondritis and related disorders, and some cutaneous adverse effects of rheumatological treatments.

History and examination

Apart from a dermatological and occupational history, direct questioning about the musculoskeletal system may suggest an underlying rheumatological diagnosis. Is there pain or stiffness? Where is it localised (e.g. specific muscles or large or small joints)? What exacerbates or relieves it? Which words best describe the pain (e.g. the burning pain of neuropathy or the steady ache of an inflammatory arthritis such as rheumatoid)? Emotive terms such as 'excruciating' or 'terrible' may indicate a chronic pain syndrome or fibromyalgia, although ethnic and cultural factors may influence the description [1]. Joint stiffness in the morning or after a period of immobility is a feature of inflammatory joint disease. An accurate history of joint swelling can be difficult to elicit. Other questions include a history suggesting serositis, e.g. pleuritic chest pain, fever and its pattern, circulatory problems such as Raynaud phenomenon, soreness and redness of the eyes and fatigue.

Examination of the musculoskeletal system begins when the patient enters the consulting room. Are posture or gait affected? Localise points of pain, e.g. to specific joints, muscles or tendon sheaths; 'trigger points' of tenderness are seen in fibromyalgia. Active and passive movements of arthritic joints are equally painful, whereas active mobilisation tends to be more painful than passive in periarticular disease. The presence of joint swelling, synovial thickening or an effusion should be assessed, and the joints that are affected should be established. Monoarthritis can be a typical presentation of gout. Psoriatic arthritis often affects the distal interphalangeal joints, with associated nail dystrophy, but it can also affect large joints such as the shoulder or the axial skeleton. Red or pink skin or temperature change near the affected joints should be assessed – often skin temperature is normal over osteoarthritic joints. Vasomotor alteration and trophic skin changes over a hand or foot occur in algodystrophy (Sudek atrophy), perhaps associated with neurological damage. The presence of a joint deformity, crepitus or restricted range of movement should be assessed. Muscle wasting or weakness should be noted. The patient's movement when getting out of the chair at the end of the consultation should be carefully analysed. Laboratory and radiological tests can support the clinical diagnosis but should not be interpreted in isolation.

INFECTIVE ARTHROPATHIES

Several infective agents are associated with specific patterns of skin and joint involvement [1] ('infection-related arthritis'); the major ones are discussed here.

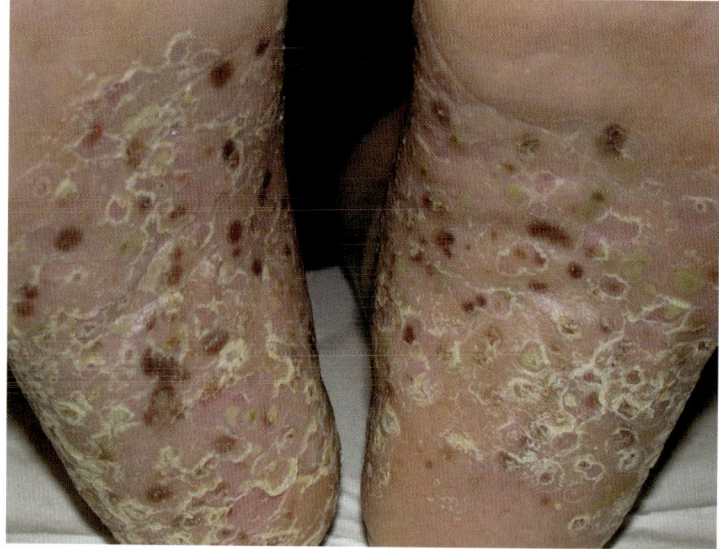

Figure 155.1 Keratoderma blennorhagicum in a patient with reactive arthritis.

Reactive arthritis

The term reactive arthritis refers to the development of an acute spondyloarthritis, often asymmetrical, following a genitourinary or gastrointestinal infection. It is strongly linked with the HLA-B27 haplotype and typically affects young men [1,2]. A range of infective organisms has been associated with the syndrome (Table 155.1). The classical clinical presentation comprises the triad of an asymmetrical large joint oligoarthritis with or without dactylitis, urethritis and ocular inflammation (conjunctivitis and anterior uveitis), manifesting 1–6 weeks after an acute sexually transmitted chlamydial infection. These may be accompanied by constitutional symptoms including fever and malaise. Skin lesions, most characteristically palmoplantar pustulosis and psoriasiform hyperkeratosis (keratoderma blennorhagicum: blennorhagia = excessive discharge of mucus), develop in around 15% of men with the syndrome. Mouth erosions, geographic tongue and circinate balanitis are common features (Figures 155.1 and 155.2). Although the condition is usually self-limiting, it can progress to a chronic arthritis in around 15–20% of patients [3]. Co-infection with human immunodeficiency virus (HIV) is common in sexually acquired cases [4] and HIV may be arthritogenic [5]. There appears to be molecular mimicry between the infective organisms and a region of the HLA-B27α-I helix [6].

A reactive arthritis occurs in 2–3% and septic arthritis in 1% [6]. Diffuse infiltrative lymphocytosis syndrome (DILS), which mimics Sjögren syndrome, may be a presenting feature of HIV infection [6]. Unlike Sjögren syndrome, males are predominantly affected and anti-ENA antibodies (Ro/SSA and La/SSB) are rarely found [7]. Since the advent of highly active antiretroviral therapy (HAART), DILS is now rare. Immune reconstitution syndrome describes a systemic inflammatory process which develops from 3 to 24 months after initiating HAART. CD4 cells are elevated, with increased circulating cytokines such as interleukin (IL)-6 and interferon γ. It is associated with a higher prevalence of autoimmune connective tissue diseases such as systemic lupus erythematosus and dermatomyositis [8–10].

Viral arthropathies (Chapters 25 and 31)

Rubella and parvovirus B19 are the most commonly implicated viruses in self-limiting arthritis in the developed world. In *rubella*, a maculopapular rash spreads cephalocaudally, followed or preceded by occipital lymphadenopathy and arthralgia in up to 50%. A few develop a symmetrical polyarthritis affecting the metacarpal and proximal interphalangeal joints, later involving the larger joints [1].

Parvovirus B19 is associated with erythema infectiosum (fifth disease), characterised by 'slapped cheek' redness on the face (and sometimes also on the cheeks of the buttocks) and a reticulate redness of the trunk and limbs (Figure 155.3). This red to pink discoloration may recur over several weeks when the child is warm. Posterior cervical lymph nodes are enlarged. Systemic symptoms, such as myalgia and a symmetrical arthritis, are much commoner in adults than in children occurring around a fortnight after infection [2]. Although parvovirus B19 infection may be associated with a chronic polyarthritis resembling rheumatoid disease [3],

Table 155.1 Infectious agents commonly and less frequently associated with reactive arthritis.

Gastrointestinal tract	Yersinia
	Salmonella
	Shigella
	Campylobacter jejuni
Uro-genital tract	Chlamydia trachomatis
	Neisseria gonorrhoea
	Mycoplasma genitalium
	Ureaplasma urealyticum
Less frequent agents	Clostridium difficile
	Campylobacter lari
	Chlamydia psittaci
	Chlamydia pneumoniae

From Selmi and Gershwin 2014 [2].

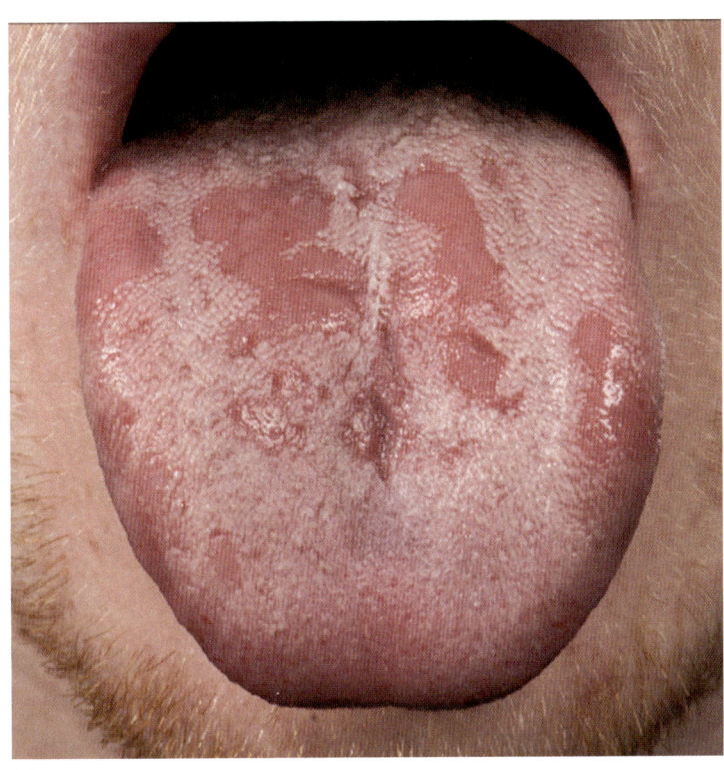

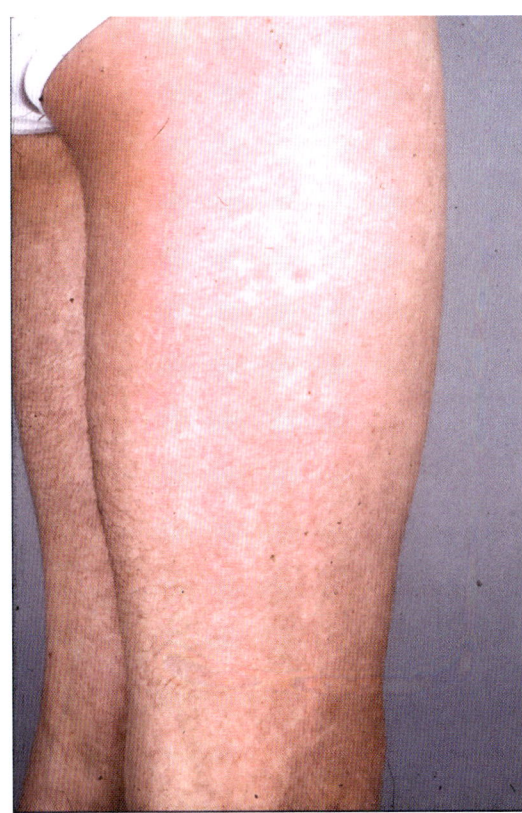

Figure 155.3 Reticulate red-to-pink discoloration of erythema infectiosum.

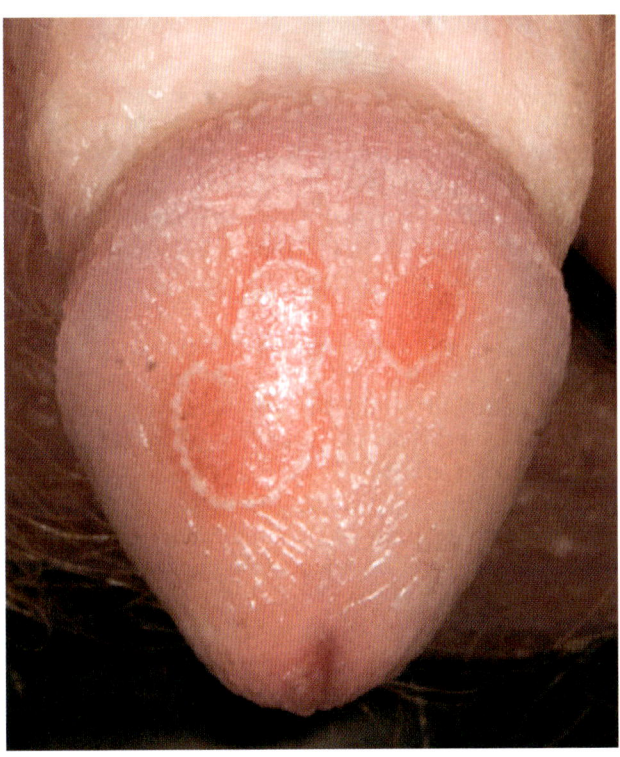

Figure 155.2 (a) Geographic tongue and (b) circinate balanitis in HLA-B27 positive adolescent.

there appears to be of little value in screening for viral infection in patients with polyarthritis persisting for more than 6 weeks [4].

Arthralgia is common in the acute phase of many viral infections. Polyarthritis, which can be migratory, and cutaneous vasculitis can be a feature of acute *hepatitis B* or C infection, usually before the icteric phase. Several rheumatological manifestations are associated with *HIV* infection. Around 10% of patients develop severe migratory joint pain at the acute seroconversion stage, chiefly affecting shoulders, elbows and knees, often persisting for fewer than 24 hours in each joint [5,6].

Alphaviruses are transmitted by mosquitoes, chiefly *Aedes* species. Specific syndromes include chikungunya (literally 'twisting up') and O'nyong-nyong virus (literally 'joint-breaker'), which are chiefly found in tropical Africa, Sindbis (chiefly in Sweden, Finland and the Baltic states), Mayaro virus (tropical South America) and Ross River virus (epidemic polyarthritis), which occurs in Australia, chiefly Queensland [7]. They are all associated with a maculopapular eruption, severe arthralgia and typically mild synovitis which resolves after weeks or months, although a rheumatoid arthritis-like syndrome may develop [8]. Chikungunya fever presents as facial or neck flushing within 1–5 days, followed by a widespread maculopapular eruption. Other features include centrofacial hyperpigmentation and oral ulcers resembling aphthae.

Coronaviruses: although Covid-19 has been associated with autoimmune thrombocytopenia, antiphospholipid syndrome and systemic lupus erythematosus, arthritis is rare; it usually presents early and is self-limiting [9].

Bacterial arthropathies (Chapters 26 and 30)

Septic arthritis, usually due to *Staphylococcus aureus*, should be considered in the differential diagnosis of synovitis, particularly if there is a recent history of trauma or joint aspiration or if the patient is immunosuppressed, e.g. HIV infection or high-dose systemic corticosteroids. In patients on immunosuppressive drugs, joint infection may be caused by opportunistic organisms. Arthralgia can be a feature of acute bacterial infection and may predominate in *brucellosis*. An intermittent migratory arthritis may follow the characteristic erythema migrans of Lyme disease or a relatively painless monoarthritis may develop, particularly targeting the knee joint. Arthritis may be episodic and may persist after antimicrobial therapy, sometimes leading to cartilage destruction and bony erosions [1]. Although arthralgia is common in syphilis, frank synovitis is rare, although neuropathy may cause joint trauma.

Neisseria gonorrhoeae and *N. meningitidis* are both associated with inflammatory arthritis. Acute infections with either organism can be followed by an acute polyarthritis within 2–3 weeks [2]. Chronic meningococcal arthritis is now chiefly seen in resource-poor regions. It can be associated with widespread macular redness and tender papular, nodular or pustular lesions (Figure 155.4), which may become purpuric. Histological changes range from perivascular inflammation to leukocytoclastic vasculitis [3]. Similarly, papular and vesicular lesions, often periarticular, occur in chronic gonococcaemia and may be misdiagnosed as papular lupus erythematosus [4]. Gonococcal arthritis can be destructive, with or without associated tenosynovitis [5]. Men are at higher risk of gonococcal arthritis and there may be co-infection with HIV. Usually, the organism can be isolated from blood culture or synovial fluid; if not, it can be identified by polymerase chain reaction (PCR) [6] (Chapter 30).

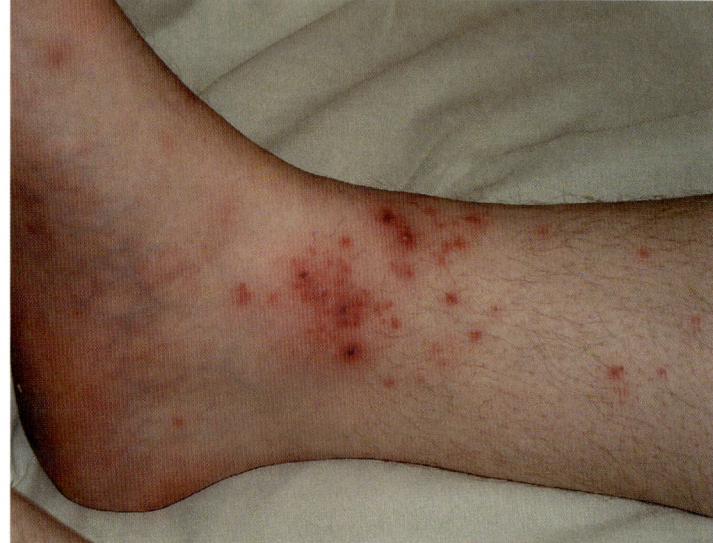

Figure 155.4 A 19-year-old man with short history of headache, nausea, vomiting and weakness: the subsequently confirmed clinical suspicion of early meningococcal septicaemia was raised by the presence of a pustular vasculitic rash over the ankles.

Mycobacterial infections (Chapters 27 and 28) may be overlooked as causes of joint disease. In borderline *leprosy* a symmetrical peripheral polyarthritis, often of insidious onset and of waxing and waning severity [7], can mimic a connective tissue disease and, confusingly, serological tests such as rheumatoid factor and antinuclear factor may be positive [8]. Extension of skin lesions on the fingers and toes can give rise to a dactylitis with leprous periostitis and eventually osteomyelitis [9]. Synovitis and dactylitis coincide with the appearance of skin lesions in the reactional state of erythema nodosum leprosum. Enthesitis and sacroiliitis occur more rarely. Chronic nerve damage leads to muscle deformity and joint contracture with eventual joint destruction. *Tuberculosis* characteristically involves the spine; it may present to the dermatologist as a paravertebral abscess (Pott disease). Peripheral septic arthritis is usually monoarticular, and may result in bony ankylosis of the joint [10]. A reactive aseptic polyarthritis (Poncet disease) may occur in active tuberculosis; it is often associated with erythema nodosum but sacroiliitis is uncommon [**11**]. Septic arthritis, bursitis, tenosynovitis and even osteomyelitis can result from subcutaneous inoculation [12,13] or as a contaminant during joint injection [14] of atypical mycobacteria such as *M. marinum* and *M. avium-cellulare*.

Rheumatic fever [15] follows infection with group A β-haemolytic *Streptococcus*, and comprises pyrexia, a very painful migratory polyarthritis, typically involving large joints, and carditis. It affects children, usually between 5 and 15 years, mostly in resource-poor countries. It may be preceded by scarlet fever or pharyngitis. Impetigo due to group A streptococci predisposes to rheumatic carditis [16]. Scabies infestation, which is commonly impetiginised, is a major risk factor for rheumatic fever and post-streptococcal glomerulonephritis [17].

The characteristic urticated annular skin lesions of erythema marginatum, with a predilection for the trunk and proximal limbs, comprise one of the major criteria for the diagnosis of rheumatic fever (Figure 151.5) [18]. However, they are evanescent, and only seen in around 10% of children. Up to 20% develop subcutaneous nodules, which often occur in crops, typically on the extensor aspects of the limbs, but also over the scapula, occiput and forehead. Nodules may last only a few weeks. They are sometimes associated with the development of vegetations on the heart valves. In the Lewis rat model of rheumatic carditis, passive transfer of T-cell lines specific to peptides of streptococcal M protein induce valvulitis with expression of CD4+ T cells and upregulation of vascular cell adhesion molecule type 1 (VCAM-1) on heart valves of naive rats. Additionally, antistreptococcal antibodies attack the valve endothelium leading to T-cell infiltration. These antibodies are also linked to the development of neuropsychiatric disease and Sydenham chorea [19].

In affluent countries, *Kawasaki disease* has replaced rheumatic fever as a prime cause of cardiovascular disease in childhood [20]. Adult cases have been reported. A specific pathogen has not been identified although an increased incidence has been noted following viral infections such as influenza and Covid-19 [**21**]. It is a systemic vasculitis. Clinical features include high swinging fever, conjunctival injection, redness of the oral mucosa with a 'strawberry tongue' and fissured lips. Skin changes include a diffuse macular redness and red discoloration of the palms and soles, which may result in desquamation of the limbs (Figure 150.4).

Up to 30% develop a self-limiting oligo- or polyarthritis of large joints [22].

Whipple disease typically affects middle-aged men who present with weight loss and diarrhoea, focal infections (e.g. endocarditis, encephalitis) and joint symptoms. The actinomycete *Tropheryma whipplei* has been identified as the causative organism, probably transmitted by the oro-oral or faeco-oral routes. It can be cultured from synovial fluid [23] or detected by PCR of skin lesions, lymph nodes or synovial fluid [24]. A chronic seronegative arthritis affects one or more large limb joints; the process is often intermittent. Spondyloarthropathy may develop [25]. Skin lesions, which are uncommon, include multiple generalised subcutaneous nodules and a septal panniculitis. A granulomatous dermal infiltrate is associated with periodic acid–Schiff (PAS) positive macrophages [26]. Treatment has been associated with the development of lesions resembling erythema nodosum leprosum [27]. Untreated, the neurological changes can be fatal, and lifelong doxycycline is recommended because of the risk of relapse [24].

Other infective arthropathies

Disseminated fungal infection (e.g. coccidioidomycosis [1]) may lead to synovitis of one or more joints, particularly in immunosuppressed individuals.

Mycetoma is a progressive tumour-like mass, often affecting the foot. It may be caused by actinomycetes (actinomycetoma; Chapter 26) or fungi, notably *Madurella mycetomatis* (eumycetoma; Chapter 32). The diagnosis can be confirmed by histology and culture of the grains that extrude from the lesion. The mass can destructively invade underlying bone and amputation is often required [2,3].

Post kala-azar dermal leishmaniasis (Chapter 33) is an inflammatory process that may be associated with arthralgia and joint contracture (Figure 155.5). *Leishmania* synovitis has been described mostly in dogs, although polyarthritis has been reported in immunosuppressed humans [4].

INFLAMMATORY ARTHROPATHIES

Seronegative arthritis and spondylitis

Seronegative arthritis and spondyloarthropathy are associated with inflammatory bowel disease (Chapter 153) and psoriasis (Chapter 35), notably in individuals possessing the HLA-B27 haplotype. Typical musculoskeletal features include back pain, with early morning stiffness, and sacroiliitis together with enthesitis. Uveitis and oral ulceration are common. There is an increased prevalence of hidradenitis suppurativa in these individuals [1]. Pyoderma gangrenosum is also characteristically associated with ulcerative colitis and spondyloarthritis. In one survey of 103 patients with spondyloarthritis, 34% had inflammatory bowel disease and 19% had pyoderma gangrenosum [2].

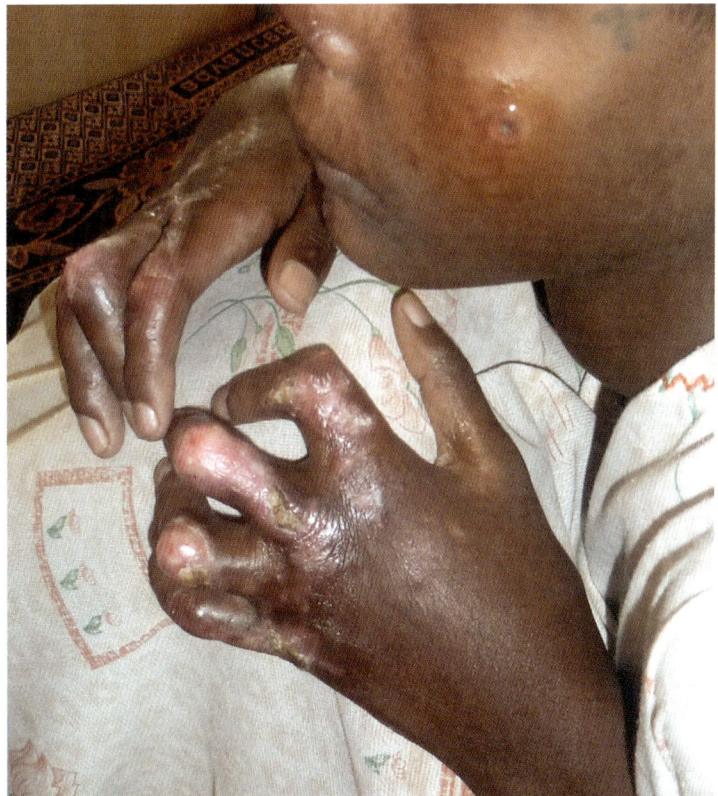

Figure 155.5 Severe joint contractures in a child with post-kala-azar dermal leishmaniasis.

Rheumatoid arthritis

Reddening of the skin and a burning sensation may be the initial manifestation of rheumatoid disease, before joint changes develop [1]. Rheumatoid arthritis is associated with several skin abnormalities, including non-segmental vitiligo [2] (Box 155.1).

Atrophic skin with rheumatoid arthritis

In rheumatoid patients over the age of 60 years, especially women, the skin on the dorsa of the hands may become thin, loose, smooth, inelastic and transparent, leading to clear visualisation of the veins and tendons. The change is generalised but is seldom conspicuous except on the hands and forearms. Histologically, the dermis is thinned but shows no distinctive changes.

There is a significant association between transparent skin, rheumatoid arthritis and osteoporosis and it is assumed to form part of a general connective tissue defect [1]. Steroid therapy is not a factor but it will potentiate the problem [2,3]. Skin collagen is structurally abnormal [4]. A reported association with pseudoxanthoma elasticum may be coincidental [5].

Rheumatoid nodules

Skin-coloured subcutaneous nodules, often multiple, occur in over 20% of patients with rheumatoid arthritis, especially in men and in seropositive disease [1]. They are usually asymptomatic unless they compress an adjacent nerve or ulcerate. Nodules are found over extensor surfaces, such as the elbows and knees

> **Box 155.1 Skin manifestations of rheumatoid arthritis**
>
> **General**
> - Skin redness, burning sensation (may precede joint changes)
> - Hyperpigmentation, especially over affected joints and on lower legs in Felty syndrome
> - Nodules (including accelerated rheumatoid nodulosis)
> - Atrophy (linked to osteoporosis)
> - Skin infections
> - Vitiligo (non-segmental)
> - Possible association with pseudoxanthoma elasticum
>
> **Vasculitis**
> - Splinter haemorrhages and periungual infarcts
> - Palpable purpura
> - Livedo reticularis
> - Atrophie blanche
>
> **Neutrophil-related disorders**
> - Pyoderma gangrenosum (often atypical)
> - Rheumatoid neutrophilic dermatosis
>
> **Leg ulcers, often multifactorial, including**
> - Vasculitis
> - Venous insufficiency
> - Lymphoedema
> - Reduced mobility
> - Skin atrophy
> - Delayed wound healing
> - Neuropathy (foot ulcers)
>
> **Miscellaneous**
> - Interstitial granulomatous dermatitis
> - Intralymphatic histiocytosis
> - Adverse effects of antirheumatic drugs

(Figure 155.6), and sites of repetitive trauma. They vary in size from a few millimetres to several centimetres. Histology is characteristic with palisading granulomata around a central area of fibrinoid necrobiosis (Figure 155.7). Necrobiosis is closely associated with the pathogenesis of rheumatoid disease including collagen degeneration, recruitment of activated neutrophils, production of pro-inflammatory cytokines and vascular injury [2].

The differential diagnosis includes knuckle pads, subcutaneous sarcoid and subcutaneous granuloma annulare. The latter (especially in children) can be associated with a positive rheumatoid factor, leading to a false diagnosis of rheumatoid arthritis (Chapter 97). Measurement of anti-citrullinated peptide antibodies is current rheumatological practice in the diagnosis of rheumatoid arthritis. These antibodies are more specific than rheumatoid factor and appear to be more predictive of progressive disease [3]. Nodules may occur also in the lung parenchyma (Kaplan syndrome). Cutaneous nodules wax and wane with treatment of the disease and rituximab has proved a beneficial treatment [4]. However, some drugs, including methotrexate, antitumour necrosis factor (TNF) agents and leflunomide may exacerbate nodulosis [1]. The term 'accelerated rheumatoid nodulosis' describes painful rheumatoid-like nodules which develop rapidly, chiefly on the ears, hands and feet [5] and often on previously unaffected sites. They are typically associated with methotrexate therapy and often regress when the drug is discontinued but recur if it is reintroduced [6]. The aetiopathogenesis is uncertain; genetic factors include an increased prevalence of HLA-DR4 [7] and the 2756GG genotype of methionine synthase reductase in affected patients [8] (Chapter 97). However, similar changes are reported with anti-TNF therapy.

Rheumatoid vasculitis and cutaneous ulceration

Digital vasculitis (Figure 155.8) presents as splinter haemorrhages and periungual infarcts, palpable purpura, livedo reticularis and atrophie blanche, especially in patients with high titres of rheumatoid factor or citrullinated peptides (CCP). Vasculitis may be associated with cutaneous and pulmonary nodulosis, episcleritis and pleural or pericardial effusions. Pyoderma gangrenosum, which may be atypical [1], can be associated with rheumatoid arthritis. It may respond to colchicine, ciclosporin or dapsone but some patients require high dose corticosteroids or even anti-TNF-α drugs such as infliximab or certolizumab pegol [2–4]. Rheumatoid vasculitis, like other systemic features of the disease, appears to be in decline, perhaps due to effective disease control with biological agents [5]. Rheumatoid patients on immunosuppressive therapy are at risk of infections that may simulate vasculitis [6,7].

Chronic leg ulcers in rheumatoid patients are often difficult to manage, and often have mixed aetiology. Causes include arterial occlusion due to vasculitis, venous insufficiency, lymphoedema, 'inactivity ulcers' linked with immobility, poor wound healing and thin skin [8,9,**10**]. Methotrexate and TNF-α inhibitor therapy appear to potentiate vasculitic ulcers in some cases [11,12], but can be beneficial in others. Loss of sensation and forefoot deformity contribute to foot ulceration in rheumatoid patients [13].

Rheumatoid neutrophilic dermatosis

Neutrophilic disorders occupy a spectrum including pyoderma gangrenosum and Sweet disease and these different conditions may coexist. They are typically associated with systemic diseases such as blood cell dyscrasias, inflammatory bowel disease and rheumatoid arthritis [1] and have also been associated with systemic lupus erythematosus [2].

Rheumatoid neutrophilic dermatosis presents as urticaria-like papules and plaques, often symmetrically on the trunk and limbs. There is probably an overlap with Sweet syndrome, although the typical plum-coloured lesions of the latter are not generally seen. Histologically, there is a heavy dermal infiltrate of neutrophils but no frank vasculitis (Figure 155.9) [3]. Tense bullae may occur on the lower legs; this variant responds to dapsone, but not to corticosteroids [4,5]. Neutrophilic dermatosis can present in patients with seropositive or seronegative rheumatoid disease. Some patients develop nodular lesions which can progress to rheumatoid nodules [6].

Other

Other conditions which may occur in association with rheumatoid arthritis include interstitial granulomatous dermatosis and intralymphatic histiocytosis (see Interstitial granulomatous dermatosis and Intralymphatic histiocytosis).

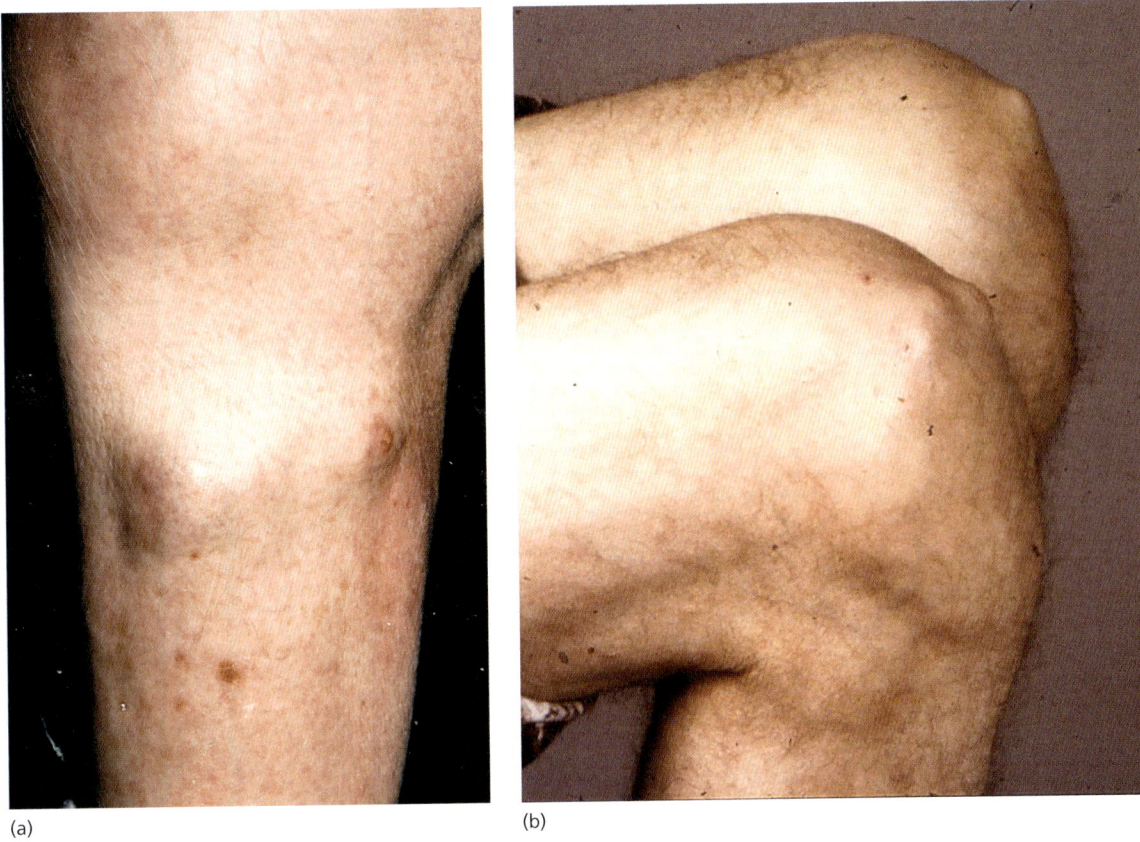

Figure 155.6 (a, b) Multiple rheumatoid nodules on the lower leg and knees.

Fibroblastic rheumatism

This rare condition occurs worldwide, primarily affecting white people of any age with equal sex incidence. Acute onset symmetrical polyarthritis is associated with multiple skin-coloured papules and nodules measuring 5–20 mm diameter on the limbs. Some patients give a history of Raynaud phenomenon; there may be sclerodactyly and palmar thickening [1–3], suggesting a *forme fruste* of a connective tissue disease such as systemic sclerosis. Histology of the skin lesions reveals increased numbers of fibroblasts with myofibroblast differentiation, diffuse dermal fibrosis and absence of elastin on orcein staining [4,5]. Myofibroblast-like cells are also seen within a collagenous stroma in the synovium [1]. Periarticular erosions may be detected on bone X-ray [1,6]. Clinically, the condition may mimic multicentric reticulohistiocytosis and it has been suggested that, like the latter condition, fibroblastic rheumatism is a form of non-Langerhans cell histiocytosis [7]. However, it fits better into the category of an inflammatory fibromatosis [1,4,6,8]. Unlike multicentric reticulohistiocytosis, fibroblastic rheumatism is not associated with systemic disease or malignant neoplasia [9]. The condition is often self-limiting [10], although immunosuppressive therapy has been used to good effect, including methotrexate [2,5], interferon-α [6] and infliximab [11]. Bony erosions may persist despite methotrexate therapy [6].

Sarcoidosis (Chapter 96)

Acute joint swelling is common in patients with Löfgren syndrome (an acute variant of sarcoidosis with erythema nodosum and bilateral hilar lymphadenopathy on chest X-ray). Joint pain is due to soft tissue swelling and tenosynovitis, affecting ankles and knees in particular; it tends to resolve in 3–6 months. Chronic sarcoid dactylitis typically affects young adults; the fingers and toes become sausage shaped with spindling (Figure 96.15; Figure 155.10). X-rays show a lace-like trabecular pattern with cystic changes in the phalanges [**1**]. There may be additional flexion deformity due to involvement of finger muscles [2]. Chronic sarcoid oligo- or polyarthritis is rare, affecting around 0.2% patients, favouring those with African ancestry [**1**,3]. Sacroiliitis and spondyloarthritis are more common than in the general population [4]. Methotrexate is beneficial for both cutaneous lesions and inflammatory joint disease [5]. Although anti-TNF drugs are associated with radiological improvement [6], there is little evidence that they are beneficial clinically for joint disease [7].

So-called 'early-onset sarcoidosis', which is associated with a chronic granulomatous polyarthritis, has been shown to be the sporadic variant of autoinflammatory granulomatosis of childhood (Blau syndrome) [8]. It is discussed in further detail in Chapter 45.

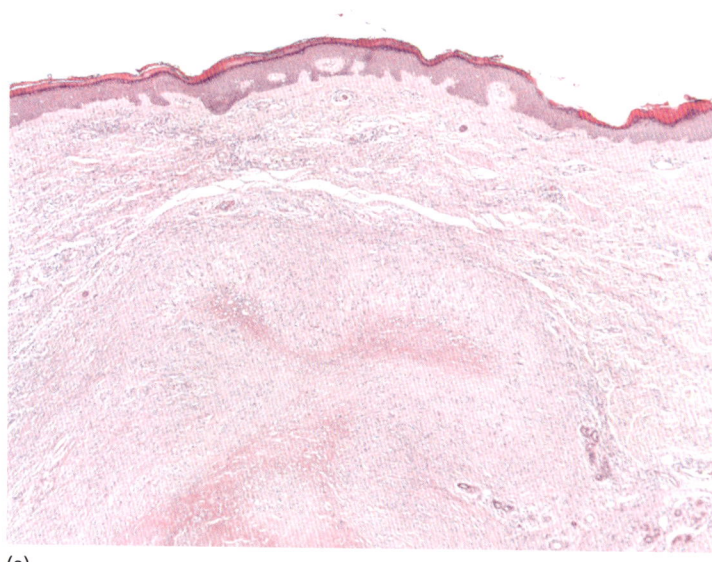

(a)

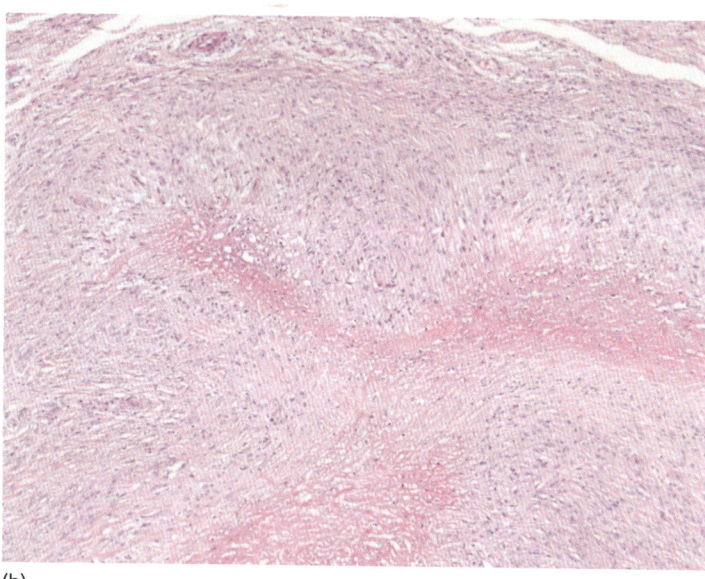

(b)

Figure 155.7 Histology of rheumatoid nodule at low power (a) and at higher power showing palisading granulomata (b).

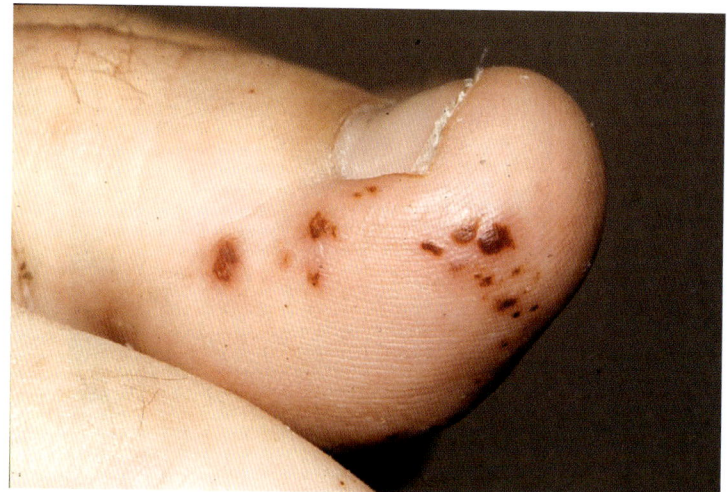

Figure 155.8 Digital vasculitis in rheumatoid arthritis.

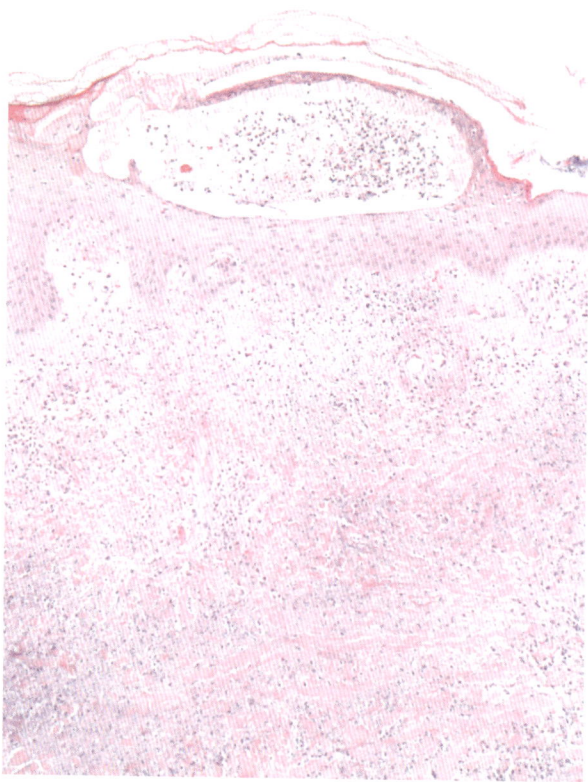

Figure 155.9 Histology of neutrophilic dermatosis in a patient with rheumatoid arthritis.

OSTEOARTHRITIS

A patient with osteoarthritis may present to the dermatologist with concerns about Heberden nodes. Additionally, two metabolic syndromes, haemochromatosis and alkaptonuria, are associated with osteoarthritis.

Heberden and Bouchard nodes

Heberden nodes [1] are posterolateral bony outgrowths affecting one or more distal interphalangeal joints. Similar changes, affecting the proximal interphalangeal joints, are termed Bouchard nodes. Both Heberden and Bouchard nodes are strongly associated with osteoarthritis, although they may be inherited independently as an autosomal dominant trait [2,3]. Characteristically, they are asymptomatic and of insidious onset, although tender nodes may develop acutely with a red swollen joint. They are commoner on the dominant hand and are associated with radiological features of osteoarthritis such as joint space narrowing [4]. The association of multiple symmetrical nodes with distal interphalangeal joint arthritis has been termed 'primary generalised osteoarthritis'. Because this is associated with the tissue types HLA-A1 and B8 and shows a marked female preponderance, it has been postulated to be an autoimmune disorder: increased amounts of immune complexes can be detected in cartilage and synovium [5].

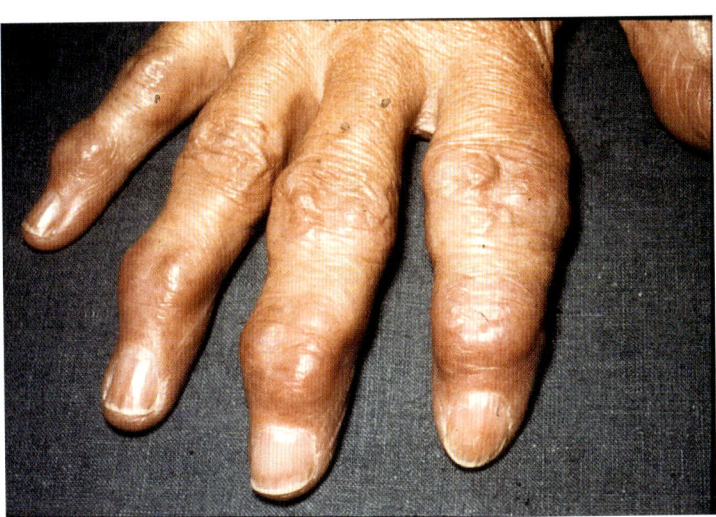

Figure 155.10 Sarcoid dactylitis.

METABOLIC DISORDERS WITH MUSCULOSKELETAL AND CUTANEOUS INVOLVEMENT

Haemochromatosis (Chapter 86)

The classic triad of diabetes, grey-brown skin hyperpigmentation (bronze diabetes) and cirrhosis is now rare but musculoskeletal symptoms are common and unresponsive to phlebotomy. The second and third metacarpophalangeal joints are typically affected with pseudogout-like attacks followed by degenerative joint changes with osteophytes. X-ray studies reveal chondrocalcinosis in 50% of cases. Most patients with the condition exhibit a C282Y homozygous mutation in the *HFE* gene [1].

Alkaptonuria (Chapter 79)

In this autosomal recessive metabolic disorder, deficiency of homogentisic acid oxidase results in deposition of homogentisic acid in connective tissue (ochronosis), causing a grey-black pigmentation most noticeable in ear and nose cartilage. Homopolymeric oxidation products of homogentisic acid bind to collagen, leading to inflammation and degenerative change. Eventually this results in calcification of intervertebral discs and osteoarthritis, chiefly affecting the knees [1,2]. Treatment with nitisinone, a potent inhibitor of 4-hydroxyphenylpyruvate dehydrogenase, arrests the deposition of homogentisic acid and reduces disease progression [3].

Gout

Gout may present at any age in adults especially in the elderly when it may be triggered by diuretic therapy. Acute gout is commoner in men. Although the clinical features are caused by deposition

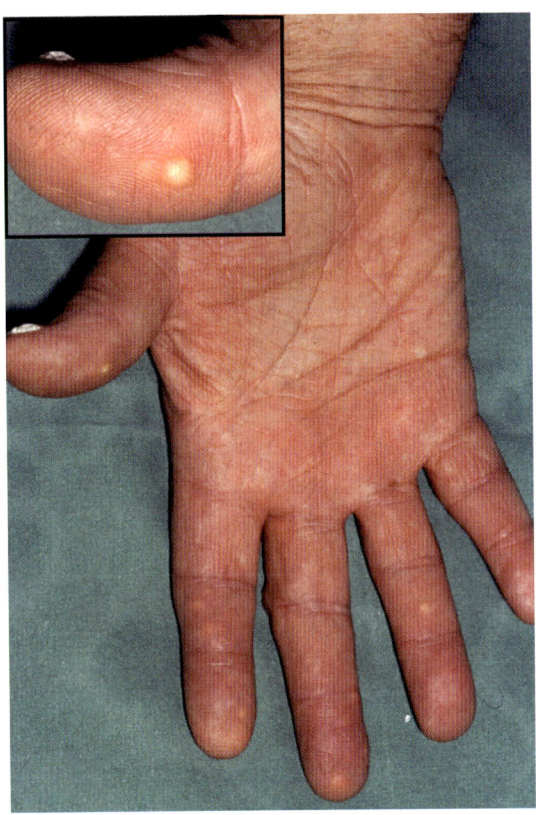

Figure 155.11 Tophaceous gout showing multiple cream-coloured papules on the palmar surfaces of the digits (inset: close-up view of thumb).

of monosodium urate in tissues, fewer than 5% of subjects with hyperuricaemia in the UK develop clinical gout. Deposition of the needle-like crystals of monosodium urate is often linked to a sudden recent rise of serum uric acid. Acute gout presents as a monoarthritis, classically affecting the metatarsophalangeal joint of the great toe. Untreated hyperuricaemia may lead to recurrent more severe attacks affecting several joints.

Tophaceous gout used to be a common presenting feature of acute symptomatic gout [1,2]. A creatinine clearance of less than 30 mL/min is strongly associated with the development of tophi [3]. Since the introduction of allopurinol therapy for hyperuricaemia and gout, tophi occur much less frequently. A tophus is a dense aggregate of monosodium urate crystals presenting as a papule or nodule in the skin [1] (Figures 155.11 and 155.12). Tophi have a predilection for the pinnae, elbows and Achilles tendons (where they may be confused with tendon xanthomata). Tophi may occur without arthritis [4]. They may ulcerate and become secondarily infected. Release of crystals in the conjunctivae cause an acute red eye. Tophi can also occur in the viscera such as the heart. The differential diagnosis includes rheumatoid nodules, neurofibromata and xanthomata. Diagnosis can be made by polarising microscopy of an aspirate; the stacks of crystals are strongly birefringent [2] (Figure 155.13). The histopathology of gout is discussed in Chapter 97.

Monosodium urate crystals stimulate IL-β secretion via cryopyrin, giving rise to the acute inflammatory response [5]. Allopurinol is the drug of choice in reducing hyperuricaemia. The drug, however, can be associated with cutaneous adverse effects including

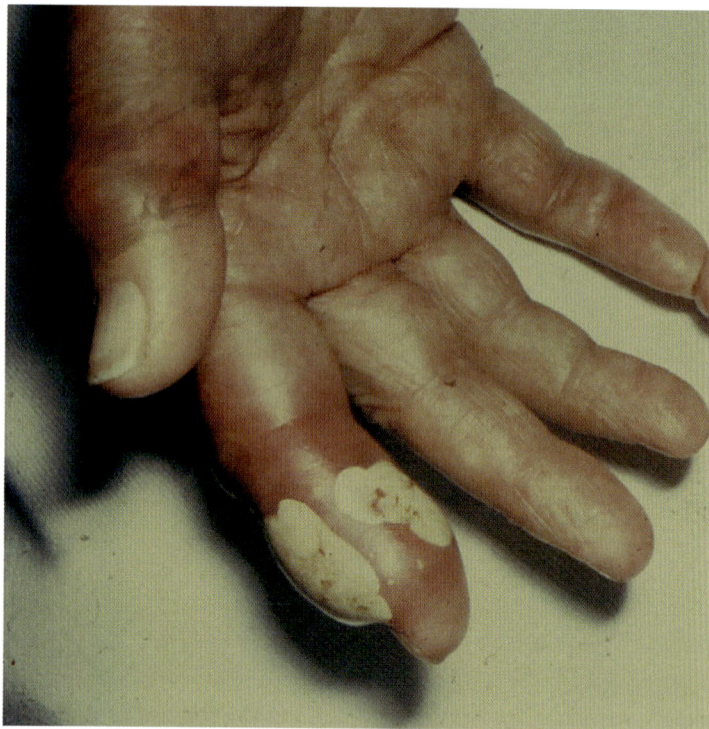

Figure 155.12 Severe tophaceous gout and acute gouty inflammation affecting the index finger and thumb.

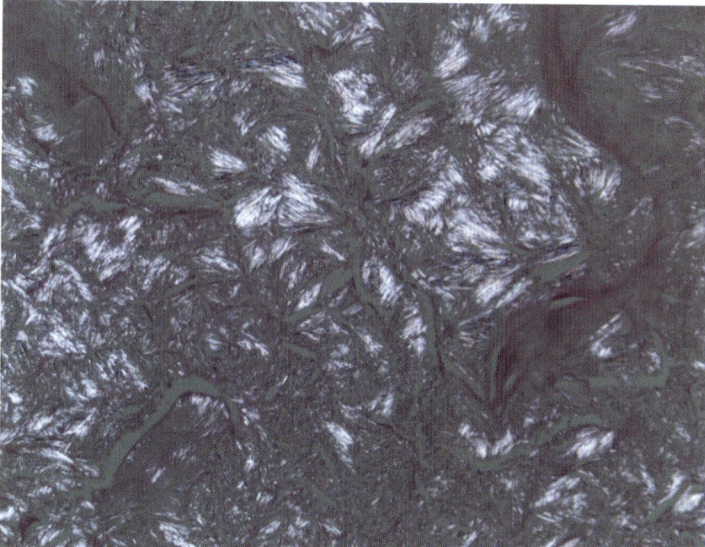

Figure 155.13 Birefringent crystals of uric acid in a gouty tophus (examined under polarising microscope).

DRESS (drug reaction or rash, eosinophilia and systemic symptoms), Stevens–Johnson syndrome and toxic epidermal necrolysis (Chapter 118). Recent pharmacogenetic studies have shown that severe reactions are associated with the (HLA)B* allele, offering the possibility of genetic testing in the future [6]. Several abnormalities in urate transporter genes have been identified in patients from South-East Asia.

AUTOINFLAMMATORY DISORDERS

Hereditary autoinflammatory disorders [1]

Several monogenic 'inflammasome' disorders have been described which result in autoactivation of the IL-β pathway. Most of them can cause arthralgia or arthritis. Most are rare and present in early childhood. They can be classified into a number of broad groups (Box 155.2)

They are discussed in greater detail in Chapter 45.

> **Box 155.2 Monogenic autoinflammatory syndromes** (Chapter 45)
>
> **Hereditary periodic fevers**
> - Cryopyrin-associated periodic syndromes (CAPS)
>   - Familial cold autoinflammatory syndrome (FCAS)
>   - Muckle–Wells syndrome (MWS)
>   - Chronic infantile neurological and articular syndrome (CINCA)
> - Tumour necrosis factor-associated periodic syndrome (TRAPS)
> - Familial Mediterranean fever (FMF)
>   - Mevalonate kinase (MVK) deficiency and hyper-IgD syndrome (HIDS)
>
> **Autoinflammatory granulomatosis of childhood** (Blau syndrome)
>
> **Autoinflammatory syndromes with pustulosis**
> - Deficiency of IL-1 receptor antagonist (DIRA)
> - Pyogenic sterile arthritis, pyoderma gangrenosum and acne (PAPA) syndrome
> - Deficiency of IL-36 receptor antagonist (DITRA)
>
> **Miscellaneous monogenic autoinflammatory syndromes**
> - Chronic atypical neutrophilic dermatosis with lipodystrophy and elevated temperature (CANDLE)
> - Majeed syndrome

Acquired autoinflammatory disorders

Schnitzler syndrome, adult-onset Still disease, systemic-onset juvenile idiopathic arthritis and SAPHO syndrome (*s*ynovitis, *a*cne, *p*ustulosis, *h*yperostosis and *o*steitis) all affect the musculoskeletal system and are discussed in Chapter 45.

Acne (Chapter 88)

Severe acne is associated with joint symptoms and arthritis.

Acne conglobata has been linked to sacroiliitis especially in young black men [1]. Associated features may include dissecting cellulitis of the scalp and hidradenitis suppurativa. In addition to sacroiliitis and axial spondylosis, there may be an asymmetrical peripheral arthritis, which develops later than the skin disease.

Unlike other spondyloarthropathies, the condition is not associated with HLA-B27 [2].

Acne fulminans is a systemic disease typically affecting adolescent white males. In addition to severe acne with abscesses and areas of ulceration, the syndrome includes fever, weight loss and arthralgia. X-rays may reveal osteolytic lesions in the clavicle, sternum, long bones or ilium [1]. Isotretinoin therapy is commonly associated with arthralgia and myalgia in both sexes; this is often trivial and therapy can be continued. Prolonged isotretinoin therapy is associated with spinal hyperostosis which may be asymptomatic [1]. In a patient with severe acne, isotretinoin therapy may precipitate acute sacroiliitis, which can be disabling [3,4]. Concomitant prednisolone therapy, and initiating isotretinoin at a low dose, may help prevent this.

Fibromyalgia is commoner in patients presenting with acne compared with the general population [5].

Significant acne is a feature of several syndromes, several of which have musculoskeletal features. These include monogenic inherited syndromes such as PAPA (*p*yogenic *a*rthritis, *p*yoderma gangrenosum and *a*cne), DIRA (*d*eficiency of *IL*-1 *r*eceptor *a*ntagonist) and SAPHO syndromes, all of which are described in Chapter 45.

Hidradenitis suppurativa (Chapter 90)

This is associated with several syndromes described earlier, as well as with inflammatory bowel disease [1]. A recent survey of hidradenitis suppurativa patients identified an association with arthralgia, back pain and enthesitis (especially in females), as well as SAPHO syndrome (Chapter 45) [2].

INFLAMMATORY CHONDROPATHIES

Relapsing polychondritis

Definition and nomenclature
In this non-infective condition, focal inflammatory destruction of cartilage is accompanied by fibroblastic regeneration. It is characterised by the following:
- Recurrent bilateral chondritis of the pinnae.
- Chondritis of the nasal cartilage.
- Chondritis of the respiratory tract.
- Ocular inflammation, including conjunctivitis, scleritis, episcleritis or uveitis.
- Cochlear or vestibular lesions.
- Seronegative non-erosive inflammatory arthritis.

Three or more of these features are required for the diagnosis [1].

Synonyms and inclusions
- Atrophic polychondritis
- Systemic chondromalacia

Aetiology
Relapsing polychondritis has been recorded as rare, with around 3.5 new cases/million/year in the UK, but recent reports suggest that it is not so uncommon but is easily overlooked. The cause is unknown but it is probably a Th1-mediated disease. Serum levels of cytokines such as interferon-γ, IL-12 and IL-2 parallel changes in disease activity whereas Th2 cytokines do not [2].

Antibodies to type II collagen have been detected in the serum in acute polychondritis, and granular deposits of immunoglobulin G (IgG), IgA, IgM and C3 at fibrochondral junctions have indicated a possible role of immune-complex deposits [3–7]. Antibody production is T-cell dependent and major histocompatibility complex (MHC) restricted; the arthritis in experimental animal models can be suppressed by synthetic type II collagen peptides [8]. The intravenous injection of papain into rabbits produces loss of cartilage rigidity, manifested by floppy ears [9]. It has been suggested that local protease activity may play some part in causing relapsing polychondritis [10]. Cartilage oligomeric matrix protein (COMP) is decreased and cartilage matrix protein (matrillin-1) increased. Both revert to normal levels during successful therapy [11]; however, in practice they are unreliable markers of disease activity [12]. A recent study suggests that the serum level of soluble triggering receptor, expressed on myeloid cells and typically associated with bacterial infections such as meningitis, more closely reflects disease activity and may be a useful biomarker [13].

Associated conditions suggest that autoimmune mechanisms may be concerned (see MAGIC syndrome). They include rheumatoid arthritis, lupus erythematosus, vasculitis, Behçet disease, Hashimoto disease, ulcerative colitis, Crohn disease, psoriasis, glomerulonephritis, Sjögren syndrome, thymoma, ankylosing spondylitis, myeloproliferative disorders and following intravenous injections [14–19]. Cutaneous manifestations have been reported in a patient treated for prostatic adenocarcinoma with goserelin, a luteinising hormone releasing analogue [20].

Relapsing polychondritis probably overlaps with granulomatosis with polyangiitis (GPA). Auricular chondritis has been described in some patients with the latter [21], and cANCA, an antibody once regarded as specific for GPA, has been reported in patients with relapsing polychondritis [22].

Pathology [23]
Areas of damaged cartilage, which have lost the normal basophilic staining, are separated by areas of predominantly lymphocytic infiltration. Later, the fragments of cartilage are surrounded and replaced by abundant granulation tissue and even nascent cartilage. Occasionally, there is evidence of vasculitis [24].

Clinical features [1,25–28] (Box 155.3)
The condition affects both sexes equally and usually begins between the ages of 30 and 50 years. Chondritis ultimately involves three or more sites in most patients but may be limited to one or two for long periods. The following tissues may be involved in decreasing order of frequency: auricular, joint, nasal, ocular, respiratory tract, heart valves and skin [29,30]. During the acute stage, the affected area is swollen, red and tender, and may be mistaken for cellulitis

Box 155.3 Clinical features of relapsing polychondritis

Cartilage
- Ears
  - 'Cellulitis' sparing lobule
  - Floppy: 'forward listening'
  - Cartilage thinning: 'blue ear'
  - Serous otitis media
- Nose
  - Obstruction
  - Deformity, e.g. sudden collapse of nasal bridge
- Larynx/trachea/bronchi
  - Airway obstruction
  - Infection

Vasculitis
- Cutaneous
  - Superficial thrombophlebitis
  - 'Toxic' erythema
  - Annular urticated eruption
- Systemic
  - Cerebral aneurysm
  - Granulomatous lung disease
  - Giant cell myocarditis
  - Heart valve rupture

Haematological, e.g. myelodysplasia

Articular, small peripheral joint arthritis (RA-like)

Eyes
- Episcleritis
- Conjunctivitis
- Iritis
- Scleromalacia
- Proptosis
- Rarely: keratoconjunctivitis sicca or chorioretinitis

Oro-genital ulceration (MAGIC syndrome)

Associated systemic autoimmune disease, e.g. SLE

RA, rheumatoid arthritis; SLE, systemic lupus erythematosus.

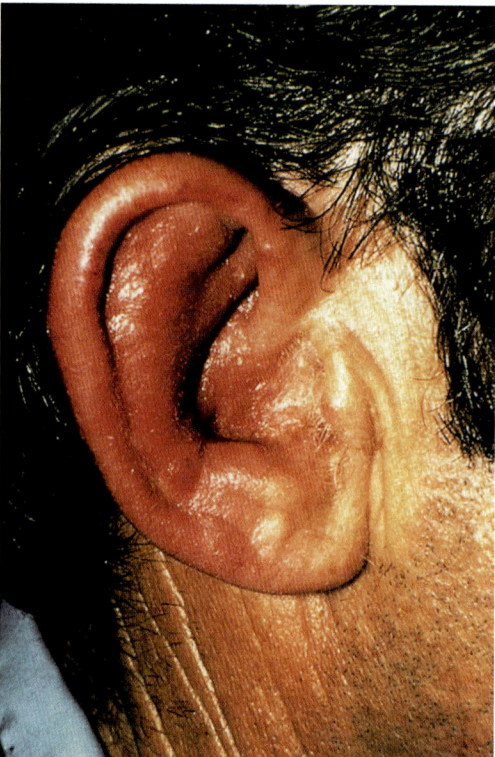

Figure 155.14 Relapsing polychondritis, showing inflammation of the pinna.

(Figure 155.14). Sparing of the ear lobule is a useful differentiating sign. The ear becomes floppy (the 'forward listening' ear). Thinning of the cartilage allows the underlying vasculature of the ear to be more visible (the 'blue ear' sign) [31]. Serous otitis media can occur and there may be loss of hearing even in the absence of chondritis [32]. Involvement of the nasal cartilage leads to obstruction and later to a saddlenose deformity, which may lead to collapse of the nasal bridge [33] (Figure 155.15). Cutaneous and systemic vasculitis, cerebral aneurysms, superficial thrombophlebitis and toxic erythema have been described [1,24,27,34]. A few patients have been described in whom an annular eruption comprising tense urticated papules precedes chondritis; histology reveals a lymphocytic vasculitis. All these patients have haematological abnormalities such as myelodysplasia. Although initially responsive to corticosteroids, this variant carries a poor prognosis [35].

The joint changes, usually affecting the smaller peripheral joints, may simulate rheumatoid arthritis [36]. Involvement of

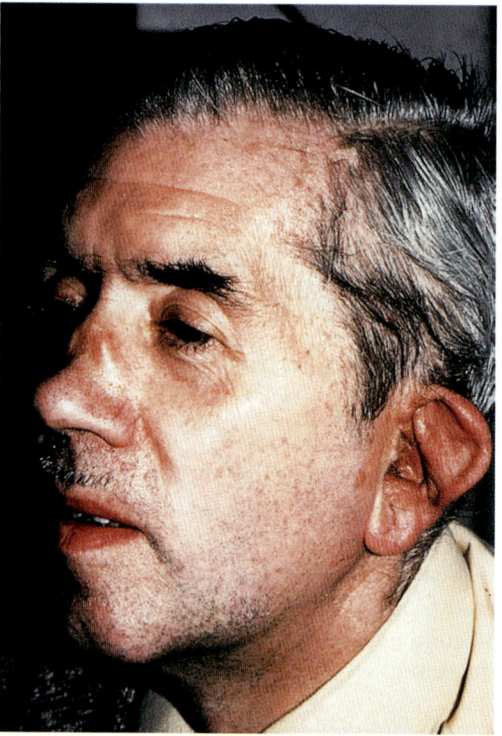

Figure 155.15 Relapsing polychondritis: late stage, showing damage to the cartilage of the ear and nose.

the larynx, trachea or bronchi produces respiratory embarrassment and recurrent infection. Permanent tracheostomy may be required [23,32]. An association with granulomatous lung disease has also been described. Ocular abnormalities are found in some

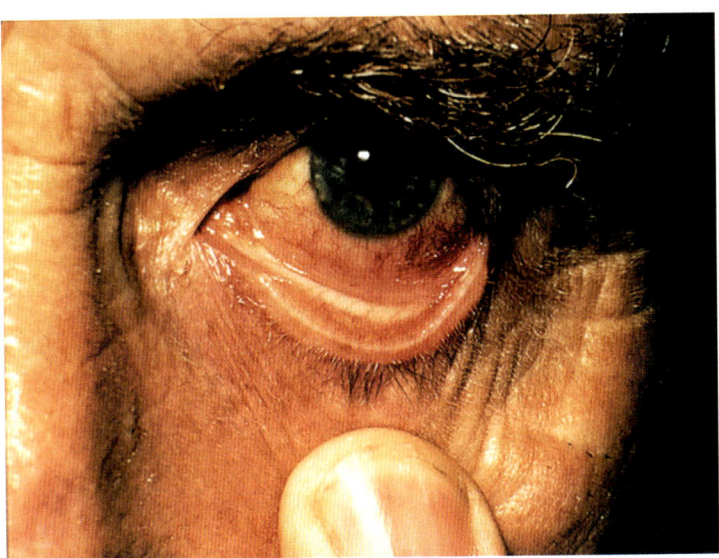

Figure 155.16 Relapsing polychondritis, showing ocular involvement.

cases: episcleritis, conjunctivitis and iritis (Figure 155.16), scleromalacia, and more rarely keratoconjunctivitis sicca or chorioretinitis. Proptosis occurs in 3% of cases [37,38]. Giant cell myocarditis is reported and involvement of the heart valves may cause serious complications including sudden valve rupture, even in a patient otherwise in remission [1,39,40].

The course of the disease is extremely variable [19,28]. Attempts have been made to devise a 'disease activity' score [41]. Relapses are the rule, but they vary in frequency and severity. Some cases continue to relapse for over 20 years but others become inactive within a short period. Pregnancy does not appear to affect the course of the disease although complications are more frequent [42]. Deformity of the ears and nose is common but in general the disease is a source of discomfort and disfigurement rather than a threat to life. Plasma viscosity or erythrocyte sedimentation rate is usually raised and anaemia is frequent. The rheumatoid factor and antinuclear factor are often positive. Leukocytosis is inconstant but eosinophilia is found in 40% of cases. A characteristic biochemical finding is the increased urinary excretion of acid mucopolysaccharides during each relapse.

Radiological abnormalities are not pathognomonic but evidence of extensive destruction of joint cartilage without changes in adjacent bone is suggestive on plain X-ray. In some cases, the changes are indistinguishable from rheumatoid arthritis. Fluorine-18 deoxyglucose uptake is increased in affected cartilage on positron emission tomography/computed tomography (PET/CT). This is a useful investigation to determine the extent of cartilage involvement [43]. Doppler echocardiography, MRI and dynamic expiratory computed tomography are of value in investigating cardiopulmonary involvement [12]. Bronchoscopy runs the risk of worsening respiratory dysfunction [12].

Diagnosis

Polychondritis may present to the dermatologist as 'chronic otitis externa with cellulitis of the pinna'. The diagnosis is established by biopsy, or by other associated changes, and appropriate radiology. GPA and lethal midline granuloma (also causes of a saddle-nose deformity [33]) can produce a similar histology but in these two conditions the involvement is more purely destructive.

Treatment

The progression of the acute relapse can be controlled with corticosteroids. An initial daily dose of 30 mg prednisolone can be gradually reduced and finally discontinued as remission develops. Indometacin and dapsone have been used [5]. Colchicine is also helpful in some patients [44]. Immunosuppressive agents such as methotrexate and ciclosporin [7,12] may have a role. Pulsed intravenous cyclophosphamide has been used for renal disease [12,45]. Intravenous immunoglobulin [46] and anti-TNF antagonists such as adalimumab and etanercept have proved to give sustained remission in several cases [47,48]. Other cytokine modulators used with success include tocilizumab [2]. Variable results have been obtained with rituximab [49]. Remission has followed autologous stem cell transplantation [50]. Surgical reconstruction of the nose or larynx is sometimes required [49].

MAGIC syndrome

Several patients have been described with features of both relapsing polychondritis and Behçet disease [1]. The term MAGIC syndrome (*m*outh *a*nd *g*enital ulcers with *i*nflamed *c*artilage) has been used for this overlap syndrome. The underlying immunological defects are still unclear but circulating immune complexes and autoantibodies to elastic tissue have been suggested as possible factors [1,2]. The nodules on the auricle affect the antihelix but, as in polychondritis, spare the lobule [3].

Aortic valve disease and aneurysmal aortitis have been associated with the syndrome [4,5] and features of the MAGIC syndrome have been described in an HIV-positive individual [6].

Several therapies have been tried including dapsone, corticosteroids and pentoxifylline. Infliximab has been successful in a severe case [7].

MISCELLANEOUS DISORDERS INVOLVING THE SKIN AND MUSCULOSKELETAL SYSTEM

Mastocytosis (Chapter 46)

Some patients with cutaneous mastocytosis (e.g. telangiectasia macularis eruptiva perstans) experience bone pain due to osteoporosis, related to release of mast cell mediators such as heparin, tryptase and IL-6. Radiological bone changes include localised osteolysis or osteosclerosis and generalised osteopenia or osteosclerosis [1]. The spine is particularly affected and pathological fractures are commoner in men; the severity of osteoporosis relates to raised levels of mast cell tryptase [1] and IL-6 [2]. Spondyloarthritis is commoner in patients with mastocytosis than in the general population [3] and increased numbers of synovial mast cells may contribute to joint symptoms [4].

Multicentric reticulohistiocytosis

This condition is characterised by destructive polyarthritis, chiefly affecting the distal interphalangeal joints. It may be misdiagnosed as rheumatoid or psoriatic arthritis. It is one of the most destructive forms of arthritis and severe changes (arthritis mutilans) occur in nearly 50% of patients, with 'pencil in cup' changes on X-ray. It is described in detail in Chapter 135.

Pachydermoperiostosis

Synonyms and inclusions
- Primary (idiopathic) hypertrophic pulmonary osteoarthropathy
- Touraine–Solente–Golé syndrome

In this rare condition [1–3], inheritance is autosomal dominant but autosomal recessive families probably also occur [4]. At least two gene mutations are implicated: HPGD and SLCO2A1 [5]. Both genes are components of prostaglandin (PG) E_2 catabolism and these mutations are associated with a failure of PGE_2 degradation.

The condition typically presents in teenage males. Digital clubbing is associated with painful cylindrical thickening of legs and forearms (which may suggest acromegaly [6]) (Figure 155.17), hyperhidrosis, seborrhoea, sebaceous gland hyperplasia and folliculitis. Arthritis may be severe with florid knee effusions. Additional clinical features include thickened skin on the forehead, carpal and tarsal tunnel syndrome, chronic leg ulceration and calcification of the Achilles tendon [7]. Cultured dermal fibroblasts synthesise increased amounts of collagen and α_1 [8] procollagen mRNA and exhibit upregulation of transcriptional activity of the $\alpha_1(I)$ procollagen gene promoter [9]. Proteoglycan synthesis is also affected [10].

X-rays reveal symmetrical, irregular periosteal ossification, predominantly affecting the distal ends of long bones [1]. Histology shows cutaneous sclerosis and hyalinosis, with perivascular infiltration by lymphoid cells in the dermis [2].

When conventional treatments (including non-steroidal anti-inflammatory drugs (NSAIDs) and corticosteroids) fail, bisphosphonates such as intravenous pamidronate inhibit osteoclast activity and may help rheumatological manifestations [11]. A recent study has demonstrated reduction in serum and urinary PGE_2 together with symptomatic improvement following the use of the COX-2 inhibitor, etoricoxib [12]. Cosmetic procedures such as facelift and botulinum toxin improve facial appearance [13].

Interstitial granulomatous dermatosis (Chapter 100)

This condition is associated with several organ-specific autoimmune disorders such as Hashimoto thyroiditis and diabetes, as well as autoimmune connective tissue diseases, inflammatory bowel disease, haematological malignancy and drugs including allopurinol. An association with rheumatoid arthritis is reported in several cases although the arthritis is often seronegative and non-erosive. In over 50% of patients, usually affecting adults, it is progressive and destructive resembling psoriatic arthritis [1,2].

Skin-coloured, red or purple papules, linear bands (the rope sign) or plaques develop symmetrically on the lateral aspects of the trunk, proximal thighs or axillae. Lesions can be painful or associated with a burning pruritus [1,2]. Palisaded neutrophilic and granulomatous dermatitis [3] is probably a variant, with papules and nodules on the extremities.

Skin histology is distinctive: there is a granulomatous interstitial and palisading infiltrate with CD68+ histiocytes showing a variable degree of phagocytosis in the mid to deep reticular dermis. The collagen bundles are thickened but there is also piecemeal fragmentation of collagen and elastic fibres [2,4,5].

It is probable that the condition is related to deposition of immune complexes in the skin. Skin and joint lesions may resolve spontaneously in a few weeks, may be recurrent or progress over many months or years [1,2]. Several drugs have been tried including NSAIDs, corticosteroids, dapsone, colchicine and tacrolimus [6]. Anti-TNF therapies such as etanercept [5] are beneficial although these agents may trigger the condition [6]. Ustekinumab has also been used successfully [7].

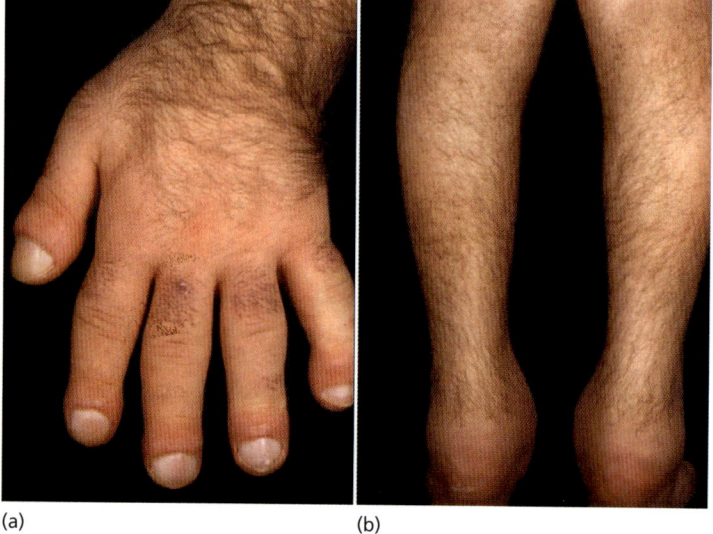

Figure 155.17 (a,b) Views of the hand (a) and the lower legs and ankles (b) in pachydermoperiostosis.

Intralymphatic histiocytosis [1–4]

Swelling and erythema resembling cellulitis occurs around the elbow or knee in some patients, often elderly women, with rheumatoid arthritis and other inflammatory disorders such as Crohn disease. It may occur in the absence of systemic disease [4]. Several cases are reported affecting the tissues adjacent to an orthopaedic metal implant [5,6,7]; this may raise concern about infection or rejection. Typically, asymptomatic poorly demarcated red plaques or livedo reticularis-like lesions develop near an elbow or knee. There may be overlying verrucous change. Histology shows dilated vascular structures in the reticular dermis, with an endothelial marker profile suggesting lymphatic origin. Some vessels contain CD68+ mononuclear histiocytes [1,4,7]; the vessel walls stain with D2-40. It has been suggested that the condition is related to reactive intravascular angioendotheliomatosis, forming part of the spectrum of cutaneous reactive angiomatosis [4,7,8]. It is a benign process and may resolve with treatment of the underlying cause [9]. Although there are reports of the use of drugs such as infliximab [10], it can respond to simple pressure bandaging, suggesting that it may be related to local lymphostasis [11].

CUTANEOUS ADVERSE REACTIONS TO ANTIRHEUMATIC THERAPIES

(Chapters 119 and 120)

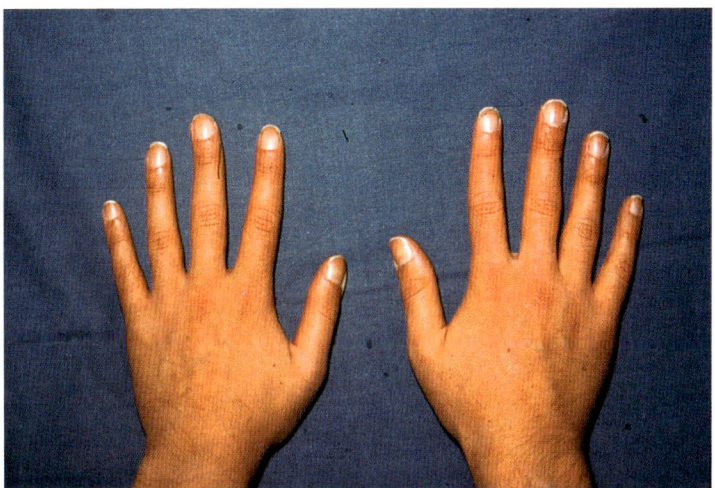

Figure 155.18 Yellow pigmentation of the skin due to mepacrine.

Skin lesions are commonly encountered in patients receiving antirheumatic therapy. Some are trivial but others may require discontinuation of treatment. Alopecia may occur in patients receiving azathioprine or methotrexate and eczema-like lesions occur with many drugs, including leflunomide.

NSAIDs and *allopurinol* are among the most frequently reported causes of severe adverse drug reactions including DRESS, Stevens–Johnson syndrome and toxic epidermal necrolysis [1]. Viraemia can be a compounding factor in an immunosuppressed patient [2]. A better understanding of pharmacogenomics may enable screening at-risk patients in the future [2,3]. This is already potentially achievable with allopurinol [4]. NSAIDs are photosensitising and can induce photo-onycholysis. A pseudoporphyria, clinically resembling porphyria cutanea tarda, is seen in patients taking naproxen. Fixed drug eruptions are associated with some NSAIDs, including piroxicam, mefenamic acid and oxyphenbutazone. Urticarial lesions may be induced by immunological or pharmacological mechanisms [3]. Topical NSAIDs, notably ketoprofen, may photosensitise. Cross-reaction with octocrylene, a sunscreen ingredient, is often seen with ketoprofen photosensitivity [5].

Antimalarials, e.g. hydroxychloroquine, should be avoided in patients with psoriasis as they may exacerbate the condition [6]. They are also implicated in lichenoid drug reactions, acute generalised exanthematic pustulosis [7] and DRESS syndrome [8]. Mepacrine causes yellow pigmentation of the skin (Figure 155.18) and sclerae and can also induce cutaneous ochronosis (Figure 155.19).

Sulfasalazine is also implicated in DRESS [9] as well as Stevens–Johnson syndrome. It is a photosensitiser and can induce or exacerbate lupus erythematosus [10].

Corticosteroids: the atrophogenic effects of systemic corticosteroids are well recognised [11] but even intralesional steroids can induce cushingoid features and an acneiform eruption [12], as well as the risk of local dermal atrophy. Systemic corticosteroids may cause hypertrichosis.

Penicillamine can induce lupus or a lichenoid reaction and its use in Wilson disease is associated with a pseudoxanthoma elasticum-like syndrome.

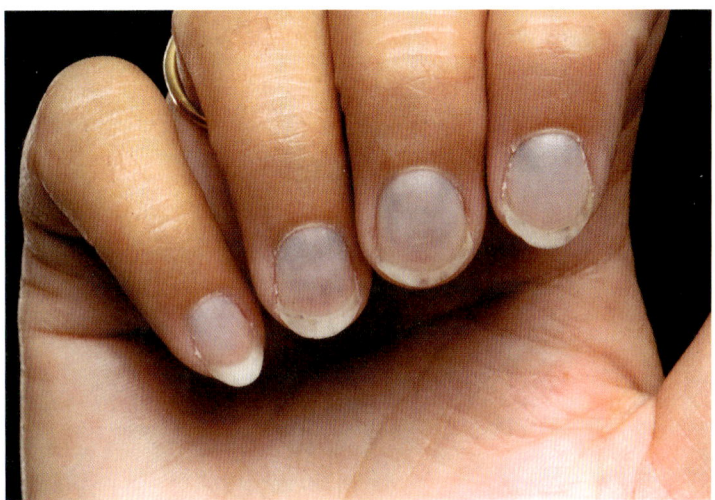

Figure 155.19 Ochronosis of the nail beds due to mepacrine.

TNF-α inhibitors may cause lichenoid eruptions. Paradoxically, they can induce an eruption clinically and histologically resembling psoriasis, particularly in patients with rheumatoid arthritis. Adalimumab may be a major culprit [13,14]. Fortunately, the eruption often responds to topical therapy and, if not, generally resolves on changing to another biological agent. The risk of serious skin and soft-tissue infections does not appear to be increased in rheumatoid patients on anti-TNF-α drugs [15].

Janus kinase (JAK) inhibitors such as baricitinib and tofacitinib are effective in monotherapy of rheumatoid arthritis but may increase the risk of herpes zoster [16].

Skin cancer promotion: non-melanoma skin cancer is commoner in rheumatoid patients than in the general population, attributable at least in part to drugs such as methotrexate, anti-TNF drugs [17] and possibly tofacitinib [16]. Multiple eruptive squamous cell carcinomata occurred in a patient on abatacept for rheumatoid arthritis [18]. Multiple eruptive keratoacanthomata have been associated with leflunomide, regressing when the drug was discontinued [19]. Lymphomatoid papulosis has been attributed to adalimumab in a patient with juvenile idiopathic arthritis [20]. Fortunately, the prevalence of melanoma is not increased in rheumatoid arthritis [21]. Historically, multiple basal cell carcinomas developed in the skin overlying sites of radiotherapy for ankylosing spondylitis, i.e. the spine and sacroiliac joints, usually many years after irradiation [22,23].

Acknowledgement

The author is grateful to Dr Leigh Biddlestone for providing the histological images.

Key references

The full list of references can be found in the online version at https://www.wiley.com/rooksdermatology10e

Infective arthropathies
1 Espinoza LR, Garcia-Valladares I. Of bugs and joints: the relationship between infection and joints. *Rheumatol Clin* 2013;9:229–38.

Reactive arthritis
2 Selmi C, Gershwin ME. Diagnosis and classification of reactive arthritis. *Autoimmune Rev* 2014;13:546–9.

Viral arthropathies
9 Novelli L, Motta F, De Santis M *et al*. The JANUS of chronic inflammatory and autoimmune diseases onset during COVID-19 – a systematic review of the literature. *J Autoimmun* 2021;117:102592.

Bacterial arthropathies
11 Sharma A, Pinto B, Dogra S *et al*. A case series and review of Poncet's disease, and the utility of current diagnostic criteria. *Int J Rheum Dis* 2016;19:1010–17.
21 Ouldali N, Pouletty M, Mariani P *et al*. Emergence of Kawasaki disease related to SARS-CoV-2 infection in an epicentre of the French COVID-19 epidemic: a time-series analysis. *Lancet Child Adolesc Health* 2020;4:662–8.

Atrophic skin with rheumatoid arthritis
Rheumatoid nodules
1 Clarke JT, Werth VP. Rheumatic manifestations of skin disease. *Curr Opin Rheumatol* 2010;22:78–84.

Rheumatoid vasculitis and cutaneous ulceration
5 Bartels C, Bell C, Rosenthal A *et al*. Decline in rheumatoid vasculitis prevalence among US veterans: a retrospective cross-sectional study. *Arthritis Rheum* 2009;60:2553–7.
10 Hasegawa M, Nagai Y, Sogabe Y *et al*. Clinical analysis of leg ulcers and gangrene in rheumatoid arthritis. *J Dermatol* 2013;40:949–54.

Rheumatoid neutrophilic dermatosis
6 Yamamoto T. Cutaneous manifestations associated with rheumatoid arthritis. *Rheumatol Int* 2009;29:979–88.

Sarcoidosis
1 Al-Kofahi K, Korsten P, Ascoli C *et al*. Management of extrapulmonary sarcoidosis: challenges and solutions. *Ther Clin Risk Manag* 2016;12:1623–34.

Alkaptonuria
3 Zatkova A, Ranganath L, Kadasi L. Alkaptonuria: current perspectives. *Appl Clin Genet* 2020;13:37–47.

Gout
1 Sapkota K, Kolade VO, Boit ML. Gouty tophi. *J Community Hosp Intern Med Perspect* 2014;4:10.3402.

Hereditary autoinflammatory disorders
1 Figueras-Nart I, Mascaró JM Jr, Solanich X, Hernández-Rodríguez J. Dermatologic and dermatopathologic features of monogenic autoinflammatory diseases. *Front Immunol* 2019;10:2448.

Acne
1 Knitzer RH, Needleman BW. Musculoskeletal syndromes associated with acne. *Semin Arthritis Rheum* 1991;20:247–55.
5 Yazmalar L, Çelepkolu T, Batmaz İ *et al*. High frequency of fibromyalgia in patients with acne vulgaris. *Arch Rheumatol* 2016;31:170–5.

Relapsing polychondritis
1 McAdam LP, O'Hanlan MA, Bluestone R *et al*. Relapsing polychondritis: prospective review of 23 patients and review of the literature. *Medicine (Baltimore)* 1976;55:193–215.
2 Arnaud L, Mathian A, Haroche J *et al*. Pathogenesis of relapsing polychondritis: a 2013 update. *Autoimmune Rev* 2014;13:90–5.
49 Borgia F, Giuffrida R, Guarneri F, Cannavò SP. Relapsing polychondritis: an updated review. *Biomedicines* 2018;6:84.

MAGIC syndrome
1 Orme RL, Nordlund JJ, Barich L *et al*. The MAGIC syndrome (mouth and genital ulcers with inflamed cartilage). *Arch Dermatol* 1990;126:940–4.

Mastocytosis
4 Polivka L, Frenzel L, Jouzeau JY *et al*. Mast cells in spondyloarthritis, more than simple inflammatory bystanders? *Ther Adv Musculoskelet Dis* 2020;12: 1759720X20971907.

Pachydermoperiostosis
8 Cantatore FP, Mancini L, Ingrosso AM *et al*. Pachydermoperiostosis. Dermatological, neurological and radiological observations. *Clin Rheumatol* 1995; 14:705–7.
12 Yuan L, Liao RX, Lin YY *et al*. Safety and efficacy of cyclooxygenase-2 inhibition for treatment of primary hypertrophic osteoarthropathy: a single-arm intervention trial. *J Orthop Translat* 2018;18:109–18.

Interstitial granulomatous dermatosis
2 Peroni A, Colato C, Schena D *et al*. Interstitial granulomatous dermatitis: a distinct entity with characteristic histological and clinical pattern. *Br J Dermatol* 2012;166:775–83.

Intralymphatic histiocytosis
7 Requena L, El-Shabrawi-Caelen L, Walsh SN *et al*. Intralymphatic histiocytosis. A clinicopathologic study of 16 cases. *Am J Dermatopathol* 2009;31:140–51.
9 Blackwell TJ, Ingersoll Z, Blackwell M. Intralymphatic histiocytosis: an unusual presentation. *Case Rep Dermatol* 2021;13:1–6.

Cutaneous adverse reactions to antirheumatic therapies
1 Jeung YJ, Lee JY, Oh MJ *et al*. Comparison of the causes and clinical features of drug rash with eosinophilia and systemic symptoms and Stevens–Johnson syndrome. *Allerg Asth Immunol Res* 2010;2:123–6.
16 Angelini J, Talotta R, Roncato R *et al*. JAK-Inhibitors for the treatment of rheumatoid arthritis: a focus on the present and an outlook on the future. *Biomolecules* 2020;10:1002.

PART 14
Aesthetic Dermatology

CHAPTER 156

Skin Ageing

Elisabeth A. Pedersen[1], Gary J. Fisher[1], John J. Voorhees[1] and Dana L. Sachs[2]

[1] University of Michigan Medical Center, Ann Arbor, MI, USA
[2] Independent scholar, MI, USA

Introduction, 156.1	Idiopathic guttate hypomelanosis, 156.5	Photoageing and natural ageing, 156.10
Clinical features, 156.1	Bateman purpura, 156.5	Implications of skin ageing, 156.10
Intrinsic ageing, 156.1	Menopausal skin ageing, 156.6	Medical implications, 156.10
Extrinsic ageing, 156.1	Genetics of skin ageing, 156.6	Barrier dysfunction, 156.10
Extrinsic ageing variants, 156.3	Grading and measurement of skin ageing, 156.6	Dermatoporosis, 156.11
Smoking and skin ageing, 156.4	Pathophysiology, 156.7	Cosmetic implications, 156.11
Cutaneous nodular elastosis with cysts and comedones, 156.4	Ultraviolet irradiation damage/episodic exposure, 156.7	Social implications, 156.11
Skin ageing of the neck, 156.4	Other environmental influences in skin ageing, 156.8	Key references, 156.11
	Collagen fibril fragmentation, 156.8	

Introduction

Ageing is inevitable in every organ system, yet no organ conveys to the outside world an aged appearance as does the skin. The implications of skin ageing are broad and include cosmetic concerns of appearance, as well as medical and social concerns. An aged appearance, especially of the face, results from the confluence of ageing bone (structural ageing), muscle, fat and skin. Although changes in skin over time account for an aged appearance, it is not possible to attribute the changes entirely to skin pathology. It is important to recognise that concomitant with skin ageing, other significant organ systems are undergoing changes that contribute to an aged appearance. Bone ageing is characterised by excess resorption leading to volume and support loss; muscle ageing can present with hypertrophy or atrophy of particular muscle groups; and fat pads, especially those of the face, age at different rates with atrophy and positional changes leading to an older appearance. In this chapter, we describe the clinical features of intrinsic and extrinsic skin ageing across various ethnicities, the molecular mechanisms of both types of skin ageing and the cosmetic, medical and social implications of aged skin.

Clinical features

Intrinsic ageing

Intrinsic skin ageing is also known as chronological ageing, natural ageing or just skin ageing and occurs inevitably, continuously and gradually in all skin types over an individual's lifetime. Intrinsic ageing is observed in its purest form on the upper inner aspects of the arms and on the hips and buttocks, sites typically protected from ultraviolet (UV) irradiation exposure. The salient clinical features of intrinsic ageing include dryness, homogenous colour, atrophy and fine wrinkling (Figure 156.1).

Extrinsic ageing

Ageing in white skin

Extrinsic ageing is commonly referred to as photoageing and results from the damaging effects of UV radiation, which is the primary cause of premature skin ageing, although other factors such as tobacco smoking, pollution, chronic psychological stress, poor sleep and a high glycaemic index (GI) diet may also have an impact. The hallmark clinical features of extrinsic ageing in white skin are rough texture, dryness, dyspigmentation, fine and coarse wrinkles and telangiectases. The dyspigmentation manifests as either hyperpigmentation or hypopigmentation. Hyperpigmentation includes, but is not limited to, solar lentigines and patchy, irregular, tan to brown discoloration which can be diffuse. Dyspigmentation also includes areas where the skin has pigment loss leading to hypopigmented and depigmented areas. Extrinsic ageing is best exemplified on anatomical sites subject to repeated solar UV irradiation exposure such as the face, upper chest (décolleté), extensor forearms, dorsal hands and neck.

Asymmetrical skin ageing has been observed, and comparison studies of left and right sides of the face have further strengthened the argument for the role of UV irradiation in the pathophysiology of ageing skin. The side of the face exposed to solar UV irradiation during driving has been shown to demonstrate more severe and extensive photoageing [1].

Rook's Textbook of Dermatology, Tenth Edition. Edited by Christopher Griffiths, Jonathan Barker, Tanya Bleiker, Walayat Hussain and Rosalind Simpson.
© 2024 John Wiley & Sons Ltd. Published 2024 by John Wiley & Sons Ltd.

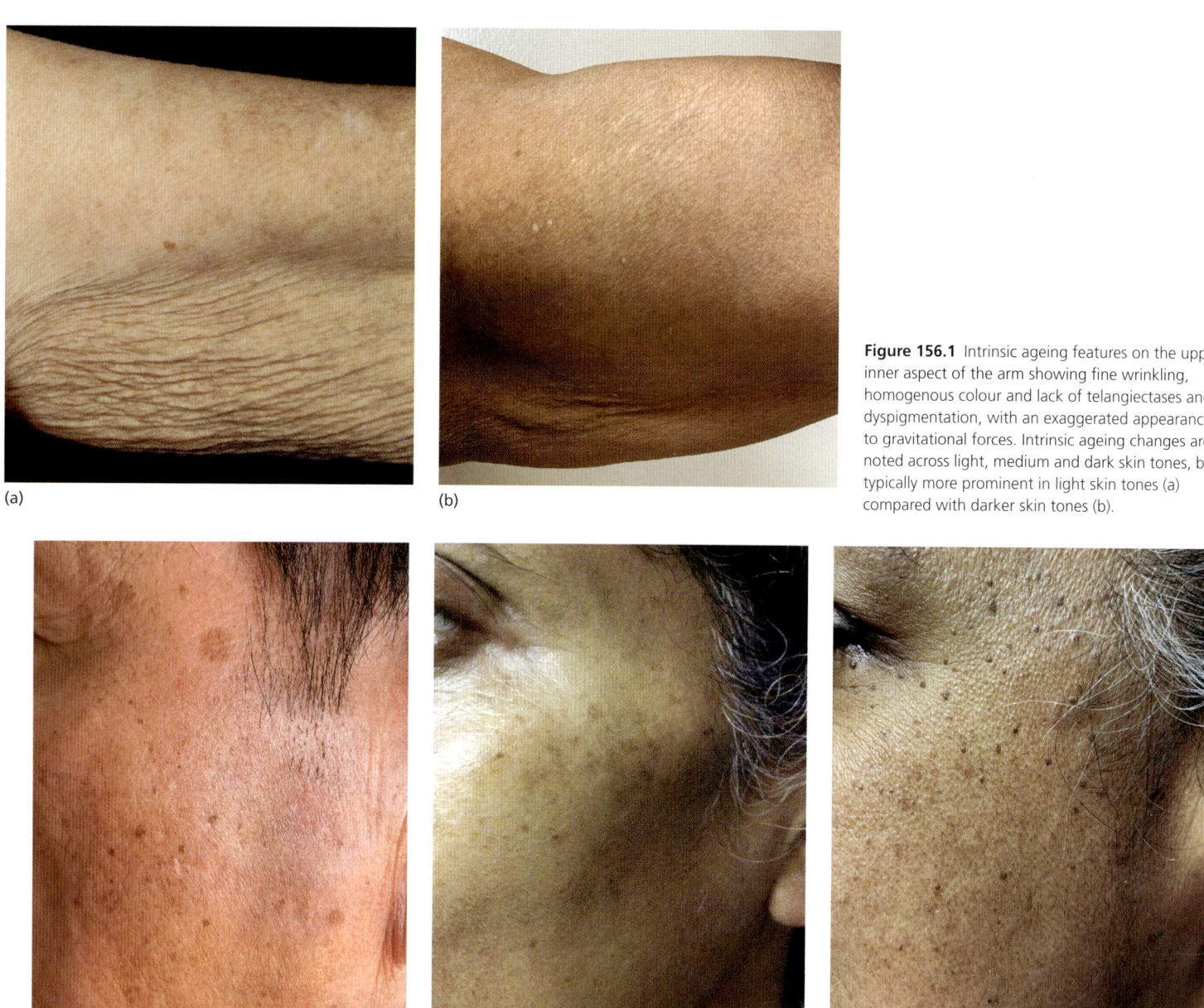

Figure 156.1 Intrinsic ageing features on the upper, inner aspect of the arm showing fine wrinkling, homogenous colour and lack of telangiectases and dyspigmentation, with an exaggerated appearance due to gravitational forces. Intrinsic ageing changes are noted across light, medium and dark skin tones, but are typically more prominent in light skin tones (a) compared with darker skin tones (b).

Figure 156.2 Dyspigmentation tends to be a more common manifestation of extrinsic skin ageing compared with wrinkling in darker skin types such as (a) East Asian, (b) Indian and (c) African descent. It is often patchy and ill defined. Judicious and consistent sun protective measures may prevent it from developing. Treatment modalities to improve appearance and even the skin tone include topical therapy with retinoids and cosmeceuticals, chemical peeling agents and laser therapy.

Ageing in skin of colour

The previous clinical descriptions of intrinsic and extrinsic ageing are based on studies and observations of white skin. Skin of colour (SOC) is a broad term used to describe many ethnic skin phenotypes and includes but is not limited to individuals of Asian, Latino and African descent. Individuals may often share features across several ethnicities making categorisation of individuals into distinct ethnic groups difficult. In general, SOC photoageing manifests differently compared with white skin. Inherent protection due to increased melanin in darker skin types confers more protection from extrinsic photoageing due to UV light damage and there may be as yet unknown genetic variations among different ethnicities that influence skin ageing rates and clinical manifestations. In addition, a thicker dermis, increased convolution of the dermal–epidermal junction and increased fibroblast number and activity have been noted in SOC, most notably in African skin, with some increase in Asian skin compared with white skin [2].

In general, photoageing in darker skin types, including East and South-East Asian skin types, is characterised by early findings of pigmentation irregularities (Figure 156.2). Wrinkling does not typically become readily apparent until after the age of 50 years and to a much lesser extent compared with fairer skin (Figure 156.3) [3]. A fairly comprehensive review of photoageing in East and South-East Asians concluded that Korean skin with severe dyspigmentation

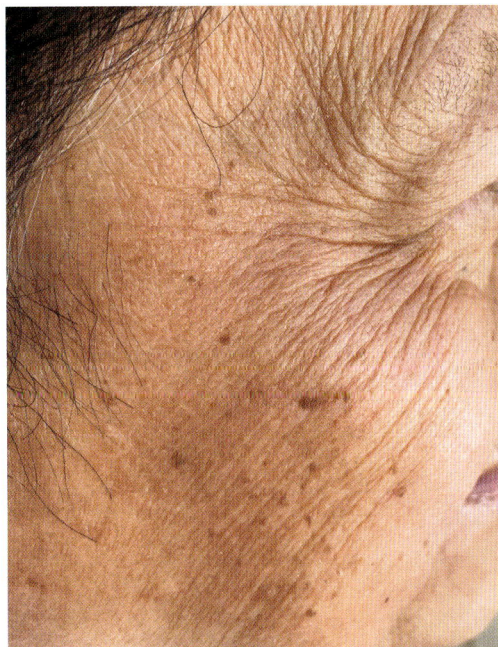

Figure 156.3 Extrinsic ageing manifesting as wrinkling in a 73-year-old Asian man.

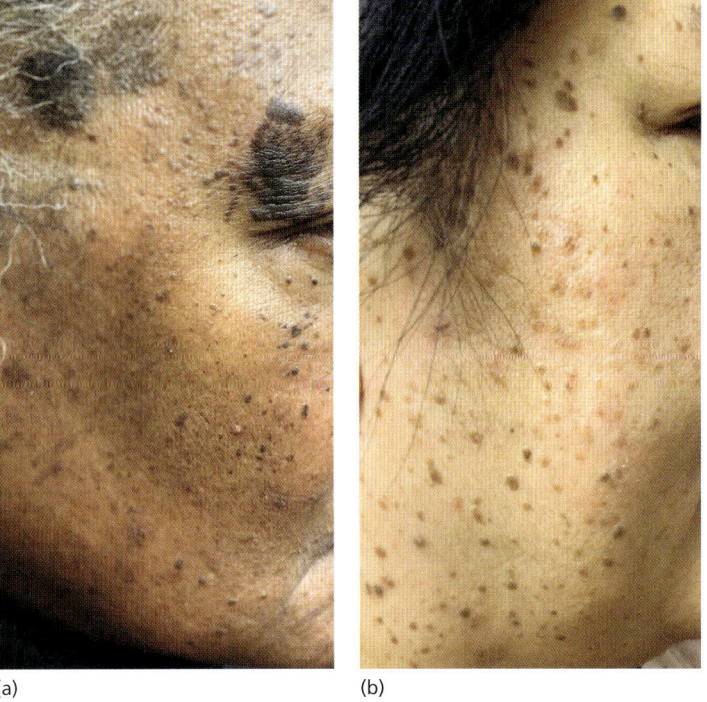

Figure 156.4 Dermatosis papulosis nigra are seborrhoeic keratosis-like lesions presenting on the face in (a) African and (b) Asian skin phenotypes. They have a predilection for the lateral aspects of the face and other sun-exposed sites. There are no known medical implications of these lesions, although they can be a source of cosmetic concern for patients.

correlated to more severe wrinkling, but the latter tended to be less of an issue compared with white skin [4]. Another difference in the manifestation of photoageing in SOC is dermatosis papulosis nigra (DPN). DPNs are small seborrhoeic keratosis-like lesions typically confined to sun-exposed sites on the lateral aspects of the face including the temples and cheeks (Figure 156.4). They are frequently noted in Asian and African skin types. In a recent survey study of 50 African American patients, 86% of DPNs were noted to be present on the face and 84% of patients had a first-degree relative with similar lesions. Although most DPNs were not symptomatic, they were noted to exert a moderate adverse effect on quality of life [5]. Treatment modalities may involve hyfrecation and curettage or Q-switched lasers.

More extensive research into darker skin ageing would enhance our understanding of the biology of ageing with respect to skin types containing more melanin than white skin. This understanding could further advance efforts in the area of rejuvenation for both cosmetic and medical purposes. More specific and precise therapy and skin care regimens could be designed targeting the specific ageing changes observed in the myriad skin types.

Extrinsic ageing variants

Several clinical variants of extrinsic ageing have been recognised and described. Gilchrest and others were among the first to describe distinct clinical variants of extrinsic ageing [6]. Atrophic photoageing, the more common variant, is characterised by individuals with numerous fine facial wrinkles, epidermal atrophy, telangiectases and/or redness, focal depigmentation and hyperpigmentation (lentigines and/or patchy hyperpigmentation) (Figure 156.5a). In this variant, there is a predisposition to the development of pre-cancerous and cancerous skin lesions. Yaar and Gilchrest originally described this variant as characterised by 'proliferative exhaustion', epidermal atrophy, focal depigmentation, pseudoscars, freckles, naevi, lentigo maligna, melanoma, actinic keratoses and basal and squamous cell carcinoma in patients with Fitzpatrick skin type I–II [6]. In support of this qualitative description of atrophic photoageing is a study of patients with basal cell carcinoma and wrinkles. In this work, discordance between facial wrinkling and the presence of basal cell carcinoma was observed, lending further credence to the observations that patients with fine wrinkles have more basal cell carcinomas than patients with coarse wrinkling [7].

The less common variant, hypertrophic photoageing, is characterised by homogenous colour, coarse wrinkling and less tendency to the development of skin cancers (Figure 156.5b). Yaar and Gilchrest originally described this variant as characterised by 'protective hyperplasia', tanning, lentigines and epidermal thickening mostly seen in Fitzpatrick skin types III–IV [6]. Although the atrophic and hypertrophic variants have been long recognised, there is increasing scientific evidence to support this clinical observation [8]. Examination and quantification of clinical and molecular features of atrophic and hypertrophic photoageing versus age-matched control subjects have demonstrated the same degree of collagen damage between the two clinical variants. However, in hypertrophic photoageing, more elastotic damage was observed compared with atrophic photoageing and controls. Hypertrophic photoageing generally occurred in younger subjects compared with atrophic photoageing. A negative correlation between solar elastosis and actinic keratoses raises the possibility that hypertrophic and atrophic photoageing develop as a result of fundamental differences in the skin's response to UV irradiation [8]. Undoubtedly, there is a great spectrum of clinical presentation between the atrophic and hypertrophic variants and most patients will in fact exhibit features of both atrophic and hypertrophic photoageing. Extrinsic ageing is

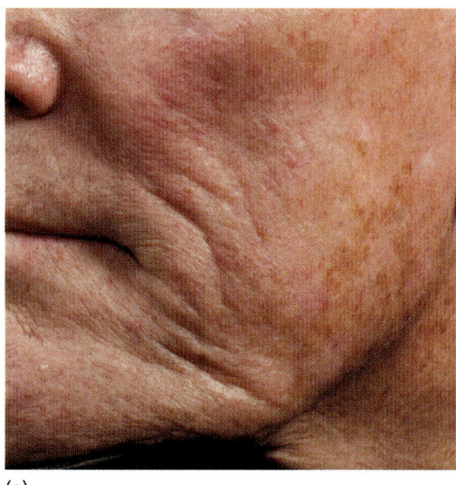
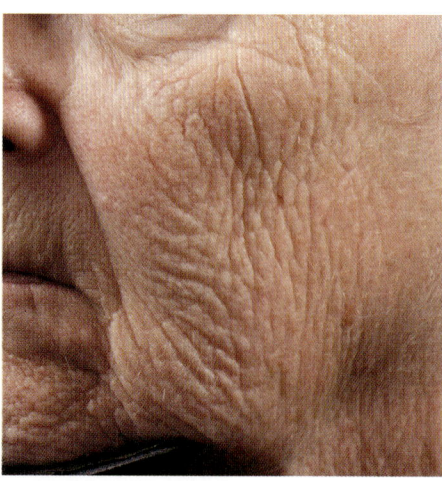

Figure 156.5 (a) Atrophic extrinsic ageing showing fine wrinkling, telangiectases, and dyspigmentation in the form of patchy, ill-defined hyperpigmentation. (b) Hypertrophic variant showing coarse wrinkling, fairly homogenous coloration tending toward a sallow or bronzed appearance, and lack of dyspigmentation and telangiectases.

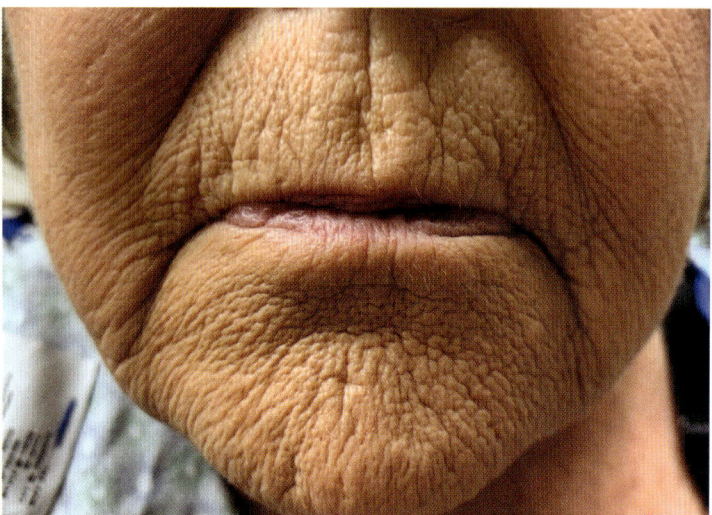

Figure 156.6 Smoker's skin is characterised by wrinkles radiating at 90-degree angles from the lips, and sallow yellow-grey discoloration.

always superimposed on intrinsic ageing since intrinsic ageing is a gradual and ongoing process. Certain clinical manifestations of extrinsic ageing deserve separate discussion.

Smoking and skin ageing

External factors, other than solar irradiation, that drive premature skin ageing include tobacco and other forms of non-ionising radiation. Individuals who are longstanding users of tobacco are readily identifiable by particular clinical features. Tell-tale signs of a smoker include the tobacco smoke odour of their skin and clothing, tobacco staining of the fingers and nails and the 'smoker's face' first described in 1971. 'Smoker's face' is characterised by wrinkles radiating at 90-degree angles from the lips and eyes, gaunt features, an uneven complexion and a greyish skin hue (Figure 156.6) [9]. In SOC, hyperpigmentation around and within the oral cavity can be observed [10,11]. A population-based study of factors associated with photoageing before the age of 55 years found that moderate to heavy smoking measured by pack-year was strongly associated with premature ageing [12]. A study of a pair of identical twins with marked differences in smoking habits (one had a 52-pack-year smoking history) further illustrated the effect of tobacco smoke on skin ageing [13].

The mechanism of tobacco smoke leading to facial wrinkling is poorly understood but is thought to involve tobacco's deleterious effects on elastic fibres – specifically an increase in the area of elastic fibres due to elastic fibre degradation rather than to newly synthesised elastic fibres [14]. Tobacco smoke is thought to have effects on new collagen synthesis and matrix metalloproteinase (MMP) induction similar to those effects resulting from UV irradiation exposure [15]. Fibroblast activity is altered by the generation of reactive oxygen species (ROS) and through the direct effects of nitrosonornicotine, which is found in high levels in tobacco and cigarettes [15–17]. Tobacco smoke also results in reduced blood flow within the microcirculation, further contributing to fibroblast dysfunction [16]. These findings suggest a process similar to that seen with fragmented and degraded collagen fibrils in aged skin.

Cutaneous nodular elastosis with cysts and comedones

Cutaneous nodular elastosis with cysts and comedones was described by Favre and Racouchot and represents another manifestation of extrinsic skin ageing [18]. It is characterised by open cysts and comedones of the lateral malar cheeks and periorbital regions and is noted more commonly in smokers (Figure 156.7). While there are no known medical implications of this condition, patients are often disturbed by the clinical appearance. Treatment modalities have not been standardised and may include comedone extraction and surgical removal.

Skin ageing of the neck

Photoageing of the neck is quite different in most cases from that of the face, even in the same individual. It assumes several different phenotypes depending on the anatomical location. Poikiloderma of Civatte is the term used to describe the findings of extrinsic photoageing of the lateral neck in white skin (Chapter 86). It is characterised by reticulated redness and dyspigmentation of the lateral aspects of the neck (Figure 156.8) but can become circumferential to involve the anterior base of the neck. Redness and dyspigmentation are usually seen in this condition; however, sometimes poikiloderma of Civatte can tend towards more redness or more dyspigmentation.

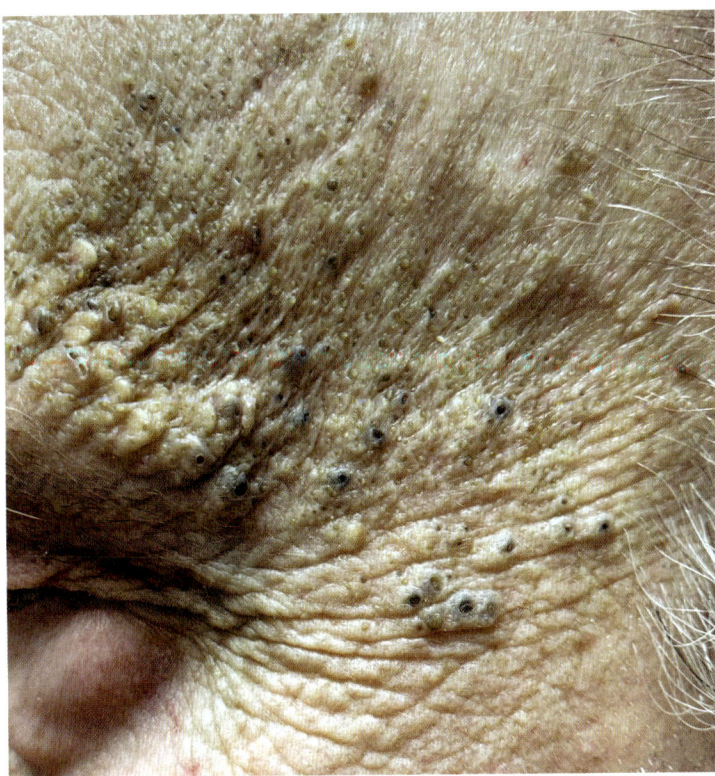

Figure 156.7 Nodular elastosis in the dermis with open comedones and cysts favoring the lateral malar cheeks and periorbital regions is seen more commonly in smokers.

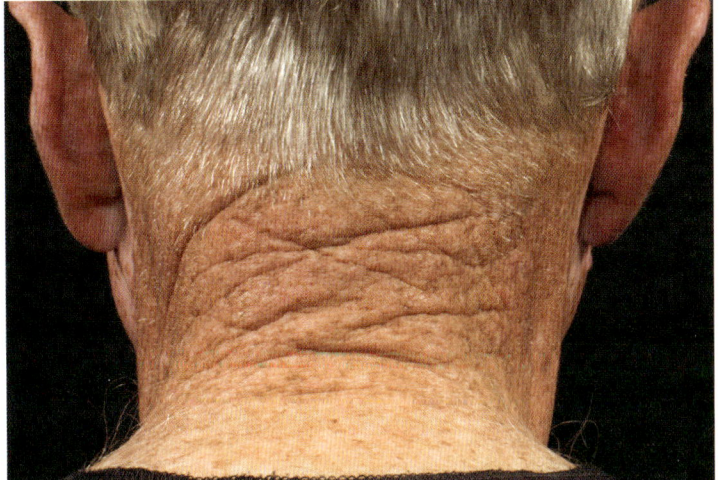

Figure 156.9 Posterior neck skin ageing known as cutis rhomboidalis nuchae showing coarse wrinkling in a cross-hatched configuration and bronzed coloration.

Interestingly, skin on the nuchal region ages in a manner that differs from that of the lateral neck. Coarse wrinkling, a bronzed or sallow coloration and minimal telangiectases – features seen in the hypertrophic variant of photoageing – are prominent at this site (Figure 156.9), compared with the lateral aspects of the neck. These findings are typically seen in men, likely due to shorter hairstyles allowing for more chronic UV irradiation exposure. It is noted anecdotally that very few skin cancers arise in this anatomical site, which is consistent with observations in patients with hypertrophic photoageing.

Idiopathic guttate hypomelanosis

Idiopathic guttate hypomelanosis is a term used to describe a form of hypopigmentation that presents as small single or numerous white macules, which tend to be most pronounced over the extensor surfaces of the upper and lower extremities (Figure 156.10) in both light and darker skin types. They may appear more exaggerated during the summer months when the surrounding skin darkens due to suntanning. These lesions are likely attributable to irreversible UV irradiation injury to melanocytes, but no formal research on these lesions has been published.

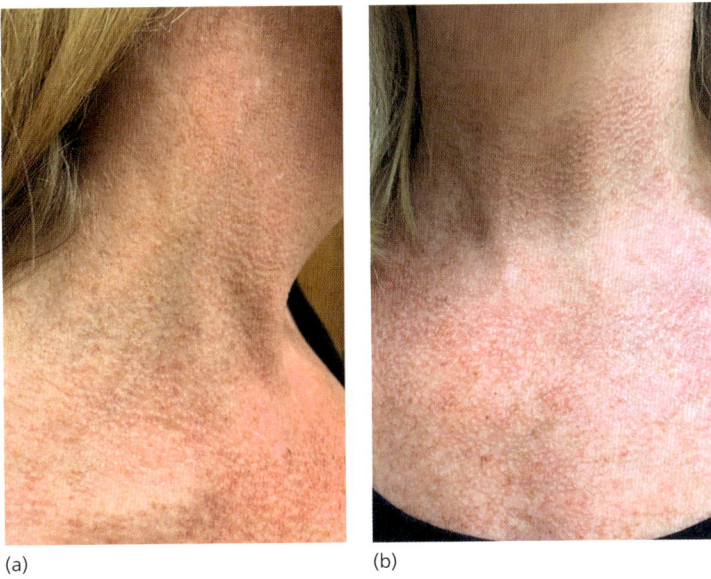

(a) (b)

Figure 156.8 Reticulated redness, dyspigmentation and fine papules of the lateral aspects of the neck sparing the submental region are characteristic of poikiloderma of Civatte.

The condition specifically spares the submental region as this area is relatively sun protected. The features of poikiloderma of Civatte are similar to those seen in the atrophic variant of extrinsic photoageing (discussed earlier in this chapter). Interestingly, patients may present with profound changes of poikiloderma on the neck with minimal extrinsic skin ageing of the face. This condition is not commonly observed in SOC. Laser and light-based therapies are useful in improving this cosmetically disturbing condition.

Bateman purpura

Bateman purpura (also known as senile purpura) are ecchymotic patches on photodamaged extensor surfaces of the arms and dorsal hands that appear with or without antecedent trauma (Figure 156.11). Clinically, they are small or extensive and may be very slow to resolve. It is striking that these lesions are not seen on the flexor surfaces of the arms nor on any sun-protected sites. This lends further credence to the concept that they are truly a hallmark lesion of the effects resulting from an overlap of intrinsic and extrinsic ageing. In addition to intrinsic and extrinsic ageing, Bateman purpura are likely attributable to antecedent trauma and anticoagulant medications such as aspirin, heparin, warfarin and other new antiplatelet agents, and oral and topical corticosteroids. Resolution is often slow, and the condition is recurrent. Patients do not like the appearance of these ecchymoses, but no good therapy

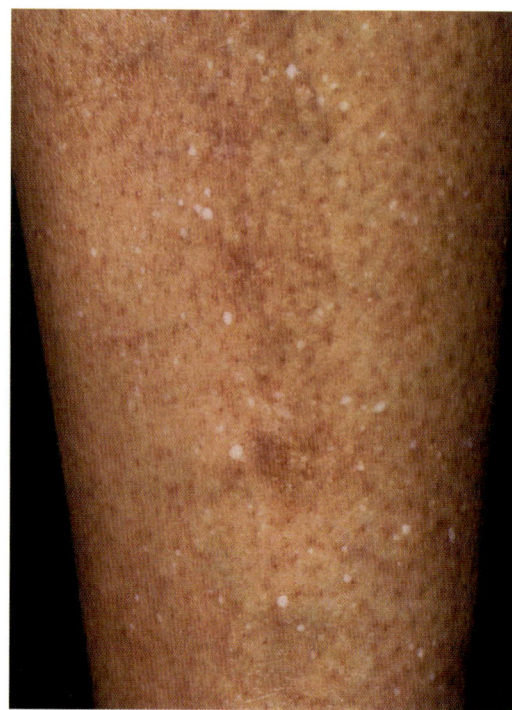

Figure 156.10 The extensor surface of the lower extremity is a common site for idiopathic guttate hypomelanosis.

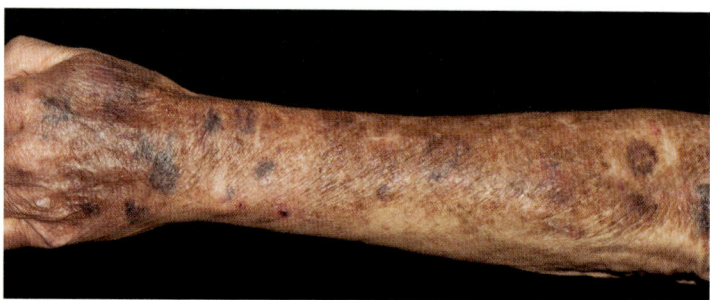

Figure 156.11 Ecchymotic patches over the extensor forearms, known as Bateman purpura, represent an extreme example of superimposed intrinsic and extrinsic ageing.

is available. Judicious sun protection starting in early life may mitigate against this condition.

Menopausal skin ageing

The study and observations of skin ageing in the menopausal population offer insight into the role that hormones may play in ageing skin. Oestrogen is known to exert its actions on skin through oestrogen receptors. The effects of oestrogen on skin are derived from studies of postmenopausal women. Oestrogens have been reported to have effects on both the epidermis and the dermis. In the epidermis, they have been associated with increased thickness, hydration and an increase in surface lipid content. In the dermis, they have been associated with increased hydration through an increase in glycosaminoglycan content as well as through increased collagen [19]. Menopause is associated with an increase in skin dryness, decreased elasticity and decreased dermal thickness [20,21]. Oestrogen-based treatments are believed to be beneficial for improving the appearance of photoaged skin, but the scientific evidence is scanty. Women who take oestrogen replacements have been observed to have better skin hydration, elasticity and fewer fine lines [22,23]. Other studies, however, have not demonstrated beneficial effects of oestrogen therapy on photoaged skin [20].

Studies of topical oestradiol applied to photoaged skin (face and forearms) and sun-protected skin (hips) revealed an increase in collagens I and III in sun-protected skin in both male and female subjects, but no change in the collagens in photoaged skin [24].

Genetics of skin ageing

There is great diversity in skin ageing even within families. However, little is known about genetic influences in skin ageing. It would seem that genes regulated by exposure of the skin to UV irradiation or those associated with particular phenotypes such as light complexion traits, blue or green eyes and light hair colour would be most implicated.

The *MCR1* (melanocortin 1 receptor) gene maps to chromosome 16q24.3 and is located on the surface of melanocytes. *MCR1* plays a critical role in skin pigmentation. When the receptor is activated, melanocytes produce eumelanin (black pigment), which is protective from UV irradiation. In contrast, when the receptor is blocked, phaeomelanin (red pigment) is synthesised, which does not confer as much protection from UV irradiation. Polymorphisms in the *MCR1* gene are responsible for the normal variability observed in populations with respect to hair and skin pigmentation [1].

In a study of over 500 middle-aged French women, logistic regressions were performed to assess the influence of *MCR1* gene polymorphisms on severe photoageing [2]. Subjects with two common major diminished function variants were at up to 5.61 times greater risk for severe photoageing compared with subjects with two wild-type alleles. Given the protective effects of eumelanin compared with phaeomelanin, these findings are consistent with what is understood about UV irradiation and the mechanisms of skin ageing. However, even after adjustment for skin colour and lifetime sun exposure, these *MCR1* polymorphisms still remained a significant risk for severe photoageing. The authors postulated that phaeomelanin is a potential source of ROS, in contrast to eumelanin, which scavenges ROS thereby leading to wrinkling [2].

In addition to inherited genetic polymorphisms, non-heritable epigenetic changes also occur with intrinsic ageing and photoageing. In intrinsically aged skin, there is a trend towards hypermethylation across the genome [3,4]. Aged and sun-exposed skin tends to be hypomethylated and hyperacetylated in areas that are important for the expression of genes that are involved in skin homeostasis, leading to changes in gene expression. These epigenetic changes are correlated with clinical measures of photoageing [4,5]. Further research into the genetic and epigenetic mechanisms of ageing may provide novel avenues for intervention and prevention.

Grading and measurement of skin ageing

Histopathology of the skin demonstrates the hallmark finding of solar elastosis in photoaged skin, which is quantifiable, along with the extent and degree of collagen fibril fragmentation and disorganisation. Skin ageing, in particular photoageing, can be quantified on a histological basis by the measurement of solar elastosis. The quantification of photoageing is desirable as it may yield important clinical information on the risk of actinic keratosis and skin cancer development. The histological quantification of skin ageing is not, however, practical in the clinic. Non-invasive tools to quantify skin ageing for the purposes of patient care and clinical research have been proposed and created for both extrinsic and intrinsic ageing.

A widely used photonumerical scale was developed to describe and quantify the clinical degree of photoageing. This scale employs nine ratings (0 to 8), each with an illustrative photograph, and was found to be much superior to a descriptive scale that did not employ photographs [1]. It specifically assesses clinical features of wrinkling and dyspigmentation, where 0 refers to no photodamage and 8 refers to severe photodamage. It is particularly relevant and useful in clinical research studies involving facial photoageing and is easy to use given the clearly illustrative examples and simple numerical grading scale.

This scale does not, however, discriminate between hypertrophic and atrophic variants of photoageing. A new version of this nine-point scale specifically addressing the atrophic variant of photoageing has been developed as a useful tool in both clinical practice and research [2]. Scales that address ageing skin specific to both sexes might also be desirable as factors such as menopause and hormones may influence the rate and degree of skin ageing. Particular clinical features of skin ageing such as perioral wrinkling, which is more prominent in women [3], are yet another reason that sex-specific scales may be useful in describing photoageing. When utilising photonumerical scales it is critical that the user remains cognisant of wrinkles caused by cutaneous ageing, as opposed to creases and skin folds due to underlying structural changes such as fat pad atrophy and skeletal resorption.

Another limitation of the photonumerical photoageing scale is that it does not take into account SOC and mainly addresses extrinsic ageing in lighter skin types. A scale that grades wrinkles and dyspigmentation in Koreans was developed with the use of subject interviews to determine cumulative sun exposure and smoking history along with measurements of skin colour [4]. Given that this study assessed 407 subjects, it is possible that these results might be relevant to other Asian skin types. Scales that assess African, Middle Eastern and mixed ethnicities are lacking. Such scales would be useful for clinical research, but would require great efforts as a number of scales would be needed in order to account for the wide spectrum of SOC across the world. The issue of mixed ethnicities introduces a greater level of complexity when trying to quantify skin ageing.

A photonumerical scale to assess photoprotected skin (intrinsically aged skin) has been developed and has shown significant correlation with patient age and history of cigarette smoking [5]. This scale employs a nine-point rating system and illustrative clinical photographs of the inner aspects of the upper arms; a 0 score represents no fine wrinkling and 8 represents severe fine wrinkling.

Tools to assess anatomical sites other than the face offer value particularly in clinical research. Skin ageing is known to be more or less accelerated depending on the particular anatomical site. As cosmetic procedures expand to include more sites off the face (neck, décolleté, hands and forearms), tools to measure and describe photoageing at these sites become desirable. Examples of such scales include a photographic global assessment of forearm sun damage [6] and a five-point, dynamic, platysmal band photonumerical assessment scale useful in cosmetic clinics [7].

Pathophysiology

Skin ageing is apparent in both the epidermis and the dermis. However, the changes observed in the extracellular matrix, particularly dermal collagen and elastic fibres, are the hallmark of aged skin and are believed to be responsible for the wrinkled appearance. Type I collagen is by far the most abundant protein in the dermis and accounts for nearly 80% of the dry weight of the dermis. Degradation and decreased production of new collagen result in the clinical phenotype of wrinkling [1]. Several decades of work focused on understanding the mechanisms of retinoids in ageing skin led to the elucidation of skin ageing pathophysiology as we understand it at the present time, especially with respect to photoageing. Also, in recent years great strides have been made in understanding the pathophysiology of intrinsic ageing. Though there are differences in the pathophysiological processes between intrinsic and extrinsic ageing, both processes culminate in a final common pathway. Extrinsic ageing is always superimposed on intrinsic ageing. The changes of extrinsic ageing tend to be more pronounced compared with intrinsic ageing.

ROS are the molecules that drive and catalyse the complex signalling cascades in ageing skin leading to (i) fragmentation of formed collagen; and (ii) reduced new collagen synthesis [2]. ROS cause direct cellular damage to the cell walls, lipid membranes, mitochondria and DNA, but more importantly ROS play critical roles in catalysing the complex cellular signalling pathways in fibroblasts and keratinocytes that are relevant to new collagen formation and breakdown of mature collagen.

Ultraviolet irradiation damage/episodic exposure

Research on the mechanism of action of retinoids in the treatment of photoageing has helped to elucidate the molecular basis of premature sun-induced skin ageing. A landmark series of publications reported the sequence of events by which solar UV irradiation leads to collagen fibril fragmentation and depression of collagen production [3–5], which are primary antecedents of the clinical phenotype of photoageing. In skin cells, the inherent energy in UV irradiation is converted to ROS, which initiates a cascade of biochemical reactions [6–8]. As little as one-tenth of minimal erythema dose (MED) UVB (280–320 nm) leads to statistically significant cellular and molecular responses that deleteriously alter the dermal collagenous extracellular matrix. These responses increase in magnitude with increasing strength of UV exposure to two MEDs, a dose that causes relatively modest skin reddening [3]. It is envisioned that repetition of these responses over a lifetime of episodic UV exposures causes accumulation of dermal damage that brings about photoageing [5,9].

ROS are generated in skin cells that are directly exposed to UV irradiation. ROS are initially produced through photochemical reactions involving molecular oxygen within skin cells. This initial oxidative stress elicits cellular responses that generate additional ROS through signal transduction and metabolic pathways. ROS directly inhibit protein tyrosine phosphatases (PTPs) [10–15], which normally function to limit the activities of protein tyrosine kinases (PTKs) and their downstream signalling pathways [16–20]. The family of growth factor and cytokine receptors depend on PTK activities for their activation [21–23]. Oxidative inhibition of PTPs and the consequent activation of growth factor and cytokine receptors occur rapidly following UV irradiation [24,25].

Activation of the epidermal growth factor receptor PTK activity resulting from oxidative inhibition of receptor PTP-κ has been found to be a key initiator of signalling pathways that drive many of the deleterious cellular and molecular responses to UV irradiation [25,26]. These pathways include mitogen-activated protein (MAP) kinases ERK, p38 and JNK, which control growth, differentiation and stress responses in skin cells [27,28,29]. MAP kinase pathways induce transcription factor AP-1, which is composed of Jun and Fos proteins. c-Jun, which is the major AP-1 protein induced by UV irradiation in human skin [4,30,31], is activated by direct phosphorylation by JNK.

AP-1 is critical to the photoageing process because it is the major regulator of gene expression of a subset of MMPs. These are a family of enzymes that are capable of degrading the structural proteins that comprise the dermal extracellular matrix. AP-1 regulates gene expression of MMP-1, MMP-3 and MMP-9, which are induced in skin following UV irradiation exposure [3–5,30,32]. Induction of MMPs occurs primarily in the epidermis and the enzymes move to the dermis where they act on collagen fibrils and other components of the dermal extracellular matrix [5,32]. MMP-1 is a key enzyme because it is specifically able to initiate collagen fibril degradation [33]. Once cleaved, collagen fibrils can be further degraded by MMP-3 and MMP-9. In combination, the three MMPs have the capacity to degrade the majority of proteins in the dermal extracellular matrix, thereby impairing the strength and resiliency of the skin. Collagen fibril degradation by MMP-1, -3 and -9, coupled with imperfect repair over a lifetime of episodic sun exposures, has been proposed to be a key mechanism giving rise to the clinical phenotype of wrinkling [9,34,35].

Induction of AP-1 by UV irradiation, in addition to stimulating the production of MMPs, has significant suppressive effects on new collagen formation [30,36]. This inhibition occurs through antagonism of the transforming growth factor β (TGF-β) pathway, which is a major regulator of collagen production [37–39]. TGF-β promotes collagen production via the activation of Smad transcription factors [40–42]. AP-1 interacts with Smad3, thereby interfering with the ability of Smad3 to stimulate collagen gene transcription [43,44]. UV exposure also leads to impairment of the Smad3 function via downregulation of the TGF-β type II receptor (TβRII), which is required for Smad3 activation [45–47]. Activation of AP-1 and reduction of TβRII act together to suppress collagen gene expression. The combined effects of enhanced collagen fibril degradation and decreased new collagen formation result in a net accumulation of fragmented collagen fibrils [9,48,49]. This accumulation increases with continued episodic UV exposures.

Other environmental influences in skin ageing

The skin exposome refers to the totality of environmental exposures over a lifetime that modify or induce skin conditions including photoageing and certain inflammatory skin conditions [50]. While UV irradiation and smoking are known contributors to photoageing, other environmental influences include traffic-related air pollution, hormones, nutrition and psychological stressors such as stress and lack of sleep [50]. A direct link between skin ageing, particularly dyspigmentation and wrinkles, and airborne particulate matter (air pollution) was discovered in an epidemiological study [51]. The proposal for this centres on the mechanism by which particulate matter exposure generates ROS. In addition, particulate matter may also serve as carriers for organic metals and chemicals that localise in mitochondria and generate ROS [52,53]. The effects of these various environmental factors result in biochemical processes including oxidation, inflammation and glycation, all of which may affect collagen degradation and production through various pathways.

Collagen fibril fragmentation

Collagen fibril fragmentation impacts not only dermal structural integrity, but also dermal fibroblast function. This latter property of collagen fibril fragmentation derives from its disruption of the normal interactions between fibroblasts and their surrounding intact collagen fibrils. Through this mechanism, collagen fibril fragmentation achieves central importance as a driving force for the perpetuation of both photoageing and natural skin ageing.

Type I collagen is the most abundant dermal protein. It forms fibrils, which associate with several additional extracellular matrix proteins including other types of collagens and proteoglycans [54,55]. Haematoxylin and eosin staining of young skin reveals eosinophilic dense bundled material occupying the dermis. The majority of this eosinophilic material is type I collagen fibrils. These fibrils serve as structural support for the skin, and as dynamic scaffolding to which dermal cells adhere and interact. Fibroblasts synthesise, secrete and promote the assembly of all the components of collagen fibrils [56].

The normal assembly of collagen fibrils involves the formation of intra- and interfibril cross-links, which are catalysed by the enzyme lysyl oxidase [57]. Cross-linking is absolutely necessary for mechanical stability of collagen fibrils. Cross-links are also highly resistant to proteolytic degradation. Normal turnover of skin collagen is exceedingly slow, with an average half-life of 15 years [58]. However, due to their relative resistance to proteolytic removal, cross-linked regions of collagen molecules accumulate within the fibrillar network throughout a lifetime. This lifelong accumulation of residual collagen cross-links represents essentially permanent disruption of the extracellular matrix in photoaged and naturally aged human skin.

As skin ages, changes in proteins that regulate collagen homeostasis occur. Dermal fibroblasts secrete a signalling protein called CCN1, and CCN1 levels become elevated in aged skin. Elevated levels of CCN1 impair TGF-β signalling and subsequent collagen formation [59]. Decreased TGF-β signalling results in decreased collagen production and subsequent dermal thinning. Elevated expression of CCN1 also results in the upregulation of the transcription factor AP-1, which contributes to collagen fibril fragmentation through elevated expression of MMPs [59]. Mice genetically engineered to express high levels of CCN1 have accelerated dermal aging [59], implicating this protein as a critical regulator of skin ageing, independent of age or UV exposure.

Fibroblasts not only produce the dermal collagenous extracellular matrix, but also are embedded within it, bound to collagen fibrils through receptors known as integrins [60–63]. This binding

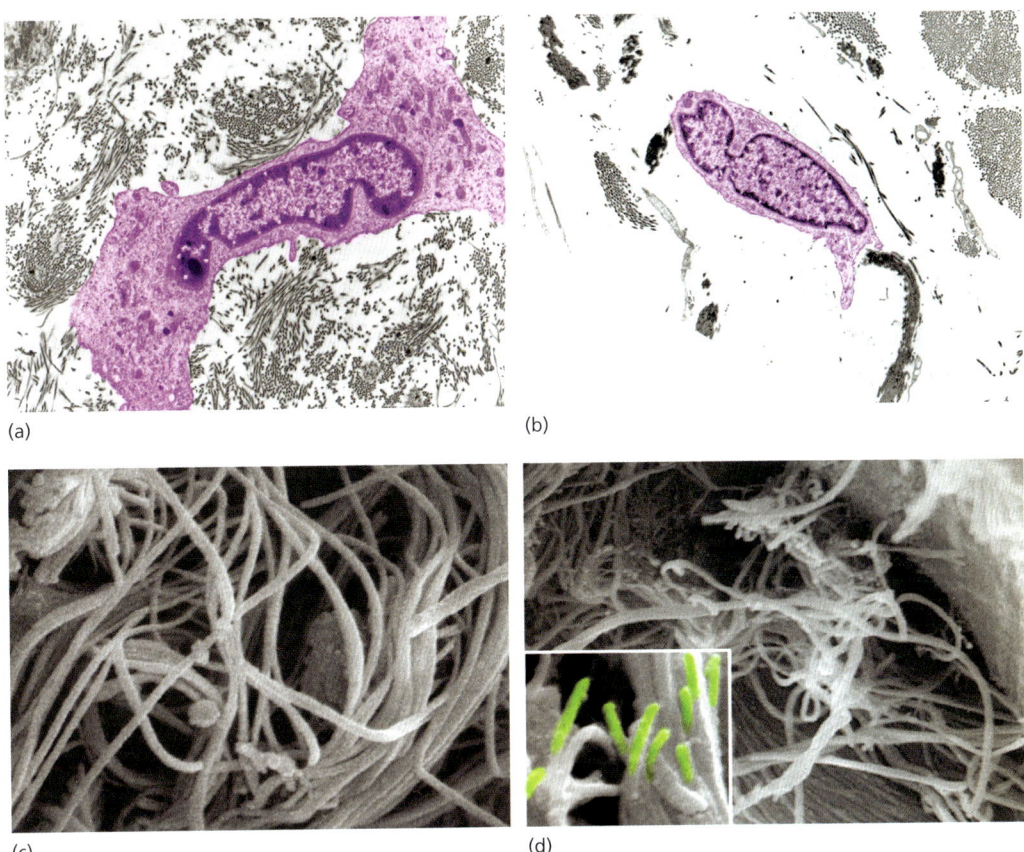

Figure 156.12 (a) Transmission electron micrograph (TEM) of a fibroblast (computer stained purple for clarity) within the dermis of sun-protected skin in a young adult. Note the elongated appearance and extended cytoplasm away from the nucleus of the fibroblast which is in close proximity to abundant collagen fibrils (original magnification 2000×). (b) TEM of a fibroblast within the dermis of photoaged skin showing the collapse of cytoplasm inwards towards the nucleus and the lack of adjacent collagen fibrils. The fibroblast is surrounded by amorphous material (original magnification 2000×). (c) Scanning electron micrograph (SEM) of collagen fibrils in young adult skin. Note that the long fibrils are closely packed and fill the space with no apparent breaks in them (original magnification 10 000×). (d) SEM of collagen fibrils in photoaged skin showing large gaps and numerous fragmented fibrils (original magnification 12 500×). The inset highlights the fragmented collagen fibrils (computer coloured green). From Fisher et al. [48], © 2008 American Medical Association; all rights reserved.

allows the fibroblast cytoskeletal machinery to exert mechanical traction forces on the surrounding collagen fibrils [61,62]. Due to their inherent mechanical properties, intact collagen fibrils provide resistive mechanical forces, thereby establishing a state of dynamic mechanical equilibrium within the dermal microenvironment. The mechanical load that is created drives the assembly of intracellular scaffolding, involving the main components of the cytoskeleton, actin filaments, intermediate filaments and microtubules. Cytoskeleton assembly causes fibroblasts to stretch and expand the area of their cytoplasm. Thus, the interaction of fibroblasts with collagen fibrils dictates the dermal mechanical microenvironment and fibroblast shape. Importantly, cellular mechanics and shape have a fundamental impact on fibroblast function. Regulation of cell function by shape is a fundamental aspect of cell biology, and the mechanistic basis that links form to function is the subject of intensive research [64,65].

In young and photoprotected skin, fibroblasts bound to intact collagen fibrils apply tension to the extracellular matrix and achieve stretch. In this stretched state, fibroblasts display a biosynthetic phenotype that maintains optimal collagen fibril homeostasis. In contrast, in aged skin, MMP-mediated collagen fibril fragmentation destroys sites for fibroblast binding. With the loss of collagen fibril binding, fibroblasts are unable to apply tension to the surrounding extracellular matrix and are unable to stretch. In this collapsed state, fibroblasts exhibit a catabolic phenotype.

Electron micrographs of fibroblasts in young photoprotected skin reveal stretched morphology and illustrate the close association of fibroblasts with the surrounding intact collagen fibrils (Figure 156.12). In aged skin, collapsed fibroblasts occupy amorphous space containing fragmented collagen fibrils.

Fibroblast collapse activates many of the same cellular stress pathways observed in cells following direct exposure to UV irradiation. These responses include increased production of ROS, activation of AP-1 and downregulation of TβRII with impairment of TGF-β/Smad pathway signalling [66–68]. As observed in UV-irradiated cells, these responses lead to elevated expression of MMPs and reduced expression of collagen. However, unlike acute UV irradiation, collagen fragmentation induces stress responses primarily in dermal cells, rather than epidermal cells. Thus, fragmented collagen is a common driving force that mediates the convergence of many of the molecular and cellular features of extrinsic and intrinsic skin ageing.

Age-related alterations of fibroblast architecture cause fibroblasts to acquire a phenotype that is characterised by reduced production of extracellular matrix proteins, increased expression of extracellular matrix-degrading enzymes and elevated expression of pro-inflammatory mediators [69]. This is a process called inflammageing [70]. The phenotype of fibroblasts in aged skin can be thought of as reflecting adaptation to the deleterious alterations in the extracellular matrix microenvironment, in contrast to cell-autonomous ageing. These adaptive responses perpetuate extracellular matrix degradation, inflammageing and create a tissue milieu conducive to cancer initiation. Thus, dermal ageing can be viewed as 'outside-in adaptation', which is reversible by targeting improvements in the composition, organisation and/or mechanical properties of the dermal extracellular matrix.

Photoageing and natural ageing

The linkage between fibroblast form and function is critically important for the ageing process in human skin, and forms a conceptual basis that unites the pathophysiology of photoageing and natural ageing. The lynchpin that connects these two forms of skin ageing is the accumulation of cross-linked collagen fibril fragments. Whether initiated by UV exposure or the passage of time, both photoageing and natural ageing cause the accumulation of fragmented collagen fibrils. This accumulation leads to both impairment of the mechanical properties of the dermis and reduced spreading of fibroblasts. Loss of stretch stimulates cellular stress responses similar to those induced by direct UV exposure. Stressed fibroblasts have altered function, epitomised by less collagen biosynthesis and more production of collagen fibril-degrading MMPs. This imbalance of collagen homeostasis becomes self-sustaining as elevated levels of MMPs and reduced collagen fibril production lead to higher amounts of fragmented collagen fibrils, which further promote excess MMPs and decreased collagen fibril synthesis (Figure 156.13). The self-perpetuating nature of this process ultimately results in permanent collagen loss, clinically manifested as photoageing of sun-exposed skin or natural ageing of sun-protected skin.

Implications of skin ageing

It is easy to view skin ageing as a purely cosmetic concern. However, as the annual amount of money spent on skin rejuvenation therapies and procedures continues to escalate worldwide, it is clear that skin ageing has broader implications pertaining to medical conditions that may arise in the setting of ageing skin and the social implications of an aged appearance.

Medical implications

A study investigating whether skin appearance plays a role in predicting disease risk determined that individuals from long-lived families (at least two siblings living to be nonagenarians) had less skin wrinkling on photoprotected sites compared with age-matched controls. The study also found that perceived facial age was a marker of longevity in men and cardiovascular disease in women independent of other factors such as smoking, sun damage and body mass index [1]. This study suggests that the implications of skin ageing surpass cosmetic concerns and may indeed be predictive of certain disease states.

Barrier dysfunction

A myriad of diseases and lesions such as bullous pemphigoid and seborrhoeic keratoses are seen in aged skin, however discussion of these entities is beyond the scope of this chapter and can be found elsewhere. The conditions of xerosis, pruritus and asteatosis in ageing skin, on the other hand, deserve special mention. With ageing these conditions become quite common and problematic. The epidermal barrier is defective in ageing and this probably accounts for many of the clinical findings. Lipids processed by enzymes requiring an acidic pH compose the epidermal water barrier. In ageing skin, the pH of the skin surface becomes less acidic such that lipid production is decreased to the degree that the barrier cannot be maintained to the same extent as in younger skin [2]. In addition, ceramides that maintain the epidermal barrier have been noted to be reduced in elderly skin [3]. Aquaporin-3 is a channel that allows for the flow of water and glycerol that maintains skin hydration. In ageing skin,

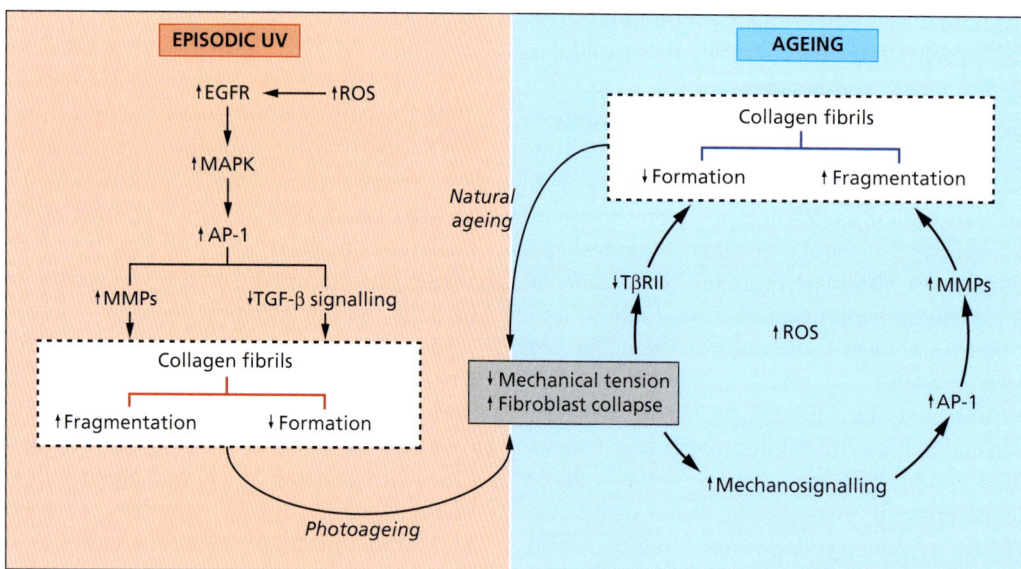

Figure 156.13 Molecular mechanisms in ageing skin. Collagen fibril fragmentation is a critical mediator that links episodic ultraviolet (UV) exposure, photoageing and natural ageing in the human skin. Episodic UV irradiation induces reactive oxygen species (ROS) mediated signalling cascades, primarily in the epidermis (shown in red), which lead to fragmentation and reduced production of collagen fibrils in the dermis. In photoageing, the accumulation of damage to collagen fibrils from episodic UV exposures causes mechanical instability, thereby promoting fibroblast collapse. This collapse leads to further fragmentation and reduced production of collagen fibrils through upregulation of matrix metalloproteinases (MMPs) and downregulation of TGF-β receptor (TβRII) signalling, respectively. In natural ageing, normal collagen fibril turnover, occurring over many years, causes the accumulation of fragmented collagen, which results in mechanical instability and fibroblast collapse, as seen in photoageing. Thus, collagen fibril damage drives a self-perpetuating cycle (shown in blue) that is common to photoageing and natural ageing. AP-1, activator protein 1 transcription factor; EGFR, epidermal growth factor receptor; MAPK, mitogen-activated protein kinase; TGF-β, transforming growth factor β.

aquaporin gene expression is reduced, leading to poor hydration [4]. These changes in lipids, ceramides and aquaporin gene expression, leading to barrier dysfunction with ageing, probably account for the resulting xerosis, asteatosis and pruritus. In addition, the altered barrier function likely results in an increased incidence of irritant and contact dermatitis in aged skin [5].

Dermatoporosis

Dermatoporosis refers to a chronic cutaneous syndrome associated with advanced age and sun exposure in which the integrity of skin is severely compromised [6]. In this syndrome, the skin appears atrophic, has lacerations, and bruises and bleeds easily. Though there are cosmetic implications of these findings, the emphasis in this syndrome is on the loss of the functional integrity of the skin to confer protection. The age-associated functional impairment in skin in dermatoporosis is similar to osteoporosis in which bone fragility can lead to significant morbidity and mortality.

Four stages of dermatoporosis have been described. In stage I disease, pronounced skin thinning, purpura and stellate pseudoscars are observed. In stage II disease, lacerations resulting from the cleavage between the epidermis and dermis are seen in addition to the lesions in stage I. In stage III disease, the lacerations are numerous and extensive, sometimes involving an entire extremity, and delays in wound healing are a pronounced feature. In stage IV disease, dissecting haematomas result from the extreme skin damage. Hyaluronic acid, the major glycosaminoglycan in skin, is decreased along with its cell surface receptor CD44 in dermatoporotic skin, as compared with young skin [7,8]. One might consider that Bateman purpura represent stage I dermatoporosis.

Cosmetic implications

Skin ageing has significant cosmetic ramifications. Many patients presenting with cosmetic concerns are specifically anxious about fine and coarse wrinkling, skin laxity, dyspigmentation, redness and telangiectases, and textural irregularities such as dullness and roughness. These concerns apply to patients of all skin types, with the exception of redness, which is a more common complaint in lighter skin types. Most of these concerns are attributable to the results of both intrinsic and extrinsic ageing. Numerous treatments and procedures are available to rejuvenate skin damage and improve facial ageing on a wider scale. These include topical therapies, various non-ablative and ablative laser procedures, as well as soft tissue injectables and neurotoxins. Prophylaxis of photoageing is achieved with stringent sun protective measures including, but not limited to, sun avoidance and sun protection through both physical and chemical means.

The mainstay of topical therapy for intrinsically and extrinsically aged skin is topical retinoids, which include both the natural and synthetic forms. The natural molecules, of which retinoic acid (tretinoin) is the gold standard, have been extensively investigated for their effects in aged skin. Retinoic acid and its metabolic precursor, retinol, are associated with clinical and histological improvement of wrinkles via their ability to increase TGF-β, leading to an increase in new collagen formation in photoaged and naturally aged skin. In addition, retinoic acid and retinol block collagenase, thereby preventing further collagen degradation in the skin. The actions of new collagen production and the reduction of further breakdown of existing collagen together lead to clinical improvement in wrinkling. Retinoic acid use, through mechanisms not completely understood, also results in improvement in dyspigmentation and lentigines. Early in retinoic acid therapy, notable epidermal spongiosis and accumulation of glycosaminoglycans are noted in the epidermis, imparting skin smoothening. Further discussion of retinoic acid is found in Chapters 157 and 160.

Emerging data also support a beneficial role for the use of synthetic retinoids including adapalene and tazarotene in skin photoageing [9–11]. The obvious prophylactic measure to prevent skin ageing is the avoidance of factors such as UV irradiation and tobacco smoke that play significant roles in the generation of ROS.

A promising treatment for both photoaged and intrinsically aged skin is the use of intradermal injections of cross-linked hyaluronic acid ('filler') [12]. Administration of intradermal cross-linked hyaluronic acid promotes the synthesis of new, undamaged collagen, which in turn promotes fibroblast stretch, and may slow the ageing process [12].

Social implications

Skin is one of the key indicators of beauty, conveying attractiveness and youth to the outside world. Features seen in ageing such as wrinkles, dyspigmentation and textural irregularities significantly detract from a youthful experience. A study of cheek images from 170 females aged 11–76 years were blind-rated for attractiveness, healthiness, youthfulness and biological age by over 350 raters. Skin colour homogeneity was found to significantly influence perception of age, attractiveness, health and youth [13]. It is well established that a youthful and attractive appearance is associated with greater success and opportunities in the work force, increased social and sexual attractiveness and overall happiness [14,15].

New knowledge about skin ageing continues to mount. Continued strides in understanding molecular mechanisms, and the development of more sophisticated tools to quantify skin ageing, will hopefully lead to substantial prevention and repair of this cosmetically and medically debilitating condition.

Key references

The full list of references can be found in the online version at https://www.wiley.com/rooksdermatology10e

Clinical features

6 Yaar M, Gilchrest BA. Photoageing: mechanism, prevention and therapy. *Br J Dermatol* 2007;157:874–87.

Pathophysiology

3 Fisher GJ, Datta SC, Talwar HS *et al*. Molecular basis of sun-induced premature skin ageing and retinoid antagonism. *Nature* 1996;379:335–9.
4 Fisher GJ, Talwar HS, Lin J *et al*. Retinoic acid inhibits induction of c-Jun protein by ultraviolet radiation that occurs subsequent to activation of mitogen-activated protein kinase pathways in human skin in vivo. *J Clin Invest* 1998; 101:1432–40.
5 Fisher GJ, Wang ZQ, Datta SC, Varani J, Kang S, Voorhees JJ. Pathophysiology of premature skin aging induced by ultraviolet light. *N Engl J Med* 1997;337:1419–28.
9 Fisher GJ, Kang S, Varani J *et al*. Mechanisms of photoaging and chronological skin aging. *Arch Dermatol* 2002;138:1462–70.

27 Chung JH, Kang S, Varani J, Lin J, Fisher GJ, Voorhees JJ. Decreased extracellular-signal-regulated kinase and increased stress-activated MAP kinase activities in aged human skin in vivo. *J Invest Dermatol* 2000;115:177–82.

30 Fisher GJ, Datta S, Wang Z et al. c-Jun-dependent inhibition of cutaneous procollagen transcription following ultraviolet irradiation is reversed by all-trans retinoic acid. *J Clin Invest* 2000;106:663–70.

48 Fisher GJ, Varani J, Voorhees JJ. Looking older: fibroblast collapse and therapeutic implications. *Arch Dermatol* 2008;144:666–72.

64 Ingber DE. Cellular mechanotransduction: putting all the pieces together again. *FASEB J* 2006;20:811–27.

Implications of skin ageing

12 Fisher GJ, Varani J, Voorhees JJ. Looking older: fibroblast collapse and therapeutic implications. *Arch Dermatol* 2008;144:666–72.

CHAPTER 157

Cosmeceuticals

Neera R. Nathan[1], Eubee Koo[2], Alexandra B. Kimball[3] and Molly Wanner[1]

[1] Department of Dermatology, Harvard Medical School, Massachusetts General Hospital, Boston, MA, USA
[2] Permanente Medical Group, Oakland, CA, USA
[3] Harvard Medical Faculty Physicians, Beth Israel Deaconess Medical Center, Boston, MA, USA

Introduction, 157.1	Kojic acid, 157.4	Green tea, 157.9
Antioxidants, 157.1	Tranexamic acid, 157.4	Lycopene, 157.9
Alpha-lipoic acid, 157.1	**Anti-ageing: rhytid reduction, 157.4**	Pomegranate, 157.10
Coenzyme Q10, 157.2	Glycosaminoglycans, 157.4	Soya, 157.10
Vitamin B, 157.2	Hydroxy acids, 157.4	**Anti-inflammatories, 157.10**
Vitamin C, 157.2	Polyunsaturated fatty acids, 157.5	Aloe, 157.10
Vitamin E, 157.3	Peptides, 157.5	Caffeine, 157.11
Anti-ageing: lightening, 157.3	Vitamin A (retinoids), 157.6	Chamomile, 157.11
Arbutin, 157.3	**Herbals and phytochemicals, 157.7**	**Conclusions, 157.11**
Cysteamine, 157.3	Carnosine, 157.7	
Hydroquinone, 157.3	Grape seed, 157.7	**Key references, 157.13**

Introduction

In the late 1970s, Albert Kligman popularised the term 'cosmeceutical', which referred to a category of skincare products that embodied characteristics of both drugs and cosmetics. Today, the term is used predominantly by the cosmetics industry to describe products that are purported to have therapeutic action capable of affecting the appearance of skin beyond the time of application [1]. However, the term cosmeceutical is not recognised by the US Food and Drug Administration (FDA), which identifies a product as either a cosmetic, which must not alter the structure or function of skin, or a pharmaceutical (https://www.fda.gov/cosmetics/cosmetics-labeling-claims/cosmeceutical; last accessed March 2023). In the European Union, cosmeceuticals are considered a subtype of cosmetics. Thus, cosmeceuticals are not subject to the stringent review and approval processes associated with drugs and, consequently, are readily made available to the public. For those looking for an accessible means of maintaining a more youthful appearance, cosmeceuticals offer an attractive alternative to expensive cosmetic treatments and surgeries without the hassle of doctors' appointments and the risks and side effects associated with prescription medications and invasive procedures.

While the demand is high for these types of products, many consumers are unaware of the limited regulatory control and often scanty scientific evidence supporting many of their claims. Additionally, perhaps as a result of the 'soft' regulatory climate, product claims are often supported by *in vitro* work or studies on 'appearance', with limited *in vivo* research due to concern that evidence for action on skin structure and function will lead to drug labelling and insurmountable regulatory barriers [2]. In other words, while marketing implies therapeutic effect, there is often limited evidence for a true effect. Additionally, a low tolerance for side effects often keeps active ingredients at ineffective concentrations, further obscuring the true efficacy of a product.

As the number of different cosmeceutical formulations on the market continues to rise, it is becoming more difficult for physicians to attest to the efficacy and safety of each. This chapter attempts to summarise the ingredients often encountered in cosmeceuticals, with attention to their proposed mechanisms and efficacy and some of their associated side effects. Here they are grouped by their primary action as either an antioxidant or 'anti-ageing' agent, although they typically confer multiple therapeutic effects that span these categories. Herbals and phytochemicals, which have greater anti-inflammatory potential, are also addressed in the chapter.

Antioxidants

Alpha-lipoic acid

Alpha-lipoic acid (ALA) is a scavenger of reactive oxygen species and a key player in the regeneration of endogenously produced antioxidants, such as vitamins C and E, glutathione and ubiquinol [1]. Taken together, these functions endow ALA with potent antioxidant properties. *In vitro* findings have been corroborated by an

Rook's Textbook of Dermatology, Tenth Edition. Edited by Christopher Griffiths, Jonathan Barker, Tanya Bleiker, Walayat Hussain and Rosalind Simpson.
© 2024 John Wiley & Sons Ltd. Published 2024 by John Wiley & Sons Ltd.

ex vivo study in which an undefined dose of ALA topically applied to porcine skin prior to ultraviolet B (UVB) exposure showed a reduction in radiation-induced cytotoxicity and apoptosis [2]. However, a similar *in vivo* study reported that there was no significant reduction in UV-induced skin redness or cellular damage in porcine skin treated with 5% ALA [3]. This contradictory evidence calls into question whether topicals containing ALA – especially commercial formulations, which typically do not exceed 2% ALA – retain the antioxidant attributes demonstrated in biochemical assays. Another limitation of the effectiveness of topical ALA may be penetration through the epidermal barrier. A recent *in vivo* study showed that a novel nanoencapsulated 3% topical ALA, designed to improve skin permeability, significantly improved UV-induced pigmentation ($P < 0.001$) after 9 days of application compared with non-encapsulated ALA [4]. While there are some conflicting data regarding the effectiveness of ALA *in vitro* or in animal models, investigators have pursued clinical studies on its anti-ageing potential. A double-blinded placebo-controlled study on 12 women demonstrated an 8.84% increase in skin thickness with the application of topical ALA cubosome gel that was statistically significant when compared to placebo at 3 months; subjective measures indicated progress in the reduction of facial lines and skin colour and texture [5]. Similarly, another placebo-controlled split-face study on a cohort of 33 women showed that 3 months of ALA cream use reduced skin roughness by 51% compared to 41% with vehicle ($P < 0.001$); it also reduced the appearance of lentigines and fine wrinkles [6]. One possible mechanism of action is explained by an *in vitro* study that showed that ALA induces collagen biosynthesis in human dermal fibroblasts [7].

Additionally, clinical studies have demonstrated ALA to be only minimally irritating and well tolerated, but several cases of contact dermatitis to ALA in antiwrinkle creams have been reported [8]. More concerning, however, is that one of the by-products of ALA oxidation, dihydrolipoic acid, may actually be a pro-oxidant capable of causing worse free radical damage than that which the ALA use is intended to prevent [9]. The clinical implications of this finding have yet to be understood fully.

Coenzyme Q10

Coenzyme Q10 (CoQ10; also known as ubiquinone) is a naturally occurring vitamin-like substance and a renowned antioxidant [10]. Various *in vitro* assays have consistently shown that both CoQ10 and its significantly more potent synthetic derivative, idebenone, are able to effectively scavenge free radicals, inhibit lipid peroxidation and protect against UV-induced DNA damage [11,12]. Formulations containing other common antioxidants, however, may be more effective in protecting skin from UV radiation. An *in vivo* study comparing CoQ10 with a formulation of vitamins C and E and ferulic acid showed that the latter was more effective in reducing skin damage in UV-exposed skin [13].

In addition to its antioxidant and photoprotective activity, CoQ10 has been suggested to have other mechanisms by which it exerts its beneficial effects on the skin. Cells treated with CoQ10 demonstrated increased fibroblast proliferation, type IV collagen expression and elastin gene expression, as well as an ability to inhibit tyrosinase activity and melanocyte-inducing transcription factor [10,12,14–16]. While *in vitro* evidence appears robust, *in vivo* evidence supporting the cosmetic use of CoQ10 has not been published. Further, CoQ10's ability to penetrate and exert its action in the skin remains to be determined; *in vitro* assays, however, have demonstrated that CoQ10 exhibits enhanced bioavailability when formulated in nano-structured lipid carriers [17].

Serious side effects have not been reported with the use of CoQ10, although there have been reports of allergic dermatitis to idebenone-supplemented over-the-counter creams [18,19].

Vitamin B

Although the mechanisms of action remain somewhat unclear, it is thought that B vitamins are potent antioxidants. Niacinamide, the amide form of vitamin B_3, is a precursor of nicotinamide adenine dinucleotide phosphate (NADH) and its reduced form NADPH – two naturally occurring antioxidants found in the body [20].

Niacinamide and other B vitamin derivatives, such as panthenol (vitamin B_5), have also been found to stimulate fibroblast proliferation and epidermal re-epithelialisation. This is probably via the promotion of lipids, fatty acids, cholesterol, ceramide and sphingolipid synthesis, which are crucial in maintaining skin barrier function and integrity [21]. Niacinamide is also known to share some properties of vitamin A, including the ability to stimulate collagen synthesis and to inhibit melanosome transfer [22]. Interestingly, topical niacinamide has also been shown to inhibit hair growth *ex vivo* [23]. It is one of the better studied ingredients, with investigations corroborating several of these *in vitro* findings clinically, demonstrating that niacinamide use can lead to visible improvements in skin tone, texture, fine lines, pigmentation and facial acne vulgaris [24,25]. Overall, vitamin B is a well-tolerated and chemically stable ingredient, which has fuelled its popularity in cosmeceutical products.

Vitamin C

Vitamin C, the most abundant antioxidant found in skin, is known to attenuate sun damage. An *in vivo* porcine study using 15% L-ascorbic acid and 1% tocopherol on pig skin yielded a fourfold increase in sun protection with fewer sunburn cells and thymine dimers following irradiation [26]. Vitamin C is also a necessary component in proper collagen synthesis and wound healing. Its involvement as both a promoter and key player in collagen synthesis as a cofactor to essential hydroxylases probably contributes to vitamin C's anti-ageing effects. One *in vivo* human study determined that 5% L-ascorbic acid produced statistically significant increases, as compared with vehicle, in mRNA levels of collagen I and III as determined from biopsies of treated forearm skin [27]. Another double-blind split-face study demonstrated an 8–18.6% improvement in wrinkles on the treatment side versus 2.5–14.5% on the placebo side with a corresponding mild increase in collagen on biopsy specimens [28].

Vitamin C inhibits elastin synthesis, and *in vitro* studies have discovered that vitamin C can inhibit tyrosinase, interrupting melanogenesis and reducing pigmentation [29]. These actions may contribute to its ability to prevent solar elastosis and diminish signs of photodamage [30]. A randomised, double-blind, vehicle-controlled study of 19 patients showed a 58% greater improvement in signs of photoageing over placebo [31]. Another study of 20 females showed similar findings with statistically significant improvements in global scores of photoageing with the use of a cream containing 5% vitamin C as compared with placebo; however, electron microscopy and biopsy did not detect any differences in the amount of collagen [32].

Despite these purported effects, however, vitamin C's action in the skin may be limited by poor penetration and stability. Investigators have found that L-ascorbic acid must be formulated at a pH of less than 3.5 to penetrate the skin [33]. A separate study found that after 2 months, 0% of L-ascorbic acid remained in various solution and topical formulations [34]. However, another group noted that more than 90% of L-ascorbic acid was present at 2 months when formulated with ferulic acid [35]. Thus, vitamin C, when properly formulated, could be feasibly used in cosmeceutical preparations with some expected benefits. Laser-assisted drug delivery may offer a solution to overcoming the epidermal barrier and appears promising in providing synergistic benefits from both topical vitamin C as well as the laser itself [36].

Vitamin E

Found naturally within cell membranes and organelles, vitamin E has generated a large amount of interest for its photoprotective, antioxidant and anti-inflammatory properties. To date, the greatest amount of evidence exists in support of vitamin E's use as a photoprotectant. Multiple animal studies, as well as human studies, have demonstrated protective effects in the setting of UV radiation as measured by decreases in skin redness [37]. Studies investigating photoageing effects have also been executed. Notably, murine studies have suggested that vitamin E – although not all of its derivatives – can attenuate skin wrinkling and sagging [38,39]. Although these findings have been well corroborated in animal models, human skin studies have largely focused on the reduction of redness and not anti-ageing effects.

Other studies have investigated the antioxidant potential of vitamin E, which appears to be the most marketed attribute of this compound. Experiments using murine and porcine *in vitro* skin models have assessed the degree of lipid peroxidation, for example, and have shown a lesser degree of oxidative damage in skin treated with topical vitamin E, corroborating *in vitro* findings of its antioxidant potential [40]. These effects have been demonstrated to be enhanced in combination formulations containing vitamin C, which regenerates oxidised vitamin E. Effects are even more pronounced when used in combination formulae containing vitamins E and C and other antioxidants such as ferulic acid and phloretin, which stabilise the vitamins and increase delivery to the skin [**41**]. In a clinical study of 15 patients artificially exposed to ozone on the forearm, the combination of vitamins C and E with ferulic acid or phloretin appeared to protect against ozone-induced collagen degradation and skin damage [42].

Finally, vitamin E is also known for its ability to act as a rather effective moisturiser, its lipophilicity acting as an effective occlusive to seal in moisture [43]. As such, vitamin E is often included in various skincare formulations. However, there have been several case reports describing local and generalised contact dermatitis, contact urticaria and erythema multiforme-like eruptions in the setting of vitamin E-containing topical agents [44], which may limit its use.

Anti-ageing: lightening

Arbutin

Arbutin is a naturally occurring plant derivative of hydroquinone that is found in the dried leaves of a variety of berry trees. Arbutin and its synthetic derivative, deoxyarbutin, competitively inhibit tyrosinase in a dose-dependent manner and are comparable, at high doses, in their lightening capacity to that of hydroquinone [1]. They are much less cytotoxic than hydroquinone, but pose the risk of paradoxical hyperpigmentation at the high doses required for their therapeutic effect. Controlled *in vivo* trials are unavailable, but some studies suggest that arbutin is less effective than other botanical compounds such as kojic acid [2].

Cysteamine

Cysteamine is an aminothiol that occurs naturally in the body as L-cysteine. Like other thiols, cysteamine can inhibit melanin synthesis and therefore can be employed as a depigmenting agent. *In vitro* studies have shown that there are several mechanisms by which cysteamine may induce depigmentation, including interfering with eumelanin synthesis and, to a lesser extent, through the direct inhibition of tyrosinase [3,4]. An animal model demonstrated that a topical cysteamine product caused marked depigmentation of black guinea pig skin [5]. There are limited clinical trials evaluating the efficacy of cysteamine, although the data are promising. In one randomised controlled clinical trial of 50 people, daily 5% cysteamine cream significantly improved the appearance of epidermal melasma compared with placebo after just 2 months of treatment [6]. It may be slightly inferior to or equivalent in efficacy to hydroquinone in the treatment of melasma [7,8].

Hydroquinone

Hydroquinone is best known and most utilised for its bleaching effect although, strictly speaking, it does not bleach the skin. Extensive studies have revealed at least a twofold mechanism of action for this whitening effect. First, hydroquinone interferes with the active site of tyrosinase, a key enzyme of melanogenesis. Second, it inhibits RNA and DNA synthesis, which is thought to further contribute to the disruption of melanocytes and their ability to form melanosomes [9]. Several clinical studies have illustrated its utility in pigmentary disorders, such as melasma [10,11] and pigmentary changes associated with photodamage [12]. Hydroquinone is one of the oldest and most effective chemical depigmenting agents and has been highly scrutinised [13]. Concerns over its safety from animal studies and case reports have generated a lengthy list of short-term and potential long-term detrimental effects, including irritant contact dermatitis, vitiligo, exogenous ochronosis, renal and hepatic toxicity and carcinogenesis [14]. Safety concerns have led to the development of regulatory limitations on the maximum allowed concentration and, in some countries, bans on hydroquinone in products. In the USA, the Coronavirus Aid, Relief and Economic Security (CARES) Act was recently passed, and as a result, over-the-counter hydroquinone is no longer available and any new drugs containing hydroquinone must undergo a formal new drug application through the FDA [15]. Countries with bans on hydroquinone include Japan, Australia and countries of the

European Union. Still, hydroquinone remains the gold standard of depigmenting agents and is often the comparator in clinical trials of skin-lightening agents. Alternative agents have emerged that may be as effective but better tolerated for the treatment of pigmentary alterations, including topical tranexamic acid (TXA) [16].

Kojic acid

Kojic acid is derived from various strains of fungal species, namely *Aspergillus* and *Penicillium*, and has been used for many years in a variety of applications. In skincare products, kojic acid has become a popular staple of skin-whitening products, including soaps, lotions and creams, and particularly so following the ban on hydroquinone in many countries. In cosmetics, kojic acid has generally been considered safe at 2% concentration [17].

In vitro studies have demonstrated kojic acid's ability to inhibit tyrosinase, a key enzyme involved in melanogenesis [18,19]. It is commonly used as a positive standard by many investigators testing new tyrosinase inhibitors [20]. Studies of kojic acid on black guinea pigs demonstrated an ability to depigment skin at 4% concentration, though not at 1%. *In vivo* animal studies have shown that kojic acid may be a safer alternative to hydroquinone for depigmentation, as the latter may disrupt the epidermis and thin the dermis [21].

Clinical studies looking at kojic acid as monotherapy continue to be limited [22]. In combination with other compounds, however, clinical studies have been able to demonstrate some efficacy in the treatment of pigmentation disorders such as melasma [22]. In one study of 40 Chinese women with melasma, 10% glycolic acid and 2% hydroquinone with 2% kojic acid showed significant improvement in melasma as measured by clinical evaluation, photography and self-assessment questionnaires [23]. Also 2% kojic acid with 5% glycolic acid was found to be comparable with a 2% hydroquinone and 5% glycolic acid formulation in another clinical study of 39 subjects with pigmentary disorders [24]. Finally, kojic acid combined with embilica extract and glycolic acid was shown to be comparable with hydroquinone 4% in 80 multiethnic patients with dyschromia of the face in a 3-month, double-blind study, suggesting that these combination topical agents may be effective alternatives to hydroquinone [25].

Other properties of kojic acid have been less publicised and have, overall, received less attention than its skin-lightening effect. Kojic acid is also an antioxidant, capable of scavenging free radicals [26], and *in vivo* studies have demonstrated its ability to prevent photodamage and related photoageing in hairless mice [18,27].

Tranexamic acid

Tranexamic acid is an antifibrinolytic drug that was incidentally noted to treat melasma in its oral form. In recent years, topical formulations have been used to treat pigmentary disorders due to its ability to inhibit melanogenesis, possibly through decreasing tyrosinase activity in the epidermis [28], blocking UV activation of plasmin [29] and activating the autophagy system [28] or targeting vascular endothelial growth factor (VEGF) receptors [30]. A prospective cohort study showed that topical 2% TXA significantly improved the melasma area and severity index (MASI) in 22 patients [29]. A randomised controlled trial comparing topical 5% TXA with 3% hydroquinone showed approximately equivalent efficacy in pigment reduction [31]. However, a randomised, placebo-controlled, split-face clinical trial of 23 women using topical 5% TXA did not show a statistically significant improvement in the MASI, and the intervention group had increased redness of the skin [32]. One hypothesis is that topical TXA does not penetrate into the dermis, and thus the inhibitory effects on vasculature and dermal structure may not be as pronounced as with oral formulations [33,34]. To overcome the epidermal barrier using topical formulations, fractional ablative laser-assisted drug delivery of topical TXA has been employed and has demonstrated clinical improvement and improved quality of life in people with melasma [35,36].

Anti-ageing: rhytid reduction

Glycosaminoglycans

Glycosaminoglycans (GAGs) are a critical part of the extracellular matrix and help regulate cell processes in the dermis that are related to skin ageing – these include hyaluronic acid, dermatan sulphate, chondroitin sulphate and keratan sulphate [1]. Both *in vitro* and clinical studies have demonstrated the potential for topical GAGs to improve skin ageing. In an *in vitro* model, chrondroitin sulphate induced collagen expression and promoted wound healing [2]. In clinical studies, another GAG, heparin sulphate, was shown to significantly reduce facial fine lines and wrinkles with daily use of a 0.5% cream after 8 weeks of use [3].

Unlike chondroitin sulphate or heparin sulphate, hyaluronic acid (HA) is not sulphated or covalently attached to core proteins. It is a major component of the extracellular matrix [4] and is incredibly hydrophilic, thus increasing tissue hydration and improving the appearance of skin. As skin ages, HA is prominently depleted from the epidermis [5]. Novel topical preparations with HA have emerged that replenish this sugar. A randomised, split-face clinical trial of 76 adult female subjects showed that 0.1% HA cream significantly improved skin hydration and elasticity [6]. This same study also showed that low-molecular-weight HA also significantly improved periorbital wrinkle depth compared with the vehicle cream, likely secondary to increased penetration. Similarly, an open label clinical study of female subjects showed that three times daily application of an HA-based serum for the lips improved lip colour, lip texture and lip plumpness after 4 weeks [7].

Hydroxy acids

Although hydroxy acids were first utilised for their beneficial effects on pathological skin conditions such as ichthyosis, xerosis and keratoses, they have become a popular staple in the cosmeceutical industry. This is due to *in vitro* studies showing an ability to increase GAGs and collagen, thereby increasing epidermal and dermal thickness [8,9]. *In vivo* studies have also suggested that they may improve the quality of elastic fibres [10]. Further, they enhance skin surface texture and colour, probably by accelerating exfoliation of the stratum corneum [11]. The specific mechanism by which hydroxy acids effect this is poorly understood, but it is speculated that chelation of calcium ions in the skin disrupts cell–cell adhesions, resulting in desquamation [12,13]. Hydroxy acids, combined with other whitening agents, such as hydroquinone, are also effective at diminishing the appearance of hyperpigmented lesions [8,14].

Three main classes of hydroxy acids often encountered in cosmeceutical formulations are α-hydroxyl acids (AHAs), β-hydroxyl acids (BHAs) and polyhydroxy acids (PHAs). The most commonly used are the AHAs glycolic acid and lactic acid, which have the smallest molecular size of the AHAs, allowing for greater skin penetration and, theoretically, better efficacy. Studies conducted on 8% AHA formulations, which is less than the typical 12% encountered in commercial products, have shown results. In a human study investigating glycolic acid, lactic acid, tartaric acid and gluconolactone, it was found that the various acids could modify stratum corneum to enhance protection against chemical and mechanical irritants [15]. A single-centre, 22-week, double-blind, vehicle-controlled, randomised clinical trial on 74 women showed that glycolic and L-lactic acid creams were superior to vehicle in reducing overall severity of photodamage and sallowness as determined by self and physician assessments using concentrations available over the counter (8% glycolic acid and 8% lactic acid) [16].

In-office glycolic acid peels in higher concentrations may also improve pigmentary disorders, such as melasma as shown in one randomised controlled trial [17], and Becker nevus as demonstrated in a single patient [18]. Other investigations with higher concentrations, such as 25% AHAs, used for 6 months, showed that treatment was associated with an increase in epidermal and papillary dermal thickness with a clinical reversal of photoageing [9,10]. Although generally well tolerated, AHAs have been associated with more skin irritation compared with other hydroxy acids. Side effects include redness, swelling, blistering, burning, pruritus, discoloration and increased photosensitivity [8,12].

BHAs found in cosmeceuticals often have elements that classify them as AHAs as well, the latter being the primary class of hydroxy acids encountered in cosmetics. Citric acid has been documented to have anti-ageing effects, potentially derived from its antioxidant properties. Salicylic acid is another commonly known BHA, although some researchers do not consider it to be a hydroxy acid due to its distinct mechanism of action [8]. Salicylic acid is very commonly encountered in over-the-counter acne treatments, but less so in anti-ageing preparations.

Of the PHAs, gluconolactone is the most commercialised in cosmeceuticals because, in addition to providing the anti-ageing benefits typical of hydroxy acids, it is thought to strengthen skin barrier function while being relatively gentle and non-irritating to the skin. One clinical study found that the benefits offered by gluconolactone as measured by silicone replicas and clinical grading were comparable to AHAs, while sallowness and pinch recoil for skin resiliency showed that it was inferior to AHAs [19]. Because of the PHAs' large molecular size, they do not penetrate the skin well.

Polyunsaturated fatty acids

The omega 6 and omega 3 fatty acids are two of the main classes of polyunsaturated fatty acids (PUFAs). Omega 6 can be encountered in a number of foods, including poultry, eggs, avocado, nuts and most vegetable oils, while omega 3 is primarily found in fish. Both fatty acids have been extensively studied to reveal benefits in all realms of medicine, ranging from oncology to psychiatry. In dermatology, PUFAs have been suggested to promote maturation and differentiation of the stratum corneum, to be involved in lamellar body formation and secretion and to interfere with inflammation by inhibiting eicosanoids, cytokines and lipoxygenase [20].

Unfortunately, *in vivo* data to support topical PUFAs and their role in cosmeceuticals are limited. One single-blind, vehicle-controlled trial in 16 participants evaluated the effects of an omega-6-enriched topical derived from chia seeds (*Salvia hispanica* L.) and showed significantly improved skin hydration over the vehicle [21]. Other investigations have centred on the effects of dietary supplementation, which is the most common route of consumption. A single-blind randomised trial of 24 females showed that with a supplement of a proprietary product containing natural fish oils, skin elasticity increased 10% after 3 months; there was no statistically significant improvement in either skin roughness or transepidermal water loss when compared with the control group [22].

Peptides

Peptides found in cosmeceuticals can be divided into three broad categories, despite some apparent overlap in peptide function. These categories are signal peptides, neurotransmitter-affecting peptides and carrier peptides.

Signal peptides

The signal peptides commonly found in cosmeceuticals consist of bioactive amino acid chains that directly stimulate human skin fibroblasts to increase dermal remodelling and decrease the action of collagenases, leading to a net increase in ground substance production [23].

The most extensively studied and commercially available signal peptide is a sequence found on type I collagen: lysine-threonine-threonine-lysine-serine (KTTKS). In cosmeceuticals it is linked to palmitic acid for better epidermal penetration, and marketed as palmitoyl pentapeptide 3 or Matrixyl® (Sederma SA, France). Within the dermis this peptide stimulates feedback regulation of new collagen synthesis, resulting in a concentration-dependent increase in the production of extracellular matrix proteins such as type I and II collagen and fibronectin, with the most pronounced effects at concentrations greater than 2.8 ppm [24]. A small, double-blind, split-face study of 16 females showed statistically significant improvement in wrinkles from baseline for pal-KTTKS that was comparable to 0.07% retinol [25]. A double-blind, placebo-controlled, randomised, split-face study of 60 females also demonstrated a trend towards improved appearance of fine lines, wrinkles and skin texture with overall improvement of aged appearance, although these findings were not statistically significant [23,26]. Current recommendations based on the results of these different studies as well as economic considerations suggest a concentration between 2 and 8 ppm for cosmetic formulations [27].

Another peptide sequence, glycine-glutamate-lysine-glycine (GEKG), has been studied in reversing the signs of ageing. Farwick *et al.* showed significant increases in the production of procollagen, hyaluronic acid synthase 1 and fibronectin, with corresponding increases in mRNA expression when human fibroblasts were treated with GEKG. A follow-up *in vivo* study on 60 volunteers demonstrated that topically applied GEKG increased skin elasticity and improved volume and skin roughness in a dose-dependent manner at 10 and 100 ppm [28]. Commercial use remains limited.

Table 157.1 Mechanisms of action of common peptides.

Peptide	Proposed mechanisms
Palmitoyl valine-glycine-valine-alanine-proline-glycine (palmitoyl-VGVAPG)	Upregulates production of collagen types I and III and tropoelastin through stimulation of elastin-binding protein receptor [34]
	Stimulates growth of human skin fibroblasts [35,36]
	Stimulates expression of pro-matrix metalloproteinase 1, which may play a role in collagen remodelling [37]
Tyrosine-tyrosine-arginine-alanine-aspartame-aspartame-alanine	Procollagen c proteinase inhibition, leading to decreased collagen breakdown [38]
Glycyl-L-histidyl-L-lysine (GHK) (biopeptide-CL)	Coupled to copper, stimulates fibroblasts to produce collagen and glycosaminoglycans [39,40]
	Promotes fibroblast and keratinocyte growth and differentiation [41]
	Scavenges free radicals and inhibits inflammatory cytokines [41]
Elaidyl-lysine-phenylalanine-lysine (elaidyl-KFK)	Downregulates matrix metalloproteinase mRNA [42]
Phenylalanine-valine-alanine-proline-phenylalanine-proline (peptamide 6)	Delays the onset of senescence in both intrinsically and extrinsically aged fibroblasts [43]
Tripeptide/hexapeptide (Alastin®)	Stimulates tropoelastin and procollagen to increase dermal collagen and dermal elastin, also anti-inflammatory to promote epidermal renewal [44–46]

More recently, a tripeptide/hexapeptide combination has been studied. The results of a small five-subject study suggested that this topical may penetrate the skin and increase elastin. This topical may be able to speed healing after treatment with energy-based devices. This product has been studied in combination with ablative fractional laser, non-ablative fractional laser, microneedling and radiofrequency [29–33]. Other signal peptides continue to be identified and a few of the more commonly studied are summarised in Table 157.1 [34–46].

Neurotransmitter-affecting peptides

One of the most effective and well-known products for the treatment of fine lines and wrinkles is the neurotransmitter-affecting peptide, botulinum neurotoxin, which is approved by the US FDA for subcutaneous, intradermal and intramuscular injection. This polypeptide inhibits acetylcholine release at the neuromuscular junction, subsequently causing a reversible paralysis that, when induced in the proper areas, reduces the appearance of wrinkles [47]. Given its efficacy, cosmeceutical companies have scrambled to create more readily accessible products that, like botulinum toxin, act on neuronal transmission to decrease facial muscle contraction.

Though several products have found their place in the market by virtue of sound theory, there remains some scepticism as to whether these compounds are able to penetrate tissue deeply enough to reach their site of action. Most of these proprietary formulations lack published data demonstrating their effect [23]. Only one peptide, acetyl hexapeptide 3 with the sequence AC-glycine-glutamate-methionine-glutamine-arginine-arginine-NH_2 (also known as argireline), has published data establishing its ability to inhibit neurotransmitter release. It does this by interfering with the formation and/or stability of the SNARE (soluble N-ethylmaleimide-sensitive factor attachment receptor) complex that is responsible for vesicular fusion [48]. One *in vivo*, small, observational study showed that argireline was able to mask iatrogenic and traumatic scar appearance by smoothing the surrounding skin and reducing the appearance of wrinkles [49].

Carrier peptides

Carrier peptides are most commonly used to stabilise and deliver important trace elements to the skin where they can be utilised for various enzymatic processes. An example of a carrier peptide is glycyl-L-histidyl-L-lysine (GHK) which complexes with copper and facilitates the transport of copper into cells; Cu-GHK is also considered a signal peptide. This peptide is available with a lipophilic attachment and as a nano carrier, and an *in vivo* study using an imaging system showed a statistically significant improvement in rhytids [50]. Its effects on the skin are summarised in Table 157.1. Like the tripeptide/hexapeptide topical, the use of Cu-GHK has been studied in combination with energy-based devices [51].

Other uses for carrier peptides continue to be investigated. Initial *in vitro* studies suggest that peptides such as Pep-1, a short amphipathic carrier peptide, coupled with elastin are capable of passing cellular membranes [52]. The transduction of different cellular components such as elastin into cells, in theory, could attenuate signs of ageing. It remains to be determined, however, whether these peptides are able to penetrate the stratum corneum to deliver their contents to target cells to produce a clinically noticeable result.

Other peptides

In vitro studies have shown that some peptides have anti-inflammatory properties [53,54]. One *in vivo* study investigating the short peptide sequences, leucine/glutamate and methionine/tyrosine, demonstrated an ability to attenuate UVB-induced redness on human skin [55].

Vitamin A (retinoids)

Retinoids, derived from vitamin A, are naturally synthesised in the body. Retinyl esters and carotenoids are hydrolysed and oxidised, respectively, into retinol in the gut, which is oxidised first into retinaldehyde then ultimately to retinoic acid, the biologically active form of vitamin A in the skin [56,57–59]. These lipophilic molecules diffuse through cellular and other phospholipid membranes to bind to nuclear receptors within cells, eventually inducing stimulatory and inhibitory changes in gene expression. These changes lead to a net increase in epidermal proliferation and differentiation and the production of epidermal GAGs and extracellular dermal matrix components [56,60–63]. Retinoids also inhibit the production of collagenase and matrix metalloproteinases (MMPs), leading to decreased collagen and elastin degradation. It is thought that this combination of stimulatory and inhibitory effects leads to the attenuation of fine lines and wrinkles [11].

Retinoids additionally provide photoprotection by absorbing UV radiation. Animal experiments on hairless mice demonstrated that retinoids prevented UVB-induced apoptosis and DNA photodamage [64]. In human studies, some topical applications of retinoids were equivalent to sunscreen with a sun protection factor of 20 [65]. For all of the aforementioned effects, retinoids have become recognised by both the medical and lay community as the gold standard for topical treatment of photoageing.

Of all the retinoids, retinoic acid is, to date, the most extensively studied. It continues to be frequently employed as topical therapy for a number of skin conditions and for cosmetic enhancement of aged skin. However, given its high potency and side effects, including dryness, scaling and redness, retinoic acid and its synthetic derivatives adapalene, tazarotene and bexarotene are registered drugs and available only by prescription. Unfortunately, side effects can be experienced with the cosmeceutical retinoids – retinaldehyde, retinol and retinyl – though often to a lesser degree inversely related to potency.

Retinaldehyde
Retinaldehyde's activity is derived from its conversion to retinoic acid. It is better tolerated than retinoic acid as it is metabolised into retinoic acid exclusively by keratinocytes, enabling a more controlled delivery of retinoic acid [64,66–68]. Although considered to be second to retinoic acid in terms of retinoid activity, retinaldehyde has been shown to be comparable to retinoic acid in its anti-ageing effects in one study. This study of 125 patients demonstrated parity in degree of surface roughness and wrinkling reduction, measured by optical profilometry of silicone replicas, between 0.05% retinaldehyde cream and 0.05% retinoic acid. Retinaldehyde in higher concentrations (0.1%) may also improve pigmentary alterations in addition to surface texture and wrinkling [69].

Retinol
Retinol, a precursor for the synthesis of endogenous retinaldehyde and retinoic acid, has been shown to have many of the beneficial effects of retinoic acid, including the induction of epidermal thickening and inhibition of UV-induced MMP production [70,71] without significant transepidermal water loss, skin redness or scaling. However, *in vivo* studies showed that topical retinol had only modest retinoid-like activity when compared with topical retinaldehyde and retinoic acid [56,71], exhibiting only modest improvement in fine wrinkles when measured by clinical assessment [63,72,73]. Of note, however, the various studies indicate that the beneficial effects of retinol are likely to occur at concentrations of 0.3% and higher, although there may be considerably more irritation at higher concentrations [74], whereas retinol concentrations found in cosmeceuticals tend to be much lower at approximately 0.08% or less [75].

Retinyl esters
Studies investigating retinyl esters, such as retinyl-palmitate and retinyl-propionate, have routinely failed to show anti-ageing properties clinically, histologically and with profilometric parameters [76,77]. As a result, retinyl esters are unlikely to be found as the sole active anti-ageing ingredient in cosmeceuticals; instead, they are usually offered in combination with other compounds, such as hydroxy acids and sunscreens [78].

Herbals and phytochemicals

Thousands of these plant- and fungus-derived compounds have been identified to date and continue to find their way into hundreds of different cosmeceutical products. Their appeal is heightened by innate anti-inflammatory, photoprotective, anticarcinogenic and anti-ageing properties and by consumer demand for 'natural' products [1]. Although these different ingredients indisputably contain various bioactive compounds, a lack of data from well-designed studies obscures the validity of these ingredients' most oft-touted claims. This sections presents several of the more commonly encountered ingredients and Table 157.2 offers a summary of other common but less studied ingredients.

Carnosine
Carnosine, or β-alanyl-histidine, is a natural dipeptide found in abundance in muscle and brain tissue [2]. To date, the majority of studies on carnosine have been on its antioxidant potential. These studies have demonstrated that carnosine is a potent hydrophilic antioxidant that can neutralise superoxide anion and hydroxide radicals [3,4]. It is also an ion chelator that can prevent the production of hydroxyl radicals by binding to heavy metal ions such as Cu^{2+} [5–8]. These antioxidant properties have also been demonstrated in *in vivo* animal models [9,10] and in one clinical study that investigated a combination of *Rhodiola rosea* and L-carnosine agent on subjects with sensitive skin [11].

Carnosine is also known for its anti-ageing potential, probably stemming from an *in vitro* discovery that it is capable of reverting senescent cells into 'younger' forms that can continue to divide [12]. Other anti-ageing mechanisms proposed involve reducing non-enzymic glycation of proteins and protein carbonyl groups and cross-links, which are events associated with ageing [13]. This was demonstrated in an *in vitro* study showing that a cream formulation containing carnosine had the ability to reduce advanced glycation end-products which have been associated with skin ageing [14]. Clinical studies continue to lag, however, and most available studies have investigated combination products that include other commonly utilised ingredients such as urea, peptides and vitamins, which all individually have been shown to have their own therapeutic benefits. Thus, despite a demonstrated ability to improve fine wrinkles and overall skin appearance, it is unknown if carnosine is the active ingredient to which these benefits can be attributed [15,16].

Grape seed
Grape seed extract (GSE), derived from the seed of the plant *Vitis vinifera*, has been highly popularised in skincare products as a moisturising agent. In the scientific community its antioxidant properties and its role in fighting oxidative stress are the primary interest [17].

GSE is one of the richest natural sources of the flavonoid proanthocyanidin – the polyphenol from which this common cosmeceutical ingredient derives its greatest antioxidant properties. Proanthocyanidin, in particular, has been shown to have potent free radical

Table 157.2 Summary of herbal and phytochemical ingredients not discussed in text.

Product (active ingredients)	Significant findings
Bakuchiol	Clinical: significantly reduced hyperpigmentation and wrinkles; no statistical difference compared with 0.5% retinol, but was less irritating [74]
Comfrey	In vitro:
	No anticollagenase or antielastase activity [75]. Little antioxidant capacity as compared with other plant extracts [75]
	In vivo and clinical: no in vivo or clinical findings to date
Feverfew (parthenolide)	In vitro:
	Inhibits the nuclear factor κB (NFκB) inflammatory pathway [76]
	Free radical scavenging activity [77]
	Clinical: reduced UV-induced skin redness, epidermal hyperplasia, DNA damage and apoptosis [77]
Frankincense	Clinical: demonstrated improvements in photoageing, tactile roughness, fine lines and increase in elasticity [78]
Jojoba oil	Clinical: supplemented moisturising effect when added to glycerol formulation [79]
Lavender (Figure 157.1)	In vitro:
	May cause damage to the cell membrane of fibroblasts [80]
	Linalyl acetate, a main component of lavender oil, forms strong contact allergens [81]
	Clinical: limited utility in the treatment of inflammatory skin disease
Licorice	In vitro:
	Glabridin inhibits tyrosinase activity [82]
	Licochalcone A inhibits cyclo-oxygenase (COX) and lipoxygenase to decrease inflammation [83]
Milk thistle (silymarin) (Figure 157.2)	In vitro: decreases inflammation by COX-2 and interleukin 1 (IL-1) inhibition [84]
	In vivo: animal studies show decreased UV-induced sunburn, DNA damage and apoptosis [84]
Pine bark extract (Pycnogenol®)	In vitro: inhibits the NFκB inflammatory pathway [85], antioxidant [86]
	Clinical:
	Human studies showed oral supplementation improved hydration and elasticity of skin [87,88]
	Decreased UV-induced skin redness and pigmentation [89]
Rose	In vitro:
	Antioxidant [90]
	Anticollagenase and antielastase activity [90]
	Rose hip found to inhibit tyrosinase activity [91]
Turmeric (curcuminoids) (Figure 157.3)	In vitro:
	Antioxidant [92]
	Inhibits inflammatory cascade [93]
	Inhibits collagenase, elastase and hyaluronidase [93]
	In vivo:
	Wound healing in animal studies model [94]
	Photoprotection in animal studies [95]
	Clinical: may improve periorbital pigmentation [96]

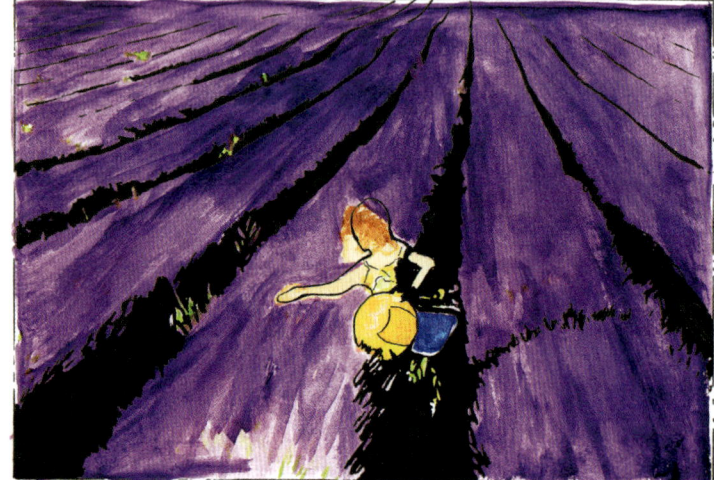

Figure 157.1 Lavender. Courtesy of Ryan Denman.

scavenging activity with the additional capacity to strongly inhibit xanthine oxidase, which generates oxygen radicals [18]. In fact, in vitro studies have shown that the antioxidant properties conferred by proanthocyanidin and other polyphenols, such as reservatrol, give GSE greater efficacy as an antioxidant than even vitamins C and E [19]. In vivo studies in mouse models have demonstrated proof of concept by showing an ability to attenuate the oxidative damage associated with ageing, UV radiation and chemical, ischaemic and hypoxic injury with oral supplementation with grape seed [19–21], and it has shown photostability in sunscreen formulation [22]. Topical studies of GSE on human skin exist. One group investigated the photoprotective effects of GSE in the setting of UV radiation and showed on both histological and immunohistochemical evaluation of biopsies that pre-treatment with GSE resulted in fewer sunburn cells [23].

Other investigators have looked at GSE's ability to moisturise skin and reverse signs of ageing. An in vitro study revealed that GSE stabilises collagen and elastin through the inhibition of MMP [24] but only one clinical study has attempted to corroborate these anti-ageing properties at the clinical level. In this study, a formulation containing GSE, lycopene, acerola extract and a proprietary compound of various marine proteins was tested on 50 women with photoaged skin. Although there were improvements noted in hydration, dermal thickness, skin fibre density and overall appearance, given that several of the other ingredients have also been associated with antioxidant and anti-ageing properties, it

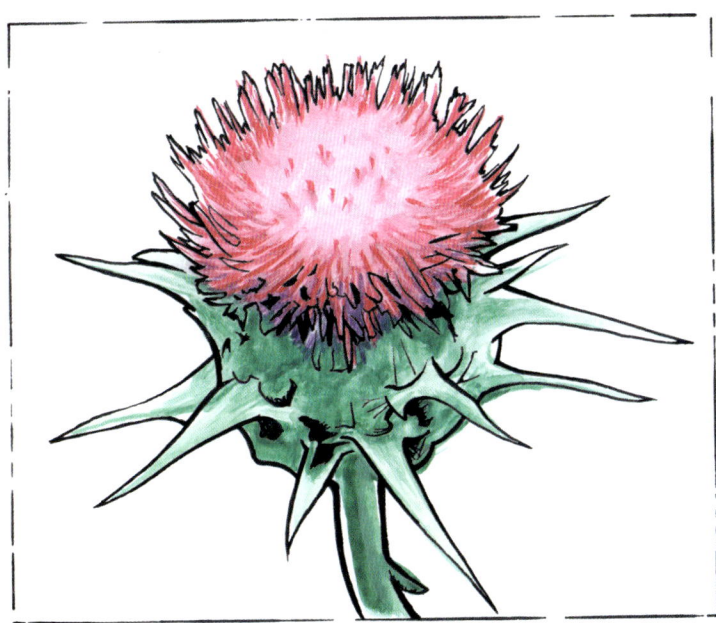

Figure 157.2 Milk thistle. Courtesy of Ryan Denman.

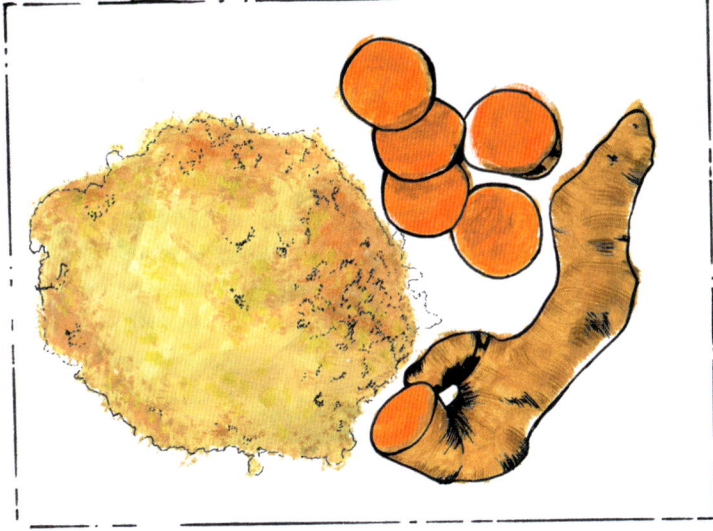

Figure 157.3 Turmeric. Courtesy of Ryan Denman.

is difficult to ascertain the specific contributions of GSE to these findings [25].

Green tea

Green tea (*Camellia sinensis*), a very popular beverage during both ancient and modern times, has been investigated extensively to show beneficial effects in various diseases including Parkinson disease, Alzheimer disease, diabetes and obesity. The polyphenols known as catechins are credited with these effects, and the various catechins found in green tea, which include (−)-epigal-locatechin-3-gallate (EGCG), (−)-epicatechin-3-gallate (ECG), (−)-epigallocatechin and (−)-epicatechin, have been tested for their respective therapeutic advantages. Of these mentioned catechins, EGCG is the predominant form of polyphenol in green tea, making up 50–80% in a 200–300 mg brew [26]. Other ingredients like proteins, amino acids, lipids, vitamins and caffeine are also purported to play a role in green tea's therapeutic effects [27]. In the cosmeceutical industry, green tea is included in various formulations for its antioxidant, anti-inflammatory and – given that it has been shown to also be effective in preventing photodamage – anti-ageing potential [28].

Multiple *in vitro* studies on human cell lines have revealed different mechanisms by which green tea components function as antioxidants. For example, green tea extracts inhibit UVB-induced lipid peroxidation and intracellular release of hydrogen peroxide, dose-dependently reduce UVB-induced cell death, scavenge reactive oxygen species and inhibit protein oxidation [29–32]. Mouse and guinea pig epidermal studies have shown similar findings, in addition to an ability to inhibit the accumulation of leukocytes that produce these deleterious effects [33,34]. Finally, *in vivo* human studies in which topical EGCG was applied prior to UVB exposure have corroborated the aforementioned protective effects [35–37].

In cultures of human fibroblasts, EGCG was shown to block UV-induced increases in collagenase mRNA levels and collagenase secretion and to inhibit the induction of inflammatory nuclear transcription factors such as nuclear factor κB (NFκB) and AP-1 [38]. Further *in vivo* human studies have revealed that topical application of green tea provides a dose-dependent inhibition of skin redness and decreases the numbers of sunburn cells and DNA damage. The polyphenols EGCG and ECG produced the best results [36].

Given the *in vivo* findings, scientists have further investigated green tea's anti-ageing potential. One clinical study on 10 healthy male volunteers showed that 2 months of green tea cream application provided no significant change in elastic or biological properties of the skin, but provided an improvement in skin viscoelasticity that was statistically significant [39]. In another randomised, double-blind control study of 40 women, green tea supplements and a 10% green tea cream were investigated for anti-ageing potential. Skin was graded based on wrinkling, roughness, coarse rhytids, skin laxity and pigmentation and was compared at baseline and at an 8-week follow-up. There was no clinically significant change noted between the treatment and control groups, although histological assessment revealed improvement in elastic tissue content of the treatment group [40]. The evidence available for green tea's use in photoageing appears preliminary at best, but continues to grow.

Additionally, *in vitro* studies have demonstrated that green tea components may have an inhibitory effect on melanin production [41,42], implying a possible whitening effect on the skin, while also promoting skin moisturisation. Although green tea extract has found its way into many skin-whitening products, there is limited evidence on this purported effect.

Lycopene

Lycopene is a commonly encountered natural carotenoid most popularly associated with tomatoes, but is also found in a myriad of produce including red carrots, watermelons and papayas [43]. Lycopene is best known for its potent antioxidant activity by both the lay and scientific community alike, the latter suggesting that lycopene is the most efficient singlet oxygen-reducing biological carotenoid [44]. When applied topically to the skin in microemulsions, the effect of lycopene appeared to amplify antioxidant activity in the skin by 10 times [45]. Unfortunately, studies of topical lycopene are limited in number as the feasibility of lycopene use is restricted secondary to its instability during processing [46].

An *in vitro* study of UVA's effects on human keratinocytes showed that lycopene alone was not photoprotective, as measured by degree of suppression of MMP-1 mRNA expression. Combined with vitamin E, however, lycopene was shown to inhibit rises in MMP-1 mRNA [47]. In a small clinical trial of 10 patients, investigators measured redness response and change in barrier function in UV-irradiated skin after the application of lycopene versus a formulation of vitamin E and C versus control. This preliminary study showed that lycopene optimally reduced both skin redness and transepidermal water loss, suggesting photoprotectivity [48].

Given lycopene's antioxidant and suggested photoprotective properties, its anti-ageing properties have also been investigated. However, these studies have been conducted on the effects of oral supplementation as opposed to topical application, and often use supplements containing several other ingredients in addition to lycopene. For example, in one study, 50 females were provided a mixture of lycopene, acerola extract, grape seed and a proprietary biomarine complex. Its use resulted in increases in cutaneous hydration, a reduction in skin pH and increases in the density of skin, and, histologically, showed a corresponding increase in collagen and elastic fibres [25]. Another study demonstrated similar findings, showing increases in skin density and thickness with corresponding clinical improvements in roughness, scaling, smoothness and wrinkling [49]. Studies designed to clearly distinguish the role of lycopene in topical formulations continue to be absent in the literature. A randomised, double-blind, placebo-controlled clinical study of 22 people with melasma showed that a lycopene–wheat bran cream combination improved melasma after 12 weeks of twice-daily application [50].

Pomegranate

Pomegranate, or *Punica granatum*, has a rich history of medicinal uses across different cultures and historical eras. In modern times, it is known best for its highly potent antioxidant capacity, but many *in vitro* and animal studies continue to suggest its ability to prevent photodamage and to lighten skin. As such, pomegranate is commonly encountered on cosmetic shelves, although human studies continue to lag in providing definitive evidence of these purported actions.

Pomegranate is comprised of anthocyanins [51], EGCG polyphenols [52], flavonoids [53], minerals, vitamins and organic acids [54]. Ellagic acid, a polyphenol, found in the highest concentrations in the juice and seed oil of the fruit, is generally accepted as the key active ingredient responsible for much of pomegranate extract's beneficial effects [55,56] including its antioxidant properties. Both *in vitro* and animal studies have shown that pomegranate extract inhibits lipid peroxidation and promotes the synthesis of naturally occurring cutaneous antioxidants [57]. Another study comparing pomegranate with the other well-known antioxidants, green tea and red wine, showed that pomegranate was consistently superior in its antioxidant capacity when measured by four different assays [58].

Pomegranate extract has also been extensively studied for its photoprotective effects. *In vitro* studies have shown that this fruit extract attenuates UVA-mediated damage in human epidermal keratinocytes [59]. Other studies investigating ellagic acid treatment prior to UVB insults, in *in vitro* and *in vivo* hairless mice models, have shown dose-dependent reductions in cell death and significantly decreased amounts of pro-inflammatory cytokines and UV radiation-associated proteins in the skin [60,61]. Another investigation on human reconstituted skin showed no significant increase in either the number or intensity of cyclopyrimidine dimers when compared with non-irradiated negative controls [62].

Although the evidence supporting pomegranate's antioxidant and photoprotective properties is substantial, evidence for an impact on clinical signs of ageing remains in preliminary phases. Thus far, *in vitro* investigations have illustrated that ellagic acid has an inhibitory effect on UVB-mediated MMP production with a corresponding decrease in mRNA transcripts for these collagenases [57]. One murine study demonstrated that skin treated with ellagic acid prior to UV irradiation had significantly fewer wrinkles. Corresponding histological assessment of the skin at study termination revealed increased levels of type I collagen in treated skin [60]. Clinical trials remain to be executed.

Soya

The most potent components of soya are the isoflavone phytoestrogens, genistein and daidzein, which are associated with increased skin thickness and collagen synthesis [63]. A study using a gel formula containing 10% bifidobacterium-fermented soya milk extract with both genistein and daidzein demonstrated significant improvement in elasticity and viscoelasticity of mouse skin. Further, the same investigators corroborated their findings on human forearm skin, suggesting possible utility in anti-ageing formulations [64].

In vitro studies and *in vivo* nude mouse studies have also shown that the phytoestrogens of soya extracts contain antioxidant properties that attenuate the carcinogenic effects of chemical and UV insults to skin cells [65–68]. Studies on human reconstituted skin demonstrated a dose-dependent inhibition of UVB-induced damage as well [69].

Another purported benefit of isoflavones includes skin lightening via soyabean trypsin and Bowman–Birk inhibitor action against melanosome transfer to keratinocytes and inhibition of ornithine decarboxylase, respectively [70]. A small trial of 30 women showed a modest effect of soya on lentigines [71]. A double-blind, placebo-controlled clinical study showed improvement in skin tone after the application of a soya-containing moisturiser [72]. Relative to the number of clinical studies investigating systemic treatment with oral supplementation, few *in vivo* human investigations studying the topical applications of soya exist. One single-centre, randomised controlled trial showed that a topical soya cream applied after laser treatment appeared to significantly reduce wrinkles in a dose-dependent fashion when used in conjunction with a neodymium:yttrium-aluminium-garnet (Nd:YAG) laser [73]. More clinical studies are needed to determine the true benefits of soya in cosmeceutical products.

Anti-inflammatories

Aloe

Several components have been identified in aloe extract that contribute to aloe's anti-inflammatory effect. *In vitro* studies have shown that the bioactive compounds aloe-emodin and aloin, for example, suppress the production of cyclo-oxygenase 2 (COX-2) mRNA and COX-2, prostaglandin E_2 (PGE_2) and nitric oxide [1]. Another compound, C-glucosyl chromone, was found to be comparable to hydrocortisone in its ability to reduce oedema in a mouse model [2]. *In vitro* studies on whole aloe extract have shown an ability to reduce interleukin 8 (IL-8), tumour necrosis factor α (TNF-α), IL-6 and IL-1β cytokine production in a dose-dependent manner [3]. Finally, others have also shown antibradykinin activity and inhibition by aloe glycoproteins of thromboxane [4]. Animal models have corroborated aloe's efficacy as an anti-inflammatory agent [5–7]. One rat study showed that ozonated aloe vera, in particular, appeared to improve wound healing in mice by increasing collagen thickness [8].

However, there remains a surprising lack of clinical studies to support cosmeceutical applications of aloe vera. Only one clinical study directly investigated aloe's most popular claim of reducing inflammation following sunburn. This study showed that aloe significantly reduced UV-induced skin redness after 48 h, but was less effective than 1% hydrocortisone cream [9]. Other studies have investigated aloe's effects on acute radiation dermatitis; these have all demonstrated little to no effect in reducing radiation-induced side effects [10–13]. Despite substantial cellular and molecular evidence of the anti-inflammatory effects of aloe, the role of aloe as a topical anti-inflammatory agent remains to be definitively determined. Overall, aloe has proven to be, however, a rather safe ingredient in topical preparations with only a few case reports of contact dermatitis and hypersensitivity, probably induced by the anthraquinone aloin [14,15].

Caffeine

Caffeine is a very commonly encountered drug, near ubiquitous in many societies and cultures – often in our beverages – and most frequently sought after for its stimulant properties. Studies have begun to reveal other potential benefits of topical caffeine.

Thus far, studies have produced substantial evidence in support of caffeine's ability to protect against damage induced by UV radiation. In one study, SKH-1 hairless mice were irradiated with UV and subsequently treated with topical caffeine. These mice, when evaluated by treatment-blind examiners for skin roughness and transverse rhytids, were significantly less affected by UV radiation than their placebo-treated counterparts. Histological examination of the skin revealed that topical caffeine promoted apoptosis in keratinocytes with damaged DNA, indicating that caffeine, in addition to its ability to prevent photoageing, may also play a role in the prevention of photocarcinogenesis [16].

Other investigators have discovered that caffeine promotes lipolysis by inhibiting phosphodiesterases within the cell, leading to intracellular accumulation of 3′,5′-cyclic adenosine monophosphate (cAMP) which is responsible for the purported effect on cellulite [17]. Studies have revealed a minor effect of caffeine on cellulite that has not been uniformly statistically significant [18,19]. Studies are often difficult to interpret because circumference change rather than cellulite improvement is evaluated and weight loss is not measured despite its effect on cellulite. The true effect is probably modest, if present at all.

Due to its vasoconstrictive effects, derived from competitive inhibition of adenosine receptors in vessels [20], caffeine is also thought to be helpful in the treatment of infraorbital dark circles. It is encountered in eye creams for this purpose and has been evaluated for the treatment of periorbital wrinkles as well; however, studies have evaluated caffeine in combination with other active ingredients, obscuring its role in product efficacy. Recent studies of *ex vivo* hair follicles have also shown that caffeine may show promise for treating hair loss due to its ability to counteract the stress-induced response [21]. While this is an exciting advancement, clinical studies are needed to confirm these findings.

Chamomile

The mechanisms of chamomile's anti-inflammatory action have been investigated in multiple *in vitro* studies [22,23] and corroborated by clinical studies. These studies have shown that chamomile is as effective as 0.25% hydrocortisone, but less effective than 1% hydrocortisone – a concentration commonly found in over-the-counter ointments – in the treatment of inflammatory conditions such as eczema [24,25]. Another study of chamomile on UV radiation and tape-stripping-induced inflammation showed that chamomile cream was less effective than 1% hydrocortisone cream in reducing skin redness [26]. The anti-inflammatory effects were further demonstrated in a clinical study that showed that a chamomile 8.35% gel delayed and potentially reduced the occurrence of radiation dermatitis in patients receiving radiation compared with standard of care [27]. Thus, while chamomile may have some utility in very mild irritation, its true effect appears modest.

Chamomile may provide other benefits via the antioxidant properties conferred to it by a variety of well-known phytochemical compounds, including terpenes, flavonoids, apigenin, α-bisabolol and quercetin, that are found in chamomile extract [28–30]. The terpenoid chamazulene, in particular, is a very strong antioxidant, inhibiting leukotriene B_4 synthesis by inhibiting lipoxygenase and COX [31]. Several *in vitro* assays have also examined whole chamomile extract. These demonstrated that chamomile extract can inhibit the formation of hydroperoxide radicals and inhibit lipid peroxidation, though to a lesser degree than other botanical extracts tested in parallel [32–34]. No *in vivo* studies have been done to corroborate these findings.

Regardless, chamomile retains significant appeal secondary to its relatively safe side effect profile. Cases of contact dermatitis [35–37] and severe allergic reactions – namely, angioedema with contact urticaria and allergic conjunctivitis – to chamomile tea rinses and compresses, however, have been reported [38,39]. Additionally, chamomile, especially when ingested, may interact with warfarin and ciclosporin metabolism, thus increasing the doses required [40]. Studies investigating cutaneous absorption have not been done.

Conclusions

The demand for cosmeceuticals is high and continues to grow, driven by a growing population of consumers seeking products with true therapeutic potential (Table 157.3). Industry has responded quickly, creating thousands of cosmeceutical products often supported by preliminary scientific data. The current structure of

Table 157.3 Summary of cosmeceutical ingredients and their potential uses.

Active ingredient	*In vitro* studies	Animal studies	Human studies	Randomised controlled trial	EWG Skin Deep® rating[a]	Potential uses
Alpha-lipoic acid	✓	✓	✓	Beitner 2003 [3]	1	Antioxidant Lightening Anti-ageing
Cysteamine	✓	✓	✓	Mansouri et al. 2015 [4]	1	Lightening
Glycosaminoglycans	✓		✓	Pavicic et al. 2011 [5]	1	Anti-ageing
Hydroquinone	✓	✓	✓	Mauricio et al. 2011 [6]	8 (primarily due to risk for skin allergy/irritation)	Lightening
Hydroxy acids	✓	✓	✓	Stiller et al. 1996 [7]; Thibault et al. 1998 [8]	1–4	Anti-ageing
Tranexamic acid	✓		✓	Janne et al. 2019 [9]; Kanechorn Na Ayutha et al. 2012 [10]	1	Lightening
Peptides:						
Signal	✓		✓	Kaczvinsky et al. 2009 [11]; Farwick et al. 2011 [12]	No rating available	Anti-ageing
Neurotransmitter affecting	✓	✓	✓	Wang et al. 2013 [13]	No rating available	Anti-ageing
Carrier	✓			Miller et al. 2006 [14]	No rating available	Anti-ageing
Polyunsaturated fatty acids	✓	✓	✓	Huber et al. 2020 [15]	No rating available	Anti-ageing
Vitamins:						
Retinal	✓	✓	✓	Creidi et al. 1998 [16]	3–6 (primarily due to risk for skin allergy/irritation)	Anti-ageing
Retinol	✓	✓	✓	Pierard-Franchimont et al. 2000 [17]	9 (primarily due to risk for skin allergy/irritation)	Anti-ageing
Retinyl esters	✓	✓	✓	Green et al. 1998 [18]	6–9 (primarily due to risk for skin allergy/irritation)	Anti-ageing
B	✓	✓	✓	Christman et al. 2012 [19]	1	Antioxidant Anti-ageing Lightening
C	✓	✓	✓	Humbert et al. 2003 [20]; Inui and Itami 2007 [21]	1	Antioxidant Lightening
E	✓	✓	✓		1	Antioxidant Anti-inflammatory Anti-ageing
Natural:						
Aloe	✓	✓	✓	Reuter et al. 2008 [22]	1–3	Antioxidant Anti-inflammatory
Arbutin	✓	✓	✓		1	Lightening
Bakuchiol	✓		✓	Dhaliwal et al. 2019 [23]	1	Anti-ageing Lightening
Caffeine	✓	✓			1	Anti-ageing
Carnosine	✓	✓			1	Antioxidant Anti-ageing
Chamomile	✓	✓	✓		1–2	Antioxidant Anti-inflammatory
Comfrey	✓				4	Antioxidant Anti-inflammatory
CoQ10	✓	✓	✓	McDaniel et al. 2005 [24]	No rating available	Anti-ageing Antioxidant
Feverfew	✓	✓	✓	Martin et al. 2008 [25]	1	Anti-ageing Lightening Antioxidant Anti-inflammatory
Frankincense	✓	✓	✓	Calzavara-Pinton et al. 2010 [26]	1	Anti-ageing
Grape seed	✓	✓			1	Antioxidant Anti-ageing
Green tea	✓	✓	✓	Chiu et al. 2005 [27]; Camouse et al. 2009 [28]	1–2	Antioxidant Anti-inflammatory Anti-ageing Lightening
Jojoba oil	✓	✓	✓	Meyer et al. 2008 [29]	1	Anti-ageing
Kojic acid	✓	✓	✓	Hermanns et al. 2002 [30]; Draelos et al. 2010 [31]	4–7 (primarily due to risk for skin allergy/irritation)	Antioxidant Lightening

Table 157.3 (continued)

Active ingredient	In vitro studies	Animal studies	Human studies	Randomised controlled trial	EWG Skin Deep® rating[a]	Potential uses
Lavender	✓	✓			1	Anti-inflammatory
Licorice	✓	✓	✓	Kolbe et al. 2006 [32]	4	Anti-inflammatory Lightening
Lycopene	✓		✓		1	Antioxidant Anti-ageing
Milk thistle	✓	✓			1	Anti-inflammatory Antioxidant
Pine bark extract	✓	✓			1	Anti-inflammatory Anti-ageing
Pomegranate	✓	✓			1	Antioxidant Anti-inflammatory Anti-ageing
Rose	✓				No rating available	Antioxidant Anti-ageing
Soya	✓	✓	✓	Hermanns et al. 2002 [30]	1	Antioxidant Lightening
Turmeric	✓	✓	✓		1	Antioxidant Anti-inflammatory Lightening

[a] The Environmental Working Group (EWG) is an independent organisation that reviews ingredients in personal care products, including cosmeceuticals, for potential hazards to health. Ratings of 1–2 denote 'low hazard', 3–6 denote 'moderate hazard' and 7–10 denote 'high hazard' (https://www.ewg.org/skindeep/; last accessed March 2023).

regulatory oversight has offered little incentive for further studies, especially well-designed human studies, the results of which could potentially place a product under the drug category and, consequently, the scrutiny of regulatory bodies. Although a low tolerance for side effects in cosmeceutical preparations has pushed companies to use very small and safe – possibly subtherapeutic – amounts of active ingredients, it remains important for dermatologists to understand and explain the implications of using such products to those patients so eagerly seeking them.

Recently, there has been significant attention dedicated to 'clean' or natural beauty and personal care products – which constitutes a multibillion dollar growing industry [1]. In addition to discussions about product efficacy, it is prudent for dermatologists to be aware of concerns about safety of personal care products, including cosmeceuticals, in the USA and globally. As the FDA does not require pre-approval or mandated safety reporting or recalls of currently marketed cosmetic and cosmeceutical products, independent groups such as the Environmental Working Group (EWG) have made determinations about ingredients included in these product types that may pose risks for health based on potential to be carcinogenic, cause endocrine disruption, or skin allergies. While the bulk of concern is over preservatives and binding agents rather than active ingredients, the EWG does rank active ingredients found in cosmeceuticals as well (Table 157.3). The ratings of 1–2 denote 'low hazard', 3–6 denote 'moderate hazard' and 7–10 denote 'high hazard'. Of note, these ratings may not fully reflect the usual dose or route of administration of the ingredient, and the degree of risk to human health depends on absorption through the skin and concentration of the ingredient [2].

Key references

The full list of references can be found in the online version at https://www.wiley.com/rooksdermatology10e

Introduction
1 Newburger AE. Cosmeceuticals: myths and misconceptions. *Clin Dermatol* 2009;27:446–52.

Antioxidants
21 Bissett DL. Common cosmeceuticals. *Clin Dermatol* 2009;27:435–45.
22 Manela-Azulay M, Bagatin E. Cosmeceuticals vitamins. *Clin Dermatol* 2009; 27:469–74.
41 Chen L, Hu JY, Wang SQ. The role of antioxidants in photoprotection: a critical review. *J Am Acad Dermatol* 2012;67:1013–24.

Anti-ageing: lightening
23 Lim JT. Treatment of melasma using kojic acid in a gel containing hydroquinone and glycolic acid. *Dermatol Surg* 1999;25:282–4.

Anti-ageing: rhytid reduction
8 Green BA, Yu RJ, Van Scott EJ. Clinical and cosmeceutical uses of hydroxyacids. *Clin Dermatol* 2009;27:495–501.
11 Bissett DL. Common cosmeceuticals. *Clin Dermatol* 2009;27:435–45.
56 Sorg O, Antille C, Kaya G, Saurat J-H. Retinoids in cosmeceuticals. *Dermatol Ther* 2006;19:289–96.
75 Manela-Azulay M, Bagatin E. Cosmeceuticals vitamins. *Clin Dermatol* 2009; 27:469–74.
77 Lupo MP. Antioxidants and vitamins in cosmetics. *Clin Dermatol* 2001;19:467–73.

Herbals and phytochemicals
1 Baumann LS. Less-known botanical cosmeceuticals. *Dermatol Ther* 2007;20:330–42.

CHAPTER 158

Soft-Tissue Augmentation (Fillers)

Berthold Rzany

Medizin am Hauptbahnhof, Wien, Austria

Introduction, 158.1
Indications, 158.1
Techniques, 158.1
Needles and cannulas, 158.1
Depot and fanning techniques, 158.2
Fillers, 158.3

Biodegradable fillers, 158.3
Non-biodegradable fillers, 158.7
Common injection errors and how to avoid them, 158.8
General errors, 158.8
Injection errors, 158.8

Adverse reactions and their treatment, 158.8
Assessing and reducing the risks, 158.9
Potential adverse reactions, 158.9
Fillers and different skin types, 158.11
Acknowledgements, 158.12

Key references, 158.12

Introduction

Although the popularity of botulinum toxin seemed initially to have overshadowed dermal filler injections in the aesthetic market, the reduction of mimetic muscle is often not enough to convincingly rejuvenate the ageing face. Injectable fillers offer an effective and versatile choice for dermal restoration by reducing wrinkles and folds, as well as for deeper volume augmentation. There are a multitude of injectable fillers available in the international marketplace, with the exception of the USA where strict regulatory guidelines limit product availability to a handful of Food and Drug Administration (FDA) approved dermal filler devices. Updated European Union directives on such products focus on safety rather than efficacy [1].

Indications

Initially, the indication for dermal filler use was to diminish and efface skin wrinkles and folds. With the advent of fillers designed for very superficial use as well as for deeper volume augmentation, the indications have expanded substantially.

Improving skin quality. When skin ages, particularly skin types I–III, it becomes atrophic with fine wrinkles. One of the indications for injectable fillers is the improvement of skin quality [1].

Wrinkles and folds. The initial indication for dermal fillers was to address wrinkles and folds, and this remains a primary indication for injectable fillers (Figure 158.1). Effacement of the naso-labial fold is the indication with the most evidence, due to the fact that the US FDA has required every major injectable filler to be tested for this indication.

Volumising. Facial ageing results in a reduction in the size of the facial fat pads, with resultant positional shifting and malalignment causing an aged facial phenotype, even in those with a high body mass index (BMI). Natural and convincing replenishment of lost volume is a skill that requires accurate patient assessment and proficient aesthetic judgement. Often patients come with advanced signs of volume loss and simple filling of the defects would incur unacceptably high costs for patients due to the expense of the product required. The answer for this challenge is 'smart filling' – that is filling the areas that will have the most visual impact. Overcorrection of volume looks unconvincing and should be avoided. The goal is less concavity, not an overblown face. This is particularly relevant in men, where volume loss in the cheeks should only be gradually corrected (Figure 158.2). Volumisation can also be used to supplement a baseline deficit where increased volume would be aesthetically desirable. A good indication for this is the upper and lower lip. Here, small lips can be augmented to a fuller state (Figure 158.3), bearing in mind that, in white people, the vermillion portion of the lower lip should remain fuller than the upper portion. In general, younger lips are easier to correct compared with older lips where elastosis might limit volumisation.

Techniques

Needles and cannulas

Fillers can be injected using needles as well as cannulas (Table 158.1). The discussion about which is best is sometimes more dogmatic than scientific. When it comes to efficacy in this author's opinion, the location of product placement remains more important than the method used to deliver it. However, there is a clear indication for the use of needles for more superficial cutaneous lines (Figures 158.4 and 158.5a), as this delivery method effectively

Rook's Textbook of Dermatology, Tenth Edition. Edited by Christopher Griffiths, Jonathan Barker, Tanya Bleiker, Walayat Hussain and Rosalind Simpson.
© 2024 John Wiley & Sons Ltd. Published 2024 by John Wiley & Sons Ltd.

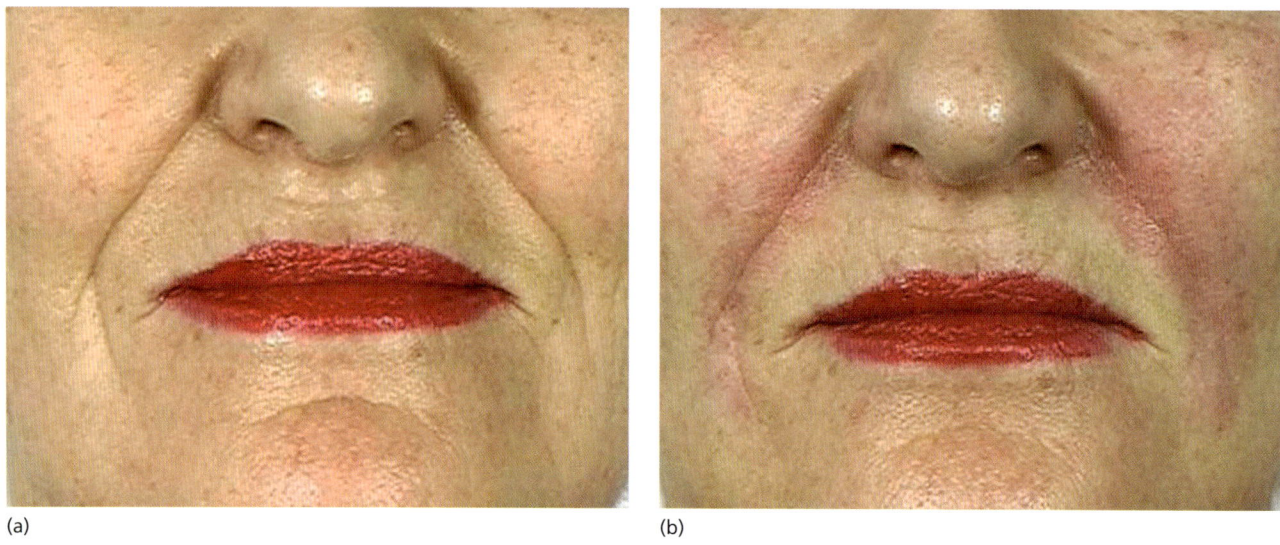

Figure 158.1 Naso-labial fold before (a) and immediately after (b) augmentation with 1.5 mL of a hyaluronic acid preparation. Note the post-injection skin redness.

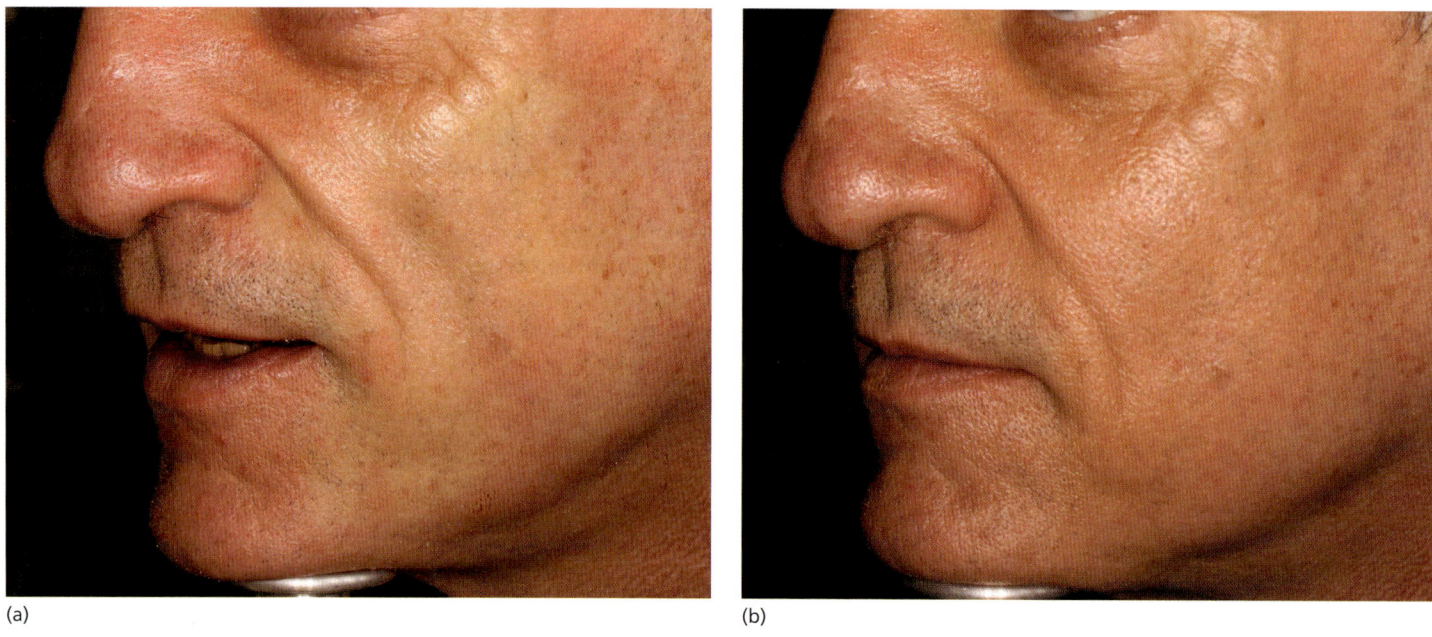

Figure 158.2 Cheeks before (a) and 16 days after (b) injections of 2 mL of a hyaluronic acid preparation per cheek.

targets intradermal layers, whereas cannulas target the subdermal plane (Figure 158.5b). Cannulas may also be unsuitable for some types of filler. For example, poly-L-lactic acid (PLLA) is best delivered using a needle as the mixture of PLLA and distilled water is prone to clogging a cannula, sometimes requiring withdrawal from the patient before continuation of the procedure.

Evidence demonstrating that the cannula technique is safer than the use of needles is scarce, although the theoretical risk of penetration of a vessel with resultant embolisation and vascular compromise seems to be reduced when using a blunt-tipped cannula compared with using a sharp needle. There are some case series favouring cannulas [1], and there is only one small randomised controlled trial where a newly designed cannula was compared with a standard 30 G needle when treating naso-labial folds [2]. In this setting, less haematoma and redness was reported for the cannula-treated site, in addition to less reported pain. However, in this study a hyaluronic acid without lidocaine was used. In a recent study by Alam et al. [3], a lower risk for vascular compromise was found when using cannulas. However, this was a retrospective study with some serious selection bias so the assumptions of the study need to be carefully weighted. Of greater importance is that the injector feels comfortable with the tool they are using.

Depot and fanning techniques

There are two basic techniques used for the injection of a dermal filler. One is the depot technique where blebs of various sizes are injected in the area of need (e.g. the tower technique [4]) and the

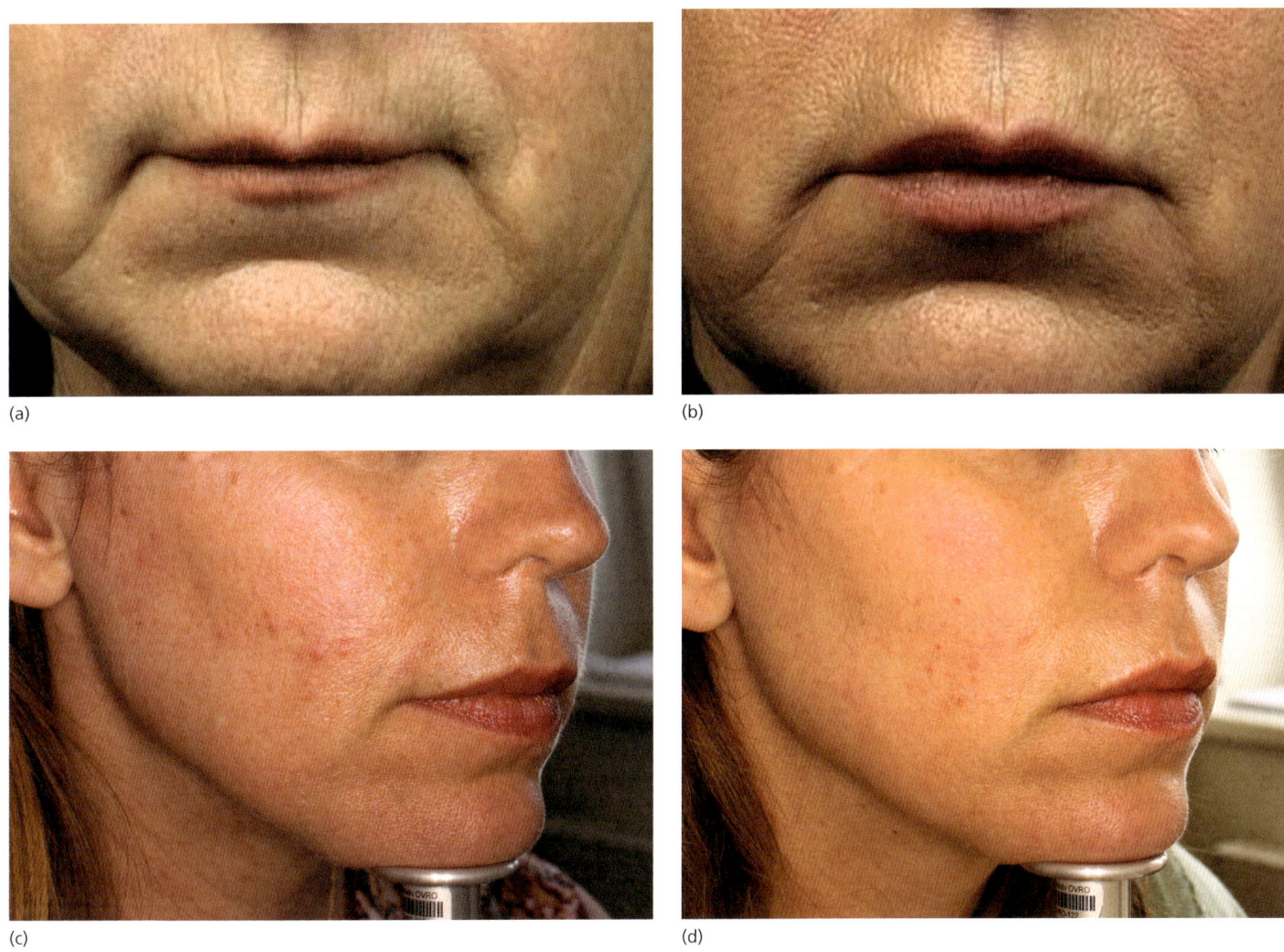

Figure 158.3 (a, b) Upper and lower lip in an older patient before (a) and after (b) reconstruction with 1.4 mL of a hyaluronic acid preparation. Note that the marionette lines were also treated and the results are very natural. (c, d) Upper and lower lip in a young patient before (c) and after (d) reconstruction with 1 mL of a hyaluronic acid preparation. Note that younger lips are much easier to treat.

Table 158.1 Indications for the use of needles and/or cannulas.

Indications	Cannula	Needle
Volume deficits	Yes	Yes
Folds and deep wrinkles	Yes	Yes
Fine wrinkles	No	Yes
Dermal restoration	No	Yes

other is the fanning technique, where some of the effect might come from the needle or cannula dissecting the subcutaneous area. In this author's opinion, the depot technique allows a more precise and probably more economical positioning of the material.

Fillers

There are a large number of injectable filler products available on the market, particularly outside the USA, most of which are biodegradable. The purpose of this overview is to summarise the various materials, to review specific fillers where good efficacy and/or safety data are available and to highlight those fillers that may pose an increased risk of adverse reactions.

Biodegradable fillers

Biodegradable fillers are non-permanent, and currently dominated by hyaluronic acid (HA) products. Collagens are not currently available in most markets, and calcium hydroxylapatite and polycaprolactone do not seem to be, at least in Europe, a mainstay of treatment.

The biodegradable fillers can be grouped into those that are inert and those where collagen stimulation is a major feature for the efficacy (i.e. PLLA, see below for the clinical trial data).

Inert fillers

All inert fillers act in a similar fashion, however there is only one product group with an antidote – the HA fillers. This is very important, not only in case of adverse events – specifically vascular occlusion – but also for overcorrection, which occurs far more commonly than adverse events.

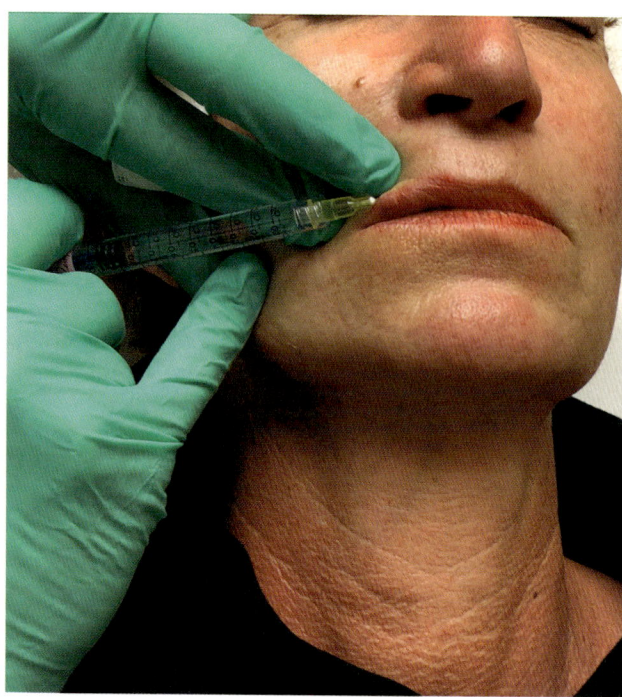

Figure 158.4 Injection of an HA in the upper lip by linear technique.

Hyaluronic acid-based filler

Hyaluronic acid fillers are overwhelmingly the most popular type of product used for injectable volume enhancement. They are long lasting with low allergenic potential and other relative risks, and have an improved safety profile compared with non-HA fillers due to the ability to reverse effects with the use of hyaluronidase. At the end of 2020, the HA dermal filler product ranges available in the USA and approved by the FDA were still very limited. However, outside the USA, a myriad of HA-based fillers are available due to a comparative laxity in manufacturing and market regulation. Products vary in concentration of HA, particle size, cross-linkage, gel consistency and hardness.

The evidence base for the use of HAs can be grouped as (i) those with a minimum of one good clinical trial (randomised, blinded, with a comparator and of sufficient size and duration); and (ii) those without good clinical data. But even with good clinical data, often studies are restricted to use in a few indications such as the naso-labial folds, cheeks and lips, and do not reflect accurately widespread use in other facial (e.g. chin) and non-facial (e.g. dorsal hands and décolletage) sites. The arena is further confused by the vast number of HA fillers available and the fast pace of product evolution.

The HA product with the longest historical use is the Restylane® NASHA™ family. It is the HA product group with the largest body of high-quality evidence as two of these products have been the comparators in several European and US FDA-approval trials. The first good trial published for the filler family was a randomised controlled clinical trial conducted to compare the efficacy and safety of Restylane and Zyplast®, a bovine collagen no longer available. A total of 137 patients were included, and after 6 months the authors concluded that Restylane was superior to Zyplast (based on the assessment of the wrinkle severity rating scale (WSRS)) [1]. The investigators rated Restylane as superior in 56.9% of patients,

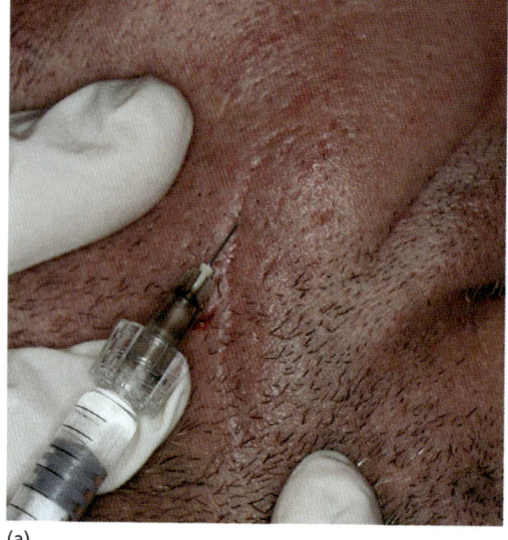

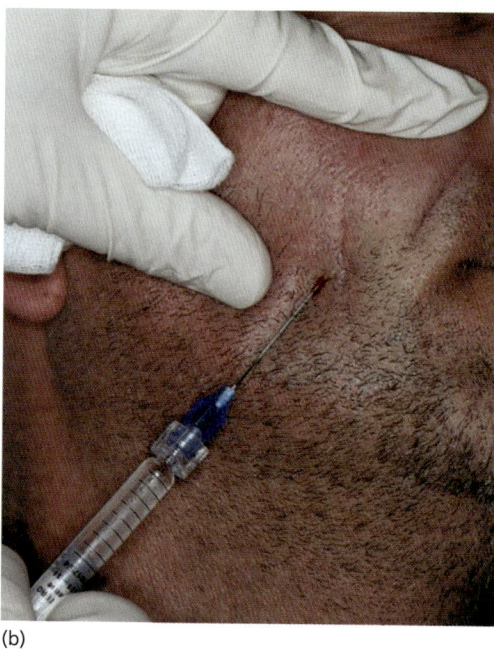

Figure 158.5 Volumisation of the cheeks. (a) Injection of a more fluid hyaluronic acid (HA) superficially with a needle to decrease the visibility of a cheek fold in a former acne patient with a thick dermis. (b) Injection of an HA for cheek volumisation using a cannula.

compared with 9.5% of patients in whom the investigators felt that Zyplast was superior ($P < 0.0001$). Those patients in whom there was no difference between these products (33.6%) were not included in the simple univariate statistics [1]. These findings were supported by further data from another randomised controlled study [2].

Due to marketing reasons, a completely different HA product, previously called Emervel®, is distributed under the name of Restylane with the addendum OBT (optimal balance technology). OBT Restylane differs from the 'old' NASHA Restylane and there are good clinical trials published comparing the efficacy and safety of the Restylane NASHA and Restylane OBT products [3–5]. Restylane Perlane® (now Restylane Lyft®) performed similarly or slightly less well than Emervel Deep® (now Restylane Defyne®) [6]. In a unique case series, patients were treated for a number of indications using a range of Restylane OBT products, reflecting realistic practice [7].

The Juvéderm® family is very large, including the new Vycross® (e.g. Voluma®, Volbella®, Volift® and Volite®) range, and offers products for different types of lines and wrinkles as well as for volumising indications. As with the Restylane products, there is strong evidence supporting the safety and efficacy for some of the products in the Juvéderm family [8–10]. The newer Vycross fillers are cross-linked with shorter chains compared with the older Juvéderm products. Voluma has the highest HA concentration at 20 mg/mL, followed by Volift at 17.5 mg/mL and Volbella with a lower concentration of 15 mg/mL. There is one good randomised clinical trial on Voluma for mid-face volumising compared with no treatment [11] and some supporting cases series [12]. There is a Volbella case series involving lip augmentation [13] that demonstrated a good duration of action (12 months). There is some evidence that points to an increased risk of inflammatory reactions when using Vycross products [**14**,15] (see 'Adverse reactions and their treatment' later in this chapter). Other HA fillers supported by at least one good clinical study involving a product in its family include the Belotero® range [16], the Croma range [17] and the Teosyal® range [18].

The safety profile of HA is improved due to the availability of hyaluronidases, soluble protein enzymes capable of degrading HA. These are used therapeutically to reverse the effects of inappropriate placement, overcorrection or adverse events associated with HA such as nodules and inflammation [19,20]. The use of hyaluronidases is essential in emergency situations such as vascular occlusion or embolisation from HA filler [21]. Local injection site reactions may occur with hyaluronidase, including redness, oedema, pruritus, pain and both immediate and delayed allergic reactions.

Non-hyaluronic acid-based fillers

All other available biodegradable fillers lack an antidote. This is a clear disadvantage which needs to be considered carefully when choosing a filler.

Calcium hydroxylapatite. Calcium hydroxylapatite (CaHa) is quite popular, particularly in the USA. It is a whitish material made from synthetically formed calcium phosphate pearls, usually mixed with lidocaine to reduce injection pain. Early studies focused on the correction of drug-induced lipoatrophy in patients with human immunodeficiency virus (HIV) [22,23]. However, there are also three randomised controlled clinical trials, one comparing CaHa with collagen [24] and two with HA products [25,26], focusing on the correction of naso-labial folds. CaHa was considered to be superior compared with human collagen in the 6-month study [24], but the two 12-month comparison studies with the HA fillers were not as clear; the larger one of these failed to show any superiority in the WSRS [25,26]. Patient preference and satisfaction with treatment favoured CaHA, however neither study was double-blinded, potentially introducing a bias towards the treatment under investigation.

There is little evidence available regarding common adverse reactions to CaHa. Sklar and White [27] and Tzikas [28] reported case series with 64 and 90 patients, respectively, treated for facial soft-tissue augmentation. Apart from mild bruising and swelling, no immediate side effects were observed. Sklar and White [27] reported five patients with complications after CaHa treatment. Three patients had palpable bumps, one had puffiness of the lower eyelid and another developed a pink-white plaque. The latter two adverse events occurred when treating the tear trough area over a treatment period of 6 months. A naso-labial fold trial of CaHa compared with human collagen found that patients treated with CaHa reported more oedema (73.9% compared with 56.4%) and had more ecchymosis (63.2% compared with 43.6%) over a period of 6 months [24]. The area where adverse reactions were quite frequently reported initially is in the lip region. In one 6-month study [28], 7 out of 90 patients developed persistent, visible mucosal lip nodules, four of whom required an intervention such as surgical extrusion. Furthermore, there are reports of CaHa causing arterial occlusion leading to local necrosis or even blindness [29,30]. In cases of adverse events or overcorrection from CaHa, no antidote exists to date [31].

Alginates. At the end of 2009, Novabel®, a filler derived from brown algae, was introduced to the European market. Based on the results of the initial large case series, which were reported at various scientific meetings, the product showed promise. Redness, swelling and even haematomas seemed to be less prevalent compared with HA products (unpublished data), and it was very easy to inject. However, subsequent adverse events such as nodule formation were reported, specifically in areas such as the infraorbital hollow, and as no corrective antidote is available the filler was removed from the market [32].

Bovine collagen. Bovine collagen was a very early injectable filler used in the aesthetic arena. Bovine enzyme-digested collagen (95% type I, 5% type III) was available in several preparations, which were distinguished by the collagen content and the addition of glutaraldehyde for stabilisation [33,34]. Different products emerged depending on the collagen content and the degree of cross-linking. Zyderm 1® and Zyderm 2®, based on non-cross-linked collagen, were designed for the superficial dermis. The cross-linked Zyplast was indicated for injection in the deeper dermis and was cleared for marketing in 1981 by the FDA. Approval was based on clinical data from a large case series of 9427 tested and 5109 treated patients [33].

The risk of collagen hypersensitivity reactions meant that pre-testing was mandatory. This consisted of an intradermal injection of Zyderm 1 collagen into the volar aspect of the forearm, which was evaluated after 28 days. The incidence of adverse reactions to bovine collagen (Zyderm 1) was approximately 3%. Most of these reactions occurred quite quickly after testing, however a negative test did not preclude the potential for subsequent reactions. An additional 1.3% of patients reported adverse reactions despite negative pre-testing [34]. Bovine collagens are no longer available in Europe and the USA due primarily to the inconvenience of the prick test requirement and poor longevity compared with HA preparations.

Porcine collagen. The only porcine collagen in wide use was Evolence®, introduced into the European market in 2004 and withdrawn in 2009. There were two preparations available, Evolence and Evolence Breeze®, both stabilised by glycation using D-ribose as a cross-linking agent. Evolence was used for naso-labial folds and Evolence Breeze was indicated for more superficial dermal injections and lip augmentation. Efficacy was supported by several good clinical trials [35,36]. The risk of hypersensitivity reactions for porcine collagen was not of clinical relevance [37], so no skin testing was required. There were, however, a few reports of foreign body reactions inducing abscess-like lesions [38]. Porcine collagen proved more difficult to inject compared with bovine collagen, although mixing lidocaine (0.2 mL) into the product syringe facilitated ease of injection in addition to reducing patient discomfort. Porcine collagen has a yellowish colour which was visible beneath the mucosal surface when injected too superficially.

Human collagen. Human collagen used for cosmetic injection was derived from natural human collagen grown under controlled laboratory conditions, and did not require pre-testing [39]. Two products became available, both containing 0.3% lidocaine: CosmoDerm® was a non-cross-linked formulation that was used in the treatment of superficial lines, whereas cross-linked CosmoPlast® was used primarily in the treatment of more pronounced wrinkles. A few clinical trials are available in which CosmoDerm was used as a comparator, for example to PLLA. Based on these trials the durability seemed to be inferior to other products [40], contributing to the subsequent withdrawal of these products from European and US markets.

Collagen-stimulating fillers

The concept of separating fillers into inert and collagen-stimulating categories is somewhat historical. PLLA was the first filler that postulated and showed collagen-stimulating properties. However, now it is recognised that even HA is not completely 'inert' and repeated injections seem to stimulate native collagen production through mechanical properties of fibroblast stretching. Direct comparative studies between a collagen-stimulating product and an HA filler for at least 12 months are needed, and as no good data currently exist such claims should be viewed with caution.

Polyl-L-lactic acid

Poly-L-lactic acid is the only injectable filler with a proven significant collagen-stimulating potential. The onset of action of PLLA is delayed and patients must be advised it is not used for immediate results. It is not an inert filler, and there is no antidote. After repeated treatments, the long-lasting effects and durability are a major advantage over some of the other products available. The manufacturer of Sculptra® recommends three initial treatment sessions, each approximately 6–8 weeks apart. After these initial treatments the result may last for up to 2 years or more. The product comes as a powder and needs to be diluted with sterile water prior to injection. The current recommendation based on a recent European consensus is a dilution volume of 9 mL or more, including 2 mL of a local anaesthetic. Even when administered using the correct injection technique and a higher dilution, in some cases the 26 G needle will become occluded during the injection, at which point the syringe has to be withdrawn and the plunger retracted until the PLLA flows again.

Before 2010, studies on the efficacy and safety of PLLA were based mainly on the treatment of HIV patients with drug-induced lipoatrophy [41,42]. In 2010, a large clinical trial was published comparing PLLA with human collagen ($n = 233$) [40], which showed at 3 months the superiority of the PLLA when using a 5 mL dilution. The mean number of treatment sessions required per subject was 3.2 in the injectable PLLA group compared with 2.6 in the collagen group. The mean (standard deviation (SD)) volume of injectable PLLA used per session for both naso-labial folds was as follows: first session 4.1 mL; second session 3.5 mL (SD 1.2); third session 3.3 mL (SD 1.2); and fourth session 3.5 mL (SD 1.1). For human collagen, the mean (SD) volume used per session was first session 3.1 mL (SD 1.1); second session 2.1 mL (SD 1.1); third session 1.9 mL (SD 1.1); and fourth session 1.7 mL (SD 1.0). Importantly, the correction with PLLA lasted for more than 13–25 months, which is why most patients preferred this product [43]. However, the grade of correction that could be achieved was less in PLLA compared with that of HA (approximately 0.66–0.85 for PLLA on a six-point scale versus approximately 1.0 on a five-point scale in HA trials) [40].

Papule/nodule formation is the main adverse reaction of PLLA, and the prevalence seems to be associated with the volume used for dilution. There is indirect evidence that papule/nodule formation can be reduced when a higher volume for dilution is used [44,45]. One reason may be that the PLLA is more evenly distributed with higher dilution, mitigating the risk of papules caused by focal areas of collagen formation around PLLA deposits. In a few patients the formation of large nodules has been reported and this may indicate an exaggerated immunological reaction to the product. There are case reports of large solitary nodular masses, for example in the temporal region [46], as well as abscess formation [47]. In most patients, nodule formation is temporary and will decrease over time [48] so aggressive treatment is not required.

Polycaprolacton

Ellansé®, which was approved for use in the European market (CE marked) in 2009, is composed of polycaprolactone (PCL) microspheres in an aqueous carboxymethylcellulose gel carrier. It is claimed to have some collagen biostimulating properties. There is only one small, clinical, randomised controlled trial comparing PCL with an HA filler (Restylane Perlane now Restylane Lyft) [49]. In this single trial PCL was shown to be slightly superior to Restylane Perlane after 12 months. However, no further comparative trials with another HA filler have been conducted so far. There is no antidote available so in case of an overcorrection or an adverse event the treatment options are limited [50,51].

Calcium hydroxylapatite as a biostimulating filler

Calcium hydroxylapatite is sometimes advocated as a biostimulating filler. However, the evidence is scarce. When injected as a filler (e.g. for naso-labial folds) there is no evidence that repetitions of injections in the same side are needed less frequently than with HA fillers. There is a small retrospective study for mid and upper face rejuvenation based on 40 patients [52] and a consensus paper on the use of diluted and hyperdiluted CaHa for skin tightening [53]. However, the evidence for the consensus paper is mostly based on expert opinion and not randomised controlled clinical studies. A randomised controlled clinical trial, for instance comparing diluted/hyperdiluted CaHa with PLLA, would be very welcome in guiding clinical practice.

Non-biodegradable fillers

In Europe and the USA there are only a few non-biodegradable or permanent fillers currently available. Several products were removed from the market due to very severe adverse reactions, both acute and delayed, which negated any potential advantages. Although their popularity has waned, it is important for practitioners to familiarise themselves with permanent fillers as there are still patients with these implanted products, who may present with adverse reactions and require management decades after initial injection. Furthermore, these or similar products could resurface on the international scene. There are no antidotes available to these fillers.

Single substance products
Silicones

Silicones are not widely used in Europe or in the USA. Medical-grade silicone is a clear, oily, colourless liquid composed of long chains of polymerised dimethylsiloxane. There are several methods of injection for this product, including the microdroplet technique [54,55]. Fluid silicone is injected into the dermis as 0.01 mL microdroplets at 1 mm intervals, with a preference for undercorrection. Silicone, particularly that with dubious provenance, has led to disastrous local and systemic effects. In general, the inflammatory reaction surrounding injected silicone is self-limited; however, the extent of the reaction is not predictable and in some cases can be quite severe. Local adverse reactions include chronic inflammation, infection, migration, extrusion, ulceration and silicone granuloma formation [56–59]. Once these complications occur, removal of the injected silicone is quite difficult, necessitating wide tissue resections and complex reconstructions [56]. As Pérez-Ruiz [60] showed, methotrexate therapy may be a good alternative to surgical intervention. The quality of the product in terms of purity has improved significantly over the last decades and in a patient record review of 916 patients treated with 1000-centistoke silicone oil, only very few adverse events were documented [61].

Polyacrylamides

There are still several polyacrylamide products in the marketplace, but only Aquamid® is available in Europe and the USA. Composed of 97.5% water and 2.5% cross-linked polyacrylamide, it is used for volume correction and is injected deeply, usually using the subcutaneous tunnelling technique [62,63]. In a large trial (N = 315) by Narins et al. [64], Aquamid was compared with an HA filler for the correction of naso-labial folds. The degree of correction was comparable between both products at 6 and 12 months and adverse effects were infrequent. In 2004, Breiting et al. reported the results of a retrospective case series of 104 patients, where 49 patients had undergone polyacrylamide gel injection for breast augmentation and 65 for facial treatment [62]. Migration of the gel was demonstrated in three women who had had their naso-labial folds treated. No long-term adverse effects were observed in this study, which reported an average observation time of 3.9 years [62].

However, when adverse effects do arise, they may be severe and a challenge to treat. In 2003, Wang et al. published a case series of 15 patients with adverse reactions assessed over 2 years and reported the following: nodules (80%), pain (60%), secondary deformity (20%), discomfort (13%) and long-lasting swelling (6.6%) [65]. Pathological examinations showed macrophagocyte infiltration (60%), capsule formation (53.3%) and granulomatous reactions (20%). In a large study comparing PLLA and polyacrylamide in HIV-positive patients with therapy-induced lipoatrophy, more severe inflammatory reactions were seen in the polyacrylamide group [66]. Bjarnsholt and colleagues postulated biofilm formation, which is a low-grade microbial colonisation adherent to the filler product, as the cause of these adverse reactions and recommended antibiotic treatment instead of immunomodulatory treatments [67]. However, as Alijotas-Reig et al. [68] point out, there is no clinical proof that a mere antibiotic treatment is beneficial in nodule formation due to polyacrylamide.

Polyalkylamide

Polyalkylamide, marketed as Bio-Alcamid®, consisted of alkylimide group networks (approximately 4%) and water (approximately 96%), in two preparations of different viscosity indicated for lip and facial augmentation. The material needed to be injected subdermally and, according to the manufacturer's information, was supposed to be easily removable when injected in larger volumes [69]. There are very few data available on this product, although an initial case series by Protopapa et al. [69] reported no adverse events in 73 patients over a follow-up period of up to 3 years. However, in an independent retrospective Dutch study on 3194 patients, 154 complications were reported, the most common being inflammation and hardening, as well as migration [70]. The authors concluded that the prevalence of these reactions was unacceptably high and that the use of the product could not be recommended. Similar conclusions were drawn from a British group of surgeons when reviewing 67 patients with HIV antiretroviral-associated lipoatrophy who had all been treated with polyalkylimide, where 50% of the treated patients experienced at least one complication (migration, hardening or irregularity) [71]. These results were supported by a Canadian group, where in 19% of 267 patients infectious complications were noted [72]. Currently the product is not available in Europe.

Multiple substance products (combination fillers)
Polymethylmethacrylate and collagen

The fixed combination of polymethylmethacrylate (PMMA) and bovine collagen (now BellaFill®, formerly ArteFill®, formerly Artecoll®) was introduced at the end of the 1980s and is the oldest available combination filler. PMMA beads are suspended in a solution of 3.5% bovine collagen as a carrier and 0.3% lidocaine for anaesthetic effect. While the collagen resorbs over a period of 2–3 months, the PMMA spheres become encapsulated by fibrotic material and remain permanently in the tissue. BellaFill is meant to be injected into the lower third of the dermis with a 26–27 G needle, using the tunnelling technique. The material should not be injected too superficially and the needle should never be visible through the overlying skin. Careful massage with a fingertip after application helps to distribute the material more evenly. Overcorrection is not advisable; however, a second implantation may be necessary after 3 months [73]. Although the preparation contains collagen, in Europe a skin test is not mandatory. This is the only permanent filler that has been subject to a large clinical trial [74]. In this clinical study 251 patients were followed up for 1 year to assess the risk of adverse reactions [74]. Even when followed for a further 4–5 years, the risk remained low [75]. This is in accordance with a review of filler complications in the FDA database. BellaFill/ArteFill nodule formation was the most commonly reported complication in five people (40.0%), and this comprised 0.01% of all ArteFill/BellaFill injections performed [76]. However, as the product is permanent, adverse reactions such as granuloma formation may develop years later [77].

Hydroxyethylmethacrylate and ethylmethacrylate microspheres suspended in hyaluronic acid

Hydroxyethylmethacrylate (HEMA) and ethylmethacrylate microspheres suspended in HA was available in Europe as DermaLive® from the end of the 1990s until 2007. This product consisted of 40% bacteria-derived HA and 60% acrylic hydrogel particles (diameter 45–65 μm). A product from the same family was marketed as DermaDeep® and was intended to be injected deeper. DermaLive was injected with a 27.5 G needle into the deeper layers of the dermis, while DermaDeep was supposed to be injected with a slightly larger 26.5 G needle deeper still, into the hypodermis or subperiosteal layer [78]. This product has the ignominious distinction as being the dermal filler product associated with the highest risk of adverse reactions, primarily nodule formation, but also abscesses and ulcerations [79]. In 2001, Bergeret-Galley *et al.* published an overview in which the overall incidence of late side effects and complications (nodules, swelling and redness, on average 6 months after injection), based on data from the manufacturer, is given as <1.2 per 1000 patients [78]. Although this product is no longer manufactured, it is highly likely that adverse reactions to this permanent product will continue to present years after its use.

Common injection errors and how to avoid them

Treatment with injectable fillers is generally very safe if administered by a properly trained practitioner. However, adverse reactions or injection mistakes may occur.

General errors

Using fillers with no antidote. Fillers with no antidote pose a challenge when they are accidentally injected into the intravascular space as they cannot be dissolved emergently. Furthermore, in slowly biodegradable or permanent fillers, products may remain implanted for years or even permanently. The patient's immunological reactivity may change over time, resulting in delayed adverse events such as large granuloma formation. Although these reactions can be addressed, they are much more challenging than the treatment of granulomatous reactions to HA-based fillers [1]. Currently there is no treatment or antidote to degrade non-HA-based biodegradable and/or permanent fillers.

Using products without good clinical data. The use of products in the absence of good clinical data increases the risk of early adverse reactions such as abscess formation. Therefore, it is desirable to use products where evidence exists. However, most clinical trials are restricted to use in the naso-labial folds. Other areas such as the lips, glabella, temple, forehead and infraorbital hollow may be less well understood [2,3]. One should be very cautious, particularly with new products and new indications.

Injection errors

Inadequate aseptic technique before injections. Early inflammation, infection and abscess formation may be consequences of non-sterile technique. Thorough local disinfection prior to the injection is mandatory.

Disregard of and/or lack of respect for anatomy. Fillers are increasingly used for volume augmentation in all kinds of patients. To avoid an aesthetically displeasing outcome (e.g. asymmetry) or more serious adverse events (e.g. arterial occlusion), a good understanding of both the surface and deeper facial anatomy is required. This includes not only the layers of the skin and subcutis but the muscles, fat compartments, ligaments, nerves, vessels and underlying bony structures.

Using deep injection fillers too superficially. Injecting a filler designed for deep injections very superficially is a common operator-dependent error. HA fillers intended for deep injections have a high G-prime rating [4], which is a marker for the hardness of the HA gel or its lifting capacity. High G-prime fillers are those used for volumisation, but if injected superficially will result in unsightly bumps or sausage-like lines. In cases where an HA was injected, these can be easily corrected with hyaluronidase.

Injecting too much volume in one session. A conservative, 'less is more' approach is safest, and aligns with a natural, gradual rejuvenation strategy which most patients desire. Large amounts (e.g. more than 3 mL per site when treating the cheeks) will lead to very visible changes and might be totally unsuitable in elastotic skin where the filler might extend the skin to an unsightly overextended face [5].

Injecting under timely constraints. Adverse events occur more frequently when the injector works under time constraints. Injecting in a relaxed manner will benefit the patient and the injector alike. Fillers should be injected slowly in small amounts. Overcorrections, asymmetries, haematomas and probably arterial occlusions through to increased injection pressure will occur less often. Similarly, caution must be used prior to a special occasion (e.g. a wedding), particularly in the novice patient, with plenty of time allowed for bruising to settle or for any necessary corrections or touch-ups.

Adverse reactions and their treatment

No injectable filler is without the potential risk of an adverse reaction. The key issues to consider are how high is the risk and can it be mitigated?

Assessing and reducing the risks

To accurately assess the risk of a specific injectable filler, the following data are required: (i) the number of adverse reactions; and (ii) the total number of patients treated. For most injectable fillers this information is not available. Data on the number of adverse reactions are dependent on adverse event reporting, and it is well recognised that there are serious lapses in the clinician–reporting interface. Often the clinician dealing with a presenting complication is not the original injector and the patient may not be aware of which product was used, or may have had a number of different products injected over time. The total number of patients treated can only be estimated based on the volume of product sold, but in contrast to the drug market, there is no reliable source reporting this information. Furthermore, the product can be purchased from a number of illegitimate and black-market sources [1].

Two attempts have been made to estimate the risk of adverse reactions. Friedman et al. [2] reviewed the data of all unwanted effects of the Restylane range of HA products reported globally (Europe, Australia, South America, Asia) to the manufacturer between 1999 and 2000. For 1999, based on 144 000 treatments, the incidence was calculated at 0.15%; for 2000, based on approximately 262 000 treatments, an incidence of 0.06% was given. The differences between these incidences were explained through changes made in the manufacturing process.

Another more recent attempt to estimate the risk for adverse reactions took place in the Netherlands in 2012. The sales of HyaCorp HS® and H1000® were temporarily stopped after several patients were reported with problems following the use of two products from the range. Based on these cases the estimated risk of adverse reaction was 1.4% [3]. Investigation by the Dutch authorities ensued and the company opted to withdraw HyaCorp HS500® and H1000 as well as HyaCorp L® from the European market in August 2013. Thus, risk can be reduced or mitigated by either modifying the production process or withdrawing the filler from the market.

The Vycross family has also come into focus for a potentially increased risk of inflammatory nodular adverse reactions. In 2019, Sadeghpour et al. published a case series of 1029 patients who received 1250 Vycross filler treatments [4]. Five patients developed delayed nodules to the Vycross Volbella filler, with an incidence of 1.0% per patient and 0.8% per syringe. Compared with other currently approved NASHA fillers, Volbella is associated with a higher incidence of nodule formation. Mu et al. [5] identified a characteristic histopathological pattern for these reactions of discrete foci of tightly cuffed palisaded granulomas with eosinophils around the Vycross fillers. Despite an increased risk of inflammatory reaction the Vycross products are still widely used.

Potential adverse reactions

In general, adverse reactions can be classified as acute, subacute or delayed, based on time of onset after the injection. Acute reactions occur immediately after the injection or after a few days. Subacute onset is somewhat vaguely defined; it generally encompasses reactions that occur weeks after an injection. Reactions can also be grouped according to the clinical diagnosis. The most severe adverse reactions are abscesses, nodule formation and arterial infarction, followed by immunological reactions [6].

The management plan for any adverse event is dependent upon the type of filler and the type of reaction. If there is uncertainty as to the type of filler, a biopsy is recommended. The biopsy may allow identification of the broad type of product (e.g. biodegradable versus permanent), as well as identification of specific fillers with a characteristic histological appearance such as PLLA. It is important to send these specimens to a dermatopathologist familiar with these reactions to avoid the vague comment of 'foreign body reaction'. Dadzie et al. described several typical reactions to different fillers that may assist the histopathologist [7].

Abscesses are usually acute or subacute (Figure 158.6a), although cases occurring after several months or years have been reported (Figure 158.6b). If the abscess is fluctuant, it should be drained and bacterial microscopy and culture undertaken, with consideration for atypical mycobacterium, followed by administration of anappropriate antibiotic.

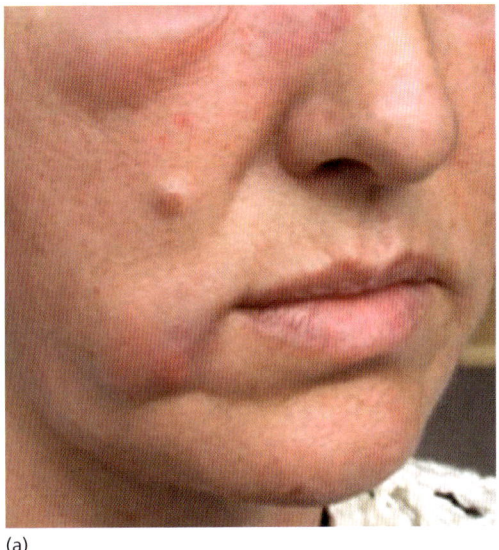

(a)

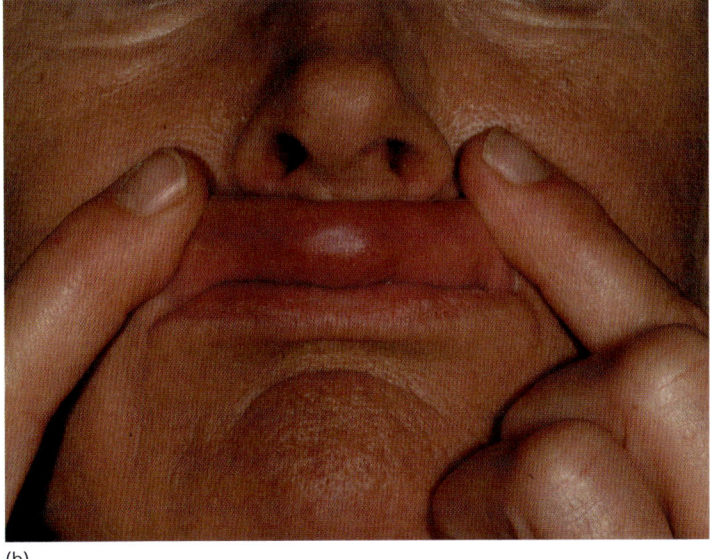

(b)

Figure 158.6 (a) Abscess 19 days after the injection of a hyaluronic acid (Matridur®). (b) Abscess several months after the injection of a porcine collagen (Evolence Breeze).

Nodule formation as a sign of an exaggerated immune response is the most common adverse reaction to all fillers (Figure 158.7). Some researchers advocate that biofilm, a low-grade bacterial colonisation, may play a significant role in nodule formation by triggering an immunological reaction [8]. When antibiotics appear to be beneficial, it is uncertain if this is due to bactericidal, anti-inflammatory or immunomodulatory effects, or a combination of these (Figure 158.8) [9]. In the last years in cases of inflammatory reactions towards permanent fillers, methotrexate therapy has

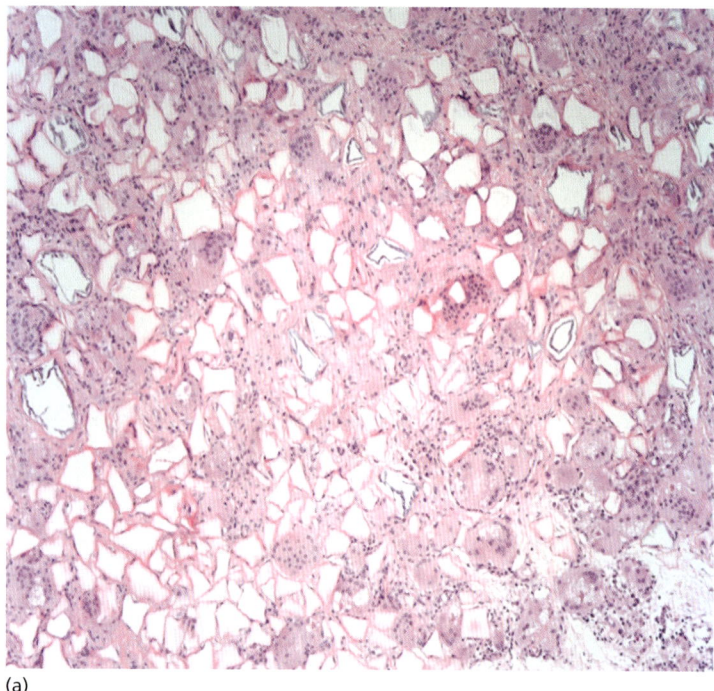

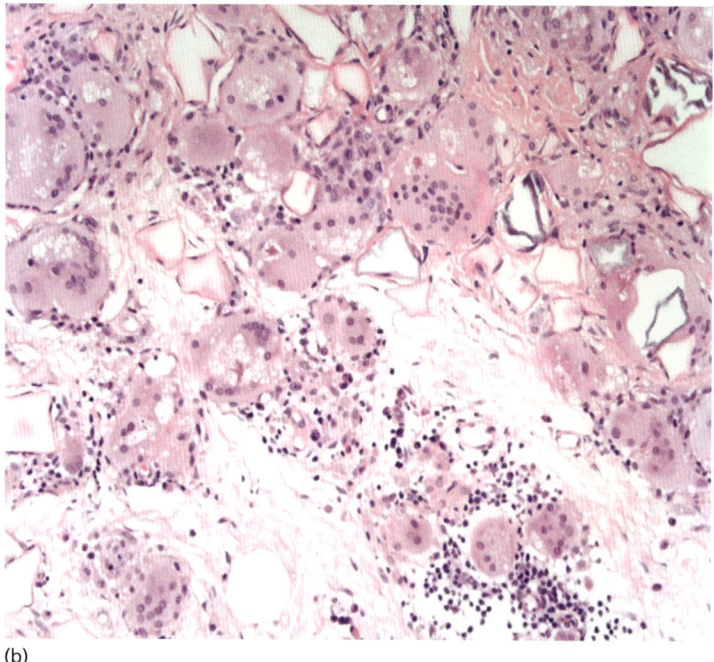

Figure 158.7 (a, b) Haematoxylin and eosin staining of a hyaluronic acid plus methacrylate (DermaLive) filler implant showing characteristic polygonal structures immersed in a granulomatous reaction. Courtesy of T. Griffiths and L. Motta.

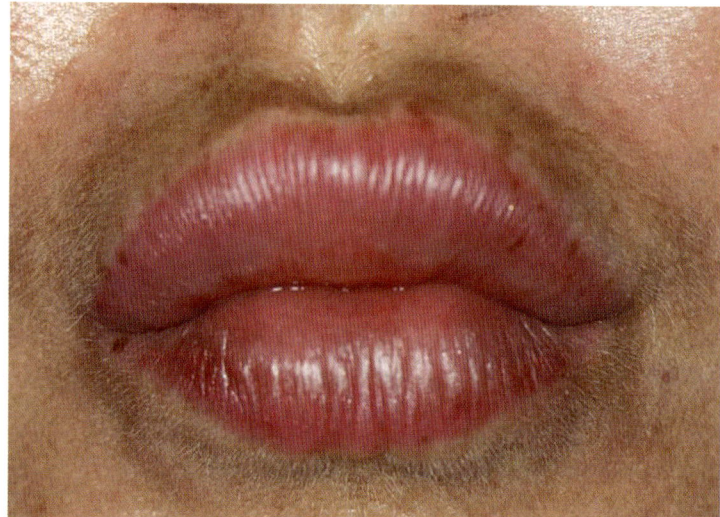

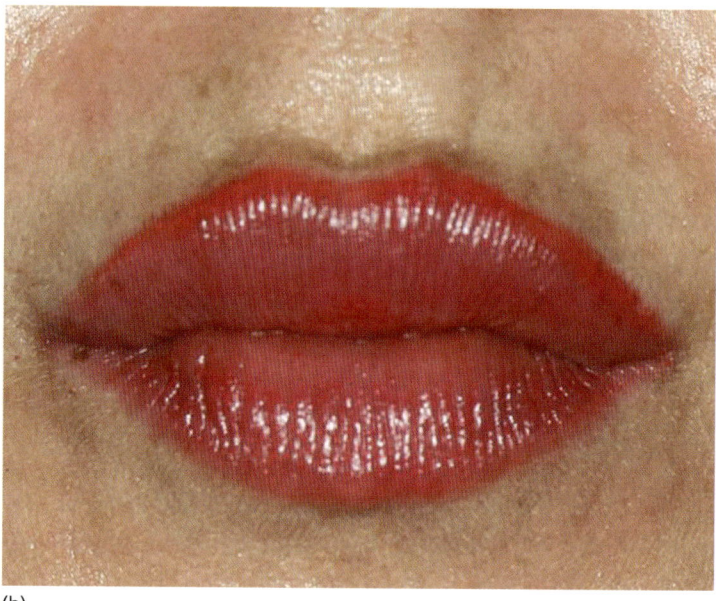

Figure 158.8 (a) Massive nodular mass formation around polyacrylamid (Aquamid) injected 5 years earlier. (b) Results after 4 months of treatment following a polypragmatic approach with oral antibiotics, steroids and fumaric acid.

been used in a couple of case series with apparently good success [10,**11**,12].

The treatment plan for such nodules is outlined in Tables 158.2 and 158.3.

The most severe adverse reaction, considered a medical emergency, is arterial occlusion due to either direct embolisation or compression. Usually this is an acute event accompanied by immediate pain and a whitish vascular reaction in the area of the occlusion. The highest-risk injection sites for this medical emergency are the glabella/forehead area, the nose and the naso-labial folds. There are several reports of blindness due to arterial occlusion following filler injection in these areas [13–17]. If HA is the culprit filler, hyaluronidase should immediately be injected around the HA depot and along the flow of the artery [18,19]. The injection of hyaluronidase is most effective in the first hours after the injection.

Table 158.2 Treatment approach for immune response nodules after hyaluronic acid (HA) fillers.

Step	Treatment	Comments
First line: hyaluronidase injection	If an HA filler has been used, inject hyaluronidase around the nodule (in the nodule if possible)	Do not forget that bovine hyaluronidase might elicit allergic reactions
Second line: immunomodulatory treatment	Inject intralesional steroids and/or 5-fluorouracil	Be careful of steroid atrophy
	Or start an oral steroid treatment as pulse (e.g. prednisolone)	Give prednisolone 60 mg for 2 days; 40 or 50 mg for 2 days; 20 mg for 2 days; then off for 1 week. Extend dosing if required
	And/or oral doxycycline 100 mg twice a day over 3 weeks[a]	
Third line: surgical treatment	Excision	Be aware of scar formation

[a] Low-dose oral doxycycline 40 or 50 mg once a day, as it is used in rosacea or acne, might be an alternative.

Table 158.3 Treatment approach for immune response after non-hyaluronic acid (non-HA) fillers.

Step	Treatment	Comments
First line: immunomodulatory treatment	Inject intralesional steroids and/or 5-fluorouracil	Be careful of steroid atrophy
	Or start an oral steroid treatment as pulse (e.g. prednisolone)	Give prednisolone 60 mg for 2 days; 40 mg for 2 days; 20 mg for 2 days; then off for 1 week. Extend dosing if required
	And/or oral doxycycline 100 mg twice a day over 3 weeks[a]	
	And/or oral methotrexate 10–15 mg once a week, with usual folic acid supplementation	Methotrexate has been shown in some case series to be highly effective in granulomatous reactions to permanent fillers [10,**11**,12]
	And/or oral fumaric acid tablets (Figure 158.8)	This is a drug used in psoriasis and has shown some effect in sarcoidal granulomas
Third line: surgical treatment	Excision	Be aware of scar formation
	Laser	Diode and CO_2 lasers are used to drill openings in the granulomas and the filler is then extruded [22]

[a] Low-dose oral doxycycline 40 mg once a day, as it is used in rosacea, might be an alternative.

Animal studies demonstrate that an occlusion was reversible in a 4 h period only [19]. After 24 h, the effects were less reversible (Table 158.4). However, expert consensus recommends treatment with hyaluronidase even after 24 h. Injections should be repeated until the pain subsides. In the case of acute blindness after an HA injection, the patient should be given an immediate hyaluronidase injection around the treated area. It is not clear whether retrobulbar injection of hyaluronidase is helpful [20]. In any case the patient should be seen as an emergency by an ophthalmologist.

In conclusion, the treatment of adverse reactions to dermal filler injections remains a significant challenge. The evidence that underpins recommendations is based on expert opinion and/or case series only. Nevertheless, adverse reactions appear to be diminishing over the years, particularly with the increasing popularity of biodegradable products where the risk of persistent sequelae is very low [21].

Table 158.4 Treatment approach for different cases of arterial occlusion.

Type of case	Treatment	Comments
Blanching and severe pain or loss of vision	Stop the filler injection immediately	
Signs of cutaneous occlusion following the use of a hyaluronic acid (HA) filler	Inject hyaluronidase around the injected area and the course of the affected artery; repeat if necessary over several days until the pain subsides	Although hyaluronidase is most effective in the first 4 h after injection, hyaluronidase should be always used in vascular occlusion even when diagnosed a couple of days after the event
Signs of cutaneous occlusion following the use of a non-HA filler	Apply topical nitroglycerine to enhance dermal blood flow[a]	
Loss of vision	In the case of an HA, inject hyaluronidase immediately where the original filler was injected. There is some controversy over whether retrobulbar injections are helpful or not [20]. Urgent ophthalmologist referral is advised	Due to the rarity of this adverse event the evidence for all treatment options is more based on theoretical considerations instead of good evidence [20]

[a] Although a recent animal study questions the use of topical nitroglycerin [23].

Fillers and different skin types

Most filler studies have been conducted on skin types I–III. This may be due to the natural photoprotection from premature skin ageing present in darker skin, with a subsequent later presentation of the signs of facial ageing. There are no known differences in cases of immunological reactions between different skin types, therefore the rate of adverse reactions can be assumed to be quite similar independent of the type of skin.

Darker skin may react with more hyperpigmentation to inflammation; some smaller studies and a data subanalysis project examining patients with skin types IV–VI are ongoing. Marmur et al. [1] could not show an increased risk of any adverse reaction in a case series of patients with skin types IV–VI treated with CaHa. Similar results were reported by Downie et al. [2] when looking at an HA (Belotero Balance®) and Grimes et al. [3] for the Juvéderm range, the latter being a subanalysis of trial data already available. In addition, there is a study from India examining 30 patients with skin type IV–VI who were treated with an HA (Restylane Perlane now Restylane Lyft). Efficacy and safety were similar compared with fair skin patients [4]. However, as there is a higher risk of postinflammatory hyperpigmentation in adverse reactions such as abscess formation, the frequency of hyperpigmentation in these selected cases might be higher.

One needs to be aware of the myths and knowledge gaps associated with aesthetic treatments in patients with skin of colour. On balance, the risks of filler treatments are similar independent of ethnicity [5].

Acknowledgements

Parts of this chapter are based on the second edition of *Injectable Fillers in Aesthetic Medicine* by de Maio and this author, published in 2014 [1]. I would like to thank Tamara Griffiths for her thorough review and the provision of the two histological photos.

Key references

The full list of references can be found in the online version at https://www.wiley.com/rooksdermatology10e

Fillers
1 Narins RS, Brandt F, Leyden J *et al*. A randomized, double-blind, multicenter comparison of the efficacy and tolerability of Restylane versus Zyplast for the correction of nasolabial folds. *Dermatol Surg* 2003;29:588–95.
7 Rzany B, Cartier H, Kestemont P *et al*. Full-face rejuvenation using a range of hyaluronic acid fillers: efficacy, safety, and patient satisfaction over 6 months. *Dermatol Surg* 2012;38:1153–61.
11 Jones D, Murphy DK. Volumizing hyaluronic acid filler for midface volume deficit: 2-year results from a pivotal single-blind randomized controlled study. *Dermatol Surg* 2013;39:1602–1.
14 Artzi O, Loizides C, Verner I, Landau M. Resistant and recurrent late reaction to hyaluronic acid-based gel. *Dermatol Surg* 2016;42:31–7.
60 Pérez-Ruiz C, Barabash-Neila R, Zulueta-Dorado T, Conejo-Mir Sánchez J. Adverse granulomatous reaction to silicone filler treated with methotrexate. *Dermatol Surg* 2019;45:489–92.
68 Alijotas-Reig J, Fernández-Figueras MT, Puig L. Late-onset inflammatory adverse reactions related to soft tissue filler injections. *Clin Rev Allergy Immunol* 2013; 45:97–108.
79 Roßner M, Roßner F, Bachmann F, Wiest L, Rzany B. Increased risk of severe adverse reactions towards an injectable filler composed of a fixed combination of methacrylate particles and hyaluronic acid (Dermalive). *Dermatol Surg* 2009;35(Suppl. 1):367–74.

Common injection errors and how to avoid them
5 Jones D, Murphy DK. Volumizing hyaluronic acid filler for midface volume deficit: 2-year results from a pivotal single-blind randomized controlled study. *Dermatol Surg* 2013;39:1602–12.

Adverse reactions and their treatment
9 Alijotas-Reig J, Fernández-Figueras MT, Puig L. Late-onset inflammatory adverse reactions related to soft tissue filler injections. *Clin Rev Allergy Immunol* 2013;45:97–108.
11 Pérez-Ruiz C, Barabash-Neila R, Zulueta-Dorado T, Conejo-Mir Sánchez J. Adverse granulomatous reaction to silicone filler treated with methotrexate. *Dermatol Surg* 2019;45:489–92.

Acknowledgements
1 De Maio M, Rzany B. *Injectable Fillers in Aesthetic Medicine*, 2nd edn. Heidelberg: Springer, 2014.

CHAPTER 159

Aesthetic Uses of Botulinum Toxins

Nicholas J. Lowe[1] and Philippa L. Lowe[2]

[1]University of Manchester, Manchester, UK; UCLA School of Medicine, Los Angeles, CA, USA
[2]Manchester, UK

Introduction, 159.1
History and early research, 159.1
History of clinical applications, 159.2
Pharmacology and action of neurotoxins, 159.2
Variation and equivalence, 159.3
Clinical applications of botulinum toxins for aesthetic indications, 159.3

Upper face, 159.4
Mid face, 159.5
Lower face, 159.5
Neck, 159.6
Ethnic diversity and botulinum toxins, 159.6
Adverse events, 159.6

Special considerations, 159.8
Acquired resistance to botulinum toxins, 159.8
Combination treatment, 159.8
Future botulinum toxins in development, 159.8

Key references, 159.9

Introduction

Botulinum neurotoxins, sometimes referred to as neuromodulators, have proven efficacy for a variety of clinical conditions resulting from neuromuscular hyperactivity, which includes spasticity and blepharospasm. The approved aesthetic and dermatological indications for type A botulinum toxins include treatment of hyperfunctional facial muscles causing facial lines and the treatment of focal hyperhidrosis.

In 1992, the seminal observation that botulinum toxin type A (BTX-A) was effective in reducing muscle-induced forehead lines was reported [1]. This was followed by double-blind, placebo-controlled, evidence-based studies confirming the efficacy of BTX-A for the reduction of dynamic facial lines [2,3,4,5]. Botox™, now designated onabotulinumtoxinA (BTX-A Ona), was developed in the USA as the first BTX-A for aesthetic treatments. It rapidly gained popularity during the 1990s and the early 21st century [1,2,3,4,5] as a paradigm shift in the treatment of facial rejuvenation. In the UK, an alternative type of BTX-A known as Dysport™, now designated abobotulinumtoxinA (BTX-A Abo), was developed for similar indications. Controlled clinical trials followed with publications in 2004 and 2006 [6,7].

Another approved indication for BTX-A Ona is the treatment of severe axillary sweating. The treatment of gustatory sweating was reported by Naumann *et al.* [8] and was followed by studies treating severe axillary hyperhidrosis with BTX-A Ona [9]. BTX-A is now a recognised treatment option for severe localised hyperhidrosis and is discussed in more detail in Chapter 92.

Three types of BTX-A currently exist and are approved in Europe and the USA for several aesthetic indications (Table 159.1). In addition, botulinum toxin type B (BTX-B) has distinct pharmacological mechanisms but similar clinical responses to those of type A toxins.

Table 159.1 Pharmaceutical terminology of some available neurotoxins in 2022.

Trade name	Pharmaceutical name
Botox	Ona botulinum toxin type A
Dysport	Abo botulinum toxin type A
Xeomin	Inco botulinum toxin type A
Myobloc/NeuroBloc	Rima botulinum toxin type B

History and early research

Botulism was first described by a German physician, Justinus Kerner, in the early 19th century when he observed outbreaks of food poisoning from contaminated sausages [10]. He noted neurological effects resulting in muscle paralysis and then death secondary to respiratory depression. In the late 19th century, van Ermengem identified the bacterium causing botulism which he named the botulinum bacterium. This terminology was later changed to *Clostridium botulinum* [10].

In the 1940s, the USA and UK developed botulinum toxins as potential biological agents to be used during the Second World War. As a corollary, vaccines were also developed in order to prevent troops from succumbing to reciprocal biological warfare from the enemy. BTX-A toxin was purified and developed by Edward J. Schantz at the US biological warfare centre in Fort Detrick, Maryland [1]. This strain later became known as Occulinum™ and then Botox, or Ona BTX-A. In the UK, at the Porton Down biological warfare centre on Salisbury Plain, research was conducted with a different serotype of BTX-A with similar characteristics to the Fort Detrick toxin, which became known as Dys*port* after *Port*on Down, now called Abo BTX-A.

Medical use of Ona BTX-A was pioneered by ophthalmologist Alan Scott in an attempt to discover a non-surgical treatment for

---

Rook's Textbook of Dermatology, Tenth Edition. Edited by Christopher Griffiths, Jonathan Barker, Tanya Bleiker, Walayat Hussain and Rosalind Simpson.
© 2024 John Wiley & Sons Ltd. Published 2024 by John Wiley & Sons Ltd.

strabismus. Scott had obtained the toxin from Fort Detrick and initially studied the effects of this toxin in the ocular muscles of monkeys [11].

In the 1980s, Scott and colleagues proved that it was possible to improve strabismus by injecting BTX-A into the appropriate periocular muscles. The trade name of this injectable toxin became Occulinum and it was utilised for the treatment of strabismus, blepharospasm and hemifacial spasm [12,13]. Another pharmaceutical company subsequently acquired Occulinum and renamed it Botox.

History of clinical applications

It was noted during the treatment of strabismus that BTX-A could reduce wrinkles in the glabellar region of the face. These seminal observations were reported by Jean Carruthers, an ophthalmologist, and Alastair Carruthers, a dermatologist, in 1992 [1]. Other researchers confirmed these findings in double-blind placebo-controlled studies, demonstrating the ability of BTX-A to reduce what were essentially hyperfunctional muscle-induced facial lines [2,3,4,5], or so-called dynamic wrinkles. In 2002, the US regulatory body, the Food and Drug Administration (FDA), approved Ona BTX-A for the treatment of glabellar lines, and regulatory body approval in a variety of other countries including the UK followed shortly thereafter. An additional approved indication, the treatment of severe axillary hyperhidrosis, has been confirmed as safe and effective in evidence-based multicentre studies [9].

In addition to the reduction of facial lines and hyperhidrosis, there are many other approved and non-approved indications for botulinum toxins in medicine. These include conditions relating to muscle hyperactivity such as focal dystonia, blepharospasm, cervical dystonia, spasmodic dysphonia, writer's cramp, occupational cramps, hemifacial spasm, spasticity of the limbs in adults and children, strabismus, nystagmus, brow ptosis, facial tics, rigidity syndromes and bruxism. Autonomic nervous system indications include focal hyperhidrosis, gustatory sweating, hyperlacrimation and sialorrhoea. Various organ systems are covered, including urological indications such as overactive bladder, vaginismus, urethrism; gastrointestinal indications such as anal fissures, outlet constipation and sphincter of Oddi dysfunction; and neurological applications for the treatment of essential tremor, parkinsonian tremor and spasticity, pain control in migraine and focal muscle pain [14].

Pharmacology and action of neurotoxins

The clinical effects of BTX-A and BTX-B result from pharmacological action at the neuromuscular junction blocking release of acetylcholine (Ach) at the neuronal endplate [15,16], with subsequent inhibition of muscular contraction (Figure 159.1). The core molecule in all botulinum toxins is a 150 kDa protein with three distinct domains, and various accessory or neurotoxin-associated proteins (NAPs) according to serotype.

The three domains of the core molecule are the binding domain, translocation domain and catalytic domain. The binding domain docks with specific receptors on the neuronal surface and the translocation domain allows for entry of the catalytic domain into

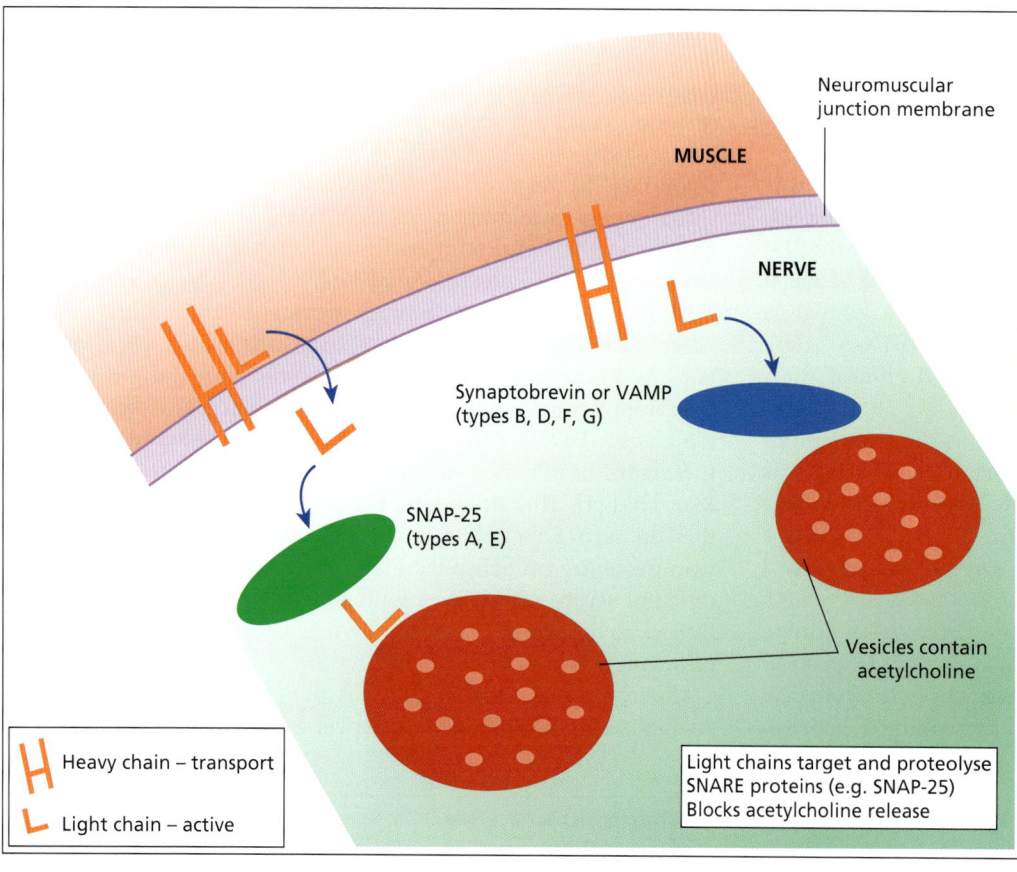

Figure 159.1 Different botulinum toxins block acetylcholine release via different synaptic proteins, BTX-A bind to SNAP-25 and BTX-B binds to synaptobrevin. VAMP, vesicle-associated membrane protein.

Table 159.2 Some characteristics of the botulinum neurotoxins.

Product (trade name)	Toxin type	Molecular weight (kDa)	pH	Approved for facial etc. lines	Approved for hyperhidrosis	Approved for some medical indications, e.g. cervical dystonia, blepharospasm
Botox[a]	A	900	7	Yes	Yes	Yes
Dysport	A	500–900	7	Yes	No	Yes
Xeomin	A	150	7	Yes	No	Yes
Myobloc/NeuroBloc	B	300–500	5.6	No	No	Yes

[a] Botox was also approved for crow's feet by the US Food and Drug Administration, October 2013.

the cell. Once inside the neuron, the catalytic domain binds to specific intracellular proteins resulting in the blockade of neurotransmitter release. The catalytic domain of BTX-A binds to intracellular SNAP-25 proteins [15] which prevents exocytosis of ACh from the synaptic vesicle, thus inhibiting muscular contraction. BTX-B binds the intracellular synaptic protein synaptobrevin [16], also referred to as vesicle-associated membrane protein (VAMP), likewise preventing ACh transportation across the neuronal cell membrane into the neuromuscular junction and blockading muscular contraction. It is thought that the limited duration of the clinical effect of botulinum toxins results from the synthesis of new synaptic proteins over time, re-establishment of ACh release and subsequent muscular activity.

Variation and equivalence

Manufacture of botulinum toxins utilises similar processes of anaerobic fermentation to those used to produce *Clostridium botulinum*. The toxin produced by the bacteria is then separated and purified by a variety of proprietary methods. It is likely that the active light chain toxin in all proprietary BTX-A products is identical, but variations in subsequent manufacturing processes result in pharmacological differences between the final products. These include differences in molecular weight, among other formulation variations (Table 159.2). Botulinum toxin potency is estimated as units of activity. These vary among the different type A toxins and have been the subject of numerous comparative studies [5,6,7,17–19]. The following summary of the comparative per unit therapeutic efficacy is based on such studies, and on anecdotal and personal experience:

Ona BTX-A 1 unit equivalent to Inco BTX-A 1.25 units equivalent to Abo BTX-A 3 units

It must be stressed that it is best practice to consider each as a different drug, the dose of which is to be individually determined.

Clinical applications of botulinum toxins for aesthetic indications

Applications for the aesthetic use of botulinum toxin have become well documented over the last two decades. The main target muscles for botulinum toxin in the face are shown in Figure 159.2, with some common sites for these injections indicated. These will vary with the individual patient and tailored treatment after careful assessment is key to an optimal outcome.

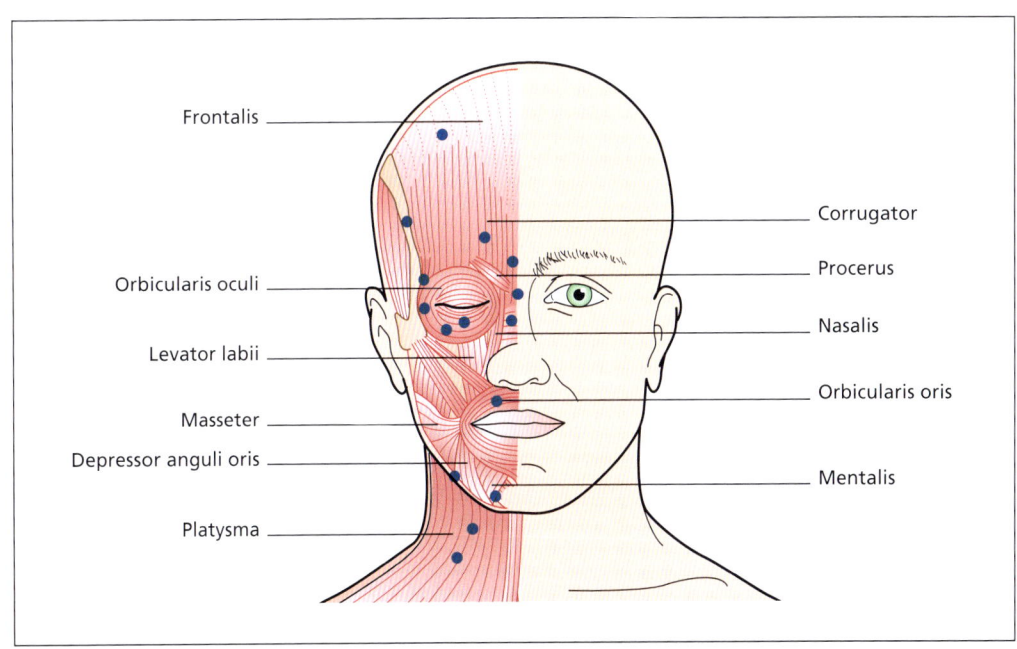

Figure 159.2 Idealised diagram of the facial muscles that create rhytides that can be injected with botulinum toxin for aesthetic changes to the face. The blue dots indicate some of the frequent sites used for such injections.

There are many variations in the selection of injection site, and treatment must be tailored according to the muscular dynamics of the patient; what is considered to be optimum placement continues to evolve over time. Industry-sponsored research studies involving botulinum toxin injections into the lower forehead utilised different injection sites in order to gain relevant regulatory approval [4,5,6,18]. Idealised diagrams can be helpful but are not necessarily relevant or optimal for individual patients, due to the frequency of facial asymmetry or imbalance in baseline muscular action.

In reality, the first and most critical aspect of cosmetic facial use of botulinum toxin injection is to learn how to accurately examine the patient. Assessment should be made at facial rest and at maximum muscle contraction. It is these authors' practice to take facial photographs at rest and at maximum muscle contraction. Many cases of facial asymmetry are found and as a result require a change from the 'standard' patterns of injection sites for botulinum toxin that are recommended in many articles.

Upper face

Most of the clinical research studies addressing the cosmetic use of botulinum toxin for forehead rhytids have focused on dividing varying doses of BTX-A over five to seven injection sites [1,2,3,4,5]. In general, one or two injection sites into the procerus and usually two each into each corrugator are the ideal injection sites frequently cited in education and training for the cosmetic use of botulinum toxin. The relevant injection sites and doses of various BTX-A serotypes must be based on a detailed knowledge of facial anatomy. The desired aesthetic outcome requires appropriate training and experience, underpinned by a fundamental knowledge of the evidence-based research and literature [1,2,3,4,5].

The muscles producing the frown or 'knitting of the brow' were those first studied for regulatory approval of the cosmetic use of BTX-A. All three commercially available BTX-A products were first approved for injection at this site. Figure 159.3 shows the injection sites from an early study on Ona BTX-A [3]. The corrugator and procerus are the most important muscles that lead to lower and central vertical forehead lines. These muscles are also responsible for eyebrow depression and ptosis (Figures 159.3, 159.4 and 159.5). It must be noted that the frontalis muscle is the main brow elevator that lifts the forehead and brows, and is responsible for horizontal forehead lines. Understanding the brow depressor/elevator muscle balance is key to successful upper face botulinum toxin rejuvenation strategies.

Glabellar area

The muscles that create vertical forehead lines in the glabellar area also often act as brow depressors and are as follows:
- Corrugator muscle.
- Procerus muscle.

Brow elevation is produced mainly by the frontalis muscle. When the corrugator and procerus muscles contract, the facial expression is that of anger or concern. Contracting the corrugator muscles also results in narrowing of the eyes. Contracting the procerus muscle induces further medial brow depression and creates horizontal lines between the eyebrows and the bridge of the nose [5,7,20].

Forehead

The frontalis muscle is employed to raise the eyebrows and to prevent eyebrow ptosis. It also creates forehead expression lines that are

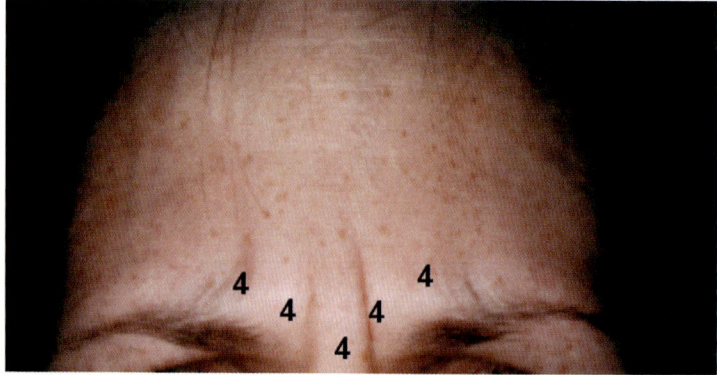

(a)

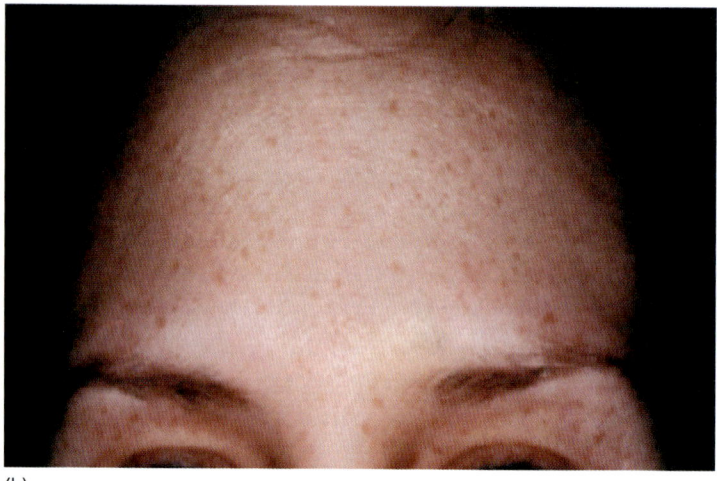

(b)

Figure 159.3 (a) Usual injection sites for a symmetrical forehead with vertical glabella lines before treatment and to correct brow ptosis: 4 Ona BTX-A units per site. (b) Patient photographed attempting to frown 7 days after injection of BTX-A.

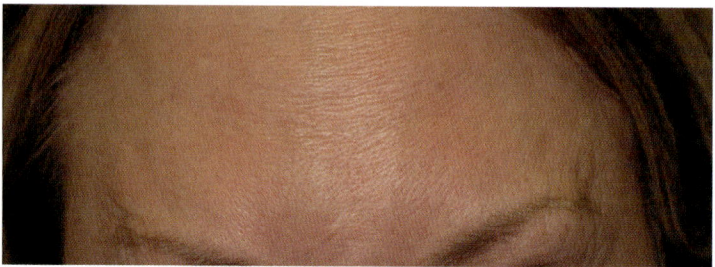

Figure 159.4 Forehead facial asymmetry. Stronger right corrugator and procerus muscles resulted in right brow ptosis compared with left.

horizontal and can express surprise or fear. Botulinum toxin treatment to the mid and lateral forehead should be performed with relatively small amounts of toxin compared with the glabellar area. Overdose of toxin across the frontalis muscle inevitably results in undesirable brow ptosis.

Individual injection site doses and the number of sites used will vary between the different proprietary brands of botulinum toxin. Complications in this area of injection are relatively rare, but occur as a result of the wrong placement of the toxin, for example too large a dose of BTX-A can result in either eyelid or eyebrow ptosis or both if placed in the lateral forehead. In some patients, there

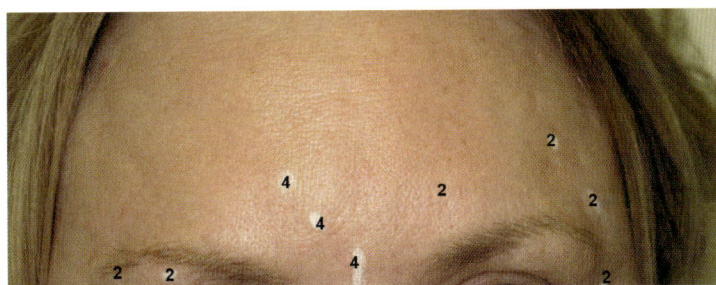

Figure 159.5 Forehead facial asymmetry using 2 BTX-A units and 4 Ona BTX-A units or equivalent. The aesthetic goal was to (i) reduce right brow depressors and give brow elevation; and (ii) maintain left brow height and shape.

is relative ptosis of one brow compared with the other and appropriate adjustment to the standard injection site and dose is required to achieve brow lift of the lower brow side. Examples of idealised injection sites in a 'symmetrical' forehead are shown in Figure 159.3. Examples of forehead facial asymmetry are shown in Figures 159.4 and 159.5.

The differences between male and female eyebrow shape should be noted. Many males prefer a flatter brow, whereas the ideal feminine brow is slightly arched mediolaterally. In men, additional injection sites and higher units can be used in the lateral forehead to achieve a more masculine brow appearance. Facial musculature also varies between sexes, with increased strength and bulk in men. Therefore, higher doses and increased number of injection sites are generally required in men in all regions of the face (Figure 159.6).

Brows

The corrugator and procerus are the primary muscles used for brow depression. There is a further contribution from the superolateral orbicularis oculi muscle. Selective reduction in the activity of these muscles with botulinum toxin can result in the elevation of the lateral and to a lesser degree the medial brow. This is often the desired aesthetic outcome in women. Overelevation of the brow resulting in unnaturally arched or pointed eyebrows is usually undesirable, but can be corrected with injections of small doses of BTX into the lateral lower frontalis muscle.

Crow's feet or lateral canthal and periorbital lines

Commonly known as crow's feet, the lateral periorbital lines radiate outwards from the lateral canthal area (Figures 159.7 and 159.8). They are caused by the contraction of the orbicularis oculi muscle; wrinkles are exacerbated by squinting and smiling. In addition, both intrinsic and extrinsic skin ageing will add to their persistence and severity [21].

In order to reduce these lines, the target muscle for the botulinum toxin is the lateral orbicularis oculi. The ideal site is determined by examination of the patient at both smiling and at rest. Typically, two to four injections are placed around the lateral canthal area on each side, 1–2 cm lateral to the ocular bony rim (Figure 159.7) [21]. If there is coexistent cutaneous photodamage exacerbating periocular lines in the crow's feet region, combination treatment with laser resurfacing can be used (Figure 159.8) [22]. Infraorbital lines can also be reduced by very small and carefully placed doses of botulinum toxin (Figure 159.9).

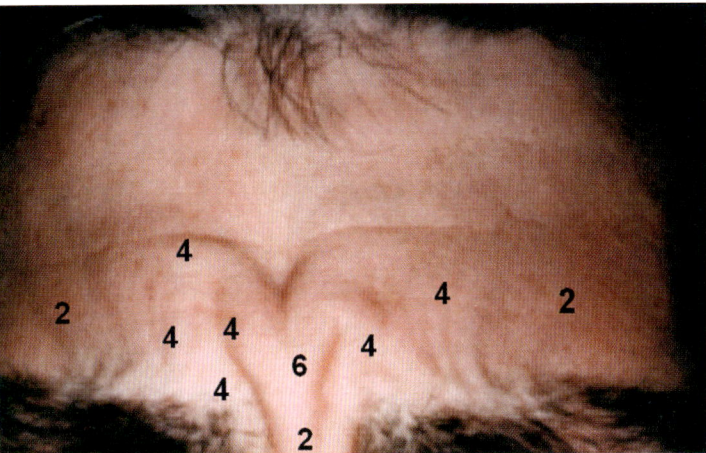

(a)

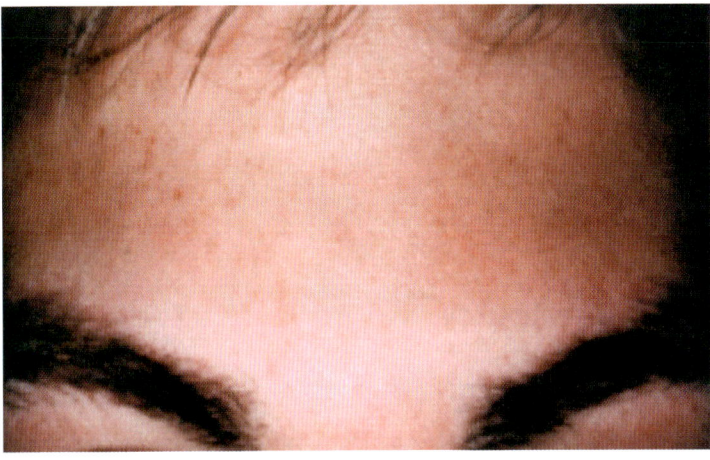

(b)

Figure 159.6 Higher total doses of BTX-A are often required in the male forehead: total of 36 Ona BTX-A units. (a) Male forehead with the corrugator and procerus muscles creating multiple vertical and horizontal lines and brow points. The location of the injection sites (and number of units at each) are indicated. (b) Seven days later showing a smooth forehead at frown plus brow elevation.

Mid face

The mid face area can be also selected as a site for cosmetic botulinum toxin injections. Lateral nasal lines can be reduced by treating the nasalis muscle [20]. Drooping of the nasal tip occurs with age and slight elevation can be achieved with small doses of botulinum toxin into the depressor septi nasi muscle. An exaggerated gum show with smiling, also referred to as a 'gummy smile', is considered unattractive in some patients, where the central upper lip is elevated excessively with smiling. This can be improved with injection into the levator labii superioris alaeque nasi muscle.

Lower face

There are several muscles targeted for aesthetic botulinum toxin treatment in the lower face. These include the depressor anguli oris muscle that depresses the angles of the mouth often leading to a 'sad' appearance (Figure 159.2). Injection is at the very lower point of this muscle where it inserts into the mandibular area. This is found by teeth clenching, and injecting just anteriorly to the anterior border of the masseter on the mandible.

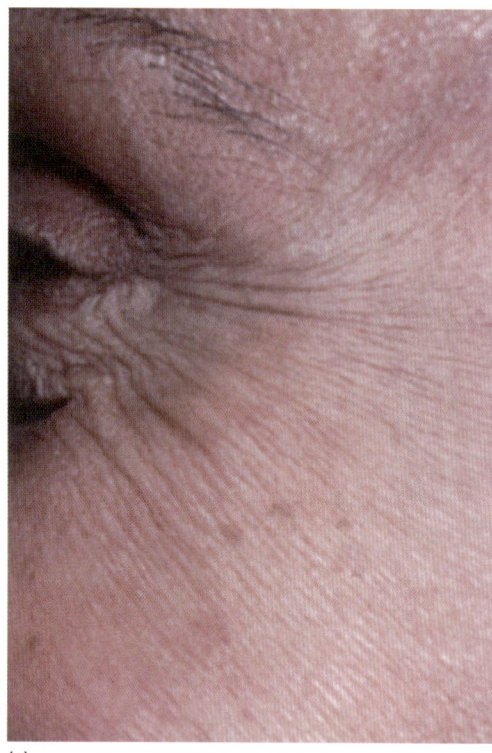
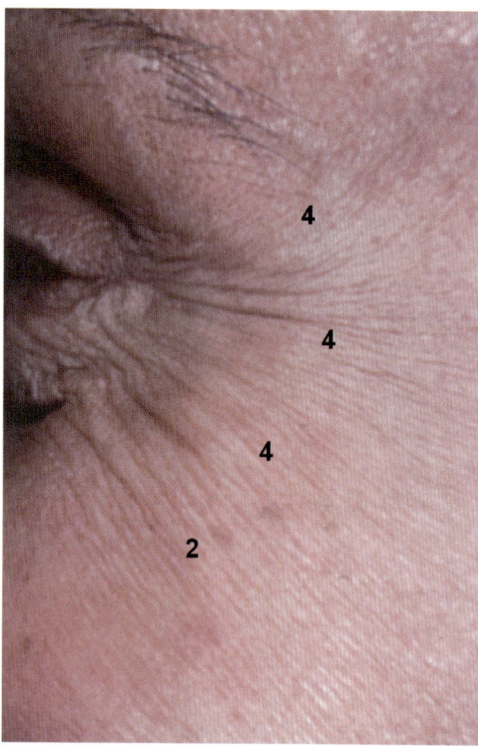

Figure 159.7 Crow's feet. (a) Wrinkles extending laterally from the periorbital area produced by contraction of the orbicularis oculi muscle. (b) BTX-A injection sites and number of Ona BTX-A units injected at each site.

The orbicularis oris muscle is responsible in part for lines between the upper lip and nose, so-called smoker's lip lines. They are caused by lip pursing and contraction and with time these lines become more severe and visible even at rest. Very small doses of botulinum toxin can be injected into the relevant part of the upper lip (Figure 159.10). Additionally, if the upper lip is atrophic, combination with hyaluronic acid filler has been described [23].

The primary chin muscle is the mentalis. Activation can lead to puckering of the chin, known as a 'peau d'orange' appearance. It can also lead to additional depression of the angles of the mouth. This pebbling or puckering of the chin can be corrected by a single injection of a relatively small dose of BTX into the centre of the mentalis muscle (Figure 159.11).

Masseter prominence and hypertrophy has been successfully treated with BTX both for aesthetic reshaping of the face and temporomandibular joint pain from teeth clenching. A reduction of masseter prominence is particularly sought in East Asian countries such as Korea to reduce the perceived over-squared lower face [24].

Neck

The main muscles of the neck appropriate for aesthetic injections of botulinum toxin are the bands of the platysma muscle. Platysmal vertical bands tend to become more notable with age because of the loss of subcutaneous fat, exposing the platysma muscle [23]. The platysma tightens the skin of the neck and in addition can produce depression of the lateral face. In some patients, activation of the platysma can produce downward pull of the perioral lateral area and the medial and lateral cheek. The injection of small doses of BTX-A into the platysma can reduce the 'bands' produced by the platysma as well as reduce downward traction of the lateral face [25].

Although there have been anecdotal claims for the value of botulinum toxin injections to reduce horizontal superficial neck lines, the impact is minimal, though some effect may be achieved by reduction of the platysma muscle action.

Ethnic diversity and botulinum toxins

Botulinum toxins have been successfully used for aesthetic indications in different ethnic groups. For example, different upper facial characteristics are important aesthetic considerations in East Asia where the idealised eye shape differs from those of most white people. One study reported on the efficacy of BTX-A Ona for lateral canthal lines in a large cohort of Chinese patients assessed using facial line outcome and facial line satisfaction questionnaires [26]. This confirmed the findings from other studies on Japanese patients [27] and suggested a faster reported improvement for lateral canthal lines in East Asian patients compared with those for white patients.

Adverse events

Serious side effects from botulinum toxin for aesthetic indications are uncommon because the total doses utilised are low. The main causes for adverse events are poor injection technique, inappropriate dose selection and incorrect injection site. Resultant side effects are listed in Box 159.1. Undesirable results and complications are usually mild and transient. Poor results may be improved by further injection (e.g. into compensatory muscles) in order to correct or minimise the unsatisfactory response. It is imperative that the practitioner understands the complexities of the relevant muscle vectors for a satisfactory and natural outcome.

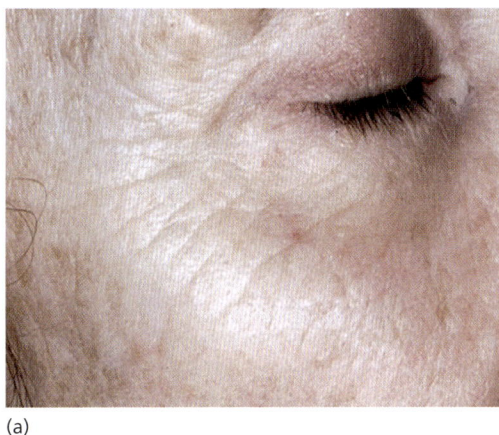

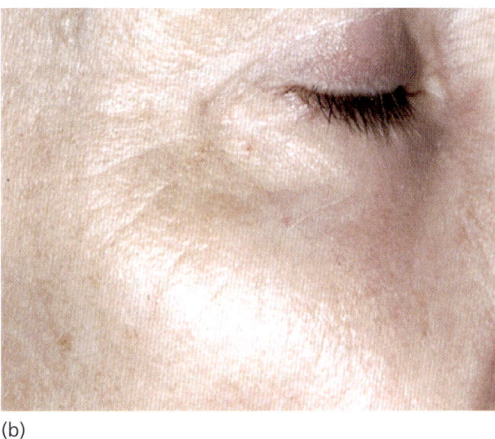

Figure 159.8 Crow's feet: treatment with a combination of BTX-A followed by ultrapulsed carbon dioxide laser. (a) Before, showing crow's feet plus multiple lentigo. (b) Six months post procedure.

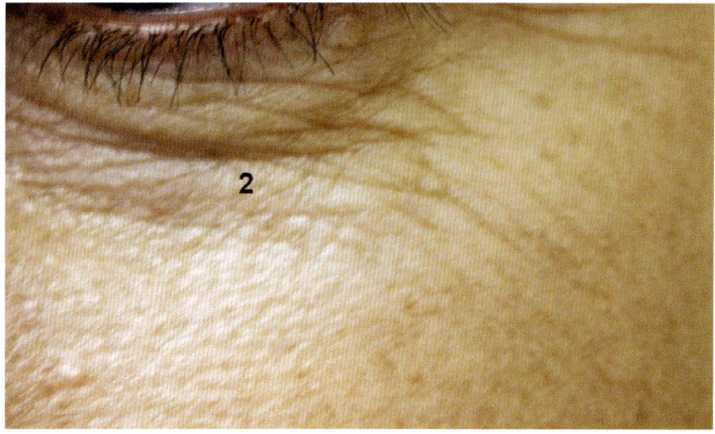

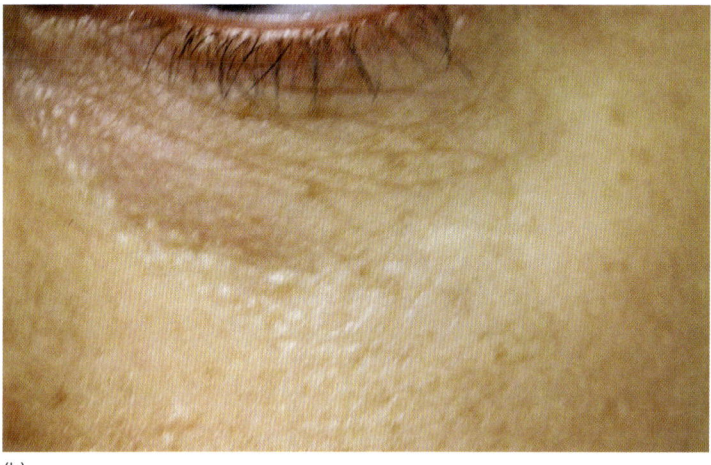

Figure 159.9 Infraorbital lines: (a) before treatment with 2 units BTX-A, and (b) 7 days later.

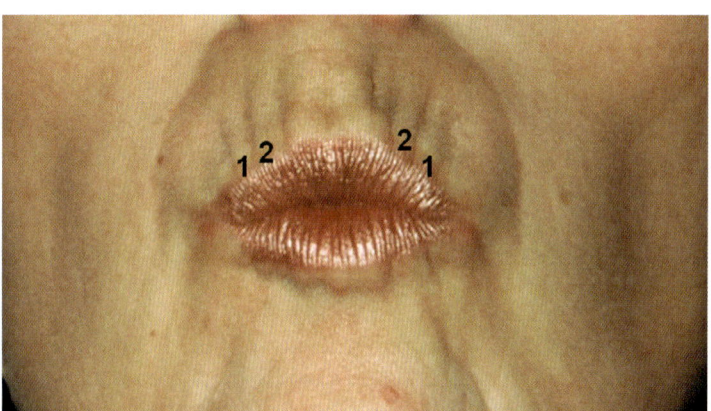

Figure 159.10 Perioral wrinkling due to contraction of the orbicularis muscle and dermal actinic elastosis. Treatment is with 1–2 Ona BTX-A units per wrinkle site, with a maximum of 4–6 units per lip per session.

> **Box 159.1 Summary of reported side effects following aesthetic treatment with botulinum toxin**
>
> **More frequent**
> - Bruising
> - Lower eyelid oedema
> - Brow ptosis and lower face asymmetry
>
> **Less frequent**
> - Headaches
> - Flu syndromes
>
> **Much less frequent**
> - Diplopia
> - Distant muscle weakness (dysarthria) with platysmal injections
> - Hypersensitivity reactions
> - Dry mouth, dry eyes

Bruising from needle injections is probably the most common side effect, occurring most frequently in the periorbital region (e.g. the lateral periocular crow's feet area). The forehead is the second most common site. Bruising can usually be avoided by close examination of the patient's cutaneous vascular network. Further mitigation of bruising risk involves avoidance of injection in those patients taking medications or supplements that increase the predisposition to bruising, such as those taking aspirin, non-steroidal anti-inflammatory agents, anticoagulant drugs or oral omega-3 and omega-6 fish oil supplements, as well as excessive ingestion of oily fish or alcohol. Local skin swelling at the injection site is usually

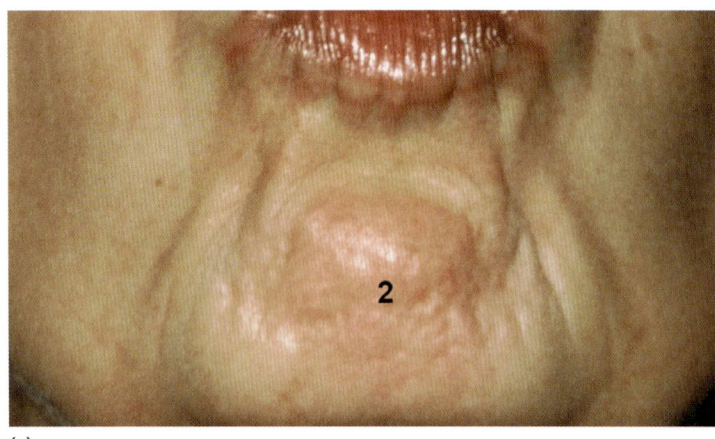

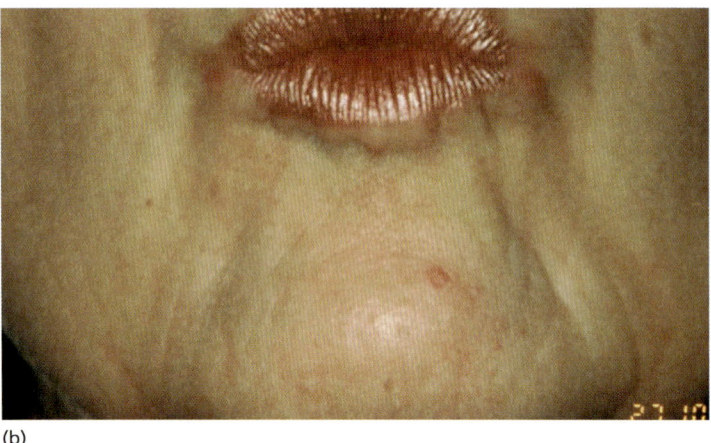

Figure 159.11 Mentalis muscle 'creases' treated with BTX-A. (a) Before treatment with 2 Ona BTX-A units. (b) 7 days later.

more visible on the forehead skin, but will clear within an hour or less.

Postinflammatory hyperpigmentation is a higher risk in darker skin phototypes following bruising.

Another common side effect is pain on injection. Rarely, patients may have a persistent headache and pain lasting several days. The mechanisms for this are not known, but may possibly be due to injection close to a subcutaneous nerve. This pain is paradoxical, as one of the medical indications for botulinum toxin is reduction in frequency and severity of migraine headaches.

Other site-specific side effects relating to botulinum toxin for aesthetic treatments are eyebrow and lower eyelid ptosis. Again, this usually results from inaccurate placement of the botulinum toxin, and is commonly the result of injection of too high a dose into the lower lateral or mediolateral forehead. The resultant diffusion of the toxin into the elevator muscles of the eye or lower fibres of the frontalis results in ptosis. Lower facial and lateral lip ptosis can also result when injections in the lower periocular area are too lateral and too low to the infraorbital areas, encroaching on the malar area. The effect of the toxin on the levator muscles of the lower face causes ptosis and lateral lip drooping. Facial asymmetry resulting from an unequal effect of the toxin is another complication which can be of considerable concern.

Less common side effects include paraesthesia, diplopia, dry eyes, dysphagia and dysarthria. These are all generally due to inappropriately high doses of toxin injection, with diffusion into either the periocular muscles or the muscles of the larynx and pharynx. Practitioners must remember the therapeutic window for a cosmetic patient is narrower than that of someone receiving medical therapy, therefore a cautious conservative approach is best, particularly for inexperienced practitioners.

Special considerations

The incidence of undesirable side effects is generally higher in older patients possibly because of increased spread of the toxin into atrophic muscles, as well as increased likelihood of weaker baseline facial musculature. Furthermore, in the older patient with more severe extrinsic and intrinsic facial ageing, it is unlikely that the use of botulinum toxin alone will be sufficient to result in an acceptable outcome.

Botulinum toxin use in the perioral area should be used with caution for professional wind musicians and singers where subtle alterations in fine muscular activity will have a significant impact. The same theoretical risk exists for the treatment of palmar hyperhidrosis in those who require very fine muscular control in the hands (e.g. for typing or for jewellers and musicians).

Contraindications to botulinum toxin injections include patients with a history of myasthenia gravis or other neuromuscular disorder. Pregnancy and breastfeeding are also contraindications (manufacturers advise avoidance unless essential for medical treatment). Some oral medication and supplements, such as oral erythromycin and zinc supplements, can also increase the therapeutic response to botulinum toxin. A careful medical history and examination are mandatory prior to botulinum toxin injection.

Acquired resistance to botulinum toxins

A rare problem is the development of acquired resistance to BTX-A. This does not appear to be related in all cases to the presence of antibodies, as resistance has been noted in patients where antibodies remain undetected. In addition, studies have demonstrated instances where antibodies to BTX-A are present, but a therapeutic response to the toxin persists. If BTX-A resistance occurs, BTX-B can be effective as it acts via a different synaptic protein [15–17].

Combination treatment

The various serotypes of botulinum toxin may be combined with selected treatments for aesthetic indications in relevant patients to enhance efficacy [20]. Such combination treatments include concomitant use with dermal fillers to facial folds and facial volume loss that may occur with age [23], with radiofrequency for skin tightening and lasers for skin rejuvenation procedures [22].

Future botulinum toxins in development

The development of a topical application of BTX-A was initially encouraging after research showed efficacy against hyperhidrosis and superficial facial lines [28]. Further research, however, did not confirm these studies and as yet there is no topical botulinum toxin approved.

A number of new type A toxins are in development or waiting regulatory approval in the UK or USA (in 2023) including prabotulinumtoxinA, daxibotulinumtoxinA and lanbotulinumtoxinA, as well as a liquid type of BTX-A Abo [29].

Another botulinum toxin is type E, which has a more rapid onset and shorter duration than type A toxins, the clinical uses of which are yet to be determined.

Key references

The full list of references can be found in the online version at https://www.wiley.com/rooksdermatology10e

1 Carruthers JD, Carruthers JA. Treatment of glabellar frown lines with C. botulinum-A toxin. *J Dermatol Surg Oncol* 1992;18:17–22.

4 Carruthers JD, Lowe NJ, Menter MA *et al.*, for the BOTOX Glabellar Lines I Study Group. A multicenter, double-blind, randomized, placebo-controlled study of the efficacy and safety of botulinum toxin type A in the treatment of glabellar lines. *J Am Acad Dermatol* 2002;46:840–9.

6 Ascher B, Zakine B, Kestemont P *et al*. A multicenter, randomized, double-blind, placebo-controlled study of efficacy and safety of 3 doses of botulinum toxin A in the treatment of glabellar lines. *J Am Acad Dermatol* 2004;51:223–33.

7 Lowe P, Patnaik R, Lowe N. Comparison of two formulations of botulinum type A for the treatment of glabellar lines: a double-blind randomized study. *J Am Acad Dermatol* 2006;55:975–80.

9 Naumann M, Lowe NJ. Botulinum toxin type A in treatment of bilateral primary axillary hyperhydrosis; randomised parallel group, double blind, placebo controlled trial. *BMJ* 2001;323:1–4.

CHAPTER 160

Chemical Peels

Chee-Leok Goh[1] and Joyce Teng Ee Lim[2]

[1] National Skin Centre, Singapore; National University of Singapore, Singapore
[2] Joyce Lim Skin and Laser Clinic, Singapore

Introduction, 160.1	Pre-peel procedure, 160.6	Premature peeling, 160.12
Basic chemistry, 160.1	Counselling, 160.6	Milia and acneform eruption, 160.12
Peels with metabolic action, 160.1	Skin priming, 160.7	Postinflammatory hyperpigmentation, 160.12
Peels with caustic action, 160.2	Consent and photo documentation, 160.8	Infection, 160.13
Peels with toxic action, 160.3	Peeling procedure, 160.8	Allergic contact dermatitis, 160.13
Depth of peels, 160.4	Equipment, 160.8	Systemic toxicity, 160.13
Superficial peels, 160.4	Peeling technique, 160.8	Postinflammatory hypopigmentation, 160.14
Medium depth peels, 160.4	Peeling agents, 160.9	Scarring, 160.14
Deep peels, 160.5	Post-peel care, 160.11	Chemical peels in patients with skin of colour, 160.15
Indications and contraindications, 160.5	Side effects and complications, 160.11	
Indications, 160.5	Persistent redness, 160.11	Key references, 160.15
Contraindications, 160.6	Chemical burns, 160.12	

Introduction

For centuries people have sought treatments to improve the appearance and texture of their skin; for example, ancient Egyptians used animal oils, salt and alabaster [1] and Cleopatra was reported to bathe in sour milk for skin rejuvenation. Dermatologists began to explore various methods for skin peeling and rejuvenation in the mid-1800s. Chemical exfoliating agents were applied onto the skin surface to destroy the epidermis and/or dermis, thus stimulating cell regeneration and creating a facial resurfacing effect. Dermatologists who pioneered the use of peeling agents include Ferdinand Hebra, Tilbury Foc and Henry Piffard [2]. In the 1970s, work began on full-face peels with trichloroacetic acids (TCAs) and phenol. The α-hydroxy acids (AHAs) were introduced in the late 1970s by Van Scott and Yu [3], and salicylic acid was introduced in the 1990s. In the ensuing years, novel and more effective skin rejuvenation procedures using mechanical abrasion, lasers and light devices have been introduced. However, the use of chemical peeling remains popular both as a monotherapy and as part of combined therapy for skin rejuvenation, due to its efficacy, low cost and potential for minimal recovery time.

Basic chemistry

Peeling agents utilise a chemical solution to remove the skin's damaged outer layers, thereby improving texture and smoothness. They can also be used to remove facial imperfections such as actinic lentigines and fine wrinkles, and can also address actinic keratoses and be used to control acne [1–4]. Commonly used peeling agents are either alcohols that contain carboxyl (-COOH) and hydroxyl (-OH) groups or regular acids. Examples of peeling agents include AHAs, TCA, Jessner solution, salicylic acid, pyruvic acid and phenol-based formulae.

The chemicals used in skin peeling agents can be classified according to their chemical action and properties. These include (i) metabolic action (e.g. AHAs and pyruvic, azelaic and retinoic acid); (ii) caustic action (e.g. TCA); and (iii) toxic action (e.g. phenol, resorcinol and salicylic acid) [5].

Peels with metabolic action
Alpha-hydroxyl acids

Alpha-hydroxyl acids (e.g. glycolic, lactic, malic, oxalic, tartaric and citric acid) are carboxylic acids derived from fruits and vegetables and have been used in cosmetic preparations and procedures for centuries. AHAs are weak acids that induce their rejuvenation activity by either metabolic or caustic effect. At low concentration (<30%), AHAs reduce sulphate and phosphate groups from the surface of corneocytes. By decreasing corneocyte cohesion, they

Rook's Textbook of Dermatology, Tenth Edition. Edited by Christopher Griffiths, Jonathan Barker, Tanya Bleiker, Walayat Hussain and Rosalind Simpson.
© 2024 John Wiley & Sons Ltd. Published 2024 by John Wiley & Sons Ltd.

induce exfoliation of the stratum corneum. At higher concentration, their effect is mainly destructive.

The most common AHA used is glycolic acid (GA), which penetrates the skin easily due to its small molecular size. GA skin peels act very superficially and are more stimulatory than destructive. They induce a relatively acid pH, thereby acting as kerato-regulators that increase corneocyte shedding and cell replacement. AHAs disrupt enzymes (sulphotransferases, phosphotransferases and kinases) that function by fixing sulphate and phosphate groups onto the surface of the corneocytes. The reduction of these groups results in decreased corneocyte cohesion and subsequent exfoliation and shedding.

Topical AHAs (up to 25% glycolic, lactic or citric acid) diminish corneocyte cohesion immediately above the granular layer and reduce the number of desmosomes and the aggregation of tonofilaments. This results in stratum corneum detachment and desquamation as early as 24 h after treatment. When used in strong concentrations (30–70% free acid in aqueous solution), a destructive effect is exerted. The highest concentration without precipitation at room temperature is 70% with a pH of 0.5. The chemical effects of the many formulations of AHA differ based on the bioavailability of the acid, its concentration and the pH. Only free acid is biologically active, therefore higher concentrations and lower pH result in a proportionally stronger biological effect. Cosmetic products containing neutralised glycolic acid as an ester must be split by esterases or hydrolysed for activation.

Because of the low acidity of AHAs, they do not induce adequate coagulation of skin proteins. Therefore, they are unable to neutralise themselves and the application of water or weak buffer (e.g. sodium bicarbonate) is required once the desired depth has been reached.

Lactic acid (10–30%)

Lactic acid (LA) is structurally identical to GA but with a methyl group at the β-carbon end; it has a lower pKa and thus a lower pH at equivalent concentrations. It causes intraepidermal and dermal–epidermal junction disruption. It has comparable efficacy for treating photodamage, superficial hyperpigmentation and fine rhytides compared with GA. A lower concentration of LA is often used to achieve an equivalent depth of kerato-coagulation compared with GA. Neutralisation is necessary, and exfoliation after treatment typically occurs over several days, with complete re-epithelialisation in 7–10 days.

Pyruvic acid

Pyruvic acid (PA), the smallest α-ketoacid, is structurally a carboxylic acid with a functional ketone moiety. It has similar keratolytic properties to salicylic acid (SA) but has less lipophilicity. It causes intraepidermal and dermal–epidermal junction disruption. It is also partially hydrophilic, giving it properties of both SA and GA. Clinically, PA peels have demonstrated efficacy in the treatment of acne vulgaris and associated disorders of excess sebum production and mild photoageing and hyperpigmentation. It is commonly used as a superficial peeling agent for inflammatory and comedonal acne, though it is not as efficacious as salicylic acid due to reduced penetration through the lipid barriers of the epidermis. Pyruvic acid is not self-neutralising and will continue to cause kerato-coagulation for the duration of exposure to the skin until it is neutralised with an alkaline solution. Exfoliation after treatment typically occurs over several days, and re-epithelialisation is complete within 5–10 days.

Azelaic acid

Azelaic acid is a saturated dicarboxylic acid produced by *Malassezia furfur* and is found naturally in wheat, rye and barley. It is active at a concentration of 20% in topical products and is used as therapy for a number of skin conditions – mainly acne and melasma. *In vitro*, azelaic acid works as a scavenger (captor) of free radicals. It normalises keratinisation and leads to a reduction in the content of free oily acids in the lipids on the skin surface.

Retinoic acid

Retinoic acid is the oxidised form of vitamin A (retinol). Retinol is present in food (β-carotene) and converts completely in the skin to retinaldehyde (retinal). Subsequently, 95% of this is converted into retinyl ester and 5% into all-*trans* and 9-*cis* retinoic acids. Retinoic acid acts by binding the retinoic acid receptor (RAR) and the retinoid X receptor (RXR) to heterodimers. These then bind to retinoic acid response elements (RAREs) in the regulatory regions of direct targets (including *Hox* genes), thereby activating gene transcription. RARs mediate transcription of different sets of genes involved in cell differentiation, normalising hyperkeratinisation for a peeling effect; it also has deeper dermal reparative impact.

Peels with caustic action
Trichloroacetic acid

Trichloroacetic acid, also referred to as trichloroethanoic acid, is an analogue of acetic acid in which the three hydrogen atoms of the methyl group have all been replaced by chlorine atoms. Its molecular structure is close to GA, but it is a much stronger acid; its pKa is 0.26, which is much closer to zero compared with the pKa of GA at 3.83. TCA is naturally found as hygroscopic and deliquescent crystals and is dissolved in distilled water to make aqueous solutions. The standard pharmaceutical method of preparing TCA solutions for dermatological use is the weight in volume (w/v) method, producing a clear and colourless liquid with no precipitate or particles. TCA has been the gold standard in chemical peeling for many decades.

By varying the concentration of TCA, one can control the depth of penetration into the skin. Concentrations of 10–25% are used for superficial peels, however the most popular TCA application is at a concentration of 35% for medium depth penetration, which can effectively treat dyschromias and early facial rhytids. There is destruction of the epidermis and upper papillary dermis, followed by epidermal and dermal regeneration, new collagen deposition and normalisation of the elastic tissue. Concentrations of more than 35% are not recommended due to less predictable results and risk of scarring.

The destructive activity of TCA is caused by its acidity in aqueous solution. The acid is rapidly neutralised through coagulation of skin proteins, which results in the clinical appearance of frosting. Like GA, TCA does not have general toxicity, even when applied in concentrated form on the skin, nor is there risk of allergic reaction.

Within a short period after application, the skin develops redness followed by a white frost, indicating coagulation of the epidermal proteins. The depth of penetration correlates with the intensity of the skin frost, which acts as a reliable clinical marker, and gives predictable results. Superficial TCA peels may demonstrate only redness or redness with irregular light frost. Higher concentrations will penetrate further into the skin as the acid seeks water for neutralisation in deeper cutaneous tissues, resulting in more intense and confluent frosting and intensifying its destructive effect. Multiple applications will also magnify impact.

There is no need to neutralise TCA; however dilution with water decreases its concentration and terminates its effect. Frosting disappears within 10–30 min and is replaced by skin redness, which may last for 1–2 days. Patients should be informed of the expected skin changes, which include redness, mild oedema, transient hyperpigmentation and occasionally symptoms of itching and tightness.

Jessner solution

Jessner solution (JS) contains 14% LA, 14% SA and 14% resorcinol in ethanol. JS provokes stratum corneum separation only, with upper epidermal intraepithelial and intercellular oedema. It is very easy to use, either alone or in combination with TCA. JS is a clear, faintly amber-coloured liquid. The depth of the peel is determined by the number of coats applied. JS is used for light peels alone or in preparation for a TCA peel.

Two or three applications of JS are typically used and the solution should be brushed uniformly over the entire surface to be peeled. On application there is an intense burning sensation, generally greater than that of GA. The first response is mild redness, followed by powdery whitening of the skin due to precipitation of the chemical compounds in the solution. This whitening is easily removed with water or by simple rubbing. An observable exfoliation may follow that lasts for 8–10 days.

Overpeel, or unintentional or inappropriate deeper skin destruction, is very rare and therefore the risk of complications is very low. Peelings can be repeated monthly.

Peels with toxic action
Phenol

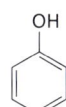

Phenol, C_6H_5OH, is an aromatic alcohol and a weak acid. Also known as carbolic acid, hydroxybenzene and phenic acid, phenol is a toxic, white, crystalline solid with a sweet tarry odour, commonly referred to as 'hospital smell'. It reacts with strong bases to form the salts called phenolates. Its pKa is high, at 9.9.

Phenol activity on the skin results from its direct toxicity to cell proteins and membranes and enzymatic inactivation. Phenol is a protoplasmic poison that works through enzymatic inactivation and protein denaturation with the production of insoluble proteinates. At a concentration of 88%, phenol causes immediate coagulation of epidermal keratin and penetrates only to the level of the upper reticular dermis. When diluted to 45–55%, phenol becomes a keratolytic, disrupting sulphur bonds, and thus has the capability to penetrate deeper to the mid-reticular dermis.

Deep chemical peels are used primarily to improve the appearance of cutaneous ageing. Changes such as deep rhytids, as well as dyschromia, solar elastosis and actinic keratoses, can be effectively treated. Phenol is partially inactivated by hepatic conjugation and is excreted by the kidney. It also has cardiotoxic effects, so for full-face peels cardiac monitoring and resuscitative equipment should be available. These risks have resulted in diminished popularity of its use.

Salicylic acid

Salicylic acid, $C_6H_4(OH)COOH$, is classified as a β-hydroxy acid. It is found naturally in certain plants (*Spiraea ulmaria*, *Andromeda leschenaultii*) and particularly in fruits. SA is essentially used alone as a topical preparation or in solution for peeling, due to its keratolytic properties. It has a high affinity for lipids and preferentially exerts its keratolytic effect inside the pores, making it a helpful therapy for acne. It also exhibits anti-inflammatory effects. A 50% SA paste has been used in the past to peel arms and hands addressing seborrhoeic keratoses, lentigines and keratosis pilaris, with good results.

Recently, SA has been formulated in concentrations of 20–30% in a hydroethanolic or polyethylene glycol vehicle for use as a superficial peeling agent. Indications for SA peeling include early to moderate photodamage, oily skin with enlarged pores, comedonal and inflammatory acne, rosacea, postinflammatory hyperpigmentation (PIH) and epidermal melasma.

Neutralisation is not necessary for SA and after application the skin can be rinsed with tap water. Redness and oedema are minimal. Desquamation is more vigorous compared with GA peels, and usually begins after 2–3 days, lasting up to 1 week. SA peels

Table 160.1 Depth of peel and histological level of controlled necrosis.

Depth of peel	Histological level of controlled necrosis
Very superficial (exfoliation)	Destruction of the stratum corneum but no wound below the stratum granulosum
Superficial (epidermal)	Necrosis of part or all of the epidermis, anywhere from the stratum granulosum to the basal cell layer
Medium depth (papillary dermis)	Necrosis of the epidermis and part or all of the papillary dermis
Deep (reticular dermis)	Necrosis of the epidermis, papillary dermis, and extending into the reticular dermis

Table 160.2 Superficial chemical peels and application methods.

Peeling agents	Peeling methods
Glycolic acid 30–50%	Single coat 2–3 min (very superficial peel)
	Neutralise with water or sodium bicarbonate
Glycoic acid 50–70%	Single coat 3–10 min, or until redness
	Neutralise with water or sodium bicarbonate
Jessner solution	1–3 coats (very superficial peel)
	4–5 coats
Salicyclic acid 30%	1–3 coats
Lipohydroxy acid	1–3 coats
Lactic acid 10–30%	1–3 coats
Mandelic acid 40%	1–3 coats
Pyruvic acid 50%	1–3 coats, or until redness
	Neutralise with water or sodium bicarbonate
Trichloroacetic acid 10–30%	1–3 coats until level 1 frosting

Table 160.3 Medium depth chemical peels and application methods.

Peeling agents	Peeling methods
35–50% trichloroacetic acid (TCA)	Until confluent light frost + redness (level 2 frost)
	Until solid white frost without redness (level 3 frost)
Solid CO_2 slush plus 35% TCA	Solid CO_2 slush for 3–15 s (transient frost)
	Followed by 35% TCA (level 2–3 frost)
Jessner solution (JS) plus 35% TCA	JS until faint pseudo-frost
	Followed by 35% TCA (level 2–3 frost)
70% glycolic acid (GA) plus 35% TCA	70% GA for 2 min and removed with water
	Followed by 35% TCA (level 2–3 frost)
88% phenol for limited areas	Unoccluded 88% phenol to localised areas

can be repeated every 4 weeks. A distinct advantage of SA is its predictability. There are no concerns about timing or overpeeling because there is very little penetration after precipitation of the active agent. SA peels are a good choice for patients with Fitzpatrick skin types V and VI. Furthermore, SA causes superficial anaesthesia so discomfort is minimal for patients. Very rarely, SA can cause systemic toxicity (salicylism).

Depth of peels

Chemical peeling is classified according to the depth of the wound created and the histological level of controlled necrosis (Table 160.1). Superficial peels produce injury limited to the epidermis, medium depth peels produce injury to the papillary dermis, while deep chemical peels produce injury extending into the reticular dermis.

The depth of the peel is dependent on the peeling agents, their concentration and the mode of application as well as the skin type and the skin condition [1,2]. In general, the depth of the peel determines the patient's downtime during and after the procedure, the overall healing time, the risk and severity of side effects and the treatment outcome [3].

Superficial peels

Superficial chemical peels (SCPs) involve the application of a chemical agent to the skin, resulting in destruction of part or all of the epidermis. Indications for SCPs include acne, epidermal dyschromia, superficial static lines and wrinkles, mild actinic keratoses and mild photoageing [4,5]. SCPs are popular as they are safe to use on all Fitzpatrick skin types, they have minimal side effects with no risk of overpeeling or irritation from multiple applications, they do not require anaesthesia and the desquamation is usually well accepted. The disadvantages of SCP are that the treatment outcome does not always meet the patient's expectations and a series of repeated peels may be required. The most commonly used chemical agents in an SCP are GA, JS, SA, lipohydroxy acid, LA, mandelic acid, pyruvic acid and TCA (Table 160.2). The end point in an SCP is mild redness with no or patchy light frosting.

Medium depth peels

Medium depth chemical peels (MDCPs) result in controlled, full-thickness epidermal necrosis and partial-thickness dermal necrosis to a level between the papillary dermis and upper reticular dermis. MDCPs are indicated for the treatment of pigmentary disorders, photodamage, skin rejuvenation, actinic keratoses, chemical reconstruction and softening of acne scars, xanthelasma and textural skin changes [4,5,6]. Following an MDCP, re-epithelialisation is usually complete in 7 days and dermal collagen remodelling may continue for more than 6 months. For patients with extensive actinic keratoses, an MDCP using TCA permits treatment of subclinical disease over the entire face, unlike localised cryotherapy or electrodesiccation and curettage of individual lesions. MDCPs can be used to treat PIH and melasma, but are associated with a higher incidence of post-peel pigmentation. MDCPs should not be performed on non-facial sites due to the relative paucity of follicular units, increasing the risk of poor healing and changes in pigmentation. Because of the risk of hyperpigmentation, MDCP should be used with caution in patients with skin of colour (SOC).

MDCPs are performed with 35–50% TCA alone, or more commonly using a combination of an initial superficial peeling agent followed by 35% TCA (Table 160.3). This allows for predictable and even penetration and increases the safety profile [7–11]. The end point is level 2–3 frost. The depth of necrosis correlates with the concentration of TCA. A 10–30% w/v TCA solution results in epidermal exfoliation, whereas a 30–40% w/v TCA solution causes 0.3–0.5 mm of dermal necrosis but spares the inferior portion of the follicular apparatus, permitting regrowth of the epidermis. TCA in a concentration of approximately 65–70% w/v results in 0.8–0.9 mm of dermal necrosis, which would probably result in scarring and is only appropriate for localised use.

Table 160.4 Formulae of two deep chemical peels.

Ingredients	Baker-Gordon peel (1962)	Hetter formula (1996): light to heavy peel
Croton oil (concentration)	2.10%	0.35–1.1%
Phenol (concentration)	49.30%	33%
Croton oil	3 drops	1–3 drops
Phenol 88%	3 mL	4 mL
Water	2 mL	6 mL
Septisol	8 drops	16 drops

Deep peels

Deep chemical peels (DCPs) involve the application of a compounded phenol-croton oil solution to produce a controlled cutaneous necrosis to the mid-reticular dermis (Table 160.4). The subsequent wound repair results in marked collagen formation and reorganisation of elastic fibres [12], which can persist for over a decade [13]. DCPs are used primarily to improve the appearance of moderate to severe photoageing, severe acne scars and actinic cheilitis. Hetter showed that the strength and depth of DCPs can be modified by lowering the concentration of croton oil and phenol and this reduces the incidence of side effects [14].

DCPs have diminished in popularity due to prolonged postoperative downtime, the increased risk of complications (which include infection, scarring, hyper- and hypopigmentation, fluid imbalance and cardiotoxic effects) and the need for cardiac monitoring. Laser resurfacing has replaced DCPs, especially in patients with darker skin, as it is safer, with more precise depth control, and is easier to use with no risk of systemic toxicity.

Indications and contraindications

Indications

Chemical peels are mainly recommended for facial skin rejuvenation and the treatment of photodamage, pigmentary dyschromia, acne vulgaris, scars, fine wrinkles and actinic keratoses. The careful selection of patients, the conditions to be treated, and a thorough knowledge of the peeling agents and the peeling procedures are critical for a good outcome [1,2,3].

Facial skin rejuvenation

Superficial chemical peels and MDCPs are useful for facial rejuvenation, improving skin texture, fine wrinkles, poikiloderma, pigmentary dyschromia and oily skin. SCPs enhance desquamation, resulting in a temporarily 'refreshed' look, while MDCPs are able to efface wrinkles and improve dyspigmentation. Usually, a series of SCP treatments is required for optimum results.

Photodamaged skin and actinic keratoses

Photodamaged skin is one of the main indications for all types of chemical peels. MDCPs are the most popular as they not only induce histological and clinical improvement in the epidermis, but they also have dermal impact including a thickening and regeneration of the papillary dermis with new collagen and elastic fibre formation [4]. SCPs are used to treat skin changes associated with mild photodamage [5–8]. Examples include SA, GA, lipohydroxy acid and TCA. They cause skin exfoliation and induce skin rejuvenation. DCPs are less popular and have been replaced by MDCPs or laser resurfacing as the latter have a better safety profile, are more predictable and have precise results and ease of use.

Medium depth TCA and phenol peels are effective in treating actinic keratoses and superficial Bowen disease [9,10,11]. Medium depth TCA peels are as effective as topical 5% fluorouracil, carbon dioxide laser resurfacing or aminolaevulinic acid photodynamic therapy in reducing the number of visible actinic keratoses at 3 months and in preventing lesion recurrence for up to 1 year [11–13].

Acne vulgaris and acne scars

Superficial chemical peels are effective for the treatment of acne vulgaris (especially non-inflammatory acne), post-acne hyperpigmentation and superficial acne scarring [14,15]. They are often used as an adjunct to the medical treatment of acne. SCPs break down the cementing substance of corneocytes promoting exfoliation, inducing keratolysis and providing comedolytic effects. It is also believed to reduce sebum production and pore size although studies have failed to confirm this [16,17]. Most SCP agents have anti-inflammatory and antibacterial properties. In addition, SCPs enhance the absorption of topical products, improve post-acne hyperpigmentation and some possess a skin whitening effect [18]. SCPs that are effective for treating acne vulgaris include SA, lipohydroxy acid, GA, mandelic acid, PA, azelaic acid and JS [19–24]. A systematic review of randomised controlled trials of chemical peels for acne vulgaris demonstrated that the different peeling agents have approximately the same efficacy and adverse event profile, all being well tolerated [25]. Figure 160.1 shows the treatment response of acne scars with chemical peeling.

Acne scars are polymorphic. MDCPs and DCPs are useful in treating moderate acne scarring but the risk of post-peel hyperpigmentation is high, especially in patients with SOC [26,27]. For these patients, safer and more effective energy-based devices have replaced MDCPs and DCPs. Atrophic and ice-pick acne scars can be treated with TCA chemical reconstruction of skin scars (TCA CROSS). This procedure uses a toothpick tip soaked with 75–100% TCA solution that is pressed hard on the entire ice-pick depressed scars (Figure 160.2) [28,29,30].

Pigmentation

Dyschromias are alterations in skin pigmentation, commonly associated with photodamage, and often observed in darker skin types. Common hyperpigmented lesions treated with chemical peels include solar lentigines (Figure 160.3), melasma (Figures 160.4 and 160.5), PIH and infraorbital hyperpigmentation.

SCPs are effective and safe in treating melasma and PIH in all skin types, and they have been shown to improve the quality of life in patients with PIH [31]. GA, JS and SA are the most popular superficial peeling agents used to treat melasma and PIH, although LA, mandelic acid, TCA and tretinoin peels are also effective. A series of SCPs, usually at monthly intervals, are needed to obtain a satisfactory outcome (Figures 160.3, 160.4 and 160.5).

SCPs are often used in combination with skin lighteners, such as 2–4% hydroquinone or 10% azelaic cream, for a synergistic effect [32–36]. Studies comparing the efficacy of various superficial peeling

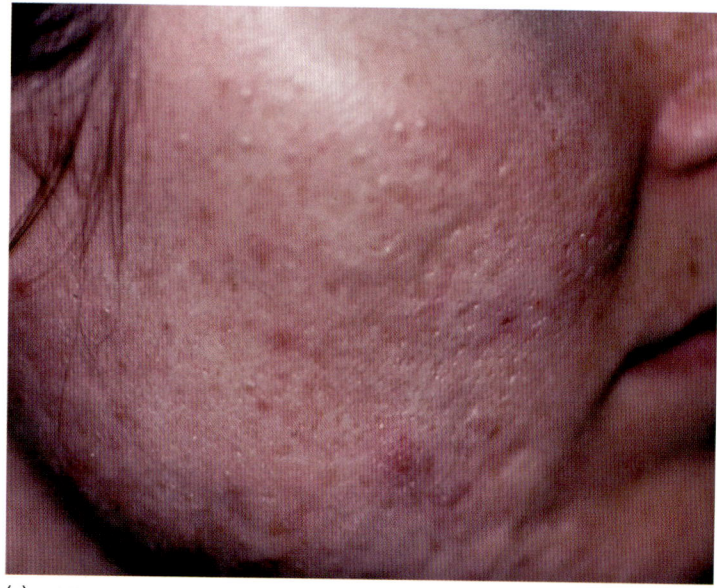

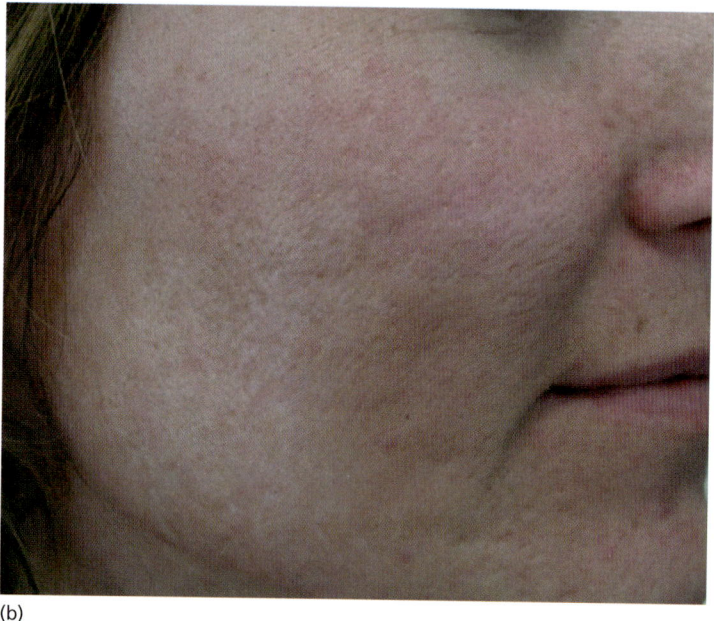

Figure 160.1 Acne and acne scars (a) before and (b) after a medium depth chemical peel. Courtesy of Richard Barlow.

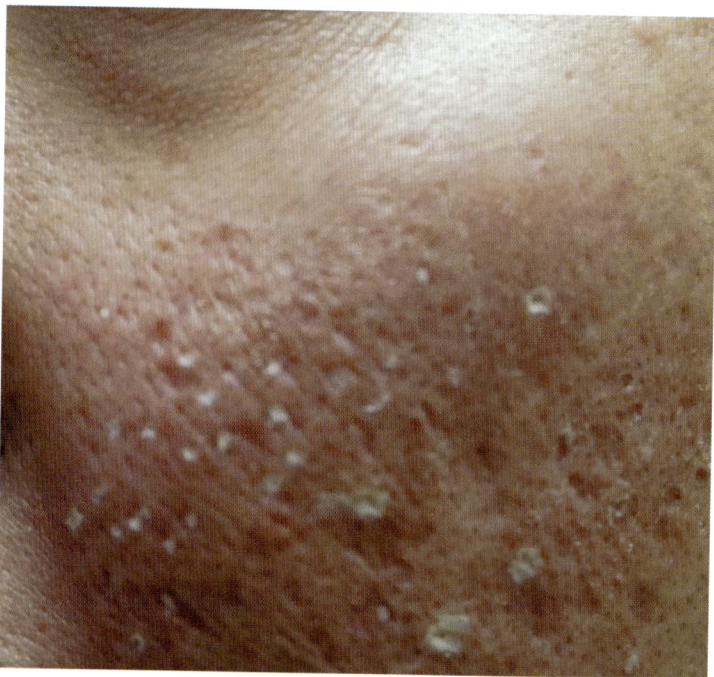

Figure 160.2 Treatment with trichloroacetic acid chemical reconstruction of skin scars (TCA CROSS) where a TCA frost is seen at base of the acne scars.

agents (LA, JS, tretinoin, GA and TCA) for the treatment of melasma and PIH demonstrate they are equally effective [37–39]. Fastidious sun protection must be adhered to in order to prevent relapse after treatment.

Infraorbital hyperpigmentation has a multifactorial aetiology and only those with periorbital melanosis may benefit from a series of SCPs. Lower concentrations of SCP using TCA, LA and GA plus adjunctive treatment with antioxidants such as topical vitamin C have been used with some success [40,41].

Contraindications

There are few contraindications for chemical peels. A thorough medical history should be taken to determine if there are medical co-morbidities rendering the patient unsuitable for chemical peels. Absolute contraindications to chemical peels include allergy to the peeling solutions or the neutralising agents as well as patients with unrealistic expectations.

Relative contraindications for chemical peels include concomitant use of some medications. For example, care must be taken in patients on oral contraceptives, tetracyclines and drugs that can induce pigmentary disorders. Concomitant oral isotretinoin should be avoided. It is common practice for isotretinoin to be discontinued 6 months prior to MDCPs and DCPs as it may interfere with effective re-epithelialisation of the peeled skin. However, a systematic review of evidence-based recommendations found insufficient evidence for this [42]. Radiotherapy irradiated skin is another relative contraindication for a similar reason, as there is a reduction in epithelial appendages which may lead to poor healing and increased risk of scarring.

Other relative contraindications include patients who work outdoors and those with photosensitivity as they risk development of photodermatitis or PIH. Pregnancy and lactation are relative contraindications, although there are no reports of teratogenesis or fetal malformation from chemical peels [43]. Patients who are prone to keloid scarring should also avoid MDCPs and DCPs. Immunosuppression, concurrent illness, recent head or neck surgery, recent facial hair removal (waxing, depilation, electrolysis), active herpes labialis, the presence of plane warts and dermatitis are also relative contraindications and chemical peeling should be postponed until they are resolved.

Pre-peel procedure

Counselling

During the first visit, identification of the patient's concerns, expectations and their acceptance of side effects and downtime is

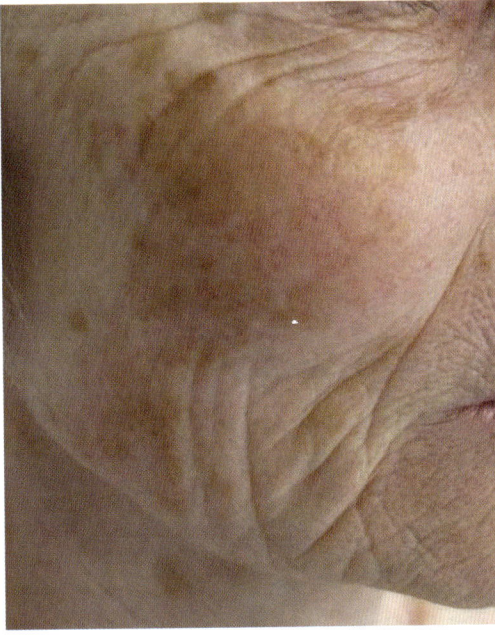

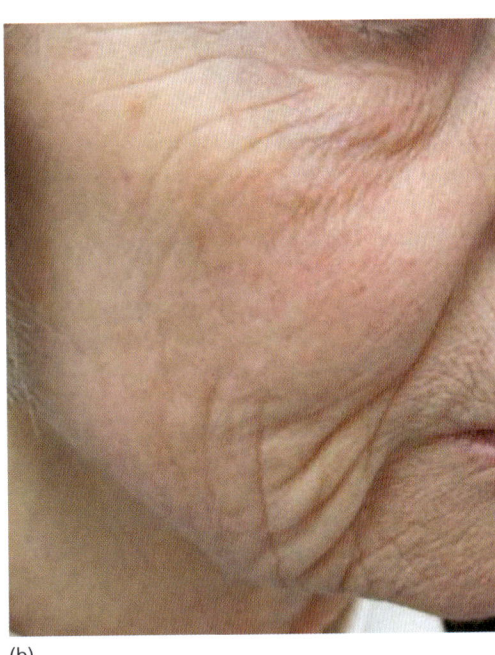

Figure 160.3 Solar lentigines (a) before and (b) after a Jessner solution peel. Courtesy of Richard Barlow.

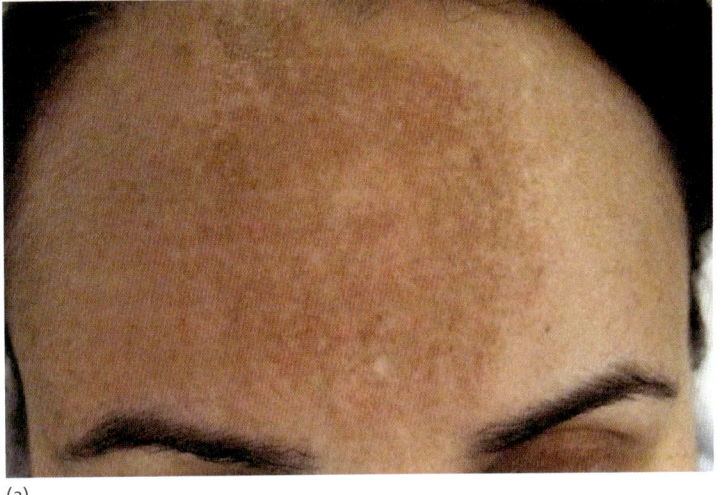

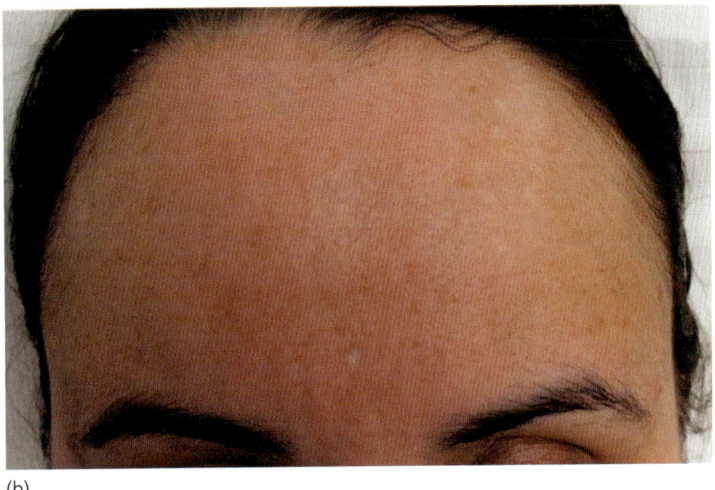

Figure 160.4 Melasma (a) before and (b) after a Jessner solution peel. Courtesy of Richard Barlow.

paramount. Various peeling options, their potential benefits, healing time and complications and alternative treatment options must be discussed. The choice of peeling agents should be recommended based on the skin pathology, patient's risk of complications, patient's attitudes towards post-peel healing time and level of intensity of treatment. Generally, SCPs address acne vulgaris, skin rejuvenation and pigmentary conditions, and are the preferred choice for patients with SOC. MDCPs and DCPs are useful for photodamage, wrinkles and some acne scars. Some patients may prefer a series of SCPs with minimal or no downtime and slow incremental improvement, while others may prefer a more aggressive MDCP requiring a week of downtime but with more dramatic outcome.

During the physical examination, it is important to note the patient's skin type, the degree of photodamage or scarring and the sebaceous quality of the skin. Generally, atrophic, dry skin is more sensitive to chemical peeling agents, while those with thicker, sebaceous-rich skin will be more tolerant. Any underlying inflammatory skin condition that may increase the absorption of the peeling agents should be established from the onset. A history of sensitive skin or allergy to the peeling agent should be sought, and any skin disorder associated with the Koebner phenomenon should be excluded.

Skin priming

Before performing chemical peels, the target skin should be primed for 2–4 weeks. The priming regimen varies with the underlying condition and the patient's skin type. The aim of skin priming is to allow a more uniform penetration of the peeling agent, to shorten wound healing time and to reduce the risk of PIH [1]. Topical retinoids are used to thin the stratum corneum and to enhance the penetration and depth of the peeling agent's action [2,3]. They enhance epidermal turnover reducing the risk of delayed epithelialisation, and also reduce epidermal melanosome transfer.

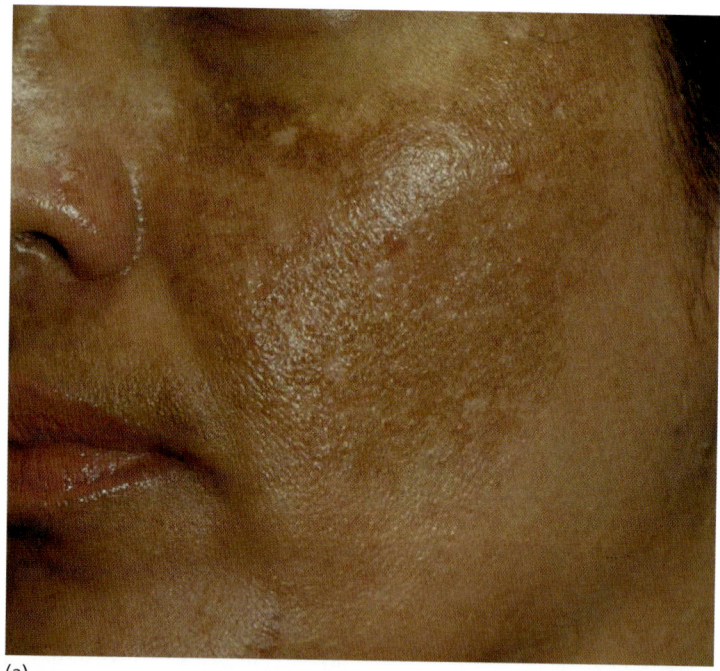

When treating pigmentary disorders or patients with darker skin, topical hydroquinone or other non-hydroquinone skin lightening agents may be used as priming agents to reduce the risk of PIH. Topical hydroquinone is preferred as a priming agent over topical tretinoin to enhance the effects of GA peels and lessen the risk of PIH [5]. In addition to preparing the skin, the priming period allows patients to become accustomed to the maintenance regimen that they will need to comply with after the peel.

Consent and photo documentation

Once the skin is primed and the patient is ready for the chemical peel, informed consent should be obtained from the patient. The procedure should be explained in detail, including the post-peel course and aftercare, potential complications of the peel and when to resume topical medications. Those patients who are unable to follow instructions are at a higher risk of complications. For MDCPs and DCPs, the patient is informed about the redness, swelling, peeling and a downtime of about 7–10 days. Strict sun avoidance is advised for at least 14 days post peel. Before and after peel photos are essential as documentation.

Peeling procedure

Equipment

The standard peel tray should include a small fan, alcohol or acetone for skin degreasing, gauze pads, sponges, cotton-tipped swabs, a spray bottle for water, a mild cleanser and a bland moisturiser (Figure 160.6). A timer and a neutralising agent are required for GA and PA peels.

Peeling technique

Chemical peels are performed in the out-patient setting. The patient should remove any make-up and wash their face with soap and water. The patient lies supine on the bed with their head elevated

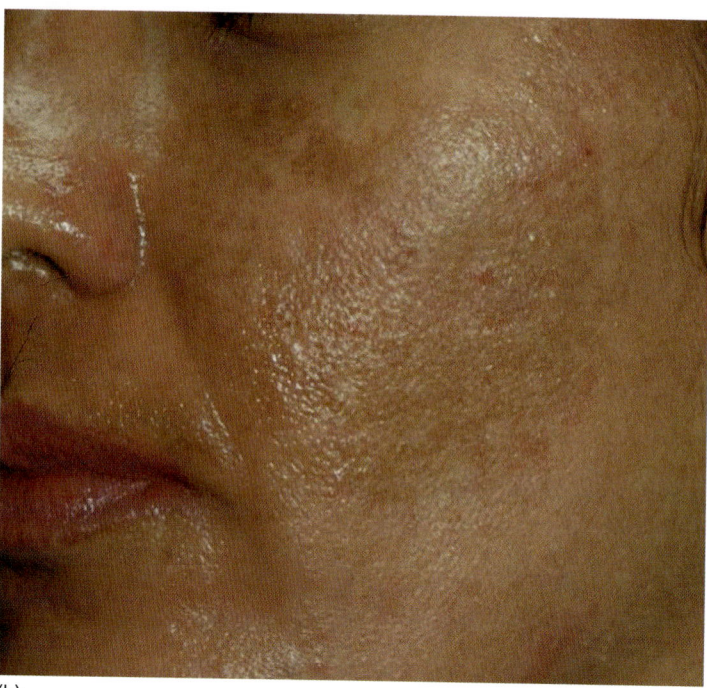

Figure 160.5 Melasma (a) before and (b) after a series of Jessner solution peels in a patient with darker skin type.

The topical retinoid is usually stopped 1–2 days before the chemical peel and is resumed post peeling. When treating patients with darker skin, topical retinoids may be omitted during the priming stage or stopped 1 week before the peel to reduce the risk of excessive peeling, prolonged redness and PIH. Topical GA products are often added as priming agents in order to thin the stratum corneum, to allow for a more uniform penetration of the peeling agent and to improve epidermal healing. It may also help improve tolerance of GA peels [4].

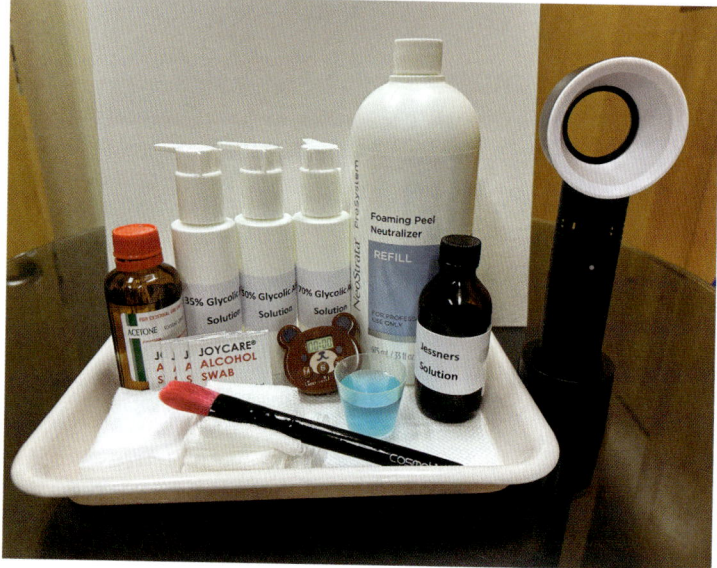

Figure 160.6 Typical equipment required for glycolic acid chemical peels. Courtesy of Dr Joyce Lim.

at 45 degrees. SCPs do not require any anaesthesia. For MDCPs, topical anaesthesia can be used without affecting the clinical or histopathological outcome [1]. Mild preoperative sedation and non-steroidal anti-inflammatory drugs may be needed in some patients. DCPs generally require sedation and analgesia. The skin is degreased with alcohol or acetone or both. Acetone is preferred for TCA and DCPs. Degreasing is necessary to facilitate a uniform penetration of the peel solution.

Petroleum jelly is applied to protect sensitive areas including the corners of the mouth, alar creases and eyelids. The peeling solution is poured into a glass or metal cup. The solution is applied with cotton-tipped applicators, sponge applicators, 4 × 4 cm gauze pads or a sable brush. For broad areas like the cheeks and forehead, two to three applicator swabs can be used together, or a gauze pad or brush used. For very sensitive areas like the perinasal and periorbital areas, one semi-dry applicator is used. The physician should always take extreme care to avoid accidental spillage of solution and never move the cotton-tipped applicators or sable brush directly over the eye area. A syringe of saline for dilution should always be available if any peel solution gets into the eye.

The peel solution is applied sequentially either clockwise or anticlockwise from the forehead to temple, down to the cheek and chin and across over to the other cheek, temple and forehead. Avoid skipping or overlapping areas. The eyelids and periocular areas are treated last as the skin in these areas is thin, more sensitive to pain and prone to oedema. Tearing dilutes the peel solutions and may cause pigmented streaks; tears should therefore be quickly wiped away with dry cotton applicators.

Infraorbital areas are treated with the eyes open and the patient gazing superiorly. The peeling solution is gently applied using cotton-tipped applicators onto the lower eyelids up to 1 mm from the ciliary margins, taking care that the solution does not enter the eyes. For the upper eyelid, the eyes are closed and the peel is applied in upward strokes with feathering into the eyebrow. When treating wrinkles around the eyes, the skin is stretched and care must be taken that the peeling solution does not enter the eye by capillary action.

In patients who do not require a full-face peel, the peeling agent is applied to the individual cosmetic units. When treating photo-damaged skin, the solution is feathered at the hairline and neck to promote blending with untreated skin. During the peeling process, the skin is cooled with a fan continuously to decrease the stinging or burning sensation.

Peeling agents
Glycolic acid peels

Glycolic acid peels are solutions of free acids ranging from 20% to 70%. Buffered solutions and gel formulations are also available and these generally cause less burning, stinging and redness and possibly less risk of uneven penetration. In using GA peels, the concentration of free acid and the time of contact will determine the results and risk of complications. A low concentration (20–30%) of GA solution should be started with a short contact time, usually 3–5 min. With subsequent treatments, the acid concentration and contact time should be increased.

Once the skin is primed and degreased with alcohol, the GA solution is applied and a timer started. Patients will feel a stinging or burning sensation. During the peel, the clinician should be alert for the development of areas of redness or epidermolysis. If these are seen they must be neutralised immediately while the rest of the peel is left to continue to act until the desired contact time. The end point depends on the skin pathology and the desired level of peeling. If a superficial epidermal peel is desired, then the end point is mild redness (Figure 160.7). If epidermolysis (or a full epidermal peel) is desired, then the end point is vesiculation or a red-white discoloration (Figure 160.8). The treated skin will heal with crusts and has a higher incidence of PIH.

Once the end point is reached, the GA solution must be neutralised with a sodium bicarbonate solution or an alkaline agent to terminate its action. It is important to neutralise the acid in the same chronological order as used during the application of the peel. Sodium bicarbonate causes an exothermic reaction, resulting in some discomfort; this can be reduced by spraying cold water on the skin prior to neutralisation. During neutralisation, a bubbling or fizzing sound occurs as carbon dioxide gas is produced. This will cease when all the GA is neutralised and indicates completion. Once the GA is neutralised, the face should be washed with water followed by the application of a mild emollient and sunscreen.

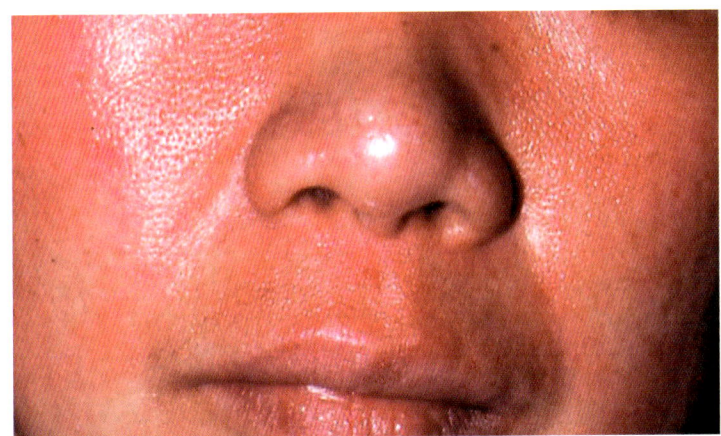

Figure 160.7 Skin redness during a glycolic acid peel.

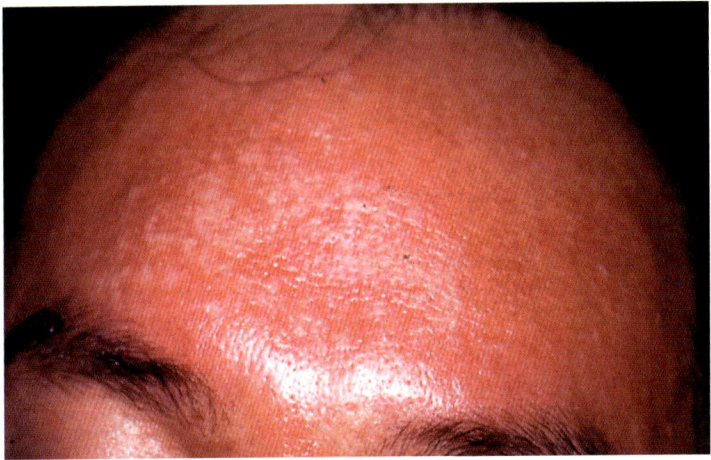

Figure 160.8 Epidermolysis with a glycolic acid peel showing full epidermal peeling indicated by the white colour and near vesiculation.

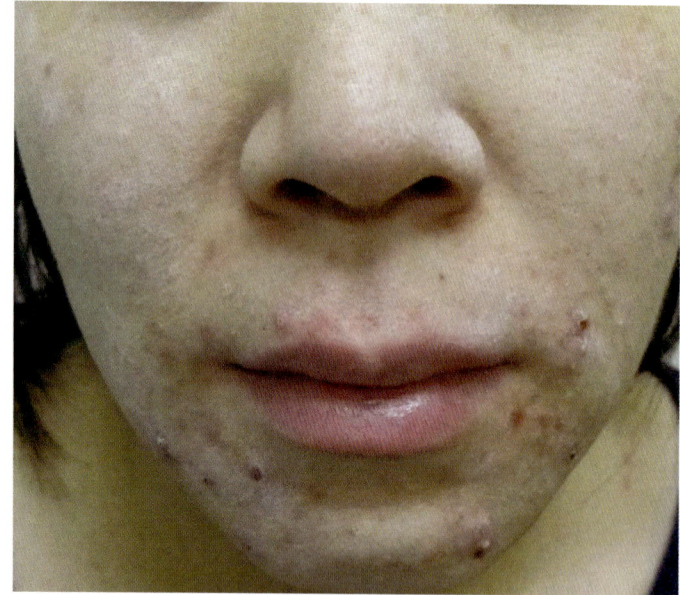

Figure 160.9 Light powdery whitening with a Jessner solution peel.

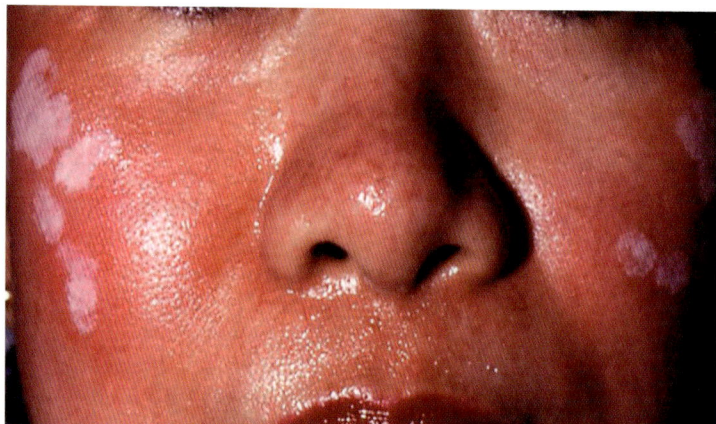

Figure 160.10 Level 3 peel demonstrating 'fridge white' frosting using a trichloroacetic acid peel.

A series of superficial GA peels are performed at 3–4-weekly intervals and the peel concentration or the contact time is increased with each subsequent treatment. For patients who are prone to PIH, a low acid concentration and a short contact time should be initiated and the intervals between subsequent peels delayed. GA peels are often used alone for an SCP or combined with a 35% TCA solution to achieve an MDCP.

Jessner peel

After cleansing and degreasing the skin, the JS is applied evenly to the treatment areas. A faint redness followed by a light, powdery whitening will appear (Figure 160.9). This is due to precipitation of the chemicals and is not a true frost from tissue coagulation. If a deeper peel is desired, additional coats of JS can be applied. With more coats the skin becomes red and there may be areas of white frost from tissue coagulation. The patient will experience a stinging or burning sensation. Unlike GA peels, there is no need for neutralisation. The powdery whitening is washed off with water and a mild moisturiser applied.

Salicylic acid peel

A 20–30% SA solution is applied to the face and, for acne, a second coat is applied to the papules and pustules. A tingling or burning sensation will be felt. A white frost of crystalline precipitation of the SA is seen within the first few minutes of application. Pustules and papules become deroofed during the process. After 3–5 min the frost is complete and the face should be washed and a moisturiser applied. The peels are repeated at 2–3-week intervals and the number of peels is dependent on the severity of the acne.

Trichloroacetic acid peel

Trichloroacetic acid 15–25% is used in SCPs and 35–50% solution is used in MDCPs. The depth of peel depends on the concentration of TCA used, the method by which the acid is applied, the number of applications and the amount of acid on the applicator. The TCA is rubbed into the skin with a 4 × 4 cm gauze. An even redness or frosting is seen. The depth of the TCA peel penetration correlates clinically with the intensity of frosting on the skin. Care should be taken to allow adequate time (approximately a minute) between TCA applications to ensure the coagulation process is complete before another coat is applied. A light frost corresponds to a superficial epidermal peel (level 1 TCA peel), a white frost with redness showing through corresponds to a full epidermal peel (level 2 TCA peel), while a solid white frost ('fridge white') corresponds to a papillary dermal peel (level 3 TCA peel) (Figure 160.10). The patient will experience a burning sensation within a minute of TCA application. When the desired end point is reached, the treated areas are washed with water and an emollient is applied.

Combined glycolic acid and trichloroacetic acid

The combination of 70% unbuffered GA peel followed by TCA 35% produces a consistent MDCP and is safer than a medium depth TCA concentration. GA 70% is applied to the face for 2 min and then washed off with water. A TCA 35% solution is applied in the usual manner. The patient will experience a burning sensation within a minute of TCA application. Once frosting is completed, the face is washed with water and an emollient applied.

Combined Jessner solution and trichloroacetic acid

The goal of combining JS followed by a 35% TCA solution (both superficial peeling agents) is to create an MDCP without the risk of using high concentrations of TCA. JS (1–4 coats) is applied to the face until a uniform redness with light powdery whitening is seen, after which TCA 35% is then applied. A white frost (of tissue coagulation) is seen following the TCA application (Figure 160.11). The face is then washed with water.

Phenol–croton oil peel

Croton oil is mixed with 88% phenol into a solution, followed by the addition of septisol and water. The peel solution is applied over the entire face or cosmetic units (segmental peels). The optimal application technique includes the correct amount of solution, the pressure and the number of passes. DCPs are performed with preoperative sedation and adequate hydration. For full-face peels, intravenous fluids should be administered to reduce cardiac complications related to phenol toxicity. Continuous cardiac monitoring is needed

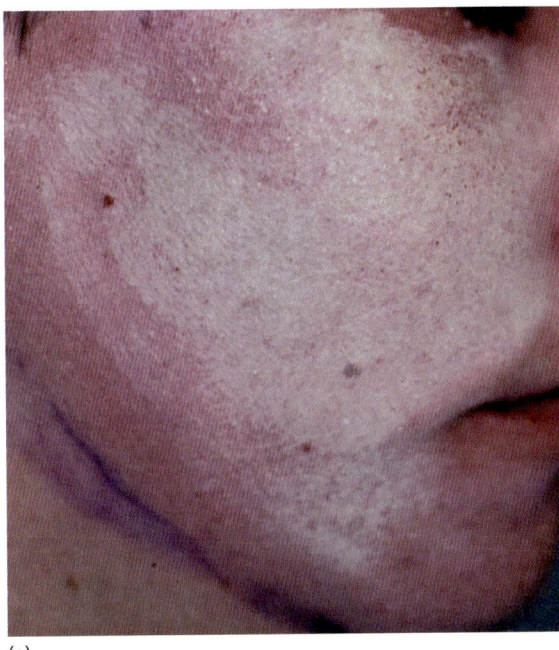

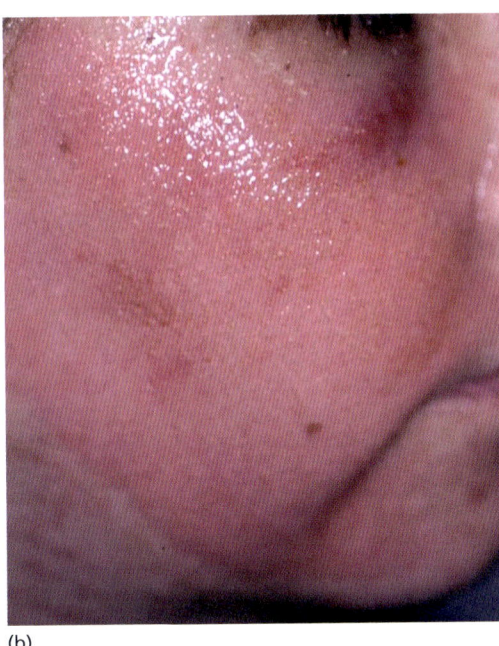

Figure 160.11 (a) Dense white frosting after a combination of Jessner solution and 35% trichloroacetic acid peel. (b) Skin redness 6 days after the peel, lasting for 14 days. Courtesy of Richard Barlow.

if peels exceed 1% of the body surface area. After completion of the DCP, occlusion is with either petrolatum jelly or zinc oxide tape and bismuth subgallate powder. A DCP can be done without occlusion and this involves more application of the peel solution and does not provide as deep a peel as the occluded method.

Post-peel care

The post-peel care regimen depends on the peeling agents used. For SCPs, no special care is required. A bland emollient is often used 2–4 times a day for 1–2 days post peel. After an SCP, the skin re-epithelialises in 3–4 days. When the skin looks and feels normal, the patients can restart their skincare.

After an MDCP, skincare consists of measures to keep the necrotic skin layer in place for as long as possible as it acts as a protective dressing, as well as maximising patient comfort. A bland emollient or ointment is dabbed (not rubbed) on the treated area to keep the skin moist and a mild soap can be used for gentle cleansing. Patients should be reminded not to pick, rub or scratch at their skin as this will result in premature peeling and delayed wound healing. Furthermore, while showering, care should be taken to avoid water spraying directly on the face. If there are exudative areas, acetic acid compresses or an antibiotic ointment may be used. Medium depth peels will re-epithelialise in 5–7 days.

After a DCP, full epidermal necrosis occurs and wound care is thus important to prevent infection. During the healing phase, dilute vinegar soaks will remove the necrotic debris and prevent crust formation. Repetitive application of an emollient enhances epithelialisation and reduces the risk of scarring.

Side effects and complications

Complications from SCPs and MDCPs are uncommon when performed by an experienced practitioner. Chemical peeling is based on controlled wounding of the skin, using an optimal peeling agent for an appropriate indication. However, side effects and complications can occur and risks are higher with MDCPs and DCPs (Box 160.1) [1,2].

> **Box 160.1 Complications from chemical peels**
>
> - Persistent redness
> - Chemical burns
> - Premature peeling
> - Milia and acneform eruption
> - Postinflammatory hyperpigmentation
> - Infection
> - Allergic contact dermatitis
> - Systemic toxicity
> - Postinflammatory hypopigmentation
> - Scarring

To minimise complications, appropriate patient and product selection together with proper skin priming, good technique, realistic patient expectations and compliance with post-peel care are of paramount importance. Patients at risk include those prone to PIH or keloid formation and those unable to adhere to post-treatment care. MDCPs and DCPs should be avoided in such individuals.

Persistent redness

Post-peeling redness usually fades over the course of a week. It is abnormal if it persists beyond 30 days post SCP and 60 days post MDCP. Persistent redness (Figure 160.12) is uncommon and is more likely to be seen in patients with rosacea or if the patient has been on topical tretinoin before and after the peel. It can persist for

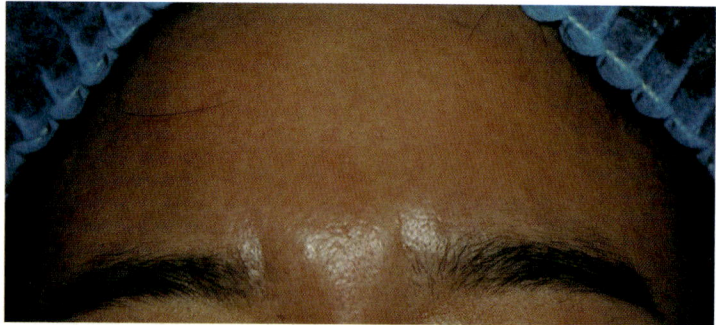

Figure 160.12 Persistent redness 2 months after a trichloroacetic acid peel which will resolve with time.

12–24 months but is rarely permanent; however, localised persistent redness may be a sign of an impending scar.

Chemical burns
Chemical peeling is a controlled chemo-exfoliation of the skin. Extensive chemical burns after superficial peels (Figure 160.13) are uncommon but can happen, especially if the GA is left on the skin for too long without neutralisation. If it occurs, burns tend to be localised and heal with PIH (Figure 160.14).

Premature peeling
Premature peeling can occur with MDCPs and DCPs (Figure 160.15) and may be accidental or intentional, caused by the patient rubbing or picking, which must be resisted. With normal healing, the superficial necrotic layer acts as a dressing while the deeper layer heals. In premature peeling, the protective superficial necrotic layer is removed and the underlying fragile healing skin may not re-epithelialise, which can lead to persistent redness, post-peel pigmentation or even scarring. The skin may look raw and moist. The open wound must be treated with a topical antibiotic ointment or covered with petroleum jelly to prevent infection until re-epithelialisation is complete. Patients should be reminded not to traumatise or pick their healing skin.

Milia and acneform eruption
Milia may be seen during the healing phase after chemical peels, likely due to the occlusive effects of the ointment used after treatment. They tend to occur approximately 3 weeks after peeling, commonly in the periorbital area, and can be removed by gentle scrubbing or using tretinoin creams.

Acneform eruptions may appear during the healing phase. Lesions are seen as tender, red, follicular papules or pustules and usually respond to topical acne medication such as a combination benzoyl peroxide–antibiotic cream. They tend to resolve within 1–2 weeks (Figure 160.16).

Postinflammatory hyperpigmentation
Postinflammatory hyperpigmentation can occur with any chemical peel agent and is more frequent in patients with SOC or if there is unprotected sun exposure after chemical peeling (Figure 160.17). It is usually seen within 1–4 weeks and up to 8 weeks after a peel. PIH will gradually clear but may take several months for complete resolution. Hence, high-risk individuals should be primed with

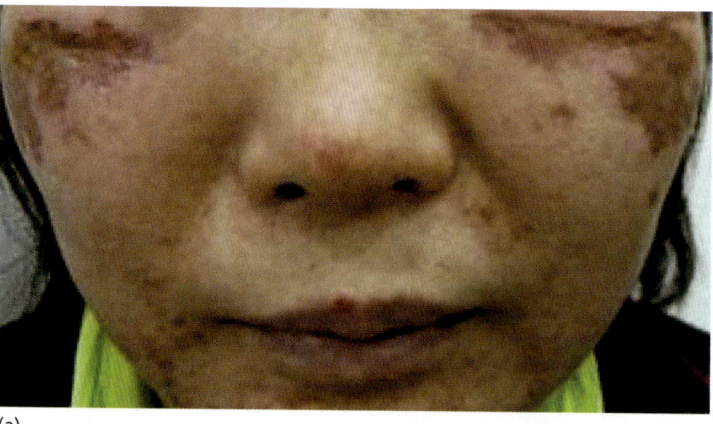

(a)

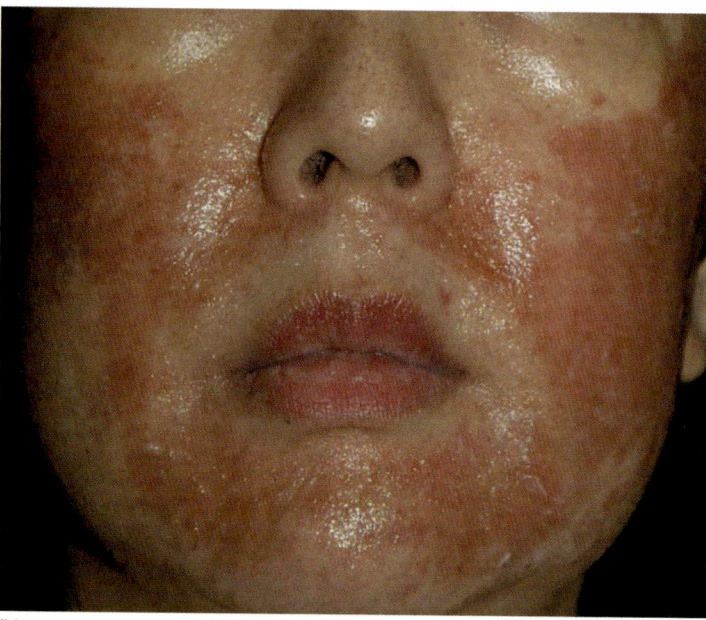

(b)

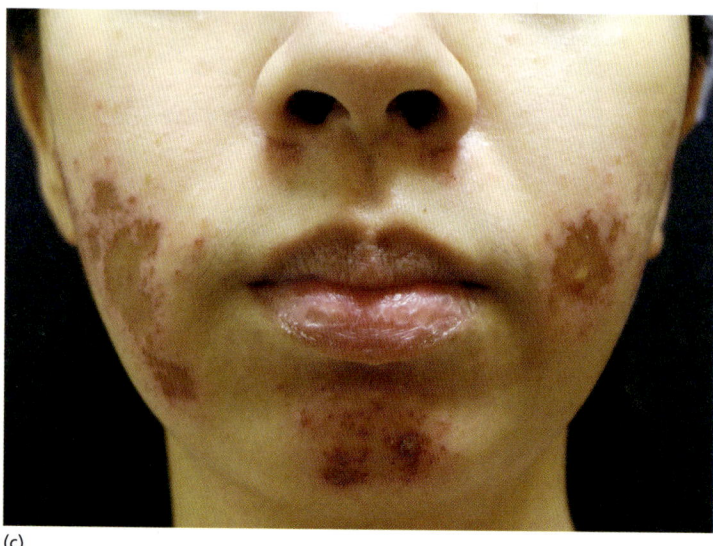

(c)

Figure 160.13 Chemical burns to (a) the periorbital skin, (b) the cheeks and (c) the chin.

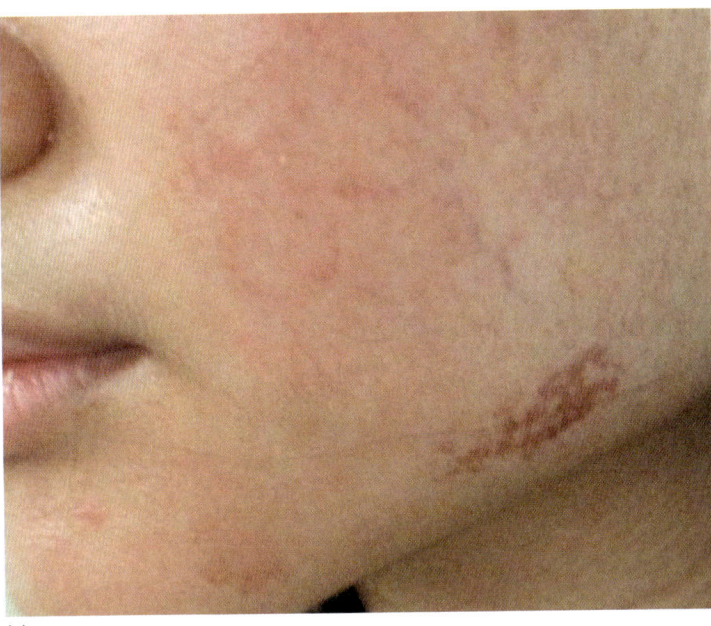

(a)

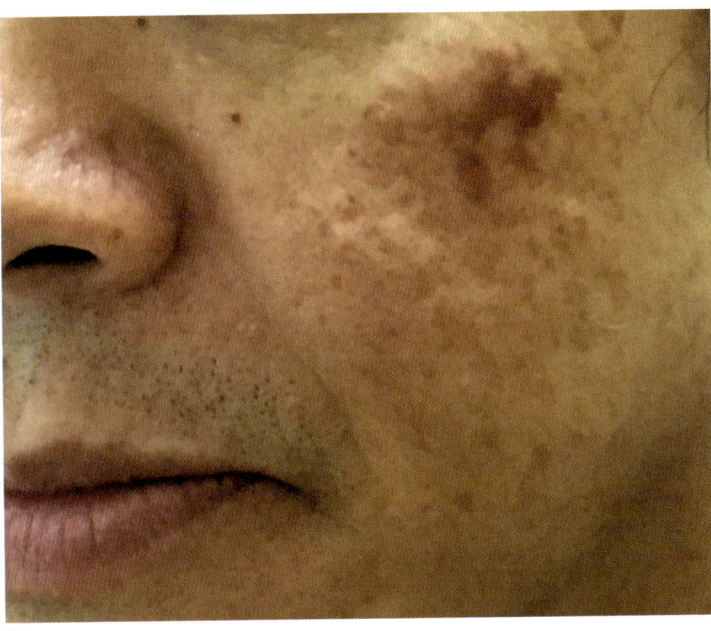

(b)

Figure 160.14 (a, b) Localised chemical burn with postinflammatory hyperpigmentation.

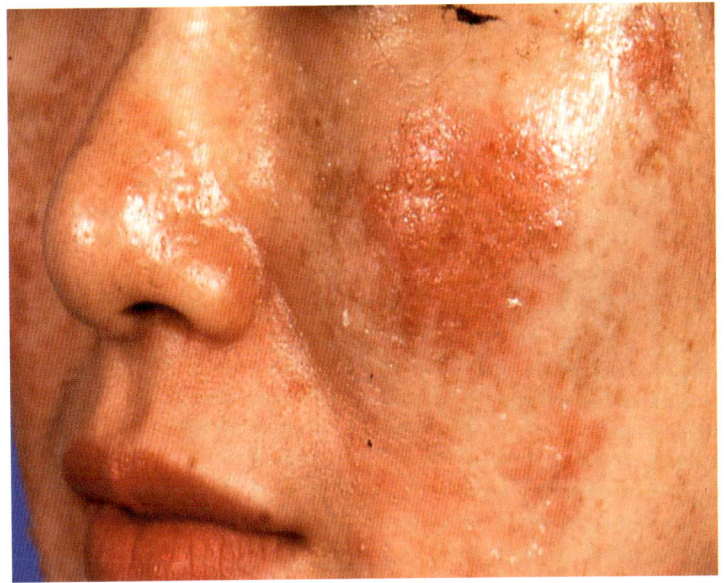

Figure 160.15 Premature peeling after a trichloroacetic acid peel with a loss of the protective necrotic layer caused by excessive scrubbing by the patient, with resultant redness.

topical hydroquinone prior to the procedure and observe fastidious sun protection and sun avoidance after the peel. PIH can be treated with a combination of a broad spectrum sunscreen and topical lightening agents, antioxidants, retinoids or fruit acids. If the response to topical treatment is slow, a very superficial peel that is non-inflammatory such as a TCA 10%, JS or GA 50% can be utilised to exfoliate the superficial epidermis and any melanin pigment within it.

Infection
Infection is not common following a chemical peel but may occur as an early postoperative complication. Skin flora such as *Staphylococcus* and *Streptococcus* species, and occasionally *Pseudomonas*, *Enterobacter* and *Candida* species, can overgrow, causing infection.

The risk of infection increases with the depth of the peel and with full-thickness epithelial necrosis. Infections must be treated early and aggressively as they may lead to scarring. Suspicion for infection must be raised if there are necrotic crusts, particularly as heavy crusts generally do not form in SCPs or MCPs, or if there is an area of persistent redness, pain or erosion. If infection is suspected, a Gram stain and culture test should be done. All infections should be managed with the appropriate topical and oral antibiotic, antifungal or antiviral therapy. Crusts should be removed and wounds dressed with acetic acid soaks or other antiseptic treatment.

Reactivation of dormant herpes simplex infection can occur and present with pain and erosions; vesicles are often not obvious. Generally, antiviral prophylaxis is not required for SCPs but is indicated for MDCPs or DCPs if the patient has a positive history of herpes simplex. Prophylactic antiviral treatment should be started 1 day prior to and for 7 days post peel or until complete epithelialisation. Active herpes simplex infection occurring after the peel should also be treated [3].

Allergic contact dermatitis
Chemical peeling agents seldom cause allergic contact dermatitis. GA and TCA are not common sensitisers but the resorcinol used in JS is a known skin sensitiser. A high index of suspicion is needed to detect contact allergy.

Systemic toxicity
Resorcinol, SA and phenol applied on the skin may be absorbed systemically to cause toxicity. The risk of toxicity is dependent on the quantity of chemical absorbed into the skin. Resorcinol toxicity from JS is rare and has not been reported even after multiple applications to large surface areas of the face, neck and chest. SA toxicity

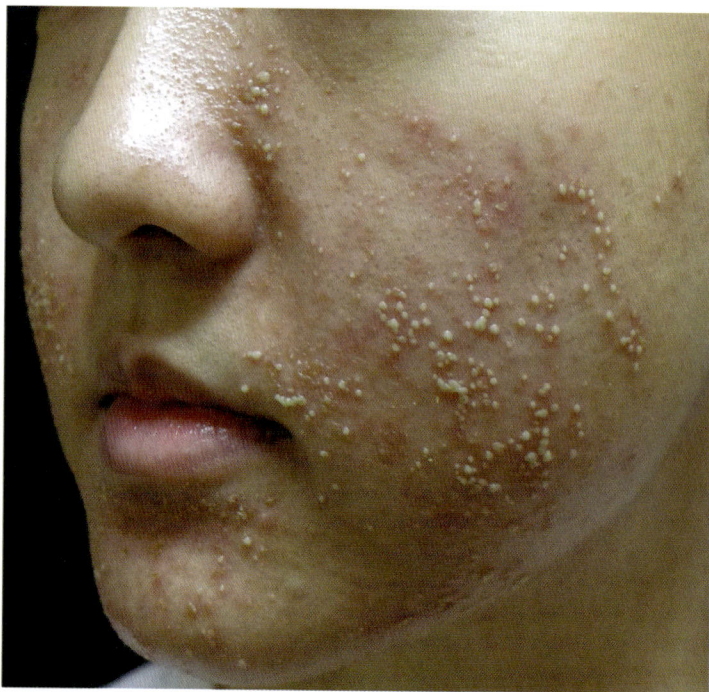

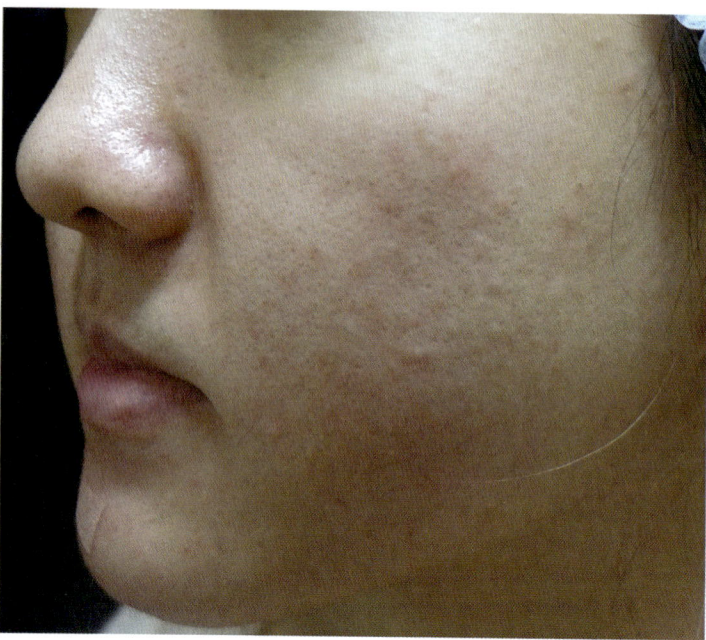

Figure 160.16 Pustules (a) seen after peels and (b) resolved within 2 weeks.

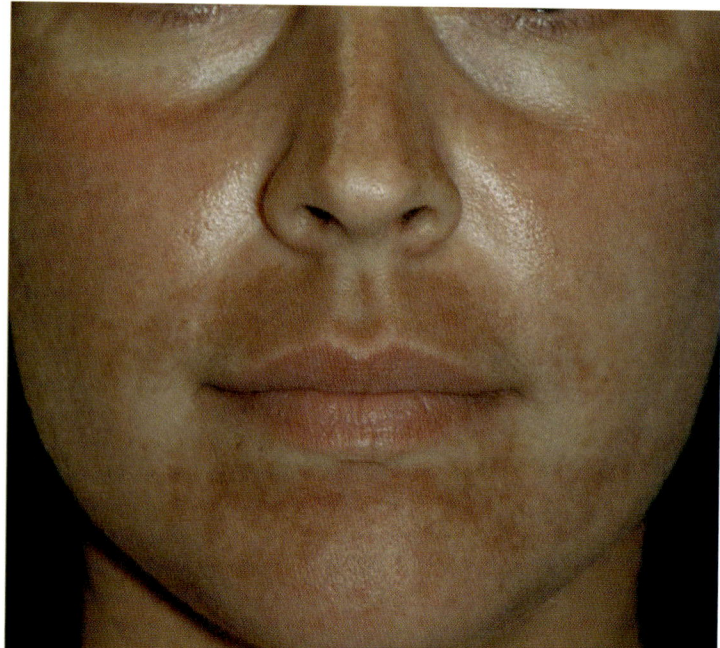

Figure 160.17 Postinflammatory hyperpigmentation to the perioral region that developed after sun exposure after a superficial chemical peel.

(salicylism) can occur when large areas of the face, chest, arms and legs are treated simultaneously.

Postinflammatory hypopigmentation

Hypopigmentation is a recognised complication of DCPs and results from melanocyte destruction in both the hair follicles and reticular dermis. Phenol peels are known to cause hypopigmentation and the degree is proportional to the amount of phenol used.

Hypopigmentation seen after MDCPs is due to necrosis of the entire epidermis and delayed repigmentation by the follicular melanocytes, and may persist for up to 2–3 months. However, hypopigmentation as a result of chemical peeling may be permanent, due to scarring and superficial fibrosis of the upper dermis. Once permanent, treatment is usually unsatisfactory and patients may require cosmetic camouflage make-up.

Scarring

Scarring is the most concerning complication of chemical peels, although it is seen rarely with SCPs. Patients at higher risk of scarring include those with an exaggerated inflammatory response, those with a history of poor or delayed wound healing and those with a tendency to form hypertrophic or keloid scars. Deeply penetrating peeling agents are risk factors, as well as inadequate time between peeling procedures. Shortened intervals will fail to allow for adequate skin healing and increase the risk for scarring.

Most scars are a result of a secondary event, such as infection, premature peeling or a premature repeat procedure. Careful monitoring during the healing phase after the peel enables early detection of infection or premature peeling and prompt treatment of these events can prevent scarring. In the early stages, scars appear as indurated red patches and plaques, usually seen within the first 3 months post peel. High-risk sites include the upper lip, inframandibular skin and glabella. Focal persistent redness may be a sign of an impending scar and early intervention with topical steroids or pulsed dye laser treatment may prevent scar formation. Once scarring is noticed, close follow-up is essential. Hypertrophic and keloidal scars can be treated with pulsed dye laser, fractional laser resurfacing and intralesional steroid.

Chemical peels in patients with skin of colour

The indications for chemical peels in patients with melanin-rich skin differ from those for people with fair skin. Common presenting problems in patients with darker skin include skin dyschromia (such as melasma, lentigines or PIH), acne vulgaris, superficial acne and scars, textural changes such as roughness, oily skin and fine wrinkles and enlarged pores. Wrinkling, rhytids and actinic keratoses are less common presenting problems

SCPs are effective and safe in treating acne, superficial acne scars, melasma and PIH [1–5]. Some of the more popular SCP in patients with SOC are GA, JS, SA and LA as they have a lower incidence of side effects compared with TCA peels. JS contains resorcinol which has a skin lightening effect while SA has a whitening effect on darker skin types. A series of superficial peels are preferred to a more aggressive single MDCP. MDCPs must be used with caution in patients due to the high risk of PIH. DCPs should not be performed in patients with SOC as the risk of complications far outweighs the benefits. Furthermore, they have been replaced with energy-based devices.

When carrying out chemical peels in patients with SOC, special consideration should be given to the pre-peel priming, peel indication, choice of chemical peel agent and post-peel care. As the incidence of post-peel pigmentary changes is high, all patients should be thoroughly counselled on adequate skin priming, sun avoidance, adequate UV protection and treatment with skin lighteners before and after the procedure. Topical retinoids, GA and SA are often used as priming agents as they can reduce epidermal melanin, increase epidermal healing and improve the penetration of the peeling agent. When treating pigmentary dyschromia, topical retinoids should be discontinued 1 week before the peel to reduce the risk of excessive redness, peeling and post-peel pigmentation. Adherence to a strict post-peel regimen is important to reduce the risk of complications.

Key references

The full list of references can be found in the online version at https://www.wiley.com/rooksdermatology10e

Introduction
2 Brody HJ, Monheit GD, Resnik SS, Alt TH. A history of chemical peeling. *Dermatol Surg* 2000;26:405–9.

Basic chemistry
5 Dewandre L, Tenenbaum A. Chemistry of peels: a hypothesis of action mechanisms and a proposal of a new classification of chemical peels. In: Tung RC, Rubin MG, eds. *Chemical Peels*, 2nd edn. London: Elsevier Saunders, 2011:1–16.

Depth of peels
5 Lee KC, Wambier CG, Soon SL *et al.* Basic chemical peeling: superficial and medium-depth peels. *J Am Acad Dermatol* 2019;81:313–24.
12 Wambier CG, Lee KC, Soon SL *et al.* Advanced chemical peels: phenol-croton oil peel. *J Am Acad Dermatol* 2019;81:327–36.

Indications and contraindications
1 Soleymani T, Lanque J, Rahman Z. A practical approach to chemical peels: a review of fundamentals and step-by step algorithmic protocol for treatment. *J Clin Aesthet Dermatol* 2018;11:21–8.
9 Sidiropoulou P, Gregoriou S, Rigopoulos D *et al.* Chemical peels in skin cancer: a review. *J Clin Aesthet Dermatol* 2020;13:53–7.
14 Castillo DE, Keri JE. Chemical peels in the treatment of acne: patient selection and perspectives. *Clin Cosmet Investig Dermatol* 2018;11:365–72.
25 Chen X, Wang S, Yang M *et al.* Chemical peels for acne vulgaris: a systemic review of randomised controlled trials. *BMJ Open Access* 2018;8:e019607.
28 Lee JB, Chung WG, Ho K *et al.* Focal treatment of acne scars with trichloroacetic acid: chemical reconstruction of skin scars method. *Dermatol Surg* 2002;28:1017–21.

Side effects and complications
2 Costa IM, Damasceno PS, Coasta MC *et al.* Review in peeling complications. *J Cosmet Dermatol* 2017;153:802–9.

CHAPTER 161

Lasers and Energy-based Devices

Nazanin Saedi[1] and Christopher B. Zachary[2]

[1]Department of Dermatology and Cutaneous Biology, Thomas Jefferson University, Philadelphia, PA, USA
[2]Department of Dermatology, University of California, Irvine, CA, USA

Introduction, 161.1
Skin resurfacing, 161.1
Carbon dioxide and Er:YAG lasers, 161.1
Fractionated non-ablative devices, 161.2
Fractionated ablative devices: carbon dioxide and Er:YAG, 161.2
Management of patients undergoing laser resurfacing procedures, 161.3
Laser-assisted drug delivery, 161.5
Hypertrophic scars, 161.5
Rhytids, 161.5

Melasma, 161.5
Clinical features, 161.5
Laser management, 161.5
Complications, 161.6
CryoModulation technology, 161.6
Skin tightening, 161.6
Methods of radiofrequency delivery, 161.7
Safety and adverse events, 161.7
Ultrasound, 161.7
Radiofrequency microneedling, 161.8
Body contouring, 161.8

Muscle definition, 161.8
Fat contouring, 161.8
Cellulite, 161.9
Rapid Acoustic Pulse (RAP) technology for improvement of cellulite, 161.9
Other cellulite treatments, 161.9
Nano-pulse stimulation technology, 161.10
Conclusion, 161.10
Key references, 161.10

Introduction

Laser, light and energy-based therapies have offered significant advances in dermatological therapy in the past several decades, having evolved from the somewhat disastrous first use of the ruby laser in 1960 [1] to the current time when such technologies have become a mainstay of treatment for a host of medical conditions. Given the large number of devices available, it is important for the laser surgeon to understand their capabilities and limitations. To provide patients with optimal treatments, one must accurately identify the target structure, select an appropriate laser, light or energy-based system and then tailor the specific parameters for the intended target. Please refer to Chapter 23 for a description of the science and general clinical applications of laser and light devices.

This chapter considers laser, light and other energy-based devices and their applications for aesthetic purposes.

Skin resurfacing

Carbon dioxide and Er:YAG lasers

Classic ablative skin resurfacing gained popularity and set the gold standard for facial rejuvenation in the 1990s. The carbon dioxide (CO_2) laser, originally developed as a surgical cutting instrument, became the prototype device for facial resurfacing largely due to the outstanding observations of Richard Fitzpatrick MD. Operating at a wavelength of 10 600 nm and targeting water, the high-energy, short-pulse CO_2 laser achieves efficient soft tissue vaporisation, such as the skin, when delivered above a vaporisation threshold of $5 J/cm^2$ and in pulses of 1 ms or less. The vaporisation achieved is time and temperature dependent, and is always associated with residual thermal damage extending 50–150 μm beyond the vaporisation zone depending on the pulse duration and number of pulses delivered. The surrounding zone of thermal coagulation results in neocollagenesis and skin tightening. If lower fluence, subvaporisation threshold pulses are delivered, tissue coagulation and desiccation occur instead.

The erbium:yttrium-aluminium-garnet (Er:YAG) laser emits light within the mid-infrared portion of the electromagnetic spectrum at a wavelength of 2940 nm. Compared with the CO_2 laser, energy from the Er:YAG laser is 12–18 times more efficiently absorbed by water-containing tissues, with a tissue ablation threshold of approximately $1.5 J/cm^2$. As such, this device induces much less thermal injury in the areas immediately surrounding the vaporised tissue, leading to faster healing, reduced redness and less delayed-onset permanent hypopigmentation. These advantages are offset by the so-called 'cold' vaporisation of the Er:YAG, because of its relatively poor ability to coagulate tissue. Hence, use of lower power Er:YAG lasers was thought to be less effective for anything more than a superficial laser peel as immediate bleeding will impede further vaporisation. However, the high-power ER:YAG devices are very efficient ablators of tissue and also have an effective coagulative component that reduces bleeding [2].

After 30 years, laser resurfacing devices still remain the gold standard for photorejuvenation, wrinkle reduction and skin tightening. Having said that, the initial fervor for fully ablative laser skin resurfacing waned somewhat based on the morbidity associated

---

Rook's Textbook of Dermatology, Tenth Edition. Edited by Christopher Griffiths, Jonathan Barker, Tanya Bleiker, Walayat Hussain and Rosalind Simpson.
© 2024 John Wiley & Sons Ltd. Published 2024 by John Wiley & Sons Ltd.

with this classic technique, especially since the post-treatment recovery requires complete re-epithelialisation, with an increased risk of superficial bacterial, viral and fungal infections. Long-term sequelae include significant post-treatment erythema that can linger months following treatment. It was not uncommon to see a line of demarcation with relative hypopigmentation between treated and untreated areas, a tell-tale sign of classic resurfacing. Furthermore, the problem of delayed-onset permanent hypopigmentation within the treatment zone occurs in approximately 15–20% of subjects.

Fractionated non-ablative devices

In an effort to maximise clinical efficacy while reducing treatment-associated morbidity and speeding up postoperative healing, fractionated photothermolysis was introduced, causing a significant paradigm shift with regard to both efficacy and safety [3]. The development of fractionated lasers has changed the way laser surgeons practise. Whereas traditional full field resurfacing treats the entirety of the skin, fractional photothermolysis treats a relatively small percentage of the skin surface.

Non-ablative fractional resurfacing (NAFR) is characterised by the delivery of narrow beams of high-energy light using a variety of wavelengths targeting tissue water. Depending on the device, depths of up to 1.5 mm can be reached. Histology of tissue immediately after treatment reveals clear zones of epidermal and dermal necrosis within the microscopic treatment zones (MTZs). Lactate dehydrogenase staining, demonstrating evidence of viable tissue, was evident adjacent to the MTZs. The microscopic epidermal necrotic debris (MEND) overlying the MTZ contained cellular components as well as melanin, which were gradually extruded over the course of 2 weeks. No histological or clinical evidence of persistence of the microthermal zones was present at 3 months. Despite visible necrosis of the epidermis and dermis in the MTZs, the stratum corneum remained histologically and functionally intact. Thus, rejuvenation with the prototype device was termed non-ablative.

The first non-ablative fractional device (Fraxel re:store®, Solta Medical Inc., Hayward, CA, USA) is the most extensively studied to date. The device uses an erbium fibre laser at a non-ablative wavelength of 1550 nm. The handpiece utilises a scanning mode based on an intelligent optical tracking system. The Fraxel re:store device creates MTZs 100–200 μm in width and 500–1400 μm in depth. Energy levels can be adjusted from 4 to 70 mJ/MTZ. Additional NAFR lasers followed.

Non-ablative fractional photothermolysis has been shown to improve photoageing on both facial and other skin surfaces. Similarly, texture, wrinkling, dyspigmentation and telangiectasis have been documented to have been improved after treatment. In 2006, Geronemus [4] showed improvement in the vertical lines of the upper lip. Since then, studies have shown efficacy in photoageing of the hands and other non-facial surfaces. NAFR has been shown to be effective for atrophic acne scars, traumatic scars, striae distensae, minocycline hyperpigmentation and residual skin redundancy following resolution of haemangioma.

The thulium 1927 nm laser (Fraxel Dual®, Solta Medical Inc., Hayward, CA, USA) increased the versatility of fractionated devices. Given this wavelength's strong absorption by water, the thulium device has a non-linear depth–energy profile, unlike the 1550 nm non-ablative device. Thus, the maximum depth of penetration of 202 μm is achieved at around 20 mJ per pulse. At this energy, the dermal thermal injury profile is similar to a superficial CO_2 laser; the main advantage is that there is no epidermal loss with the thulium device, and thus no exudation or bleeding. With this minimal depth of penetration, one can effectively perform superficial treatments aimed primarily at targeting epidermal processes. In addition to applications for dermatoheliosis and dyschromia, this device is relatively effective at removing widespread actinic keratoses and actinic cheilitis. It is considered a significant advance as a treatment modality associated with successful outcome and lower risk, especially in darker skin types.

Fractionated ablative devices: carbon dioxide and Er:YAG

Following the success of fractionated non-ablative rejuvenation came the development of fractionated ablative rejuvenation [5]. Three wavelengths – 10 600 nm (CO_2 laser), 2940 nm (Er:YAG laser) and 2790 nm (yttrium-scandium-gallium-garnet (YSGG) laser) – were selected because their wavelengths are so well absorbed by water content in tissues. The Fraxel re:pair® (Solta Medical Inc., Hayward, CA, USA) was the first ablative fractional device. The device employs a 10 600 nm CO_2 laser delivered by scanning handpiece technology and has the ability to place 2000 microablative MTZs per second.

The Active/Deep FX™ system (Lumenis Aesthetic, Santa Clara, CA, USA) is another well-studied ablative fractional laser device. The Active FX utilises the original computer pattern generator handpiece with updated technology to create random patterns of injury while preventing bulk heating. The second technology, known as Deep FX, utilises a narrower spot diameter but achieves greater penetration into the dermis. When the two treatments are used together, the first pass with Deep FX and the second pass with Active FX, the procedure is termed 'Total FX'. Unlike the scanning delivery method in the Fraxel re:pair, the Deep FX system uses a stamping method. It is important to note that the parameters of energy and density are not interchangeable between the two devices.

Fractional ablative technology using Er:YAG lasers include the ProFractional™ (Sciton Inc., Palo Alto, CA, USA), the Pixel® (Alma Lasers, Buffalo Grove, IL, USA) and the StarLux2940™ (Palomar Medical Technologies, Burlington, MA, USA), among others. These devices vary from one another, but are based on the 2940 nm wavelength. More recently, the fractionated 2910 nm fibre laser has recently become available. This delivers light at the peak of water absorption and maximises tissue ablation while minimising the incidence of postinflammatory hyperpigmentation (PIH) or post-inflammatory erythema (PIE) (UltraClear™, Acclaro Corporation, Rhode Island, RI, USA).

A more recent addition to the fractionated group of lasers is a hybrid system commercially known as Halo® (Sciton Inc., Palo Alto, CA, USA). This system combines non-ablative 1470 nm diode wavelength with an ablative 2940 nm Er:YAG wavelength in a single handpiece that has the ability to deliver both wavelengths in a single pass. The 1470 nm wavelength is absorbed by water and is capable of penetrating the dermis up to 700 μm. Unique to the Halo

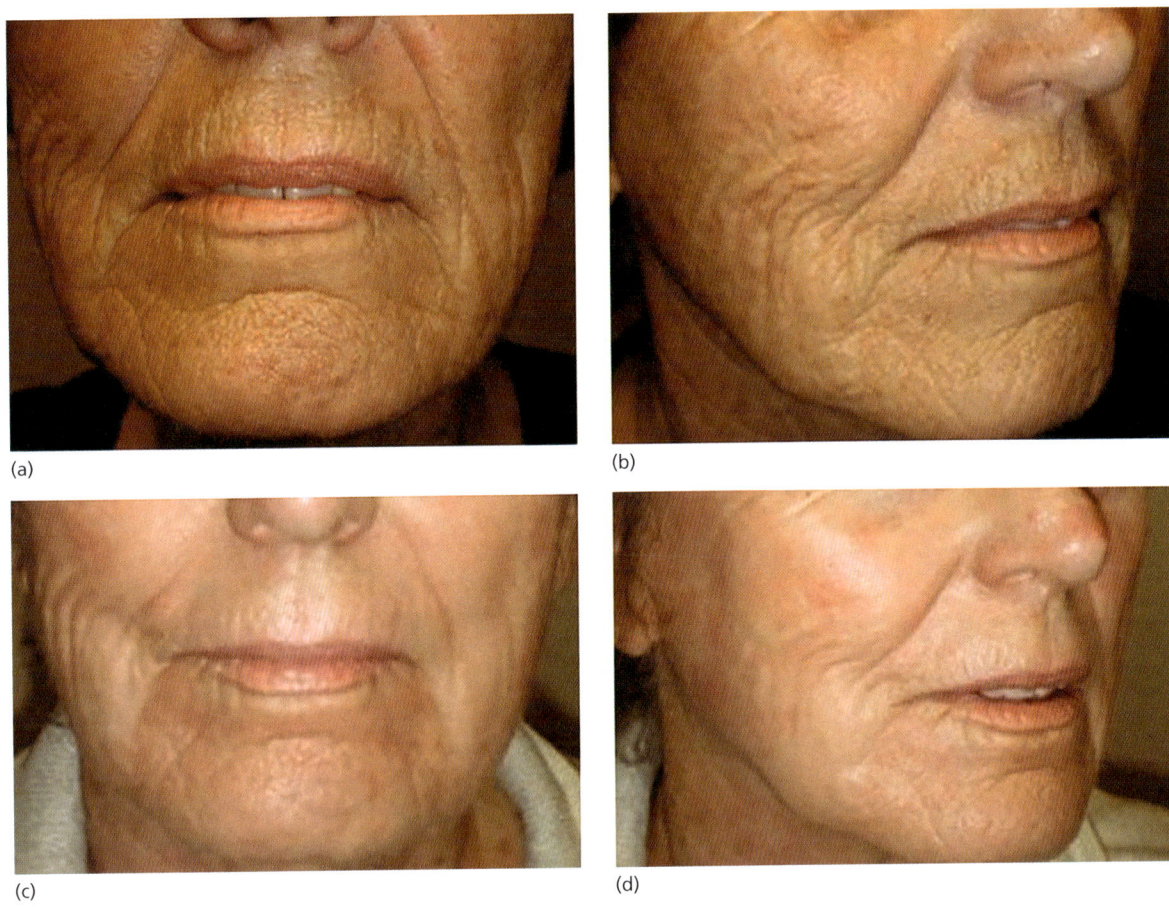

Figure 161.1 Treatment with ablative fractional resurfacing for photodamage: (a,b) before treatment and (c,d) 3 months after treatment.

is the ability to adjust the penetration depth to as little as 100 μm, thus allowing for less aggressive treatment options, but also the ability to more precisely target actinic damage at the 300–400 μm level. This device is significantly less painful than the 1550 nm non-ablative devices and is becoming popular with patients and practitioners alike.

Immunohistochemical studies demonstrate neocollagenesis after ablative fractional resurfacing with the expression of markers for heat shock proteins, collagen III, proliferating cell nuclear antigen and α-smooth muscle actin in treatment areas. Heat shock protein 47, required for collagen remodelling and maturation, persists for nearly 3 months following treatment, suggesting ongoing collagen synthesis long after the immediate recovery phase.

Ablative fractional photothermolysis offers the opportunity for relatively safe treatment of anatomical regions that were notoriously difficult to rejuvenate with conventional ablative resurfacing, and has been shown to be effective in treating photodamage and acne scarring (Figures 161.1 and 161.2).

In a reversal of recent trends, the prevailing concepts in facial rejuvenation are that the traditional full field CO_2 and Er:YAG lasers provide the best outcomes in terms of improvement per treatment. These fully ablative treatments are gaining popularity in the perioral and periorbital region while treating the rest of the face with the fractional counterpart.

Table 161.1 provides a partial list of devices.

Management of patients undergoing laser resurfacing procedures

Patient selection

Caution should be exercised in treating those with a history of delayed wound healing secondary to tobacco or alcohol abuse, diabetes or any other systemic medical condition, malnutrition, a history of connective tissue disease or an immunocompromised status. Isotretinoin use in the prior 6–12 months could impair wound healing, though recently this concept has been challenged. The majority of laser surgeons will require their patients to have a 3–6 month washout period prior to performing laser surgery, even though this is probably unnecessary [5]. Special consideration should be given to any patient with active local or systemic infections and those with a history of keloid scarring. Patients with a personal or family history (first-degree relative) of vitiligo should avoid any aesthetic laser surgery as this might activate a latent tendency.

Preoperative management and anaesthesia

Both ablative and non-ablative fractional resurfacing can be quite painful without appropriate anaesthesia, particularly when using high energies at high density. The application of a topical anaesthetic ointment such as lidocaine/tetracaine 23/7% for approximately 1 hour is a simple and effective method for increasing patient comfort. Cooling strategies such as forced cold air or contact cooling can

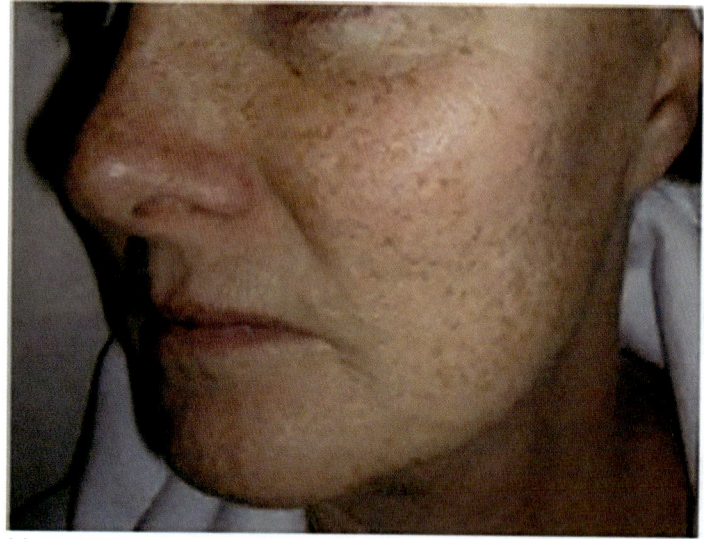

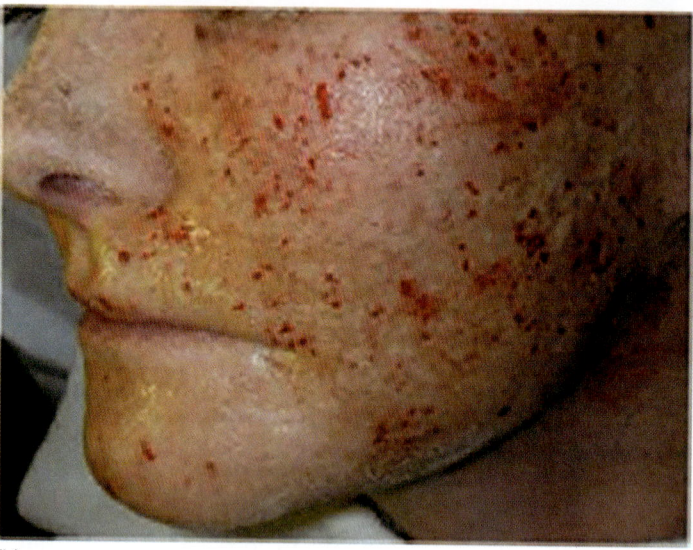

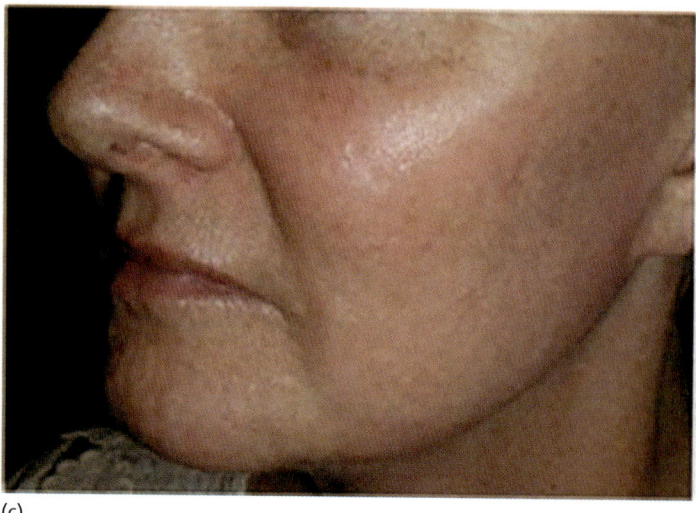

Figure 161.2 Ablative fractional resurfacing for acne scarring: (a) before treatment, (b) immediately after treatment and (c) 3 months after treatment.

enhance patient tolerance. For more aggressive ablative procedures, additional anaesthesia (with nerve blocks, tumescent anaesthesia or systemic narcotics) with anxiolytics is often used.

Oral antiviral therapy is generally recommended for herpes simplex virus prophylaxis. Acyclovir or valaciclovir is typically given anywhere starting the day of treatment for 7–10 days post treatment. For ablative procedures, patients may also receive antibacterial prophylaxis, usually in the form of penicillins or macrolides.

Postoperative course

Following ablative fractional resurfacing, punctate bleeding and serosanguinous drainage are expected side effects, which dry into a thin keratinaceous crust within 24–48 h. Significant oedema and erythema of treated skin is observed with both ablative and non-ablative fractionated therapies, although the latter is much less evident and its duration shorter. A single application of a topical potent corticosteroid ointment immediately following the procedure can reduce these side effects.

In cases of ablative laser resurfacing, either full field or fractional, careful attention to wound care is important. The skin should be cleaned gently with either dilute vinegar or hydrogen peroxide and kept moist with petroleum jelly until fully epithelialised. For ablative fractional photothermolysis, the erythema dramatically improves within 1 week, but mild erythema and oedema can persist for 3–6 weeks. Most patients are able to return to their normal activities, including work, and can apply make-up approximately 7 days after ablative fractional photothermolysis, depending on the depth and density of treatment. Unsightly lines of demarcation between treated and untreated skin can be easily avoided by feathering treatment at the borders with low energy and density settings.

Non-ablative fractional photothermolysis typically requires little 'downtime' for healing, as the oedema and erythema resolve within a few days.

Since the areas of vaporisation are so minute and with rapid skin healing, fractionated ablative systems offer an unparalleled safety margin compared with traditional ablative lasers. Up to 50% of facial skin can be treated with these devices and yet the skin heals within 5 days with no evident scarring. However, infection remains a significant complication and can lead to permanent scarring if not recognised and treated early. Furthermore, laser surgeons should be cautious when treating 'underprivileged' areas such as the neck and chest where the dermis is relatively thin with fewer adnexal structures such as follicular units, resulting in less robust healing [6]. For example, skin on the cheek has a thicker dermis with abundant adnexal structures and can therefore tolerate high energies and densities; much lower densities of fractionated treatment should be employed on less privileged areas. The laser surgeon should have a thorough understanding of relative skin thicknesses and an appreciation the composition of the skin structures in all potential treatment sites.

Another important strategy to minimise the risk of scarring is the avoidance of bulk heating. These devices lay down discrete packages of injury, each separated from the other by normal untreated skin. Scanning or stamping repeatedly over the same area will induce bulk heating, which might induce full-thickness skin loss, and subsequent scarring. The use of a non-overlapping technique

Table 161.1 Ablative and non-ablative fractional devices.

Device	Company	Type	Wavelength (nm)
Ablative fractional lasers			
Harmony™	Alma Lasers	Er:YAG	2940
Lux2940™	Palomar	Er:YAG	2940
ProFractional™	Sciton	Er:YAG	2940
Active FX™	Lumenis	CO_2	10 600
Deep FX™	Lumenis	CO_2	10 600
Fraxel re:pair® SST	Solta	CO_2	10 600
MiXto SX®	Lasering USA	CO_2	10 600
Pixel® CO_2	Alma Lasers	CO_2	10 600
SmartXide DOT®	DEKA	CO_2	10 600
Non-ablative fractional lasers			
LuxIR Fractional™	Palomar	IPL-powered infrared	825–1350
Emerge™	Palomar	Erbium fibre	1410
Fraxel re:fine®	Solta	Erbium fibre	1410
Clear + Brilliant®	Solta	Nd:YAG/fibre	1440/1927
Lux1540™	Palomar	IPL-powered laser	1540
Fraxel Dual®	Solta	Erbium fibre/thulium	1550/1927
Sellas1550™	Benev	Erbium fibre	1550
Hybrid ablative and non-ablative laser			
Halo®	Sciton	Erbium	1470/2940

CO_2, carbon dioxide; Er:YAG, erbium:yttrium-aluminium-garnet; IPL, intense pulsed light; Nd:YAG, neodymium:yttrium-aluminium-garnet; YSGG, yttrium-scandium-gallium-garnet.

allows the treated skin sufficient time to cool before the application of a subsequent pass in the same area.

Laser-assisted drug delivery

Laser-assisted drug delivery (LADD) uses the vertical cone-shaped channels known as micoablation zones (MAZ) from the ablative or non-ablative fractionated lasers to create a viable path for drug delivery. The application of topical agents to the MAZ allows for dramatically increased penetration and bioavailability of the medications (e.g. triamcinolone, 5-fluorouracil). Low percentage fractional laser treatment densities (coverage of the skin should be less than 5%) are used to prevent toxic systemic absorption of topically applied medications. The holes created by microneedling or radiofrequency microneedling tend to close immediately and hence are less able to facilitate percutaneous delivery of topical agents. One should also understand that the rapid rate of absorption through the skin should limit the agents used to those that are FDA approved for injection *into* the skin.

Hypertrophic scars

Combining ablative fractional resurfacing with both intralesional and topical medications has shown promise for the treatment of keloids and hypertrophic scars. The most commonly used medications include intralesional triamcinolone, topical triamcinolone and topical 5-fluorouracil. A recent review of 10 randomised controlled trials involving 329 patients indicated improvement when LAAD was compared with the medication alone. Waibel and colleagues demonstrated successful treatment of hypertrophic scars using a fractionated carbon dioxide laser and LAAD of either triamcinolone or 5-fluorouracil [7]. There was no statistically significant difference between triamcinolone and 5-fluorouracil. However, 5-fluorouracil had fewer side effects such as atrophy or telangiectasia formation.

Rhytids

Perioral rhytids can be stubborn to treat and often require multiple treatment modalities to achieve the desired outcomes. Ibrahim and colleagues demonstrated the efficacy of three treatments with a low density fractional ablative CO_2 laser and the topical application of poly-L-lactic acid (PLLA) for upper cutaneous lip rhytids had a 47% decrease in their severity [8]. This is a similar technique as described with atrophic acne scarring. For limited areas, fully ablative laser treatments could be more effective and less costly for patients, but they do require an experienced practitioner.

Melasma

Clinical features
Melasma remains a challenging disorder to treat (Chapter 86) and laser therapy is no exception. It commonly involves the face and presents as tan to dark brown patches with sparing of photo-protected sites. Current treatment regimens show varying degrees of improvement and recurrence is expected despite precautionary measures such as strict sun protection.

Laser management
Early reports using fractionated non-ablative lasers were initially encouraging. A preliminary case report described clinical improvement of treatment-resistant facial melasma after two treatments [9]. A subsequent study demonstrated that 60% of patients

with skin phototypes III–V achieved 75–100% improvement. The clinical improvements correlated with appropriate histological findings of melanin extrusion in the dermal and epidermal necrotic debris. Also, post-treatment electron microscopy revealed fewer melanocytes and less melanin in the surrounding keratinocytes than in the pre-treatment specimens. While these initial studies showed promise for the treatment of melasma, more recent reports have suggested some limitations in efficacy, with high recurrence rates after treatment, especially in those patients with darker skin types. Fractionated treatments can be useful for melasma when used in combination with topical 'bleaching' agents by increasing absorption, for example, of hydroquinone. However, as with all treatments for melasma, recurrence is customary unless subjects remain fastidious about sun protection measures.

Given that melasma is a disorder of hyperpigmentation with increased melanin in epidermal melanocytes and dermal melanophages, there is some rationale for the use of very short pulsed (Q-switched or QS) lasers. Low-fluence treatments with the QS 1064 nm Nd:YAG laser is currently used for melasma with repeated sub-photothermolytic energy pulses causing fragmentation of melanin granules and facilitating their removal without cellular destruction.

Choi et al. [10] studied the effects of low-fluence (2.0–3.5 J/cm^2) QS 1064 nm laser in 20 melasma patients, performed at 1-week intervals. After five treatments, the pigmentation was significantly decreased, and the investigators also noticed a decrease in the degree of wrinkling. Goldberg et al. [11] treated 20 melasma patients with a QS 1064 nm laser employing a 6 mm spot size at 2 J/cm^2. The patients underwent eight treatments at 1–2-week intervals, and all subjects showed improvement in their melasma. Kauvar [12] treated 27 female melasma patients with a combination of microdermabrasion followed immediately by treatment with a low-fluence QS 1064 nm laser. The treatment was repeated at 4-week intervals and the patients began applying hydroquinone, tretinoin and sunscreen 2 days following the laser treatment. After an average of 2.6 treatment sessions, 81% of the patients had greater than 75% clearance of melasma. As always, caution is advised as there are some reports of depigmentation associated with the QS Nd:YAG lasers for melasma and photorejuvenation, as well as an unmasking of previously subclinical melasma.

More recently, there has been increased use of picosecond lasers for the treatment of melasma and in particular with low frequency (repetition rate) and density. The picosecond alexandrite laser has been studied for treating refractory melasma, and there is increased efficacy in using the fractionated (diffractive lens) with a slow, low density treatment to minimise the thermal injury [13]. When comparing the fractionated lens with the regular handpiece, higher rates of clearance and less recurrence have been noted.

As mentioned, lasers and light-based devices are not the first line of treatment for melasma and caution should be taken when using any device that applies too much heat to the skin. Of note, while the intense pulsed light (IPL) is often used, it can exacerbate melasma.

Complications

Depending on the selected modality used, adverse effects such as scarring with irregular hypopigmentation, postinflammatory hyperpigmentation, post-treatment purpura, mottled appearance,

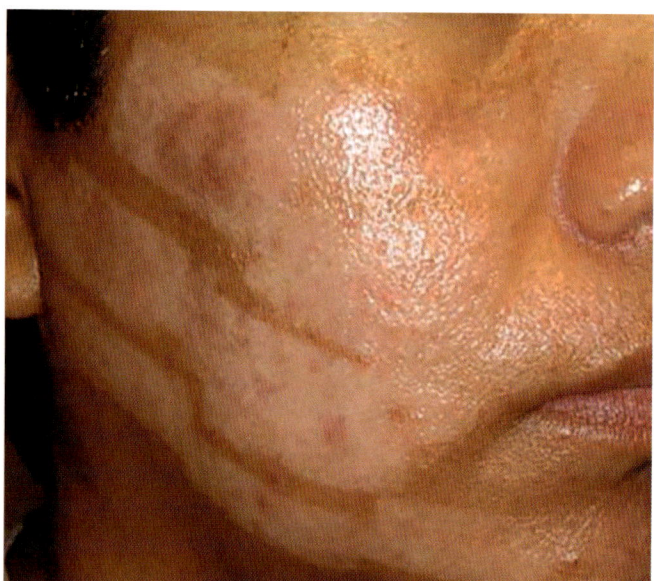

Figure 161.3 Footprinting following intense pulse light treatment in type IV skin individual.

crusting and erythema can occur, particularly when used by inexperienced professionals or those without adequate training, and is a common cause for litigation due to an aesthetic procedure (Figure 161.3).

CryoModulation technology

CryoModulation technology (R2, Blossom Innovations, MA, USA) provides an intriguing new way to lighten, brighten and rejuvenate skin. This novel approach treats benign lesions with precision, using a controlled cryo-based technology to reduce melanin production while maintaining melanocyte viability [14]. The skin barrier remains intact, ensuring effective treatment without the disadvantages commonly associated with comparable treatments.

Skin tightening

The consumer demand for non-invasive skin tightening is continually growing, although the US Food and Drug Administration has had some difficulty in defining this process. Significant research has focused on the science of radiofrequency (RF) and ultrasound. Other research has investigated the role of bulk cooling and deoxycholic acid, both of which provide limited evidence of skin tightening as part of their fat reduction process. Shockwave therapy is used in some spas for skin tightening but has little scientific basis of relevance. Further, traditional spa-type shockwave therapy is a far cry from the new Soliton RAP^{TM} acoustic wave technology referred to below.

Traditionally, the best-understood treatments for non-surgical skin tightening have been traditional laser resurfacing with the CO_2 and hot Er:YAG resurfacing. Of note, these successful skin tightening procedures only delve 300–400 μm into the skin; newer RF and ultrasound technologies attain 2–6 mm, reaching the superficial musculo-aponurotic system (SMAS). When comparing the relative benefits of depth vs density, it is the latter which is more important for skin tightening.

Having said that, RF can be used to induce volumetric heating at selected depths by changing the frequency and the configuration of the electrodes. Water is the target of this process, with depth of penetration being inversely proportional to the frequency, ranging from 3 kHz to 24 GHz. The configuration of these devices can be either bipolar or unipolar. Localised heat injury at a specific depth will induce an inflammatory reaction resulting in neocollagenesis and neoelastogenesis to achieve wrinkle reduction and tissue tightening. Of note, care must be taken to avoid excessive heating of the subcutaneous fat, which can result in localised fatty depressions in the skin.

Methods of radiofrequency delivery

Monopolar devices utilise a grounding plate so that energy is delivered through the skin of the patient, into the body, and then ultimately to the grounding plate. Other popular RF devices use a continuous (dynamic) delivery technique with constant gyration of the handpiece by the operator while the pulse fires continuously. Sophisticated devices include constant surface temperature monitoring while delivering the RF to avoid overheating, though the patients' own protective sensory mechanisms for pain are very effective as temperatures above 41°C are generally not well tolerated. For this reason, topical anaesthesia is not given prior to treatment.

The first monopolar RF device cleared by the FDA was Thermage® (Solta Medical Inc., Hayward, CA, USA). In 2004, it was approved for treating periocular wrinkles and the initial indication that was promoted for eyebrow elevation. Soon after, the device was used for the treatment of sagging jowls and skin tightening in other body areas such as the abdomen and thighs.

Through a process called capacitative coupling, the device can heat the dermis to between 65 and 75°C at a depth of 2–6 mm while maintaining epidermal temperatures between 35 and 45°C. Electrodes (tips) are available for the face, body and eyes. The technology provides transcutaneous electrical nerve stimulation (TENS)-like interruption of RF energy interspersed with hot/cold skin stimulation, as well as vibration (acting on the gate theory of pain), a modulated RF profile and a more distributive electrode. Electron microscopy has shown an increase in the diameter of collagen fibres in post-treatment biopsies compared with pretreatment biopsies [15]. Non-randomised, non-blinded studies have shown subjective improvement in lower face skin tightening, submental laxity and cheek laxity [16].

Bipolar RF devices use two electrodes within the handpiece, so that the RF travels between alternating positive and negative poles. Spacing the electrodes at a certain distance determines the depth of penetration. Studies have shown a 25–50% improvement in wrinkles, skin smoothness and texture. The objective of combined light and bipolar RF devices is to create more efficient tissue heating. The synergistic effects may increase the efficacy of each, but further studies need to be performed to substantiate a benefit beyond RF alone. It is important that we physicians determine the credibility of these devices.

Safety and adverse events

High quality RF devices have an excellent safety profile, largely attributed to advances in real-time monitoring of tissue impedance. By adjusting the power according to the impedance, the operator can avoid overheating and blistering. Keeping the energy flow controlled and having automatic heating power adjustment allows for precise and even treatment over areas of high impedance variability. The practitioner should be aware that there are multiple inferior 'copy-cat' devices purporting to be as effective and safe.

A retrospective study on 600 treatments with monopolar RF found that the most common side effect was erythema and oedema lasting for fewer than 24 hours. Significant side effects of superficial crusting, atrophic depression on the cheek, erythematous papules and neck tenderness only occurred with first generation devices and were absent in the multiple-pass lower energy treatment algorithms of newer generation devices. It must be kept in mind that all RF devices are indicated for mild to moderate skin laxity and excess subcutaneous fat tissue. Reasonable expectations must be set in place prior to the procedures. In appropriate settings, the options of more invasive methods such as surgery should be discussed.

Ultrasound

Ultrasound is established as a technique for non-invasive tissue tightening, though the enthusiasm for this depends on the experience of the provider. The primary mechanism is the tissue absorption of either very brief focused or longer diffuse acoustic energy. Skin pigmentation does not impact ultrasound, it is described as 'colourblind' and thus can be used on all skin types.

High Intensity microfocused ultrasound (HIFU)

Ultherapy™ (Merz, Raleigh, NC, USA) is FDA approved for improvement in appearance of the face, neck and décolletage. Depth-specific transducers induce millisecond pulses of focal injury within the skin without damage to the epidermis. Early results indicated significant skin tightening, with a 1 mm eyebrow lift in >75% of treated subjects. In cadaveric skin, damage was noted at a depth of 4.2 mm, including damage to the SMAS. This targeted approach was met with significant enthusiasm, and a number of investigators have observed good clinical improvement. However, some clinicians remain skeptical about the long-term benefits. Side effects include focal bruising and significant pain during treatment. Anecdotal evidence suggests high patient motivation is required to endure this procedure.

SofWave™ (SofWave Inc, Irvine, CA, USA) provides more diffuse ultrasound mid dermal heating at 60–70°C, maximally targeting a depth of 1.5 mm for 5 seconds without damage to the underlying structures including bone, nerves, fat and blood vessels. Advantages of this device are related to its relative simplicity; it has no disposables, no moving parts and no optics. The parallel delivery of more diffuse ultrasound beams, integrated cooling and a large contact area allow for less discomfort and faster treatments. The large zone of volumetric heating measuring 1.5 × 4 mm from each of seven transducers target the mid dermis, and as such the speed of treating an entire face is about 30 minutes. Anecdotal experience suggests there are both immediate and delayed responses; initial plumping of the skin with better reflectance and general appearance followed by tightening. Reports of significant brow lifting after treatment of the forehead are encouraging. This process can take several weeks to months. Patients should understand that these devices cannot replace surgical skin tightening and it may take multiple treatments to achieve the desired outcome.

As with most cosmetic treatments, photographic evidence of improvement is critical for acceptance of real benefit. Thus all patients should be appropriately photographed with good focus and lighting, consistent positioning, avoidance of neck extension, and other features that allow good and reproducible comparison. Ultimately, it is the patient who decides whether the benefit is worth the time and financial investment, but accurate photo documentation will facilitate their ability to do so in a realistic manner.

Radiofrequency microneedling

RF microneedling devices have become popular treatments for facial rejuvenation, especially since they are inexpensive and effective. Furthermore, they have become the 'go-to' device for some physicians for the treatment of acne scarring, especially in darker-skinned patients. Fractional RF microneedling devices have become prolific. Whereas microneedling as a stand-alone treatment is of questionable benefit, when combined with RF the results are more convincing. Devices can be monopolar or bipolar; also the electrodes are either insulated or non-insulated. Most disposable tips have approximately 50 electrodes in a square configuration. Careful analysis of each system should be performed before considering purchase as many of these devices are not FDA or European Commission CE cleared.

The original device (Profound®, Candela, MA, USA) has been demonstrated to induce new collagen and elastin in the mid dermis, and has demonstrated improvement in skin laxity on and off the face. However, it is quite uncomfortable, requiring topical anaesthetic, nerve blocks, and possibly nitrous oxide and injectable pain control. In general, RF microneedling devices are performed 4–6 times at one-month intervals using only topical anaesthetic. The needle density and length are sufficient to provide both superficial and deep controlled thermal injury. The low downtime and lack of postinflammatory hyperpigmentation in all skin types are making these devices quite popular among both aesthetic surgeons and the spa industry.

Microneedling devices without RF have been manufactured at breakneck speed, most without any FDA clearance. Just as rapid are the social media representations about their often unsubstantiated benefits. There is some evidence to support the benefit of microneedling as a stand-alone device for acne scarring, although there remains little evidence to support touted skin tightening benefits. It is evident that RF and/or the immediate use of topical agents following treatment can provide real benefits.

The first such fractionated RF system (eMatrix™, Candela Medical Ltd, Wayland, MA, USA) used numerous bipolar mini-electrodes specifically arranged to create a pattern of selective microthermal injury with adjacent tissue sparing. This technology is used for skin rejuvenation and subjects have seen improvement in skin tightening, smoothness and wrinkles. Pre-procedure anaesthesia should be utilised 30–60 min prior to beginning the treatment.

Body contouring

Body contouring refers to the optimisation of the definition, smoothness and shape of the human physique [17]. Apart from the underlying skeletal frame, this mainly involves muscular definition and distribution of subcutaneous fat. While diet and exercise remain the mainstay of 'looking your best', there are several non-surgical aids that can provide convincing improvements in appearance. These include both muscle toning and subcutaneous fat redistribution or elimination.

Muscle definition

Electromagnetic muscle stimulation (EMMS) selectively delivers strong electrical pulses to muscle tissue, dramatically increasing muscle contractile force, thereby conditioning the muscle in a non-invasive manner. The field generates a current when in range with a conductive material at a given intensity and frequency. Whereas skin and fat are poor conductors, muscle is an excellent conductor. Sensory nerves are bypassed. As the electrical current penetrates the muscle tissue, the motor units are stimulated resulting in intense involuntary muscular contractions. Post treatment, this results in strengthening, toning, and firming of the muscles in the abdomen, buttocks and thighs. Patients will notice an almost immediate improvement in contractility, although this is not permanent. There is some debate regarding the role of EMMS in reducing localised fat after muscle stimulation sessions. These devices are manufactured and sold by Emsculpt® (BTL, Marlborough, MA, USA), CoolTone® (Allergan, Irvine, CA, USA) and Physiq® (Cartessa, Melville, NY, USA).

Fat contouring

Historically, the approach to body contouring has largely involved invasive procedures such as liposuction and abdominoplasty. Liposuction is among the most popular of cosmetic surgery procedures performed in the USA, but it is an invasive procedure with attendant downtime and rare but significant risks, including complications from anaesthesia, infections and even death. With the rising demand for body contouring, non-invasive devices for fat reduction have become increasingly popular.

In recent years, increasing numbers of non-obese patients have sought procedures with minimal downtime and little or no associated risk, despite the fact that such procedures are less effective than traditional surgical approaches and, unlike surgery, may require repeated treatments. Current non-surgical body contouring devices including those inducing bulk cooling (cryolipolysis) [18] and bulk heating (thermolipolysis). Low-level laser therapy, low-energy non-thermal ultrasound and HIFU have also met with some success in fat reduction but are regarded by many as relics on the long road of redundancy.

Bulk cooling/cryolipolysis

The concept of cryolipolysis was introduced in 2007 and cleared by the FDA in 2010. Cryolipolysis applies controlled cold exposure with cup suction to induce targeted apoptotic reduction of subcutaneous fat. The technology is based on the concept of 'popsicle panniculitis', which has long been reported as a form of cold-induced inflammation with subsequent apoptotic fat loss [19]. By controlling and

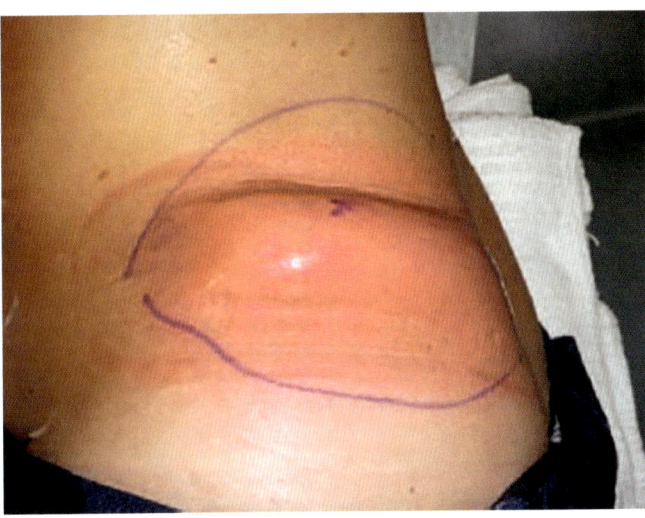

Figure 161.4 Appearance of skin immediately after cryolipolysis.

modulating the cold exposure, it is possible to damage adipocytes selectively, while avoiding damage to the overlying epidermis and dermis. The decrease in fat thickness occurs gradually over 3 months following treatment and it is most pronounced in patients with limited, discrete fat bulges.

Multiple clinical trials have demonstrated the efficacy of cryolipolysis. In one study, 32 patients with localised fat accumulation in the flanks ('love handles') demonstrated clinical improvement as measured by digital photography, physician assessment and subject satisfaction. Of these patients, 10 underwent ultrasonography of their treatment area with an average 22.4% reduction of fat layer thickness.

The known risks of this procedure include modest discomfort during the procedure, erythema of the skin, bruising and temporary numbness at the treatment site. Figure 161.4 demonstrates the appearance of the skin immediately after treatment. Coleman et al. [20] reported that there are no long-term effects on the function of the peripheral nerves. To date, there have been no reports of scarring, ulceration or alterations in blood lipid or liver function profiles. It should be noted that caution should be exercised when treating patients with cold-induced dermatological syndromes, including cryoglobulinaemia, cold-induced urticaria, Raynaud syndrome and paroxysmal cold-induced haemoglobinuria, until further studies have been done. There have been rare reports of severe pain and also paradoxical fat hypertrophy at the treatment site, but these have been ameliorated with the new design of applicators which require less negative pressure and limited cooling time.

Bulk heating/thermolipolysis

Localised bulk heating of fat has been demonstrated to effectively induce an apoptotic reduction in adipose thickness. The two best developed devices are the 1060 nm laser (SculpSure™, Cynosure, Westford, MA, USA) and the RF devices (truSculpt™ Cutera Inc., Brisbane, CA, USA). These have successfully been employed to sculpt body fat, although without the same success as bulk cooling devices. One marked difference between the two concepts is that heating tends to cause pain whereas cooling simply results in the sensation of skin numbing. Unfortunately there are rampant 'copy-cat' imitations of bulk cooling devices, with resultant dangerous practice and a litany of tissue burns and scars.

Cellulite

Rapid Acoustic Pulse (RAP) technology for improvement of cellulite

Rapid Acoustic Pulse (RAP™ Soliton Inc, Houston, TX, USA) technology has recently been developed and found to be useful both for tattoo removal and in the treatment of cellulite. This device uses ultrashort high-energy acoustic pulses (shockwaves) to induce a sheering stress on tissues that are relatively solid and fixed in comparison to surrounding structures (Figure 161.5). Indeed, its major use in the future will be for the disruption of subcutaneous fibrous septae and the smoothing of the rippled and dimpled appearance of cellulite. It is a cosmetic 'condition' which is almost universal in women and felt to be a variant of normal physiology represented by the appearance of dimpling of the skin aggravated with a certain pose or movement, although may eventually occur at rest. It can vary from a slight rippling irregularity of the skin surface to major depressions in the soft tissues, most frequently on the thighs and buttocks, but also other locations. It is related to tethering of the fat compartments to the underlying fascia. There is good evidence that high intensity, high frequency, ultrashort acoustic wave pulses are capable of disrupting these fascial connections, rendering the dimpling less evident.

The treatment of tattoos is addressed elsewhere (Chapter 23), but it is worthwhile to mention here that RAP technology was originally developed to be used in conjunction with short pulsed lasers for tattoo removal, by clearing the epidermal and intradermal vacuolar whitening associated with Q-switched laser treatment. This enables the use of multiple laser passes in a single session to efficiently remove tattoos. It should be noted that RAP technology is not the same as other traditional shockwave treatments, which have neither the power nor the ultrashort (nanosecond) pulses required to induce these specific changes referenced above (Figure 161.6).

Other cellulite treatments

Another FDA cleared treatment for cellulite includes Cellulaze™ (Cynosure Westford, MA, USA). Cellulaze is a minimally invasive 1440 nm laser procedure designed to interrupt the fibrous structures responsible for the development and persistence of cellulite. This side-firing SideLaze™ laser involves the insertion of a cannular directly under the skin. It is said to increase the thickness of skin, while simultaneously releasing the fibrous bands.

Furthermore, Cellfina® (MERZ, Raleigh NC, USA) has achieved FDA clearance as a semiautomated invasive cellulite reduction treatment. It works by detaching fibrous septae using a very thin blade, inserted through a tiny incision with local anaesthetic. The dimpled skin is suctioned up into the Cellfina device, allowing a stable platform under which the blade mechanically separates the fibrous septae. To date, Cellfina is indicated as a long-lasting cellulite treatment, particularly for larger/deeper cellulite depressions, with results lasting up to 3 years. There is some swelling and bruising, but results are noticeable within a few days of treatment.

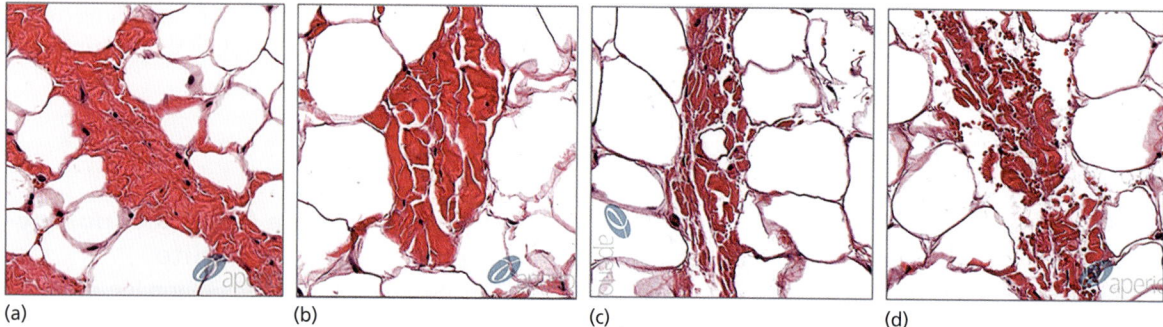

Figure 161.5 Time dose response to rapid acoustic pulse: (a) Control – 20×; (b) 1 min – 20×; (c) 2 min – 20×; (d) 3 min – 20×.

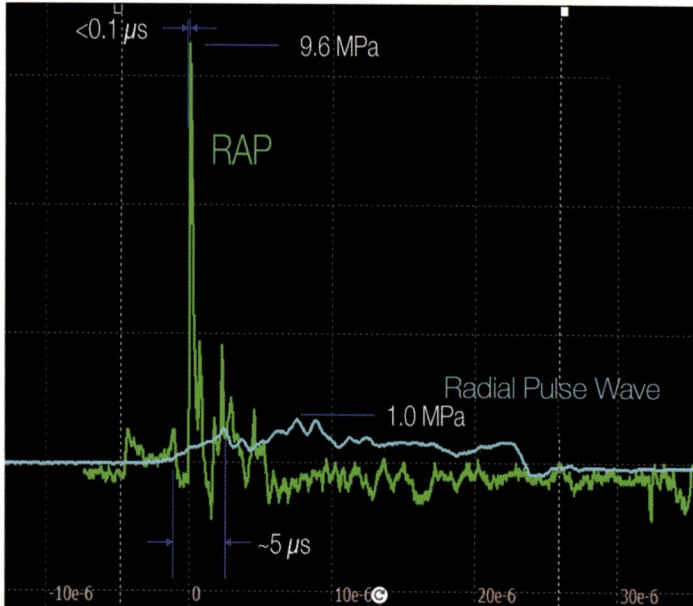

Figure 161.6 Hydrophone measurements using an Onda Corporation (Sunnyvale, CA, USA) AIMS III (Acoustic Intensity Measurement System) (green) vs a Z-Wave handpiece (blue).

Nano-pulse stimulation technology

Nano-pulse stimulation (NPS) technology (Pulse Biosciences, Inc Hayward, CA, USA) is a novel energy modality that has demonstrated a unique mechanism of action that targets only cellular morphology while sparing the non-cellular stroma. Each electrical pulse is delivered over an ultrashort (billionths of a second) time-period via microneedle arrays, resulting in internal organelle disruption and cellular apoptosis (regulated cell death). The cell-specific effect is non-thermal, with a typical nano-pulse delivering about 0.1 joules of energy distributed across a significant volume of tissue.

Early human studies have established safe threshold doses, which have been demonstrated in clinical trials to clear non-genital warts, seborrhoeic keratoses and sebaceous hyperplasia, as well as superficial basal cell carcinomas. The NPS mechanism of inducing regulated cell death has also been demonstrated in animal models of induced malignant tumours to eliminate these tumours safely while stimulating a secondary immune response that results in cytosine deaminase (CD) mediated rejection of similar malignant cells subsequently introduced to the same animal. Initial results indicate high rates of benign lesion clearance with a low incidence of scarring.

Conclusion

The rapid advances in laser, light and other energy-based devices are a testament to several factors including the engineers who design these technologies, the enquiring minds of the physicians who seek better devices for their patients, consumer demand, and the availability of funding for research and development.

Consumer demand is likely to grow, resulting in increased market share and financial incentivisation. The new paradigms of health care delivery will mean that a host of new providers will seek to offer these procedures. Although the indications for the use of these devices are cosmetic in nature, many were originally developed for medical conditions. This does not mitigate the inherent risks of the procedure itself, and it is clear that adverse events can be disfiguring and debilitating. Adequate training, education and regulation is paramount for the safe and effective use of lasers and other devices. Our first commitment is always the wellness of our patients.

Key references

The full list of references can be found in the online version at https://www.wiley.com/rooksdermatology10e

1 Maiman TH. Stimulated optical radiation in ruby. *Nature* 1960;187:493–4.
5 Hantash BM, Bedi VP, Kapadia B *et al.* In vivo histological evaluation of a novel ablative fractional resurfacing device. *Lasers Surg Med* 2007;39:96–107.
7 Waibel J, Wulkan A, Rudnick A. Treatment of hypertrophic scars using laser-assisted corticosteroid versus laser-assisted 5-fluorouracil delivery. *Dermatol Surg* 2019;45:423–30.
8 Ibrahim O, Ionta S, Depina J *et al.* Safety of laser-assisted delivery of topical poly-l-lactic acid in the treatment of upper lip rhytides: a prospective, rater-blinded study. *Dermatol Surg* 2019;45:968–74.
13 Polnikorn N, Tanghetti E. Treatment of refractory melasma in Asians with the picosecond alexandrite laser. *Dermatol Surg* 2020;46:1651–6.
14 Vazirnia A, Oritz AE. Treatment of benign pigmented lesions using a novel dermal cooling system. *Lasers Surg Med* 2019;51:59–61.

Index

Note: Page numbers in *italics* refer to figures and those in **bold** refer to tables and boxes, where they fall outside the main text range. References are to pages within chapters, thus 58.10 is page 10 of Chapter 58.

22q11 deletion syndrome *see* velocardiofacial syndrome
25-hydroxy vitamin D_3 88.19

A

AA *see* Amyloid A
AAE *see* acquired angio-oedema
AAS *see* angioedema activity score
abacavir, hypersensitivity reactions to **14.6**, 14.7
ABA criteria *see* American Burn Association criteria
abatacept, psoriatic arthritis treatment 35.46
ABC *see* atopic blepharoconjunctivitis; avidin–biotin–peroxidase complex method
ABCA12 gene
    harlequin ichthyosis 63.8
    ichthyosis 63.7
ABCD algorithm, melanoma diagnosis 142.9
ABCD mnemonic, melanoma diagnosis limitations 145.1
A-B-C model of habit disorders 84.12
ABD *see* Adamantiades–Behçet disease
abdomen
    atrophoderma of Pasini–Pierini *55.19*
    connective tissue naevus *73.18*
    Crohn disease, metastatic *95.15*, 95.16
    heparin necrosis *99.10*
    IgM pemphigoid *50.54*
abdominal fistula *112.3*
abdominal wall lymphoedema *103.51–103.52*
ABHD5 gene, neutral lipid storage disease with ichthyosis 63.36
ablative fractional resurfacing 161.1–161.3
    for acne scarring *161.4*
    avoidance of bulk heating 161.4
    device names **161.5**
    laser types **161.5**
    for photodamaged skin *161.3*
    for rhytids 161.5
    wound care 161.4
ablative lasers, hidradenitis suppurativa treatment 90.11
ABPI *see* ankle brachial Doppler pressure index
ABQOL *see* Autoimmune Bullous Disease Quality of Life
abrasions, sports injuries 122.16
ABS *see* acrylonitrile butadiene styrene
abscesses 3.43
    acne conglobata *88.66*

dental abscess 108.9
dermal fillers, adverse reactions *158.9*
see also furuncles
abscopal effects, radiotherapy on melanoma metastases 24.14
absorption, distribution, metabolism and elimination (ADME) 13.1–13.4
absorption of a drug
    clinical pharmacology 13.2
    topical medication 18.3, 18.5
AC *see* acne conglobata
acantholysis 3.38–3.39, 50.3
acanthomas
    benign proliferations of keratinocytes 132.1–132.8
    clear cell acanthoma 132.6–132.7
acanthome cellules claires of Degos and Civatte *see* clear cell acanthoma
acanthosis 3.39
    chronic actinic dermatitis 126.14, *126.15*
    sensitisation 127.8
acanthosis nigricans (AN) 85.3–85.6, 148.14–148.15
    dermatoendocrinology **150.10**, *150.11*, **150.11**, *150.13*
    diabetic patients 62.3
    female genitalia 110.22
    oral lesions 108.67
acanthosis palmaris 148.15–148.16
acanthotic and ichthyotic epidermal disorders 148.14–148.17
acanthotic lesions, elastosis perforans serpiginosa *94.55*, *94.56*
Acari 34.37–34.57
ACC *see* American College of Chemosurgery
accelerated rheumatoid nodulosis (ARN) 97.16
accessory tragus *106.8*
access to health care, initiatives for 7.8–7.11
ACD *see* allergic contact dermatitis
ACD by-proxy dermatitis ('conubial' dermatitis) 109.12
ACE *see* angiotensin-converting enzyme
acetylacetone test, formaldehyde 127.34
acetylcholine 2.9
    botulinum toxins, aesthetic use of *159.2*
    pruritus 81.3, 81.4
acetylsalicylic acid, urticaria 117.5
ACH *see* acrodermatitis continua of Hallopeau
Achenbach syndrome (paroxysmal finger haematoma) *94.19*, 99.5–99.6, 122.13–122.14
aciclovir
    pharmacological properties 19.49

topical therapies 18.13
acid phosphatase 2.42
acids, burns 128.11
Acinetobacter 26.51
acitretin
    ichthyoses management 63.44–63.45
    psoriasis treatment 35.25–35.26
ACL *see* acquired cutaneous lymphangiectasia
aclovir-resistant herpes simplex virus 149.20, 149.21
ACMS *see* American College of Mohs Surgery
acne 88.1–88.74
    acneform naevi 88.31
    agminata 88.34
    antiandrogens in management of *88.50*
    assessment tools 16.4
    causative organisms 88.15–88.18
    chemical peel side effect 160.12
    comedonal *4.19*, 88.1–88.2, *88.3*, 88.14, *88.26*, *88.27*, *88.28*, 88.45–88.47, **88.45**, **88.65**
        familial comedones 88.32
        prepubertal comedones 88.69
        senile comedones 88.31–88.32
    comprehensive acne severity system 88.38, **88.39**
    cosmetics use 88.25
    Cutibacterium 26.43
    depression 88.39
    detergent 88.25
    and diet **88.20–88.24**, 88.26
    drug-induced 88.11–88.14
        drug classes **88.12**
    ear dermatoses 106.22
    ectopic 88.31
    endocrinopathy 88.42
    environmental and lifestyle factors 88.18–88.26
    granulomatous 88.30
    heritable traits **88.18**
    hormonal investigations **88.42**
    infantile 88.68–88.74, 115.4–115.5
    inflammation 88.14–88.15, *88.17*
    inflammatory *88.3*, *88.27*
    isotretinoin treatment 5.3
    joint symptoms and arthritis association 155.10–155.11
    keloid-like 88.30, *94.50*
    mechanical 88.30
    neonatal 88.68–88.74
    nodular *88.29*
    and nutrition **88.20–88.24**, 88.26
    occupational 88.66–88.68, **88.66**

    chloracne-inducing chemicals **88.66**
    contaminated oil ingestion **88.68**
    differential diagnosis **88.67**, **88.68**
    dioxin accidents **88.68**
    papulopustular *88.3*
    penile 109.24
    photodynamic therapy 22.7
    pomade acne 88.25, *88.26*
    predisposing medical conditions **88.6**
    prepubertal 88.68–88.74
        associated diseases 88.70
        clinical features 88.70–88.71
        complications and co-morbidities 88.72
        differential diagnosis **88.71**
        disease course and prognosis 88.72
        epidemiology 88.69–88.70
        investigations **88.72**
        isotretinoin treatment **88.73**
        management 88.72–88.74
        pathophysiology 88.70
    psychological factors 15.3–15.4
    psychosocial effects 88.39
    pyogenic granulomas 88.41
    pyogenic sterile arthritis, pyoderma gangrenosum and acne syndrome **45.6**, 45.13
    quality of life measurement 16.8, 88.38–88.39
    scarring
        ablative fractional resurfacing *161.4*
        chemical peels 160.5, *160.6*
    severity measures 5.4
    suicide risk 88.39
    synovitis, acne, pustulosis, hyperostosis and osteitis syndrome 45.22, 88.7
    treatment options **88.44**
    vulval 110.45
    see also chloracne
acne of chemical origin 129.7, 129.12–129.13
acne conglobata (AC) 87.50, *88.29*, 88.62–88.66
    abscesses and cysts *88.66*
    associated diseases 88.63
    differential diagnosis 88.64
    features of **88.65**
    genetics 88.64
    management 88.65–88.66, **88.67**
    predisposing factors 88.63
    sacroiliitis 155.10–155.11
    treatment options **88.67**
Acne Core Outcomes Research Network (ACORN) 16.3
acné excoriée 84.20–84.22, 88.28–88.29, *88.30*

Rook's Textbook of Dermatology, Tenth Edition. Edited by Christopher Griffiths, Jonathan Barker, Tanya Bleiker, Walayat Hussain and Rosalind Simpson.
© 2024 John Wiley & Sons Ltd. Published 2024 by John Wiley & Sons Ltd.

Index

acne fulminans 88.59–88.62
  associated diseases 88.59
  causative organisms 88.60
  differential diagnosis 88.61
  features of **88.61**
  genetics 88.60
  investigations 88.61–88.62
  management 88.62, **88.63**
  musculoskeletal features 155.11
  presentation 88.60
  systemic treatments **88.63**
acneiform eruptions *91.3*
Acne Inversa Severity Index (AISI) 16.4–16.5
acne keloidalis *93.3–93.4*
acne keloidalis nuchae (AKN) 87.50–87.51, 122.16–122.17
Acne Lesion Score Scale system (Echelle de Cotation des Lésions d'Acné/ECLA) 16.4
acne mechanica 122.15, 122.16
acne necrotica varioliformis *93.4–93.5*
Acne-QoL *see* Acne-specific Quality of Life Questionnaire
Acne Quality of Life Scale (AQOL) 16.8
Acne-specific Quality of Life Questionnaire (Acne-QoL) 16.8
Acne Symptom and Impact Scale (ASIS) 16.8
acne tarda *88.4*
acne treatment, use during pregnancy 113.20
acne vulgaris 88.1–88.59
  acne agminata *88.34*
  acneform naevi *88.31*
  acromegaly association 88.7
  in adolescence *88.5*
  age and sex 88.1–88.2, *88.4*
  alcohol use 88.25
  androgen receptor blockers 88.51
  anorexia nervosa association 88.30
  antiandrogen treatment *88.50*
  antibiotic therapy 88.46, 88.47, 88.48–88.49, 88.52
    adverse effects **88.49**
    gram-negative folliculitis 88.36
    interactions with oral contraceptives 88.49
    prescribing policies **88.50**
    resistance to antibiotics **88.50**
  Apert syndrome association 88.10–88.11
  associated diseases 88.4–88.11
  azelaic acid treatment 88.47
  benzoyl peroxide treatment 88.46, 88.47
  and birth weight 88.26
  blue light therapy 88.58
  body dysmorphic disorder 88.30
  body mass index association 88.19
  causative organisms 88.15–88.18
  chemical peels 88.58–88.59, 160.5, *160.6*
  chloracne *88.14*
  clinical features 88.26–88.28
  clinical variants 88.28–88.30
  comedo extractor *88.58*
  complementary therapies 88.57–88.58
  congenital adrenal hyperplasia association 88.5–88.7, **88.10**
  corticosteroid treatment 88.57
  cosmetics use 88.25
  Cushing disease association 88.7
  dapsone treatment 88.46–88.47
  detergent acne 88.25
  devices and physical treatment 88.58
  diagnosis **88.42**
  and diet **88.20–88.24**, 88.26
  differential diagnosis 88.30–88.39
  disability-adjusted life years *88.5*
  disease course and prognosis 88.41
  drug-induced 88.11–88.14
    diagnosis **88.16**
    drug classes **88.12**
  eating disorders 88.30
  endocrinopathy **88.42**
  environmental and lifestyle factors 88.18–88.26

epidemiology 88.1–88.14
ethnicity 88.2–88.3
female patients
  acne tarda *88.4*
  hirsutism and hyperandrogenism *88.45*
  polycystic ovary syndrome 88.4–88.5, **88.7**–**88.8**, *88.9*
  premenstrual flare of acne **88.25**
genetics 88.18
granulomatous acne 88.30
HAIR-AN syndrome association 88.7–88.8, *88.11*
hirsutism *88.45*
hormonal investigations **88.42**
hormonal therapy 88.49–88.52
25-hydroxy vitamin D_3 88.19
hyfrecation of macrocomedones *88.57*
hyperandrogenism *88.45*
hypercortisolism association 88.7
inflammation 88.14–88.15, *88.27*, 88.28
  inflammatory cascades *88.17*
inflammatory papules 88.12
investigations 88.41–88.42
isotretinoin treatment 88.51, 88.52–88.57
  adverse effects 88.54–88.57
  prescribing guidelines **88.53**
  relative success of **88.53**
keloidalis *88.30*
light therapy 88.58
management 88.42–88.59
  aims of **88.43**
  comedonal acne 88.45–88.47
  complementary therapies 88.57–88.58
  devices and physical treatment 88.58
  first line therapy 88.44–88.45
  fixed combination therapy 88.46, 88.47
  general principles 88.42–88.43
  papulopustular acne **88.46**, 88.47–88.52
  poor response to treatment **88.50**
  side effects of topical treatments 88.48
  systemic therapy 88.48
  treatment options **88.44**
mechanical acne 88.30
and menstrual cycle 88.25
metformin treatment 88.57
neurophysiology 88.15–88.18
nicotinamide treatment 88.57
nodular 88.29
and nutrition **88.20–88.24**, 88.26
obesity association **88.23–88.24**
occupational hazards 129.12
oestrogen treatment 88.50–88.51
PAPA (pyogenic sterile arthritis, pyoderma gangrenosum and acne) association **88.8**–88.10
papulopustular acne, treatment **88.46**, 88.47–88.52
pathogenesis 88.17
pathophysiology 88.14–88.15
photodynamic therapy 88.58
pigment changes *88.3*
polycystic ovary syndrome association 88.4–88.5, **88.7**, **88.8**, *88.9*
pomade acne 88.25, *88.26*
postinflammatory macules *88.3*
predisposing heritable traits **88.18**
predisposing medical conditions **88.6**
in pregnancy 88.26, 113.11–113.12
premenstrual flares **88.25**
presentation 88.26–88.28
progestin treatment 88.50–88.51
Propionibacterium acnes effect on human sebocytes *88.17*
psychological problems 88.28–88.29
psychosocial effects 88.39
pustules *88.12*
pyogenic granulomas 88.41
quality of life measurement 88.38–88.39, **88.40**
retinoid treatment 88.45–88.46, 88.47
salicylic acid treatment 88.57
SAPHO synovitis syndrome association 88.7
scarring *88.3*, *88.4*, *88.29*, 88.39–88.41

  duration correlation *88.4*
  immune responses *88.40*
  mimics 88.38
sebaceous glands, neuropeptide–cytokines/chemokine signalling *88.17*
Sebutape analysis *88.28*, *88.43*
severe acne *88.3*, **88.42**
  management 88.52–88.57
  treatment algorithm *88.52*
severity classification/definition 88.38–88.39, **88.43**
in skin of colour 88.43–88.44, *88.45*
sleep deprivation impact 88.25
and smoking 88.19
spironolactone treatment 88.51
and stress 88.25
sulphur treatment 88.57
systemic therapy 88.52
treatment options **88.44**
UV radiation impact 88.25–88.26
visible light treatment 88.58
vitamin C treatment 88.57
zinc treatment 88.51–88.52, 88.57
ACORN *see* Acne Core Outcomes Research Network
acquired angio-oedema (AAE) 43.1, 43.3, **43.6**
acquired autoinflammatory disorders 155.10
acquired cutaneous lymphangiectasia (ACL) 103.6
acquired cutis laxa 94.21–94.23
acquired digital fibrokeratoma 136.4
acquired disorders
  dermal connective tissue 94.1–94.58
  elastic tissue deposition 94.32–94.33
  epidermal keratinisation 85.1–85.31
  of hair 87.1–87.102
  pilosebaceous unit 93.1–93.13
acquired disorders with skin and renal involvement 154.6
acquired elastotic haemangioma 136.29
acquired epidermodysplasia verruciformis (AEV) 25.66, 25.71–25.72, *25.73*, **25.73**
acquired generalised lipodystrophy (AGL) 98.1–98.4
acquired hypermelanosis 86.9–86.33
acquired hypertrichosis 87.86–87.87
acquired hypomelanosis 86.34–86.47
acquired ichthyosis 63.47–63.50, 63.73, 85.1–85.3, 148.17
acquired idiopathic generalised anhidrosis 92.12
acquired idiopathic livedo reticularis 124.9–124.10
acquired immune deficiency syndrome *see* AIDS
acquired immunodeficiency diseases 149.18–149.20, **149.21**
  cytokine and signalling protein mutations **149.20**
  human papillomavirus infection 25.65–25.73, **25.66**, 25.71–25.73
  primary 149.18–149.20, **149.21**
  skin cancer 147.2–147.5
  skin manifestations 149.20–149.22
  see also AIDS; inherited immunodeficiency
acquired keratodermas 63.71–63.79
acquired lipodystrophy 98.1–98.13
acquired melanocytic naevi 131.17–131.21
  clinical presentation **131.16**
  compound naevus *131.19*, *131.21*
  dermoscopic presentation **131.16**
  junctional naevus *131.18*, *131.20*
  naevomelanocytic nests *131.18*, *131.20*
  naevus cell types *131.19*, *131.20*
  pathology **131.16**
acquired non-infective disorders, pilosebaceous unit 91.1–91.20
acquired pachydermatoglyphia (acanthosis palmaris) 148.15–148.16
acquired partial lipodystrophy (APL) 98.4–98.6, *98.5*

  renal failure 154.2
acquired perforating dermatoses 63.76–63.77, 94.53–94.57
  renal failure and dialysis complications 154.3–154.4
acquired pigmentary disorders 86.1–86.56
acquired poikiloderma 94.13
acquired progressive kinking of the hair 87.81
acquired progressive lymphangioma 136.38
acquired pseudo-ainhum 94.48
acquired pseudoxanthoma elasticum 94.30–94.31
acquired resistance, glucocorticoids 19.19
acquired resistance to insecticides, head lice 34.21–34.22
acquired syndromic hypomelanosis 86.42–86.47
acral acanthosis nigricans 85.5
acral arteriovenous tumour *see* cirsoid aneurysm
acral blistering
  epidermolysis bullosa simplex *69.10*, *69.11*
  self-improving dystrophic epidermolysis bullosa *69.17*
acral fibromyxoma 136.59
acral lentiginous melanoma (ALM)
  melanoma classification 142.7, 142.8
  presentation 142.10, *142.14*, *142.15*, *142.17*, 142.19
acral lesions, PJT syndrome 68.13
acral melanoma (volar skin of palms and soles), dermoscopy 145.9, 145.11–145.13
acral naevi 131.23–131.24
  compound acral naevus *131.23*
  on sole of foot *131.24*
acral peeling skin syndrome (APSS) 63.29, 69.19, *69.20*
  genes/proteins linkage 69.5–69.6
acral persistent papular mucinosis 57.6–57.7
Acremonium, skin lesions 32.93
acroangiodermatitis, purpura 99.4
acrocyanosis 79.9, 124.6–124.7
acrodermatitis 69.24
  Lyme disease/*Borrelia burgdorferi* role in B-cell lymphoma 139.37–139.38
acrodermatitis chronica atrophicans 94.15–94.16
acrodermatitis continua of Hallopeau (ACH) 35.39–35.41
  clinical features 35.40
  differential diagnosis 35.40–35.41
  genetics 35.40
  management 35.41
acrodermatitis enteropathica 79.15–79.16
  oral involvement 108.20
  zinc deficiency 61.25, 61.26
acrodermatitis pustulosa *see* infantile acropustulosis
acrodynia 121.5, 121.6
acrofacial purpura and necrosis, Covid-19 association 25.111
acrogeria (Grotton syndrome) 70.28
  clinical features of *70.26*
acro-ischaemia, Covid-19 association 25.111
acrokeratoelastoidosis 63.59, 63.60, 94.31–94.32
acrokeratosis paraneoplastica 148.19
acrokeratotic poikiloderma of Weary **75.2**, 75.7
acromegaly 86.18
  acne vulgaris association 88.7
  dermatoendocrinology **150.11**, *150.12*, *150.15*, 150.16
  ear dermatoses **106.22**
acromelia, congenital pseudo-ainhum 94.48
acro-osteolysis with keratoderma (Bureau–Barrière syndrome) 63.71
acrospiroma
  use of term/hidradenoma relationship 137.23, 137.28

see also hidradenocarcinoma; hidradenoma
acrosyringeal naevus *see* eccrine syringofibroadenoma
acrosyringium, keratinisation of   63.71
acrylate resins   127.69–127.70
acrylates, contact allergy   127.47
acrylic nail systems   127.61
acrylonitrile butadiene styrene (ABS)   122.21
ACTG *see* AIDS Clinical Trial Group
ACTH *see* adrenocorticotrophic hormone
actin   3.25
actinic cheilitis (solar cheilosis)
   lip lesions   108.58
   photothermal ablation   23.21
actinic comedonal plaque   94.3
actinic elastosis   94.2–94.4
actinic folliculitis   91.6–91.8, 93.6
actinic granuloma and annular elastolytic giant cell granuloma   94.27–94.29
actinic keratoses (AK)   63.74, 141.1–141.12
   with Bowen disease, immunocompromised people   147.11–147.12
   chemical peels   160.5
   photodynamic therapy   22.4–22.6
   squamous cell carcinoma relationship   141.1
actinic lentigo (solar lentigo)   131.5–131.7, 160.7
actinic lichen planus   37.7, 37.17
actinic prurigo (AP)   126.2, 126.4, 126.10–126.21
   lip lesions   108.58–108.59
   photopatch testing   126.36
   polymorphic light eruption differentiation   126.7
actinic purpura   99.5
   ageing of skin   156.5, *156.6*
actinic reticuloid   126.13
Actinomyces israelii, actinomycosis   26.84–26.86
Actinomyces keratolytica, pitted keratolysis   26.42–26.43
Actinomyces pyogenes see Trueperella pyogenes
actinomycetes   26.84–26.87
   mycetoma   32.73–32.75
   nocardiosis   26.86–26.87
actinomycosis   26.84–26.86
   botryomycosis similarity   26.77
actinophytosis *see* botryomycosis
action spectroscopy   10.4–10.5
active psoriasis *see* unstable psoriasis
active sensitisation, patch testing   127.32, 127.61
active sweating   2.9
acute adverse effects, photodynamic therapy   22.12–22.14
acute alcohol sensitivity   **104.9**
acute arsenical dermatitis   121.2
acute atrophic oral candidiasis *see* acute erythematous candidiasis
acute candidiasis
   oral involvement   32.61, 108.20, 108.31, *108.32*
   see also oral candidiasis
acute contact dermatitis   127.12
   arsenic   121.2
acute cutaneous lupus erythematosus   89.8
acute cutaneous miliary tuberculosis   27.17
acute dermatolymphangioadenitis (ADLA)   103.16, 103.34–103.35
acute dermatomyositis   52.3, 52.5
acute diffuse otitis externa   106.16–106.17, 106.18
acute disseminated histoplasmosis   32.82–32.83
acute epidermal distension   85.28–85.30
acute erythema, solar urticaria   126.22
acute erythematous candidiasis   32.61
acute febrile neutrophilic dermatosis *see* Sweet syndrome
acute generalised exanthematous pustulosis (AGEP)   14.4, 118.1–118.4, 118.10
acute generalised pustular psoriasis of von Zumbusch   35.33–35.34, 118.4

acute genital ulcers *see* Lipschutz ulcers
acute graft versus host disease (aGvHD)   38.1, 38.2, 38.3–38.7
   clinical features   38.3–38.5
   epidemiology   38.1–38.2
   management   38.5–38.7
   pathology   38.2–38.3
   severity classification   38.4, **38.5**
acute guttate psoriasis   35.12–35.13
   lesions   *35.13*
acute haemorrhagic oedema, infants   115.9, *115.10*
acute herpetic neuralgia (AHN)   82.4
acute inflammation, sports injuries   122.16
acute intermittent porphyria (AIP)   58.5
acute limb ischaemia, treatment options   **101.5**
acute liver disease, cutaneous features   153.4–153.5
acute localised exanthematous pustulosis (ALEP)   118.4
acute necrotising eosinophilic myocarditis (ANEM)   118.9
acute necrotising (ulcerative) gingivitis and noma (ANUG)   108.54–108.55
acute oedema
   allergic contact dermatitis   *127.15*
   blisters   85.28–85.30
acute otitis externa   106.15
acute perihepatitis (Fitz-Hugh-Curtis syndrome)   30.5
acute phototoxicity, PUVA phototherapy adverse effects   21.13
acute physiological reactions, heat/IR radiation   124.14
acute pseudomembranous candidiasis   32.61, 108.31, *108.32*
acute pulmonary histoplasmosis   32.82
acute pulmonary insufficiency   125.4
acute radiation dermatitis   119.14
acute radiodermatitis   24.18, *24.19*
acute scrotum   109.23, 109.25–109.26
acute selenium exposure   121.7
acute SJS/TEN   118.17
acute spongiotic dermatitis   126.15
acute spontaneous urticaria   42.5, 42.15–42.16
acute telogen effluvium   87.54, *87.56*
AD *see* atopic eczema (dermatitis); autosomal dominant
ADA *see* adenosine deaminase
adalimumab
   hidradenitis suppurativa treatment   90.10
   psoriasis treatment   35.28
   psoriatic arthritis treatment   35.45
   scalp folliculitis   *91.14*
ADAM17 deficiency   45.16
Adamantiades-Behçet disease (ABD)   48.1–48.11, 97.9, 97.25, 97.51–97.52
   aphthous ulcers   *48.5*, **48.8**
   articular involvement   48.4, **48.8–48.11**
   autoimmune mechanisms   48.3
   bacterial agents   48.2
   causative organisms   48.2
   central nervous system involvement   **48.11**
   clinical features   48.4–48.6
   cytokine mediators   48.3
   differential diagnoses   **48.7**
   disease course and prognosis   48.6–48.7
   drug treatment   **48.9–48.10**
   endothelial cells   48.3–48.4
   epidemiology   48.1–48.2
   gastrointestinal involvement   **48.11**
   genetics   48.2–48.3
   genital ulcers   *48.5*, 109.23
   heat shock proteins   48.3
   immunogenetic factors   48.3–48.4
   international criteria for   **48.4, 108.40**
   International Study Group for Behçet syndrome   **108.40**
   investigations   48.7
   MAGIC syndrome   155.13
   management   48.7–48.8
   mechanical stimuli   122.3

   mucocutaneous involvement   48.4, **48.8**
   ocular disease   48.4, *48.6*, **48.8**
   oral ulceration   *48.2*, 48.5, 108.40–108.41
      treatment   **48.8**
   pathology   48.2
   positive pathergy test   *4.25*
   prevention   48.11
   severity classification   48.6
   sex ratio   48.1
   skin and pulmonary involvement   152.4, *152.5*
   systemic lesions   48.4–48.6
   treatment ladder   **48.8–48.11**
   uveitis   48.4, *48.6*
   vascular involvement   **48.11**
   viral agents   48.2
   vulval ulceration   110.20
   see also Behçet-like disease entries
adamantinoid trichoblastoma   137.12
Adams-Oliver syndrome   **79.10**
ADAMTS metalloproteinases   2.32, *2.33*
adapalene   18.25
AD (atopic dermatitis) *see* atopic eczema (dermatitis)
ADCs *see* AIDS defining cancers
ADCT *see* Atopic Dermatitis Control Test
addiction, illicit drugs   120.1
Addison disease   86.7, 86.17, *86.18*
   adrenal function   86.17
   cytotoxic drugs   86.26
   ear dermatoses   **106.22**
   skin pigmentation changes   150.7, **150.10, 150.11**, *150.13*, *150.15*, 150.18
adenoid cystic carcinoma   137.39–137.40
adenoma sebaceum   88.32
adenopathy and extensive skin patch overlying a plasmacytoma (AESOP) syndrome   149.11, *149.12*
adenosine deaminase (ADA) deficiency   80.8
adenosine triphosphate (ATP) synthesis   121.2
adermatoglyphia   70.36
ADHD *see* attention-deficit hyperactivity disorder
adherens junctions   2.19–2.20
   keratinocytes   *2.19*
adipocytes   2.42, 97.1–97.2, 97.4
   cytotoxic T lymphocytes interaction   97.6–97.7
   erythema nodosum   97.22
   insulin sensitivity   97.5
   necrosis of   97.7–97.8, *97.44*, *97.55*
adipocytic necrosis, cold panniculitis   97.36
adipocytokines, obesity link   98.27
adipogenesis   97.5
adipokines   97.5–97.6
adiponecrosis e frigore   97.35
adiponectin   97.5
adipophilin   97.7
adipose tissue
   acquired generalized lipodystrophy   98.2
   CLOVES syndrome   72.9
   congenital (familial) lipodystrophies   72.1–72.3
   familial lipoedema   72.12
   familial partial lipodystrophies   72.3, **72.4**
   fibroadipose hyperplasia   72.9
   functions   98.27
   genetic disorders   72.1–72.13
   hemihyperplasia–multiple lipomatosis syndrome   72.9, *72.11*
   hereditary obesity   72.3–72.9
   hereditary panniculitis   **72.11**
   lipodystrophies   72.1–72.3
   lipomatoses, hereditary   **72.10**
   pain   98.17
   physiology   97.3–97.4
   PIK3CA-related overgrowth spectrum   72.9–72.11
   types of   72.1
   see also obesity
adipose triglyceride lipase   63.36
adiposis dolorosa (Dercum disease)   **72.10**, 98.17–98.20

   benign symmetric lipomatosis contrast   98.16
   obesity association   98.17–98.18, 98.28
adjuvant and salvage radiotherapy, skin cancer   24.9–24.10
adjuvant systemic treatment, melanoma   144.6
ADLA *see* acute dermatolymphangioadenitis
ADLI *see* autosomal dominant lamellar ichthyoses
ADME *see* absorption, distribution, metabolism and elimination
adnexal carcinoma NOS   137.37–137.38
adnexal polyps, neonatal   114.19
adnexal structures   2.5–2.7
adolescents
   acne vulgaris   *88.5*
   measuring impact of skin disease   16.10
   psychological and social factors   15.3
   Skindex-Teen Dermatology Life Quality Index   16.10
   skin picking disorder   84.19
   trichotillosis   84.22–84.23, 87.32, 87.33
adrenal hyperfunction
   dermatoendocrinology   150.17–150.18
   see also congenital adrenal hyperplasia; Cushing disease/syndrome; hyperaldosteronism; hypercortisolism
adrenal insufficiency *see* Addison disease
adrenal steroid genesis pathway   *88.9*
adrenal suppression, systemic glucocorticoid therapy   19.19
adrenergic nerve supply, eccrine sweating   92.3
adrenocortical carcinoma   87.91
adrenocorticotrophic hormone (ACTH)
   ACTH administration, hypermelanosis   86.18–86.19
   hair follicle   87.11
adult colloid milium   94.5–94.6
adult eosinophilic pustular folliculitis   91.4
adult haemangiopericytoma   136.40
   see also myopericytoma
adult myofibroma   136.39–136.40
   see also myopericytoma
adult-onset Still disease (AOSD)   45.21, 53.8, 53.9, 100.29
adult progeria *see* Werner syndrome
adult T-cell leukaemia–lymphoma (HTLV-1 associated)   139.34–139.36
advanced glycation end-products (AGEs)   62.1
advancement flaps, surgical reconstruction   20.23, **20.24**, 20.25
adverse effects
   critical appraisal for evidence based medicine   17.17–17.18
   drug-induced pruritus   81.10–81.11
   drug-related   13.6, 13.9–13.11
   extracorporeal photochemotherapy   21.15
   isotretinoin acne treatment   84.42, 155.11
   patient education   21.16
   patient selection and assessment   21.15–21.16
   photodynamic therapy   22.12–22.14
   phototherapy   21.11–21.17
   pseudolymphoma   134.1, 134.2–134.3
   PUVA phototherapy   21.13–21.15, 21.16
   topical calcipotriol plus steroids   18.28, *18.29*
   topical corticosteroids   18.15, 18.17–18.20
   topical therapy   18.4–18.5
   UVA-1 phototherapy   21.15
   UVB phototherapy   21.11–21.13
   see also cutaneous adverse drug effects; drug reactions
adverse immune reactions to drugs *see* immunological reactions to drugs
AE *see* atopic eczema (dermatitis)
aEDS *see* arthrochalasia Ehlers–Danlos syndrome
AEGCG *see* annular elastolytic giant cell granuloma
AEI *see* annular epidermolytic ichthyosis; annular erythema of infancy

AEIOU acronym, clinical characteristics of Merkel cell carcinoma 146.5, **146.7**
AEP *see* atopic eruption of pregnancy
AE-QoL *see* Angioedema Quality of Life Questionnaire
aerosolised cleaning fluid, inhalation of 120.4
AESOP syndrome *see* adenopathy and extensive skin patch overlying a plasmacytoma syndrome
aesthetic therapies
    laser resurfacing 161.1–161.6
    photodynamic therapy 22.8
    skin tightening 161.6–161.8
    see also cosmeceuticals; cosmetic treatments
AEV *see* acquired epidermodysplasia verruciformis
Africa, access to dermatologists 7.4
African eye worm (*Loa loa*) *see* loiasis
African histoplasmosis (*duboisii* form) 32.82, 32.83
African skin phenotypes, photoageing 156.2–156.3, 156.7
African trypanosomiasis (sleeping sickness) 33.39–33.43
    clinical features 33.40–33.41, *33.42*
    investigations 33.42
    management 33.43
    pathophysiology 33.39, *33.40*
Africa Teledermatology Project (ATP) 7.9
AFX *see* atypical fibroxanthoma
AGA *see* androgenetic alopecia
age
    drug pharmacokinetics and pharmacodynamics 13.7–13.8
    pruritus 81.2, 81.11
age effects
    basal cell carcinoma 140.2
    Merkel cell carcinoma risk 146.1–146.2
    seborrhoeic keratosis 132.1
ageing of skin 2.45–2.46, 156.1–156.12
    air pollution 156.8
    Barrier dysfunction 156.10–156.11
    Bateman purpura 156.5, *156.6*
    cellular changes 2.45
    chronic inflammation 2.45
    clinical features 156.1–156.6
    collagen fibril fragmentation 156.8–156.9
    cosmetic implications 156.11
    cutaneous nodular elastosis with cysts and comedones 156.4
    cutis rhomboidalis nuchae *156.5*
    dermal connective tissue changes 94.1–94.6
    dermatoporosis 156.11
    dermatosis papulose nigra, skin of colour *156.3*
    DNA damage/repair 2.46
    dyspigmentation *156.2, 156.5*
    extrinsic ageing 156.1–156.4
    variants 156.3, *156.4*
    genetic diseases 2.46
    genetics of 156.6
    grading and measurement 156.6–156.7
    idiopathic guttate hypomelanosis 156.5, *156.6*
    implications of 156.10–156.11
    intrinsic ageing 2.46, 156.1, *156.2*
    medical implications 156.10
    menopausal skin ageing 156.6
    molecular mechanisms *156.10*
    neck 156.4–156.5
    nodular elastosis with comedones and cysts *156.5*
    pathophysiology 156.7–156.10
    photoageing 2.45, 2.46, 156.1–156.4
    and natural ageing 156.10
    reactive oxygen species 156.4, 156.6
    sensory perception 2.45
    skin of colour 156.1–156.3
    skin structure and function 2.45–2.46
    smoking 156.4
    social implications 156.11

telomere shortening 2.45–2.46
transcriptomic analysis 2.46
UV exposure 2.46, 156.7–156.8, *156.10*
white skin 156.1
see also cosmeceuticals; premature ageing syndromes
AGEP *see* acute generalised exanthematous pustulosis
AGEs *see* advanced glycation end-products
aggrecan *2.38*
aggressive angiomyxoma *see* deep ('aggressive') angiomyxoma
aggressive digital papillary adenocarcinoma 137.34–137.35
aggressive systemic mastocytosis (ASM) 46.1, *46.9*, 46.10
AGL *see* acquired generalised lipodystrophy
agminated or segmental lentiginosis 131.3
agranulocytosis
    acute generalised exanthematous pustulosis 118.3
    dapsone 19.14
    oral involvement 108.71
AGS *see* Aicardi–Goutières syndrome
aGvHD *see* acute graft versus host disease
AHN *see* acute herpetic neuralgia
AI *see* artificial intelligence
Aicardi syndrome *72.10*
Aicardi–Goutières syndrome (AGS) **45.5, 45.6**, 45.13
AIDS
    case definition 31.5–31.6
    dermatological involvement 31.1
    eye disease **107.35**
    Kaposi sarcoma-associated herpesvirus 25.42, 25.43
    see also HIV infection
AIDS-associated eosinophilic pustular folliculitis 93.8
AIDS-associated Kaposi sarcoma 25.42, 25.43, 31.30–31.31, 31.35, 138.1, **138.2**, 138.4, 138.5, 138.6
AIDS Clinical Trial Group (ACTG), Kaposi sarcoma staging 138.4, **138.5**
AIDS defining cancers (ADCs) 147.2
AIDS patients
    biopsies 3.38
    hypermelanosis 86.25
AIDS wasting syndrome 98.7
AIN *see* anal intraepithelial neoplasia
ainhum 94.47–94.48
AIP *see* acute intermittent porphyria
airborne allergens 127.17–127.18
airborne contact dermatitis 126.18, 128.4
Aircast Walker's boot *83.16*
air pollution
    ageing of skin 156.8
    atopic eczema 41.7
airway oedema, burn injuries 125.2, 125.5
AISI *see* Acne Inversa Severity Index
AK *see* actinic keratoses
AKC *see* atopic keratoconjunctivitis
AKN *see* acne keloidalis nuchae
ALA *see* alpha-lipoic acid; 5-aminolaevulinic acid
Alagille syndrome (arteriohepatic dysplasia) 153.5
albinism 7.2, 68.5–68.8
    Griscelli–Pruniéras syndrome 68.9
    partial albinism in Chediak–Higashi syndrome 80.14
    skin cancer prevention and management 7.10–7.11, 7.12, *7.13*
albinism–deafness syndrome 68.9
Albright hereditary osteodystrophy **72.7**
    in infancy *72.9*
ALCL *see* anaplastic large-cell lymphoma
alcohols, topical therapies 18.9
alcohol sensitivity flushing **104.9**
alcohol services, psychosocial diseases 120.8
alcohol use
    and acne 88.25

BSL association 98.15, 98.16
cutaneous disease 84.39–84.40
oral squamous cell carcinoma 108.46
psoriasis association 35.4, 120.3
rosacea risk 89.3
Alcyonidium diaphanum stings 130.4
aldehydes, topical therapies 18.10
ALEP *see* acute localised exanthematous pustulosis
Alexandrite lasers, vascular lesions 23.7
alexithymia, identification and treatment importance 15.3
Alezzandrini syndrome 86.42
alginate dermal filler 158.5
ALHE (angiolymphoid hyperplasia with eosinophilia) *see* epithelioid haemangioma
Alibert, Jhaemmean-Louis 1.4, *1.5*
alitretinoin (9-cis retinoic acid) 41.29
    topical 18.25
ALK *see* anaplastic lymphoma kinase
alkalis, burns 128.11
alkali tests, irritant contact dermatitis 129.5
alkaptonuria 79.12, 86.50, 106.24
alkyl glucosides 127.59
Allegemeines Krankenhaus, Vienna 1.6
alleles 8.3, 8.4–8.5, 8.9
Allen test 122.13
allergens 127.36–127.78
    arthropods 34.2
    bedbug bites 34.26–34.27
    beetle larval hairs 34.31–34.32
    binding to skin components 127.6–127.7
    contact cheilitis association **108.60**
    horse fly bites 34.9
    house dust mites 34.51
    hymenoptera venom 34.9, 34.16–34.18
    locusts 34.32
    mites 34.50, 34.51
    patch testing 129.7
    prevention strategies 127.2
    Reduviidae bug bites 34.29
    standard series lists **127.30**
    stings 130.4
    venom immunotherapy 34.18
allergic components, chemicals 128.6
allergic contact dermatitis (ACD) 9.10, 39.3, 39.21, 127.1–127.88, 128.2, 128.3, 128.5, 128.12, 129.5–129.7
    atopic eczema relationship 41.12, 41.22
    chemical peels, side effect of 160.13
    drug-induced eczema 117.3–117.5
    epidemiology 127.2–127.4
    erythroderma 39.35
    eyelids *39.22*
    male genitalia 109.12, **109.13**
    occupational 16.12, 129.5–129.7
    pathophysiology 127.6–127.7
    perianal skin 111.9
    peristomal skin 112.7–112.8
    population studies 127.3–127.4
    prevalence 127.3
    sensitising chemicals 127.6
    stings 130.4
    vulval 110.15
    see also contact dermatitis
allergic contact urticaria 127.82–127.86
    vulval 110.16
allergic disorders, involving respiratory system 152.1–152.2
allergic occupational hazards 129.8–129.11
allergic reactions 9.9–9.10
    clinical pharmacology 13.6
    dermatophyte infections 32.50
    IgE-related type 1 skin hypersensitivity 9.9–9.10
    patch testing technique 1.8
    sensitising agents used in topical therapies 18.33–18.34
    to insulin and glucose monitors 62.4
    topical therapy adverse effects 18.4, 18.5
    urticaria 42.5
allergic rhino-conjunctivitis, and atopic eczema 41.20
allergic transfusion reactions 149.15

allogeneic haematopoietic stem cell transplantation, graft versus host disease 38.1–38.12
allopurinol
    cutaneous adverse effects 155.9–155.10, 155.15
    hypersensitivity reactions **14.6**
allylamines, topical therapies 18.12
ALM *see* acral lentiginous melanoma
aloe, cosmeceutical use of 157.10–157.11
alopecia
    alopecia totalis 105.12
    biopsy 3.7
    cancer treatment 87.71–87.74
    chemotherapy-induced 119.5–119.6
    cicatricial *68.11*, 87.37, 87.38–87.53, 88.37
    secondary 105.6–105.9
    cosmetic approaches 87.69, 87.97–87.101
    Covid-19 association 25.113
    cutaneous lesions 96.13
    cutaneous manifestations of Hodgkin disease 139.49
    diagnosis 87.13
    incontinentia pigmenti *68.11*
    lichen planopilaris 37.11
    linear morphoea en coup de sabre *55.24*
    lipoedematous 98.24–98.25, 105.10–105.11
    medical traumatic hair loss 87.30
    metastases to the scalp 148.5, 148.6
    monitoring/assessment 87.16–87.18
    neonatal 114.4
    non-scarring 87.28–87.35
    psoriatic 87.34, *105.3*
    radiotherapy-associated 119.14
    scarring 87.13–87.14, *87.19–87.20*, 87.36–87.38, 91.11, 107.4
    syphilis 29.10, *29.12*
    systemic lupus erythematosus *51.26*
    thallium poisoning 121.9
    topical use of sensitising agents 18.33–18.34
    vitamin D deficiency 61.10
    X-linked syndromes 63.69
    see also hair loss
alopecia areata (AA) 87.13–87.14, 87.16, 87.18–87.28
    Covid-19 association 25.113
    dupilumab 87.35
    eyebrows 107.4
    pigmentary disorders *87.92, 87.93*
    psychodermatology 84.3
alopecia areata incognita 87.23–87.24, 87.58–87.59
alopecia mucinosa (AM) 57.15–57.18, 87.47, 105.8, 139.14–139.15
alopecia neoplastica 148.5
alopecia totalis 87.24–87.27
alopecia universalis 87.24–87.27
ALOXE3 mutations 63.12, 63.13
alpha-1 antitrypsin deficiency **72.11**
alpha-1 antitrypsin deficiency panniculitis 97.43–97.45
α_1-antitrypsin deficiency 152.5
alpha-hydroxyl acids, chemical peels 160.1–160.2
α-keratin intermediate filaments (α-KIF) 87.6
alpha-lipoic acid (ALA), cosmeceutical use of 157.1–157.2
alpha-mannosidosis, glycoproteinoses 79.3
alpha-N-acetyl-galactosaminidase deficiency 79.4
α_5-reductase inhibitors 87.96
alphaviruses
    mosquito borne togavirus infections 25.87–25.91
    viral arthropathies 155.3
Alstroemeriaceae dermatitis 127.73
Alström syndrome **72.7**
alternative treatments *see* complementary/alternative/traditional therapies; herbals
aluminium, allergic contact dermatitis 127.41

aluminium acetate 18.9
aluminium chloride, hyperhidrosis treatment 92.9
aluminium chloride hexahydrate
 caustic agent for skin surgery 20.47
 topical 18.9
ALUs *see* arterial leg ulcers
AM *see* alopecia mucinosa
amalgam fillings 127.41
amalgam tattoos 108.15
Ambras-type congenital hypertrichosis 87.85
ambulatory photodynamic therapy 22.11
AMD3100, wound healing *11.12*
amelanosis 86.8
amelanotic melanomas 142.14, *142.16*, *142.17*
Amerchol L101 127.58
American Academy of Dermatology Resident International Grant Scheme 7.14
American Burn Association (ABA) criteria, burn injuries 125.2
American College of Chemosurgery (ACC) 20.32, 20.37
American College of Mohs Surgery (ACMS) 20.37
American cutaneous leishmaniasis 33.44, 33.45, 33.46, 33.49, 33.50–33.51
American Joint Committee on Cancer (AJCC), Merkel cell carcinoma staging 146.5, 146.7, **146.8**
American Society of Tropical Medicine and Hygiene (ASTMH) 7.6
American trypanosomiasis (Chagas disease) 33.39–33.43
 clinical features 33.41–33.42
 investigations 33.43
 management 33.43
 pathophysiology 33.39–33.40, *33.41*
amicrobial, *see also* sterile
amicrobial pustulosis of the skin folds 49.20–49.21
 erosions and crusts involving the retro-auricular region *49.20*
amino acid metabolism and transport disorders **79.2**, 79.10–79.15
 alkaptonuria 79.12
 argininosuccinic aciduria 79.13–79.14
 dermatological features **79.11**
 Hartnup disease 79.14
 phenylketonuria 79.10–79.11
 prolidase deficiency 79.12–79.13
 serine, proline and glutamine synthesis defects 79.14–79.15
 tyrosinaemia type 2 79.11–79.12
amino acids, alpha-1 antitrypsin 97.43
amino acid supplements 88.12
amino formaldehyde resins 127.71
5-aminolaevulinic acid (ALA)
 contact allergy 22.13, *22.14*
 in photodynamic therapy 22.2–22.3, 22.4–22.6
amiodarone 86.25, 86.27–86.28
amnion, burn treatment 125.6
amniotic bands, and lymphoedema 103.29–103.30
amniotic membrane transplantation (AMT) 118.20
amobiasis 33.36–33.38
 clinical features 33.37
 epidemiology 33.36
 investigations 33.37–33.38
 management 33.38
 pathophysiology 33.37
amoebiasis, perianal skin 111.16
amorphous basophilic material, actinic elastosis 94.2
amphetamines, dermatoses induced by 120.2, *120.5*
ampicillin, exanthem caused by *117.2*
amputation stump neuromas 136.43
AMT *see* amniotic membrane transplantation
amylase, pancreatic panniculitis 97.41
Amyloid A (AA) amyloidosis, renal and skin involvement 154.2

amyloidoses 56.1–56.14, 86.22–86.23
 amyloid deposition in papillary dermis *56.5*
 amyloid, electron microscopy of *56.6*
 amyloidogenesis 56.1–56.2
 cardiac involvement 151.4
 classification 56.2
 clinical presentation 56.2
 cutaneous amyloidoses due to systemic disease 56.10–56.13
 ear dermatoses **106.22**
 electron microscopy 56.5, *56.6*
 eye disease **107.35**
 functional and disease-causing amyloids 56.2
 hereditary localised cutaneous amyloidosis **56.3**
 hereditary systemic amyloidoses with cutaneous involvement **56.4**
 hereditary systemic diseases with secondary cutaneous amyloidosis **56.4**
 histology 56.3–56.4
 immunohistochemistry 56.4, *56.5*, *56.6*
 investigations 56.2–56.6
 localised cutaneous amyloidoses **56.3**, 56.6–56.10
  associated diseases 56.8–56.9
  clinical features 56.9–56.10
  clinical variants 56.10
  complications and disease course 56.10
  differential diagnosis 56.10
  epidemiology 56.7
  ethnicity 56.7–56.8
  pathophysiology 56.9
 management 56.13–56.14
 non-hereditary localised cutaneous amyloidosis **56.3**
 non-hereditary systemic amyloidoses with cutaneous involvement **56.4**
 oral involvement 108.69–108.70
 penile 109.25
 respiratory involvement 152.6
 systemic amyloidoses with cutaneous involvement 56.10–56.13
 ultrastructure 56.1
amyloidosis 86.22–86.23
amyopathic dermatomyositis 52.1
 see also clinically amyopathic dermatomyositis
amyotrophic lateral sclerosis 122.2
AN *see* acanthosis nigricans; atypical naevi
ANA *see* antinuclear antibody test
anabolic steroids, urticaria treatment 42.19
anaemia
 ancylostomiasis 33.15
 epidermolysis bullosa 69.26
 fanconi anaemia 76.11, **80.5**, 80.12–80.13
 skin signs 149.15–149.16
anaerobic bacteria 26.67–26.69
 aerotolerant coryneforms 26.37, 26.43
 Bacteroidaceae 26.67–26.68
 classification 26.67–26.68
 clostridia 26.48
 Eikenella corrodens 26.67
 normal skin flora 26.3, 26.4
 Peudomonas aeruginosa 26.51–26.53
 tropical ulcers 26.68–26.69
anaesthesia
 biopsy 3.2–3.3
 peripheral nerve damage in leprosy 28.3, 28.7
 photothermal ablation 23.21
 in pregnancy 113.24
anagen hair bulb *87.5*, 87.8
anagen hair follicles 87.3, 87.7–87.8, *87.57*
 appearance *87.57*
 dermal papilla 87.5
 pathology 87.21
 pigmentation disorders *87.12*
 suprabulbar region 87.4
anagen release, telogen effluvium 87.53

anal canal 111.2
 internal haemorrhoids *111.32*
anal cancer 111.21–111.24
 clinical features 111.22–111.23
 epidemiology 111.22
 management 111.24
 pathophysiology 111.22
 perianal carcinoma *111.23*
anal fissure 111.30–111.31
anal fistula 111.28–111.30
 conditions associated with **111.29**
 development of an intersphincteric fistula *111.29*
 Parks classification *111.30*
analgesia
 hidradenitis suppurativa treatment 90.9
 SJS/TEN treatment 118.20
anal intraepithelial neoplasia (AIN) 111.19–111.21, 141.26
 histopathology *111.20*
anal orifice 111.2–111.3
anal/perianal/genital intraepithelial carcinomas 141.24, 141.26
anal sphincter 111.2–111.3
anal tags 111.32, *111.33*
anaphylaxis
 drug-induced 14.1–14.2, 117.5–117.7
 flushing 104.8
 rubber latex allergy 127.84–127.85
 urticaria 42.1
anaplasia 3.39
Anaplasma phagocytophilum, tick-borne zoonotic infection 26.66–26.67
anaplasmosis 26.66–26.67
anaplastic large-cell lymphoma (ALCL) 139.28–139.29
anaplastic lymphoma kinase (ALK) 3.28
 positive/negative cutaneous lymphomas 139.1, 139.26, 139.28, 139.34
ANA screening *see* antinuclear antibody test
anatomical considerations, skin surgery 20.1–20.4
anatomy of skin 9.1
ANCA *see* antineutrophil cytoplasmic antibody
anchoring fibrils 2.26–2.27
ancient medical texts 1.1–1.3
Ancylostoma brasiliense see cutaneous larva migrans
Ancylostoma caninum see cutaneous larva migrans
Ancylostoma ceylonicum see cutaneous larva migrans
Ancylostoma duodenale, ancylostomiasis 33.15–33.17
ancylostomiasis 33.15–33.17
 clinical features 33.17
 epidemiology 33.15
 management 33.17
 pathophysiology 33.16–33.17
androgenetic alopecia (AGA) 87.10, 87.60–87.71
 children/adolescents 87.66–87.67
 COVID-19 association 25.113
 FPHL with **87.67**
 treatment 87.68–87.70
androgen excess 87.88
androgen insensitivity syndrome 87.10
androgen receptor 87.10
androgen receptor blockers, acne vulgaris treatment 88.51
androgens
 for dyskeratosis congenita 67.15
 hair growth 87.9–87.10
 nail–patella syndrome 67.15
androgen-secreting tumours, hirsutism association 87.91
androgen-stimulated hair growth 87.10
androgen synthesis 87.10
ANEM *see* acute necrotising eosinophilic myocarditis
anetoderma 94.23–94.25
 of prematurity 114.9–114.10
aneurysmal fibrous histiocytoma 136.20, 136.21

anger, emotional effects of skin conditions 15.2
angina bullosa haemorrhagica, oral involvement 108.20
angioedema 152.2, *152.3*
 assessment tools 16.5, 16.9
 drug-induced 117.5–117.7
 oral involvement 108.10
 reactions to COVID-19 (mRNA) vaccines 25.117
angioedema activity score (AAS) 16.5
Angioedema Quality of Life Questionnaire (AE-QoL) 16.9
angioedema swellings, urticaria 42.1, *42.3*
angioedema without weals 43.1–43.7
 clinical features 43.4
 clinical variants 43.4–43.5
 definition and nomenclature 43.1
 disease course and prognosis 43.5
 epidemiology 43.2–43.3
 genetics 43.4
 investigations 43.5
 laboratory profiles *43.5*
 management 43.5–43.6
 pathophysiology 43.3–43.4
 treatment 43.5–43.6
angiofibromas
 non-ablative laser therapies 23.11
 photothermal ablation 23.21, *23.22*
 tuberous sclerosis complex 78.8, *78.10*
angiogenesis 101.1
 wound healing 11.5–11.6
angioimmunoblastic T-cell lymphoma 139.45
angiokeratoma circumscriptum 101.13–101.14
angiokeratoma corporis diffusum *see* Fabry disease
angiokeratomas 101.13–101.14, **101.17**
 dermoscopic view of *101.14*
 labia majora 110.3, *110.4*
 laser therapies 23.11, *23.12*
 lysosomal diseases associated with **79.7**
 male genitalia 109.6–109.7
 subtypes of **101.15**
angiolipoma 136.56
angiolupoid sarcoidosis 96.12
angiolymphoid hyperplasia with eosinophilia *106.24*
 ear dermatoses **106.22**
angiolymphoid hyperplasia with eosinophilia (ALHE) *see* epithelioid haemangioma
angiomas, laser therapies 23.11
angioma serpiginosum 71.4–71.5, 101.16, **101.17**, *101.18*, **101.18**
angiomatoid fibrous histiocytoma 136.62–136.63
angiomatosis, diffuse dermal *4.11*
angiomyofibroblastoma 136.9
angiomyolipomas, tuberous sclerosis complex 78.9
angiosarcoma 119.15, 136.34–136.36
 epithelioid angiosarcoma 136.37
 lymphangiosarcoma *103.7*
angiotensin-converting enzyme (ACE) 127.10
angiotensin-converting enzyme (ACE) inhibitor-induced angio-oedema 43.2, 43.3, 43.4
angora hair naevus 73.21–73.22
angular cheilitis/angular stomatitis 32.62–32.63, 108.20, 108.59–108.60
angulated lines dermoscopy patterns, melanoma 145.7, *145.8*
anhidrosis
 eccrine gland disorders **92.11**
 hyperhidrosis and 92.11–92.12
animal bites *see* bites
animal parasites
 Cimicidae bugs 34.25–34.26
 mites 34.50, 34.54–34.55
animals, exposure to, and atopic eczema 41.8

animal-type melanoma *see* pigmented epithelioid melanocytoma/pigment synthesising melanoma
ankle
  familial Mediterranean fever 45.10
  hypertrophic lichen planus 37.7
  lichen planus pemphigoides 37.9
  lichen simplex 39.29
  lipoatrophic panniculitis in childhood 97.56–97.57
  primary localised cutaneous amyloidosis 56.7
  venous eczema 39.20
ankle brachial Doppler pressure index (ABPI) 101.4, **101.4**
  lower leg eczema 39.21
ankle flare (corona phlebectatica paraplantaris) 101.43, *101.44*
ankyloglossia
  epidermolysis bullosa 69.25
  oral involvement 108.87
annular elastolytic giant cell granuloma (AEGCG) 62.5, 94.27–94.30
annular epidermolytic ichthyosis (AEI) 63.16
annular erythema of infancy (AEI) 47.9
  histopathology of lesional skin *47.10*
annular lesions 4.7, *4.10*, 4.15, *63.75*
annular lichen planus 37.8
annular purpura 122.16
annular sarcoidosis *96.10*
ano-genital cellulitis 111.14
ano-genital infections 32.63–32.65
ano-genital mammary-like gland tumours 137.40
ano-genital pilonidal sinus 122.23
ano-genital region
  allergic contact dermatitis 127.16–127.17, 127.22
  anatomy 109.3–109.4
  child abuse, signs of 109.9
  ecthyma gangrenosum 109.26
  embryogenesis of 111.3, *111.4*
  HIV 31.35–31.36
  hypo- and hyperpigmentation **109.42**
  irritants **109.11**
  staphylococcal cellulitis 109.26
  structure and function of 111.1–111.3
  see also perineal and perianal skin
ano-genital tumours
  anal/vulval/penile and perianal intraepithelial carcinoma 141.24, 141.26
  hidradenoma papilliferum 110.31–110.33, 137.20–137.21
ano-genital warts 25.61–25.64, 109.9
  cervical intraepithelial neoplasia association 25.65
  clinical features 25.62–25.64
  cutaneous squamous cell carcinoma association 25.65
  epidemiology 25.61
  male genitalia 109.29
  management 25.64
  pathophysiology 25.61–25.62
  vulva *110.30*
  see also condylomata acuminata
ano-rectal abscess 111.27–111.28
  classification of *111.28*
anorexia nervosa 84.26–84.27, 88.30
ANS *see* autonomic nervous system
antenatal procedures, neonatal complications arising from **114.10**
anterolateral lower leg alopecia 87.29–87.30
Anthocidae (minute pirate/flower bugs) 34.29–34.30
Anthozoa, stings from 130.1–130.2
anthrax 26.44–26.45
  clinical features 26.44–26.45
  epidemiology 26.44
  management 26.45
  pathophysiology 26.44
anthropophilic dermatophytes 32.19–32.20
anthroquinone dyes 127.65–127.66
anti-ageing cosmeceuticals 157.3–157.7

rhytid reduction 157.4–157.7
skin lightening 157.3–157.4
antiandrogens 87.70
  acne vulgaris treatment *88.50*
  hair disorder treatment 87.95–87.97
  in pregnancy **113.23**
antibiotics
  acne vulgaris treatment 88.46, 88.47, 88.48–88.49, 88.52
    adverse effects of **88.49**
    interactions with oral contraceptives 88.49
  allergic contact dermatitis 127.45
  anti-inflammatory effects 19.48
  atopic eczema association 41.9
  atopic eczema treatment 41.27
  eye, side effects on 107.43
  'happenstance therapy' 29.12
  in pregnancy **113.21**
  syphilis 29.12, 29.20–29.21
  systemic 19.46–19.48
  topical therapies 18.10–18.12
antibiotic sore tongue *see* acute erythematous candidiasis
antibody deficiencies 80.13
  inherited immunodeficiency 80.5
antibody probes, epidermolysis bullosa diagnosis 69.21
anticholinergic agents 18.38
anticonvulsant hypersensitivity syndrome 118.5
antidepressants 84.43–84.44
  prescribing 84.43
  selective serotonin reuptake inhibitors 84.43, **84.44**, 117.3
  switching 84.44
  tricyclic antidepressants 84.44, **84.45**
  types 84.43–84.44
antiepileptic drugs, acneform reaction 88.13
antifungal agents
  dermatophyte infections 32.32–32.34
  in pregnancy **113.20**
  seborrhoeic dermatitis management 40.8, 40.9
  skin cancer risks in immunocompromised people 147.8
  systemic drugs 19.48, 40.9
  topical therapies 18.12–18.13, 32.33–32.34, 40.8
anti-GBM *see* antiglomerular basement membrane vasculitis
antigenic tests 4.24–4.25
antigen mapping 69.21
antigen-presenting cells (APCs) 127.7, 135.2
  histiocytoses 135.1
  immune system 9.4–9.5
  T-cell receptors 118.5
antigens, epidermolysis bullosa 69.4
antiglomerular basement membrane vasculitis (anti-GBM) 100.19–100.20
antihistamines
  adverse effects 42.17–42.18
  atopic eczema treatment 41.27
  in childhood 42.18
  mastocytosis treatment 46.9
  pharmacokinetic and clinical properties **42.18**
  in pregnancy 42.18, 113.19, **113.22**
  solar urticaria 126.24
  systemic 19.3–19.4
    cautions 19.4
    dose and regimens 19.4
    drug–drug interactions 19.4
    pharmacological properties 19.3–19.4
    potential adverse effects 19.4
  topical therapies 18.37
  urticaria treatment 42.17–42.18, 42.19
anti-inflammatory agents
  antibiotics 19.48
  cosmeceuticals 157.10–157.11
  mastocytosis treatment 46.9
  in pregnancy **113.20**
  systemic therapy 19.2–19.46

antimalarial agents 19.4–19.7
  adverse effects 155.15
  cautions 19.6
  contraindication 19.6
  dermatological uses 19.4–19.5
  discoid lupus erythematosus treatment **51.11**
  dose and regimens 19.7
  drug–drug interactions 19.6
  hypermelanosis 86.26, 86.27–86.28
  monitoring 19.7
  ocular side effects 19.6, 107.43
  pharmacological properties 19.5
  potential adverse effects 19.5–19.6
  pre-treatment screening 19.7
  side effects **51.11**, *51.25*
  systemic lupus erythematosus treatment 51.37
antimicrobial agents
  allergic contact dermatitis 127.49–127.58
  burn injuries 125.10
  fast growing *Mycobacterium* species **27.45**
  genital contact dermatitis **109.13**
  in pregnancy 113.23–**113.24**
  systemic therapies 19.46–19.49
antimicrobial peptides, possible seborrhoeic dermatitis therapies 40.9
antimicrobial resistance
  corynebacteria 26.38
  gonococcus/*Neisseria gonorrhoeae* 30.1, 30.2, 30.7, **30.8**
  impetigo management 26.16
  multidrug-resist tuberculosis 27.10
  Mycoplasma genitalium 30.24, 30.25
  STI coinfections 30.13
  topical fusidic acid use 18.11
  see also methicillin-resistant *Staphylococcus aureus*
antineoplastic and cytotoxic agents 18.29–18.31
antineutrophil cytoplasmic antibody (ANCA) associated small vessel vasculitis 100.9, 100.13, 100.20–100.28, 152.3–152.4
antinomy, dermatological reactions 121.1–121.2
antinuclear antibody (ANA) test 126.6
  systemic lupus erythematosus 51.34–51.36
antioxidants
  allergies 127.59
  cosmeceuticals 157.1–157.3
  resuscitation use 125.4
  topical medication 18.8
anti-p200 pemphigoid 50.38–50.42
  clinical features 50.40
  epidemiology 50.39
  histopathology *50.40*
  investigations and diagnosis 50.40
  management 50.40–50.42
  pathophysiology 50.39–50.40
  serum autoantibodies against p200 antigen *50.42*
  treatment ladder 50.42
antiparasitic agents, topical therapies 18.13–18.14
antiparasitic treatment
  lice 34.22, 34.25
  scabies 34.45–34.48, 34.50
  tungiasis 34.15
antiperspirants 18.37–18.38
antiphospholipid antibody syndrome (APLS) 51.42–51.45, 99.17–99.19
  associated diseases 51.42–51.43
  cardiac involvement 151.4
  clinical features 51.43
  complications and co-morbidities 51.43–51.44
  criteria for **99.17**
  cutaneous findings 99.18
  disease course and prognosis 51.44
  investigations 51.44
  management 51.44–51.45
  pathophysiology 51.43
  treatment ladder 51.45

antipsychotics 84.44–84.46
  body dysmorphic disorder 84.14
  delusional infestation management 84.7, 84.8–84.9, 84.44
  types 84.45–84.46
antiretroviral-induced alopecia 87.35
antiretroviral therapy (ART)
  cutaneous side effects **31.13**
  drug reactions 31.2, 31.8, 31.10, **31.13**, 31.19, 31.20
  HIV/AIDS 31.2, 31.8, 31.9–31.10
  HIV-associated lipodystrophy 98.6–98.8
  reduction in AIDS defining cancers 147.2
antiseptics
  allergic contact dermatitis 127.45
  pressure ulcer treatment 123.11
  topical therapies 18.9–18.10
antistreptolysin O titre (ASOT) 26.11, 26.12, 26.36
antisynthetase syndrome 52.8
anti-TNF-α treatment, mycobacterial infections 27.11–27.12
anti-TNF biologic therapy, pyoderma gangrenosum 49.7
α$_1$-antitrypsin deficiency 152.5
anti-type IV collagen pemphigoid 50.53
antivenom, cnidarian stings 130.3
antiviral agents 19.49
  adverse cutaneous effects, hepatitis treatments 25.75, 25.76–25.77
  hepatitis B treatment 25.75
  hepatitis C treatment 25.76–25.77
  herpes simplex infections 25.22, 25.23–25.24, 25.26, 25.27
  human herpesvirus 6 and 7 25.40
  pox viruses 25.7, 25.11, 25.18
  in pregnancy **113.24**
  prophylaxis for immune suppressed patients 25.31, 25.42, 25.75
  prophylaxis for perinatal transmission 25.31, 25.75
  prophylaxis to prevent HSV reactivation 25.23, 25.24, 25.26, 25.27, 25.28
  topical therapies 18.13
  varicella-zoster virus 25.31, 25.32, 25.35
ants 34.16
ANUG *see* acute necrotising (ulcerative) gingivitis and noma
anus
  mucosal melanomas 142.11, *142.16*
  see also anal entries
anxiety
  acne vulgaris 88.39
  morphoea 55.29
  psoriasis 35.19
  skin-related health anxieties 15.2, 84.25–84.26
anxiolytics 84.46
AOSD *see* adult-onset Still disease
AP *see* actinic prurigo
APCs *see* antigen-presenting cells
APECED *see* autoimmune polyendocrinopathy Candida ectodermal dystrophy syndrome
Apert syndrome 106.7
  acne vulgaris association 88.10–88.11
aphonia, vitamin B1 deficiency 61.14
aphthous-like ulcers
  oral ulceration 108.38–108.39
  systemic factors associated with **108.39**
aphthous ulcers
  Adamantiades–Behçet disease *48.5*, **48.8**
  female genitalia 110.19
  treatment **48.8**
Aphthovirus infections 25.93
APL *see* acquired partial lipodystrophy
APLAID *see* autoinflammation and PLCG2-associated antibody deficiency and immune dysregulation
aplasia
  congenital pseudo-ainhum 94.48
  ocular features **107.41**
aplasia cutis 87.30
APLS *see* antiphospholipid antibody syndrome

apocrine carcinoma 137.22–137.23
apocrine cystadenoma *see* apocrine hidrocystoma
apocrine glands 2.9, 2.43, 92.15–92.17
 changes in during pregnancy 113.2–113.3
 disorders 92.16–92.19
 function 92.1
 tumours 137.1, 137.2, 137.18–137.23
apocrine hidrocystoma 137.18–137.19
apocrine miliaria 92.18–92.19
apocrine tubular adenoma 137.22
apoeccrine glands 2.9, 92.1
apoptosis 3.39
appearance, social impacts 15.1
appendageal tumours *see* tumours of skin appendages
application sparganosis 33.35
applicators, brachytherapy 24.3
apps
 diagnosis 4.26, 5.13
 NLR SkinApp 7.12
apremilast
 discoid lupus erythematosus treatment 51.12
 immunomodulatory therapy 19.7–19.8
 psoriasis treatment 35.26
apron eczema 39.14, *39.15*, 128.4
APS-1 *see* autoimmune polyendocrinopathy syndrome type 1
APSEA *see* Assessments of the Psychological and Social Effects of Acne
APSS *see* acral peeling skin syndrome
apthous lesions, autoinflammatory diseases **80.19**
AQOL *see* Acne Quality of Life Scale
AQP5 mutations, non-epidermolytic palmoplantar keratoderma 63.54
AQPs *see* aquaporins
aquagenic keratoderma 63.61–63.62
aquagenic urticaria **42.9**, 42.12, *42.13*
aquaporins (AQPs) 63.54
 eccrine glands 92.2
AR *see* autosomal recessive
Arachnida 34.34–34.57
 mites 34.41–34.57
 scorpions 34.36–34.37
 spiders 34.34–34.36
 ticks 34.37–34.41
Araneae (spiders) 34.34–34.36
Arao–Perkins bodies 87.64
arboviruses *see* arthropod-borne viruses
arbutin
 cosmeceutical use 157.3
 topical depigmenting agents 18.32
Arcanobacterium haemolyticum 26.43
ARCI *see* autosomal recessive congenital ichthyosis
ARC syndrome *see* arthrogryposis–renal dysfunction–cholestasis syndrome
arcuate lesions *4.11*
arenavirus infections 25.81–25.83
areola, microscopic examination of 3.33
Argentina, community dermatology 7.8
Argentinian haemorrhagic fever 25.82–25.83
argininosuccinic aciduria 79.13–79.14, 87.76
argyria 86.51–86.52, 121.8
ARIH *see* autosomal recessive ichthyosis with hypotrichosis
arm
 acne scarring 88.40
 acute generalised pustular psoriasis 35.33
 ageing of skin 156.2
 allergic contact dermatitis 127.14, 127.22
 Apert syndrome 88.11
 atopic eczema 41.19
 Bateman purpura 156.6
 bullous pemphigoid 50.16
 capillary malformations 71.5
 carcinoma telangiectatica *103.15*
 cicatricial pemphigoid 50.53
 dermatitis herpetiformis 50.57
 eczema *39.2*
 elephantine psoriasis 35.14

eosinophilic fasciitis 55.22
erythema multiforme *47.2*
IgA vasculitis 100.15
interstitial granulomatous dermatitis 53.6
keratosis pilaris *88.35*
lichenification of in patient with atopic eczema *39.28*
linear morphoea *55.26*
linear psoriasis with guttate psoriasis 35.15
lymphatic malformations *71.22*
miliaria *114.7*
mucous membrane pemphigoid 50.29
necrolytic migratory erythema *47.15*
pansclerotic morphoea 55.21
pemphigus vulgaris 50.5
psoriasis vulgaris *35.7*, 35.11
Rothmund–Thomson syndrome 75.5
subcutaneous fat necrosis of the newborn *114.16*
swelling due to oedema 103.44–103.46
systemic lupus erythematosus *51.23*, 51.24
systemic sclerosis *54.4, 54.5*
urticaria *42.2, 42.11*
see also digital entries; finger; hand
armpit *see* axillary entries
ARN *see* accelerated rheumatoid nodulosis
arochordons *see* skin tags
arrector pili muscle
 degeneration in pattern hair loss 87.64
 hamartoma 136.52–136.53
 leiomyoma 136.53–136.54
arsenic
 acute toxicity 121.2–121.3
 agricultural chemicals 141.18
 dermatological reactions 121.1, 121.2–121.3
 groundwater contamination 141.13, 141.18
 historic medications 141.18
 hypermelanosis 86.25
 pigmentation effects 86.52
 predisposition to Bowden disease 141.18
 routes of exposure 141.13, 141.18
arsenical keratosis 141.13–141.14
arsenite 121.2
ART *see* antiretroviral therapy
artefacts 3.31–3.32
 due to blocking and sectioning 3.32
 due to poor biopsy technique 3.31–3.32
 due to staining techniques 3.32
 and fixation media 3.32
arterial/arteriolar disorders 101.1–101.31
 angiogenesis 101.1
 arterial leg ulcers 102.7–102.10
 arteriogenesis 101.1
 arteriovenous malformations 101.22–101.24
 cutaneous vascular malformations 101.26–101.31
 hypertensive ischaemic leg ulcers 102.10–102.13
 Klippel–Trenaunay syndrome 101.27–101.30
 livedo reticularis *124.9*
 mixed leg ulcers 102.4–102.7
 neurovascular disorders 101.6–101.9
 Parkes Weber syndrome **101.28**, 101.30–101.31
 peripheral vascular disease 101.2–101.3
 telangiectases 101.10–101.22
 thromboangiitis obliterans 101.3–101.6
 ulceration 102.1–102.13
 vasculogenesis 101.1
 verrucous haemangioma 101.26, *101.27*
arterial leg ulcers (ALUs) 102.7–102.10
 clinical features 102.8–102.9
 epidemiology 102.8
 management 102.9–102.10
 pathophysiology 102.8
arterial occlusion, dermal filler, adverse reaction 158.10, **158.11**
arterial tortuosity syndrome **70.16**

arteries
 anatomy of head and neck 20.1–20.2
 subcutaneous fat 97.7
arteriogenesis 101.1
arteriohepatic dysplasia (Alagille syndrome) 153.5
arterioles *2.40, 2.41*
arteriolosclerosis, subcutaneous, hypertensive ischaemic leg ulcer *102.11*
arteriovenous disorders 71.11–71.14
 arteriovenous malformation 71.11–71.12
 hereditary haemorrhagic telangiectasia 71.12–71.13
 PTEN hamartoma tumour syndrome 71.13–71.14
arteriovenous malformations (AVM) 71.11–71.12, 101.22–101.24
 clinical features **101.23**
 conditions associated with **101.22**
 in infants *101.23*
 investigations 101.23
 management 101.24
 pathophysiology 101.23
arthritis
 acne association 88.63
 NLRP1-associated autoinflammation with arthritis and dyskeratosis 45.18
 osteoarthritis 155.8
 pachydermoperiostosis 155.14
 systemic lupus erythematosus 51.30
 systemic-onset juvenile idiopathic arthritis 45.21–45.22
 see also mixed connective tissue disease; psoriatic arthritis; reactive arthritis; rheumatoid arthritis; sexually acquired reactive arthritis
arthritis mutilans *35.42*
arthrochalasia Ehlers–Danlos syndrome (aEDS) **70.4**, 70.9
Arthroderma species 32.18, 32.25–32.26
 see also Microsporum gypseum
arthrogryposis–renal dysfunction–cholestasis (ARC) syndrome 63.30
arthropathies
 infective 155.2–155.5
 inflammatory 155.5–155.7, *155.8, 155.9*
arthropod bites, pseudolymphoma 134.2
arthropod-borne viruses (arboviruses)
 Bunyavirus infections 25.83–25.84
 flavivirus infections 25.85–25.87
 togavirus infections 25.87–25.91
arthropods 34.1–34.58
 arachnids 34.34–34.57
 attraction to humans 34.3
 centipedes and millipedes 34.57
 classification 34.1
 clinical and epidemiological features 34.3–34.4
 disease transmission 34.2
 environmental factors in exposure 34.2–34.3
 insects 34.6–34.34
 investigations of skin disease 34.4–34.5
 larval invasion of tissues/myiasis 34.2, **34.7**, 34.9–34.13
 management of skin disease 34.6
 pathology of skin effects 34.3
 pathophysiology of skin disease 34.2–34.3
 protective clothing and repellents 34.5
 see also louse-borne diseases
artificial hair implantation 122.23
artificial intelligence (AI) 4.26–4.27
 melanoma detection 142.16
 objective measures of skin properties 16.5
Ascher syndrome 94.27
Asclepius 1.2
ascorbic acid (vitamin C), topical depigmenting agents 18.33
aseptic abscess syndrome 49.21
Ashkenazi Jews, hyperhidrosis 92.5
ash-leaf-shaped macules, tuberous sclerosis complex 78.8

ashy dermatosis 86.32–86.33
Asian skin phenotypes, photoageing 156.2–156.3, 156.7
ASIS *see* Acne Symptom and Impact Scale
ASM *see* aggressive systemic mastocytosis
ASOT *see* antistreptolysin O titre
aspartylglucosaminuria 79.3–79.4
aspergillosis
 oral ulceration 108.56–108.57
 panniculitis due to 97.60–97.61
Aspergillus
 A. niger, otomycosis 32.17
 A. terreus, superficial onychomycosis 32.54–32.55
Aspergillus species, skin lesions 32.93
aspirin, urticaria 117.6
ASPRV1 encoding, autosomal dominant lamellar ichthyoses 63.20–63.21
assassin bugs 34.29
assessment *see* measurement
Assessments of the Psychological and Social Effects of Acne (APSEA) questionnaire 16.8
asteatosis 85.26–85.28
asteatotic eczema *see* eczema, asteatotic
asteroid bodies, sarcoidosis 96.3
asthma, and atopic eczema 41.11, 41.20
ASTMH *see* American Society of Tropical Medicine and Hygiene
Astrakhan fever *see* tick typhus
astringents 18.9
Astruc, Jean 1.3–1.4
asymmetrical cell division 2.44
asymmetrical hyperhidrosis 92.6–92.7
asymmetric periflexural exanthem of childhood 25.123
asymptomatic neurosyphilis 29.15
AT *see* ataxia telangiectasia
ataxia-pancytopenia syndrome 149.14
ataxia telangiectasia (AT) 76.10–76.11, **78.13**, **80.4**, 148.13–148.14
 bulbar telangiectasia *80.11*
 pulmonary involvement 152.5
ataxia with vitamin E deficiency (AVED) 61.11–61.12
atherosclerosis 101.2–101.3
athletes foot, *see also* tinea peddis
athlete's nodules 122.16
atlases, dermatology 1.4
atopic blepharoconjunctivitis (ABC) 107.16, 107.18, *107.22*
atopic cataract 41.21, *107.19*
atopic dermatitis (AD) *see* atopic eczema (dermatitis)
Atopic Dermatitis Control Test (ADCT) 16.3
atopic disease, hair loss presentation 87.20
atopic eczema/dermatitis (AE) 41.1–41.33
 acute 41.13
 adult phase 41.15
 age and sex 41.3
 air pollution 41.7
 allergens 127.12–127.13
 allergic contact dermatitis 41.12, 41.22, 127.10, 127.72, 127.83
 allergic rhino-conjunctivitis association 41.20
 allergy association 41.11
 animal exposure 41.8
 antibiotics association 41.9
 assessment tools 16.3–16.4, **16.4**
 asthma 41.11, 41.20
 'atopic march' 41.11
 atopic and non-atopic eczema 41.2–41.3
 autoimmune disease association 41.22
 autoimmunity 41.12
 bacterial infections 41.20
 bathing and showering 41.26
 biologic therapies 9.8–9.9
 breastfeeding and delayed weaning 41.7, 41.23
 calcineurin inhibitors 41.27
 cancer risk association 41.21–41.22
 cardiovascular disease association 41.21
 cheilitis 128.4–128.5

atopic eczema/dermatitis (AE) (continued)
　childhood infections and vaccinations 41.8–41.9
　childhood phase 41.15
　classification 41.1
　climatic conditions 41.6
　clinical features **41.1, 41.2,** 41.12–41.16
　clinical variants 41.16
　community survey 5.2
　complications and associated diseases 41.20–41.22
　corticosteroids, topical 41.26–41.27
　cost studies 5.6
　developmental delay association 41.21
　diagnosis 5.4, **41.2,** 41.3
　diet 41.7, 41.23
　differential diagnosis 41.22
　discoid eczema lesions *41.17*
　disease endotypes 41.15
　disease prevention 41.23
　disease severity 41.3, 41.16, **41.18**
　drug endotypes 41.15
　dry skin 41.15
　ear dermatoses **106.22**
　economic burden of 6.10, 41.3–41.4
　　psoriasis comparison *6.10*
　emollients 41.26, 41.27
　endocrine factors 41.19
　endotoxin exposure 41.8
　endotypes 41.15
　environmental risk and protective factors 41.6–41.9
　epidemiology 5.4, 41.3–41.4
　and epidermal barrier 41.5–41.6
　erythema, papules, excoriations, crusting and secondary infection *41.15*
　ethnicity 5.10
　Filaggrin genetics and epidermal barrier 41.5–41.6
　financial cost of 5.6
　first line treatment 41.24, **41.25**
　flexural dermatitis *41.13, 41.14*
　food allergy 41.11–41.12, 41.20
　general advice and education 41.24
　genetic factors 41.4–41.5
　global distribution **7.3**
　global prevalence *41.4*
　glucocorticoid sensitivity 41.19
　growth delay association 41.21
　gut microbiome 41.9
　habit reversal therapy 84.47–84.48
　hand involvement 41.16–41.17, *41.19,* 41.23
　helminth parasites 41.8
　history 41.12–41.13, **41.12**
　HIV 31.15
　house dust mite avoidance 41.23
　hygiene hypotheis 5.14, 41.7–41.8
　hyperpigmentation *41.14, 41.17*
　ichthyosis vulgaris association 41.15
　immune dysregulation 41.9–41.10
　immunoglobulin E role 41.11
　incidence of 7.2
　infant feeding 41.23
　infantile phase 41.15, 115.2–115.3
　infantile seborrhoeic dermatitis 41.22
　infection and antibiotics 41.27
　inflammation in 2.17, 9.8
　initial assessment **41.12,** 41.24
　innate immune cells 41.11
　investigations 41.23–41.24
　itch and antihistamines 41.27
　JAK inhibitors 41.27, 41.30–41.33
　KP association 85.9
　lichenification *41.14, 41.16, 41.17, 41.19*
　lipids 41.6
　lip-lick cheilitis 41.22
　maintenance therapy 41.27
　male genitalia 109.12
　malignancy risk association 41.21–41.22
　management 41.24–41.33
　mast cell role 2.16, 2.17
　maternal smoking during pregnancy 41.7
　microbial colonisation 2.13
　microbial exposure 41.7–41.8

　microbial responses 41.10
　mimics of atopic eczema **41.22**
　morbidity and cost 41.3–41.4
　novel therapies 41.30–41.33
　obesity 41.7
　occupational aspects 41.23
　ocular surface disorders 41.20–41.21
　papulovesicules *41.13*
　pathophysiology 41.3, 41.4–41.12, *41.32*
　pets, exposure to 41.8
　phototherapy 21.4, *21.5,* 41.28
　physical inactivity 41.7
　pityriasis alba 41.17
　prevalence of 5.10, 5.11, 6.1, 41.4
　pruritus 41.12, 81.7–81.8
　psychodermatology 84.3
　psychological factors 15.4, 41.19
　psychosocial aspects 41.19–41.20
　quality of life impact 16.8, **41.18**
　as risk factor for allergic contact dermatitis 9.10
　sex steroids 41.19
　skin barrier dysfunction 41.23
　skin of colour 41.16
　skin microbiome 9.8, 41.9
　staphylococci/streptococci role 26.13
　subtypes 5.4
　subtypes of 5.4
　sweating 41.18–41.19
　synonyms and inclusions **41.2**
　targeting of pathophysiological pathways *41.32*
　third line therapy 41.28–41.33
　　biologic therapy 41.29–41.30, **41.31,** *41.32*
　　conventional systemic agents **41.31**
　tobacco smoke, exposure to 41.7
　topical therapy 41.26–41.27, **41.32**
　　intensive topical treatment 41.28
　treatment algorithm **41.25**
　trigger factors *41.12,* 41.24–41.26
　unresponsive disease 41.28
　urban versus rural living 41.6–41.7, 41.8
　urticaria association 41.22
　UVA-1 phototherapy 21.4, 21.6
　viral infections 41.20
　and water hardness 41.23
　wet-wrap technique for control of 41.28
　white dermographism 41.17–41.18
atopic eruption of pregnancy (AEP) 113.15–113.16
　pruritus 81.11
atopic eye disease 107.16–107.23
　associated diseases 107.16
　clinical characteristics **107.21**
　clinical variants 107.17–107.18
　diagnosis **107.21**
　future therapeutic agents 107.23
　investigations 107.22
　management 107.22–107.23
　pathology 107.16–107.17
　severity classification 107.21
atopic hand eczema 128.2
atopic keratoconjunctivitis (AKC) 107.16, 107.17, 107.18, *107.19–107.20,* 107.21, 107.22
　with atopic eczema localised to eyelids *107.19*
　bacterial keratitis *107.19*
　inferior fornix and plical scarring *107.19*
　'polar bear rug' cataract *107.19*
　pseudogerontoxon *107.19*
　tarsal conjunctiva *107.19*
atopy 41.2, 41.23
　allergic contact dermatitis 127.10
　atopic eye disease 107.16–107.23
　Netherton syndrome 63.26
　obesity link 98.28
ATP *see* adenosine triphosphate; Africa Teledermatology Project
atrichia with papular lesions (APL) 87.28–87.29
atrophic morphoea, 'coup de sabre' paramedian form 94.21
atrophic parapsoriasis *see* large plaque parapsoriasis

atrophic photoageing 156.3, *156.4*
atrophic scars 94.13–94.15
atrophic skin
　Huriez syndrome 63.67
　rheumatoid arthritis 155.5
atrophic stria *94.8*
atrophie blanche
　chronic venous insufficiency **101.43,** *101.44*
　discoid lupus erythematosus *51.8*
　purpura 99.20–99.21
atrophies, ocular features **107.41**
atrophodermas 94.16–94.19
　follicular 94.16–94.17
　linear atrophoderma of Moulin 55.25–55.27, 73.22, 94.17
　of Pasini–Pierini 55.17, *55.19,* 94.18–94.19
　vermiculatum 85.11
atrophy of skin
　causes 94.6–94.21
　due to corticosteroids 94.6–94.9
　onchocerciasis 33.4
atropine-like drugs, hyperhidrosis treatment 92.9
attention-deficit hyperactivity disorder (ADHD) 63.6–63.7
ATTS *see* atypical trigeminal trophic syndrome
atypical adult-onset pityriasis rubra pilaris (type II) 36.2–36.4
atypical blotches, melanoma 145.7, *145.8,* 145.9
atypical decubitus fibroplasia 136.6
atypical dermal melanocytosis 73.21
atypical dots and globules, melanoma 145.7, *145.8*
atypical/dysplastic naevus syndrome 142.3–142.4
　see also dysplastic naevus syndrome
atypical fibrous histiocytoma 136.20, 136.21
atypical fibroxanthoma (AFX) 24.21, 136.22–136.23
atypical genital naevi, vulva 110.33
atypical intradermal smooth muscle neoplasm *see* leiomyosarcoma
atypical juvenile pityriasis rubra pilaris (type V) 36.4
atypical lipomatous tumour 136.58–136.59
atypical lymphocytes, chronic actinic dermatitis 126.14, *126.15*
atypical mycobacteria *see* non-tuberculous mycobacteria
atypical naevi (AN) **131.17,** 131.40–131.46
　clinical features 131.42–131.43
　dermoscopic images *131.44–131.45*
　disease course and prognosis 131.43
　epidemiology 131.41
　investigations 131.43
　management 131.43–131.46
　as melanoma precursors 142.2–142.3
　pathophysiology 131.41–131.42
　Spitz naevi **131.36**
atypical network patterns
　melanomas 145.7, *145.8,* 145.10
　Spitz neavi 145.7
atypical (non-classical) epidermodysplasia verruciformis 25.66, 25.69
atypical post-radiation vascular lesion *see* atypical vascular proliferation after radiotherapy
atypical progeroid syndrome **72.5**
atypical smooth muscle tumour (dermal and subcutaneous type leiomyosarcoma) 136.54–136.55
atypical streaks, melanoma 145.7, *145.8, 145.10*
atypical trigeminal trophic syndrome (ATTS) 82.8, *82.9*
atypical vascular lesions 103.32, 119.15
atypical vascular proliferation after radiotherapy (AVPRs) 136.38–136.39
atypical vascular structures/vessels, melanoma 145.8, 145.9, 145.14
auricle (pinna) *see* ear, auricle

auricular haematoma 122.16
Auspitz sign, in psoriasis vulgaris 35.9
Australia, skin cancer 6.1, 6.6, **6.7**
Austria, dermatology history 1.6
autoantibody screens, cutaneous photosensitivity diseases 126.6
autocrine factors, pigmentation regulation 86.5–86.7
autografts, burn wounds 125.5, 125.6
Autoimmune Bullous Disease Quality of Life (ABQOL) 108.8
autoimmune disorders
　acquired ichthyosis association 85.2
　APL association 98.4
　atopic eczema association 41.22
　bullous disease 85.30, 108.8
　dermatomyositis 52.1–52.13
　diabetic patients 62.4
　drug reaction with eosinophilia and systemic symptoms 118.11
　hair loss presentation 87.19–87.20, 87.22
　interstitial granulomatous dermatosis with musculoskeletal involvement 155.14
　involving respiratory system 152.2–152.3
　morphoea 55.7
　pregnancy 113.7–113.9
　skin and digestive system 153.3
　sweat glands 92.12
　urticaria association 42.3
　vitiligo association 86.35
autoimmune lymphoproliferative syndrome **72.11,** 80.14–80.15
autoimmune polyendocrinopathy Candida ectodermal dystrophy syndrome (APECED) 32.67
autoimmune polyendocrinopathy syndrome type 1 (APS-1) 87.20
autoimmune reactions, hair loss 87.74
autoimmunity
　in atopic eczema 41.12
　morphoea 55.8–55.9
autoimmunity defects, complement diseases 80.18–80.19
autoinflammation
　hidradenitis suppurativa 90.2–90.3
　panniculitis and dermatosis syndrome **72.11**
autoinflammation and PLCG2-associated antibody deficiency and immune dysregulation (APLAID) **45.5, 45.7,** 45.12
autoinflammatory diseases with granuloma 45.11–45.12
　autoinflammation and PLCG2-associated antibody deficiency and immune dysregulation 45.12
autoinflammatory disorders 45.1–45.23, 80.17–80.18
　clinical features 45.1
　cutaneous manifestations **80.19**
　hereditary monogenic autoinflammatory syndromes 45.2–45.19
　urticarial or maculopapular rash 45.20–45.22
autoinflammatory granulomatosis of childhood (Blau syndrome) **45.5, 45.7,** 45.11–45.12
autologous stem cell therapies 87.95
autonomic nervous system (ANS) 83.4–83.5
　adipose tissue 97.4
autosomal chromosome defects 74.1–74.3
　Behçet-like disease associated with trisomy 8 myelodysplasia 149.8
　chromosome 4, short-arm deletion syndrome 74.3
　chromosome 5, short-arm deletion syndrome 74.3
　chromosome 18, long-arm deletion syndrome 74.3
　Edwards syndrome (trisomy 18) 74.2
　Patau syndrome (trisomy 13) 74.2–74.3
　see also Down syndrome
autosomal dominant (AD) inheritance 8.3
autosomal dominant cutis laxa 77.5–77.6

autosomal dominant disorders
　disseminated superficial actinic
　　porokeratosis 141.15–141.18
　Loeys-Dietz syndrome 141.42
　Muir–Torre syndrome 141.44–141.45
　multiple self-healing squamous
　　epithelioma 141.41–141.42
autosomal dominant dystrophic
　epidermolysis bullosa 69.16
autosomal dominant epidermolysis bullosa
　simplex
　with migratory circinate redness
　　69.9–69.10
　with mottled pigmentation 69.9
autosomal dominant familial partial
　lipodystrophy, AGL differentiation
　98.3
autosomal dominant IFAP2 syndrome
　63.25–63.26
autosomal dominant intermediate
　epidermolysis bullosa 69.15–69.16
autosomal dominant intermediate
　epidermolysis bullosa simplex
　69.8–69.9
　with cardiomyopathy 69.10
autosomal dominant lamellar ichthyoses
　(ADLI) 63.20–63.21
autosomal dominant localised epidermolysis
　bullosa simplex 69.8
autosomal dominant punctate porokeratosis
　63.59
autosomal dominant striate palmoplantar
　keratoderma 63.57
autosomal recessive agammaglobulinaemia
　80.5
autosomal recessive (AR) inheritance 8.3
autosomal recessive congenital ichthyosis
　(ARCI) 63.7–63.10
　management of 63.41, 63.44
autosomal recessive cutis laxa 77.6–77.7
autosomal recessive deafness, palmoplantar
　keratodermas 63.63
autosomal recessive dystrophic
　epidermolysis bullosa 69.16
autosomal recessive epidermolysis bullosa
　69.15–69.16
autosomal recessive epidermolysis bullosa
　simplex 69.10
　with BP230 deficiency 69.10
autosomal recessive ichthyosis with
　hypotrichosis (ARIH) 63.40
autosomal recessive intermediate
　epidermolysis bullosa simplex, with
　exophilin-5 deficiency 69.10–69.11
autosomal recessive localised epidermolysis
　bullosa simplex
　with exophilin-5 deficiency 69.10–69.11
　with muscular dystrophy 69.11
　with nephropathy 69.11
autosomal recessive mutations,
　erythrokeratoderma variabilis
　63.18
autosomal recessive PPK, gene mutations
　63.54
autosomal recessive severe epidermolysis
　bullosa simplex, with pyloric
　atresia 69.11
AVED *see* ataxia with vitamin E deficiency
avidin–biotin conjugate, immunoenzyme
　methods 3.15–3.16
avidin–biotin–peroxidase complex (ABC)
　method 3.16
AVM *see* arteriovenous malformations
AVPRs *see* atypical vascular proliferation
　after radiotherapy
axes of endocrine signalling 150.2
axilla
　abscess 90.4
　allergic contact dermatitis 127.16
　anti-p200 pemphigoid 50.41
　ectopic plaque 90.7
　hidradenitis suppurativa 88.38, 90.4
　microbiome 26.3, 26.4, 26.5
　staphylococcal scalded skin syndrome
　　26.29

surgical treatment 90.11
axillary apocrine miliaria 92.19
axillary dermatitis, textile allergy 127.66
axillary fold, amicrobial pustulosis of the
　skin folds 49.20
axillary hair
　androgen-stimulated growth 87.10
　trichomycosis axillaris 26.41–26.42
axillary hyperhidrosis 92.3, 92.5–92.6
　management 92.9
　surgical treatment 92.10
axillary malodour 92.16–92.17
axillary skin
　childhood linear IgA disease 80.15
　microscopic examination of 3.33
　neurofibromatosis type 1 78.2
　pseudoxanthoma elasticum 70.32
azathioprine (AZA) 19.8–19.10
　atopic eczema treatment 41.29
　cautions 19.9
　contraindication 19.9
　dermatological uses 19.8
　dose and regimens 19.10
　drug–drug interactions 19.9
　monitoring 19.10
　pemphigus treatment 50.8
　pharmacological properties 19.8–19.9
　potential adverse effects 19.9
　pre-treatment screening 19.10
　systemic sclerosis treatment 54.24
azelaic acid
　acne vulgaris treatment 88.47
　chemical peels 160.2
　topical depigmenting agents 18.32
azo dyes 127.60, 127.61, 127.65–127.66

B
BA *see* benzyl alcohol; bioavailability
babies *see* infants; neonates
Baboon syndrome (BS) **117.4**, 117.5, 121.6
BAC *see* benzalkonium chloride
bacillary angiomatosis 26.62, 26.64–26.65,
　109.28
bacille Calmette–Guérin (BCG)
　infection 27.1–27.4, 27.6, 27.11, *27.12*,
　　80.8–80.9
　leprosy protection 28.16
　lupus vulgaris 27.23, *27.24*
　tuberculosis vaccination 5.3, 27.3–27.5,
　　27.10–27.11, 27.20, 27.21, 27.25,
　　27.27–27.29, 27.40, 80.8
　see also BCG vaccination
Bacillus anthracis 26.44–26.45
Bacillus cereus 26.44–26.45
*Bacillus pyocyaneus see Pseudomonas
　infections, P. aeruginosa/P. pyocyanea*
bacitracin 18.10
back
　acne conglobata 88.64
　acne fulminans 88.61
　acne-induced hyperpigmentation 88.41
　acne scarring 88.40
　acne vulgaris 88.27, 88.28
　annular erythema of infancy 47.10
　atopic eczema 41.17
　bullous pemphigoid 50.17, 50.18, 50.20
　diffuse cutaneous mastocytosis 46.6
　dysplastic naevus syndrome 131.41
　epidermolysis bullosa acquisita 50.45
　erythrodermic psoriasis 35.14
　linear morphoea 55.23
　naevus comedonicus 88.32
　pansclerotic morphoea 55.21
　pemphigus vulgaris 50.4
　pigmentary mosaicism 115.13
　pityrosporum folliculitis 88.37
　psoriasis vulgaris 35.8, 35.14
　roseola infantum 115.6
　spina bifida, tuft hair association 83.18
　steatocystoma multiplex 88.34
　subacute cutaneous lupus erythematosus
　　51.15
　systemic lupus erythematosus 51.23,
　　51.28
　systemic sclerosis 54.4

urticaria 42.10, *42.12*, 42.13
bacteria
　adherence to the skin 26.5
　antibiotic resistance 18.11, 26.8
　dermatoses possibly attributable to
　　infection 26.87–26.90
　molecular genetic identification methods
　　26.2, 26.3
　normal skin microbiome 26.3–26.5
　possible role in chancriform pyoderma
　　26.87–26.88
　sampling methods for skin microbes
　　26.3
　temporary residents on skin 26.2
　see also microbial ecology of the skin; skin
　　microbiome
bacterial antigen tests 4.24–4.25
bacterial arthropathies 155.4–155.5
bacterial colonisation, burn injuries
　125.9–125.10
bacterial decomposition, apocrine glands
　92.16
bacterial dysbiosis, lichen planus 37.3
bacterial infections 26.1–26.91
　actinomycetes 26.84–26.87
　anaerobic bacteria 26.67–26.69
　botryomycosis 26.76–26.77
　burn injuries 125.9
　chlamydiae 26.79
　ear piercing 106.11
　eyelids 107.38–107.39
　female genitalia 110.25–110.27
　gram-negative bacteria 26.49–26.67
　gram-positive bacteria 26.6–26.49
　HIV coinfection 31.20–31.22
　immunosuppressed renal allograft
　　recipients 154.5
　legionellosis 26.79
　mycobacteria 27.1–27.46
　Mycoplasma 26.78–26.79
　necrotising subcutaneous infections
　　26.77–26.78
　non-syphilitic sexually transmitted
　　diseases 30.1–30.26
　opportunistic pathogens from skin 26.2,
　　26.4, 26.17, 26.51, 26.55, 26.86
　perineal and perianal skin 111.13–111.15
　possible role in dermatoses 26.87–26.90
　protective role of normal skin flora
　　26.4–26.5
　rickettsiae 26.80–26.84
　secondary to varicella 25.30
　skin defence mechanisms 26.5–26.6
　skin manifestations of primary
　　immunodeficiencies 149.19
　spirochaetes 26.69–26.76, 109.27
　staphylococci and streptococci
　　26.12–26.37
bacterial interference 26.6
bacterial isolates 90.3
bacterial panniculitis 97.47
bacterial pseudomycosis *see* botryomycosis
bacterial toxins
　diphtheria 26.38
　recurrent toxin-mediated perineal
　　erythema 26.32
　scarlet fever 26.35
　streptococcal toxin-mediated disease
　　26.35–26.37
Bacteroidaceae 26.67–26.68
Bacteroides 26.19, 26.67, 26.68, 26.78
　B. bacilliformis, Oroya fever and verruga
　　peruana 26.65–26.66
　B. henselae, bacillary angiomatosis
　　26.64–26.65
　cat scratch disease 26.62–26.64
BAD *see* British Association of
　Dermatologists
BADAS *see* bowel-associated
　dermatitis–arthritis syndrome
Bailey nylon monofilament 83.15
balanitis 109.4, 109.5
　Zoon balanitis 109.14
balanoposthitis 109.4–109.5
　non-specific balanoposthitis
　　109.21–109.22

non-syphilitic spirochaetal ulcerative
　109.27
baldness cure, ancient Egypt 1.2
ballooning degeneration 3.40
balsam allergies 127.41–127.45
bandaging, lymphoedema therapy 103.58,
　103.59
band patterns, melanoma involving nail unit
　145.13
Bannayan–Riley–Ruvalcaba syndrome
　101.28
BAP-1 *see* BRAC1-associated protein
BAP1-inactivated melanocytic neoplasms
　(BIM), as melanoma precursor
　142.2
BAP1-inactivated naevus, scalp 131.34
BAP1 tumour suppressor gene, melanoma
　risk 142.4–142.5, 142.7
Barainelli–Seip syndrome *see* congenital
　generalised lipodystrophies
barber's hair sinus 122.22
Bardet–Biedel syndrome **72.6**
baricitinib, atopic eczema treatment 41.30,
　41.31
Barmah Forest virus (BFV) 25.90–25.91
Barr body 8.7
barrier creams, allergic contact dermatitis
　127.35
Barrier dysfunction, ageing of skin
　156.10–156.11
Bartholin abscess
　chlamydia 30.11
　gonorrhoea 30.5
Bartholin cyst, vulval 110.31
Bartonella
　B. quintana, bacillary angiomatosis
　　26.64–26.65
　infections 26.62–26.66
　trench fever 26.62
Bart–Pumphrey syndrome 63.64, 94.37
basal cell carcinoma (BCC) 140.1–140.21
　advanced/high risk disease 140.9,
　　140.14, **140.15**, 140.16–140.17, 140.19
　ano-genital region 111.24
　auricle 106.21–106.27
　　epidemiology 106.21–106.24
　　management 106.26–106.27
　　pathophysiology 106.25–106.26
　Bazex–Dupré–Christol syndrome
　　140.20–140.21
　biopsy 3.4
　diagnosis 3.30, 3.31
　differential diagnosis 140.9–140.10
　drug/chemical photosensitivity 126.30
　epidemiology 140.1–140.2
　eyelid 107.47–107.48
　female genitalia 110.39
　histopathology 140.3, *140.4*
　immunocompromised people
　　147.12–147.13, 147.16
　incidence of, in UK 6.1
　investigations 140.10, *140.11, 140.12*,
　　140.14
　lip 108.43–108.44
　male genitalia 109.42
　management 140.11–140.18
　margin assessment 140.14, **140.15**, 140.16
　Merkel cell carcinoma misdiagnosis
　　146.5
　naevoid basal cell carcinoma syndrome
　　140.3–140.4, 140.18–140.20
　pathophysiology 140.2–140.10
　photodynamic therapy 140.11,
　　140.12–140.13
　　contraindications 22.8
　　Gorlin naevoid syndrome 22.2, 22.7
　　superficial and thin nodular BCC
　　　22.6–22.7
　radiotherapy 24.12–24.13, *24.14*
　　for ankylosing spondylitis as cause
　　　155.16
　　indications 24.8–24.10
　risk factors **140.2**
　risk stratification 140.11, **140.14**
　spectacle-frame acanthoma distinction
　　122.14

basal cell carcinoma (BCC) (continued)
　superficial treatments　140.11, 140.12–140.14
　surgical treatments　140.14–140.16
　types　140.3
　see also keratinocyte cancer; naevoid basal cell carcinoma syndrome
basal cell papilloma see seborrhoeic keratosis
basal cells
　division of　2.44
　terminal differentiation　2.44
basal lamina　3.39
basaloid follicular hamartoma　137.12–137.13
Basan syndrome　63.66
base excision repair (BER)　10.6
baseline patch test series　127.29–127.30
basement-membrane region　122.4–122.5
basidiobolomycosis　32.79–32.80
Basidiobolus ranarum　32.79–32.80
basophilic, round tumour cell proliferations, Merkel cell carcinoma　146.3
basophilic amorphous deposits　97.61
basophilic fat necrosis　97.8
basosquamous (metatypical) basal cell carcinoma　140.3, 140.9
BAT see brown adipose tissue
Bateman purpura see actinic purpura
Bateman, Thomas　1.4
bathing, atopic eczema　41.26
'bathing cap' distribution, multivoltage X-ray techniques　24.3, 24.5
bathing suit ichthyosis (BSI)　63.7, 63.8, 63.11
Bazex syndrome, ear dermatoses　**106.22**
Bazex–Dupré–Christol syndrome　**78.12**, 140.20–140.21
Bazin disease see erythema induratum of Bazin
BB-UVB see broad-band UVB
BCC see basal cell carcinoma
B-cell differentiation, lymphoid markers　3.29
B-cell directed biologic therapies　19.37–19.39
B-cell lymphoma
　external ear　106.34
　radiotherapy　24.18
B-cell pseudolymphoma (lymphocytoma cutis)　134.1, 134.2, 134.8–134.10
B cells, immune system　9.6, 103.3
BCH see benign cephalic histiocytosis
BCS see brittle cornea syndrome
BD see Bowen disease
BDD see body dysmorphic disorder
BDI see Beck Depression Inventory
BDP see Bowen disease of the penis
BE see bioequivalence
beards
　pseudofolliculitis barbae　91.8, 91.9, 122.23
　ringworm of the beard/tinea barbae　32.40–32.41
　sycosis　26.26–26.27
Beare–Stevenson syndrome　85.4
Beau lines　119.7, 119.8
becaplermin　18.39
Beck, Aaron T.　15.1–15.2
Beck Depression Inventory (BDI)　16.11
Becker melanosis, laser therapies　23.15–23.16
Becker naevus (or Becker melanosis)　73.18, 87.85, 87.86
Beckwith–Wiedemann syndrome　106.6
bed bugs　34.25–34.29
　clinical features　34.27
　epidemiology　34.26
　management　34.27–34.28, 34.29
　pathophysiology　34.26–27
'bed sores'　123.1
Beer's law, light absorption by skin　23.3
bees　34.16
Beetles (Coleoptera)　34.30–34.32
　allergenic species of　34.31–34.32

behaviour
　links to emotions and beliefs　15.1–15.3
　psychological factors in patients　15.2
Behçet disease see Adamantiades–Behçet disease
Behçet-like disease associated with trisomy 8 myelodysplasia　149.8
Behçet-like disease or inflammatory bowel disease-like autoinflammatory syndromes　45.15–45.16
Beighton score　**70.8**
bejel (endemic syphilis)　26.70
beliefs
　links to emotions and behaviours　15.1–15.3
　psychological factors in patients　15.2–15.3
belimumab　51.12
Bell palsy　25.23
Belostomatidae (giant water bugs)　34.30
benign adnexal lesions, eyelid　107.45
benign calcifying epithelioma of Malherbe see pilomatricoma
benign cephalic histiocytosis (BCH)　135.17–135.18
benign cutaneous adverse reactions to drugs　117.1–117.9
benign cutaneous tumours and proliferations
　photothermal ablation　23.21
　see also capillary haemangiomas
benign cysts, eyelid　107.45–107.47
benign essential telangiectasia see hereditary benign telangiectasia
benign fibrous cutaneous nodules　94.43
benign keratinocytic acanthomas　132.1–132.8
　clear cell acanthoma　132.6–132.7
　dermatosis papulosa nigra　132.4–132.5
　lichenoid keratosis　132.7–132.8
　seborrhoeic keratosis　132.1–132.4
　stucco keratosis　132.4
　warty dyskeratoma　132.5–132.6
　see also inverted follicular keratosis
benign lesions
　dermoscopic patterns of naevi　145.1–145.7
　ear　106.33
　eyelid　107.44–107.47
benign lymphangioendothelioma　103.29
benign lymphoid proliferations see pseudolymphoma
benign melanocytic naevi, in pregnancy　113.9
benign nodular calcification　154.2
　see also metastatic cutaneous calcification
benign papillomatosis of the nipple see nipple, adenoma
benign proliferations　132.1–132.10
　benign keratinocytic acanthomas　132.1–132.8
　pseudoepitheliomatous hyperplasia　132.9–132.10
　skin tags　132.8–132.9
benign symmetrical lipomatosis (BSL)　98.15–98.17, 103.46
benign tumours, male genitalia　109.29–109.31
benign vascular tumours　136.25–136.32
　classification　**116.1**
benzalkonium chloride (BAC)　127.57
　topical therapies　18.10
1,2-Benzisothiazolin-3-one (BIT)　127.53, 127.54
benzo(a)pyrene　129.15
benzocaine, patch testing　127.47
benzothiazole contact allergy　127.64
benzoyl peroxide (BPO)　88.46, 88.47
benzyl alcohol (BA)　127.58
BER see base excision repair
beriberi, vitamin B1 deficiency　61.14
Berloque dermatitis　86.28–86.30
beryllium, dermatological reactions　121.9
best evidence, evidence based medicine　17.4–17.8
β-adrenergic blockers, burn treatment　125.14

β-Carotene therapy　126.8
β rays　24.1
　see also electron beam therapy
beta-lactam allergy　117.7
beta-mannosidosis, glycoproteinoses　79.3
betamethasone, dose-vasoconstriction response profiles for　12.5
betel nut chewing
　oral hyperpigmentation　108.17
　oral lichen planus　37.3
　oral squamous cell carcinoma　108.46
　teeth staining　108.15
bexarotene　18.25
BFLS see Börjeson–Forssman–Lehmann syndrome
BFS see burning feet syndrome
BFV see Barmah Forest virus
BHA see butylated hydroxyanisole
BHD see Birt–Hogg–Dubé
bias
　Cochrane Collaborations risk of bias tool　17.9
　epidemiological studies　5.14
　types of bias in research studies　17.9–17.10
Bible, leprosy　1.3
'bib-sign', redness on chest in dermatomyositis　52.4, 52.6
bicalutamide　87.96
Biett, Laurent　1.4–1.5
bilateral lymphoedema, lower legs　98.27
bilharziasis see schistosomiasis
biliary tract disease　153.5
bilirubin　86.49
BIM see BAP1-inactivated melanocytic neoplasms
bimatoprost　18.39
bimekizumab
　psoriasis treatment　35.30
　psoriatic arthritis treatment　35.46
bioavailability (BA)
　clinical pharmacology　13.2–13.3, **13.2**
　of topical drugs　12.7–12.8
biobanking　8.1
biochemical functions, mechanical forces　122.1
biocides, formaldehyde-releasing　127.51–127.52
biodegradable dermal fillers　158.3–158.7
bioequivalence (BE), of topical drugs　12.7–12.8
biological dosimetry　10.2
biological elasticity　122.5
biologic registries, psoriasis treatment　35.29
biologic therapies　19.31–19.34
　atopic eczema　41.29–41.30, **41.31, 41.32**
　C1-esterase inhibitor replacement therapy　19.39
　clinical pharmacology　13.1, 13.2
　definition　13.1
　directed against B-cells　19.37–19.39
　directed against cytokines　19.32–19.37
　eye, side effects on　107.44
　hidradenitis suppurativa　90.10, 90.11
　intravenous immunoglobulins　19.31, 19.40–19.41
　monoclonal antibodies (mAbs)　19.31–19.32
　morphoea　55.38–55.42
　omalizumab　19.39
　in pregnancy　113.21, **113.22**
　psoriasis treatment　35.27–35.31
　pyoderma gangrenosum　49.7
biomarkers　8.8–8.9
　prenatal testing and diagnosis　8.11
biomechanical properties of skin　122.5–122.6
biomedical literature, evidence based medicine　17.2
biopsy of skin　3.2–3.10
　AIDs patients　3.38
　alopecia　3.7
　artefacts due to poor technique　3.31–3.32
　basal cell carcinoma　3.4
　blocking of specimens　3.6, 3.32

　curettage　3.3–3.4
　cysts　3.31
　Darier disease　3.39
　direct immunofluorescence studies　3.12, 3.17
　division of specimen　3.2, 3.4
　electron microscopy　3.4
　elliptical surgical biopsy　3.3, 3.6
　epidermolysis bullosa diagnosis　69.20–69.21, 69.23
　excisional biopsy　3.2
　fetal skin　8.10
　fixatives　3.4, **3.5**, 3.32
　frozen sections　3.5
　histochemistry　3.7–3.10
　histological sections with little or no abnormality　3.44–3.45
　identification labels　3.5
　inadequate biopsy　3.1
　inclusional/exclusional elliptical biopsies　20.8–20.9
　indications for　3.2
　information provided with specimen　3.4
　instruments for　3.3
　interpretation problems　3.1
　labelling of specimen　3.6
　laboratory methods　3.5–3.10
　little or no abnormality in histological sections　3.44–3.45
　local anaesthetic　3.2
　melanoma　143.1, 143.4–143.5
　Michel medium　3.4–3.5, 3.12
　microscopic examination of tissue sections　3.32–3.38
　multiple biopsies　3.2
　needle biopsy　3.4
　painting margins of specimen　3.5–3.6
　palm skin　3.33
　photocopy procedure, blocking of specimens　3.6
　planning　20.8–20.9
　punch biopsy　3.3, 20.9–20.10
　request form　3.4
　retention of tissue specimens　3.6
　section types　3.38
　shave biopsy　3.4, 20.10–20.11
　site selection　3.2, 3.12
　skin surface　4.22
　sole skin　3.33
　specimen preparation　3.4–3.7
　squamous cell carcinoma　3.4
　staining techniques　3.7–3.10
　techniques　3.2, 3.3–3.4, 20.8–20.11
　tissue processing　3.7
　topical anaesthetic　3.2–3.3
　transport media　3.4–3.5, **3.5**
　urticaria　3.45
　urticaria pigmentosa　3.2
　see also histopathology of skin
biosimilars, psoriasis treatment　35.29
biotin
　deficiency　61.22–61.24
　metabolism disorders　79.15
　see also avidin–biotin conjugate
bipolar disorder　84.40
Bipolaris species　32.78
Birbeck granules　135.2
birthmarks
　naevus flammeus　101.10
　see also naevi
birth weight, acne association　88.26
Birt–Hogg–Dubé (BHD) syndrome　**78.14**, 78.15
　differential diagnosis　88.30–88.31
　lesions of hair follicle mesenchyme　137.15–137.16
　pulmonary involvement　152.5
　renal/skin involvement　154.2
　skin tags　132.8
BIT see 1,2-Benzisothiazolin-3-one
bites　130.5–130.8
　animal bite injuries on infants/children　130–136, 115.14
　arthropods　14.2, 34.2–34.3, **34.4**, 34.14–34.15

by humans 130.6–130.7
clinical features 34.8–34.9
dogs/cats 130.6
infants 115.14
rodents 130.5
snakes 130.5–130.6
black death 26.59–26.60
blackflies 34.7
onchocerciasis vector 33.1, 33.2, *33.3*
Blackfoot disease 121.3
black hairy tongue 108.16, *108.17*
black heel/palm 99.6, 122.10–122.11, 122.16
black piedra 32.15–32.16
black rubber mix (sensitisers) **127.63**
black skin *see* skin of colour
blanchable redness 123.4
Blaschko lines 8.7, *8.8*
congenital epidermal naevi 73.5
Conradi–Hünermann–Happle syndrome 63.22
hypomelanosis of Ito 68.10
incontinentia pigmenti 68.11
keratinopathic ichthyoses 63.14
keratosis follicularis spinosa decalvans 63.24
linear and whorled hypermelanosis 68.12
Blashkoid lesions 4.16, *4.19*
blastic plasmacytoid dendritic cell neoplasm (CD4+/CD56+haematodermic neoplasm) 139.45–139.47
Blastomyces dermatitidis 32.85–32.86
blastomycosis 32.84–32.86, 109.28
oral lesions 108.57
Blau syndrome (autoinflammatory granulomatosis of childhood) **45.5**, **45.7**, 45.11–45.12
bleeding, complications after skin surgery 20.40–20.42
bleeding in skin and mucosa (purpura/petechiae/ecchymoses/epistaxis/gingival bleeding), liver disease association 153.9
Blegvad–Haxthausen syndrome 94.24
bleomycin, topical therapies 18.29–18.30
bleomycin-induced flagellate hyperpigmentation 119.8–119.9
blepharitis 107.7–107.15
associated skin disease **107.8**
causes *107.12*, 107.13
classification of chronic blepharitis **107.8**
complications and co-morbidities 107.13
conjunctival and corneal signs **107.8**
cutaneous *Leishmania* infection of eyelid 107.12
demodex folliculorum infestation 107.10
diagnosis **107.13**
disease course and prognosis 107.13–107.14
eyelid signs **107.8**
incidence and prevalence 107.7–107.10
investigations 107.14
management 107.14–107.15
meibomian seborrhoea **107.8**
meibomitis **107.8**
ocular rosacea **107.8**, **107.10**, 107.11–107.12
pathology 107.10–107.12
Phthirus pubis causation *107.12*
predisposing factors 107.10
sebaceous carcinoma of eyelid *107.12*
seborrhoeic blepharitis **107.8**
staphylococcal blepharitis **107.8**, *107.9*, 107.10
symptoms **107.8**
treatment of chronic blepharitis **107.14**
ulcerative blepharitis *107.9*
blepharochalasis 94.26–94.27, 107.5
blepharoconjunctivitis *107.6*
blinding filariasis *see* onchocerciasis
blistering disorders 69.1–69.28
drug/chemical photosensitivity *126.29*
heat-associated diseases 124.15, *124.16*
internal malignancy association 148.22
juvenile springtime eruption 126.9

mechanical injuries 122.6, 122.8, 122.9–122.10, 122.16
PUVA phototherapy adverse effects 21.13
Stevens–Johnson syndrome/toxic epidermal necrolysis *118.14–118.15*
Tzanck smear 3.29
UVB phototherapy adverse effects 21.12
see also bullous diseases; paraneoplastic pemphigus; pemphigus
blistering distal dactylitis 26.34, 115.8
blisters
friction 122.6, 122.9–122.10
on the lips 108.60
oral ulceration **108.36**
'string of pearls' ring pattern *4.8*
vesicating beetles 34.30–34.31
Bloch, Bruno 127.1
blocking techniques, biopsy 3.6
blood eosinophilia 93.7, 93.9
blood-letting 1.3
blood supply, cones 124.8
blood tryptase, raised level of
mastocytosis 46.8
in patient without skin lesions **46.6**, *46.7*
blood vessels 2.40–2.42
anatomy of head and neck 20.1–20.2
Bloom syndrome **75.2**, **77.2**, 77.3–77.4, **78.13**, **80.5**, 148.12, 148.13
hyperpigmentation 80.11
blueberry muffin baby (dermal erythropoiesis) 114.21
blue-black lesions, melanoma 145.14
blue light therapy, acne vulgaris 88.58
blue naevus 3.44, **131.17**, 131.38–131.40
cellular *131.39*, *131.40*
common blue naevus *131.38*
congenital 73.15, *73.16*
dermoscopic image *131.40*
see also malignant blue naevus
blue rubber bleb naevus syndrome (BRBN) **71.2**, **71.17**–71.18, 136.42
blue toe syndrome *see* cholesterol embolus
blue-white veil, melanoma 145.7, *145.8*, *145.10*
blushing 104.1–104.13
clinical presentation 104.10
epidemiology 104.1
investigations 104.11
management 104.12
physiology 104.1
psychosocial aspects 104.2–104.3
typical distribution *104.2*
BMI *see* body mass index
BMPs *see* bone morphogenic proteins
BMS *see* burning mouth syndrome
BMZ *see* dermal–epidermal basement membrane zone
BNPD *see* 2-Bromo-2-nitropropane-1, 3-diol
body art 108.15–108.16
body/clothing lice 34.23–34.24
body contouring 161.8–161.9
body dysmorphic disorder (BDD) 84.12–84.15
and acne 88.30
by proxy 84.14
complaints and litigation 84.15
dislike of mole and freckles 84.26
male genitalia 109.6, 109.44
olfactory delusions 84.10
scales and screening questions **84.13**
body image 15.1
body mass index (BMI), and acne 88.19
body odour, olfactory delusions 84.10–84.11
Bohan and Peter classification, dermatomyositis 52.1
boils *see* carbuncles; furuncles
Bolivian haemorrhagic fever 25.82–25.83
bone disorders
diffuse lymphangiomatosis involving bone 136.39
Langerhans cell histiocytosis 135.8
systemic lupus erythematosus 51.30

bone dysplasia, nail–patella syndrome 67.15
bone marrow, mastocytosis 46.3, *46.4*, 46.8, *46.9*
bone marrow failure, dyskeratosis congenita 67.14–67.15
bone marrow transplantation
mastocytosis treatment 46.10
oral complications of 108.48
bone metastases, metastatic calcinosis cutis 59.5
bone morphogenic proteins (BMPs) 2.3, 2.4
bone scintigraphy, frostbite investigation 124.2
bony abnormalities, epidermolysis bullosa 69.26
borderline leprosy (BL/BB/BT) 28.2–28.3, 28.4, 28.6, 28.8, **28.9**, 28.10, 28.11, 28.13, *28.14*
Börjeson–Forssman–Lehmann syndrome (BFLS) **72.6**
Borrelia 26.72–26.74
B. afzelii 26.72, 26.73, 94.15–94.16
B. garinii 26.72, 26.73
B. recurrentis, louse-borne epidemic relapsing fever 26.72
Lyme disease 26.72–26.73
necrobiotic xanthogranuloma 97.17
Borrelia burgdorferi
complex of species 26.72
infective panniculitis 97.46
possible cutaneous B-cell lymphoma link 139.37–139.38
borreliosis 94.15–94.16
bosentan 124.12
botryomycosis 26.76–26.77
Botswana–UPENN partnership 7.7
botulinum toxin
aesthetic uses of 159.1–159.9
acetylcholine release blocking 159.2
acquired resistance to botulinum toxins 159.8
adverse events 159.6–159.8
combination treatment 159.8
ethnic diversity and botulinum toxins 159.6
future botulinum toxins in development 159.8–159.9
history of clinical applications 159.2
history and early research 159.1–159.2
lower face 159.5–159.6
mid face 159.5
neck 159.6
side effects summary **159.7**
upper face 159.4–159.5
characteristics of **159.3**
clinical applications of for aesthetic conditions 159.3–159.6
eye, side effects on 107.44
pharmaceutical terminology **159.1**
pharmacology and action of neurotoxins 159.2–159.3
variation and equivalence 159.3
botulinum toxin A injection, hyperhidrosis treatment 92.9
botulism 159.1
Bouchard nodes 155.8
Bourneville disease *see* tuberous sclerosis complex
boutonneuse fever 26.82–26.83
bovine collagen dermal filler 158.5, 158.7–158.8
bowel-associated dermatitis–arthritis syndrome (BADAS) 49.15–49.17, 97.52, 153.3–153.4
acute inflammatory distal arthritis 49.16
clinical features 49.15–49.16
episcleritis 49.17
investigations 49.16
lesion appearance *49.16*
management 49.16–49.17
pathology 49.15
predisposing factors 49.15
pustules on trunk *49.16*
urticarial plaques *49.16*

bowel carcinoma, colostomy for *112.5*
bowel disease, dermatoses associated with 112.12–112.15
Bowen disease (BD) 141.18–141.24, *141.25*
and actinic keratoses, immunocompromised people 147.11–147.12
discoid skin lesions **39.10**
epidemiology 141.18
first line treatments 141.22–141.24
male genitalia 109.31–109.34
management 141.22–141.24, *141.25*
pathophysiology 141.18–141.22, *141.25*
perianal skin 111.20–111.21
photodynamic therapy 22.6
photothermal ablation 23.21
radiotherapy 24.14
second/third line treatments 141.24
see also anal/perianal/genital intraepithelial carcinomas; *in situ* carcinoma of the skin
Bowen disease of the penis (BDP) 109.31–109.34
bowenoid papulosis
Bowen disease comparison 141.19, 141.20–141.21, *141.22*
human papilloma virus 141.21
male genitalia 109.31–109.34
see also anal/perianal/genital intraepithelial carcinomas
box jellyfish stings 130.1–130.2
BP230 *see* bullous pemphigoid antigen
BP230 deficiency, autosomal recessive epidermolysis bullosa simplex with 69.10
BP *see* bullous pemphigoid
BPO *see* benzoyl peroxide
BRAC1-associated protein (BAP-1), germline mutations in 3.24
brachioradial pruritus (BRP) 81.12, 83.6–83.7
Brachycera (biting flies) 34.8
brachytherapy 24.3
bradykinin-induced angio-oedema 43.1, **43.2**, *43.3*, **43.6**
BRAF inhibitors
causing keratoacanthoma 141.38, 141.41
melanoma systemic therapy 144.4–144.5, *144.11*, **144.11**, 144.12
BRAF mutations, lobular capillary haemangioma/pyogenic granuloma within port-wine stains 136.26
BRAF-positive tumours 85.9
BRAF therapy *see* B-rapidly accelerated fibrosarcoma protein inhibitor therapy
BRAF V600E mutation
Erdheim–Chester disease 135.21
histiocytoses 135.3, 135.7, 135.9
juvenile xanthogranuloma 135.16
brain metastases 144.7
brain–skin axis
neuroendocrine stress response in skin 150.8–150.9
psychological factors in patients 15.2
branchial cyst *106.4*
branchio-oto-renal syndrome *106.4*, **106.7**
B-rapidly accelerated fibrosarcoma protein (BRAF) inhibitor therapy 85.23
Brazilian haemorrhagic fever 25.82–25.83
BRBN *see* blue rubber bleb naevus syndrome
breast
abscess, neonatal 114.25
diffuse dermal angiomatosis *4.11*
lymphangiomatous papules, benign *103.32*
lymphoedema 103.43–103.44
melanocytic naevi 131.22
morphoea *55.18*
pansclerotic morphoea *55.21*
swollen 103.43–103.44
breast cancer
breast lymphoedema *103.44*
carcinoma telangiectatica on arm *103.15*

breast cancer (*continued*)
 radiotherapy side effects   119.15
 recurrent cellulitis in lymphoedema   103.14
 skin involvement   148.2–148.3
breastfeeding, and atopic eczema   41.7, 41.23
breast surgery, Mondor disease after   101.37
breathing exercises, lymphoedema   103.59
BRESEK/BRESHEK syndrome   63.24–63.25
Breslow thickness, melanomas   142.2, 142.8, 142.15–142.16, 142.21, 142.22, 142.24
Brevibacterium mcbrellneri, synergistic role with *Trichosporon* yeast in white piedra   32.16
Brief Symptom Inventory (BSI)   16.11
Brill–Zinsser disease   26.81
brimonidine   18.39
Britain, dermatology history   1.6–1.7
British Association of Dermatologists (BAD)   7.14
brittle cornea syndrome (BCS)   **70.6–70.7**, 70.10
broad-band UVB (BB-UVB)
 phototherapy
  carcinogenesis risk   21.13
  efficacy   21.3–21.4, 21.7
  principles   21.1, 21.2
Brocq's acné excoriée   84.20–84.22
brodalumab
 psoriasis treatment   35.30
 psoriatic arthritis treatment   35.46
bromhidrosis   92.16–92.17
bromides, acneform reaction   88.13
bromidrosiphobia *see* olfactory delusions
2-bromo-2-nitropropane-1, 3-diol (BNPD)   127.52
bronchial epithelium, SJS/TEN involvement   118.20
bronchiolitis obliterans   118.17
bronchopneumonia, inhalation injury   125.4–125.5
bronchopulmonary injuries   125.5
bronze baby syndrome   86.49–86.50
Brooke's tumour *see* trichoepithelioma
Brooke–Spiegler syndrome
 cylindroma   137.30
 spiradenoma   137.31
 trichoepithelioma   137.10
brown adipose tissue (BAT)   72.1
brown fat   97.1–97.2
brown fat hypertrophy   98.15
brown pseudoscars, diabetic dermopathy   94.14
brown recluse spiders (Sicariidae)   34.35–34.36
brown tongue   108.16
brows
 botulinum toxin use   159.5
 see also eyebrows
BRP *see* brachioradial pruritus
Brucella   26.60–26.62
brucellosis   26.60–26.62
bruises/bruising *see* ecchymosis
Brunsting–Perry pemphigoid   50.51–50.52, 50.53
Bruton disease (X-linked agammagobulinaemia)   **80.5**, 80.13
Bryozoa, stings from   130.4
BS *see* Baboon syndrome
BSI *see* bathing suit ichthyosis; Brief Symptom Inventory; Burma Skincare Initiative
BSL *see* benign symmetrical lipomatosis
BSLE *see* bullous systemic lupus erythematous
bubble hair   87.77–87.78
buboes *see* inguinal buboes; lymphadenitis
bubonic plague   26.59–26.60
Bubostumum phlebotomum see cutaneous larva migrans
buccal fat-pad herniation   108.10
buccal mucosa
 cheek biting   108.32

epidermolysis bullosa acquista   50.45
erythroplakia   108.24
examination of   108.7
Fordyce spots   108.29
homogeneous leukoplakia   108.34
leiomyoma   108.13
leukoedema   108.29, *108.30*
lichen planus   37.5, 37.6, *108.76*
sarcoidosis   108.67
 see also cheek
Buddhist texts   1.2–1.3
Buerger test, peripheral vascular disease   *101.3*
buffalo hump, HIV-associated lipodystrophy   98.7
bugs (Hemiptera)   34.25–34.30
bulbar telangiectasia   80.11
bulge region, hair follicle   87.4
bulimia nervosa   84.26–84.27
Bulkley, Henry D.   1.7
bullae   3.39
bullous dermatoses   4.8
 IP differential diagnosis   68.11
bullous diseases
 autoimmune, assessment   108.8
 diagnosis   3.11, 3.29, 3.30
 digestive system   153.6
 direct immunofluorescence   *3.18*
 ear dermatoses   **106.22**
 electron microscopy studies   3.30, 69.21–69.22
 female genitalia   110.20, **110.21**
 flexural sites   **4.18**
 internal malignancy association   148.21–148.22
 microscopic appearance   3.29
 renal failure and dialysis complications   154.4
bullous eruptions, reactions to COVID-19 vaccines   25.118
bullous impetigo   2.19, 26.13–26.15
 neonates   114.24
bullous lesions, autoinflammatory diseases   **80.19**
bullous lichen planus   37.8–37.9, 37.17
bullous lupus erythematosus   51.28–51.29
bullous pemphigoid (BP)   50.10–50.22, 148.22
 acute oedema blisters   85.30
 age of onset   50.11
 antigens   69.4, 69.5, **69.8**, 69.10
 associated diseases   50.11
 autoantibodies   50.11–50.12
 blisters, erosions, and haemorrhagic crusts   *50.11, 50.16*
 cellular immune response   50.12
 in childhood   50.20
 clinical features   50.15–50.16
 clinical variants   50.16–50.17
 cytokines and chemokines   50.12
 diagnosis   50.20, *50.21*, **50.22**, *50.24*
 differential diagnosis   50.17–50.18
 direct immunofluorescence microscopy   *50.14*
 disease course and prognosis   50.18–50.19
 epidemiology   50.10–50.11
 genetics   50.15
 histopathology   50.13
 investigations   50.20, *50.21*, **50.22**
 localised bullous pemphigoid   50.17, *50.19*
 management   50.20–50.22
 oral involvement   108.81–108.82
 papule appearance   50.17
 pathogenic mechanisms   50.12–50.13
 pathophysiology   50.11–50.13
 predisposing factors   50.13
 randomised controlled trials   50.20–50.21, **50.23**
 renal effects   154.6
 serum autoantibodies   50.14–50.15
  serological screening   *50.14, 50.15*
 severity classification   50.18
 tissue-bound autoantibodies   50.13–50.14

treatment guidelines   50.21–50.22
urticarial and erythematous plaques   *50.18*
vulval   **110.21**
bullous porphyrias
 histopathology   58.4–58.5
 samples for laboratory testing   58.7
 typical subepidermal bulla in   *58.6*
bullous pyoderma gangrenosum   49.4–49.5
bullous systemic lupus erythematous (BSLE)   50.48–50.51
 blisters on erythematosus   *50.49*
 differential diagnosis   50.50
 epidemiology   50.48–50.49
 investigations and diagnosis   50.50
 management   50.50–50.51
 pathophysiology   50.49
 presentation   50.49–50.50
 serum autoantibodies   *50.50*
 treatment ladder   50.51
 violaceous maculae   *50.50*
Bunyaviruses, haemorrhagic fevers   25.83–25.84
buprenorphine, addiction prevalence   120.2
burden of skin disease   5.5, 5.6–5.7, *5.8, 5.9*
Bureau–Barrière syndrome   63.71
Burkholderia   26.53–26.55
 B. mallei, glanders   26.55
 B. pseudomallei, melioidosis   26.53–26.54
Burkitt lymphoma   25.38
Burma Skincare Initiative (BSI)   7.11
burn depth
 assessment of   125.2
 clinical appearances   **125.3**
 evaluation of   125.5–125.8
burning feet syndrome (BFS)   83.10–83.11
burning mouth syndrome (BMS)   82.1–82.3, 108.64–108.65, 127.18
 causes   **108.64**
 epidemiology   82.2
 management   82.3
 pathophysiology   82.2–82.3
burning sensation, irritation   128.10–128.12
burns   125.1–125.15
 first-degree burns   125.5
 grafts   11.12
 hospital care   125.1
 oral lesions   108.31
 shock   125.2–125.4
Burton's lead line   121.5
Buruli ulcer   97.47
 genital   109.28
Buschke disease *see* scleroedema
Buschke–Löwenstein tumour
 male genitalia   109.39–109.40
 perianal skin   *111.23*
Buschke–Ollendorff syndrome   94.43
butterflies (Lepidoptera)   34.32–34.34
butterfly erythema pattern on face, dermatomyositis   52.3, *52.5*
butterfly sign (mid-back sparing), nodular prurigo   84.15
buttock
 bullous pemphigoid   *50.16*
 capillary malformations   *71.5*
 cryoglobulinaemic vasculitis   100.16
 dermatitis herpetiformis   *50.57*
 eruptive xanthomas   60.4
 hemihyperplasia–multiple lipomatosis syndrome   *72.11*
 herpes simplex   *4.8*
 linear IgA disease   *50.37*
 morphoea   55.16
 mucous membrane pemphigoid   *50.29*
 necrolytic migratory erythema   *47.15*
butylated hydroxyanisole (BHA)   127.59

C

C&C (curettage and cautery) *see* curettage and electrodessication
C1-esterase inhibitor (C1-INH) deficiency, angio-oedema due to   43.1, 43.4, 43.5–43.6
C1-esterase inhibitor (C1INH) replacement therapy   19.39

C3 nephritic factor, APL pathology   98.4
cacosmia *see* olfactory delusions
CACP (camptodactyly, arthropathy, coxa vara, pericarditis) syndrome   94.40–94.41
CAD *see* chronic actinic dermatitis; computer-aided diagnostic systems
CADIS *see* Childhood Atopic Dermatitis Impact Scale
CADM *see* clinically amyopathic dermatomyositis
café-au-lait macules (CALMs)   78.3, **131.1**
café-au-lait patches, laser therapies   23.15, *23.16*
caffeine
 cosmeceutical use of   157.11
 rosacea risk   89.3
 topical therapies   18.39
CAG repeats, hirsutism   87.88
CAH *see* congenital adrenal hyperplasia
CaHa *see* calcium hydroxylapatite
CAIN *see* CCAAT enhancer binding protein ε-associated autoinflammation and immune impairment of neutrophils
Calabar swellings *see* loiasis
calcaneal petechiae   122.16
calcification, lupus panniculitis   97.38
calcification of blood vessels *see* calciphylaxis
calcification of skin and subcutaneous tissues   59.1–59.10
 calciphylaxis   59.6–59.9
 dystrophic calcification   59.1–59.4
 idiotrophic calcification   59.4–59.5
 metastatic calcification   59.5–59.6
 secondary to trauma or injection/infusion of calcium-containing materials   59.3
 secondary to tumours and genetic disease   59.3–59.4
calcific panniculitis   154.2
 see also metastatic cutaneous calcification
calcific uraemic arteriolopathy *see* calciphylaxis
calcified cutaneous nodules of the heels, infants   115.15
calcifying aponeurotic fibroma   136.7–136.8
calcifying epithelioma of Malherbe (benign) *see* pilomatricoma
calcifying fibrous tumours/pseudotumours   136.7
calcifying nodules, ear dermatoses   **106.22**, *106.24*
calcifying panniculitis *see* calciphylaxis
calcineurin inhibitors
 atopic eczema treatment   41.27
 mastocytosis treatment   46.10
 psoriasis treatment   35.22
 topical therapies   18.22–18.26, 41.27
calcinosis
 dermatomyositis   52.6
 systemic sclerosis   **54.3**, 54.17, **54.26**
 see also calcification of skin and subcutaneous tissues
calcinosis, scrotal   59.4, *59.5*, 109.30
calciphylaxis   59.6–59.9, 97.32–97.35, 99.23, 154.2, *154.3*
 penile   109.24
calcipotriol   18.28–18.29
calcitriol   18.28
calcium-containing injections/infusions   59.3
calcium enhancement indirect technique   3.14
calcium homeostasis, systemic abnormalities   59.5–59.6
calcium hydroxylapatite (CaHa) dermal filler   158.5, 158.6–158.7
calcium pump disorders   69.23–69.24
calibre-persistent artery, lip lesions   108.63
callosities   122.7–122.9
calluses   122.7–122.9, 122.16
CALMs *see* café-au-lait macules
calpains   94.38
calpastatin (*CAST*), skin fragility disorders   69.6

calponin 3.25
Calymmatobacterium granulomatis see Klebsiella granulomatis
Cambodia, clinical officer training 7.7–7.8
camouflage options
  alopecia 87.18, 87.69, 87.97–87.101
  hair disorders 87.101
camphor 18.38
camptodactyly 94.40–94.41
camptodactyly, arthropathy, coxa vara, pericarditis (CACP) syndrome 94.40–94.41
camptodactyly, tall stature and hearing loss (CATSHL) 94.40
CA-MRSA *see* community-acquired MRSA
CAMs *see* cellular adhesion molecules
Canada, psoriasis, economic burden of 6.8
Canale–Smith syndrome *see* autoimmune lymphoproliferative syndrome
cancer
  ectodermal dysplasias 69.18, 69.26–69.27
  hypermelanosis association 86.19, 86.20
  morphoea 55.7
  oral cancer 108.43–108.50
  palmoplantar keratodermas and 63.65–63.68
  photodynamic therapy 22.2
  radiotherapy principles 24.1–24.24
  systemic sclerosis 54.9–54.10
  urticaria association 42.3
cancer phobia 84.26
cancer-related lymphoedema 103.37–103.38
cancer risk, atopic eczema association 41.21–41.22
cancer treatment
  cutaneous side effects 119.1–119.15
  hair loss 87.71–87.74
Candida
  allergy 32.67
  antigen test 4.24
  classification 32.55
  colonisation sites in body 32.56–32.57
  cutaneous carriage 32.56
  identification 32.58–32.60
  intertrigo 32.63
  onychomycosis 32.66
  paronychia 32.65–32.66
  see also candidiasis
Candida albicans
  biology 32.55, 32.56
  identification 32.58–32.59
  versus other *Candida* species 32.55, 32.56
Candida infection
  hyper-IgE syndrome due to STAT3 loss of function mutations 80.17
  infants 115.8
  male genitalia 109.5, 109.11, 109.27
  peristomal skin 112.8, 112.9
  pustular psoriasis 118.4
candidal balanitis 32.64
candidal stomatitis *see* acute pseudomembranous candidiasis
candidal vulvo-vaginitis 110.27–110.28
candidiasis/candidosis 32.55–32.69
  biology 32.56–32.57
  chronic mucocutaneous candidiasis 80.17
  chronic oro-perineal candidiasis 80.7
  congenital candidiasis 114.28
  endocrine factors 32.58
  histology 32.60
  HIV/AIDS 31.6, 31.26, 31.34, 31.37, 32.58
  host factors 32.57–32.58
  identification 32.58–32.59
  immunological factors 32.58
  infants 32.65
  management 32.60–32.61
  nails and paronychium 32.65–32.66
  neonatal 114.28
  oral lesions 108.20–108.22, 108.31–108.32, 108.34, 108.57, 108.71
  oral mucous membranes 32.61–32.63
  organisms 32.55, 32.57
  pathophysiology 32.57–32.58
  penile 109.27
  perineal and perianal skin 111.15

  in pregnancy 113.7
  skin and genital mucous membranes 32.63–32.65
  systemic 32.92–32.93
  types of 108.57
CANDLE *see* chronic atypical neutrophilic dermatosis with lipodystrophy and elevated temperature
canities (hair greying) 87.91–87.93
cannabis
  dermatoses induced by 120.4–120.6
  drug interactions 120.3
  prevalence of use 120.2
  psychodermatology 120.2
cannabis arteritis 120.4
canthal lines, reduction of by botulinum toxin application 159.5
cantharidin (Spanish fly), vesicating beetles 34.30
Cantu syndrome 87.85
canula injection, dermal fillers 158.1–158.2, **158.3**, 158.4
capecitabine, palmoplantar erythrodysaesthesia 119.2
capillaries 2.40, 2.41
capillaritis 86.47, 86.48, 86.49
capillary disorders 71.3–71.11
  angioma serpiginosum 71.4–71.5
  capillary marmorata telangiectatica congenita 71.6
  CLOVES syndrome 71.9, 71.10
  disseminated capillary malformation with overgrowth 71.7–71.8
  Klippel–Trenaunay–Weber syndrome 71.8–71.9
  macrocephaly–capillary malformation syndrome 71.8
  microcephaly–capillary malformation syndrome 71.7
  PI3K-related overgrowth syndromes 71.7–71.11
  Proteus syndrome 71.10-11child
  Sturge–Weber syndrome 71.3–71.4
capillary filtration, chronic oedema **103.4**
capillary haemangiomas
  laser therapies, infants 23.8
  strawberry naevus on eyelid 107.46–107.47
  see also infantile haemangiomas; pyogenic granuloma
capillary loops 2.41
capillary malformation with dilated veins (CMDV) 71.4
capillary malformation with overgrowth (CMO) 71.7
capillary malformations (CMs) 71.3
capillary malformation–arteriovenous malformation (CM–AVM) 71.5–71.6
capillary marmorata telangiectatica congenita (CMTC) 71.6
capilleroscopy, acrocyanosis investigation 124.7
Capnocytophaga canimorsus 130.6
CAPS *see* cryopyrin-associated periodic syndrome
capsaicin 18.39
caput medusae 112.9
carbamazepine, hypersensitivity reactions **14.6**, 14.7
carba mix (sensitisers) 127.63, 127.64
carbapenems 19.46
carbohydrate disorders **79.2**
carbon dioxide lasers
  photothermal ablation 23.20–23.21
  skin resurfacing 161.1–161.3, **161.5**
carbon monoxide (CO) inhalation 125.4
carbuncles 26.25–26.26
carcinogenesis
  heat/IR radiation 124.14
  PUVA phototherapy risks 21.14
  skin cancer surveillance after phototherapy 21.16–21.17
  UVA-1 phototherapy risks 21.15
  UVB phototherapy risks 21.13

carcinogenicity, azathioprine 19.9
carcinogens
  arsenic 141.13
  occupational skin cancer 129.14
  palmoplantar keratodermas 63.73
carcinoid syndrome (CS) 86.19–86.20
  flushing 104.1, **104.6**, 148.25–148.26
carcinoid tumours
  dermatoendocrinology **150.10**, *150.12*, 150.19
  flushing **104.6**
carcinoma
  apocrine carcinoma 137.23
  basal cell 4.22, 110.39
  causative viral agents, MCPyV human polyomavirus 146.2, 146.3
  extramammary Paget disease, female genitalia 110.37–110.39
  heat-associated 124.15
  keratinocytes *see* basal cell carcinoma; squamous cell carcinoma
  Merkel cell carcinoma 2.12, 146.1–146.10
  metastatic to the skin from other primaries, radiotherapy 24.15
  penile 109.35–109.39
  pilomatrical carcinoma 137.14–137.15
  sebaceous 88.33
  sweat glands 137.33–137.40
  trichilemmal 137.7
  verrucous carcinoma, female genitalia 110.37
carcinoma cells, carcinoma erysipeloides 148.3, *148.4*
carcinoma en cuirasse 148.2, *148.3*
carcinoma erysipeloides 148.2, *148.4*
  genito-crural region 111.24
cardiac complications, drug reaction with eosinophilia and systemic symptoms 118.9
cardiac disorders 151.1–151.6
cardiac dysfunction, systemic sclerosis **54.23**
cardiac embolus, purpura 99.15
cardiac function, striate keratoderma 63.63
cardiac pacemakers, cutaneous reactions 151.5–151.6
cardiac rhabdomyomas, tuberous sclerosis complex 78.9
cardiac-valvular Ehlers–Danlos syndrome (cvEDS) **70.3**, 70.9
cardio-facio-cutaneous syndrome **78.9**
cardiomyopathy
  autosomal dominant intermediate epidermolysis bullosa simplex with 69.10
  palmoplantar keratodermas and 63.62–63.63
cardiopulmonary disorders, systemic sclerosis 54.17–54.18
cardiorespiratory pulmonary fibrosis, systemic sclerosis **54.23**
cardiotoxicity, antimalarials 19.6
cardiovascular disease
  atopic eczema association 41.21
  hidradenitis suppurativa association 90.2, 90.8
  psoriasis 35.19
  systemic lupus erythematosus 51.30
  systemic sclerosis 54.17–54.18
  UV radiation exposure 10.9
cardiovascular syphilis 29.14, *29.16*
Carney complex **72.7**, **78.13**, 108.16, **131.3**, *131.4*, 148.11, 151.3–151.4
carnosine 157.7
carotenaemia 61.9
carotene 86.50
carotenoderma 61.9, 86.50
carotenoids 86.2
CARP *see* confluent and reticulated papillomatosis
Carpenter syndrome **72.6**
carriage
  Staphylococcus aureus 26.7–26.8
  Streptococcus pyogenes 26.11–26.12

carrier peptides, cosmeceutical use of 157.6
cartilage, inflammatory chondopathies 155.11–155.13
cartilage excision, auricle melanoma 106.32
cartilage hair hypoplasia **78.14**, **80.4**, 80.11–80.12
Carvajal-Huerta syndrome 63.28, 63.63
Casal's necklace, pellagra 61.17
case–control studies about adverse events 17.17, 17.18
caseous necrosis 97.27
CASPAR *see* Classification of Psoriatic Arthritis
CASS *see* comprehensive acne severity system
catabolic states, adiponectin system 97.5
catagen phase of hair root 87.7, 87.8, *87.9*, 87.57
cataract, atopic *41.21*, *107.19*
cat bites 130.6
catecholamines 97.4
caterpillar dermatitis 34.32–34.34
cathepsin B (*CTSB*), skin fragility disorders 69.6
cathepsin C 63.68
catheter-related bloodstream infections (CRBSI) 125.10
catheter-related infection (CRI) 125.10
cathinone derivatives 120.3
cationic detergents 87.98
cat scratch disease, *Bartonella henselae* 26.62–26.64
CATSHL *see* camptodactyly, tall stature and hearing loss
causative agents of disease 5.8–5.10
caustic agents, skin surgery 20.47, 20.50
CBAs *see* computer-based assessments
CBCL *see* cutaneous B-cell lymphoma
CBLL *see* chilblain-like lesions
CBT *see* cognitive behavioural therapy
CCA *see* clear cell acanthoma
CCAAT enhancer binding protein ε-associated autoinflammation and immune impairment of neutrophils (CAIN) 45.16–45.17
CCCA *see* central centrifugal cicatricial alopecia
CCLA *see* central conducting lymphatic anomaly
CCMs *see* cerebral cavernous malformation-associated cutaneous lesions
CCPDMA *see* complete circumferential peripheral and deep margin assessment
CCPWA *see* Comprehensive Care Programme with Persons with Albinism
CCTR *see* Cochrane Controlled Trials Registry
CD4+/CD56+haematodermic neoplasm (blastic plasmacytoid dendritic cell neoplasm) 139.45–139.47
CD8+ mycosis fungoides variant, epidermotropic/cytotoxic CD8+ T-cell lymphoma distinction 139.5
CD10 (endothelial cell marker) 3.26
CD30+ anaplastic large-cell lymphomas
  anaplastic lymphoma kinase expression 139.1
  primary cutaneous 139.28–139.29
CD30+ lymphoproliferative disorders
  Hodgkin disease relationship 139.26, 139.44
  primary cutaneous 139.25–139.29
  see also primary cutaneous CD30+ lymphoproliferative disorders
CD30-positive lymphoproliferative disorders 3.28
CD31 (glycoprotein) 3.26
CD34 (glycosylated transmembrane protein) 3.25, *3.26*
CD34-positive fibrous tumours 136.7, 136.8, 136.9, 136.14, 136.15, 136.16, 136.17, 136.18

CD34-positive superficial fibroblastic tumour   136.16–136.17
CD40 deficiencies   80.9
CD56 (neural cell adhesion molecule)   3.28
CD151 antigen/tetraspanin (*CD151*)   69.4
CDAGS syndrome   85.22
CDC *see* Centers for Disease Control and Prevention
CDK4 *see* cyclin-dependent kinase 4 gene
CDKN2A *see* cyclin-dependent kinase inhibitor 2A gene
CDLE *see* chronic discoid lupus erythematosus
CDLQI *see* Children's Dermatology Life Quality Index
CDSN protein, peeling skin syndromes   63.28–63.29
CEA *see* cultured epithelial autografts
CEDNIK syndrome *see* cerebral dysgenesis–neuropathy–ichthyosis–palmoplantar keratoderma syndrome
cEDS *see* classical Ehlers–Danlos syndrome
CeHV-1 (cercopithecine herpesvirus 1) *see* herpes B virus infection
cell damage, pressure ulcers   123.2
Cellfina, cellulite laser treatment   161.9
'cellist's chest'   122.12
cell markers, immunocytochemistry panels of   3.10
cell-mediated immunity (CMI), leprosy   28.2, 28.3, 28.4–28.5
cell therapy, epidermolysis bullosa   69.27–69.28
cellular adhesion molecules (CAMs)   127.7
cellular angiofibroma   136.9
cellular digital fibromyxoma *see* acral fibromyxoma
cellular fibrous histiocytoma   136.20, 136.21
cellular identification, electron microscopy studies   3.30
cellular neurothekeoma   136.48
Cellulaze, cellulite laser treatment   161.9
cellulite   98.25–98.27, **98.26**
  treatments   161.9, 161.10
cellulitis   103.13–103.17
  ano-genital cellulitis   111.14
  definition and relationship to erysipelas   26.18
  gangrenous   26.78
  lymphadenitis   103.15
  lymphangitis   103.14–103.15
  perianal cellulitis   109.26, 111.14
  perianal streptococcal   26.33–26.34
  recurrent cellulitis (erysipelas)   103.13–103.14
  X-linked agammaglobulinaemia   80.13
cellulitis/erysipelas   26.18–26.22
  clinical features   26.19, 26.20–26.21
  clinical investigations   26.19
  epidemiology   26.18
  investigations   26.19
  management   26.19, 26.21–26.22
  pathophysiology   26.18–26.19
  Staphylococcus aureus role   26.19
  Streptococcus role   26.18–26.19
cement-induced chromate sensitivity   127.40
CEN *see* congenital epidermal naevi
Centers for Disease Control and Prevention (CDC)   7.6
centipedes (Chilopoda)   34.57
CENTRAL *see* Cochrane Central Register of Controlled Trials
central centrifugal cicatricial alopecia (CCCA)   87.46–87.47, 87.68
central conducting lymphatic anomaly (CCLA)   103.32
central line associated infections, burn injuries   125.10
central nervous system (CNS)
  control of endocrine signalling axes   150.2
  drug reaction with eosinophilia and systemic symptoms   118.9

Erdheim–Chester disease   135.22
  incontinentia pigmenti   68.11
centrifugal lipodystrophy (CLD)   98.12–98.13
CEP *see* congenital erythropoietic porphyria
cephalic pustulosis, neonatal   88.69
Cephalopoda class, molluscs   130.4
cephalosporins   19.46
Ceratopogonidae (midges)   34.7–34.8, 34.9
cercarial dermatitis   33.29–33.30
cercarial organisms, jellyfish stings   130.2
cercopithecine herpesvirus 1 (CeHV-1) *see* herpes B virus infection
cerebral cavernous malformation-associated cutaneous lesions (CCMs)   71.2, 71.19
cerebral dysgenesis–neuropathy–ichthyosis–palmoplantar keratoderma (CEDNIK) syndrome   63.30
cerebro-oculo-facio skeletal syndrome (COFS)   76.8
cerebrospinal fluid examination, syphilis   29.20, 29.21
cerebrotendinous xanthomatosis   60.10
CERS3 deficiency   63.15
CERS3 gene, congenital ichthyosiform erythroderma   63.11
certolizumab pegol, psoriasis treatment   35.28–35.29
cerumen (wax), external ear   106.2–106.3
ceruminous glands, tumours of   106.34–106.35
cervical cancer   25.51, 25.64–25.65
  vulval lymphangiectasia   103.31
cervical intraepithelial neoplasia (CIN)   25.52, 25.65
cervical lymph nodes, drainage areas of   108.6
cervical trophic syndrome (CTS)   82.8–82.9
cestodes, infections   33.31–33.35
cetearyl alcohol   127.59
cetrimide   18.10
cetuximab, papulopustular eruptions   119.3
CEVD *see* congenital erosive and vesicular dermatosis
CGH *see* comparative genomic hybridisation; congenital generalised hypertrichosis
CGL *see* congenital generalised lipodystrophies
CGPD *see* childhood granulomatous periorificial dermatoses
cGvHD *see* chronic graft versus host disease
CH *see* chlorhexidine
Chagas disease *see* American trypanosomiasis
chalazion (meibomian gland cyst)   107.11
  eyelid   107.45–107.46
chamomile   157.11
chancriform pyoderma   26.87–26.88
chancroid   30.18–30.21
  clinical features   30.19–30.20
  epidemiology   30.19
  investigations   30.20–30.21
  management   30.21
  pathophysiology   30.19
Chapare (Bolivian) haemorrhagic fever   25.82–25.83
chapping of the lips   108.60
Charcot arthropathy, diabetic patients   62.2
Charcot (neuropathic) joints, syphilis   29.15–29.16
CHARGE (coloboma, heart defects, atresia of the nasal choanae, retardation of growth/development, genital/urinary abnormalities and ear abnormalities and deafness) syndrome   80.4, 80.8, 106.4, **106.7**
CHB *see* congenital heart block
checkpoint inhibitors *see* immune checkpoint inhibitors
Chédiak–Higashi syndrome   68.8–68.9, **80.5**, 148.13
  partial albinism in   80.14

cheek
  biting   108.32
  dermal fillers   158.2, 158.4
  discoid lupus erythematosus   51.8
  erythropoietic protoporphyria   58.15
  impetigo   115.7
  pseudofolliculitis   93.2
  solar lentigo   131.6
  spontaneous atrophic scarring   94.14–94.15
  venous malformation   71.15
  volumisation of   158.4
  see also buccal mucosa
cheilitis   108.60–108.63, 127.15, 127.80, 128.4–128.5
  actinic cheilitis   108.58
  actinic prurigo   126.10, 126.11
  angular cheilitis   108.20, 108.59–108.60
  contact cheilitis   108.60–108.61
  drug-induced cheilitis   108.61
  eczematous cheilitis   108.61
  exfoliative cheilitis   108.61–108.62
  foreign body cheilitis   108.62
  glandular cheilitis   108.62–108.63
  granulomatous cheilitis   108.73
  infective cheilitis   108.63
  plasma cell cheilitis   108.63
  retinoid-induced   88.56
  Stevens–Johnson syndrome/toxic epidermal necrolysis   118.16
cheiroarthropathy, diabetic patients   62.5, 62.7
chemical burns   128.11–128.12
  oral lesions   108.31
chemical depigmentation   86.45
chemical exposure, scleroderma-like syndromes   94.45
chemical peels   160.1–160.15
  acne treatment   88.58–88.59, 160.5, *160.6*
  actinic keratoses   160.5
  alpha-hydroxyl acids   160.1–160.2
  azelaic acid   160.2
  caustic action peels   160.2–160.3
  chemistry of   160.1–160.4
  consent   160.8
  contraindications   160.6
  counselling   160.6–160.7
  deep peels   160.5
  depth of   160.4–160.5
  equipment for   160.8
  facial skin rejuvenation   160.5
  glycolic acid   160.2, *160.8*, 160.9–160.10
  histological level of controlled necrosis   **160.4**
  indications   160.5–160.6
  Jessner solution   160.3, *160.7*, *160.8*, 160.10, *160.11*
  lactic acid   160.2
  medium depth peels   160.4
  metabolic action peels   160.1–160.2
  peeling agents   160.9–160.11
  peeling technique   160.8–160.11
  phenol   160.3
  phenol-croton oil peel   160.10–160.11
  photodamaged skin   160.5
  photo documentation   160.8
  pigmentation   160.5–160.6
  post-peel care   160.11
  pre-peel procedure   160.6–160.8
  pyruvic acid   160.2
  retinoic acid   160.2
  salicylic acid   160.3–160.4, 160.10
  side effects and complications   160.11–160.14
    allergic contact dermatitis   160.13
    chemical burns   160.12, *160.13*
    infection   160.13
    milia and acneform eruption   160.12
    postinflammatory hyperpigmentation   160.12–160.13, *160.14*
    postinflammatory hypopigmentation   160.14
    premature peeling   160.12, *160.13*
    redness, persistent   160.11–160.12
    scarring   160.14

    systemic toxicity   160.13–160.14
  skin of colour   160.15
  skin pigmentation   160.5–160.6
  skin priming   160.7–160.8
  superficial peels   160.4
  toxic action peels   160.3–160.4
  trichloroacetic acid   160.2–160.3, 160.10, *160.11*
chemical photosensitivity   126.1, 126.27–126.32
chemical protection, glove materials   **128.8**
chemicals
  acne-inducing   129.7, 129.12–129.13
  allergic components   128.6
  irritant properties   128.2–128.3, 128.6, 129.5
  occupational leukoderma   129.13–129.14
  phototoxic properties   128.9
  sensitisation   127.6
chemokines, bullous pemphigoid   50.12
chemoprophylaxis, leprosy   28.16
chemotactic factors, eosinophilic pustular folliculitis   93.7
chemotherapy
  cutaneous side effects   119.1–119.15
  cutaneous T-cell lymphoma   139.24
  hair changes   119.5–119.6
  hyperpigmentation   119.8–119.9
  hypertrichosis   119.6
  hypopigmentation   119.10–119.11
  leprosy   28.13–28.14
  Mee's lines   *121.3*
  nail changes   119.6–119.8
  systemic sclerosis   54.25–54.26
  toxic erythema   119.1–119.2
chemotherapy-induced alopecia (CIA)   87.71–87.74, 119.5–119.6
chemotherapy-related eccrine syringosquamous metaplasia   92.15
ChemSex, drugs with sex   120.2–120.3
cherry angiomas   101.12–101.13, **101.17**
chest
  acne fulminans   88.61, 88.62
  acne vulgaris   88.12, 88.13
  Brunsting–Perry pemphigoid   50.53
  IgM pemphigoid   50.54
  linear morphoea   55.23
  lithium-induced acne   88.13
  macular cutaneous amyloidosis   56.7
  morphoea   55.5, 55.20, 55.21, 55.23
  pansclerotic morphoea   55.21
  plaque morphoea   55.20
  segmental psoriasis   35.15
  subacute cutaneous lupus erythematosus   51.15
  systemic sclerosis   54.4
chest wall, Mondor disease on   101.37
cheveux incoiffables *see* uncombable hair syndrome
Cheyletiella mites   34.53, *34.54*
CHHS *see* Conradi–Hünermann–Happle syndrome
chickenpox *see* varicella infection
chicken-wire reticulate erythema/urticaria   43.4
Chikungunya fever
  mosquito-borne togavirus infection   25.89
  oral involvement   108.50
chilblain-like lesions (pseudo-perniosis)
  COVID-19 association   25.108–25.109, 25.113–25.114
  COVID-19 vaccines   25.118
  internal malignancy association   148.25
chilblain lupus   51.6–51.7, *51.9*, 51.25
chilblains (perniosis)   97.37, 124.6
CHILD *see* congenital hemidysplasia–ichthyosiform naevus–limb defect syndrome
child abuse
  ano-genital signs of sexual abuse   109.9
  non-accidental injury   115.14
childhood, psychological and social factors   15.3, 15.4
Childhood Atopic Dermatitis Impact Scale (CADIS)   16.8

childhood granulomatous periorificial dermatoses (CGPD)   89.18–89.19
childhood HIV-associated lipodystrophy   98.6
childhood linear IgA disease   50.36, 80.14, 80.15, 108.81
childhood lipoatrophic panniculitis   97.56–97.57
childhood NEH   92.14, 92.15
childhood rosacea   89.3
   idiopathic facial aseptic granuloma   89.16
   management   89.14–89.15
   ocular   89.6
children
   acne, prepubertal   88.68–88.74
   acrodermatitis enteropathica   61.26
   actinic lichen planus   37.7
   acute scrotum   109.23, 109.25–109.26
   agminated or segmental lentiginosis   131.3
   antihistamine treatment   42.18
   argininosuccinic aciduria   79.13
   arteriovenous malformation   71.11
   atopic eczema   41.13, 41.14, 41.15, 41.16, 41.17, 41.18, 41.26
      psychodermatology   84.3
   autoinflammatory granulomatosis of childhood   45.5, 45.7, 45.11–45.12
   blistering distal dactylitis   26.34
   Bloom syndrome   77.3
   bullous pemphigoid   50.20
   calcifying aponeurotic fibroma   136.7–136.8
   calcifying fibrous tumour/pseudotumour   136.7
   capillary malformations   71.3, 71.5
   cellular fibrous histiocytoma   136.21
   choanal atresia and lymphoedema   71.27
   chronic bullous dermatosis   50.36, 80.14, 80.15, 108.81
   congenital blue naevi   73.16
   congenital melanocytic naevi   73.12
   cranial (nodular) fasciitis   136.5
   cutis laxa   70.17
   DOCK8 deficiency   80.10
   dog and cat bites   130.6
   epidermolysis bullosa acquista   50.45, 50.46
   erythema infectiosum/fifth disease   25.77–25.78, 115.6, 155.2, 155.3
   erythropoietic protoporphyria   58.14
   factitious nail disease   84.33
   flushing   104.10
   fucosidosis   79.4
   giant cell fibroblastoma   136.15–136.16
   granuloma annulare   95.5, 95.7
   Griscelli syndrome   80.14
   hair follicle naevus   137.7–137.8
   Hartnup disease   61.16
   impact of skin disease assessment   16.8, 16.9–16.10
   inherited immunodeficiency   80.2
   juvenile dermatomyositis   52.8–52.9
   juvenile plantar dermatosis   39.23–39.24
   juvenile springtime eruption, external ear   106.25
   Langerhans cell histiocytosis   115.15–115.16, 135.4, 135.5–135.7, 135.9
   late-onset primary lymphoedema   103.24–103.25
   lichen nitidus   37.10
   lichen striatus   37.18
   lip-lick cheilitis   41.22
   lipofibromatosis   136.13–136.14
   lymphangioma   108.13
   Maffucci syndrome   71.20
   malnutrition   61.2, 61.3, 61.4
      severity classification   61.5–61.6
   mastocytosis   46.9
   microbial ecology of the skin   26.4
   midface toddler excoriation syndrome due to pain insensitivity   83.12–83.13
   morphoea, diagnosis, assessment and treatment   55.39

mucopolysaccharidoses   79.3
Münchausen syndrome by proxy   84.37–84.38
neurocutaneous disorders, subgroups   83.2
neurofibromatosis type 1, Manchester checklist   78.5
normophosphataemic familial tumoral calcinosis   79.18
paediatric HIV/AIDS   31.36–31.37
paediatric inflammatory multisystem syndrome temporally associated with SARS-CoV-2 infection   25.114
paediatric IRIS/IRD/IRAD   31.8
pansclerotic morphoea   55.19–55.21
papular acrodermatitis/Gianotti-Crosti syndrome   25.74
perianal streptococcal cellulitis   26.33–26.34
perianal viral warts   111.18, 111.19
phosphomannomutase 2 deficiency   79.10
pilomatricoma   137.13
pityriasis rubra pilaris   36.4, 36.5
plexiform fibrohistiocytic tumour   136.22
primary herpetic gingivostomatitis   25.21
pro-opiomelanocortin deficiency   72.8
pruritus, idiopathic   111.6
psoriasis vulgaris   35.15
PTEN hamartoma tumour syndrome   71.13
purpura artefact   84.33
roseola infantum   25.39–25.40, 115.5–115.6
Rothmund–Thomson syndrome   75.5
scarlet fever   26.35–26.36
severe combined immunodeficiency   80.8
spindle cell haemangioma   136.31
staphylococcal scalded skin syndrome   26.27, 26.28, 26.28, 114.24–114.25, 115.7–115.8
streptococcal vulvovaginitis in prepubescent girls   26.33
sun exposure as melanoma risk   142.6
syphilis, congenital   114.27–114.28
systemic juvenile idiopathic arthritis   53.8, 53.9
systemic juvenile xanthogranuloma   135.17
systemic lupus erythematosus   51.32
systemic-onset juvenile idiopathic arthritis   45.21–45.22
telangiectasia   75.5
tinea capitis   32.31–32.32, 32.37–32.38, 115.8–115.9
topical therapy application quantities   18.3, 18.4
trichotillosis   84.22–84.23, 87.24, 87.32, 87.33
urticaria pigmentosa   46.4, 46.5
Williams–Beuren syndrome   70.18
Wiskott–Aldrich syndrome   80.9
wound healing   11.2
xeroderma pigmentosum   76.4
X-linked lymphoproliferative diseases   80.11
see also infants; juvenile...; neonates
Children's Dermatology Life Quality Index (CDLQI)
   atopic eczema   16.8
   questions   16.10
   usage   16.9–16.10
chillblains (perniosis)   97.36, 124.5–124.6
   type I cryoglobulinaemia   149.13, 149.14
Chilopoda (centipedes)   34.57
CHIME (coloboma–heart defect–ichthyosiform dermatosis–mental retardation–ear anomalies) syndrome   63.38–63.39
chin
   impetigo   115.7
   numb chin syndrome/mental neuropathy   148.23
   sinus related to dental abscess   108.9
China, ancient medical texts   1.2
Chi-square test, statistical analysis of clinical studies   17.22

Chlamydia
   C. pneumoniae   26.79
   C. psittaci   26.79
Chlamydia pneumoniae, skin features   26.79
Chlamydia trachomatis   26.79
   life cycle   30.10
   serovars L1-L3, lymphogranuloma venereum   30.14–30.18
   strains D-K, genital infection   30.8–30.14
   see also genital chlamydia
chloracne (MADISH)   88.14, 88.15, 88.66–88.68, 129.7, 129.12–129.13, 133.1, 133.7
   chemicals causing   88.66, 129.12
chlorhexidine (CH)   127.57–127.58
chlorine-releasing agents   18.10
chloroacetate esterase stain   3.9
chlorocresol   127.56
chlorophenols   129.12
chloroquine
   drug-induced pruritus   81.11
   eye, side effects on   107.43
   pruritus   117.3
   sarcoidosis management   96.16
chloroquine pigmentation   86.26
chloroxylenol   18.10, 127.55–127.56
chlorpromazine
   hypermelanosis   86.26–86.27
   photosensitivity   126.30
choanal atresia and lymphoedema   71.27
cholera, epidemiology   5.9–5.10
cholestasis   60.11–60.12, 153.5
cholestatic pruritus   81.9–81.10
cholesteatoma   106.21
cholesterol embolus, purpura   99.14–99.15
cholesterol sulphate
   acquired ichthyosis   63.47
   recessive X-linked ichthyosis   63.5
cholinergic urticaria   42.9, 42.11–42.12
chondrodermatitis nodularis (CN)   106.9–106.11
   clinical features   106.10
   epidemiology   106.9
   management   106.10–106.11
chondroid cells, juvenile hyaline fibromatosis   94.42
chondroid syringoma *see* mixed tumour of the skin
chondroitin sulphate (CS)   2.38, **2.39**
chorionic villi, DNA-based prenatal diagnosis   8.10
chromate allergy   127.23
chromatograms, patch testing   127.33
chromhidrosis   92.18
chromium allergy   127.36, 127.39–127.41
chromium VI (CrVI) exposure   127.2
chromoblastomycosis   32.75–32.77
chromomycosis *see* chromoblastomycosis
chromophores
   light absorption by skin   23.3–23.4
   selective photothermolysis   23.5–23.6
chromophytosis *see* pityriasis versicolor
chromosomal disorders   8.6, 74.1–74.5
   autosomal chromosome defects   74.1–74.3
   chromosomal mosaicism   74.5
   sex chromosome defects   74.3–74.5
chromosomal mosaicism   74.5
chromosome 4, short-arm deletion syndrome   74.3
chromosome 5, short-arm deletion syndrome   74.3
chromosome 18, long-arm deletion syndrome   74.3
chromosomes   8.3, 8.4
chronica atrophicans, cutaneous B-cell lymphoma   139.37–139.38
chronic acral dermatitis   39.14–39.15
chronic actinic dermatitis (CAD)   126.4, 126.13–126.21, 126.31, 126.32–126.35, 126.37, 127.81
chronic active Epstein–Barr virus infection   25.38
chronically sun-damaged skin   145.9, 145.11, **145.11**

chronically swollen limb   103.9–103.10
chronic arsenic poisoning   121.2
chronic atrophic candidiasis *see* chronic erythematous candidiasis
chronic atypical neutrophilic dermatosis with lipodystrophy and elevated temperature (CANDLE)   45.5, 45.6, 45.14–45.15, **72.11**, 72.12
chronic bulbous disease of childhood *see* childhood linear IgA disease
chronic bullous dermatosis (linear IgA disease of children)   108.81
chronic candidiasis   108.31–108.32
chronic cholestasis   60.11–60.12
chronic contact dermatitis   127.13
chronic cutaneous leishmaniasis   33.47–33.48
chronic diffuse telogen effluvium   87.54
chronic discoid lupus erythematosus (CDLE)   87.43–87.44
chronic disseminated histoplasmosis   32.83
chronic erythema nodosum   97.25
chronic erythematous candidiasis   32.62
chronic graft versus host disease (cGvHD)   38.1, 38.2, 38.3, 38.7–38.11
   clinical features   38.7–38.9
   epidemiology   38.2
   management   38.9–38.11
   pathology   38.3
   predisposing factors   38.2
   severity classification   38.9, 38.10
   skin cancer risks   147.4–147.5
chronic granulomatous disease   **80.5**
   eyelid, papular lesions around   80.15
   malar erythematous photosensitive macular skin lesions   80.16
chronic hyperplastic candidiasis *see* chronic plaque-like candidiasis
chronic infantile neurological cutaneous and articular syndrome (CINCA)   45.5, 45.6
chronic inflammation, and skin ageing   2.45
chronicity of disease   5.10
chronic kidney disease (CKD), pruritus association   81.8–81.9
chronic liver disease
   skin lesions   **153.4**
   vascular changes   153.8–153.9
chronic (long) COVID-19   25.113
chronic lymphocytic leukaemia (CLL)
   immunocompromised patients   147.1, 147.3
   insect bite-like reactions   149.8–149.9
   skin infiltration as first sign   149.2
   see also non-Hodgkin lymphoma
chronic metabolic disease, acquired ichthyosis association   85.1
chronic mucocutaneous candidiasis (CMC)   32.67–32.69, 80.17
   clinical features   32.68, 32.69
   management   32.69
   oral lesions   108.32
   pathophysiology   32.67–32.68
chronic nodular candidiasis   32.62
chronic non-scarring folliculitis   91.13–91.14
chronic oedema   103.2, 103.3–103.5
   causes   **103.4**
   clinical features   103.4
   epidemiology   103.3
   investigations   103.4–103.5
   lymphoedema comparison   103.3
   management   103.5
   pathophysiology   103.3–103.4
   penis   109.19–109.21
chronic oro-perineal candidiasis   80.7
chronic otitis externa   106.16, 106.17, 106.18–106.19
chronic pain syndromes, male genitalia   109.43–109.44
chronic panniculitis   97.30–97.32
chronic papillomatous dermatitis (CPD)   112.8
chronic physiological reactions   124.14
chronic plaque-like candidiasis   32.62
chronic plaque psoriasis *see* psoriasis vulgaris

chronic pruritus (CP) 81.1–81.14
    atopic eczema 81.7–81.8
    clinical variants 81.7–81.12
    drug-induced pruritus 81.10–81.11
    epidemiology 81.1–81.2
    history taking 81.6
    inflamed skin/dermatoses 81.7
    investigations 81.13
    management 81.13–81.14
    presentation 81.6–81.7
    psoriasis vulgaris 81.8
    severity rating 81.12–81.13
    uncontrollable scratching 81.15
chronic pseudomembranous candidiasis 32.61
chronic pulmonary histoplasmosis 32.83
chronic radiation dermatitis 119.14
chronic radiodermatitis 24.18–24.20
chronic/recurrent self-healing eruptions, lymphomatoid papulosis 139.26–139.28
chronic red leg 103.16–103.17
chronic sarcoidosis 96.6
chronic scalp pain and dysaesthesia 82.12
chronic selenium toxicity 121.7
chronic spontaneous urticaria (CSU) 16.5
chronic superficial dermatitis, discoid skin lesions **39.10**
chronic superficial scaly dermatitis *see* small plaque parapsoriasis
chronic telogen effluvium 87.59–87.60
chronic ulcerative stomatitis 108.79
chronic ulcers, radiotherapy-associated 119.15
chronic urticaria 84.3
Chronic Urticaria Quality of Life Questionnaire (CU-Q$_2$oL) 16.9
chronic venous disease (CVD), venous leg ulcers 102.1–102.4
chronic venous insufficiency 101.40–101.46
    categories 101.40–101.41
    causes **101.41**
    clinical features **101.43**
    investigations **101.45**
    management 101.45–101.46
    pathogenesis **101.42**
    risk factors **101.41**
    treatment **101.45**
chronic wounds, elderly people 6.1
chrysiasis 86.52, 121.4
chrysoderma 86.52
Chrysops (tabanid flies) 33.12
    see also loiasis
Churg–Strauss syndrome *see* eosinophilic granulomatosis with polyangiitis
chylous disease 103.32
chymase 2.17
CIA *see* chemotherapy-induced alopecia
cicatricial alopecia 87.37, 87.38–87.53, 88.37
    central centrifugal 87.46–87.47, 87.68
    incontinentia pigmenti 68.11
    marginal 87.32
    non-specific 87.51
    secondary 87.52–87.53, 105.6–105.9
cicatricial pemphigoid 50.51–50.52, 50.53, 105.6
    diagnosis *50.24*
    penile 109.25
cicatrising conjunctivitis 107.24–107.34
    management 107.29–107.32
ciclopirox olamine 18.12
ciclosporin 19.10–19.12
    dermatological uses 19.10
    dose and regimens 19.12
    drug–drug interactions 19.11–19.12
    monitoring 19.12
    morphoea treatment 55.38
    pharmacological properties 19.10–19.11
    potential adverse effects 19.11
    pre-treatment screening 19.12
    psoriasis treatment 35.25
    Stevens–Johnson syndrome/toxic epidermal necrolysis 118.11–118.12, 118.21

topical therapies 18.23
    urticaria treatment 42.18
CIC-rearranged sarcoma (CIC-DUX4 sarcoma) 136.52
CIE *see* congenital ichthyosiform erythroderma; International Commission on Illumination
'cigarette face' 94.2
cigarette-induced keratoses 108.33
cigarette paper-like wrinkling 94.26
cigarette smoking *see* smoking
Cimicidae (including bed bugs) 34.25–34.29
CIN *see* cervical intraepithelial neoplasia
CINCA *see* chronic infantile neurological cutaneous and articular syndrome
circumcision, male 109.7
circumferential hyperkeratosis 63.64
circumscribed alopecias 87.30
circumscribed hyperhidrosis 92.6–92.7, 92.9
circumscribed juvenile pityriasis rubra pilaris (type IV) 36.4, *36.5*
circumscribed palmoplantar hypokeratosis 63.78
circumscribed plaque morphoea 55.17
    differential diagnosis **55.27**
cirrhosis 153.5, 153.8, 153.9
    hypermelanosis 86.22
cirsoid aneurysm 136.27
Civatte bodies *118.13*
CKD *see* chronic kidney disease
CK syndrome 63.23
CLA *see* cutaneous lymphocyte antigen
Cladophialophora carrionii 32.77
clam digger's itch *see* cercarial dermatitis
CLAPO syndrome **101.28**
'clarinettist's cheilitis' 122.12
Clarkson syndrome 43.4
CLAs *see* complicated lymphatic anomalies
clascoterone, acne vulgaris treatment 88.49–88.50
Class A drugs 120.3
Class B drugs 120.3
Class C drugs 120.3
classic adult-onset pityriasis rubra pilaris (type I) 36.2, 36.4, *36.6*
classical adult eosinophilic pustular folliculitis 91.4
classical Ehlers–Danlos syndrome (cEDS) 70.2, **70.3**, *70.8*
classical eosinophilic pustular folliculitis 93.7, 93.8
classical epidermodysplasia verruciformis 25.66, 25.69
classical-like Ehlers–Danlos syndrome (clEDS) **70.3**, 70.9–70.10
classical-like type 2 Ehlers–Danlos syndrome (clEDS2) **70.3**
classic epidermolysis bullosa
    clinical subtypes 69.8–69.11
    genes/proteins implicated in 69.2–69.8
    molecular pathology 69.11–69.15
classic juvenile-onset pityriasis rubra pilaris (type III) 36.4, *36.5*
classic Sweet syndrome (CSS) 49.8, *49.11*
Classification of Psoriatic Arthritis (CASPAR) criteria **35.41**
classification of skin diseases 1.4, *1.6*
claudication, peripheral vascular disease **101.5**
claudin-1 junction, neonatal ichthyosis–sclerosing cholangitis 63.41
claudins 2.20
    gene mutations 2.21
CLCI *see* cumulative life course impairment
CLD *see* centrifugal lipodystrophy
cleansing of skin, neonates 114.2
clearance, clinical pharmacology **13.2**
clear cell acanthoma (CCA) 132.6–132.7
clear-cell hidradenoma *see* hidradenoma
clear cell sarcoma 136.64
cleavage resistant RIPK1-induced autoinflammatory syndrome 45.17
clEDS2 *see* classical-like type 2 Ehlers–Danlos syndrome

clEDS *see* classical-like Ehlers–Danlos syndrome
cleft lip/palate 108.83–108.85
    clinical features 108.84
    management 108.84–108.85
    pathophysiology 108.83–108.84
    predisposing factors 108.83–108.84
    syndromes associated with **108.84**
clenched fist injuries 130.6–130.7
Clericuzio-type poikiloderma with neutropenia 149.14
climate, and atopic eczema 41.6
climate change, and skin health 7.3–7.4
climatic bubo *see* lymphogranuloma venereum
clindamycin 18.10
clinical decision-making 16.6
clinical end point studies, topical bioavailability/bioequivalence assessment 12.7
clinically amyopathic dermatomyositis (CADM) 52.1, 52.7, 52.9, 52.11
clinical margins, melanoma excision 143.2–143.3
clinical officer training, Cambodia 7.7–7.8
clinical pharmacology 13.1–13.13
    absorption, distribution, metabolism and elimination of a drug 13.1–13.4
    adherence to treatment 13.9
    bioavailability 13.2–13.3, **13.2**
    clearance **13.2**
    drug actions, mechanisms underlying **13.4**, 13.5–13.6
    drug choice and medical decision making 13.7
    drug development and licensing 13.11–13.13
    drug interactions 13.9
    drug toxicity and adverse effects 13.6, 13.9–13.11
    drug types 13.1
    ethics and drug trial reporting 13.13
    medication errors 13.9–13.11
    molecular mechanisms underlying drug actions 13.5–13.6
    novel methods of drug delivery 13.3
    oral drug administration 13.2, 13.3
    'orphan' status of drugs 13.13
    parenteral drug administration 13.2–13.3
    personalised medicine 8.1, 13.11
    pharmacists' role 13.11
    pharmacodynamics **13.2**, 13.4–13.6
        factors affecting 13.7–13.9
    pharmacogenomics 13.11
    pharmacokinetics 13.1–13.4
    polypharmacy 13.8
    prescription-writing, medication errors 13.10, 13.11
    regulatory approval of drug applications 13.13
    'Swiss cheese model', drug-related patient harm *13.10*
    terminology 13.1, **13.2**
    therapeutic outcome, factors affecting 13.7–13.11
    therapeutic window **13.2**
clinical questions, well-built questions in evidence based medicine 17.3–17.4
clinical research, evidence based medicine 17.1–17.2
clinical research papers
    adequate reporting 17.18–17.20
    data evaluation 17.18–17.25
    shortcut method for reading 17.24–17.25
    statistical methods 17.20–17.24
clinical trials
    critical appraisal for evidence based medicine 17.12–17.15
    see also randomised controlled clinical trials
clioquinol, patch testing 127.47
clitoris, structure and function of 110.2, 110.3
CLL *see* chronic lymphocytic leukaemia

CLND *see* completion lymph node dissection
clofazimine 86.26
clostridia 26.48–26.49
clostridial myonecrosis (gas gangrene) 26.48–26.49
Clostridium botulinum 120.7
Clostridium histolyticum, myonecrosis 26.48–26.49
Clostridium novyi, myonecrosis 26.48–26.49
Clostridium perfringens, myonecrosis 26.48–26.49
Clostridium septicum, myonecrosis 26.48–26.49
Clostridium sodellii, myonecrosis 26.48–26.49
clothing
    allergens *127.64*, 127.65–127.67
    callosities 122.8
    dermatitis 127.16–127.17
    photoprotection 10.12
Clouston syndrome 63.68, 67.12, **78.13**
    oral lesions 108.28
    pachyonychia congenita 67.12
CLOVES (congenital lipomatous overgrowth, vascular malformations, epidermal naevi and skeletal/spinal anomalies) syndrome 71.2, 71.9, 71.10, 72.9, 72.11, 73.6–73.7, **101.28**, 103.23
clubbing of nails, internal malignancy links 148.18
clutton joints, congenital syphilis 29.25
CM *see* cutaneous mastocytosis
CMC *see* chronic mucocutaneous candidiasis
CMDV *see* capillary malformation with dilated veins
CMI *see* cell-mediated immunity
CMN *see* congenital melanocytic naevi
CMO *see* capillary malformation with overgrowth
CMs *see* capillary malformations
CMTC *see* capillary marmorata telangiectatica congenita
CMV *see* cytomegalovirus
CM–AVM *see* capillary malformation–arteriovenous malformation
CN *see* chondrodermatitis nodularis; cyanide
cnidarian stings 130.1–130.5
CNS *see* central nervous system; Comèl–Netherton syndrome
coagulase negative *Staphylococcus* 26.3, 26.9–26.10
coagulase positive *Staphylococcus* 26.3, 26.8, 93.2
coagulation defects, liver disease association 153.9
coagulopathies, HIV 31.12
coal tar 18.36–18.37, 35.21–35.22
cobalamin (vitamin B12) deficiency 61.19–61.21
cobalt allergy 127.38–127.39
cobalt spot test 127.33–127.34
cocaine
    death rates 120.1
    dermatoses induced by 120.2, 120.5
    pharmaceutical drug interactions 120.3
    prevalence of use 120.2
    soft-tissue infections 120.7
cocamide diethanolamide 127.59
coccidioidal granuloma *see* coccidioidomycosis
Coccidioides
    C. immitis 32.86, 32.87
    C. posadasii 32.86, 32.87
coccidioidin test 4.25
coccidioidomycosis 32.86–32.88
Cochrane, Archie 17.1, 17.6
Cochrane Central Register of Controlled Trials (CENTRAL) 17.6, 17.7
Cochrane Collaboration 17.2, 17.6–17.7
    risk of bias tool 17.9
Cochrane Controlled Trials Registry (CCTR) 17.9

Cochrane Library 17.6–17.7
Cochrane Skin Core Outcomes Initiative (CS-COUSIN) 17.14
cockade naevus 131.30, *131.31*
Cockayne syndrome (CS) 75.6, 76.5, 76.6–76.8, **77.2**
   bird-like facial appearance 76.7
   clinical features 76.7–76.8
   clinical variants 76.8
   genes and protein products **76.7**
   investigations 76.8
   management 76.8
   pathophysiology 76.7
cockroaches (Dictyoptera) 34.32
COCs *see* combined oral contraceptives
coding systems, diagnostic 4.2
coefficient of friction 122.6
coeliac disease
   oral involvement 108.72
   psoriasis association 35.18
   skin manifestations 153.3
coenzyme Q10 (CoQ10), cosmeceutical use of 157.2
Coffin–Lowry syndrome **72.7**
COFS *see* cerebro-oculo-facio skeletal syndrome
cognitive behavioural therapy (CBT) 84.47
cognitive models, beliefs/emotions/behaviours 15.1–15.3
Cohen syndrome **72.6**
cohort studies, adverse events 17.17–17.18
CO inhalation *see* carbon monoxide inhalation
COL1A1-USP6 gene rearrangement 136.6
colchicine 19.12–19.13
   dermatological uses 19.12
   pharmacological properties 19.12–19.13
   potential adverse effects 19.13
   safety precautions 19.13
cold
   cutaneous reactions to 124.1–124.16
   diseases caused/aggravated by 124.1–124.14
cold abscesses 33.24, 33.33, *33.35*
cold agglutinins 124.13–124.14
   cryogelling/cryoagglutination disorders 99.11–99.14
cold contact urticaria 42.9, 42.10–42.11
cold-induced sweating syndrome 92.7
cold-induced vasoconstriction 124.1
cold-induced vasodilation 83.5
cold injury, neonatal 114.15, **114.18**
cold panniculitis 97.35–97.37, 114.14
cold sores *see* herpes labialis
Cole disease 63.61
Coleoptera (beetles) 34.30–34.32
collagen 2.2, 2.27–2.29
   basement membrane collagen 2.22–2.23
   biosynthesis 2.29–2.31, *2.30*
   cross-linking 2.31
   degradation 2.31–2.32, 10.10–10.11
   elastin interdependence 122.5
   epidermolysis bullosa 69.5, 69.16, 69.18–69.19, 69.21, *69.22*, 69.27
   fibril fragmentation in ageing 156.8–156.9
   gene expression 2.29–2.31
   genetic disorders 70.1–70.14
      Ehlers–Danlos syndromes 70.1 70.11
      osteogenesis imperfecta 70.12–70.14
      prolidase deficiency 70.11–70.12
   genetic heterogeneity **2.27**
   hydroxylation reactions 2.29, *2.30*
   light absorption/scattering by skin 23.4
   periodicity in collagen fibres *2.23*
   scarring 11.8
   type I 2.22, 2.23, 2.28, 2.32
   type III 2.28, 2.32
   type IV 2.22–2.23, 2.28
   type V 2.28
   type VI 2.28
   type VII 2.26–2.27, 2.28, 2.32
   type XVII 2.28–2.29
   wound healing 11.7, 11.8

collagen bundles
   deep morphoea 97.13
   granuloma annulare 97.14
collagen dermal filler 158.5–158.6, 158.7–158.8
collagenoma 94.43
   Cowden syndrome *78.11*
collagenosis nuchae *see* nuchal-type fibroma
collagenous colitis 153.3
collagenous fibroma *see* desmoplastic fibroblastoma
collagenous marginal plaques of the hands 94.4–94.5
collagen peptide supplements 122.6
collagen-stimulating dermal fillers 158.6–158.7
collarette scale *4.13*
collective teloptosis 87.53
Colliers' stripes 86.53
collodion baby 63.8, 63.12–63.13, 63.43–63.44, 114.19–114.21
collodions, vehicle choice for topical therapies 18.2
colloid body 3.40
colloid degeneration 94.5–94.6
   penile 109.31
colloid milium 94.5–94.6
coloboma–heart defect–ichthyosiform dermatosis–mental retardation–ear anomalies (CHIME) syndrome 63.38–63.39
colon, gastrointestinal polyposis 78.11
colophony 127.17–127.18, 127.45, 127.74–127.78
colostomy **112.3**
   Crohn ulceration *112.13*, *112.14*
   inflammatory polyps *112.6*
   irritant skin reaction *112.2*
   leakage and faecal dermatitis *112.4*, *112.5*
   localised bullous pemphigoid *112.12*
colour dyes, specimen preparation 3.5–3.6
colour of skin *see* skin of colour
CoLQ *see* Course of Life Questionnaire
combined dyslipidaemia **60.2**
   type III hyperlipoproteinaemia 60.8–60.9
combined immunodeficiencies **80.4**, 80.7–80.13
   associated/syndromic features 80.11–80.13
combined melanocytic naevi 131.24–131.26
combined oral contraceptives (COCs)
   androgenic effect **88.13**
   antibiotic interactions 88.49
   hair disorder treatment 87.89, 87.95, **87.96**
comedo extractor 88.58
comedo naevus 73.7, 88.31, *88.32*, 137.5
comedonal acne 4.19, 88.1–88.2, *88.3*, 88.14, *88.26*, *88.27*, *88.28*, 88.45
   in acne conglobata 88.65
   comedo extractor 88.58
   cutaneous nodular elastosis with 156.4
   management 88.45–88.47
   nodular elastosis *156.5*
   prepubertal 88.69
   submarine comedones *88.28*
   treatment algorithm *88.45*
   see also chloracne
Comèl–Netherton syndrome (CNS) 63.26–63.28, **80.4**, 80.11
commensal skin flora 26.2–26.5
common acquired naevi **131.16**, 131.17–131.21
common naevi, low melanoma risk 142.2
common variable immunodeficiency (CVID) 80.1, **80.5**, 80.13, 147.2
common warts (verruca vulgaris) 25.52, 25.53, 25.54
   see also cutaneous warts
communication, holistic management of skin disease 15.6, 15.7
community-acquired MRSA (CA-MRSA) 26.6–26.7
community dermatology 7.7, 7.8, 7.11
community diagnosis 5.2
company-sponsored clinical trials 17.3

comparative genomic hybridisation (CGH), melanoma diagnosis 142.21
compensatory hyperhidrosis 92.7
   surgical treatment 92.10
complaints and litigation
   body dysmorphic disorder 84.15
   delusional infestation 84.9–84.10
   factitious skin diseases by proxy 84.38
complementary/alternative/traditional therapies
   acne vulgaris 88.57–88.58
   cosmeceuticals 157.7–157.10
   metal poisoning 121.1
   psychiatric problems 84.48
   topical 18.38
   wart treatments 25.60
   see also herbals
complement diseases, inherited immunodeficiency 80.18–80.20
complete circumferential peripheral and deep margin assessment (CCPDMA), basal cell carcinoma 140.16
completion lymph node dissection (CLND), melanoma 143.4, 143.5
complex aphthosis, oral ulceration 108.39–108.40
complex regional pain syndrome (CRPS) 83.20–83.23
   dermatological manifestations **83.22**
   diagnostic criteria **83.21**
   management 83.22–83.23
   treatment ladder 83.23
   triggers of **83.21**
complicated lymphatic anomalies (CLAs) 71.1, 71.22–71.23
Compositae (Asteraceae) allergy 127.11, 127.16–127.17, 127.19–127.20, 127.71–127.74
composite haemangioendothelioma 136.33–136.34
compound allergy 127.29
compound follicles 87.84
compound naevi
   acquired melanocytic naevi *131.19*, *131.21*
   acral naevi *131.23*
   conjunctival naevus *131.25*
   definition **131.1**
   dysplastic melanocytic naevi *131.42*
   Spitz naevus *131.33*
comprehensive acne severity system (CASS) 88.38, **88.39**
Comprehensive Care Programme with Persons with Albinism (CCPWA) 7.10–7.11
compression syndromes, BSL association 98.15, 98.17
compression therapy, venous leg ulcer *102.5*
computed tomography (CT) scans
   foreign body reactions 122.18
   morphoea 55.31
computer-aided diagnostic systems (CAD), melanoma diagnosis 142.10
computer-aided image analysis, skin properties 16.5
computer-based assessments (CBAs) 16.2
computerised dermoscopy devices, melanoma diagnosis 142.9
conception, drug pharmacokinetics and pharmacodynamics 13.8
conditioners (hair), alopecia management 87.98–87.99
condoms, genital contact dermatitis **109.13**
condyloma acuminata, human papillomavirus infection *113.4*
condylomas, penis 109.39–109.40
condylomata acuminata 25.61–25.64
   see also ano-genital warts
condylomata lata, syphilis 29.5, 29.10, 29.11, 29.17
cones, blood supply 124.8
confetti ichthyoses 63.16, *63.18*
confetti-like macular atrophy 94.25

confidence intervals
   epidemiological studies 5.14
   statistical analysis of clinical studies 17.22–17.23
confluent hyperkeratosis *63.59*
confluent and reticulated papillomatosis (CARP) 85.6–85.8
confocal microscopy, basal cell carcinoma 140.10, *140.13*
congenital adrenal hyperplasia (CAH) 87.90–87.91
   acne vulgaris association 88.5–88.7
   adrenal steroid genesis pathway *88.9*
   clinical features **88.10**
   dermatoendocrinology 150.17–150.18
congenital alopecias 87.30
congenital anomalies, oral involvement 108.87–108.88
congenital biliary tract hypoplasia with consecutive cholestasis, jaundice 153.5
congenital candidiasis 32.66–32.67, 114.28
congenital cyanotic heart disease, associated finger clubbing 151.1, *151.3*
congenital cytomegalovirus infection 25.41
congenital dermatosis with reticulate scarring 94.14
congenital disorders
   and genetic syndromes, involving respiratory system and skin 152.5
   prenatal diagnosis 8.9–8.10
congenital epidermal naevi (CEN) 73.3–73.8
   Blaschko linear distribution *73.5*
   classification 73.2
   clinical features 73.4–73.5
   clinical variants 73.5–73.7
   complications and co-morbidities 73.7–73.8
   eccrine naevus 73.6
   epidermal thickening with hyperkeratosis and inflammatory reaction *73.4*
   genetic basis of **73.3**
   investigations 73.8
   management 73.8
   pathophysiology 73.3–73.4
   sebaceous naevus 73.5, *73.6*, *73.7*, 73.8
   verrucous epidermal naevus *73.4*, *73.5*
congenital erosive and vesicular dermatosis, healing with reticulated supple scarring 114.9
congenital erosive and vesicular dermatosis (CEVD), neonates 114.9
congenital erythropoietic porphyria (CEP) 58.9–58.11
   clinical features 58.9–58.10
   genetic counselling 58.11
   investigations 58.10
   scarring of skin with resorption of terminal phalanges 58.10
   treatment 58.10–58.11
congenital generalised fibromatosis *see* infantile myofibromatosis
congenital generalised hypertrichosis (CGH) 87.85
congenital generalised lipodystrophies (CGL) 72.2–72.3, 98.3
congenital haemangiomas, infants 116.7–116.9
congenital haemolytic anaemias 86.48–86.49
congenital heart block (CHB) 51.39–51.42
congenital hemidysplasia–ichthyosiform naevus–limb defect (CHILD) syndrome 63.23–63.24
congenital hypertrichosis 87.85
   lanuginosa 87.85
congenital ichthyoses
   management 63.41–63.46
   non-syndromic 63.7–63.13
   psychosocial aspects 63.46
   trichothiodystrophy 63.37
congenital ichthyosiform erythroderma (CIE) 63.10–63.13, *63.12*, *63.27*
congenital lax skin 94.21

congenital leptin deficiency 97.5
congenital lesions, oral involvement 108.28–108.31
congenital lipodystrophy 72.1–72.3, 98.2
congenital livedo reticularis 124.9
congenital localised hypertrichosis 87.85–87.86
congenital melanocytic naevi (CMN) 73.8–73.15, 131.15–131.17
  associated diseases 73.9
  benign proliferative nodule 73.11
  bland naevus cells 73.9, 73.10
  clinical features 73.11
  clinical presentation **131.16**
  clinical variants 73.11–73.12
  complications and co-morbidities 73.12–73.13
  dermoscopic presentation **131.16**
  differential diagnosis 73.12
  environmental factors 73.11
  facial features characteristic of 73.13
  genetics 73.10–73.11
  laser therapies 23.16
  management 73.14–73.15
  melanoma development 73.10
  as melanoma precursors 142.2
  melanoma risk 73.13
  neurological abnormalities 73.12–73.13
  neurological investigation and patient follow-up 73.14
  pathology **131.16**
  pathophysiology 73.9–73.10
  severity classification 73.12
  speckled lentiginous naevus 131.15–131.17
congenital midline hamartoma see rhabdomyomatous congenital hamartoma
congenital muscle hamartoma 73.19
congenital naevi 73.1–73.18
  blue naevus 73.15, 73.16
  classification 73.1–73.2
  congenital epidermal naevi 73.2, 73.3–73.8
  congenital melanocytic naevi 73.8–73.15
  congenital naevus spilus 73.15–73.16
  connective tissue naevi 73.2, 73.16–73.18
  fat naevus 73.2, 73.16–73.18
  genetic classification 73.2
  histological classification 73.2
  inheritance of naevus mutations 73.3
  muscle 'naevi' 73.2
  naevus phenotypes 73.1
  pigment cell naevi **73.2**
  Spitz naevi 73.15
  terminology **73.2**
congenital naevus spilus 73.15–73.16
congenital-onset primary lymphoedema 103.24
congenital palmoplantar and periorificial keratoderma with corneal epithelial dysplasia (Olmsted syndrome) 63.69–63.70, 108.30
congenital pilar/smooth muscle naevus see smooth muscle hamartoma
congenital poikiloderma 94.13
congenital pseudo-ainhum 94.48
congenital reticular ichthyosiform erythroderma (CRIE) 63.16, 63.18
congenital rubella syndrome 25.92, 114.23
congenital self-healing reticulohistiocytosis (CSHRH) 135.5, 135.6–135.7
congenital Spitz naevi 73.15
congenital superficial capillary malformations (port-wine stains) 73.20
  eyelids 107.47
  laser therapies 23.8–23.9, 23.10, 23.11
  lobular capillary haemangioma/pyogenic granuloma within 136.26
  phakomatosis pigmentovascularis 73.22
congenital syphilis (CS) 29.2, 29.22–29.29
  clinical features 29.23–29.26
  definition 29.22–29.23
  early manifestations 29.23–29.25, 29.27
  epidemiology 29.23
  investigations 29.26–29.27
  late manifestations 29.25–29.26, 29.27
  management 29.27–29.29
  neonatal 114.27–114.28
  pathophysiology 29.23
congenital tuberculosis, neonates 114.28
congenital vellus hamartoma, hair follicle naevus 137.7
congestive heart failure, oedema 85.29
conglobate acne see acne conglobata
conidiobolomycosis 32.79–32.80
Conidiobolus coronatus 32.79–32.80
conjunctiva
  bulbar telangiectasia 80.11
  UV radiation-exposure damage 76.5
conjunctival hyperaemia, mucous membrane pemphigoid 50.30
conjunctival naevi 131.24, 131.25
conjunctivitis, actinic prurigo 126.10
connective tissue diseases (CTD) 3.44, 53.1–53.3
  acquired ichthyosis 63.47
  autoimmune disorders affecting skin and respiratory system 152.2
  direct immunofluorescence findings 3.19
  dystrophic calcification 59.1
  investigations 53.3
  management 53.3
  mechanical injuries 122.2
  ocular features 107.41
  papular and nodular mucinosis 57.13–57.14
  skin fragility 69.20
  systemic sclerosis 54.8–54.9
connective tissue naevi 73.2, 73.16–73.18
  haematoxylin and eosin stain 3.8
  tuberous sclerosis complex 78.8
connective tissues, malignancy and rheumatological disorders 148.20–148.21
connective tissue septa 97.3, 97.6
connexin 26, Vohwinkel syndrome 63.64
connexins, KID syndrome 63.33
connexons, gap junction 2.20
Conradi syndrome, follicular atrophoderma 94.17
Conradi–Hünermann–Happle syndrome (CHHS) 63.22–63.23
COnsensus-based Standards for the selection of health Measurement INstruments (COSMIN) checklist 16.3
Consolidated Standards of Reporting Trials (CONSORT) 17.14
constitutive pigmentation 68.1, 86.8–86.9
constitutive skin colour 86.1–86.2
constricting bands of the extremities 94.46–94.48
constriction artefact, oedema induction 84.33
consultants, referral rates 5.13
contact allergies
  musical instruments 122.12
  purpura **99.9**
  topical therapy 18.5
contact brucellosis 26.61
contact cheilitis 108.60–108.61
contact dermatitis 105.5, 127.1
  arsenic 121.2, 121.4
  cannabis-induced 120.4
  drug-induced eczema 117.3–117.5
  ear dermatoses **106.22**
  ear piercing 106.11–106.12
  erythromelalgia 101.9
  eyelid 107.6
  irritants 128.1–128.13, 129.1–129.5
  lichen planus-like contact dermatitis 37.3
  patch testing technique 1.8
  perianal skin 111.12
  pseudolymphoma 134.1, 134.2
  vulval 110.14–110.15
  see also allergic contact dermatitis
contact hypersensitivity, Langerhans cells 2.14
contact immunotherapy, alopecia treatment 87.27
contact urticaria (CU) 42.13–42.14, 127.82–127.86
  non-immune 128.8–128.9
  occupational hazards 129.8–129.11
contagious pustular dermatitis see orf virus
contingency tables, statistical analysis of clinical studies 17.22
contour, principles of surgical design 20.19–20.20
contraception
  systemic lupus erythematosus 51.32
  see also combined oral contraceptives
contrite reaction, olfactory reference syndrome 84.10
contusion, external ear 106.8
conubial dermatitis (ACD by-proxy dermatitis) 109.12
Conus genus, stings from 130.4
conventional photodynamic therapy, actinic keratosis 141.10
cooling management,
  chemotherapy-induced alopecia 87.72
Copenhagen Psoriasis Severity Index 16.3
copper allergy 127.41
copper deficiency 2.34, 61.27–61.29
CoQ10 see coenzyme Q10
coral stings 130.1–130.3
core outcome measures 16.3
Core Outcome Set (COS), eczema outcome measures **16.3**
corkscrew hairs, vitamin C deficiency 61.21, 61.22
cornea
  brittle cornea syndrome 70.6–70.7, 70.10
  UV radiation-exposure damage 76.5
  vascularisation and scarring, herpes simplex virus 107.37
corneal argyria, silver exposure 121.8
corneal transplant, ocular rosacea 107.11
corneocytes 2.1, 2.6
corneodesmosin 69.6
cornification
  exfoliative disorders 63.26–63.30
  inherited disorders 63.1–63.80
cornoid lamella 85.20–85.21
  porokeratoses 63.75–63.76
corns 122.7–122.9, 122.16
corona phlebectatica paraplantaris (ankle flare), chronic venous insufficiency **101.43**, 101.44
coronary artery disease 51.30, 151.5
coronavirus see COVID-19
cortex, hair fibres 87.6, 87.7
cortical cells 2.9
corticosteroid-induced rosacea-like facial dermatosis 89.17
corticosteroid injection, localised lipoatrophy due to 98.11–98.12
corticosteroid purpura 99.5
corticosteroids 1.8, 12.3, 12.8
  acneform reaction 88.11–88.12
  acne treatment 88.57, 129.12
  allergic contact dermatitis 127.45, 127.47
  allergic reactions 127.4
  atopic eczema treatment 41.26–41.27
  atrophy due to 94.6–94.10
  bronchopneumonia treatment 125.5
  chemical structure **18.14**
  cutaneous adverse effects 155.15
  drug reaction with eosinophilia and systemic symptoms 118.11–118.12
  eye, side effects on 107.40–107.43
  genital contact dermatitis **109.13**
  indications 18.15, **18.17**
  inflammatory peristomal skin diseases **112.4**
  intralesional injection 18.21–18.22
  local adverse effects 18.15, 18.17–18.19
  mastocytosis treatment 46.10
  mechanism of action 18.15
  morphoea treatment 55.36–55.37
  occlusion 18.21
  patch testing 127.47
  pemphigus treatment 50.8
  poststeroid panniculitis 97.58–97.59
  potency classification 18.14–18.15, **18.16**
  in pregnancy 113.19, **113.22**
  primary localised cutaneous amyloidosis treatment 56.13, 56.14
  psoriasis treatment 35.20, 35.21
  side effects 18.15, 18.17–18.20
  Stevens–Johnson syndrome/toxic epidermal necrolysis 118.21
  systemic adverse effects 18.19–18.20
  tinea (ringworm) infections 32.49–32.50
  topical therapies 18.14–18.22
  urticaria treatment 42.18
corticosteroid-sparing agents, sarcoidosis management 96.15–96.16
corticotrophin-releasing hormone (CRH), hair follicle 87.11
Corynebacterium
  C. diphtheriae, diphtheria 26.38–26.39
  C. flavescens, trichomycosis axillaris 26.41–26.42
  C. minutissimum, erythrasma 26.39
  C. propinquum, trichomycosis axillaris 26.41–26.42
  C. pseudotuberculosis, diphtheria 26.38
  C. tenuis, trichomycosis axillaris 26.41–26.42
  C. ulcerans, diphtheria 26.38
  pitted keratolysis 26.42–26.43
Corynebacterium acnes see Cutibacterium
Corynebacterium haemolyticum see Arcanobacterium haemolyticum
Corynebacterium kroppenstedtii, rosacea 89.4
Corynebacterium pyogenes see Trueperella pyogenes
coryneform bacteria 26.37–26.43
  found on skin 26.4
  general description 26.37–26.38
  types 26.37
COS see Core Outcome Set
cosmeceuticals 157.1–157.13
  aloe 157.10–157.11
  alpha-lipoic acid 157.1–157.2
  anti-ageing
    rhytid reduction 157.4–157.7
    skin lightening 157.3–157.4
  anti-inflammatories 157.10–157.11
  antioxidants 157.1–157.3
  arbutin 157.3
  caffeine 157.11
  carnosine 157.7
  carrier peptides 157.6
  chamomile 157.11
  coenzyme Q10 157.2
  'cosmeceutical' term 157.1
  cysteamine 157.3
  efficacy of 157.1, 157.13
  glycine-glutamate-lysine-glycine 157.5
  glycosaminoglycans 157.4
  grape seed extract 157.7–157.9
  green tea (Camellia sinensis) 157.9
  herbals and phytochemicals 157.7–157.10
  hydroquinone 157.3–157.4
  hydroxy acids 157.4–157.5
  ingredients and potential uses, summary of **157.12–157.13**
  kojic acid 157.4
  lycopene 157.9–157.10
  neurotransmitter-affecting peptides 157.6
  origin of 157.1
  peptides 157.5–157.6
    mechanism of action **157.6**
  polyunsaturated fatty acids 157.5
  pomegranate 157.10
  regulation of 157.1, 157.13
  retinaldehyde 157.7
  retinoids 157.6–157.7
  retinol 157.7
  retinyl esters 157.7
  risks of using 157.13
  safety of 157.13
  signal peptides 157.5–157.6

soya 157.10
tranexamic acid 157.4
vitamin A (retinoids) 157.6–157.7
vitamin B 157.2
vitamin C 157.2–157.3
vitamin E 157.3
see also cosmetic treatments
cosmesis, alopecia treatment 87.18
cosmetic allergens 127.4–127.5, 127.12, 127.47–127.58, 127.59–127.60
EU directives/regulations 127.35
cosmetic dermatitis 128.4
cosmetic exhaustion 128.4
cosmetic fillers, factitious panniculitis 97.48–97.49
cosmetic products, seborrhoeic dermatitis effects 40.4
cosmetics
 and acne 88.25, 129.12
 lead poisoning 121.5
 metal poisoning 121.1, 121.5
 photocontact facial melanosis 86.12
cosmetic subunit junction lines, principles of surgical design 20.20
cosmetic treatments 1.8, 1.9
 alopecia 87.69, 87.97–87.101
 APL management 98.6
 fat hypertrophy 98.15
 laser resurfacing 161.1–161.6
 in pregnancy 113.21, 113.24
 skin photoageing 156.11
 skin tightening 161.6–161.8
 see also cosmeceuticals
cosmetic vehicles/excipients 127.58–127.60
COSMIN *see* COnsensus-based Standards for the selection of health Measurement INstruments checklist
cost-benefit analysis, health economics 6.4
cost of disease *see* economic burden of disease
Costello syndrome 70.16, **78.9**
cost-minimisation studies, health economics 6.4
counselling, chemical peels 160.6–160.7
Course of Life Questionnaire (CoLQ) 16.11
covert injections, dermatitis artefacta 84.33
COVID-19-induced perniosis, type I cryoglobulinaemia 149.14
COVID-19/SARS-CoV-2 (severe acute respiratory syndrome coronavirus 2) 1.8, 1.9, 25.100–25.120
 altered dermatological healthcare during pandemic 25.120
 clinical features 25.102
 cutaneous manifestations 152.4
 epidemiology 25.100
 exacerbation of pre-existing mucocutaneous diseases 25.115
 infants 115.5
 investigations 25.102
 irritant contact dermatitis 129.2
 mucocutaneous manifestations of infection 25.103–25.115
  children 25.113–25.115
  clinical features 25.104–25.115
  clinical variants **25.105–25.107**, 25.108–25.113
  epidemiology 25.103–25.104, 25.113
  hair and nail disorders 25.113
  management **25.105–25.107**
  pathophysiology 25.104
  relationship to disease severity 25.108
  timeline relative to systemic features 25.108
 mucocutaneous manifestations of treatment 25.116
 mucocutaneous reactions to vaccines 25.117
 occupational dermatoses 127.4
 outcomes in patients with pre-existing mucocutaneous diseases 25.115
 pathophysiology 25.100–25.101
 perniosis 124.5
 PPE-occupational dermatoses 25.119
 sexually transmitted infections, effect on 29.2
 treatment, mucocutaneous manifestations 25.116
 vaccination considerations 25.117–25.119
 virology 25.101
 vitamin D deficiency 61.10
'Covid toes/fingers', chilblain-like lesions/pseudo-pernio associated with COVID-19 25.108–25.109
Cowden syndrome (PTEN hamartoma tumour syndrome) 71.2, 71.13–71.14, **72.10**, *78.11*, **78.14**, 148.11–148.12
 oral involvement 108.85
 storiform collagenoma 136.3
 trichilemmoma 137.6
cowpox virus 25.12–25.13
 vaccinia virus relationship 25.7
coxsackieviruses 25.93–25.95
 vesicular exanthem 25.5
 see also eczema coxsackium
CP *see* chronic pruritus
CPD *see* chronic papillomatous dermatitis; cyclobutane pyrimidine dimer
crab lice 34.24–34.25
crack cocaine 120.1, 120.5
cradle cap 40.5, 115.1, *115.2*
cranial dysraphism 87.86
cranial nerves, anatomical positions 20.2–20.4
cranial neuropathies 82.6
cranial (nodular) fasciitis 136.5
cranio-facial hyperhidrosis 92.6
craniosynostosis syndromes **70.17**
CRBSI *see* catheter-related bloodstream infections
creams, topical drugs 12.3–12.4, 18.2
creep 122.3
creeping hair 122.22
CRH *see* corticotrophin-releasing hormone
CRI *see* catheter-related infection
cri du chat syndrome 74.3
CRIE *see* congenital reticular ichthyosiform erythroderma
crinkles 94.2, 94.26
crisaborole, atopic eczema treatment 41.27
Crisponi syndrome 94.40
Crohn disease (CD)
 cutaneous Crohn disease 95.13–95.16
 hidradenitis suppurativa association 90.2, 90.6, 90.7
 ileostomy for 112.5, *112.9*
 leukonychia 121.7
 mucocutaneous features of **111.27**
 oral involvement 108.72
 perianal 95.14, 111.26–111.27
 peristomal 112.13–112.15
 psoriasis in 35.18
 pyoderma gangrenosum *112.15*
 skin involvement 153.2–153.3
 ulcerative colitis distinction 153.1–153.2
 vulval 110.23–110.24
cromoglicate 18.39
Cronkhite–Canada syndrome 87.58
Cross syndrome 68.9
croton oil, chemical peels 160.10–160.11
Crouzon syndrome 85.4, **106.7**
Crown vessels, sebaceous gland hyperplasia *91.17*
crow's feet (lateral periorbital lines), botulinum toxin injection 159.5, *159.6*, *159.7*
CRPS *see* complex regional pain syndrome
crude petroleum, acne 129.12
crust 3.40
crustacean vectors of parasitic disease, *Cyclops* species and dracunculiasis 33.13
CrVI *see* chromium VI
cryofibrinogenaemia, purpura 99.11–99.14
cryoglobulinaemia 124.13
 purpura 99.11–99.14
cryoglobulinaemic vasculitis 100.15–100.17, 124.13
 serum protein electrophoresis *100.17*
cryoglobulins,
 cryogelling/cryoagglutination disorders 99.11–99.14
cryolipolysis, fat contouring 161.8–161.9
CryoModulation technology 161.6
cryopyrin-associated periodic syndrome (CAPS) 45.8–45.9
cryosurgery 20.46–20.47
 basal cell carcinoma treatment 140.11, 140.14–140.16
cryotherapy
 actinic keratosis 141.9
 Bowen disease 141.22–141.23
 cutaneous squamous cell carcinoma 141.35
 cutaneous warts 25.58–25.59
cryptococcosis 32.90–32.92
 oral involvement 108.57
cryptococcus infection, HIV 31.28
Cryptococcus neoformans 32.91, 32.92
crystal globulin vasculopathy 99.15
crystalloids, resuscitation use 125.3
crystal meth 120.4–120.5
crystal violet, tattoos 86.53
CS *see* carcinoid syndrome; chondroitin sulphate; Cockayne syndrome; congenital syphilis
cSCC *see* cutaneous squamous cell carcinoma
CS-COUSIN *see* Cochrane Skin Core Outcomes Initiative
CSHRH *see* congenital self-healing reticulohistiocytosis
CSS *see* classic Sweet syndrome; cultured skin substitute
CSU *see* chronic spontaneous urticaria
CSVV *see* cutaneous small-vessel vasculitis
CT *see* computed tomography
CTCL *see* cutaneous T-cell lymphoma
CTD *see* connective tissue diseases
CTLs *see* cytotoxic T lymphocytes
CTS *see* cervical trophic syndrome
CU *see* contact urticaria
Cubozoa (box jellyfish), stings 130.1
'cuff sign', lipoedema 99.22
cultured epithelial autografts (CEA) 125.6
cultured skin substitute (CSS) 125.6
culture-independent microbial studies, molecular genetic methods 26.2, 26.3
culturing samples
 quantitative bacterial studies 26.4
 skin flora 26.3
cumulative life course impairment (CLCI) 16.11
 impact of a long-term health condition over time 15.3
cupping, discoid hyperpigmentation 4.12
CU-Q$_2$oL *see* Chronic Urticaria Quality of Life Questionnaire
curettage 3.3–3.4
 Bowen disease treatment 141.23
 treating skin lesions 20.48
 unsuitable for basal cell carcinomas 20.35, **20.37**
curettage and cautery (C&C) *see* curettage and electrodessication
curettage and electrodessication
 actinic keratosis 141.9
 basal cell carcinoma 140.14
 cutaneous squamous cell carcinoma 141.34–141.35
Curie, Marie 1.9
curlicue (storiform) pattern 3.40
Curry–Jones syndrome 73.7, **78.12**
Cushing disease/syndrome 86.7, 86.18
 acne vulgaris association 88.7
 dermatoendocrinology 150.11, *150.13*, 150.17
 striae 94.0, 94.11
cutaneo-mucosal venous malformation *see* venous mucocutaneous malformation
cutaneous adnexal tumours *see* tumours of skin appendages
cutaneous adverse drug effects
 allopurinol 155.9–155.10, 155.15
 antimalarials 19.5–19.6, 155.15
 antirheumatic therapies 155.15–155.16
 NSAIDs 155.15
cutaneous adverse events, reactions to COVID-19 vaccines 25.117
cutaneous amyloidoses *see* amyloidoses
cutaneous arteriovenous haemangioma *see* cirsoid aneurysm
cutaneous arteritis 97.9–97.11, 100.28–100.30
cutaneous atrophy
 causes 94.6–94.21
 perineal and perianal 111.12
 vascular Ehlers–Danlos syndrome *70.8*
cutaneous B-cell lymphoma (CBCL)
 diffuse large B-cell lymphoma 139.37, 139.41–139.43
 follicle centre cell 139.37, 139.40–139.41
 marginal zone lymphoma 139.37–139.39
 primary 139.37–139.43
 secondary 139.43–139.45
 treatment algorithm **139.38**
cutaneous bleeding
 causes **99.5**
 see also ecchymosis (bruises); purpura
cutaneous burns, treatment **125.7–125.8**
cutaneous Crohn disease 95.13–95.16
 clinical features 95.16
 lip swelling due to oro-facial granulomatosis 95.14
 management 95.16
 metastatic Crohn disease, 'knife-cut' fissures *95.15*, 95.16
 pathology 95.14–95.16
 peno-scrotal lymphoedema *95.15*
 peri-anal skin tags 95.14
 perivascular dermal infiltrates *95.15*
 vulval swelling *95.15*
cutaneous cylindroma, CYLD cutaneous syndrome *78.11*
cutaneous cysts *see* chloracne; comedonal acne; cysts; dermoid cysts; metabolising acquired dioxin-induced skin hamartoma; vellus hair cyst
cutaneous effects of systemic therapies
 antimalarials 19.5–19.6, 155.15
 glucocorticoids *19.19*
 hydroxycarbamide 19.21–19.22
cutaneous endometriosis, vulva 110.33
cutaneous epithelioid angiomatous nodule 136.28–136.29
cutaneous erythema *see* redness (erythema)
cutaneous Ewing sarcoma 136.51–136.52
cutaneous haemosiderosis 86.47–86.49
cutaneous histiocytoses 135.1–135.32
cutaneous histoplasmosis 32.82, 32.83
cutaneous horn 141.12–141.13
cutaneous hyperextensibility, classical Ehlers–Danlos syndrome *70.8*
cutaneous infections
 panniculitis 97.46
 SJS/TEN complications 118.20
cutaneous juvenile xanthogranuloma 135.17
cutaneous keratocysts 133.6–133.7
cutaneous larva migrans *4.16*
 clinical features 33.19–33.20
 definition/nomenclature 33.18–33.19
 management 33.20
 nematodes of other animals 33.18–33.20
 pathophysiology 33.19
 perineal skin 111.16
 see also ancylostomiasis
cutaneous laser therapy 23.1–23.24
cutaneous leishmaniasis 33.43–33.51
 chronic 33.47–33.48
 clinical features 33.46–33.49
 clinical variants **33.45**, 33.46–33.49
 diffuse 33.48–33.49
 epidemiology 33.43–33.45
 investigations 33.49–33.50

cutaneous leishmaniasis (continued)
  management 33.50–33.51
  pathophysiology 33.45–33.46
cutaneous lesions 96.13, 96.15
  juvenile xanthogramuloma 135.16
  liver disease association 153.9
  panniculitis 97.6
  progressive nodular histiocytosis 135.19
cutaneous lupus 126.32, 126.33
cutaneous lymphadenoma see adamantinoid trichoblastoma
cutaneous lymphangiectasia 103.31–103.32
cutaneous lymphocyte antigen (CLA), primary cutaneous T-cell lymphomas 139.2
cutaneous lymphoid hyperplasia see pseudolymphoma
cutaneous lymphomas 139.1–139.50
  blastic plasmacytoid dendritic cell neoplasm 139.45–139.47
  classification 139.1, **139.2**, 139.37
  leukaemia cutis 139.47–139.48
  post-transplant lymphoproliferative disorder 139.47
  primary B-cell lymphoma 139.37–139.43
  primary T-cell lymphomas 139.1–139.37
  radiotherapy 24.15–24.18
  secondary B-cell lymphoma 139.43–139.45
  secondary T-cell lymphoma 139.45
  see also haematological malignancies
cutaneous macroglobulinosis 149.13
cutaneous markers of internal malignancy 148.1–148.28
cutaneous mastocytosis (CM) **46.2**, 46.3–46.5
  musculoskeletal involvement 155.13
cutaneous melanomas see malignant melanoma
cutaneous meningioma see meningothelial heterotopias
cutaneous metastases 148.4–148.6
cutaneous miliary tuberculosis, acute 27.17
cutaneous mucinosis 57.1–57.19
  classification 57.1, **57.2**
  connective tissue diseases 57.13–57.14
  dermal mucinoses 57.2–57.15, 57.16
  detection for research 57.1
  digital myxoid cyst 57.15, 57.16
  facial 57.14–57.15
  focal 57.14–57.15
  follicular mucinoses 57.15–57.18
  of infancy 57.6, 57.7
  lichen myxoedematosus 57.1–57.8
  myxoedema in thyroid diseases 57.11–57.14
  pinkus follicular mucinosis 57.16, 57.17
  primary mucinoses 57.2–57.18
  reticular erythematous mucinosis 57.8–57.9
  scleroedema 57.9–57.11
  secondary mucinoses 57.1, **57.2**, 57.18
  self-healing cutaneous mucinoses 57.14
  urticaria-like follicular mucinosis 57.16–57.17
cutaneous myoepithelioma 137.32–137.33
cutaneous necrosis, intravenous drug administration 120.7
cutaneous neoplasia, photodynamic therapy 22.6–22.7, 22.8
cutaneous neoplasms 3.21–3.29
  cytokeratin markers 3.21–3.22
  epithelial markers 3.21–3.23
  histiocytic markers 3.27
  keratin markers 3.21–3.23
  Langerhans cell markers 3.27, 3.28
  lymphoid markers 3.27–3.29
  melanocytic markers 3.23–3.25
  mesenchymal markers 3.25–3.26
  metastatic cutaneous tumours 3.26–3.27
  neuroendocrine markers 3.23
cutaneous (neuro-) endocrine signalling mechanism, key components **150.4**
cutaneous neurofibromas 78.3

cutaneous nodular elastosis with cysts and comedones, ageing of skin 156.4
cutaneous photosensitivity diseases 126.1–126.39
cutaneous polyarteritis nodosa 97.9–97.11
cutaneous porphyrias see porphyria
cutaneous radiation recall reactions, chemotherapy 119.12
cutaneous reactions
  cold and heat 124.1–124.16
  implanted metals 127.19
  surgical implants 151.5–151.6
cutaneous rhabdomyosarcoma 136.55–136.56
cutaneous rosacea 89.3, 89.13
cutaneous sarcoid-like reactions, tattoos 122.22
cutaneous sarcoidosis 96.3, 96.4, 96.6–96.7, 96.16
  rare forms 97.53–97.54
  treatment ladder **96.17**
cutaneous sarcoid reaction 96.17–96.18
cutaneous schwannoma 106.35
cutaneous small-vessel vasculitis (CSVV) 100.5–100.8
  blisters **100.7**
  causes **100.5**
  leukocytoclastic vasculitis 100.6
cutaneous squamous cell carcinoma (cSCC) 106.27–106.28, 141.26–141.37
  associated diseases 141.1, 141.27
  causative organisms 141.30
  clinical features 141.30–141.34
  clinical variants 141.31
  definitions/nomenclature 141.26
  disease course and prognosis 141.32–141.34
  epidemiology 141.26–141.27
  first line treatment
    high/very high-risk disease 141.35, 141.37
    low-risk disease 141.34–141.35
  human papillomavirus association 25.65
  immunocompromised people
    clinicopathological features 147.10–147.11
    management 147.16–147.18
  investigations 141.34
  as a keratinocyte cancer 141.1
  management 141.34–141.37
  multiple self-healing **78.13**, 141.41–141.42
  pathology 141.29–141.30
  pathophysiology 141.27–141.30
  predisposing factors 141.29
  second line treatment 141.37
  severity classification/staging systems 141.31–141.32
  signalling pathways/networks 141.27–141.28, 141.29
  verrucous carcinoma of the foot/epithelioma cuniculatum 141.31
  see also keratinocyte cancer
cutaneous T-cell lymphoma (CTCL) 86.44
  acquired ichthyosis 63.48
  combination therapy 139.23–139.24
  extracorporeal photochemotherapy 21.7
  management 139.20–139.25
  origin of term 139.1
  phototherapy 21.4, 21.7
  primary 139.1–139.25
  rare primary cutaneous variants (non-MF) 139.29–139.37
  secondary 139.45
  systemic therapies 139.22–139.25
  topical therapies 139.21–139.22
  see also mycosis fungoides
cutaneous tuberculosis see tuberculosis of the skin
cutaneous tumours, WHO classification 142.8
cutaneous vascular malformations 101.26–101.31
  disorders associated with **101.28**

see also vascular disorders
cutaneous vasculitis see vasculitis, cutaneous
cutaneous warts
  clinical features 25.53–25.57
  cryotherapy 25.58–25.59
  epidemiology 25.52
  human papillomavirus 25.52–25.61
  hyperthermic therapy 25.59
  investigations 25.57
  laser therapy 25.59
  management 25.57–25.61
  pathophysiology 25.52–25.53
  photodynamic therapy 25.59
  surgery 25.59
  topical pharmacology 25.57–25.58, 25.59
cutibacteria
  in follicles and sebaceous glands 26.3
  infections 26.43
Cutibacterium (previously Propionibacterium)
  C. acnes 26.43
    effect on human sebocytes 88.17
    necrotising lymphocytic folliculitis 93.4
    sarcoidosis causation 96.4
    scalp folliculitis 93.5
  C. avidum 26.43
  C. granulosum 26.43
cuticle, hair fibres 87.6
cuticle defects, trichorrhexis nodosa 87.76
cuticular cells 2.9
cutis laxa 70.14–70.17, 77.5–77.7, 94.21–94.23
  autosomal dominant cutis laxa 70.17, 77.5–77.6
  autosomal recessive cutis laxa 77.6–77.7
  autosomal recessive type 1A cutis laxa 70.17
  causative genes 77.6
  clinical features 70.15, **70.16**
  craniosynostosis syndromes **70.17**
  differential diagnosis 70.15
  elastin gene mutations 2.33–2.34
  glycosylation disorders **79.10**
  investigations 70.15
  management 70.17, 77.7
  molecular defect **70.16**
  pathophysiology 70.14–70.15, 77.5
  phenotypes **77.6**
  related syndromes **70.16**
  subtypes **77.6**
  types of **70.16**
cutis marmorata 114.3, 124.9
cutis marmorata telangiectatica congenita 124.9
cutis rhomboidalis nuchae, ageing of skin 156.5
cutis verticis gyrata (CVG) 98.25, 105.10
  dermatoendocrinology **150.10**, 150.12
CVD see chronic venous disease
cvEDS see cardiac-valvular Ehlers–Danlos syndrome
CVG see cutis verticis gyrata
CVID see common variable immunodeficiency
cyanide (CN), inhalation injury 125.4
cyanoacrylates 127.70
cyclin-dependent kinase 4 gene (CDK4), melanoma risk 142.4
cyclin-dependent kinase inhibitor 2A gene (CDKN2A) 3.24
  melanoma risk 142.4, 142.7
cyclobutane pyrimidine dimer (CPD), UV radiation exposure 10.6
cyclodopa 86.5
cyclophosphamide
  mucous membrane pemphigoid, management of 107.31
  pemphigus treatment 50.8
  systemic lupus erythematosus treatment 51.38
cyclo-phosphamide-induced alopecia 119.5
cyclophyllidea, infections 33.31–33.34
CYLD cutaneous syndrome 78.11, **78.12**

cylindroadenocarcinoma 137.35
cylindroma 137.29–137.30
  familial 137.30, 137.35
  malignant 137.35
  spiradenoma relationship 137.31
CYP1B1 variant 87.41
cyproterone acetate 87.96
cystatin A (CSTA), skin fragility disorders 69.6
cysteamine, cosmeceutical use of 157.3
cysticercosis 33.32–33.34
  clinical features 33.32–33.33
  management 33.33–33.34
  pathophysiology 33.32
cystic fibrosis
  sweat glands 92.3
  transient aquagenic keratoderma 63.62
cysts
  acne conglobata 88.66
  biopsy 3.31
  classification of cutaneous cysts 133.1, **133.2**
  cutaneous 133.1–133.7
  cutaneous keratocysts 133.6–133.7
  cutaneous nodular elastosis with 156.4
  dermoid cysts, infants 115.12, 115.13
  epidermoid 78.11, 88.33–88.34, 133.1–133.3
  with infundibular epithelial walls 133.1–133.4
  with isthmic epithelial walls 133.4–133.6
  milia 133.4
  mucocele 57.15, 57.16, 108.12, 109.30, 110.31
  nodular elastosis with 156.5
  pachyonychia congenita 63.52
  preauricular cysts, infants 115.12
  with sebaceous duct epithelial walls 133.6–133.7
  trichilemmal cysts 105.11, 133.4–133.5, 133.6, 137.5–137.6
  see also chloracne; comedonal acne; cysts; dermoid cysts; metabolising acquired dioxin-induced skin hamartoma; vellus hair cyst
cytodiagnosis 3.29–3.30
cytokeratin markers, cutaneous neoplasms 3.21–3.22
cytokine directed biologic therapies 19.32–19.37
cytokine mediators, Adamantiades–Behçet disease 48.3
cytokine mutations, immunodeficiencies **149.20**
cytokines
  antigen-presenting cells 127.7
  bullous pemphigoid 50.12
  hormone relationship 150.3
  macrophage secretion 97.5–97.6
  morphoea 55.10
  pruritus **81.3**, 81.4–81.5
  radiation dermatitis 119.14
  wound healing **11.4**, **11.5**
cytomegalovirus (CMV) 25.41–25.42
  HIV 31.24–31.25, 31.38
  infiltrating lipomatosis of the face association 98.19
  oral ulceration 108.51
  perianal skin 111.15
cytophagic histiocytic panniculitis 97.61–97.63
cytoreductive treatment, for mastocytosis 46.10
cytotoxic agents 18.29–18.31
  cutaneous T-cell lymphoma therapy 139.25
  factitious panniculitis 97.48
  hypermelanosis 86.26, 86.28
  intralesional treatment of cutaneous warts 25.60
cytotoxicity, UVA-1 phototherapy 21.2
cytotoxic protein expression, primary cutaneous aggressive epidermotropic CD8+ T-cell lymphoma 139.31–139.32

cytotoxic T lymphocytes (CTLs)
   adipocytes interaction   97.6–97.7
   drug-induced   118.12
   macrophages interaction   97.6–97.7

D

dabrafenib   141.38
Dabska tumour *see* papillary intralymphatic angioendothelioma
dactylitis, psoriatic arthritis   35.41
DADA2 *see* deficiency of adenosine deaminase 2
DALY *see* disability adjusted life year
DALYs *see* disability adjusted life years
danazol   97.32
dandruff   40.1, 40.4
   Malassezia yeast   32.14
dapsone   19.12–19.15
   acne vulgaris treatment   88.46–88.47
   adverse effects   19.14–19.15
   dermatological uses   19.13
   dose and regimens   19.15
   hypersensitivity syndrome   14.6, 19.15
   pharmacological properties   19.13–19.14
   safety precautions   19.15
   topical therapies   18.11
daptomycin   19.47
DARE (database of abstracts of systematic reviews)   17.7
Darier disease   3.41, 69.23–69.24, 110.6
   biopsy   3.39
   male genitalia   109.25
   oral lesions   108.28
Darier's sign, mastocytosis   46.5
dark-field microscopy, syphilis   29.18
Darling disease *see* histoplasmosis
database of abstracts of systematic reviews (DARE)   17.7
databases of controlled clinical trials   17.6–17.7
data protection, computer-based assessments   16.2
daylight photodynamic therapy   22.11–22.12, 141.10–141.11
DC *see* dissecting cellulitis; dyskeratosis congenita
DCMO *see* diffuse capillary malformation with overgrowth
DCOIT *see* dichloro-octylisothiazolinone
DCPs *see* deep chemical peels
DCs *see* dendritic cells
deafness
   albinism with   68.9
   congenital syphilis   29.26
   mitochondrial keratoderma with   63.65
   otic syphilis   29.16
   palmoplantar keratodermas with   63.63–63.65
   systemic lupus erythematosus   51.32
   Waardenburg syndrome   68.5
debridement, pressure ulcers   123.10
deceptive behaviour, factitious skin disease   84.29–84.38
decision making, holistic management of skin disease   15.6, 15.7
decongestion therapy, lipoedema management   98.23
decorin   2.38
'decubitus ulcers'   123.1
dEDS *see* dermatosparaxis Ehlers–Danlos syndrome
deep ('aggressive') angiomyxoma   136.62
deep burn wounds   125.6, 125.8
deep chemical peels (DCPs)   160.5
deep fibromatoses   94.33–94.34, 94.35
deep folliculitis   91.8–91.15
deep morphoea   97.12–97.14, 97.30
   lupus panniculitis contrast   97.39, 97.64
deep partial-thickness burns   128.12
deep penetrating naevus (DPN)   142.2
deep perniosis   124.5
deep subcutaneous fat   97.3
deep-vein thrombosis (DVT)   101.31–101.34
   clinical features   101.32, **101.33**
   investigations   101.32–101.33
   management   101.33–101.34
   neoplasia association   148.26
   risk factors   **101.32**
   treatment   **101.34**
deer fly *see Chrysops*
deerfly fever *see* tularaemia
deficiency of adenosine deaminase 2 (DADA2)   **45.5**, **45.7**, 45.17
deficiency of interleukin 1 receptor antagonist (DIRA) syndrome   **45.5**, **45.6**, 45.12
deficiency of interleukin 36 receptor antagonist (DITRA)   45.12
deficiency states, oral features   108.70
degenerations
   dermal   3.40
   epidermal   3.40–3.41
degos acanthoma *see* clear cell acanthoma
Degos disease   99.21–99.22
dehydroepiandrosterone A (DHEA) supplements, acneform reaction   88.12
De Lange syndrome, oral involvement   108.85
delayed inflammatory reactions (DIRs), to COVID-19 vaccines   25.118
delayed pressure urticaria   **42.9**, 42.10
delayed reaction time, use of term   127.7
delayed tanning (DT), UV radiation exposure   10.8
delayed-type bacterial antigen tests   4.25
delayed-type stinging   128.10–128.11
deliberate self-harm   84.38–84.39
   with suicidal ideation   84.38
   without suicidal intent   84.38–84.39
deltanoids *see* vitamin D analogues
delusional beliefs
   Morgellons syndrome   84.11–84.12
   olfactory delusions   84.10–84.11
   psychodermatology   84.5–84.12
delusional disease by proxy, delusional infestation   84.5
delusional infestation (DI)   84.5–84.10
   associated diseases   **84.6**, 84.7
   clinical features   84.6–84.7
   complaints and litigation   84.9–84.10
   epidemiology   84.5–84.6
   investigations   84.7–84.8
   management   84.8–84.9
   pathophysiology   84.6
   thrip infestation confusion   34.30
demeclocycline, phototoxicity to   126.29
Demodex
   eosinophilic pustular folliculitis   93.7
   folliculorum infestation   107.10
   rosacea   89.3, 89.4–89.5, 89.10
dendrite surveillance extension and retraction cycling habitude (dSEARCH)   2.13
dendritic cells (DCs)
   allergic contact dermatitis   9.10
   dermal   2.15
   histiocytoses   135.1, 135.3
   immune system   9.3, 9.4
   subtypes   9.4–9.5
dendritic epidermal T cells (DETCs)   9.7
dendritic keratitis, eyelid   107.37
dendritic melanocytes, naevus of Ota   131.14
dendrocytes, immune system   9.5
dengue, oral involvement   108.50
dengue haemorrhagic fever   25.86–25.87
denileukin diftitox (DAB389–IL-2 fusion toxin - Onzar/Ontak), cutaneous T-cell lymphoma   139.25
Denmark, non-melanoma skin cancer, incidence of   6.1
de novo post-transplant melanoma   147.13
dental abscesses   108.9
dental amalgam, oral lichen planus   37.3
dental care, epidermolysis bullosa   69.25
dental malformations, ectodermal dysplasias   69.18
dental plaque   108.5
dental sinus, acne nodule distinction   88.38
dental treatments, amalgam fillings   121.6, 121.8
dentition loss, Papillon–Léfèvre syndrome   63.69
dentogingival junction, anatomy of   108.4
denture-induced hyperplasia   108.10
denture sore mouth/denture stomatitis   32.62, 108.20–108.21
depigmentation   86.8
   acquired hypomelanosis differentiation   86.42
   allergic contact dermatitis   127.20–127.21
   melasma   86.45
   see also hypopigmentation
depigmenting agents, topical therapies   18.31–18.33
depilatories   18.33
deposition disorders, internal malignancy association   148.22–148.23
depot technique, dermal filler injection   158.2–158.3
depressed plaques
   centrifugal lipodystrophy   98.13
   insulin injection   98.11
depression
   acne vulgaris   88.39
   antidepressants   84.43–84.44, **84.44**, **84.45**, 117.3
   assessment   84.41
   dermatological patients   84.40–84.42
   emotional effects of skin conditions   15.2
   isotretinoin acne treatment   84.42
   morphoea   55.29
   psoriasis   35.19
   types   84.40
depth dose curves
   electron beam therapy   24.1–24.2
   proton beam therapy   24.2
   superficial X-ray therapy   24.1
Dercum disease (adiposis dolorosa)   **72.10**, 98.16, 98.17–98.18
   benign symmetric lipomatosis contrast   98.16
   obesity association   98.17–98.18, 98.28
dermal artefact   84.33
dermal atypical smooth muscle tumour (leiomyosarcoma)   136.54–136.55
dermal burns   125.6
dermal connective tissue, acquired disorders of   94.1–94.58
dermal degenerations   3.40
dermal deposition disorders, internal malignancy association   148.22–148.23
dermal deposits   3.30–3.31, 3.44
dermal–epidermal basement membrane zone (BMZ)   2.21–2.22
   basement membrane collagen   2.22–2.23
   hemidesmosomes   2.25–2.26
   immunofluorescence staining   2.23
   laminins   2.23–2.25
   molecular components   2.21
   structural components   2.22
   transmission electron microscopy image   2.22
dermal erythropoiesis (blueberry muffin baby)   114.21
dermal fillers   158.1–158.12
   adverse reactions and treatment for   108.62, 158.8–158.12
      management plan for   158.9
   alginate filler   158.5
   antidotes   158.8
   arterial occlusion   158.10
      treatment for   **158.11**
   biodegradable fillers   158.3–158.7
   bovine collagen filler   158.5, 158.7–158.8
   calcium hydroxylapatite filler   158.5, 158.6–158.7
   canula injection   158.1–158.2, **158.3**, 158.4
   collagen-stimulating fillers   158.6–158.7
   combination fillers   158.7–158.8
   depot technique   158.2–158.3
   and different skin types   158.11–158.12
   fanning technique   158.2–158.3
   filler products   158.3–158.8
   human collagen filler   158.6
   hyaluronic acid filler   158.9
      immune response after   **158.11**
   hydroxyethlmethacrylate and ethylmethacrylate microspheres suspended in hyaluronic acid   158.8
   indications   158.1, **158.3**
   inert fillers   158.3–158.6
   injection errors   158.8
   medical emergency following adverse reaction   158.10, **158.11**
   multiple substance products   158.7–158.8
   needle injection   158.1–158.2, **158.3**, 158.4
   non-biodegradable fillers   158.7–158.8
   non-hyaluronic acid-based fillers   158.5–158.6
      immune response after   **158.11**
   polyacrylamides   158.7
   polyalkylamide   158.7
   polycaprolacton filler   158.6
   poly-L-lactic acid filler [replace capital L with small cap L**]   158.6
   polymethylmethacrylate and collagen   158.7–158.8
   porcine collagen filler   158.5–158.6
   risk assessment/reduction   158.9
   silicones   158.7
   single substance products   158.7
   techniques   158.1–158.3
      injection errors   158.8
   types of   **108.62**
dermal hyperneury   136.42–136.43
dermal infiltrate   3.44–3.45
dermal inflammatory infiltrate   126.3
   photothermal ablation   23.22
dermal leishmanoid *see* post-kala-azar dermal leishmaniasis
dermal mucin   94.44
dermal mucinoses   57.2–57.15, 57.16
dermal nerve sheath myxoma   136.47–136.48
dermal non-neural granular cell tumour   136.60
dermal papilla   87.5, 87.8, 87.11
dermal pigmentation, laser therapies   23.16–23.17
dermal plaque, sarcoidosis   96.8
dermal plaque-like fibromatosis *see* dermatomyofibroma
dermal sheath, hair follicle   87.5
dermal-subcutaneous interface   98.24, 98.25–98.26
dermal substitutes, burn treatment   125.6
dermatan sulphate (DS)   **2.39**
dermatitis
   chronic actinic   4.6
   financial cost of   7.2
   'flaky paint' dermatitis in kwashiorkor   61.4
   herpetiformis   4.8
   Wilkinson's triangle (chronic actinic dermatitis)   4.6
   see also allergic contact dermatitis; atopic eczema (dermatitis); contact dermatitis; eczema; hand eczema; irritant contact dermatitis; photoallergic contact dermatitis
dermatitis artefacta   84.29–84.36
   by proxy (witchcraft syndrome)   84.33
   clinical features   84.31–84.35
   epidemiology   84.30
   male genitalia   109.9
   management   84.35–84.36
   pathophysiology   84.30–84.31
   skin picking disorder relationship   84.19
Dermatitis Family Impact questionnaire (DFI)   16.8, 16.10
dermatitis gangrenosa infantum   26.88–26.89
dermatitis herpetiformis (DH)   50.54–50.59
   associated diseases   50.56
   coeliac disease   153.3

dermatitis herpetiformis (DH) (continued)
  direct immunofluorescence microscopy 3.18, *3.19*, *50.58*
  disease course and prognosis 50.57
  epidemiology 50.55–50.56
  genetics 50.56
  histopathology *50.58*
  internal malignancy association 148.22
  investigations 50.58
  management 50.58–50.59
  oral involvement 108.81
  pathophysiology 50.56
  presentation 50.56
  treatment ladder 50.59
dermatitis neglecta *see* dermatitis passivata
dermatitis passivata 84.36
dermatitis simulata 84.36
dermatitis veineuse *see* venous eczema
dermatochalasis 107.5
dermatoendocrinology 150.1–150.22
  biological basis 150.2–150.10
  clinical practice 150.10–150.21
  complexity of intraepithelial endocrine and neuroendocrine signalling milieu 150.8
  endocrinological considerations in skin therapy 150.12–150.14
  future perspectives 150.21
  key components in cutaneous (neuro-) endocrine signalling mechanism **150.4**
  (neuro-)endocrine contributions to cutaneous pathogenesis 150.5–150.8
  patient evaluation for (neuro-) endocrine disorders 150.10–150.15
  signs and symptoms
    general endocrine disease seen in skin **150.7**
    hormone-based skin disease **150.7**
    indicative of endocrine disease **150.10**, **150.11**
  skin and appendages as (neuro-) endocrine organs 150.3, **150.4**, 150.5
  skin and appendages as research models for general neuroendocrinology 150.9
  specific endocrine conditions 150.15–150.21
  stress responses 150.8–150.9
  see also endocrine disorders; hormones
dermatoepidemiology 5.1–5.2, 5.15–5.16
  see also epidemiology
dermatofibroma 4.19, 136.19–136.21
dermatofibrosarcoma protuberans (DFSP) 3.25, *3.26*, 24.15, 136.2, 136.14–136.15
dermatological pathomimicry 84.36
dermatology atlases 1.4
dermatology history 1.1–1.10
  ancient medical texts 1.1–1.3
  dermatology as global speciality in 20th century 1.7–1.10
  rational medicine, growth of 1.2–1.4
  scientific dermatology 1.4–1.7
Dermatology Index of Disease Severity 16.3
Dermatology Life Quality Index (DLQI/Skindex) 6.4, 15.3, 16.6–16.7, 35.17
  adolescents 16.10
  descriptive score bandings **16.7**
  questions **16.7**
  usage 16.3, 16.7, 16.8, 16.12
Dermatology Quality of Life Scales 16.7
dermatomycosis furfuracea *see* pityriasis versicolor
dermatomyofibroma 136.8
dermatomyositis-associated panniculitis 97.39, 97.40
dermatomyositis (DM) 52.1–52.13, 86.21, 89.8
  cardiac involvement 151.4
  clinical features 52.3–52.8
  clinical variants 52.8–52.10
  definitions 52.1
  differential diagnosis 52.10

dystrophic calcification 59.1–59.2
epidemiology 52.1–52.2
eye disease **107.35**
internal malignancy association 148.20–148.21
investigations 52.10–52.12
management 52.12, **52.13**
myositis-specific antibodies 52.2, 52.5, 52.6, 52.11
oral involvement 108.67–108.68
pathophysiology 52.2–52.3
respiratory disease 152.2–152.3
severity classification 52.10
dermatopathia pigmentosa reticularis 68.12
dermatopathology
  examinations/national societies for 3.1
  terminology 3.38–3.43
dermato-pharmacokinetic (DPK) method 12.8
Dermatophilus congolensis, pitted keratolysis 26.42–26.43
dermatophyte infection
  perineal and perianal skin 111.15
  in pregnancy 113.7
dermatophytes 32.6–32.69
  anthropophilic 32.19
  asexual–sexual states **32.18**
  classification 32.18, **32.19**, 32.22–32.30
  collecting material 32.7–32.8
  geophilic 32.19
  identification 32.6–32.10
  non-dermatophyte hyphal fungi 32.51–32.52
  Wood's light examination 32.6–32.7
  zoophilic 32.19
dermatophytide reaction (allergic response) 32.50
dermatophytosis 39.34
  biology 32.20–32.21
  co-morbidities 32.22
  epidemiology 32.22
  HIV 31.26–31.27
  identification 32.22–32.30
  immunity 32.21
  management 32.30–32.34
  pathophysiology 32.21–32.22
  preventing spread 32.30–32.32
  therapeutic agents 32.32–32.34
dermatophytosis (ringworm) 32.18–32.34
dermatoporosis 94.1, 156.11
dermatoscopy *see* dermoscopy
dermatoses
  bullous dermatosis *4.8*
  chronic superficial scaly dermatosis *4.17*
  flexural sites **4.18**
  malignancy association 148.19–148.20
  in occupational groups **4.4**
  pruritus in inflamed skin 81.7
  sun-related 7.8
dermatosis papulosa nigra (DPN) 132.4–132.5, *156.3*
dermatosparaxis Ehlers–Danlos syndrome (dEDS) **70.5**, 70.9
dermis 2.2
  anatomy 9.1
  chronological ageing/photoageing **10.10**
  collagen fibres *2.27*
  embryonic development 2.3, 2.5
  immune cells 9.4–9.6
  immune surveillance 2.15, *2.16*
  mechanical properties 122.5
  microvessels in *2.41*
dermographism, urticaria 42.9–42.10
dermoid cysts
  infantile 115.12, *115.13*
  mouth 108.12
  penis 109.31
dermopathy, diabetic 62.2
dermoscopy 4.20–4.21
  acquired and small congenital naevi 145.2, *145.3*, 145.4–145.6
  basal cell carcinoma 140.10, *140.11*
  benign patterns of naevi 145.1–145.7
  facial skin/chronically sun-damaged skin melanoma 145.9, *145.11*, **145.11**

intradermal naevi 145.6
melanoma diagnosis 142.9, 145.1–145.16
organised patterns in melanoma 145.13–145.14, *145.15*
Spitz naevi 145.6
volar skin of palms and soles (acral) melanoma 145.9, 145.11–145.13
deroofing, lesions 90.10
desert rheumatism *see* coccidioidomycosis
designated patient irradiance (DPI) 21.3
desmin 3.25
desmocollin 3 (*DSC3*) 69.7
desmoglein-1 (*DSG1*) 69.6
desmoglein 3 (*DSG3*) 69.7
desmoglein (DSG) autoantibodies 3.14, *3.21*
Desmons syndrome 63.35
desmoplakin 69.7
  mutations, Carvajal-Huerta syndrome 63.63
desmoplasia 3.41
desmoplastic basal cell carcinoma *see* morphoeic basal cell carcinoma
desmoplastic fibroblastoma 136.11–136.12
desmoplastic trichoepithelioma *73.7*, 137.10–137.11
desmosines 2.33, 2.34, *2.35*
desmosomal disorders 69.20
desmosomes 2.18–2.19, *2.19*, 63.57–63.58
desquamation, neonates 114.3–114.4
desquamative gingivitis 108.23, *108.82*
destructive/pro-inflammatory topical treatments, molluscum contagiosum infection 25.18
detached epidermis 118.14, 118.19
  Stevens–Johnson syndrome/toxic epidermal necrolysis *118.15*
DETCs *see* dendritic epidermal T cells
detergent acne 88.25
detergents
  alopecia management 87.98
  exposure regulations 127.2
  irritant properties 128.3
developing countries *see* low and middle income countries
developmental delay, atopic eczema association 41.21
dew itch *see* ancylostomiasis
dexpanthenol 127.59–127.60
DFI *see* Dermatitis Family Impact questionnaire
DFSP *see* dermatofibrosarcoma protuberans
DGEBF novolac resins *see* diglycidyl ether of bisphenol F resins
DH *see* dermatitis herpetiformis
DHA *see* dihydroxyacetone
DHEA *see* dehydroepiandrosterone A
dhobie itch *see* tinea cruris
DHT *see* dihydrotestosterone
DI *see* diabetes insipidus
diabetes 62.1–62.8
  acanthosis nigricans association 85.5
  acquired ichthyosis association 85.1–85.2
  acquired perforating dermatosis 94.53, *94.54*
  AGL association 98.2
  autoimmune disease 62.4
  bullae 62.7
  calluses 122.7
  cutaneous complications **150.11**
  dermopathy 62.2
  disease associations 62.4, *62.5*
  drug reaction with eosinophilia and systemic symptoms 118.9, 118.11
  eruptive xanthomas 62.3, *62.4*
  erysipelas-like reaction 62.2
  foot ulcer 62.2–62.3
  genetic syndromes 62.4–62.5
  granulomatous disorders 62.5
  hyperlipidaemia 62.3, *62.4*
  infections 62.3
  leg ulceration 62.1
  metabolic syndrome 62.4
  necrobiosis lipoidica *62.6*, 95.12
  neurological damage 62.2–62.3
  obesity association 62.3, 98.28

perforating collagenosis (folliculitis)4 *62.5*
pressure ulcers 123.4
pruritus 81.10
psoriasis association 35.18
retinopathy *62.5*
rubeosis 62.2
secondary dyslipidaemia 60.11
skin tags 62.3
stiff skin and joints 62.5–62.6
systemic allergic contact dermatitis 117.4
treatment-related skin manifestations 62.4
types of 62.1
vascular damage 62.1–62.2
wet gangrene of the foot 62.2
wound healing 11.9
see also insulin resistance
diabetes insipidus (DI), Langerhans cell histiocytosis 135.5, 135.8
diabetes mellitus *see* diabetes
diabetic bullae 62.7, 85.30
diabetic dermopathy 62.2
  brown pseudoscars *94.14*
diabetic foot ulcer 62.2–62.3
diabetic retinopathy *62.5*
diabetic scleroedema 57.9, 57.10, 62.5–62.6, *62.7*
diabetic thick skin 94.45
diacetylmorphine *see* heroin
diagnosis 4.1–4.27
  apps 4.26, 5.13
  artificial intelligence 4.26–4.27
  atopic eczema 5.4
  clinical investigations 4.19–4.20
  coding systems 4.2
  community diagnosis 5.2
  diascopy 4.19
  disease definition 4.1–4.2
  examination of skin 4.5
  fine-needle aspiration of lymph nodes 4.22
  fundamentals 4.1
  history taking 4.2–4.5
  imaging examination 4.22–4.23
  imaging systems 4.20–4.22
  lesions, description of 4.5–4.20
  microscopy 4.20–4.22
  mobile smartphone applications 4.26, 5.13
  palpation 4.17–4.18, *4.19*
  photography 4.19
  preimplantation genetic diagnosis 8.10–8.11
  prenatal diagnosis 8.9–8.11
  presenting complaint 4.2–4.5
  in primary and secondary care 5.13
  quality of life assessment 4.5
  radiological examination 4.22–4.23
  simple clinical examination 4.18
  skin testing 4.23–4.25
  smartphone apps 4.26, 5.13
  store-and-forward consultations 4.25–4.26
  teledermatology 4.25–4.26
  Wood's light 4.19–4.20
'Diagnostic Handbook', Mesopotamian 1.2
diagnostic test studies, critical appraisal for evidence based medicine 17.15–17.17
diaper area *see* nappy/diaper/napkin area
diascopy 4.19
diazolidinyl urea 127.51
DIC *see* disseminated intravascular coagulation
dichloro-octylisothiazolinone (DCOIT) 127.54
diclofenac 18.30
Dictyoptera (cockroaches) 34.32
diet
  and acne **88.20–88.24**, 88.26
  and atopic eczema 41.7
  diagnosis 4.4
  epidemiology 5.11
  and flushing **104.3**

low pseudoallergen diet **42.6**
seborrhoeic dermatitis 40.4
and urticaria **42.6**, 42.8
see also nutrition
dietary management
  allergic contact dermatitis 127.35, 127.38
  epidermolysis bullosa 69.25
  lipoedema 98.23
  Refsum disease 63.32
  Sjögren–Larsson syndrome 63.33
  subcutaneous fat disorders 98.26
  trimethylaminuria 92.18
DIF *see* direct immunofluorescence
differentiated vulval intraepithelial neoplasia (VIN) 110.34, 110.35
diffuse alopecia areata 87.23–87.24
diffuse alopecias 87.28–87.35, 87.64
diffuse arterial disease 124.9
diffuse capillary malformation with overgrowth (DCMO) 101.28
diffuse cutaneous mastocytosis 46.6
diffuse/disseminated cutaneous leishmaniasis 33.48–33.49
diffuse fibrosis, causes 94.33–94.48
diffuse keratodermas 63.50–63.51
  ectodermal dysplasias 63.68, *63.69*
  woolly hair 63.63
diffuse large B-cell lymphoma (DLBCL) 25.39
diffuse lymphangiomatosis 136.39
diffuse melanosis 86.20, 86.22
diffuse neurofibroma 136.46–136.47
diffuse pigmentation, arsenic exposure 121.3
diffuse reticular pattern naevi *145.2*, *145.3*, 145.4
diffuse telogen effluvium 87.54, *87.55*
diffusion enhancers, topical drug delivery 12.6
DiGeorge syndrome **80.4**, 80.8
digestive system disorders 153.1–153.9
digital clubbing, pachydermoperiostosis 155.14
digital fibromyxoma *see* acral fibromyxoma
digital ischaemia, internal malignancy association 148.24–148.25
digital mucous cyst 136.60
digital myxoid (mucous) cysts 57.15, *57.16*
digital necrosis, cannabis-induced 120.4
digital papillary adenocarcinoma 137.34–137.35
digital papular calcific elastosis 63.60
digital pathology 3.32
digital technology 1.9, 5.13
digital vasculitis, rheumatoid arthritis 155.6, *155.8*
digitate dermatitis *see* small plaque parapsoriasis
digitate hyperkeratoses 63.77
digitate lesions *4.17*
digits
  blistering distal dactylitis 26.34
  see also finger; toe
diglycidyl ether of bisphenol F (DGEBF novolac) resins 127.68
DIHS *see* drug-induced hypersensitivity syndrome
5α-dihydrotestosterone (DHT) 87.10
dihydroxyacetone (DHA) 18.39
dilated pore lesions, expanded follicular infundibulum 137.3
dimethylglyoxime test, nickel allergy 127.33, *127.34*
dimethylol dimethyl (DMDM) hydantoin 127.52
dimethyl sulfoxide (DMSO), irritant responses 128.3
dimeticone 18.14
dimorphic fungi, morphology and diseases **32.3**
dimples, commissural pit distinction 108.86
dinitrochlorobenzene (DNCB), allergic reactions 127.5–127.6
dioxin intoxication/poisoning

acne 88.68
acne vulgaris *88.15*
1,3-Diphenylguanidine (DPG) 127.63, *127.64*
diphtheria 26.38–26.39
diploid/triploid mosaicism **72.7**
Diplopoda (millipedes) 34.57
Diptera 34.6–34.13
  classification 34.6–34.8
  clinical features of bites 34.8–34.9
  myiasis 34.9–34.13
DIRA *see* deficiency of interleukin 1 receptor antagonist
direct immunofluorescence (DIF) 3.11–3.12, 3.17–3.19
  bullous pemphigoid 50.14
  connective tissue diseases 3.19
  dermatitis herpetiformis 3.18, *3.19*, *50.58*
  disease findings **3.17**
  epidermolysis bullosa acquisita 3.18, *3.19*, *50.35*
  lichen planus 3.18, *3.19*, 37.15
  linear IgA bullous dermatosis 3.18
  linear IgA disease *50.35*
  mucous membrane pemphigoid 107.28
  pemphigoid 3.17–3.18
  pemphigus 3.17, *3.18*, *50.3*, 50.7
  serration pattern analysis 3.17
direct tissue deformation damage, pressure ulcers 123.2
dirofilariasis 33.23–33.24
DIRs *see* delayed inflammatory reactions
disability, caused by skin disease 5.5–5.6
disability adjusted life years (DALYs) 5.6, 5.9, 6.3, 6.4, 7.2, 16.9
  acne vulgaris **88.5**
disappearing/vanishing/phantom bone disease 136.39
  see also Gorham syndrome; Gorham–Stout disease
discoid lesions *4.12*
discoid lupus erythematosus (DLE) 51.1–51.12, 87.43–87.44, *87.45*, 89.10, 97.38
  antimalarial treatment **51.11**
  associated diseases 51.2
  atrophy of the epidermis 51.2
  basal layer degeneration 51.2, *51.3*
  chilblain lupus 51.6–51.7, *51.9*
  clinical features 51.3–51.6
  clinical variants 51.6–51.9
  differential diagnosis 51.9–51.10
  disease course and prognosis 51.10
  disseminated DLE 51.4–51.6
  emerging therapies 51.12
  epidemiology 51.1–51.2
  genetics 51.3
  gyrate erythema *51.8*
  histology *51.2*, *51.3*, **51.3**
  inflammatory infiltrate *51.2*
  investigations 51.10
  lesion appearance *51.4*, *51.5*, *51.6*, *51.24*
  lichen planus 37.8, 37.16
  lip lesions 108.64
  localised disease 51.3–51.4
  lupus erythematosus profundus (panniculitis) 51.7–51.8, *51.9*
  lymphocytic infiltration *51.3*
  management 51.10–51.12
  oral agents in treatment of chronic DLE **51.11**
  oral involvement *108.78*, *108.79*
  pathology 51.2–51.3
  pathophysiology 51.2
  predisposing factors **51.2**
  rosaceous pattern *51.5*
  scarring 51.4, *51.5*, *51.7*, *51.8*
  severity classification 51.10
  stem cells *51.3*
  systemic lupus erythematosus relationship/comparison 51.6, *51.9*
discoid skin lesions
  diagnosis of **39.10**
  retinoid-induced *88.56*

discrete papular lichen myxoedematosus *57.6*, *57.7*
discrimination, institutionalised 1.9
disease, definition 5.4–5.5
disease associations 5.14
  epidemiology 5.11–5.12
disease burden, global 7.2
disease frequency 5.7–5.11, 5.14
disease-modifying antirheumatic drugs (DMARDs), morphoea treatment 55.38
disease transmission, arthropods 34.2, **34.3**
disfigurement 4.3, 5.5
disorders of sexual development (DSDs) 110.5
disperse dyes 127.65–127.66
displaced persons camps (DPCs) 7.13
  skin diseases diagnosed in **7.14**
dissecting cellulitis (DC) 87.50
  localised swellings over the crown *105.7*
  scalp 88.37, 105.7–105.8
disseminated blastomycosis 32.85
disseminated capillary malformation with overgrowth (DCMO) 71.7–71.8
disseminated disease
  Mycobacterium tuberculosis complex 27.11, 27.13, 27.17–27.18, 27.21, 27.32, 27.33, 27.34, 27.35–27.36, 27.38, 27.40, 27.44
  non-tuberculous mycobacteria 27.32–27.36, 27.38, 27.40–27.45
  skin involvement 135.6
disseminated gonococcal infection 30.2, *30.4*, 30.5–30.6
disseminated infundibulofolliculitis 91.14–91.15, 93.6–93.7
disseminated intravascular coagulation (DIC)
  haemorrhage in patients with 99.17
  neonatal purpura fulminans 114.21
disseminated palmoplantar porokeratosis 85.20, 85.22
disseminated superficial actinic porokeratosis (DSAP) 63.74–63.75, 85.20–85.22, 141.15–141.18
distal arthritis, in bowel-associated dermatitis–arthritis syndrome *49.16*
distal and lateral subungual onychomycosis (DLSO) 32.47
distal nose, actinic prurigo *126.11*
distal symmetrical polyneuropathy **83.9**
distichiasis, lymphoedema–distichiasis syndrome 151.2
dithiocarbamates 127.63, 127.64
dithranol 18.39–18.41
  psoriasis treatment 35.21
DITRA *see* deficiency of interleukin 36 receptor antagonist
DLBCL *see* diffuse large B-cell lymphoma
DLE *see* discoid lupus erythematosus
D-limonene 127.42–127.43
DLQI *see* Dermatology Life Quality Index
DLSO *see* distal and lateral subungual onychomycosis
DM *see* dermatomyositis
DMARDs *see* disease-modifying antirheumatic drugs
DMDM hydantoin *see* dimethylol dimethyl hydantoin
DM skin severity index (DSSI) 52.10
DMSO *see* dimethyl sulfoxide
DN *see* dysplastic naevi
DNA
  human genome sequencing 8.8–8.9
  methylation machinery 8.6
  mutations and disease 8.5–8.7
  prenatal diagnosis 8.9–8.11
DNA damage
  skin ageing 2.46
  tanning association 86.9
DNA photodamage, repair of 10.5–10.6
DNA repair disorders 76.1–76.12, **76.2**
  ataxia telangiectasia 76.10–76.11
  Cockayne syndrome 76.6–76.8

fanconia anaemia 76.11
inherited immunodeficiency **80.4–80.5**, 80.11
Muir–Torre syndrome 76.11
trichothiodystrophy syndrome 76.9–76.10
xeroderma pigmentosum 76.1–76.6
DNA sequencing, epidermolysis bullosa diagnosis 69.22–69.23
DNA viruses 25.6–25.78
  hepatitis 25.73–25.77
  herpesviruses 25.19–25.46
  human papillomaviruses 25.49–25.73, **25.50–25.51**
  parvoviruses 25.77–25.78
  pathogenesis 25.2, 25.5
  polyomaviruses 25.46–25.49
  poxviruses 25.6–25.19
DNCB *see* dinitrochlorobenzene
DNS *see* dysplastic naevus syndrome
docetaxol treatment, palmoplantar erythrodysaesthesia *119.2*
DOCK8 deficiency 80.9, *80.10*
documentation/record keeping
  biopsy information request form 3.4
  ethics and drug trial reporting 13.13
  histopathology skin report 3.38
  phototherapy 21.17
dog bites 130.6
'dog ear' repair 20.22, *20.23*
Doll, Sir Richard 5.1
dominant dystrophic epidermolysis bullosa 94.43
donation of medicines 7.13
donor transmitted melanoma 147.13–147.14
donovanosis (granuloma inguinale), perineal skin 111.17
dopaquinone 86.5
Doppler ultrasound 4.22, *101.4*, **101.4**
dorsal hands, neutrophilic dermatosis of 49.12, *49.13*
dorsal nose, actinic prurigo 126.10, *126.12*
dosimetry, UV radiation measurement 10.2
dots and globules dermoscopy patterns, melanoma 145.7
double lip 108.85
Dowling–Degos disease 68.13, 85.24
  vulval lesions 110.23
Down syndrome (trisomy 21) 74.1–74.2, **106.7**
  elastosis perforans serpiginosa 94.55, *94.56*
  hair loss presentation 87.20
  hidradenitis suppurativa association 90.2
  oral involvement 108.85
doxepin, urticaria treatment 42.19
DPCs *see* displaced persons camps
D-penicillamine, cutaneous adverse effects 155.15
DPG *see* 1,3-Diphenylguanidine
DPI *see* designated patient irradiance
DPK *see* dermato-pharmacokinetic method
DPN *see* deep penetrating naevus; dermatosis papulosa nigra
dracontiasis *see* dracunculiasis
dracunculiasis 33.12–33.13
  clinical features 33.13
  management 33.13
Dracunculus medinensis (dracunculiasis) 33.12–33.13
dragon worm *see* dracunculiasis
draining lesions, Hurley stage III disease *90.9*
draining tunnels, hidradenitis suppurativa *90.5*
DRESS *see* drug reaction with eosinophilia and systemic symptoms
dressings
  SJS/TEN treatment 118.19
  skin surgery 20.37–20.38, 20.41
'drip sign', intentional damage by corrosive liquids 84.32, *84.34*
drug actions, mechanisms underlying **13.4**, 13.5–13.6
  extracellular mechanisms 13.5

drug actions, mechanisms underlying (*continued*)
  intracellular mechanisms 13.5–13.6
  transmembrane mechanisms 13.5
drug allergens 127.4, 127.45–127.47, 127.54–127.58
  ano-genital region 127.16–127.17
  applied medicaments 127.45–127.47
drug-associated NEH 92.14–92.15
drug choice, and medical decision making 13.7
drug concentrations, topical therapies 18.1–18.2
drug delivery
  clinical pharmacology 13.2–13.3
  see also topical drug delivery
drug dependence, illicit drugs 120.1
drug development 13.11–13.13
  ethics and trial reporting 13.13
  preclinical drug identification 13.11–13.12
drug–drug interactions
  antibiotics with combined oral contraceptives 88.49
  antihistamines 19.4
  antimalarial agents 19.6
  azathioprine 19.9
  ciclosporin 19.11–19.12
  glucocorticoids 19.20
  hydroxycarbamide 19.22
  methotrexate 19.27
  mycophenolate mofetil 19.29
  pharmaceutical drugs with recreational drug 120.3
  polypharmacy 13.8
  retinoids systemic therapy 19.44
  tumour necrosis factor antagonist systemic therapy 19.34
drug hypersensitivity *see* immunological reactions to drugs
drug-induced hypersensitivity syndrome (DIHS) 118.5
drug injections, panniculitis 97.50
drug metabolism 13.3
drug reaction with eosinophilia and systemic symptoms (DRESS) 14.3–14.4, 14.7, 117.2, 118.1, 118.4–118.22
  musculoskeletal therapy effects 155.10, 155.15
drug reactions
  acanthosis nigricans 85.5
  acne vulgaris 88.11–88.14, **88.16**
  acrocyanosis 124.7
  anaphylaxis 117.5–117.7
  angioedema 117.5–117.7
  antiretroviral therapy 31.2, 31.8, 31.10, **31.13**, 31.19, 31.20
  benign cutaneous adverse reactions 117.1–117.9
  cheilitis 108.61
  chronic oedema 103.12–103.13
  clinical pharmacology 13.9
  dermatomyositis 52.9–52.10
  dermatoses, illicit drugs 120.4–120.6
  ear dermatoses **106.22**
  eczema 117.3–117.5
  erythema multiforme 47.3–47.4
  exanthems 117.1–117.2
  HIV
    antiretroviral therapy 31.2, 31.8, 31.10, **31.13**, 31.19, 31.20, **31.36**
    non-antiretroviral therapy 31.18–31.20, **31.36**
  hypermelanosis 86.25–86.31, 86.53–86.54
  hyperpigmentation
    laser therapies 23.17
    oral involvement 108.17
  hypertrichosis 87.86–87.87
  lichen planus 37.3
  lupus erythematosus 117.7–117.9
  male genitalia 109.24–109.25
  morphoea 55.14–55.15
  neutrophilic eccrine hidradenitislsquo 149.7

neutrophilic panniculitis 97.52, **97.53**
oedema 103.12–103.13
oral ulcers 108.41
pemphigus 50.4
perineal and perianal skin 111.12–111.13
pruritus 81.10–81.11, 117.2–117.3
psoriasis vulgaris 35.3–35.4
purpura **99.4**
scleroderma 94.45–94.46
seborrhoeic dermatitis 40.6–40.7
severe cutaneous adverse reactions 118.1–118.22
subacute cutaneous lupus erythematosus **51.13–51.14**
Sweet syndrome 49.8, 49.10–49.11, 149.6
systemic lupus erythematosus 51.21, **51.22**
systemic therapy 19.2
telogen effluvium 87.56
urticaria 42.5, 42.8, 117.5–117.7
see also adverse effects; cutaneous adverse drug effects; drug–drug interactions; immunological reactions to drugs
drug-related links between skin and liver **153.9**
drugs
  eccrine glands and 92.15
  and flushing **104.3**
  licensing procedures 13.11–13.13
  ocular complications of drug therapy 107.40–107.44
  photosensitivity 126.1, 126.27–126.32
  secondary dyslipidaemia due to 60.12
  toxicity and adverse effects 13.6, 13.9–13.11
  types of 13.1
  see also clinical pharmacology; narcotic drugs
drug services, psychosocial diseases 120.8
dry beriberi, vitamin B1 deficiency 61.14
dry skin *see* xerosis cutis
DS *see* dermatan sulphate
DSAP *see* disseminated superficial actinic porokeratosis
DSDs *see* disorders of sexual development
dSEARCH *see* dendrite surveillance extension and retraction cycling habitude
DSG *see* desmoglein autoantibodies
DSH *see* dyschromatosis symmetrica hereditaria
DSSI *see* DM skin severity index
DT *see* delayed tanning
Duane reaction syndrome **106.7**
Duckett Jones criteria, rheumatic fever diagnosis **47.11**
duckhunter's itch, *see also* cutaneous larva migrans
duck itch *see* cercarial dermatitis
Ducreyi disease *see* chancroid
DUH *see* dyschromatosis universalis hereditaria
Duhring, Louis 1.7
dumping syndrome flush **104.9**
Duncan disease *see* X-linked lymphoproliferative diseases
Dunnigan-type familial partial lipodystrophy (FPLD2) 98.9
dupilumab
  alopecia areata 87.35
  chronic actinic dermatitis 126.21
  systemic therapy 19.36
Dupuytren contracture (Dupuytren disease) *see* palmar fibromatosis
Durand–Nicholas–Favre disease *see* lymphogranuloma venereum
dutasteride 87.69, 87.96
DVT *see* deep-vein thrombosis
dye allergens 127.60–127.61, 127.65–127.67
  see also hair dyes
dyes
  antiseptic applications 18.38
  specimen preparation 3.5–3.6
dynein 86.4

dysaesthesia 83.7
  male genitalia 109.43–109.44
  neuropathic 83.5–83.6
dysaesthetic syndromes 82.1
  with/without neurological deficit **82.2**
  see also mucocutaneous pain syndromes
dyschromatoses 68.1, 68.14–68.15
dyschromatosis symmetrica hereditaria (DSH) 68.14–68.15
dyschromatosis universalis hereditaria (DUH) 68.15
'dyshidrotic' eczema 129.1
dyskeratosis 3.41
dyskeratosis congenita (DC) 67.12–67.15, 68.12, 75.1–75.4, **78.12**, **80.5**, 80.12, 148.14, 149.14
  causative genes and modes of inheritance **75.2**
  clinical features **75.2**, 75.3–75.4
  co-morbidities 75.4
  cutaneous changes 67.13
  genetics 75.1–75.3
  investigations and diagnosis 75.4
  leukoplakia development 75.3
  management 75.4
  oral lesions 108.29
  skin cancer 147.2
  see also puritic and dyskeratotic dermatoses
dyskeratotic follicular epithelium, necrotising lymphocytic folliculitis 93.4
dyslipidaemias
  cerebrotendinous xanthomatosis 60.10
  classification 60.1, **60.2**
  combined dyslipidaemia **60.2**, 60.8–60.9
  cutaneous features **60.2**
  hypercholesterolaemia **60.2**, 60.6–60.8
  hypertriglyceridaemias **60.2**, 60.9–60.10
  primary dyslipidaemias **60.2**, 60.6–60.10
  secondary dyslipidaemias **60.2**, 60.11–60.12
  sitosterolaemia 60.11
dyslipidaemic plane (planar) xanthomas 60.4–60.6
dysmorphic disorders *see* body dysmorphic disorder
dyspigmentation
  ageing of skin 156.2, 156.5
  chemotherapy-induced 119.8–119.11
  occupational 129.13–129.14
dysplasia 3.41
  ocular features **107.41**
  penis 109.38
dysplastic melanocytic naevi 131.41, 131.42
  histological criteria **131.43**
  microscopic images 131.45
dysplastic naevi (DN), as melanoma precursors 142.2–142.3
dysplastic naevus syndrome (DNS) 142.3–142.4, 142.7
  see also atypical/dysplastic naevus syndrome
dysproteinaemic purpura 99.6–99.7
dysthymia 84.40
dystonin epidermal isoform (BP230) (DST) 69.4
dystrophic anagen hairs 119.5
dystrophic calcification
  secondary to inflammatory disease/infections 59.1–59.3
  secondary to trauma or injection/infusion of calcium-containing materials 59.3
  secondary to tumours and genetic disease 59.3–59.4
dystrophic calcinosis, in systemic lupus erythematosus 51.28
dystrophic epidermolysis bullosa 69.2, 69.15–69.18
  cancer and 69.26–69.27
  connective tissue disorders 69.20
  diagnosis 69.21, *69.22*
  management 69.25–69.26

molecular-based approaches 69.18–69.19
systemic treatment 69.26
type VII collagen 69.5
dystrophy *see* fingernail dystrophy; nail dystrophy; toenail dystrophy

E
EAC *see* erythema annulare centrifugum; external auditory canal
ear 106.1–106.35
  ageing changes 106.7–106.8
  allergic contact dermatitis 127.15–127.16
  anatomy 106.1–106.2, *106.3*
  antiphospholipid antibody syndrome 99.18
  arterial blood supply 106.2
  arteriovenous malformation 71.11
  auricle
    ageing changes 106.7–106.8
    anatomy *106.1*, *106.3*
    basal cell carcinoma 106.21–106.27
    developmental anatomy *106.3*
    infections 106.19–106.21
    lumpy scalp syndrome 106.6
    melanoma of 106.31–106.33
    pre-auricular anomalies 106.6–106.7, *106.8*
    squamous cell carcinoma 106.27–106.29
    terminal hair *106.3*
    tumours of 106.21–106.35
    variations in shape of 106.5–106.6
  basal cell carcinoma of the auricle 106.21–106.27
  benign lesions 106.33
  cerumen (wax) 106.2–106.3
  cholesteatoma 106.21
  cicatricial pemphigoid *50.52*
  cryofibrinogenaemia 99.13
  developmental disorders 106.3–106.7
    low-set ears 106.5
    macrotia (large ears) 106.5
    microtia (small ears) 106.4, *106.5*
  discoid lupus erythematosus *51.5*, *51.7*
  earlobe creases 106.8
  elastotic nodules 94.3
  external auditory canal 106.1–106.3
    microbiome 26.5
    tumour management 106.29–106.31
  granuloma annulare 95.7
  ichthyoses 63.45
  infections 106.15–106.21
    otitis externa 106.15–106.19
    of the pinna 106.19–106.21
  inflammatory chondopathy effects 155.12
  involvement in skin disease and systemic disease 106.21, **106.22–106.23**
  keratosis obturans 106.21
  low-set ears 106.5
  macrotia (large ears) 106.5
  microbiology 106.2
  microtia (small ears) 106.4, *106.5*
  nerve supply *106.2*
  otomycosis 32.17–32.18
  perforating disorders **106.23**
  petrified ear 106.21
  physiology 106.1–106.2
  piercing
    keloids 106.14
    traumatic conditions 106.11–106.12
  premalignant lesions 106.33–106.34
  radiotherapy for skin cancer 24.11, *24.12*, *24.20*
  rheumatoid nodules *53.6*
  squamous cell carcinoma of the auricle 106.27–106.29
  systemic lupus erythematosus 51.32
  traumatic conditions 106.8–106.15
    chondrodermatitis nodularis 106.9–106.11
    contusion 106.8
    ear piercing 106.11–106.12
    haematoma 106.8
    keloids 106.14–106.15

pseudocyst 106.8–106.9
split earlobe 106.12–106.14
tympanic membrane 106.2
see also perioral area
ear canal samples, superficial mycoses identification 32.8
earlobe
creases 106.8
keloid 94.50
piercing 106.11–106.12
split earlobe 106.12–106.14
repair techniques 106.13
early adulthood, psychological and social factors 15.3
early detection strategies, melanoma 142.15–142.18
EASI see Eczema Area and Severity Index
eating disorders 84.26–84.27
and acne 88.30
cutaneous co-morbidities 84.27
oral lesions 108.83
EB see epidermolysis bullosa
EBA see epidermolysis bullosa acquisita
Ebers Papyrus 1.2
EBM see evidence based medicine
Ebola haemorrhagic fever 25.84–25.85
EBP gene
Conradi–Hünermann–Happle syndrome 63.22–63.23
MEND syndrome 63.23
EBS see epidermolysis bullosa simplex
EBV see Epstein–Barr virus
ECCA see Echelle d'évaluation Clinique des Cicatrice d'Acné
ecchymosis (bruises)
causes **99.2**, **99.5**
diagnosis by lesion size **99.3**
primary ecchymotic haemorrhage syndromes 99.4–99.7
scurvy *61.22*
trauma injury 99.6
see also purpura
ecchymotic lesions, Hermansky–Pudlak syndrome *68.8*
ECCL see encephalocraniocutaneous lipomatosis
eccrine angiomatous hamartoma 137.23
eccrine or apocrine/follicular carcinomas 137.35–137.40
eccrine or apocrine gland/follicular tumours 137.28–137.33
eccrine carcinoma, eyelid 107.49
eccrine dermal duct tumour 137.25
eccrine duct-blocking agents, hyperhidrosis 92.8–92.9
eccrine duct epithelium tumours, hidroacanthoma simplex 137.24–137.25
eccrine gland ablation, hyperhidrosis treatment 92.10
eccrine gland carcinomas 137.33–137.35
eccrine gland hamartomas and tumours 137.23–137.28
eccrine glands 2.2, 2.8–2.9, 92.1–92.4
disorders 92.4–92.15, **92.11**
drugs and 92.15
duct 92.2, 92.16
embryonic development 2.5
peptide histidine methionine immunoreactive fibres *83.4*
in pregnancy 113.2–113.3
tumours 137.2
vasoactive intestinal peptide immunoreactive fibres *83.4*
eccrine hidrocystoma 137.24
eccrine naevus *73.6*
eccrine poroma *4.13*, 137.25–137.26
see also hidroacanthoma simplex
eccrine spiradenoma see spiradenoma
eccrine sweating
control of 92.3–92.4
neonates 114.3
eccrine syringofibroadenoma 137.26
eccrine syringosquamous metaplasia 92.15
ECD see Erdheim–Chester disease

ECDS see en coup de sabre
Echelle de Cotation des Lésions d'Acné (ECLA) 16.4
Echelle d'évaluation Clinique des Cicatrice d'Acné (ECCA) 16.4
echinocandin antifungals 19.48
echinococcosis 33.31–33.32
clinical features 33.32
management 33.32
pathophysiology 33.31–33.32
Echinoidea, stings from 130.3
echoviruses 25.93–25.94
ECLA see Echelle de Cotation des Lésions d'Acné
ECM see extracellular matrix
economic burden of disease 5.6, 6.5–6.10
definition 6.1
skin cancer 6.5–6.8
ECP see extracorporeal photopheresis
ecstasy (MDMA) 120.2, 120.4
'ecstasy pimples' 120.4
ecthyma
management 26.17–26.18
pathophysiology 26.17
role of *Staphylococcus aureus* and *Streptococcus pyogenes* 26.17–26.18
ecthyma contagiosum see orf virus
ecthyma gangrenosum
ano-genital region 109.26, 111.15
neonates 114.27
Pseudomonas aeruginosa 26.51, 26.52–26.53
ectodermal dysplasias (ED), palmoplantar keratodermas in **63.65**, 63.68–63.70
ectodermal dysplasia–electrodactyly–macular dystrophy (EEM) syndrome 2.20
ectomesenchymal chondromyxoid tumour see cutaneous myoepithelioma
ectopic ACTH syndrome 148.17
ectopic calcification and abnormal mineralisation 70.31–70.36
fibrodysplasia ossificans progressiva 70.35
primary hypertrophic osteoarthropathy 70.35–70.36
pseudoxanthoma elasticum 70.31–70.35
ectopic disease, hidradenitis suppurativa association 90.6
ectopic glands 92.15
ectopic lesions, penis 109.6
ectopic plaque, axillae *90.7*
ectopic sebaceous glands 88.31
ectothrix type tinea capitis 32.38–32.39
eczema 39.1–39.7
acrodermatitis enteropathica 79.16
acute phase *39.2*, *39.3*, 39.4, 39.6
age and sex 39.2
allergic contact testing 1.8
asteatotic 39.9–39.12, 85.27, *85.28*, *85.29*, 85.30
associated diseases 39.10
clinical features and variants 39.11
craquelé appearance *39.11*
ear dermatoses **106.22**
environmental factors 39.11
management 39.11
pathology 39.10–39.11
predisposing factors 39.10
treatment 39.11
causative organisms 39.4
chronic *39.2*, *39.3*, 39.6–39.7
classification 39.1, **39.2**
clinical features 39.4–39.5
complications and co-morbidities 39.5, 127.22–127.23
conditioned hyperirritability 39.5
definition and nomenclature 39.1
discoid *4.12*
drug-induced 117.3–117.5
endogenous **39.2**
environmental factors 39.4, 39.11
epidemiology 39.1–39.2
exogenous **39.2**
genetics 39.4
house dust mites 34.51

investigations 39.5
male genitalia 109.11–109.13
management 39.6–39.7
patch testing 39.5–39.6
pathology 39.3–39.4
pathophysiology 39.3
psychological and social factors 15.4
secondary dissemination 39.4–39.5
severity classification 39.5
subacute *39.3*, 39.6
therapeutic agents **39.6**
treatment 39.7
unclassified 39.1
Wiskott–Aldrich syndrome *80.9*
see also atopic eczema; hand eczema; pompholyx eczema
Eczema Area and Severity Index (EASI) 16.3–16.4
eczema coxsackium 25.44, 25.94
eczéma craquelé see eczema, asteatotic
eczema herpeticum 25.43–25.46, *108.53*
and atopic eczema 41.10, *41.20*
clinical features 25.44–25.46
management 25.46
pathophysiology 25.44
eczema marginatum see tinea cruris
eczematous cheilitis 108.61
eczematous dermatoses
contact dermatitis distinction 129.6
scrotum 109.11
eczematous disorders 39.1–39.36
apron eczema 39.14, *39.15*
assessment, investigation and management 39.1–39.24
chronic acral dermatitis 39.14–39.15
chronic superficial scaly dermatitis 39.27
discoid skin lesions, diagnosis of **39.10**
erythroderma 39.31–39.35
eyelid eczema 39.22–39.23
fingertip eczema 39.15
'gut'/slaughterhouse eczema 39.15–39.16
halo dermatitis 39.28
hyperkeratotic palmar eczema 39.14
infective dermatitis 39.24–39.26
juvenile plantar dermatosis 39.23–39.24
lichenification 39.28–39.31
lichenoid chronic dermatitis 39.8, *39.9*
lichen simplex 39.28–39.31
lower leg eczema 39.19–39.22
Murray Williams warts 39.28
nummular dermatitis 39.7–39.9, **39.10**
patchy vesiculosquamous eczema 39.16
pityriasis alba 39.26–39.27
pompholyx eczema 39.14
recurrent focal palmar peeling 39.16
ring eczema 39.16
see also atopic eczema; eczema; hand eczema
eczematous skin diseases
primary immunodeficiencies 149.19–149.20
xerosis cutis in 85.26
eczema vaccinatum 25.44
ED see ectodermal dysplasias
EDC see epidermal differentiation complex
EDS see Ehlers–Danlos syndromes
education, see also patient education
educational partnerships 7.1–7.2, 7.14
see also training programmes/resources
education of general public, early melanoma detection 142.18
Edwards syndrome 74.2
Edwards syndrome (trisomy 18) 74.2
EECDRG see European Environmental and Contact Dermatitis Research Group
EEC syndrome **106.7**
EED see erythema elevatum diutinum
EEM see ectodermal dysplasia–electrodactyly–macular dystrophy syndrome
EFAD see essential fatty acid deficiency
EFFC see erythromelanosis follicularis faciei et colli
efficacy, influences on topical therapies 18.2

EGFR see epidermal growth factor receptor
EGPA see eosinophilic granulomatosis with polyangiitis
Egypt, ancient medical texts 1.2
eHFSCs see epithelial HF stem cells
Ehlers–Danlos syndromes (EDS) 70.1–70.11
arthrochalasia type **70.4**, 70.9
atrophic scars 94.13
Beighton score **70.8**
brittle cornea syndrome **70.6–70.7**, 70.10
cardiac-valvular type **70.3**, 70.9
classical 70.2, **70.3**, *70.8*, 70.9–70.10
clinical variants 70.2–70.10
cutis laxa 94.22
dermatosparaxis type **70.5**, 70.9
diagnostic clinical criteria **70.3–70.7**
differential diagnosis 70.10
elastosis perforans serpiginosa 94.55, *94.56*
epidemiology 70.1
hypermobility type 70.2–70.8, **70.3**
inheritance mode **70.3–70.7**
investigations 70.10–70.11
kyphoscoliotic type **70.4**, 70.9
lax skin 94.27
management 70.11
molecular defect **70.3–70.7**
molecular subtypes **70.3–70.7**
musculocontractural type **70.6**, 70.9
myopathic Ehlers–Danlos syndrome **70.7**, 70.10
pathophysiology 70.2
periodontal Ehlers–Danlos syndrome **70.5**, *70.10*
piezogenic pedal papules 122.26
in pregnancy 70.11, 113.9
spondylodysplastic type **70.5–70.6**, 70.9
ultrastructural findings **70.3–70.7**
vascular type **70.4**, 70.8–70.9, 70.11
Ehrlichia, tick-borne zoonotic infection 26.66–26.67
ehrlichiosis 26.66–26.67
Ehrlich, Paul 1.7
eighth nerve deafness (neurolabyrinthitis), congenital syphilis 29.26
Ekbom disease see delusional infestation
EKV see erythrokeratoderma variabilis
elastic fibres 2.2, 2.32–2.33
assembly and cross-linking 2.35
degradation disorders 2.34–2.35, 94.21–94.32
genetic disorders 70.14–70.21
cutis laxa 70.14–70.17
Marfan syndrome 70.20–70.21
Michelin tyre baby syndrome 70.19, 73.17
Williams–Beuren syndrome 70.18–70.19
transmission electron microscopy image 2.34
elastic tissue deposition, acquired disorders 94.32–94.33
elastin 2.33–2.35
collagen interdependence 122.5
gene mutations 2.33–2.34
elastin-associated microfibrils 2.35–2.36
elastin degradation, UV radiation exposure 10.10–10.11
elastinopathies 70.14–70.19
cutis laxa 70.14–70.17
Michelin tyre baby syndrome 70.19
Williams–Beuren syndrome 70.18–70.19
elastoderma 94.33
elastofibroma dorsi 94.33, 136.10
elastogenesis 94.32
elastolytic conditions 94.27–94.30
elastolytic giant cell granuloma 94.27–94.29
elastorrhexis 94.31
annular elastolytic giant cell granuloma 94.29
elastosis perforans serpiginosa *4.11*, 63.76, 94.30, 94.55–94.57
renal failure and dialysis complications 154.3–154.4
elastotic degeneration 3.40

elastotic marginal plaques of the hands 94.4–94.5
elastotic nodules of the ear 94.3
elbow
   atrophic scarring, classical Ehlers–Danlos syndrome 70.8
   dermatitis herpetiformis 4.8
   lichenification of 39.30
   mixed connective tissue disease 53.4
   rheumatoid nodules 53.5
   Rothmund–Thomson syndrome 75.5
   tufted angioma 116.11
   xanthoma excised from 60.3
elderly people
   chronic wounds, incidence of 6.1
   microbial ecology of the skin 26.4
   pityriasis rubra pilaris 36.4
   psoriasis vulgaris 35.15
   psychological and social factors at older age 15.3
   systemic lupus erythematosus 51.32
   wound healing 11.10
electrocautery 20.42–20.43
electrochemotherapy (ECT) 20.48
   basal cell carcinoma 140.17
   melanoma 144.2
electrocoagulation 20.44
electrodesiccation 20.44
electrofulguration 20.44, 20.45
electromagnetic muscle stimulation (EMMS) 161.8
electromagnetic spectrum 10.1
electron beam therapy 24.1–24.2
   see also total skin electron beam therapy
electronic health records 5.11–5.12
electronic records
   disease outcome measurements 16.2
   see also computer-based assessments
electron microscopy 3.30–3.31
   amyloidoses 56.5, 56.6
   biopsy 3.4
   epidermis image 2.6
   epidermolysis bullosa diagnosis 69.21–69.22
   see also transmission electron microscopy
electrosection 20.44–20.45
electrosurgery 20.42–20.46
   characteristics 20.43
   effects 20.44–20.45
   equipment 20.43–20.44
   hazards and risks 20.45–20.46
   hidradenitis suppurativa treatment 90.11
   terminology 20.43
Elejalde syndrome 68.9
elephantiasis, ear dermatoses **106.22**
elephantiasis nostra verrucosa (ENV) 103.6
elephantine psoriasis 35.14
elicitation 127.6–127.7
elimination of a drug, clinical pharmacology 13.3–13.4
ELISA see enzyme-linked immunosorbent assay
elliptical surgical biopsy 3.3, 3.6
   principles 20.8–20.9
   technique 20.11–20.12
ELOVL4 deficiency 63.35
EM see erythema multiforme
EMA see epithelial membrane antigen
emapalumab 135.13–135.14
EMBASE (Elsevier's biomedical database) 17.7
embedding procedure, tissue processing 3.7
Emberger syndrome 103.25
emboli, purpura 99.14–99.19
embolic metastasis to digits 148.5, 148.6
embryonic development of skin 2.3–2.5
embryos, wound healing 11.2, 11.10
emergency treatment, burn injuries 125.1–125.2
Emergomyces infections, rare endemic mycoses 32.90
EMM see erythema multiforme major
EMMS see electromagnetic muscle stimulation

emollients 12.3, 18.3–18.4, 18.8–18.9
   atopic eczema treatment 41.26, 41.27
   ichthyoses management 63.42, **63.43**, 63.44
emotional disturbances, necrotising lymphocytic folliculitis 93.4
emotional sweating 2.9
emotions
   links to beliefs and behaviours 15.1–15.3
   psychological factors in patients 15.2
EMPD see extramammary Paget disease
emperipolesis, sinus histiocytosis with massive lymphadenopathy 135.27
emulsifiers, topical medication vehicles 18.5, 18.7
emulsions, topical drugs 12.3–12.4
EN see erythema nodosum
encephalitis, herpes simplex virus 25.23
encephalocraniocutaneous lipomatosis (ECCL) **72.10**, 98.20–98.21, 98.25
enchondromas, Maffucci syndrome 71.20
ENCODE see Encyclopedia of DNA Elements
en coup de sabre (ECDS) 87.52
   morphoea 55.23–55.24
Encyclopedia of DNA Elements (ENCODE) Project 8.1–8.2
endemic mycoses
   rare, systemic *Emergomyces* infections 32.90
   rare systemic *Emergomyces* infections 32.90
endemic (non-venereal) treponematoses 26.69–26.72
endemic relapsing fever, *Borrelia* spp. 26.72
endemic syphilis (bejel) 26.70
endocrine disorders 150.1–150.22
   causes 150.2
   hirsutism 87.91
   hypermelanosis 86.17–86.19
   lipodystrophy 98.8
   oral involvement 108.83
   signs and symptoms of general endocrine disease seen in skin **150.7**
   specific endocrine conditions 150.15–150.21
   tuberous sclerosis complex 78.9
   see also dermatoendocrinology; hormones
endocrine dysregulation, obesity 98.27–98.28
endocrine factors
   melanocyte regulation 86.7
   pigmentation regulation 86.5–86.7
endocrine mucin-producing sweat gland carcinoma 137.39
endocrine system
   drug reaction with eosinophilia and systemic symptoms 118.9
   nervous system relationship 150.2
endocrine therapies, hair loss 87.73
endocrinology
   principles 150.2–150.3
   role of skin and hair follicles 150.3
   signalling axes 150.2
   see also dermatoendocrinology
endocrinopathy
   acquired ichthyosis association 85.1
   chronic mucocutaneous candidiasis 32.68
endogenous eczema, contact dermatitis distinction 129.6
endogenous non-melanin pigmentation 86.47–86.51
endogenous ochronosis 86.50–86.51
endo-MT see endothelial-to-mesenchymal transition
endonyx onychomycosis 32.48
endophytic seborrhoeic keratosis see inverted follicular keratosis
endoplasmic reticulum (ER) 63.21
endothelial cells 2.40, 2.41, 2.42
   Adamantiades–Behçet disease 48.3–48.4
   microscopic examination of 3.37
   wound healing 11.6
endothelial-to-mesenchymal transition (endo-MT), systemic sclerosis 54.10

endothelin-1 86.10
   pruritus **81.3**, 81.5
endothelins 86.7
endothrix infection, periodic acid–Schiff stain 3.8
endotoxin exposure, and atopic eczema 41.8
endovascular lymphatic angioendothelioma see papillary intralymphatic angioendothelioma
energy fluence of lasers, selective photothermolysis 23.5
energy homeostasis, adipose tissue 97.4
England, skin cancer, economic burden of 6.5–6.6, **6.7**
enhancers, topical drug delivery 12.5–12.6
ENKTCL-NT see extranodal NK/T-cell lymphoma, nasal type
ENL see erythema nodosum leprosum
The Enlightenment 1.3–1.4
Entamoeba histolytica, amoebiasis 33.36–33.38
enterobiasis 33.14–33.15
   clinical presentation 33.15
   definition/nomenclature 33.14
   epidemiology 33.14
   management 33.15
   pathophysiology 33.14–33.15
Enterobius vermicularis 33.14–33.15
enteroviral vesicular stomatitis with exanthem see hand, foot and mouth disease; herpangina
enterovirus infections 25.93–25.96
   oral involvement 108.50
ENV see elephantiasis nostra verrucosa
envenomation see venoms
environmental acne see occupational acne
environmental allergens 127.4
environmental and drug-induced scleroderma 94.45–94.46
environmental factors
   acne 88.18–88.26
   arthropod exposure 34.2–34.3
   atopic eczema 41.6–41.9
   congenital melanocytic naevi 73.11
   eczema 39.4, 39.11
   epidemiology of skin disease 5.10–5.11
   generalised pustular psoriasis 35.32–35.33
   lichen planus 37.2–37.3
   melanoma 142.5–142.6
   neonatal lupus erythematosus 51.40
   nummular dermatitis 39.8
   palmoplantar pustulosis 35.37
   pemphigus 50.3–50.4
   psoriasis vulgaris 35.3–35.4
   pyoderma gangrenosum 49.4
   rural and urban environments 41.6–41.7, 41.8
   scleroderma 94.45–94.46
   seborrhoeic dermatitis 40.4, 40.7
   Sweet syndrome 49.10–49.11
   systemic lupus erythematosus 51.21
   systemic sclerosis 54.14–54.15
   urticaria 42.7
environmental mycobacteria see non-tuberculous mycobacteria
enzymatic fat necrosis 97.8, 97.42
enzyme-linked immunosorbent assay (ELISA) 3.16, 3.20–3.21
EORTC see European Organization of Research and Treatment of Cancer
EORTC QLQ-C30 see European Organisation for Research and Treatment of Cancer Core Questionnaire
eosinophilia
   drug reaction 118.1, 118.4–118.12
   gold toxicity 121.4
   HIV primary infection 31.7–31.8
eosinophiliamyalgia syndrome 94.30
eosinophilic cellulitis (Wells syndrome) 47.16
eosinophilic fasciitis (Shulman syndrome) **54.20**, 55.2, **55.3**, **55.4**, 55.21–55.23, 55.22, **55.27**, 97.13
eosinophilic folliculitis, HIV 31.17

eosinophilic globules 3.42
eosinophilic granulomatosis with polyangiitis (EGPA) 100.25–100.28, 152.3–152.4
eosinophilic pustular folliculitis 91.3–91.5, 93.7–93.10, 115.12
eosinophils
   lupus panniculitis 97.37–97.38
   microscopic examination of 3.35–3.36
EPDS see erosive pustular dermatosis of the scalp
ephelides 78.3, 86.2, 86.15–86.16, 131.1–131.3
   epidermis of 131.2
   hyperpigmentation 131.2
   melanoma risk 142.3
   oculocutaneous albinism 68.8
epidemic arthritic erythema see *Streptobacillus moniliformis*
epidemic polyarthritis see Ross River virus
epidemic typhus
   human body louse transmitted rickettsial infection 26.80–26.81
   rodent flea transmitted rickettsial infection (murine typhus) 26.81
epidemiology of skin disease 5.1–5.17
   association and causation 5.7–5.10
   burden of skin disease 5.5, 5.6–5.7, 5.8, 5.9
   causative agents of disease 5.8–5.10
   chronicity of disease 5.10
   clinical epidemiology 5.1
   community diagnosis and control 5.2
   comparisons and inferences 5.3
   continuum of disease 5.2–5.3
   definition 5.1
   dermatoepidemiology 5.1–5.2, 5.15–5.16
   diagnostic criteria 5.4
   dietary factors 5.11
   digital technologies 5.13
   disease associations 5.11–5.12, 5.14
   disease definition 5.4–5.5
   disease frequency 5.7–5.11, 5.14
   disease severity assessment 5.5
   early and later environment 5.10–5.11
   electronic health records 5.11–5.12
   epidemiological studies 5.15
   ethnicity 5.10
   genetic epidemiology 5.10
   Global Burden of Disease study 5.6–5.7, 5.8, 5.9
   health services research 5.12–5.14
   impairment, disability and handicap caused by disease 5.5–5.6
   incidence of disease 5.10, 5.14
   interpretation of results 5.14–5.15
   leisure factors 5.11
   medical need/supply and demand relationship 5.13–5.14
   and migration 5.10
   natural history of skin diseases 5.11–5.12
   needs assessments 5.12
   occupational groups 5.11
   population approach 5.2–5.4, 5.5
   prevalence of disease 5.10, 5.14
   prevention paradox 5.3–5.4
   public health approach 5.2, 5.4–5.7
   regional distribution of burden of disease 5.9
   relevance to dermatology 5.1–5.2
   risk factors 5.7–5.10, 5.14
   skin diseases as 'entities' in population 5.2–5.3
   Snow's epidemiological research 5.9–5.10
   socioeconomic factors 5.10–5.11
   terminology 5.14–5.15
   validity and repeatability 5.15
epidermal cysts
   formation, foreign body reactions 122.17
   vulva **110.32**
epidermal degenerations 3.40–3.41
epidermal detachment, in SJS/TEN 118.17, 118.20
epidermal differentiation complex (EDC) 2.7

epidermal dysplasia, photothermal ablation 23.21
epidermal growth factor receptor (EGFR) 87.73
epidermal growth factor receptor (EGFR) inhibitors 119.3–119.5, 119.7–119.8
　acneform reaction 88.14, *88.16*
epidermal growth factor receptor (EGFR) signalling 2.4
epidermal hyperplasia, calluses 122.7
epidermal inclusion cysts *see* epidermoid cysts
epidermal keratinisation, acquired disorders 85.1–85.31
epidermal keratins 63.13–63.18
epidermal lesions 3.44
epidermal melanin pigments **86.5**
epidermal melanin unit 86.2–86.3
epidermal naevi **73.2, 73.3**, *73.4*
　see also congenital epidermal naevi
epidermal necrosis *118.13–118.14*
epidermal neoplasia, photothermal ablation 23.21
epidermal pigmentation, Q-switched laser treatments 23.12–23.17, *23.18*
epidermal spongiosis, chronic actinic dermatitis 126.14, *126.15*
epidermal thickening, palmoplantar keratodermas 63.49
epidermis 2.1, *2.2*
　anatomy 9.1, *9.2*
　chronological ageing/photoageing 10.10
　cornified cell envelope *2.7*
　dendritic epidermal T cells 9.7
　desmosomes 2.18–2.19
　differentiation *2.6, 2.7*, 2.8
　electron micrograph *2.6*
　embryonic development 2.3
　granular layer 2.5–2.6
　hyperproliferation 2.8
　immune cells 9.3–9.4
　lipids *2.8*
　Merkel cells 2.2, 2.11–2.12
　mesenchymal cells 2.4
　nail bed 2.11, 119.7
　stem cell proliferation *2.43*, 2.44
　stratum basale 2.5
　stratum corneum 2.1, 2.6
　stratum lucidum 2.7
　structures of 2.5–2.7
　substance P immunoreactive nerve endings in *83.3*
epidermodysplasia verruciformis (EV) 2.13, 25.65–25.66, **25.67**, 25.69–25.71
　classical/non-classical types 25.66, 25.69
　clinical features 25.69, *25.70*
　management 25.69–25.70
　pathophysiology 25.66, 25.69
　skin cancer 147.1–147.2
　see also acquired epidermodysplasia verruciformis
epidermoid cysts 78.11, 88.33–88.34, 133.1–133.3
　epidemiology 133.1
　management 133.2–133.3
　pachyonychia congenita *67.11*
　pathophysiology/clinical features 133.2
　sebaceous duct epithelial walled cutaneous cysts 133.6–133.7
　surgical treatment 20.49
epidermolysis
　with glycolic acid peel *160.9*
　use of term 69.2
epidermolysis bullosa (EB) *8.8*, 8.10, 69.1–69.28, 94.43, 110.5
　clinical subtypes 69.8–69.11
　diagnosis 69.20–69.23
　digestive system 153.6
　friction blisters 122.10
　genes implicated in 69.2–69.8
　genito-urinary involvement 154.6
　innovative therapies 69.27–69.28
　oral involvement 108.23
　proteins implicated in 69.2–69.8
　sweat glands 92.8
　treatment 69.24–69.28
epidermolysis bullosa acquisita (EBA) 50.42–50.48
　associated diseases 50.43
　in childhood *50.45, 50.46*
　clinical features 50.44–50.46
　clinical variants 50.46
　diagnosis *50.24*
　differential diagnosis 50.46
　direct immunofluorescence findings 3.18, *3.19, 50.35*
　epidemiology 50.43
　IgA EBA 50.36
　inflammatory variant *50.45, 50.46*
　internal malignancy association 148.22
　investigations and diagnosis 50.46–50.47
　management 50.47–50.48
　mechanobullous variant *50.44, 50.45*
　oral involvement 108.81
　pathophysiology 50.43–50.44
　perioral crusts and erosions *50.46*
　treatment ladder 50.48
　vulval **110.21**
epidermolysis bullosa simplex (EBS) 2.8, 69.2, 69.8–69.11
　management 69.25
　molecular pathology 69.11–69.15
epidermolytic hyperkeratosis 3.41, *63.16–63.17*
epidermolytic ichthyosis 63.14–63.16
epidermolytic palmoplantar keratoderma (EPPK) 63.50–63.51
epidermophytide, dermatophytide reaction 32.50
Epidermophyton, dermatophytosis 32.18, **32.19**, 32.21, 32.30, *32.32*
Epidermophyton floccosum **32.19**, 32.21, 32.30, *32.32*
epigenomics 8.6
epiluminescence microscopy *see* dermoscopy
epinephrine, urticaria treatment 42.18
episcleritis, BADAS-associated *49.17*
episodic angio-oedema with eosinophilia syndrome (Gleich syndrome) 43.4–43.5
Epistemonikos, finding systemic reviews 17.7
epithelial cysts *see* epidermoid cysts
epithelial HF stem cells (eHFSCs) 87.4
epithelial keratinocyte necrosis, drug-induced 118.12
epithelial markers, cutaneous neoplasms 3.21–3.23
epithelial membrane antigen (EMA) 3.22
epithelial necrolysis, acute SJS/TEN 118.17
epithelial sheath neuroma 136.50
epithelial stem cells *2.43*
　inflammatory memory 9.9
epithelioid angiosarcoma 136.37
epithelioid (bacillary) angiomatosis, oral infection 108.55
epithelioid haemangioendothelioma 136.36–136.37
epithelioid haemangioma 136.27–136.28
epithelioid sarcoma 97.15, 136.63–136.64
Epithelioid sarcoma-like haemangioendothelioma *see* composite haemangioendothelioma
epithelioma adenoides cysticum *see* trichoepithelioma
epithelioma cuniculatum (verrucous carcinoma of the foot) 141.31, **141.32**
epithiloid fibrous histiocytoma 136.20–136.21
epoxy resin, allergic contact dermatitis *127.14*, 127.68–127.69
EPP *see* erythropoietic protoporphyria
EPPK *see* epidermolytic palmoplantar keratoderma
Epstein–Barr virus (EBV) 14.4, 25.36–25.39, 126.25, 135.11
　angioimmunoblastic T-cell lymphoma 139.45
　CD30+ lymphoproliferative disorders 139.26
　diffuse large B-cell lymphoma 25.39
　extranodal NK/T-cell lymphoma (nasal type) 139.36–139.37
　lymphomatoid granulomatosis 139.44
　lymphoproliferative disorders and malignancy 25.38–25.39
　oral involvement 108.32, 108.51
　post-transplant lymphoproliferative disorder 139.47
Epstein pearls, neonates 114.4
equestrian cold panniculitis *97.35*, 97.36, *97.37*
equestrian panniculitis 124.6
equine disease, glanders 26.55
Er:YAG, photothermal ablation 23.21
Er:YAG lasers, skin resurfacing 161.1–161.3, **161.5**
ER *see* endoplasmic reticulum
erbium:yttrium-aluminium-garnet (Nd:YAG) lasers
　absorption spectra *23.4*
　tattoo removal 23.15
　vascular lesions 23.7, 23.10
Erdheim–Chester disease (ECD) 135.21–135.22
　BRAF V600E mutation 135.9
erectile dysfunction, systemic sclerosis 54.28
erethism 121.6
erisipeloid 26.46–26.48
erlotinib, papulopustular eruptions 119.3, 119.4
erosions, oral ulceration 108.36
erosive adenomatosis of the nipple *see* nipple, adenoma
erosive pustular dermatosis of the scalp (EPDS) 105.13–105.14
erosive skin fragility disorders 69.20
erucism *see* caterpillar dermatitis
eruption cyst, over a primary tooth 108.10
eruptions
　diagnosis 4.3
　quinine-induced photo-lichenoid eruption *4.7*
　see also lesions
eruptive inflammatory psoriasis *see* unstable psoriasis
eruptive lentiginoses 86.17
eruptive melanocytic naevi 147.14
eruptive pseudoangiomatosis and eruptive hypomelanosis 25.123
eruptive vellus hair cyst 137.8
eruptive xanthomas 60.4
　diabetic patients 62.3, *62.4*
erysipelas 103.13–103.14, 106.19
　definition and relationship to cellulitis 26.18
　eyelid 107.38
　sclerosing panniculitis differentiation 97.32
erysipelas-like changes in skin, carcinoma erysipeloides 148.2–148.3, *148.4*
erysipelas-like reaction, diabetes mellitus 62.2
Erysipelothrix rhusiopathiae 26.46–26.48
erythema (redness)
　acne vulgaris *88.27, 88.29*
　atopic eczema *41.15*
　chemical peels, side effect of 160.11–160.12
　chronic venous insufficiency **101.43**
　dermatomyositis 52.3, 52.4, *52.5, 52.6*
　differential diagnosis 89.7
　disease course 89.11
　drug/chemical photosensitivity *126.29*
　epidermolysis bullosa acquista *50.45*
　grading of in psoriasis vulgaris **35.17**
　hereditary angio-oedema *43.4*
　indicator of pressure ulcers 123.4
　irritant contact dermatitis 128.6
　laser therapies 23.9–23.11, *23.12, 23.13*
　lichen planus *110.12*
　linear IgA disease *50.37*
　morphoea *55.18*
　non-blanchable 123.4, **123.5**, 123.8
　transient *see* flushing
　ultraviolet radiation *10.3, 10.4*
　UVB phototherapy adverse effects 21.11–21.12
　UVR exposure 10.7
　venous leg ulcer *102.5*
　see also flushing; rosacea
erythema ab igne *4.16*, 124.14–124.16
erythema annulare centrifugum (EAC) *4.11*, 47.6–47.8
　associated diseases 47.7
　causes and associations **47.7**
　differential diagnosis 47.8
　histology *47.8*
　investigations 47.8
　lesion appearance *47.7*
　pathology 47.8
　predisposing factors 47.7
　treatment 47.8
erythema chronicum migrans (ECM) 47.9
　Lyme disease 26.69, 26.72, 26.73, *26.73*, 26.74
erythema dyschromicum perstans 86.32–86.33
erythema elevatum diutinum (EED) 100.8–100.10
　fibrosis *100.8*
　inflammatory cell infiltrate *100.8*
erythema gyratum repens 47.11–47.12
erythema induratum of Bazin 27.29–27.31, 97.26–97.30
　clinical features 27.30
　epidemiology 27.29–27.30
　investigations 27.30–27.31
　management 27.31
　pathophysiology 27.30
erythema infectiosum (fifth disease) 25.77–25.78, 115.6, 155.2, *155.3*
erythema marginatum 47.9–47.11
　associated diseases 47.10
　clinical features 47.11
　complications and co-morbidities 47.11
　Duckett Jones criteria for diagnosis of rheumatic fever **47.11**
　investigations 47.11
　pathology 47.10
　treatment 47.11
erythema multiforme (EM) 47.1–47.6, 127.19–127.20, 127.72
　classic target lesion *47.2*
　clinical features 47.5–47.6
　differential diagnosis 47.6
　drug reactions 47.3–47.4
　　with eosinophilia and systemic symptoms 118.6
　epidermal necrosis 47.5
　erythema multiforme minor *47.5*
　eye involvement *47.3*
　herpes simplex virus 25.23
　histopathology of a subepidermal blister *47.5*
　immunology 47.2–47.3
　management 47.6
　mucosal lesions *47.2*
　oral involvement 108.75
　pathology 47.5
　target lesions in *4.15*
　topical agents triggering erythema multiforme-like reactions 47.4–47.5
　triggering factors 47.3
erythema multiforme-like lesions, COVID-19 association 25.111
erythema multiforme-like PLE *126.4, 126.5*
erythema multiforme major (EMM) 118.15
erythema neonatorum 114.3
erythema nodosum (EN) 27.31, 96.14, 97.18–97.25
　aetiological factors **97.19–97.20**, 97.21
　in pregnancy 113.12
erythema nodosum leprosum (ENL) 28.3, 28.4, *28.5*, 28.11, *28.12*, 28.15, 97.25–97.26

erythema nodosum-like lesions 97.51–97.52
erythematotelangiectatic rosacea 89.1
　microbiome 89.4
erythematous candidiasis
　acute 32.61
　chronic 32.62
　oral lesions 32.62, 108.20–108.22
erythematous rosacea, pathology 89.3
erythem (redness) 4.13, 126.1
erythrasma 26.39–26.41
　clinical features 26.39–26.41
　of groin *4.20*
　investigations 26.41
　management 26.41
　pathophysiology 26.39
erythrocyanosis 124.7–124.8
erythrocytosis *see* polycythaemia vera; TEMPI syndrome
erythroderma 39.31–39.35
　allergic contact dermatitis 39.35
　causes of and prevalence in adults **39.31**
　chronic actinic dermatitis 126.18
　clinical features 39.32
　clinical variants 39.32–39.35
　complications and co-morbidities 39.35
　dermatophytosis 39.34
　disease course and prognosis 39.35
　drug reactions 39.33
　　with eosinophilia and systemic symptoms 118.7, *118.8*
　eczematous dermatoses 39.32
　epidemiology 39.31
　HIV 31.12
　ichthyosiform erythroderma 39.33
　internal malignancy association 148.23
　leukaemia 39.32–39.33
　lichen planus 39.34
　lymphoma 39.32–39.33
　management 39.35
　Norwegian scabies 39.34
　papuloerythroderma of Ofuji 39.34–39.35
　pathology 39.31–39.32
　pemphigus foliaceus 39.34
　pityriasis rubra pilaris 39.33–39.34
　predisposing factors 39.31
　psoriasis 39.32
　severe combined immunodeficiency 80.7
　Sézary syndrome *39.33*
　treatment 39.35
　unknown origin 39.33
erythrodermatous exfoliative 127.72
erythrodermic psoriasis 35.14, **35.16**
erythrodermic sarcoidosis 96.13
erythrogenic toxin, scarlet fever 26.35
erythrokeratodermas 63.18–63.20
erythrokeratoderma variabilis (EKV) 63.18–63.19
erythromelalgia 82.12–82.13, 101.6–101.9
　age of onset 101.7
　clinical features **101.8**
　ear dermatoses **106.22**
　epidemiology 101.7
　internal malignancy association 148.25
　investigations 101.9
　irritant contact dermatitis *101.9*
　management 101.9
　pathophysiology 101.7–101.8
　primary erythromelalgia 101.7–101.8
　secondary erythromelalgia 101.8
　associated diseases in 101.7
erythromelanosis follicularis of the face and neck 85.10, 86.14–86.15
erythromelanosis follicularis faciei et colli (EFFC) 85.10, 86.14–86.15
erythromycin 18.11, 19.47, 19.48
erythroplakia, oral involvement 108.23, *108.24*
erythroplasia of Queyrat
　penis 109.31–109.34
　see also anal/perianal/genital intraepithelial carcinomas
erythropoietic protoporphyria (EPP) 58.4, 58.14–58.17, *94.3*, 99.24, 126.7, 126.32–126.33
　acute reactions 58.15

bone health 58.16
clinical features 58.14–58.15
genetic counselling 58.16
investigations 58.15
liver disease in 58.16–58.17
oral involvement 108.85
osteoporosis 58.16
pathophysiology 58.14
photoprotection 58.15
escharotomy, burn management 125.8
essential fatty acid deficiency (EFAD) 61.31–61.34
　clinical features 61.32–61.33
　epidemiology 61.32
　genetics 61.32
　investigations 61.33
　management 61.33–61.34
　pathophysiology 61.32–61.33
essential thrombocythaemia (ET) thrombocytosis 99.10–99.11
etanercept
　psoriasis treatment 35.28
　psoriatic arthritis treatment 35.45
ethical issues
　drug trials, reporting of 13.13
　medical volunteer trips **7.15**
Ethiopia, medical schools 7.8
ethnicity
　botulinum toxins, aesthetic uses of 159.6
　chemical peels 160.15
　cutaneous squamous cell carcinoma in white and non-white populations 141.27
　dermatosis papulosa nigra 132.5
　diagnosis 4.4
　epidemiology 5.10
　mucocutaneous manifestations of COVID-19 infection 25.104
　neurobiological differences in pruritus 81.2
　rosacea 89.2
　seborrhoeic keratosis 132.1
ethylenediamine 127.19
ethylhexylglycerin 127.56–127.57
ethylmalonic encephalopathy 124.7
EU directives/regulations
　allergens 127.35
　MCI/MI preservatives 127.54
eumelanin 2.17, *2.18*, 86.5
Europe, skin cancer, economic burden of 6.6–6.8
European Environmental and Contact Dermatitis Research Group (EECDRG) 127.1–127.2
European Hidradenitis Suppurativa Foundation (EHSF) 16.5
European Organisation for Research and Treatment of Cancer Core Questionnaire (EORTC QLQ-C30) 16.9
European Organization of Research and Treatment of Cancer (EORTC), cutaneous lymphoma classifications 139.1, **139.2**, 139.6
EV *see* epidermodysplasia verruciformis
evidence based medicine (EBM) 17.1–17.25
　adverse events study evaluation 17.17–17.18
　applying evidence to specific patients 17.12, 17.16, 17.17
　clinical trial evaluation 17.12–17.15
　critically appraising evidence and applying it to individual patients 17.8–17.18
　definition 17.1
　diagnostic test study evaluation 17.15–17.17
　evaluating the data in clinical research papers 17.18–17.25
　experience-based decisions by physicians 17.5–17.6
　finding best evidence 17.2, 17.6–17.8
　five steps of practising 17.2
　formulating questions and finding evidence 17.3–17.8

hierarchy of evidence 17.4
levels of evidence **17.5**
limitations 17.2–17.3
meta analysis 17.4–17.5
presentation of data and basic statistics in clinical research papers 17.18–17.20
shortcut method for appraising clinical research papers 17.24–17.25
statistical methods in clinical research papers 17.20–17.24
systematic review evaluation 17.8–17.12
threats 17.3
validity of research 17.8–17.10, 17.12–17.16, 17.17
see also randomised controlled clinical trials
Ewing sarcoma, cutaneous 136.51–136.52
EWSR1-SMAD3-rearranged fibroblastic tumour 136.4
examination of skin 4.5
exanthema subitum *see* roseola infantum
exanthematous pustulosis 118.1–118.4
exanthems (rashes)
　COVID-19 association 25.109
　diagnosis 4.2
　drug-induced 117.1–117.2
　drug reaction with eosinophilia and systemic symptoms 118.7
　HIV acute primary infection 31.6, 31.7
　Langerhans cell histiocytosis 135.4, 135.6
　secondary syphilis 29.7–29.10
　viral infections 25.4–25.5, **25.4**
excessive hair growth 87.84–87.91
excessive washing
　obsessive–compulsive behaviour 84.26
　olfactory delusions 84.10
excisional biopsy 3.2
exclamation mark hairs 87.14–87.15, 87.23, *87.24*
excoriated nodular prurigo *see* prurigo nodularis
excoriée acné 84.20–84.22, 88.28–88.29, *88.30*
exercise, lymphoedema therapy 103.58
exercise-induced purpura 99.5, **99.9**
exercise-induced urticaria 42.12
exfoliative cheilitis 108.61–108.62
exfoliative dermatitis
　cutaneous manifestations of Hodgkin disease 139.49
　drug reaction with eosinophilia and systemic symptoms 118.7, *118.8*
　internal malignancy association 148.23
exfoliative disorders, cornification 63.26–63.30
exfoliative erythroderma, drug reaction with 118.10
exfoliative ichthyosis (EXI) 63.21–63.22
exocytosis 3.41
exogen 87.8
exogenous agents, perforating disease due to 94.55
exogenous androgens 87.91
exogenous drug- and chemical-induced photosensitivity 126.27–126.32
exogenous ochronosis 86.50–86.51
exogenous pigmentation 86.51–86.54
Exophiala jeanselmei 32.78
exophilin-5 deficiency, autosomal recessive EB simplex with 69.10–69.11
exophilin-5 epidermolysis bullosa 69.4
extensive dermal melanocytosis 73.21
external auditory canal (EAC) 106.1–106.3
　microbiome 26.5
　tumour management 106.29–106.31
external auditory meatus *see* external auditory canal
external carotid artery, anatomy of head and neck 20.1–20.2
external otitis, otomycosis 32.17–32.18
external root sheath tumours 137.5–137.7
　see also trichilemmal cyst
extracellular matrix (ECM) 2.27–2.28, 2.40
　wound healing 11.5

extracorporeal photochemotherapy *see* extracorporeal photopheresis
extracorporeal photopheresis (ECP)
　administration 21.11
　adverse effects 21.15
　conditions treated 21.7
　cutaneous T-cell lymphoma 21.7, 139.24–139.25
　graft-versus-host disease 21.7
　history 21.2
　principles 21.1
extracts
　allergic contact dermatitis 127.49
　patch testing 127.33
extracutaneous pyoderma gangrenosum 49.5
extracutaneous tumours, familial adenomatous polyposis 78.11
extragenital lichen sclerosus 94.25
extramammary Paget disease (EMPD) 110.37–110.39, 137.42–137.43, 148.7
　classification **110.38**
　immunocytochemical markers **110.38**
　male genitalia 109.40–109.41
　perianal skin 111.24
extramedullary haematopoiesis 149.5
extranodal NK/T-cell lymphoma, nasal type (ENKTCL-NT) 108.70, 139.36–139.37
extrapulmonary sarcoidosis 96.5
extravascular paraprotein deposition 149.13
extremities, constricting bands of 94.46–94.48
extremity escharotomies 125.8
eye 107.1–107.50
　acquired immune deficiency syndrome **107.35**
　amyloidosis **107.35**
　anatomy and physiology 107.1–107.2
　antibiotics, side effects 107.43
　antimalarials, side effects 19.6, 107.43
　atopic eye diseases 107.16–107.23
　biologic agents, side effects 107.44
　botulinum toxin, side effects 107.44
　cicatrising conjunctivitis 107.24–107.34
　conjunctival hyperaemia *50.30*
　contact dermatitis 107.6
　corticosteroids, side effects 107.40–107.43
　dermatomyositis **107.35**
　drug side effects 107.40–107.44
　epidermolysis bullosa 69.25–69.26
　episcleritis, BADAS-associated *49.17*
　erythema multiforme *47.3*
　extrapulmonary sarcoidosis 96.5
　filariasis (onchocerciasis) 107.40
　graft-versus-host disease 107.34
　granulomatosis with polyangiitis **107.35**
　herpes infection *1.10*
　histiocytoses **107.35**
　hypopyon, Adamantiades–Behçet disease *48.6*
　ichthyoses 63.45
　inflammatory bowel disease **107.35**
　inherited disorders **107.41–107.42**
　juvenile xanthogranuloma *135.16*, 135.17
　Kaposi sarcoma 107.49–107.50
　lacrimal apparatus *107.4*
　lacrimal glands 107.3
　leprosy 28.13, 107.39
　lupus erythematosus **107.35**
　Lyme disease 107.40
　malignant melanoma 107.49
　mucous membrane pemphigoid *50.30*, 107.24–107.32
　mycobacterial infections 107.39–107.40
　ocular complications of drug therapy 19.6, 19.15–19.16, *19.19*, 107.40–107.44
　ocular syphilis 29.16, 107.39–107.40
　onchocerciasis 33.2, 33.5
　ophthalmological terms **107.5**
　polyarteritis nodosa **107.35**
　porphyria **107.35**
　precorneal tear film 107.3

protozoal infections   107.40
pseudoxanthoma elasticum   70.33
psoralens, side effects   107.43–107.44
psoriasis   107.6
reactive arthritis   **107.35**
retinoids, side effects   107.43
river blindness (onchocerciasis)   107.40
sarcoidosis   **107.35**
Sjögren syndrome   **107.35**
Stevens–Johnson syndrome   107.32–107.34
syphilis   107.39–107.40
systemic diseases   **107.35**
systemic lupus erythematosus   51.32
toxic epidermal necrolysis   107.32–107.34
treponemal infections   107.39–107.40
tuberculosis   107.39
uveitis, Adamantiades–Behçet disease   48.4, 48.6
see also conjunctival entries; cornea; corneal entries; macular; ocular entries
eye area, use of lead shielding in radiotherapy for skin cancer   24.3, 24.4, 24.10–24.11
eyebrows
  anatomy and role   107.2
  disorders of   107.3–107.4
  hair density reduction   107.4
  hypertrichosis   107.4
  hypoplasia   107.4
  linear morphoea en coup de sabre   55.24
  synophrys   107.4
  syphilis of   105.12
  thinning of   107.4
  see also brows
eye colour, melanoma risk   142.3
eyelashes
  anatomy and physiology   107.2
  disorders of   107.4–107.5
  hordeolum   107.38, 107.39
  hypotrichosis   107.4
  madarosis   107.4–107.5
  Phthiriasis (lice) infestation   107.40
  trichomegaly   107.4
eyelids   107.1–107.50
  abnormalities of   107.5–107.6
  anatomy and physiology   107.2–107.3
  angioedema   42.3
  atopic eczema   41.20–41.21
  bacterial infections   107.38–107.39
  basal cell carcinoma   107.47–107.48
  benign adnexal lesions   107.45
  benign cysts   107.45–107.47
  benign lesions   107.44–107.47
  blepharitis   107.7–107.15
  blepharoconjunctivitis   107.6
  chalazion   107.45–107.46
  chronic granulomatous disease   80.15
  dendritic keratitis   107.37
  dermatitis   107.6, 127.15, 127.37
  eccrine carcinoma   107.49
  eczema of   39.22–39.23
  erysipelas   107.38
  haemangioma   107.46–107.47, 116.6
  herpes simplex virus infection   107.34–107.36, 107.37
  herpes zoster   107.36–107.38
  hordeolum   107.38, 107.39
  impetigo   107.38
  infantile haemangioma   116.6
  infections   107.34–107.40
  juvenile xanthogranuloma   107.45
  Kaposi sarcoma   107.49–107.50
  keratoacanthoma   107.47
  lipoid proteinosis   70.37
  malignant lesions   107.47–107.50
  malignant melanoma   107.49
  melanocytic naevi   107.46
  Merkel cell carcinoma   107.49
  microcystic adnexal carcinoma   107.49
  molluscum contagiosum   107.34, 107.36
  naevus of Ota   107.46
  necrotising fasciitis   107.39
  neonatal lupus erythematosus   51.40
  oedema   103.46, 103.47

ophthalmological terms   **107.5**
papular lesions around   80.15
parasitic infections   107.40
periorbital oedema   107.6–107.7
pigmentation changes   107.7
port-wine stain   107.47
psoriasis   107.6
scarring, long-term SJS/TEN   118.17
sebaceous carcinoma   107.49
seborrhoeic keratosis   107.44
skin cancer treatment   24.10, 24.11
squamous cell carcinoma   107.47, 107.48
swelling
  allergic contact dermatitis   129.6
  Stevens–Johnson syndrome/toxic epidermal necrolysis   118.14, 118.16
syringomas   4.8
urticaria   42.3
UV radiation-exposure damage   76.5
viral infections   107.34–107.38
warts   107.34, 107.36
xanthelasma   107.44
xanthelasma palpebrarum   60.4
eye protection, phototherapy   21.3, 21.10, 21.12, 21.15, 21.16
eye therapy, SJS/TEN   118.19–118.20

F

fabricated and induced illness, see also Münchausen syndrome by proxy
Fabry disease   79.6–79.8, 79.7, 79.8, 151.2–151.3, 154.1
fucosidosis   79.4
face
  acne tarda   88.4
  acne vulgaris   88.3, 88.27, 88.28
  anti-p200 pemphigoid   50.41
  atopic eczema   41.15, 41.17
  blood vessels, position of   20.1–20.2
  bullous lupus erythematosus   51.28
  congenital adrenal hyperplasia   88.10
  discoid lupus erythematosus   51.5, 51.6
  eosinophilic pustular folliculitis   93.8
  granuloma faciale   100.12
  infantile acne   88.70
  infiltrating lipomatosis of the face   98.19–98.20
  Kikuchi–Fujimoto disease   51.33
  lichen planus actinicus   37.7
  linear morphoea, Blaschkoid nature of   55.23
  lupus erythematosus profundus   51.9
  motor nerves, position of   20.3–20.4
  neonatal acne   88.71
  neonatal lupus erythematosus   114.13
  oedema   103.46–103.49
  papular rashes, differential diagnosis   88.37–88.38
  pityriasis alba   39.27
  pityriasis rubra pilaris   36.4
  prepubertal acne   88.69, 88.70, 88.71
  progressive hemifacial atrophy   55.23, 55.24–55.25
  pyoderma faciale   88.36
  radiotherapy for skin cancer   24.10–24.12, 24.13, 24.14, 24.19
  rosacea   88.35
  sensory nerves, position of   20.2–20.3
  solid facial lymphoedema   88.41, 89.10, 89.16, 89.17, 103.47, 103.48
  Sweet syndrome   49.12
  swelling   98.19, 103.46–103.49
  systemic lupus erythematosus   51.23, 51.24
  systemic sclerosis   54.4
facial acne scar quality of life (FASQoL)   16.4
facial allergic contact dermatitis   127.14–127.15, 127.48
facial contact dermatitis   89.8
facial deformity, congenital syphilis   29.24, 29.26, 29.27
facial dermatoses, with uncertain nosological relationship to rosacea   89.15–89.17

facial dysmorphic features, Waardenburg syndrome   68.5
facial erythema, clinical features   89.5
facial hair, androgen-stimulated   87.10
facial hemiatrophy   94.20–94.21
facial hirsutism   87.90
facial hypertrichosis, porphyria cutanea tarda   87.87
facial infiltrating lipomatosis   72.11
facial lipoatrophy   98.7
facial lipomatosis, infiltrating   98.19–98.20
facial melanoses   86.9–86.15, 86.51
facial muscles, botulinum toxin injection sites   159.3
facial necrobiosis, atypical   95.12
facial nerve (CN VII), anatomy of head and neck   20.3–20.4
facial oedema
  drug reaction with eosinophilia and systemic symptoms   118.8
  minor features   89.6–89.7
facial pain syndromes   108.64–108.67
  burning mouth syndrome   108.64–108.65
  persistent idiopathic facial pain   108.65–108.66
  post-herpetic neuralgia   108.66
  trigeminal neuralgia   108.66–108.67
  trigeminal trophic syndrome   108.67
facial palsy, zoster   25.34
facial rejuvenation, laser resurfacing   161.1–161.6
facial sarcoidosis, photothermal ablation   23.22
facial skin
  ageing of skin   156.2, 156.3
  botulinum toxins, aesthetic uses of   159.3–159.6
  infantile haemangioma   116.3, 116.4
  melanoma, dermoscopy   145.9, 145.11, **145.11**
  microscopic examination of   3.33
  pyogenic granuloma   116.11
  see also chemical peels
facial surgery   20.1–20.52
facial telangiectasia, Rothmund–Thomson syndrome   75.5
facility-acquired pressure ulcers   123.1
FACS see fluorescence activated cell sorting
factitious disorders   84.29–84.38
  cheilitis   84.33, 108.61
  dermatitis artefacta   84.29–84.36
  dermatitis passivata   84.36
  dermatitis simulata   84.36
  dermatological pathomimicry   84.36
  malingering   84.36–84.37
  Münchausen syndrome by proxy   84.37–84.38
  Münchausen syndrome and pseudologia fantastica   84.37
  nails   84.33
  panniculitis   97.48–97.50
FACT-M see Functional Assessment of Cancer Therapy-Melanoma
facultative anaerobic bacteria   26.10
facultative (inducible) pigmentation   68.1, 86.2
FAE see fumaric acid esters
faecal dermatitis, colostomy leakage   112.4, 112.5
FALDH deficiency see fatty aldehyde dehydrogenase deficiency
false negative reactions, patch testing   127.28–127.29, 129.7
false positive reactions, patch testing   127.28, 129.7
famciclovir   19.49
familial acanthosis nigricans   85.4–85.5
familial adenomatous polyposis (FAP)   78.10–78.11
familial atypical/dysplastic naevus syndrome   142.4
familial body dysmorphic disorder   84.14
familial cerebelloretinal angiomatosis (von Hippel–Lindau syndrome)   148.9, 154.2

familial cold autoinflammatory syndrome (FCAS)   **45.5**, **45.6**, 45.9
familial comedones   88.32
familial dysautonomia, respiratory system involvement   152.5
familial haemophagocytic lymphohistiocytosis (FHL)   135.11, 135.13
familial hypercholanaemia   2.21
familial hypercholesterolaemia (FH)   60.2, 60.6–60.8
  diagnosis of   **60.7**
  lipid concentrations in   **60.7**
familial infantile myofibromatosis   136.40
familial lipoedema   72.12
familial mandibuloacral dysplasia   70.28–70.29
  'tree-frog' appearance   70.29
familial Mediterranean fever (FMF)   **45.5**, **45.6**, 45.9–45.10
  renal involvement   154.2
  Tel Hashomer criteria for diagnosis of   **45.10**
familial melanoma syndrome   142.3, 148.8–148.9
familial multiple KAs see multiple self-healing squamous epithelioma
familial partial lipodystrophy (FPL)   72.3, **72.4**
  Dunnigan-type   98.9
familial primary localised cutaneous amyloidosis   **56.3**, 56.9, 56.9
familial progressive hyper-hypopigmentation   68.10
familial progressive hyperpigmentation (FPH)   68.10
familial reactive perforating collagenosis   94.54–94.55
familial sea-blue histiocytosis   135.22–135.23
familial trichoepitheliomas, photothermal ablation   23.21
familial tumoral calcinosis   79.17–79.18
family
  measuring impacts of skin disease   16.10–16.11
  see also 'the Greater Patient' concept
Family Dermatology Life Quality Index (FDLQI)   16.10
family history, diagnosis   4.4
FamilyPso questionnaire   16.10
Family Reported Outcome Measure (FROM-16)   16.10
Fanconi anaemia   68.12, 76.11, **80.5**, 80.12–80.13, 148.14
FAP see familial adenomatous polyposis
FAPD see fibrosing alopecia in a pattern distribution
Farber disease   79.5–79.6
farcy see glanders
farm environments, and atopic eczema   41.8
fascial fibromatoses   94.34–94.36
Fas-Fas ligand, TEN interaction   118.21
FASQoL see facial acne scar quality of life
fat cell tumours   136.56–136.59
fat contouring   161.8–161.9
  bulk cooling/cryolipolysis   161.8–161.9
  bulk heating/thermolipolysis   161.9
fat homeostasis, lymphatic system   103.2
fat hypertrophy   98.13–98.15
fatigue, cold agglutinins   124.13
fat naevus   **73.2**, 73.16–73.18
fat necrosis, necrotic adipocytes   97.55
fat organ, adipokines   97.5
fat pads, glycosylation disorders   **79.10**
FATP gene, ichthyosis–prematurity syndrome   63.39
fat, subcutaneous see subcutaneous fat
fat tissue, composition   97.1–97.3
fatty acids
  acne   129.12
  and alcohols, topical medication vehicles   18.7
  energy homeostasis   97.4
fatty aldehyde dehydrogenase (FALDH) deficiency   63.32

fauces, examination of   108.7
Favre–Racouchot syndrome   88.31–88.32, 94.3–94.4
favus (favic type tinea capitis)   32.38, 32.39
FCAS *see* familial cold autoinflammatory syndrome
FCL *see* follicle centre cell lymphoma
FD *see* Flegel disease
FDEs *see* fixed drug eruptions
FDLQI *see* Family Dermatology Life Quality Index
febrile ulceronecrotic Mucha–Habermann disease (FUMHD)   134.3, 134.4
feet *see* foot
female androgenetic alopecia   87.68–87.70
female androgen physiology   87.88
female genital mutilation (FGM)   110.43
female pattern hair loss (FPHL)   87.13, 87.61, 87.62–87.66, *87.67*
Female Sexual Function Index (FSFI)   16.12
Ferguson-Smith disease *see* multiple self-healing squamous epithelioma
Ferriman–Gallwey scoring system, hirsutism   87.88–87.89
ferritin   87.59, 87.70–87.71
fetal skin biopsy   8.10
fetal varicella syndrome   114.23
fetus
  hydrops fetalis   103.23
  lymphatic-related hydrops fetalis   103.23
feverfew (parthenolide)   **157.8**
FFA *see* frontal fibrosing alopecia
FGFR3 epidermal naevus syndrome   73.7
FGFRs *see* fibroblast growth factor receptors
FGFs *see* fibroblast growth factors
FGM *see* female genital mutilation
FH *see* familial hypercholesterolaemia; fibrous histiocytoma
FHL *see* familial haemophagocytic lymphohistiocytosis
fibreglass dermatitis   122.21, 129.1
fibrillinopathy   70.20–70.21
fibrillins   2.35–2.36
fibrinoid degeneration   3.40
fibroadipose hyperplasia   72.9
fibroblast growth factor receptors (FGFRs), acanthosis nigricans   85.4
fibroblast growth factors (FGFs)   2.3, 2.4
  wound healing   11.6
fibroblastic rheumatism (FR)   53.7–53.8, 155.7
  multicentric reticulohistiocytosis differentiation   135.25
fibroblastic tumours, EWSR1-SMAD3-rearrangement   136.4
fibroblasts   2.3, 2.39–2.40, 2.45
  collagen fibril fragmentation   156.8–156.9
  gene expression   2.40
  hair follicles   2.40
  microscopic examination of   3.37
  morphoea   55.10–55.11
  palmar fascial fibromatosis   94.34
  reactive oxygen species   156.4
  transmission electron microscopy   *2.40, 156.9*
  wound healing   *11.6*, 11.7–11.8
fibrodysplasia ossificans progressiva   70.35
fibroepithelial polyp *see* skin tags
fibrofolliculoma   137.16
  Birt–Hogg–Dubé syndrome   *78.15*
  differential diagnosis   88.30–88.31
fibrohistiocytic tumours   136.19–136.23
  diagnosis   3.25–3.26
  reclassification of angiomatoid malignant fibrous histiocytoma   136.17
fibroma
  tendon sheath   136.11
  vulval   **110.32**
fibroma-like epithelioid sarcoma *see* pseudomyogenic haemangioendothelioma
fibromatoses   94.33–94.48
  keloids association   94.49
fibromatous nodule, tuberous sclerosis complex   *78.10*

fibromyalgia, acne relationship   155.11
fibromyxoid sarcoma, low grade   136.18–136.19
fibro-osseous pseudotumour of the digits   136.6
fibrosing alopecia in a pattern distribution (FAPD)   87.43
fibrosis
  erythema elevatum diutinum   *100.8*
  mucous membrane pemphigoid   107.25, 107.32
  oral tissues   108.68
  in phyma   89.3
  subcutaneous sarcoidosis   96.3, 97.54
  systemic sclerosis   54.11–54.13
fibrous digital nodules   94.43
fibrous hamartoma of infancy   136.6–136.7
fibrous histiocytoma (FH)   *4.19*, 136.19–136.21
fibrous long-spacing collagen, CLD association   98.13
fibrous and myofibroblastic tumours   136.1–136.19
fibrous papules of the face   136.2–136.3
fibrous papulosis of the neck   94.39–94.40
fibroxanthoma, atypical   *106.34*
fibulins   2.36
fiddleback/violin spiders (Sicariidae)   34.35–34.36
'fiddler's neck'   122.12
fifth disease *see* erythema infectiosum
'fight bites'   130.6–130.7
filaggrin 2
  peeling skin syndromes   63.30
  skin fragility disorders   69.6
filaggrin   2.6
  deficiency   85.2
filaggrin mutations
  allergic contact dermatitis   127.10
  ichthyosis vulgaris   63.3–63.4
  occupational contact dermatitis   129.3, 129.6
filarial elephantiasis *see* lymphatic filariasis
filarial worms   33.7–33.10
  see also lymphatic filariasis
filariasis (onchocerciasis)   107.40
filiform keratosis   63.77
filivirus infections, haemorrhagic fevers   25.85–25.87
fillers *see* dermal fillers
filovirus infections, haemorrhagic fevers   25.84–25.85
financial costs of disease *see* economic burden of disease
finasteride   87.69, 87.96–87.97
fine-needle aspiration of lymph nodes   4.22
finger
  acquired digital fibrokeratoma   136.4
  acral fibromyxoma   136.59
  allergic contact dermatitis   127.13, *127.14*
  Apert syndrome   *88.11*
  arthritis mutilans   *35.42*
  atopic eczema   *41.18*
  blistering distal dactylitis   26.34
  bluish discoloration of fingertip   *54.3*
  callosities   122.12
  digital mucous cyst   136.60
  digital ulceration   *54.3*, 54.17, **54.25**
  discoid lupus erythematosus   *51.4*, *51.9*
  fibroblastic rheumatism   53.8
  fibro-osseous pseudotumour of the digits   136.6
  'finger pebbles', diabetes   62.5
  flexion contractures and calcinosis   *54.3*
  florid lichen planus   *4.16*
  fungal infection   80.12
  granulomatosis with polyangiitis   *100.25*
  hand, foot and mouth disease   115.6
  Kawasaki disease   115.10
  Orf-induced pemphigoid   50.55
  paroxysmal haematoma   94.19, 99.5–99.6, 122.13–122.14
  pompholyx eczema   39.15
  spindling, in discoid lupus erythematosus   *51.9*

  systemic sclerosis   *54.3*, *54.4*, *54.5*, 54.17, **54.25**
  ulceration and necrosis   *54.3*, 54.17, **54.25**
  vesicular eczema   129.6
  see also digits; phalanges
fingernail dystrophy
  nail–patella syndrome   67.15–67.16
  pachyonychia congenita   67.1, *67.11*
  see also nails
fingertip
  eczema   39.15
  topical therapy application measure   18.3, *18.4*
Finn patch test chamber   127.24–127.25
fire, hazards and risks of electrosurgery   20.45–20.46
FISH *see* fluorescence in situ hybridisation
fish odour syndrome (trimethylaminuria)   84.11, 92.17–92.18
fish stings   130.4–130.5
fish tank granuloma (*Mycobacteria marinum*)   27.32–27.35
fissured dermatitis   129.3
fissures
  hand eczema   128.4
  lip fissure   108.63–108.64
fistulae, complications of   112.1–112.16
Fitz-Hugh–Curtis syndrome   30.5
Fitzpatrick classification, acute and carcinogenic effects of UV radiation exposure   10.7
Fitzpatrick skin types I/II, cutaneous squamous cell carcinoma   141.30
fixatives
  biopsy   3.4, **3.5**, 3.32
  fragrances   127.42
fixed drug eruptions (FDEs)   14.4, 86.28, *86.29*, 86.30–86.31
fixed-effects models   17.10
flagellate dermatitis   *119.10*
flagellate hyperpigmentation   119.8–119.9, *119.10*
'flaky paint' dermatitis, kwashiorkor   61.4
flaps, surgical   20.22–20.29, **20.24–20.25**
flashlamps
  epidermal pigmentation   23.15
  selective photothermolysis   23.5
  therapeutic devices   23.3
  vascular lesion treatment   23.7, 23.10
flatworms *see* trematodes
flavouring agents, allergic contact dermatitis   127.41–127.45
flea-borne bacterial infections
  cat scratch disease   26.62–26.63
  murine typhus   26.81
  plague   26.59–26.60
  spotted fever   26.83, 26.84
fleas
  classification   34.13
  clinical features/investigations of bites   34.14
  epidemiology   34.13–34.14
  management of bites   34.14–34.15
  tungiasis   34.15
  see also Tunga penetrans (sand fleas)
Flegel disease (FD)   63.77–63.78, 85.17–85.18
flexibility (hypermobility), Beighton score   70.8
flexural Dowling–Degos disease   68.13
flexural psoriasis (inverse psoriasis)   35.8, *35.9*, **35.16**
flexures, allergic contact dermatitis   127.22
Florida horse leech *see Pythium insidiosum* infection
florid cutaneous papillomatosis   148.16, *148.17*
  AN association   85.3–85.4
florid oral papillomatosis   108.45
florid papillomatosis of the nipple ducts *see* nipple, adenoma
flow cytometry, peripheral blood cell analysis   9.2
flucytosine antifungals   19.48
'fluid creep', resuscitation   125.3
fluid homeostasis, lymphatic system   103.2

fluid replacement, SJS/TEN treatment   118.20
flukes *see* trematodes
fluocinolone acetonide gel   12.3
fluorescence activated cell sorting (FACS)   9.2
fluorescence microlymphangiography   103.56
fluorescence in situ hybridisation (FISH), melanoma diagnosis   142.21
fluorescent lamps, cutaneous photosensitivity diseases   126.34
fluoroquinolones   19.47
5-fluorouracil (5-FU)
  basal cell carcinoma topical treatment   140.12
  Bowen disease topical treatment   141.23
  intralesional for keloids   94.52
  topical therapies   18.29, 140.12, 141.23
flushing (transient erythema)   89.6, 89.8–89.9, 89.12, 104.1–104.13
  associated disorders   **104.4–104.9**
  causes of   **104.3**
  characteristics of   **104.4–104.9**
  in children   **104.10**
  clinical presentation   104.10–104.11
  drug-induced   **104.3**
  epidemiology   104.1
  food-induced   **104.3**
  'geographical' pattern due to carcinoid tumour   *150.12*
  harlequin colour change   **104.10**
  in infants   *104.10*, **104.10**
  internal malignancy association   148.25–148.26
  investigations   **104.4–104.9**, 104.11
  management   104.11–104.12
  pathogenesis   **104.4–104.9**
  pathophysiology   104.1–104.2
  physiology   104.1
  rosacea   89.1, **89.2**, 89.6, 89.8–89.9, 89.12, **89.14**
  symptoms and signs   **104.4–104.9**
  treatment   **89.14**, **104.4–104.9**
flutamide   87.70, 87.96
flux measurement, topical drug delivery   12.3, 12.4, 12.5
FMF *see* familial Mediterranean fever
focal acantholytic dyskeratoma *see* warty dyskeratoma
focal adhesions (focal contacts)   2.26
focal dermal elastosis, late-onset   94.32
focal epithelial hyperplasia, oral involvement   108.11
focal hyperhidrosis *see* gustatory hyperhidrosis
focal keratoderma, pachyonychia congenita   63.52
focal mucinosis, oral involvement   108.85–108.86
focal palmoplantar keratoderma   63.56–63.58
focal palmoplantar and oral hyperkeratosis syndrome   108.29
focal plantar keratoderma   63.52
foetal programming, maternal stress impacts   150.8
folate deficiency   61.18–61.19, 86.23–86.24
folate supplementation   19.27
folate synthesis inhibitors   19.47
folds, dermal fillers, indication for   158.1, **158.3**
foliaceus, in pregnancy   113.8–113.9
foliate papillae, anatomy of   108.4
foliate papillitis, oral involvement   108.11
folic acid depletion, UVB phototherapy adverse effects   21.12
follicle centre cell lymphoma (FCL)   139.37
follicle mites   34.55–34.57
follicular atrophoderma   94.16–94.17
follicular canal, eosinophilic pustular folliculitis   *93.8*
follicular eruptions, systemic medications   91.2–91.3

follicular hyperkeratoses
  keratosis circumscripta 85.13
    KP association 85.10
  pachyonychia congenita 67.12
follicular hyperkeratosis 3.41–3.42
follicular inflammation 93.7
follicular infundibulum
  dilated pore lesions 137.3
  tumours 137.3–137.4
follicular lichen planus 87.38–87.50
follicular miniaturisation 87.64, *87.65*
follicular mucinosis 57.15–57.18, 87.47, 105.8, 139.14–139.15
follicular naevus 73.7
follicular occlusion tetrad 90.2
follicular papules 93.7
follicular pattern, hidradenitis suppurativa 90.6
follicular psoriasis 35.7, *35.9*
follicular pustules 93.6
follicular units 87.64
folliculitis 26.22–26.23
  clinical features 26.22–26.23
  decalvans 87.48–87.50, 88.36–88.37
  deep 91.8–91.15
  diabetic patients 62.4, *62.5*
  differential diagnosis 88.34–88.35
  HIV infection 87.35
  keloidalis 88.35–88.36, *88.37*, 91.10–91.12, 93.3–93.4
  lymphocytic 91.12–91.13
  Malassezia yeast 32.13
  management 26.23
  pathophysiology 26.22
  perineal and perianal skin 111.13–111.14
  scalp 91.13–91.14
  superficial 91.1–91.8
folliculosebaceous cystic hamartoma 106.35
Fonsecaea pedrosoi 32.77
food allergies
  atopic eczema 41.11–41.12, 41.20, 41.23
  contact urticaria 127.84
  Netherton syndrome 63.26, 63.28
  oral allergy syndrome 42.13, 108.12, 127.84
  see also diet; nutrition
foot
  acral naevi 131.24
  allergic contact dermatitis 127.17, 127.22
  annular erythema of infancy 47.10
  anti-p200 pemphigoid 50.41
  arteriovenous malformation 71.11
  atrophie blanche 99.21
  blue naevus 131.40
  callosities 122.8
  calluses 122.7–122.8
  carotenoderma 61.9
  chronic acral dermatitis 39.14–39.15
  congenital blue naevi 73.16
  cryofibrinogenaemia 99.13
  cutaneous small-vessel vasculitis 100.7
  deformities 122.7
  diabetic 62.2–62.3
  discoid eczema 4.12
  discoid lupus erythematosus 51.4
  erysipelas-like reaction, diabetic patients 62.2
  erythromelalgia 82.12–82.13
  forefoot dermatitis 127.67
  freeze-induced damage 124.4
  glomuvenous malformation 71.18
  granuloma annulare 95.5
  granulomatosis with polyangiitis 100.25
  hair sinuses 122.22
  juvenile plantar dermatosis 39.23–39.24
  lichen planus pemphigoides 50.51
  lymphoedema 71.28
  mixed connective tissue disease 53.4
  neurofibroma, extensive plexiform 78.2
  neuropathic ulcer 83.13, 83.14, 83.15
  palisaded and neutrophilic granulomatous dermatitis 53.7
  pansclerotic morphoea 55.21
  podoconiosis 7.3, 103.36

pretibial myxoedema *103.42*
serpiginous lesions *4.16*
STING-associated vasculopathy with onset in infancy *45.14*
wet gangrene in diabetes 62.2
see also heel; sole; toe
foot calluses 122.7
foot and mouth disease 25.94
foot ringworm *see* tinea peddis
footwear
  allergies 127.67–127.68
  calluses caused by 122.7
Footwork: the International Podoconiosis Initiative 7.9–7.10
Fordyce, scrotal angiokeratoma of 109.6
Fordyce spots 91.15–91.17, 93.10–93.12
  labia minora/majora 110.3, *110.4*
  oral lesions 108.29
forehead
  botulinum toxins, aesthetic uses of 159.4–159.5
  comedonal acne 88.2, 88.27, 88.28
  haemangioma, infantile *116.3*, 116.6
  scarring, classical Ehlers–Danlos syndrome *70.8*
  sebaceous gland hyperplasia 88.32
foreign bodies, hair as 91.10–91.11
foreign bodies/deposits
  detection of 3.38
  male genitalia 109.8
foreign body reactions 122.17–122.24
  cheilitis 108.62
  inflammatory 93.1–93.3
foreskin *see* prepuce
forest plots, meta-analysis of clinical trials 17.11
formaldehyde
  acetylacetone test method 127.34
  allergic contact dermatitis 127.49–127.51, 127.66
  cosmetic allergies 127.49–127.50
  resins 127.70–127.71
formaldehyde-releasing biocides 127.51–127.52
formaldehyde-releasing preservatives **127.50**, 127.51–127.52
formalin, specimen preparation 3.5
formication, drug-induced 120.5
formulations, topical medication vehicles 18.2–18.3, 18.5–18.8, 18.21
fornix meter, ocular disease assessment 50.30
four humours theory, Galen 1.3
Fournier gangrene 26.77, 26.78
  male genitalia 109.26–109.27
Fox-Fordyce disease *see* axillary apocrine miliaria
FPH *see* familial progressive hyperpigmentation
FPHL *see* female pattern hair loss
FPL *see* familial partial lipodystrophy
FPLD2 *see* Dunnigan-type familial partial lipodystrophy
fractional ablative lasers
  for acne scarring 161.4
  device names **161.5**
  laser types **161.5**
  for photodamaged skin *161.3*
  resurfacing 23.24
  for rhytids 161.5
  wound care 161.4
fractional non-ablative resurfacing 23.23–23.24
fractionated ablative lasers, skin resurfacing 161.2–161.3, **161.5**
fragile X syndrome *72.7*, 74.5, 106.7
fragrances *see* perfumes
framycetin 18.11
France
  dermatology history 1.4–1.5
  skin cancer, economic burden of 6.6, **6.7**
Francisella tularensis, tularaemia 26.57–26.58
Franklin disease 108.70
freckles *see* ephelides

Fredrickson classification, dyslipidaemias 60.1
free margins, principles of surgical design 20.19
freeze-induced damage 124.2–124.4
Frey syndrome *see* gustatory hyperhidrosis
friction
  acne mechanica 122.15
  effects 122.6–122.7
  pressure ulcers 123.2, 123.3
  psoriasis 129.2
  sports injuries 122.16–122.17
  stratum corneum 122.4
frictional hypermelanosis *86.11*
frictional trauma, mechanical stimuli 122.3
friction blisters 122.6, 122.9–122.10
FROM-16 *see* Family Reported Outcome Measure
frontal fibrosing alopecia (FFA) 87.41–87.43
frostbite 97.37, 124.2–124.4
frostnip 124.2
FSFI *see* Female Sexual Function Index
5-FU *see* 5-fluorouracil
fucosidosis
  angiokeratoma corporis diffusum *79.4*
  glycoproteinoses 79.3
fugitive swellings *see* loiasis
fulminant liver failure 118.11
fumarates 19.15–19.17
  dermatological uses 19.16
  pharmacological properties 19.17
  potential adverse effects 19.17
  safety precautions 19.17–19.18
fumaric acid esters (FAE)
  discoid lupus erythematosus treatment 51.12
  psoriasis treatment 35.26
FUMHD *see* febrile ulceronecrotic Mucha–Habermann disease
Functional Assessment of Cancer Therapy-Melanoma (FACT-M) 16.9
fungal arthropathies 155.5
fungal biology 32.2–32.3
fungal cultures, superficial mycoses identification 32.8–32.9
fungal dysbiosis, lichen planus 37.3
fungal infections 3.44, 32.1–32.95
  burn injuries 125.10
  female genitalia 110.27–110.28
  hand dermatitis differentiation 128.5
  HIV coinfections 31.26–31.29, 31.35
  immunosuppressed renal allograft recipients 154.5–154.6
  inherited immunodeficiency 80.12
  male genitalia 109.28
  oral infections 108.56–108.57
  perineal and perianal skin 111.8, 111.15
  in pregnancy 113.7
fungal nail disease *see* onychomycosis
fungal panniculitis 97.47–97.48, 97.60–97.61
fungi
  asexual reproduction 32.4, *32.5*
  classification/taxonomy 32.3–32.4
  morphology and diseases **32.3**
  reproduction 32.3
  sexual reproduction 32.4–32.5
  spore formation 32.4–32.5
furocoumarins 86.29–86.30
furuncles (boils/abscesses) 26.23–26.25
  clinical features 26.24–26.25
  definitions 26.23
  epidemiology 26.23–26.24
  investigations 26.25
  management 26.25
  pathophysiology 26.24
furunculosis, perineal and perianal skin 111.13–111.14
Fusarium species
  skin lesions 32.93
  superficial onychomycosis 32.54–32.55
fusidic acid 18.11
Fusobacterium 26.67–26.68
  tropical ulcers 26.68

G
GA *see* glycolic acid; granuloma annulare
gadolinium chelates 94.44
GAGs *see* glycosaminoglycans
gain-of-function STAT1 mutation, oro-pharyngeal mucocutaneous *Candida* infection 80.17
Gaiter-like sclerosis 94.16
galactosialidosis 79.5
GALEF *see* Global Alliance to Eradicate Lymphatic Filariasis
Galen 1.3, 1.5
gallates 127.59
gall bladder, cutaneous features of biliary tract disease 153.5
Galli–Galli disease 68.13, 85.24
Gamasida mites 34.54–34.55
gamma heavy chain disease (Franklin disease) 108.70
gamma-hydroxybuyrate (GHB) 120.3
gangrene
  peripheral vascular disease **101.5**
  peristomal skin 112.10
  see also gas gangrene; necrotising subcutaneous infections; pyoderma gangrenosum
gap junctions 2.20
Gardner disease 108.86
GARFIELD acronym 80.2
garlic allergy 127.71, 127.73
gas gangrene 26.48–26.49
gastrointestinal bleeding 153.6–153.7
gastrointestinal cancer, syndromes linked with **78.14**
gastrointestinal diseases
  cutaneous features 153.1–153.4, **153.7**
  oral involvement 108.72–108.74
  systemic lupus erythematosus 51.31
  systemic sclerosis 54.17, **54.23**
gastrointestinal hamartomas 68.13–68.14
gastrointestinal involvement
  drug reaction with eosinophilia and systemic symptoms 118.9
  long-term SJS/TEN 118.17
gastrointestinal malabsorption
  associated skin conditions 153.6–153.7, **153.8**
  causes **153.8**
gastrointestinal polyposis, familial adenomatous polyposis 78.11
gastrointestinal symptoms, syndromic ichthyoses **63.39**
gastrointestinal toxicity
  antimalarials 19.6
  glucocorticoids *19.19*
  methotrexate 19.26
gastrointestinal tract, epidermolysis bullosa 69.25
gastrointestinal ulcers 149.8
gastrointestinal venous malformations 71.17
gastro-oesophageal reflux disease 108.74
gastrostomy (G-Tube), bullous pemphigoid 50.19
GATA2 deficiency 149.14
Gaucher disease 79.5
  type II 63.30
GBD *see* global burden of disease
GBFDE *see* generalised bullous fixed drug eruption
GC *see* glucocorticoids
GCA *see* giant cell arteritis
GCs *see* glucocorticoids
GEH *see* generalised eruptive histiocytosis
GEKG *see* glycine-glutamate-lysine-glycine
gel nails 127.61
gels 12.3, 18.2
gender
  melanoma, trends in incidence and mortality 142.1
  women with HIV/AIDS 31.36
gender effects, Merkel cell carcinoma risk 146.1–146.2
gene mutations
  arsenic toxicity 121.2

gene mutations (continued)
    autosomal dominant lamellar ichthyoses 63.20–63.21
    autosomal recessive PPK 63.54
    CHILD syndrome 63.23–63.24
    Cole disease 63.61
    congenital ichthyoses 63.7–63.13
    Conradi–Hünermann–Happle syndrome 63.22–63.23
    Desmons syndrome 63.35
    disease 8.5–8.7
    dyskeratosis congenita **67.13**
    epidermolytic ichthyosis 63.15, *63.17*
    epidermolytic palmoplantar keratoderma 63.50
    exfoliative ichthyosis 63.21
    ichthyosis vulgaris 63.4
    ichthyosis–prematurity syndrome 63.39
    keratinopathic ichthyoses 63.13
    KID syndrome 63.33
    loricrin keratoderma 63.56
    Neu–Laxova syndrome 63.38
    pachyonychia congenita 63.51–63.52
    palmoplantar keratodermas 63.68
    recessive X-linked ichthyosis 63.5, 63.6
    Refsum disease 63.31
    see also genes; genetic disorders; genetics/genetic factors
General Health Questionnaire (GHQ-12), psychological impacts assessment 16.11
generalised anhidrosis, acquired 92.12
generalised bullous fixed drug eruption (GBFDE) 14.4
generalised cutaneous atrophy *94.10*
generalised diffuse Dercum disease 98.18
generalised Dowling–Degos disease 68.13
generalised elastolysis 94.21
generalised eruptive histiocytosis (GEH) 135.18
generalised eruptive keratoacanthoma 141.43–141.44
generalised essential telangiectasia **101.17**, 101.18–101.19
    branching with pressure *101.19*
    in pigmented skin *101.19*
generalised hyperhidrosis 92.4–92.5
generalised hypertrichosis 87.86–87.87
generalised lentiginosis without associated systemic symptoms 68.10
generalised lymphadenopathy, syphilis 29.10
generalised lymphatic anomaly (GLA) 103.28–103.29
generalised lymphatic dysplasia (GLD) 103.22
generalised nodular Dercum disease 98.18
generalised pigmentation, systemic sclerosis *86.21*
generalised plaque morphoea **55.3**, **55.4**, 55.17–55.19
generalised pruritus, neoplasia association 148.27
generalised pustular psoriasis (GPP) 35.31–35.36
    acute generalised pustular psoriasis of von Zumbusch 35.33–35.34
    age of onset 35.32
    clinical features 35.33–35.34
    co-morbidities 35.35
    differential diagnosis 35.34
    disease course and prognosis 35.35
    environmental factors 35.32–35.33
    epidemiology 35.32
    genetic factors 35.32
    histology 35.34
    investigations 35.35
    management 35.35–35.36
    pathogenic mechanisms 35.33
    in pregnancy 113.10–113.11
    severity classification 35.34–35.35
    subacute annular generalised pustular psoriasis 35.34
    systemic therapy 35.36
    topical treatment 35.36

generalised skin disease, linear manifestations of 73.22–73.23
general practitioners (GPs) 5.12–5.13
genes 8.3–8.4, *8.6*
    autosomal 8.4
    features of typical human gene *8.6*
gene therapy, epidermolysis bullosa 69.27
genetic counselling 8.9, 8.11
genetic disorders/syndromes
    adermatoglyphia 70.36
    of adipose tissue 72.1–72.13
        familial lipoedema 72.12
        fibroadipose hyperplasia 72.9
        hereditary panniculitis **72.11**
        lipomatoses **72.10**
        PIK3CA-related overgrowth spectrum 72.9–72.11
        basal cell carcinoma as an ancillary feature **140.7**
    Bazex–Dupré–Christol syndrome 140.20–140.21
    blistering diseases 69.1–69.28
    BSL differential diagnosis 98.16
    chromosomal disorders 74.1–74.5
        autosomal chromosome defects 74.1–74.3
        chromosomal mosaicism 74.5
    of collagen 70.1–70.14
        dystrophic calcification 59.3–59.4
        Ehlers–Danlos syndromes 70.1–70.11
        osteogenesis imperfecta 70.12–70.14
        prolidase deficiency 70.11–70.12
    congenital muscle hamartomas 73.19
    congenital naevi 73.1–73.18
    cornification 63.2
    DNA repair disorders with cutaneous features 76.1–76.12
    dystrophic calcification of skin and subcutaneous tissues 59.3–59.4
    of ectopic calcification and abnormal mineralisation 70.31–70.36
        fibrodysplasia ossificans progressiva 70.35
        primary hypertrophic osteoarthropathy 70.35–70.36
        pseudoxanthoma elasticum 70.31–70.35
    of elastic fibres 70.14–70.21
        cutis laxa 70.14–70.17
        Marfan syndrome 70.20–70.21
        Michelin tyre baby syndrome 70.19, 73.17
        Williams–Beuren syndrome 70.18–70.19
    genetic disorders/syndromes, sex chromosome defects 74.3–74.5
    heterotrimeric G-protein mosaic disorders 73.19–73.21
    immunodeficiency, inherited 80.1–80.20
    infantile stiff skin syndromes 70.21–70.24
        hyaline fibromatosis syndrome 70.21–70.22
        restrictive dermopathy 70.24
        stiff skin syndrome 70.22–70.23
        Winchester syndrome 70.23–70.24
    inherited immunodeficiency 80.1–80.20
    inherited metabolic diseases 79.1–79.18
    inherited skin tumour syndromes 78.1–78.15
        familial adenomatous polyposis 78.10–78.11
        mosaic neurofibromatosis type 1 78.4–78.7
        neurofibromatoses 78.1–78.7
        RASopathies 78.7, *78.8*, **78.9**
        tuberous sclerosis complex 78.7–78.10
    keratins 2.8
    lipoid proteinosis 70.36–70.37
    metabolic diseases, inherited 79.1–79.18
    midface toddler excoriation syndrome 82.9
    miscellaneous dermal disorders 70.36–70.38
    naevi, congenital 73.1–73.18
    Naevoid basal cell carcinoma syndrome 140.3–140.4, 140.18

    nails/nail growth 67.1–67.17
    neutral lipid storage disease with ichthyosis 63.36
    pigmentation 68.1–68.15
    poikiloderma syndromes 75.1–75.8
    premature ageing syndromes 70.25–70.31, 77.1–77.7
        acrogeria **70.26**, 70.28
        familial mandibuloacral dysplasia 70.28–70.29
        Mulvihill–Smith syndrome 70.29–70.30
        neonatal progeroid syndrome 70.30–70.31
        progeria 70.25–70.26, **70.26**
        Werner syndrome 70.26–70.27, **70.26**
    pterygium syndromes 70.37–70.38
    skin ageing 2.46
    vascular disorders 71.1–71.28
        arteriovenous disorders 71.11–71.14
        capillary disorders 71.3–71.11
        lymphatic disorders 71.21–71.28
        venous disorders 71.14–71.21
genetic epidemiology 5.10
genetic mosaicism, lymphoedema 103.23
genetic risk score *see* polygenic risk score
genetics/genetic factors 1.9, 8.1–8.11
    adenoid cystic carcinoma 137.39
    angioma serpiginosum 101.16
    angiomatoid fibrous histiocytoma 136.63
    angiosarcoma 136.35
    apocrine carcinoma 137.23
    apocrine tubular adenoma 137.22
    arteriovenous malformations 101.23
    atypical lipomatous tumour 136.58–136.59
    autosomal dominant inheritance *8.3*
    autosomal recessive inheritance *8.3*
    basal cell carcinoma 140.3–140.5, 140.18
    basaloid follicular hamartoma 137.13
    biomarkers, prenatal testing and diagnosis 8.11
    Blaschko lines 8.7, *8.8*
    BRAF mutations, lobular capillary haemangioma/pyogenic granuloma within port-wine stains 136.26
    calcifying aponeurotic fibroma 136.7
    cellular angiofibroma 136.9
    chromosomal disorders 8.6
    chronic mucocutaneous candidiasis 32.67
    CIC-rearranged sarcoma 136.52
    classical epidermodysplasia verruciformis 25.66, 25.69
    clear cell sarcoma 136.64
    comedo naevus 137.5
    composite haemangioendothelioma 136.34
    congenital disorders 8.2
    cutaneous Ewing sarcoma 136.52
    cutaneous myoepithelioma 137.33
    cutaneous squamous cell carcinoma 141.27–141.28
    cylindroma 137.29, 137.30
    deep ('aggressive') angiomyxoma 136.62
    dermatofibrosarcoma protuberans 136.15
    desmoplastic fibroblastoma 136.12
    disseminated superficial actinic porokeratosis 141.15–141.17
    eccrine gland carcinomas 137.34
    eccrine poroma 137.25
    elastofibroma 136.10
    epithelioid angiosarcoma 136.37
    epithelioid haemangioendothelioma 136.37
    epithelioid haemangioma 136.28
    epithelioid sarcoma 136.63
    erythromelalgia 101.8
    EWSR1-SMAD3-rearranged fibroblastic tumour 136.4
    extramammary Paget disease 137.43
    fibroma of tendon sheath 136.11
    fibro-osseous pseudotumour of the digits 136.6
    fibrous hamartoma of infancy 136.7

    gain-of-function mutations 8.6
    genetic heterogenity 8.5
    genetic linkage 8.9
    genetic markers 8.8–8.9, *8.11*
    gene tracking 8.9
    genome sequencing 8.8–8.9
    genomic imprinting 8.5
    giant cell fibroblastoma 136.16
    glomus tumours 136.42
    granular cell tumours 136.49
    haemosiderotic fibrolipomatous tumour 136.61
    hidradenocarcinoma 137.36
    hidradenoma 137.29
    hidradenoma papilliferum 137.21
    human genome *8.5*
    Human Genome Project 8.1
    human leukocyte antigens 8.7
    inborn errors of immunity disposing to HPV 25.65, **25.66**, 25.67–25.68, 25.70–25.71
    infantile myofibromatosis/adult myofibroma 136.40
    inherited disorders 8.8–8.9
    Kaposi sarcoma 138.3
    keratoacanthoma 141.39–141.40
    Klippel–Trenaunay syndrome 101.27–101.28
    leiomyoma 136.54
    lichen planus 110.11
    lipofibromatosis 136.14
    Lyonisation 8.7–8.8
    malignant peripheral nerve sheath tumour 136.51
    melanoma risk 142.3–142.5
        familial atypical/dysplastic naevus syndrome 142.4
        identification of at risk population 142.7
        intermediate penetrance susceptibility genes 142.5
        major/high penetrance susceptibility genes 142.4–142.5
        phenotypic traits 142.3–142.4
    microcystic adnexal carcinoma 137.37
    mitochondrial disorders 8.5
    mixed tumour of the skin 137.32
    mosaicism 8.7–8.8
    Muir–Torre syndrome 141.44
    multifactorial disorders 8.2
    multiple self-healing squamous epithelioma 141.41–141.42
    mutations and disease 8.5–8.7
    myoepithelial tumours 137.33
    myopericytoma 136.41
    nipple adenoma 137.22
    nodular fasciitis 136.5
    nosology 8.2–8.5
    Paget disease of the nipple 137.41
    Parkes Weber syndrome 101.30
    perivascular epithelioid cell tumour 136.61
    preimplantation genetic diagnosis 8.10–8.11
    preimplantation genetic haplotyping 8.11
    prenatal diagnosis 8.9–8.11
    principles of medical genetics 8.2–8.5
    pseudomyogenic haemangioendothelioma 136.34
    reactive angioendotheliomatosis 136.24–136.25
    rosacea risk 89.4–89.5
    schwannoma 136.45
    sebaceous adenomas and sebaceomas 137.17
    secretory carcinoma 137.40
    single-cell genomics 8.2
    single-gene disorders 8.2, *8.3*, *8.4*
    spindle cell haemangioma 136.31
    spindle cell lipoma 136.58
    spiradenoma 137.31
    tenosynovial giant cell tumour 136.19
    trichodiscoma 137.15
    urticarial vasculitis 44.3
    varicose veins 101.38–101.39, 101.42

venous malformations 101.25
X-linked dominant inheritance 8.4
X-linked recessive inheritance 8.4
genital area
  amicrobial pustulosis of the inguinal folds 49.20
  lymphoedema 103.49–103.51, *103.52*
  melanocytic naevi 131.22
  Stevens–Johnson syndrome/toxic epidermal necrolysis 118.17, 118.18
  swollen genitalia and mons pubis 103.49–103.51, *103.52*
genital chlamydia 30.8–30.14
  clinical features 30.10–30.11
  epidemiology 30.9–30.10
  gonorrhoea coinfection 30.7
  investigations 30.11–30.13
  management 30.13–30.14
  pathophysiology 30.10
genital dermatology 1.8
genital herpes 25.24–25.26, 109.28
genitalia, female 110.1–110.48
  acne, vulval 110.45
  angiokeratomas 110.3, *110.4*
  bacterial infections 110.25–110.27
    malakoplakia 110.26
    Mycobacterial infections 110.26
    Staphylococcal infections 110.25
    Streptococcal infections 110.25–110.26
  benign tumours 110.31–110.33
    atypical genital naevi 110.33
    Bartholin cysts 110.31
    cutaneous endometriosis 110.33
    mucinous cysts 110.31
    papillary hidradenoma 110.31–110.33, 137.20–137.21
  bullous disease 110.20, **110.21**
  clitoral variations 110.3
  congenital abnormalities 110.5
  Darier disease 110.6
  differentiated vulval intraepithelial neoplasia 110.34, 110.35
  disorders of sexual development 110.5
  epidermolysis bullosa 110.5
  female genital mutilation 110.43
  Fordyce spots 110.3, *110.4*
  fungal infections 110.27–110.28
    Candidal vulvo-vaginitis 110.27–110.28
    Tinea cruris 110.28
    Tinea incognito *110.28*
  genital papular acantholytic dyskeratosis 110.45
  genodermatoses 110.5–110.6
  graft-versus-host disease 110.43–110.44
  Hailey–Hailey disease 110.5–110.6
  high-grade squamous intraepithelial lesions 110.34–110.36
  history and examination 110.2
  immunobullous disease 110.20, **110.21**
  inflammatory dermatoses of the vulva 110.6–110.18
    allergic contact dermatitis 110.15
    allergic contact urticaria 110.16
    irritant eczema 110.14–110.15
    lichen planus 110.10–110.13
    lichen sclerosus 110.6–110.10
    lichen simplex 110.16–110.17
    psoriasis 110.17–110.18
    reactive arthritis 110.18
    seborrhoeic eczema 110.14
    zoon vulvitis 110.13–110.14
  investigations 110.2
  labial variations 110.3
  malignant neoplasms 110.36–110.40
    basal cell carcinoma 110.39
    extramammary Paget disease 110.37–110.39
    Langerhans cell histiocytosis 110.40
    squamous cell carcinoma 110.36–110.37
    verrucous carcinoma 110.37
    vulval melanoma 110.39–110.40
  necrolytic migratory erythema 110.44–110.45

non-sexually transmitted infections 110.24–110.31
normal flora 110.3
normal variants 110.3–110.4
pain disorders 110.40–110.42
  classification of vulval pain **110.41**
papular acantholytic dyskeratosis 110.45
pigmentary disorders 110.20–110.23
  acanthosis nigricans 110.22
  Dowling–Degos disease 110.23
  vitiligo 110.20–110.21
  vulval melanosis 110.21–110.22
premalignant conditions 110.34–110.36
structure and function 110.2–110.3
traumatic lesions 110.42–110.43
  female genital mutilation 110.43
  mechanical hymenal fissures 110.42–110.43
ulcerative disorders 110.18–110.20
  aphthous ulcers 110.19
  Behçet disease 110.20
  causes of vulval ulcers **110.19**
  non-sexually acquired genital ulcers 110.19–110.20
vaginal discharge, diagnosis of 110.24–110.25
varicosities 110.4
vestibular papillomatosis 110.4
viral infections 110.28–110.31
  herpes simplex virus infections 110.29–110.30
  human papillomavirus infections 110.30–110.31
  poxvirus infections 110.28–110.29
  vulval warts *110.30*
vulval acne 110.45
vulval oedema 110.23–110.24
vulvo-vaginal adenosis 110.44
see also vagina; vulvo-vaginal
genitalia, male 109.1–109.51
acne 109.24
acute scrotum 109.23
allergic contact dermatitis 109.12, **109.13**
amyloidosis 109.25
anatomy 109.2–109.4
angiokeratomas 109.6–109.7
ano-genital warts 109.9
artefactual conditions 109.8–109.9
atopic eczema 109.12
bacillary angiomatosis 109.28
balanitis 109.4
balanoposthitis 109.4–109.5
basal cell carcinoma 109.42
benign tumours 109.29–109.31
body dysmorphic disorder 109.6, 109.44
Bowen disease of the penis 109.31–109.34
bowenoid papulosis 109.31–109.34
Buschke–Löwenstein tumour/giant condyloma 109.39–109.40
Candida infection 109.5, 109.11, 109.27
carcinoma of the penis 109.35–109.39
child abuse, signs of 109.9
chronic pain syndromes 109.43–109.44
cicatricial (mucous membrane) pemphigoid 109.25
condylomas of penis 109.39–109.40
congenital and developmental abnormalities 109.7–109.8
cutaneous genital conditions 109.42–109.44
Darier disease 109.25
dermatitis artefacta 109.9
dermoid cysts 109.31
drug reactions 109.24–109.25
dysaesthesia 109.43–109.44
ecthyma gangrenosum 109.26
ectopic lesions on penile shaft 109.6
eczema 109.11–109.13
eczematous dermatoses 109.11
erythroplasia of Queyrat 109.31–109.34
extramammary Paget disease 109.40–109.41
foreign body 109.8
Fournier gangrene 109.26–109.27
fungal infection 109.28

genital herpes simplex 109.28
genital pruritus, causes of **109.2**
genito-crural intertrigo **109.3**
haematoma and rupture, penile 109.8
history and examination 109.4–109.5
HIV infection 109.29
human papillomavirus infection 109.29
hyperpigmentation **109.42**
hypopigmentation 109.28, **109.42**, 109.43
idiopathic lipogranuloma 109.43
inflammatory dermatoses 109.9–109.26
intraepithelial neoplasia, penile 109.31–109.34
investigations 109.5
irritant contact dermatitis 109.11
Kaposi sarcoma 109.42
keloid 109.31
koro syndrome 109.44
leishmaniasis 109.28
lichen planus 109.18–109.19
lichen sclerosus 109.15–109.18
lichen simplex 109.11
lipogranuloma 109.8–109.9, 109.43
malignant melanoma 109.41
median raphe cysts 109.30
melanocytic naevi 109.6
melanosis, penile 109.42–109.43
Melkersson–Rosenthal syndrome 109.25
metastases to the penis 109.42
molluscum contagiosum 109.29
MRSA 109.28
mucoid cysts 109.30
mutilation 109.9
mycosis fungoides 109.42
naevi on the penis 109.6
non-sexually transmitted infections 109.26–109.28
non-specific balanoposthitis 109.21–109.22
non-syphilitic spirochaetal ulcerative balanoposthitis 109.27
normal variants 109.5–109.7
oedema, chronic penile 109.19–109.21
pearly penile papules 109.6
pemphigus 109.25
penile horn 109.35
penile lymphoma 109.42
penile necrosis 109.22–109.24
penoscrotal swelling **109.20**
perianal cellulitis 109.26
perineal streptococcal dermatitis 109.26
Peyronie disease 109.24
phimosis 109.4, 109.16–109.17
phthiriasis 109.29
pilonidal sinus 109.24
pityriasis rosea 109.28
porokeratosis of Mibelli 109.35
porokeratosis ptychotropica 109.35
pre-cancerous dermatoses and carcinoma *in situ* 109.31–109.35
pseudoepitheliomatous micaceous and keratotic balanitis 109.35
psoriasis 109.9–109.10
psychiatric disorders 109.44
pubic hair 109.4, 109.27
pyoderma gangrenosum 109.9, 109.23
radiodermatitis 109.12
sacral herpes zoster 109.28
scabies 109.29, *109.30*
sclerosing lymphangitis 109.8
scrotal calcinosis 109.30
scrotal panniculitis 109.23
sebaceous gland prominence 109.6
seborrhoeic dermatitis 109.12, 109.13
self-instrumentation of 109.8
self-mutilation of 109.9
sexually transmitted diseases 109.28–109.29
skin tags 109.5–109.6
squamous carcinoma and malignant neoplasms 109.35–109.42
squamous cell carcinoma, penile 109.31–109.34
squamous hyperplasia 109.34–109.35
squamous intraepithelial lesions 109.34–109.35

staphylococcal cellulitis 109.26
strangulation of the penis 109.8
striae of Wickham *109.19*
structure and function 109.2–109.4
syphilis 109.28
tinea 109.27–109.28
trauma 109.8–109.9
trichomycosis pubis 109.27
tuberculosis 109.27
ulceration 109.5, 109.22–109.24, 109.28
  causes **109.22**
verruciform xanthoma 109.30–109.31
viral warts 109.29
warts 109.9, 109.29
white patches and plaques, causes of **109.34**
yaws 109.27
zoon balanoposthitis 109.14–109.15
see also penis; scrotum
genital lentiginosis, laser therapies 23.15, *23.16*
genital melanosis 131.10
genital mucosa, lichen planus 37.6
genital mucosal lesions, COVID-19 association 25.113
genital pain
  penoscrotodynia 82.11–82.12
  vulvodynia 82.9–82.11
genital porokeratosis 85.21, *85.22*
genital psoriasis 35.10
genital sarcoidosis 96.14–96.15
genital skin, bowenoid papulosis 141.20–141.21
genital ulceration 30.18–30.19
  Adamantiades–Behçet disease *48.5*
  Behçet-like syndrome associated with trisomy 8 myelodysplasia 149.8
  granuloma inguinale 30.21–30.23
  Lipschütz ulcers 25.37, 25.41, 25.113
  see also chancroid
genital warts see ano-genital warts
genito-femoral area
  Hurley stage I disease *90.7*
  Hurley stage II disease *90.8*
genitofemoral neuropathic pain/neuralgia 83.7
genito-urinary tract abnormalities 69.26
genodermatoses 8.2, *8.3*, *8.4*, 149.14
  associated with internal malignancies 148.7–148.13, 148.14
  blistering 69.1–69.28
  female genitalia 110.5–110.6
  with nail anomalies *67.2–67.3*, *67.9*
genome-wide score see polygenic risk score
genomic analysis of neoplasms, naevae as melanoma precursors 142.2
genomic analysis of squames, melanoma diagnosis 142.10
genomic imprinting 8.5
genomic medicine 8.1
genomics
  epigenomics 8.6
  immune system 9.2
  pharmacogenomics 13.11
  single-cell genomics 8.2
  skin ageing 2.46
  see also comparative genomic hybridisation
genophotodermatoses 126.1
genotype–phenotype correlations, congenital ichthyosiform erythroderma 63.7, 63.12
gentamicin 18.11
geographical factors, diagnosis 4.4
geographic tongue 108.24
geotrichosis, oral involvement 108.57
Germany
  health economic evaluations 6.2
  psoriasis, economic burden of 6.8–6.9
  skin cancer, economic burden of 6.6, **6.7**
germ line mosaicism, keratinopathic ichthyoses 63.14
gerodermia osteodysplastica **70.16**
GG-NER *see* global genome nucleotide excision repair
GHB *see* gamma-hydroxybuyrate

ghost adipocytes
  infective panniculitis 97.46
  pancreatic panniculitis 97.41, 97.43
GHQ-12 *see* General Health Questionnaire
Gianotti–Crosti syndrome 25.121–25.123, 25.221–25.223
  Epstien-Barr virus association 25.37
  hepatitis B association 25.74
  infants 115.11
giant cell arteritis (GCA) 100.32–100.34
  oral involvement 108.69
  ultrasonographic image of superficial temporal artery 100.33
  vessel wall involvement by granulomatous reaction 100.32
giant cell fibroblastoma 136.15–136.16
giant cell granuloma 94.27–94.29
giant cells
  microscopic examination of 3.36, 3.37
  multicentric reticulohistiocytosis 135.25
giant juvenile xanthogranuloma 135.16
giant porokeratoses 63.75
Giemsa stain 3.8
Gieson stain 3.8
Gilchrist disease *see* blastomycosis
gingiva
  anatomy 108.4
  homogeneous keratosis *108.33*
  hypoplasminogenaemia 108.70
  melanotic macule 108.18
  oral lichen planus *108.77*
  proliferative verrucous leukoplakia *108.35*
gingival erythema 110.12
gingival lichen planus 108.77
gingival recession, lip/tongue piercing 108.16
gingival ulceration 108.55
gingivitis
  acute necrotising (ulcerative) gingivitis and noma 108.54–108.55
  desquamative gingivitis 108.23, *108.82*
  plasma cell gingivitis 108.25
  vitamin C deficiency 61.21–61.22
gingivostomatitis, primary herpetic 25.20–25.22
Girimananda Sutra 1.2–1.3
GJB2 gene
  associated disorders 63.34
  KID syndrome 63.33, **63.34**
GLA *see* generalised lymphatic anomaly
glabella, botulinum toxins, aesthetic uses of 159.4
glabrous skin 2.43
glanders, *Burkholderia mallei* 26.55
glands of Tyson, Fordyce spots 93.11
glandular cheilitis 108.62–108.63
glandular fever *see* infectious mononucleosis
GLD *see* generalised lymphatic dysplasia
Gleich syndrome 43.4–43.5
glial heterotopic nodules 136.50
Global Alliance to Eradicate Lymphatic Filariasis (GALEF) 7.10
global burden of disease (GBD) 5.6–5.7, *5.8, 5.9*, 7.2
global genome nucleotide excision repair (GG-NER) 76.2
global health dermatology 7.1–7.15
  academic capacity building 7.12
  access to health care initiatives 7.8–7.11
  burden of disease 7.2
  capacity development 7.7–7.8
  climate change and skin health 7.3–7.4
  community dermatology 7.7
  concept of global health 7.1
  educational capacity building 7.11–7.12
  educational partnerships 7.1–7.2, 7.14
  history of global health 7.1
  impact of common skin diseases **7.3**
  key stakeholders 7.4–7.6
  medical volunteerism 7.13, **7.15**
  migrant health dermatology 7.13, **7.14**
  needs assessments 7.12–7.13
  Sustainable Development Goals 7.1, 7.6–7.7

sustainable educational and health care partnerships 7.14
teledermatology 7.8–7.9
terminology 7.6–7.7
volunteering opportunities 7.13, **7.15**
Global Programme to Eliminate Lymphatic Filariasis (GPELF) 103.35
globular patterns
  dermoscopy
    melanomas 145.7, *145.8*, 145.10
    naevi *145.2, 145.3*, 145.4–145.5, 145.6
GLODERM (International Alliance for Global Health Dermatology) 7.6
glomangioma/glomangiomyoma *see* glomus tumour
glomeruloid haemangioma 136.25
glomovenous malformations, oral involvement 108.25
glomus tumour 136.41–136.42
  diagnosis 3.25
glomuvenous malformation (GVM) 71.2, 71.18–71.19
glossitis 108.24–108.25
  atrophic glossitis *108.25*
  median rhomboid glossitis 108.22
glossodynia/glossopyrosis/glossalgia *see* burning mouth syndrome
glove materials, chemical protection **128.8**
GLP-1 *see* glucagon-like peptide-1
GLPLS *see* Graham-Little–Piccardi–Lassueur syndrome
glucagon and glucagonoma, dermatoendocrinology **150.10**, 150.12, 150.19
glucagon-like peptide-1 (GLP-1) 125.14
glucagonoma syndrome, necrolytic migratory erythema 153.6
glucocorticoids (GCs) 19.17–19.21
  cautions 19.19–19.20
  contraindications 19.18
  dermatological uses 19.17
  dose and regimens 19.20–19.21
  drug–drug interactions 19.20
  monitoring 19.21
  pharmacological properties 19.17–19.18
  potential adverse effects 19.18, *19.19*
  pre-treatment screening 19.20
  sensitivity to, atopic eczema 41.19
glucocorticosteroids 2.31
glucose levels, burn injuries 125.14
glucose monitors, allergic reactions to 62.4
glue sniffer's rash 120.4
glutamine supplementation, hypermetabolism treatment 125.11–125.12
glutamine synthesis defects 79.14–79.15
glutathione-S-transferases (GSTs) 127.10
gluteal region *see* buttock
glyceryl trinitrate 18.41
  Raynaud phenomenon treatment 124.12
glycine-glutamate-lysine-glycine (GEKG) 157.5
glycine substitutions, dystrophic epidermolysis bullosa 69.19
glycolic acid (GA), chemical peels 160.2, *160.8*, 160.9–160.10
glycopeptides 19.47
glycoproteinoses 79.3–79.4, **79.4**
glycosaminoglycans (GAGs) 2.36–2.39
  cosmeceutical use 157.4
  gene location **2.39**
  molecular structure 2.36, *2.37*
  tissue distribution **2.39**
glycosaminoglycan synthesis 94.42
glycosylation
  CHIME syndrome 63.38
  congenital disorders of 79.9–79.10
glycyrrhetinic acid, topical therapies 18.41
glyphic wrinkles 94.2
glypicans 2.38
G_{M1} gangliosidosis 79.5
gnathostomiasis 33.21–33.23
  clinical features 33.22–33.23
  epidemiology 33.21

management 33.23
pathophysiology 33.21–33.22
gold
  allergic contact dermatitis 127.40–127.41
  dermatological manifestations 121.3–121.4
Goldenhar syndrome **106.7**
golimumab, psoriatic arthritis treatment 35.45
gonadal mosaicism 8.7
gonococcal conjunctivitis 30.3, *30.4*, 30.8
gonococcal ophthalmia neonatorum 30.3, *30.4*
gonococcal vaccine 30.7
gonorrhoea 30.1–30.8
  antimicrobial resistance 30.7
  clinical features 30.3–30.6
  disseminated disease 30.5–30.6
  epidemiology 30.1
  gonococcal vaccine 30.7
  investigations 30.6–30.7
  management 30.7–30.8
  oral involvement 108.55
  pathophysiology 30.1–30.2
  perianal skin 111.16
gonosomal mosaicism 8.7
Gordon syndrome 103.24
Gorham syndrome
  diffuse lymphangiomatosis involving bone 136.39
  see also disappearing/vanishing/phantom bone disease
Gorham–Stout disease (GSD) 71.2, 103.28
  diffuse lymphangiomatosis involving bone 136.39
  see also disappearing/vanishing/phantom bone disease
Gorlin syndrome *see* naevoid basal cell carcinoma syndrome
gout **106.22**, 155.9–155.10
gouty panniculitis 97.60, *97.61*
gouty tophi *106.24*
Gower panatrophy 94.19–94.20
GPA *see* granulomatosis with polyangiitis
GPCRs *see* G-protein-coupled receptors
GPELF *see* Global Programme to Eliminate Lymphatic Filariasis
GPP *see* generalised pustular psoriasis
G-protein-coupled receptors (GPCRs), transmembrane drug mechanisms 13.5
GPs *see* general practitioners
GR *see* granulomatous rosacea
Grading of Recommendations, Assessment, Development and Evaluations (GRADE) working group 17.11
grafts
  burn injuries *125.13*
  skin surgery 20.29–20.30, *20.34*, 20.35
  wound healing 11.11–11.12
graft-versus-host disease (GvHD) 38.1–38.12, 98.9, 107.34
  acute 38.2, 38.3–38.7
  versus chronic distinction 38.1
  chronic 38.2, 38.3, 38.7–38.11
  clinical features 38.3–38.5, 38.7–38.9
  epidemiology 38.1–38.2
  extracorporeal photochemotherapy 21.7
  female genitalia 110.43–110.44
  management 38.5–38.7, 38.9–38.11
  oral involvement 108.48–108.49, 108.70
  pathology 38.2–38.3
  predisposing factors 38.2
  severity classification 38.4, **38.5**, 38.9, **38.10**
  skin cancer
    pathogenesis 147.9–147.10
    risks of chronic disease 147.4–147.5
  transfusion-associated 149.15
Graham-Little–Piccardi–Lassueur syndrome (GLPLS) 87.43
Gram-negative bacteria 26.49–26.67
Gram-negative folliculitis **88.36**
  Pseudomonas aeruginosa 26.51–26.53
  sports association 122.16

Gram-negative organisms
  burn wound infections 125.10
  Papillon–Lefèvre syndrome 63.68
Gram-positive bacteria 26.6–26.49
Gram-positive organisms, burn wound infections 125.10
Gram stain 3.9
granular cell myoblastoma, vulva **110.32**
granular cell tumours 108.45
  neural cells 136.48–136.49
granular fat 97.1–97.2
granulating wounds, postoperative care 20.37, 20.38–20.39
granulation tissue, peristomal skin *112.6*
granulocytic (myeloid) sarcoma
  infiltration of skin with malignant granulocyte precursor cells 149.2
  oral involvement 108.70
  see also leukaemia cutis
granuloma 3.41
  denture-induced granuloma 108.10
  erythema nodosum 97.22
  foreign body reactions 122.17, 122.21
  mercury 121.6
  peristomal skin *112.6*
  sarcoidosis 96.2–96.3
  subcutaneous tissue 97.12, *97.54*
granuloma annulare (GA) 3.44, 4.10, 95.1–95.8, 97.14–97.15
  associated diseases 95.1–95.2
  complications and co-morbidities 95.7
  diabetes association 62.5, *62.7*
  differential diagnosis 95.7
  disease course and prognosis 95.7–95.8
  drug-induced 95.2
  ear dermatoses **106.22**
  epidemiology 95.1
  generalised or disseminated 95.5, *95.6*
  HIV 31.18
  incidence and prevalence 95.1
  internal malignancy association 148.23
  interstitial or diffuse pattern *95.3*
  investigations 95.8
  localised 95.4–95.5
  management 95.8
  necrobiotic xanthogranuloma 97.18
  pathology 95.2–95.4
  pathophysiology 95.2
  perforating 95.3, *95.4*, 95.6, *95.7*
  presentation and clinical variants 95.4–95.7
  sarcoidal pattern 95.3, *95.4*
  subcutaneous 95.6–95.7
  sunlight exposure 95.2
  treatment ladder 95.8
granuloma faciale 89.10, 100.11–100.12
  ear dermatoses **106.22**
  inflammatory cell infiltrate *100.12*
  photothermal ablation 23.22
granuloma inguinale 30.21–30.23
  clinical features 30.22–30.23
  epidemiology 30.21
  investigations 30.23
  management 30.23
  pathophysiology 30.21–30.22
  perineal skin 111.17
granuloma multiforme 94.29–94.30
granuloma telangiectaticum *see* pyogenic granuloma
granulomatosis, orofacial 103.48, 108.72–108.74, 127.21
granulomatosis with polyangiitis (GPA) 100.22–100.25
  bilateral nodules *100.26*
  collagen degeneration *100.24*
  ear dermatoses **106.22**
  eye disease **107.35**
  inflammatory infiltrate *100.24*
  involving respiratory system 152.3–152.4
  oral involvement 108.69
  ulcerated lesions of cutaneous small-vessel vasculitis *100.26*
granulomatous acne 88.30
granulomatous disorders 95.1–95.16
  cutaneous Crohn disease 95.13–95.16

diabetic patients 62.5
granuloma annulare 95.1–95.8
necrobiosis lipoidica 95.8–95.13
orofacial granulomatosis 103.48, 108.72–108.74, 127.21
sarcoidosis 105.9
scalp 105.9
see also sarcoidosis
granulomatous (or nodular) candidiasis of the napkin area 32.65
granulomatous periorificial dermatoses, childhood 89.18–89.19
granulomatous reactions
allergens 127.21
annular elastolytic giant cell granuloma 94.29
bacterial infection 26.76–26.77
granulomatous rosacea (GR) 88.34, 89.7, *89.8*, 89.9
granulomatous skin lesions
necrotising skin *80.10*
severe combined immunodeficiency 80.8
granulomatous slack skin disease 94.30, 139.16
granulomatous superficial pyoderma gangrenosum 49.5, *49.6*
granulosis rubra nasi 92.10–92.11
grape seed extract (GSE) 157.7–157.9
Graves disease **150.7**, **150.10**, **150.11**, *150.14*, 150.20
gravitational purpura 99.4
'the Greater Patient' concept 16.10
Greece
ancient medical texts 1.2
Hippocrates 1.3
green tea (*Camellia sinensis*) 157.9
green zone 3.41
Grenz rays, kilovolt X-ray therapy 24.4, 24.7
grey lesions, melanoma 145.14
Griscelli syndrome 80.14
Griscelli–Pruniéras syndrome types I and II 68.9
griseofulvin antifungals 19.48
see also aciclovir; famciclovir; penciclovir; valaciclovir
groin
chancroid 30.18–30.21
erythrasma *4.20*
hidradenitis suppurativa 88.38
Langerhans cell histiocytosis 115.16
linear IgA disease 115.11
lymph drainage, obstruction of *103.8*
microbiome 26.4, 26.5
necrolytic migratory erythema *47.14*
subcorneal pustular dermatosis *49.18*
groin rash, Langerhans cell histiocytosis 135.4
Grotton papules 52.5, *52.7*
Grotton syndrome **70.26**, 70.28
ground itch *see* ancylostomiasis; strongyloidiasis
groundwater contamination, by arsenic 141.13, 141.18
Group A streptococcus *see Streptococcus pyogenes*
Group B streptococci 26.12, 26.36–26.37
Group C streptococci 26.12, 26.36–26.37
Grover disease *see* transient acantholytic dermatosis
growth delay, atopic eczema association 41.21
growth factors
hair disorder treatment 87.95
wound healing **11.4**, *11.5*, **11.5**, *11.6*, 11.11
growth failure, ichthyoses 63.46
growth hormone, central nervous system controlled endocrine signalling axis 150.2
growth hormone deficiency, Netherton syndrome 63.26
growth hormone treatment, burn injuries 125.13
Grzybowski syndrome 141.43–141.44
GSD *see* Gorham–Stout disease

GSE *see* grape seed extract
GSTs *see* glutathione-S-transferases
G-Tube (gastrostomy), bullous pemphigoid *50.19*
GUD (genital ulcer disease) *see* genital ulceration
guinea pig maximisation test 127.8–127.9
Guinea worm *see* dracunculiasis
'guitar nipple' 122.12
gummas, syphilis 108.56
gummatous neurosyphilis 29.15
gummatous syphilide *29.13, 29.14, 29.15*
gums *see* gingiva
gustatory hyperhidrosis 83.24, 92.5–92.6, 92.8
flushing in children **104.10**
management 92.9
gut microbiome, and atopic eczema 41.9
'gut'/slaughterhouse eczema 39.15–39.16
guttate lichen planus 37.8, *37.9*
guttate morphoea 55.17
guttate psoriasis 35.15, **35.16**, 35.19
GvHD *see* graft-versus-host disease
GVM *see* glomuvenous malformation
gynaecomastia **150.10**, *150.12*, *150.13*, 150.14, 150.16, 150.17, 150.18

H
H&E *see* haematoxylin and eosin stain
HA20 *see* haploinsufficiency of A20
HA *see* hyaluronic acid
HAART *see* highly active antiretroviral therapy
habit disorders
A-B-C model 84.12
onychotillomania and onychophagia 84.25
trichotillomania/trichotillosis 84.22–84.25, 87.14, 87.24, 87.32–87.34
see also obsessive–compulsive behaviour/disorder
habit reversal therapies, psychodermatology 84.12, 84.15, 84.17, 84.18, 84.20, 84.21, 84.25, 84.47
HADS *see* Hospital Anxiety and Depression Scale
HAE *see* hereditary angio-oedema
haem
biosynthesis of 58.2, *58.3, 58.4*
chemistry of 58.1–58.2
molecular structure *58.2*
haemangiomas 136.25–136.32
capillary, laser therapies 23.8
eyelid 107.46–107.47
infants 23.8, 116.1–116.9
oral involvement 108.25–108.26
haemangiosarcoma *see* angiosarcoma
haematological abnormalities, dyskeratosis congenita 75.4
haematological diseases
necrobiotic xanthogranuloma association 135.24
oral involvement 108.69–108.72
skin manifestations 149.1–149.16
haematological malignancies
eosinophilic pustular folliculitis 91.4
graft-versus-host disease following allogenic haematopoietic stem cell transplantation 38.1–38.12
human papillomavirus 25.71
rare syndromes 149.14–149.15
see also cutaneous lymphomas
haematological neoplasms
infiltration of skin with neoplastic cells 149.2–149.5
skin manifestations 149.1–149.15
haematological syndromes, ocular features **107.42**
haematoma
external ear 106.8
penile 109.8
skin surgery 20.41–20.42
haematopoiesis 149.5
haematopoietic malignancies 148.2
haematopoietic stem cell transplantation (HSCT) 98.8–98.9

complications of 108.48
graft-versus-host disease 38.1–38.12
skin cancer risks 147.4–147.5
haematoporphyrin, photodynamic therapy history 22.2
haematoxylin and eosin (H&E) stain 3.7, *3.8, 3.9*
haem disorders **79.2**
haemochromatosis 86.22, *86.23*, 86.48–86.49, 153.5
haemodialysis
arteriovenous shunt site complications 154.5
calciphylaxis 154.2
cutaneous complications 154.4–154.5
cutaneous signs 154.3–154.4
haemoglobin
light absorption by skin 23.3–23.4
vascular lasers 23.6
haemoglobinopathies 149.15–149.16
haemolytic anaemia/methaemoglobinaemia, dapsone side effect 19.14
haemophagocytic lymphohistiocytosis (HLH) 135.11–135.14
infectious mononucleosis complication 25.37
haemophilia, HIV/AIDS 31.37
Haemophilus ducreyi, chancroid 30.18–30.21
haemorrhagic bulla, primary systemic amyloidosis 56.13
haemorrhagic crusting, hydroa vacciniforme 126.25, *126.26*
haemorrhagic fevers
Bunyavirus infections 25.83–25.84
filivirus infections 25.85–25.87
filovirus infections 25.84–25.85
haemorrhagic lesions *4.12*
haemorrhagic onychomadesis, selenium exposure 121.7
haemorrhagic polymorphic light eruption 126.4, *126.5*
haemorrhagic proctitis, lymphogranuloma venereum 30.16
haemorrhagic rashes, measles 25.99
haemorrhoids 111.31–111.33
origin of internal and external haemorrhoids *111.32*
perianal skin tags 111.32, *111.33*
positions of internal haemorrhoids *111.32*
prolapsed internal haemorrhoids *111.32*
severity classification **111.33**
haemosiderin 86.47, *86.48*
haemosiderosis 94.10
haemosiderotic fibrolipomatous tumour 136.60–136.61
haemostasis
open wounds 20.48
wound healing 9.6
Hailey–Hailey disease (HHD) 69.24, 110.5–110.6
ano-genital region 111.10
perineal and perianal skin 111.10
Haim–Munk syndrome 63.68
hair 91.10–91.11, 122.22–122.24
acquired disorders of 87.1–87.102
anagen phase *87.8*
colour 86.5, 87.12–87.13, 87.73–87.74, 87.88, 87.99–87.101, 127.60–127.61, 142.3
corkscrew hairs, vitamin C deficiency 61.21, *61.22*
crab lice 34.24–34.25
cyclical behaviour 87.9
density on scalp 87.3
external ear *106.3*
follicular psoriasis 35.7, *35.9*
foreign-body reactions 91.10–91.11, 93.1–93.2, 122.22–122.24
fragility of 87.75–87.90
greying 87.91–87.93
head lice 34.18–34.23
inherited immunodeficiency **80.4–80.6**
internal malignancy effects 148.17–148.18
iron deficiency 61.3, 61.4, 61.24, 87.59, 87.63, 87.70–87.71

keratins 2.10
lichen planopilaris 37.5, 37.6, 37.11
metal poisoning signs 121.1
in pregnancy 113.1, **113.2**
psoriasis vulgaris 35.7, *35.9*
reddening of in protein-energy malnutrition *61.4*
regrowth, topical use of sensitising agents 18.33–18.34
sample collection in fungal infection 32.7
systemic lupus erythematosus 51.25–51.26
transplantation 87.97
types 87.2
variants, explanation for 2.10
see also arrector pili muscle; hirsutism; trichi...
HAIR-AN syndrome 85.4–85.5
acne vulgaris association 88.7–88.8, *88.11*
hair artefact, cutting/shaving to simulate disease 84.33
hair balls *see* trichobezoar
hair-bearing skin 2.43
hair bulb 87.4–87.5, 87.8
scarring alopecia 87.37
hair changes
associated with liver disease 153.9
chemotherapy-induced 119.5–119.6
hair colour 87.99–87.101, 127.60–127.61
melanoma risk 142.3
pigmentation 87.12–87.13, 87.88
trichochromes 86.5
tyrosine kinase inhibitors 87.73–87.74
hair curl, classification 87.7
hair cycle 87.7–87.9
dynamics 87.63
hair discs 2.12
hair disorders 87.1–87.102
assessment/management 87.13–87.18
common treatments 87.94–87.101
cosmetic approaches 87.69, 87.97–87.101
COVID-19 association 25.113
excessive hair growth 87.84–87.91
HIV 31.33–31.34
ichthyoses 63.45
ocular features **107.41**
pigmentation disorders 68.6–68.7, 68.9, 87.91–87.94
structural defects 87.75–87.84
syndromic ichthyoses **63.39**, 63.40–63.46
hair dyes, allergic reactions 127.5, 127.16, 127.33, 127.60–127.61
hair fall, increase in 87.53–87.71
hair fibres 87.6–87.7
hair-filled sinuses 122.23
hair follicle pigmentary unit (HFPU) 87.12–87.13
hair follicles (HF) 2.43, 87.2
androgen action mechanism 87.10–87.11
cysts and tumours, dystrophic calcification 59.3–59.4
degeneration and regeneration 2.45
density **87.3**
development/distribution 87.2–87.3
embryonic development 2.3–2.5, *2.5*
fibroplasts 2.40
growth phase 2.45
as hormone-sensitive mini-organs 150.1, 150.3
innervation 87.7
light absorption 23.5–23.6
melanocytes 2.17
Merkel cells 2.12
mesenchyme lesions 137.15–137.16
miniaturisation 87.64, *87.65*
naevi 137.7–137.8
neuroendocrinology 87.11–87.13
resting phase 2.45
staphylococcal infections 26.22–26.27
stem cells in 2.44–2.45
suprabulbar region 87.4, 87.6
tumours 137.2–137.5
see also carbuncles; folliculitis; furuncles; sycosis
hair germ tumours and cysts 137.7–137.13

hair growth 87.9–87.11
  excessive 87.84–87.91
  phases of 2.10
hair immune system 87.11
hair loss
  assessment/management 87.13–87.18
  increased hair fall-associated 87.53–87.71
  infants 115.15
  infections 87.35–87.36
  presentations 87.18–87.74
  psychological and social factors 15.4
  scalp psoriasis 105.3
  see also alopecia
hair matrix tumours 137.13–137.15
hair presentation, Netherton syndrome 63.26–63.27
hair products
  allergic contact dermatitis 127.48
  effects on dandruff 40.4
hair pulling disorders (trichotillomania/trichotillosis) 84.22–84.25, 87.14, 87.24, 87.32–87.34
hair pull test 87.54–87.55, 87.65
hair reduction, laser treatment 23.5–23.6, 23.17–23.20
hair removal
  folliculitis keloidalis 93.4
  hidradenitis suppurativa treatment 90.11
  laser assisted 23.17–23.20, 93.4
  principles of light-assisted removal 23.5–23.6
  pseudofolliculitis 91.10, 93.1–93.2
hair shaft abnormalities, trichoscopy 87.74
hair shaft (HS)
  disorders of 87.14–87.15, 87.74–87.84
  fungal infections 32.15–32.16
  suprabulbar region 87.4
  white piedra 32.16–32.17
hair shedding, in infancy 114.4
hair sinus 122.22
hair styling, alopecia 87.99
hair systems 87.101
hair-thread tourniquet syndrome 122.23
  foot involvement 122.22
hairy leukoplakia, oral lesions 108.32–108.33, 108.34
half-and-half nails 154.3
halitosis, olfactory delusions 84.10–84.11
Hallermann–Streiff syndrome 77.2
hallucinations, delusional infestation 84.6
halo dermatitis 39.28
halo eczema naevus see Myerson naevus
halogen acne 129.12
halogenated aromatic hydrocarbons 129.12
halogenated salicylanilides 127.79–127.80
halo naevi 86.40–86.42, 131.27–131.28, 131.28, 131.29
  vitiligo association 86.34–86.35, 86.41
hamartoma of cutaneous adnexa and mesenchyme see rhabdomyomatous congenital hamartoma
hamartoma of the pilosebaceous follicle 137.8–137.9
hamartomas
  basaloid follicular 137.12–137.13
  dermoid cyst, mouth 108.12
  sclerosing epithelial see desmoplastic trichoepithelioma
hamartomatous polyps, PJT syndrome 68.13
Hamilton–Norwood scale, hair loss 87.65, 87.66
hand
  atopic eczema 41.16–41.17, 41.19, 41.23
  bullous eczema 39.14
  bullous pemphigoid 50.16
  callosities 122.8
  cheiroarthropathy 62.7
  cicatricial pemphigoid 50.52
  collagenous and elastotic marginal plaques 94.4–94.5
  deformity, epidermolysis bullosa 69.17–69.18, 69.26
  dermatomyositis 52.5, 52.7, 52.8
  discoid lesions, systemic lupus erythematosus 51.23

discoid lupus erythematosus 51.8
epidermolysis bullosa acquista 50.44
erythema elevatum diutinum 100.9
erythema multiforme 4.15, 47.2
erytropoietic protoporphyria 99.24
glomuvenous malformation 71.18
granuloma annulare 95.2, 95.5
Grotton papules in dermatomyositis 52.5, 52.7
IgA vasculitis 100.15
infrared thermograms 54.22
lichen planus 39.17
lichen striatus 37.18
Maffucci syndrome 71.20
mixed connective tissue disease 53.4
mucocutaneous venous malformation 71.16
mucous membrane pemphigoid 50.29
Nékam disease 37.11
neutrophilic dermatosis of dorsal hands 49.12, 49.13
oedema 103.21
palisaded and neutrophilic granulomatous dermatitis 53.7
pellagra, niacin deficiency 61.17
psoriasis vulgaris 35.11
Rothmund–Thomson syndrome 75.6
spindle cell haemangiomas 71.20
STING-associated vasculopathy with onset in infancy 45.14
systemic lupus erythematosus 51.23, 51.24
tinea nigra palmaris 32.14–32.15
tyrosinaemia type 2 79.12
xanthomatosis 60.6
see also palm
hand eczema 39.12–39.19, 127.13–127.14, 128.1–128.2, 128.3–128.4
  acute 39.19
  advice to patients 128.7
  aetiology 39.12
  apron eczema 39.14, 39.15
  associated diseases 39.13
  chronic 39.14–39.15, 39.18–39.19
  clinical features 39.14
  clinical variants 39.14–39.16
  complications and co-morbidities 39.17
  differential diagnosis 39.16–39.17, 127.22, 128.5
  disease course and prognosis 39.17–39.18
  environmental factors 39.13–39.14
  epidemiology 39.12–39.13
  fingertip 39.15
  genetics 39.13
  'gut'/slaughterhouse eczema 39.15–39.16
  hyperkeratotic 39.14
  inflammatory pathways 39.13
  investigations 39.18
  management 39.18–39.19
  morphological patterns 39.12
  nickel allergy 127.37–127.38
  occupational contact dermatitis 129.2, 129.6
  patchy vesiculosquamous eczema 39.16
  plant allergies 127.72
  pompholyx eczema 39.14
  population studies 127.3
  predisposing factors 39.13, 127.7
  preservatives 127.53–127.54
  prognosis 127.23
  recurrent focal palmar peeling 39.16
  ring eczema 39.16
  severity classification 39.17
  treatment 39.19
  Trichophyton infection 39.17
hand, foot and mouth disease 25.94–25.95, 108.50
  infants 115.6
handicap, caused by skin disease 5.5–5.6
hand–arm vibration syndrome (HAVS) 122.24–122.26
Hand–Schüller–Christian syndrome 135.6
Hansen, Gerhard 1.8
Hansen's disease/Hanseniasis see leprosy
Hapalochlaena maculosa, stings from 130.4

haploinsufficiency of A20 (HA20) 45.5, 45.7, 45.15
haplotypes, mal de Meleda 63.55
Happle–Tinschert syndrome 73.7, 78.12
haptenisation 118.5
hapten/pro-hapten model, T-cell recognition of drugs 14.5–14.6
haptens 127.8
harlequin colour change
  flushing in children 104.10, 104.10
  neonates 114.3
harlequin ichthyosis (HI) 63.7–63.8, 63.9–63.10
  management of 63.43
Harmonising Outcome Measures for Eczema (HOME) 16.3
Hartnup disease 61.16, 79.14
harvest mites 34.54
Hashimoto–Pritzker disease 135.5, 135.7
HAVS see hand–arm vibration syndrome
Haxthausen disease 63.71–63.72
HBV see hepatitis B virus
HC see hereditary coproporphyria
HCCVM see hyperkeratotic cutaneous capillary–venous malformations
HCoVs see human coronaviruses
HCV see hepatitis C virus
HDM see house dust mite
HD-OCT see high-definition optical coherence tomography
head, allergic contact dermatitis of 127.14, 127.21
Headington's anagen release 87.53
head lice 34.18–34.23
  clinical features 34.20–34.21
  epidemiology 34.18–34.19
  investigations 34.21
  management 34.21–34.23
  on mummified body 1.2
  pathophysiology 34.20
head and neck, anatomical considerations for skin surgery 20.1–20.4
head oedema 103.46–103.49, 103.47
Heaf test 4.24
healing see wound healing
health anxieties, irrational/obsessional fears of skin problems 84.25–84.26
health care partnerships 7.14
health care settings 5.12–5.13
health economics 6.1–6.11
  decision-making in dermatology practice 6.10–6.11
  economic burden of disease 6.5–6.10
    atopic eczema 6.10
    definition 6.1
    psoriasis 6.8–6.10
    skin cancer 6.5–6.8
    studies on 6.10
  holistic perspective 6.2
  methods and approaches 6.1–6.5
    bottom-up/top-down approaches 6.3
    comparative/non-comparative studies 6.3, 6.4–6.5
    cost-benefit analysis 6.4
    cost-effectiveness analysis 6.4
    cost-minimisation studies 6.4
    cost-utility analysis 6.4
    evaluation perspectives 6.2
    friction cost approach 6.3
    human capital approach 6.3
    implementation of health economic findings in decision-making 6.5
    indirect costs 6.3
    intangible costs 6.3
    physician perspective 6.2
    prioritisation 6.5
    productivity costs 6.3
    rationalisation 6.5
    scaling 6.5
    secondary research 6.2–6.3
    types of health economic evaluation 6.2–6.5
    willingness to pay 6.4
  patient perspective 6.2
  psoriasis, economic burden of 6.8–6.10

skin cancer, economic burden of 6.5–6.8
societal perspective 6.2
third-party payer perspective 6.2
health related quality of life (HRQoL) 6.2, 16.5–16.6
health services research 5.12–5.14
Health Systems Evidence (HSE) database 17.6, 17.7
hearing impairment
  palmoplantar keratodermas and 63.63–63.65
  see also deafness
heart
  congenital heart block 51.39–51.42
  Libman–Sacks endocarditis 51.18
  sarcoidosis 96.6
  systemic lupus erythematosus 51.30
  see also cardio ... entries
heat
  cutaneous reactions to 124.1–124.16
  diseases caused by 124.14–124.16
  physiological reactions to 124.14
heat-associated carcinomas 124.15
heat contact urticaria 42.9, 42.10
heat injuries 125.1–125.15
heat rash see miliaria
heat shock proteins (HSP), Adamantiades–Behçet disease 48.3
heavy coal-tar distillates 129.12
heavy metals, oral hyperpigmentation 108.17
Heberden nodes 155.8
Hebra, Ferdinand Ritter von 1.6
Heck's disease 108.11
hedgehog pathway inhibitors, hair loss 87.74
hEDS see hypermobile Ehlers–Danlos syndromes
heel
  black heel 99.6
  calcified cutaneous nodules of the heels 115.15
  mechanical injuries 122.10–122.11
  pedal papules of infancy 115.15
  piezogenic pedal papules 122.26
heel prick calcinosis 59.3
HEH see neutrophilic eccrine hidradenitis
Helicobacter pylori infection 153.1
heliodermatitis 89.7–89.8
heliotrope rash 52.3
helminth infestations
  and atopic eczema 41.8
  perineal and perianal skin 111.16
  see also cestodes; nematodes; trematodes
HEMA see hydroxyethlmethacrylate
2-HEMA see 2-hydroxyethylmethacrylate
hematidrosis 92.18, 92.19
hemidesmosomal inner plaques, keratins 69.4
hemidesmosomes 2.25–2.26
hemihyperplasia–multiple lipomatosis syndrome 72.9, 72.11
Hemiptera (bugs) 34.25–34.30
henna 87.100
Hennekam lymphangiectasia–lymphoedema syndrome 71.26
heparan 2.37
heparan sulphate (HS) 2.39
heparan sulphate proteoglycans (HSPGs) 2.25
heparin 2.37
heparin-induced thrombocytopenia (HIT) 99.9–99.10
heparin necrosis, purpura 99.9–99.10
hepatic, see also liver disease
hepatic gummata, syphilis 29.15
hepatic haemangioma (HH), infants 116.5
hepatic sarcoidosis 96.5
hepatitis 25.73–25.77
  and lichen planus 37.2
  oral involvement 108.74
hepatitis A virus 25.96–25.97
  cutaneous features 153.4

hepatitis B virus (HBV) 25.74–25.75
   arthropathies 155.3
   cryoglobulinaemia 124.13
   cutaneous features 153.4–153.5
   human bite transmission 130.7
hepatitis C virus (HCV) 25.75–25.77
   cryoglobulinaemia 124.13
   cutaneous features 153.5
   human bite transmission 130.7
   polymorphic light eruption 126.2
   viral arthropathies 155.3
hepatobiliary disease 153.4–153.5
   cholestatic pruritus 81.9–81.10
   and psoriasis 35.19
hepatocellular carcinoma, PR association 85.8
hepatotoxicity, methotrexate 19.26
herbals
   acne vulgaris 88.57–88.58
   cosmeceutical use of 157.7–157.10
   psychodermatological uses 84.48
   traditional topical therapies 18.38
   wart treatments 25.60
   see also complementary/alternative/traditional therapies; plant extracts
hereditary angio-oedema (HAE) 43.1–43.2, 43.3–43.4
   clinical features 43.4
   reticulate prodromal erythema *43.4*
   treatment 43.6
hereditary anonychia 67.16–67.17
hereditary autoinflammatory disorders/syndromes
   arthralgia/arthritis 155.10
   renal involvement 154.2
hereditary benign intraepithelial dyskeratosis 108.29
hereditary benign telangiectasia **101.17**, 101.20, *101.21*
   aborising pattern *101.20*
hereditary coproporphyria (HC) 58.5, 58.7, 58.9, 58.12, 58.17
hereditary disorders/syndromes 8.2–8.5, 8.8–8.9
   acne plus musculoskeletal features 155.11
   cardiac involvement 151.1, 151.2–151.4
   pachydermoperiostosis 155.14
   prenatal diagnosis 8.9–8.11
   skin and renal involvement 154.1–154.2
hereditary fibrosing poikiloderma with tendon contractures, myopathy and pulmonary fibrosis 75.2, 75.7
hereditary haemorrhagic telangiectasia (HHT) 71.2, 71.12–71.13, **78.14**, 153.7
   oral involvement 108.26
hereditary leiomyomatosis and renal cell cancer (HLRCC/Reed syndrome) **78.14**, *78.15*, 148.12, 154.2
hereditary lymphoedema type 1A (LMPH1A) 71.24–71.25
hereditary monogenic autoinflammatory syndromes 45.2–45.19, **155.10**
   autoinflammatory diseases with granuloma 45.11–45.12
   Behçet disease-like or inflammatory bowel disease-like autoinflammatory syndromes 45.15–45.16
   clinical features **45.6–45.7**
   dermatological signs and entities **45.3–45.4**
   epidemiology 45.2, **45.6–45.7**
   hereditary periodic fevers 45.8–45.11
   miscellaneous monogenic autoinflammatory syndromes 45.16–45.19
   pathophysiology 45.2–45.8
   related acquired sporadic or complex disorders **45.3–45.4**
   skin and/or mucosal manifestation **45.3–45.4**
   terminology **45.5**
   treatment **45.6–45.7**
   type 1 interferonopathies 45.13–45.15

hereditary mucoepithelial dysplasia (HMD) 63.25–63.26
hereditary neuropathies 83.11–83.24
hereditary non-polyposis colorectal cancer *see* Muir–Torre syndrome
hereditary obesity 72.3–72.9
   monogenic obesity with cutaneous features 72.4, **72.7**
   monogenic obesity without cutaneous features 72.3, **72.6**
   Prader–Willi syndrome 72.6–72.9
   pro-opiomelanocortin and prohormone convertase deficiency 72.4–72.6
   secondary skin complications of primary obesity **72.4**
hereditary panniculitis **72.11**, *72.12*
hereditary papulotranslucent acrokeratoderma 63.62
hereditary periodic fevers 45.8–45.11
   cryopyrin-associated periodic syndrome 45.8–45.9
   familial Mediterranean fever **45.5**, **45.6**, 45.9–45.10
   mevalonate kinase deficiency with recurrent fever and hyper-IgD syndrome 45.11
   pyrin-associated autoinflammation with neutrophilic dermatosis 45.10–45.11
   tumour necrosis factor associated periodic syndrome **45.5**, **45.6**, 45.9
hereditary progressive mucinous histiocytosis 135.23
hereditary sensory and autonomic neuropathies (HSANs) 83.12
hereditary syndromes *see* hereditary disorders/syndromes
Hermansky–Pudlak syndrome 68.8, **78.13**, **80.5**, 80.14
hermaphroditism 63.67
heroin
   addiction prevalence 120.2
   death rates 120.1
   dermatoses induced by 120.5–120.7
herpangina 25.95–25.96, 108.50
herpes-associated erythema multiforme 25.23
herpes B virus infection 25.43
herpes genitalis
   primary 25.24–25.25
   recurrent 25.26
herpes infection
   of eye *1.10*
   hair loss 87.35–87.36
herpes labialis
   primary herpetic gingivostomatitis 25.20–25.22
   recurrent oro-facial and cutaneous herpes 25.22–25.24
herpes simplex virus (HSV) *4.8*, 25.19–25.28, **25.44**
   antigenic types 25.19–25.20
   and atopic eczema 41.10
   cytology 3.29, *3.30*
   eyelid 107.34–107.36, *107.37*
   female genitalia 110.29–110.30
   genetically engineered for oncolytic virus therapy 144.1
   gingivostomatitis 25.20–25.22, 108.51–108.53
   guanosine analogue antivirals 19.49
   HIV 31.5, 31.23, *31.38*
   lingual recurrence *108.71*
   neonatal 114.22
   perineal and perianal skin 111.15, 111.16
   in pregnancy 113.4–113.5
   primary herpes genitalis 25.24–25.25
   primary herpetic gingivostomatitis 25.20–25.22
   primary/recurrent infections 25.19–25.20
   reactivation, PUVA phototherapy adverse effects 21.12, 21.13
   recurrent genital herpes 25.26
   recurrent oro-facial and cutaneous herpes 25.22–25.24

   subclinical viral shedding 25.20
herpes stromal keratitis (HSK), eyelid *107.37*
herpesviruses 1 and 2, human bite transmission 130.7
herpesviruses 6, 7 and 8, oral infection 108.53
herpesvirus infections 25.19–25.46, **25.20**
   Kaposi sarcoma 25.42, 25.43, 31.30
   oral infection 108.50–108.54
   reactivation of 14.4
   see also cytomegalovirus; eczema herpeticum; Epstein-Barr virus; human herpesvirus 6 and 7; human herpesvirus 8; inoculation herpes simplex; varicella-zoster virus; zoster
herpesvirus reactivation, drug reaction with eosinophilia and systemic symptoms 118.5–118.6
herpes zoster 25.32–25.36
   acute herpetic neuralgia 82.4
   clinical features 25.33–25.34
   cutaneous manifestations of Hodgkin disease 139.49
   epidemiology 25.32
   eyelid 107.36–107.38
   hair loss 87.35–87.36
   investigations 25.34–25.35
   management 25.35
   neuralgia 108.66
   neurogenic bladder dysfunction 154.6
   neurological complications 25.32, 25.33–25.34
   oral infection 108.53–108.54
   oticus 25.33–25.34
   pathophysiology 25.32
   postherpetic neuralgia 82.4–82.5
   reactivation after COVID-19 vaccination 25.118
   reactivation in COVID-19 patients 25.111
herpetic gingivostomatitis 25.21
herpetic whitlow 25.28
herpetiform ulceration 108.38, *108.39*
HES *see* hydroxyethyl starch
heterotopic sebaceous glands 91.15–91.17, 93.10–93.12
heterotrimeric G-protein mosaic disorders 73.19–73.21
   McCune–Albright syndrome 73.19–73.20
   phakomatosis pigmentovascularis 73.20–73.21
   Sturge–Weber syndrome 73.20
hexachlorophene 18.10
Hexathelidae (funnel web spider) 34.35
HF *see* hair follicles; hydrops fetalis
HFPU *see* hair follicle pigmentary unit
HFTC *see* hyperphosphataemic familial tumoral calcinosis
HGPS *see* Hutchinson–Gilford progeria syndrome
HH *see* hepatic haemangioma
HHD *see* Hailey–Hailey disease
HHT *see* hereditary haemorrhagic telangiectasia
HHV *see* human herpesvirus
HI *see* harlequin ichthyosis
hibernoma 136.57
hidradenitis suppurativa (HS) 87.50, 88.37, 88.38, 90.1–90.11, 111.10–111.12
   acne conglobata association 88.63
   assessment tools 16.4–16.5
   clinical features 111.11–111.12
   epidemiology 111.10–111.11
   facial 23.23
   Hurley staging system 111.11, **111.12**
   inflammed nodules *90.5*
   management 90.10, 111.12
   pathophysiology 111.11
   psychological factors 15.4
   quality of life assessment 16.8
   scarring *111.11*, *111.12*
   sexual function measures 16.12
Hidradenitis Suppurativa, Patient-Reported Outcome Measures 16.8

Hidradenitis Suppurativa Burden of Disease (HSBOD) 16.8
Hidradenitis Suppurativa Clinical Response (HiSCR) 16.4–16.5
HIdradenitis SuppuraTiva cORe outcomes set International Collaboration (HISTORIC) 16.3, 16.8
Hidradenitis Suppurativa Impact Assessment (HSIA) 16.8
hidradenitis suppurativa lesion, area and severity index (HS-LASI) 16.4
Hidradenitis Suppurativa Physician's Global Assessment (HS-PGA) 16.4
Hidradenitis Suppurativa Quality of Life (HiSQOL) questionnaire 16.8
Hidradenitis Suppurativa Quality of Life instrument (HS-QoL) 16.8
Hidradenitis Suppurativa Symptom Assessment (HSSA) 16.8
hidradenocarcinoma 137.35–137.40
hidradenoma 137.28–137.29
hidradenoma papilliferum (papillary hidradenoma) 110.31–110.33, 137.20–137.21
hidradénomes eruptifs *see* syringoma
hidroacanthoma simplex 137.24–137.25
hidrotic ectodermal dysplasia *see* Clouston syndrome
HIDS (hyperimmunoglobulinaemia-D syndrome) *see* mevalonate kinase deficiency
HID syndrome *see* hystrix-like ichthyosis and deafness
HIFU *see* high intensity microfocused ultrasound
high-definition optical coherence tomography (HD-OCT), basal cell carcinoma 140.10, *140.12*
high-grade squamous intraepithelial lesions (HSIL), female genitalia 110.34–110.36
high intensity microfocused ultrasound (HIFU) 161.7–161.8
highly active antiretroviral therapy (HAART) 91.5
   fibrous histiocytoma 136.21
   HIV-associated lipodystrophy 98.6–98.8
   lobular capillary haemangioma 136.26
high-molecular-weight kininogen (HMWK), bradykinin-induced angio-oedema *43.3*
high-performance liquid chromatography (HPLC), porphyrias *58.8*
hindfoot anomaly 122.7
Hippocrates 1.3
Hirschsprung disease 68.5
hirsutism 87.84, 87.87–87.90
   acne vulgaris *88.45*
   depilatories 18.33
   disorders associated with 87.90–87.91
   laser-assisted hair removal 23.17, 23.19
HiSCR *see* Hidradenitis Suppurativa Clinical Response
HiSQOL *see* Hidradenitis Suppurativa Quality of Life
histamine 4 (H4) receptor, atopic eczema treatment 41.30–41.32
histamine
   release of in skin 14.1
   solar urticaria 126.21–126.23
histamine-evoked 'geographical' pattern of flushing, carcinoid tumours *150.12*
histamine receptors, pruritus **81.3**, 81.4
histiocytes
   function 135.1–135.2
   microscopic examination of 3.36
histiocytic disorders 149.16–149.17
histiocytic lymphoma 135.30–135.31
histiocytic markers, cutaneous neoplasms 3.27
histiocytic sarcoma (HS) 135.31–135.32
histiocytoid haemangioma *see* epithelioid haemangioma
histiocytoid Sweet syndrome 49.12, *49.14*, 97.22–97.23, 149.6

histiocytoma cutis *see* fibrous histiocytoma
histiocytoses 135.1–135.32
  eye disease **107.35**
histochemistry, biopsy 3.7–3.10
histone deacetylase inhibitor therapy 139.25
histopathology of skin 3.1–3.46
  artefacts 3.31–3.32
  biopsy 3.2–3.10
  cytodiagnosis 3.29–3.30
  descriptive terms 3.38–3.43
  digital pathology 3.32
  electron microscopy 3.30–3.31
  foreign body reactions 122.18–122.19
  graft versus host disease 38.2, 38.3
  histological sections with little or no abnormality 3.44–3.45
  immunogenotyping 3.31
  immunopathology 3.10–3.29
  microscopic examination of tissue sections 3.32–3.45
  pseudoepitheliomatous hyperplasia mimicking squamous cell carcinoma 132.9–132.10
  reporting of 3.38
  Tzanck smears 3.29–3.30
  viral disease diagnosis 3.31
  see also biopsy of skin
Histoplasma capsulatum 32.81, 32.82, 32.84
histoplasmin test 4.25
histoplasmosis 32.81–32.84
  clinical features 32.82–32.84
  epidemiology 32.81–32.82
  HIV 31.27
  management 32.84
  oral lesions 108.57
  pathophysiology 32.82
HISTORIC *see* HIdradenitis SuppuraTiva cORe outcomes set International Collaboration
history of dermatology *see* dermatology history
history taking 4.2–4.5, 81.6
HIT *see* heparin-induced thrombocytopenia
hives *see* urticaria
HIV infection 31.1–31.39
  acute primary infection 31.6–31.7
  ano-genital disorders 31.35–31.36
  aphthous-like ulceration *108.71*
  arthropathies 155.3, 155.4
  associated infections 31.20–31.30
  atopic eczema 31.15
  bacterial infections 31.20–31.23
  candidiasis 31.6, 31.26, 31.34, 31.37, 32.58, 108.21–108.22
  children 31.36–31.37
  clinical features 31.5–31.8
  coagulopathies 31.12
  coinfections 31.20–31.31
  complications and co-morbidities 31.7–31.8, 31.20–31.31
  as a continuum 31.6
  cryoglobulinaemia 124.13
  cryptococcus infection 31.28
  cytomegalovirus infection 31.24–31.25
  definition 31.1
  dermatological manifestations 31.11–31.39
    acute primary infection 31.6–31.7
    coinfections 31.20–31.31
    common conditions **31.11**
    neoplasms 31.30–31.33
  dermatophytosis 31.26–31.27
  diagnosis 31.7
  drug reaction with eosinophilia and systemic symptoms 118.5–118.6
  eosinophilic folliculitis 31.17, 93.7, 93.8, 93.9
  eosinophilic pustular folliculitis 91.4–91.5
  epidemiology 31.2
  erythroderma 31.12
  fungal infections 31.26–31.29
  granuloma annulare 31.18
  hair abnormalities 31.33–31.34

hair loss 87.35
hairy leukoplakia, oral lesions 108.32, *108.33*
herpes simplex infection 31.23
histoplasmosis 31.27
history 31.1
HIV-associated lipodystrophy 98.2, 98.6–98.8
HIV-induced or exacerbated psoriasis 35.15–35.16
HIV-related pityriasis rubra pilaris (type VI) 36.4
human bite transmission 130.7
human papillomavirus infection 25.71, 31.25–31.26
immunology 31.3–31.5
immunosuppression causing lymphoproliferative disorders 139.47
infection and course 31.1–31.10
infection prevention 31.9
inflammatory dermatoses 31.12–31.20
initial diagnosis 31.7, 31.11
investigations 31.8–31.9, 31.11–31.12
Kaposi sarcoma 31.30–31.31, 31.35
leprosy 28.10
lip, warts on *108.14*
male genitalia 109.29
management 31.9–31.10
mollusca/molluscipoxvirus infection 31.26
mycobacterial infections 27.2–27.3, 27.9, 27.10, 31.22
nail abnormalities 31.33–31.34
neonates 114.24
neoplasms 31.30–31.33
  photodynamic therapy 22.7–22.8
non-AIDS defining cancers 31.31
normalisation of testing 31.2, 31.11
oral hyperpigmentation 108.17
oral lesions 108.54
oro-pharyneal abnormalities 31.34–31.35, **31.36**
pathophysiology 31.2–31.5
penicilliosis 31.28
perineal and perianal skin 111.17
pigmentary disorders 31.12
porphyria cutanea tarda 31.18
posinophilic folliculitis 31.17–31.18
protozoal infections 31.29
pruritic conditions 31.12
psoriasis 31.15–31.17
recurrent genital herpes risk 25.26
scabies 31.29
scalp infection 105.12
seborrhoeic dermatitis 31.12, 31.15
seroconversion symptoms 31.5, 31.6–31.7, 31.11
skin cancer risks 147.2–147.3
skin manifestations of infection 149.20
staphylococcal infections 31.20–31.21
STI relationship 29.1, 29.3
striae 94.10
syphilis relationship 29.17, 29.21
trichodysplasia spinulosa 85.15
varicella-zoster infection 31.23–31.24
viral coinfections 31.23–31.26
viral warts, photodynamic therapy 22.7–22.8
virology 31.2–31.3, *31.4*
visceral leishmaniasis 33.52–33.53
women 31.36
see also people living with HIV
HIV-negative MSM (men who have sex with men), Kaposi sarcoma 138.1, **138.2**, 138.4
HLA *see* human leukocyte antigens
HLA-B* genes, drug reactions 118.6, 118.7
HLA-B27 haplotype 155.2, *155.3*, 155.5
HLA class II typing, cutaneous photosensitivity diseases 126.7
HLA-DR4 tissue type, actinic prurigo 126.10
HLH *see* haemophagocytic lymphohistiocytosis

HLRCC *see* hereditary leiomyomatosis and renal cell cancer
HLTS *see* hypotrichosis–lymphoedema–telangiectasia syndrome
HMD *see* hereditary mucoepithelial dysplasia
HMWK *see* high-molecular-weight kininogen
hoarseness
  disorders with skin and systemic manifestations 152.7
  pachyonychia congenita 67.12
hobnail endothelial cells 136.33
hobnail haemangioendothelioma *see* retiform haemangioendothelioma
hobnail haemangioma 136.29–136.30
Hodgkin disease
  cutaneous lymphoproliferative disorder relationship 139.26, 139.27, 139.34, 139.49
  cutaneous manifestations 139.48–139.49
  Epstein–Barr virus association 25.49
  infiltration of skin with malignant cells 149.4
  sarcoidosis association 96.1
Hoigne reactions, procaine penicillin 29.22
HOIL-1 deficiency 45.17–45.18
holistic management of skin disease 15.4–15.7
  effective communication 15.6
  key practical skills 15.6, **15.6**, *15.7*
  physical considerations 15.4–15.5
  psychological considerations 15.5
  social considerations 15.5
  spiritual considerations 15.5–15.6
holoprosencephaly **106.7**
holster sign, erythema on hips/lateral thighs in dermatomyositis 52.5, *52.9*
Holy Bible, leprosy 1.3
HOME *see* Harmonising Outcome Measures for Eczema
homeostasis 2.43–2.45, 9.4, 9.6–9.7
home phototherapy 21.3, 21.8, 21.15, 21.18
homogeneous naevi *145.4*, 145.5–145.6
homogentisic acid 86.51
honey, topical application 18.38
honeycomb keratoderma 63.56
  Vohwinkel syndrome 63.63
hooking thumb 122.17
hookworm larvae
  ancylostomiasis 33.15–33.17
  see also cutaneous larva migrans
L'Hôpital St Louis, Paris 1.4–1.5
hordeolum 107.38, *107.39*
hormones
  effects on allergic contact dermatitis 127.6
  hidradenitis suppurativa 90.2
  lipoedema 98.21
  neuropeptide/neurotransmitter/cytokine distinctions 150.2–150.3
  secondary mediator generation in skin 150.7
  skin/appendage production *150.3*, **150.4**, 150.5
  skin as target *150.3*, 150.5–150.8
  treatment for acne vulgaris 88.49–88.52
  types of signalling 150.2
  see also dermatoendocrinology; endocrine disorders; endocrinology
hormone therapy-induced alopecia (HTIA) 87.73
Horner syndrome 83.23–83.24, 94.20
Hornstein–Knickenberg syndrome *see* Birt–Hogg–Dubé syndrome
horse fly *see* Chrysops
horseradish peroxidase 3.14, 3.15
Hortaea werneckii, tinea nigra 32.14–32.15
Hospital Anxiety and Depression Scale (HADS) 16.11
host defence, skin as barrier to pathogens 26.3
host–parasite relationship shift, erythrasma 26.38

house dust mite (HDM) 34.51
  atopic eczema association 41.23
housework dermatitis 129.3
housework-typeeczema 128.3
Howel–Evans syndrome 63.66, 148.7
Hoyeraal–Hreidarsson syndrome 67.15
HPA axis *see* hypothalamic–pituitary–adrenal axis
HPeV *see* human parechoviruses
HPLC *see* high-performance liquid chromatography
HPT axis *see* hypothalamic–pituitary–thyroid axis
HPV *see* human papillomavirus
HPyV *see* human polyomavirus
HRAS/KRAS mosaicism 73.5–73.6
  see also Schimmelpenning–Feuerstein–Mims syndrome
HR gene, atrichia with papular lesions 87.29
HRQoL *see* health related quality of life
HS *see* hair shaft; heparan sulphate; hidradenitis suppurativa; histiocytic sarcoma
HSANs *see* hereditary sensory and autonomic neuropathies
HSBOD *see* Hidradenitis Suppurativa Burden of Disease
HSCT *see* haematopoietic stem cell transplantation
HSE *see* Health Systems Evidence database
HSIA *see* Hidradenitis Suppurativa Impact Assessment
HSIL *see* high-grade squamous intraepithelial lesions
HSK *see* herpes stromal keratitis
HS-LASI *see* hidradenitis suppurativa lesion, area and severity index
HSP *see* heat shock proteins
HS-PGA *see* Hidradenitis Suppurativa Physician's Global Assessment
HSPGs *see* heparan sulphate proteoglycans
HS-QoL *see* Hidradenitis Suppurativa Quality of Life instrument
HSSA *see* Hidradenitis Suppurativa Symptom Assessment
HSV *see* herpes simplex virus
HTIA *see* hormone therapy-induced alopecia
HTLV *see* human T-cell lymphotropic virus
Hughes syndrome *see* antiphospholipid antibody syndrome
human bites 130.6–130.7
human body louse (*Pediculus humanus corporis*) 26.62, 26.64, 26.72, 26.80
  see also louse-borne diseases
Human Cell Atlas project 8.2
human coronaviruses (HCoVs) 25.100–25.120
  see also COVID-19/SARS-CoV-2
human genome 8.5
  sequencing of 8.8–8.9
Human Genome Project 8.1
human herpesvirus 6 and 7 (HHV-6/HHV-7) 25.39–25.40
  reactivation 25.40
  roseola infantum 25.39–25.40, 115.5–115.6
human herpesvirus 8 (HHV-8) 25.42–25.43
  Kaposi sarcoma 138.1–138.3, *138.4*, 138.5
  post-transplant lymphoproliferative disorder 139.47
human immunodeficiency virus *see* HIV infection
human leukocyte antigens (HLA) 8.7
  drug hypersensitivity reactions 14.6–14.7, **14.6**
  gold reactions 121.4
  rheumatoid nodules 97.15
human monocytic/granulocytic ehrlichiosis *see* ehrlichiosis
human papillomavirus (HPV) 2.13, 25.49–25.73, **25.50–25.51**
  acquired immunodeficiencies 25.65, **25.66**, 25.71–25.73
  Bowen disease 141.19

bowenoid papulosis 141.21
cutaneous squamous cell carcinoma 141.30, 141.31
epidermodysplasia verruciformis 25.65–25.66, 25.69–25.71
female genitalia 110.30–110.31
HIV 31.25–31.26, 31.31–31.32, 31.35–31.36
inborn errors of immunity 25.65–25.71
male genitalia 109.29
neoplasia associations 25.64–25.65
oral squamous cell carcinoma 108.46
perineal and perianal skin 111.16, 111.17–111.19
in pregnancy 113.4
see also ano-genital warts; cutaneous warts
human parechoviruses (HPeV) 25.96
human polyomavirus (HPyV), Merkel cell carcinoma 146.2, 146.3, *146.4*
human polyomavirus-6 and -7 (HPyV-6 and HPyV-7) 25.48–25.49
human polyomavirus-8 (HPyV-8) *see* trichodysplasia spinulosa polyomavirus
human polyomavirus-9 (HPyV-9) 25.49
human polyomavirus-10 (HPyV-10) 25.49
human retrovirus infections 25.78–25.80
human T-cell lymphotropic virus 1 (HTLV-1)
  adult T-cell leukaemia–lymphoma association 139.3, 139.34–139.36
  haematological and neurological disease association 25.79
  infective dermatitis 25.79–25.80
human T-cell lymphotropic viruses 2/3/4 (HTLV-2-4) 25.79
humectants
  allergies 127.59
  topical medication vehicles 18.5, 18.7
hunter gatherer groups 1.1
hunting reaction of Lewis 124.1
Huriez syndrome 63.66, *63.67*, **78.13**
Hurley stage I disease
  chronicity 90.8
  genito-femoral area *90.7*
Hurley stage II disease
  genito-femoral area *90.8*
  inflamed nodules *90.5*
  non-inflamed nodules *90.4*
Hurley stage III disease, lesions *90.9*
Hurley staging system 90.1, 90.6
  definition of stages **90.7**
  hidradenitis suppurativa 16.4, 111.11, **111.12**
Hutchinson lupus 124.6
Hutchinson sign 145.13
Hutchinson, Sir Jonathan 1.6–1.7
Hutchinson triad, congenital syphilis 29.26
Hutchinson–Gilford progeria syndrome (HGPS) 70.25–70.26, **72.5**, 77.4–77.5
HUV *see* hypocomplementaemic urticarial; hypocomplementaemic urticarial vasculitis
HV *see* hydroa vacciniforme
HVLL *see* hydroa vacciniforme-like lymphoma
hyaline degeneration 3.40
hyaline fibromatosis syndrome 70.21–70.22, 94.42–94.43
hyalinising fat necrosis 97.8
hyaluronic acid (HA) *2.37*, 2.39
  dermal filler 158.2, 158.3, 158.4–158.6, 158.8
  adverse reaction *158.9*, **158.11**
  haematoxylin and eosin staining of *158.10*
  skin elasticity 122.5
hydantoin, hypermelanosis 86.26–86.27
hydatid disease *see* echinococcosis
hydration
  irritant contact dermatitis 128.6
  mechanical injuries 122.6–122.7
hydroarsenicism 121.2
hydroa vacciniforme (HV) 126.24–126.27, *126.33*
hydroa vacciniforme-like lymphoma (HVLL) 139.36

hydrocarbon-based formulations, topical drugs 12.3
hydrocortisone
  allergy 127.19
  topical therapies 18.14
hydrogels 12.3
hydrogen cyanide inhalation 125.4
hydrogen peroxide, topical therapies 18.10
hydropic degeneration 3.40
hydrops fetalis (HF) 103.23
hydroquinone
  cosmeceutical use of 157.3–157.4
  topical depigmenting agents 18.31–18.32
hydrotherapy, ichthyoses management 63.43
hydroxy acids 157.4–157.5
hydroxybenzoates 127.54–127.58
hydroxycarbamide 19.21–19.22
  dermatological uses 19.21
  drug–drug interactions 19.22
  potential adverse effects 19.21–19.22
  psoriasis treatment 35.26
  safety precautions 19.22
hydroxychloroquine
  eye, side effects on 107.43
  morphoea treatment 55.38
  sarcoidosis management 96.16, *96.17*
hydroxyethlmethacrylate (HEMA) and ethylmethacrylate microspheres suspended in hyaluronic acid, dermal fillers 158.8
hydroxyethyl acrylate 127.70
2-hydroxyethylmethacrylate (2-HEMA) 127.70
hydroxyethyl starch (HES), pruritus induction 81.11, 117.3
hydroxylation reactions, collagens 2.29, *2.30*
Hydrozoa, stings from 130.1
hyfrecation treatment, acne vulgaris 88.57
hygiene
  atopic eczema 5.14, 41.7–41.8
  COVID-19 considerations 20.6–20.7
  pressure ulcer prevention 123.9
  skin surgery 20.5–20.7
hymenal fissures, mechanical 110.42–110.43
hymenoptera 34.15–34.18
  classification 34.16
  clinical features 34.17
  management 34.17–34.18
  pathophysiology of venom reactions 34.16–34.17
  systemic anaphylactic reactions 34.17–34.18
  venom immunotherapy 34.18
hyperacute dermatomyositis 52.5
hyperaldosteronism 150.17
hyperandrogenism 87.68, 87.88–87.89
  acne vulgaris 88.45
  dermatoendocrinology 150.18
  pseudofolliculitis 91.9
hyperbaric oxygen (HBO), lymphoedema therapy 103.59–103.60
hypercalcaemia
  cutaneous metastatic calcification 59.5–59.6
  subcutaneous fat necrosis 97.57–97.58
hypercholanaemia, familial 2.21
hypercholesterolaemia **60.2**, 60.6–60.8
hypercoagulable states
  resulting in venous and arterial thrombosis 25.111
  superficial thrombophlebitis 97.9
hypercortisolism *see* Cushing disease/syndrome
hypereosinophilic syndrome, oral involvement 108.70
hypergammaglobulinaemic purpura 99.6–99.7
hyperglycaemia, burn injuries 125.14
hypergranulosis 3.41
hyperhidrosis 92.4–92.10
  anhidrosis 92.11–92.12
  eccrine gland disorders **92.11**
  epidermolysis bullosa simplex 69.8

gustatory 83.24, 92.5–92.6, 92.8, 92.9, **104.10**
  internal malignancy links 148.18–148.19
  management 92.8–92.10
  pachyonychia congenita 67.12
  shoe allergy 127.68
  skin disorders 92.8
  surgical treatment 92.9–92.10
  therapeutic use of antiperspirants 18.37–18.38
hyper/hypothyroidism **150.7**, **150.10**, **150.11**, 150.19–150.20
hyper-IgE syndrome due to STAT3 loss of function mutations 80.17
hyperimmunoglobulinaemia-D syndrome (HIDS) *see* mevalonate kinase deficiency
hyperinsulinaemia, obesity association 98.28
hyperkeratosis 3.41
  congenital epidermal naevi 73.4
  dermatomyositis 52.3, *52.8*
  'hystrix' like 63.17–63.18, *63.19*
  in ichthyoses 63.2, 63.10, 63.20
  inverted follicular keratosis 137.2–137.3
  of the nipple 63.79
hyperkeratosis lenticularis perstans *see* Flegel disease
hyperkeratotic cutaneous capillary–venous malformations (HCCVM) 71.2
hyperkeratotic disorders with skin fragility 69.20
hyperkeratotic lesions
  autoinflammatory diseases **80.19**
  elastosis perforans serpiginosa 94.55
  human polyomavirus-9 infection in organ transplant recipients 25.49
  tyrosinaemia type 2 *79.12*
hyperkeratotic palmar eczema 39.14
hyperkeratotic papules
  keratosis circumscripta *85.14*
  peristomal skin *112.7*
hyperkeratotic spicules, multiple minute digitate hyperkeratoses 63.77, *85.19*
hyperlipidaemia
  diabetes association 62.3, *62.4*
  granuloma annulare 95.1
  psoriasis association 35.18
hyperlipoproteinaemias
  classification **60.1**
  type I 60.9
  type III 60.8–60.9
  type IV 60.10
  type V 60.9–60.10
hypermelanosis 86.8
  acquired disorders 86.9–86.33
  drug origin 86.25–86.31, 86.53–86.54
  endocrine disorders 86.17–86.19
  solid malignant tumours 86.19, 86.20
  systemic disorders 86.19–86.25
  vitamin A deficiency 86.23–86.24
  see also hyperpigmentation
hypermetabolism, burn injuries 125.11–125.14
hypermobile Ehlers–Danlos syndromes (hEDS) 70.2–70.8, **70.3**
hypermobility (flexibility), Beighton score **70.8**
hyperoestrogenism 150.18
hyperparathyroidism
  dermatoendocrinology 150.20
  metastatic calcinosis cutis 59.5
hyperphosphataemia, cutaneous metastatic calcification 59.6
hyperphosphataemic familial tumoral calcinosis (HFTC) **79.10**, 79.17–79.18
hyperpigmentation
  acanthosis nigricans *62.3*
  acne 88.41
  atopic eczema *41.14*, *41.17*
  autoinflammatory diseases **80.19**
  Bloom syndrome *80.11*
  chemical peels, side effect of 160.12–160.13, *160.14*

chemotherapy-induced 119.8–119.9
chronic venous insufficiency **101.43**, *101.44*
compound naevus 131.21
dermal fillers, adverse reaction to 158.11–158.12
disorders of 68.1, 68.10–68.14
due to cupping *4.12*
dyskeratosis congenita 67.13, *80.12*
freckle 131.2
from sun exposure in Whipple disease 153.4
HIV 31.12
ink-spot lentigo 131.8
lentigo simplex 131.4
linear morphoea en coup de sabre 55.24
male genitalia **109.42**
melasma 86.10
  laser therapy 161.5–161.6
morphoea *55.18*, 86.20–86.21
mucosal melanosis 131.10
Nelson syndrome *86.7*
neonates 114.4
oral hyperpigmentation 108.14–108.19
penile lentiginosis 131.10
peristomal skin 112.5
pigmentary mosaicism 115.13
pityriasis versicolor 32.11
rheumatic diseases 86.20
simple lentigo 131.4
systemic sclerosis 54.17
vitamin B12 deficiency 61.20
see also hypermelanosis
hyperpituitarism 150.16–150.17
hyperplasia 97.5
  denture-induced hyperplasia 108.10
  Merkel cells 2.12
  ocular features **107.41**
  papillary hyperplasia 108.12, 136.23–136.24
  pseudoepitheliomatous 132.9–132.10
  Raynaud phenomenon 124.11
  sebaceous glands 91.17–91.18
  squamous 109.34–109.35
  see also PIK3CA-related overgrowth spectrum
hypersensitivity syndromes
  azathioprine 19.9
  dapsone 19.15
hypersensitivity to drugs *see* immunological reactions to drugs
hypertension
  nail–patella syndrome 67.16
  psoriasis association 35.18
hypertensive ischaemic leg ulcers (HYTILUs) 102.10–102.13
  clinical features 102.11–102.12
  epidemiology 102.10
  investigations 102.12–102.13
  management 102.13
  pathophysiology 102.10–102.11
hyperthermia, drug-induced 120.4
hyperthermic therapy, cutaneous warts 25.59
hyperthyroidism 86.19
  flushing **104.5**
hypertrichosis 87.84–87.87
  alopecia areata 87.35
  chemotherapy-induced 119.6
  congenital melanocytic naevi 73.12
  eyebrows 107.4
  medical disorders 87.87
  paradoxical hypertrichosis following laser-assisted hair removal 23.20
hypertriglyceridaemia **60.2**, 60.9–60.10
  haemophagocytic lymphohistiocytosis 135.12
  management 98.3
  type I hyperlipoproteinaemia 60.9
  type IV hyperlipoproteinaemia 60.10
  type V hyperlipoproteinaemia 60.9–60.10
hypertrophic photoageing 156.3
hypertrophic scars 11.9, 94.48–94.53
  laser therapies 23.12, 161.5
hypertrophy 97.5

hypoandrogenism 150.18
hypocalcaemia, vitamin D deficiency 61.10
hypocomplementaemic urticarial vasculitis (HUV) syndrome 44.1, 44.2, 44.3–44.4, 44.5, 100.18–100.19
hypoglycaemia, burn injuries 125.14
hypoglycaemic drugs, allergic reactions 62.4
hypohydrosis, ichthyoses 63.46
hypomelanosis 86.8
   acquired 86.34–86.47
   idiopathic guttate hypomelanosis-like hypopigmented macules and lentigines 21.12
hypomelanosis of Ito 68.9–68.10
hyponychial pigmentation, melanoma involving nail unit 145.13
hyponychium 2.11
hypo-oestrogenism 150.18–150.19
hypoparathyroidism 150.20–150.21
hypopigmentation
   actinic prurigo 126.12
   chemical peels, side effect of 160.14
   chemotherapy-induced 119.10–119.11
   Cole disease 63.61
   disorders of 68.1, 68.3–68.10
   HIV 31.12
   infantile seborrhoeic dermatitis *115.2*
   male genitalia 109.28, **109.42**, 109.43
   onchocerciasis 33.4–33.5
   patch testing 127.31
   pityriasis versicolor 32.11, *32.12*
   systemic lupus erythematosus 51.28
hypopigmented sarcoidosis 96.12–96.13
hypopituitarism **150.7, 150.10, 150.11,** *150.13*, 150.15–150.16
hypoplasia
   congenital pseudo-ainhum 94.48
   eyebrows 107.4
hypoplasminogenaemia, oral involvement 108.70
hypopyon, iritis 48.6
hyposensitisation, allergic contact dermatitis 127.35
hypostatic eczema *see* venous eczema
hypostatic haemosiderosis 86.47–86.49
hypothalamic–pituitary–adrenal (HPA) axis 87.11, 150.2
hypothalamic–pituitary–thyroid (HPT) axis, hair follicle 87.11
hypothalamopituitary–thyroid (HPT) axis 150.2
hypothenar hammer syndrome 122.13, 122.24
hypothyroidism
   acquired ichthyosis 85.2
   diffuse telogen effluvium *87.55*
   granuloma annulare 95.1
   heat-associated carcinomas 124.15–124.16
hypotrichosis
   eyelashes 107.4
   ichthyosis with 63.40
hypotrichosis–lymphoedema–telangiectasia syndrome (HLTS) 71.26, 103.23
hypoxia, neonates 114.3
hysteresis, stress-strain relationship 122.3
hystrix-like hyperkeratosis 63.17–63.18, *63.19*
hystrix-like ichthyosis and deafness (HID) syndrome 63.34–63.35
HYTILUs *see* hypertensive ischaemic leg ulcers

I

iatrogenic calcinosis 59.3
iatrogenic hypercarotenaemia 86.50
iatrogenic immunosuppression
   human papillomavirus 25.71
   viral infections 149.20, *149.21*
IBD *see* inflammatory bowel disease
ibuprofen, flux measurement *12.6*
ICAS *see* International Alliance for the Control of Scabies
ICD *see* irritant contact dermatitis

ice pack dermatosis 97.37
ICH-GCP *see* International Conference on Harmonisation Good Clinical Practice
ichthyoses 63.2–63.3
   acquired forms 63.47–63.49
   common forms 63.3–63.7
   congenital forms 63.41–63.79
   glycosylation disorders 79.10
   hypotrichosis 63.40
   keratinopathic forms **63.4**, 63.13–63.18
   management 63.41–63.46
   neuro-ichthyotic syndromes 63.30–63.39
   non-syndromic **63.3**, 63.20–63.22
   syndromic 63.3, 63.39–63.47, *63.39*
   trichothiodystrophy *76.10*
ichthyosiform atrophy 139.49
ichthyosiform erythroderma 39.33, *63.36*
ichthyosiform sarcoidosis 96.13
ichthyosis
   acquired 63.47–63.50, 63.73, 85.1–85.3, 148.17
   syndromic **63.3**, 63.22–63.62
ichthyosis Curth–Macklin (ICM) 63.16–63.17
ichthyosis follicularis–atrichia–photophobia (IFAP) syndrome 63.24–63.25
ichthyosis linearis circumflexa *63.27*
ichthyosis vulgaris 2.6, 63.3–63.5
   atopic eczema association 41.15
   KP association 85.9
ichthyosis–follicular atroderma–hypotrichosis–hypohidrosis (IFAH) 63.40
ichthyosis–prematurity syndrome (IPS) 63.39–63.40
ichthyotic disorders 3.44
ichthyotic epidermal disorders 148.17
ICI *see* immune checkpoint inhibitors
ICM *see* ichthyosis Curth–Macklin
ICU *see* immune contact urticaria
IDEOM *see* International Dermatology Outcome Measures
idiopathic acrocyanosis 124.7
idiopathic AGL 98.3
idiopathic circumscribed hyperhidrosis 92.7, 92.9
idiopathic cutaneous mucinoses 57.1, 57.2–57.18
idiopathic dermatitis 112.5
idiopathic facial aseptic granuloma (IFAG) 89.16
idiopathic generalised anhidrosis 92.12
idiopathic guttate hypomelanosis (IGH) 86.45–86.47
   ageing of skin 156.5, *156.6*
idiopathic guttate hypomelanosis-like hypopigmented macules and lentigines 21.12
idiopathic hirsutism 87.88, 87.90
idiopathic inflammatory myopathies (IIMs) 52.1–52.13
idiopathic livedo reticularis 124.8, 124.9–124.10
idiopathic lymphadenopathies 149.16–149.18
idiopathic mid-dermal elastolysis *94.25*, 94.26
idiopathic photodermatoses 126.1, 126.2–126.27
idiopathic thrombocytopenic purpura, oral involvement 108.70
idiotrophic calcification 59.4–59.5
IDN *see* intradermal naevi
idoxuridine 18.13
IDQoL *see* Infants' Dermatitis Quality of Life Index
IEI (inborn errors of immunity) *see* inherited immunodeficiency
IFAG *see* idiopathic facial aseptic granuloma
IFAH *see* ichthyosis–follicular atroderma–hypotrichosis–hypohidrosis
IFAP syndrome *see* ichthyosis follicularis–atrichia–photophobia syndrome

IFD *see* International Foundation for Dermatology
IFN-α2a *see* interferon α2a
IFN-α2b *see* intralesional interferon α2b
IFN α *see* interferon α
IgA pemphigus 50.6–50.7
IgA vasculitis 100.13–100.15
   fibrin deposition *100.14*
   leukocytoclasis *100.14*
   see also antineutrophil cytoplasmic antibody associated small vessel vasculitis
IgE *see* immunoglobulin E
IgE-related type 1 skin hypersensitivity 9.9–9.10
IgE test *see* immunoglobulin E test
IGF-1 *see* insulin-like growth factor
IgG4 disease, oral involvement 108.67
IgG4-related skin disease, ear dermatoses **106.22**
Iggo discs 2.12
IGH *see* idiopathic guttate hypomelanosis
IgM pemphigoid 50.53–50.54
IGRAs *see* interferon γ release assays
IHS4 *see* International Hidradenitis Suppurativa Severity Score System
IIEF *see* International Index of Erectile Function
IIF *see* indirect immunofluorescence
IIMs *see* idiopathic inflammatory myopathies
IL-1 antagonists, systemic therapy 19.37
IL-4/IL-13 antagonists, systemic therapy 19.36–19.37
IL-4/IL-13 inhibitors, atopic eczema treatment 41.29–41.30
IL-10 signalling disorders 45.16
IL-12/IL-23 p40 inhibitor, psoriasis treatment 35.29
IL-17 antagonists, systemic therapy 19.34, 19.35–19.36
IL-17 inhibitors, psoriasis treatment 35.30
IL-23 antagonists, systemic therapy 19.34, 19.35
IL-23/IL-17 antagonists, systemic therapy 19.34–19.35
IL-23p 19 inhibitors, psoriasis treatment 35.30–35.31
IL36RN gene, pustular psoriasis 118.2, 118.3
ILCs *see* innate lymphoid cells
ILD *see* interstitial lung disease
ILDS *see* International League of Dermatological Societies
ILE *see* lipid injectable emulsion
ileal metaplasia, urostomy 112.7
ileostomy **112.3**
   Candida infection 112.8, 112.9
   Crohn ulceration 112.13, 112.14
   granulation tissue with bowel metaplasia 112.6
   'granulomas' beneath the stoma 112.6
   leakage and eroded dermatitis due to corrosive faecal contents 112.4
   leakage and hyperkeratotic papules 112.7
   length of 112.5
   nicorandil ulceration 112.12
   portal hypertension affecting peristomal skin 112.9
   postinflammatory hyperpigmentation 112.5
   pyoderma gangrenosum 112.14, 112.15
   synergic gangrene 112.10
   see also stomas
ILEP *see* International Federation of Anti-Leprosy Associations
IL-F *see* infiltrating lipomatosis of the face
ILFAD *see* intestinal failure-associated liver disease
iliac horns, nail–patella syndrome 67.16
iliohypogastric neuropathic pain/neuralgia 83.7
ilioinguinal neuropathic pain/neuralgia 83.7
illicit drugs
   ChemSex 120.2–120.3

dermatoses induced by 120.1–120.9
   legal aspects 120.3–120.4
iloprost 124.12
ILP *see* isolated limb perfusion
IMACS *see* International Myositis Assessment and Clinical Studies
images, digital 1.9
imaging, melanoma diagnosis 142.9–142.10
imaging examination 4.22–4.23
imaging systems, diagnosis 4.20–4.22
imatinib, Erdheim–Chester disease treatment 135.22
imidazoles 18.12, 19.48
imidazolidinyl urea 127.51–127.52
IMIDs *see* immune-mediated inflammatory diseases
imiquimod 18.30
   basal cell carcinoma topical treatment 140.12, *140.16*
5% imiquimod cream, Bowen disease 141.23
immediate pigment darkening (IPD) 86.9
   UV radiation exposure 10.7
immediate-type reactions, contact urticaria 128.8
immediate-type stinging 128.10
immediate-weal tests 4.24
immobility, lymphoedema due to 103.40
immune cells 9.2–9.6
   chemical staining of 9.2
   dermal immune cells 9.4–9.6
   embryonic development of skin 2.3, *2.4*
   epidermal immune cells 9.3–9.4
   lymphoid lineage cells 9.5
   mucosal associated invariant T (MAIT) cells 9.5
   myeloid lineage cells 9.4–9.5
   peripheral blood 9.6
   plasma cells 9.6
   skin draining lymph node 9.6
   T cells 9.4, 9.5–9.7, 14.4, 14.5, 50.2, 127.9
immune checkpoint inhibitors (ICI) 87.74
   cutaneous side effects of cancer immunotherapy 144.9–144.12
   cutaneous squamous cell carcinoma 141.33–141.34
   melanoma systemic therapy 144.2, *144.3*, 144.4, **144.6, 144.8**, 144.9
immune complex small-vessel vasculitis 152.4
immune contact urticaria (ICU) 127.83–127.84, 127.86
immune dysregulation 80.13–80.15
   inherited immunodeficiency 80.2, **80.5**
immune ecosystem 2.12–2.13
immune function
   hidradenitis suppurativa predisposition 90.2–90.3
   and skin ageing 2.45
immune mechanisms, allergic contact dermatitis 127.6
immune-mediated inflammatory diseases (IMIDs)
   skin cancer risks 147.5
   systemic sclerosis 54.10–54.11
immune-modulating treatments, molluscum contagiosum infection 25.18
immune privilege, hair follicle 87.11, 87.22
immune reconstitution-associated disease (IRAD), antiretroviral HIV therapy effects 31.8, **31.38**
immune response, wound healing 11.2–11.3
immune suppression, UV radiation in Merkel cell carcinoma 146.3
immune surveillance 2.15, *2.16*
immune system
   dermatophytosis 32.21
   human papillomavirus 25.52
   in pregnancy 113.3–113.4
   skin disorders 149.16–149.22
   skin microbiome 26.5, 26.6
   see also immunology
immunoadsorption, pemphigus treatment 50.9

immunobullous disease 50.1–50.60
 anti-p200 pemphigoid 50.38–50.42
 bullous systemic lupus erythematous 50.48–50.51
 cicatrising conjunctivitis association 107.24–107.34
 dermatitis herpetiformis 50.54–50.59
 epidermolysis bullosa acquista 50.42–50.48
 female genitalia 110.20, **110.21**
 immunopathology **50.2**
 linear IgA disease 50.33–50.38
 mucous membrane pemphigoid 50.22–50.33
 oral involvement 108.80–108.82
 pemphigus 50.1–50.9
 rare pemphigoid disorders 50.51–50.54
 serological diagnosis *3.20*
 subepidermal diseases 50.9–50.59
immunocompromised patients
 antiviral agent prophylaxis 25.31, 25.42, 25.75
 cutaneous squamous cell carcinomas 147.10–147.11, 147.16–147.18
 cytomegalovirus infection 25.41
 haemophagocytic lymphohistiocytosis with infectious mononucleosis 25.37
 HPyV9 infection and hyperkeratotic skin lesions in organ transplant recipients 25.49
 Kaposi sarcoma 138.1, 147.2, 147.3, 147.14, 147.20–147.21, 147.23
 Kaposi sarcoma-associated herpesvirus 25.42, 25.43
 keratinocyte cancers 147.10–147.11, 147.16–147.21
 melanoma 147.13–147.14, 147.21, 147.23
 mpox infection 25.10
 non-tuberculous mycobacteria disseminated disease 27.32–27.36, 27.38, 27.40–27.45
 reactivation of human herpesvirus 6 and 7 25.39, 25.40
 reduced tumour immune surveillance, UV radiation related skin cancers 147.5–147.6
 skin cancer 147.1–147.26
  clinicopathological features 147.10–147.16
  management 147.16–147.24
  organisations 147.25
  pathogenesis 147.5–147.10
  primary and acquired immunodeficiencies 147.1–147.5
  risk of, drug effects on 147.5–147.8
  screening and surveillance 147.24–147.25
  ultraviolet radiation effects 147.5–147.6
 vaccinia infection 25.7–25.8
 varicella infection 25.30–25.31
immunodeficiency
 acquired *see* acquired immunodeficiency diseases
 neoplasia syndromes 148.13–148.14
immunodeficiency-associated eosinophilic pustular folliculitis 91.5
immunodeficiency, inherited *see* inherited immunodeficiency
immunodysregulation polyendocrinopathy enteropathy X-linked syndrome (IPEX) 80.14
immunoenzyme methods 3.14–3.16
 avidin–biotin coupling of antibody and enzyme 3.15–3.16
 chemical conjugation of peroxidase to antibody 3.14–3.16
 conjugates, use of 3.14–3.15
 controls 3.15
 enzyme-linked immunosorbent assay 3.16
 fixed frozen sections, examination of 3.15
 immunofluorescence comparison **3.14**
 paraffin sections 3.15
 technical limitations 3.14

immunofluorescence methods 3.10–3.14
 calcium enhancement indirect technique 3.14
 dermal–epidermal basement membrane zone 2.23
 direct immunofluorescence 3.11–3.12
 epidermolysis bullosa diagnosis 69.21, *69.22*
 and histopathology 3.11
 immunoenzyme methods comparison **3.14**
 indirect immunofluorescence 3.12–3.13
 photobleaching (fading) limitation 3.11
 specimen preparation
  DIF analysis 3.11–3.12
  IIF analysis 3.13
 specimen processing
  DIF analysis 3.12
  split-skin indirect technique 3.13–3.14
 specimen selection, DIF analysis **3.11**
 split-skin indirect technique 3.13–3.14
 types of 3.11
immunogenotyping 3.31
immunoglobulin E (IgE)
 atopic eczema 41.11
 IgE-mediated drug hypersensitivity 14.1–14.2
immunoglobulin E (IgE) test, contact dermatitis 129.7
immunoglobulin E test, contact dermatitis 129.7
immunoglobulin G4-related disease 149.17–149.18
immunoglobulin variable domains, naming conventions 19.31, **19.32**
immunohistochemistry, Merkel cell carcinoma 146.3, *146.4*, **146.5**
immunological abnormalities, chronic mucocutaneous candidiasis 32.68
immunological dysregulation, obesity 98.27–98.28
immunological photodermatoses 126.1, 126.2–126.27
immunological reactions to drugs 14.1–14.7
 clinical phenotype 14.6–14.7
 erythroderma 39.33
 hypersensitivity reaction, mechanisms and clinical correlations **14.2**
 IgE-mediated drug hypersensitivity 14.1–14.2
 pseudoallergic reactions 14.2–14.3
 T-cell-mediated drug hypersensitivity 14.3–14.4
 T-cell recognition of drugs 14.4–14.6
 type 4 hypersensitivity reaction, mechanisms and clinical correlations **14.2**
immunological tolerance, allergic contact dermatitis 127.9
immunology 9.2–9.8
 atopic eczema 41.9–41.10
 erythema multiforme 47.2–47.3
 HIV 31.3–31.5
 immune cells in human skin 9.2–9.6, *103.14*
 and lymphatic system 103.2
 skin immune network in humans and mice 9.7
 and skin microbiota 9.7–9.8, *103.2*, 103.3
 systemic lupus erythematosus 51.20–51.21
 tissue homeostasis 9.6–9.7
 see also immune system
immunomodulation, UV radiation exposure 10.8–10.9
immunomodulators, in pregnancy **113.22–113.23**
immunomodulatory therapy 1.8
 risk reduction 19.3
 systemic therapy 19.2–19.46
 terminology 19.2
immunopathogenesis, sarcoidosis 96.3–96.4
immunopathology 3.10–3.29
 applications of 3.16–3.29
  cutaneous neoplasms 3.21–3.29

direct immunofluorescence 3.17–3.19
 enzyme-linked immunosorbent assay 3.20–3.21
 indirect immunofluorescence 3.19–3.20
cell markers, immunocytochemistry panels **3.10**
immunocytochemistry panels of cell markers **3.10**
immunoenzyme methods 3.14–3.16
immunofluorescence methods 3.10–3.14
immunophenotyping, ichthyoses 63.45
immunostaining, oral mucosal vesiculobullous disorders **108.81**
immunosuppression
 actinic keratoses 141.1, 141.3
 Bowen disease 141.18
 ciclosporin 19.10–19.12
 cutaneous squamous cell carcinoma 141.3, 141.27, 141.29
 eosinophilic pustular folliculitis 91.3, 91.4–91.5, 93.7, 93.8–93.9
 infective panniculitis 97.46–97.47
 joint infections 155.4
 Merkel cell carcinoma 146.2, 146.9
 mucous membrane pemphigoid *107.31*
 oral candidiasis 32.58, 32.61
 renal transplantation, dermatological consequences of 154.5–154.6
 squamous cell carcinoma 141.6, 141.27, 141.29
 systemic amyloidoses treatment 56.14
 systemic lupus erythematosus treatment 51.37–51.38
 trichodysplasia spinulosa 85.15–85.16
 versus immunomodulatory drugs 19.2–19.3
 see also organ transplant recipients
immunosuppressive therapy
 acneform reaction 88.12–88.13
 post-transplant lymphoproliferative disorder 139.47
 skin cancer risks 147.5–147.8, 147.19–147.20
immunotherapy
 checkpoint inhibitors for melanoma therapy 144.2, *144.3*, 144.4, **144.6, 144.8**
 combination therapies for melanoma 144.2–144.3
 cutaneous T-cell lymphoma 139.22–139.23
 melanoma 144.2–144.4
 Merkel cell carcinoma 146.9
 systemic, cutaneous warts 25.60
 topical, cutaneous warts 25.59–25.60
Impact of Chronic Skin Disease on Daily Life (ISDL) 16.7
Impact of Psoriasis Questionnaire (IPSO) 16.8
impacts of skin disease, measurement 16.5–16.13
impairment, caused by skin disease 5.5–5.6
impetigo
 clinical features 26.14–26.16
 epidemiology 26.13–26.14
 eyelid 107.38
 infants 115.7
 management 26.16
 oral infection 108.53
 pathophysiology 26.14
 Staphylococcus aureus and *Streptococcus pyrogenes* role 26.13–26.16
 see also bullous impetigo
implantable defibrillators, cutaneous reactions 151.5–151.6
implanted metals, cutaneous reactions 127.19
implants
 brachytherapy 24.3
 types of **108.62**
IMPSG *see* International Melanoma Pathology Study Group
IMRT *see* intensity modulated radiotherapy
inborn errors of immunity (IEI) *see* inherited immunodeficiency

inborn errors of metabolism *see* inherited metabolic diseases
incidence of disease 5.10, 5.14
inclusional/exclusional elliptical biopsies 20.8–20.9
inclusion body (digital) fibromatosis 136.10–136.11
incontinentia pigmenti (IP) *4.19*, 68.10–68.11, 69.24
indeterminate leprosy 28.4
indeterminate lymphocytic lobular panniculitis 97.39
index lesions, hidradenitis suppurativa 90.3–90.5
India, ancient medical texts 1.2–1.3
Indiana vesiculovirus *see* vesicular stomatitis virus
Indian skin phenotypes, photoageing 156.2
indirect immunofluorescence (IIF) 3.12–3.13, 3.19–3.20
 mucous membrane pemphigoid 107.28
 negative and positive controls 3.14
 serological diagnosis of immunobullous disorders *3.20*
 substrates for 3.13
indolent systemic mastocytosis (ISM) 46.2–46.3, 46.10
infantile acropustulosis 114.8, 115.4
infantile digital fibromatosis 136.10–136.11
 see also inclusion body (digital) fibromatosis
infantile eosinophilic pustular folliculitis 91.3, 91.5–91.6, 93.7, 93.9–93.10
 differential diagnosis 93.**10**
infantile gluteal granuloma 115.3
infantile haemangiomas 116.1–116.7
 classification 116.2
 clinical variants 116.3–116.5
 complications and co-morbidities 116.5–116.6
 deep infantile haemangioma involving lateral neck 116.3
 facial and neck plaque-type haemangiomas, evolution of *116.3*
 haemangioma precursor 116.2
 hepatic haemangioma 116.5
 laser therapies 23.8
 management 116.6–116.7
 multifocal cutaneous infantile haemangioma 116.5
 pathophysiology 116.2
 presentation 116.2–116.3
 propranolol treatment, protocol for 116.8
 segmental infantile haemangioma **116.2**, 116.3–116.4
 treatment ladder for **116.7**
 ulceration 116.5, *116.6*
 vascular malformation comparison **116.1**
infantile haemangiopericytoma *see* infantile myofibromatosis
infantile/juvenile fibromatosis variant (non-desmoid type) *see* lipofibromatosis
infantile myofibromatosis 94.41–94.42, 136.39–136.40
infantile papular acrodermatitis *see* Gianotti–Crosti syndrome
infantile perianal pyrimidal protusion 111.3
infantile Refsum disease 63.31
infantile sclerema neonatorum 97.60
infantile seborrhoeic dermatitis (ISD) 40.5, 41.22, 115.1–115.2
infantile stiff skin syndromes 70.21–70.24
 hyaline fibromatosis syndrome 70.21–70.22
 restrictive dermopathy 70.24
 stiff skin syndrome 70.22–70.23
 Winchester syndrome 70.23–70.24
infants 115.1–115.17
 acne 88.68–88.74, 115.4–115.5
 acropustulosis 114.8, 115.4
 acute haemorrhagic oedema 115.9, *115.10*
 acute scrotum 109.25–109.26
 Albright hereditary osteodystrophy 72.9
 animal bite injuries 115.14

infants (*continued*)
  annular erythema of infancy 47.9, *47.10*
  arteriovenous malformations *101.23*
  atopic eczema *41.13, 41.14, 41.15, 41.26*, 115.2–115.3
  benign vascular tumours, vascular malformation distinction **116.1**
  bite injuries 115.14
  blistering distal dactylitis 115.8
  bronze baby syndrome 86.49–86.50
  bullous pemphigoid *50.20*
  calcified cutaneous nodules of the heels 115.15
  Candida infection 115.8
  candidiasis of the napkin area 32.65
  capillary malformations *71.4*
  chickenpox (varicella) 115.6–115.7
  chronic infantile neurological cutaneous and articular syndrome **45.5, 45.6**
  circumcision, male 109.7
  CLOVES syndrome *71.9, 72.11*
  cold panniculitis 97.36–97.37, 114.14
  collodion baby phenotype 79.5
  congenital candidiasis 32.66–32.67
  congenital haemangiomas 116.7–116.9
  congenital melanocytic naevi *73.12*
  COVID-19/SARS-CoV-2 115.5
  cradle cap 115.1, *115.2*
  cutis laxa *70.17*
  definition of infancy 115.1
  dermoid cysts 115.12, *115.13*
  developmental/genetic conditions 115.12–115.13
  discrete papular lichen myxoedematosus 57.6
  Ehlers–Danlos syndromes 70.11
  eosinophilic pustular folliculitis 115.12
  epidermolysis bullosa 69.24–69.25
  eruption cyst, over a primary tooth 108.10
  fibrous hamartoma of infancy 136.6–136.7
  fifth disease/erythema infectiosum 115.6
  flushing in *104.10*, **104.10**
  Gaucher disease 79.5
  genetic conditions 115.12–115.13
  Gianotti–Crosti syndrome 115.11
  gluteal granuloma 115.3
  haemangiomas 116.1–116.9
  hair loss 114.4, 115.15
  hand, foot and mouth disease 115.6
  hepatic haemangioma 116.5
  hereditary lymphoedema type 1A *71.24*
  human bite injuries 115.14
  hyaline fibromatosis syndrome 70.21–70.22
  impetigo 115.7
  inclusion body (digital) fibromatosis 136.10–136.11
  infective conditions 115.5–115.9
  inflammatory conditions 115.1–115.5
  iron deficiency 61.24, 61.25
  JAK3-deficient severe combined immunodeficiency *80.7*
  juvenile xanthogranuloma 115.15
  Kaposiform haemangioendothelioma 116.9–116.10
  Kasbach–Merritt phenomenon 116.9–116.10
  Kawasaki disease 115.9–115.11
  koilonychia 115.14
  Langerhans cell histiocytosis 115.15–115.16, 135.4, 135.5–135.7
  linear IgA disease 115.11
  linear morphoea 115.13
  lipofibromatosis 136.13–136.14
  lymphangioma 108.13
  lymphangioma circumscriptum 103.25–103.28
  lymphatic malformations *71.22*
  mastocytoma *46.5*
  mastocytosis 115.16–115.17
  measles 115.7
  Menkes disease 79.17
  Michelin tyre baby syndrome 70.19, 73.17
  midface toddler excoriation syndrome 82.9, 83.12–83.13
  milia 115.13–115.14
  molluscum contagiosum 115.9
  multifocal cutaneous infantile haemangioma 116.5
  napkin (diaper) dermatitis 115.3
  neonatal lupus erythematosus 114.12–114.14
  noma neonatorum (oro-facial gangrene) 114.27
  non-accidental injury 115.14
  non-malignant tumours 116.1–116.11
  Omenn syndrome 80.7–80.8
  papular urticaria 115.11–115.12
  pedal papules of infancy 115.14, *115.15*
  perianal pyrimidal protusion 111.3
  perianal streptococcal dermatitis 115.8
  perianal ulcers, leukocyte adhesion deficiency type I *80.16*
  perianal viral warts 111.18, *111.19*
  pigmentary mosaicism 115.13
  pigmented neuroectodermal tumour 136.50–136.51
  pityriasis alba 115.4
  preauricular cysts and sinuses 115.12
  psoriasis 115.3–115.4
  pyogenic granuloma 116.10–116.11
  raised linear bands of infancy 114.18–114.19
  reactive conditions 115.9–115.12
  restrictive dermopathy 70.24
  roseola infantum 25.39–25.40, 115.5–115.6
  scabies 115.9
  seborrhoeic dermatitis 115.1–115.2
  segmental infantile haemangioma **116.2**, 116.3–116.4
  severe combined immunodeficiency *80.7*
  staphylococcal scalded skin syndrome 114.24–114.25, 115.7–115.8
  stiff skin syndrome 70.22–70.23
  STING-associated vasculopathy **45.5, 45.6**, 45.13–45.14, *80.18*
  Sturge–Weber syndrome *71.4*
  tinea capitis 115.8–115.9
  tinea corporis 115.8
  tinea faciei *115.8*
  trichothiodystrophy syndrome *76.10*
  tufted angioma 116.10, 116.11
  Turner syndrome *71.28*
  urticaria 115.5
  varicella 115.6–115.7
  viral exanthems 115.5–115.7
  Winchester syndrome 70.23–70.24
  see also children; neonates
Infants' Dermatitis Quality of Life Index (IDQoL) 16.8, 16.10
Infants and Toddlers Quality of Life instrument (InToDermQoL) 16.10
infections
  acquired ichthyosis 63.47, 85.1
  burns 125.8–125.11, **125.10**
  complications after skin surgery 20.41, 20.42
  cutaneous lesions related to heart disease 151.5
  dermatitis *39.25*
  dystrophic calcification 59.1
  flexural sites **4.18**
  hair loss and 87.35–87.36
  Helicobacter pylori associated with skin disorders 153.1
  hidradenitis suppurativa differential diagnosis 90.5
  HIV coinfections **31.7**, 31.20–31.31
  immune reconstitution-associated disease 31.8, 31.37–31.39
  immunosuppressed renal allograft recipients 154.5–154.6
  scalp 105.12
    human immunodeficiency virus 105.12
    syphilis 105.12
  sexually transmitted infection overview 29.1–29.2
  skin associated effects of respiratory tract infections 152.4
  skin-related health anxieties 84.26
  syphilis 29.1–29.29
  Tropheryma whippelii/Whipple disease 97.47, 153.4, 155.5
infections of soft tissues, intravenous drug administration 120.7
infectious mononucleosis 25.36–25.37
infectious NEH 92.14
infective arthropathies 155.2–155.5
infective cheilitis 108.63
infective dermatitis 39.24–39.26
  clinical features and variants 39.26
  human T-cell lymphotropic virus 1 25.79–25.80
  pathophysiology 39.25
  treatment 39.26
infective eczematoid dermatitis 106.19
infective endocarditis, cutaneous lesions 151.5
infective panniculitis 97.46–97.48
infestations *see* myiasis; tungiasis
infiltrating lipomatosis of the face (IL-F) 98.19–98.20
infiltrative basal cell carcinoma 140.3, *140.4*
inflamed nodules, hidradenitis suppurativa 90.5
inflamed phyma, treatment **89.13–89.14**
inflammation 9.8–9.9
  acne vulgaris **88.3**, 88.14–88.15, **88.27**, *88.28*
  allergic inflammation 9.9–9.10
  focal regression of melanoma 142.14
  hand eczema 39.13
  infants 115.1–115.5
  inflammatory memory 9.9
  pathological skin inflammation 9.8–9.9
  pyoderma gangrenosum 49.3
  viral exanthems 25.4–25.5
  wound healing 9.6
  see also delayed inflammatory reactions; multisystem inflammatory syndrome; pro-inflammatory topical treatments
inflammatory arthritides, oral involvement 108.68–108.69
inflammatory arthropathies 155.5–155.7, *155.8*, *155.9*
inflammatory bowel disease (IBD)
  arthropathies 155.5
  BADAS-associated 49.16
  erythema nodosum in 97.21
  eye disease **107.35**
  neonatal onset 45.16
  psoriasis 112.10
  skin complications of stomas 153.7
  skin manifestations 153.1–153.3, **153.7**
  see also Crohn disease; ulcerative colitis
inflammatory chondropathies 155.11–155.13
  musculoskeletal features 155.11
inflammatory cutaneous lesions, laser therapies 23.12
inflammatory dermatoses
  flexural sites **4.18**
  graft-versus-host disease 38.1–38.12
  HIV 31.12–31.20
  male genitalia 109.9–109.26
  perineal and perianal skin 111.8–111.12
  seborrhoeic dermatitis 40.1–40.10
  transient acantholytic dermatosis 85.23–85.25
  urticarial vasculitis 44.1–44.6
inflammatory diseases 1.8
  Dermatology Index of Disease Severity 16.3
  dystrophic calcification of skin and subcutaneous tissues 59.1–59.3
  hidradenitis suppurativa association 90.2, 90.5–90.6
  hypopigmentation 68.4
  subcutaneous fat 97.6
inflammatory fibrosing conditions, internal malignancy association 148.21
inflammatory lesions, mouth 108.20–108.25
inflammatory myxohyaline tumour of the distal extremities with virocyte or Reed–Sternberg-like cells *see* myxoinflammatory fibroblastic sarcoma
inflammatory peeling skin syndromes 63.28, *63.29*
inflammatory plaques **80.19**
inflammatory response
  allergen exposure 127.7
  melanoma 142.18
  wound healing 11.2–11.3
inflammatory skin blistering, epidermolysis bullosa *69.16*
infliximab
  psoriasis treatment 35.27–35.28
  psoriatic arthritis treatment 35.45
infraorbital lines, reduction of by botulinum toxin application *159.7*
infrared (IR) radiation
  disease causation 124.14–124.16
  physiological reactions to 124.14
infudibulo-isthmicoma *see* pilar sheath acanthoma
infundibular cyst *see* epidermoid cysts
infundibular epithelial walled cutaneous cysts 133.1–133.4
infundibulofolliculitis 91.14–91.15, 93.6–93.7
infundibuloma, lesions/tumours of follicular infundibulum 137.3–137.4
infundibulomatosis, tumour of follicular infundibulum 137.3–137.4
infundibulum 87.3–87.4
ingenol mebutate 18.30–18.31
inguinal buboes, lymphogranuloma venereum 30.14, 30.15, 30.16, **30.17**, *30.18*
inguinal hyperhidrosis 92.6
inhalation injuries 125.4–125.5
inhalent-induced dermatoses 120.2, 120.4
inherited disorders 8.2–8.5, 8.8–8.9
  cornification 63.1–63.80
  of pigmentation **68.2–68.3**
  prenatal diagnosis 8.9–8.11
  skin fragility 69.1–69.28
  see also congenital entries; genetic disorders/syndromes; *hereditary entries*; inherited immunodeficiency; inherited metabolic diseases
inherited immunodeficiency 80.1–80.20
  10 warning signs 80.2
  antibody deficiencies **80.5**, 80.13
  autoinflammatory diseases **80.19**
  classification 80.3–80.4
  clinical features 80.1–80.2
  combined immunodeficiencies **80.4**, 80.7–80.13
  complement diseases **80.6**, 80.18–80.20
    autoimmunity defects 80.18–80.19
    complement activation regulation defects 80.20
    recurrent pyogenic infection 80.18
  diagnostic laboratory tests 80.3
  DNA repair defects **80.4–80.5**
  epidermodysplasia verruciformis 25.65–25.66, 25.69–25.71
  GARFIELD acronym 80.2
  human papillomavirus infection 25.65–25.71
  immune dysregulation 80.2, **80.5**, 80.13–80.15
  infectious disease-related manifestations 80.2
  innate immunity defects **80.6**, 80.16–80.18
  management 80.3
  neutrophil differentiation and adhesion defects 80.15–80.16
  non-infectious non-specific manifestations 80.2–80.3
  phagocytic defects **80.5–80.6**, 80.15
  severe combined immunodeficiency **80.4**, 80.7–80.9
  skin cancer 147.1–147.2

skin manifestations **80.4–80.6**, 149.18–149.20
warning signs 80.2
inherited metabolic diseases 79.1–79.18
  amino acid metabolism and transport disorders 79.10–79.15
  dermatological features **79.2**
  glycosylation disorders 79.9–79.10
  lipid metabolism disorders 79.15
  lysosomal storage disorders 79.1–79.8
  mitochondrial respiratory chain disorders 79.8–79.9
  vitamin and mineral disorders 79.15–79.18
inherited patterned lentiginosis 86.16
  oral hyperpigmentation 108.17
inherited skin tumour syndromes 78.1–78.15
  familial adenomatous polyposis 78.10–78.11
  neurofibromatoses 78.1–78.7
  skin syndromes linked with cancers **78.12–78.14**
  tuberous sclerosis complex 78.7–78.10
inherited syndromes, Alagille syndrome 153.5
injecting drug use
  HIV 31.37
  localised lipoatrophy due to 98.10
  in pregnancy **113.21**
injections
  calcium-containing materials, dystrophic calcification of skin and subcutaneous tissues 59.3
  corticosteroid, localised lipoatrophy due to 98.11–98.12
  dermatitis artefacta 84.33
  insulin, fat hypertrophy due to 98.13–98.15
  intralesional corticosteroids 18.21–18.22
  sterile furuncles (abscesses) 26.23
injection techniques, local anaesthetics 20.8
injury healing see wound healing
ink-spot lentigo 131.8–131.9
  dermoscopic image 131.9
  epidermis with lentiginous hyperplasia 131.8
  hyperpigmentation 131.8
innate immune cells, atopic eczema 41.11
innate immunity defects 80.6, 80.16–80.18
innate lymphoid cells (ILCs) 2.12–2.13
  immune system 9.5
inner canthus, radiotherapy for skin cancer 24.10–24.11
inner root sheath (IRS) 2.9–2.10
  hair follicle 87.3–87.5
inoculation herpes simplex 25.28
insect bite-like reactions
  haematological malignancy association 148.23
  paraneoplastic manifestations of lymphoproliferative neoplasms 149.8–149.9
insecticides
  flea management 34.15
  head lice 34.21–34.22
insects 34.6–34.34
  bugs (Hemiptera) 34.25–34.30
  Diptera 34.6–34.13
  fleas/Siphonaptera 34.13–34.15
  hymenoptera 34.15–34.18
  larval invasion of tissues/myiasis **34.7**, 34.9–34.13
  lice (Phthiraptera) 34.18–34.25
  myiasis **34.7**, 34.9–34.13
  tungiasis 34.15
  see also mosquitoes
insensible sweating 2.9
in situ carcinoma of the skin 141.18–141.26
  anal/vulval/penile and perianal intraepithelial carcinoma 141.24, 141.26
  Bowen disease 141.18–141.24, *141.25*
  male genitalia 109.31–109.35
  see also Bowen disease

in situ melanomas, surgery 143.3
insulin
  allergic reactions to in diabetes 62.4
  lipodystrophy 62.4
insulin-induced fat hypertrophy 98.13
insulin-induced localised fat hypertrophy 98.14–98.15
insulin-induced localised lipoatrophy 98.10
insulin-like growth factor (IGF-1), burn treatment 125.13
insulin resistance (IR) 97.5
  acanthosis nigricans 85.3–85.6, **150.10**, *150.11*, *150.13*
  hirsutism association 87.90
  hypermetabolism 125.11
  secondary dyslipidaemia 60.11
insulin secretion 97.5
insulin sensitivity, adipocytes 97.5
integrins 2.24, *2.25*
  epidermolysis bullosa 69.4–69.5
intense pulsed light (IPL), hidradenitis suppurativa treatment 90.11
intensity modulated radiotherapy (IMRT) 24.3
intensive care treatment, and vitamin K deficiency 61.13
intention-to-treat (ITT) analysis, randomised controlled trials 17.12, 17.14
interdigital irritant contact dermatitis 128.4
interface dermatitis
  lichenoid exanthema *37.19*
  lichen planus *37.14*
interferon α2a (IFN-α2a), polymorphic light eruption 126.2
interferon α (IFN-α) therapy, cutaneous T-cell lymphoma 139.15, 139.16, 139.22–139.23, 139.25
interferon γ release assays (IGRAs), tuberculosis 27.4–27.5
interferons, melanoma immunotherapy 144.2
interleukin-16 polymorphisms 127.10
interleukins (2/4/13/31), pruritus **81.3**, 81.4–81.5
intermediate dystrophic epidermolysis bullosa 69.15
intermediate epidermolysis bullosa simplex 69.8–69.11
intermediate junctional epidermolysis bullosa, molecular pathology 69.12–69.13, 69.14
internal malignancy
  cutaneous markers 148.1–148.28
  PUVA phototherapy adverse effects 21.14
International Alliance for the Control of Scabies (ICAS) 7.9
International Conference on Harmonisation Good Clinical Practice (ICH-GCP) guidelines 13.13
International Criteria for Behçet Disease (ICBD) **108.40**
International Dermatology Outcome Measures (IDEOM) 16.3
International dermatomyositis classification of severity 52.10
International Federation of Anti-Leprosy Associations (ILEP) 7.10
International Foundation for Dermatology (IFD) 7.6
international health see global health dermatology
International Hidradenitis Suppurativa Severity Score System (IHS4) 16.5
International Index of Erectile Function (IIEF) 16.12
International League of Dermatological Societies (ILDS) 7.5–7.6
International Melanoma Pathology Study Group (IMPSG) 142.3
International Myositis Assessment and Clinical Studies (IMACS) group 52.7, 52.10, 52.12
International Society for Pharmacoeconomics and Outcomes Research (ISPOR) 16.2

International Study of Asthma and Allergies in Childhood (ISAAC) 41.3
internet phenomena, Morgellons syndrome 84.11–84.12
interpolation flaps 20.27
interstitial collagenase 2.31
interstitial granulomatous dermatitis
  musculoskeletal involvement 155.14
  rheumatoid arthritis involvement 53.6
interstitial keratitis, congenital syphilis 29.25
interstitial lung disease (ILD)
  dermatomyositis 52.1, 52.2, 52.7, 52.11–52.12
  junctional epidermolysis bullosa with 69.15
intertriginous eruption associated with chemotherapy 119.2
intertrigo **109.3**
intestinal failure-associated liver disease (ILFAD) 61.32
intestinal lymphangiectasia 103.32
intestinal polyposis disorders 153.4
intestinal worms, enterobiasis 33.14–33.15
InToDermQoL see Infants and Toddlers Quality of Life instrument
intracutaneous neurohormone metabolism 150.7
intradermal injection 4.23
intradermal naevi (IDN), dermoscopic patterns 145.6
intradermal tests, for detection of delayed sensitivity to antigens 4.24–4.25
intraepidermal cleavage, epidermolysis bullosa diagnosis *69.22*
intraepidermal sweat unit 92.2
intraepithelial carcinomas, anal/perianal/genital areas 141.24, 141.26
intraepithelial neoplasia
  human papillomavirus association 25.64
  see also cervical intraepithelial neoplasia
intrahepatic cholestasis of pregnancy 113.13–113.14
intra-individual comparative analysis of naevi
  dermoscopy 145.2
  melanoma diagnosis 142.9
intralesional corticosteroids 20.47
  reactions to 122.19–122.21
  surgical indications 20.47
intralesional cytotoxics, cutaneous warts 25.60
intralesional injection, corticosteroids 18.21–18.22
intralesional interferon α2b (IFN-α2b) 140.13–140.14
intralesional therapies
  hidradenitis suppurativa 90.9
  skin malignancies 20.47–20.48
intralymphatic histiocytosis 155.14–155.15
intranodal MR lymphography **103.56**
intravascular large B-cell lymphoma 139.43–139.44
intravascular papillary endothelial hyperplasia 136.23–136.24
intravascular paraprotein deposition 149.13–149.14
intravascular thrombi, Raynaud phenomenon 124.11
intravenous immunoglobulin (IVIG) 19.31, 19.40–19.41, 118.12, 118.21
  dose and regimen 19.41
  pemphigus 50.8
  pharmacological properties 19.40
  potential adverse effects 19.40–19.41
  pyoderma gangrenosum 49.7
  safety considerations 19.41
  systemic lupus erythematosus treatment 51.38
intravenous (IV) drug administration
  dermatoses induced by 120.6–120.8
  see also injecting drug use
invasive carcinoma, human papillomavirus association 25.65

invasive wound infection, burn injuries 125.9–125.10
inversa junctional epidermolysis bullosa 69.14
inversa recessive dystrophic epidermolysis bullosa 69.18
invertebrate vectors of disease
  blackfly (*Simulium* species) and onchocerciasis 33.1, 33.2, *33.3*
  Cyclops species and dracunculiasis 33.13
  leishmaniasis 33.43, **33.45**
  mosquitoes 25.87–25.91, 33.36, *103.34*
  sandflies and cutaneous leishmaniasis 33.43, 33.45, 33.52
  tabanid flies and loiasis 33.12
  triatomidae bugs and American trypanosomiasis 33.39–33.40
  tsetse flies and African trypanosomiasis 33.39, *33.41*, *33.42*
inverted follicular keratosis 137.2–137.3
inverted nipple, glycosylation disorders **79.10**
in vitro tests 127.33
involucrin 2.7
involuting lichenoid plaque see lichenoid keratosis
iodides, acneform reaction 88.13
iodine, topical therapies 18.10
iodism, potassium iodide (systemic therapy) 19.30
iodopropynyl butylcarbamate (IPBC) 127.57
ion channels, transmembrane drug mechanisms 13.5
ionising radiation
  post-ionising radiation keratosis 141.14–141.15
  see also radiotherapy
iontophoresis, hyperhidrosis treatment 92.9
IP see incontinentia pigmenti
IPBC see iodopropynyl butylcarbamate
IPD see immediate pigment darkening
IPEX see immunodysregulation polyendocrinopathy enteropathy X-linked syndrome
IPL see intense pulsed light
IPPD see N-isopropyl-N-phenyl-p-phenylenediamine
IPS see ichthyosis–prematurity syndrome
IPSO see Impact of Psoriasis Questionnaire
IR see insulin resistance
IRAD see immune reconstitution-associated disease
iris
  juvenile xanthogranuloma of *135.16*
  Lisch nodules *78.2*
iritis, hypopyon *48.6*
iron, hair loss 87.59, 87.63, 87.70–87.71
iron deficiency 61.3, 61.4, 61.24–61.25, 87.59, 87.63, 87.70–87.71, 153.1
iron salts, tattoos 86.53
IR radiation see infrared radiation
irritable bowel disease (IBD) see inflammatory bowel disease
irritant contact dermatitis (ICD) 39.3, 128.1–128.13
  cannabis-induced 120.4
  male genitalia 109.11
  occupational 129.1–129.5
  occupational skin disease 16.12
  perineal skin 111.9
  peristomal skin 112.2–112.7
  prevalence 127.3
  vulval 110.14–110.15
irritant folliculitis 91.1
irritant occupational hazards 129.8–129.11
irritant reactions, topical therapy 18.4
irritants
  arthropod effects 34.2
  common types 128.2
  mechanism of action 128.3
IRS see inner root sheath
ISAAC see International Study of Asthma and Allergies in Childhood
ischaemic disorders, peripheral see peripheral vascular disease

ischaemic fasciitis 136.6
ischaemic fat necrosis 97.8
ischaemic heart disease 151.5
ischaemic toes, thromboangiitis obliterans 101.6
ischaemic ulcers 101.44, 123.1
   hypertensive ischaemic leg ulcers 102.10–102.13
ISD see infantile seborrhoeic dermatitis
ISDL see Impact of Chronic Skin Disease on Daily Life
Islamic medicine 1.3
island pedicle flaps, surgical reconstruction **20.24**, 20.25–20.26
ISM see indolent systemic mastocytosis
isobornyl acrylate 127.70
isocyanates, in polyurethanes 127.71
isolated dyskeratosis follicularis see warty dyskeratoma
isolated limb perfusion (ILP), melanoma 144.2
isolated striate palmoplantar keratoderma 63.56–63.57
isomorphic phenomenon see Koebner (isomorphic) phenomenon
isomorphic response, mechanical injuries 122.2
isoniazid, acneform reaction 88.13
isopropyl myristate 12.3
N-isopropyl-N-phenyl-p-phenylenediamine (IPPD) 127.63–127.64
isothiazolinones 127.53, 127.54
isotretinoin
   acne treatment 5.3, 88.51, 88.52–88.57
   adverse effects 88.54–88.57
   musculoskeletal adverse effects 155.11
   neuropsychological adverse effects 84.42
   prescribing guidelines **88.53**
   relative success of **88.53**
   childhood acne treatment **88.73**
   ichthyoses management 63.44–63.45
   prepubertal acne treatment **88.73**
   topical therapies 18.25
ISPOR see International Society for Pharmacoeconomics and Outcomes Research
isthmic epithelial walled cutaneous cysts 133.4–133.6
isthmus region of hair root 87.4
Italy
   psoriasis, economic burden of **6.8**, 6.9
   Renaissance medicine 1.3
itching
   antihistamines 41.27
   assessment tools 4.2, 16.5
   see also pruritus
itching purpura 99.7, 99.8, **99.9**
ITGA6, epidermolysis bullosa 69.4–69.5
ITGB4, epidermolysis bullosa 69.4–69.5
Ito, naevus of 68.9–68.10, 131.14–131.15
itraconazole 32.32
ITT see intention-to-treat
IV see intravenous
ivermectin 18.14
IVIG see intravenous immunoglobulin
ixekizumab
   psoriasis treatment 35.30
   psoriatic arthritis treatment 35.46

J

Jackson–Lawler type, pachyonychia congenita 67.1
Jacob disease, oral involvement 108.86
Jadassohn–Lewandowsky type, pachyonychia congenita 67.1
Jadassohn–Pellizzari-type anetoderma 94.23
JAK see janus kinases
JAKi see Janus kinase inhibitors
Janus kinase inhibitors (JAKi) 19.22–19.24, 87.27
   atopic eczema treatment 41.27, 41.30–41.33
   cautions 19.24
   cutaneous adverse effects 155.15
   dermatological uses 19.22
   dose and regimens 19.24
   monitoring 19.24
   pharmacological properties 19.22–19.23
   potential adverse effects 19.23–19.24
   pre-treatment screening 19.24
   pyoderma gangrenosum treatment 49.7
Janus kinases (JAK) 19.22–19.23
   transmembrane drug mechanisms 13.5
Japanese-form eosinophilic pustular folliculitis 93.8
Jarisch–Herxheimer reaction, penicillin 29.22
jaundice 86.49–86.50
   hepatitis A infection 25.97
   liver disorders 153.4, 153.5
   malaria 33.36
   yellow fever 25.85
jaws
   examination 108.6
   Gardner syndrome 108.86
   Gorlin syndrome 108.86
   pseudofolliculitis 93.2
JDM see juvenile dermatomyositis
Jeffrey Modell Foundation, warning signs of inherited immunodeficiency 80.2
jellyfish stings 130.1–130.3
Jessner's lymphocytic infiltrate 89.10, 134.10–134.11
   ear dermatoses **106.22**
Jessner solution (JS), chemical peels 160.3, 160.7, 160.8, 160.10
Job syndrome see hyper-IgE syndrome due to STAT3 loss of function mutations
Jod–Basedow phenomenon, potassium iodide systemic therapy 19.30
jogger's nipples 122.16
jogger's toe 122.16
joint hypermobility (flexibility), Beighton score **70.8**
joint stiffness, in diabetes 62.5–62.6
JPHT see juvenile polyposis/HHT syndrome
JS see Jessner solution
JSE see juvenile springtime eruption
Jujin haemorrhagic fever (Argentinian haemorrhagic fever) 25.82–25.83
junctional epidermolysis bullosa 69.2
   laminin-332 69.5
   management of 69.25
   molecular pathology 69.12–69.15
   with pyloric atresia 69.13–69.14
junctional naevus
   acquired melanocytic naevi 131.18, 131.20
   definition 131.1
JUP mutations, skin fragility disorders 69.7
juvenile chronic myeloid leukaemia 149.14
juvenile dermatomyositis (JDM) 52.6, 52.8–52.9, 52.11, 52.12
juvenile fibromatosis 94.41–94.43
juvenile hyaline fibromatosis 94.42–94.43
juvenile plantar dermatosis 39.23–39.24
juvenile polyposis/HHT syndrome (JPHT) 71.2
juvenile springtime eruption (JSE) 126.8–126.9
   external ear 106.25
juvenile xanthogranuloma (JXG) 115.15, 135.14–135.17, 135.20, 149.14
   eyelid 107.45
juxta-articular Dercum disease 98.18
JXG see juvenile xanthogranuloma

K

KA see keratoacanthoma
Kabuki syndrome **106.7**
Kamino bodies 3.42
   compound naevus of Spitz 131.33
kaposiform haemangioendothelioma (KHE), infants 116.9–116.10
kaposiform lymphangiomatosis (KLA) 71.2, 103.29
Kaposi sarcoma-associated herpesvirus (KSHV/HHV-8) 25.42, 25.43, 31.30
Kaposi sarcoma (KS) 25.42, 138.1–138.6
   clinical features 138.3–138.5
   epidemiology **138.2**
   eyelid 107.49–107.50
   HIV/AIDS 25.42, 25.43, 31.30–31.31, 31.35, 138.1, **138.2**, 138.4, 138.5, 138.6
   immunocompromised patients
     clinicopathological features 147.14
     management 147.23
     non-Hodgkin lymphoma/chronic lymphocytic leukaemia patients 147.3
     people living with HIV 147.2
     systemic chemoprevention 147.20–147.21
     Wiskott–Aldrich syndrome 147.2
   male genitalia 109.42
   management 138.6
   oral involvement 108.26
   pathophysiology 138.1–138.3
   radiotherapy 24.15
   subtypes 138.1, **138.2**, 138.4
Kaposi varicelliform eruption see eczema herpeticum
Kaposi–Stemmer sign **103.6**
kappa light chains, dermal deposition 56.6
Karelian disease see Sindbis virus
karyorrhexis 3.42
Kasbach–Merritt phenomenon (KMP) 116.9–116.10
Kashin–Beck disease 61.29–61.30
Kawasaki disease 100.30–100.32, 155.3–155.4
   cardiac involvement 151.4–151.5
   clinical features 26.89–26.90
   epidemiology 26.89
   infants 115.9–115.11
   management 26.90
   oral ulceration 108.41–108.42
   pathophysiology 26.89
   perineal and perianal skin 111.16
   possible bacterial role 26.89
Kaya and Saurat's classification of cutaneous adnexal cysts 133.2
Kazal-type-related inhibitor, skin fragility disorders 69.6
KC see keratosis circumscripta
KCMC see Kilimanjaro Christian Medical Centre
KCs see keratinocyte carcinomas
kEDS see kyphoscoliotic Ehlers–Danlos syndrome
Kelch-like genes, epidermolysis bullosa 69.3–69.4
keloid 94.48–94.53
   penis 109.31
   radiotherapy 24.7–24.8
keloidal blastomycosis see lobomycosis
keloidalis, folliculitis 91.10–91.12
keloidal/nodular morphoea 55.15–55.16
keloidal papules 93.3
keloid-like scars, folliculitis 91.11
keloid reaction, tattoos 86.54
keloid scarring 11.9
   external ear 106.14–106.15
   hidradenitis suppurativa 111.12
Kenya, teledermatology 7.9
Keppen–Lubinsky syndrome **72.5**
keratan sulphate (KS) 2.37, 2.38, **2.39**
keratin aggregates, ichthyoses 63.13
keratin-associated proteins, hair follicle 87.6
keratin gene expression 2.7–2.8
α-keratin intermediate filaments (α-KIF) 87.6
keratinisation disorders 63.73–63.76, 85.18
   ocular features **107.41**
keratinised tissues, dermatophytes 32.20
keratin markers, cutaneous neoplasms 3.21–3.23
keratinocyte carcinomas (KCs)
   definition 141.1
immunocompromised patients
   clinicopathological features 147.10–147.11
   management 147.16–147.18
   prevention 147.18–147.21
   see also basal cell carcinoma; squamous cell carcinoma
keratinocytes 2.1, 2.5, 2.7–2.8
   adherens junction **2.19**
   Cole disease 63.61
   differentiation process 9.1
   elatin gene expression 2.33
   grafts 11.12
   keratin filament network **2.8**
   mechanical stretching 122.1
   melanocyte interface 86.3
   melanosome transfer to 86.4
   porokeratosis 85.19–85.20
   wound healing 11.4–11.5, 11.12
keratinocyte terminal differentiation, melanosomes 68.1
keratinocytic acanthomas, benign proliferations 132.1–132.8
keratinocytic disadhesion
   Carvajal-Huerta syndrome 63.63
   striate palmoplantar keratoderma **63.57**, 63.58
keratinopathic ichthyoses (KPIs) **63.4**, 63.13–63.18
   skin fragility 69.20
keratins
   epidermolysis bullosa 69.2–69.3, 69.7
   hair 2.10, 87.99
   hemidesmosomal inner plaques 69.4
   pachyonychia congenita 67.1
keratitis–ichthyosis–deafness (KID) syndrome 63.33–63.35, 108.29
keratoacanthoma (KA) 141.38–141.41
   associated conditions 141.38–141.45
   eyelid 107.47
   generalised eruptive keratoacanthoma 141.43–141.44
   lip 108.44
   multiple self-healing squamous epithelioma 141.41–141.42
   visceral malignancy 148.12
keratoderma blennorhagicum, reactive arthritis 155.1
keratoderma climactericum (Haxthausen disease) 63.71–63.72
keratodermas
   acquired forms 63.71–63.79
   NIPAL4 mutations **63.14**
   pachyonychia congenita 67.12
   palmoplantar keratodermas 63.49–63.71
   syndromic forms 63.62–63.71
keratoelastoidosis marginalis 63.60
keratolysis exfoliativa 85.25–85.26
keratolytics, ichthyoses management 63.42–63.43, **63.43**
keratolytics (topical), seborrhoeic dermatitis 40.8
keratolytic winter erythema 63.73–63.74
   genes/proteins linked to 69.6
keratomycosis nigricans palmaris see tinea nigra
keratoses
   NLRP1-associated autoinflammation with arthritis and dyskeratosis **45.18**
   oral lesions 108.33
   PUVA phototherapy adverse effects 21.14
   seborrhoeic 132.1–132.4
   see also hyperkeratosis; seborrhoeic keratosis
keratosis alba see stucco keratosis
keratosis circumscripta (KC) 85.13–85.14, **85.14**
keratosis follicularis spinulosa decalvans (KFSD) 63.24–63.25, 85.11, 87.48
keratosis linearis–ichthyosis congenita–sclerosing keratoderma 63.21
keratosis obturans 106.21
keratosis pilaris atrophicans 85.10–85.11

keratosis pilaris atrophicans faciei 85.10, *85.11*
keratosis pilaris (KP) 85.9–85.12, 88.34, *88.35*
keratosis pilaris rubra faciei 85.10
keratotic lichenification, KID syndrome 63.33
keratotic papules
   Flegel disease 85.17, *85.18*
   lichen spinulosus 85.12
   palmoplantar keratoderma punctata 63.58, *63.59*
keratotic plug, phrynoderma 85.14–85.15
kerion
   allergic reactions 32.50
   tinea capitis type 32.39
kerotic spicules, trichodysplasia spinulosa *85.16*
Keshan disease, selenium deficiency 61.29
ketoprofen allergy 127.79
KFD *see* Kikuchi–Fujimoto disease
KFSD *see* keratosis follicularis spinulosa decalvans
KHE *see* kaposiform haemangioendothelioma
KID *see* keratitis–icthyosis–deafness syndrome
kidneys *see* nephropathy; *renal entries*
α-KIF *see* α-keratin intermediate filaments
Kikuchi–Fujimoto disease (KFD) 51.33, 149.16–149.17
Kilimanjaro Christian Medical Centre (KCMC) 7.7
kilovoltage X-ray therapy 24.1, 24.3, 24.4, 24.7
Kimura disease 136.27, 149.17
Kindler epidermolysis bullosa (Kindler syndrome) 69.5, 69.19, **75.2**, 75.6, 108.86
Kindlin-1 (*KIND1/FERMT1*) 69.5
kinesin 86.4
kissing bugs 34.29
KIT gene 2.15
KIT receptor mutations, mastocytosis 46.1, 46.2
KLA *see* kaposiform lymphangiomatosis
Klebsiella (Calymmatobacterium) granulomatis 30.21–30.23
Klebsiella pneumoniae subsp. *rhinoscleromatis* 26.56–26.57
Klein–Waardenburg syndrome 68.5
KLHL24, epidermolysis bullosa 69.3–69.4
Kligman cream, topical depigmenting agents 18.32
Klinefelter syndrome 74.4
Klippel–Trenaunay syndrome (KTS) 101.27–101.30, 103.23
   spindle cell haemangioma 136.31
Klippel–Trenaunay–Weber syndrome 71.2, 71.8–71.9
   oral involvement 108.26
KMP *see* Kasbach–Merritt phenomenon
knee
   atopic eczema *41.16*
   calcinosis *79.18*
   epidermolysis bullosa acquista *50.44*
   erythema elevatum diutinum *100.9*
   Gianotti–Crosti syndrome *115.11*
   nail–patella syndrome 67.16
   necrotising granulomatous lesions *80.10*
   sarcoidosis 96.7
   tuberous xanthomas *60.3*
knuckle pads (subcutaneous fibroma) 94.37–94.38
   Bart–Pumphrey syndrome 63.64
   sports injuries 122.16
knuckles, granuloma annulare 95.5
Koebner (isomorphic) phenomenon/Koebnerisation 86.36, 86.38, 119.14, 121.9, 128.5
   lichen planus induced by mechanical irritation 37.3
   linear lesions 4.7
   necrobiosis lipoidica 95.11, *95.12*
   psoriasis vulgaris *35.8*

Koebner (isomorphic) response, mechanical injuries 122.2–122.3, 122.22
Koenen tumours (periungual fibromas), tuberous sclerosis complex 78.8
koganbyo *see* cercarial dermatitis
Kogoj spongiform pustule 3.43
koilonychia, infants 115.14
kojic acid
   cosmeceutical use of 157.4
   topical depigmenting agents 18.32
Koplik spots
   measles 25.98, *25.99*
   oral lesions 108.33
koro syndrome, male genitalia 109.44
Kosaki overgrowth syndrome **72.5**
KP *see* keratosis pilaris
KPIs *see* keratinopathic ichthyoses
Kramer syndrome 68.9
Krokodil 120.5–120.6
KRT genes, epidermolysis bullosa 69.2–69.3, 69.7
KS *see* Kaposi sarcoma; keratan sulphate
KSHV *see* Kaposi sarcoma-associated herpesvirus
KTP *see* potassium titanyl phosphate lasers
KTS *see* Klippel–Trenaunay syndrome
Küster, Wolfgang 63.43
kwashiorkor 61.2, 61.3
   erythrodermic findings in *61.4*
   peripheral oedema and 'flaky paint' dermatitis *61.4*
   presentation 61.4
kyphoscoliotic Ehlers–Danlos syndrome (kEDS) **70.4**, 70.9
Kyrle disease *63.76*, 63.77, 94.53, 154.3–154.4
Kytococcus sedentarius, pitted keratolysis 26.42–26.43

L

L *see* lichenoid keratosis
LA *see* lactic acid
labelling of tissue specimens 3.6
labial melanotic macules (labial lentigo) 131.11–131.12
labial mucosa 108.3, 108.6–108.7
labia majora
   angiokeratomas 110.3, *110.4*
   Fordyce spots 110.3
   structure and function of 110.2
labia minora
   Fordyce spots 110.3, *110.4*
   structure and function of 110.2
   vestibular papillomatosis 110.4
Lacazia loboi 32.78–32.79
lacrimal glands 107.3
lactate, eccrine sweating 92.3–92.4
lactation
   drug pharmacokinetics and pharmacodynamics 13.8–13.9
   rosacea and 89.15
   safe treatments in pregnancy 113.19–113.24
   transfer of toxic substances in 114.14
lactic acid (LA), chemical peels 160.2
lactiferous ducts of the nipple, nipple adenoma 137.21–137.22
LAD *see* linear IgA disease
LADD *see* laser-assisted drug delivery
lake itch *see* cercarial dermatitis
LAM *see* linear atrophoderma of Moulin; lymphangioleiomyomatosis
lambda light chains, dermal deposition of 56.6
LAMB (lentigines, atrial myxoma, blue nevi) syndrome *see* Carney complex
lamellar bodies, harlequin ichthyosis 63.8, 63.10
lamellar granules/bodies 2.6
lamellar ichthyosis (LI) 63.10–63.13, *63.12*
lamellar scaling, trichothiodystrophy *63.37*
laminin-332 (*LAMA3*), (*LAMB3*), (*LAMC2*) 69.5, 69.14
laminin 411, wound healing 11.6

laminins 2.23–2.25
   chain composition **2.24**
   isoforms and domain organisations *2.24*
   laminin 332 2.25, 2.44
lamotrigine, hypersensitivity reactions to **14.6**
Langerhans cell histiocytoses (LCH) 2.15, 135.1, 135.2–135.11
   female genitalia 110.40
   infants/children 115.15–115.16, 135.4, 135.5–135.7, **135.9**
   oral involvement 108.70–108.71
Langerhans cell markers, cutaneous neoplasms 3.27, *3.28*
Langerhans cells (LCs) 2.1–2.2, 2.13–2.15
   antigen exchange 2.13, *2.15*
   epidermal immune cells *9.4*
   imaging of 2.13
   immune system 9.3
   skin ageing 2.45
   structure of 2.14, *2.16*
langerin 135.2
lanolin, topical medication vehicles 18.6–18.7
lanolin alcohols 127.58
lanolin allergy 127.58
large B-cell lymphoma (LBCL) 139.37, 139.41–139.44
large-cell lymphomas
   primary cutaneous anaplastic large-cell lymphoma 139.28–139.29
   primary cutaneous diffuse large B-cell lymphoma 139.37, 139.41–139.43
   secondary intravascular large B-cell lymphoma 139.43–139.44
large congenital melanocytic naevi, as melanoma precursors 142.2, *142.3*
large congenital naevi, melanoma detection 142.11
large plaque parapsoriasis (LPP) 134.6, *134.7–134.8*
large-vessel vasculitis 100.32–100.35
larimal duct scarring, in erosive lichen planus *110.12*
larva currens *see* strongyloidiasis
larval taeniasis *see* cysticercosis
larva migrans *see* ancylostomiasis; cutaneous larva migrans; visceral larva migrans
laryngo-onycho-cutaneous syndrome 69.14–69.15
laser-assisted drug delivery (LADD) 161.5
laser-assisted hair removal 23.17–23.20
   complications 23.19–23.20
   folliculitis keloidalis 93.4
   indications 23.19
laser-assisted lipolysis 23.24
Laser Doppler flowmetry (LDF) 128.6
laser resurfacing 161.1–161.6
   ablative and non-ablative fractional devices **161.5**
   for acne scarring *161.4*
   adverse effects 161.6
   avoidance of bulk heating 161.4
   carbon dioxide lasers 161.1–161.3, **161.5**
   device names **161.5**
   Er:YAG lasers 161.1–161.3, **161.5**
   fractionated ablative lasers 161.2–161.3, **161.5**
   management of patients 161.3–161.5
   non-ablative fractional resurfacing 161.2, **161.5**
   patient selection 161.3
   for photodamaged skin *161.3*
   postoperative course 161.4–161.5
   preoperative management and anaesthesia 161.3–161.4
   skin tightening 161.6
   wound care 161.4
lasers
   history 23.1
   principles 23.1–23.3
laser therapies 23.1–23.24
   basal cell carcinoma 140.16
   clinical applications 23.6–23.24

   cutaneous warts 25.59
   hair disorders 87.71, 87.95
   keloids/hypertrophic scars 94.52
   light-tissue interactions 23.4–23.5
   mechanical injuries 122.6
   selective photothermolysis 23.5–23.6
   theory 23.1–23.6
   tissue cooling to avoid epidermal heat damage 23.6
   tissue optics 23.3–23.4
   unrealistic expectations 23.6
   vascular lesions 23.6–23.12
   see also photothermal ablation
Lassa fever 25.81–25.82
latent syphilis 29.12
latent transforming growth factor beta binding proteins (LTBPs) 2.36
latent viral infections *see* reactivation of viruses; subclinical and latent viral infections
late-onset chronic mucocutaneous candidiasis 32.68
late-onset focal dermal elastosis 94.32
late-onset ichthyosis 63.47–63.50
late-onset junctional epidermolysis bullosa 69.14
late-onset primary lymphoedema 103.24–103.25
lateral canthal lines, reduction of by botulinum toxin application 159.5
latex *see* natural rubber latex; rubber allergy
latex–fruit syndrome 127.84
Latino skin phenotypes, photoageing 156.2–156.3
Lattice System Global Assessment, psoriasis 16.3
Laugier–Hunziker syndrome, oral involvement 108.18
lavender, cosmeceutical use of **157.8**
lax skin 94.21–94.23
   Ehlers–Danlos syndrome 94.27
lazy leukocyte syndrome *see* periodic fever, immunodeficiency and thrombocytopenia
LBCL *see* large B-cell lymphoma
LCH *see* Langerhans cell histiocytoses
LCs *see* Langerhans cells
LDF *see* Laser Doppler flowmetry
LDS *see* lipodermatosclerosis; Loeys-Dietz syndrome
LE *see* lupus erythematosus
lead, dermatological reactions 121.2, 121.4–121.5
lead shielding mask, radiotherapy for skin cancer near eyes 24.3, *24.4*, 24.10–24.11
leather
   chromium allergy 127.39–127.40
   shoe allergy 127.67–127.68
ledderhose disease *see* plantar fibromatosis
Leeds Acne Grading System 16.4
leg
   acquired cutaneous lymphangiectasia *103.6*
   acute haemorrhagic oedema in infancy 115.10
   allergic contact dermatitis of 127.17, 127.22
   amniotic bands and lymphoedema *103.30*
   annular erythema of infancy 47.10
   atopic eczema *41.14, 41.17*, 115.3
   bandaging, lymphoedema therapy *103.59*
   chronic red leg 103.16–103.17
   chronic venous oedema 103.10
   congenital generalised lipodystrophies 72.2
   congenital haemangioma *116.9*
   cutaneous polyarteritis nodosa 100.29
   cutaneous small-vessel vasculitis 100.7
   dermatitis herpetiformis *50.57*
   eczema of the lower legs 39.19–39.22
      clinical features 39.20
      clinical variants 39.21

leg (*continued*)
    complications and co-morbidities 39.21
        disease course and prognosis 39.21
        management 39.21–39.22
        pathology 39.20
        treatment for 39.22
    elephantiasis nostra verrucosa 103.6
    eosinophilic fasciitis 55.22
    eosinophilic granulomatosis with polyangiitis 100.27
    eruptive xanthomas 60.4
    granuloma annulare 95.6
    hyperglobulinaemic purpura in patient with Sjögren syndrome 53.11
    hypertrophic lichen planus 37.7
    keloidal morphoea 55.16
    laser therapies on veins 23.11
    lichen simplex 39.29
    linear IgA disease 50.37
    linear morphoea 55.26
    lipodermatosclerosis 103.17
    lipoedema 72.12, 98.21–98.23, 103.54
    livedo reticularis 4.11, 51.27, 53.3
    lymphangioma malformation 103.27
    lymphoedema–distichiasis syndrome 71.25
    mixed connective tissue disease 53.3
    morphoea 55.18, 55.20
    necrolytic migratory erythema 47.15
    Nékam disease 37.11
    nummular dermatitis 39.8
    palisaded and neutrophilic granulomatous dermatitis 53.7
    pemphigus foliaceus 50.6
    plaque morphoea 55.18, 55.20
    podoconiosis (non-filarial lymphoedema) 103.36
    psoriasis vulgaris 35.8, 35.13
    pyoderma gangrenosum 49.2
    rheumatoid arthritis-associated medium vessel vasculitis 53.8
    small-vessel vasculitis 100.2, 100.3
    STING-associated vasculopathy with onset in infancy 45.14
    Sweet syndrome 49.12
    swelling 103.9–103.10
    ulcerated necrotic lesions 100.3
    varicose veins 101.39
    vasculitis 100.2, 100.3
    veins, laser therapies 23.11
    venous malformation 71.15
    see also ankle; knee; shin; thigh
legal issues
    drug use 120.3–120.4
    litigation by psychologically disturbed patients 84.9–84.10, 84.15, 84.36–84.38
Legionella pneumophila (legionellosis) 26.76
Legius syndrome 72.10, 78.9
leg ulcers 1.3
    aetiologies 102.1, **102.2**
    arterial leg ulcers 102.7–102.10
    diabetic patients 62.1
    hypertensive ischaemic leg ulcers 102.10–102.13
    mixed leg ulcers 102.4–102.7
    rheumatoid arthritis-associated 53.7, 155.6
    systemic lupus erythematosus 51.26
    venous leg ulcers 102.1–102.4
leiomyoma 136.53–136.54
    oral involvement 108.13
    vulva **110.32**
leiomyomatosis *see* hereditary leiomyomatosis and renal cell cancer; lymphangioleiomyomatosis
leiomyosarcoma/atypical smooth muscle tumour 136.54–136.55
leishmaniasis 33.43–33.54
    blepharitis 107.12
    cutaneous 33.43–33.51
    ear dermatoses **106.23**
    HIV 33.52–33.53
    male genitalia 109.28
    oral involvement 108.57
    parasitic organisms 33.45, 33.46–33.49, 33.52
    vectors 33.43, **33.45**, *33.52*
    visceral 33.51–33.54
    see also cutaneous leishmaniasis; visceral leishmaniasis
leishmaniasis cutis diffusa (diffuse/disseminated cutaneous leishmaniasis) 33.48–33.49
leishmaniasis recidivans (chronic/lupoid cutaneous leishmaniasis) 33.47–33.48
leisure factors
    diagnosis 4.4
    epidemiology 5.11
LEKTI *see* lymphoepithelial Kazal-type-related inhibitor
lentigines 131.3–131.9
    agminated or segmental lentiginosis 131.3
    familial lentiginosis syndromes **131.3**
    ink-spot lentigo 131.8–131.9
    lentiginosis profusa 131.3
    photochemotherapy (PUVA) lentigo 131.7–131.8
    PUVA phototherapy adverse effects 21.14
    RASopathies 151.3
    simple lentigo 131.3–131.5
    solar (or actinic) lentigo 131.5–131.7
    xeroderma pigmentosum 76.4
    see also mucosal melanotic lesions
lentiginoses 86.16–86.17, **131.3**
    oral involvement 108.17–108.18
lentiginosis profusa 131.3
lentigo, definition **131.1**
lentigo maligna (LM)
    facial and chronically sun-damaged skin 145.9, *145.11*
    presentation 142.19
    radiotherapy 24.14–24.15
lentigo maligna melanoma (LMM) 106.33
    melanoma classification 142.7, 142.8
    presentation 142.10, *142.13*, 142.19
    radiotherapy 24.14–24.15
    surgery 143.3–143.4
lentigo senilis (solar/actinic lentigo) 131.5–131.7
lentigo simplex 131.3–131.5
    dermoscopic image *131.5*
    hyperpigmentation *131.4*
Lenz–Majewski syndrome 70.16
LEOPARD syndrome (Noonan with multiple lentigines) **131.3**, 151.3
Lepidoptera (butterflies and moths) 34.32–34.34
lepidopterism
    use of term 34.33
    see also caterpillar dermatitis
lepromatous leprosy (LL) 28.2, 28.3–28.4, 28.5, 28.7–28.8, *28.9*, 97.26
leprosy 28.1–28.17
    clinical features 28.6–28.13
    delayed diagnosis in non-endemic settings 28.10
    differential diagnosis of lesions 28.10–28.11
    drug treatments 1.8
    ear dermatoses **106.23**
    epidemiology 28.1
    erythema nodosum leprosum 28.3, 28.4, 28.5, 28.11, *28.12*, 28.15
    eye infection 107.39
    genetic factors 28.1–28.2
    granuloma multiforme resemblance 94.30
    hair loss 87.36
    history 28.1
    HIV 28.10
    International Federation of Anti-Leprosy Associations 7.10
    investigations 28.13
    management 28.13–28.16
    oral involvement 108.55
    pathophysiology 28.1–28.6
    predisposing factors 28.1–28.2
    pregnancy 28.10
    in pregnancy 113.6
    prevention and control 28.16
    stigma 28.1, 28.16
    variants 28.2–28.3, 28.6–28.10
leprosy reactions, erythema nodosum leprosum 97.25–97.26
leptin, role of 97.4–97.5
leptin deficiency **72.7**
leptin receptor syndrome **72.6**
leptospirosis/*Leptospira* spp. 26.74–26.75
Leser–Trélat, sign of 148.16
lesional blistering, UVB phototherapy adverse effects 21.12
lesional erythema, versus persistent/diffuse erythema of rosacea 89.7
lesions
    annular lesions 4.7, 4.15
        granuloma annulare *4.10*
        keratotic lesions 63.75
        porokeratosis *4.10*
        tinea corporis *4.10*
    arcuate lesions *4.11*
    autoinflammatory diseases **80.19**
    Blashkoid lesions 4.16, *4.19*
    cocaine-induced 120.5
    colour of skin 4.13–4.15
    dermatomal distribution 4.16
    deroofing 90.10
    description of 4.5–4.20
        anatomical factors 4.5–4.6
        border of lesion 4.15
        colour of lesion 4.15
        distribution pattern and arrangement 4.6–4.12
        external factors 4.6
        nomenclature 4.10–4.15, *4.16*, *4.17*
        shape of lesion 4.6–4.7, *4.8–4.10*, **4.12**, *4.15*, *4.16*, *4.17*
        size of lesion 4.10
    digitate lesions *4.17*
    discoid lesions *4.12*
    distribution of 4.16, **4.17**, **4.18**, *4.19*
        anatomical factors 4.16
        Blashkoid distribution 4.16, *4.19*
        dermatomal distribution 4.16
        external factors 4.16
    duration 4.3
    erythema 4.13
    erythrokeratoderma variabilis 63.18, *63.19*
    flexural sites **4.18**
    haemorrhagic lesions *4.12*
    hidradenitis suppurativa 90.3, 90.5
    history taking 4.2
    Hurley stage III disease *90.9*
    linear lesions 4.15
        anatomical and causative factors **4.13**
        Koebner/isomorphic phenomenon 4.7
    livedoid lesions *4.11*
    malar erythematous photosensitive macular skin lesions *80.16*
    periodicity 4.3
    pityriasis rotunda 63.48
    polycyclic lesions *4.11*
    reticulate lesions 4.16
    sarcoidosis 96.1, 96.6–96.7
    surface features 4.13
    target lesions *4.15*
    tuberous sclerosis complex 78.8
le tic des lèvres (factitious cheilitis) 84.33, *108.61*
Letterer–Siwe disease 135.6
leucocytoclastic vasculitis, urticarial vasculitis 44.1, 44.3
leucomelanoderma, drug/chemical photosensitivity 126.30
leukaemia cutis 139.47–139.48
    infiltration of skin with neoplastic cells 149.2–149.4
    purpura 148.2
    see also myeloid sarcoma
leukaemias
    erythroderma 39.32–39.33
    oral involvement 108.71
leukocyte antigen markers 3.27–3.28
leukocytoclasis, IgA vasculitis 100.14
leukocytoclastic vasculitis 100.6, 100.8
leukoderma 86.8
    hypomelanosis 86.45–86.47
    occupational 129.13–129.14
leukoderma acquisitum centrifugum 86.40
leukoedema, oral lesions 108.29, *108.30*
leukonychia 119.7, 121.7
leukopenias, oral involvement 108.71
leukoplakia, dyskeratosis congenita 67.14, 75.3
leukoplakia, oral lesions 108.33–108.35
    chronic hyperplastic candidiasis (candidal leukoplakia) 108.34
    hairy leukoplakia 108.34
    malignancy risk **108.35**
    speckled leukoplakia 108.34
    sublingual keratosis 108.34
    syphilitic leukoplakia 108.34
leukotriene C4 (LTC4), release of in skin 14.1, 14.2
leukotriene receptor antagonists, urticaria treatment 42.19
leukotrienes, melanocyte regulation 86.7
levamisole-induced vasculitis 120.5, *120.6*
Levulan®
    Kerastick®, Ameluz®, Alacare® 22.1
    see also 5-aminolaevulinic acid
Lewandowski and Lutz dysplasia *see* epidermodysplasia verruciformis
LF *see* lymphatic filariasis
LGV *see* lymphogranuloma venereum
LH3 *see* lysyl hydroxylase
LI *see* lamellar ichthyosis
Libman–Sacks endocarditis 51.18
lice (Phthiraptera) 34.18–34.25
    body/clothing lice 34.23–34.24
    classification 34.18
    crab lice 34.24–34.25, *34.25*, 107.12, 107.40
    head lice 1.2, 34.18–34.23
    on mummified body 1.2
    see also louse-borne diseases
lichen amyloidosus 56.3
lichen aureus 3.9, 99.7, 99.8, **99.9**
lichen exanthematicus 37.4
lichenification/lichenoid reactions 3.42, 39.28–39.31
    allergens 127.20
    atopic eczema 41.14, 41.16, 41.17, 41.19
    familial primary localised cutaneous amyloidosis 56.9
    in ichthyoses 63.11
    irritant contact dermatitis 128.5
    nail changes 119.7
    pathogenesis 37.2
    tattoos 86.54
lichenified onchodermatitis (LOD) 33.3–33.4
lichen myxoedematosus (LM) 57.1–57.8
lichen nitidus 37.9–37.10
lichenoid chronic dermatitis 39.8, *39.9*
lichenoid exanthema 37.19
lichenoid infiltrate, drug reaction with eosinophilia and systemic symptoms 118.6
lichenoid keratosis (LK) 132.7–132.8
lichenoid primary localised cutaneous amyloidosis 56.7
lichenoid sarcoidosis 96.13
lichen planopilaris (LPP) 37.5, 37.6, 37.11, 87.38–87.42
lichen planus-like drug eruptions 117.7–117.9
lichen planus-like keratosis *see* lichenoid keratosis
lichen planus (LP) 37.1–37.17, 127.20, 127.22
    actinic lichen planus 37.7, 37.17
    acute and subacute lichen planus with confluence of lesions 37.8
    amalgam fillings 127.41

annular lichen planus 37.8
associated conditions 37.13
associated with liver disease 153.4, 153.5, 153.9
bacterial or fungal dysbiosis 37.3
betel chewing 37.3
buccal mucosa *37.5, 37.6*
bullous lichen planus 37.8–37.9, 37.17
classic eruption on wrist *37.3*
clinical features 37.3–37.5
clinical variants 37.5–37.11, 37.16–37.17
complications and co-morbidities 37.11–37.12
dental amalgam 37.3
dermoscopy image of *37.13*
direct immunofluorescence 37.15
direct immunofluorescence findings 3.18, *3.19*
disease course and prognosis 37.13
drug causation 37.3
ear dermatoses **106.23**
environmental factors 37.2–37.3
epidemiology 37.1
erythrodermic lichen planus 39.34
florid *4.16*
genetics 37.2
genital mucosa 37.6
guttate lichen planus 37.8, *37.9*
hair 37.5, 37.6, 37.11
hand *39.17*
hepatitis B association 25.75
hepatitis C association 25.76
hepatitis and other viruses 37.2
histology *37.13*
hypertrophic lichen planus 37.6–37.7
interface dermatitis 37.14
internal malignancy association 148.23
investigations 37.13–37.15
keratoderma climactericum 63.72
lichen exanthematicus *37.4*
lichen nitidus 37.9–37.10
lichen planopilaris *37.5, 37.6*
lichen planus-like contact dermatitis 37.3
lichen planus pemphigoides 37.8–37.9, 37.17
lichen planus pigmentosus 37.7
male genitalia 109.18–109.19
management 37.15–37.17
mechanical irritation (Koebner phenomenon) 37.3
'mixed' lichen planus/discoid lupus erythematosus disease patterns 37.8, 37.16
mucous membranes 37.12
nails 37.11–37.12
Nékam disease 37.10–37.11, 37.16
palm *37.5, 37.7*
pathology 37.1–37.2
penis *37.4*
perianal skin 111.10
photomicrograph of *37.15*
reticulate *4.16*
scalp 37.5, 37.6
sole 37.7
treatment 37.15–37.16
vulva 110.10–110.13
 clinical features 110.11
 complications and co-morbidities 110.12
 epidemiology 110.10
 glazed erythema *110.12*
 histology *110.10*
 pathophysiology 110.10–110.11
 plaques *110.11*
 vulvo-vaginal-gingival syndrome *110.12*
 Wickham striae *110.11*
Wickham striae *37.3, 37.13*
wrist *39.17*
see also oral lichen planus
lichen planus pemphigoides 37.8–37.9, 37.17, 50.51
 oral involvement 108.78
lichen planus pigmentosus 37.7

lichens, allergic contact dermatitis 127.73, 127.74
lichen sclerosus (LS) 55.7
 ano-genital region 111.9–111.10
 liquefaction degeneration *3.40*
 male genitalia 109.15–109.18
 perineal and perianal skin 111.9–111.10
 peristomal skin 112.10, *112.11*, 112.12
 vulva 110.6–110.10
  clinical features 110.7–110.9
  complications and co-morbidities 110.8–110.9
  histology *110.7*
  management of 110.9–110.10
  plaques *110.7*
  scarring *110.9*
  squamous cell carcinoma *110.9*
lichen sclerosus morphoea **55.4**, *55.5, 55.6*, 55.7
lichen scrofulosorum (tuberculosis cutis lichenoides) 27.25–27.27
 clinical features 27.26–27.27
 epidemiology 27.25
 investigations 27.27
 management 27.27
 pathophysiology 27.25–27.26
lichen simplex 39.28–39.31
 male genitalia 109.11
 perineal and perianal skin 111.8
 vulva 110.16–110.17
lichen simplex chronicus (LSC) 81.18–81.20, 84.15, 105.5
 clinical features 81.20
 epidemiology 81.18
 management *81.19*, 81.20
 pathophysiology 81.18–81.20
lichen simplex-like eczema *127.16*
lichen spinulosus (LS) 85.12–85.13
lichen striatus *4.9*, 37.17–37.19, 86.44
 management 37.18–37.19
 presentation 37.17–37.18
life course impairment assessment 16.11
Life Quality Index Occupational Dermatoses (LIOD) 16.12
lifestyle factors
 acne 88.18–88.26
 seborrhoeic dermatitis 40.4, 40.7
lifting flaps 20.26–20.27
LIG4 syndrome **80.4**
light
 absorption by skin 23.3–23.4
 amplification 23.2
 energy 23.4
 spontaneous and stimulated emission 23.1–23.2
 transmission through skin 23.4
 see also lasers; ultraviolet
light-assisted hair removal 23.5–23.6
 see also laser-assisted hair removal
light exposure
 Bowen disease 141.18, 141.19
 mechanical injuries 122.5
light therapy *see* laser therapies; phototherapy
light-tissue interactions 23.4–23.5
lilac, *see also* violaceous
lilac erythema, upper eyelids in dermatomyositis 52.3, *52.5*
Liliaceae dermatitis *127.73*
limbs
 anatomical considerations for skin surgery 20.4
 calciphylaxis 59.7
 dermatomyositis 52.5, 52.6, *52.9*
 swelling 103.9–103.10, 103.16–103.17, 103.44–103.46
limonene 127.42–127.43, 127.44
linalool 127.44
lincosamides 19.47–19.48
Lind, James 5.1
linear atrophoderma of Moulin (LAM) 55.25–55.27, 73.22, 94.17
linear closure, skin surgery 20.21–20.22
linear epidermal naevus, oral lesions 108.30
linear furrows 94.2

linear IgA disease (LAD) 50.33–50.38, 149.13
 associated diseases 50.34
 bullous dermatosis 3.18, 50.36
 in childhood *50.36*, 108.81
 clinical features 50.36
 clinical variants 50.36
 'cluster of jewels'/'string of pearls' sign *50.37*
 diagnosis *50.24*
 differential diagnosis 50.36
 direct immunofluorescence microscopy *50.35*
 epidemiology 50.33–50.34
 histopathology 50.35
 infants 115.11
 internal malignancy association 148.22
 investigations and diagnosis 50.36–50.38
 management 50.38
 mixed immunobullous disease 50.36
 oral involvement in adults 108.81–108.82
 pathophysiology 50.34
 predisposing factors 50.34–50.35
 sub-lamina densa variant 50.36
 treatment ladder 50.38
 vesicle pattern along edge of lesion *50.37*
 vulva **110.21**
linear IgA/IgG bullous dermatosis 50.36
linear keloids 94.50
linear lesions 4.7, **4.13**, 4.15
linear morphoea ('en coup de sabre') **55.3**, **55.4**, 55.23–55.27, 105.8–105.9
linear naevus syndrome (naevus sebaceous of Jadassohn) 108.29–108.30
linear porokeratosis 63.75, 85.20–85.21, 85.22
linear psoriasis 35.15
linear and whorled naevoid hypermelanosis (LWNH) 68.12
lines of Blaschko 8.7, *8.8*
lingual erythema migrans *108.24*
lingual thyroid 108.11
lingual tonsil 108.11
Linuche unguiculata stings 130.2
LIOD *see* Life Quality Index Occupational Dermatoses
lip
 actinic cheilitis (solar cheilosis) 108.58
 actinic prurigo 108.58–108.59
 acute/chronic enlargement of, differential diagnoses **108.74**
 allergic contact dermatitis of 127.15
 anatomy of 108.3
 angioedema 108.10
 angular cheilitis 108.59–108.60
 basal cell carcinoma 108.43–108.44
 blisters 108.60
 calibre-persistent artery 108.63
 'chapping' of 108.60
 cheilitis 108.60–108.63
 cleft lip/palate 108.83–108.85
 commissural pits 108.86
 contact cheilitis 108.60–108.61
 dermal fillers *158.3, 158.4*
  adverse reaction to *158.9, 158.10*
 dermal fillers and implants **108.62**
 discoid lupus erythematosus *108.64*
 double lip 108.85
 drug-induced cheilitis 108.61
 enlargement of, acute/chronic **108.74**
 examination of 108.6–108.7
 factitious cheilitis 84.33, *108.61*
 fissures 108.63–108.64
 granulomatous cheilitis *108.73*
 haemorrhagic crusting of *108.61*
 herpes labialis *108.53*
 herpetic stomatitis *108.52*
 HIV infection *108.14*
 impetigo 115.7
 Kawasaki disease *115.10*
 keratoacanthoma 108.44
 lesions 108.57–108.64
 lupus erythematosus 108.64
 mast cell mediator-induced angio-oedema *43.2*

melanotic macule 108.18
melanotic macules 131.11–131.12
mucocutaneous venous malformation *71.16*
multiple endocrine neoplasia 108.13–108.14, *108.13*, 148.10
oedema 103.46, *103.48*
Orf-induced pemphigoid *50.55*
pits and sinuses 108.86
radiotherapy for skin cancer 24.12, *24.13*
reactive perforating collagenosis 108.64
reticulate lichen planus *4.16*
sarcoidosis 108.64
Sturge–Weber syndrome *108.27*
swelling due to oro-facial granulomatosis *95.14*
systemic amyloidosis with mucotaneous involvement *56.12*
tattooing of 108.15–108.16
ulcerative lichen planus *108.77*
venous lake *4.14*, 108.28
vermilion 108.3
vermilionectomy repair 20.22
lipase, pancreatic panniculitis 97.41
lipid injectable emulsion (ILE), parenteral nutrition 61.32, 61.33–61.34
lipid metabolism disorders 60.1–60.12, 79.15
 dyslipidaemias, classification 60.1, **60.2**
 histiocytosis 135.22–135.23
 hypercholesterolaemia 60.6–60.8
 hyperlipoproteinaemias **60.1**, 60.8–60.10
 primary dyslipidaemias 60.6–60.10
 xanthomas 60.2–60.6
lipids
 atopic eczema 41.6
 barrier to prevent irritant contact dermatitis 128.3
 epidermal 2.8
 topical medication vehicles 18.5, 18.6–18.7
lipid vascules, neutral lipid storage disease with ichthyosis 63.36
lip-lick cheilitis 41.22
lipoatrophic panniculitis of the ankles in childhood 97.56–97.57
lipoatrophy 62.4
 HAART regimes 98.7
 localised 98.9–98.13
lipoblastoma and lipoblastomatosis 136.57–136.58
lipodermatosclerosis (LDS) 39.21, 103.16–103.17
 champagne bottle leg appearance *103.17*
 chronic venous insufficiency **101.43**
 mixed leg ulcer *102.7*
lipodystrophies 72.1–72.3
 acquired 98.1–98.13
 localised 98.9–98.13
 total body irradiation association 98.8–98.9
lipoedema 98.21–98.25, 103.53–103.55
 clinical features 103.53–103.54
 differential diagnosis **98.22**, 103.54–103.55
 familial 72.12
 imaging characteristics **98.23**
 investigations 103.55
 of the lower limbs 98.21–98.23
 lymphoedema in 98.23
 management 103.55
 pathophysiology 103.53
 of the scalp 98.24–98.25
 stages of **103.55**
lipoedematous alopecia 98.24–98.25, 105.10–105.11
lipofibromatosis 136.13–136.14
lipofuscins secretion, chromhidrosis 92.18
lipogenesis 97.4
lipogranuloma, male genitalia 109.8–109.9, 109.43
lipohypertrophy 62.4
lipoid proteinosis 70.36–70.37
lipo-lymphoedema 98.23
lipolysis, regulation 97.4

lipoma 136.56–136.57
  oral involvement 108.13
  pain 98.18
  surgical treatment 20.49
  vulva **110.32**
lipomatoses
  benign symmetrical 98.15–98.17
  of the face 98.19–98.20
  fat hypertrophy distinction 98.13
  hereditary 72.10
lipomembranous fat necrosis **97.32**
lipomyelomeningocele 72.10
lipophagic granulomas, sclerosing postirradiation panniculitis 97.63
lipophagic granulomatous inflammation 97.8
lipophagic necrosis 97.7
liposarcoma 136.59
  see also atypical lipomatous tumour; well-differentiated liposarcoma
liposcution (suction lipectomy), lymphoedema 103.60–103.61
liposomes, vehicle choice for topical therapies 18.3
liposuction
  cellulite management 98.26
  fat hypertrophy 98.15, 98.16
  subcutaneous tissue 97.3
Lipschütz ulcers
  COVID-19 association 25.113
  cytomegalovirus infections 25.41
  infectious mononucleosis complication 25.37
liquefaction degeneration *3.40*
liquefactive fat necrosis 97.8
liquid nitrogen, cryosurgery 20.46
liquiritin, topical depigmenting agents 18.32
Lisch nodules (pigmented iris hamartomas) 78.2, 78.3
Listeria monocytogenes 26.46
listeriosis 26.46
listeriosis, neonatal 114.26–114.27
lithium-induced acne *88.13*
litigation *see* complaints and litigation; legal issues
livedo, sarcoidosis 96.13
livedoid lesions *4.11*
livedoid vasculopathy 124.10
  purpura 99.20–99.21
livedo racemosa *45.17,* 124.9
  COVID-19 association 25.111
livedo reticularis *4.11,* 124.8–124.10
  COVID-19 association 25.111
  in patient with mixed connective tissue disease 53.3
  in systemic lupus erythematosus 51.26–51.27
liver, *see also hepatic entries*
liver disease
  arsenic 121.2
  cirrhosis 153.5, 153.8, 153.9
  cutaneous features 153.4–153.5, 153.7–153.9
  drug-related issues **153.9**
  in erythropoietic protoporphyria 58.16–58.17
  in porphyria cutanea tarda 58.13
  systemic lupus erythematosus 51.31
  see also hepatic entries; hepatitis; intestinal failure-associated liver disease
liver dysfunction
  drug reaction with eosinophilia and systemic symptoms 118.8–118.9
  juvenile xanthogranuloma 135.17
  sarcoidosis 96.5
liver failure, drug reaction with eosinophilia and systemic symptoms 118.9, 118.11
liver spots *see* lentigines; pityriasis versicolor
liver transplantation, alpha-1 antitrypsin 97.45
LL *see* lepromatous leprosy
LLLT *see* low-level laser light therapy
LM *see* lentigo maligna; lichen myxoedematosus

LMDF *see* lupus miliaris disseminatus faciei
LMIC *see* low and middle income countries
LMM *see* lentigo maligna melanoma
LMPH1A *see* hereditary lymphoedema type 1A
LMs *see* lymphatic malformations
LMWH *see* low-molecular-weight heparin
LMWK *see* low-molecular-weight kininogen
LMX1B mutations, nail–patella syndrome 67.15
LN *see* lupus nephritis
Loa loa filariasis *see* loiasis
loath *see* endemic syphilis
lobomycosis (lobo disease) 32.78–32.79
lobular capillary haemangioma *see* pyogenic granuloma
lobular panniculitis 97.8, 97.22, 97.50–97.53
local anaesthetics
  allergic contact dermatitis 127.45
  biopsy 3.2
  injection techniques 20.8
  skin surgery 20.7–20.8
  toxic reactions 20.7–20.8
local flaps, surgical reconstruction 20.22–20.23
localised anetoderma 94.23
localised atrophy, steroid injections *94.9*
localised blistering, epidermolysis bullosa simplex *69.11*
localised bullous pemphigoid 50.17, *50.19*
  peristomal skin 112.10, *112.12*
localised circumscribed hyperhidrosis 92.6–92.7
localised cutaneous amyloidoses 56.6–56.10
  associated diseases 56.8–56.9
  clinical features 56.9–56.10
  clinical variants 56.10
  complications and disease course 56.10
  differential diagnosis 56.10
  epidemiology 56.7
  ethnicity 56.7–56.8
  insulin injections 98.14
  pathophysiology 56.9
  types of amyloidosis **56.3**
localised dermatitis, plant allergies 127.72
localised dystrophic epidermolysis bullosa, molecular pathology 69.15–69.16
localised elastolysis 94.21
localised epidermolysis bullosa 69.8
localised epidermolysis bullosa simplex 69.11
localised hypertrichosis 87.85–87.87
localised junctional epidermolysis bullosa, molecular pathology 69.14
localised lichen myxoedematosus 57.6–57.8
localised lipoatrophy 98.9–98.13
  due to injected corticosteroid 98.11–98.12
  due to injected drugs 98.10
localised lipodystrophy 98.9–98.13
localised nodular Dercum disease 98.18
localised (pretibial) myxoedema, hyperthyroidism 57.11
localised pruritus, neoplasia association 148.27
localised scleroderma cutaneous assessment tool (LoSCAT) 55.33–55.34
locally injected agents, use during pregnancy **113.21**
local wound care, pressure ulcers 123.10
locusts (Orthoptera) 34.32
LOD *see* Lichenified onchodermatitis
Loeys-Dietz syndrome (LDS) 141.42
Löfgren syndrome 97.21, 155.7
  sarcoidosis 96.1, 96.4, 96.5–96.6, 96.15
loiasis 33.7–33.12
  clinical features 33.11
  definition/nomenclature 33.10
  epidemiology 33.10
  investigations 33.11
  management 33.11–33.12
  pathophysiology 33.10–33.11
long-arm deletion syndrome, chromosome 18 74.3
long Covid (chronic COVID-19), mucocutaneous manifestations 25.113

long-delayed (6-week) intradermal reactions 4.25
loose anagen syndrome 87.82–87.83, *87.83*
loricrin keratoderma 63.56
LoSCAT *see* localised scleroderma cutaneous assessment tool
loss-of-function mutations, results of 69.27
lotions, vehicle choice for topical therapies 18.2
Louis–Bar syndrome *see* ataxia telangiectasia
louse-borne diseases
  bacillary angiomatosis 26.64
  epidemic relapsing fever 26.72
  rickettsial epidemic typhus 26.80–26.81
  trench fever 26.62
lower limbs *see* leg
low-grade fibromyxoid sarcoma 136.18–136.19
low-level laser light therapy (LLLT) 87.71, 87.95, 103.59–103.60
low and middle income countries (LMIC)
  access to dermatological health services 5.13–5.14, 7.3, *7.4*
  scabies, incidence of 7.2
low-molecular-weight heparin (LMWH), management of Klippel–Trenaunay–Weber syndrome 71.9
low-molecular-weight kininogen (LMWK), bradykinin-induced angio-oedema 43.3
low power laser therapy 23.24
LP *see* lichen planus
LPP *see* large plaque parapsoriasis; lichen planopilaris
LS *see* lichen sclerosus; lichen spinulosus
LSC *see* lichen simplex chronicus
LTBPs *see* latent transforming growth factor beta binding proteins
LTC4 *see* leukotriene C4
lubricants, genital contact dermatitis **109.13**
Lucio phenomenon 97.26
Ludwig scale, hair loss 87.65, 87.67
Lujo virus haemorrhagic fever 25.82
lumbosacral area, Mongolian spot *131.12*
lumbo-sacral hypertrichosis 87.86
lumpy scalp syndrome 106.6
Lund and Browder chart, burn injuries 125.2, *125.3*
lungs *see* interstitial lung disease; *pulmonary entries*
lupus, dystrophic calcification 59.1, 59.2
lupus anticoagulant syndrome 99.17–99.19
lupus erythematosus (LE) 51.1–51.46, 86.21, 87.55, 106.24, 106.25, 126.2
  antiphospholipid antibody syndrome 51.42–51.45
  cardiac involvement 151.4
  discoid lupus erythematosus 51.1–51.12, *51.24*
  drug-induced 117.7–117.9
  ear dermatoses **106.23**
  eye disease **107.35**
  internal malignancy association 148.21
  keratoderma association 63.72
  lip lesions 108.64
  neonatal 114.12–114.14
  neonatal lupus erythematosus 51.39–51.42
  papular and nodular cutaneous mucinosis 57.13
  periodic acid–Schiff stain *3.8*
  perniosis 124.5–124.6
  subacute cutaneous lupus erythematosus 51.12–51.16
  systemic lupus erythematosus 51.1, 51.16–51.38
  UVA-1 phototherapy 21.6
lupus erythematosus profundus (lupus panniculitis) 51.7–51.8, *51.9,* 94.21, 97.37–97.40
lupus miliaris disseminatus faciei (LMDF) 27.31, 89.7, 89.10, 89.19
lupus nephritis (LN), classification **51.20**
lupus panniculitis *see* lupus erythematosus profundus

lupus pernio *89.10,* 96.8–96.11, 96.15, *96.17*
lupus vulgaris 27.20–27.24
  clinical features 27.21–27.23
  epidemiology 27.21
  management 27.23–27.24
  pathophysiology 27.21
  sarcoidosis differential diagnosis 96.3
LVA *see* lymphatico-venous anastomosis surgery
LWNH *see* linear and whorled naevoid hypermelanosis
lycopene, cosmeceutical use 157.9–157.10
Lyell syndrome *see* toxic epidermal necrolysis
Lyme disease (Lyme borreliosis) 26.73–26.74
  acrodermatitis chronica atrophicans 94.15–94.16
  Borrelia burgdorferi complex 26.72–26.73
  clinical features/variants 26.73–26.74
  cutaneous B-cell lymphoma 139.37
  definition/description 26.72–26.73
  epidemiology 26.73
  erythema chronicum migrans 26.69, 26.72, 26.73, *26.73,* 26.74
  eye involvement 107.40
  investigations 26.74
  management 26.74
  pathophysiology 26.73
lymphadenitis (buboes) 103.15
  chancroid 30.18, 30.19, 30.20, 30.21
  lymphogranuloma venereum 30.14, 30.15, 30.16, **30.17,** 30.18
lymphadenoma, *see also* adamantinoid trichoblastoma
lymphadenopathy, syphilis 29.10
lymphadenosis benigna cutis of Bafverstedt *see* lymphocytoma cutis/B-cell pseudolymphoma
lymphangiectasia 103.30–103.33
lymphangiogenesis 103.3
lymphangioleiomyomatosis (LAM) 103.28–103.29
  tuberous sclerosis complex 78.9
lymphangioma
  acquired progressive 136.38
  oral involvement 108.13
lymphangioma circumscriptum 103.25–103.28
  atruncular lymphatic malformation without lymphoedema *103.27*
  clinical features 103.26–103.27
  differential diagnosis 103.27
  fluid-filled vesicles (frogspawn resemblance) *103.26*
  genetics 103.26
  investigations 103.27
  management 103.27–103.28
  pathophysiology 103.26
  truncular lymphatic malformation with lymphangiectasia and lymphoedema *103.27*
lymphangiomatosis *71.2,* 103.28–103.29, 136.39
lymphangiomatous papules, benign 103.32
lymphangiosarcoma 119.15
lymphangitis 103.14–103.15
lymphatic filariasis (LF) 7.10, 33.7–33.10, 103.33–103.36
  causative organisms 103.34
  clinical features 33.9, 103.34–103.35
  definition/nomenclature 33.7
  differential diagnosis 103.35
  epidemiology 33.7–33.8, 103.33
  investigations 33.9–33.10, 103.35
  lifecycle of filarial nematodes in human and mosquito hosts *103.34*
  management 33.10, 103.35–103.36
  pathophysiology 33.8–33.9, 103.33
lymphatic-like vascular channels, atypical vascular proliferation after radiotherapy 136.38–136.39
lymphatic malformations (LMs) *71.2,* 71.21–71.22, 103.25–103.30
  amniotic band constriction-induced lymphoedema 103.29–103.30

lymphangioleiomyomatosis 103.28–103.29
non-malignant lymphatic tumours 103.28–103.29
lymphatic obstruction, neoplasia association 148.27
lymphatico-lymphatic anastomosis surgery 103.61
lymphatico-venous anastomosis (LVA) surgery 103.61
lymphatic-related hydrops fetalis 103.23
lymphatic system
 anatomy of head and neck 20.2
 fat homeostasis 103.2
 fluid homeostasis 103.2
 function and structure 103.1–103.2
 and immunity 103.2
 lymphatic involvement in skin disease 103.2–103.3
 lymphatic vessel 103.14
 lymph drainage routes 103.8
 nutrition 103.2
 oedema and 103.2
 peripheral fat 103.2
lymphatic system disorders 71.21–71.28, 103.1–103.62
 abdominal wall lymphoedema 103.51–103.52
 acute dermatolymphangioadenitis 103.16
 arm swelling due to oedema 103.44–103.46
 atypical vascular lesions 103.32
 breast lymphoedema 103.43–103.44
 cancer-related lymphoedema 103.37–103.38
 cellulitis 103.13–103.17
 chronically swollen limb 103.9–103.10
 chronic oedema 103.2, 103.3–103.5
 chronic red leg 103.16–103.17
 chylous disease 103.32
 complicated lymphatic anomalies 71.1, 71.22–71.23
 congenital-onset primary lymphoedema 103.24
 cutaneous lymphangiectasia 103.31–103.32
 drug induced oedema 103.12–103.13
 facial oedema 103.46–103.49
 fluorescence microlymphangiography 103.56
 generalised lymphatic dysplasia 103.22
 genital lymphoedema 103.49–103.51, 103.52
 hand oedema 103.21
 head oedema 103.46–103.49
 histopathology 103.57
 hypotrichosis–lymphoedema–telangiectasia syndrome 103.23
 imaging techniques 103.7, 103.8, 103.55–103.57
 immobility-induced lymphoedema 103.40
 intestinal lymphangiectasia 103.32
 intranodal MR lymphography 103.56
 late-onset primary lymphoedema 103.24–103.25
 limb swelling 103.6, 103.9–103.10, 103.16–103.17, 103.44–103.46
 lipodermatosclerosis 103.16–103.17
 lipoedema 103.53–103.55
 lymphadenitis 103.15
 lymphangiectasia 103.30–103.33
 lymphangioma circumscriptum 103.25–103.28
 lymphangitis 103.14–103.15
 lymphatic filariasis 7.10, 33.7–33.10, 103.33–103.36
 lymphatic involvement in skin disease 103.2–103.3
 lymphatic malformations 71.2, 71.21–71.22, 103.25–103.30
 lymph fistula 103.32, 103.33
 lymphoceles 103.32, 103.33
 lymphography 103.55, 103.56

lymphoscintigraphy (isotope lymphography) 103.7, 103.8, 103.55, 103.56, 103.56
lymphovenous oedema 103.10–103.12
magnetic resonance lymphangiography 103.56, 103.57
massive localised lymphoedema 103.52–103.53
mosaic lymphoedema associated with disturbed growth and/or cutaneous/vascular anomalies 103.23–103.24
multisegmental lymphatic dysplasia with systemic involvement 103.22
near infrared lymphangiography (ICG lymphography) 103.56–103.57
neck oedema 103.46–103.49
obesity-related lymphoedema 103.38–103.39
phlebolymphoedema 103.10–103.12
podoconiosis (non-filarial lymphoedema) 103.36–103.37
pretibial myxoedema 103.41–103.43
recurrent cellulitis (erysipelas) 103.13–103.14
regional swelling 103.43–103.53
Schimmelpenning–Feuerstein–Mims syndrome 71.23–71.24
secondary lymphoedema 103.33–103.43
seromas 103.32, 103.33
swollen breast 103.43–103.44
swollen limb 103.6, 103.9–103.10, 103.16–103.17, 103.44–103.46
syndromic lymphoedema 103.20–103.22
trauma-induced lymphoedema 103.40
venouos oedema 103.10–103.12
WILD syndrome 103.22
yellow-nail syndrome 103.21–103.22
 see also lymphoedema
lymphatic tumours 136.37–136.39
 see also lymphangioma circumscriptum
lymph drainage
 chronic oedema 103.4
 management 103.57–103.61
lymph fistula 103.32, 103.33
lymph node metastasis, squamous cell carcinoma of the auricle 106.27–106.28
lymph nodes
 antigen-presenting cell migration 127.7
 drainage areas of cervical lymph nodes 108.6
 examination of 108.6
 fine-needle aspiration of 4.22
 immune system 9.6
 Kikuchi–Fujimoto disease 51.33
 lymphadenitis 103.15
lymph nodes and lymphatic drainage basins, in neck 106.28
lymph node transfer surgery 103.61
lymphoceles 103.32, 103.33
lymphocytes
 adipocytes interaction 97.6–97.7
 drug reaction with eosinophilia and systemic symptoms 118.5, 118.8
 microscopic examination of 3.34, 3.35
 wound healing 11.3
lymphocytic alopecia 87.37, 87.38–87.50
lymphocytic folliculitis, scalp margin 91.12–91.13
lymphocytic infiltrates 134.1–134.11
 Jessner lymphocytic infiltrate 134.10–134.11
 lymphocytoma cutis 134.1, 134.2, 134.8–134.10
 parapsoriasis 134.6–134.8
 pityriasis lichenoides 134.3–134.5, 134.6
 pseudolymphoma 134.1–134.3
lymphocytic lobular panniculitis 97.39
lymphocytic panniculitis, in childhood 97.56, 97.57
lymphocytic perifollicular, necrotising lymphocytic folliculitis 93.4
lymphocytic vasculitis 97.38

lymphocytoma cutis (B-cell pseudolymphoma) 89.10, 134.1, 134.2, 134.8–134.10
lymphoedema 103.5–103.9
 abdominal wall 103.51–103.52
 acquired cutaneous lymphangiectasia 103.6
 and amniotic bands 103.29–103.30
 bacterial/fungal infection 103.6, 103.7
 bandaging 103.58, 103.59
 breast lymphoedema 103.43–103.44
 breathing exercises 103.59
 cancer-related lymphoedema 103.37–103.38
 chronic oedema comparison 103.3
 chronic venous insufficiency 101.43
 chronic venous oedema association 103.10
 clinical features 103.6
 complications and co-morbidities 103.6
 diagnosis of 103.3
 elephantiasis nostra verrucosa 103.6
 elevation and rest 103.59
 epidemiology 103.5
 excisional surgery 103.60
 exercise and movement 103.58
 external compression 103.58–103.59
 facial lymphoedema 103.46–103.49
 genital 109.19–109.21
 genitalia and mons pubis 103.49–103.51, 103.52
 hyperbaric oxygen therapy 103.59–103.60
 imaging characteristics 98.23
 immobility-induced lymphoedema 103.40
 infection 103.6, 103.7
  prevention of 103.58
 intensive and maintenance treatment 103.60
 investigations 103.7
 Kaposi–Stemmer sign 103.6
 limb swelling 103.6, 103.9–103.10, 103.16–103.17, 103.44–103.46
 in lipoedema 98.23
 lipoedema differential diagnosis 98.22
 liposuction (suction lipectomy) 103.60–103.61
 low-level laser therapy 103.59–103.60
 lymphangiosarcoma 103.7
 lymphatico-lymphatic anastomosis surgery 103.61
 lymph node transfer surgery 103.61
 lymphovenous bypass (lymphatico-venous anastomosis) surgery 103.61
 macerated web-space skin 103.7
 malignancy 103.7
 management 103.7–103.9, 103.57–103.61
 massage (manual lymphatic drainage therapy) 103.59
 massive localised lymphoedema 103.52–103.53
 medical assessment 103.58
 obesity 98.27
 obesity-related lymphoedema 103.38–103.39
 palmoplantar keratodermas with 63.72–63.73
 pathophysiology 103.5–103.6
 penoscrotal swelling 109.20
 pharmacological therapies 103.60
 physical therapies 103.58–103.60
 postural exercises 103.59
 psychosocial issues 103.7
 skin care and infection prevention 103.58
 skin changes 103.6
 surgery 103.60–103.61
 syndromes associates with 103.20
 systemic/visceral involvement 103.22–103.23
 trauma-induced lymphoedema 103.40
 weight loss 103.59
 see also primary lymphoedema
lymphoedema–distichiasis syndrome 71.25–71.26, 103.25, 151.2

lymphoepithelial Kazal-type-related inhibitor (LEKTI) 63.26–63.27, 69.6
lymphoepithelioma-like carcinoma 137.43–137.44
lymphogranuloma inguinale see lymphogranuloma venereum
lymphogranuloma venereum (LGV) 30.14–30.18
 clinical features/stages 30.15–30.17
 epidemiology 30.15
 investigations 30.17
 management 30.18
 pathophysiology 30.15
 perineal and perianal skin 111.16
lymphography, lymphatic system 103.55, 103.56
lymphoid aggregates
 lupus panniculitis 97.37, 97.38
 necrobiotic xanthogranuloma 97.18
lymphoid lineage cells, immune system 9.5
lymphoid malignancies, skin manifestations of paraneoplastic syndromes 149.8–149.9
lymphoid markers, cutaneous neoplasms 3.27–3.29
lymphoma
 acquired ichthyosis 85.2
 B-cell lymphoma, external ear 106.34
 ear dermatoses 106.23
 erythroderma 39.32–39.33
 external ear 106.34
 follicular mucinosis, association with 105.8
 HIV 31.32–31.33
 hypermelanosis in 86.19–86.20
 oral involvement 108.71
 panniculitis-like 97.61–97.63
 pseudolymphoma relationship 134.1, 134.2
 see also cutaneous lymphomas
lymphomatoid eruptions 127.20
lymphomatoid granulomatosis
 respiratory involvement 152.6
 secondary cutaneous B-cell lymphoma 139.44–139.45
lymphomatoid papulosis 139.26–139.28, 149.9
 clinical features 139.27–139.28
 management 139.27
 pathophysiology 139.26–139.27
lymphomatous skin infiltrates 149.4
lymphoproliferative disorders
 Epstein–Barr virus association 25.38–25.39
 necrobiotic xanthogranuloma association 135.24
 post-transplant/immunodeficiency 139.47
 sarcoidosis association 96.1
lymphorrhoea 103.6
lymphoscintigraphy (isotope lymphography), lymphatic system 103.7, 103.8, 103.55, 103.56, 103.56
lymphovenous bypass (lymphatico-venous anastomosis) surgery 103.61
lymphovenous oedema 103.10–103.12
lymph vessels, subcutaneous tissue 97.2
lympthatic network 2.42
Lynch syndrome 78.14, 148.12
 see also Muir–Torre syndrome
Lyonisation 8.7–8.8
Lyral allergy 127.44
lysosomal storage disorders 79.1–79.8
 Fabry disease 79.6–79.8
 glycoproteinoses 79.3–79.4
 mucolipidoses types II and III 79.4–79.5
 mucopolysaccharidoses 79.1–79.3
 sphingolipidoses 79.5–79.6
lysyl hydroxylase 3 (LH3) 69.7
lysyl oxidases 2.34, 2.35

M

mAbs see monoclonal antibodies
macacine herpesvirus 1 see herpes B virus infection

McCune–Albright syndrome **72.7**, 73.19–73.20
machine learning, melanoma diagnosis 142.21
Machupo (Bolivian) haemorrhagic fever 25.82–25.83
macrocephaly–capillary malformation syndrome (M–CM) 71.8
macrocyclic chelating agents 94.44
macroglossia 108.11–108.12
  in amyloidosis *56.12*, *108.69*
macrolides 19.47
macrophages 135.1–135.3
  cytotoxic T lymphocytes interaction 97.6–97.7
  immune system 9.4, 9.5
  sarcoidosis 96.4
  secretion of cytokines 97.5–97.6
  tissue homeostasis *9.4*, 9.7
  wound healing 11.3
macrophage–monocyte lineage, histiocytoses 135.1
macrotia (large ears) 106.5
macular effects, pseudoxanthoma elasticum 70.33
macular lymphocytic arteritis 97.9
macular primary localised cutaneous amyloidosis **56.3**, *56.7*, 56.9
macular syphilide (roseolar rash) *29.8*, 29.9
  see also roseola infantum
macules
  ash-leaf-shaped macules, tuberous sclerosis complex 78.8
  café-au-lait macules 78.3
  hypopigmented macules *76.4*
maculopapular rash
  autoinflammatory diseases **80.19**
  complex and polygenic autoinflammatory diseases presenting with urticarial or maculopapular rash 45.20–45.22
  COVID-19 association 25.109, *25.110*
  drug-induced exanthems 117.2
maculopapular sarcoidosis 96.7
MADA *see* mandibulo-acral dysplasia with type A lipodystrophy
madarosis 107.4–107.5
MADB *see* mandibulo-acral dysplasia with type B lipodystrophy
Madelung disease (multiple symmetrical lipomatosis) **72.10**, 79.8, 98.15, *103.46*
MADISH *see* metabolising acquired dioxin-induced skin hamartoma
madura foot *see* mycetoma
Madurella mycetomatis 32.75
maduromycosis *see* mycetoma
Maffucci syndrome 71.20–71.21, 101.24, **101.25**, **101.28**, 103.29, 136.31
MAGIC (mouth and genital ulcers with inflamed cartilage) syndrome 108.41, 155.11, 155.13
magnetic resonance imaging (MRI) 4.22, 4.23
  foreign body reactions 122.18
  morphoea 55.31, *55.32*
magnetic resonance lymphangiography (MRL), lymphatic system **103.56**, 103.57
MAGPs *see* microfibril-associated glycoproteins
Majeed syndrome 45.18
Majocchi disease *see* purpura annularis telangiectodes
major depressive disorder 84.40
major histocompatibility complex (MHC)
  class I deficiency 80.10
  class I-restricted drug presentation 118.12
  drug-binding 118.5
  histiocytoses 135.2
  molecule 14.4, 14.5, 14.6
Major Life Changing Decision Profile (MLCDP) 16.11

MAL *see* methyl aminolevulinate
malabsorption, acquired ichthyosis 63.47
malabsorption syndromes, hypermelanosis 86.23
malakoplakia 135.23–135.24
  female genitalia 110.26
  perianal skin 111.15
malaria 33.36
  clinical features 33.36
  epidemiology 33.36
  management 33.36
  see also antimalarial agents
Malassezia yeast species 86.43
  confluent and reticulated papillomatosis 85.6–85.7
  eosinophilic pustular folliculitis 93.7
  folliculitis 32.13, 88.35
  pustulosis in neonates 114.28–114.29
  scalp itch 105.15–105.16
  superficial mycoses 32.10–32.14
malathion, topical therapies 18.14
Malawi polyomavirus (human polyomavirus-10) 25.49
mal de Meleda 63.54–63.56
male angiomyofibroblastoma-like tumour 136.9
male *EBP* disorder with neurological defects (MEND syndrome) 63.23
male fertility, safe treatments in pregnancy 113.19–113.24
male pattern hair loss (MPHL/male androgenetic alopecia) 87.61–87.62, 87.64, *87.66*, 87.68–87.70
malignancies
  associated with dermatomyositis 2
  associated with seborrhoeic keratosis 132.1–132.2
  basal cell carcinoma 140.1–140.21
  Epstein–Barr virus association 25.38–25.39
  eyelid lesions 107.47–107.50
  human papillomaviruses 25.71
  immunosuppressants/immunomodulatory drug risks 19.2, 19.3, 19.8, 19.9, 19.11, 19.18, 19.21–19.22, 19.24, 19.26, 19.29
  Kaposi sarcoma-associated herpesvirus 25.42, 25.43
  paraneoplastic pruritus 81.10
  radiotherapy indications for skin disorders 24.8
  skin lesions with uncertain/unpredictable malignant potential 141.1–141.18
  zoster risks 25.34
malignancy, acquired ichthyosis 63.73
malignancy-associated generalised hypertrichosis 87.86
malignant acrospiroma *see* hidradenocarcinoma
malignant atrophic papulosis 99.21–99.22
malignant blue naevus, melanomas 142.14, 142.20, *142.21*
malignant cylindroma 137.35
malignant eccrine poroma 137.33–137.34
malignant fibrous histiocytoma *see* undifferentiated soft tissue sarcoma
malignant haemangioendothelioma *see* angiosarcoma
malignant hidradenoma *see* hidradenocarcinoma
malignant histiocytosis (MH) 135.29–135.32
malignant melanoma (MM)
  adjuvant systemic treatment 144.6
  ambiguous lesions 142.18–142.19
  ano-genital region 111.24
  atypical melanocytes in epidermis *3.24*
  of the auricle 106.31–106.33
  basis for diagnosis 142.18–142.22
  biopsy 143.1
  blocking of transverse sections of *3.6*
  BRAF inhibitors (vemurafenib and dabrafenib) treatment leading to keratoacanthoma 141.38
  classification 142.7–142.9
  clinical features 142.8–142.9

clinicopathology 142.1–142.25
colour of *4.14*
combination therapies with immunotherapy 144.2–144.3
combination therapies with targeted therapy 144.5
complete response after systemic therapy 144.8–144.9
completion lymph node dissection 143.4, 143.5
congenital melanocytic naevi *73.10*, 73.13, 142.2
cost-of-illness meta-analysis **6.7**
cutaneous side effects of systemic therapies 144.9–144.12
cyclin-dependent kinase 4 gene 142.4
definition 142.1
dermoscopy 145.1–145.16
  benign naevus pattern comparison 145.1–145.7
  facial and chronically sun-damaged skin 145.9, *145.11*, **145.12**
  non-glabrous/non-facial skin 145.7–145.9
  organised patterns 145.13–145.14, *145.15*
  special locations 145.9–145.13
  volar skin of palms and soles 145.9, 145.11–145.13
detection 143.1
diagnostic tools 142.9–142.10, 142.18–142.21, 145.1–145.16
disease process 5.3
drug/chemical photosensitivity 126.30
early detection strategies 142.8–142.9, 142.15–142.18
electrochemotherapy 144.2
environmental factors 142.5–142.6
epidemiological classification 142.8
epidemiology 142.1–142.2
eyelid 107.49
follow-up 142.24–142.25
genetics 142.3–142.5
genomic link to naevi 142.2
histological subtypes 142.7
histopathological diagnosis 142.18–142.21
HIV 31.31–31.32
identification of at risk individuals 142.6–142.7
immunocompromised people
  clinicopathological features 147.13–147.14
  management 147.21, 147.23
immunotherapy 144.2–144.4
in situ, surgery 143.3
isolated limb perfusion 144.2
local therapies 144.1–144.2
macroscopic specimen of *3.6*
management after surgery 142.22–142.25
metastatic disease systemic treatment 144.6–144.7
mole and cancer phobias 84.26
molecular classification 142.9
mortality rate 5.7
mucosal system treatment 144.7
neoadjuvant systemic treatment 144.6
oculocutaneous albinism 68.7
oncolytic virus therapy 144.1–144.2
oral melanoma 108.18
palmoplantar keratodermas 63.65
pathological criteria of malignancy 142.18–142.19
penis 109.41
phenotypic traits 142.3–142.4, 142.7
PRAME (PReferentially expressed Antigen in Melanoma) 3.25
precursors 142.2–142.3
predisposing factors 142.2–142.3
in pregnancy 113.9–113.10
presentation 142.10–142.15
prevention 142.6–142.7
prognostic markers 142.21–142.22
PUVA phototherapy adverse effects 21.14

radiotherapy 24.14, *24.15*, 144.2
sentinel lymph node biopsy 143.4–143.6
skin cancer, prevalence of 5.10
special circumstances for systemic treatment 144.7–144.9
staging 142.21–142.24
surgery 143.1–143.6
systemic treatment 144.1–144.12
targeted therapies 144.4–144.5, *144.11*, **144.11**, 144.12
therapeutic approach for systemic management 144.5–144.12
tissue sampling during surgery 144.1
trends in incidence and mortality 142.1
tumour kinetics and aggressiveness classification 142.8
uveal, system treatment 144.7–144.8
UVR exposure 10.9–10.10
vulval melanoma 110.39–110.40
wide local excision surgery 143.1–143.4
malignant otitis externa 106.19
malignant peripheral nerve sheath tumours (MPNSTs) 78.3, 136.51
malignant schwannoma *see* malignant peripheral nerve sheath tumour
malignant soft-tissue tumours 136.2, 136.14–136.15, 136.17–136.18
  see also sarcomas
malignant spiradenoma *see* spiradenocarcinoma
malignant Spitz tumour/malignant spitzoiid neoplasm *see* Spitzoid melanoma
malignant syringoma *see* microcystic adnexal carcinoma
malignant tumours
  misdiagnosed benign tumours 136.2, 136.5
  neurofibromatosis type 1 78.3–78.4
  sebaceous carcinoma 137.18
  uncertain malignancy of keratoacanthoma 141.38
  vascular 136.35–136.37
malingering
  definition 84.36
  factitial disease distinction 84.29, 84.36
  falsifying dermatological symptoms 84.36–84.37
malnutrition 61.1–61.7
  adiponectin system 97.5
  assessment 61.2
  in children 61.2, 61.3, *61.4*, 61.5–61.6
  classification 61.2, 61.5–61.6
  clinical features 61.3–61.4
  complications and co-morbidities 61.6
  diagnosis 61.5
  disease course and prognosis 61.6
  epidemiology 61.2
  ethnicity role 61.2–61.3
  incidence and prevalence 61.2
  investigations 61.5
  management 61.6–61.7
  predisposing factors 61.3
  protein-energy malnutrition 61.2, 61.3
  severity classification 61.5–61.6
  skin signs of nutritional disease **61.5**
MALT *see* mucosa associated lymphoid tissue
Malta fever *see* brucellosis
mammary glands 92.15
mammary-like gland adenoma of the vulva *see* hidradenoma papilliferum
mammary-like glands, tumours of ano-genital glands 137.40
mammary-type secretory carcinoma of the skin *see* secretory carcinoma
Manchester checklist, neurofibromatosis type 1 78.4, *78.5–78.6*
mandibuloacral dysplasia 98.3
mandibuloacral dysplasia with type A lipodystrophy (MADA) **72.5**, 77.5
mandibuloacral dysplasia with type B lipodystrophy (MADB) **72.5**, 77.5
manganese deficiency and excess 61.31
mangrove fly *see* *Chrysops*
MANIAC *see* melanocytic acral naevus with intraepidermal ascentof cells

mansonelosis 33.6–33.7
 definition 33.6
 epidemiology 33.6
 management 33.7
 pathophysiology 33.6–33.7
MAP kinase (MAPK) see mitogen-activated protein kinase
marantic endocarditis 99.15
marasmic kwashiorkor syndrome 61.2
marasmus 61.2, 61.3, *61.4*
Marburg haemorrhagic fever, filovirus infection 25.84–25.85
Marfan syndrome (MFS) 70.20–70.21, 94.11
marginal papular keratoderma (MPK) 63.60–63.61
marginal zone lymphoma (MZL)
 primary cutaneous B-cell lymphoma type 139.37
 see also primary cutaneous marginal zone lymphoma
marijuana see cannabis
marionette lines, dermal fillers *158.3*
Marshall syndrome 94.22
MART-1 see Melan-A
mascular amyloidosis 86.22, *86.23*
masking in clinical trials, evidence based medicine 17.12, 17.13
Mas-related G-protein-coupled receptor agonists (Mrgpr family), pruritus **81.3**, 81.5
Mas-related G protein–coupled receptor member X2 (MRGPRX2) 117.6
massage, manual lymphatic drainage therapy 103.59
massive localised lymphoedema 103.52–103.53
Masson ammoniacal silver nitrate technique 3.8
Masson pseudoangiosarcoma see intravascular papillary endothelial hyperplasia
Masson vegetant intravascular haemangioendothelioma see intravascular papillary endothelial hyperplasia
mast cell activation syndrome 46.7
mast cell degranulating stimuli, mastocytosis **46.9**
mast cell disorders 3.45
mast cell leukaemia (MCL) 46.1
mast cell mediator-induced angio-oedema without weals 43.1, **43.2**
 clinical features 43.4
 incidence and prevalence 43.2
 pathophysiology 43.3
mast cells 2.15–2.17
 allergic-type response 9.9
 fibrosis 89.3
 granules 2.15, *2.17*
 immune cells in homeostasis *9.4*
 immune system 9.5
 immunity role 2.16–2.17
 microscopic examination of 3.37
 stabilising drugs 46.9
 staining technique 3.8–3.9
 urticaria 42.3–42.4
mast cell sarcoma **46.2**
mastitis
 neonates 114.25
 tuberculous 27.31–27.32
mastocytoma *46.3*, 46.5–46.6
mastocytosis 46.1–46.10
 aetiopathogenesis 46.2
 associated diseases 46.2–46.3
 children *46.4, 46.5, 46.9*
 classification 46.1, **46.2**
 clinical features 46.3–46.7
 co-morbidities 46.7
 diagnostic work-up **46.8**
 disease course and prognosis 46.7
 epidemiology 46.2–46.3
 flushing **104.5**, 148.26
 genetics 46.3
 histopatholgy of skin lesions *46.3*
 infants 115.16–115.17
 investigations 46.7–46.8
 management 46.8–46.10
 mast cell degranulating stimuli **46.9**
 musculoskeletal involvement 155.13
 pathophysiology 46.3
maternal autoantibodies, transplacental transfer 114.11–114.12
maternal malignant disease, transplacental transfer 114.14
maternal milk see lactation
maternal transfer, see also teratogenicity
matrix metalloproteinases (MMPs) 2.31, 2.32
 collagen and elastin degradation, UVR exposure 10.10–10.11
 skin ageing 2.46
 wound healing 11.4, *11.5*, 11.8, **11.9**
mattress skin sutures 20.17–20.18
Mayaro virus (MAYV), Mayaro/Uruma fever 25.91
May–Gruenwald stain 135.22–135.23
MBT see 2-mercaptobenzothiazole
MC see mixed cryoglobulinaemia; molluscum contagiosum
MCAP see megalencephaly–capillary malformation syndrome
MCC see Merkel cell carcinoma
mcEDS see musculocontractural Ehlers–Danlos syndrome
MCI see methylchloroisothiazolinone
MCI/MI see methylchloroisothiazolinone and methylisothiazolinone
MCL see mast cell leukaemia
MCLID see microcephaly with or without chorioretinopathy, lymphoedema or intellectual disability
MCLMR see microcephaly with or without chorioretinopathy, lymphoedema and mental retardation
M–CM see macrocephaly–capillary malformation syndrome
MCPs see mucocutaneous pain syndromes
MCPyV see Merkel cell polyomavirus
MCTD see mixed connective tissue disease
MCV see molluscipoxvirus
MDA see Misuse of Drugs Act 1971
MDBGN see methyldibromoglutaronitrile
MDCPs see medium depth chemical peels
MDMA (N-methyl-3,4-methylenedioxymetamphetamine) see ecstasy
MDR see multidrug-resistant
MDTs see multidisciplinary teams
Meado Syndrome see Münchausen syndrome by proxy
measles 1.3, 25.97–25.98
 clinical features 25.98–25.99
 epidemiology 25.98
 infants 115.7
 management 25.99
 pathophysiology 25.98
measles/mumps/rubella vaccine see MMR
measurement 16.1–16.13
 aspects of most concern to patients 16.1–16.2
 challenges 16.1
 core outcome measures 16.3
 disease assessment tools 16.3–16.5
 disease impacts 16.5–16.13
 electronic delivery 16.2
 method validation 16.2–16.3
 objective measures of skin properties 16.5
 objective tools 16.2
 psychological impacts 16.11–16.12
 quality of life measures 16.5–16.11
 role in decision making 16.1
 self-assessment 16.2
 sexual functioning 16.12
 skin disease severity 16.1–16.3
 work impacts 16.12–16.13
mechanical acne 88.30
mechanical boundary-related risk factors, pressure ulcers 123.3–123.4
mechanical hymenal fissures 110.42–110.43
mechanical injuries 122.1–122.29
 biomechanical considerations 122.3–122.7
 foreign material effects 122.17
 reactions to 122.7–122.17
 vibration injuries 122.13, 122.24–122.26
mechanical irritation
 contact dermatitis 129.1
 lichen planus 37.3
 psoriasiform contact dermatitis **128.4**
 see also Koebner (isomorphic) phenomenon
mechanical load, pressure ulcers 123.2
mechanical properties of skin 122.4
mechanical stimuli, use of 122.3
mechanobullous diseases 69.2
mechlorethamine, topical therapies 18.31
MED see minimal erythema dose
medallion-like dermal dendrocyte hamartoma, neonates 114.11
median raphe cysts 109.30
median rhomboid glossitis 32.63, 108.22
medical devices, pressure ulcers 123.2
medical texts, ancient cultures 1.1–1.3
medical volunteerism 7.13, **7.15**
medicament contact dermatitis *127.11*, 127.12, 127.18–127.19
medication, see also clinical pharmacology; drug entries
medication adherence, behavioural effects of skin conditions 15.2
medication errors, clinical pharmacology 13.9–13.11
medication history, diagnosis of drug eruptions 4.3–4.4
medicines, donation of 7.13
Medicines Act 1968 120.4
Medina worm see dracunculiasis
Mediterranean fever see brucellosis
Mediterranean spotted fever see tick typhus
medium depth chemical peels (MDCPs) 160.4
medium-vessel vasculitis *100.3*, 100.28–100.32
MEDLINE (National Library of Medicine's bibliographic database) 17.7
MEDNIK syndrome see mental retardation–enteropathy–deafness–neuropathy–ichthyosis–keratodermia syndrome
MeDOCs see Mendelian disorders of cornification
mEDS see myopathic Ehlers–Danlos syndrome
medulla, hair fibres 87.7
medullary thyroid cancer (MTC), flushing **104.7**, 148.26
medusa stings 130.1
Mee's lines 121.2, *121.3*, 121.9
megalencephaly–capillary malformation syndrome (MCAP) 71.2
megavoltage X-ray therapy 24.1, 24.3
meibomian gland cyst (chalazion) *107.11*
meibomian gland dysfunction (MGD) 107.7–107.15
meibomian seborrhoea **107.8**
meibomitis **107.8**, *107.11*
Meige disease 103.25
Meirowsky phenomenon 86.9
Meissner corpuscles, substance P fibres ending in *83.3*
MEK inhibitors see mitogen-activated protein kinase inhibitors
Melan-A (MART-1) (melanocyte marker) 3.23–3.24
melanin 2.42, 86.1
 biological significance 86.7–86.8
 disorder classification 86.8
 light absorption 23.3–23.4, 23.12
 photoprotection 10.11
 pigmentation disorders 68.1, 68.6, 87.93
 synthesis of 2.17
 trichochromes synthesis *86.6*
melanoblasts, migration/differentiation 86.3–86.4
melanocanthoma, oral melanocanthoma 108.18
melanocortin-4 receptor deficiency **72.6**
melanocortins, Addison disease 86.7
melanocytes 2.1, 2.5, 2.11, 2.17–2.18, 68.1, 86.1–86.9
 Cole disease 63.61
 culture 86.4–86.5
 differentiation *2.18*
 distribution 86.3
 endocrine regulation 86.7
 hair pigmentation 87.12
 skin pigmentation 86.1–86.9
 UV radiation response 86.5–86.7
melanocyte-stimulating hormone (MSH) 86.4, 86.10
melanocytic acral naevus with intraepidermal ascentof cells (MANIAC), use of term 142.19
melanocytic lesions 131.12–131.15
 histological sectioning of 3.7
 see also Mongolian spot
melanocytic markers, cutaneous neoplasms 3.23–3.25
melanocytic naevi 131.15–131.46
 acquired melanocytic naevi 131.17–131.21
 acral naevi 131.23–131.24
  compound acral naevus *131.23*
  on sole of foot *131.24*
 atypical naevi **131.17**, 131.40–131.46
 BAP1-inactivated naevus of the scalp *131.34*
 blue naevus **131.17**, 131.38–131.40
 breast 131.22
 cancer phobias 84.26
 clinical presentation **131.16–131.17**
 cockade naevus 131.30, *131.31*
 combined melanocytic naevi 131.24–131.26
 combined naevus *131.26*
 common acquired naevi **131.16**, 131.17–131.21
 compound naevus **131.1**, *131.19, 131.21, 131.25, 131.42*
 congenital melanocytic naevi 73.8–73.15, 131.15–131.17
 conjunctival naevi 131.24, *131.25*
 dermoscopic presentation **131.16–131.17**
 dysplastic melanocytic naevi *131.41, 131.42, 131.45*
 histological criteria of definition of **131.43**
 eyelid 107.46
 genital area 131.22
 halo naevus 131.27–131.28
  dermoscopic image *131.29*
  lymphocytic infiltrate with disruption of naevomelanocytic aggregates *131.28*
 intradermal/dermal naevus **131.1**, *131.21*
 junctional naevus **131.1**, *131.18, 131.20*
 laser therapies 23.16–23.17
 male genitalia 109.6
 Myerson naevus 131.28–131.29, *131.30*
 naevomelanocytic nests **131.1**, *131.18, 131.20*
 naevus cell types *131.19, 131.20*
 naevus of Ito 68.9–68.10, 131.14–131.15
 naevus of Ota 23.16, *23.17*, 107.46, 131.12–131.14
 oral melanocytic naevi, hyperpigmentation 108.19
 pathology **131.16–131.17**
 recurrent melanocytic naevi 131.26–131.27
 Reed naevus *131.34, 131.37*
 scalp 131.22–131.23, *131.34*
 Spitz naevus **131.16**, 131.32–131.37
 subtypes **131.16–131.17**
 targetoid haemosiderotic naevus 131.30–131.32
 with unusual morphology **131.16**, 131.24–131.32
 in unusual sites **131.16**, 131.21–131.24

melanocytic neoplasms
　diagnosis and classification 3.23–3.25
　terminology **131.1**
melanocytic tumours of uncertain malignant potential (MELTUMP), use of term 142.19
melanocytoma, melanoma precursor 142.2
melanocytosis, dermal 73.21, *73.22*
melanogenesis
　biochemistry 86.5
　UVR exposure 10.8
melanoma *see* malignant melanoma
melanoma of soft parts *see* clear cell sarcoma
melanoma–astrocytoma syndrome 148.9
melanoses, facial 86.9–86.15, 86.51
melanosomes
　keratinocyte terminal differentiation 68.1
　racial groups 86.8
　transport 86.4
melanotic macule, oral involvement 108.18
melanotic neuroectodermal tumour *see* pigmented neuroectodermal tumour of infancy
melanotic progonoma *see* pigmented neuroectodermal tumour of infancy
melasma 86.9–86.12
　depigmentation *86.45*
　on the face, dermatoendocrinology **150.6**, **150.10**, *150.14*, 150.18
　Jessner solution peel *160.7*, *160.8*
　laser therapies 23.17, *23.18*, 161.5–161.6
　treatment 86.33
melatonin, hair growth 87.9
Meleney synergistic gangrene 26.77, 26.78
melioidosis, *Burkholderia pseudomallei* 26.53–26.54
Melkersson–Rosenthal syndrome 109.25
MELTUMP *see* melanocytic tumours of uncertain malignant potential
membrane-bound transporters, drug pharmacokinetics 13.5
membranes, burn treatment 125.6
membranous fat necrosis 97.8, 97.12, 121.6
MEN *see* multiple endocrine neoplasia
Mendelian disorders of cornification (MeDOCs) 63.20–63.21, 63.45
Mendelian randomisation 5.8
MEND syndrome *see* male *EBP* disorder with neurological defects
meningeal involvement, xanthoma disseminatum 135.20
meningeal neurosyphilis 29.15
meningism, primary genital herpes infection 25.25
meningitis
　Acinetobacter 26.51
　anthrax 26.44
　listeriosis 26.46
　Neisseria meningitidis 26.49, 26.50
　streptococci 26.12
meningococcal infection 26.49–26.50
meningothelial heterotopias 136.49–136.50
meningovascular syphilis 29.15
Menkes syndrome/disease 2.34, 61.28, 61.29, 79.16, *79.17*, 87.93
menopause
　ageing of skin 156.6
　flushing **104.4**
menstrual cycle
　acne flares 88.25
　urticaria 42.8
mental/emotional sweating 2.9
mental health 1.9
　hair loss 87.21
　hidradenitis suppurativa association 90.2, 90.11
　psychiatric side-effects of systemic therapies 19.7, 19.18, *19.19*, 19.20, 19.43, 19.45
mentalis muscle 'creases', reduction of by botulinum toxin application *159.8*
mental neuropathy (numb chin syndrome), internal malignancy association 148.23
mental retardation–enteropathy–deafness–neuropathy–ichthyosis–keratodermia (MEDNIK) syndrome 63.30, 63.35, 79.17
menthol, traditional topical therapy 18.38
men who have sex with men (MSM)
　ChemSex 120.2–120.3
　Kaposi sarcoma in HIV-negative men 138.1, **138.2**, 138.4
　lymphogranuloma venereum 30.15
ME-PPD *see* 2-methoxymethyl-p-phenylenediamine
meralgia paraesthetica 83.7
2-mercaptobenzothiazole (MBT) 127.63–127.64
mercapto mix (sensitisers) 127.63
Mercurialis (Geronimo Mercuriale) 1.3
mercury
　allergic contact dermatitis 127.18, 127.41
　dermatological reactions 121.5–121.6
　pigmentation effects 86.52–86.53
Merkel cell carcinoma (MCC) 2.12, 146.1–146.10
　AEIOU diagnostic acronym 146.5, **146.7**
　clinical features 146.5–146.8
　course and prognosis 146.5
　diagnosis of *3.22*, 3.23
　epidemiology 146.1–146.2
　eyelid 107.49
　human polyomavirus-MCPyV 146.2, *146.3*
　immunocompromised people
　　clinicopathological features 147.14–147.15
　　management 147.23–147.24
　　non-Hodgkin lymphoma/chronic lymphocytic leukaemia patients 147.3
　　people living with HIV 147.2
　investigations 146.7–146.8
　management 146.8–146.10
　pathogenesis 146.2
　pathology 146.3–146.5
　polyomavirus infection 25.46–25.47
　predisposing factors 146.2
　radiotherapy 24.15
　staging 146.5, 146.7
Merkel cell polyomavirus (MCPyV) 25.46–25.47
　MCPyV-negative Merkel cell carcinoma 146.2, 146.3, *146.4*, 146.5, 146.9
　MCPyV-positive Merkel cell carcinoma 25.46–25.47, 146.2, 146.3, *146.4*
Merkel cells 2.2, 2.11–2.12
　disputed origins of Merkel cell carcinoma 146.2
　embryonic development 2.5
　hyperplasia 2.12
Merkel cell–neurite complexes 2.12
mesenchymal cells 2.4, 2.5
mesenchymal markers 3.25–3.26
mesenchyme, pre-adipocytes 97.1
mesoderm 2.3
Mesopotamia, ancient medical texts 1.2
meta analysis
　evidence based medicine 17.4–17.5
　see also systematic reviews
metabolic disorders
　acquired ichthyosis 63.47, 85.1
　AGL association 98.2
　blistering 69.24
　hair disorders 87.93
　ocular features **107.42**
　primary dyslipidaemias 60.6–60.10
　xanthomas 60.2–60.6
　see also amino acid metabolism and transport disorders; inherited metabolic diseases; lipid metabism disorders
metabolic syndrome
　diabetic patients 62.4
　hidradenitis suppurativa association 90.2
metabolising acquired dioxin-induced skin hamartoma (MADISH/chloracne) 88.14, 88.15, 88.66–88.68, 129.7, 129.12–129.13, 133.1, **133.2**, 133.7
metabolism
　androgen synthesis 87.10
　burn-induced changes 125.11
　hypermetabolic response to burn injuries 125.11–125.14
metabolism of drugs, clinical pharmacology 13.3
metabolism of prohormones to active metabolites 150.7
metabolism of steroid hormones *150.3*
metabolism of vitamins 59.5, 79.15
metaherpetic keratitis, eyelid *107.37*
metalloprotiens *see* ADAMTS metalloproteinase; matrix metalloproteinases; tissue inhibitors of metalloproteinases
metals
　allergies 127.19, 127.36–127.41
　oral hyperpigmentation 108.17
　pigmentation effects 86.51–86.53
　toxicity 121.1–121.10
metaplasia 3.42
　ileostomy *112.6*
metastases
　from primary epidermal tumours 148.3
　penis 109.42
　scalp metastases 105.11–105.12
　to the skin from internal cancer 24.15, 148.4–148.6
metastatic calcinosis cutis 59.5–59.6, 154.2
　see also metastatic cutaneous calcification
metastatic carcinomas of skin *148.4*
metastatic cutaneous calcification 97.33–97.34
　uraemic patients with combined hyperphosphataemia and hypercalcaemia 154.2
metastatic cutaneous tumour diagnosis 3.26–3.27
metastatic melanoma, systemic therapy 144.6–144.7
metastatic Merkel cell carcinoma 146.7, 146.9
metastatic oral neoplasms 108.45
metastatic pregnancy-associated melanoma (MPAM) 113.10
metastatic regressive melanoma 142.14
metastatic tuberculous abscess 27.17–27.19
metatypical (basosquamous) basal cell carcinoma 140.3
metformin
　acne vulgaris treatment 88.57
　hidradenitis suppurativa treatment 90.10
methacrylate allergic contact dermatitis 127.13, *127.14*
methacrylate nail systems 127.61–127.62
(meth)acrylate-related contact allergy 127.47
methaemoglobinaemia, dapsone side effect 19.14
methamphetamine, dermatoses 120.4–120.5
methicillin-resistant *Staphylococcus aureus* (MRSA) 26.8–26.9
　age effects 26.7
　community-acquired 26.6–26.7
　genetics 26.9
　HIV 31.21, 31.37
　male genitalia 109.28
methicillin-sensitive *Staphylococcus aureus* (MSSA), age effects 26.7
methotrexate (MTX) 19.24–19.28
　alopecia treatment 87.27
　atopic eczema treatment 41.29
　cautions 19.27
　contraindications 19.26
　dermatological uses 19.24–19.25
　dose and regimens 19.27
　drug–drug interactions 19.27
　folate supplementation 19.27
　monitoring 19.27–19.28
　morphoea treatment 55.37
　pemphigus treatment 50.9
　pharmacological properties 19.25–19.26
　potential adverse effects 19.26
　pre-treatment screening 19.27
　psoriasis treatment 35.23–35.25
　sarcoidosis treatment 96.16
　systemic lupus erythematosus treatment 51.38
2-methoxymethyl-p-phenylenediamine (ME-PPD) 127.61
N-methyl-3,4-methylenedioxymethamphetamine (MDMA) *see* ecstasy
methyl acrylate 127.70
methyl aminolevulinate (MAL), use in photodynamic therapy 22.2–22.3, 22.4, 22.5–22.7
methylchloroisothiazolinone (MCI) 127.53–127.54
methylchloroisothiazolinone and methylisothiazolinone (MCI/MI) 127.53–127.54
methyldibromoglutaronitrile (MDBGN) 127.55
methylisothiazolinone (MI) 127.53–127.54
methyl methacrylate (MMA) 127.70
metronidazole, topical therapies 18.11
Metvixia® *see* methyl aminolevulinate
Metvix® *see* methyl aminolevulinate
mevalonate kinase deficiency (MKD) **45.5**, **45.6**, 45.11
mevalonate kinase (*MVK*) genes 85.20
mevalonic aciduria 63.74
Mexico
　community dermatology 7.8
　teledermatology training 7.9
MF *see* mycosis fungoides
MFAPs *see* microfibril-associated proteins
mFGS *see* modified Ferriman–Gallwey score
MFS *see* Marfan syndrome
MGD *see* meibomian gland dysfunction
MGUS *see* monoclonal gammopathy of uncertain significance
MH *see* malignant histiocytosis
MHC *see* major histocompatibility complex
MI *see* methylisothiazolinone
Mibelli porokeratosis 63.74, 63.75, 85.20, 85.21, 109.35
Michelin tyre baby syndrome 70.19, 73.17
Michel medium, biopsy 3.4–3.5, 3.12
microabscesses 3.43
microbial ecology of the skin 26.3–26.5
　age/sex/ethnic difference 26.4
　bacterial adherence 26.5
　modifying factors 26.4
　normal flora 26.3–26.5
　quantitative cultural studies 26.4
　role of normal flora 26.4–26.5
　sampling methods 26.3
　specialised areas 26.5
　temporary residents on skin 26.2, 26.3
microbial exposure, atopic eczema 41.7–41.8
microbiome
　gut 26.4, 26.5
　oral 108.5
　see also skin microbiome
microcephalic osteodysplastic primordial dwarfism type II **72.7**
microcephaly with or without chorioretinopathy, lymphoedema or intellectual disability (MCLID) 103.24
microcephaly with or without chorioretinopathy, lymphoedema and mental retardation (MCLMR) 71.27
microcephaly–capillary malformation syndrome (MIC–CAP) 71.7
microchimerism, rheumatoid nodules 97.15
microclimate 123.3
Micrococcus spp., normal skin flora 26.3
microcystic adnexal carcinoma 107.49, 137.36–137.37
microdialysis, topical bioavailability/bioequivalence assessment 12.8
microfibril-associated glycoproteins (MAGPs) 2.36

microfibril-associated proteins (MFAPs) 2.36
microneedling
  hair disorder treatment 87.95
  skin tightening 161.8
micronodular basal cell carcinoma 140.3, *140.4*
micronutrients, hypermetabolism treatment 125.12
microorganisms
  rosacea 89.4
  staining techniques 3.9–3.10
micropapular polymorphic light eruption 126.4, *126.5*
microscopic examination
  diagnosis 4.20–4.22
  superficial mycoses identification 32.8
microscopic examination of tissue sections 3.32–3.45
  areola 3.33
  axillary skin 3.33
  biopsy site and normal histological variation 3.33
  endothelial cells 3.37
  eosinophils 3.35–3.36
  examination of sections 3.33
  facial skin 3.33
  fibroblasts 3.37
  foreign bodies/deposits 3.38
  giant cells 3.36, *3.37*
  high-magnification examination 3.34
  histiocytes 3.36
  histopathology skin reports 3.38
  low-magnification histological pattern diagnosis 3.34
  lymphocytes 3.34, *3.35*
  mast cells 3.37
  monocytes 3.36
  mucous membranes 3.33
  myofibroblasts 3.37
  neutrophils 3.35
  palm and sole skin 3.33
  pericytes 3.37
  plasma cells 3.35
  preparing for microscopy 3.32–3.33
  rhabdomyocyte (striated muscle cell) 3.37
  scalp skin 3.33
  Schwann cells 3.37
  scrotum skin 3.33
  smooth muscle cells 3.37
  tissue macrophages 3.36
  truncal skin 3.33–3.34
microscopic polyangiitis (MPA) 100.20–100.22, 152.4
microsponges, vehicle choice for topical therapies 18.2–18.3
microsporide *see* dermatophytide reaction
Microsporum infections, Wood's light examination 32.6
Microsporum species
  dermatophytosis 32.18–32.20, **32.19**, 32.24–32.26
  M. audouinii 32.24–32.25
  M. canis 32.25
  M. gypseum 32.25–32.26
microtia (small ears) 106.4, *106.5*
microvascular occlusion disorders, purpura 99.9–99.24
microvenular haemangioma 136.30
MIC–CAP *see* microcephaly–capillary malformation syndrome
mid-dermal elastolysis 94.25–94.26
middle age, psychological and social factors 15.3
midface toddler excoriation syndrome (MiTES) 82.9, 83.12–83.13
midges 34.7–34.8
Miescher radial granulomas 97.22–97.23
migrant health dermatology 7.13, **7.14**
migration, epidemiology 5.10
migratory circinate redness, autosomal dominant epidermolysis bullosa simplex with 69.9–69.10
migratory erythemas, internal malignancy association 148.19–148.20

migratory thrombophlebitis
  adenocarcinoma of the pancreas 153.6
  neoplasia association 148.26
milia
  chemical peel side effects 160.12
  cysts 133.4
  differential diagnosis 88.30, *88.31*
  infants 115.13–115.14
  neonates 114.4
miliaria 92.12–92.14
  management 92.13–92.14
  neonates 114.6–114.7
miliaria crystallina (sudamina) 92.12–92.13
miliaria profunda 92.12–92.13, 92.14
miliaria rubra (prickly heat) 92.12–92.13, 92.14
miliary calcinosis cutis 59.4, 59.5, 59.6
miliary tuberculosis, acute cutaneous 27.17
milk alkali syndrome, metastatic calcinosis cutis 59.5
milker's nodule 25.15
milker's sinuses 122.22–122.23
milk thistle (silymarin), cosmeceutical use of **157.8**, *157.9*
millipedes (Diplopoda) 34.57
Milroy disease 103.24
Milroy-like lymphoedema 103.24
mineral disorders 61.24–61.31, **79.2**, 79.15–79.18
  acrodermatitis enteropathica 79.15–79.16
  copper deficiency 2.34, 61.27–61.29
  familial tumoral calcinosis 79.17–79.18
  hair loss 59
  iron deficiency 61.3, 61.4, 61.24–61.25, 87.59, 87.63, 87.70–87.71, 153.1
  manganese deficiency and excess 61.31
  MEDNIK syndrome 79.17
  Menkes disease 79.16, *79.17*
  occipital horn syndrome 79.16
  selenium deficiency and excess 61.29–61.31
  skin manifestations of impaired absorption 153.1
  Wilson disease 79.17
  zinc deficiency 61.25–61.27, 69.24, 108.20, 153.9
mineralisation, abnormal 70.31–70.36
mineral oils/greases, topical medication vehicles 18.6
miner's anaemia *see* ancylostomiasis
'miniature puberty', neonates 114.4
miniaturised follicles 87.64, *87.65*
minimal erythema dose (MED), phototherapy 21.7–21.8
minimal phototoxic dose, PUVA 21.9
minocycline, sarcoidosis management 96.16
minocycline-induced hyperpigmentation 86.27–86.28
minoxidil 87.69–87.70, 87.73, 87.94
minoxidil acid, topical therapies 18.41
MIS-A *see* multisystem inflammatory syndrome in adults
MIS-C *see* multisystem inflammatory syndrome in children
Misuse of Drugs Act 1971 (MDA) 120.3–120.4
MiTES *see* midface toddler excoriation syndrome
mites (Acari) 34.41–34.57
  animal diseases 34.50
  bird/rodent/reptile mites 34.54–34.55
  Cheyletiella mites 34.53, *34.54*
  follicle mites 34.55–34.57
  harvest mites 34.54
  house dust mites 34.51
  plant mites 34.52
  Pyemotes mites 34.51–34.52
  rickettsial infection transmission 26.84
  scabies 34.41–34.50
  stored products 34.50–34.51
mitochondrial disorders 8.5
mitochondrial palmoplantar keratoderma 63.64–63.65
mitochondrial respiratory chain disorders **79.2**, 79.8–79.9

mitochrondria, damage from UVR exposure 10.11
mitogen-activated protein kinase (MAPK) pathway, targeted therapy for melanoma 144.4
mitogen-activated protein kinase (MEK) inhibitors
  chemotherapy cutaneous side-effects 119.3, 119.7–119.8
  melanoma systemic therapy 144.4–144.5, *144.11*, **144.11**, 144.12
mitogen-activated protein (MAP) kinase 87.73
mitten hand deformity, epidermolysis bullosa 69.17, 69.26
mixed connective tissue disease (MCTD) 53.1–53.3
  acral lesions *53.4*
  cardiac involvement 151.4
  clinical features 53.2
  diagnostic criteria **53.2**
  investigations 53.3
  management 53.3
  pathophysiology 53.1–53.2
  and retiform purpura 53.4
mixed cryoglobulinaemia (MC) 25.76, 124.13
mixed immunobullous disease 50.36
mixed inflammatory infiltrate 87.50–87.52
mixed leg ulcers (MLUs) 102.4–102.7
  clinical features 102.7
  disorders associated with **102.6**
  epidemiology 102.5–102.6
  lipodermatosclerosis *102.7*
  management of *102.8*
  predisposing factors 102.6
mixed tumour of the skin 137.32
Mkar disease 94.30
MKD *see* mevalonate kinase deficiency
MLCDP *see* Major Life Changing Decision Profile
MLDSI *see* multisegmental lymphatic dysplasia with systemic involvement
MLUs *see* mixed leg ulcers
MM *see* malignant melanoma
MMA *see* methyl methacrylate
MMDK *see* multiple minute digitate keratoses
MMF *see* mycophenolate mofetil
MMP *see* mucous membrane pemphigoid
MMPs *see* matrix metalloproteinases
MMR (measles/mumps/rubella) vaccine
  intralesional immunotherapy for human papillomavirus infections 25.59–25.60
  prophylaxis 25.92, 25.99
  uptake of 115.7
MMR-V (measle/mumps/rubella/varicella) vaccine 25.92, 25.99
MMS *see* Mohs micrographic surgery
modified Ferriman–Gallwey score (mFGS), hirsutism 87.88–87.89
modified hidradenitis suppurativa score 16.4
modified Parkland resuscitation formula 125.2–125.3
modified Rodnan skin score (MRSS), systemic sclerosis **54.17**
modified Sartorius Score (MSS) 16.4
'Mogul skier's palm' 122.17
Mohs micrographic surgery (MMS) 20.30–20.37, 90.11
  basal cell carcinoma 140.16
  Boden disease 141.21
  cutaneous squamous cell carcinoma 141.33, 141.35, 141.37
  defect closure procedures 20.20–20.22, 20.26–20.29
  defect reconstruction 20.20–20.22, 20.26–20.29, 20.30–20.37
  definition 20.30–20.31
  history 20.31–20.32
  practical aspects and indications 20.35–20.37

  procedure 20.33–20.34, *20.36*
  results 20.34–20.35
  skin cancer treatment comparisons 20.32–20.33
  types of tumours **20.37**
moisture-associated skin damage 123.4
moisturisers, ichthyoses management 63.42
molecular amplification tests, syphilis 29.18
molecular-based approaches
  classic epidermolysis bullosa simplex 69.11–69.15
  classic junctional epidermolysis bullosa 69.15
  dystrophic epidermolysis bullosa 69.18–69.19
  pigmentation disorders 68.14
molecular diagnosis, superficial mycoses identification 32.9
molecular genetic methods, culture-independent microbial studies 26.2, 26.3
moles *see* melanocytic naevi
Moll, cyst of 107.45
mollicutes, *Mycoplasma genitalium* infection 30.23–30.25
mollusca, stings 130.4
molluscipoxviruses (MCV-1 to MCV-4), HIV 31.26
molluscum contagiosum (MC) 25.15–25.19
  clinical features 25.16–25.17
  eczematisation around lesions *39.25*
  epidemiology 25.15–25.16
  eyelid 107.34, *107.36*
  infants 115.9
  investigations 25.18
  management 25.18
  pathophysiology 25.16
  penis 109.29
  perianal skin *111.13*, 111.15
molluscum sebaceum *see* keratoacanthoma
moluscipoxviruses **25.6**, 25.15–25.18
molybdenum, dermatological reactions 121.9
MOMES syndrome **72.7**
MOMO syndrome **72.6**
'Mona Lisa smile', dermatitis artefacta 84.31, *84.32*
Mondor disease 101.36–101.37
  neoplasia association 148.26–148.27
  subtypes **101.38**
monetary costs of disease *see* economic burden of disease
Mongolian spot 73.22, 79.3, 86.2, 131.12
monilethrix 87.78
monkey oesophagus substrate, indirect immunofluorescence *3.12*, 3.13–3.14, 3.19
monkeypox virus (MPXV) *see* mpox
monobenzyl ether of hydroquinone, topical depigmenting agents 18.32
monochromator phototesting 126.5–126.6, 126.12, 126.19, *126.20*, 126.23, *126.27*, 126.31, *126.35*
monoclonal antibodies (mAbs) 19.31–19.32
  cutaneous T-cell lymphoma therapy 139.25
  WHO naming conventions 19.31, **19.32**
monoclonal gammopathy of clinical or cutaneous significance 149.10
monoclonal gammopathy of uncertain significance (MGUS)
  disorders of paraprotein activity 149.9–149.13
  disorders of paraprotein deposition 149.13, 149.14
  necrobiotic xanthogranuloma 135.24
  pyoderma gangrenosum 149.7
  skin disorders from cell infiltration 149.2, 149.4–149.5
monoclonal mast cell activation syndrome 46.6
monocytes
  immune system 9.5
  microscopic examination of 3.36

monogenic autoinflammatory syndromes *see* hereditary monogenic autoinflammatory syndromes
monogenic inherited pigmentation disorders 68.2–68.3
monogenic obesity with cutaneous features 72.4, **72.7**
monogenic obesity without cutaneous features 72.3, **72.6**
monomorphic follicular papules, infundibulofolliculitis 93.7
monomorphic follicular papules/pustules, actinic folliculitis 93.6
monomorphic polymorphic light eruption 126.4
monosymptomatic delusional hypochondriasis
　delusional infestation 84.5–84.10
　olfactory reference syndrome 84.10–84.11
mons pubis
　cutaneous Crohn disease 95.15
　lymphoedema 103.49–103.51, *103.52*
mood disorders
　dermatological patients 84.40–84.42
　types 84.40
mood stabilisers 84.46–84.47
Moraxella spp. 26.51
Morbihan disease (solid facial lymphoedema) 88.41, 89.10, 89.16, *89.17*, 103.47, *103.48*
morbilliform eruption, drug reaction 118.7
morbillivirus 25.97–25.99
　see also measles
Morgellons syndrome 84.11–84.12
MORM syndrome **72.6**
morphine
　death rates 120.1
　drug-induced pruritus 81.11
　topical therapies 18.41
morphoea 55.1–55.42, 105.8
　age of onset 55.6–55.7
　associated diseases 55.7
　atrophoderma of Pasini–Pierini 55.17, *55.19*
　atrophodermas 94.18
　autoantibodies in relation to clinical features 55.9
　autoimmune diseases 55.7
　autoimmunity 55.8–55.9
　biologic therapies 55.38–55.42
　blood tests 55.30–55.31
　Borrelia antibodies 94.16
　cancer association 55.7
　causative organisms 55.12
　in childhood **55.39**
　circumscribed plaque morphoea 55.17, **55.27**
　classification 55.2–55.3
　clinical assessment **55.31**
　clinical features *55.9*, 55.15–55.27
　complications and co-morbidities 55.28–55.29
　CT scans 55.31
　cytokines and cellular signatures 55.10
　deep morphoea **55.3**, 55.16–55.17
　differential diagnosis 55.27
　disease course and prognosis 55.29–55.30
　disease modifiers **55.4**, 55.15–55.17
　drug reactions 55.14–55.15
　en coup de sabre 55.23–55.24
　environmental factors 55.13–55.15
　eosinophilic fasciitis **55.4**, 55.21–55.23, **55.27**
　epidemiology 55.6–55.7
　epidermal–dermal interaction 55.9
　erythematous plaque with telangiectases *55.6*
　extracutaneous manifestations 55.28–55.29
　fibroblast activation and sclerosis 55.10–55.11
　generalised plaque morphoea **55.3**, **55.4**, 55.17–55.19
　genetics 55.12–55.13
　guttate morphoea 55.17

　histology *55.5*
　histopathology 55.11–55.12
　hyperpigmentation *55.18*, 86.20–86.21
　imaging modalities 55.31–55.32
　immunopathology 55.9–55.11
　incidence and prevalence 55.6
　investigations 55.30–55.35, **55.31**
　keloidal/nodular morphoea 55.15–55.16
　lichen sclerosus morphoea **55.4**, *55.5*, *55.6*, 55.7
　limited morphoea **55.3**, **55.4**, 55.17
　linear morphoea **55.3**, **55.4**, 55.23–55.27
　　differential diagnosis **55.27**
　　head/neck variant 55.23–55.24
　　linear atrophoderma of Moulin 55.25–55.27
　　linear deep atrophic morphoea 55.27
　　morphoea en coup de sabre 55.24
　　progressive hemifacial atrophy 55.24–55.25
　　trunk/limb variant 55.25
　localised scleroderma cutaneous assessment tool 55.33–55.34
　management 55.35–55.42
　　biologic therapies 55.38–55.42
　　corticosteroids 55.36–55.37
　　phototherapy 55.36
　　therapeutic algorithm *55.41*
　　topical therapies 55.35–55.36
　　treatments and levels of evidence **55.40**
　mixed type morphoea **55.4**, 55.27
　MRI imaging 55.31, *55.32*
　outcome measures 55.32–55.35
　paediatric morphoea **55.39**
　pansclerotic morphoea **54.20**, **55.4**, 55.19–55.21, **55.27**
　pathophysiology 55.8–55.15
　patient reported outcomes **55.35**
　plaque morphoea **55.3**
　predisposing factors 55.8
　presentation 55.15
　pressure sites from clothing *55.5*
　psychological manifestations 55.29
　radiation 55.14
　radiotherapy-associated 119.15
　redness (erythema) *55.18*
　sclerosis, causes of **55.14**
　severity assessment and classification 55.27–55.28
　skin biopsy 55.31
　synonyms and inclusions 55.1
　terminology 55.1–55.2
　therapeutic algorithm *55.41*
　topical therapies 55.35–55.36
　and trauma to skin 55.13–55.14
　and vaccination 55.13
　vascular activation and damage 55.9
　waxy plaques *55.5*
morphoeaform sarcoidosis 96.13
morphoea profunda 97.12–97.13
morphoeic basal cell carcinoma 140.3, 140.6, *140.8*, 140.9
morphogenesis 87.2
morpholines, topical therapies 18.12
Morton neuroma/metatarsalgia 136.43
mosaic acral keratosis 63.61
mosaicism 8.7–8.8, 74.5
mosaic lymphoedema associated with disturbed growth and/or cutaneous/vascular anomalies 103.23–103.24
mosaic neurofibromatosis type 1 78.4–78.7, **78.7**
mosaic pattern, piebaldism 68.4
mosaic RASopathies, lymphatic abnormalities 103.24
mosquitoes 34.6–34.7, 34.8–34.9
　lymphatic filariasis 103.34
　malaria 33.36
　togaviruses infections 25.87–25.91
mossy foot *see* podoconiosis (non-filarial lymphoedema)
moths (Lepidoptera) 34.32–34.34
motor nerves, anatomy of head and neck 20.3–20.4

mottled pigmentation, autosomal dominant epidermolysis bullosa simplex 69.9
mottling effect, livedo reticularis 124.9, *124.10*
moulds
　brachytherapy 24.3
　identification of isolates 32.10
　morphology and diseases **32.3**
Moulin, linear atrophoderma of 55.25–55.27, 73.22, 94.17
moult cycle, hair 87.2
Moulting ('Mauserung') phenomenon, superficial epidermolytic ichthyosis 63.18
moult waves 87.9, 87.53
mouse studies, immune system 9.3, 9.7
mouth *see* oral cavity
Mozart ear 106.5
MPA *see* microscopic polyangiitis
MPAM *see* metastatic pregnancy-associated melanoma; *Mycoplasma pneumoniae*-associated mucositis
MPHL *see* male pattern hair loss
MPK *see* marginal papular keratoderma
M-plasty, skin surgery 20.21, *20.22*
MPNSTs *see* malignant peripheral nerve sheath tumours
mpox (formerly monkeypox) 25.8–25.12
　2022 outbreak 25.9–25.10
　clinical features 25.9, *25.10*
　complications and co-morbidities 25.10
　epidemiology 25.8–25.9
　investigations 25.10
　management 25.10–25.12
　pathology 25.10
　pathophysiology 25.9
　risk increased with waning smallpox immunity 25.6
MPSs *see* mucopolysaccharidoses
MPXV (monkeypox virus) *see* mpox
Mrgpr family *see* Mas-related G-protein-coupled receptor agonists
MRGPRX2 *see* Mas-related G protein–coupled receptor member X2
MRH *see* multicentric reticulohistiocytosis
MRI *see* magnetic resonance imaging
MRL *see* magnetic resonance lymphangiography
MRSS *see* modified Rodnan skin score
MSAs *see* myositis-specific antibodies
MSH *see* melanocyte-stimulating hormone
MS-LCH *see* multisystem Langerhans cell histiocytoses
MSM *see* men who have sex with men
MSS *see* modified Sartorius Score
MSSE *see* multiple self-healing squamous epithelioma
MTC *see* medullary thyroid cancer
MTS *see* Muir–Torre syndrome
MTX *see* methotrexate
muccous membrane changes, dyskeratosis congenita 67.14
Mucha–Haberman disease, oral ulceration 108.41
mucin
　skin deposition 57.1–57.19
　structure 57.1
　see also cutaneous mucinoses
mucinosis
　systemic lupus erythematosus 51.28
　see also cutaneous mucinoses
mucinous carcinoma 137.38
mucin-producing sweat gland carcinoma *see* endocrine mucin-producing sweat gland carcinoma
Muckle–Wells syndrome (MWS) **45.5**, **45.6**, 154.2
mucocele (mucous cysts)
　digital myxoid cysts 57.15, *57.16*
　male genitalia 109.30
　mouth 108.12
　vulva 110.31
mucocutaneous candidiasis, primary immunodeficiencies 149.18–149.19

mucocutaneous leishmaniasis
　New-World 33.43, *33.44*, 33.45, 33.46, 33.49
　Old-World 33.47, *33.48*
mucocutaneous lymph node syndrome *see* Kawasaki disease
mucocutaneous pain syndromes (MCPs) 82.1–82.14
　atypical trigeminal trophic syndrome 82.8, *82.9*
　burning mouth syndrome 82.1–82.3
　cervical trophic syndrome 82.8–82.9
　chronic scalp pain and dysaesthesia 82.12
　erythromelalgia 82.12–82.13
　midface toddler excoriation syndrome 82.9
　penoscrotodynia 82.11–82.12
　postherpetic neuralgia 82.4–82.5
　trigeminal neuropathic pain syndrome 82.5–82.7
　trigeminal trophic syndrome 82.7–82.8
　trophic syndromes 82.7–82.9
　vulvodynia 82.9–82.11
mucocutaneous venous malformation 71.16–71.17
mucoepithelial dysplasia 108.26–108.27
mucolipidoses types II and III 79.4–79.5
mucopolysaccharidoses (MPSs) 79.1–79.3
mucormycosis (zygomycosis) 32.93, 109.28
　oral involvement 108.57
　panniculitis due to 97.60–97.61
mucosa associated lymphoid tissue (MALT) lymphomas 139.37, 139.38
mucosal advancement flap, vermilionectomy repair 20.22
mucosal associated invariant T (MAIT) cells 9.5
mucosal lesions
　COVID-19 association 25.112–25.113
　psoriasis vulgaris 35.11–35.12
　systemic lupus erythematosus 51.29
mucosal melanoma
　presentation 142.11, *142.16*
　systemic treatment 144.7
　vaginal *145.12*, 145.13
mucosal melanotic lesions 131.9–131.12
　pigmented melanotic macules 131.9–131.11
　see also lentigines
mucositis (mucosal barrier injury), oral involvement 108.49–108.50
mucous cysts *see* mucocele
mucous membrane pemphigoid (MMP) 3.17, 50.22–50.33, 105.6, 107.24–107.32
　associated diseases 50.24
　biochip mosaic for detection of serum anti-laminin 332 IgG *50.31*
　classification of severity 107.26
　clinical features 50.26
　clinical features of ocular MMP 107.26
　clinical variants 50.26
　complications and co-morbidities 107.26
　conjunctival hyperaemia 50.30
　diagnosis *50.24*, *50.32*, 107.26
　diagnostic problems in ocular MMP 107.26–107.28
　differential diagnosis 50.26
　direct immunofluorescence for 107.28
　epidemiology 50.24, 107.24–107.25
　European Consensus criteria for diagnosis of 107.28–107.29
　fibrosis prevention 107.32
　genital involvement 50.28
　histopathology 50.25
　immunosuppression in *107.31*
　indirect immunofluorescence in 107.28
　investigations 107.26–107.28
　investigations and diagnosis 50.28–50.30, *50.31*
　lesions *50.29*
　management 50.30–50.31, 107.29–107.32
　ocular disease in *50.30*
　ocular pemphigoid 50.26
　　classification **50.28**

ocular signs of   107.27–107.28
oral involvement   108.82
oral lesions   50.27
pathology   107.25–107.26
pathophysiology   50.24–50.25
predisposing factors   107.25
randomised controlled trials   50.30–50.31
serum autoantibodies   50.25–50.26
severity classification   50.26–50.28
tissue-bound autoantibodies   50.25
treatment guidelines   50.31
treatment ladder   50.31–50.33
vulva   **110.21**
vulvar pemphigoid   50.26
mucous membranes
    allergic contact dermatitis   127.18
    congenital syphilis   29.23
    lichen planus   37.12
    microscopic examination of   3.33
    samples for superficial mycoses identification   32.8
    syphilis   29.10, 29.14, *29.15*
mudi-chood, ear dermatoses   **106.23**
Muir–Torre syndrome (MTS/Lynch II syndrome)   76.11, **78.14**, 141.44–141.45
    sebaceous adenomas and sebaceomas   137.17
    sebaceous carcinoma   137.18
multicentric reticulohistiocytosis (MRH)   135.25–135.27, 155.14
    internal malignancy association   148.24
    oral involvement   108.71–108.72
    pleural effusion   152.6
multidisciplinary teams (MDTs)
    psychodermatology   84.2, 84.7, 84.8, 84.9, 84.12, 84.18, 84.35
    SJS/TEN treatment   118.19
multidrug-resistant (MDR) tuberculosis   27.10
multifocal cutaneous infantile haemangioma   116.5
multifocal epithelial hyperplasia (focal epithelial hyperplasia), oral involvement   108.11
multifocal venous malformation (MVM)   *71.2*
multiple cutaneous neuromas *see* dermal hyperneury
multiple cutaneous and uterine leiomyomas syndrome *see* hereditary leiomyomatosis and renal cell cancer
multiple endocrine neoplasia (MEN)   108.13–108.14, 148.10–148.11
multiple endocrine neoplasia type 1 (MEN1)   148.10
multiple endocrine neoplasia type 2A (MEN2A)   148.10
multiple endocrine neoplasia type 2B (MEN2B)   108.13–108.14, 148.10–148.11
multiple glomangioma   136.42
multiple haemorrhagic sarcoma *see* Kaposi sarcoma
multiple hamartoma and neoplasia syndrome
    renal/urinary tract involvement   154.2
    trichilemmoma   137.6
multiple minute digitate hyperkeratoses   63.77
multiple minute digitate keratoses (MMDK)   85.18–85.19
multiple mucosal neuroma syndrome   108.13–108.14
multiple organ failure, hypermelanosis   86.21–86.22
multiple pigment sarcoma *see* Kaposi sarcoma
multiple primary hypersensitivities, patch testing   127.32
multiple self-healing squamous epithelioma (MSSE)   **78.13**, 141.41–141.42
multiple symmetrical lipomatosis *see* Madelung disease

multipotent stem cell transplantation, *see also* haematopoietic stem cell transplantation
multisegmental lymphatic dysplasia with systemic involvement (MLDSI)   103.22
multisystem inflammatory syndrome in adults (MIS-A), COVID-19 association   25.112
multisystem inflammatory syndrome in children (MIS-C), COVID-19 association   25.114–25.115
multisystem Langerhans cell histiocytoses (MS-LCH)   135.2–135.9
multisystem sarcoidosis, acquired ichthyosis   *63.48*
multisystem tumours, associated skin conditions   148.2
multivoltage X-ray techniques
    'bathing cap' distribution   24.3, *24.5*
    'stocking' distribution   24.3–24.4, *24.6–24.7*
Mulvihill–Smith syndrome   70.29–70.30
Münchausen syndrome   84.37
Münchausen syndrome by proxy   84.37–84.38
Munro microabscess   3.43, *35.6*
mupirocin, topical therapies   18.11
murine typhus   26.81
Murray Williams warts   39.28
muscle, *see also* dermatomyositis
muscle cells, smooth   2.40–2.41
muscle cell tumours   136.52–136.56
    skeletal muscle   136.55–136.56
    smooth muscle   136.52–136.55
muscle definition, electromagnetic muscle stimulation   161.8
muscle 'naevi'   **73.2**
muscle signs, dermatomyositis   52.7
muscular dystrophy, autosomal recessive epidermolysis bullosa simplex with   69.11
musculocontractural Ehlers–Danlos syndrome (mcEDS)   **70.6**, 70.9
musculoskeletal system   155.1–155.16
    epidermolysis bullosa   69.26
    history and examination   155.1–155.2
    ichthyoses   63.46
    sarcoidosis   96.5–96.6
    systemic sclerosis   54.18
musical instruments, skin reactions   122.11–122.13
mutations *see* gene mutations; genetic disorders/syndromes
mutilation, male genitalia   109.9
MVK genes *see* MeValonate Kinase genes
MVM *see* multifocal venous malformation
MWS *see* Muckle–Wells syndrome
Myanmar, skincare initiative   7.11
mycetoma   32.72–32.75
    clinical features   32.73–32.74
    epidemiology   32.72–32.73
    investigations   32.74–32.75
    management   32.75
    pathophysiology   32.73
mycobacterial infections   27.1–27.46
    eyelid   107.39–107.40
    female genitalia   110.26
    HIV coinfection   27.2–27.3, 27.10, 31.22
    non-tuberculous mycobacteria   27.3, 27.32–27.45
    panniculitides   97.46
    sarcoidosis causation   96.4
    superficial   32.6–32.69
    systemic   32.80–32.94
    types/classification   27.1, 27.2
    see also tuberculosis
Mycobacterium
    histology   28.3–28.4, *28.5*
    M. abscessus group   27.2, 27.43–27.45
    M. avium complex   27.2, 27.3, 27.32, 27.40–27.41
    M. balnei see M. marinum
    M. bovis   27.1, 27.2, 27.5, 27.6, *27.12*
        see also bacillus Calmette–Guérin
    M. chelonae   27.2, 27.43–27.45, *97.47*
    M. fortuitum group   27.2, 27.43–27.45

M. goodii   27.2, 27.32
M. gordonae   27.3
M. haemophilum   27.41–27.42
M. intracellulare   27.1, 27.2, 27.40
M. kansasii   27.2, 27.3, 27.35–27.36
M. leprae   27.1, 27.2, 28.1–28.6, *97.27*
    histology   28.3–28.4, *28.5*
    immunology   28.4–28.5
    serology   28.6
    see also leprosy
M. malmoense   27.3
M. marinum   27.2, 27.5, 27.20, 27.32–27.35
    sporotrichoid distribution   *4.10*
M. mucogenicum   27.2, 27.42, 27.43
M. platypoecilus see M. marinum
M. scrofulaceum   27.42–27.43
M. simiae   27.3
M. smegmatis   27.2, 27.32, 27.43–27.45
M. szulgai   27.3
M. tuberculosis   27.1, 27.2
    complex   27.5–27.24
    complex tuberculids   27.24–27.32
    erythema induratum   97.26, *97.29*
    HIV combination   31.22
    nucleic acid amplification tests   27.8–27.9
    protective immunity   27.3–27.4
M. ulcerans   27.36–27.40
    clinical features   27.38
    epidemiology   27.37
    investigations   27.38–27.39
    management   27.39–27.40
    pathophysiology   27.37–27.38
M. wolinskyi   27.2, 27.32
M. xenopi   27.3
rapid growing species   27.2, 27.43–27.45
slow growing species   27.2, 27.5–27.43
see also tuberculosis of the skin
mycophenolate, morphoea treatment   55.37–55.38
mycophenolate mofetil (MMF)   19.28–19.30
    atopic eczema treatment   41.29
    dermatological uses   19.28
    dose and regimen   19.30
    drug–drug interactions   19.29
    monitoring   19.30
    pemphigus treatment   50.8
    pharmacological properties   19.28–19.29
    potential adverse effects   19.29
    safety precautions   19.29
    systemic lupus erythematosus treatment   51.38
Mycoplasma pneumoniae associated mucositis (MPAM)   118.16
Mycoplasma spp.   26.78–26.79
    M. genitalium   30.23–30.25
        clinical features   30.24–30.25
        epidemiology   30.24
        investigations   30.25
        management   30.25
        pathophysiology   30.24
    M. pneumoniae, in SJS/TEN   118.20
    Stevens–Johnson syndrome   118.15–118.16
mycoses (fungal infections)   32.1–32.95
    fungal biology and reproduction   32.2–32.5
    morphology of fungi   *32.3*
    nomenclature   32.5–32.6
    pinna infection   106.21
    subcutaneous   32.69–32.80
    superficial   32.6–32.69
    systemic   32.80–32.94
mycosis fungoides
    discoid skin lesions   **39.10**
    extracorporeal photochemotherapy   21.7
    male genitalia   109.42
    oral involvement   108.72
    phototherapy indications   21.4
    radiotherapy   24.15–24.16
    UVA-1 phototherapy   21.7
mycosis fungoides (MF)   139.2–139.25
    clinical features   139.8–139.12
    clinical variants/related conditions   139.9, 139.14–139.19

    epidemiology   139.3
    investigations   139.12–139.14
    management   139.20–139.25
    molecular features   139.19–139.20
    parapsoriasis relationship   134.6
    pathophysiology   139.3–139.8
    predisposing factors   139.3–139.4
    prognosis   139.10–139.12, *139.13–139.14*, **139.13**
    relationship to other lymphomas   139.1
    relationship to Sézary syndrome   139.2, 139.19–139.20
    staging/classification   139.6, **139.7**, **139.8**, 139.9–139.10
    T-cell receptor gene analysis   139.6–139.8
    typical   139.2–139.14
mycotic otitis externa *see* otomycosis
myelodysplasia
    oral involvement   108.72, 149.8
    VEXAS syndrome   45.19, 149.6, 149.7
myeloid disorders, leukaemia cutis   149.2–149.5
myeloid lineage cells   9.4–9.5
myeloid malignancies, skin manifestations of paraneoplastic syndromes   149.5–149.8
myeloid sarcoma (granulocytic sarcoma)
    infiltration of skin with malignant granulocyte precursor cells   149.2
    oral involvement   108.70
    see also leukaemia cutis
myeloma, oral involvement   108.72
myeloproliferative disorders, associated skin conditions   148.2
myelosuppression/myelotoxicity
    antimalarials   19.5
    azathioprine   19.9, 19.10
    hydroxycarbamide   19.21, 19.22
    methotrexate   19.26
Myerson naevus   131.28–131.29, *131.30*
MYH9-USP6 fusion gene, nodular fasciitis   136.5
myiasis, insect larvae   **34.7**, 34.9–34.13
myoepithelial cells, eccrine glands   92.2
myoepithelial tumours   137.32–137.33
myofibroblasts   2.40
    microscopic examination of   3.37
    palmar fascial fibromatosis   94.34
    wound healing   11.7
myofibroma (adult)   136.39–136.40
myofibromatosis (infantile)   94.41–94.42, 136.39–136.40
myopathic Ehlers–Danlos syndrome (mEDS)   **70.7**, 70.10
myopericytoma   136.40–136.41
myositis-specific antibodies (MSAs), dermatomyositis   52.2, 52.5, 52.6, 52.11
MYT1L deficiency   **72.6**
myxoedema
    palmoplantar keratodermas with   63.72–63.73
    in thyroid diseases   57.11–57.14
myxofibrosarcoma   136.18
myxoid degeneration   3.40
myxoid liposarcoma, pleomorphic liposarcoma   136.59
myxoid malignant fibrous histiocytoma *see* myxofibrosarcoma
myxoid tumours, dermal nerve sheath myxoma   136.47–136.48
myxoinflammatory fibroblastic sarcoma   136.17
myxoma, mouth   108.14
Myxoma syndrome (Carney complex)   **72.7**, **78.13**, 108.16, **131.3**, *131.4*, 148.11, 151.3–151.4
MZL *see* marginal zone lymphoma

N

NAC *see* N-acetylcysteine
N-acetylcysteine (NAC)   63.42–63.43
N-acetyltransferases (NATs)   127.10
NADCs *see* non-AIDS-defining cancers
NAE *see* necrolytic acral erythema

Naegeli–Franceschetti–Jadassohn syndrome 68.12
naevi
- acneform naevi 88.31
- Becker naevus 73.18
- blue naevus 3.44, 73.15, *73.16*, **131.17**, 131.38–131.40
- cancer phobias 84.26
- classification 73.1–73.2
- common dermoscopic patterns *145.2, 145.3*, 145.4–145.6
- congenital epidermal naevi 73.2, 73.3–73.8
- congenital naevi 73.8–73.16
- dermoscopy, benign patterns 145.1–145.7
- dynamic analysis for melanoma diagnosis 142.9
- epidermal 4.9
- fat naevus **73.2**, 73.16–73.18
- genetic classification 73.2
- hair follicles 137.7–137.8
- histological classification 73.2
- inheritance of naevus mutations 73.3
- intradermal, dermoscopic patterns 145.6
- intra-individual comparative analysis, melanoma diagnosis 142.9
- linear epidermal naevus, oral lesions 108.30
- linear naevus syndrome (naevus sebaceous of Jadassohn), oral lesions 108.29–108.30
- melanoma precursors 142.2–142.3
- melanoma presentation 142.10
- muscle 'naevi' **73.2**
- naevus phenotypes 73.1
- pigment cell naevi **73.2**
- prophylactic surgical excision to prevent melanoma not recommended 142.3
- reticular pattern naevi *145.2, 145.3*, 145.4, 145.6
- Spitz naevi 73.15, *145.5*, 145.6–145.7
- terminology **73.2**
- white sponge naevus, oral lesions 108.31
- *see also* melanocytic naevi; naevus-like entities

naevoid basal cell carcinoma syndrome (NBCCS/Gorlin syndrome) 22.2, 22.7, **78.12**, 140.3–140.4, 140.18–140.20, 148.7
- clinical features 140.18–140.20
- diagnostic criteria 140.19, **140.20**
- epidemiology 140.18
- genetics 140.3–140.4, 140.18
- management 140.20
- oral involvement 108.86

naevoid congenital hypertrichosis 87.85–87.86
naevoid hyperkeratosis 63.79
'naevoid melanoma', use of term 142.19
naevus acneiformis unilateralis *see* comedo naevus
naevus comedonicus 73.7, 88.31, *88.32*, 137.5
naevus depigmentosus 86.38
naevus flammeus 101.10
naevus folliculoris keratosus *see* comedo naevus
naevus of Ito 68.9–68.10, 131.14–131.15
naevus-like entities **73.2**, 73.21–73.23
naevus lipomatosus 98.25
naevus of Ota 131.12–131.14
- eyelid 107.46
- laser therapies 23.16, 23.17

naevus phenotype (number and features of naevi), melanoma risk 142.3–142.4
naevus sebaceous (organoid naevus) 73.5, 73.6, 73.7, 73.8, 87.30, 88.32, 105.11, *106.33*, 137.19–137.20
naevus spilus (speckled lentiginous naevus) *4.8*, 23.16, 73.15–73.16, 131.15–131.17
naevus zoniforme *see* comedo naevus
NAFR *see* non-ablative fractional resurfacing
Nagashima PPK 63.54
Nager syndrome **106.7**

NAI *see* non-accidental injury
NAIAD *see* NLRP1-associated autoinflammation with arthritis and dyskeratosis
Nail Assessment in Psoriasis and Psoriatic Arthritis (NAPPA) 16.3
nail bed epithelium 2.11, 119.7
nail biting (onychophagia) 84.25
nail changes
- chemotherapy-induced 119.6–119.8
- COVID-19 25.113
- during pregnancy 113.1, **113.2**
- HIV 31.33–31.34
- liver disease 153.9
- selenosis 121.7

nail disease, alopecia areata 87.23, 87.25, 87.28
nail dysplasia 67.15
- nail–patella syndrome 67.15
- with triangular lunula 67.15, *67.16*

nail dystrophy
- dyskeratosis congenita 67.13, *67.14*
- epidermolysis bullosa *69.11, 69.13*, 69.15, *69.16*
- gold toxicity 121.4
- melanoma 145.13
- pachyonychia congenita 63.51, 67.11
- peeling skin syndromes 69.20
- pigmentation disorders 68.12
- primary systemic amyloidosis 56.13

nail fold, mixed connective tissue disease 53.2
nail fold capillaroscopy 54.16
nail fold infection, candidiasis 32.65–32.66
nail fold necrosis, systemic lupus erythematosus 51.25
nail growth, genetic defects of 67.1–67.17
nail matrix epithelium 119.7
nail-patella-like renal disease 67.15, 154.1–154.2
nail–patella syndrome (NPS) 67.15–67.16, 154.1–154.2
nail picking (onychotillomania) 84.25
nail plate fungal infections *see* onychomycosis
Nail Psoriasis Severity Index (NAPSI) 16.3
nails 2.10–2.11
- acrodermatitis continua of Hallopeau 35.40
- allergic reactions 127.13, 127.15, 127.21, 127.47, 127.48, 127.49, 127.61–127.62
- anatomy and structure 2.11
- atopic eczema 41.18
- basal keratinocyte layers 2.11
- blue nail discoloration due to antimalarial therapy 51.25
- chloroquine pigmentation, systemic lupus erythematosus 51.23
- clubbing, internal malignancy links 148.18
- dermatomyositis 52.5, *52.9*
- embryonic development 2.5
- factitious nail disease 84.33
- genetic defects of 67.1–67.17
- hyperpigmentation, vitamin B12 deficiency 61.20
- inherited immunodeficiency **80.4–80.6**
- iron deficiency 61.24
- lichen planus 37.11–37.12
- lichen striatus 37.18
- melanoma 142.10–142.11, *142.15, 145.12*, 145.13
- metal poisoning signs 121.1
- mixed connective tissue disease 53.2
- nail bed 2.11, 119.7
- nail matrix 2.11, 119.7
- pigmentation effects of renal failure and dialysis 154.3
- pitting, psoriatic 35.12
- pityriasis rubra pilaris 36.3
- psoriasis vulgaris 35.10–35.11, *35.12*
- psoriatic subungual hyperkeratosis with distal onycholysis 35.12
- rheumatoid arthritis 53.7
- role of 2.43

salmon patches ('oil drops'), psoriasis vulgaris *35.12*
sarcoidosis 96.13
selenium excess 61.30
subungual hyperkeratosis and splinter haemorrhages 36.3
syphilis 29.10
systemic lupus erythematosus 51.23, 51.25
systemic sclerosis 54.16
yellow-nail syndrome 103.21–103.22, 152.6
see also onychomycosis
nail samples, superficial mycoses identification 32.7
'naked granuloma' 96.2
NAME (nevi, atrial myxoma, ephelides) *see* Carney complex
Nannizia species (*Microsporum*) **32.19**, 32.26
nano-pulse stimulation (NPS) technology 161.10
NAPPA *see* Nail Assessment in Psoriasis and Psoriatic Arthritis
nappy/diaper/napkin area
- dermatitis 40.5, 115.3, 128.5
- perianal candidiasis of infancy 32.65

NAPSI *see* Nail Psoriasis Severity Index
narcotic drugs, recreational use 120.1
narrow-band UVB (NB-UVB/TL-01) phototherapy
- adverse effects/risks 21.11–21.13, 21.15, 21.17
- combination therapy 21.10
- indications/efficacy 21.3–21.4, 21.5, 21.7
- polymorphic light eruption 126.7–126.8, *126.36*
- principles 21.1, 21.2–21.3
- psoriasis treatment 35.22–35.23
- regimen 21.8

nasal alar ulceration, trigeminal trophic syndrome 82.7, *82.8*
nasal glioma *see* glial heterotopic nodules
nasal type extranodal NK/T-cell lymphoma 139.36–139.37
nasal vestibule
- carriage of *Staphylococcus aureus* 26.4, 26.7–26.8
- microbiome 26.5

naso-labial fold, dermal fillers 158.2
nasopalpebral lipoma–coloboma syndrome **72.10**
nasopharyngeal carcinoma, Epstein–Barr virus association 25.49
natal teeth, pachyonychia congenita 67.12
National Cancer Registration and Analysis Service (NCRAS), basal cell carcinoma incidence 140.1
national and international organisations, psychodermatology 17.7
National Library of Medicine's bibliographic database (MEDLINE) 17.7
NATs *see* N-acetyltransferases
natural gene therapy 8.8
natural history of skin diseases 5.11–5.12
natural killer (NK)/T cell extranodal lymphoma 139.36–139.37
natural rubber latex (NRL)
- allergy testing 4.24, 129.7
- allergy to rubber gloves 39.14, 127.63
- contact urticaria 127.84–127.85
- genital contact dermatitis 109.13

nausea, PUVA phototherapy adverse effects 21.13
Naxos syndrome 63.62–63.63, 69.7
NBCCS *see* naevoid basal cell carcinoma syndrome
NB-UVB *see* narrow-band UVB
NCRAS *see* National Cancer Registration and Analysis Service
Nd:YAG *see* erbium:yttrium-aluminium-garnet lasers
near infrared lymphangiography (ICG lymphography), lymphatic system 103.56–103.57

neat (insoluble) cutting oils 129.12
Necator americanus, ancylostomiasis 33.15–33.17
neck
- ageing of skin 156.4–156.5
- allergic contact dermatitis of 127.14, 127.16
- atopic eczema 41.18
- botulinum toxins, aesthetic uses of 159.6
- bullous lupus erythematosus 51.28
- 'dirty neck', atopic 41.18
- dyskeratosis congenita 75.3
- folliculitis keloidalis 88.37, 93.3
- granuloma annulare 95.2
- infantile haemangioma 116.3
- Kaposiform haemangioendothelioma 116.9
- lymph nodes and lymphatic drainage basins 106.28
- morphoea 55.23–55.24
- oedema 103.46–103.49
- perforating granuloma annulare 95.7
- plane xanthomatosis 60.5
- progressive hemifacial atrophy 55.25
- reticulate pigmentation, atopic eczema 41.18
- systemic lupus erythematosus 51.23
- white fibrous papulosis of 94.39–94.40

necrobiosis 3.42
necrobiosis-lipoidica-like lesions 96.13
necrobiosis lipoidica (NLD) 95.8–95.13, 97.11–97.12, 97.15
- associated diseases 95.9
- atrophy 95.11, *95.13*
- atypical facial necrobiosis 95.12
- clinical features 95.11
- diabetic patients 62.5, *62.6*, 95.12
- differential diagnosis 95.11–95.12
- epidemiology 95.9
- incidence and prevalence 95.9
- management 95.12–95.13
- necrobiotic inflammation 95.10
- pathology 95.10, *95.11*
- pathophysiology 95.9–95.10
- rheumatoid nodule differentiation 97.16–97.17
- telangiectasia 95.11
- treatment ladder 95.13

necrobiotic palisading granulomas 95.2–95.3
necrobiotic xanthogranuloma (NXG) 97.17–97.18, 135.24–135.25, 149.11
necrolysis 3.42
necrolytic acral erythema (NAE), hepatitis C 25.76, 153.5
necrolytic migratory erythema (NME) 47.12–47.16, 110.44–110.45, 153.6
- clinical features 47.13–47.14
- clinical variants 47.15
- dermatoendocrinology **150.10**, 150.12, *150.14*, 150.19
- disease course and prognosis 47.16
- epidemiology 47.13
- histology *47.13*
- investigations 47.14, 47.16
- pathology 47.13
- presentation 47.14
- treatment for 47.16

necrosis 3.42
- chemical peels **160.4**
- diabetic foot with neurotrophic ulceration and necrosis ('mal perforans') 62.2
- drug-induced 120.7
- penis 109.22–109.24

necrotic adipocytes 97.7–97.8
- alpha-1 antitrypsin *97.44*
- cold panniculitis 97.36
- fat necrosis 97.55

necrotic keratinocytes, acute generalised exanthematous pustulosis 118.2
necrotising fasciitis 26.77, 26.78, 111.15, 130.7
- eyelid 107.39
- neonates 114.26

necrotising granulomatous lesions 80.10

necrotising infundibular crystalline folliculitis 63.76
necrotising lymphocytic folliculitis, scalp margin 91.12–91.13, 93.4–93.5
necrotising otitis externa 106.19
necrotising sarcoid granulomatosis, respiratory involvement 152.6
necrotising sialometaplasia, oral ulceration 108.42
necrotising soft-tissue infections, perineal and perianal skin 111.15
necrotising subcutaneous infections 26.77–26.78
needle biopsy 3.4
needle injection, dermal fillers 158.1–158.2, **158.3**, *158.4*
needs assessments
  access to dermatological health services 5.12
  global health dermatology 7.12–7.13
NEFAs *see* non-esterified fatty acids
negative network dermoscopy patterns
  melanomas 145.7, *145.8*
  naevi 145.6
Neglected Tropical Disease Non-Governmental Organisation Network (NNN) 7.6
neglected tropical diseases (NTDs) 7.2, 7.6, 7.7
  training guide for frontline health workers 7.11–7.12
NEH *see* neutrophilic eccrine hidradenitis
Neisser, Albert 1.6, 1.8
Neisseria gonorrhoeae 30.1–30.2, 30.8
Neisseria meningitidis 26.49–26.50
Nékam disease 37.10–37.11, 37.16
Nelson syndrome 86.7, 86.18, *86.19*
Nematocera 34.6–34.7
nematocysts, stings 130.1–130.2
nematodes
  infection with human nematodes 33.1–33.18
  infection with other animal nematodes 33.18–33.26
NEMO, pigmentation disorders 68.10
neoadjuvant systemic treatment, melanoma 144.6
neoangiogenesis 101.1
neomycin
  patch testing 127.47
  topical therapies 18.11
neonatal acne 88.68–88.74
neonatal candidiasis 114.28
neonatal candidiasis *see* congenital candidiasis
neonatal cold panniculitis 97.36–97.37
neonatal erythroderma 63.40
neonatal herpes, primary HSV infection in mother 25.27
neonatal ichthyosis–sclerosing cholangitis (NISCH) 63.41
neonatal lupus erythematosus (NLE) 51.39–51.42
  associated diseases 51.39
  cardiac involvement 151.4
  cardiac problems 51.41
  clinical features 51.40–51.41
  disease course and prognosis 51.41
  environmental factors 51.40
  genetics 51.39–51.40
  haematological and hepatic problems 51.41
  pathophysiology 51.39
  pregnancy 51.41–51.42
  in pregnancy 113.7–113.8
  'racoon' eyelid lesions *51.40*
neonatal onset of pancytopenia, autoinflammation, rash and episodes of hemophagocytic lymphohistiosis syndrome 45.18–45.19
neonatal progeria syndrome **77.2**
neonatal progeroid syndrome 70.30–70.31
neonates 114.1–114.30
  acute pseudomembranous candidiasis 108.31

ADAM17 deficiency 45.16
adnexal polyp 114.19
alopecia 114.4
anetoderma of prematurity 114.9–114.10
antenatal procedures, complications arising from **114.10**
atrophic lesions of 114.11
bacterial infections 114.24–114.28
'blueberry muffin' baby 114.21
breast abscesses 114.25
bullous impetigo 114.24
cervico-facial oedema *71.28*
cleansing and moisturising of skin 114.2
cold injury 114.15, **114.18**
cold panniculitis 114.14
collodion baby 63.8, 63.12–63.13, 63.43–63.44, 114.19–114.21
congenital cytomegalovirus infection 25.41
congenital erosive and vesicular dermatosis 114.9
congenital heart block 51.39–51.42
congenital rubella 114.23
congenital syphilis 114.27–114.28
congenital tuberculosis 114.28
cutis marmorata 114.3
desquamation 114.3–114.4
eccrine sweating 114.3
ecthyma gangrenosum 114.27
epidermolysis bullosa 69.23–69.25
Epstein pearls 114.4
erosions in, differential diagnosis **114.24**
erythema neonatorum 114.3
fetal varicella syndrome 114.23
fungal infections 114.28–114.29
gonococcal ophthalmia neonatorum 30.3, *30.4*
gonorrhoea 30.3, 30.4, 30.5
harlequin colour change 114.3
herpes simplex virus infection 25.21, 25.27, 114.22
human immunodeficiency virus infection 114.24
hyperpigmentary disorders 114.4
hypoxia 114.3
infantile acropustulosis 114.8
infections 114.22–114.29
lentiginosis profusa 131.3
listeriosis 26.46, 114.26–114.27
lupus erythematosus 51.39–51.42, 114.12–114.14
Malassezia pustulosis 114.28–114.29
mastitis 114.25
maternal autoantibodies, transplacental transfer of 114.11–114.12
maternal malignant disease, transplacental transfer of 114.14
maternal milk, transfer of toxic substances in 114.14
medallion-like dermal dendrocyte hamartoma 114.11
medical procedures, complications arising from **114.10**
Michelin tyre baby syndrome 70.19, 73.17
microbial ecology of the skin 26.4, 26.5, 26.7
milia 114.4
miliaria 114.6–114.7
'miniature puberty' 114.4
necrotising fasciitis 114.26
noma neonatorum (cancrum oris/oro-facial gangrene) 114.27
nomenclature 114.1
Noonan syndrome *71.28*
occipital alopecia 114.4
omphalitis 114.26
oral findings 114.4
orbital cellulitis 114.26
pemphigoid gestationis, transplacental 114.12
pemphigus vulgaris 114.12
percutaneous absorption, toxicity risk 114.2
peripheral cyanosis (acrocyanosis) 114.3

periporitis staphylogenes 114.25
phytotherapy-induced rashes **114.11**
pityriasis rubra pilaris 36.4
postmature neonates 114.4
prematurity, complications of 114.9–114.10
preorbital cellulitis 114.26
purpura fulminans 114.21–114.22, 114.27
pustular eruptions **114.8**
raised linear bands of infancy 114.18–114.19
sclerema neonatorum 97.59–97.60, 114.17–114.18
sebaceous gland hypertrophy 114.4
sebaceous gland secretion 114.3
sepsis risk 114.2
skin appearance 114.3–114.4
skin barrier function 114.1–114.3
skin blistering 69.24
skin disorders 114.5–114.9, 114.18–114.22
small-for-dates 114.4
staphylococcal cold abscesses of the large folds 114.25
staphylococcal scalded skin syndrome 114.24–114.25
subcutaneous fat disorders 114.14–114.18
subcutaneous fat necrosis 114.15–114.17, **114.18**
subcutaneous fat necrosis of 97.57–97.58
succulent gums 114.4
suction blisters 114.4
sweat gland abscesses 114.25
sweating 114.3
terminology 114.1
toxic erythema of the newborn 114.5–114.6
transepidermal water loss 114.2
transient myeloproliferative disorder 114.8
transient pustular melanosis 114.7–114.8
transplacental transfer/maternal milk-induced disorders 114.11–114.14
umbilical cord care 114.2–114.3
vernix caseosa 114.3, 114.4
viral infections 114.22–114.24
vitamin K deficiency 61.13
see also infants
neoplasia 86.19–86.20
  acquired ichthyosis association 85.1
  cutaneous metastases from gastrointestinal tract 153.1
  gastrointestinal and skin manifestations **153.7**
  infiltration of skin with neoplastic cells from haematological malignancies 149.2–149.5
  Merkel cell carcinoma 146.1–146.10
  musculoskeletal therapy relationship to skin cancer 155.15–155.16
  renal tumours related to hereditary syndromes 154.2
  rosacea 89.10
  skin manifestations of haematological neoplasms 149.1–149.15
  skin tumours in immunosuppressed renal allograft recipients 154.6
  umbilical metastases 153.1
neoplastic process, epithelioid sarcoma 97.15
neoprene allergy 127.64
Neoscytalidium species, superficial mycoses 32.51–32.52
nephritic factors, APL pathology 98.4
nephrocalcinosis 97.58
nephrogenic pruritus 81.8–81.9
nephrogenic systemic fibrosis **54.20**, 94.43–94.45
  differences from scleromyxoedema **57.5**
  renal dysfunction 154.5
nephropathic cystinosis, flushing in children **104.10**
nephropathy, autosomal recessive epidermolysis bullosa simplex with 69.11

nephrotic syndrome
  junctional epidermolysis bullosa with 69.15
  secondary dyslipidaemia and 60.12
  zinc deficiency associated with *61.26*
nephrotoxicity
  ciclosporin 19.11
  methotrexate 19.26
NEPPK *see* non-epidermolytic palmoplantar keratoderma
NER *see* nucleotide excision repair
nerve damage, skin surgery 20.42
nerve endings
  hair follicle 87.7
  hyperplasia 2.12
nerve entrapment syndromes 83.6–83.8
nerve sheath myxoma 136.47–136.48
nervous system
  anatomical considerations for skin surgery 20.2–20.4
  anatomy of head and neck 20.2–20.4
  anatomy of limbs 20.4
  autonomic 2.2–2.3, 83.4–83.5
  cutaneous innervation 83.2–83.4
  endocrine system relationship 150.2
  sensory innervation 83.2–83.4
  see also neurological disorders
NESS *see* Nottingham Eczema Severity Score
Netherton syndrome 63.26–63.28, **78.14**, 87.79, *87.80*
  pruritus in 63.46
  skin cancer 147.2
  SPINK5 69.6
  target therapy 63.45
network naevi *see* reticular pattern naevi
neuralgia
  genitofemoral neuropathic pain/neuralgia 83.7
  iliohypogastric neuropathic pain/neuralgia 83.7
  ilioinguinal neuropathic pain/neuralgia 83.7
  post-herpetic neuralgia 108.66
  pudendal neuropathic pain/neuralgia 83.7, 83.8
  trigeminal neuralgia 108.66–108.67
neural tissue tumours/neuromas *see* peripheral neuroectodermal tumours
neurocutaneous syndromes, ocular features **107.42**
neurodermatitis 127.15
neurodermatitis circumscripta *see* lichen simplex chronicus
neuroendocrine markers, cutaneous neoplasms 3.23
neuroendocrine stress response in skin, brain–skin axis 150.8–150.9
neuroendocrinology
  hair follicle 87.11–87.13
  (neuro-)endocrine contributions to cutaneous pathogenesis 150.9–150.10
  skin and hair as research models 150.9
neurofibromas 136.45–136.47
  cutaneous neurofibromas 78.3
  plexiform neurofibromas 78.3
  vulva **110.32**
neurofibromatoses 78.1–78.7
  mosaic neurofibromatosis type 1 78.4–78.7
  RASopathies 78.7, *78.8*, **78.9**
neurofibromatosis type 1 (NF1/von Recklinghausen disease) 78.1–78.4, **78.9**, 108.87, 148.9, 149.14
  clinical features 78.3
  diagnostic criteria **78.2**
  investigations 78.4
  lung disease 152.5
  malignant tumours in 78.3–78.4
  management 78.4, *78.5–78.6*
  Manchester checklist 78.4, *78.5–78.6*
  neurological disease 78.3
  oral involvement 108.87
  pathophysiology 78.1–78.3

neurofibromatosis type 1 (NF1/von Recklinghausen disease) (continued)
  renal involvement 154.1
  skeletal abnormalities 78.3
neurofibromatosis type 2 148.9
neurofibromin, juvenile xanthogranuloma 135.15
neurofibrosarcoma *see* malignant peripheral nerve sheath tumour
neurofilament, Merkel cell carcinoma 3.23
neurogenic pathways, rosacea 89.3
neuro-ichthyotic syndromes 63.30–63.39, **63.31**
neurokinin 1 receptor (NK1R), pruritus 81.4
neurolabyrinthitis (eighth nerve deafness), congenital syphilis 29.26
neurological abnormalities
  congenital melanocytic naevi 73.12–73.13
  secondary syphilis 29.10, 29.12
  xeroderma pigmentosum 76.5
neurological causes
  anhidrosis **92.11**
  hyperhidrosis **92.11**
neurological complications
  varicella infection 25.30
  zoster infection 25.32, 25.33–25.34
neurological disorders 83.1–83.25
  antibodies and targeted structures in skin biopsies 83.6
  autonomic nervous system 83.4–83.5
  brachioradial pruritus 83.6–83.7
  burning feet syndrome 83.10–83.11
  of childhood 83.2
  cold-induced vasodilation 83.5
  complex regional pain syndrome 83.20–83.23
  cutaneous innervation 83.2–83.4
  diagnosis 83.5
  distal symmetrical polyneuropathy, causes 83.9
  dysaesthesia 83.5–83.6, 83.7
  genetic neurocutaneous disorders 83.1–83.6
  genitofemoral neuropathic pain/neuralgia 83.7
  gustatory hyperhidrosis 83.24
  hereditary neuropathies 83.11–83.24
  hereditary sensory and autonomic neuropathies 83.12
  Horner syndrome 83.23–83.24
  iliohypogastric neuropathic pain/neuralgia 83.7
  ilioinguinal neuropathic pain/neuralgia 83.7
  mechanical injuries 122.1
  meralgia paraesthetica 83.7
  midface toddler excoriation syndrome due to pain insensitivity 83.12–83.13
  motor polyneuropathy **83.8**
  nerve entrapment syndromes 83.6–83.8
  nervous system and the skin 83.1–83.6
  neuropathic pruritus 81.11–81.12
  neuropathic ulcer 83.13–83.19
  neurophysiological testing for skin innervation 83.5
  NF1-related tumours, secondary to 78.3
  notalgia paraesthetica 83.7
  oral involvement 108.83
  peripheral neuropathy 83.8–83.10
  pruritus 83.5–83.6
  pudendal neuropathic pain/neuralgia 83.7, 83.8
  restless leg syndrome 83.10–83.11
  scalp pruritus **105.15**
  sensory innervation 83.2–83.4
  sensory polyneuropathy **83.8**
  skin biopsy 83.5, **83.6**
  small fibre neuropathy **83.9**
  spinal cord injury 83.19–83.20
  spinal dysraphism 83.17–83.19
  substance P immunoreactive nerve endings in the epidermis 83.3
  sympathetic nerve injury 83.20

sympathetic skin response 83.5
syringomyelia 83.16–83.17
systemic lupus erythematosus 51.31–51.32
triple response of Lewis 83.5
tuberous sclerosis complex 78.8–78.9
neurological manifestations
  BSL association 98.15
  palmoplantar keratodermas 63.71
neuromuscular blocking agents (NMBA) 117.7
neuromuscular hamartoma 136.42
neuromuscular toxicity
  antimalarials 19.6
  glucocorticoids *19.19*
neuropathic changes, burning mouth syndrome 82.2
neuropathic pain 123.10
  acute herpetic neuralgia 82.4
  IASP definition 82.5
  leprosy 28.16
  somatosensory system lesions/disease 82.5–82.6
  trigeminal neuropathic pain syndrome 82.5–82.7
neuropathic ulcer 83.13–83.19
  Aircast Walker's boot *83.16*
  clinical features 83.13–83.14
  investigations 83.14
  management 83.14–83.16
  probing a neuropathic wound *83.15*
  sensory loss assessment *83.15*
  severity classification 83.14
  treatment ladder 83.16
  Wagner foot ulcer classification **83.14**
neuropathy, *see also* peripheral neuropathy
neuropeptides
  pruritus 81.3, 81.4, 81.5, 81.8, 81.15, 81.20
  see also endothelin 1; substance P
neuropeptides/neurotransmitters, hormone relationship 150.2–150.3
neurosarcoidosis 96.5
neurosyphilis 29.15–29.16, 29.21
  congenital 29.26
neurothekeoma *see* cellular neurothekeoma; dermal nerve sheath myxoma
neurotransmitter-affecting peptides, cosmeceutical use of *157.6*
neurotrophins, pruritus 81.3, 81.4
neurovascular disorders 101.6–101.9
neutral lipid storage disease with ichthyosis (NLSDI) 63.35–63.36
neutral lipid storage disease with myopathy (NLSDM) 63.36
neutropenia, haemophagocytic lymphohistiocytosis 135.12
neutrophil adhesion defects, inherited immunodeficiency 80.15–80.16
neutrophil differentiation defects, inherited immunodeficiency 80.15
neutrophilic cicatricial alopecias 87.48–87.50
neutrophilic dermatoses 49.1–49.22
  amicrobial pustulosis of the skin folds 49.20–49.21
  aseptic abscess syndrome 49.21
  bowel-associated dermatitis–arthritis syndrome 49.15–49.17
  internal malignancy association 148.23–148.24
  involving respiratory system 152.5
  pyoderma gangrenosum 49.1–49.8
  pyodermatitis-pyostomatitis vegetans 49.19–49.20
  subcorneal pustular dermatosis 49.17–49.19
  see also Sweet syndrome
neutrophilic dermatosis, rheumatoid arthritis 155.6, *155.8*
neutrophilic eccrine hidradenitis (NEH) 92.14–92.15, 119.2, 149.7–149.8
neutrophilic folliculitis 91.13
neutrophilic genital ulceration, Behçet-like syndrome associated with trisomy 8 myelodysplasia 149.8

neutrophilic granulomatous dermatitis, in patient with rheumatoid arthritis *53.7*
neutrophilic lobular panniculitis 97.50–97.53
neutrophils 2.32
  immune cells in homeostasis *9.4*
  microscopic examination of 3.35
  wound healing 11.2–11.3
neutrophil–macrophage colony-forming unit (NM-CFU) 135.1
Neu–Laxova syndrome (NLS) 63.38
nevoid basal cell carcinoma syndrome, basaloid follicular hamartoma 137.13
newborns *see* neonates
Newton law, viscoelastic materials 122.3
New-World cutaneous leishmaniasis *33.44*, 33.45, 33.46, 33.49, 33.50–33.51
next generation sequencing (NGS) 69.23
NF1 *see* neurofibromatosis type 1
NF-kB pathway-related primary immunodeficiencies 80.16
NFTC *see* normophosphataemic familial tumoral calcinosis
NGS *see* next generation sequencing
niacinamide, topical depigmenting agents 18.33
niacin (vitamin B3) deficiency 61.15–61.17
NICH *see* non-involuting congenital haemangioma
nickel allergy 127.36–127.39
  dimethylglyoxime test 127.33, *127.34*
  prevention strategies 127.2
  prognosis 127.23
  sites of 127.16
  social factors 127.4–127.5
nicorandil ulceration, peristomal skin 112.10, *112.12*
nicotinamide 88.57, 121.3
nicotinamide-adenine dinucleotide (NAD), niacin deficiency 61.15, 61.16
nicotinamide and nicotinic acid, topical therapies 18.41
NICU *see* non-immune contact urticaria
nidogens 2.25
Niemann–Pick disease 79.5
Nightcliff gardener's disease *see* melioidosis
Nijmegen breakage syndrome **80.4**
Nikolsky sign 118.14, 122.2–122.3
nintedanib, systemic sclerosis treatment 54.24
NIPAL4 mutations
  congenital ichthyosiform erythroderma 63.11, 63.12
  keratinopathic ichthyoses 63.14
nipple
  adenoma 137.21–137.22
  'guitar nipple' 122.12
  hyperkeratosis of 63.79
  inverted, glycosylation disorders **79.10**
  jogger's nipples 122.16
  Paget disease 137.41
NISCH *see* neonatal ichthyosis–sclerosing cholangitis
nitrite and nitric oxide, topical therapies 18.41
'nitritoid' reaction, gold toxicity 121.4
nivirapine, hypersensitivity reactions **14.6**
nivolumab, panniculitis induced by *97.53*
NK1R *see* neurokinin 1 receptor
NK *see* natural killer
NLD *see* necrobiosis lipoidica
NLE *see* neonatal lupus erythematosus
NLRC4-associated autoinflammatory disease (NLRC 4-AID) **45.5**, **45.7**, 45.16
NLRP1-associated autoinflammation with arthritis and dyskeratosis (NAIAD) 45.8, 45.18
NLR SkinApp 7.12
NLS *see* Neu–Laxova syndrome
NLSDI *see* neutral lipid storage disease with ichthyosis
NLSDM *see* neutral lipid storage disease with myopathy

NM *see* nodular melanoma
NMBA *see* neuromuscular blocking agents
NM-CFU *see* neutrophil–macrophage colony-forming unit
NME *see* necrolytic migratory erythema
N-methyl-3,4-methylenedioxymetamphetamine (MDMA) *see* ecstasy
NMSC *see* non-melanoma skin cancer
NNN *see* Neglected Tropical Disease Non-Governmental Organisation Network
NNN Skin NTD CCG *see* Skin Related NTDs Cross Cutting Group
NNTs *see* numbers needed to treat
Nocardia spp., nocardiosis 26.86–26.87
NOCARH *see* neonatal onset of pancytopenia, autoinflammation, rash and episodes of hemophagocytic lymphohistiosis syndrome
nociceptive pain 123.10
nodular actinic elastosis 94.3–94.4
nodular basal cell carcinoma 140.3, *140.4*, *140.8*, *140.11*
nodular fasciitis 94.43, 108.12, 136.5
nodular or granulomatous candidiasis of the napkin area 32.65
nodular histiocytosis 135.19
nodular lesions, Langerhans cell histiocytosis 135.6
nodular lichen myxoedematosus 57.6, 57.7
nodular melanoma (NM)
  dermoscopic patterns 145.13, *145.14*
  melanoma classification 142.7
  presentation 142.10, *142.12*, 142.19
nodular morphoea 55.15–55.16
nodular prurigo *see* prurigo nodularis
nodular sarcoidosis 96.7–96.8
nodular (tubercular) syphilide 29.12–29.14
nodular (tumefactive) primary localised cutaneous amyloidosis **56.3**, 56.5, *56.8*
nodular vasculitis
  as a tuberculid 27.29, 27.31
  see also erythema induratum of Bazin
nodular–cystic fat necrosis 97.55
nodules
  hidradenitis suppurativa *90.6*
  Merkel cell carcinoma 146.5, *146.6*
  onchocerciasis 33.5
  sarcoidosis 96.8–96.9
nodulocystic hidradenoma *see* hidradenoma
noma neonatorum (cancrum oris/oro-facial gangrene) 114.27
non-ablative fractional resurfacing (NAFR) 161.2, **161.5**
non-ablative lasers, hidradenitis suppurativa treatment 90.11
non-ablative resurfacing, laser therapy 23.23–23.24
non-accidental injury (NAI), infants 115.14
non-adherence to medical regimes 15.2
non-AIDS-defining cancers (NADC), people living with HIV 147.2–147.3
non-blanchable erythema 123.4, **123.5**, 123.8
non-bullous impetigo 26.13, 26.14
non-classical (atypical) epidermodysplasia verruciformis 25.66, 25.69
non-draining lesions, Hurley stage III disease *90.9*
non-draining tunnel, hidradenitis suppurativa *90.4*
non-eczematous responses, allergens 127.17–127.21
non-epidermolytic palmoplantar keratoderma (NEPPK) 63.53–63.56
non-esterified fatty acids (NEFAs) 97.4
non-follicular pustules, acute generalised exanthematous pustulosis 118.3
non-formaldehyde-releasing preservatives 127.52–127.53

non-Hodgkin lymphoma (NHL)
  AIDS defining cancer   147.2
  immunocompromised patients   147.1, 147.3
  infiltration of skin with neoplastic cells   149.4
  oral involvement   108.71
  see also chronic lymphocytic leukaemia
non-hyaluronic acid (non-HA) dermal fillers   158.5–158.6, **158.11**
non-immune contact urticaria (NICU)   127.83, 127.86, 128.8–128.9
non-inflamed nodules, Hurley stage II disease   *90.4*
non-inflamed phyma, treatment   **89.14**
non-inflammatory disorders of subcutaneous fat   98.1–98.30
non-involuting congenital haemangioma (NICH)   *71.2*
non-Langerhans cell histiocytoses (non-LCHs)   135.14–135.21
non-LSH lesions   135.6
non-malignancy, generalised hypertrichosis association   87.86–87.87
non-malignant tumours, infants   116.1–116.11
non-melanin pigmentation   86.47–86.54
non-melanoma skin cancer (NMSC)
  arsenic exposure   121.3
  incidence of in Denmark/Slovakia   6.1
  PUVA phototherapy adverse effects   21.14
  recurrence in   6.5
  rheumatoid patients   155.15
non-scarring alopecia   87.28–87.35, 98.24
non-segmental vitiligo   86.34, 86.38
non-sexually acquired genital ulcers   110.19–110.20
non-sexually transmitted infections, male genitalia   109.26–109.28
non-specific balanoposthitis   109.21–109.22
non-specific cicatricial alopecia   87.51
non-specific hyperreactivity, patch testing   127.32
non-steroidal anti-inflammatory drugs (NSAIDs)
  allergic contact dermatitis   127.45, 127.79
  cutaneous adverse effects   155.15
  frostbite   124.3
  photosensitivity   126.27, 126.29, 126.31
  urticaria   117.6
non-syndromic autosomal recessive deafness   63.63
non-syndromic congenital ichthyoses   63.7–63.13
non-syndromic genodermatoses with nail anomalies   **67.9**
non-syndromic ichthyoses   **63.3**, 63.20–63.22
non-syndromic palmoplantar keratodermas   63.50–63.62
non-syphilitic bacterial sexually transmitted diseases   30.1–30.26
non-syphilitic spirochaetal ulcerative balanoposthitis   109.27
non-tuberculous mycobacteria (NTM)   27.1, 27.2, 27.3, 27.32–27.45
  classification   27.32
  disseminated disease   27.32–27.36, 27.38, 27.40–27.45
  disseminated tuberculous disease   27.32, 27.33, 27.34, 27.35–27.36, 27.38, 27.40, 27.42, 27.43, 27.44, 27.45
  infection diagnosis   27.5
Noonan with multiple lentigines syndrome (LEOPARD syndrome)   **131.3**, 151.3
Noonan syndrome   78.9, 103.21, **106.7**
  granular cell tumours   136.49
  neonates   *71.28*
  oral involvement   108.86
noradrenergic and specific serotonergic antidepressants (NaSSAs)   84.43, **84.45**
norepinephrine reuptake inhibitors (SNRIs)   84.43

normocomplementaemic urticarial vasculitis (NUV)   44.1, 44.3, 44.4, 44.5
normolipaemic plane xanthoma   97.18
normolipaemic xanthoma, paraprotein activity   149.11
normophosphataemic familial tumoral calcinosis (NFTC)   79.17
North American blastomycosis   32.84, *32.86*
Norwegian scabies   39.34, *63.72*
nose
  fibrous papules   136.2–136.3
  granuloma faciale   *100.12*
  inflammatory chondopathy effects   155.12
  primary localised cutaneous amyloidosis   *56.8*
  radiotherapy for skin cancer   24.11–24.12, *24.20*
  see also nasal entries; olfactory entries
nosological relationship, to rosacea   89.15–89.17
nosology   8.2–8.5
notalgia paraesthetica   83.7
  pruritus   81.12
notch signalling, hidradenitis suppurativa genetics   90.3
Nottingham Eczema Severity Score (NESS)   16.4
NPS *see* nail–patella syndrome; nano-pulse stimulation technology
NRL *see* natural rubber latex
NRS-11 *see* Numeric Rating Scale
NRTI *see* nucleoside reverse transcriptase inhibitor
NSAIDs *see* non-steroidal anti-inflammatory drugs
NSDHL mutations, CHILD syndrome   63.23–63.24
NTDs *see* neglected tropical diseases
NTM *see* non-tuberculous mycobacteria
nuchal-type fibroma   136.12
nuclear factor kappa-light-chain enhancer of activated B cells-autoinflammatory disease   45.16
nuclear hormone receptors
  hair growth   87.10
  intracellular drug mechanisms   13.5
nucleic acid amplification tests, *Mycobacterium tuberculosis*   27.8–27.9
nucleoside reverse transcriptase inhibitor (NRTI), HAART regimes   98.6–98.7
nucleotide excision repair (NER)   10.5–10.6, 76.2
numb chin syndrome (mental neuropathy), internal malignancy association   148.23
numbers needed to treat (NNTs), evidence based medicine   17.11, **17.12**
Numeric Rating Scale (NRS-11), peak itch over past 24 hours   16.3
nummular dermatitis   39.7–39.9
  associated diseases   39.7
  causative organisms   39.8
  clinical features   39.8, *39.9*
  differential diagnosis   39.8–39.9
  discoid skin lesions   **39.10**
  environmental factors   39.8
  epidemiology   39.7
  infected dermatitis   *39.25*
  investigations   39.9
  management   39.9
  treatment for   39.9
nutrition
  acne   **88.20–88.24**, 88.26
  epidermolysis bullosa   69.25
  hair disorders   87.93
  hypermetabolism treatment   125.11–125.12
  ichthyoses   63.46
  lymphatic system   103.2
  pressure ulcer prevention   123.9–123.10
  SJS/TEN management   118.20
  see also diet; dietary management; mineral disorders; vitamins

nutritional anaemias, skin signs   149.15
nutritional disorders   61.1–61.35
  essential fatty acid deficiency   61.31–61.34
  malnutrition   61.1–61.7
    assessment   61.2
    in children   61.2, 61.3, *61.4*
    classification   61.2, 61.5–61.6
    clinical features   61.3–61.4
    complications and co-morbidities   61.6
    diagnosis   61.5
    disease course and prognosis   61.6
    epidemiology   61.2
    ethnicity role   61.2–61.3
    incidence and prevalence   61.2
    investigations   61.6
    predisposing factors   61.3
    protein-energy malnutrition   61.2, 61.3
    severity classification   61.5–61.6
    skin signs of nutritional disease   **61.5**
  ocular features   **107.41**
  see also mineral disorders; vitamins
NUV *see* normocomplementaemic urticarial vasculitis
NXG *see* necrobiotic xanthogranuloma

O

OA *see* ocular albinism
OAS *see* oral allergy syndrome
obesity
  acne association   **88.23–88.24**
  adiposis dolorosa/Dercum disease   98.17–98.18, 98.28
  and atopic eczema   41.7
  BSL differential diagnosis   98.16
  cutaneous consequences   98.27–98.28
  diabetes patients   62.3
  hereditary obesity   72.3–72.9
  hidradenitis suppurativa association   90.2, 90.10
  lipoedema differential diagnosis   98.22, 98.23
  monogenic obesity with cutaneous features   72.4, **72.7**
  monogenic obesity without cutaneous features   72.3, **72.6**
  Prader–Willi syndrome   72.6–72.9
  pro-opiomelanocortin and prohormone convertase deficiency   72.4–72.6
  psoriasis association   35.18
  secondary skin complications of primary obesity   **72.4**
  skin effects   98.27–98.28
  subcutaneous tissue   97.3
  visceral adipose tissue   97.5
obesity-related lymphoedema   103.38–103.39
obesity-related striae   94.11
objective measures, skin properties   16.5
Objective Severity Assessment Atopic Dermatitis (OSAAD)   16.4
obsessive–compulsive behaviour/disorder (OCD)
  acné excoriée   84.20–84.22
  body dysmorphic disorder   84.12–84.15
  hair loss   87.32
  lichen simplex chronicus   84.15
  nodular prurigo   84.15–84.18
  olfactory delusions   84.10
  psychodermatology   84.12
  skin picking disorder   84.19–84.20
  skin-related health anxieties   84.25–84.26
  trichotillomania/trichotillosis   84.22–84.25, 87.14, 87.24, 87.32–87.34
obstetric risk, pseudoxanthoma elasticum   70.33–70.34
obstetric trauma, perineal skin   *111.7*, **111.8**
OCA *see* oculocutaneous albinism
occipital alopecia, neonates   114.4
occipital horn syndrome   2.34, 79.16
occipital scalp, hair transplantation   87.97
occludins   2.20
occlusive patch testing   127.32
occupational acne   88.66–88.68
  chloracne-inducing chemicals   **88.66**, 129.12

contaminated oil ingestion   **88.68**
differential diagnosis   **88.67**, **88.68**
dioxin accidents   **88.68**
occupational allergic contact dermatitis   129.5–129.7
  methylisothiazolinone   127.53
occupational argyria   86.52
occupational dermatology   129.1–129.17
  workplace visits   129.3–129.4
occupational dermatoses   127.12
  cement-induced   127.40
  classification   1.4
  data collection   127.3
  population studies   127.4
occupational dyspigmentation   129.13–129.14
occupational factors, epidemiology   5.11
occupational groups
  dermatoses occurring in   **4.4**
  history taking   4.4
occupational irritant contact dermatitis   128.2, 128.6, 129.1–129.5
occupational leukoderma   86.45, 129.13–129.14
occupationally-induced skin tumours   129.14–129.15
occupational skin disease, work impact measures   16.12
occupational skin protection programme   128.7
occupational vitiligo   *86.46*
ochronosis   86.50–86.51
Ockelbo disease *see* Sindbis virus
OCP *see* oral contraceptive pill
OCT *see* optical confocal tomography; optimum cutting temperature
octopus stings   130.4
2-*n*-Octyl-4-isothiazolin-3-one (OIT)   127.53, 127.54
ocular albinism (OA)   68.6
ocular anomalies, infiltrating lipomatosis of the face association   98.21
ocular complications of drug therapy   19.6, 19.15–19.16, *19.19*, 107.40–107.44
ocular dermatoses *see* eye
ocular disorders
  Adamantiades–Behçet disease   48.4, *48.6*, **48.8**
  ophthalmic zoster   25.33, 25.34
  ophthalmological terms   **107.5**
  tuberous sclerosis complex   78.9
ocular effects
  congenital syphilis   29.25, *29.28*
  extrapulmonary sarcoidosis   96.5
  long-term SJS/TEN   118.17
  palmoplantar keratodermas   63.70–63.71
  PUVA phototherapy adverse effects   21.14–21.15
  UVB phototherapy adverse effects   21.12–21.13
ocular juvenile xanthogramuloma   135.17
ocular larva migrans   33.21
ocular melanoma   142.11–142.12
ocular pemphigoid   50.26, **50.28**
ocular rosacea   89.1, *89.8*, **107.8**, 107.11–107.12
  clinical signs of   **107.10**
  co-morbidities   89.10–89.11
  complications   89.10–89.11
  major features   89.6
  pathology   89.4
  treatment   89.13, **89.14**, **89.15**
ocular rosacea-like cutaneous rosacea   89.11
ocular signs, phrynoderma   85.15
ocular surface disorders
  atopic eczema   41.20–41.21
  cancers, xeroderma pigmentosum   76.5
  systemic lupus erythematosus   51.32
ocular syphilis   29.16, 107.39–107.40
oculocerebral syndrome with hypopigmentation   68.9
oculocutaneous albinism (OCA)   68.5–68.8, **78.13**
oculocutaneous tyrosinaemia (tyrosinaemia type II)   63.70–63.71

oculomucocutaneous syndromes **108.41**
oculotoxicity
    antimalarials 19.6, 107.43
    dapsone 19.15–19.16
    glucocorticoids *19.19*
odds ratios (ORs), number needed to treat derivation 17.11, **17.12**
Odland bodies 85.17, 85.19
odonto-onycho-dermal dysplasia 63.68
ODSS *see* oral disease severity score
OE *see* otitis externa
oedema
    arm swelling 103.44–103.46
    chronic oedema 103.2, 103.3–103.5, 109.19–109.21
    chronic venous insufficiency **101.43**
    congestive heart failure 85.29
    constriction artefact 84.33
    drug induced oedema 103.12–103.13
    drug reaction with eosinophilia and systemic symptoms 118.8
    erythropoietic protoporphyria *58.14*
    eyelids 103.46
    facial oedema 103.46–103.49
    hand oedema *103.21*
    head oedema 103.46–103.49
    intravenous drug administration *120.7*
    kwashiorkor *61.4*
    lips 103.46, *103.48*
    lymphatic-related hydrops fetalis 103.23
    lymphovenous oedema 103.10–103.12
    neck oedema 103.46–103.49
    penis 109.19–109.21
    venouos oedema 103.10–103.12
    venous leg ulcer *102.5*
    vulval 110.23–110.24
    see also angioedema without weals; lymphoedema
oedema blisters 85.28–85.30
oedematous appearing striae *94.12*
oesophageal atresia, flushing in children **104.10**
oesophageal cancer, tylosis with 63.66, *63.67*, **78.13**
oesophageal involvement, epidermolysis bullosa 69.17–69.18, 69.25
oesophagus, gastro-oesophageal reflux disease 108.74
oesophagus tissue, monkey oesophagus substrate used in indirect immunofluorescence *3.12*, 3.13–3.14, 3.19
oestrogens
    acne vulgaris treatment 88.50–88.51
    pigmentation effects 86.7, 86.25
OFD1 *see* oro-facial–digital syndrome type 1
OFG *see* orofacial granulomatosis
Ofuji disease 91.3, 93.7
OHIP *see* Oral Health Impact Profile
oil hyperkeratoses 129.15
oils, contaminated, occupational acne **88.68**
ointments, vehicle choice for topical therapies 18.2
OIT *see* 2-*n*-Octyl-4-isothiazolin-3-one
old age spot *see* solar lentigo
older people *see* elderly people
Old-World cutaneous leishmaniasis 33.43–33.51
olfactory delusions 84.10–84.11
olfactory reference syndrome (ORS) 84.10–84.11
Olmsted syndrome (congenital palmoplantar and periorificial keratoderma with corneal epithelial dysplasia) 63.69–63.70, 108.30
OLP *see* oral lichen planus
omalizumab
    mastocytosis treatment 46.10
    systemic therapy 19.39
Omenn syndrome **80.4**, 80.7–80.8
omphalitis, neonates 114.26
Onchocerca volvulus 33.1–33.6
onchocerciasis (river blindness) 33.1–33.6, 94.13, 107.40
    ano-genital consequences 109.28

clinical features 33.2–33.5
    epidemiology 33.2
    investigations 33.5–33.6
    management 33.6
    pathophysiology 33.2
oncogenic viruses, skin cancer risks in immunocompromised people 147.8–147.9
oncolytic virus therapy, melanoma 144.1–144.2
Ontak *see* denileukin diftitox
onycholysis 127.21
onychomadesis 119.7
onychomycosis
    caused by *Candida* species 32.66
    caused by dermatophytes 32.47–32.49
    caused by miscellaneous moulds 32.55
    caused by *Neoscytalidium* species 32.51
    caused by non-dermatophyte moulds 32.52–32.55
    caused by *Onychocola canadensis* 32.55
    caused by *Scopulariopsis* species 32.53–32.55
    chronic mucocutaneous candidiasis *32.69*
    identification of causative organism 32.53
    patterns 32.47–32.48
    superficial 32.47–32.48, 32.54–32.55
onychophagia (nail biting) 84.25
onychotillomania (nail picking) 84.25
O'Nyong–Nyong fever, togavirus infections 25.89–25.90
Onzar *see* denileukin diftitox
open tests, allergic contact dermatitis 127.33, 127.86
ophthalmic zoster 25.33, 25.34
ophthalmological effects *see* eye; ocular effects
ophthalmological terms **107.5**
opiates
    pruritus **81.3**, 81.4–81.5, 117.3
    psychodermatology 120.2
opportunistic bacteria on skin 26.2, 26.4, 26.17, 26.51, 26.55, 26.86
opportunistic mycobacteria *see* non-tuberculous mycobacteria
opportunistic systemic mycoses 32.93
optical coherence tomography
    basal cell carcinoma 140.10, *140.12*
    epidermal thickness measurement 16.5
optical confocal tomography (OCT)
    high-definition for basal cell carcinoma 140.10, *140.12*
    melanoma diagnosis 142.9
optimism, adjusting to long-term health conditions 15.3
optimum cutting temperature (OCT) compound, biopsy for DIF examination 3.12
oral allergy syndrome (OAS) 42.13, 108.12, 127.84
oral cancer 108.43–108.50
    basal cell carcinoma of the lip 108.43–108.44
    complications of cancer treatment 108.48–108.50
    florid oral papillomatosis 108.45
    granular cell tumours 108.45
    keratoacanthoma of the lip 108.44
    metastatic oral neoplasms 108.45
    squamous cell carcinoma of the lip 108.44–108.45
    verrucous carcinoma 108.48
oral candidiasis 108.20–108.22, 108.31–108.32, 108.57, *108.71*
    acute pseudomembranous candidiasis 32.61, 108.31, *108.32*
    chronic candidiasis 108.31–108.32
    chronic hyperplastic candidiasis (candidal leukoplakia) 108.34
    chronic mucocutaneous candidiasis 32.68, 108.32
    HIV 31.6, 31.26, 31.34, 31.37
    oral lesions 108.20–108.22, 108.31–108.32, 108.34, 108.57, *108.71*

types of **108.57**
oral cavity 108.1–108.88
    abscesses 108.9
    acanthosis nigricans 108.67
    acquired lesions 108.31–108.35
    acrodermatitis enteropathica 108.20
    actinic cheilitis (solar cheilosis) 108.58
    actinic prurigo 108.58–108.59
    acute candidiasis 108.20
    acute necrotising (ulcerative) gingivitis and noma 108.54–108.55
    acute pseudomembranous candidiasis 108.31, *108.32*
    agranulocytosis 108.71
    allergic reactions in 127.18
    amalgam tattoos 108.15
    amyloidosis 108.69–108.70
    anatomical variants 108.7
    anatomy of 108.3–108.5
    angina bullosa haemorrhagica 108.20
    angioedema 108.10
    angular cheilitis 108.20, 108.59–108.60
    ankyloglossia 108.87
    aphthous-like ulcers 108.38–108.39
    aspergillosis 108.56–108.57
    bacterial infections 108.54–108.56
    basal cell carcinoma of the lip 108.43–108.44
    Behçet syndrome 108.40–108.41
    betel staining *108.15*, 108.17
    biology of 108.3–108.5
    black hairy tongue 108.16, *108.17*
    blastomycoses 108.57
    blisters, causes of **108.36**
    body art 108.15–108.16
    bone marrow transplantation, oral complications of 108.48
    brown tongue 108.16
    buccal fat-pad herniation 108.10
    buccal mucosa, examination of 108.7
    bullous pemphigoid 108.81
    burning mouth syndrome 108.64–108.65
    burns, oral lesions 108.31
    calibre-persistent artery, lip lesions 108.63
    cancer treatment, complications of 108.48–108.50
    Carney complex 108.16
    cervical lymph nodes, drainage areas of **108.6**
    'chapping' of the lips 108.60
    cheek biting 108.32
    cheilitis 108.60–108.63, *108.73*
    chemical burns, oral lesions 108.31
    chickenpox (varicella) 108.51
    chikungunya 108.50
    chronic bullous dermatosis of childhood 108.81
    cleft lip/palate 108.83–108.85
    Clouston syndrome 108.28
    coated tongue 108.16
    coeliac disease 108.72
    complex aphthosis 108.39–108.40
    congenital anomalies 108.87–108.88
    congenital lesions 108.28–108.31
    contact urticaria 42.13
    Cowden syndrome 108.85
    Crohn disease 108.72
    cryptococcosis 108.57
    cytomegalovirus infection 108.51
    Darier disease 108.28
    De Lange syndrome 108.85
    deficiency states 108.70
    dengue 108.50
    dental abscesses 108.9
    dentogingival junction, anatomy of 108.4
    denture-induced hyperplasia 108.10
    denture-induced stomatitis 32.62, 108.20–108.21
    dermatitis herpetiformis 108.81
    dermatological diseases 108.74–108.80
    dermatomyositis 108.67–108.68
    dermoid cyst 108.12
    desquamative gingivitis 108.23
    diagram of *108.4*

double lip 108.85
Down syndrome 108.85
drug-induced hyperpigmentation 108.17
dyskeratosis congenita 108.29
endocrine disorders 108.83
enteroviruses 108.50
epidermolysis bullosa 69.25, 108.23
epidermolysis bullosa acquisita *50.45*, 108.81
epithelioid (bacillary) angiomatosis 108.55
Epstein–Barr virus infections 108.51
erosions 108.36
eruption cyst 108.10
erythema multiforme *47.2*, *47.5*, 108.75
erythematous candidiasis 108.20–108.22
erythroplakia 108.23, *108.24*
erythropoietic protoporphyria 108.85
examination of 108.5–108.8
examinations 118.20
extranodal NK/T-cell lymphoma, nasal type 108.70
facial pain syndromes 108.64–108.67
fauces, examination of 108.7
fibrosis of oral tissues 108.68
fissured tongue 108.87–108.88
floor of mouth, examination of 108.7
florid oral papillomatosis 108.45
focal epithelial hyperplasia 108.11
focal mucinosis 108.85–108.86
focal palmoplantar and oral hyperkeratosis syndrome 108.29
foliate papillae, anatomy of 108.4
foliate papillitis 108.11
Fordyce spots 108.29
fungal infections 108.56–108.57, **108.56**
gamma heavy chain disease (Franklin disease) 108.70
Gardner syndrome 108.86
gastrointestinal diseases 108.72–108.74
gastro-oesophageal reflux disease 108.74
geographic tongue (benign migratory glossitis/erythema migrans) 108.24
geotrichosis 108.57
giant cell arteritis 108.69
gingiva (gums), anatomy of 108.4
gingival lichen planus 108.77
gingival recession, lip/tongue piercing 108.16
gingivitis
    acute necrotising (ulcerative) gingivitis and noma 108.54–108.55
    desquamative gingivitis 108.23, *108.82*
glomovenous malformations 108.25
glossitis 108.22, 108.24–108.25
gonorrhoea 108.55
Gorlin syndrome 108.86
graft-versus-host disease 108.48–108.49, 108.70
granular cell tumours 108.45
granulocytic sarcoma (myeloid sarcoma) 108.70
granulomatosis with polyangiitis 108.69
granulomatous cheilitis *108.73*
haemangioma 108.25–108.26
haematological diseases 108.69–108.72
haematopoietic stem cell transplantation, complications of 108.48
hairy leukoplakia 108.32–108.33, 108.34
hand, foot and mouth disease 108.50
hard tissue benign tumours 108.14
heavy metal induced hyperpigmentation 108.17
hepatitis 108.74
hereditary benign intraepithelial dyskeratosis 108.29
hereditary haemorrhagic telangiectasia (Osler–Rendu–Weber syndrome) 108.26
herpangina 108.50
herpes simplex gingivostomatitis 108.51–108.53
herpes simplex infections 25.20–25.24
herpesviruses 6, 7 and 8 108.53

herpesviruses 108.50–108.54
herpes zoster 108.53–108.54
herpetiform ulceration 108.38, *108.39*
histoplasmosis 108.57
HIV-associated candidiasis 108.21–108.22
HIV infection 108.17, 108.54
hypereosinophilic syndrome 108.70
hyperpigmentation 108.14–108.19
  causes of **108.15**
  drug, food, habits and heavy metal induced 108.16–108.17
hypoplasminogenaemia 108.70
idiopathic thrombocytopenic purpura 108.70
IgG4 disease 108.67
immune defects 108.25
immunity in 108.5
immunobullous disorders 108.80–108.82, **108.81**
impetigo 108.53
infections of 25.20–25.24, 108.50–108.57
inflammatory arthritides 108.68–108.69
inflammatory lesions 108.20–108.25
inherited patterned lentiginosis 108.17
intraoral examination 108.6–108.7
Jacob disease 108.86
jaws, examination of 108.6
Kaposi sarcoma 108.26
keratitis, icthyosis and deafness syndrome 108.29
keratocanthoma of the lip 108.44
keratoses 108.33
Kindler syndrome 108.86
Klippel–Trenaunay–Weber syndrome 108.26
Koplik spots 108.33
Langerhans cell histiocytosis 108.70–108.71
Laugier–Hunziker syndrome 108.18
leiomyoma 108.13
leishmaniasis 108.57
lentiginoses 108.17–108.18
leprosy 108.55
lesions 78.3
lesions presentation 108.5
lesions that may cause lumps or swellings in the mouth **108.9**
leukaemias 108.71
leukoedema 108.29, *108.30*
leukopenias 108.71
leukoplakia *75.3*, 108.33–108.35
linear epidermal naevus 108.30
linear IgA disease of adults 108.82
linear IgA disease of children 108.81
linear naevus syndrome (naevus sebaceous of Jadassohn) 108.29–108.30
lingual thyroid 108.11
lingual tonsil 108.11
lipoma 108.13
lumps and swellings 108.8–108.14
  lesion types **108.9**
  plant allergies 127.72
lupus erythematosus, lip lesions 108.64
lymphangioma 108.13
lymph nodes, examination of 108.6
lymphomas 108.71
macroglossia 108.11–108.12
MAGIC syndrome 108.41, 155.11, 155.13
malignant neoplasms 108.43–108.50
median rhomboid glossitis 108.22
melanocanthoma 108.18
melanoma 108.18
melanotic macule 108.18
metastatic oral neoplasms 108.45
microbiome 108.5
mixed connective tissue disease *53.3*
mucocele 108.12
mucoepithelial dysplasia 108.26–108.27
mucormycosis 108.57
mucosal immune system 108.5
mucosal melanomas 142.11, *142.16*
mucosal melanosis *131.10*
mucositis (mucosal barrier injury) 108.49–108.50

mucous membrane pemphigoid *50.27*, 108.82
multicentric reticulohistiocytosis 108.71–108.72
multiple endocrine neoplasia type 2B *108.13*, 148.10
multiple mucosal neuroma syndrome 108.13–108.14
mycosis fungoides 108.72
myelodysplastic syndromes 108.72, 149.8
myeloma 108.72
myxoma 108.14
neurological diseases 108.83
nodular fasciitis 108.12
non-Hodgkin lymphoma 108.71
Noonan syndrome 108.86
Olmsted syndrome 108.30
orocutaneous syndromes 108.83–108.87
orofacial granulomatosis 103.48, 108.72–108.74, 127.21
osteoma mucosae 108.14
pachyonychia congenita 108.30
papillary hyperplasia 108.12
papilloma 108.14
paraproteinaemias 108.72
pemphigoid (subepithelial immune bullous diseases) 108.81–108.82
pemphigus 108.80–108.81
perioral region, examination of 108.5–108.8
persistent idiopathic facial pain 108.65–108.66
Peutz–Jeghers syndrome 108.19
pigmentary incontinence 108.19
pigmented lesions 108.14–108.19
  causes of **108.15**
  drug, food, habits and heavy metal induced 108.16–108.17
plasma cell gingivitis 108.25
polyarteritis nodosa 108.69
post-herpetic neuralgia 108.66
premalignant lesions 108.42–108.43
presentation of oral lesions 108.5
protozoal infestations 108.57
pseudolymphoma 108.72
psoriasis 108.35
psychiatric disorders 108.83
purpura 108.27
pyodermatitis-pyostomatitis vegetans *49.19*
pyostomatitis vegetans 108.74
reactive arthritis (Reiter's syndrome) 108.68
reactive perforating collagenosis 108.64
recurrent labial HSV infection 108.52–108.53
red lesions 108.19–108.28
renal diseases 108.83
rhabdomyoma 108.14
rheumatoid arthritis 108.68
rheumatological diseases 108.67–108.69
salivary glands
  anatomy of 108.4
  examination of 108.6
sarcoidosis 108.64, 108.67
scarring of oral tissues 108.68
scleroderma 108.68–108.69
scrotal tongue *108.87*
sebaceous adenoma 108.30
soft tissue benign tumours 108.12–108.14
soft tissue swelling 108.9–108.12
squamous cell carcinoma of the lip 108.44–108.45
Stevens–Johnson syndrome 108.61, 108.79, 118.20
stomatitis 25.97, 32.62–32.63, 108.20–108.21, *108.52*, 108.59–108.60
strawberry tongue 108.25
Sturge–Weber syndrome 108.27
Sweet syndrome 108.41
swelling 108.8–108.14, **108.9**, 127.72
syphilis 108.56
systemic diseases, oral manifestations 108.67–108.83
systemic lupus erythematosus 51.29

systemic sclerosis *54.4*
tattoos
  amalgam tattoos 108.15
  body art 108.15–108.16
teeth, anatomy of 108.4
telangiectasia 108.27
  hereditary haemorrhagic telangiectasia (Osler–Rendu–Weber syndrome) 108.26
tongue
  anatomy of 108.4
  examination of 108.7
trigeminal neuralgia 108.66–108.67
trigeminal trophic syndrome 108.67
tuberculosis 108.56
tuberous sclerosis 108.87
tylosis 108.35
Van der Woude syndrome 108.87
varicosities 108.27
vascular lesions 108.25–108.28
vascular proliferative lesions 108.27
vasculitides 108.69
velocardiofacial syndrome (22q11 deletion syndrome) 108.87
venous lake 108.28
venous mucocutaneous malformation 108.28
verruciform xanthoma 108.14
verrucous carcinoma 108.48
viral infections 25.20–25.24, 108.50–108.54
von Recklinghausen neurofibromatosis 108.87
Waldenström macroglobulinaemia 108.72
warty dyskeratoma (focal acantholytic dyskeratosis) 108.30–108.31
white lesions 108.28–108.35
white sponge naevus 108.31
Wiskott–Aldrich syndrome 108.28
xeroderma pigmentosum 108.87
see also lip; palate; perioral area; teeth; tongue
oral commissures, lips 108.3
oral contraceptive pill (OCP), hair disorder treatment 87.89, 87.95, **87.96**
oral disease severity score (ODSS) 108.8
oral drug administration 13.2, 13.3
oral dysaesthesia *see* burning mouth syndrome
oral epithelium, anatomy 108.3
oral hairy leukoplakia, reactivated Epstein–Barr virus 25.37–25.38
Oral Health Impact Profile (OHIP) 108.8
oral isotretinoin management, sebaceous gland hyperplasia 93.13
oral leukokeratoses, pachyonychia congenita *67.12*
oral leukoplakia, dyskeratosis congenita *67.14*
oral lichen planus (OLP) 37.3, 37.5–37.6, 108.76–108.79
  atrophic and ulcerative OLP 108.77
  betel chewing 37.3
  bullous OLP 108.78
  clinical features 108.76–108.78
  dental amalgam 37.3
  desquamative gingivitis 108.77
  differential diagnoses 108.78–108.79
  management of 108.78
  papular or plaque OLP 108.77
  pathophysiology 108.76
  postinflammatory hyperpigmentation *108.19*
  reticular OLP 108.76
  topical therapies **108.79**
oral melanocytic naevi 108.19
oral microbiome 108.5
oral minoxidil 87.70, 87.73, 87.94
oral mucosa
  acquired pigmentary disorders 86.24
  anatomy of 108.4
oral mucosal lesions 96.13
  COVID-19 association 25.113
  tylosis with oesophageal cancer *63.67*

oral pain, trigeminal neuropathic pain syndrome 82.5–82.7
oral pyogenic granuloma *113.3*
oral scarring, long-term SJS/TEN 118.17
oral squamous cell carcinoma (OSCC) 108.45–108.48
  classification of severity 108.47
  disease course and prognosis 108.47
  epidemiology 108.45–108.46
  features suggestive of **108.47**
  grades of carcinoma **108.47**
  history 108.46
  investigations 108.47–108.48
  management 108.48
  potentially malignant disorders **108.47**
  predisposing factors 108.46
  presentation 108.47
  TNM (tumour, node, metastases) classification 108.47, **108.48**
oral submucous fibrosis 108.42–108.43
oral therapy *see* systemic therapy
oral thrush *see* acute candidiasis
oral ulcers 108.36–108.42
  Adamantiades–Behçet disease *48.2*, *48.5*, **48.8**
  agranulocytosis 108.71
  aphthous-like ulceration *108.71*
  aphthous-like ulcers 108.38–108.39, *108.71*
  aspergillosis 108.56–108.57
  Behçet-like syndrome associated with trisomy 8 myelodysplasia 149.8
  Behçet syndrome 108.40–108.41
  causes of **108.36**
  chronic ulcerative stomatitis 108.79
  complex aphthosis 108.39–108.40
  cryptococcosis 108.57
  drug-induced ulcers 108.41
  gingival ulceration *108.55*
  immune defects 108.25
  leukaemias 108.71
  leukopenias 108.71
  MAGIC syndrome 108.41, 155.11, 155.13
  mucormycosis 108.57
  necrotising sialometaplasia 108.42
  oral lichen planus 108.77
  recurrent aphthous stomatitis 108.37–108.38
  recurrent (episodic) ulceration 108.37–108.42
  single episode of ulceration 108.36–108.37
  superficial mucocoeles 108.42
  Sweet syndrome 108.41
  systemic disease association 108.41–108.42
  tongue *108.52*
  traumatic ulcerative granuloma with stromal eosinophilia 108.37
  treatment **48.8**
  ulcerative colitis 108.74
  ulcers of local aetiology 108.36–108.37
orange peel appearance (*peau d'orange*), infiltrative carcinoma skin 148.2, *148.3*
ORAS *see* otulin-related autoinflammatory syndrome
orbital cellulitis, neonates 114.26
orcein–Giemsa stain 3.8
Orf-induced pemphigoid 50.54, *50.55*
orf virus (ORFV) 25.13–25.14
organoid naevus (naevus sebaceous) *73.5*, *73.6*, *73.7*, *73.8*, 87.30, 88.32, 105.11, *106.33*, 137.19–137.20
organ transplant recipients (OTRs)
  keratinocyte cancer risk factors 147.10
  melanoma 147.13–147.14
  pigmentation gene effects on skin cancer risks 147.4
  predisposition to cutaneous squamous cell carcinoma 141.3, 141.27, 141.29
skin cancer
  management protocols **147.22, 147.23**
  radiotherapy 24.15
  risks 147.3–147.5

orificial tuberculosis 27.16–27.17
orocutaneous syndromes 108.83–108.87
oro-facial and cutaneous herpes, recurrent 25.22–25.24
orofacial granulomatosis (OFG) 103.48, 108.72–108.74, 127.21
oro-facial–digital syndrome type 1 (OFD1), abnormalities and renal involvement 154.2
orofaciodigital syndrome **106.7**
oro-genital ulceration, MAGIC syndrome 108.41, 155.11, 155.13
oro-pharyngeal abnormalities, HIV 31.26, 31.34–35, **31.36**
oro-pharyngeal mucocutaneous *Candida* infection, gain-of-function STAT1 mutation 80.17
oropyrosis *see* burning mouth syndrome
Oroya fever, *Bartonella bacilliformis* 26.65–26.66
'orphan' status of drugs, clinical pharmacology 13.13
ORs *see* odds ratios
ORS *see* outer root sheath
orthopoxviruses 25.6–25.13, **25.6**
see also mpox; smallpox
Orthoptera (locusts) 34.32
OSAAD *see* Objective Severity Assessment Atopic Dermatitis
OSCC *see* oral squamous cell carcinoma
Osler–Rendu–Weber syndrome *see* hereditary haemorrhagic telangiectasia
osteoarthritis 155.8
osteogenesis imperfecta 70.12–70.14
  clinical variants 70.13
  differential diagnosis 70.13–70.14
  management 70.14
osteoma cutis 88.41
osteoma mucosae, oral mucosa 108.14
osteoporosis
  erythropoietic protoporphyria 58.16
  systemic lupus erythematosus 51.30
ostraceous psoriasis 35.14
Ota, naevus of 23.16, *23.17*, 107.46, 131.12–131.14
otic syphilis 29.16
otitis externa (OE) 106.15–106.19
  acute diffuse OE 106.16–106.17, 106.18
  acute localised OE 106.19
  acute OE *106.15*
  causative organisms 106.16
  chronic OE 106.16, 106.17, 106.18–106.19
  clinical features 106.16–106.17
  complications and co-morbidities 106.17–106.18
  investigations for 106.18
  necrotising OE 106.19
  pathophysiology 106.16
otomycosis 32.17–32.18, 106.20–106.21
otophyma, ear dermatoses **106.23**
OTRs *see* organ transplant recipients
otulin-related autoinflammatory syndrome (ORAS) 45.19
Oudtshoorn disease 63.73, *63.74*
outcomes
  core outcome measures 16.3
  digital recording 16.2
  see also measurement
outer root sheath (ORS), hair follicle 2.10, 2.44, 87.3–87.6
outlier lesions, atypical naevi for that individual 145.2
ovarian hyperthecosis 87.90
ovarian tumours, hirsutism association 87.91
overgrowth syndromes, infiltrating lipomatosis of the face differential diagnosis 98.19
overlap/coincident alopecias 87.51
overlap syndromes, dermatomyositis 52.8
OX40 deficiency 80.9–80.10
oxalate ebmolus, purpura 99.15
oxandrolone 97.32
  burn treatment 125.13–125.14

oxazolidinones 19.48
oxygenation factors, pressure ulcers 123.4
oxyhaemoglobin, erythema 128.6
oxyuriasis *see* enterobiasis
ozenoxacin, topical therapies 18.11

P

P4 (predictive, personalised, preventative, participatory) medicine 8.1
P13K/AKT/mTOR pathway, gene abnormalities within, lymphoedema association 103.23–103.24
PA *see* pyruvic acid
PAAND *see* pyrin-associated autoinflammation with neutrophilic dermatosis
PAC *see* perennial allergic conjunctivitis
PACD *see* photoallergic contact dermatitis
pachydermatoglyphy (acanthosis palmaris) 148.15–148.16
pachydermodactyly 94.38–94.39
pachydermoperiostosis 155.14
pachyonychia congenita (PC) 63.51–63.52, 67.1, 67.11–67.12
  friction blisters 122.10
  oral lesions 108.30
  skin fragility 69.20
  sweat glands 92.8
PAD13 gene 87.46
PAD (peripheral arterial disease) *see* peripheral vascular disease
paediatric autoimmune neuropsychiatric disorders associated with streptococcal infections (PANDAS) 26.11
paediatric dermatology 1.9
  see also adolescents; childhood; children; infants; neonates
paediatric inflammatory multisystem syndrome temporally associated with SARS-CoV-2 infection (PIM-TS) 25.114
PAF *see* platelet-activating factor
Paget disease 3.22, 137.40–137.42, 148.6–148.7
  see also extramammary Paget disease
pagetoid reticulosis 139.15–139.16
pagetoid spread of melanoma 142.18
pailloma 3.42
pain
  adipose tissue 98.17
  chemical burns 128.11
  diagnosis 4.3
  ectodermal dysplasias 69.27
  lipomas 98.18
  pressure ulcers 123.10
  PUVA phototherapy adverse effects 21.13
  stomas 112.6
pain disorders, female genitalia 110.40–110.42
painful hereditary callosities 63.52–63.53
painful plantar keratoderma, pachyonychia congenita 67.11
painful post-traumatic trigeminal neuropathy *see* trigeminal neuralgia
paints, vehicle choice for topical therapies 18.2
palaeodermatology 1.1
palate (roof of mouth)
  cleft lip/palate 108.83–108.85
  examination of 108.7
  leiomyoma 108.13
  melanotic macule 108.18
  mixed connective tissue disease 53.3
  papillary hyperplasia 108.12
  systemic lupus erythematosus *51.29*
  torus palatinus 108.7, *108.8*
pale acanthoma *see* clear cell acanthoma
palisaded granulomatous dermatitis in patient with rheumatoid arthritis 53.7
palisading granulomas

classification 97.16–97.17
  necrobiotic xanthogranuloma 97.18
palisading necrobiotic granulomas 96.3
palladium allergy 127.40
palm
  acanthosis palmaris 148.15–148.16
  annular lesions of discoid lupus erythematosus *51.24*
  anti-p200 pemphigoid *50.41*
  black palm 99.6
  congenital generalised lipodystrophies 72.2
  discoid lupus erythematosus *51.24*
  eccrine poroma 137.25–137.26
  hyperkeratotic palmar eczema 39.14
  keratolytic winter erythema 63.73, *63.74*
  lichen planus of 37.5, 37.7
  microscopic examination of 3.33
  non-pustular palmoplantar psoriasis 35.10, *35.11*
  palmoplantar pustulosis 35.36–35.39
  pityriasis rubra pilaris *36.3*, *36.5*
  pompholyx eczema 39.14, *39.15*
  recurrent focal palmar peeling 39.16
  xerosis cutis *85.26*
palmar creases
  ichthyosis vulgaris 63.4, *63.5*
  punctate keratosis of 63.60
palmar erythema
  internal malignancy association 148.25
  liver disease association 153.9
palmar fascial fibromatosis 94.34–94.35
palmar fibromatosis 93.34, 94.41–94.42, 136.12–136.13
palmar hyperhidrosis, surgical treatment 92.10
palmar keratoderma, pachyonychia congenita 67.12
palmar and plantar fibromatosis, superficial fibromatoses 136.12–136.13
palmar xanthomas 60.5–60.6
palmoplantar erythrodysaesthesia 119.2
palmoplantar hyperhidrosis 92.5, 92.6
palmoplantar hyperkeratosis 63.49
palmoplantar hyperlinearity, *ALOXE3* mutations 63.13
palmoplantar keratoderma punctata (PPKP) 63.58–63.59
palmoplantar keratodermas (PPKs) *36.3*, *36.5*, 63.49–63.62, 79.8–79.9
  cancer and 63.65–63.68
  cardiomyopathy and 63.62–63.63
  in ectodermal dysplasias 63.68–63.70
  hearing impairment and 63.63–63.65
  neurological manifestations 63.71
  opthalmic manifestations 63.70–63.71
  sex reversal and 63.67–63.68
palmoplantar lesions, Stevens–Johnson syndrome/toxic epidermal necrolysis 118.14
palmoplantar phenotype, non-syndromic ichthyoses 63.20
palmoplantar porokeratosis (of Mantoux) 63.75
palmoplantar pustulosis (PPP) 35.36–35.39, 93.8
  acute palmoplantar pustulosis *35.38*
  biologic therapy 35.39
  clinical features 35.37
  co-morbidities 35.38–35.39
  differential diagnosis 35.37
  environmental factors 35.37
  genetics 35.36–35.37
  histopathology 35.37
  management 35.39
  pathogenic mechanisms 35.37
  phototherapy 35.39
  pustulation in *35.38*
  severity classification 35.37–35.38
  systemic therapy 35.39
  topical treatment 35.39
palpation 4.1, 4.17–4.18, *4.19*
PAMS *see* paraneoplastic autoimmune multiorgan syndrome

PAN *see* polyarteritis nodosa
Panama, scabies, prevalence of **5.2**, 5.3
panatrophy 94.19–94.20
panatrophy of Gower 94.19–94.20
pancreatic carcinoma 97.41–97.42
pancreatic disease, cutaneous features 153.5–153.6
pancreatic enzymes, panniculitis 97.41
pancreatic neuroendocrine tumours (PNET) **104.8**
pancreatic panniculitis 97.41–97.43
pancreatitis 97.41–97.42
pancreatitis, panniculitis and polyarthritis (PPP) syndrome 97.42
pangeria (Werner syndrome) 70.26–70.27, **72.5**, 75.6, 77.1–77.3, **78.12**, 148.12, 148.13
panniculitis 97.1–97.64
  autoinflammatory diseases **80.19**
  biopsy 3.2
  classification **97.7**
  dermatomyositis 52.6
  hereditary **72.11**, *72.12*
  localised lipodystrophy secondary to 98.12
  pancreatic disease 153.6
  radiotherapy-associated 119.15
  of scleroderma 97.30
  scrotal panniculitis 109.23
  see also lupus erythematosus profundus
pansclerotic morphoea **54.20**, **55.4**, 55.19–55.21, **55.27**, 97.13
panthenol *see* dexpanthenol
Panton–Valentine leukocidin (PVL) virulence factor, Staphylococcal infections 111.13–111.14
PAP *see* peroxidase–antiperoxidase complexes
PAPA *see* pyogenic sterile arthritis, pyoderma gangrenosum and acne syndrome
papillary adenocarcinoma, aggressive digital 137.34–137.35
papillary dermis, anatomy 9.1
papillary eccrine adenoma *see* tubular adenoma
papillary endothelial hyperplasia, intravascular 136.23–136.24
papillary haemangioma 136.25
papillary hidradenoma (hidradenoma papilliferum) 110.31–110.33, 137.20–137.21
papillary hyperplasia, mouth 108.12
papillary intralymphatic angioendothelioma (PILA) 136.33
papillary tip microabscesses 3.43
papillomas
  milker's nodule/paravaccinia 25.15
  oral involvement 108.14
  see also human papillomavirus
papillomatosis 3.42
Papillon–Lefèvre syndrome 63.68, *63.69*
papular acrodermatitis *see* Gianotti–Crosti syndrome
papular elastorrhexis 94.33
papular facial rashes, differential diagnosis 88.37–88.38
papular keratoderma 63.60–63.61
papular lesions
  atrichia with 87.28–87.29
  drug-induced exanthems 117.2
papular (lichenoid) primary localised cutaneous amyloidosis **56.3**
papular mucinosis 57.6–57.7, 57.13–57.14
papular polymorphic light eruption 126.4, *126.5*
papular-pruritic gloves and socks syndrome, viral infections 25.120–25.121
papular syphilide 29.9–29.10
papular urticaria, infants 115.11–115.12
papular xanthoma 135.18–135.19
papules
  actinic prurigo 126.11
  conjunctival naevus 131.25
  eyelid 70.37

rosacea 89.6, *89.7*, *89.8*, 89.12, **89.14–89.15**
sarcoidosis 96.7–96.8
papuloerythroderma of Ofuji 39.34–39.35
papulonecrotic tuberculid (tuberculosis papulonecrotica) 27.27–27.29
papulopustular eruptions 119.3–119.5
  drug triggers **119.3**
  severity grading **119.4**
papulopustular rosacea 89.1
papulovesicular eruptions, COVID-19 association 25.109
papulovesicular polymorphic light eruption 126.4, *126.5*
parabens
  cosmetic allergies 127.52–127.53
  medicament allergies 127.54–127.58
parabens paradox 127.52–127.53, 127.55
parachlorometaxylenol (PCMX) 127.55–127.56
parachordoma *see* cutaneous myoepithelioma
paracoccidioidal granuloma *see* paracoccidioidomycosis
Paracoccidioides brasiliensis 32.89
paracoccidioidomycosis 32.88–32.89, 109.28
paracrine factors, pigmentation regulation 86.5–86.7
paradoxical hypertrichosis, following laser-assisted hair removal 23.20
paraesthetica, hypermelanosis *86.31*
paraffinoma 97.48, 97.49, 122.19
paraffin sections, immunoenzyme methods 3.15
paraffin wax, tissue processing 3.7
paragonimiasis 33.30–33.31
parakeratosis 3.42
parakeratosis ('shoulder parakeratosis'), pityriasis rubra pilaris *36.3*
parakeratosis variegata *see* large plaque parapsoriasis
parakeratotic hyperkeratosis 63.75
paramyxovirus infections 25.97–25.100
paraneoplastic acanthosis nigricans 85.5
paraneoplastic autoimmune multiorgan syndrome (PAMs) 50.6
paraneoplastic dermatoses 148.14–148.15, 148.19–148.20
paraneoplastic hypertrichosis lanuginosa 148.17–148.18
paraneoplastic pemphigus 50.3, 50.6, 148.21–148.22, 149.9
  oral involvement 108.81
paraneoplastic pemphigus (PNP), respiratory involvement 152.6–152.7
paraneoplastic phenomena involving the skin 148.14–148.20
paraneoplastic pigmentation 148.17, **148.18**
paraneoplastic pruritus 81.10, 148.27, 149.9
paraneoplastic syndromes
  lymphoid malignancies 149.8–149.9
  myeloid malignancies 149.5–149.8
  Sweet syndrome 149.6–149.7
paranichia (nail fold infection), candidiasis 32.65–32.66
paraphimosis 109.4, 109.16–109.17
parapoxviruses **25.6**, 25.13–25.15
paraproteinaemia
  granuloma annulare 97.18
  oral involvement 108.72
paraprotein-associated vasculitis 149.14
paraproteins
  plasma cell disorders 149.9–149.10
  skin manifestations/syndromes due to biological activity 149.10–149.13
  skin manifestations/syndromes due to paraprotein deposition 149.13–149.14
parapsoriasis 39.27, 134.6–134.8
'parasarcoidosis' syndromes 96.6
parasitic diseases 33.1–33.55
  cestodes 33.31–33.35
  nematodes - animal 33.18–33.26
  nematodes - human 33.1–33.18
  protozoa 33.35–33.55

trematodes 33.26–33.31
parasitic infections, eyelid 107.40
parasitophobia *see* delusional infestation
parastomal pyoderma gangrenosum 49.4, *49.5*
para-tert-butylphenolformaldehyde resin (PTBPFR) 127.67–127.68, 127.70–127.71
paravaccinia *see* milker's nodule
paraviral cutaneous eruptions 25.120–25.127
parechovirus infection 25.96
parenchymal injury 125.5
parenchymatous syphilis 29.15
parenteral drug administration 13.2–13.3
parenteral nutrition (PN), essential fatty acid deficiency 61.32, 61.33–61.34
Parents' Index of Quality of Life in Atopic Dermatitis (PIQoL-AD) 16.8
Parkes Weber syndrome 71.5, 71.7, 71.11, **101.28**, 101.30–101.31, 103.24
Parkland resuscitation formula 125.2–125.3
Parks classification of anal fistulae 111.30
paronychia 119.7–119.8, **119.9**
paronychial herpes simplex *see* inoculation herpes simplex
paroxysmal finger haematoma 94.19, 99.5–99.6, 122.13–122.14
Parry–Romberg syndrome *see* progressive hemifacial atrophy
partial lipodystrophy, TBI/HSCT association 98.8
partial-thickness burns 125.6, 125.8
particulate matter (air pollution)
  ageing of skin 156.8
  atopic eczema 41.7
partitioning enhancers, topical drug delivery 12.5
parvovirus infections 25.77–25.78, 155.2–155.3
PAS *see* periodic acid–Schiff stain; pre-auricular sinus
PASH syndrome, acne conglobata association 88.63
PASI *see* Psoriasis Area and Severity Index
Pasini–Pierini, atrophoderma of 55.17, *55.19*, 94.18–94.19
PASS syndrome, acne conglobata association 88.63
pastes, vehicle choice for topical therapies 18.2
Pasteurella multocida 26.59, 130.6
Patau syndrome (trisomy 13) 74.2–74.3
patch test artefacts, dermatitis artefacta 84.33
patch testing 127.1, 127.23–127.33
  age-related factors 127.5
  allergic contact eczema 1.8
  chronic actinic dermatitis 126.19, *126.21*, 126.34–126.35
  contact urticaria 127.86
  cosmetic allergens 127.49, 127.61
  drug impacts 127.6
  eczema 1.8, 39.5–39.6
  fragrance allergies 127.44–127.45
  medicament allergens 127.46–127.47
  metal allergies 127.41
  occupational contact dermatitis 129.7
  population studies 127.4
  sensitivity threshold 127.9
  stomas **112.9**
patchy alopecia 87.24, 87.26–87.27, 87.28–87.35
patchy reticular pattern naevi, dermoscopy *145.2*, *145.3*, 145.4
patchy vesiculosquamous eczema 39.16
patellar involvement, nail–patella syndrome 67.16
pathergy/pathergy testing 4.25, 122.2
Patient Benefit Index (PBI) 16.5
patient-centred care, key practical skills 15.6, **15.6**, *15.7*
patient education
  leprosy 28.15
  phototherapy 21.16

systemic therapy 19.2
patient follow-up, skin cancer surveillance after phototherapy 21.16
Patient Generated Index 16.9
patient involvement, measurement of disease state 16.1–16.2
patient organisations, ichthyoses 63.46, **63.47**
Patient-Oriented Eczema Measure (POEM) 16.3, 16.4
patient preparation for skin surgery 20.11
Patient-Reported Outcome Measures (PROMs) 16.2, 16.8
patient safety, phototherapy 21.16
patient selection
  sentinel lymph node biopsy for melanoma 143.5–143.6
  systemic therapy 19.1–19.2
patient specific measures, quality of life assessment 16.9
pattern hair loss 87.13–87.14, 87.60–87.71
  see also female pattern hair loss; male pattern hair loss
pattern recognition, melanoma diagnosis 142.9
paucibacillary cutaneous tuberculosis, lupus vulgaris 27.20–27.24
Paul of Aegina 1.3
Pautrier microabscesses 3.43
PB *see* pseudopelade of Brocq
PBI *see* Patient Benefit Index
PC1 deficiency **72.7**
PC *see* pachyonychia congenita
PCAs *see* primary cicatricial alopecias
PCBs *see* polychlorinated biphenyls
PCD *see* protein contact dermatitis
PCFCL *see* primary cutaneous follicle centre cell lymphoma
pCIA *see* persistent chemotherapy-induced alopecia
PCMX *see* parachlorometaxylenol
PCMZL *see* primary cutaneous marginal zone lymphoma
PCOS *see* polycystic ovary syndrome
PCPV (pseudocowpox) *see* milker's nodule
PCR *see* polymerase chain reaction
PCT *see* porphyria cutanea tarda
PD *see* periorificial facial dermatitis
PDCD *see* programmed cell death
PDD *see* puritic and dyskeratotic dermatoses
PDGF *see* platelet-derived growth factor
PDI *see* Psoriasis Disability Index
PDLs *see* pulsed dye lasers
PD-PSV *see* pyodermatitis-pyostomatitis vegetans
PDS *see* pleomorphic dermal sarcoma
PDT *see* photodynamic therapy
PEAG *see* pustulose exanthemique aiguë generalisés
peak itch over past 24 hours, NRS-11 16.3
pearly penile papules 109.6
peau d'orange (orange peel appearance), infiltrative carcinoma skin 148.2, *148.3*
'pebbling' of skin, mucopolysaccharidoses 79.3
PECL *see* postinflammatory elastolysis and cutis laxa
PEComa *see* perivascular epithelioid cell tumour
pedal papules of infancy 115.14, *115.15*
Pediatric Symptom Checklist 16.10
Pediculus capitis (head lice) 34.18–34.23
Pediculus corporis (body/clothing lice) 34.23–34.24
pEDS *see* periodontal Ehlers–Danlos syndrome
peeling skin, leukonychia, acral punctate keratoses, cheiliti and knuckle pads syndrome (PLACK) 94.37–94.38
peeling skin syndromes (PSSs) 63.28–63.30, 69.5–69.6, 69.19–69.20
PeIN *see* penile intraepithelial dysplasia; penile intraepithelial neoplasia
pellagra 5.1–5.2, 86.23–86.24

Casal's necklace *61.17*
niacin deficiency 61.16, *61.17*
pelvic floor, muscles of (female) 111.3
pelvic inflammatory disease (PID)
  chlamydia 30.10, 30.11, 30.14
  gonorrhoea 30.5, 30.7
PEM *see* pigmented epithelioid melanocytoma/pigment synthesising melanoma
PEMKB *see* pseudoepitheliomatous micaceous and keratotic balanitis
pemphigoid diseases
  autoantibodies **50.10**
  direct immunofluorescence findings 3.17–3.18
  oral involvement 108.81–108.82
  see also bullous pemphigoid
pemphigoid gestationis (PG) 113.17–113.19
  blister formation 113.18
  transplacental 114.12
  urticated red plaques *113.18*
pemphigus 50.1–50.9
  acantholysis 50.3
  age of onset 50.2
  antibodies 50.2–50.3
  associated diseases 50.2
  bullous pemphigoid 50.10–50.22
  clinical features 50.4–50.5
  clinical variants 50.5–50.7
  diagnosis **50.10**
  differential diagnosis 50.7
  direct immunofluorescence findings 3.17, *3.18*
  direct immunofluorescence microscopy *50.3*, 50.7
  disease course and prognosis 50.7
  division of 5.4
  drug-induced 50.4
  ELISA analysis 3.20, *3.21*
  environmental factors 50.3–50.4
  epidemiology 50.1–50.2
  genetics 50.3
  histopathology 50.7
  IgA pemphigus 50.6–50.7
  internal malignancy association 148.22
  investigations 50.7–50.8
  lesions in skin folds *50.5*
  management 50.8–50.9
    azathioprine 50.8
    corticosteroids 50.8
    cyclophosphamide 50.8
    immunoadsorption 50.9
    intravenous immunoglobulin therapy 50.8
    methotrexate 50.9
    mycophenolate mofetil 50.8
    plasmapherisis 50.9
    rituximab 50.9
    topical therapy 50.8
  oral involvement 108.80–108.81
  paraneoplastic 50.3
  pathophysiology 50.2–50.3
  penis 109.25
  serological assays 50.7–50.8
  severity classification 50.7
  T cells in 50.2
  see also paraneoplastic pemphigus
pemphigus foliaceus (PF) 39.34, 50.5, *50.6*, 50.7
pemphigus herpetiformis 50.6
pemphigus vegetans 50.5–50.6, 108.81
pemphigus vulgaris (PV) 50.4–50.5
  differential diagnosis 50.7
  neonatal 114.12
  oral involvement 108.80–108.81
  in pregnancy 113.8–113.9
  vulva **110.21**
PEN *see* porokeratotic eccrine ostial duct naevus
penciclovir, topical therapies 18.13
penetration enhancers, topical medication vehicles 18.5, 18.7–18.8
penetration injury, foreign bodies 122.17–122.18
D-penicillamine, cutaneous adverse effects 155.15

penicillamine, pseudoxanthoma elasticum 94.30
penicillin 1.8, 19.46
  cellulitis/erysipelas management 26.19, 26.21–26.22
  congenital syphilis 29.23, 29.28, 29.29
  cutaneous adverse effects of D-penicillamine 155.15
  reactions and allergies 29.21–29.22, 29.29, 117.7
  syphilis 29.20–29.22
penicilliosis (*Talaromyces marneffei* infections) 31.28, 32.89–32.90
penile fibromatosis 94.36–94.37, 136.13
penile horn 109.35
penile intraepithelial dysplasia (PeIN) 141.26
penile intraepithelial neoplasia (PeIN) 109.31–109.34
penile lentiginosis 131.10
penile psoriasis 35.10
penile squamous cell carcinoma (PSCC) 109.31–109.34
penis
  acne 109.24
  amyloidosis 109.25
  anatomy 109.2–109.3
  balanitis 109.4, 109.5
  Bowen disease of the penis 109.31–109.34
  bowenoid papulosis 109.31–109.34
  Buruli ulcer 109.28
  candidiasis 109.27
  carcinoma of 109.35–109.39
    classification **109.37**
    dysplasia and squamous carcinoma *109.38*
    risk factors **109.36**
  cellulitis 109.26
  chronic oedema 109.19–109.21
  cicatricial (mucous membrane) pemphigoid 109.25
  colloid degeneration 109.31
  condylomas 109.39–109.40
  dermoid cysts 109.31
  drug reactions 109.24–109.25
  ecthyma gangrenosum 109.26
  ectopic lesions 109.6
  erythroplasia of Queyrat 109.31–109.34
  fixed drug eruption 109.24
  Fordyce spots 93.11, 93.12
  foreign body 109.8
  haematoma and rupture 109.8
  keloid 109.31
  lentiginosis *131.10*
  lichen planus 37.4
  lichen sclerosus *109.16*
  linear IgA disease *50.37*
  lipogranuloma 109.8–109.9
  lymphoedema 103.49–103.51, 109.19–109.21
  lymphoma 109.42
  malignant melanoma 109.41
  median raphe cysts 109.30
  melanosis 109.42–109.43
  Melkersson–Rosenthal syndrome 109.25
  metastases 109.42
  molluscum contagiosum 109.29
  mucous membrane pemphigoid *50.28*
  naevi on 109.6
  necrosis 109.22–109.24
  pearly papules 109.6
  pemphigus 109.25
  Peyronie disease 109.24
  pilonidal sinus 109.24
  porokeratosis of Mibelli 109.35
  psoriasis vulgaris 35.10
  sclerosing lymphangitis 109.8
  squamous hyperplasia 109.34–109.35
  squamous intraepithelial lesions 109.34–109.35
  strangulation of 109.8
  striae of Wickham *109.19*
  tinea 109.27–109.28
  tuberculosis 109.27
  ulceration 109.22–109.24, 109.28

peno-scrotal lymphoedema, cutaneous Crohn disease 95.15
penoscrotodynia (PSD) 82.11–82.12
PENS syndrome 73.7
Pentatomidae (stink bugs) 34.30
pentazocine panniculitis 97.48, 97.50
pentazocine ulcers 122.19, 122.21
Pentinnen syndrome **72.5**
people with albinism (PWA) 7.2, 7.10–7.11, 7.12, *7.13*
people living with HIV (PLWH)
  global trends 31.2
  infections 31.20–31.30
  inflammatory dermatoses 31.12–31.20
  Kaposi sarcoma 147.2
  Merkel cell carcinoma 147.2
  neoplasms 31.30–31.33
  non-AIDS-defining cancers 147.2–147.3
  pruritic skin conditions 31.12
  skin cancer risks 147.2–147.3, 147.12–147.16
PEP *see* polymorphic eruption of pregnancy
peptide repertoire model, T-cell recognition of drugs 14.6
peptides, cosmeceutical use 157.5–157.6
percentage concentrations of drugs, weight in weight or weight in volume 18.1
percutaneous absorption
  mechanisms of 12.1–12.2
  neonates 114.2
perennial allergic conjunctivitis (PAC) 107.16, 107.17, 107.18
perforating collagenosis *see* perforating folliculitis
perforating dermatoses 94.53–94.55
perforating disease due to exogenous agents 94.55
perforating disorders, renal failure and dialysis complications 154.3–154.4
perforating folliculitis (perforating collagenosis)
  diabetic patients 62.4, *62.5*
  renal failure and dialysis complications 154.3–154.4
perforating keratotic disorders 63.76–63.77
perforating pseudoxanthoma elasticum 94.30
perforin 135.11–135.12
perfumes
  allergies 127.41–127.45, 127.48, 127.79
  genital contact dermatitis **109.13**
perfusion factors, pressure ulcers 123.4
perianal abscess 111.27–111.28
perianal candidiasis 32.64–32.65
perianal candidiasis of infancy 32.65
perianal carcinoma *111.23*
perianal cellulitis 109.26
perianal conditions, *see also* perineal and perianal skin
perianal dermatitis 128.5
perianal skin tags 111.32, *111.33*
perianal streptococcal cellulitis (dermatitis) 26.33–26.34
perianal streptococcal dermatitis, infants 115.8
perianal ulcers, leukocyte adhesion deficiency type I *80.16*
peribuccal pigmentation of Brocq 86.15
pericytes *see* perivascular myoid cells
periderm 2.3
perieccrine calcium deposition, calcific arteriolopathy 97.33
perifollicular fibroma 137.15–137.16
perifollicular inflammation, rosacea 89.3
perifollicular papules, mid-dermal elastolysis 94.26
perifollicular purpura, scurvy *61.22*
perineal and perianal skin 111.1–111.34
  amoebiasis 111.16
  anal abscess 111.27–111.28
  anal fissure 111.30–111.31
  anal fistula 111.28–111.30
  anal intraepithelial neoplasia 111.19–111.21

  anal and perianal malignancy 111.21–111.24
  bacterial infections 111.13–111.15
    ano-genital cellulitis 111.14
    ecthyma gangrenosum 111.15
    folliculitis 111.13–111.14
    furunculosis 111.13–111.14
    necrotising soft-tissue infections 111.15
    perianal cellulitis 111.14
    perianal malakoplakia 111.15
    perianal tuberculosis 111.15
    Streptococcal dermatitis 111.14
  basal cell carcinoma 111.24
  Bowen disease 111.20–111.21
  carcinoma erysipeloides 111.24
  congenital and developmental abnormalities 111.3
  Crohn disease 95.14, 111.26–111.27
  drug reactions 111.12–111.13
  embryogenesis of ano-genital region 111.3, *111.4*
  extramammary Paget disease 111.24
  fungal infection 111.8
  fungal infections 111.15
  haemorrhoids 111.31–111.33
  helminth infestations 111.16
  hidradenitis suppurativa 111.10–111.12
  history and examination 111.1
  human papillomavirus infection 111.16, 111.17–111.19
  infantile perianal pyrimidal protusion 111.3
  inflammatory dermatoses 111.8–111.12
    deep inflammatory dermatoses 111.10–111.12
    superficial inflammatory dermatoses 111.8–111.10
  investigations for 111.1
  melanoma 111.24
  obstetric trauma *111.7*, **111.8**
  perianal carcinoma *111.23*
  perianal sensory disturbances 111.3–111.8
  perianal skin tags 111.32, *111.33*
  perianal trauma 111.7–111.8
  perianal viral warts 111.18, *111.19*
  perineal and perianal pain 111.6–111.7
  pilonidal sinus 111.25–111.26
  pressure sores 111.7–111.8
  pruritus ani 111.3–111.6
  scabies infection 111.16
  sexually transmitted diseases 111.16–111.17
  squamous cell carcinoma 111.21–111.24
  structure and function of ano-genital region 111.1–111.3
  surgical management of conditions 111.25–111.33
  ulceration 111.12–111.13, 111.30–111.31
    HIV infection **111.17**
  viral infections 111.15–111.16
    cytomegalovirus infection 111.15
    herpes simplex virus infections 111.15
    Kawasaki disease 111.16
    molluscum contagiosum infection 111.13, 111.15
perineal streptococcal dermatitis 109.26
perineum 111.1, *111.2*
  formation of *111.4*
  microbiome 26.3, 26.4, 26.5
  see also perineal and perianal skin
perineural invasion (PNI), advanced basal cell carcinoma 140.9
perineurioma 136.47
periodic acid–Schiff (PAS) stain *3.7, 3.8*
periodic fever, immunodeficiency and thrombocytopenia (PFIT) 45.19
periodicity of lesion/eruption, diagnosis 4.3
periodontal Ehlers–Danlos syndrome (pEDS) **70.5**, *70.10*
perioral area, allergic contact dermatitis 127.15
perioral dermatitis 88.34, *88.36*, 89.10, *89.18*
perioral wrinkling, reduction of by botulinum toxin application *159.7*

periorbital bleeding, primary systemic amyloidosis with cutaneous involvement 56.11
periorbital dermatitis *41.20*
periorbital lines, reduction of by botulinum toxin application 159.5, *159.6*, *159.7*
periorbital oedema, eyelids 107.6–107.7
periorbital syringomas, photothermal ablation 23.21, 23.22
periorificial facial dermatitis (PD) 89.10, 89.17–89.18
periostin, keloids 94.50
peripheral blood, immune system 9.6
peripheral cyanosis (acrocyanosis), neonates 114.3
peripheral fat, lymphatic system 103.2
peripheral globules, naevi 145.2, *145.3*, 145.4–145.5
peripheral light brown structureless areas, melanoma 145.7
peripheral network naevi with central hypo- or hyperpigmentation 145.2, *145.3*, 145.4
peripheral neuroectodermal tumours 136.42–136.52
peripheral neuropathy 83.8–83.10
  dapsone 19.14
  leprosy 28.1, *28.2*, 28.3–28.4, 28.6, 28.7, 28.9–28.10, 28.11, 28.12, 28.13, 28.15–28.16
  thallium poisoning 121.9
peripheral primitive neuroectodermal tumour *see* cutaneous Ewing sarcoma
peripheral streak patterns
  melanoma 145.7, *145.8*
  Spitz naevi 145.6, 145.7
peripheral tan structureless areas, melanoma 145.9, 145.10
peripheral vascular disease (PVD) 101.2–101.3
  arterial leg ulcer 102.9
  clinical features **101.2**
  investigations for **101.4**
  ischaemic foot *101.3*
  mixed leg ulcers 102.4–102.7
  platelet emboli *101.3*
  radiological investigations **101.4**
  treatment options **101.5**
  trophic changes *101.3*
  ulceration *101.3*
periporitis staphylogenes, neonates 114.25
peristomal dermatitis 128.5
peristomal pyoderma gangrenosum 49.4, *49.5*
peritonitis, acute scrotum 109.25
periungual allergic contact dermatitis *127.62*
periungual fibromas (Koenen tumours), tuberous sclerosis complex 78.8
perivascular adipocytes 97.6
perivascular cell tumours 136.39–136.42
perivascular epithelioid cell tumour (PEComa) 136.61
perivascular myoid cells (pericytes) 2.40
  microscopic examination of 3.37
  myopericytoma 136.40–136.41
perlèche *see* angular cheilitis
perniosis *see* chilblain-like lesions; chilblains
peroxidase–antiperoxidase (PAP) complexes 3.14–3.16
per protocol analysis, randomised controlled trials 17.14
persistent chemotherapy-induced alopecia (pCIA) 87.72–87.74
persistent dento-alveolar pain disorder *see* trigeminal neuralgia
persistent erythema
  diagnostic features 89.5, 89.12
  diffuse 89.7
  treatment **89.13**
persistent human papillomavirus infections, primary immunodeficiencies 149.19

persistent idiopathic facial pain (PIFP) 108.65–108.66
persistent light reaction 126.29, 127.80–127.81
persistent light reactors 126.13–126.14
persistent pigment darkening (PPD) 86.9, 87.100
   UVR exposure 10.8
persistent superficial scaly dermatitis *see* small plaque parapsoriasis
persistent viral infections 25.4
   Epstein–Barr virus 25.36, 25.38
   herpesviruses 25.19
   human herpesvirus 6 and 7 25.39, 25.40
   see also recurrent entries
personal care products, genital contact dermatitis 109.13
personalised medicine, clinical pharmacology 8.1, 13.11
personality traits, beliefs/emotions/behaviours 15.3
personal protective equipment (PPE)
   allergic reactions 127.4
   irritant contact dermatitis 129.4
   occupational dermatoses in COVID-19 pandemic 25.119
persons with albinism (PWA) 7.2, 7.10–7.11, 7.12, *7.13*
perspiration, types of 2.9
PEST *see* Psoriasis Epidemiology Screening tool
petechiae
   COVID-19 association 25.109
   diagnosis by lesion size 99.3
   reactions to COVID-19 vaccines 25.118
   sports injuries 122.16
petrified ear 106.21
petrolatum, patch testing 127.25, *127.26*
pets
   arthropod infestation 34.4, 34.5, *34.6*, 34.13, 34.14
   atopic eczema 41.8
Peutz–Jeghers syndrome **78.14**, **131.3**
   oral hyperpigmentation 108.19
Peutz–Jeghers–Touraine (PJT) syndrome 68.13–68.14
Peyronie disease 94.37, 109.24
PF *see* pemphigus foliaceus
PFIT *see* periodic fever, immunodeficiency and thrombocytopenia
PFR *see* phenol formaldehyde resin
PFS *see* post-finasteride syndrome
PG *see* pemphigoid gestationis; propylene glycol; pyoderma gangrenosum; pyogenic granuloma
PGA *see* Physician's Global Assessment
PGD2 *see* prostaglandin D2
PGD *see* preimplantation genetic diagnosis
PGH *see* preimplantation genetic haplotyping
PGs *see* proteoglycans
PHA *see* progressive hemifacial atrophy
PHACES syndrome (posterior fossa malformations, haemangiomas, arterial anomalies, cardiac anomalies, eye abnormalities, sternal pit and supraumbilical raphe) 116.3
phaeochromocytoma 86.19–86.20
   dermatoendocrinology 150.19
   flushing **104.7**
   pallor and rebound flushing 148.26
phaeohyphomycosis 32.77–32.78
phaeomelanin 2.17, *2.18*, 86.5
phaeomycotic subcutaneous cyst *see* phaeohyphomycosis
phagedena/phagedenic ulcer, *see also* tropical ulcer
phagocytes 135.1
phagocytic defects, inherited immunodeficiency **80.5–80.6**, 80.15
phagocytosis 135.2
phakomatosis pigmentokeratotica 73.5–73.6

see also HRAS/KRAS mosaicism; Schimmelpenning–Feuerstein–Mims syndrome
phakomatosis pigmentovascularis (PPV) 73.20–73.21
   phenotypic subclassifications **73.21**
   port-wine stain 73.22
phalanges
   congenital erythropoietic porphyria 58.10
   familial mandibuloacral dysplasia 70.29
   see also finger; toe
phantom tooth pain (trigeminal neuropathic pain) 82.5–82.7
phantosmia *see* olfactory delusions
pharmacists, clinical pharmacology 13.11
pharmacodynamics **13.2**, 13.4–13.6
   age 13.7–13.8
   conception, pregnancy and lactation 13.8–13.9
pharmacogenomics, clinical pharmacology 13.11
pharmacokinetics (PK) 13.1–13.4
   age 13.7–13.8
   conception, pregnancy and lactation 13.8–13.9
   topical bioavailability/bioequivalence assessment 12.8
pharmacological interaction (p-i) model, T-cell recognition of drugs 14.5, 14.6
pharmacological modalities, burn injuries 125.13–125.14
pharmacotherapy (topical and systemic agents), phototherapy combination 21.10
pharmionics, clinical pharmacology 13.9
pharyngitis, *Streptococcus pyogenes* 26.10
phenol
   burns 128.11
   chemical peels 160.3
phenol-croton oil peel 160.10–160.11
phenol derivatives of hydroquinone, topical depigmenting agents 18.32
phenol formaldehyde resin (PFR), allergy 127.70–127.71
'phenoplastics' 127.70
phenothiazines, eczema 117.4
phenotype
   rosacea 89.1
   sweat glands 92.8
p-phenylenediamine (PPD) 127.60–127.61, 127.63–127.64, 127.66
p-phenylenediamine and toluene-2,5-diamine (PTD) 127.60–127.61
phenylketonuria (PKU) 79.10–79.11
phenytoin, palmar fascial fibromatosis 94.34
Phialophora verrucosa 32.77
philtrum 108.3
phimosis 109.4, 109.16–109.17
phleboliths, Maffucci syndrome *71.20*
phlebolymphoedema 103.10–103.12
PHN *see* postherpetic neuralgia
PHO *see* primary hypertrophic osteoarthropathy
phobias
   moles/skin cancer 84.26
   topical corticosteroids 84.26
   see also delusional infestation
pholcodeine hypothesis 117.7
phosphatase and tensin homologue (PTEN) hamartomatous syndromes **131.3**
   see also PTEN hamartoma tumour syndrome
phosphomannomutase 2 deficiency 79.10
photoablation, UV radiation 23.5
photoactivation 127.79
photoageing 2.45, 2.46
   atrophic photoageing 156.3, *156.4*
   chemical peels 160.5
   collagen fibril fragmentation 156.8–156.9
   grading and measurement of 156.6–156.7
   hypertrophic photoageing 156.3

   implications of 156.10–156.11
   molecular mechanisms in *156.10*
   and natural ageing 156.10
   PUVA phototherapy adverse effects 21.13
   in skin of colour 156.1–156.3
   UVB phototherapy adverse effects 21.13
   UV irradiation damage/episodic exposure 156.7–156.8, *156.10*
   UVR exposure 10.10–10.11
   in white skin 156.1
photoaggravated diseases 126.1, 126.32, *126.33*
photoallergic contact dermatitis (PACD) 127.78–127.82
photoallergic reactions
   chemotherapy 119.11–119.12
   polymorphic light eruption 126.2
   systemic drug-induced photosensitivity 126.28
   UV filters 127.62
photobiology 10.1–10.14
   normal effects of UVR on skin 10.5–10.11
   personal and population exposure to UVR 10.12–10.14
   photoprotection 10.11–10.12
   principles of 10.1–10.5
photobleaching, immunofluorescence 3.11
photochemical changes in skin
   laser therapies 23.4
   see also photodynamic therapy
photochemotherapy (PUVA)
   adverse effects 21.13–21.15
   history 21.2
   lentigo 131.7–131.8
   light source units 21.3
   mastocytosis treatment 46.10
   minimal phototoxic dose 21.9
   photosensitivity management 126.37
   PLE management 126.7–126.8
   principles 21.1
   psoralen choice and regimen 21.9
   UVA delivery 21.10
   UVB phototherapy comparison 21.5–21.6
   see also extracorporeal photopheresis
photocontact allergy 126.35, 127.11
photocontact facial melanosis 86.12–86.15
photodamage
   ablative fractional resurfacing therapy *161.3*
   dermal connective tissue 94.1–94.6
photodermatoses **106.23**
   acquired non-infective disorders 91.6–91.8
   pilosebaceous unit disorders 93.6
   PUVA phototherapy adverse effects 21.13
photodistributed erythema 89.9
photo documentation, chemical peels 160.8
photodynamic reactions, pigmentation 86.28–86.30
photodynamic therapy (PDT) 22.1–22.15
   acne vulgaris 88.58
   actinic keratosis 141.10–141.11
   acute adverse effects 22.12–22.14
   adverse effects **22.12**
   ambulatory 22.11
   basal cell carcinoma 140.11, 140.12–140.13
   Bowen disease 141.24
   chronic adverse effects 22.14
   clinical governance 22.15
   contraindications 22.8
   conventional methodology 22.9–22.11
   cutaneous squamous cell carcinoma 141.35
   cutaneous warts 25.59
   daylight 22.11–22.12
   history 22.1–22.2
   indications 22.4–22.8
   light sources 22.3–22.4
   methodology 22.8–22.12
   patient selection 22.8–22.9
   photosensitisers 22.2–22.3
   principles 23.4

   process 22.1
   see also phototherapy
photoepilation 23.17
   see also laser-assisted hair removal
photo-exposed skin, Jessner lymphocytic infiltrate 134.10
photographic assessment methods
   acne 16.4
   challenges 16.5
   diagnosis 4.19
   psoriasis 16.3
photography, development of dermatology 1.9
photomechanical interactions, laser therapies 23.5
photo-onycholysis 119.12
photopatch testing 126.34–126.35, 127.31, 127.78–127.79, 127.81–127.82
   chronic actinic dermatitis 126.19
   sunscreen chemicals *126.31*
photopheresis
   principles 21.1–21.2
   see also extracorporeal photopheresis
photophoresis *see* extracorporeal photopheresis
photoprotection 10.11–10.12
   cutaneous photosensitivity diseases 126.36
   erythropoietic protoporphyria 58.15
   keratinocyte cancer prevention in immunocompromised people 147.18
photosensitisation
   mechanisms 127.79
   photodynamic therapy 22.2–22.3
   see also 5-aminolaevulinic acid; methyl aminolevulinate
photosensitive eczema 126.13
   plant allergies 127.72
photosensitive psoriasis 126.2
photosensitivity 126.1
   allergic contact dermatitis 127.21
   chemotherapy-induced 119.11–119.12
photosensitivity diseases 126.1–126.39
   clinical assessment/management 126.32–126.37
   ocular features **107.42**
photostimulation/photobiomodulation, laser therapies 23.4
phototesting, extracorporeal photochemotherapy 21.11
phototherapy 1.8, 21.1–21.18
   acne vulgaris 88.58
   adverse effects 21.11–21.15
      PUVA 21.13–21.15
      UVA-1 21.15
      UVB 21.11–21.13
   alopecia treatment 87.27
   at home 21.3, 21.8, 21.15, 21.18
   atopic eczema 21.4
   atopic eczema treatment 41.28
   audits 21.17
   carcinogenesis risks 21.13, 21.14, 21.15
   clinical governance 21.17
   combination therapy 21.10
   conditions treated 21.3–21.5
   contraindications 21.6
   cutaneous photosensitivity diseases 126.37
   cutaneous T-cell lymphoma 21.4
   delivery methods 21.8
   documentation/record keeping 21.17
   dosimetry 21.3, *21.4*, 21.17
   equipment maintenance 21.17
   equipment types 21.2–21.3
   history 21.2
   indications 21.3–21.5
   mastocytosis treatment 46.10
   minimal erythema dose 21.7–21.8
   modality choices 21.5–21.7
   morphoea 55.36
   new developments 21.18
   palmoplantar pustulosis 35.39
   patient education 21.16
   patient follow-up/skin cancer surveillance 21.16

phototherapy (continued)
  patient selection/assessment 21.15–21.16
  polymorphic light eruption 21.5
  principles 21.1–21.18
  psoriasis 21.3–21.4
  regimen variables 21.8
  risk management 21.16, 21.17
  safety of patients and staff 21.16
  setting up a phototherapy unit 21.17–21.18
  starting dose/increments/frequency and number of exposures 21.8
  topical and systemic agents combination 21.10
  types 21.1–21.2
  UVB versus PUVA 21.5–21.6
  UV calibration/dosimetry 21.3, 21.4
  vitiligo 21.4
  see also laser therapies; photodynamic therapy
phototherapy and photochemotherapy, cutaneous T-cell lymphoma 139.22
photothermal ablation
  complications 23.23
  devices 23.20–23.21
  indications 23.21–23.23
  skin disorder treatments 23.20–23.23
photothermal reactions, laser therapies 23.4–23.5
photothermolysis, selective 23.5–23.6
phototoxic contact dermatitis 127.78, 128.9–128.10
phototoxic drugs, photosensitivity diseases 126.28
phototoxic reactions
  chemotherapy 119.11–119.12
  pigmentation 86.28–86.30
  porphyrias 58.1
phototrichogram 87.14, 87.56
phrynoderma 61.8, 85.14–85.15
Phthiraptera (lice) 34.18–34.25
Phthiriasis pubis (crab lice) 34.24–34.25
  blepharitis due to 107.12
  eyelashes 34.25, 107.40
  male genitalia 109.29
PHTS see PTEN hamartoma tumour syndrome
phycomycosis see mucormycosis
phyma, fibrosis in 89.3
phymatous rosacea 89.1
  diagnostic features 89.5–89.6, 89.12
  differential diagnosis 89.10
  treatment 89.13–89.14
Physalia, stings 130.1–130.3
physical dosimetry 10.2
physicians, experience based decisions versus evidence based 17.5–17.6
Physician's Global Assessment (PGA), psoriasis 16.3
physiological functions of skin 2.42–2.43
physiological hypermelanosis 86.9
physiological livedo reticularis 124.8, 124.9
physiological reactions, heat/IR radiation 124.14
phytanic acid 63.31
phytochemicals, cosmeceutical use of 157.7–157.10
phytophotodermatitis 86.28–86.30, 126.29–126.30
phytophotodermatosis 4.9
phytotherapy, psoriasis treatment 35.22–35.23
phytotherapy-induced rashes, neonates 114.11
PI3Kδ deficiency 80.13
PI3K-related overgrowth syndromes 71.7
PI see protease inhibitor
piano paronychia 122.12
picker's acne see acné excoriée
picker's nodules see lichen simplex chronicus
PICO/PICOT acronyms of components for formulating well-built clinical questions 17.3, 17.4
Picornavirus infections 25.93–25.97

PID see pelvic inflammatory disease
piebaldism 68.3–68.4
Piedraia hortae, black piedra 32.15–32.16
piezogenic pedal papules 122.26–122.27
PIFP see persistent idiopathic facial pain
pigmentary disorders 3.44, 86.1–86.56
  electron microscopy studies 3.30
  female genitalia 110.20–110.23
  genetic disorders 68.1–68.15
  glycosylation disorders 79.10
  haemochromatosis 153.5
  hair 87.12, 87.91–87.94
  HIV 31.12
  laser therapies 23.12–23.17, 23.18
  ocular features 107.42
  xeroderma pigmentosum 76.4–76.5
  see also hyperpigmentation; hypopigmentation
pigmentary incontinence 3.43
  incontinentia pigmenti 4.16, 4.19, 4.22
  oral hyperpigmentation 108.19
pigmentary mosaicism, infants 115.13
pigmentation
  basal cell carcinoma 140.3, 140.4, 140.6, 140.8, 140.9, 140.10, 140.18, 140.21
  changes in during pregnancy 113.1, 113.2, 113.2
  chemical peels 160.5–160.6
  cutaneous manifestations of Hodgkin disease 139.49
  internal malignancy links 148.17, 148.18
  liver disease association 153.8
  Merkel cell carcinoma risk 146.2
  pancreatic disease 153.5–153.6
  renal failure and dialysis effects 154.3
  seborrhoeic dermatitis effects 40.4–40.5
  UV light exposure 10.7–10.8
  UV light regulation 86.5–86.7
  variation in 2.18
  see also melanocytes; skin colour
pigmentation genes, skin cancer risks in immunocompromised people 147.6
pigmentation of hair 87.12–87.13, 87.88
pigmentation of hair nodules, trichomycosis axillaris 26.41–26.42
pigmentation of nails, renal failure and dialysis effects 154.3
pigment cell naevi 73.2
pigmented dermatitis 127.20
pigmented epithelioid melanocytoma/pigment synthesising melanoma (PEM/animal-type melanoma) 142.2, 142.20
pigmented lesions
  surgical treatment 20.50
  see also malignant melanoma
pigmented melanotic macules 131.9–131.11
  genital melanosis 131.10
  labial melanotic macules 131.11–131.12
    dermoscopic image 131.11
  penile lentiginosis 131.10
  squamous epithelium of oral cavity 131.10
pigmented neuroectodermal tumour of infancy 136.50–136.51
pigmented purpura see capillaritis
pigmented purpuric dermatoses 99.7–99.9
pigmented purpuric lichenoid dermatosis of Gougerot and Blum 99.7, 99.8, 99.9
pigment lasers
  complications 23.17
  tattoo and pigmented lesion treatments 23.12–23.17, 23.18
PIK3CA-related overgrowth spectrum (PROS) 72.9–72.11, 98.19
  CLOVES syndrome 72.9
  facial infiltrating lipomatosis 72.11
  fibroadipose hyperplasia 72.9
  hemihyperplasia–multiple lipomatosis syndrome 72.9, 72.11
PILA see papillary intralymphatic angioendothelioma
pilar cysts see trichilemmal cysts

pilar leiomyoma tumour see leiomyosarcoma/atypical smooth muscle tumour
pilar sheath acanthoma 137.4
pilar tumour of the scalp see proliferating trichilemmal tumour
pili annulati 87.80, 87.81
pili multigemini 87.84
pili torti 87.78–87.79
pili triangular et canaliculi 87.46
pilomatrical carcinoma 137.14–137.15
pilomatricoma 137.13–137.14
  dystrophic calcification 59.4
  familial pilomatrixoma 78.13
pilomatrix carcinoma see pilomatrical carcinoma
pilomatrixoma see pilomatricoma
pilonidal sinus 87.50, 122.23
  penis 109.24
  perineal and perianal skin 111.25–111.26
pilosebaceous apparatus, tumours of skin appendages 137.1
pilosebaceous cysts, pachyonychia congenita 67.12
pilosebaceous naevoid disorders 88.31
pilosebaceous unit 2.9–2.10
  acquired disorders 93.1–93.13
  acquired non-infective disorders 91.1–91.20
  tumours of 105.11
pimecrolimus, topical therapies 18.23
p-i model see pharmacological interaction model
pinkus follicular mucinosis 57.16, 57.17
pinna (auricle) see ear, auricle
pinta 26.71–26.72
  clinical features 26.71–26.72
  investigations 26.72
pin worm see enterobiasis
PIQoL-AD see Parents' Index of Quality of Life in Atopic Dermatitis
PiS allele 97.43–97.44
pited lips 108.86
pitted keratolysis 26.42–26.43
pitted skin, prolidase deficiency 70.12, 79.13
pityriasis alba 39.26–39.27, 86.43–86.44
  atopic eczema 41.17
  discoid skin lesions 39.10
  infants 115.4
  treatment for 39.27
pityriasis amiantacea 105.4
pityriasis capitis (dandruff) 40.1, 40.4
  Malassezia yeast 32.14
pityriasis circinata et maculata of Vidal see pityriasis rosea
pityriasis folliculorum 89.10
pityriasis lichenoides 134.3–134.5, 134.6
pityriasis lichenoides chronica (PLC) 134.3–134.5, 134.6
pityriasis lichenoides et varioliformis acuta (PLEVA) 134.3–134.4, 134.5
pityriasis nigra see tinea nigra
pityriasis rosea 25.123–25.127
  clinical features 25.124–25.126
  discoid skin lesions 39.10
  epidemiology 25.123–25.124
  male genitalia 109.28
  management 25.126–25.127
  pathophysiology 25.124
  in pregnancy 113.6–113.7
  reactions to COVID-19 vaccines 25.119
pityriasis rosea-like eruption, COVID-19 association 25.111
pityriasis rotunda 63.47–63.49, 85.8–85.9, 148.17
pityriasis rubra pilaris (PRP) 36.1–36.6, 39.33–39.34
  associated diseases 36.1
  atypical adult-onset PRP (type II) 36.2–36.4
  atypical juvenile PRP (type V) 36.4
  circumscribed juvenile PRP (type IV) 36.4, 36.5
  classic adult-onset PRP (type 1) 36.2, 36.4, 36.6

classic juvenile-onset PRP (type III) 36.4, 36.5
  clinical features 36.2
  clinical variants 36.2–36.4
  differential diagnosis 36.4
  disease course and prognosis 36.5
  epidemiology 36.1
  erythroderma 39.33–39.34
  genetics 36.2
  HIV-related PRP (type VI) 36.4
  hyperkeratosis with follicular plugging and parakeratosis 36.3
  hyperkertotic follicular papules 36.3
  irregular psoriasiform acanthosis showing alternating ortho- and parakeratosis ('checkerboard' pattern) 36.3
  islands of sparing (areas of normal skin) 36.3, 36.4, 36.6
  management 36.5–36.6
  palmoplantar keratoderma 36.3
  pathophysiology 36.1–36.2
  psoriasis comparison 36.2
  treatment ladder 36.6
pityriasis versicolor (tinea versicolour) 32.10–32.13, 86.43–86.44
  clinical features 32.12
  clinical investigations 32.12
  epidemiology 32.11
  management 32.12–32.13
  pathophysiology 32.11–32.12
pityrosporal dermatitis see seborrhoeic dermatitis
Pityrosporum see Malassezia
pityrosporum folliculitis 88.37
PiZ allele 97.43–97.44
PJT syndrome see Peutz–Jeghers–Touraine syndrome
PK see pharmacokinetics
PKDL see post-kala-azar dermal leishmaniasis
PKU see phenylketonuria
PL see primary lymphoedema
PLACK see peeling skin, leukonychia, acral punctate keratoses, cheiliti and knuckle pads syndrome
placode 87.3
plague, Yersinia pestis 26.59–26.60
PLAID see PLCG2-associated antibody deficiency and immune dysregulation syndrome
plain radiography, foreign body reactions 122.18
plakoglobin (JUP) 69.7
plakoglobin loss, palmoplantar keratodermas 63.63
plakophilin-1 (PKP1), skin fragility disorders 69.7
planar xanthomas 60.4–60.6
plane warts (verruca plana) 25.52, 25.53–25.54
  see also cutaneous warts
plant allergies 127.13, 127.16–127.17, 127.19–127.22, 127.43, 127.71–127.74
plantar callosities 63.52
plantar fascial fibromatosis 94.35–94.36
plantar fibromatosis 136.12–136.13
plantar hyperhidrosis 92.7
plantar keratoderma 63.51
  pachyonychia congenita 67.11–67.12
plantar pain, pachyonychia congenita 63.51–63.52
plantar phenotype, mal de Meleda 63.55
plant contact
  allergic contact dermatitis 129.6
  irritants 128.2
  photosensitivity 126.29
  poison ivy dermatitis 127.5–127.6, 127.20, 127.22, 127.71
plant extracts
  allergic contact dermatitis 127.49
  cutaneous wart therapy 25.60
  see also herbals
plant mites 34.52
plaque, dental 108.5
plaque-like CD34-positive dermal fibroma 136.8

plaque polymorphic light eruption 126.4, *126.5*
plaque psoriasis *see* psoriasis vulgaris
plaques
 actinic prurigo *126.11*
 in periodontal Ehlers–Danlos syndrome *70.10*
plaque sarcoidosis 96.7–96.8, *96.8–96.9*
plasma cell cheilitis 108.63
plasma cell disorders, skin manifestations 149.9–149.14
plasma cell gingivitis 108.25
plasma cell malignancies, infiltration of skin with neoplastic cells 149.4–149.5
plasma cells
 immune system 9.6
 microscopic examination of 3.35
plasmacytoid dendritic cells, blastic neoplasm 139.45–139.47
plasmacytoma-associated systemic amyloidosis with cutaneous involvement *56.11*
plasmapheresis, pemphigus treatment 50.9
plastics, allergy to 127.68–127.71
plat dermatitis 127.11
platelet-activating factor (PAF), disease pathogenesis role 14.1, 14.2
platelet-derived growth factor (PDGF), wound healing 11.6
platelet disorders, purpura due to 99.2–99.4
platelet emboli, peripheral vascular disease *101.3*
platelet plugging
 heparin necrosis 99.9–99.10
 thrombocytosis 99.10–99.11
platelet-rich plasma (PRP), hair treatment 87.27, 87.71, 87.95
platelets, wound healing 11.2–11.3
platinum, dermatological reactions 121.9
PLC *see* pityriasis lichenoides chronica
PLCA *see* primary localised cutaneous amyloidosis
PLCG2-associated antibody deficiency and immune dysregulation (PLAID) syndrome **45.5, 45.7**
PLE *see* polymorphic light eruption
plectin (*PLEC*), epidermolysis bullosa 69.4
Plenck, Joseph Jacob 1.4
pleomorphic dermal sarcoma (PDS) 136.22–136.23
pleomorphic fibroma 136.4
pleomorphic lipoma 136.58
pleomorphic liposarcoma 136.59
pleomorphism 3.43
pleuropneumonia-like organisms *see* *Mycoplasma* spp.
PLEVA *see* pityriasis lichenoides et varioliformis acuta
plexiform fibrohistiocytic tumour (plexiform fibrous histiocytoma) 136.22
plexiform neurofibroma 78.3, 136.46
PLLA *see* poly-L-lactic acid [replace capital L with small cap L**]
plumber's itch *see* cutaneous larva migrans
Plumbe, Samuel 7.3
Plummer–Vinson syndrome, iron deficiency 61.24
PLWH *see* people living with HIV
plymers, isocyanates in polyurethanes 127.71
PMH *see* progressive macular hypomelanosis
PMMA *see* polymethylmethacrylate
PN *see* parenteral nutrition; prurigo nodularis
PNET *see* pancreatic neuroendocrine tumours
Pneumocystis jiroveci infections 32.93–32.94
pneumonia
 inhalation injury 125.4–125.5
 skin features 26.79
pneumonic plague *see* plague
PNH *see* progressive nodular histiocytosis
PNI *see* perineural invasion
PNP *see* paraneoplastic pemphigus
PNPLA2 gene, neutral lipid storage disease with ichthyosis 63.36

podoconiosis 7.3
 Footwork initiative 7.9–7.10
podoconiosis (non-filarial lymphoedema) 103.36–103.37
podophyllin/podophyllotoxin, topical therapies 18.13, 25.59, 25.64
POEM *see* Patient-Oriented Eczema Measure
POEMS syndrome (polyneuropathy, organomegaly, endocrinopathy, monoclonal protein and skin changes) 86.24–86.25, 149.11–149.12
Pogosta disease *see* Sindbis virus
poikiloderma of Civatte 86.13–86.14, 94.13
poikiloderma syndromes 75.1–75.8, 94.13
 acrokeratotic poikiloderma of Weary **75.2**, 75.7
 dyskeratosis congenita *67.14*, 67.15, 75.1–75.4
 hereditary fibrosing poikiloderma with tendon contractures, myopathy and pulmonary fibrosis **75.2**, 75.7
 Kindler epidermolysis bullosa 69.5, 69.19, **75.2**, 75.6, 108.86
 poikiloderma with neutropenia, Clericuzio type **75.2**, 75.7
 Rothmund–Thomson syndrome 75.4–75.6
poikilodermatous mycosis fungoides 94.13
poikilodermatous parapsoriasis *see* large plaque parapsoriasis
poikilodermatous plaque-like haemangioma 136.32
point mutations 8.6
poison ivy dermatitis 127.5–127.6, 127.20, 127.22, 127.71
poison/poisonous *see* toxic...; toxins
'polar bear rug' cataract, atopic keratoconjunctivitis *107.19*
polar gel formulations, topical drugs 12.3
polarisable foreign bodies 122.17
poliosis 87.93
pollen allergy 127.84
pollen-fruit allergy syndrome *see* oral allergy syndrome
polyalkylamide, dermal fillers 158.7
polyangiitis, involving respiratory system 152.3–152.4
polyarteritis nodosa (PAN) 100.28–100.30
 eye disease **107.35**
 hepatitis B 25.74
 hepatitis B virus infection 153.5
 oral involvement 108.69
 scrotal pain 109.26
polyarthritis, viral infections 155.2–155.3
polybrominated biphenyls 129.12
polycaprolacton dermal filler 158.6
polychlorinated biphenyls (PCBs), chloracne 129.12
polychondritis, relapsing/atrophic 155.11–155.13
polycyclic hydrocarbons, occupational skin cancer 129.15
polycyclic lesions *4.11*
polycystic ovary syndrome (PCOS) 87.62, 87.88
 acne vulgaris association 88.4–88.5, **88.7, 88.8**, *88.9*
 diagnosis criteria **88.7**
 hidradenitis suppurativa association 90.2
 hirsutism association 87.90
 subtypes **88.7**
polycythaemia vera (PV)
 pruritus 81.10
 thrombocytosis 99.10–99.11
polyendocrine disease 150.19
 see also autoimmune polyendocrinopathy
polyene antifungals 19.48
polyenes, topical therapies 18.12
polygenic risk score (PRS) 8.1
polyhydramion, Neu–Laxova syndrome 63.38
poly-L-lactic acid (PLLA), collagen-stimulating filler [replace capital L with small cap L**] 158.2, 158.6

polymerase chain reaction (PCR) test 3.9
polymers, allergic contact dermatitis 127.68–127.71
polymethylmethacrylate (PMMA) and bovine collagen, dermal fillers 158.7–158.8
polymicrobial flora, human bite wounds 130.7
polymorphic eruption of pregnancy (PEP) 113.16–113.17
polymorphic light eruption (PLE) 126.2–126.8, 126.32–126.33, *126.36*
 phototherapy 21.5, 21.12
 and psoriasis vulgaris 35.4
polymorphisms 3.43, 8.6
 HIV-associated lipodystrophy 98.7
 interleukin-16 127.10
 skin cancer risks 147.6
 thiopurine methyl transferase 19.8–19.9, 19.10
polymyositis
 dermatomyositis relationship 52.1
 internal malignancy association 148.20–148.21
polymyxin B, topical therapies 18.11
polyneuropathy, organomegaly, endocrinopathy, monoclonal protein and skin changes (POEMS) syndrome 86.24–86.25, 149.11–149.12
polyomaviruses (PyVs) 25.46–25.49, **25.47**, 85.15
 Merkel cell polyomavirus-positive carcinoma 25.46–25.47, 146.2, 146.3, *146.4*
 trichodysplasia spinulosa polyomavirus 25.48, 85.15–85.17, 87.36
polypharmacy 13.8
 see also drug–drug interactions
Polypodium leucotomos treatment 126.8
polypoid lesions *see* skin tags
polyposis disorders 153.4, **153.7**
 familial adenomatous polyposis 78.10–78.11
 gastrointestinal polyposis 78.11, 153.4
polyps
 hamartomatous polyps in PJT syndrome 68.13
 inflammatory intestinal polyps *112.6*
 neonatal adnexal polyps 114.19
 see also skin tags
polytrichia 87.49
polyunsaturated fatty acids (PUFAs), cosmeceutical use of 157.5
polyurethanes (PUs), isocyanates in 127.71
pomade acne 88.25, *88.26*
POMC *see* pro-opiomelanocortin deficiency
pomegranate, cosmeceutical use of 157.10
pompholyx eczema 39.14
POP *see* progesterone-only pill
popsicle panniculitis 97.35
population approach, epidemiology 5.2–5.4, 5.5
poradenitis inguinalis *see* lymphogranuloma venereum
porcine collagen dermal filler 158.5–158.6
porcine dermal matrices 125.6
pore of Winer *see* dilated pore lesions
pork tapeworm, cysticercosis 33.32–33.34
porocarcinoma *see* malignant eccrine poroma
porokeratosis 3.44, *4.10*, 63.74–63.76, 85.19–85.23
 autosomal dominant punctate porokeratosis 63.59
 discoid skin lesions **39.10**
 disseminated palmoplantar porokeratosis 85.20, 85.22
 disseminated superficial actinic porokeratosis 63.74–63.75, 85.20–85.22, 141.15–141.18
 genital 85.21, *85.22*, 109.35
 keratinocytes 85.19–85.20
 linear 63.75, 85.20–85.21, *85.22*, 109.35
 ptychotropic 63.75, 85.21, *85.22*, 109.35
 punctate palmoplantar 85.20–85.21

porokeratosis of Mantoux (palmoplantar porokeratosis) 63.75, 85.20–85.21
porokeratosis of Mibelli 63.74, 63.75, 85.20, 85.21, 109.35
porokeratotic eccrine ostial duct naevus (PEN) 63.33–63.34
poromas
 eccrine *4.13*
 eccrine versus apocrine 137.25
porphyria 58.1–58.20
 acute attacks of 58.5–58.7
  precipitants of 58.6
  treatment 58.7
 bullous porphyrias, typical subepidermal bulla in *58.6*
 causing cutaneous disease and acute attacks 58.17–58.18
 causing cutaneous disease but not acute attacks 58.9–58.17
 chemistry of porphyrins 58.1–58.2
 classification 58.2–58.4
 ear dermatoses **106.23**, *106.25*
 enzyme deficiencies and 58.2
 eye disease **107.35**
 haem
  biosynthesis of 58.2, *58.3*, *58.4*
  chemistry of 58.1–58.2
  molecular structure *58.2*
 high-performance liquid chromatography analysis *58.8*
 histopathology 58.4–58.5, *58.6*
 individual porphyrias 58.9–58.19
  acute intermittent porphyria 58.5
  congenital erythropoietic porphyria 58.9–58.11
  erythropoietic protoporphyria 58.4, 58.14–58.17
  hereditary coproporphyria 58.5, 58.7, 58.9, 58.12, 58.17
  porphyria cutanea tarda 58.11–58.14
  pseudoporphyria 58.18–58.19
  variegate porphyria 58.5, 58.7, 58.9, 58.12, 58.17–58.18
 laboratory testing 58.7–58.9
  biochemical findings in cutaneous porphyrias **58.8**
  interpretation of results 58.8–58.9
  porphyrin analysis 58.8
  sample analysis 58.7
  screening of relatives 58.9
 management of skin disease 58.5
 pathogenesis 58.5
 pathophysiology 58.4
 photochemistry of porphyrins 58.2
 phototoxicity of porphyrins 58.1
 and the skin 58.4
 theoretical basis for understanding 58.1–58.2
porphyria cutanea tarda (PCT) 58.11–58.14, 126.7, 127.22
 associated with liver disease 153.7, 153.9
 clinical features 58.11
 clinical variants 58.11–58.12
 epidemiology and pathophysiology 58.11, *58.12*
 erosions, blisters, pigmentary changes and scarring *58.12*
 facial hypertrichosis *87.87*
 genetic counselling 58.14
 hepatitis C 25.76
 HIV 31.18
 investigations 58.12
 liver disease in 58.13
 mortality in 58.14
 renal failure and dialysis complications 154.4
 risk factors for 58.12–58.13
 scleroderma-like syndromes *94.46*
 treatment 58.13–58.14
 see also pseudoporphyria
porphyrin/protoporphyrin, photodynamic therapy 22.2, 22.3, 22.4
porphyrins
 chemistry of 58.1–58.2
 photochemistry of 58.2
 phototoxicity of 58.1

port-wine stains (PWS)   73.20
  eyelid   107.47
  laser therapies   23.8–23.9, *23.10*, *23.11*
  lobular capillary haemangioma   136.26
  phakomatosis pigmentovascularis   *73.22*
posinophilic folliculitis, HIV   31.17–31.18
posterior fossa malformations *see* PHACES syndrome
post-finasteride syndrome (PFS)   87.96–87.97
post-herpetic neuralgia (PHN)   82.4–82.5, 108.66
  zoster   25.32, 25.34, 25.35
posthitis   109.4, 109.16–109.17
postinflammatory elastolysis and cutis laxa (PECL)   94.22, *94.23*
postinflammatory hypermelanosis   86.30–86.31
postinflammatory hyperpigmentation, laser therapies   23.17, *23.18*
postinflammatory hypomelanosis   86.43–86.44
post-ionising radiation keratosis   141.14–141.15
post-irradiation morphoea   119.15
post-kala-azar dermal leishmaniasis (PKDL)   33.51–33.52, 33.53–33.54, 155.5
post-operative care, skin surgery   20.37–20.40
postpartum telogen effluvium   87.56
post-radiotherapy alopecia   87.74
poststeroid panniculitis   97.37, 97.58–97.59
poststreptococcal glomerulonephritis (PSGN), scabies association   26.10
postsurgical artefact, induced non-healing for psychological reasons   84.33, *84.34*
postsurgical wounds, induced non-healing for practical gain   84.37
post-thrombotic syndrome, venous leg ulcer   102.6
post-transfusion purpura   149.15
post-transplant lymphoproliferative disorder (PTLD)   25.39, 139.47
post-traumatic trigeminal neuropathy *see* trigeminal neuralgia
postural exercises, lymphoedema   103.59
potassium, thallium substitution   121.9
potassium iodide (systemic therapy)   19.30–19.31
  dermatological uses   19.30
  potential adverse effects   19.30
  safety issues   19.30–19.31
potassium permanganate, topical therapies   18.9
potassium sorbate (PS)   127.58
potassium titanyl phosphate (KTP) lasers
  absorption spectra   *23.4*
  tattoo removal   23.15
  vascular lesions   23.6, 23.7, 23.9, 23.12
povidone panniculitis   97.48, 97.50
powders, topical medication vehicles   18.2, 18.8
power of clinical trials, statistical analysis   17.22–17.23
poxvirus infections   25.6–25.19
  vulva   110.28–110.29
PPD *see* persistent pigment darkening; (*p*-)phenylenediamine
PPE *see* personal protective equipment
PPKP *see* palmoplantar keratoderma punctata
PPKs *see* palmoplantar keratodermas
PPP *see* palmoplantar pustulosis
PPP syndrome *see* pancreatitis, panniculitis and polyarthritis syndrome
PPV *see* phakomatosis pigmentovascularis
Prader–Willi syndrome (PWS)   72.6–72.9, **72.7**
  obesity association   98.28
  piezogenic pedal papules   122.26
PRAME (PReferentially expressed Antigen in Melanoma)   3.25
pravastatin-induced lichenoid drug eruption   *117.8*

pre-adipocytes   2.40, 97.1
pre-auricular cysts and sinuses, infants   115.12
pre-auricular sinus (PAS)   106.6–106.7
Preferred Reporting Items for Systematic Reviews and Meta-analyses (PRISMA), systemic review assessment   17.8
pregnancy   113.1–113.25
  acne   88.26
  acne vulgaris   113.11–113.12
  antihistamines in   42.18
  apocrine gland activity   113.2–113.3
  atopic eruption of pregnancy   113.15–113.16
  autoimmune skin diseases   113.7–113.9
  benign melanocytic naevi   113.9
  candidiasis   113.7
  cytomegalovirus infection   25.41
  dermatophyte infections   113.7
  drug pharmacokinetics and pharmacodynamics   13.8
  eccrine gland activity   113.2–113.3
  Ehlers–Danlos syndrome   70.11, 113.9
  eosinophilic pustular folliculitis   93.7
  erythema nodosum   113.2
  foliaceus   113.8–113.9
  fungal infections   113.7
  generalised pustular psoriasis   113.10–113.11
  glandular function   113.2
  hair and nail changes in   113.1, **113.2**
  herpes simplex virus infection   113.4–113.5
  HIV   31.36
  human papillomavirus infection   113.4
  immune system changes in   113.3–113.4
  inflammatory skin diseases   113.10–113.12
  intrahepatic cholestasis of pregnancy   113.13–113.14
  itching   113.13–113.24
  leprosy   28.10, 113.6
  malignant melanoma   113.9–113.10
  maternal smoking during, and atopic eczema   41.7
  melasma   86.10, 86.12
  metastatic pregnancy-associated melanoma   113.10
  neonatal lupus erythematosus   51.41–51.42, 113.7–113.8
  obstetric trauma to perineal skin   111.7, **111.8**
  pemphigoid gestationis   113.17–113.19
  pemphigus vulgaris   113.8–113.9
  physiological skin changes in   113.1–113.4
  pigmentation changes in   113.1, *113.2*, **113.2**
  pityriasis rosea   113.6–113.7
  polymorphic eruption of pregnancy   113.16–113.17
  postpartum telogen effluvium   87.56
  pregnancy-specific dermatoses and itching   113.13–113.24
  prenatal diagnoses   8.9–8.11
  pruritus   81.11, 113.13–113.14
  pseudoxanthoma elasticum   70.33–70.34
  psoriasis   35.19, 113.10–113.11
  rosacea   89.15, 89.16, 113.11–113.12
  rubella infection   25.92
  safe treatments in   113.19–113.24
  scabies   113.5–113.6
  sebaceous gland activity   113.2–113.3
  skin infections and infestations   113.4–113.7
  skin tumours   113.9–113.10
  STIs   30.6, 30.11, 30.14
  striae   94.11
  striae distensae   *113.2*, 113.3
  syphilis   113.6
  syphilis management   29.21, 29.22
  systemic lupus erythematosus   51.32, 113.7–113.8
  systemic therapies in   113.19–113.21, **113.22–113.24**
  topical therapies in   113.19, **113.20–113.21**

transplacental transfer of maternal autoantibodies   114.11–114.12
transplacental transfer of maternal malignant disease   114.14
urticaria   42.8, 42.18, 113.12
varicella zoster virus infection   113.5
vascular changes in   **113.2**, 113.3
yeast infections   113.7
  see also congenital…; teratogenicity
pre-haptens   127.8
preimplantation genetic diagnosis (PGD)   8.10–8.11
preimplantation genetic haplotyping (PGH)   8.11
prejudice regarding skin diseases   1.9
prelymphomatous eruption, discoid skin lesions   39.10
premalignant lesions
  external ear   106.33–106.34
  oral cavity   108.42–108.43
  vulva   110.34–110.36
premature ageing syndromes   70.25–70.31, 77.1–77.7
  acrogeria (Grotton syndrome)   **70.26**, 70.28
  Bloom syndrome   **77.2**, 77.3–77.4
  clinical features of   **70.26**
  cutis laxa   77.5–77.7
  familial mandibuloacral dysplasia   70.28–70.29
  Hutchinson–Gilford progeria syndrome   70.25–70.26, **72.5**, 77.4–77.5
  mandibulo-acral dysplasia with type A lipodystrophy   77.5
  mandibulo-acral dysplasia with type B lipodystrophy   77.5
  Mulvihill–Smith syndrome   70.29–70.30
  neonatal progeroid syndrome   70.30–70.31
  pangeria (Werner syndrome)   70.26–70.27, **70.26**, **72.5**, 75.6, 77.1–77.3, **78.12**, 148.12, 148.13
  progeroid laminopathies and related conditions   77.4
premature greying of hair   87.92
premature teloptosis   87.53
prenatal diagnoses   8.9–8.11
preoperative preparation, skin surgery   20.11
preorbital cellulitis, neonates   114.26
prepubertal acne   88.68–88.74
  associated diseases   88.70
  clinical features   88.70–88.71
  complications and co-morbidities   88.72
  differential diagnosis   88.71
  disease course and prognosis   88.72
  epidemiology   88.69–88.70
  investigations   **88.72**
  isotretinoin treatment   **88.73**
  management   88.72–88.74
  pathophysiology   88.70
prepubescent girls, streptococcal vulvovaginitis   26.33
prepuce
  anatomy   109.3
  balanoposthitis   109.4–109.5
  circumcision   109.7
  dorsal perforation   **109.5**
  dorsal perforation of   **109.5**
  paraphimosis   109.4, 109.16–109.17
  posthitis   109.4, 109.16–109.17
  structure and function   109.7
prescribing, topical therapies   18.1–18.4
prescription-writing, medication errors   13.10, 13.11
preservatives
  allergic contact dermatitis   127.48, 127.49–127.58
  genital contact dermatitis   **109.13**
  topical medication   18.8
pressure-associated ulceration and necrosis, COVID-19 association   25.111
pressure dressings, skin surgery   20.38, 20.41
pressure erythema, chronic venous insufficiency   **101.43**

pressure-induced alopecia   87.30–87.31
pressure injuries   123.1–123.12
pressure perception   2.12
pressure sores
  ischaemic fasciitis   136.6
  perineal and perianal skin   111.7–111.8
pressure ulcers   123.1–123.12
  classification systems   123.4–123.6
  COVID-19 association   25.111
  prevalence/incidence   123.1–123.2, **123.3**
  preventative measures   123.6–123.10
  risk factors   123.3–123.4, 123.6
pretibial myxoedema (PTM)   103.41–103.43
  clinical features   103.42–103.43
  hyperthyroidism   57.11
  investigations   103.43
  management   103.43
  pathophysiology   103.42
pre-transplant skin cancers   147.13, 147.18
prevalence of disease   5.10, 5.14
prevention paradox   5.3–5.4
prickly heat *see* miliaria rubra
prick tests   4.23–4.24
primary anetoderma   94.23–94.25
primary biliary cirrhosis (PBC)   86.21–86.22, 153.5
primary care   5.12–5.13
primary CD30+ lymphoproliferative disorders   139.25–139.29
primary chronic telogen effluvium   87.59–87.60
primary cicatricial alopecias (PCAs)   87.37, 87.38–87.50
primary congenital hypertrichosis   87.85–87.86
primary cutaneous acral CD8+ T-cell lymphoma (provisional)   139.33–139.34
primary cutaneous adenocystic carcinoma *see* adenoid cystic carcinoma
primary cutaneous aggressive epidermotropic CD8+ T-cell lymphoma   139.31–139.32
  CD8+ mycosis fungoides variant distinction   139.5
primary cutaneous anaplastic (CD30+) large-cell lymphoma   139.28–139.29
primary cutaneous B-cell lymphomas   139.37–139.43
primary cutaneous blastomycosis   32.85
primary cutaneous CD4+ small/medium pleomorphic T-cell lymphoproliferative disorder (provisional)   139.33
primary cutaneous CD30+ lymphoproliferative disorders   139.25–139.29
primary cutaneous diffuse large B-cell lymphoma   139.37, 139.41–139.43
primary cutaneous follicle centre cell lymphoma (PCFCL)   139.37, 139.40–139.41
primary cutaneous γδT-cell lymphoma   139.32–139.33
primary cutaneous histoplasmosis   32.82, 32.83
primary cutaneous lymphomas (PCLs), immunocompromised people   147.15–147.16
primary cutaneous mammary analogue secretory carcinoma *see* secretory carcinoma
primary cutaneous marginal zone lymphoma (PCMZL)   139.37–139.39
  clinical features/investigations   139.39
  definition   139.38
  management   139.39
  pathogenesis   139.37
  pathophysiology   139.37–139.38
primary cutaneous mucinoses   57.1, 57.2–57.18
primary cutaneous T-cell lymphomas   97.61, 97.62–97.63, 139.2–139.37

see also cutaneous T-cell lymphoma; mycosis fungoides
primary erythromelalgia   101.7–101.8
primary haemophagocytic lymphohistiocytosis   135.11, 135.13
primary herpetic gingivostomatitis   25.20–25.24
primary hypertrophic osteoarthropathy (PHO)   70.35–70.36
primary (idiopathic) cutaneous mucinoses   57.1, 57.2–57.18
primary immunodeficiency diseases *see* inherited immunodeficiency
primary localised cutaneous amyloidosis (PLCA)   56.2, **56.3**
  on ankle   *56.7*
  on chest   *56.7*
  management   56.13–56.14
  on nose   *56.8*
  staining of amyloid   *56.5*
  on toes   *56.8*
  treatment   56.13–56.14
primary lymphoedema (PL)   71.24–71.28, 103.17–103.20
  causative genes and phenotypes   **103.19**
  choanal atresia and lymphoedema   71.27
  clinical features   103.20
  congenital-onset primary lymphoedema   103.24
  epidemiology   103.19
  Hennekam lymphangiectasia–lymphoedema syndrome   71.26
  hereditary lymphoedema type 1A   71.24–71.25
  hypotrichosis–lymphoedema–telangiectasia syndrome   71.26
  late-onset primary lymphoedema   103.24–103.25
  lymphoedema–distichiasis syndrome   71.25–71.26
  microcephaly with or without chorioretinopathy, lymphoedema and mental retardation   71.27
  with myelodysplasia   71.27–71.28
  pathophysiology   103.19–103.20
  St George's classification algorithm   *103.18*
  terminology   **103.18**
primary (naevoid) congenital hypertrichosis   87.85–87.86
primary neutrophilic cicatricial alopecias   87.48–87.50
primary Raynaud phenomenon   124.10–124.12
primary syphilis   29.6–29.7, 29.17
primary systemic or amyloid light-chain amyloidosis (extravascular)   149.13
primary systemic amyloidosis
  haemorrhagic bulla   *56.13*
  macroglossia   *56.12*
  nail dystrophy   *56.13*
  periorbital bleeding   *56.11*
primary telangiectasias   101.16, **101.17**, **101.18**
primary tumours, Merkel cell carcinoma   146.6, 146.8
primin allergy   127.71, 127.73
primitive polypoid/non-neural granular cell tumour *see* dermal non-neural granular cell tumour
Primula dermatitis   127.5, *127.14–127.15*, 127.20–127.22, 127.71, 127.72–127.73
prioritisation, health economics   6.5
PRISMA *see* Preferred Reporting Items for Systematic Reviews and Meta-analyses
procollagen-lysine, 2-oxoglutarate 5-dioxygenase 3 (*PLOD3*)   69.7–69.8
proctitis/proctocolitis syndrome, lymphogranuloma venereum   30.15, 30.16, 30.17
productivity costs, health economic evaluation   6.3

proflavine, topical therapies   18.10
progeroid laminopathies   77.4
progeroid syndromes *see* premature ageing syndromes
progesterone-only pill (POP)   87.95
progestins
  acneform reaction   88.13
  acne vulgaris treatment   88.50–88.51
programmed cell death (PDCD)   *71.2*
progressive bacterial synergistic gangrene   26.77, 26.78
progressive hemifacial atrophy (PHA)   55.23, *55.24–55.25*
progressive hyperpigmentation   68.10
progressive macular hypomelanosis (PMH)   86.44–86.45
progressive mucinous histiocytosis   135.23
progressive nodular histiocytosis (PNH)   135.19
progressive symmetrical erythrokeratoderma (PSEK)   63.19–63.20
pro-haptens   127.8
prohormones, transformation into active metabolite   *150.7*
pro-inflammatory cytokines, antigen-presenting cells   127.7
pro-inflammatory topical treatments, molluscum contagiosum infection   25.18
prolactin
  central nervous system controlled endocrine signalling axis   *150.2*
  hair follicle   87.11–87.12
prolidase deficiency   70.11–70.12, **72.7**, 79.12–79.13
proliferating trichilemmal tumour   137.5–137.6
proline synthesis defects   79.14–79.15
PROMs *see* Patient-Reported Outcome Measures
pro-opiomelanocortin deficiency (POMC)   **72.7**
  C202T mutation   *72.8*
  gene structure and post-translational processing   *72.8*
pro-opiomelanocortin and prohormone convertase deficiency   72.4–72.6
prophylactic dressings, pressure ulcer prevention   123.9
prophylactic phototherapy, PLE management   126.7–126.8
prophylactic skin treatments, papulopustular eruptions   119.4
prophylactic surgical excision of naevi, not recommended to prevent melanoma   142.3
Propionibacterium see Cutibacterium
propolis   127.59, 127.74–127.78
propranolol
  burn treatment   125.14
  infantile haemangioma treatment   *116.8*
propylene glycol (PG)   12.3, 12.5, 127.59
PROS *see* PIK3CA-related overgrowth spectrum
Prospective Register of Systematic Reviews (PROSPERO)   17.8, 17.9
prostaglandin D2 (PGD2), release in skin   14.1
prostaglandins
  hair disorders   87.94–87.95
  male hair loss   87.62
prosthetic implants, cutaneous reactions   127.19
prosthetics, hair loss cover   87.69, 87.101
protease inhibitor (PI), HAART regimes   98.6–98.7
proteases
  Mas-related G-protein-coupled receptor agonists, endothelin   81.1
  pruritus   **81.3**, 81.5
protein contact dermatitis (PCD)   127.10, 127.83, 127.85
protein C/protein S-related disease, purpura   99.15–99.17

protein-energy malnutrition   61.2, 61.3
  hair reddening   *61.4*
  skin signs of nutritional disease   **61.5**
protein fibre, types of   2.2
proteins
  in epidermolysis bullosa   69.2–69.8
  skin fragility link   69.5–69.8
proteinuria, nail–patella syndrome   67.16
protein–hyaluronic acid complex
  normal component of the dermal extracellular matrix   57.1
  see also cutaneous mucinoses; mucin
proteoglycans (PGs)   2.36–2.39
  functions of   2.38–2.39
  gene location   **2.39**
  molecular characteristics and tissue distribution   2.38, **2.39**
Proteus syndrome   71.10–71.11, **72.10**, 73.6, **101.28**, 103.23–103.24
proton beam therapy   24.2–24.3
protothecosis   32.94
protozoal infestations/infections   33.35–33.55
  eye   107.40
  HIV coinfections   31.29
  oral involvement   108.57
provocation testing, cutaneous photosensitivity diseases   126.4–126.6, 126.12, 126.19, 126.34
proximal subungual onychomycosis   32.48
PRP *see* pityriasis rubra pilaris; platelet-rich plasma
PRS *see* polygenic risk score
pruriginosa dystrophic epidermolysis bullosa   69.16
prurigo
  cutaneous manifestations of Hodgkin disease   139.49
  terminology   81.14
prurigo-like morphology, chronic actinic dermatitis   126.17
prurigo nodularis (PN)   81.14–81.18, 84.15–84.18
  clinical features   81.16–81.17, 84.16–84.17
  epidemiology   81.14, 84.16
  investigations   81.17–81.18
  lichen simplex chronicus relationship   84.15
  management   81.18, 84.17–84.18
  pathophysiology   81.15–81.16
  underlying diseases   **81.17**
pruritic conditions (pruritus/xerosis/ichthyosis/prurigo)
  hepatitis C   25.76
  HIV   31.12
pruritus   81.1–81.21
  acetylcholine   **81.3**, 81.4
  antihistamines   41.27
  atopic eczema   41.12, 81.7–81.8
  brachioradial   81.12, 83.6–83.7
  central transmission of itch   81.3
  chronic   81.1–81.14
  chronic kidney disease related   81.8–81.9
  clinical features   81.6–81.13
  cutaneous induction of itch   81.2–81.3
  cutaneous manifestations of Hodgkin disease   139.49
  definitions/nomenclature   81.1
  diabetes   81.10
  diabetic patients   62.6–62.7
  drug-induced   81.10–81.11, 117.2–117.3
  fibreglass dermatitis   122.21
  friction blisters   *122.9*
  genital pruritus   **109.2**
  gold toxicity   121.4
  hepatobiliary disease/cholestasis   81.9–81.10
  histamine/histamine receptors   **81.3**, 81.4
  in ichthyoses   63.46, 63.47
  inflamed skin/dermatoses   81.7
  itching purpura   99.7, 99.8, **99.9**
  lichen simplex   81.18–81.20
  lichen simplex chronicus   84.15
  liver disease association   153.8
  localised   81.12

malignancy manifestation   81.10
mediators of itching in skin diseases   **81.3**, 81.4–81.8
methamphetamine-induced   120.5
neoplasia association   148.27
neurological aspects   81.2–81.4, 81.11–81.12
neuropathic   83.5–83.6
neuropathic pruritus   81.11–81.12
non-atopic causes   84.16
notalgia paraesthetica   81.12
opioid peptides   **81.3**, 81.4–81.5
peripheral and central neuronal sensation   81.4
phototherapy adverse effects   21.12
polycythaemia vera   81.10
in pregnancy   81.11, 113.13–113.24, **113.20**
prurigo nodularis   81.14–81.18
psoriasis vulgaris   81.8
psychiatric and psychosomatic diseases/psychogenic pruritus   81.12
psychogenic   84.27–84.29
PUVA phototherapy adverse effects   21.13
renal failure and dialysis complications   154.3, *154.4*
scalp   105.14–105.17
scratching   81.3–81.4
senescence   81.11
systemic diseases   81.8–81.10
systemic sclerosis   54.16, **54.26**
tachykinins   **81.3**, 81.4
thyrotoxicosis   81.10
trophic syndromes   82.7–82.9
see also itching
pruritus ani   111.3–111.6
  clinical features   111.5–111.6
  epidemiology   111.5
  excoriations and lichenification, idiopathic pruritus   111.6
  management of   111.6
  medicament allergens   *127.46*
  pathophysiology   111.5
  secondary causes of   **111.4–111.5**
PS *see* potassium sorbate
PSCC *see* penile squamous cell carcinoma
PSD *see* penoscrotodynia
PSEK *see* progressive symmetrical erythrokeratoderma
Pseudallescheria boydii see Scedosporium apiospermum
pseudo-ainhum   63.55, 63.56, *63.64*, 94.48
pseudoallergic reactions
  drug hypersensitivity   14.2–14.3
  urticaria   42.5, 42.6, 42.8
pseudochromhidrosis   92.18
pseudocowpox (PCPV) *see* milker's nodule
pseudocyst, external ear   106.8–106.9
pseudoedematous-appearing striae   *94.12*
pseudoepitheliomatous hyperplasia   132.9–132.10
pseudoepitheliomatous micaceous and keratotic balanitis (PEMKB)   109.35
pseudofolliculitis   26.27, 91.8–91.10, 93.1–93.2
pseudofolliculitis barbae   91.8, *91.9*, 122.23
pseudohypoaldosteronism, miliaria association   92.13
pseudo-Kaposi syndrome *see* acroangiodermatitis
pseudologia fantastica   84.37
pseudolymphoma   134.1–134.3
  B-cell/lymphocytoma cutis   134.1, 134.2, 134.8–134.10
  external ear   106.34
  oral involvement   108.72
  pathophysiology   134.1–134.2
  T-cell origin   134.1–134.2
pseudomembranous candidiasis   32.61
Pseudomonas infections   26.51–26.53
  botryomycosis   26.76–26.77
  clinical features and variants   26.52–26.53
  colonisation of wounds, colour   *4.14*

Pseudomonas infections (*continued*)
  epidemiology 26.51
  management 26.53
  P. aeruginosa/*P. pyocyanea* 26.51–26.53
  pathophysiology 26.51
  see also ecthyma gangrenosum;
    Stenotrophomonas maltophilia
pseudomyogenic haemangioendothelioma 136.34
pseudopelade of Brocq (PB) 87.44–87.46
pseudo-pernia *see* chilblain-like lesions
pseudophotodermatitis 127.72
Pseudophyllidea, infections 33.31, 33.34–33.35
pseudopods, melanomas 145.7, 145.8
pseudoporphyria 58.18–58.19
  bullous eruption due to renal failure/dialysis 154.4, 154.5
  drug-induced 126.29
pseudopyogenic granuloma *see* epithelioid haemangioma
pseudosarcomatous fasciitis/pseudosarcomatous fibromatosis *see* nodular fasciitis
pseudosarcomatous fibroblastic/myofibroblastic proliferations, ischaemic fasciitis 136.6
pseudoxanthoma elasticum (PXE) 70.31–70.35, 94.30–94.31, 97.30
  associated diseases 70.31
  of axillary skin 70.32
  cardiovascular changes 70.33
  'chicken skin' appearance 70.32
  clinical variants 70.34
  diagnostic criteria **70.32**
  differential diagnosis 70.34
  gastrointestinal changes 70.33
  investigations 70.34
  management of 70.34–70.35
  obstetric risk 70.33–70.34
  ocular changes 70.33
  pathophysiology 70.31–70.32
  skin changes 70.32–70.33
PSI *see* Psoriasis Symptom Inventory
psittacosis 26.79
psoralen photosensitisers
  adverse effects 21.9, 107.43–107.44
  development of PUVA 21.2
  natural sunlight therapies 21.2
  oral and topical regimens 21.9
  photochemotherapy principles 21.1
  used in PUVA 21.9
psoralen and ultraviolet A (PUVA) 86.17, 126.6
  cutaneous T-cell lymphoma 139.21, 139.22, 139.23
  development 21.2
  lentigines 86.17, 131.7–131.8
  mastocytosis treatment 46.10
  palmoplantar pustulosis 35.39
  psoriasis treatment 35.23
  UVB phototherapy comparison 21.5–21.6
  see also phototherapy
psoriasiform dermatitis 85.14
psoriasiform irritant contact dermatitis 128.4
psoriasiform palmar phenotype, Papillon–Léfèvre syndrome 63.69
psoriasiform plaques, zinc deficiency 61.26
psoriasiform sarcoidosis 96.13
psoriasis 35.1–35.48
  acute generalised exanthematous pustulosis distinction **118.4**
  alcohol misuse relationship 84.40
  alopecia 87.34, 105.3
  ano-genital psoriasis 109.9–109.10
  assessment tools 16.3, **16.3**
  atopic eczema cost comparison 6.10
  biologic therapies 9.8–9.9
  classification **35.2**
  diagnosis 4.1
  disease associations 5.11
  ear dermatoses **106.23**, 106.25
  economic burden of 6.8–6.10

erythrodermic psoriasis 39.32
eyelid 107.6
genetic factors 8.1
global distribution **7.3**
gold reactions 121.4
hand dermatitis differentiation 127.22, 128.5
HIV 31.15–31.17
hypopigmentation 86.44
infantile psoriasis 115.3–115.4
inflammation mechanism 9.8
irritant contact dermatitis 129.1, 129.2
keratoderma climactericum 63.72
male genitalia 109.9–109.10
mechanical injuries 122.2
oral lesions 108.35
perineal and perianal skin 111.8
peristomal skin 112.9, 112.10, 112.11
phototherapy 21.3–21.4
pityriasis rubra pilaris comparison **36.2**
polymorphic light eruption 126.2
in pregnancy 113.10–113.11
psychodermatology 84.4
psychological and social factors 15.4
PUVA-induced lentigines in patient with 131.7
quality of life assessment 16.7–16.8
radiation dermatitis differentiation 119.14
recreational drug-related 120.3
scalp 105.2–105.4
susceptibility genes and pathways **35.3**
vitamin D analogue topical treatment 18.27–18.28
vulva 110.17–110.18
see also psoriasis vulgaris (chronic plaque psoriasis); psoriatic arthritis; pustular psoriasis
Psoriasis Area and Severity Index (PASI) 16.3, 35.16–35.17, **35.27**
Psoriasis Disability Index (PDI) 16.8
Psoriasis Epidemiology Screening tool (PEST) 16.3
Psoriasis Family Impact 16.10
psoriasis gyrata 1.5
Psoriasis Symptom Inventory (PSI) 16.5
psoriasis vulgaris (chronic plaque psoriasis) 35.1–35.31
  acute guttate psoriasis 35.12–35.13
  age at onset 35.2
  alcohol misuse 35.4
  atypical forms of 35.14
  Auspitz sign 35.9
  biologic therapy 35.27–35.31
    adalimumab 35.28
    bimekizumab 35.30
    biosimilars 35.29
    brodalumab 35.30
    certolizumab pegol 35.28–35.29
    etanercept 35.28
    IL-12/IL-23 p40 inhibitor 35.29
    IL-17 inhibitors 35.30
    IL-23p 19 inhibitors 35.30–35.31
    infliximab 35.27–35.28
    ixekizumab 35.30
    registries 35.29
    secukinumab 35.30
    short-term efficacy in randomised trials **35.27**
    TNF-alpha inhibitors 35.27
  cancer association 35.18
  cardiovascular disease 35.19
  in childhood 35.15
  cigarette smoking 35.4
  clinical features 35.6–35.12
  clinical variants 35.12–35.14
  complications and co-morbidities 35.17–35.19
  differential diagnosis 35.16
  disease course and prognosis 35.19
  drug reactions 35.3–35.4
  elephantine psoriasis 35.14
  environmental factors 35.3–35.4
  epidemiology 35.1–35.2
  epidermal hyperplasia with suprapapillary thinning 35.6

erythema, scaling and induration, grading of **35.17**
erythrodermic psoriasis 35.14, **35.16**
flexural psoriasis (inverse psoriasis) 35.8, 35.9, **35.16**
follicular psoriasis 35.7, 35.9
genetics 35.2–35.3
genital psoriasis 35.10
guttate psoriasis 35.15, **35.16**, 35.19
hepatobiliary disease 35.19
histopathology 35.5, 35.6
history 35.6
HIV-induced or exacerbated psoriasis 35.15–35.16
immune-mediated inflammatory disease association 35.18
incidence and prevalence 35.1–35.2
infection 35.3, 35.18
intraepidermal spongiform pustule 35.5
investigations 35.19–35.20
linear psoriasis 35.15
management 35.20–35.31
metabolic syndrome association 35.18
molecular genetics 35.2–35.3
mucosal lesions 35.11–35.12
Munro microabscess formation in lesional stratum corneum 35.6
nail psoriasis 35.10–35.11, 35.12
non-pustular palmoplantar psoriasis 35.10, 35.11
in older age groups 35.15
ostraceous psoriasis 35.14
pathogenic mechanisms 35.4–35.5
physical trauma 35.4
phytotherapy 35.22–35.23
pityriasis rubra pilaris comparison **36.2**
plaques
  changes in fully developed plaques 35.5
  encircled by clear peripheral zone (halo or ring of Woronoff) 35.7
  fiery red plaques of unstable psoriasis 35.13
  with gross hyperkeratosis 35.14
  red scaly plaques 35.7
  silvery white scaling 35.8
pregnancy outcomes 35.19
presentation 35.6
pruritus 81.8
psychological distress 35.4
psychological/psychiatric morbidity 35.19
PUVA photochemotherapy 35.23
remissions from 35.19
scalp psoriasis 35.7, 35.9
seborrhoeic psoriasis (sebopsoriasis) 35.7–35.8
segmental psoriasis 35.15
severity classification 35.16–35.17
sunlight exposure 35.4
systemic therapy 35.23–35.27
  acitretin 35.25–35.26
  apremilast 35.26
  ciclosporin 35.25
  fumaric acid esters 35.26
  hydroxycarbamide (hydroxyurea) 35.26
  methotrexate 35.23–35.25
  properties of **35.24**
  tofacitinib 35.27
  tyrosine kinase 2 inhibitor 35.27
topical treatment 35.20–35.22
  calcineurin inhibitors 35.22
  coal tar 35.21–35.22
  corticosteroids 35.20, 35.21
  dithranol 35.21
  novel agents 35.22
  vitamin D analogues 35.20–35.21
unstable psoriasis 35.13, 35.14, 35.35
vascular bleeding points 35.9
psoriatic alopecia 87.34, 105.3
psoriatic arthritis 35.41–35.46
  age at onset 35.42
  assessment tools 16.3
  associated diseases 35.42

biologic treatment 35.45–35.46
Classification of Psoriatic Arthritis (CASPAR) criteria **35.41**
clinical features 35.43
distal interphalangeal involvement 35.42
epidemiology 35.42
genetics 35.42
investigations 35.43
management 35.44
pathophysiology 35.42–35.43
severity classification 35.43
systemic therapy 35.44–35.45
treatment 35.43–35.46
PSS-AD *see* Psychosomatic Scale for Atopic Dermatitis
PSSs *see* peeling skin syndromes
psychiatric disorders
  male genitalia 109.44
  oral effects 108.83
  see also anxiety; body dysmorphic disorder; depression; stress
psychiatric side-effects of systemic therapies 19.7, 19.18, 19.19, 19.20, 19.43, 19.45
psychiatric therapies
  alternative therapies 84.48
  combined somatic/psychological disorders 84.47–84.48
  drug therapies 84.43–84.47
  psychological therapies 84.47–84.48
  use in dermatology 84.42–84.43
  see also talk therapies
psychoactive drugs *see* psychotropic drugs
Psychoactive Substances Act 2016 120.4
psychodermatolgy
  atopic eczema 41.19
  urticaria 42.8
psychodermatology 1.8–1.9, 84.1–84.49
  "by proxy" disorders 84.5, 84.14, 84.26, 84.29, 84.33, 84.37–84.38
  classification 84.2
  deliberate self-harm 84.38–84.39
  delusional beliefs 84.5–84.12
  eating disorders 84.26–84.27, 108.83
  factitious skin disease 84.29–84.38, 97.48–97.50, 108.61
  'golden rules' 84.2–84.3
  illicit drug use 120.2
  models of service provision 84.2
  multidisciplinary teams 84.2
  national and international organisations 84.2
  obsessive–compulsive behaviour 84.12–84.26
  psoriasis 35.19
  psychoemotional stress role in skin disease 150.8
  psychogenic itch 84.27–84.29
  psychogenic pruritus 81.12
  quality of life assessment 84.4–84.5
  skin-related health anxieties 84.25–84.26
  stigmatisation 1.9, 5.5, 16.8, 28.1, 28.16, 84.3–84.4
  therapies for psychological disorders 84.42–84.48
  treating skin condition concomitantly with psychological disease 84.2, 84.14
  see also suicidality
psychoemotional stress, role in skin disease 150.8
psychogenic itch 84.27–84.29
psychogenic pruritus 81.12, **105.15**
psychological care, stepped approach **15.5**
psychological distress
  acne 88.28–88.29
  morphoea 55.29
  psoriasis vulgaris 35.4
psychological and emotional factors, exacerbating cutaneous disorders 84.1, 84.2
psychological factors, diagnosis 4.5
psychological impacts, measurement 16.11–16.12
psychological methods, cutaneous wart therapy 25.60–25.61
psychological and social factors

atopic eczema 41.19–41.20
  beliefs/emotions/behaviours 15.1–15.3
  childhood and adolescence 15.3, 15.4
  co-morbidities of recreational drug use 120.8
  holistic management of skin disease 15.5–15.7
  ichthyoses 63.46
  impacts of long-term conditions 15.1–15.5
  lymphoedema 103.7
  specific conditions 15.3–15.4
psychopharmacological treatments
  antidepressants 84.43–84.44, **84.44**, **84.45**, 117.3
  antipsychotics 84.44–84.46
  anxiolytics 84.46
  body dysmorphic disorder 84.14
  mood stabilisers 84.46–84.47
Psychosomatic Scale for Atopic Dermatitis (PSS-AD) 16.8
psychotherapies *see* psychiatric therapies
psychotropic drugs
  acneform reaction 88.13
  hypermelanosis 86.26–86.27
  recreational use 120.1
PTBPFR *see para*-tert-butylphenolformaldehyde resin
PTD *see* (*p*-)phenylenediamine and toluene-2,5-diamine
PTEN *see* phosphatase and tensin homologue
PTEN hamartoma tumour syndrome (PHTS) 71.2, 71.13–71.14, *72.10*, *78.11*, **78.14**, 148.11–148.12
  oral involvement 108.85
  storiform collagenoma 136.3
  trichilemmoma 137.6
pterygium syndromes 70.37–70.38
PTLD *see* post-transplant lymphoproliferative disorder
PTM *see* pretibial myxoedema
ptosis 107.6
ptychotropic porokeratosis 63.74, 85.21, *85.22*, 109.35
pubertal growth striae *94.10*, 94.11
pubic hair
  androgen-stimulated growth 87.10
  male 109.4, 109.27
  trichomycosis 26.41–26.42, 109.27
public health approach, epidemiology 5.2, 5.4–5.7
pudendal neuropathic pain/neuralgia 83.7, 83.8
PUFAs *see* polyunsaturated fatty acids
puffy hand syndrome *120.7*
pulley sutures 20.18
pulmonary blastomycosis 32.85
pulmonary disorders
  fungal diseases 32.81–32.88
  interstitial lung disease 52.1, 52.2, 52.7, 52.11–52.12, 69.15
  junctional epidermolysis bullosa with interstitial lung disease 69.15
  Mycobacterium kansasii 27.35
  tuberculosis 27.2, 27.5, 27.6
  tuberous sclerosis complex 78.9
pulmonary involvement
  drug reaction with eosinophilia and systemic symptoms 118.9, 118.11
  Erdheim–Chester disease 135.22
  methotrexate toxicity 19.26
  microscopic polyangiitis 100.21–100.22
  systemic lupus erythematosus 51.31
  systemic sclerosis 54.18, **54.26**
pulmonary oedema, inhalation injury 125.4–125.5
pulmonary sarcoidosis 96.5, 96.15–96.16
pulpitis *128.5*
pulsed dye lasers (PDLs), vascular lesions 23.6–23.12
punch biopsies 3.3, 20.9–20.10
punctate autosomal dominant porokeratosis 63.59
punctate keratosis of the palmar creases 63.60

punctate lesions, palmoplantar keratoderma punctata 63.59
punctate palmoplantar porokeratosis 85.20–85.21
punctuate keratotic projections 63.59
pure diffuse leprosy 28.8
pure neural leprosy 28.10
puritic and dyskeratotic dermatoses (PDD), human polyomavirus-6 and -7 25.48–25.49
purpura 99.1–99.25
  acroangiodermatitis 99.4
  actinic purpura 99.5
  annularis telangiectodes 99.7, 99.8, **99.9**
  antiphospholipid antibody syndrome 99.17–99.19
  associated diseases **100.4**
  atrophie blanche 99.20–99.21
  bacterial infections 99.14
  blood vessels, abnormal or decreased support of 99.5–99.7
  calcific uraemic arteriolopathy 99.23
  cardiac embolus 99.15
  causes **99.2**, **99.5**
  cholesterol embolus 99.14–99.15
  classification 99.1, 99.2
  coagulation disorders **99.2**
  contact allergy **99.9**
  corticosteroid purpura 99.5
  cryogelling/cryoagglutination disorders 99.11–99.14
  cryoglobulinaemia 124.13
  Degos disease 99.21–99.22
  diagnosis by lesion size of macular non-retiform haemorrhage/petechiae **99.3**
  drug-induced purpura **99.4**
  dysproteinaemic purpura 99.6–99.7
  emboli 99.14–99.19
  exercise-induced purpura 99.5, **99.9**
  fungal infections 99.14
  gravitational purpura 99.4
  heparin-induced thrombocytopenia 99.9–99.10
  heparin necrosis 99.9–99.10
  hypergammaglobulinaemic purpura 99.6–99.7
  infections 99.14
  with inflammation **99.2**
  intravascular causes **99.2**, 99.4–99.5
  itching purpura 99.7, 99.8, **99.9**
  lichen aureus 99.7, 99.8, **99.9**
  livedoid vasculopathy 99.20–99.21
  lupus anticoagulant syndrome 99.17–99.19
  malignant atrophic papulosis 99.21–99.22
  mechanical vascular causes **99.2**
  microvascular occlusion disorders 99.9–99.24
  non-thrombocytopenic vascular causes 99.4–99.7
  oral involvement 108.27
  oxalate ebmolus 99.15
  paroxysmal finger haematoma 99.5–99.6
  physical and artefactual bleeding 99.6
  pigmented purpuric dermatoses 99.7–99.9
  pigmented purpuric lichenoid dermatosis of Gougerot and Blum 99.7, 99.8, **99.9**
  platelet disorders 99.2–99.4
  primary ecchymotic haemorrhage syndromes 99.4–99.7
  protein C/protein S-related disease 99.15–99.17
  purpura fulminans 99.15–99.17
  retiform/stallate 25.111, *53.4*, 99.16
  Schamberg disease 99.7, 99.8, **99.9**
  scurvy 99.6
  in Sjögren syndrome 53.10–53.11
  Sneddon syndrome 99.19–99.20
  solar purpura 99.23–99.24
  systemic coagulopathies 99.15–99.19
  thrombocytopenia 99.2–99.4
  thrombocytosis 99.3–99.4, 99.10–99.11

  trauma injury 99.6
  vascular coagulopathies 99.19–99.24
  Waldenström hypergammaglobulinaemic purpura 99.6–99.7
  warfarin-induced necrosis 99.15–99.17
purpura annularis telangiectodes (Majocchi disease) 99.7, 99.8, **99.9**
purpura artefact, induced bruising 84.33
purpura fulminans, neonatal 114.21–114.22, 114.27
purpuric lesions, calciphylaxis 59.7
purpuric macules, Stevens–Johnson syndrome/toxic epidermal necrolysis 118.14
purpuric polymorphic light eruption 126.4, *126.5*
purpuric reactions
  allergens 127.20
  COVID-19 infection 25.109, 25.111, *25.112*
  COVID-19 vaccines 25.118
purse string sutures 20.18
PUs *see* polyurethanes
pustular conditions of the scalp 105.12–105.14
  diagnosis *105.13*
  erosive pustular dermatosis of the scalp 105.13–105.14
pustular drug rash 118.1
pustular folliculitis 91.3–91.5, 93.8
pustular miliaria 92.13
pustular patch test reactions 127.27
pustular psoriasis 35.31–35.41, 118.4
  acrodermatitis continua of Hallopeau 35.39–35.41
  diagnosis of **35.32**
  generalised pustular psoriasis 35.31–35.36
  IL36RN gene 118.2, 118.3
  palmoplantar pustulosis 35.36–35.39
  von Zumbusch variant 35.33–35.34, 118.4
pustular pyoderma gangrenosum 49.4
pustular ulcerative syphilide 29.10
pustules 3.43
  chemical peels, side effect of *160.14*
  rosacea 89.6, *89.7*, 89.12, **89.14–89.15**
pustulose exanthemique aiguë generalisés (PEAG)
PUVA *see* psoralen and ultraviolet A
PV *see* pemphigus vulgaris; polycythaemia vera
P-values, incompatibility of data with a statistical model 17.20–17.21
PVD *see* peripheral vascular disease
PVL *see* Panton–Valentine leukocidin virulence factor
PWA *see* persons with albinism
PWS *see* port wine stains; Prader–Willi syndrome
PXE *see* pseudoxanthoma elasticum
Pyemotes mites 34.51–34.52
pyknosis 3.43
pyloric atresia
  junctional epidermolysis bullosa with 69.13–69.14
  severe recessive epidermolysis bullosa simplex with 69.11
pyoderma, global distribution **7.3**
pyoderma faciale, differential diagnosis 88.34, *88.36*
pyoderma gangrenosum (PG) 49.1–49.8, 53.6, 120.5
  acne conglobata association 88.63
  associated diseases 49.2
  associated with liver disease 153.9
  biologic therapy 49.7
  bullous pyoderma gangrenosum 49.4–49.5
  causative organisms 49.4
  clinical features 49.4
  clinical variants 49.4–49.5
  complications and co-morbidities 49.6
  differential diagnosis 49.5–49.6
  environmental factors 49.4
  epidemiology 49.1–49.2
  extracutaneous pyoderma gangrenosum 49.5

  genetics 49.3, 49.4
  granulomatous superficial pyoderma gangrenosum 49.5, *49.6*
  haematological neoplasms 149.7
  healing ulcer and scarring *49.5*
  immune system activation 49.3
  inflammatory pathways recruitment 49.3
  internal malignancy association 148.23, *148.24*
  intravenous immunoglobulin therapy 49.7
  investigations 49.6
  lesion appearance *49.4*, *49.5*
  male genitalia 109.9, 109.23
  management 49.6–49.8
  Maverakis diagnostic criteria **49.2**
  neutrophil activation 49.3
  parastomal pyoderma gangrenosum 49.4, *49.5*
  pathology 49.3
  pathomechanism of 49.3
  peristomal skin *112.10*, 112.13–112.15
  predisposing factors 49.2
  pustular pyoderma gangrenosum 49.4
  sarcoidosis association 96.15
  severity classification 49.6
  tissue destruction 49.3–49.4
  treatment for **49.7**
  vegetative pyoderma gangrenosum 49.5, *49.6*
pyodermatitis-pyostomatitis vegetans (PD-PSV) 49.19–49.20
pyoderma vegetans, possible bacterial/viral roles 26.88
pyogenic arthritis-pyoderma gangrenosum-acne (PAPA) syndrome **45.5**, **45.6**, 45.13, 88.8–88.10, **88.11**, 88.63
pyogenic granuloma (PG) (lobular capillary haemangioma) 71.2, 136.25–136.27
  in acne 88.41
  infants 116.10–116.11
  laser therapies 23.11
  oral *113.3*
  within port-wine stains 136.26
pyogenic infection
  external ear 106.19
  recurrent 80.18
pyogenic sterile arthritis, pyoderma gangrenosum and acne syndrome *see* pyogenic arthritis-pyoderma gangrenosum-acne syndrome
pyostomatitis vegetans, oral involvement 108.74
pyrethroids, topical therapies 18.14
pyridoxine (vitamin B6) deficiency 61.17–61.18
pyrin-associated autoinflammation with neutrophilic dermatosis (PAAND) 45.10–45.11
pyruvic acid (PA), chemical peels 160.2
Pythium insidiosum infection 32.94
PyV *see* polyomaviruses

Q
QALY *see* Quality-Adjusted Life Year
QES *see* Questionnaire on Experience with Skin complaints
Q fever 97.46
QoL *see* quality of life
Q-switched lasers, tattoo and pigmented lesion treatments 23.12–23.17
Quality-Adjusted Life Year (QALY) *6.3*, *6.4*, 16.9
quality of life (QoL) assessment 4.5, 16.5–16.11
  acne 88.38–88.39, **88.40**
  adolescents 16.10
  children 16.9–16.10
  dermatology specific measures 16.6
  disease specific measures 16.7–16.9
  evaluation 6.3
  families 16.10–16.11
  general health measures 16.6
  Harmonising Outcome Measures for Eczema 16.3

quality of life (QoL) assessment (continued)
  informing clinical decisions 16.6
  meaning 16.5–16.6
  measurement 6.4
  methods 16.6
  occupational skin disease 16.12
  practical use of measures 16.11
  psychodermatology 84.4–84.5
  purpose 16.6
  rosacea 89.5
Quality of Reporting of Meta-analyses (QUOROM), systemic review assessment 17.8
quaternium-15 127.51
quenching effects, patch testing 127.29
Questionnaire on Experience with Skin complaints (QES) 16.8
quinine-induced photo-lichenoid eruption 4.7
quinines, allergic contact dermatitis 127.80
quintana fever see trench fever
QUOROM see Quality of Reporting of Meta-analyses

R

RA see rheumatoid arthritis
Rab GTPase Rab27B, epidermolysis bullosa 69.4
racial factors
  dermatomyositis 52.1
  facial melanoses 86.9
  see also skin of colour
radial streak patterns see peripheral streak patterns; starburst patterns
radiation dermatitis see radiodermatitis
radiation-induced angiosarcoma, atypical vascular proliferation after radiotherapy comparison 136.38–136.39
radiation-induced carcinogenesis 24.4, 24.21
  latent period 24.4, 24.21
  management 24.21
  rare tumours 24.21
  risk in treatment of benign conditions 24.4, 24.21
  sarcomas 24.21
  tumour risks in immunocompromised people 147.9
radiation reactions
  early/acute 24.18, 24.19
  late/chronic 24.18–24.20
radiation recall phenomena 119.12–119.13
radiculoneuropathy, primary ano-genital herpes infection 25.25
radiodermatitis 105.5–105.6, 109.12, 119.13–119.15
radiofrequency (RF), skin tightening 161.6
  methods of delivery 161.7
  microneedling devices 161.8
  safety and adverse events 161.7
radiological examination 4.22–4.23
radiological investigations, peripheral vascular disease 101.4
radio-responsiveness, radiotherapy 24.4
radiotherapy 24.1–24.24
  associated skin side effects 119.13–119.15
  atypical vascular proliferation after radiotherapy 136.38–136.39
  basal cell carcinoma 140.16–140.17
  benign skin conditions 24.4, 24.7
  Bowen disease 141.24
  brachytherapy 24.3
  causing post-ionising radiation keratosis 141.14–141.15
  compared to surgery for skin cancer 24.8, **24.10**
  cutaneous side effects 119.1–119.15
  cutaneous squamous cell carcinoma 141.35, 141.37
  cutaneous T-cell lymphoma 139.15, 139.16, 139.21, 139.22
  dose fractionation and treatment regimens 24.10
  early/acute reactions 24.18, 24.19

electron beam therapy 24.1–24.2
hypofractionated regimens for melanoma 24.14
indications 24.4, 24.7–24.10
melanoma 144.2
morphoea 55.14
multivoltage X-ray techniques 24.3–24.4
particular skin sites with basal cell or squamous cell carcinomas 24.9, 24.10–24.12
proton beam therapy 24.2–24.3
radio-curability and radio-responsiveness 24.4
superficial techniques 24.33
tumour recurrence 24.20–24.21
tumours induction see radiation induced carcinogenesis
types 24.1–24.3
raised linear bands of infancy 114.18–114.19
Rajka Langeland severity classification, atopic eczema 16.4
RAK see reticulate acropigmentation of Kitamura
Ramazzini, Bernadino 1.4
random-effects models, systematic reviews 17.10
randomisation sequence assessment, evidence based medicine 17.12, 17.13
randomised controlled clinical trials (RCTs)
  bullous pemphigoid 50.20–50.21, **50.23**
  mucous membrane pemphigoid 50.30–50.31
  see also evidence based medicine
rapid acoustic pulse (RAP) technology, cellulite treatment 161.9
Rapunzel syndrome 84.24
RAS see recurrent aphthous stomatitis
RASA1 mutations see RASopathies
rashes see exanthems
Ras-MAPK signalling pathway 78.7, *78.8*, **78.9**
RASopathies 78.7, *78.8*, **78.9**
  cardiac and cutaneous malformations 151.3
  lymphatic abnormalities 103.24
  neurofibromatoses 78.7, *78.8*, **78.9**
Ras–mitogen activated protein kinase (Ras-MAPK) signal transduction pathway 78.7, *78.8*
  genetic syndromes of **78.9**
rat-bite fevers 26.75–26.76, 130.5
  Spirillum minus 26.75
  Streptobacillus moniliformis 26.75–26.76
rationalisation, health economics 6.5
rational medicine
  growth of 1.2–1.4
  see also evidence based medicine
rat transitional epithelium, antibody detection 3.20
Raynaud phenomenon (RP) 53.1, 124.10–124.13, 129.15–129.16
  acrocyanosis distinction 124.7
  cannabis-induced 120.4
  causes **54.19**
  clinical features **54.19**
  fingertip rewarming in patient with *54.22*
  fish stings 130.4
  internal malignancy association 148.24–148.25
  investigation and management **54.25**
  in systemic lupus erythematosus 51.26
  systemic sclerosis *54.3*, 54.15, **54.19**
  vibration white finger 122.24
al-Razi, Muhammad ibn Zakariya ('Rhazes') 1.3
RCM see reflectance confocal microscopy
RCTs see randomised controlled clinical trials
RD see Refsum disease
RDD see Rosai–Dorfman–Destombes disease
RDTC see Regional Dermatology Training Centre, Moshi, Tanzania
reactivation of viruses 25.4
  after COVID-19 vaccination 25.118
  in COVID-19 patients 25.111

human herpesvirus 6 and 7 25.40
immunomodulatory drug effects 19.3
zoster 25.32–25.36
reactive angioendotheliomatosis 136.24–136.25
reactive arthritis (Reiter's syndrome) 155.2, *155.3*
  eye disease **107.35**
  oral involvement 108.68
  vulva 110.18
reactive cutaneous lymphoid hyperplasia see lymphocytoma cutis/B-cell pseudolymphoma
reactive diluents, resins 127.69
reactive granulomatous dermatitis (RGD) 53.5
reactive inflammatory erythemas 47.1–47.17
  annular erythema of infancy 47.9, *47.10*
  erythema annulare centrifugum 47.6–47.8
  erythema chronicum migrans 47.9
  erythema gyratum repens 47.11–47.12
  erythema marginatum 47.9–47.11
  erythema multiforme 47.1–47.6
  necrolytic migratory erythema 47.12–47.16
  rheumatic fever, Duckett Jones criteria for diagnosis of **47.11**
reactive material, removal techniques 122.19
reactive oxygen intermediates (ROIs), erythema nodosum 97.21
reactive oxygen species (ROS)
  ageing of skin 156.4, 156.6
  hair pigmentation 87.12–87.13
reactive perforating collagenosis 63.76
  lip lesions 108.64
  renal failure and dialysis complications 154.3–154.4
reactive vascular lesions 136.23–136.25
rebound phenomena, discontinuation of corticosteroids 18.21
recalcitrant irritant dermatitis, excessive hand washing 84.26
recall reaction dermatitis 119.12–119.13
RECAP see Recap of Atopic Eczema
Recap of Atopic Eczema (RECAP) 16.3
ReCell 125.6
receptor–effector system, drug action mechanisms 13.5
receptor tyrosine kinases (RTKs), transmembrane drug mechanisms 13.5
recessive dystrophic epidermolysis bullosa 69.5, 69.16–69.18, *69.16*, **78.14**
  cancer and 69.26–69.27
  combined with dominant 69.18
  management of 69.25–69.26
recessive X-linked ichthyosis 63.5–63.7
recombinant human growth hormone (rhGH), burn treatment 125.13
recombinant protein therapy, ectodermal dysplasias 69.27
record keeping, systemic therapy 19.2
recreational drug use 120.1–120.9
  delusional infestation 84.5, 84.6, 84.7, 84.8, 84.9
  olfactory delusions 84.10
  pharmaceutical drug interactions 120.3
recto-vaginal fistula *111.7*
rectum
  ano-rectal abscess 111.27–111.28
  gastrointestinal polyposis 78.11
recurrent angioedema without weals see angioedema without weals
recurrent aphthous stomatitis (RAS) 108.37–108.38
recurrent cellulitis see erysipelas
recurrent cutaneous necrotising eosinophilic vasculitis 100.10–100.11
recurrent focal palmar peeling 39.16
recurrent genital herpes 25.26
recurrent infundibulofolliculitis 91.14–91.15, 93.6–93.7

recurrent labial HSV infection (RHL) 108.52–108.53
recurrent lymphocytic meningitis, herpes simplex virus 25.23
recurrent melanocytic naevi 131.26–131.27
recurrent oro-facial and cutaneous herpes 25.22–25.24
recurrent toxin-mediated perineal erythema 26.32, 26.33
recurring digital fibrous tumour of childhood see inclusion body (digital) fibromatosis
red ear syndrome 106.23
redness (erythema) 4.13, 126.1
  acne vulgaris 88.27, 88.29
  atopic eczema 41.15
  chemical peels, side effect of 160.11–160.12
  chronic venous insufficiency **101.43**
  dermatomyositis 52.3, 52.4, *52.5*, *52.6*
  differential diagnosis 89.7
  disease course 89.11
  drug/chemical photosensitivity *126.29*
  epidermolysis bullosa acquista *50.45*
  grading of in psoriasis vulgaris **35.17**
  hereditary angio-oedema 43.4
  indicator of pressure ulcers 123.4
  irritant contact dermatitis 128.6
  laser therapies 23.9–23.11, *23.12*, *23.13*
  lichen planus *110.12*
  linear IgA disease *50.37*
  morphoea *55.18*
  non-blanchable 123.4, **123.5**, 123.8
  ultraviolet radiation 10.3, *10.4*
  UVB phototherapy adverse effects 21.11–21.12
  UVR exposure 10.7
  venous leg ulcer *102.5*
  see also erythema...; flushing; rosacea
α5-reductase inhibitors 87.96
Reduviidae (kissing bugs/assassin bugs/cone-nosed bugs) 34.29
Reed naevi *131.34, 131.37*, **145.5**, **145.6**
Reed naevi see Spitz naevi
Reed naevus *131.34, 131.37*, **145.2**, 145.5, 145.6
Reed syndrome (hereditary leiomyomatosis and renal cell cancer) 78.14, *78.15*, 148.12, 154.2
reference listed drug (RLD), topical bioavailability/bioequivalence assessment 12.7, 12.8
reflectance confocal microscopy (RCM) 4.21, *4.22*, 142.9
Refsum disease (RD) 63.30–63.32
refugee camps see displaced persons camps
Regional Dermatology Training Centre, Moshi, Tanzania (RDTC) 7.7
RegiSCAR drug reactions **118.9**
regression structures, melanoma 145.7, *145.8*
regressive melanoma 142.14, *142.17*, 142.20
regulations, drug application approval 13.13
regulatory T cells (Tregs) 127.9
Reiter's syndrome see reactive arthritis
RELA haploinsufficiency 45.15
relapsing fever (epidemic), *Borelia recurrentis* 26.72
relapsing polychondritis 155.11–155.13
  ear dermatoses **106.23**
  respiratory disease 152.2
relaxed skin tension lines, principles of surgical design 20.20–20.21
REM see reticular erythematous mucinosis
Renaissance medicine 1.3
renal abnormalities/dysfunction
  drug reaction with eosinophilia and systemic symptoms 118.9, 118.11
  systemic lupus erythematosus 51.31
renal cancer, syndromes linked with **78.14**
renal cell carcinoma, flushing **104.8**
renal cell carcinoma syndrome, hereditary cutaneous leiomyomatosis links 154.2

renal disorders 154.1–154.7
  calcific arteriolopathy 97.32–97.33
  calciphylaxis involving the penis 109.24
  chronic kidney disease 81.8–81.9
  nail–patella syndrome 67.15, 67.16
  oral involvement 108.83
  skin involvement 154.2, *154.3*
  systemic lupus erythematosus 51.31
  systemic sclerosis 54.18, **54.24**
  see also nephropathy
renal failure, hypermelanosis 86.21–86.22
renal failure and dialysis, cutaneous signs 154.3–154.5
renal failure and dialysis complications, Kyrle disease 154.3–154.4
renal function, drug elimination 13.3
renal transplantation
  dermatological consequences of immunosuppression 154.5–154.6
  see also organ transplant recipients
repeat open application tests (ROATs), allergen testing 127.28, 127.33, 127.49, 127.50
reperfusion injury 123.2
repetitive behaviour disorders 84.22–84.26
repigmentation pattern, piebaldism *68.4*
repositioning interventions, pressure ulcers 123.6–123.8, 123.10
reproductive toxicity, methotrexate 19.26
resin contact allergy 127.65–127.66
resins, allergy to 127.68–127.71
resin systems, allergy to 127.18
respiratory fungal diseases 32.82–32.88
respiratory support, SJS/TEN management 118.20
respiratory symptoms
  BSL management 98.15, 98.16
  dermatomyositis 52.7–52.8
  syndromic ichthyoses **63.39**
  yellow nail syndrome 152.6
respiratory syncytial virus (RSV) 25.99–25.100
respiratory system 152.1–152.7
respiratory tract infections, skin features 26.79
restless leg syndrome (RLS) 83.10–83.11
restrictive dermopathy 63.38, 70.24, **77.2**
resuscitation, burn shock 125.2–125.4
resuscitation fluids
  inhalation injuries 125.5
  types 125.3–125.4
resuscitation formulae 125.2–125.3
resveratrol, topical depigmenting agents 18.33
retapamulin, topical therapies 18.11
reticular degeneration 3.40–3.41
reticular dermis, mechanical strength 122.4–122.5
reticular erythematous mucinosis (REM) 57.8–57.9
reticular hyperpigmentation, heat-associated carcinomas *124.15*
reticular pattern naevi
  dermoscopy *145.2, 145.3*, 145.4
  Spitz naevi 145.6
reticular variant, mid-dermal elastolysis 94.26
reticulate acropigmentation of Kitamura (RAK) 68.13, *68.14*
reticulate hyperpigmentation, drug/chemical photosensitivity 126.30
reticulate scarring, congenital erosive and vesicular dermatosis with 94.14
reticuloendothelial system, sarcoidosis 96.5
reticulohistiocytoma 135.22
reticulohistiocytosis 135.25–135.27
retiform haemangioendothelioma 136.32–136.33
retiform parapsoriasis *see* large plaque parapsoriasis
retiform purpura 99.16
  COVID-19 association 25.111
  in patient with mixed connective tissue disease *53.4*

retina, pseudoxanthoma elasticum 70.33
retinal anlage tumour *see* pigmented neuroectodermal tumour of infancy
retinaldehyde, cosmeceutical use of 157.7
retinoic acid (tretinoin) 18.23, 18.24
  chemical peels 160.2
  topical depigmenting agents 18.32
  topical therapies 18.25
retinoids
  acne vulgaris treatment 88.45–88.46, 88.47
  chemical structure *18.24*
  cosmeceutical use of 157.6–157.7
  dermatitis reactions *88.55*
  eye, side effects on 107.43
  hidradenitis suppurativa treatment 90.10
  keratinocyte cancer chemoprevention 147.20
  synthetic 19.41–19.42
  topical therapies 18.23–18.26
  use during pregnancy 63.44–63.45, 113.22–113.23
retinoids (systemic therapy) 19.42–19.44
  cautions 19.44
  contraindications 19.44
  cutaneous T-cell lymphoma 139.16, 139.23
  dermatological uses 19.42
  drug–drug interactions 19.44
  monitoring 19.44
  pharmacological properties 19.42
  potential adverse effects 19.43–19.44, 63.44–63.45
  pre-treatment screening 19.44
retinol (vitamin A)
  cosmeceutical use of 157.7
  deficiency 61.7–61.8, 85.14–85.15, 86.23–86.24
  excess 61.8–61.9
  metabolic production 18.23–18.24
  topical therapies 18.24
retinyl esters, cosmeceutical use of 157.7
retrovirus infections 25.78–25.80
reverse smoking (bidi), keratoses 108.33
revertant mosaicism 8.8
Revesz syndrome 67.15
rexinoid oral therapy, cutaneous T-cell lymphoma 139.15, 139.23
RF *see* radiofrequency
RGD *see* reactive granulomatous dermatitis
rhabdomyocyte (striated muscle cell), microscopic examination of 3.37
rhabdomyoma 136.55
  oral involvement 108.14
rhabdomyomatous congenital hamartoma 136.55
rhabdovirus infections 25.97
rheumatic diseases
  calluses 122.7
  hyperpigmentation 86.20
rheumatic fever 53.12, 155.3
  cutaneous lesions 151.5, *151.6*
  Duckett Jones criteria for diagnosis of **47.11**
rheumatoid arthritis (RA) 53.3–53.8, 155.5–155.6, *155.7*
  callosities 122.9
  clinical features 53.4, **53.5**
  clinical variants 97.16
  epidemiology 53.4
  fibroblastic rheumatism 53.7–53.8
  gold treatment 121.3–121.4
  interstitial granulomatous dermatitis 53.6
  investigations 53.8
  leg ulcers 53.7
  management 53.8
  medium vessel vasculitis *53.8*
  oral involvement 108.68
  panniculitis 97.52
  pathophysiology 53.4
  pyoderma gangrenosum 53.6
  reactive granulomatous dermatitis 53.5
  rheumatoid neutrophilic dermatosis 53.5–53.6

rheumatoid nodules 53.5
rheumatoid vasculitis 53.6–53.7
skin manifestations 155.5–155.6, *155.7*
systemic lupus erythematosus comparison **51.30**
vascular lesions associated with 53.6
rheumatoid disease 155.1–155.16
  ear dermatoses **106.23**
  oral involvement 108.67–108.69, **108.68**
rheumatoid neutrophilic dermatosis (RND) 53.5–53.6, 155.6, *155.8*
rheumatoid nodules (RN) 53.5, 97.15–97.17, 155.5–155.6, *155.7, 155.8*
rheumatoid vasculitis (RV) 53.6–53.7, 155.6
rhGH *see* recombinant human growth hormone
rhinoentomophthoromycosis 32.79–32.80
rhinophyma
  disease course 89.11
  photothermal ablation 23.22
  sex prevalence 89.2
  treatment *89.13*
rhinoscleroma, *Klebsiella pneumoniae* subsp. *rhinoscleromatis* 26.56–26.57
rhinosporidiosis 32.79
RHL *see* recurrent labial HSV infection
RHSF *see* European Hidradenitis Suppurativa Foundation
rhytids (wrinkles)
  ablative fractional resurfacing 161.5
  ageing of skin *156.2, 156.5*
  cosmeceuticals 157.4–157.7
  dermal fillers, indication for 158.1, **158.3**
  glyphic wrinkles 94.2
  laser-assisted drug delivery 161.5
  mid-dermal elastolysis 94.26
  reduction of by botulinum toxin application 159.5, *159.6, 159.7*
  smoker's skin *156.4*
riboflavin (vitamin B2) deficiency 61.14–61.15
rickets, hair disorders 87.29
rickettsial infections 26.80–26.84
  scrub typhus group 26.84
  spotted fever group 26.81–26.83
  transitional group 26.83–26.84
  typhus group 26.80–26.81
rickettsialpox 26.83–26.84
Rickettsia prowazekii, epidemic typhus 26.80–26.81
rifamycins 19.47
ring eczema 39.16, 128.3
ringworm of the beard *see* tinea barbae
ringworm of the body *see* tinea corporis
ringworm of the face *see* tinea faciei
ringworm of the foot *see* tinea peddis
ringworm of the groin *see* tinea cruris
ringworm of the hand *see* tinea manuum
ringworm of the nails (onychomycosis caused by dermatophytes) 32.47–32.49
ringworm of the scalp *see* tinea capitis
risk reduction for systemic therapy 19.1–19.2, 19.3
Ritter disease *see* staphylococcal scalded skin syndrome
rituximab 135.29
  mucous membrane pemphigoid, management of 107.31–107.32
  pemphigus treatment 50.9
  systemic sclerosis treatment 54.24–54.25
river blindness *see* onchocerciasis
RLD *see* reference listed drug
RLS *see* restless leg syndrome
RN *see* rheumatoid nodules
RNA editing, dyschromatoses 68.14–68.15
RNA profiling, immune cell analysis 9.2
RNA sequencing, melanoma diagnosis 142.21
RNA viruses 25.78–25.120
  human coronavirus 25.100–25.119
  human retroviruses 25.78–25.80
  paramyxoviruses 25.97–25.100
  pathogenesis 25.2, 25.5
  Picornaviruses/enteroviruses 25.93–25.97

rhabdoviruses 25.97
togaviruses 25.80, 25.87–25.92
viral haemorrhagic fevers 25.80–25.87
RND *see* rheumatoid neutrophilic dermatosis
ROATs *see* repeat open application tests
Robles disease *see* onchocerciasis
Rocky Mountain spotted fever, rickettsial infection 26.82
rodent bites 26.75–26.76, 130.5
rodent borne viruses, haemorrhagic fevers 25.81–25.83
rodent flea disease transmission
  plague 26.59–26.60
  rickettsial infection/murine typhus 26.81
roflumilast, psoriasis treatment 35.22
ROIs *see* reactive oxygen intermediates
Roman Empire, rational medicine 1.3
ROS *see* reactive oxygen species
rosacea 89.1–89.20
  causative organisms 89.4
  classification 89.1
  clinical features 89.5
  definition 89.1
  diagnostic features **89.2**, 89.5–89.6, 89.12
  differential diagnosis 88.34
  disease course 89.11
  epidemiology 89.2
  flushing **104.4**
  laser therapies 23.9, *23.12*
  major features **89.2**, 89.6
  management 89.11–89.12
  on mid-face *88.35*
  minor features **89.2**, 89.6–89.7
  pathology 89.3–89.5
  pathophysiology 89.2–89.4
  in pregnancy 113.11–113.12
  prognosis 89.11
  sarcoidosis differential diagnosis 96.3
  treatment **89.13–89.14**
rosacea fulminans 89.16
rosacea-like dermatoses due to medication 89.10
rosacea-like erythema of the face, dermatomyositis 52.3, *52.5*
Rosai–Dorfman disease 3.23, 135.1
Rosai–Dorfman–Destombes disease (RDD) 135.27, *135.28*, 149.17
rose, cosmeceutical use of **157.8**
roseola infantum (sixth disease) 25.39–25.40, 115.5–115.6
roseolar rash (macular syphilide) *29.8*, 29.9
Ross River virus (RRV) 25.90
Ross syndrome 92.7, 92.9, 92.12
rotations flaps, surgical reconstruction **20.24**, 20.25
Rothmann–Makai disease 97.8
Rothmund–Thomson syndrome (RTS) 75.4–75.6, **78.12**, 148.12, 148.13
  clinical features **75.2**, 75.5–75.6
  differential diagnosis 75.6
  genetics 75.5
  management 75.6
round cell liposarcoma 136.59
roundworms *see* nematodes
Royal Society of Tropical Medicine and Hygiene (RSTMH) 7.6
RP *see* Raynaud phenomenon
RRV *see* Ross River virus
RSPO4 gene, hereditary anonychia 67.16
RSTMH *see* Royal Society of Tropical Medicine and Hygiene
RSV *see* respiratory syncytial virus
RTKs *see* receptor tyrosine kinases
RTS *see* Rothmund–Thomson syndrome
rubber allergy 127.17, 127.62–127.65, 127.68; 127.84–127.85
rubber gloves, allergies 39.14, 127.63
rubber products, genital contact dermatitis 109.13
rubella 25.91–25.92
  clinical features 25.92
  congenital rubella 114.23
  epidemiology 25.91
  managements 25.92
  pathophysiology 25.91–25.92

rubeosis, diabetic patients 62.2
Rubinstein–Taybi syndrome **72.7**
rufous albinism 68.6
Ruijs–Aalfs syndrome **72.5**
running intradermal suture 20.19
rural versus urban environments, atopic eczema 41.6–41.7
RV *see* rheumatoid vasculitis

S

S-100 protein (melanocyte marker) 3.23, 3.25
SA *see* salicylic acid; sorbic acid
SABR *see* stereotactic ablative radiotherapy
SAC *see* seasonal allergic conjunctivitis
SACD *see* systemic allergic contact dermatitis
sacral herpes zoster 109.28
SADSS *see* Six Area Six Sign Atopic Dermatitis severity score
safety issues
  electrosurgery 20.45–20.46
  phototherapy 21.16
  radiofrequency skin tightening 161.7
  skin surgery 20.6–20.7, 20.11
  treatments in pregnancy 113.19–113.24
SAHA *see* seborrhoea, acne, hirsutism and/or androgenic alopecia syndrome
salbutamol, topical therapies 18.41
salicylic acid (SA) 63.44
  acne vulgaris treatment 88.57
  chemical peels 160.3–160.4, 160.10
salicylism, ichthyoses 63.42
salivary glands 108.4, 108.6
SALT *see* severity of alopecia tool
saltpetre disease 94.31
salt-split human skin substrate, subepithelial blistering disease diagnosis 3.20
salvage therapy, haemophagocytic lymphohistiocytosis 135.13–135.14
sampling errors, epidemiological studies 5.14
SAM syndrome *see* severe dermatitis–multiple allergies–metabolic wasting syndrome
sandflies 33.43, 33.45, *33.52*, 34.3, 34.7
sand worm eruption, *see also* cutaneous larva migrans
Sanger sequencing 69.22–69.23
San Joaquin valley fever *see* coccidioidomycosis
SAPHO *see* synovitis, acne, pustulosis, hyperostosis and osteitis
saprophytic moulds, superficial mycoses 32.18
sarcoidal granulomas, subcutaneous sarcoidosis 97.54
sarcoidal granulomatous inflammation, tattoos 122.22
sarcoid dactylitis 96.12, 155.7, *155.9*
sarcoidosis 89.10, 89.19, 96.1–96.18, 105.9
  arthropathies 155.7, *155.9*
  cardiac involvement 151.4
  ear dermatoses **106.23**
  erythema nodosum with 97.21–97.22
  eye disease **107.35**
  facial, photothermal ablation 23.22
  foreign body reactions 122.17
  induced by drugs 96.4
  lip lesions 108.64
  metastatic calcinosis cutis 59.5
  neuroendocrinology 150.16
  oral lesions 108.67
  panniculitis 97.53–97.54
  pulmonary involvement 152.5
  systemic manifestations 96.5
sarcomas
  clear cell 136.64
  fat cells 136.58–136.59
  low-grade fibromyxoid sarcoma 136.18–136.19
  malignant vascular tumours 136.34–136.37

neural origins 136.51–136.52
non Kaposi in immunocompromised people 147.16
radiation-induced 24.21
undifferentiated soft tissue sarcoma 136.17–136.18
see also dermatofibrosarcoma protuberans; Kaposi sarcomas; myxofibrosarcoma; myxoinflammatory fibroblastic sarcoma; pseudosarcomatous fibroblastic/myofibroblastic proliferations
Sarcoptidae (mites)
  animal scabies 34.50
  human classical scabies 34.41–34.48
  human crusted scabies 34.48–34.50
SARS-CoV-2 spike protein stains perniosis 124.5
  see also COVID-19/SARS-CoV-2
SART3 *see* Squamous Cell Carcinoma Antigen Recognized by T-cells
Sartorius Score, hidradenitis suppurativa 16.4
SASH *see* Severity and Area Score for Hidradenitis
Sata, Sarachiro 1.7
SAVI *see* STING-associated vasculopathy with onset in infancy
sawah itch *see* cercarial dermatitis
saw-toothing 3.43
sBCC *see* superficial basal cell carcinoma; superficial basal cell carcinomas
SC *see* stratum corneum
scabies 34.41–34.50, 127.22
  animal scabies 34.50
  diagnosis 4.22
  global control measures 7.9
  global distribution **7.3**
  HIV 31.29
  human classical scabies 34.41–34.48
  human crusted scabies 34.48–34.50
  incidence of 7.2
  infants 115.9
  male genitalia 109.29, *109.30*
  in Panama **5.2**, 5.3
  perineal and perianal skin 111.16
  population approach to 5.2
  in pregnancy 113.5–113.6
  pseudolymphoma 134.1, 134.2
  secondary infections 26.10, 26.11
  treatment during pregnancy **113.20**
scabs, wound healing 11.10
scalded mouth syndrome *see* burning mouth syndrome
scaling
  acquired ichthyosis 63.47
  collarette scaling *4.13*
  health economics 6.5
  ichthyosis vulgaris 63.4, *63.5*
  recessive X-linked ichthyosis 63.5, *63.6*
  scalp disorders 105.1–105.6
scalp
  cooling treatments for chemotherapy-induced alopecia 119.6
  microscopic examination of skin 3.33
  scalp desquamation, ichthyoses 63.45
scalp disorders 3.45, 105.1–105.18
  allergic contact dermatitis of 127.16
  BAP1-inactivated naevus *131.34*
  Brunsting–Perry pemphigoid *50.53*
  chronic non-scarring folliculitis 91.13–91.14
  chronic pain/dysaesthesia/tenderness without obvious cause 82.12
  contact dermatitis 105.5
  cutis verticis gyrata 105.10
  dermatomyositis 52.3–52.4, *52.5*
  discoid lupus erythematosus *51.4*
  dissecting cellulitis 88.37
  follicular plugging, discoid lupus erythematosus *51.4*
  folliculitis 88.35, 93.5–93.6
  folliculitis keloidalis 93.3

human immunodeficiency virus infection 105.12
infections of the scalp 105.12
lichen planopilaris *37.5*, 37.6
lichen simplex chronicus 105.5
linear morphoea en coup de sabre *55.24*
lipoedema of 98.24–98.25
melanocytic naevi 131.22–131.23, *131.34*
mucous membrane pemphigoid *50.29*
pityriasis amiantacea 105.4
pityriasis amiantacea in psoriasis *35.9*
pruritus 105.14–105.17
  associated diseases 105.14–105.15
  causative organisms 105.15–105.16
  classification 105.16
  clinical features 105.16
  cutaneous sensory receptors and mediators *105.16*
  epidemiology 105.14
  investigations *105.16*
  management 105.16–105.17
  pathophysiology 105.15
psoriasis 105.2–105.4
psoriasis vulgaris 35.7, *35.9*
pustular conditions 105.12–105.14
  diagnosis *105.13*
  erosive pustular dermatosis of the scalp 105.13–105.14
radiodermatitis 105.5–105.6
scaling disorders 105.1–105.6
  contact dermatitis 105.5
  lichen simplex chronicus 105.5
  pityriasis amiantacea 105.4
  psoriasis 105.2–105.4
  radiodermatitis 105.5–105.6
  seborrhoeic dermatitis 105.1–105.2
scalp dyaesthesia 105.17–105.18
seborrhoeic dermatitis 105.1–105.2
secondary cicatricial alopecia 87.52–87.53, 105.6–105.9
  causes **105.6**
  cicatricial (mucous membrane) pemphigoid 105.6
  dissecting cellulitis of scalp 105.7–105.8
  follicular mucinosis 105.8
  granulomatous conditions 105.9
  sarcoidosis 105.9
  sclerosing conditions 105.8–105.9
syphilis 105.12
thickened scalp disorders 105.10–105.11
  cutis verticis gyrata 105.10
  lipoedematous alopecia 105.10–105.11
tumours of the scalp 105.11–105.12
  pilosebaceous unit 105.11
  scalp metastases 105.11–105.12
  sebaceous naevus 105.11
  syringocystadenoma papilliferum 105.11
scalp hair
  anagen phase *87.8*
  cyclical behaviour 87.9
  density 87.3
scalp margin
  necrotising lymphocytic folliculitis 91.12–91.13, 93.4
  varioliform scars *93.4*
SCARF syndrome **70.16**
scarlet fever 26.35–26.36
  clinical features 26.35–26.36
  epidemiology 26.35
  management 26.26
  pathophysiology 26.35
scarring
  acne scars, chemical peels 160.5, *160.6*
  acne vulgaris **88.3**, *88.4*, *88.29*, 88.39–88.41
  actinic prurigo *126.12*
  chemical peels, side effect of 160.14
  chronic wounds 11.8–11.9
  discoid lupus erythematosus 51.4, *51.5*, *51.7*, *51.8*
  external ear 106.14–106.15
  formation of scar tissue 9.7
  hidradenitis suppurativa 90.4, 90.6, 90.8, *111.11*, *111.12*

hypertrophic scars 11.9
  initiation of *11.7*
  intermediate recessive epidermolysis bullosa *69.16*
  intravenous drug administration 120.6–120.7
  inversa recessive dystrophic epidermolysis bullosa *69.18*
  keloid scars 11.9, 106.14–106.15
  larimal duct scarring, in erosive lichen planus *110.12*
  lichen sclerosus *110.9*
  mimics of acne scarring 88.38
  oral tissues 108.68
  skin folds 93.1
  trichloroacetic acid chemical reconstruction of skin scars *160.6*
  unsatisfactory outcomes of skin surgery **20.41**, 20.42
scarring alopecia 87.13–87.14, 87.36–87.38, 96.13, 98.24
  folliculitis 91.11
  monitoring/assessment 87.19–87.20
scarring psoriasis 87.34
SCARS *see* self-assessment of clinical acne-related scars; severe cutaneous adverse reactions
scar-sarcoidosis 96.11
SCC *see* squamous cell carcinoma; squamous cell carcinomas
Scedosporium apiospermum (*Pseudallescheria boydii*) 32.75
SCF *see* stem cell factor
SCFN *see* subcutaneous fat necrosis of the newborn
Schamberg capillaritis 86.49
Schamberg disease 99.7, 99.8, **99.9**
Schaumann bodies, sarcoidosis 96.3
Schilder disease 86.21
Schimmelpenning–Feuerstein–Mims syndrome (SFM) 71.23–71.24, 73.5–73.6
  see also HRAS/KRAS mosaicism; phakomatosis pigmentokeratotica
schistosomes, cercarial dermatitis 33.29–33.30
schistosomiasis (bilharziasis) 33.26–33.29, 111.16
  clinical features 33.27–33.28
  management 33.28–33.29
  pathophysiology 33.26–33.27
Schnitzler syndrome 45.20–45.21
  paraprotein activity 149.12–149.13
  Strasbourg diagnostic criteria **45.20**
Schöpf–Schulz–Passarge syndrome 63.68, **78.13**
Schwann cells, microscopic examination of 3.37
schwannoma 136.44–136.45
Schweninger–Buzzi-type anetoderma 94.23
SCI *see* Skin Cancer Index
SCID *see* severe combined immunodeficiency
SCLE *see* subacute cutaneous lupus erythematosus
sclera, in osteogenesis imperfecta *70.13*
sclerema neonatorum 97.37, 97.59–97.60, 114.17–114.18
scleroderma
  meaning 55.1
  see also morphoea; systemic sclerosis
scleroderma spectrum disorders **54.19**, 55.1
sclerodermatous processes, digestive system 153.6
sclerodermiform basal cell carcinoma *see* morphoeic basal cell carcinoma
sclerodermiform reaction, vitamins K and B_{12} 122.19
scleroedema **54.20**, 57.9–57.11
  diabetic and non-diabetic types 57.9
  diabetic patients 57.9, 57.10, 62.5–62.6, *62.7*
  differences from scleromyxoedema **57.5**
  neonates 97.60
scleroedema of Buschke, paraprotein activity 149.10–149.11

scleroma see rhinoscelroma
scleromyxoedema **54.20**, 57.2–57.6
   lung disease 152.6
   paraprotein activity 149.10
sclerosing angioma see fibrous histiocytoma
sclerosing cholangitis 63.41
sclerosing collagenoma, Cowden syndrome 78.11
sclerosing epithelial hamartoma see desmoplastic trichoepithelioma
sclerosing lipogranuloma 97.49, 97.50
sclerosing lymphangitis, penis 109.8
sclerosing panniculitis 97.30–97.32
sclerosing post-irradiation panniculitis 97.63–97.64, 119.15
sclerosing skin conditions, UVA-1 phototherapy 21.6
sclerosing/syringomatous sweat duct carcinoma see microcystic adnexal carcinoma
sclerosis
   causes **55.14**
   localised form see morphoea
   systemic see systemic sclerosis
   terminology 55.1
sclerotic collagen bundles, deep morphoea 97.13
sclerotic panatrophy 94.19–94.20
Scopulariopsis brevicaulis, onychomycoses 32.53–32.55
SCORing Atopic Dermatitis (SCORAD) 16.3, 16.4
scorpions 34.36–34.37
SCORTEN scoring system, SJS/TEN 118.18
SCPs see superficial chemical peels
scratching
   habit reversal therapy 84.37–84.38
   lichen simplex chronicus 81.18–81.20, 84.15
   nodular prurigo 84.16
   prurigo nodularis 81.14–81.18
   pruritus 81.3–81.4
   see also chronic pruritus; pruritus
scratch tests 4.24, 127.86
screening, early melanoma detection 142.18
scRNA-seq see single-cell RNA sequencing
scrofuloderma (tuberculosis colliquativa cutis) 27.13–27.16
scrotal calcinosis 59.4, 59.5, 109.30
scrotal candidiasis 32.64–32.65
scrotal lymphoedema, hidradenitis suppurativa 90.9
scrotal squamous carcinoma 129.14
scrotal tongue 108.87
scrotum
   acute scrotum 109.23, 109.25–109.26
   calcinosis 109.30
   carcinoma of 109.39
   eczematous dermatoses 109.11
   examination of 109.4
   Fordyce spots 93.11
   inflammation 109.26
   microscopic examination of skin 3.33
   panniculitis 109.23
   polyarteritis nodosa 109.26
   porokeratosis of Mibelli 109.35
   psoriasis vulgaris 35.10
   scrotal angiokeratoma of Fordyce 109.6
   squamous cell carcinoma 109.39
   swelling, causes of **109.20**
   tinea 109.27–109.28
scrub typhus group (STG), Rickettsiae 26.80, 26.84
scurvy
   purpura 99.6
   vitamin C deficiency 61.21, *61.22*
Scyphozoa, stings from 130.1
SD see seborrhoeic dermatitis
SDGs see Sustainable Development Goals
SDRIFE see symmetrical drug-related intertriginous and flexural exanthema
SDTI see suspected deep tissue injury
sea anemone stings 130.1–130.3
seabather's eruption 130.2

sea-blue histiocytosis 135.22–135.23
sea mat stings 130.4
seasonal allergic conjunctivitis (SAC) 107.16, 107.17, 107.18
seasonal hair shedding 87.9, 87.56
seatworm see enterobiasis
sea urchin injuries (SUIs) 130.3
sebaceous adenomas 88.32–88.33
   oral lesions 108.30
   and sebaceomas 137.16–137.17
sebaceous carcinomas 88.33, 137.18, 147.16
   eyelid 107.12, 107.49
sebaceous cysts see epidermoid cysts
sebaceous duct epithelial walled cutaneous cysts 133.6–133.7
sebaceous gland disorders 91.15–91.18
sebaceous gland hyperplasia 88.32, 91.17–91.18, 93.12–93.13
sebaceous gland hypertrophy, neonates 114.4
sebaceous glands 2.43
   changes in during pregnancy 113.2–113.3
   embryonic development 2.5
   eosinophilic pustular folliculitis 93.7
   male genitalia 109.6
   neuropeptide–cytokines/chemokine signalling 88.17
sebaceous gland secretion, neonates 114.3
sebaceous gland tumours 88.32
   carcinomas in immunocompromised people 147.16
   visceral malignancy 148.12
sebaceous hyperplasia, photothermal ablation 23.21–23.22
sebaceous naevus (organoid naevus) *73.5, 73.6, 73.7, 73.8*, 87.30, 88.32, 105.11, *106.33*, 137.19–137.20
sebopsoriasis see seborrhoeic psoriasis
seborrhoea 88.41
   in quadriplegic patients 83.19
seborrhoea, acne, hirsutism and/or androgenic alopecia (SAHA) syndrome 88.11
seborrhoeic blepharitis **107.8**
seborrhoeic dermatitis 127.21
   vulva 110.14
seborrhoeic dermatitis (SD) 40.1–40.10, 89.8, 105.1–105.2
   alcohol misuse relationship 84.40
   causative organisms 40.2–40.4
   clinical features 40.4–40.7
   clinical variants 40.5–40.6
   differential diagnosis 40.6
   drugs inducing or exacerbating condition 40.6–40.7
   ear dermatoses **106.23**
   environment and lifestyle factors 40.4, 40.7
   epidemiology 40.1–40.2
   genetic factors 40.4
   HIV 31.12, 31.15
   HIV association 40.7
   infants 40.5, 41.22, 115.1–115.2
   Langerhans cell histiocytosis 135.6–135.7
   Malassezia yeast 32.14
   male genitalia 109.12, 109.13
   management 40.8–40.9
   pathophysiology 40.2–40.4
   perineal and perianal skin 111.8, *111.9*
   in quadriplegic patients 83.19
   systemic treatments 40.9
   thickened yellow adherent scales 105.2
   topical antifungals 40.8
   topical keratolytics 40.8
   topical treatment agents 40.8–40.9
   see also infantile seborrhoeic dermatitis
seborrhoeic eczema see seborrhoeic dermatitis
seborrhoeic keratosis (SK) 132.1–132.4
   eyelid 107.44
   inverted follicular keratosis 137.2–137.3
   laser therapies 23.16
   malignancy association 132.1–132.2
   management 132.3–132.4
   pathophysiology 132.2–132.3

seborrhoeic melanosis 40.5, *040.6*
seborrhoeic psoriasis (sebopsoriasis) 35.7–35.8, 40.1, 40.6, 40.7
seborrhoeic wart see seborrhoeic keratosis
Sebutapes, sebum analysis 88.28, 88.43
secondary anetoderma 94.23, 94.24–94.25
secondary care 5.13
secondary cicatricial alopecia 87.52–87.53, 105.6–105.9
   causes **105.6**
   dissecting cellulitis of scalp 105.7–105.8
   follicular mucinosis 105.8
   granulomatous conditions 105.9
   linear morphoea ('en coup de sabre) 105.8–105.9
   morphoea 105.8
   mucous membrane pemphigoid 105.6
   sarcoidosis 105.9
   sclerosing conditions 105.8–105.9
secondary cutaneous B-cell lymphomas 139.43–139.45
   intravascular large B-cell lymphoma 139.43–139.44
   lymphomatoid granulomatosis 139.44–139.45
secondary cutaneous mucinoses 57.1, **57.2**, 57.18
secondary cutaneous T-cell lymphoma 139.45
   angioimmunoblastic lymphoma 139.45
secondary erythromelalgia 101.7, 101.8
secondary haemophagocytic lymphohistiocytosis 135.11, 135.14
secondary infections, arthropod bites and stings 34.2
secondary infections of skin lesions, nodular prurigo 84.15
secondary intention healing, skin surgery 20.21, *20.22*
secondary livedo reticularis 124.8
secondary localised cutaneous amyloidosis (SLCA) 56.2, **56.3**, 56.9
secondary Raynaud phenomenon 124.10–124.12
secondary syphilis 29.7–29.12, 29.17–29.18
   nephrotic syndrome 154.6
secondary to inflammatory disease/infections 59.1–59.3
second-degree burns 125.6
second primary cancers, increase risk in Merkel cell carcinoma 146.2
secosteroids (vitamin D analogues), topical therapies 18.26–18.29
Secretan's syndrome 97.50
secretory carcinoma 137.40
secretory coil, eccrine glands 92.2, 92.16
secukinumab
   psoriasis treatment 35.30
   psoriatic arthritis treatment 35.45–35.46
sedge pool itch see cercarial dermatitis
segmental infantile haemangioma **116.2**, 116.3–116.4
segmental lentiginosis 86.16
segmental odonto-maxillary dysplasia 73.18
segmental psoriasis 35.15
segmental vitiligo 86.34, 86.36, *86.37*, 86.38–86.39, *86.40*
SEI see superficial epidermolytic ichthyosis
selective photothermolysis, theory 23.3–23.6
selective serotonin reuptake inhibitors (SSRIs) 84.43, **84.44**, 117.3
selenium deficiency 61.29–61.30
selenium excess (selenosis) 61.30–61.31, 121.6–121.7
Self-Administered Psoriasis Area and Severity Index 16.3
self-assessment, *see also* Patient-Reported Outcome Measures
self-assessment of clinical acne-related scars (SCARS) 16.4
self-esteem 15.1
self-examination, early melanoma detection 142.18

self-healing collodion baby (SHCB) 63.8
self-healing cutaneous mucinosis 57.14
self-help 5.12
self-improving congenital ichthyosis (SICI) 63.7, 63.8, *63.11*, 63.12
self-improving dystrophic epidermolysis bullosa 69.16
self-induced traumatic panniculitis 97.50
self-mutilation, male genitalia 109.9
self-mutilation of the skin
   deliberate self-harm 84.38–84.39
   delusional infestation 84.7
   factitious skin disease 84.29–84.36, 84.37
   malingering 84.36–84.37
   obsessive–compulsive behaviour 84.15–84.22
self-neglect, lack of skin cleaning 84.36
semicircular lipoatrophy (SL) 97.55, 98.9–98.10, 122.15
semi-open tests, allergic contact dermatitis 127.33
senescence, pruritus 81.11
senescent alopecia 87.67–87.68
senile freckle see solar lentigo
senile keratosis/senile wart see seborrhoeic keratosis
senile purpura see actinic purpura
sensitisation 127.6–127.9
   acanthosis facilitation 127.8
   patch testing 127.32
   potential of allergens 127.8–127.9
   risk 127.9
sensitising agents
   antihistamines 18.37
   hair regrowth in alopecia 18.33–18.34
   occupational hazards 129.8–129.11
   reactions to topical therapy 18.5
   use in topical therapies 18.33–18.34
   see also allergic reactions
sensitive skin 128.10–128.11
sensory irritation 128.10–128.11
sensory nerves, anatomy of head and neck 20.2, *20.3*
sensory perception, and skin ageing 2.45
sentinel lymph node biopsy (SLNB) 106.29, 106.32–106.33, 143.4–143.6
sentinel (lymph) node status, melanoma, prognostic markers 142.21, 142.22
sepsis
   burn injuries 125.11
   drug reaction distinction 118.10
   risk for neonates 114.2
   SJS/TEN complications 118.20
   vasculitis 100.7
septal panniculitis 97.11, 97.23
septicaemia, acute SJS/TEN 118.17
septic arthritis 155.4
serine protease inhibitor Kazal-type 5 (*SPINK5*) 69.6
serine synthesis defects 79.14–79.15
seroconversion, HIV 31.5, 31.6–31.7, 31.11
serological diagnosis, of immunobullous disorders 3.20
serological tests, viral infections 25.5–25.6
seromas 103.32, 103.33
seronegative arthritis 155.5
serotoninergic syndromes, cocaine use 120.3
serpiginous lesions, on foot 4.16
serpin B8 (*SERPINB8*), skin fragility disorders 69.6
serration pattern analysis, direct immunofluorescence findings 3.17
serum autoantibodies
   bullous pemphigoid 50.14–50.15
   mucous membrane pemphigoid 50.25–50.26
serum protein electrophoresis, cryoglobulinaemic vasculitis *100.17*
serum sickness-like reaction (SSLR), hepatitis B 25.74
Servelle–Martorelle syndrome **101.28**
sesquiterpene lactone mix (SLM) 127.73
sesquiterpene lactones (STLs) 127.71

severe acute respiratory syndrome coronavirus-2 *see* COVID-19/SARS-CoV-2
severe autosomal recessive epidermolysis bullosa simplex 69.10
severe combined immunodeficiency (SCID) **80.4**, 80.7–80.9
  skin cancer 147.2
severe cutaneous adverse reactions (SCARs)
  to COVID-19 vaccines 25.119
  to drugs 118.1–118.22
severe dermatitis–multiple allergies–metabolic wasting (SAM) syndrome 63.28, 63.63
severe epidermolysis bullosa simplex 69.9
severe erythroderma, Desmons syndrome *63.35*
severe junctional epidermolysis bullosa
  management of 69.25
  molecular pathology *69.13*
severe recessive dystrophic epidermolysis bullosa 69.16–69.18
  management of 69.25–69.26
severe recessive epidermolysis bullosa simplex, with pyloric atresia 69.11
severity of alopecia tool (SALT) 87.24, *87.25*
Severity and Area Score for Hidradenitis (SASH) 16.5
severity rating, types of scales 81.12–81.13
sex chromosome defects 74.3–74.5
  fragile X syndrome 74.5
  Klinefelter syndrome 74.4
  Turner syndrome 74.3–74.4
  XXXXY syndrome 74.4–74.5
  XXYY syndrome 74.4
  XYY syndrome 74.4
sex differences
  burning mouth syndrome 82.2
  dermatomyositis 52.2
  hormone responses in skin/appendages 150.8
  urticarial vasculitis 44.2
sex reversal, palmoplantar keratodermas and 63.67–63.68
sex steroids, and atopic eczema 41.19
sexual abuse of children, ano-genital signs of 109.9
sexual behaviour, ChemSex/drugs with sex 120.2–120.3
sexual development, disorders of 110.5
sexual hair growth 87.2
sexually acquired reactive arthritis (SARA)
  genital chlamydia 30.9, 30.10, 30.11, 30.12, 30.13, 30.14
  gonorrhoea 30.5–30.6
sexually transmitted infections (STIs)
  ano-genital warts 25.61–25.64
  genital herpes 25.24–25.26
  global overview 29.1–29.2
  gonorrhoea 30.1–30.8
  illicit drug-related 120.3
  male genitalia 109.28–109.29
  non-syphilitic bacterial diseases 30.1–30.26
  perineal and perianal skin 111.16–111.17
  recurrent genital herpes increasing risk of HIV and other STIs 25.26
  see also HIV; syphilis
sexual functioning, impact measures 16.12
Sézary syndrome (SS) 139.16–139.25
  clinical features 139.18–139.19
  definition 139.16
  erythroderma in *39.33*
  management 139.20–139.25
  molecular features 139.19–139.20
  pathophysiology 139.16–139.18
  relationship to mycosis fungoides 139.2, 139.19–139.20
  staging **139.8**
SFM *see* Schimmelpenning–Feuerstein–Mims syndrome
SFN *see* small fibre neuropathy
Shah–Waardenburg syndrome 68.5
shame, emotional effects of skin conditions 15.2

shampoos
  allergic reactions 127.16, 127.50
  alopecia management 87.98
shared decision making, holistic management of skin disease 15.6, 15.7
shared delusions, delusional infestation 84.5
shave biopsy 3.4
  epidermolysis bullosa diagnosis 69.21
  principles 20.10–20.11
shave excisions 20.10–20.11, *20.45*
shaving practices, pseudofolliculitis 91.9–91.11
'shawl-sign', redness on back in dermatomyositis 52.4, *52.6*
SHCB *see* self-healing collodion baby
shear force, pressure ulcers 123.2, 123.3
shearing stresses 122.3
SHH *see* sonic hedgehog
SHHis *see* sonic hedgehog pathway inhibitors
shin
  diabetic bulla on *62.7*
  diabetic dermopathy *62.2*
  granuloma annulare *95.7*
  necrobiosis lipoidica *62.6*, *95.9*
shingles *see* herpes zoster
shiny white line dermoscopy patterns, melanoma 145.7, 145.14, *145.15*
SHML *see* sinus histiocytosis with massive lymphadenopathy
shockwave therapy, skin tightening 161.6
shoes
  allergic contact dermatitis 127.17, 127.67–127.68
  callosities 122.8
short anagen syndrome 87.53, 87.83
short-arm deletion syndrome, chromosome 4 74.3
short-arm deletion syndrome, chromosome 5 74.3
short stature/lipoedema syndrome **72.12**
SHORT syndrome **72.5**
shoulder
  granuloma annulare *95.2*
  naevus of Ito *131.15*
  subcutaneous fat necrosis of the newborn *114.16*
SHP *see* Specific Health Problem
Shulman syndrome (eosinophilic fasciitis) **54.20**, 55.2, **55.3**, **55.4**, 55.21–55.23, *55.22*, **55.27**, 97.13
sialidosis, glycoproteinoses 79.3
Sicariidae (fiddleback/violin spiders) *34.35–34.36*
SICI *see* self-improving congenital ichthyosis
sideroblastic anaemia with B-cell immunodeficiency, periodic fevers and developmental delay (SIFD) 45.19
signalling disorders
  blistering 69.24
  IL-10 45.16
signalling protein mutations, acquired immunodeficiency diseases **149.20**
signal peptides, cosmeceutical use of 157.5–157.6
signal transducer and activator of transcription (STAT) proteins
  STAT1 gain-of-function mutation, oro-pharyngeal *Candida* infection 80.17
  STAT3 loss of function mutations, hyper-IgE syndrome 80.17
  STAT inhibitor medication for pyoderma gangrenosum treatment 49.7
signal transduction pathway, drug action mechanisms 13.5
sign of Leser–Trélat 148.16
SIL *see* squamous intraepithelial lesions
sildenafil 124.12
silicone
  reactions to 122.21
  topical therapies 18.41

silicone implants, factitious panniculitis *97.48*
silicones, dermal fillers 158.7
Silk Road 1.2
silver, dermatological reactions 121.7–121.8
silver nitrate
  caustic agent for skin surgery 20.47
  topical therapies 18.9
silver sulfadiazine, topical therapies 18.11–18.12
SIM1 deficiency **72.6**
Simon Broome Register Group, familial hypercholesterolaemia diagnosis **60.7**
simple interrupted skin sutures 20.14–20.17
Simplified Psoriasis Index (SPI) 16.3, 16.8
simulated skin disease (dermatitis simulata) 84.36
Simuliidae (blackflies) 34.7, 34.9
Simulium species (blackfly), onchocerciasis vector 33.1, 33.2, 33.3
Sinclair scale, hair grading *87.58*, 87.65
Sindbis virus (SINV) 25.88
single-cell genomics 8.2
single-cell RNA sequencing (scRNA-seq) 9.2
single-gene disorders 8.2, *8.3*, *8.4*
single nuclei RNA sequencing (snRNA-seq) 9.2
single nucleotide polymorphisms (SNPs), skin cancer risks 147.6
single-organ small-vessel vasculitis 100.5–100.12
single system Langerhans cell histiocytoses (SS-LCH) 135.2–135.8
sinonasal melanoma 142.14–142.15
sinuses, lips 108.86
sinuses, preauricular, infants 115.12
sinus histiocytosis with massive lymphadenopathy (SHML) 135.27–135.29
sinusoidal haemangioma 136.30–136.31
SINV *see* Sindbis virus
siphonaptera *see* fleas
Siphonophora, stings from 130.1
Sipple syndrome *see* multiple endocrine neoplasia type 2A
sitosterolaemia 60.11
Six Area Six Sign Atopic Dermatitis severity score (SASSAD) 16.4
sixth disease *see* roseola infantum
SJIA *see* systemic juvenile idiopathic arthritis
Sjögren syndrome (SS) 53.9–53.11
  classification criteria **53.10**
  clinical features 53.10
  eye disease **107.35**
  investigations 53.11
  management 53.11
  mucocutaneous features of 53.10–53.11
  respiratory disease 152.3
Sjögren–Larsson syndrome (SLS) 63.32–63.33
SJS *see* Stevens–Johnson syndrome
SJS/TEN *see* Stevens–Johnson syndrome/toxic epidermal necrolysis
SK *see* seborrhoeic keratosis
skeletal abnormalities 78.3
skeletal muscle tumours 136.55–136.56
skeletal osteomas, familial adenomatous polyposis 78.11
skin ageing *see* ageing of skin
skin anatomy 9.1, *9.2*
skin appendage tumours 137.1–137.49
  immunocompromised people 147.16
skin barrier dysfunction, irritant contact dermatitis 128.2
skin biopsy *see* biopsy of skin
skin cancer 1.8, 7.2
  acquired immunodeficiency diseases 147.2–147.5
  clinicopathological features, immunocompromised people 147.10–147.16
  direct, mortality and morbidity costs of melanoma **6.7**

  economic burden of 6.1, 6.5–6.8
  effects of altered healthcare during COVID-19 pandemic 25.120
  factors influencing treatment choice 24.8, **24.10**
  global distribution **7.3**
  HIV/AIDS 147.2–147.3
  host genetic predisposition, immunocompromised people 147.6
  immunocompromised people 147.1–147.26
    clinicopathological features 147.10–147.16
    drug effects on cancer risk 147.6–147.8
    management 147.16–147.24
    organisations 147.25
    pathogenesis 147.5–147.10
    screening and surveillance 147.24–147.25
  intralesional therapies 20.47–20.48
  management
    immunocompromised people 147.16–147.24
    protocols for organ transplant recipients **147.22**, **147.23**
    treatment comparisons 20.32–20.33
    see also Mohs micrographic surgery
  occupationally-induced 129.14–129.15
  oculocutaneous albinism 68.7
  pathogenesis, immunocompromised people 147.5–147.10
  persons with albinism 7.10–7.11, 7.12, *7.13*
  and photoageing 10.11
  prevalence of 5.10
  primary immunodeficiency diseases/inborn errors of immunity 147.1–147.2
  psychological and social factors 15.4
  quality of life assessment 16.9
  resources used and persons affected by **6.6**
  screening and surveillance, immunocompromised people 147.24–147.25
  solid-organ transplant recipients 147.3–147.4, **147.22**, **147.23**
  surveillance after phototherapy 21.16–21.17
  ultraviolet radiation effects in immunocompromised people 147.5–147.6
  UVR exposure 10.9–10.10
  xeroderma pigmentosum *76.4*, 76.5
Skin Cancer Index (SCI) 16.9
skincare creams, irritant contact dermatitis 129.4
skincare principles, occupational dermatology **129.4**
skin cleaning neglect 84.36
skin cleansing, neonates 114.2
skin colour 86.1–86.2
  changes as signs of cardiac disease 151.1
  lightening cosmeceuticals 157.3–157.4
  malaria 33.36
  melanoma risk in fair skin 142.3
  see also jaundice; pigmentation
skin of colour (SOC) 4.13–4.15, 86.1–86.2
  acne vulgaris **88.45**
  acne vulgaris treatment 88.43–88.44
  ageing in 156.1–156.3
  atopic eczema 41.16
  chemical peels 160.15
  discoid lupus erythematosus *51.7*
  facial melanoses 86.9
  geographic distribution of pigmentation 86.7–86.8
  inherited patterned lentiginosis 86.16
  matching principles in surgical design 20.21
  mucocutaneous manifestations of COVID-19 infection 25.104
  photoageing scale 156.7
  sun exposure responses 86.8

Skindex (dermatology life quality index) 6.4, 15.3, 16.3, 16.6–16.8, 16.12, 35.17
Skindex-Teen 16.10
skin extensibility 122.5
skin folds
  amicrobial pustulosis 49.20–49.21
  scarring 93.1
skin fragility disorders 69.1–69.28
skin grafting
  ectodermal dysplasias 69.27
  full-thickness grafts 20.30, 20.35
skin hydration
  effects on skin bacteria 26.4, 26.5
  pressure ulcers 123.3
skin infections 1.7–1.8
  effects on urinary tract 154.6
  immunosuppressed renal allograft recipients 154.5–154.6
skin injuries, mechanical 122.1–122.29
skin lesions with uncertain/unpredictable malignant potential 141.1–141.18
  actinic keratoses 141.1–141.12
  arsenical keratosis 141.13–141.14
  cutaneous horn 141.12–141.13
  disseminated superficial actinic porokeratosis 141.15–141.18
  post-ionising radiation keratosis 141.14–141.15
skin lightening, cosmeceuticals 157.3–157.4
skin microbiome 2.13, 2.14, 26.2–26.6
  atopic eczema 9.8, 41.9
  erythematotelangiectatic rosacea 89.4
  hair follicle 87.11
  immune system 9.7–9.8, 26.5, 26.6, 103.2, 103.3
  Malassezia yeast species 32.10
  normal 26.3–26.5
skin necrosis, calciphylaxis 154.2, 154.3
skin-only Langerhans cell histiocytoses 135.3–135.4, 135.9–135.10
skin picking disorders 82.7–82.9, 84.19–84.20
  see also acné excoriée; lichen simplex chronicus
'skin popping' 120.6–120.7
skin prick test, contact dermatitis 129.7
skin properties, objective measures 16.5
skin protection, pressure ulcer prevention 123.9
skin-related health anxieties 84.25–84.26
Skin Related NTDs Cross Cutting Group (NNN Skin NTD CCG) 7.6
skin samples, superficial mycoses identification 32.7
skin, structure and function 2.1–2.47
  adherens junctions 2.19–2.20
  adnexal structures 2.5–2.7
  ageing of skin 2.45–2.46
  anchoring fibrils 2.26–2.27
  blood vessels 2.40–2.42
  cellular progression 2.1
  collagens 2.27–2.29
    basement membrane collagen 2.22–2.23
    biosynthesis 2.29–2.31, 2.30
    cross-linking 2.31
    degradation 2.31–2.32
    gene expression 2.29–2.31
    genetic heterogeneity **2.27**
    hydroxylation reactions 2.29, 2.30
    periodicity in collagen fibres 2.23
  components of normal skin 2.1–2.3, 2.2
  dermal–epidermal basement membrane zone 2.21–2.22
    basement membrane collagen 2.22–2.23
    hemidesmosomes 2.25–2.26
    laminins 2.23–2.25
  dermis 2.2
    collagen fibres 2.27
    embryonic development 2.5
    immune surveillance 2.15, 2.16
    microvessels in 2.41
  desmosomes 2.18–2.19
  development of skin 2.3–2.5

elastic fibres 2.32–2.33, 2.34
  assembly and cross-linking 2.35
  degradation 2.34–2.35
elastin 2.33–2.35
elastin-associated microfibrils 2.35–2.36
embryonic development of skin 2.3–2.5
epidermis 2.1, 2.2
  cornified cell envelope 2.7
  desmosomes 2.18–2.19
  differentiation 2.6, 2.7, 2.8
  embryonic development 2.3
  hyperproliferation 2.8
  Merkel cells 2.2, 2.11–2.12
  mesenchymal cells 2.4
  nail bed 2.11
  structures of 2.5–2.7
extracellular matrix 2.27–2.28, 2.40
fibroblasts 2.3, 2.39–2.40, 2.45
focal adhesions 2.26
gap junctions 2.20
glabrous skin 2.43
glycosaminoglycans 2.36–2.39
hair-bearing skin 2.43
hair follicles, embryonic development 2.3–2.5, 2.5
hemidesmosomes 2.25–2.26
immune ecosystem 2.12–2.13
immune surveillance 2.15, 2.16
keratinocytes 2.1, 2.7–2.8
laminins 2.23–2.25
Langerhans cells 2.1–2.2, 2.13–2.15
  skin ageing 2.45
lymphatic network 2.42
mast cells 2.15–2.17
melanocytes 2.1, 2.17–2.18
Merkel cells 2.2, 2.11–2.12
  embryonic development 2.5
microbiome 2.13
motor innervation 2.2–2.3
nails 2.10–2.11
physiological functions of skin 2.42–2.43
pilosebaceous units 2.9–2.10
proteoglycans 2.36–2.39
skin homeostasis 2.43–2.45
subcutaneous fat 2.42, 2.43
sweat glands 2.2, 2.8–2.9
tight junctions 2.20–2.21
types of human skin 2.43
skin substitutes, wound healing 11.12, 11.13
skin surface electrical properties, stratum corneum hydration measurement 16.5
skin surgery 20.1–20.52
  anatomical considerations 20.1–20.4
  biopsies 20.8–20.11
  caustic agents 20.47, 20.50
  complications 20.33, 20.40–20.42, **20.41**
    flaps 20.29, 20.33
  cryosurgery 20.46–20.47
  curettage 20.48
  dressings 20.37–20.38
  electrosurgery 20.42–20.46
  equipment, needles and suture materials 20.12
  equipment requirements 20.4–20.5
  flaps 20.22–20.29, **20.24–20.25**, 20.30–20.33
  grafts 20.29–20.30, 20.34, 20.35
  haemostasis for open wounds 20.48
  hygiene and sterilisation 20.5–20.7
  local anaesthetics 20.7–20.8
  Mohs micrographic surgery 20.30–20.37
  pharmacological complications 20.40
  post-operative care 20.37–20.40
  preoperative preparation 20.11
  presurgical procedures and techniques 20.4–20.11
  snip excision 20.48
  specific conditions 20.49–20.50
  suture removal 20.40
  suturing 20.12–20.19
  undermining levels and tissue planes 20.4, **20.6**
  unsatisfactory outcomes 20.42
  see also surgical treatment

skin tags 132.8–132.9
  diabetic patients 62.3
  male genitalia 109.5–109.6
  pre-auricular 106.8
  vulval **110.32**
skin testing 4.23–4.25
  delayed (4–8 h) tests 4.24
  immediate-weal tests 4.24
  intradermal tests for detection of delayed sensitivity to antigens 4.24–4.25
  techniques 4.23–4.24
skin thickening, lichen simplex chronicus 84.15
skin thickness, irritant contact dermatitis 128.6
skin tightening therapies 161.6–161.8
skin tumours
  immunosuppressed renal allograft recipients 154.6
  occupationally-induced 129.14–129.15
  see also benign proliferations; skin cancer
skin tunnels, hidradenitis suppurativa 90.4, 90.6, 90.11
skin-window technique 4.24
SL *see* semicircular lipoatrophy
slapped cheek syndrome *see* erythema infectiosum (fifth disease)
slaughterhouse eczema 39.15–39.16
SLBN *see* sentinel lymph node biopsy
SLCA *see* secondary localised cutaneous amyloidosis
SLE *see* systemic lupus erythematosus
sleep deprivation, and acne 88.25
sleeping sickness *see* African trypanosomiasis
SLE-like vasculopathy 80.18
sliding flaps, surgical reconstruction 20.23
SLM *see* sesquiterpene lactone mix
SLN *see* speckled lentiginous naevus
SLNB *see* sentinel lymph node biopsy
Slovakia, non-melanoma skin cancer, incidence of 6.1
SLS *see* Sjögren–Larsson syndrome
SM *see* steatocystoma multiplex; systemic mastocytosis
small fibre neuropathy (SFN) **83.9**
small molecule therapy, epidermolysis bullosa 69.28
small plaque parapsoriasis (SPP) 39.27, 134.6–134.7
smallpox (variola virus) 1.3, 25.6–25.7
small-vessel ANCA-associated vasculitis 100.9, 100.13, 100.20–100.28, 152.3–152.4
small-vessel immune complex-associated vasculitis 100.13–100.20
small-vessel vasculitis, involving respiratory system 152.3–152.4
smartphone apps 5.13
  diagnosis 4.26
  disease outcome measurement and recording 16.2
SMC *see* smooth muscle cell
Smith–Lemli–Opitz syndrome 79.15
smoke, hazards and risks of electrosurgery 20.45–20.46
smoker's melanosis 108.16–108.17
smoking 5.10
  acne 88.19
  ageing of skin 156.4
  dermal connective tissue damage 94.2
  hidradenitis suppurativa association 90.2, 90.9
  keratoses 108.33
  oral hyperpigmentation 108.16–108.17
  oral squamous cell carcinoma 108.46
  penile carcinoma, risk factor for 109.36
  psoriasis association 120.3
  psoriasis vulgaris 35.4
  rosacea risk 89.3
smooth muscle cells (SMCs) 2.40–2.41
  microscopic examination of 3.37
  venous malformations 71.14
smooth muscle hamartoma 73.19, 136.52–136.53

smooth muscle tumours 136.52–136.55
SmPC *see* summary of product characteristics
SMS *see* sodium metabisulphite
snake bites 130.5–130.7
Sneddon syndrome 99.19–99.20
Sneddon–Wilkinson disease 118.4
Snow, John 5.9–5.10
snRNA-seq *see* single nuclei RNA sequencing
snuff dipper's keratosis 108.33
SO *see* superficial onychomycosis
SOC *see* skin of colour
social factors
  diagnosis 4.5
  see also psychological and social factors
social impacts of long-term conditions 15.1–15.4
social inclusion 15.1
social medicine 1.8–1.9
socioeconomic factors, epidemiology 5.10–5.11
sodium bicarbonate, ichthyoses management 63.43
sodium hypochlorite, topical therapies 18.10
sodium metabisulphite (SMS) 127.56
sodium thiosulphate, calciphylaxis treatment 59.8
soft chancre *see* chancroid
soft fibromas *see* skin tags
soft-tissue augmentation *see* dermal fillers
soft-tissue tumours 136.1–136.68
  fat cells 136.56–136.59
  fibrohistiocytic tumours 136.19–136.23
  fibrous/myofibroblastic 136.2–136.19
  lymphatic tumours 136.37–136.39
  muscle tumours 136.52–136.56
  peripheral neuroectodermal tumours 136.42–136.52
  perivascular cells 136.39–136.42
  skeletal muscle cells 136.55–136.56
  smooth muscle cells 136.52–136.55
  uncertain histogenesis 136.59–136.64
  vascular tumours 136.23–136.37
SofWave, ultrasound skin tightening 161.7
SoJIA *see* systemic-onset juvenile idiopathic arthritis
solar cheilitis/cheilosis *see* actinic cheilitis
solar lentigo (actinic lentigo) 131.5–131.7, 160.7
solar purpura 99.23–99.24
solar urticaria (SU) **42.9**, 42.12, 126.21–126.24, 126.32–126.33
sole of foot
  acral naevi 131.24
  blue rubber bleb naevus syndrome 71.17
  congenital generalised lipodystrophies 72.2
  eccrine poroma 137.25–137.26
  lichen planus of 37.7
  microscopic examination of skin 3.33
  non-pustular palmoplantar psoriasis 35.10, 35.11
  pompholyx eczema 39.14
  recurrent focal palmar peeling 39.16
solid facial (lymph)oedema (Morbihan disease) 88.41, 89.10, 89.16, 89.17, 103.47, 103.48
solid-organ transplant recipients (SOTRs)
  skin cancer risks 147.3–147.4
  see also organ transplant recipients
solitary circumscribed neuroma 136.43–136.44
solitary lichen planus *see* lichenoid keratosis
solitary neurofibroma 136.45–136.46
solitary venous malformations 101.24–101.25
soluble oils 129.1
  irritant contact dermatitis 129.2
solvent fumes, inhaling 120.4
somatic mutation 8.5
somatic RASopathies associated with lymphatic abnormalities 103.24
somatosensory system lesions/disease, neuropathic pain definition 82.5

somatostatin analogue octreotide 97.43
sonic hedgehog pathway inhibitors (SHHis), basal cell carcinoma treatment 140.17–140.18
sonic hedgehog (SHH) pathway, basal cell carcinoma pathogenesis 140.3, *140.5*, 140.17, 140.18
sorbic acid (SA) 127.58
sorbisan sesquioleate 127.44
Sotos syndrome *72.12*
SOTRs *see* solid-organ transplant recipients
South American blastomycosis *see* paracoccidioidomycosis
SOX-10 (transcription factor) 3.24
soya, cosmeceutical use of 157.10
SP *see* substance P
Spain, psoriasis, economic burden of **6.8**, 6.9
Spanish fly *see* cantharidin
sparganosis 33.34–33.35
 clinical features and variants 33.35
 pathophysiology 33.34–33.35
sparganum proliferum 33.35
spastic diplegia, KID syndrome *63.33*
spatial genomics technologies, immune system 9.2
spatial transcriptomics, immune system 9.2–9.3
specialists *see* multidisciplinary teams
Specific Health Problem (SHP) versions, work productivity assessment instruments 16.13
'specimen sign', delusional infestation 84.7–84.8
speckled lentiginous naevus (SLN/naevus spilus) *4.8*, 23.16, 73.15–73.16, 131.15–131.17
speckled leukoplakia, oral lesions 108.34
spectacle-frame acanthoma 122.14–122.15
spectrophotometric image analysis 4.21
spEDS *see* spondylodysplastic Ehlers–Danlos syndrome
'speedballs' 120.7
SPF *see* sun protection factor
sphincter, anal 111.2–111.3
sphingolipidoses 79.5–79.6
SPI *see* Simplified Psoriasis Index
spice allergies 127.41–127.45
spiders (Araneae) 34.34–34.36
spider telangiectases 101.10–101.12, **101.17**, 153.8
 associated diseases 101.11
 clinical features **101.11**
 investigations for **101.12**
 laser therapies 23.9
 management of **101.12**
 pathophysiology 101.11
Spiegler's tumour *see* cylindroma
Spiegler–Fendt sarcoid *see* lymphocytoma cutis/B-cell pseudolymphoma
spina bifida, tuft hair association 83.18
spinal cord injury, dermatoses associated with 83.19–83.20
spinal dysraphism 83.17–83.19
 localised hypertrichosis 87.86
spindle cell haemangioma (haemangioendothelioma) *71.20*, 136.31
spindle cell lipoma 136.58
spindle cell naevi *see* Spitz naevi
SPINK5, skin fragility disorders 69.6
spinulosis of the face 85.13
spiny keratoderma 63.59–63.60
spiradenocarcinoma 137.36
spiradenoma 137.31–137.32
 cylindroma relationship 137.30
Spirillum minus (*Spirillum minor*), rat-bite fever 26.75
spirochaetes 26.69–26.76
 Borrelia spp. 26.72–26.74
 Leptospira spp. 26.74–26.75
 non-syphilitic spirochaetal ulcerative balanoposthitis 109.27
 rat-bite fevers 26.75–26.76
 treponemes 26.69–26.72

spironolactone 87.70, 87.95–87.96
 acne vulgaris treatment 88.51
spironolactone treatment, hidradenitis suppurativa 90.10
Spitz naevi 3.36, *3.37*, **131.16**, 131.32–131.37
 atypical Spitz tumours *131.36*, **131.36**
 BAP1-inactivated naevus of the scalp *131.34*
 classic Spitz naevus *131.35*, **131.36**
 clinical features 131.33–131.34
 compound naevus *131.33*
 congenital 73.15
 dermoscopic patterns *145.2*, 145.5, 145.6–145.7
 differential diagnosis 131.34
 disease course and prognosis 131.35
 genetics 131.33
 investigations 131.35–131.37
 management 131.37
 pathology 131.32–131.33
 pigmented Spitz naevus *131.35*
 Reed naevus *131.34*, *131.37*, *145.2*, 145.5, 145.6
Spitzoid melanoma (malignant Spitz tumour/malignant spitzoiid neoplasm) 142.8, 142.20, 142.21
S-plasty, skin surgery 20.21–20.22, *20.23*
split-skin indirect technique, immunofluorescence 3.13–3.14
split-thickness skin grafts 20.30, *20.34*
spondyloarthritis 155.2, 155.5, 155.7, 155.13
spondylodysplastic Ehlers–Danlos syndrome (spEDS) **70.5–70.6**, 70.9
sponge stings 130.3
spongiosis 3.43, 126.14, *126.15*
spontaneous atrophic scarring of cheeks 94.14–94.15
spontaneously regressing tumours, keratoacanthoma 141.38–141.41
spontaneous urticaria
 acute 42.5, 42.15–42.16
 chronic 42.5, *42.6*, 42.7, 42.16, *42.17*
sporadic MMDK 85.18, 85.19
sporadic typhus (Brill–Zinsser disease) 26.81
Sporothrix schenckii 32.72
sporotichosis 32.70–32.72
 clinical features 32.71–32.72
 epidemiology 32.70
 management 32.72
 pathophysiology 32.70–32.71
 systemic form 32.71
sports, traumatic effects 122.16–122.17
spotted fever group (SFG), Rickettsiae 26.80, 26.81–26.83
spot tests, allergic contact dermatitis 127.33–127.34
SPP *see* small plaque parapsoriasis
SPPK *see* striate palmoplantar keratoderma
SPTCL *see* subcutaneous panniculitis T-cell lymphomas
squamoid eccrine ductal carcinoma 137.34–137.35
Squamous Cell Carcinoma Antigen Recognized by T-cells (*SART3*) 85.20
squamous cell carcinoma (SCC) 141.1–141.46
 anal cancer 111.21–111.24
 arsenic poisoning 121.2
 associated conditions 141.1–141.27
 biopsy 3.4
 definitions/nomenclature 141.26
 diagnosis of 3.21
 drug/chemical photosensitivity 126.30
 dyskeratosis congenita 67.14
 ear/auricle 106.27–106.29
 ectodermal dysplasias 69.18, 69.26–69.27
 eyelid 107.47, 107.48
 female genitalia 110.36–110.37
 heat-associated 124.15
 hidradenitis suppurativa co-morbidity 90.7
 incidence compared to basal cell carcinoma

 as a keratinocyte cancer 141.1
 keratoacanthoma relationship 141.38
 KID syndrome *63.34*
 lichen sclerosus *110.9*
 lip 108.44–108.45
 male genitalia 109.35–109.42
 metastatic risk 141.26
 pilonidal sinus 122.23
 possible precursors
  actinic keratoses 141.1–141.12
  arsenical keratosis 141.13–141.14
  cutaneous horn 141.12–141.13
  disseminated superficial actinic porokeratosis 141.15–141.18
  post-ionising radiation keratosis 141.14–141.15
 pseudoepitheliomatous hyperplasia mimicking 132.9–132.10
 radiotherapy 24.13–24.14
 radiotherapy indications 24.8–24.10
 well-differentiated/keratoacanthomatous type 141.38
 see also Bowen disease; cutaneous squamous cell carcinoma; *in situ* carcinoma of the skin; oral squamous cell carcinoma
squamous cell epithelioma *see* cutaneous squamous cell carcinoma
squamous hyperplasia, penis 109.34–109.35
squamous intraepithelial lesions (SIL), anal/perianal/genital areas 109.34–109.35, 110.34–110.36, 141.24, 141.26
SRs (systemic retinoids) *see* retinoids (systemic therapy)
SS *see* Sézary syndrome; Sjögren syndrome
SSc *see* systemic sclerosis
SS-LCH *see* single system Langerhans cell histiocytoses
SSLR *see* serum sickness-like reaction
SSM *see* superficial spreading melanoma
SSR *see* sympathetic skin response
SSRIs *see* selective serotonin re-uptake inhibitors
SSSS *see* staphylococcal scalded skin syndrome
staining techniques
 artefacts 3.32
 avidin–biotin staining method *3.16*
 biopsy 3.7–3.10
standardisation of terminology 1.4, *1.5*
standing cutaneous deformity ('cone' or 'dog ear') repair 20.22, *20.23*
staphylococcal infections 26.8–26.10, 26.12–26.32
 ano-genital cellulitis 109.26
 blepharitis **107.8**, *107.9*, 107.10
 cold abscesses of the large folds in neonates 114.25
 external ear 106.19
 female genitalia 110.25
 HIV 31.20–31.21
 non-bullous impetigo 26.13
 Panton–Valentine leukocidin virulence factor 111.13–111.14
 see also methicillin-resistant *Staphylococcus aureus*
staphylococcal scalded skin syndrome (SSSS) 2.19, 26.6, 26.27–26.30
 children 26.27, 26.28, *26.28*
 clinical features 26.28–26.29
 infants 115.7–115.8
 management 26.29, **26.30**
 neonates 114.24–114.25
 pathophysiology 26.28
staphylococcal toxic shock syndrome 26.30–26.32
Staphylococcus spp.
 causing infections 26.8–26.10
 coagulase negative 26.9–26.10
 immune responses 9.7
 normal skin flora 26.3
 S. aureus
  antibiotic resistance, impetigo management 26.16

  atopic eczema 41.10
  botryomycosis 26.76–26.77
  colonisation of skin 26.2, 26.3, 26.4, 26.6
  co-pathogen in dermatophytosis 32.22
  discoid eczema colonisation *88.56*
  EGFR inhibitors 119.3
  epidemiology 26.6–26.7
  follicular infections 26.22–26.27
  folliculitis decalvans 87.48–87.49
  folliculitis keloidalis 93.3
  genetics 26.9
  impetigo 26.14
  infections 26.6–26.9
  methicillin-resistant 26.8–26.9, 31.21, 31.37, 109.28
  necrotising lymphocytic folliculitis 93.4–93.5
  pathophysiology 26.7–26.9
  perianal cellulitis type dermatitis 26.34
  recurrent toxin-mediated perineal erythema 26.32
  resident on skin 26.3
  scalp itch 105.16
  skin infections 26.12–26.13, 26.28–26.29
  toxic shock syndrome 26.30–26.32
  see also methicillin-resistant *Staphylococcus aureus*
 S. epidermidis 9.7, 26.9–26.10
 S. hominis 26.3, 26.9
 S. lugdunensis 26.9
 S. saccharolyticus 26.3
 S. saprophyticus 26.3, 26.9
starburst pattern
 melanoma 145.13, *145.15*
 Reed (Spitz) naevi *145.2*, 145.5, 145.6
'starfish' keratoses, Vohwinkel syndrome *63.64*
starvation
 adiponectin system 97.5
 see also malnutrition
stasis dermatitis/eczema *see* venous eczema
STAT *see* signal transducer and activator of transcription
static friction, laws of 122.6
statin treatment, pachyonychia congenita 63.52, 67.12
statistical methods, clinical research papers 17.20–17.24
statistical summary presentation, clinical research papers 17.18–17.20
Staurozoa, stings from 130.2
steatocystoma multiplex (SM) 88.33–88.34, 133.6, *133.7*
stelae, hair loss 87.64
stellate pseudoscars 94.13, *94.14*
stellate purpura *see* retiform purpura
stem cell factor (SCF) 2.15
 KIT receptor mutations 46.1, 46.2
stem cells 2.43–2.45
 burn treatment 125.8
 epidermal proliferation of *2.43*, 2.44
 epithelial stem cells *2.43*
 hair disorder treatment 87.95
 proliferative potential of *2.44*
 wound healing therapy 11.11
Stemmer's sign, lipoedema differential diagnosis 98.22, 98.23
Stenotrophomonas maltophilia 26.55–26.56
stereotactic ablative radiotherapy (SABR), and stereotactic radiosurgery for melanoma 24.14
sterile, *see also* amicrobial
sterile furuncles (abscesses) 26.23
sterile pustules
 eosinophilic pustular folliculitis 93.9, *93.10*
 infantile eosinophilic pustular folliculitis *91.7*
sterilisation, skin surgery 20.5–20.7
steroid hormones
 metabolism and synthesis in skin *150.3*
 signalling effects in skin 150.7
steroid-modified tinea 32.49–32.50

steroids
  colloid milium   94.6–94.9
  rosacea induction   89.17
  withdrawal syndrome   19.18
  see also corticosteroids
Stevens–Johnson syndrome (SJS)
  acute conjunctivitis with mucus discharge   107.33
  erythema multiforme   47.1–47.2
  haemorrhagic crusting of lips   108.61
  history   118.12
  management   107.33–107.34
  musculoskeletal therapy effects   155.10, 155.15
  ocular complications of   107.32–107.33
  oral involvement   108.61, 108.79, 118.20
  T-cell-mediated drug hypersensitivity   14.3, 14.7
  toxic epidermal necrolysis relationship   47.1–47.2, 118.12
  varicella infection/vaccination   25.30
Stevens–Johnson syndrome/toxic epidermal necrolysis (SJS/TEN)   47.1–47.2, 107.32–107.34, 108.79, 118.1–118.2, 118.10, 118.12–118.22
stiff skin syndrome   70.22–70.23
stigma/sigmatization/stigmatisation   1.9, 5.5
  assessment measures   16.8
  leprosy   28.1, 28.16
  psychodermatology   84.3–84.4
  see also Questionnaire on Experience with Skin complaints
stigmata, congenital syphilis   29.26
Still disease   45.21–45.22, 53.8–53.9, 100.29
STING-associated vasculopathy with onset in infancy (SAVI)   45.5, 45.6, 45.13–45.14
stinging potential, sensory irritation   128.10–128.11
stingray stings   130.4
stings
  hymenoptera   34.15–34.18
  marine/aquatic animals   130.1–130.5
stippled calcification, Conradi–Hünermann–Happle syndrome   63.23
STIs *see* sexually transmitted infections
StK *see* stucco keratosis
STLs *see* sesquiterpene lactones
'stocking' distribution, multivoltage X-ray techniques   24.3–24.4, 24.6–24.7
stomas   112.1–112.16
  allergic contact dermatitis   112.7–112.8
  appliance types   112.1, **112.3**
  assessment of patient   112.1
  corticosteroids for inflammatory peristomal skin diseases   **112.4**
  Crohn ulceration   112.13–112.15
  definition   112.1
  dermatological assessment   **112.3**
  dermatoses associated with underlying bowel disease   112.12–112.15
  infections   112.8–112.10
  irritant skin reactions   112.2–112.7
  lichen sclerosus   112.10
  localised bullous pemphigoid   112.10, 112.12
  nicorandil ulceration   112.10, *112.12*
  pain   *112.6*
  patch test series   **112.9**
  psoriasis   *112.9*, 112.10, 112.11
  pyoderma gangrenosum   *112.10*, 112.13–112.15
  skin complications   153.7
  streptococcal cellulitis   *112.10*
  treatment for   112.1
  types of   112.1, **112.3**
  ulceration   112.10, 112.12–112.15
stomatitis
  angular   32.62–32.63, 108.20, 108.59–108.60
  candidal *see* acute pseudomembranous candidiasis; chronic erythematous candidiasis

denture-induced   32.62, 108.20–108.21
herpetic   108.52
  primary herpetic gingivostomatitis   25.20–25.24
  vesicular stomatitis virus   25.97
stomatodynia *see* burning mouth syndrome
stored product mites   34.50–34.51
storiform collagenoma   136.3–136.4
storiform patterning   3.43
storiform perineural fibroma *see* perineurioma
stork bite *see* naevus flammeus
Stormorken syndrome   63.30
STP *see* superficial thrombophlebitis
strain   122.3
strangulation of the penis   109.8
Strasbourg diagnostic criteria, Schnitzler syndrome   **45.20**
stratum basale, epidermis   2.5
stratum corneum (SC)   122.4
  black heel   *122.11*
  calluses   122.7
  epidermis   2.1, 2.6
  friction blisters   122.9
  function of   12.1, 12.8–12.9
  hydration measurement, surface electrical properties   16.5
  irritant contact dermatitis   128.2
  percutaneous absorption mechanisms   12.1–12.2
  permeability coefficient of water across   12.2
  sampling of by tape-stripping   12.8
  sensitising chemicals   127.6
stratum granulosum, epidermis   2.5–2.6
stratum lucidum, epidermis   2.7
strawberry naevus, eyelid   107.46–107.47
strawberry tongue   108.25
streblodactyly   94.41
Streptobacillus moniliformis   26.75–26.76
streptocerciasis (*Mansonella streptocerca* infection)   33.6–33.7
streptococcal cellulitis
  necrotising   26.78
  perianal   26.33–26.34, 111.14
  peristomal skin   *112.10*
streptococcal impetigo, post-streptococcal glomerulonephritis   154.6
Streptococcal infections of female genitalia   26.33, 110.25–110.26
streptococcal toxic shock-like syndrome (STSLS)   26.30, 26.36–26.37
Streptococcus
  groups   26.12
  infections   26.10–26.12
  S. agalactiae (group B)
    diseases   26.12
    toxic shock-like syndrome   26.36–26.37
    scarlet fever   26.35–26.36
  S. dysgalactiae (group C)
    diseases   26.12
    toxic shock-like syndrome   26.36–26.37
    skin infections   26.13
  S. pyogenes (group A)   26.10–26.12
    antibiotic resistance, impetigo management   26.16
    diseases   26.12
    epidemiology   26.10–26.11
    M antigens   26.35
    pathophysiology   26.11–26.12
    recurrent toxin-mediated perineal erythema   26.32
    toxic shock-like syndrome   26.30, 26.36–26.37
    vulvovaginitis   26.33, 110.25
  S. suis, toxic shock-like syndrome   26.36–26.37
  toxin-mediated disease   26.32, 26.35–26.37
  transients on skin   26.3, 26.4
stress   122.3
  and acne   88.25
  associated hormones   150.8–150.9
  emotional effects of skin conditions   15.2
  relaxation   122.3
  systemic lupus erythematosus   51.21

urticaria   42.8
see also psychodermatology
stretch marks *see* striae
striae   *4.9, 94.7, 94.8,* 94.9–94.12
striae distensae   94.32
  in pregnancy   *113.2,* 113.3
  sports injuries   122.17
striae of Wickham, penis   *109.19*
striated muscle hamartoma *see* rhabdomyomatous congenital hamartoma
striate palmoplantar keratoderma (SPPK)   63.56–63.58, 63.62–63.63, 69.7
'strimmer phytophotodermatosis   *4.9*
Strongyloides stercoralis
  ancylostomiasis   33.15–33.17
  perineal and perianal skin   111.16
strongyloidiasis   33.17–33.18
  clinical features   33.17–33.18
  management   33.18
  pathophysiology   33.17
structure of skin *see* skin, structure and function
strumous bubo *see* lymphogranuloma venereum
stucco keratosis (StK)   132.4
Sturge–Weber syndrome (SWS)   71.3–71.4, 73.20, **101.28**, 108.27
SU *see* solar urticaria
subacute annular generalised pustular psoriasis   35.34
subacute cutaneous lupus erythematosus (SCLE)   51.12–51.16
  associated diseases   51.12
  autoantibody status   51.13
  clinical features   51.14
  clinical variants   51.14
  complications and co-morbidities   51.15
  differential diagnosis   **51.15**
  drug-induced SCLE   51.13
  drugs associated with development of   **51.13–51.14**
  epidemiology   51.12
  genetics   51.14
  investigations   51.15
  lesion appearance   *51.15*
  management   51.15–51.16
  pathology   51.14
  pathophysiology   51.12–51.13
  predisposing factors   51.13–51.14
subacute nodular migratory panniculitis   97.25
subacute panniculitis-like T-cell lymphoma   **72.11**
subareolar duct papillomatosis *see* nipple, adenoma
subcision, cellulite management   98.26
subclinical and latent viral infections
  herpes simplex   25.19–25.20
  human papillomaviruses   25.51–25.52
subcorneal haematoma, black heel   *122.11*
subcorneal pustular dermatosis   49.17–49.19, 49.19, 118.4
  associated diseases   49.17
  histology   *49.17*
  management   49.18–49.19
  pathophysiology   49.17
  presentation   49.18
  pustule appearance   *49.18*
subcorneal pustules   3.43
subcutaneous atypical smooth muscle tumour (leiomyosarcoma)   136.54–136.55
subcutaneous calcification *see* calcification of skin and subcutaneous tissues
subcutaneous drug administration, dermatoses induced by   120.6–120.8
subcutaneous fat
  anatomy   97.1–97.5
  necrosis and pancreatic disease   153.6
  physiology   97.1–97.5
  role of   2.43
subcutaneous fat disorders   2.42
  arteries   97.7

fungal infections   97.47
inflammatory diseases   97.6
miscellaneous disorders   98.25–98.27
neonates   97.37, 97.57–97.58, 114.14–114.18, **114.18**
non-inflammatory disorders   98.1–98.30
subcutaneous fat necrosis of the newborn (SCFN)   97.37, 97.57–97.58, 114.15–114.17, **114.18**
subcutaneous γ/δ T-cell lymphoma   97.61–97.63
subcutaneous glatiramer acetate injections   97.48–97.49
subcutaneous granuloma annulare   97.14–97.15
  rheumatoid nodule differentiation   97.16–97.17
subcutaneous granulomas   97.12, 97.54
subcutaneous lipomatosis   98.15–98.21
subcutaneous mycoses   32.69–32.80
Subcutaneous mycosis due to *Basidiobolus* and *Conidiobolus*   32.79–32.80
subcutaneous necrobiosis lipoidica   97.11
subcutaneous necrotising infections   26.77–26.78
subcutaneous nodules
  autoinflammatory diseases   **80.19**
  progressive nodular histiocytosis   135.19
  rheumatoid arthritis   155.5–155.6
  in systemic lupus erythematosus   51.28
subcutaneous panniculitis-like T-cell lymphoma   97.61–97.63, 139.29–139.31
subcutaneous panniculitis T-cell lymphoma (SPTCL)   97.39–97.40, 97.46, 97.61–97.63, 139.29–139.31
subcutaneous phycomycosis   32.79–32.80
subcutaneous sarcoidosis   96.3, 96.11–96.12, 97.53–97.54
subcutaneous Sweet syndrome   49.12, 97.51
subcutaneous tissue
  anatomy   97.2–97.3
  cellular composition   97.1–97.2
  vascularisation   97.6
subcutaneous tumours, juvenile hyaline fibromatosis   94.42
subcutaneous zygomycosis   32.79–32.80
subepidermal blistering   85.28
  heat-associated diseases   124.15, *124.16*
subepidermal nodular fibrosis *see* fibrous histiocytoma
subjective sensory irritation   128.10–128.11
sublamina densa blistering, antigen mapping   69.21
submammary flexural psoriasis   35.9
Sub-Saharan Africa, persons with albinism   7.10–7.11, 7.12, *7.13*
substance P (SP), pruritus   **81.3**, 81.4
subungual haematoma, sports injuries   122.16
subungual melanoma, presentation   142.10–142.11, *142.15*
succulent gums, neonates   114.4
suction blisters, neonates   114.4
sudamina *see* miliaria crystallina
sudoriparous angioma *see* eccrine angiomatous hamartoma
suicidality
  acne patients   88.39
  body dysmorphic disorder   84.13
  delusional infestation   84.7, 84.8, 84.9
  dermatological patients   84.41–84.42
  eating disorders   84.27
  isotretinoin acne treatment   84.42
  psychodermatology   84.2, 84.41–84.42
  recalcitrant itch   84.28
  risk assessment   84.41–84.42
  risk factors   **84.41**
  self-harm   84.38
  SSRI antidepressants   84.43
SUIs *see* sea urchin injuries
sulfasalazine, cutaneous adverse effects   155.15
sulphites, allergic reactions   127.56
sulphonamides, urticaria treatment   42.19

sulphonylureas, eczema 117.4
sulphur, acne vulgaris treatment 88.57
summary of product characteristics (SmPC), systemic therapy 19.2, 19.3
sunbed UVR exposure 10.13
 polymorphic light eruption 126.4
sunburn
 melanoma risk 142.6
 xeroderma pigmentosum 76.4
sun-damaged skin, melanomas 145.9, *145.11*, **145.11**
sunlight exposure
 children melanoma risk 142.6
 granuloma annulare 95.2
 infantile eosinophilic pustular folliculitis 91.7
 mechanical injuries 122.5
 melanoma risk 142.5–142.6, 145.9
 Merkel cell carcinoma risk 146.2–146.3
 occupational skin cancer 129.14
 pigmentation response 86.8–86.9, *86.44*, 86.46
 psoriasis vulgaris 35.4
 solar purpura 99.23–99.24
 sun-related dermatoses 7.8
 suppressing immune responses and permitting progression of immunogenic tumours 146.3
 UVR exposure 10.12–10.13
 UVR path lengths *10.3*
 see also ultraviolet radiation
sun protection factor (SPF), sunscreens 10.11–10.12
sunscreens 18.34–18.36
 photoallergic reactions 127.62, 127.79
 photopatch testing *126.31*
 photoprotection 10.11–10.12
 photosensitivity management 126.36–126.37
 porphyria, management of 58.5
superantigen toxins, recurrent perineal erythema 26.32
superficial actinic porokeratosis 85.21, 85.22–85.23
superficial angiomyxoma 136.59–136.60
superficial basal cell carcinoma (sBCC) 140.3, *140.4*, 140.6, *140.8*, 140.9, *140.11*
 mimicking Bowen disease *141.20*
 photodynamic therapy 22.6–22.7
 photothermal ablation 23.21
superficial burn wounds 125.6, 128.12
superficial chemical peels (SCPs) 160.4
superficial epidermolytic ichthyosis (SEI) 63.15–63.16, *63.18*
superficial fibromatoses 94.33
 palmar and plantar fibromatosis 136.12–136.13
superficial folliculitis 91.1–91.8
superficial haemosiderotic lymphovascular malformation *see* hobnail haemangioma
superficial mucocoeles, oral ulceration 108.42
superficial mycoses *see* dermatophytes
superficial onychomycosis (SO)
 caused by dermatophytes 32.47–32.48
 caused by non-dermatophyte moulds 32.54–32.55
superficial papillary adenomatosis *see* nipple, adenoma
superficial radiotherapy, basal cell carcinoma/squamous cell carcinoma 24.8–24.10
superficial spreading melanoma (SSM)
 melanoma classification 142.7, 142.8
 presentation 142.10, *142.11*, *142.12*, 142.20
superficial subcutaneous fat 97.3
superficial thrombophlebitis (STP) 97.8–97.9, *97.10*, 97.24
superficial ulceration, striae *94.8*
superficial venous thrombosis 101.34–101.35
 clinical features **101.35**
 investigations for **101.35**
 treatment **101.36**
 see also thrombophlebitis migrans
superficial X-ray therapy
 depth dose curves 24.1
 principles 24.1
 techniques and equipment 24.3
superinfections
 ichthyoses 63.46
 mal de Meleda 63.55
supernumerary ribs, Waardenburg syndrome 68.5
support surfaces, pressure ulcer prevention 123.8–123.9, 123.10
suppressor T cells, sensitisation reaction 127.9
suprabasal keratins, gene expression 2.8
suprabulbar region, hair follicles 87.4, 87.6
surfactants, allergies 127.59
surgeons, preoperative preparation 20.11
surgical complications 20.29, 20.33, 20.40–20.42, **20.41**
surgical smoke, hazards and risks of electrosurgery 20.45–20.46
surgical treatment 1.8
 auricle melanoma 106.32
 basal cell carcinoma 140.14–140.16
 body dysmorphic disorder 84.15
 burns 125.8
 compared to radiotherapy for basal cell or squamous cell carcinomas 24.8, **24.10**
 cutaneous squamous cell carcinoma 141.35
 cutaneous tuberculosis 27.10
 cutaneous warts 25.59
 during pregnancy 113.24
 hidradenitis suppurativa 90.10–90.11
 hyperhidrosis 92.9–92.10
 induced non-healing of wounds 84.33, *84.34*, 84.37
 lymphoedema 103.60–103.61
 melanoma 143.1–143.6
 perineal and perianal skin conditions 111.25–111.33
 pressure ulcers 123.11–123.12
 reconstruction principles of design 20.19–20.21
 tissue sampling for molecular genetic profiling of melanoma 144.1
 see also skin surgery
suspected deep tissue injury (SDTI), pressure ulcers **123.6**
Sustainable Development Goals (SDGs) 7.1, 7.6–7.7
sutural alopecia 87.30
sutures
 removal after skin surgery 20.40
 wound healing 11.10
suturing for skin surgery
 knot tying 20.12–20.14
 needles and materials 20.12
 techniques 20.14–20.19
swamp cancer *see* Pythium insidiosum infection
sweat duct carcinoma *see* adnexal carcinoma NOS
sweat gland abscesses, neonates 114.25
sweat gland carcinomas 137.33–137.40
sweat gland cellular inclusions, disorders with 92.15
sweat glands 2.2, 2.8–2.9, 2.43
 apoeccrine glands 2.9, 92.1
 disorders 92.1–92.22
 embryonic development 2.5
 inherited immunodeficiency **80.4–80.6**
 perspiration types 2.9
 tumours of skin appendages 137.1–137.2
 see also apocrine glands; eccrine glands
sweating
 atopic eczema 41.18–41.19
 cholinergic urticaria 42.11–42.12
 mechanical injuries 122.1
 neonates 114.3
 obesity 98.27
 thermal 2.9
 thermoregulation 92.3, 92.4
 see also hyperhidrosis
Sweden
 health economics, holistic perspective 6.2
 skin cancer, economic burden of 6.6, **6.7**
Sweet syndrome 49.8–49.15, 97.51
 associated diseases 49.8–49.10
 causative organisms 49.10
 classic Sweet syndrome 49.8, *49.11*
 clinical features 49.11–49.12
 clinical variants 49.12
 dermal infiltrate in lesional skin *49.14*
 diagnostic criteria **49.13**
 differential diagnosis 49.13
 disease course and prognosis 49.14
 drug-induced Sweet syndrome 49.8, 49.10–49.11
 drug reactions 49.8, 49.10–49.11, 149.6
 environmental factors 49.10–49.11
 epidemiology 49.8
 erythema nodosum with 97.21–97.23
 on face 49.12
 genetics 49.10
 histiocytoid Sweet syndrome 49.12, *49.14*, 97.22–97.23, 149.6
 histology 49.11
 investigations 49.14
 on leg 49.12
 malignancy association 148.23–148.24, 149.6, 149.7
 management 49.14–49.15
 neutrophilic dermatosis of dorsal hands 49.12, *49.13*
 oral ulceration 108.41
 paraneoplastic forms 149.6–149.7
 pathology 49.10
 predisposing factors 49.10
 pseudovesicles within inflammatory plaques *49.11*
 reactivation in COVID-19 patients 25.112
 sarcoidosis association 96.15
 severity classification 49.14
 subcutaneous Sweet syndrome 49.12
 treatment for 49.14–49.15
 see also VEXAS syndrome
swelling
 eyelids 118.14, *118.16*, 129.6
 face 98.19, 103.46–103.49
 limbs 103.9–103.10, 103.16–103.17, 103.44–103.46
 mouth 95.14, 108.8–108.14, **108.9**, 127.72
 penoscrotal **109.20**
 vulva *95.15*
 see also loiasis; oedema
'swimmer's' itch *see* cercarial dermatitis
'swimmer's shoulder' 122.17
swimming pool granuloma (*Mycobacteria marinum*) 27.32–27.35
'Swiss cheese model', drug-related patient harm 13.10
Switzerland, psoriasis, economic burden of 6.8
SWS *see* Sturge–Weber syndrome
sycosis 26.26–26.27
symmetrical acrokeratoderma 63.20
symmetrical drug-related intertriginous and flexural exanthema (SDRIFE) 127.46
symmetrical dyschromatoses 68.14–68.15
sympathectomy, hyperhidrosis treatment 92.9–92.10
sympathetic nerve endings, sweat glands 2.9
sympathetic nerve injury 83.20
sympathetic nerves, gustatory hyperhidrosis 92.8
sympathetic skin response (SSR), neurophysiological testing for skin innervation 83.5
symplastic haemangioma 136.31–136.32
symptoms, measurement tools 16.5
synaptophysin 3.23
syndecans 2.38
syndromic congenital ichthyosis 63.22–63.62
syndromic genodermatoses with nail anomalies **67.2–67.3**
syndromic hidradenitis suppurativa 90.2
syndromic ichthyosis **63.3**, 63.22–63.62
syndromic keratodermas 63.62–63.71
syndromic lymphoedema 103.20–103.22
syndromic palmoplantar keratoderma **63.57**
synophrys 107.4
synovitis, acne, pustulosis, hyperostosis and osteitis (SAPHO) syndrome 45.22, 88.7, 88.63
synthetic cannabinoid receptor agonists 120.2
synthetic coolants 129.1
synthetic retinoids 19.41–19.42
syphilis 29.1–29.29
 clinical features 29.5–29.20
 congenital 29.2, 29.22–29.29, 114.27–114.28
 congenital neonatal 114.27–114.28
 definition and nomenclature 29.2
 differential diagnoses 29.17–29.18
 endemic syphilis (bejel) 26.70
 epidemiology 29.2–29.3
 of eyebrows *105.12*
 eye involvement 107.39–107.40
 hair loss 29.10, *29.12*, 87.35
 HIV coinfection 31.21–31.22
 HIV relationship 29.16, 29.17
 investigations and tests 29.18–29.20
 latent stage 29.12
 late skin forms 29.12–29.14
 male genitalia 109.28
 management 29.20–29.22
 nephrotic syndrome 154.6
 ocular syphilis 29.16, 107.39–107.40
 oral involvement 108.34, 108.56
 pathophysiology 29.3–29.5
 perianal skin 111.16
 in pregnancy 113.6
 primary stage 29.6–29.7, 29.17
 pustule 'grape cluster' *1.6*
 rashes 29.7–29.10
 scalp infection 105.12
 secondary stage 29.7–29.12, 29.17–29.18
 sexual contact identification and treatment 29.22
 stages and course 29.5–29.6
 systemic features 29.10, 29.12
 tertiary/late stage 29.12–29.17, 29.18
 treatment for 1.7–1.8
syphilitic alopecia 29.10, *29.12*, 87.35
syphilitic leukoplakia 108.34
syringocystadenoma
 papilliferum 105.11, 137.19–137.20
 in sebaceous naevus *73.8*
 see also syringoma
syringocystoma *see* syringoma
syringoid eccrine carcinoma (adnexal carcinoma NOS) 137.37
syringoma *4.8*, 4.10, 137.27–137.28
 differential diagnosis 88.30
 malignant *see* microcystic adnexal carcinoma
 vulva **110.32**
syringomyelia 83.16–83.17
systematic reviews, critical appraisal for evidence based medicine 17.8–17.12
systematised linear porokeratosis 85.22
systemic absorption of topical therapies
 adverse effects 18.5
 application quantity 18.3
 corticosteroids 18.19–18.20
systemic allergic contact dermatitis (SACD), drug-induced eczema 117.3–117.5
systemically reactivated contact dermatitis 127.18–127.19
systemic amyloidoses with cutaneous involvement **56.3**, 56.10–56.13
 macroglossia *56.12*
 periorbital bleeding *56.11*

plasmacytoma-associated systemic amyloidosis *56.11*
   treatment 56.14
systemic antibiotics 19.46–19.48
   hidradenitis suppurativa treatment 90.9–90.10
systemic antihistamines 19.3–19.4
systemic autoimmune diseases, skin and renal involvement 154.6
systemic calcium homeostasis, cutaneous metastatic calcification 59.5–59.6
systemic candidiasis 32.92–32.93
systemic capillary leak syndrome (Clarkson syndrome) 43.4
systemic chondromalacia, *see also* relapsing polychondritis
systemic coagulopathies, purpura 99.15–99.19
systemic component, histiocytosis 135.14–135.29
systemic contact dermatitis, medicament allergens 127.46
systemic disorders
   acquired ichthyosis 63.48
   cardiac involvement 151.4–151.5
   causing pruritus 81.8–81.10
   changes in microbial ecology of the skin 26.4
   hypermelanosis 86.19–86.25
   involving respiratory system 152.5–152.6
   liver disease with cutaneous features 153.7–153.8
   mechanical injuries 122.1–122.2
systemic drug-induced photosensitivity 126.27–126.28
systemic drug reactions 118.1, 118.4–118.12
systemic drug-related intertriginous and flexural exanthema (SDRIFE) 117.5, 127.18
systemic drug treatment
   antifungal therapy 19.48, 40.9
   follicular eruptions 91.2–91.3
   hyperhidrosis 92.9
   phototherapy combination 21.10
   sarcoidosis 96.17
systemic features
   dermatomyositis 52.7–52.8
   sarcoidosis 96.5
systemic immunotherapy, cutaneous warts 25.60
systemic juvenile idiopathic arthritis (SJIA/Still disease) 45.21–45.22, 53.8, 53.9
systemic juvenile xanthogranuloma 135.17
systemic lupus erythematosus (SLE) 51.1, 51.16–51.38, *87.55*, 89.8
   age at onset 51.18
   antinuclear antibody (ANA) test 51.34–51.36
   arthritis 51.30
   assessment of disease activity 51.36
   association with other diseases 51.32–51.33
   autoantibodies 51.20–51.21
   bone changes 51.30
   bullous lesions 51.28–51.29
   cardiac involvement 151.4
   cardiovascular disease 51.30
   cell appearance *51.18*
   'chilblain' lesions *51.9*, 51.25
   in children 51.32
   classification **51.16**
   clinical features 51.21–51.29
   complications and co-morbidities 51.30–51.32
   in contraception 51.32
   coronary artery disease 51.30
   cutaneous features **51.23**
   cutaneous vascular reactions 51.26–51.27
   Degos-like lesions *51.27*
   diagnosis criteria *51.17*
   differential diagnosis 51.29–51.30
   discoid lupus erythematosus relationship/comparison 51.6, **51.9**
   disease course and prognosis 51.34
   drug-induced SLE 51.21, **51.22**
   dystrophic calcinosis 51.28
   ear 51.32
   in elderly people 51.32
   environmental factors 51.21
   epidemiology 51.17–51.18
   eye 51.32
   gastrointestinal tract 51.31
   genetics 51.19–51.20
   hair changes 51.25–51.26
   hearing loss 51.32
   heart 51.30
   hepatic lesions 51.31
   hormonal factors 51.21
   and immune system 51.20–51.21
   immunohistology 51.19
   infections 51.21
   internal malignancy association 148.21
   internal organs 51.19
   investigations 51.34–51.36
   and Kikuchi–Fujimoto disease 51.33
   leg ulcers *51.26*
   liver disease 51.31
   lungs 51.31
   'lupus hair' with diffuse alopecia *51.26*
   lupus nephritis, classification **51.20**
   lupus non-specific changes 51.25
   lupus-specific changes 51.23–51.25
   macroscopic/microscopic appearances 51.18, *51.19*
   management 51.36–51.38
   mucinosis 51.28
   mucous membrane lesions 51.29
   muscle changes 51.30
   nail changes 51.25
   neurological disease 51.31–51.32
   ocular changes 51.32
   oral involvement 108.78
   pathological features **51.18**
   pathophysiology 51.18–51.19
   pigmentary changes 51.28
   in pregnancy 51.32, 113.7–113.8
   pulmonary system 51.31
   renal changes 51.31
   respiratory disease 152.2
   rheumatoid arthritis comparison **51.30**
   skin features 51.19
   stress 51.21
   subcutaneous nodules 51.28
   susceptible genes and pathways **51.20**
   thyroid disease 51.31
   treatment of non-renal SLE 51.37
   ultraviolet radiation 51.21
   urticarial lesions 51.27–51.28
   vasculitis 51.26
   vasculopathy 51.26–51.27
systemic mastocytosis (SM) **46.2**, *46.4*, 46.6
systemic mucormycosis 32.93
systemic mycoses 32.80–32.94
   identification 32.80–32.81
   pathophysiology 32.80
systemic neoplasia
   associated skin conditions 148.1–148.28
   see also internal malignancy
systemic non-eczematous reactions to allergens 127.21
systemic-onset juvenile idiopathic arthritis (SoJIA/Still disease) 45.21–45.22, 53.8, 53.9
systemic photodynamic therapy 22.2
systemic retinoid therapy *see* retinoids (systemic therapy)
systemic sarcoidosis 96.7, 96.15–96.16
systemic sclerosis (SSc) 3.44, 54.1–54.29, 86.20–86.21, 94.45
   age of onset 54.7–54.8
   associated diseases 54.8–54.10
   autoantibodies
      and clinical associations **54.5–54.6**
      type and frequency **54.9**
   calcinosis 54.17, **54.26**
   cancer risk 54.9–54.10
   cardiac involvement 54.17–54.18, **54.23**, 151.4
   cardiopulmonary manifestations 54.17–54.18
   cardiorespiratory pulmonary fibrosis **54.23**
   causative organisms 54.13
   cellular and molecular pathogenesis *54.12*
   chemotherapy 54.25–54.26
   classification 54.1–54.2, **54.7**
   clinical features **54.2**, **54.5–54.6**, 54.15–54.18
   clinical variants 54.18
   complications and co-morbidities 54.21
   connective tissue disease 54.8–54.9
   critical digital ischaemia/ulceration **54.25**
   cutaneous manifestations 54.15–54.17
   diagnosis 54.21–54.22
   differential diagnosis 54.18–54.20
   diffuse cutaneous **54.2**
   digital ulceration 54.17, **54.25**
   disease assessment **54.17**
   disease course and prognosis 54.21
   disease modifying drugs, targets for *54.27*
   dyspigmentation 54.17
   dystrophic calcification 59.1, 59.2
   endothelial-to-mesenchymal transition 54.10
   environmental and drug-induced 94.45–94.46
   environmental factors 54.14–54.15
   epidemiology 54.7–54.8
   erectile dysfunction 54.28
   fibrosis 54.11–54.13
   gastrointestinal manifestations 54.17, **54.23**
   genetics 54.13–54.14
   histopathology *54.12*
   history 54.15
   immune-mediated inflammation 54.10–54.11
   incidence and prevalence 54.7
   internal malignancy association 148.21
   investigations 54.21, 54.22, **54.23–54.24**, **54.26**
   limited cutaneous SSc **54.2**
   localised scleroderma cutaneous assessment tool **55.33–55.34**
   lung involvement **54.26**
   malignancy risk 54.9–54.10
   management 54.22–54.29, **54.26**, *54.28*
      targets for disease modifying drugs *54.27*
   mechanical properties 122.5
   modified Rodnan skin score **54.17**
   muscle involvement 54.18
   musculoskeletal manifestations 54.18
   oral involvement 108.68–108.69
   organ-based disease assessment 54.22
   pathogenesis *54.27*
   pathophysiology 54.10–54.13
   predisposing factors 54.10
   presentation 54.15–54.18
   pruritus 54.16, **54.26**
   pulmonary manifestations 54.18, **54.26**
   Raynaud phenomenon *54.3*, 54.15, *54.22*
      causes and clinical features **54.19**
      investigation and management **54.25**
   renal manifestations 54.18, **54.24**
   respiratory disease 152.2
   scleroderma spectrum disorders **54.19**, 55.1
   scleromyxoedema comparison **57.5**
   severity classification 54.20–54.21
   skin thickening 54.15–54.16
   synonyms and inclusions 54.1
   telangiectasia 54.16–54.17, **54.26**
   tendon friction rubs 54.18
   terminology 55.1
   vasculopathy 54.10, **54.25**
   see also morphoea; sclerosis
systemic therapy 19.1–19.50
   anti-inflammatory and immunomodulatory drugs 19.2–19.46
   drug interactions 19.2
   hidradenitis suppurativa 90.9–90.10
   ichthyoses 63.44–63.45
   melanoma 144.1–144.12
   patient education 19.2
   patient selection 19.1–19.2
   prescribing and monitoring practice 19.2
   recessive dystrophic epidermolysis bullosa 69.26
   record keeping 19.2
   risk reduction 19.1–19.2, 19.3
   standards of care 19.1
   versus topical therapy 19.1
   vitiligo 86.39–86.40

T

TA *see* tufted angioma
tabanid flies (*Chrysops* species) 33.12
   see also loiasis
tabetic neurosyphilis 29.15–29.16
tacalcitol, topical therapies 18.28
tachykinins, pruritus **81.3**, 81.4
tachyphylaxis
   corticosteroids 18.20
   systemic glucocorticoid therapy 19.19
tacrolimus
   topical therapies 18.22, **18.23**
   wound healing *11.12*
TAD *see* transient acantholytic dermatosis
Taenia solium, cysticercosis 33.32–33.34
TAK *see* transient aquagenic keratoderma
Takayasu arteritis 100.34–100.35
Talaromyces marneffei (penicilliosis) 31.28, 32.89–32.90
Talimogene laherparepvec (T-vec), oncolytic virus therapy 144.1
talk therapies
   body dysmorphic disorder 84.14
   cognitive behavioural therapy 84.47
   combined somatic/psychological disorders 84.47–84.48
   habit reversal therapies 84.12, 84.15, 84.17, 84.18, 84.20, 84.21, 84.25, 84.47
   nodular prurigo *84.18*
   skin related health anxieties 84.26
tanapox virus (TANV) 25.19
tanning
   ability variation/skin types 2.18, **86.9**, 142.3
   melanoma risk 142.3
   physiology of 68.1, 86.9
   sunbed use 10.13
   sun-reactive skin types **86.9**
   UVR exposure 10.7–10.8
TANV *see* tanapox virus
Tanzania, Regional Dermatology Training Centre 7.7
tapeworms *see* cestodes
tapinarof, psoriasis treatment 35.22
targeted oncology therapies *87.73*, 144.4–144.5, *144.11*, **144.11**, 144.12
target lesions *4.15*
targetoid haemosiderotic haemangioma *see* hobnail haemangioma
targetoid haemosiderotic naevus 131.30–131.32
tars, topical therapies 18.36–18.37
tattoo granulomas, photothermal ablation 23.23
tattoos
   allergic granulomatous reactions 127.21
   amalgam tattoos, mouth 108.15
   body art, mouth 108.15–108.16
   foreign body reactions 122.21–122.22
   hair disorders 87.101
   hypermelanosis 86.53–86.54
   mercury allergy 127.41
   p-phenylenediamine allergy 127.60
   pseudoepitheliomatous hyperplasia 132.9, *132.10*
   removal by laser treatment 23.12–23.15
tattoo sarcoidosis 96.11
taxane, palmoplantar erythrodysaesthesia 119.2
tazarotene, topical therapies 18.25–18.26

TBHQ *see* t-butylhydroquinone
TBI *see* total body irradiation
TBSA *see* total body surface area
t-butylhydroquinone (TBHQ)   127.59
TCA CROSS *see* trichloroacetic acid chemical reconstruction of skin scars
TCDD *see* 2,3,7,8-Tetrachlorodibenzo-p-dioxin-p-dioxin
T-cell leukaemia–lymphomas, cells of origin   139.3
T-cell lymphoma
  panniculitis-like   97.61–97.63
  positive staining of atypical cells   *3.28*
  radiotherapy   24.16, 24.18
  see also cutaneous T-cell lymphoma
T-cell-mediated drug hypersensitivity   14.3–14.4
  acute generalised exanthematous pustulosis   14.4
  drug reaction with eosinophilia and systemic symptoms   14.3–14.4, 14.7
  Stevens–Johnson syndrome   14.3, 14.7
  toxic epidermal necrolysis   14.3, 14.7
T-cell pseudolymphoma   134.1–134.2
T-cell receptor gene analysis, mycosis fungoides   139.6–139.8
T-cell recognition of drugs   14.4–14.6
  altered peptide repertoir model   14.6
  hapten/pro-hapten model   14.5–14.6
  MHC–peptide–TCR interaction   14.4, *14.5*
  pharmacological interaction model   *14.5*, 14.6
T cells   9.4, 9.5–9.7, 14.4, 14.5, 50.2, 127.9
T-cells
  activation   2.12, 14.4
  allergens binding to   127.7
  allergic contact dermatitis   9.10
  dermis   2.15
  immune system   9.3–9.6, 103.3
  in pemphigus   50.2
T-cell theory, drug-specific   118.5
TCI *see* topical calcineurin inhibitors
TDT *see* thermal damage time
TE *see* telogen effluvium
tear film, precorneal   107.3
tea tree oil, allergy to   127.71
TEC *see* toxic erythema of chemotherapy
Technetium-99 bone scintigraphy   124.2, *124.3*
Tedania ignis, stings from   130.3
TEE *see* transepidermal elimination; transepithelial elimination
Teenagers' Quality of Life Index (T-QoL)   16.10
teenagers, *see also* adolescents
teeth
  anatomy of   108.4
  betel staining   *108.15*
  congenital syphilis   29.26, *29.28*
  dental plaque   108.5
  epidermolysis bullosa presentation   69.17, *69.18*
  eruption cyst   108.10
  eruption cyst over a primary tooth   108.10
  incontinentia pigmenti presentation   68.11
  methamphetamine-induced tooth decay   120.5
  pachyonychia congenita presentation   67.12
  periodontal Ehlers–Danlos syndrome   **70.5**, 70.10
  phantom tooth pain/trigeminal neuropathic pain   82.5–82.7
  tooth decay, methamphetamine-induced   120.5
teething, flushing in children   104.10
telangiectases   101.10–101.22, *101.39*, *101.44*
  angiokeratomas   101.13–101.14, **101.17**
  angioma serpiginosum   101.16, **101.17**, *101.18*, **101.18**
  causes of   **101.10**
  cherry angiomas   101.12–101.13, **101.17**
  facial   23.9–23.10
  generalised essential telangiectasia   **101.17**, 101.18–101.19
  hereditary benign telangiectasia   **101.17**, 101.20, *101.21*
  histology   **101.10**
  laser therapies   23.6, 23.9–23.11, *23.12*
  leg veins   23.11
  pathophysiology   101.10
  primary telangiectasias   101.16, **101.17**, **101.18**
  spider telangiectases   101.10–101.12, **101.17**
  unilateral naevoid telangiectasia syndrome   101.20–101.22
  venous lakes   101.14–101.16, **101.17**
telangiectasia
  atrophic stria with   *94.8*
  hereditary haemorrhagic telangiectasia   71.12–71.13
  hereditary haemorrhagic telangiectasia (Osler–Rendu–Weber syndrome)   108.26
  metastatic carcinoma   148.3–148.4
  necrobiosis lipoidica   *95.11*
  oral involvement   108.27
  Rothmund–Thomson syndrome   *75.5*
  skin lesions associated with gastrointestinal disorders   **153.7**
  systemic sclerosis   54.16–54.17, **54.26**
  see also hereditary haemorrhagic telangiectasia; spider telangiectases
telangiectasia, elevated erythropoietin and erythrocytosis, monoclonal gammopathy, perinephric fluid collections and intrapulmonary shunting (TEMPI) syndrome   149.12
telangiectasia macularis eruptiva perstans (TMEP)   *46.1*, 46.5
telangiectatic metastatic carcinoma   148.3–148.4
telangiectatic rosacea   *89.9*
  major features   89.6, *89.7*, 89.12
  pathology   89.3
  treatment   **89.14**
teledermatology   1.9, 4.25–4.26, 5.13, 7.8–7.9
Tel Hashomer criteria, familial Mediterranean fever diagnosis   45.10
telogen effluvium (TE)   87.13, 87.53–87.60
  COVID-19 association   25.113
  telogen (hair follicle resting phase)   87.7–87.8, 87.21, *87.57*
telogen release, hair fall   87.53
telomeres, dyskeratosis congenita   67.13
telomere shortening, skin ageing   2.45–2.46
'telomeropathies'   67.13
temperature-dependent urticaria   **42.9**, 42.10–42.11
TEMPI (telangiectasia, elevated erythropoietin and erythrocytosis, monoclonal gammopathy, perinephric fluid collections and intrapulmonary shunting) syndrome   149.12
temporal triangular alopecia (TTA)   87.28
TEN *see* toxic epidermal necrolysis
tendon friction rubs, systemic sclerosis   54.18
tendon xanthomas   60.2–60.3
tennis toe   122.16
tenosynovial fibroma   136.11
tenosynovial giant cell tumour   136.19
tensile strength, elastic tissue   94.21
teratogenicity
  methotrexate   19.26
  mycophenolate   19.29
  retinoid therapy   19.43, 19.44
  thalidomide   19.45, 19.46
terbinafine, dermatophytosis treatment   32.32
terminology
  commonly used dermatopathological terms   3.38–3.43
  standardisation of   1.4, *1.5*
terpenes, allergic contact dermatitis   127.42–127.43

terra firme forme *see* dermatitis passivata
tertiary syphilis   29.12–29.17, 29.18
'tertiary teledermatology'   4.26
TERT telomerase gene, melanoma risk   142.5
testis, torsion of   109.25
testosterone, hair growth stimulation   87.10
tetanus immunisation, bites   130.6
2,3,7,8-tetrachlorodibenzo-p-dioxin-p-dioxin (TCDD)   129.12
tetracyclines   19.47, 19.48
  hypermelanosis   86.27–86.28
  topical therapies   18.12
tetraethylthiuram disulphide, eczema   117.4
tetraspanins, epidermolysis bullosa   69.4
TEWL *see* transepidermal water loss
Texier disease   97.50
textile dermatitis   127.65–127.67
textile dyes, genital contact dermatitis   109.13
texture of skin, matching principles in surgical design   20.21
TFIIH *see* transcription/DNA repair factor IIH
TGF *see* transforming growth factor
TGF-β binding proteins *see* latent transforming growth factor beta binding proteins
TGM1 mutations, congenital ichthyosiform erythroderma   63.12
TH2 activity, alopecia areata   87.22
thalidomide   19.44–19.45
  dermatological uses   19.44
  pharmacological properties   19.44–19.45
  potential adverse effects   19.45
  safety considerations   19.45–19.46
  sarcoidosis treatment   96.17
thallium, dermatological reactions   121.8–121.9
theque, definition   *3.43*
therapeutic relationship between clinician and patient   84.47
therapeutic window, clinical pharmacology   **13.2**
therapy
  assessing benefit to patients, Patient Benefit Index tool   16.5
  decisions, appraising clinical trials   **17.12–17.13**
  principles of topical therapy   18.1–18.42
Theridiidae (widow spiders)   34.34–34.35
thermal damage time (TDT), light assisted hair removal   23.5–23.6
thermal relaxation time (TRT), of skin chromophores   23.5
thermal sweating   2.9
thermokinetic selectivity, laser treatments   23.6
thermolipolysis, fat contouring   161.9
thermoplastics, allergic contact dermatitis   127.68
thermoregulation   2.9, 2.42–2.43
thermoregulatory sweating   92.3, 92.4
THET *see* Tropical Health and Education Trust
thiamine (vitamin B1) deficiency   61.13–61.14
thickening of skin, diabetic patients   62.5–62.6
thigh
  cicatricial pemphigoid   *50.52*
  cryopyrin-associated periodic syndrome   *45.9*
  cutaneous small-vessel vasculitis   *100.7*
  erythema multiforme   *47.2*
  hemihyperplasia–multiple lipomatosis syndrome   *72.11*
  lichen striatus   *37.18*
  linear IgA disease   *50.37*
  massive localised lymphoedema   *103.53*
  microtrauma to   *98.9*
  urticaria pigmentosa   *46.4*
thiomersal, allergic reactions   127.3–127.5
thiopurine methyl transferase (TPMT), polymorphism affecting

azathioprine metabolism   19.8–19.9, 19.10
thioureas   *127.65*
thiuram mix (sensitisers)   127.63–127.64
thiurams   127.64
thorax, pulmonary haemorrhage, microscopic polyangiitis   *100.21*
Thost–Unna keratoderma   63.53
threadworm *see* enterobiasis
Three Item Severity Score (TIS)   16.4
thrips (Thysanoptera)   34.30
thromboangiitis obliterans   101.3–101.6
  causative organisms   101.6
  clinical features   **101.6**
  epidemiology   101.4
  investigations for   101.6
  ischaemic toes   *101.6*
  management of   **101.7**
  pathophysiology   101.5–101.6
  vascular occlusion and corkscrew collaterals   *101.7*
thrombocytopenia, purpura   31.12, *31.14*, 99.2–99.4
thrombocytosis, purpura   99.3–99.4, 99.10–99.11
thrombophlebitis, neoplasia association   148.26
thrombophlebitis migrans   101.35–101.36
thrombosis *see* venous thrombosis
thrush *see* candidiasis
thumbnail, lichen planus   *37.12*
thymol, traditional topical therapy   18.38
thyroid disease
  myxoedema   57.11–57.14
  systemic lupus erythematosus   51.31
thyroid dysfunction, drug reaction with eosinophilia and systemic symptoms   118.9, 118.11
thyroid dysfunction (hyper/hypothyroidism), dermatoendocrinology   **150.7**, **150.10**, **150.11**, 150.19–150.20
thyroiditis, granuloma annulare   95.1
thyroid medullary cancer, flushing   **104.7**, 148.26
thyrotoxicosis, pruritus   81.10
thyroxine, urticaria treatment   42.19
Thysanoptera (thrips)   34.30
ticks (Acari)   34.37–34.41
  anaphylactic reactions to bites   14.2
  carried diseases   26.66–26.67, 26.72, 26.82–26.83, 34.39–34.41
  'tick typhus', rickettsial infections   26.82–26.83
'tiger-tail pattern', trichothiodystrophy   63.37
tight junctions   2.20–2.21
Time Trade-Off (TTO), quality of life assessment   16.9
TIMPs *see* tissue inhibitors of metalloproteinases
tinea
  allergic reactions   32.50
  granuloma annulare mistaken for   *95.5*
  penis/scrotum   109.27–109.28
  steroid-modified infections   32.50
  see also dermatophytosis
tinea barbae   32.40–32.41
tinea capitis   32.37–32.40, 87.24
  clinical features   32.38
  clinical variants   32.38–32.39
  epidemiology   32.37–32.38
  infants   115.8–115.9
  infection control   32.31–32.32, 32.40
  late sequelae of radio treatment   24.4, *24.8*, 24.21
  management   32.40
  pathophysiology   32.38
tinea circinata *see* tinea corporis
tinea corporis   4.10, 32.35–32.37
  clinical features   32.35–32.37
  corticosteroid effects   32.49–32.50
  discoid skin lesions   *39.10*
  infants   115.8

management 32.37
pathophysiology 32.35
tinea cruris 32.45–32.46
  female genitalia 110.28
tinea faciei 32.41–32.42, 89.10
  infants 115.8
tinea incognito, female genitalia 110.28
tinea manuum 32.44–32.45
tinea nigra (pityriasis nigra) 1
tinea nigra (tinea nigra palmaris/pityriasis nigra) 32.14–32.15
tinea nodosa see black piedra
tinea peddis 32.42–32.44
  clinical features 32.43–32.44
  epidemiology 32.42
  management 32.44
  pathophysiology 32.42–32.43
  sports association 122.16
tinea tonsurans see tinea capitis
tinea unguium (onychomycosis caused by dermatophytes) 32.47–32.49
tinea versicolor/tinea flavea see pityriasis versicolor
TIS see Three Item Severity Score
tissue-bound autoantibodies
  bullous pemphigoid 50.13–50.14
  mucous membrane pemphigoid 50.25
tissue cooling, avoiding epidermal heat damage during laser therapies 23.6
tissue engineering, wound healing 11.11–11.13
tissue inhibitors of metalloproteinases (TIMPs) 2.32
  wound healing 11.5
tissue injury, alpha-1 antitrypsin 97.44
tissue macrophages, microscopic examination of 3.36
tissue optics, fate of incident light on skin 23.3–23.4
tissue-processing machine 3.7
tissue tightening therapies 161.6–161.8
tixocortol pivalate, allergic reactions 127.47
TKIs see tyrosine kinase inhibitors
TL-01 UVB see narrow-band UVB
TLR-4 see Toll-like receptor
TMD see transient myeloproliferative disorder
TMEP see telangiectasia macularis eruptiva perstans
TN see trichorrhexis nodosa; trigeminal neuralgia
TNF-α, sarcoidosis 96.4
TNF-α inhibitors
  cutaneous adverse effects 155.15
  psoriasis treatment 35.27
  sarcoidosis treatment 96.17
TNF-inhibitor-associated alopecia 87.34–87.35
TNM (tumour, node, metastases) classification, oral squamous cell carcinoma 108.47, **108.48**
tobacco smoke exposure
  ageing of skin 156.4
  atopic eczema 41.7
tobacco use
  keratoses 108.33
  oral hyperpigmentation 108.16–108.17
  oral squamous cell carcinoma 108.46
  types 108.33
  see also smoking
tocilizumab
  morphoea treatment 55.39
  systemic sclerosis treatment 54.24
tocopherol 127.59
toe
  acquired digital fibrokeratoma 136.4
  acral fibromyxoma 136.59
  bandaging, lymphoedema therapy 103.59
  'chilblain' lesions 51.9
  discoid lupus erythematosus 51.8
  epidermolysis bullosa acquisita 50.45
  fibro-osseous pseudotumour of the digits 136.6

frostbite 124.2, *124.3*
lymphoedema 103.6
neuropathic ulcer 83.14, 83.15
perniosis *124.6*
pretibial myxoedema 103.42
primary localised cutaneous amyloidosis 56.8
psoriatic arthritis 35.41
systemic sclerosis 54.4
see also phalanges
toe cleft intertrigo (athletes foot), see also tinea peddis
toe clefts, microbiome 26.3, 26.5
toenail dystrophy 63.51
  epidermolysis bullosa 69.17
  pachyonychia congenita 67.1, 67.11
toenails
  lichen planus 37.12
  metal poisoning signs 121.1
  see also nails
toe systolic BP, peripheral vascular disease **101.4**
tofacitinib, psoriasis treatment 35.27
togaviruses 25.80, 25.87–25.93
Toll-like receptor 4 (TLR-4) 127.7
Toll-like receptors, transmembrane drug mechanisms 13.5
Toll-like receptor signalling, skin defence against pathogens 26.5, 26.6
tolnaftate, topical therapies 18.12–18.13
toluene-2,5-diamine 127.60–127.61
tombstone comedones, hidradenitis suppurativa 90.5
tongue
  amyloidosis 108.69–108.70
  anatomy of 108.4
  angioedema 108.10
  ankyloglossia 108.87
  black hairy tongue 108.16, *108.17*
  brown tongue 108.16
  candidiasis *108.32*
  circumvallate papillae *108.7*
  coated tongue 108.16
  dorsum, examination of 108.7
  examination of 108.7
  fissured tongue 108.87–108.88
  fungiform papillae *108.7*
  furred tongue *108.52*
  geographic tongue (benign migratory glossitis/erythema migrans) 108.24
    in patient with psoriasis 35.13
  glossitis 108.22, 108.24–108.25
  herpes simplex lingual recurrence *108.71*
  herpetic stomatitis *108.52*
  Kawasaki disease *115.10*
  leiomyoma 108.13
  leukoplakia 75.3
  linear IgA disease *50.37*
  lingual erythema migrans *108.24*
  lingual thyroid 108.11
  lingual tonsil 108.11
  macroglossia 108.11–108.12, *108.69*
    primary systemic amyloidosis *56.12*
  median rhomboid glossitis *108.22*
  multiple endocrine neoplasia 108.13–108.14, *108.13*, 148.10
  oral lichen planus *108.77*
  osteoma mucosae 108.14
  piercing of (body art) *108.16*
  pigmented lesions 108.15
  polyarteritis nodosa 108.69
  scrotal tongue *108.87*
  squamous cell carcinoma *108.46*
  strawberry tongue 108.25
  strawberry tongue, Kawasaki disease *115.10*
  venous malformation *71.15*
  ventrum, examination of 108.7
tongue cancer patient, facial lymphoedema *103.48*
tonofilament aggregates, pachyonychia congenita 63.52
'tonotubular' PPK 63.50
tophaceous gout 155.9, *155.10*

topical anaesthetics, biopsy 3.2–3.3
topical calcineurin inhibitors (TCI), atopic eczema treatment 41.27
topical dressings, burn management 125.8
topical drug delivery 12.1–12.9
  absorbed dose 12.4
  advice/instructions for patients 18.4
  application quantity and frequency 18.3–18.4
  bioavailability/bioequivalence assessment 12.7–12.8
    in vitro methods 12.7
    in vivo methods 12.7–12.8
  creams 12.3–12.4
  drug concentration 18.1–18.2
  drug structure/properties and skin permeation 12.2–12.3
  efficacy influences 18.2
  efficiency of 12.4
  flux measurement *12.3*, 12.4, 12.5
  formulation design and dosage choice 12.5
  formulation 'metamorphosis' 12.6–12.7
  formulations 12.3–12.4
  hazards 18.4–18.5
  hydrocarbon-based formulations 12.3
  'metamorphosis' of formulation 12.6–12.7
  non-volatile residual phase design 12.6–12.7
  patient-centred optimisation 12.4–12.7
  percutaneous absorption mechanisms 12.1–12.2
  polar gel formulations 12.3
  saturated solutions
    with partitioning and diffusion enhancers 12.6
    with partitioning enhancers 12.5–12.6
    simple solutions 12.5
  skin barrier function 12.1
topical photosensitisation, photodynamic therapy 22.2
topical therapies
  acne 129.12
  actinic keratosis 141.8–141.10
  acute herpetic neuralgia 82.4
  advice/instructions for patients 18.4
  antibiotics 18.10–18.12
  antifungal agents 18.12–18.13, 32.33–32.34, 40.8
  anti-inflammatory agents 40.8–40.9
  antineoplastic agents 18.29–18.31
  antiparasitic agents 18.13–18.14
  antiseptics 18.9–18.10, 123.11
  antiviral agents 18.13, 25.23–25.24
  application frequency 18.3
  application quantity 18.3–18.4
  astringents 18.9
  atopic eczema 41.27
  basal cell carcinoma 140.11, 140.12
  Bowen disease 141.23, 141.24
  calcineurin inhibitors 18.22–18.26, 41.27
  corticosteroids/glucocorticoids 18.14–18.22, 46.10, 129.12
  cutaneous T-cell lymphoma 139.21–139.22
  cutaneous warts 25.59–25.60
  cytotoxic agents 18.29–18.31
  depigmenting agents 18.31–18.33
  drug concentration 18.1–18.2
  efficacy influences 18.2
  emollients 18.8–18.9
  erythema multiforme-like reactions to 47.4–47.5
  formulations 18.5–18.8
  hazards 18.4–18.5
  herpes simplex infections 25.23–25.24
  hidradenitis suppurativa 90.9
  hyperhidrosis 92.8–92.9
  immunotherapy 25.59–25.60
  impetigo 26.16
  keratolytics 40.8
  lidocaine 82.4
  mastocytosis 46.10
  minoxidil 87.70, 87.73, 87.94

occlusion 18.21
phototherapy combination 21.10
potency classification of corticosteroids 18.14–18.15, **18.16**
prescribing 18.1–18.4
pressure ulcers 123.11
primary localised cutaneous amyloidosis 56.13–56.14
principles 18.1–18.42
prostaglandins 87.94–87.95
retinoids 18.23–18.26
seborrhoeic dermatitis 40.8
systemic absorption and effects 18.3, 18.5
traditional remedies 18.38
vehicles 12.3–12.4, 18.2–18.3, 18.5–18.8
vitamin D analogues 18.26–18.29
TORCH syndrome, viral infections 25.221
tori mandibularis 108.7, *108.8*
torso involvement, dermatomyositis 52.4–52.5, *52.6*
torus palatinus 108.7, *108.8*
total body irradiation (TBI), lipodystrophy association 98.8–98.9
total body surface area (TBSA), burn size 125.1–125.2
totally dystrophic onychomycosis 32.48
total skin electron beam therapy (TSEBT)
  cutaneous T-cell lymphoma 139.20–139.21, 139.22
  mycosis fungoides 24.16, *24.17*
touch domes 2.12
touch perception 2.12
Touton cells, juvenile xanthogranuloma 135.15
Touton giant cell 3.36
Townes–Brocks syndrome **106.7**
toxic epidermal necrolysis (TEN) 47.1–47.2
  arsenic 121.2
  management 107.33–107.34
  ocular complications 107.32–107.33
  renal effects 154.6
  and Stevens–Johnson syndrome 47.1–47.2, 107.32–107.34, 108.79, 118.1–118.2, 118.10, 118.12–118.22
  T-cell-mediated drug hypersensitivity 14.3, 14.7
toxic erythema of chemotherapy (TEC) 119.1–119.2
toxic erythema of the newborn 114.5–114.6
Toxicodendron species dermatitis 127.5, 127.11, 127.71–127.72, 127.73–127.74
toxic pustuloderma 118.1
toxic reactions, local anaesthetics 20.7–20.8
toxic shock syndrome (TSS) 26.30–26.32
  clinical features 26.30–26.31
  epidemiology 26.30
  management 26.32
  pathophysiology 26.30
  streptococcal 26.30, 26.36–26.37
  see also streptococcal toxic shock-like syndrome
toxins
  bacterial 26.32, 26.35–26.37, 26.38
  botulinum 26.43, 159.1–159.9
  cutaneous T-cell lymphoma therapy 139.25
  metals 121.1–121.10
  see also cytotoxic agents
Toxocara canis see visceral larva migrans
Toxocara cati see visceral larva migrans
Toxocara malayensis see visceral larva migrans
toxocariasis (visceral larva migrans) 33.20–33.21
toxoplasmosis 33.54–33.55
  clinical features 33.54
  management 33.54–33.55
  pathophysiology 33.54
TPMT see thiopurine methyl transferase
T-QoL see Teenagers' Quality of Life Index
trace elements
  hypermetabolism treatment 125.12
  resuscitation use 125.4
traction alopecia 87.31–87.32, 87.42
traditional remedies see complementary/alternative/traditional therapies; herbals

training programmes/resources
  for dermatologists 7.8
  for dermatology 7.11–7.12
  health care workers 7.8
  teledermatology 7.9
  see also educational partnerships; patient education
tralokinumab, systemic therapy 19.36–19.37
tranexamic acid
  cosmeceutical use of 157.4
  urticaria treatment 42.19
transaldolase deficiency **70.16**
transaminitis, haemophagocytic lymphohistiocytosis 135.12
transcription/DNA repair factor IIH (TFIIH) 63.37
transcriptomics
  immune system 9.2–9.3
  skin ageing 2.46
transepidermal elimination (TEE) 94.53–94.55
transepidermal water loss (TEWL) 12.1, 128.2–128.3, 128.6
  atopic eczema 41.23
  irritant contact dermatitis 129.5
  neonates 114.2
  skin barrier function assessment 16.5
  xerosis cutis 85.26
transepithelial elimination (TEE), pseudoxanthoma elasticum 94.30
transforming growth factor (TGF) 71.2
transfusion-associated graft-versus-host disease 149.15
transfusion reactions, skin involvement 149.15
transgender patients, hair loss 87.71
transglutaminase-1, congenital ichthyosiform erythroderma 63.11
transglutaminase 1 deficient skin 63.15
transglutaminase 5 (*TGM5*), skin fragility disorders 69.5
transient acantholytic dermatosis (TAD/Grover disease) 85.23–85.25, 148.17
transient aquagenic keratoderma (TAK) 63.61–63.62
transient erythema *see* flushing
transient myeloproliferative disorder (TMD), neonatal pustulosis of 114.8
transient pustular melanosis, neonates 114.7–114.8
transmission electron microscopy
  dermal–epidermal basement membrane zone 2.22
  elastic fibres 2.34
  epidermolysis bullosa diagnosis 69.21–69.22
  fibroblasts 2.40, 156.9
transplants *see* graft versus host disease; organ transplant recipients
transport media, biopsy 3.4–3.5, **3.5**
transposition flaps, surgical reconstruction **20.24**, 20.26
TRAPS *see* tumour necrosis factor receptor-associated periodic syndrome
trauma
  dystrophic calcification of skin and subcutaneous tissues 59.3
  male genitalia 109.8–109.9
  morphoea association 55.13–55.14
  scratching/manipulating skin, trigeminal trophic syndrome 82.7–82.8
trauma-induced lymphoedema 103.40
traumatic lesions, female genitalia 110.42–110.43
traumatic neuroma 136.43
traumatic panniculitis 97.50, 97.54–97.56
traumatic ulcerative granuloma with stromal eosinophilia (TUGSE), oral ulceration 108.37
travel abroad, cutaneous leishmaniasis 33.51
Treacher Collins syndrome 106.5, **106.7**

treadmill test, peripheral vascular disease **101.4**
tree balsams 127.42
tree moss allergy 127.45, 127.73
tregeminal neuralgia *see* trigeminal neuralgia
Tregs (regulatory T cells) 127.9
trematodes 33.26–33.31
trench fever, *Bartonella quintana* 26.62
trench foot 124.4–124.5
trench mouth *see* acute necrotising (ulcerative) gingivitis and noma
Treponema pallidum
  subsp. *carateum*, pinta 26.71–26.72
  subsp. *endemicum*, endemic syphilis 26.70
  subsp. *pertenue*, yaws 26.70–26.71
Treponema pallidum subsp. *pallidum* 29.2, 29.3–29.5
treponematoses
  differential diagnosis 29.4, 29.12, 29.19
  endemic/non-venereal 26.69–26.72
  eye 107.39–107.40
  microbiology 29.5
  see also syphilis; yaws
tretinoin, *see also* retinoic acid
triangular lunula, nail dysplasia with 67.15, 67.16
triangular shape melanonychia, melanoma involving nail unit 145.13
Triatominae (assassin bugs) 34.29
triazole antifungals 19.48
trichiasis 119.6
trichilemmal carcinoma 137.7
trichilemmal cysts (pilar cysts) 105.11, 133.4–133.5, *133.6*, 137.5–137.6
trichilemmal tumour proliferating 137.5–137.6
trichilemmoma 137.6–137.7
trichinelliasis *see* trichinosis
trichinellosis *see* trichinosis
trichiniasis *see* trichinosis
trichinosis 33.24–33.26
  clinical features 33.25
  management 33.25–33.26
  pathophysiology 33.24–33.25
trichloroacetic acid
  caustic agent for skin surgery 20.47
  chemical peels 160.2–160.3, 160.10
trichloroacetic acid chemical reconstruction of skin scars (TCA CROSS) 160.6
trichoadenoma 137.4–137.5
trichobacteriosis *see* trichomycosis
trichobezoar 84.24
trichoblastic fibroma *see* trichoblastoma
trichoblastoma 137.11–137.12
trichoblastoma spectrum, trichoepithelioma 137.9–137.10
trichochrome B *86.7*
trichochromes 86.5, *86.6*
trichodiscomas 137.15
  histology of *78.15*
trichodynia 87.54
  COVID-19 association 25.113
trichodysplasia spinulosa polyomavirus (TSPyV/TSV/HPyV-8) 25.48, 85.15–85.17, 87.36
trichoepithelioma 105.11, 137.9–137.10
  photothermal ablation 23.21
trichofolliculoma 137.8–137.9
trichogenic fibroma *see* trichoblastoma
trichograms 87.14, 87.55
trichokinesis 105.14
tricholemmal cysts *see* trichilemmal cysts
tricholemmoma *see* trichilemmoma
trichomatricoma *see* pilomatricoma
trichomegaly 107.4
trichomoniasis 33.38–33.39
  clinical features 33.38
  epidemiology 33.38
  management 33.38–33.39
trichomycosis axillaris 26.41–26.42
trichomycosis nodularis (black piedra) 32.15–32.16
trichomycosis pubis 109.27
trichophytide, dermatophytide reaction 32.50

trichophytin test 4.25
Trichophyton spp.
  dermatophytosis 32.18–32.20, **32.19**, 32.26–32.30
  hand eczema 39.17
  T. rubrum 32.27–32.28, 32.29, *32.29*
trichoptilosis 87.75
trichorrexis invaginata 63.27
trichorrhexis invaginata 87.79, *87.80*
trichorrhexis nodosa (TN) 87.75–87.77, 87.93–87.94
  argininosuccinic aciduria 79.13
trichoscopy 4.21, 87.65–87.66, 87.74
Trichosporon yeasts 32.66–32.67, 32.93
trichosporosis nodosa *see* white piedra
trichostasis spinulosa 87.83–87.84
trichothiodystrophy (TTD) 63.36–63.38, 76.5, 76.9–76.10, **77.2**, 87.80
trichotillomania (TTM)/trichotillosis 84.24–84.25, 87.14, 87.24, 87.32–87.34
trichrome stains 3.8
trichrome vitiligo 86.36, *86.38*
triclosan 127.58
triclosan/triclocarban, topical therapies 18.10
tricone ('dog ear') repair 20.22
tricyclic antidepressants 84.44, **84.45**
trifarotene, topical therapies 18.26
trigeminal cranial nerve (CN V), anatomy of head and neck 20.2, *20.3*
trigeminal nerve, ophthalmic zoster 25.33
trigeminal neuralgia (TN)/trigeminal neuropathic pain syndrome 82.5–82.7, 108.66–108.67
trigeminal trophic syndrome (TTS) 82.7–82.8, 108.67
triglycerides 97.4
trimethylaminuria (fish odour syndrome) 84.11, 92.17–92.18
tripe palms *see* acanthosis palmaris
triple response of Lewis, testing for skin innervation 83.5
trisomy 8 myelodysplasia, Behçet-like disease association 149.8
trisomy 13 (Patau syndrome) 74.2–74.3
trisomy 18 (Edwards syndrome) 74.2
trisomy 21 *see* Down syndrome
Triton tumour *see* neuromuscular hamartoma
TrkB deficiency **72.6**
trophic syndromes, skin picking disorders 82.8–82.9
tropical bubo *see* lymphogranuloma venereum
Tropical Dermatology: A Syndrome-Based Approach (online course) 7.12
tropical disorders
  actinic lichen planus 37.7
  lymphatic filariasis 103.33–103.36
  neglected tropical diseases 7.2, 7.6, 7.7, 7.11–7.12
tropical elephantiasis *see* lymphatic filariasis
Tropical Health and Education Trust (THET) 7.14
tropical ulcers 26.68–26.69
tropoelastin 2.33
Trousseau sign 97.9
TRT *see* thermal relaxation time
true histiocytic lymphoma 135.30–135.31
Trueperella pyogenes, infection 26.43
trunk
  atrophoderma of Pasini–Pierini 55.19
  bowel-associated dermatitis–arthritis syndrome 49.16
  bullous pemphigoid 50.18
  keratolytic winter erythema lesions 63.73, 63.74
  linear IgA disease 50.36
  linear morphoea trunk/limb variant 55.25
  lithium-induced acne 88.13
  microscopic examination of skin 3.33–3.34
  morphoea 55.5, 55.20
  pansclerotic morphoea 55.21
  pityriasis rubra pilaris, type I 36.4, 36.6

  plaque morphoea 55.20
  psoriasis vulgaris 35.7, *35.13*
  pustules, bowel-associated dermatitis–arthritis syndrome 49.16
  toxic erythema of the newborn 114.5
trypanosomiasis 33.39–33.43
  clinical features 33.40–33.42
  epidemiology 33.39
  investigations 33.42–33.43
  management 33.43
  pathophysiology 33.39–33.40, *33.41*
  see also African trypanosomiasis; American trypanosomiasis
trypsin, pancreatic panniculitis 97.41
TSC *see* tuberous sclerosis complex
TSEBT *see* total skin electron beam therapy
tsetse flies, trypanosomiasis 33.39–33.40, *33.41, 33.42*
TSPyV *see* trichodysplasia spinulosa polyomavirus
TST *see* tuberculosis skin test
TSV *see* trichodysplasia spinulosa polyomavirus
TTA *see* temporal triangular alopecia
TTD *see* trichothiodystrophy
t-test, statistical analysis of clinical studies 17.21
TTM *see* trichotillomania
TTO *see* Time Trade-Off
TTS *see* trigeminal trophic syndrome
tubercles of Montgomery, Fordyce spots 93.12
tuberculids 27.24–27.32
  erythema induratum of Bazin 27.29–27.31
  lichen scrofulosorum 27.25–27.27
  other nodular lesions 27.31–27.32
  papulonecrotic tuberculid 27.27–27.29
tuberculin test 4.24
tuberculoid/borderline tuberculoid leprosy 28.1, 28.2–28.3, 28.4, 28.6, 28.7, **28.7**, 28.8, 28.9, 28.10
tuberculoid granulomas 96.3
tuberculoid leprosy 94.30
tuberculosis 27.2–27.5
  acute cutaneous miliary 27.17
  BCG vaccination 5.3, 27.3–27.5, 27.10–27.11, 27.20, 27.21, 27.25, 27.27–27.29, 27.40, 80.8
  congenital tuberculosis 114.28
  cutaneous manifestations 152.4
  diagnostic tests 27.4–27.5, 27.8–27.9
  ear dermatoses **106.23**
  epidemiology 27.2–27.4
  erythema induratum of Bazin 97.26, 97.29
  erythema nodosum 97.25
  eye infection 107.39
  oral lesions 108.56
  penis 109.27
  perianal skin 111.15
  sarcoidosis causation 96.4
  see also mycobacterial infections; *Mycobacterium tuberculosis*; tuberculosis of the skin
tuberculosis colliquativa cutis (scrofuloderma) 27.13–27.16
tuberculosis cutis indurativa *see* erythema induratum of Bazin
tuberculosis cutis lichenoides *see* lichen scrofulosorum
tuberculosis cutis miliaris acuta generalisata *see* acute cutaneous miliary tuberculosis
tuberculosis cutis miliaris disseminate *see* acute cutaneous miliary tuberculosis
tuberculosis papulonecrotica (papulonecrotic tuberculid) 27.27–27.29
tuberculosis of the skin (cutaneous tuberculosis) 27.5–27.24
  acute cutaneous miliary tuberculosis 27.17
  classification 27.5–27.6

diagnosis 27.7–27.9
HIV 31.22
lupus vulgaris 27.20–27.24
metastatic tuberculous abscess 27.17–27.19
orificial tuberculosis 27.16–27.17
pathophysiology 27.6–27.7
primary inoculation 27.12–27.13
scrofuloderma 27.13–27.16
treatment 27.9–27.10
warty tuberculosis 27.19–27.20
tuberculosis skin test (TST) 27.4
tuberculosis verrucosa cutis (warty tuberculosis) 27.19–27.20
tuberculous mastitis 27.31–27.32
tuberous sclerosis complex (TSC) 78.7–78.10, 148.10
  cardiac rhabdomyomas 78.9
  clinical features 78.7–78.9
  diagnostic criteria **78.10**
  endocrine disorders 78.9
  investigations 78.10
  management 78.10
  mosaic forms of 78.8
  neurological features 78.8–78.9
  ocular signs 78.9
  oral involvement 108.87
  pulmonary involvement 78.9, 152.5
  renal involvement 154.2
tuberous xanthomas 60.3
tubular adenoma 137.28
tubular apocrine adenoma 137.28
tufted angioma (TA), infants 116.10, *116.11*
tufted folliculitis 87.49, 87.84
TUGSE *see* traumatic ulcerative granuloma with stromal eosinophilia
tularaemia, *Francisella tularensis* 26.57–26.58
tumefactive primary localised cutaneous amyloidosis 56.5
  tumour resemblance 56.8
tumour classification, melanoma 142.8
tumour necrosis factor, allergic contact dermatitis 127.10
tumour necrosis factor antagonists (systemic therapy) 19.32–19.34
  cautions 19.33–19.34
  contraindications 19.33
  dermatological uses 19.32
  drug–drug interactions 19.34
  pharmacological properties 19.32–19.33
  potential adverse effects 19.33
  pre-treatment screening 19.34
tumour necrosis factor inhibitor-associated alopecia 87.34–87.35
tumour necrosis factor receptor-associated periodic syndrome (TRAPS) **45.5, 45.6**, 45.9
tumour necrosis receptor associated periodic syndrome, renal involvement 154.2
tumours
  acanthosis nigricans association 85.3, 85.4–85.5
  acquired ichthyosis association 85.2
  dystrophic calcification of skin and subcutaneous tissues 59.3–59.4
  spread to skin 148.2–148.7
tumours of ano-genital mammary-like glands 137.40
tumours of fat cells 136.56–136.59
tumour spillage (direct contamination of wounds with tumour cells during a laparoscopy or surgical procedure) 148.3–148.4
tumours of the scalp 105.11–105.12
  pilosebaceous unit tumours 105.11
  scalp metastases 105.11–105.12
  sebaceous naevus 105.11
  syringocystadenoma papilliferum 105.11
tumours of skin appendages 137.1–137.49
  apocrine gland tumours 137.18–137.23
  classification 137.2
  eccrine or apocrine gland/follicular tumours 137.28–137.33
  eccrine gland hamartomas and tumours 137.23–137.28

external root sheath tumours 137.5–137.7
from eccrine and apocrine glands 137.1–137.2
hair follicle mesenchyme lesions 137.15–137.16
hair follicle tumours 137.2–137.5
hair matrix tumours 137.13–137.15
hamartomas and hair germ tumours and cysts 137.7–137.13
miscellaneous 137.40–137.44
sebaceous gland tumours 137.16–137.18
sweat gland carcinomas 137.33–137.40
tumours of uncertain malignancy, keratoacanthoma 141.38
Tunga penetrans (sand flea/jigger/chigoe) 34.15
tungiasis 34.15
tunnel disease *see* ancylostomiasis
turban tumour *see* cylindroma
'turf toe' 122.16
turmeric (curcuminoids), cosmeceutical use of **157.8**, *157.9*
Turner, Daniel *1.3*, *1.4*
Turner syndrome 74.3–74.4, 86.41, 103.20, **106.7**
  infant with *71.28*
turpentine allergy 127.74–127.78
T-vec *see* Talimogene laherparepvec
'two-hit' hypothesis of genetic disorders, disseminated superficial actinic porokeratosis 141.16
tylosis, oral lesions 108.30
tylosis with oesophageal cancer 63.66, *63.67*, **78.13**
tympanic membrane *106.2*
type 1 interferonopathies 45.13–45.15
  Aicardi–Goutières syndrome (AGS) 45.5, **45.6**, 45.13
  chronic atypical neutrophilic dermatosis with lipodystrophy and elevated temperature 45.5, **45.6**, 45.14–45.15
  STING-associated vasculopathy with onset in infancy 45.5, **45.6**, 45.13–45.14
type I cryoglobulinaemia (intravascular) and perniosis 149.13–149.14
type III hypersensitivity reactions, urticarial vasculitis 44.2
type VII collagen (*COL17A1*) 69.5, 69.16, 69.18–69.19, 69.21, *69.22*, 69.27
type XVII collagen (*COL17A1*) 69.5
typhus group Rickettsiae 26.80–26.81
typical (classical) epidermodysplasia verruciformis 25.66, 25.69
tyrosinaemia type II 63.70–63.71, 79.11–79.12
tyrosine 68.1
tyrosine kinase inhibitors (TKIs)
  hair pigmentation 87.73–87.74
  hypertrichoses 119.6
  mastocytosis treatment 46.10
  psoriasis treatment 35.27
Tzanck smears 3.29–3.30

U

UAS *see* urticarial activity scores
ubiquinone *see* coenzyme Q10
UCT *see* urticaria control test
UCTD *see* undifferentiated connective tissue disease
'ugly duckling' sign *see* intra-individual comparative analysis of naevi
UK *see* United Kingdom
ulceration 102.1–102.13
  anal fissure 111.30–111.31
  arterial leg ulcers 102.7–102.10
  Behçet-like syndrome associated with trisomy 8 myelodysplasia 149.8
  calciphylaxis 59.7
  chemical burns 128.12
  dermatomyositis 52.5, 52.6, *52.8*, 52.9, 52.11
  diabetic patients 62.1, 62.2–62.3
  diphtheria 26.38–26.39
  female genitalia 110.18–110.20

herpes simplex virus infection, neonatal *114.22*
human immunodeficiency virus infection **111.17**
hypertensive ischaemic ulcers 102.10–102.13
infantile haemangiomas 116.5, *116.6*
intravenous drug administration 120.6–120.7
ischaemic ulcer *101.44*
male genitalia 109.5, 109.22–109.24, 109.28
melanoma 142.7, 142.10, 142.11, 142.20, 142.21, 142.22, **142.23**, 145.14
mixed leg ulcers 102.4–102.7
Mycobacterium ulcerans infection 27.36–27.40
neuropathic ulcer 83.13–83.19
perineal and perianal skin 111.12–111.13, 111.30–111.31
peripheral vascular disease *101.3*
peristomal skin 112.10, 112.12–112.15
prolidase deficiency *79.13*
rheumatoid arthritis-associated 53.7, 155.6
striae *94.8*
tropical ulcers 26.68–26.69
venous leg ulcers 102.1–102.4
wound healing 11.2, 11.12
see also granuloma inguinale; leg ulcers; oral ulcers
ulcerative basal cell carcinoma 140.8–140.9
ulcerative colitis (UC)
  Crohn disease distinction 153.1–153.2
  oral involvement 108.74
  psoriasis in 35.18
  skin involvement 153.2, 153.3
ulcerative sarcoidosis 96.13
ulcus molle *see* chancroid
ulerythema ophryogenes 89.8
ulnar-mammary syndrome **72.7**
ultrasound 4.22
  foreign body reactions 122.18
  peripheral vascular disease *101.4*, **101.4**
  psoriatic plaque thickness measurements 16.5
  skin tightening 161.6–161.8
  superficial temporal artery, giant cell arteritis *100.33*
ultraviolet filters, allergies 127.62, 127.79, 127.80, 127.82
ultraviolet index (UVI) 10.13
ultraviolet light, Wood's light examination for superficial mycosis 32.6–32.7
ultraviolet radiation (UVR) 10.1–10.14
  absorption spectrum *10.4*
  and acne 88.25–88.26
  action spectroscopy 10.4–10.5
  acute and carcinogenic effects of UVR exposure **10.7**
  ageing of skin 10.10–10.11, 156.7–156.8, *156.10*
  allergic contact dermatitis 127.11
  artificial sources 10.2–10.3, 21.1, 21.2–21.3, 142.6
  calibration/dosimetry 21.3, *21.4*
  chronic effects of 10.9–10.11
  clinical effects of 10.7–10.11
  cutaneous squamous cell carcinoma 141.27, 141.30
  damaging effects 86.8
  emission spectra *10.3*
  erythema response 126.1
  Fitzpatrick classification of acute and carcinogenic effects **10.7**
  Flegel disease 85.17
  genetic changes 147.5
  history of phototherapy 21.2
  interactions with skin 10.3–10.4
  measurement 10.2
  melanocyte number 2.18
  melanocytes response to 86.5–86.7
  melanoma risk 142.5–142.6
  Merkel cell carcinoma risk 146.2–146.3
  molecular and cellular effects 10.5–10.6

non-solar sources 10.13
normal effects on skin 10.5–10.11
occupational skin cancer 129.14
oral squamous cell carcinoma 108.46
path lengths for differing solar elevations *10.3*
personal and population exposure to 10.12–10.14
photon absorption *10.4*
photoprotection 10.11–10.12
phototherapy 1.8
  use during pregnancy 113.21–113.24
physicochemical aspects 10.3–10.4
pigmentation regulation 86.5–86.7
PLE manifestation 126.3
porokeratosis 85.22–85.23
principles 21.2–21.3
production and sources 10.1–10.2
reduced tumour immune surveillance, skin cancer risks 147.5–147.6
risks versus benefits of population UVR exposure 10.13–10.14
rosacea risk 89.11
skin ageing 2.46
skin cancer risks
  immunocompromised people 147.5–147.6
  occupational 129.14
  solar urticaria 126.21–126.24
  subcategories 10.2
suppressing immune responses and permitting progression of immunogenic tumours 146.3
systemic lupus erythematosus 51.21
tanning response 86.9
terrestrial UVR 10.2
transient acantholytic dermatosis 85.23
UVA-1 phototherapy 126.7–126.8
UVA/UVB wavelength ranges 21.1
UV index 10.13
xeroderma pigmentosum 76.3–76.5
see also photoageing; photochemotherapy; phototherapy; sunlight
ultraviolet recall reaction 119.11
ultraviolet-sensitive syndrome (UVSS) 76.8
umbilicus
  angiokeratoma corporis diffusum *79.7*
  bacterial infections 26.5
  bullous pemphigoid *50.19*
  flexural psoriasis *35.9*
  neonatal care 114.2–114.3
UN *see* United Nations
uncinarial dermatitis *see* ancylostomiasis
uncombable hair syndrome 87.46, 87.82, *87.83*
undecenoic acid, topical therapies 18.13
undernutrition *see* malnutrition
undifferentiated connective tissue disease (UCTD) 53.1–53.3
undifferentiated soft tissue sarcoma (USTS) 136.17–136.18
undulant fever *see* brucellosis
Unicararia stenocephala see cutaneous larva migrans
unifocal bone disease, Langerhans cell histiocytosis 135.8
unilateral acanthosis nigricans 85.5
unilateral lentiginosis 86.16
unilateral naevoid telangiectasia syndrome 101.20–101.22
  clinical features **101.21**
  grouped lesions *101.21*
United Kingdom (UK)
  basal cell carcinoma incidence 6.1
  Biobank 3.1
  Ethiopia Residents Programme 7.8
  global health activities 7.14
  skin cancer, economic burden of 6.1
United Nations (UN) 7.4–7.5
United States
  dermatology history 1.7
  economic burden of disease 6.5
  psoriasis, economic burden of **6.8**, 6.9
  skin cancer, economic burden of 6.5, **6.7**
unsatisfactory outcomes of skin surgery **20.41**, 20.42

unstable psoriasis 35.13, *35.14*, 35.35
upadacitinib, atopic eczema treatment 41.30, **41.31**
upper dermal elastolysis 94.26
upper dermal perivascular lymphohistiocytic infiltrate, chronic actinic dermatitis 126.14, *126.15*
uraemia, cutaneous signs 154.3
uraemic pruritus 81.8–81.9
urban versus rural environments, atopic eczema 41.6–41.7, 41.8
urethral caruncle, vulva **110.32**
urethral involvement, Stevens–Johnson syndrome/toxic epidermal necrolysis *118.17*, 118.18
urinary tract
 effects of skin diseases 154.6
 see also renal disorders
urinary tract abnormalities, epidermolysis bullosa 69.26
uro-genital tract examination, SJS/TEN 118.20
urostomy **112.3**
 chronic papillomatous dermatitis *112.8*
 ileal metaplasia *112.7*
 irritant skin reaction *112.2*
 lichen sclerosus *112.11*
urticaria 42.1–42.20
 acute spontaneous urticaria 42.5, 42.15–42.16
 aetiology 42.4–42.5, **42.13**
 aggravating factors **42.7**
 allergic 42.5, 127.82–127.86
 anaphylaxis 42.1
 ancient Chinese medical text 1.2
 anetoderma 94.25
 angioedema swellings 42.1, *42.3*
 antihistamine treatment 42.17–42.18, 42.19
 aquagenic urticaria **42.9**, 42.12, *42.13*
 assessment tools 16.5
 associated diseases 42.3
 atopic eczema association 41.22
 autoallergic reactions 42.5–42.6
 autoimmune urticaria 42.6
 autoinflammatory diseases **80.19**
 biopsy 3.45
 burden on patient and society 42.14
 causes 42.4–42.5, **42.13**
 cholinergic urticaria **42.9**, 42.11–42.12
 chronic condition associated with genital herpes 25.26
 chronic spontaneous urticaria 42.5, *42.6*, *42.7*, 42.16, *42.17*
 classification 42.1, **42.8**
 clinical features 42.7–42.14
 cold contact urticaria **42.9**, 42.10–42.11
 complications and co-morbidities 42.14
 contact urticaria 42.13–42.14
 COVID-19 association 25.109, *25.111*
 delayed pressure urticaria **42.9**, 42.10
 dermal oedema *42.6*
 dermographism 42.9–42.10
 and diet **42.6**, 42.8
 dietary pseudoallergens 42.8
 differential diagnosis **42.1**, 42.14
 disease course and prognosis 42.14–42.15
 drug-induced 42.5, 42.8, 117.5–117.7
 environmental factors 42.7
 epidemiology 42.2–42.3
 exercise-induced urticaria 42.12
 genetics 42.7
 heat contact urticaria **42.9**, 42.10
 histology *42.6*
 idiopathic urticaria 42.5
 immunological and non-immunological stimuli 42.3–42.4
 immunomodulatory and immunosuppressive treatments 42.19
 inducible urticarias 42.8–42.14
  challenge procedures 42.9
  classification **42.8**
 infants 115.5
 and infection 42.3, 42.5, 42.6, 42.8
 infestation-related urticaria 42.6
 investigations 42.15–42.16
 malignancy association 42.3, 148.23
 management 42.16–42.19
  adverse effects of antihistamines 42.17–42.18
  first line treatment 42.16–42.17
  second line treatment 42.18
  third line treatment (targeted therapies) 42.19
 mast cell role 42.3–42.4
 mechanical forces, reactions to 42.9–42.10
 and menstrual cycle 42.8
 natural history of urticaria in hospital patients study 42.15
 non-allergic urticaria 42.5, 42.13–42.14
 non-pharmacological treatments 42.19
 oral allergy syndrome 42.13
 pathology 42.6–42.7
 pathophysiology 42.3–42.4
 pharmacological treatments 42.19
 predisposing factors 42.4
 pregnancy 42.8, 42.18, 113.12
 pseudoallergic reactions 42.5, 42.6, 42.8
 psychological factors 15.4, 42.8
 quality of life assessment 16.9
 reactions to COVID-19 (mRNA) vaccines 25.117
 rescue medication 42.18
 severity classification 42.14
 solar urticaria **42.9**, 42.12
 stress 42.8
 symptomatic dermographism 42.9–42.10
 in systemic lupus erythematosus 51.27–51.28
 temperature-dependent urticaria **42.9**, 42.10–42.11
 terminology 42.1
 UVR exposure 126.21–126.24
 vibratory urticaria **42.9**, 42.10, 45.19
 vulva 110.16
 weals/wealing 42.1, *42.2*, *42.6*, 42.7, *42.11*, *42.13*, 94.25
urticaria control test (UCT) 16.5
urticarial activity scores (UAS/UAS7/UAS$_{ID}$) 16.5
urticaria-like follicular mucinosis 57.16–57.17
urticarial like rash, complex and polygenic autoinflammatory diseases presenting with urticarial or maculopapular rash 45.20–45.22
urticarial vasculitis 44.1–44.6
 clinical features 44.3–44.4
 clinical variants 44.3–44.4
 drugs implicated in development 44.3
 epidemiology 44.1–44.2
 genetics 44.3
 histopathology 44.1, *44.5*
 infections implicated in development 44.3
 investigations 44.4–44.5
 leucocytoclastic vasculitis 44.1, 44.3
 management 44.5–44.6
 pathology 44.2–44.3
urticaria pigmentosa
 biopsy 3.2
 in children *46.4*, 46.5
 Darier's sign 46.5
 maculopapular cutaneous mastocytosis *46.1*
 mast cell infiltrates *46.3*
 mastocytomas *46.3*
 mastocytosis 46.3–46.5
 treatment 46.10
 wealing *46.5*
Uruma fever *see* Mayaro virus
ustekinumab, systemic therapy 19.34–19.35
USTS *see* undifferentiated soft tissue sarcoma
uterine leiomyoma 154.2
 see also hereditary leiomyomatosis and renal cell cancer
utility measures, quality of life assessment 16.9

UV *see* ultraviolet radiation
UVA-1 phototherapy
 administration 21.10–21.11
 adverse effects 21.15
 atopic eczema 21.4, 21.6
 conditions treated 21.6–21.7
 history 21.2
 lupus erythematosus 21.6
 mycosis fungoides 21.7
 principles 21.1, 21.2
 sclerosing skin conditions 21.6
UVA exposure
 allergic contact dermatitis 127.11
 photopatch tests 127.81
UVB exposure, allergic contact dermatitis 127.11
UVB phototherapy
 administration 21.7–21.9
 adverse effects 21.11–21.13
 polymorphic light eruption 126.7–126.8, *126.36*
 principles 21.1
 PUVA comparison 21.5–21.6
 vitiligo 86.39
uveal melanoma
 genetic factors 142.4
 system treatment 144.7–144.8
uveitis, Adamantiades–Behçet disease patients 48.4, *48.6*
UVI *see* ultraviolet index
UV light *see* ultraviolet radiation
UVR *see* ultraviolet radiation
UVSS *see* ultraviolet-sensitive syndrome

V

vaccination
 and atopic eczema 41.8–41.9
 complications 25.8–25.9
 COVID-19 25.117–25.119
 development of vaccinia virus 25.7
 and morphoea 55.13
 mpox 25.12
 recombinant hepatitis B associated skin conditions 25.75
 smallpox 25.6, 25.7
vaccinia virus (VAVC) 25.7–25.8
 cowpox virus relationship 25.7, 25.12
Vagabonds' disease 86.23–86.24
vagina, recto-vaginal fistula *111.7*
vaginal adenosis 110.44
vaginal candidiasis *see* vulvo-vaginal candidiasis
vaginal discharge, diagnosis of 110.24–110.25
vaginal infections
 amoebiasis 33.37
 enterobiasis 33.15
 streptococcal 26.33, 110.25
 trichomoniasis 33.38–33.39
valaciclovir, pharmacological properties 19.49
validation, measurement methods 16.2–16.3
validity of research
 evidence based medicine 17.8–17.10, 17.12–17.16, 17.17
 strengthening validity of trials 17.14–17.15
valley fever *see* coccidioidomycosis
vancomycin, hypersensitivity reactions to **14.6**
Van der Woude syndrome 108.87
VAP *see* ventilator-associated pneumonia
variable-vessel vasculitis, involving respiratory system 152.4
varicella infection 25.28–25.32
 clinical features 25.29–25.30
 complications and co-morbidities 25.30–25.31
 epidemiology 25.29
 infants 115.6–115.7
 investigations 25.31
 management 25.31–25.32
 oral involvement 108.51
 pathophysiology 25.29

varicella-zoster virus (VZV) 25.28–25.36, 87.35–87.36
 fetal varicella syndrome 114.23
 HIV 31.23–31.24
 in pregnancy 113.5
 see also varicella; zoster
varicose eczema 39.19–39.22
varicose veins 101.38–101.39, 101.42
 on abdomen, associated with liver disease 153.9
 clinical features **101.40**
 management of **101.40**
 pathogenesis **101.39**
varicosities
 labial veins 110.4
 oral involvement 108.27
variegate porphyria (VP) 58.5, 58.7, 58.9, 58.12, 58.17–58.18
 clinical features 58.17–58.18
 genetic counselling 58.18
 investigations 58.18
variola virus (VARV; smallpox) 25.6–25.7
varioliform atrophy 94.15–94.16
varioliform scars
 hydroa vacciniforme 126.25, *126.26*
 necrotising lymphocytic folliculitis 91.12
 scalp margin 93.4
VARV *see* variola virus
VAS *see* visual analogue scale
vascular calcification, calcific arteriolopathy 97.32–97.33
vascular changes
 during pregnancy **113.2**, 113.3
 liver disease association 153.8–153.9
vascular coagulopathies, purpura 99.19–99.24
vascular disorders 71.1–71.28
 arteriovenous disorders 71.11–71.14
 capillary disorders 71.3–71.11
 classification of 71.1
 genetic mutations 71.1, *71.2*
 internal malignancy association 148.24–148.26
 lymphatic disorders 71.1, 71.21–71.28
 protein mutations in *71.2*
 venous disorders 71.14–71.21
 see also peripheral vascular disease
vascular Ehlers–Danlos syndrome (vEDS) **70.4**, 70.8–70.9, 70.11
vascular endothelial growth factor receptor (VEGFR) *71.2*
vascular endothelial growth factor (VEGF) *71.2*
 loricrin keratoderma 63.56
 wound healing *11.6*
vascularised composite tissue allografts (VCAs), skin cancer risks 147.4
vascular lasers 23.6–23.12
 complications 23.12
 devices 23.7
 indications 23.7
 light–tissue interactions 23.6
 tests and assessments 23.7–23.8
vascular lesions
 atypical vascular proliferation after radiotherapy 136.38–136.39
 laser therapies 23.6–23.12
 mouth 108.25–108.28
 proliferative 108.27
 rheumatoid arthritis 53.6
vascular malformations
 classification **116.1**
 cutaneous 101.26–101.31
 infantile haemangioma comparison **116.1**
vascular syndromes, ocular features **107.42**
vascular tumours 136.23–136.37
 benign types 136.25–136.32
 intermediate malignancy types 136.32–136.34
 malignant types 136.34–136.37
 reactive lesions 136.23–136.25
vasculature 2.40–2.42
vasculitides *see* vasculitis
vasculitis
 autoinflammatory diseases **80.19**

cardiac involvement 151.4
drug-induced 120.5
erythema induratum 97.28–97.29
erythema nodosum 97.24
gastrointestinal and skin manifestations 153.7
internal malignancy association 148.25
lupus panniculitis 97.38
nodular as a tuberculid 27.29, 27.31
nomenclature and classification 154.6
oral involvement 108.69
panniculitis 97.6
paraprotein-associated 149.14
relapsing polychondritis 155.11, 155.12
renal and skin involvement 154.6
respiratory system involvement 152.3–152.4
rheumatoid arthritis 53.8, 155.6, *155.8*
rheumatoid nodules 97.16
in Sjögren syndrome 53.10
in systemic lupus erythematosus 51.26
urticarial 44.1–44.6
see also erythema induratum of Bazin; urticarial vasculitis
vasculitis, cutaneous 100.1–100.37
ANCA-associated vasculitis 100.9, 100.13, 100.20–100.28, 152.3–152.4
antiglomerular basement membrane vasculitis 100.19–100.20
classification **100.2**
clinical features 100.1–100.3
clinical variants 100.3–100.4
cocaine-induced 120.5
cryoglobulinaemic vasculitis 100.15–100.17
cutaneous arteritis 100.28–100.30
cutaneous small-vessel vasculitis 100.5–100.8
due to infection *100.7*
due to sepsis *100.7*
eosinophilic granulomatosis with polyangiitis 100.25–100.28
erythema elevatum diutinum 100.8–100.10
giant cell arteritis 100.32–100.34
granuloma faciale 100.11–100.12
granulomatosis with polyangiitis 100.22–100.25
history 100.1–100.2
hypocomplementaemic urticarial vasculitis 100.18–100.19
IgA vasculitis 100.13–100.15
investigations 100.4
Kawasaki disease 100.30–100.32
large-vessel vasculitis 100.32–100.35
leukocytoclastic *100.6*, 100.8
management 100.5
medium-vessel vasculitis *100.3*, 100.28–100.32
microscopic polyangiitis 100.20–100.22
physical signs **100.3**
polyarteritis nodosa 100.28–100.30
presentation 100.2–100.3
purpura pattern **100.4**
recurrent cutaneous necrotising eosinophilic vasculitis 100.10–100.11
single-organ small-vessel vasculitis 100.5–100.12
small-vessel ANCA-associated vasculitis 100.9, 100.13, 100.20–100.28, 152.3–152.4
small-vessel immune complex-associated vasculitis 100.13–100.20
systemic examination **100.3**
Takayasu arteritis 100.34–100.35
ulcerated necrotic lesions *100.3*
urticarial 100.18–100.19
vasculogenesis 101.1
vasculopathic ulcers, dermatomyositis 52.5, 52.6, *52.8*, 52.9, 52.11
vasculopathy
autoinflammatory diseases **80.19**
calciphylaxis 59.6–59.9
systemic lupus erythematosus 51.26–51.27

systemic sclerosis 54.10, **54.25**
vasoactive intestinal peptide (VIP) 2.9
vasoconstriction, cold-induced 124.1, 124.12
vasoconstriction assay, topical bioavailability/bioequivalence assessment 12.8
vasoconstrictors, Raynaud phenomenon 124.12
vasodilatation, perniosis 124.5
vasodilatory substances, Raynaud phenomenon 124.12
vasomotor symptoms, hand–arm vibration syndrome 122.25
vaso-occlusive disorders, COVID-19 association 25.111
VAT adipocytes *see* visceral adipose tissue adipocytes
VAVC *see* vaccinia virus
VCAs *see* vascularised composite tissue allografts
VDDRIIa *see* vitamin D-dependent rickets type 2a
Vedic writings 1.2
vEDS *see* vascular Ehlers–Danlos syndrome
vegetable oils, topical medication vehicles 18.6
vegetative pyoderma gangrenosum 49.5, *49.6*
VEGF *see* vascular endothelial growth factor
VEGFR *see* vascular endothelial growth factor receptor
vehicles for topical therapies
choice and formulations 18.2–18.3, 18.5–18.8
corticosteroids 18.21
veins
intravenous drug administration 120.7
subcutaneous fat 97.7
superficial thrombophlebitis 97.10
veins in the periorbital and temple area, laser therapies 23.11, *23.14*
vellus hair cyst 137.8
velocardiofacial syndrome (22q11 deletion syndrome) 108.87
Velpeau, Aristide Auguste Stanislas 90.1
vemurafenib (RAF inhibitor)
causing keratoacanthoma 141.38, 141.41
Langerhans cell histiocytoses therapy 135.9
radiation recall *119.13*
Venezuelan haemorrhagic fever 25.82–25.83
venoms
allergic reactions 34.9, 34.16–34.18
antivenoms 130.3
aquatic and marine animal stings 130.1–130.5
arachnids 34.34–34.37
centipedes/millipedes 34.57
cnidarian stings 130.2
fish stings 130.4
hymenoptera 34.2, 34.9, 34.16–34.18
immunotherapy 34.18
lepidoptera/caterpillars 34.33–34.34
management 34.6
pharmacologically active agents 34.2
snake bites 130.5
venouos oedema 103.10–103.12
venous, venous thrombosis 101.31–101.38
venous disorders 71.14–71.21, 101.31–101.46
anatomy 101.31
arteriovenous malformations 101.22–101.24
blue rubber bleb naevus syndrome *71.2*, 71.17–71.18
cerebral cavernous malformation-associated cutaneous lesions *71.2*, 71.19
chronic venous insufficiency 101.40–101.46
cutaneo-mucosal venous malformation 71.16–71.17
cutaneous vascular malformations 101.26–101.31

glomuvenous malformation *71.2*, 71.18–71.19
haemangioma 101.26, *101.27*
Klippel–Trenaunay syndrome 101.27–101.30
Maffucci syndrome 71.20–71.21
mixed leg ulcers 102.4–102.7
Parkes Weber syndrome **101.28**, 101.30–101.31
physiology 101.31
telangiectases 101.10–101.22
ulceration *101.44*, 102.1–102.13
varicose veins 101.38–101.39, **101.40**
varicosities, labial veins 110.4
venous macrocirculation 101.31
see also verrucous...
venous eczema
allergic contact dermatitis 127.45
chronic venous insufficiency **101.43**
lower leg eczema 39.19–39.22
venous hypertension 97.30
venous lakes 101.14–101.16, **101.17**
larger venous lake *101.16*
laser therapies 23.11
lip *4.14*, 108.28
small venous lake *101.15*
venous leg ulcers (VLUs) 102.1–102.4
chronic venous disease *102.5, 102.6*
clinical features 102.3
compression therapy *102.5*
disorders associated with **102.2**
epidemiology 102.2
ethnicity 102.2
histology *102.3*, 102.4
investigations for 102.3–102.4
management of 102.4, *102.6*
pathophysiology 102.2–102.3
post-thrombotic syndrome *102.6*
wound histology 102.4
venous macrocirculation 101.31
venous malformations (VMs) 71.14–71.16, 101.24–101.25
clinical features **101.25**
investigations for **101.25**
management of 101.25
treatment options **101.26**
verrucous 71.19–71.20
venous mucocutaneous malformation (VMCM) 71.16–71.17, 108.28
venous obstruction, neoplasia association 148.27
venous system 101.31
venous thromboembolism *102.6*
venous thrombosis 101.31–101.38
deep-vein thrombosis 101.31–101.34
Mondor disease 101.36–101.37
neoplasia association 148.26–148.27
superficial veins 97.8–97.9
superficial venous thrombosis 101.34–101.35
thrombophlebitis migrans 101.35–101.36
venous ulceration 39.21
ventilator-associated pneumonia (VAP) 125.10–125.11
verapamil 94.52
vermilionectomy, mucosal advancement flap repair 20.22
vermilion (outer lip) 108.3
vernal keratoconjunctivitis (VKC) 107.16, 107.17, *107.18*, 107.22
Verneuil's disease 90.1
vernix caseosa, neonates 114.3, 114.4
verruca plana (plane warts) 25.52, 25.53, 25.54
see also cutaneous warts
verruca vulgaris (common warts) 25.52, 25.53, 25.54
see also cutaneous warts
verruciform xanthoma
ear dermatoses **106.23**
male genitalia 109.30–109.31
oral 108.14
vulva **110.32**
verrucous carcinoma 108.48
female genitalia 110.37

verrucous carcinoma of the foot (epithelioma cuniculatum) 141.31
verrucous dermatitis *see* chromoblastomycosis
verrucous epidermal naevus *73.4, 73.5*
verrucous haemangioma 101.26, *101.27*
verrucous perforating collagenoma 94.55
verrucous sarcoidosis 96.13
verrucous-stage incontinentia pigmenti *68.11*
verrucous venous malformation (VVM) 71.19–71.20
verruga peruana, *Bartonella bacilliformis* 26.65–26.66
versican 2.38, *2.39*
vertebrate vectors of disease
dog/cat bites 130.6
leishmaniasis 33.43, **33.45**
nematode infection from non-human animals 33.18–33.26
rat bites 26.75–26.76, 130.5
vertex binding, pattern hair loss 87.61
vesicating species of beetle 34.30–34.31
vesicular dermatosis with reticulate scarring 94.14
vesicular eczema
allergic contact dermatitis *127.13*
hand 127.38
irritant contact dermatitis 129.6
vesicular stomatitis virus 25.97
vesiculobullous eruptions, COVID-19 association 25.109
vesiculobullous-stage incontinentia pigmenti *68.11*
vestibular papillomatosis, labia minora 110.4
vestibule, structure and function of 110.2–110.3
VEXAS (vacuoles, E1 enzyme, X-linked, autoinflammatory, somatic) syndrome (Sweet syndrome) 45.19, 149.6, 149.7
VHFs *see* viral haemorrhagic fevers
vibration, definition 122.24
vibration white finger 122.24, 129.15–129.16
vibratory angioedema 122.25
vibratory urticaria **42.9**, 42.10, 45.19
Vibrio vulnificus infections 26.66
villi 3.43
vimentin 3.25
VIN *see* vulval intraepithelial neoplasia
Vincent's angina *see* acute necrotising (ulcerative) gingivitis and noma
vinegar treatment, cnidarian stings 130.2–130.3
vinyl chloride-induced osteolysis 94.46
violaceous (lilac) colouring of the skin, upper eyelids in dermatomyositis 52.3
VIP *see* vasoactive intestinal peptide
viral arthropathies 155.2–155.3
viral carcinogenesis
Kaposi sarcoma 138.1–138.6
lymphoepithelioma-like carcinoma 137.43, 137.44
Merkel cell carcinoma 146.2, *146.3*
possible role in keratoacanthoma 141.39
skin cancer risks in immunocompromised people 147.8–147.9
viral haemorrhagic fevers (VHFs) 25.80–25.87, **25.81**
viral infections 25.1–25.129
burn injuries 125.10
classification 25.3–25.4
diagnosis of 3.29–3.31
DNA viruses 25.2, **25.3**, 25.5, 25.6–25.78
drug-induced exanthems 117.1–117.2
exanthems 25.4–25.5
exanthems in infants 115.5–115.7
external ear 106.20
eyelid 107.34–107.38
female genitalia 110.28–110.31
general pathology 25.2, 25.4–25.6
HIV coinfections 31.23–31.26
iatrogenic immunosuppression 149.20, *149.21*

viral infections (continued)
  immunosuppressed renal allograft recipients 154.5
  laboratory diagnosis 25.5
  perineal and perianal skin 111.15–111.16
  persistent infection/latency/reactivation 25.4
  postherpetic neuralgia 82.4–82.5
  psoriasis associated with antiviral immune pathways 31.16
  RNA viruses 25.2, 25.3–25.4, 25.5, 25.78–25.120
  serological tests 25.5–25.6
  skin infection effects on urinary tract 154.6
  see also COVID-19/SARS-CoV-2; Epstein–Barr virus; HIV infection; human herpesvirus; human papillomavirus
viral warts (verrucae)
  immunosuppressed renal allograft recipients 154.5, *154.6*
  laser therapies 23.12, *23.14*
  male genitalia 109.29
  photodynamic therapy 22.7–22.8
  primary immunodeficiencies 149.19
  see also ano-genital warts; cutaneous warts; human papillomavirus
Virchow, Rudolf 56.1
virilism 87.91
virocyte-like cells, myxoinflammatory fibroblastic sarcoma 136.17
virus-negative Merkel cell carcinoma 146.2, 146.3, *146.4*, 146.5, 146.9
visceral adipose tissue (VAT) adipocytes 97.5
visceral larva migrans
  clinical features 33.21
  management 33.21
  pathophysiology 33.20–33.21
visceral leishmaniasis 33.51–33.54
  clinical features 33.51–33.53
  clinical variants **33.45**, 33.51–33.52
  epidemiology **33.45**, 33.51
  investigations 33.53–33.54
  management 33.54
  pathophysiology 33.51
visceral tumour metastases to skin 24.15, 148.4–148.6
viscoelastic materials 122.3
visual analogue scale (VAS), itch assessment tool 16.5
vitamin D analogues
  psoriasis treatment 35.20–35.21
  topical therapies 18.26–18.29
vitamin D-dependent rickets type 2a (VDDRIIa) 87.29
vitamin K deficiency bleeding (VKDB) 61.12–61.13
vitamin and mineral disorders, inherited metabolic diseases 79.15–79.18
vitamins 61.7–61.24
  ascorbic acid as topical depigmenting agents 18.33
  biochemistry 18.26–18.27
  biotin deficiency 61.22–61.24
  biotin metabolism disorders 79.15
  cosmeceutical use of 157.2–157.3, 157.6–157.7
  deficiencies 61.13–61.19
  disorders **79.2**
  hair loss 87.63
  hypermelanosis 86.23–86.24
  ichthyoses 63.46
  metabolism, metastatic calcinosis cutis 59.5
  niacin deficiency 61.15–61.17, *61.17*
  oral features 108.70
  photosensitivity management 126.37
  phrynoderma *61.8*, 85.14–85.15
  pigmentary disorders 86.8
  resuscitation use 125.3–125.4
  sclerodermiform reaction 122.19
  skin manifestations of impaired absorption 153.1

and sunscreen use 10.12
supplement for hypermetabolism treatment 125.12
topical therapies 18.24, 18.26–18.29
UVR exposure 10.9
vitamin A
  cosmeceutical use of retinol 157.6–157.7
  deficiency 61.7–61.8, 85.14–85.15, 86.23–86.24
  excess 61.8–61.9
  hypermelanosis 86.23–86.24
  metabolic production 18.23–18.24
  topical retinol therapies 18.24
  see also retinoids
vitamin B complex, cosmeceutical use of 157.2
vitamin B1, deficiency 61.13–61.14
vitamin B2
  acneform reaction 88.13
  deficiency 61.14–61.15
vitamin B3, deficiency 61.15–61.17
vitamin B6
  acneform reaction 88.13
  deficiency 61.17–61.18
vitamin B7 (biotin)
  deficiency 61.22–61.24
  metabolism disorders 79.15
vitamin B9 deficiency 61.18–61.19
vitamin B12
  acneform reaction 88.13
  deficiency 61.19–61.21, 86.23–86.24, 108.25, 108.70
  atrophic glossitis 108.25
vitamin C
  acne vulgaris treatment 88.57
  ascorbic acid as topical depigmenting agents 18.33
  deficiency 61.21–61.22
vitamin D$_3$ (25-hydroxy), acne vulgaris 88.19
vitamin D
  and acne 88.19
  alopecia areata 87.23
  deficiency 61.9–61.11, 86.8, 87.23, 87.29
vitamin D analogue therapies 18.26–18.29, 35.20–35.21
vitamin deficiencies, folate deficiency 61.18–61.19, 86.23–86.24
vitamin E
  cosmeceutical use of 157.3
  deficiency 61.11–61.12
  excess 61.12
vitamin K$_1$ panniculitis 97.48
vitamin K
  deficiency 61.12–61.13
  sclerodermiform reaction 122.19
vitiligo 68.4, 86.34–86.41, 87.93
  dermatoendocrinology **150.6**, **150.11**, *150.16*, 150.18
  female genitalia 110.20–110.21
  koebnerisation of 127.20–127.21
  mechanical injuries 122.2
  occupational 86.46
  phototherapy 21.4
  psychological and social factors 15.4
  radiotherapy-associated 119.15
  treatment 86.33, 86.39–86.40
VKC *see* vernal keratoconjunctivitis
VKDB *see* vitamin K deficiency bleeding
VKHS *see* Vogt–Koyanagi–Harada syndrome
VLUs *see* venous leg ulcers
VMCM *see* venous mucocutaneous malformation
VMs *see* venous malformations
Voerner–Unna–Thost keratoderma 63.51
Vogt–Koyanagi–Harada syndrome (VKHS) 86.42, 87.93
Vohwinkel syndrome 63.63–63.64
Voigt–Futcher lines 86.2
volar skin of palms and soles, acral melanoma 145.9, 145.11–145.13
volatile substances
  inhaling 120.4
  irritant contact dermatitis 128.4

volumisation, dermal filler injection 158.1, *158.4*
volunteering opportunities 7.13, **7.15**
von Hippel–Lindau syndrome (familial cerebelloretinal angiomatosis) 148.9, 154.2
von Kossa method staining technique 3.9
von Recklinghausen disease *see* neurofibromatosis type 1
von Zumbusch variant, pustular psoriasis 35.33–35.34, 118.4
voriconazole photosensitivity *126.31*
VP *see* variegate porphyria
'V-sign', redness on chest in dermatomyositis 52.4
vulva
  acne 110.45
  bacterial infections 110.25–110.27
  benign tumours 110.31–110.33
  cutaneous Crohn disease *95.15*
  Fordyce spots 93.11
  fungal infections 110.27–110.28
  genital papular acantholytic dyskeratosis 110.45
  graft-versus-host disease 110.43–110.44
  hidradenoma papilliferum 110.31–110.33, 137.20–137.21
  inflammatory dermatoses of 110.6–110.18
  lymphangiectasia *103.31*
  malignant neoplasms 110.36–110.40
  melanoma 110.39–110.40, 142.11
  melanosis 110.21–110.22, 131.10
  microbiome 26.5
  mucous membrane pemphigoid *50.28*
  necrolytic migratory erythema 110.44–110.45
  non-sexually acquired genital ulcers 110.19–110.20
  oedema 110.23–110.24
  pain disorders 110.40–110.42
  premalignant conditions 110.34–110.36
  psoriasis vulgaris 35.10
  structure and function of 110.2–110.3
  tumours, hidradenoma papilliferum 110.31–110.33, 137.20–137.21
  viral infections 110.28–110.31
  warts 110.30
  see also genitalia, female; vulvo-vaginal
vulval intraepithelial neoplasia (VIN) 110.34, 110.35, 141.26
vulval swelling, cutaneous Crohn disease *95.15*
vulval ulcers
  aphthous ulcers 110.19
  Behçet disease 110.20
  causes of **110.19**
  non-sexually acquired genital ulcers 110.19–110.20
vulvar pemphigoid 50.26
vulvodynia 82.9–82.11, 110.40–110.42
vulvo-vaginal adenosis 110.44
vulvo-vaginal candidiasis 32.63–32.64, 110.27–110.28
  HIV 31.26
vulvodynia misdiagnosis 82.10
vulvo-vaginal-gingival syndrome *110.12*
vulvovaginitis
  streptococcal/bacterial 26.33, 110.25
  see also vulvo-vaginal candidiasis
VVM *see* verrucous venous malformation
VZV *see* varicella-zoster virus

W
Waardenburg syndrome 68.5, 86.4
Wade–Fite stain 3.9
Wagner foot ulcer classification **83.14**
Waldenström hypergammaglobulinaemic purpura 99.6–99.7
Waldenström macroglobulinaemia, oral involvement 108.72
warfarin-induced necrosis, purpura 99.15–99.17
Wars, Hypogammaglobulinemia, Infections, Myelocathexis syndrome (WHIM) 80.16–80.17

warts (verrucae) 4.7
  eyelid 107.34, *107.36*
  on lip, HIV infection *108.14*
  treatment during pregnancy **113.21**
  see also ano-genital warts; cutaneous warts; genital warts; seborrhoeic keratosis; viral warts
warts, immuno-deficiency, lymphoedema and ano-genital dysplasia (WILD syndrome) 103.22
warty dyskeratoma (WD) 108.30–108.31, 132.5–132.6
warty tuberculosis (tuberculosis verrucosa cutis) 27.19–27.20
wasps 34.16
WAT *see* white adipose tissue
water, light absorption by skin 23.4
water fleas, *Cyclops* species and dracunculiasis 33.13
water hardness, and atopic eczema 41.23
wavelength of laser light, selective photothermolysis 23.5
wax (cerumen), external ear 106.2–106.3
waxes, topical medication vehicles 18.7
waxy keratoses of childhood 63.78–63.79
WBS *see* Williams–Beuren syndrome
WD *see* warty dyskeratoma
weals/wealing
  immediate-weal tests 4.24
  jellyfish stings 130.2
  urticaria 42.1, *42.2*, 42.6, 42.7, *42.11*, *42.13*
  urticaria pigmentosa *46.5*
weathering of hair 87.6, 87.75–87.80, 87.93
weathering nodules, ear dermatoses **106.23**, *106.26*
Weber–Christian disease 97.8
Weber–Cockayne disease 122.10
wedge excision, lip/eyelid/ear surgery 20.22
weeverfish stings 130.4–130.5
Weibel–Palade bodies 2.41, *2.42*
Weidermann–Rautenstrauch syndrome **72.5**
weight gain, cellulite 98.26
Weil disease 26.74, 26.75
Weisse, Faneuil 1.7
well-differentiated liposarcoma 136.58–136.59
well-differentiated SCC (keratoacanthomatous type) 141.38
  see also keratoacanthoma
Wells syndrome 47.16
Wermer syndrome *see* multiple endocrine neoplasia type 1
Werner syndrome (pangeria) 70.26–70.27, **72.5**, 75.6, 77.1–77.3, **78.12**, 148.12, 148.13
wet beriberi, vitamin B1 deficiency 61.14
wet gangrene of the foot, diabetic patients 62.2
wet-wrap technique, atopic eczema treatment 41.28
WHIM (Wars, Hypogammaglobulinemia, Infections, Myelocathexis) syndrome 80.16–80.17
Whipple disease (*Tropheryma whippelii* infection) 97.47, 153.4, 155.5
whisker hair 87.81
white adipose tissue (WAT) 72.1
white dermographism, atopic eczema 41.17–41.18
white fat 97.1–97.2
white fibrous papulosis of the neck 94.39–94.40
white finger skin patches 129.15–129.16
White, James 1.7
white piedra 32.16–32.17, 32.66–32.67
white shiny line dermoscopy patterns, melanoma 145.7, 145.14, *145.15*
white sponge naevus, oral lesions 108.31
white structures
  melanoma 145.14, *145.15*
  see also blue-white veil

whitlow-like lesions
  inoculation herpes simplex   25.28
  mpox   25.9, 25.10
Whitmore disease *see* melioidosis
WHO *see* World Health Organization
whole body cabins/cabinets, equipment for phototherapy delivery   21.2–21.3, 21.8, *21.9*, 21.10, 21.16
Wickham striae
  lichen planus   37.3, 37.13, *110.11*, *111.10*
  penis   *109.19*
wide local excision (WLE), melanoma   143.1–143.4
widow spiders (Theridiidae)   34.34–34.35
Wiedemann–Rautenstrauch syndrome (neonatal progeria syndrome)   **77.2**
wigs   87.28, 87.69, 87.101
Wildemuth ear   106.5
WILD syndrome (warts, immuno-deficiency, lymphoedema and ano-genital dysplasia)   103.22
Wilkinson's triangle (chronic actinic dermatitis)   4.6
Willan, Robert   1.4, *1.5*
Williams–Beuren syndrome (WBS)   70.18–70.19, **72.12**
Williams syndrome   2.34
willingness to pay (WTP)
  health economics   6.4
  utility measure   16.9
Wilson disease   79.17
Wilson, Sir Erasmus   1.6, *1.7*
Winchester syndrome   70.23–70.24
Wiskott–Aldrich syndrome   80.9, 148.13
  oral involvement   108.28
  skin cancer   147.2
Wissler–Fanconi syndrome *see* adult-onset Still disease
witchcraft syndrome   84.33
WLE *see* wide local excision
Wnt signalling   2.3, 2.4
Wolff–Chaikoff effect, potassium iodide systemic therapy   19.30
women with HIV/AIDS   31.36
wood allergies   127.74–127.78
wood dust allergy   127.17
Wood's light examination, superficial mycosis identification   4.19–4.20, 32.6–32.7, 32.12
wood tars, topical therapies   18.36
Woolf syndrome   68.9
woolly hair   87.80–87.82
  palmoplantar keratodermas   63.62–63.63
Woringer–Kolopp disease *see* pagetoid reticulosis
work impacts, measures   16.12–16.13
work productivity, impact assessment   16.12–16.13
Work Productivity and Activity Impairment: General Health (WPAI:GH)   16.13
World Health Organization (WHO)   7.5
  classification of cutaneous tumours
    lymphoma   139.1, **139.2**, 139.6, 139.37
    melanoma   142.8
  Global Programme to Eliminate Lymphatic Filariasis   103.35
  neglected tropical diseases roadmap   7.7
Woronoff, halo/ring of, psoriasis vulgaris   35.7
wound care
  bites   130.6, 130.7
  pressure ulcers   123.10–123.11
wound healing   11.1–11.13
  abnormal healing and scarring   11.8–11.9
  acute wounds
    cytokine/growth factor role   **11.5**
    healing stages   *11.1*

age-related changes   11.2, 11.10
angiogenesis   11.5–11.6
chronic wounds   11.2
  abnormal healing and scarring   11.8–11.9
  causes of   11.11
collagenous cross-linking   11.7
cytokines   **11.4**, **11.5**
diabetes   11.9
excessive healing   11.2
fibroblasts   *11.6*, 11.7–11.8
grafts   11.11–11.12
growth factors   **11.4**, *11.5*, **11.5**, *11.6*, 11.11
hyaluronan role   2.39
impairment of   11.2
inflammatory memory   9.9
inflammatory response   11.2–11.3
keratinocytes   11.4–11.5
lymphangiogenesis   103.3
matrix metalloproteinases   11.4, *11.5*, 11.8, **11.9**
matrix synthesis   11.7–11.8
novel therapies   11.11–11.13
regulation of   11.2
revascularisation of wound   11.6
scarring   11.8–11.9
  initiation of   *11.7*
skin substitutes   11.12, *11.13*
stages of   11.1
stem cell therapy   11.11
tissue engineering   11.11–11.13
tissue homeostasis   9.6–9.7
treatment of   11.10–11.11
wound infection, pressure ulcers   123.10–123.11
wounds, *Pseudomonas* colonisation   4.14
WPAI:GH *see* Work Productivity and Activity Impairment: General Health
wrinkles (rhytids)
  ablative fractional resurfacing   161.5
  ageing of skin   *156.2*, *156.5*
  cosmeceuticals   157.4–157.7
  dermal fillers, indication for   158.1, **158.3**
  glyphic wrinkles   94.2
  laser-assisted drug delivery   161.5
  mid-dermal elastolysis   94.26
  reduction of by botulinum toxin application   159.5, *159.6*, *159.7*
  smoker's skin   *156.4*
wrist
  anti-p200 pemphigoid   50.41
  atopic eczema   41.13
  lichen planus   37.3, 39.17
  Nékam disease   37.11
  psoriasis vulgaris   35.8
WTP *see* willingness to pay

X

xanthelasmas   60.4–60.5, 107.44
xanthoerythroderma perstans *see* small plaque parapsoriasis
xanthogranuloma   97.17–97.18, **106.23**
xanthoma disseminatum (XD)   135.19–135.21
xanthomas   60.2–60.6
  classification   60.2
  colour of   4.14
  dyslipidaemic plane (planar) xanthomas   60.4–60.6
  ear dermatoses   **106.23**
  eruptive xanthomas   60.4
  palmar xanthomas   60.5–60.6
  plane xanthomas   60.5
  tendon xanthomas   60.2–60.3
  tuberous xanthomas   60.3
  xanthelasmas   60.4–60.5

xanthomatosis   *60.6*
X chromosome   8.4, 74.3–74.5
XD *see* xanthoma disseminatum
xeroderma pigmentosum/Cockayne syndrome complex (XP/CS)   76.5
xeroderma pigmentosum/trichothiodystrophy (XP/TTD) syndrome   76.5
xeroderma pigmentosum variant (XP-V)   **76.3**, 76.5
xeroderma pigmentosum (XP)   76.1–76.6, **78.12**, 126.32–126.33, 148.9
  clinical features   76.3–76.5
  clinical variants   76.5
  complementation groups   76.1, 76.3
  differential diagnosis   76.5–76.6
  epidemiology   76.2
  exaggerated sunburn and pigmentary changes   76.4–76.5
  genes, chromosomal locations and protein functions   **76.3**
  investigations   76.6
  management   76.6
  neurodegeneration   76.5
  ocular manifestations   76.5
  oral involvement   108.87
  pathophysiology   76.2–76.3
  skin cancer   *76.4*, 76.5
xerosis cutis (dry skin)   85.26–85.28
  atopic eczema association   41.15
  methamphetamine-induced   120.5
  renal failure and dialysis complications   154.3
X-linked agammaglobulinaemia (Bruton disease)   **80.5**, 80.13
X-linked congenital generalised hypertrichosis   87.85
X-linked dominant (XLD) inheritance   *8.4*
X-linked keratosis follicularis spinulosa decalvans   63.24–63.25, 85.11, 87.48
X-linked lymphoproliferative diseases   80.10–80.11
X-linked recessive (XLR) inheritance   *8.4*
X-linked skin disease, linear manifestations of   73.22
X-linked syndromes
  alopecia   63.69
  distal cholesterol biosynthesis   63.22–63.26
XP *see* xeroderma pigmentosum
XP/CS *see* xeroderma pigmentosum/Cockayne syndrome complex
XP/TTD *see* xeroderma pigmentosum/trichothiodystrophy syndrome
XP-V *see* xeroderma pigmentosum variant
X-ray photon beams   24.1
X-ray therapy
  intensity modulated radiotherapy   24.3
  kilovoltage and megavoltage modalities   24.1
  principles   24.1
  superficial treatment causing bone and cartilage necrosis   24.2
XXXXY syndrome   74.4–74.5, **106.7**
XXYY syndrome   74.4
XYY syndrome   74.4

Y

Yao syndrome   45.22
yatapoxviruses   **25.6**, 25.19
  see also tanapox virus
yaws   26.70–26.71
  clinical features   26.71
  epidemiology   26.70–26.71
  male genitalia   109.27
  presentations   29.12
  syphilis similarities   29.5, 29.12

Y chromosome   8.4, 74.3–74.5
years lost due to disability (YLD)   5.6, *5.7*, *5.8*
yeast infections
  burn injuries   125.10
  in pregnancy   113.7
yeasts
  biology   32.2–32.3
  identification of isolates   32.9–32.10
  morphology and diseases   **32.3**
  see also Candida; Malassezia; Trichosporon
yellow fever, filivirus haemorrhagic fever   25.85
yellow-nail syndrome (YNS)   103.21–103.22, 152.6
Yersinia enterocolitica   26.60
Yersinia pestis   26.59–26.60
YLD *see* years lost due to disability
YNS *see* yellow-nail syndrome
Yushchenko, Viktor, dioxin poisoning-induced acne   *88.15*

Z

Zambian haemorrhagic fever   25.82
Zeis, cyst of   107.45
Ziehl–Neelsen method   3.9
Zika virus (ZIKV)   25.87
Zimmermann–Laband syndrome   106.5, **106.7**
zinc
  acne vulgaris treatment   88.51–88.52, 88.57
  telogen effluvium treatment   87.59
zinc deficiency   61.25–61.27
  acrodermatitis enteropathica   108.20
  blistering diseases   69.24
  chronic liver disease   153.9
  hair loss   *87.55*, 87.59
Ziprkowski–Margolis syndrome   68.9
zoon balanoposthitis   109.14–109.15
zoonotic bacterial infections
  anthrax   26.44–26.45
  brucellosis   26.60–26.62
  cat scratch disease   26.62–26.64
  corynebacteria causing diphtheria   26.38
  glanders   26.55
  leptospirosis   26.74–26.75
  Pasteurella multocida   26.59
  rat-bite fevers   26.75–26.76, 130.5
  streptococcal toxic shock-like syndrome   26.37
  tick-borne, ehrlichiosis and anaplasmosis   26.66–26.67
  tularaemia   26.57–26.58
  Yersinia pestis/plague   26.59–26.60
zoonotic viral infections
  foot and mouth disease   25.95
  herpes B virus   25.43
  orthopoxviruses   25.8–25.13
  pseudocowpox/paravaccinia   25.15
  SARS-CoV-2   25.100
  vesicular stomatitis virus infection   25.97
  viral haemorrhagic fevers   25.80
zoon vulvitis   110.13–110.14
zoophilic dermatophytes   32.19, 32.20
zoster *see* herpes zoster
zosteriform lentiginosis   86.16
zosteriform lentiginous naevus *see* speckled lentiginous naevus
z-plasty   20.26–20.27, *20.30*
Zurhausenvirales (papillomaviruses)   25.49
  see also human papillomavirus
zygomycosis *see* mucormycosis